Practical
Small Animal
Internal
Medicine

Michael S. Leib, DVM, MS, Diplomate ACVIM
Professor of Small Animal Medicine
Virginia-Maryland Regional College of Veterinary Medicine
Virginia Polytechnic Institute and State University
Blacksburg, Virginia

William E. Monroe, DVM, MS, Diplomate ACVIM
Associate Professor of Small Animal Medicine
Virginia-Maryland Regional College of Veterinary Medicine
Virginia Polytechnic Institute and State University
Blacksburg, Virginia

W.B. SAUNDERS COMPANY

A Division of Harcourt Brace & Company
Philadelphia   London   Toronto
Montreal   Sydney   Tokyo

W.B. SAUNDERS COMPANY
A Division of Harcourt Brace & Company

The Curtis Center
Independence Square West
Philadelphia, Pennsylvania 19106

Library of Congress Cataloging-in-Publication Data

Practical small animal internal medicine / [edited by] Michael S.
Leib, William E. Monroe.—1st ed.
    p.   cm.
  ISBN 0-7216-4839-8
  1. Dogs—Diseases. 2. Cats—Diseases. 3. Veterinary internal
medicine.   I. Leib, Michael S.   II. Monroe, William E.
  [DNLM: 1. Veterinary Medicine.   SF 745 P895 1997]
SF991.P73 1997
636.089'6—dc20
DNLM/DLC   96-32059

PRACTICAL SMALL ANIMAL INTERNAL MEDICINE   ISBN 0-7216-4839-8

Printed in the United States of America.

Last digit is the print number: 9   8   7   6   5   4   3   2   1

We would like to dedicate this volume to the students of veterinary medicine and the small animal practitioners who will utilize its contents for the treatment of their small animal patients. We would also like to dedicate this volume to our families, who have supported us throughout our careers and during all of the nights, weekends, holidays, etc., that were spent with writing and editorial responsibilities, instead of with family activities: To my mother, Esther Leib, and to the memory of my departed father, Venty Leib, who guided me through my first 40 years of life and taught me the lessons necessary for success; to our wives, Laura Nelson and Lois Monroe; and to our children who have come along since starting this task, Alyssa Leib, Jacob Monroe, and Maya Monroe.

Contributors

Betsy R. Bond, DVM, Diplomate ACVIM (Cardiology)

Staff Cardiologist, The Animal Medical Center, New York, New York

Erin S. Champagne, DVM, Diplomate ACVO

Assistant Professor of Ophthalmology, Virginia-Maryland Regional College of Veterinary Medicine, Virginia Polytechnic Institute and State University, Blacksburg, Virginia

Rafael Ruiz de Gopegui, DVM, PhD

Veterinary Medical Teaching Hospital, Assistant Professor, Unit of Experimental Thrombosis, Faculty of Veterinary Science, Universidad Autónoma Barcelona, Barcelona, Spain

Karen R. Dyer, DVM, PhD, Diplomate ACVIM (Neurology)

Associate Professor, Virginia-Maryland Regional College of Veterinary Medicine, Virginia Polytechnic Institute and State University, Blacksburg, Virginia

Bernard F. Feldman, DVM, PhD

Professor of Clinical Hematology and Biochemistry, Chief of Laboratory Services and Director, Clinical Pathology Laboratory; Virginia-Maryland Regional College of Veterinary Medicine, Virginia Polytechnic Institute and State University; Blacksburg, Virginia

S. Dru Forrester, DVM, MS, Diplomate ACVIM

Associate Professor, Virginia-Maryland Regional College of Veterinary Medicine, Virginia Polytechnic Institute and State University, Blacksburg, Virginia

Spencer A. Johnston, VMD, Diplomate ACVS

Associate Professor, Virginia-Maryland Regional College of Veterinary Medicine, Virginia Polytechnic Institute and State University, Blacksburg, Virginia

Michael R. Lappin, DVM, PhD, Diplomate ACVIM

Associate Professor, College of Veterinary Medicine and Biomedical Sciences, Colorado State University, Fort Collins, Colorado

Michael S. Leib, DVM, MS, Diplomate ACVIM

Professor of Small Animal Medicine, Virginia-Maryland Regional College of Veterinary Medicine, Virginia Polytechnic Institute and State University, Blacksburg, Virginia

Michael E. Matz, DVM, Diplomate ACVIM

Southwest Veterinary Internal Medicine, Tucson, Arizona

William E. Monroe, DVM, MS, Diplomate ACVIM

Associate Professor of Small Animal Medicine, Virginia-Maryland Regional College of Veterinary Medicine, Virginia Polytechnic Institute and State University, Blacksburg, Virginia

Martha L. Moon, DVM, MS, Diplomate ACVR

Associate Professor of Radiology, Virginia-Maryland Regional College of Veterinary Medicine, Virginia Polytechnic Institute and State University, Blacksburg, Virginia

Wallace B. Morrison, DVM, MS, Diplomate ACVIM

Associate Professor of Small Animal Medicine, Director of Continuing Education, School of Veterinary Medicine, Purdue University, West Lafayette, Indiana

James O. Noxon, DVM

Professor, College of Veterinary Medicine, Iowa State University, Ames, Iowa; Adjunct Professor, Atlantic Veterinary College, University of Prince Edward Island, Charlottetown, Prince Edward Island, Canada

Nikola A. Parker, DVM, MS

Assistant Professor of Theriogenology, Virginia-Maryland Regional College of Veterinary Medicine, Virginia Polytechnic Institute and State University, Blacksburg, Virginia

J. Phillip Pickett, DVM, Diplomate ACVO

Associate Professor of Ophthalmology, Virginia-Maryland Regional College of Veterinary Medicine, Virginia Polytechnic Institute and State University, Blacksburg, Virginia

Beverly J. Purswell, DVM, PhD, Diplomate ACT

Associate Professor, Virginia-Maryland Regional College of Veterinary Medicine, Virginia Polytechnic Institute and State University, Blacksburg, Virginia

Linda G. Shell, DVM, Diplomate ACVIM (Neurology)

Professor, Virginia-Maryland Regional College of Veterinary Medicine, Virginia Polytechnic Institute and State University, Blacksburg, Virginia

Alice M. Wolf, DVM, Diplomate ACVIM, ABVP

Professor of Small Animal Medicine, College of Veterinary Medicine, Texas A&M University, College Station, Texas

The field of small animal internal medicine has grown enormously during the last two decades. Not only have many new diseases been discovered, but information about "older" diseases, diagnostic capabilities, and therapeutic alternatives have increased dramatically. It is now routine for practitioners to obtain a complete blood count, biochemical profile, urinalysis, and other specialized laboratory tests for most sick patients, and results are usually available in 24 hours or less. In the past, diagnostic capabilities such as endoscopy and ultrasonography were limited to select specialty practices or teaching hospitals; now they are available in many small animal practices.

While these developments have benefited patient care and animal health, they have created a problem for the practitioner and the veterinary student: how to obtain and utilize all this information. Many quick reference texts that allow the practitioner to view a concise differential diagnosis and specific therapy have been produced to help with this information explosion. However, these texts often lack the background information (anatomy, physiology, and pathophysiology) necessary for veterinarians to thoroughly understand the diseases. Such understanding is necessary to properly assess an animal's response to treatment and to adjust therapy to the individual needs of the patient.

The purpose of *Practical Small Animal Internal Medicine* is to provide veterinary students and practitioners with all the information necessary to logically diagnose and manage the majority (>90%) of the dogs and cats presented to their hospitals with medical problems. The remaining animals have uncommon or extremely complicated disorders that may be best managed at a referral center. The emphasis throughout the text has been placed on the practical aspects of small animal internal medicine.

Because animals present with problems and not diagnoses, a practical and logical approach to many of the common diagnostic problems encountered in small animal practice is discussed within the problem identification section in each chapter. When pursuing a diagnostic problem, the reader first should review the Problems Index found in the front of the book. Under each problem is a list of the common rule-outs and the pages within the book where they are discussed. Adjacent to the problem name is the location of the detailed discussion of that problem, including a diagnostic plan.

Besides using the Problems Index, readers will also utilize this volume in two other ways. First, students and practitioners may read and study an entire section that covers a body system or a single chapter focusing on a specific organ. Including only practical information has kept most of the chapters relatively short, allowing them to be read in a short period of time. Second, because this is a complete text, readers may use the book index to locate information concerning a specific disease or diagnostic procedure.

The book is divided into body systems. One author, sometimes with a co-author, has written each chapter within a body system section, allowing consistency among chapters. The chapters are divided into topics, such as the anatomy and physiology necessary to understand the diseases, diagnostic procedures, and therapies discussed within that chapter. The information under the heading Problem Identification covers the major problems associated with the diseases discussed in that chapter. This heading also alerts the readers to some of the less common problems that can be associated with the diseases found in that chapter; a cross reference is provided to refer the reader to the in-depth description of that problem, which is found elsewhere. The next topic describes the practical diagnostic tests necessary for diagnosis of diseases found within that chapter. Detailed descriptions of procedures are limited to those procedures that can be performed or obtained in private practice. Discussion of the common diseases follows. Each disease discussion includes an introduction that defines the disease, describes its incidence, and presents common signalment of affected animals; a section describing the pathophysiology that is important for understanding the disease; a description of the clinical signs of the disease; a diagnostic plan; information on treatment; and the prognosis. Finally, at the end of each chapter is a brief section covering uncommon diseases, citing references for the interested reader to pursue. Each chapter has been thoroughly referenced not only to document its accuracy but to provide the reader with a complete source of further reading.

We have expanded the traditional field of internal medicine by including sections on ophthalmic manifestations of systemic disease, diseases of the reproductive system, and diseases of the integument. These are nonsurgical areas commonly encountered by small animal practitioners. The sections on cardiovascular diseases, diseases of the integument, infectious diseases, and ophthalmic manifestations of systemic disease differ in their organization from the other sections because of the unique systems they cover. It is our hope that this book will provide both the veterinary practitioner and the veterinary student with the practical information necessary to practice small animal medicine in the 1990s and into the 21st century.

We are thankful to all the authors, who gave generously of their time, experience, and knowledge to contribute to this text. Besides their impressive academic credentials, all of the authors bring the experience of years of specialty practice to this project. Even though they are specialists or subspecialists, they have retained their perspective about general internal medicine. We are appreciative of their willingness to work within this new and unusual format, which at times was difficult to follow. All the authors were receptive to our editorial revisions. We would like to also thank Dr. Mike Matz and Dr. Laura Nelson for their review and critique of many manuscripts. We are also grateful to the entire staff at W.B. Saunders for initiating and completing this text. Linda Mills was the senior editor who initiated this project and convinced us to proceed. After she left the company, her efforts were followed and completed by Raymond Kersey. Our two developmental editors, Nellie McGrew and Hazel Hacker, have been invaluable in the collection and organization of manuscripts. Mrs. Hacker has constantly provided the support, positive reinforcement, and motivation to move us forward, even when deadlines were quickly passing or the tasks ahead of us looked insurmountable. Finally, we thank the entire production staff that helped turn this idea into a reality, including Denise LeMelledo, Production Manager; Amy Norwitz, Project Supervisor; Lisa Lambert, Illustration Specialist; and Nicholas Rook, Designer.

We would also like to thank the administration, faculty, staff, and students at the Virginia-Maryland Regional College of Veterinary Medicine who provided the encouragement, motivation, justification, and time to take on and complete this task.

MICHAEL LEIB
ED MONROE

Contents

Problems Index

William E. Monroe
Michael S. Leib

---

* These disorders are not discussed in this
text. See textbooks on surgery for more
information.

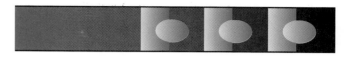

Diseases of the
Integument

Chapter 1

Clinical Approach to Dermatologic Disorders

James O. Noxon

Anatomy and Physiology

The skin is the largest organ in the body. It is uniquely designed to carry out a variety of functions (Table 1–1), including protection of the animal from physical, chemical, and microbial injury; inhibition of water, electrolyte, and nutrient loss; absorption and protection from radiation; and immunologic surveillance. In addition, the skin is a sensory organ containing several types of sensory receptors. It assists in temperature regulation; provides shape and form to the animal; acts as a storage depot for water, protein, and electrolytes; has excretory functions; may be involved in blood pressure control through changes in the vascular beds; is responsible for the production of adnexal structures such as hair, claws, hooves, and foot pads; and has endocrine functions. The skin also reflects the general health of the animal and is an indicator of internal disease.

Functions of hair include ornamentation, camouflage, insulation and thermal protection, sensory perception, and physical protection. The important functions of the skin and hair are most easily understood by considering the anatomy of its various components.

Epidermis

The epidermis is the outermost layer of the skin. It consists of a constantly renewing population of cells and varies in thickness with species and location. The majority of the epidermal cells are keratinocytes (KCs), which produce the filamentous protein keratin and are attached to neighboring cells by structures called desmosomes. The major role of KCs is to develop a protective layer of the epidermis by the process known as cornification. However, KCs have other functions. They act as immunoregulatory cells and produce cytokines, which act as growth factors and modulate the cutaneous immune system.[1] KCs may serve as antigen-presenting cells and are thought to have phagocytic properties.

KCs are arranged in several layers, which are named for their structural or functional properties. These layers represent different levels of differentiation. The deepest layer, resting on the basement membrane, is the stratum germinativum or basal cell layer. KCs composing this layer differentiate into the stratum spinosum, which further differentiates into the stratum granulosum. The outermost layer is the stratum corneum (SC). In the normal dog, a KC moves from the basal cell layer into the SC in approximately 22 days.[2, 3]

The goal of KC differentiation is production of the SC by a process called cornification. The four steps in this process are synthesis of keratin filaments (keratinization), production of the protein filaggrin (keratohyalin synthesis), formation of an insoluble envelope around the cornified cells, and production of lipid-rich material (by cells of the stratum spinosum) that is dispersed into the intracellular spaces.

The SC provides the greatest tensile strength of the epidermis and is the layer responsible for most of the protective effects of the epidermis. The SC protects against physical injury by virtue of the interdigitation of the cells and the high tensile strength of this epidermal layer. The SC also controls the entrance of chemical, toxic, and pharmacologic substances. Pharmacokinetically, it functions as a two-compartment

Table 1–1
Functions and Major Effector Mechanisms of the Skin

FUNCTION	MECHANISMS/INVOLVED STRUCTURES
Physical protection	Cornification of epidermis, hair, interdigitation of keratinocytes, nerves and receptors in skin, dermal collagen, subcutis (adipose tissue)
Chemical protection (toxic, pharmacologic)	Two-compartment system of the stratum corneum, cellular turnover, cornified cell envelope
Microbial protection	Desiccation, cellular turnover, resident microflora, keratinization, sebaceous/sweat emulsion, immunoglobulin secretion
Immunologic surveillance	Langerhans cells, keratinocyte production of cytokines, lymphocytes
Enclosing barrier	Two-compartment system of the stratum corneum
Protection from radiation	Melanocyte production of pigments, hair
Sensory organ	Merkel cells, nerves, various sensory receptors, vibrissae
Temperature regulation	Sweat production, vascular plexuses, hair and arrectores pilorum muscle, subcutis
Shape and form	Dermis, subcutis, adipose tissue
Storage depot	Dermal ground substance, subcutis, stratum corneum
Excretory function	Sweat glands
Blood pressure control	Vascular plexuses
Endocrine functions	Keratinocytes

model with polar (intracellular) and nonpolar (intercellular) compartments. This design influences the entrance of chemicals, drugs, and toxins from the exterior of the body and impedes the external movement of water and electrolytes through the epidermis.

In addition, a water gradient exists between the inner cell layers of the SC and the outer cell layers, where water content is governed by the relative humidity of the environment. The water gradient reduces the diffusion constant for water and is partially responsible for the barrier properties of the SC. The outer layers of the SC are too dry to permit colonization by microbial agents. If colonization does occur, bacteria rarely invade the intact SC, but they may enter the hair follicle and sebaceous ducts. Some organisms, such as filamentous fungi, produce keratolytic enzymes that damage the SC and facilitate invasion. However, the intact SC is an effective barrier against microbial invasion.

Interspersed with the KCs are Langerhans cells, melanocytes, Merkel cells, and lymphocytes. The Langerhans cells, derived from precursor cells in the bone marrow, have many functions in immunoregulation. They are the major antigen-presenting cells of the epidermis and produce cytokines that influence the immune system of the skin. Langerhans cells are involved in graft-versus-host reactions. The Langerhans cells interact with the KCs to regulate many immunologic reactions.

Melanocytes function primarily to protect the skin from ultraviolet radiation. They perform this function by producing melanin pigments and then transferring them to the KCs. In the skin, melanocytes are located in the basal cell layer, in the outer root sheaths of hair follicles, in the ducts of sebaceous and sweat glands, and perivascularly in the superficial dermis. The pigments produced in organelles called melanosomes are responsible for coloration of the hair and skin. Production of melanin pigments is mediated by the copper-containing enzyme tyrosinase. Albinism is the result of tyrosinase deficiency. Melanin formation is under genetic and hormonal (melanocyte-stimulating hormone) influences and is increased locally by inflammation and by ultraviolet irradiation. Melanocytes also produce interleukin-1 and may modulate inflammatory reactions at the cellular level.

Merkel cells are also found within the epidermis and are located in specialized structures called tylotrich pads. Merkel cells are considered to be part of the amine precursor uptake and decarboxylation system (APUD) cells, a group of specialized endocrine cells located throughout the body. They function as slow-adapting mechanoreceptors.[4–6]

Other cells found in the epidermis include neutrophils, eosinophils, lymphocytes, and macrophages.

Basement Membrane

The basement membrane zone is the interface of the epidermis and the underlying dermis. Ultrastructurally, it contains several layers. The basement membrane serves as a structural support and as a barrier. It is a site of immune complex deposition and may be structurally altered and actively involved in pathologic processes.

Dermis

The dermis is the largest component of the skin. It provides structural support, protection, nutrition, and storage for water and electrolytes. It is an integrated system of fibrous, filamentous, and amorphous connective tissue. It contains nerve and vascular networks, appendages (hair follicles, sweat glands, sebaceous glands), and numerous cell types, including fibroblasts, macrophages, and mast cells. The vascular network plays a role in thermoregulation and regulation of blood pressure, and receptors and nerves provide a sensory role for this structure. The dermis is dynamic and undergoes constant turnover and remodeling.

The main component of the dermis is the ground substance, which consists of proteoglycans and glycosaminoglycans. The term mucopolysaccharide is occasionally used as an all-inclusive name for these substances. Ground substance, collagen, elastin, and other glycoproteins make up the matrix of the dermis. The ground substance stores water and electrolytes and provides support, lubrication, and malleability to the skin.

Collagen is the main fibrillar protein of connective tissue. Fibroblasts make procollagen, which undergoes enzymatic modifications before being deposited in the extracellular fibers known as collagen. Collagen is the substance responsible for most of the tensile strength of the dermis and the skin. At least 10 types of collagen are present in the different connective tissues, type I being the most abundant. Collagen is very resistant to degradation by proteases, except by a specific enzyme, collagenase.

Elastic fibers are responsible for the elastic properties of the skin. These fibers are composed of elastin and a microfibrillar protein. Elastic fibers are well-visualized microscopically with special stains, such as Verhoeff stain. They are more numerous in the superficial dermis, where they are seen as fine, branching fibers.

Several types of cells are found in the dermis. Fibroblasts are responsible for collagen and elastin production and are distributed throughout the dermis. Mast cells are abundant around dermal blood vessels and appendages. These cells play a central role in many immunologic and inflammatory reactions.

Plasma cells, lymphocytes, neutrophils, macrophages (histiocytes), and eosinophils also are found in the dermis in varying numbers. There are species and seasonal differences in the distribution and concentration of these cells.

Vascular endothelial cells of the postcapillary venules play an important role in recruitment of inflammatory cells to the skin. After induction of an inflammatory reaction in the skin, endothelial cells express adhesion molecules, which bind marginating leukocytes and facilitate movement through the capillary.

Other dermal elements include nerves, blood vessels, lymphatic vessels, and a variety of specialized receptors.

Epidermal Appendages

The epidermal appendages include the hair follicle and its associated sebaceous glands, sweat glands, and arrectores pilorum muscles. Dogs and cats have compound hair follicles, with one primary (guard) hair and several secondary (undercoat) hairs. The density of hair follicles is affected by genetic factors, age, body site, environmental influences, and general body condition. Tactile hairs found in mammals include sinus hairs (or vibrissae) and tylotrich hairs, which are single hairs located throughout the skin that are surrounded by nerve plexuses and function as mechanoreceptors. Various hair coat types and color patterns are found in the dog and cat.[4] The term pelage refers to all the hairs of the body.

The hair follicle has a specific growth cycle.[4] Anagen is the period of active hair growth. It is followed by catagen, a period of transition leading into telogen, the resting phase. Telogen hairs are eventually lost from the follicle. The hair cycle is influenced by many factors, including genetics, nutrition, photoperiods, ambient temperature, hormone concentrations, and the overall health of the animal.[7] Collectively, hair growth occurs in a mosaic pattern, meaning that hair follicles in close proximity may be in different phases of the cycle at any given time. Shedding occurs if a large proportion of hairs are synchronized in the growth cycle. Shedding is governed by breed variations as well as the other factors that affect the growth cycle. Systemic illness can cause alopecia by driving hairs into the telogen phase, when hairs are most easily removed from the follicle. Arrectores pilorum muscles are smooth muscles that are associated with hair follicles. These muscles originate in the superficial dermis and insert on the hair follicle. Arrectores pilorum muscles vary in size in different locations of the body but are largest over the dorsal thoracic and lumbar areas. Contraction of these muscles causes piloerection, the process of standing the hairs up in

the follicle to improve the insulating qualities of the hair coat.[4]

Sebaceous glands are holocrine glands that usually open into the hair follicle at the junction of the upper and middle thirds of the follicle. The oily secretions are composed of triglycerides, cholesterol, cholesterol esters, unesterified fatty acids, and phospholipids. Some fatty acids present in sebum are known to have antimicrobial actions. Secretion is thought to be mainly under hormonal control: androgens cause glandular hypertrophy, and glucocorticoids and estrogens lead to glandular involution.[8] Hormonal and nutritional imbalances have been shown to alter the secretory volume and the composition of sebum in some instances. The sebaceous secretions form an emulsion with apocrine secretions; they also serve to soften the skin and help form the intercellular lipid layer of the SC.

Apocrine sweat glands are distributed throughout hair-bearing skin and usually open into the hair follicle at approximately the same level as the sebaceous glands. They vary in composition, number, size, shape, and distribution in different species. Apocrine glands function in thermoregulation, excretion of waste products, surface protection (sebum-sweat emulsion), and scent signaling. In addition, immunoglobulin A is found in apocrine sweat of dogs.[8]

Eccrine sweat glands are tubular glands similar to apocrine glands. They are found only in the foot pads in the dog and cat. Secretion of the sweat produced by these glands is under neurologic control, which explains the sweating from foot pads of nervous dogs and cats.

Subcutis

The subcutis (hypodermis) is composed of fibrous and adipose tissue. It provides cushioning against blunt trauma, insulation, reserve energy, shape and form, and structural support for vessels, nerves, and the dermis and epidermis.

Problem Identification

Dermatologic problems readily lend themselves to an organized diagnostic approach that employs a problem-solving format. Dermatologic problems are usually either historical behavioral abnormalities (e.g., pruritus) or lesions observed by the owner or veterinarian (Table 1–2). Recognition of the common clinical lesions is the first step in the problem-solving process. Dermatologic lesions are often classified as primary or secondary lesions: primary lesions have major diagnostic significance, whereas secondary lesions are less specific and can occur in association with many disease

Table 1–2
Classification of Common Dermatologic Conditions*

	PRIMARY LESION†	SECONDARY LESION‡	DERMATOLOGIC PROBLEMS
Pruritus			X
Alopecia		X	
Papules	X		
Pustules	X		
Scales		X	
Crusts		X	
Pigmentary changes		X	
Erosions	X		
Ulcers	X		
Lichenification		X	
Pododermatitis			X
Malodor			X
Fistulous tracts			X
Claw abnormalities			X
Wheals	X		

*Listed in frequency of occurrence (most frequent to less frequent).
†Classically defined problems include papules, pustules, tumors, nodules, vesicles, bullae, and wheals.
‡Classically defined lesions include alopecia, scales, crusts, lichenification, hyperpigmentation, excoriations, comedones, and ulcers.

processes that affect the skin. Although this method of classification is somewhat useful for understanding lesions, in a practical sense both primary and secondary lesions can provide key diagnostic information regarding the disease process present in any given patient.

Pruritus

Pruritus is defined as the unpleasant sensation that evokes the desire to scratch.

Pathophysiology

Pruritus is caused by irritation of the nerve endings of myelinated and unmyelinated nerve fibers in the superficial dermis.[9] The irritation is elicited by inflammation. Mast cells are of primary importance in cutaneous hypersensitivity reactions. On activation by immunologic or nonimmunologic mechanisms, these cells release substances referred to as preformed mediators of inflammation (e.g., proteolytic enzymes) and synthesize and release other inflammatory mediators.[10, 11] Physical factors, such as dehydration of the skin and increased environmental temperature, can potentiate pruritus.

Pruritus is associated with many dermatologic disorders; however, the underlying cause in most cases is pyoderma, allergies, or ectoparasites. Dermatophytosis, autoimmune diseases, keratinization disorders, and neoplastic disorders can also induce pruritus.

Clinical Signs

Pruritus is manifested clinically as scratching, chewing (or biting), licking, and rubbing of affected areas. Mild pruritus in dogs is manifested as licking or rubbing of the affected area, and severe pruritus is manifested as scratching or chewing at the area. Evidence of pruritus in a dog includes saliva-stained hair (e.g., reddish brown stains on light-colored hair), broken hairs caused by scratching or chewing, and excoriations. An excoriation (scratch or abrasion) is a self-induced linear lesion resulting in removal of superficial layers of the epidermis.

Cats manifest mild pruritus by licking, which is often mistaken by pet owners as normal grooming. However, close examination of the skin and hair may reveal excoriations or broken hairs. Severe pruritus in cats, for example in otoacariasis (ear mites), is usually manifested by scratching or biting at the affected area.

Diagnostic Plan

The key diagnostic procedures to help rule in or rule out etiologic categories of pruritic disorders include history collection, physical examination, skin scrapings, allergy testing, and biopsy. Other diagnostic procedures may be indicated in some cases. Because bacterial dermatitis, allergies, and ectoparasites account for at least 90% of all cases of pruritus, evidence of these conditions should be sought during the history and physical examination process. Ectoparasites are more likely in animals younger than 1 year of age and in animals from kennels. Bacterial dermatitis may be seen in animals of any age but is more common during the first year of life. Allergic causes of pruritus are more prevalent in animals 1 to 3 years of age. Patients with severe, continuous pruritus should be evaluated specifically for scabies, flea allergy dermatitis, primary seborrhea, and *Malassezia* dermatitis.

Skin scrapings should be performed on all pruritic patients, and they should be repeated at each examination in undiagnosed cases. Skin scrapings, fungal evaluation, and yeast preparations make up the minimum dermatologic database. Fecal flotation is always indicated to help rule out ectoparasitism. Allergy testing should be performed in those patients that fit the patient profile for allergies (see Chap. 5). Histopathologic evaluation of the skin may be helpful, but it is not likely to provide a clear diagnosis in many of the diseases characterized by pruritus.

Alopecia

Alopecia is the lack of hair where hair is normally present.

Pathophysiology

Alopecia is caused by either decreased hair growth or hair loss. Decreased hair growth may be genetic (e.g., aplasia, follicular dysplasias). It may also result from dermatologic diseases associated with scarring and destruction of hair follicles or from altered follicle activity caused by changes in concentrations of hormones or growth factors. Hair loss is responsible for the alopecia associated with pruritic dermatologic problems. Hair loss usually occurs whenever there is follicular disease, because follicular inflammation induces the hair follicle to enter the telogen phase. Hairs from follicles in telogen are easily dislodged or epilated from the follicle.

Although it is classified as a secondary lesion, alopecia is a common presenting complaint. Alopecia may be caused by pruritus, with the animal removing its hair by scratching, chewing, or biting. Common nonpruritic causes of alopecia include ectoparasitic infections (primarily demodicosis) and endocrine imbalances.

In the past, the condition referred to as feline symmetrical alopecia was assumed to be caused by endocrine imbalance. However, it is now known that symmetrical hair loss in a cat is usually traumatic in origin and represents the response of the cat to a pruritic stimulus. Underlying diseases include ectoparasitism, dermatophytosis, atopy, adverse reactions to food, and psychogenic factors.

Clinical Signs

Alopecia is a clinical lesion, but the pattern of hair loss varies from case to case. Patchy hair loss is associated more with follicular diseases, such as demodicosis, dermatophytosis, bacterial folliculitis, and follicular dysplasias. Symmetrical alopecia is most commonly associated with endocrine (hormonal) diseases, specifically hypothyroidism, hyperadrenocorticism, or imbalances of the adrenal or gonadal sex hormones. Growth hormone–responsive alopecia has also been described in the dog. The patient's hairs should be evaluated for ease of epilation, which is the ease with which hairs can be removed from the follicle. Hair that epilates easily is associated with hormonal disease, follicular diseases, and abnormalities of hair development. Broken hairs are evidence of structural damage to the hair, which can result from developmental problems (e.g., congenital disease) or from physical damage (e.g., dermatophyte invasion, scratching).

Feline Symmetrical Alopecia. In the past, symmetrical alopecia in the cat was commonly referred to as feline endocrine alopecia. The syndrome characterized by symmetrical alopecia is often first noticed on the ventral abdominal area but may involve the lateral aspects of the trunk and proximal thighs.[12] Treatment is directed at controlling the underlying disease or at reducing pruritus, if a primary process cannot be identified. Glucocorticoid therapy (e.g., methylprednisolone acetate) can be given to determine the response of the condition to antipruritic therapy. Behavioral modification or progestin therapy helps to alleviate some psychogenic problems, such as anxiety caused by moving or the introduction of a baby into the household.

Diagnostic Plan

It is useful to classify alopecia as inflammatory or noninflammatory. Inflammatory alopecia, or hair loss associated with inflammatory lesions, is probably caused by self-induced damage or removal of the hairs by scratching, licking, or chewing. Feline symmetrical alopecia is caused by excessive licking. Skin scrapings, fungal culture, fecal flotation, allergy testing, and histopathologic evaluation of the skin are useful diagnostic procedures in patients with inflammatory alopecia. Noninflammatory alopecia is more likely a result of demodicosis, dermatophytosis, genetic abnormalities of hair development, or endocrine disease. Skin scrapings, fungal evaluation, hematology, endocrine function tests, and histopathologic evaluation of the skin are useful in these patients. Key diagnostic procedures to clarify the cause of alopecia include collection of the history, the physical examination (including careful evaluation of the follicles and hair), the dermatologic database (i.e., skin scraping, fungal culture), and biopsy of the affected areas to determine the extent and nature of follicular damage.

Papules and Pustules

Papules are solid, elevated lesions of the skin that are less than 1 cm in diameter. Pustules are small elevations of the skin filled with inflammatory cells.

Pathophysiology

Most papules are the result of infiltration of the skin by inflammatory cells. Pustules are usually located within the epidermis. Papules and pustules are most commonly associated with bacterial skin infections (see Chap. 3), but they may be present in patients with other infectious diseases (e.g., dermatophytosis), autoimmune skin disorders, or other diseases of the skin.

Clinical Signs

Papules and pustules are common clinical lesions. They may be solitary but are most commonly multiple. They can appear at any location on the body, depending on the underlying disease.

Diagnostic Plan

Cytologic evaluation of the contents of a pustule is very helpful in identifying the cause. Samples should be examined for the predominant cell type and the presence of infectious agents. Histopathologic evaluation of the skin is also useful to identify the cause or pathologic mechanism if these lesions are present. As pustules dry, they leave a circular ring of scale and crust that is referred to as an epidermal collarette.

Scales

Scales are accumulations of epithelial cells on the surface of the skin. A small amount of scale is considered normal on the skin, but excessive accumulations can occur if there is a change in the metabolic activity of the epidermis or a lack of normal removal of KCs (exfoliation). Generalized scaling is seen in seborrheic diseases, in sebaceous adenitis, and as a secondary feature in many ectoparasitic infections. Key diagnostic procedures to help clarify the cause of scaling include collection of the history, careful physical examination, and skin scrapings. Ultimately, histopathologic examination of the skin may be required to identify or clarify the cause of the scaling disorder. See Chapter 6 for a complete discussion of scales.

Crusts

Crusts are accumulations of cellular debris, serum, blood cells, or medications on the surface of the skin. Crusts are often described by their content; for example, serocellular crusts contain serum and cells.

Pathophysiology

Crusts form as inflammatory cells are discharged through the epidermis by exocytosis and accumulate on the surface of the skin. Cells, debris, medications, and serum form the crust. These lesions are associated with ectoparasitic infections, pyoderma and other infectious diseases, and many immune-mediated dermatoses.

Clinical Signs

Crusts may be tightly adhered to the skin, or they may be fragile and easily removed. Crusts are often present in pruritic skin diseases, and evidence of pruritus may also be present.

Diagnostic Plan

Histopathologic examination provides the most information about the origin of a crust. Crusts should not be removed from skin before excision for histopathologic examination, because they often contain valuable information pertaining to the cause of a dermatologic disorder.

Pigmentary Changes

Hypopigmentation is the loss of pigment from the hair or skin where pigment is normally present. The term vitiligo refers to the loss of pigment from the skin, and the term poliosis describes pigment loss from hairs. Hyperpigmentation is the increased deposition or accumulation of pigment in the skin or hair.

Pathophysiology

Pigment loss can occur secondary to hormonal influences or inflammatory diseases directed at the melanin-producing cells of the skin. Loss of pigment into the underlying dermis (pigmentary incontinence) can occur if the lower levels of the epidermis or basement membrane zone are destroyed.

Pigment deposition is influenced by genetic factors, hormonal variations, and inflammation. Pigmentary changes occur commonly with infectious diseases of the skin, autoimmune skin disorders, and hormonal imbalances. Inflammatory disorders generally cause hypopigmentation in areas in which pigment is normally present and hyperpigmentation in areas not heavily pigmented.

Clinical Signs

Depigmentation is most easily noticed on the planum nasale or mucous membranes. As these areas lose pigment, they develop a slate-gray color, which eventually becomes white as progressively more pigment is lost.

Hyperpigmentation first appears, especially to clients, as dirty areas of skin. As the pigmentation increases, the affected areas become dark brown to black. Hyperpigmentation is commonly associated with lichenification.

Diagnostic Plan

Histopathologic evaluation of affected skin may be helpful to clarify the cause of the pigmentary change.

Erosions and Ulcers

An ulcer is an area of complete disruption of the epidermis. Erosion is partial damage and loss of integrity of the epidermis.

Pathophysiology

An erosion may result from trauma, inflammation of the skin, destructive or infiltrative disorders, or the loss of superficial epidermal layers (e.g., pemphigus foliaceus). An ulcer may develop from an erosion if the damage to the epidermis is extensive. Ulcers are commonly associated with bacterial diseases of the skin, autoimmune diseases, intermediate and deep mycotic infections of the skin, and cutaneous neoplasia. Ulcers are significant because they represent a break in the continuity of the epidermis, the protective barrier of the skin. Consequently, secondary infections may follow ulceration.

Clinical Signs

Erosions appear as erythematous areas. Ulcers appear as crater-like lesions of the skin. There may be exudation of the lesion, depending on the cause of the ulcer and the presence of secondary infections.

Diagnostic Plan

An extensive diagnostic evaluation is necessary to determine the cause of an ulcer. Histopathologic evaluation of an ulcer is occasionally useful if marginal areas are included in the biopsy specimen. Other tests should investigate the general health of the patient.

Lichenification

Lichenification is a chronic condition characterized by thickening of the epidermis.

Pathophysiology

Lichenification may result from external forces, such as friction or repeated licking, or from internal factors, such as changes in epidermal kinetics or inflammation. Ectoparasitism, chronic allergic dermatitis, cutaneous yeast infections, and seborrhea are commonly associated with lichenification.

Diagnostic Plan

The history and physical examination should determine whether manifestations of pruritus (e.g., rubbing, scratching) are the cause of the lichenification. If so, the diagnostic process should be identical to that for patients with pruritus. If not, histopathologic examination of skin may provide additional evidence about the cause of lichenification.

Pododermatitis

Pododermatitis is the term used to describe any disease condition involving the feet and pads. Pododermatitis is not a specific lesion but rather a collection of changes that are localized or more pronounced on the feet.

Pathophysiology

Like most other dermatologic problems, pododermatitis has many possible causes. The most common causes are ectoparasites (especially *Demodex* spp.), infectious agents (pyoderma, dermatophytosis, *Malassezia* dermatitis), and allergic conditions (atopy, adverse reactions to food, contact allergic dermatitis). Foreign bodies, especially grass awns, are common causes of pododermatitis in the western United States. Other common causes of pododermatitis include autoimmune disorders and keratinization disorders. The pathologic mechanisms may vary slightly, but the inflammation induced by these disorders contributes to the pruritus and discomfort seen in patients with pododermatitis.

Clinical Signs

Clinical lesions range from mild erythema to severe ulceration. Pustules, papules, nodules, fistulous tracts, alopecia, and lichenification are common. Lesions may be solitary or may involve all four feet.

Diagnostic Plan

Key diagnostic procedures include evaluation of the clinical history, physical examination, skin scrapings, fungal evaluation, allergy testing, and histopathologic evaluation of biopsy specimens from the affected areas. If a single foot is involved, the diagnostic approach should concentrate on a foreign body reaction or trauma. If all four feet are involved, allergies, metabolic disorders, and parasites should be considered more closely.

Malodor

Malodor is defined as an abnormal or putrid smell. Malodor may be the first clinical sign of a dermatologic problem in a dog or cat. Owners frequently comment on a bad odor arising from their pet.

Pathophysiology

Malodor is caused by excessive accumulation of body secretions and subsequent breakdown by microorganisms. Malodor commonly arises in the oral cavity, ears, perineum, skin folds, and genital areas. Dermatologic conditions commonly associated with malodor include pyoderma, demodicosis, otitis externa from any cause, anal sacculitis, and scaling disorders.

Clinical Signs

Lesions vary with the cause of the odor. If the ears are the source of the odor, they are often severely inflamed and very painful.

Diagnostic Plan

A thorough physical examination should reveal the source of the odor. Subsequent diagnostic procedures are indicated to identify the underlying cause of the lesion or disease producing the odor.

Miliary Dermatitis

Miliary dermatitis is a cutaneous reaction pattern of cats characterized by the development of crusted papules over the trunk, extremities, and head. Cutaneous reaction patterns represent the pathologic response of feline skin to various pathogenic mechanisms of disease.[13] These reaction patterns are nonspecific and are associated with a variety of diseases. The underlying cause may be ectoparasitism, dermatophytosis, bacterial skin infection, flea infestation or hypersensitivity, atopy, food hypersensitivity, or behavioral problems. Flea allergy dermatitis and allergic skin diseases are the most common underlying disorders in all feline reaction patterns.

Pathophysiology

Underlying diseases that can induce this reaction pattern include flea infestation and allergy, dermatophytosis, ectoparasitism, bacterial folliculitis, biotin deficiency, and adverse reactions to food.[14-18]

Clinical Signs

These lesions are crusted papules that are often difficult to see because of the thick hair coat of most cats. They are easily felt when the skin is palpated. The lesions are most numerous over the dorsal trunk area but may be found on the head, extremities, and ventral aspects of the body. The pattern may be mildly to severely pruritic, reflecting the degrees of pruritus associated with the various underlying diseases.

Diagnostic Plan

Because these lesions represent a reaction pattern or clinical sign, the diagnostic plan should be focused on the most common diseases underlying this condition. Skin scrapings, fungal culture, careful evaluation for fleas, and allergy testing are considered key diagnostic procedures for cats with miliary dermatitis. Histopathologic evaluation of the lesion confirms the reaction pattern, but specific diagnostic procedures are needed to identify the underlying disorder.

Diagnostic Procedures

It is important to consciously consider the age, breed, and sex of a patient presenting with a dermatologic problem. Certain diseases, such as ectoparasitism and dermatophytosis, are seen more commonly in young patients, and others, such as cutaneous neoplasia, are more likely to occur in older animals. Certain breeds are known to be predisposed to specific dermatologic conditions. A comprehensive list of these breeds and conditions is available in many dermatologic textbooks and should be consulted whenever the clinician is faced with a confusing dermatologic condition.[19] The sex of the patient influences consideration of some diseases, such as the sex hormone–related dermatoses.

History

Collection of an accurate clinical history is the single most important diagnostic procedure in dermatology. The history should include the following points.

1. **History of the present problem.** This aspect of the history should be taken in chronologic order, beginning with the owner's first impression or observation of the disease. This component includes previous treatments, by the owner or by other veterinarians, and the response to those treatments. Some owners tend to provide information in a haphazard fashion, and the veterinarian must keep the owner focused to collect a chronologic history.

2. **Past medical history.** This component of the history should include routine health care, such as heartworm prophylaxis, internal parasite control, and vaccination status. The owner must be questioned about previous health problems of the pet, even problems the owner does not believe are related to the present dermatologic

condition, because past or concurrent systemic disease may contribute to dermatologic disease.

3. **Environmental history.** This section of the history has two components. The first is the local environment of the pet, which includes the presence of other pets in the household and their health status. It also includes a description of the home environment, the percentage of time the animal spends indoors, and exposure to other animals. The second component of the environmental history is the travel history. Many pet owners travel extensively with their pets. Because there are endemic diseases in different parts of the world, it is important to know the geographic environments to which the patient has been exposed.

4. **Dietary history.** The dietary history may be taken as part of the past medical history, but it is too important to be overlooked. The type of food given to the pet, the amount, and the feeding schedule are important considerations in the diagnosis and management of many dermatologic conditions.

It is beneficial to have the owner fill out a dermatologic history form (questionnaire) when he or she arrives at the hospital. The form should include questions to clarify the important points just listed. The written questionnaire ensures a complete history of the problem. It also helps the client to focus on the pet's problem. A written history by the owner may also give the veterinarian a different perspective of the problem than the verbal history obtained during the examination process.

Physical Examination

A complete physical examination should be performed on all patients with dermatologic disease. The dermatologic signs may be part of a multisystem disorder or cutaneous manifestations of a systemic illness. Occasionally, the physical examination reveals a problem far more serious than the dermatologic condition for which the animal was presented. It is the clinician's responsibility to prioritize problems and inform clients of all problems in their pets.

Dermatologic Examination

The dermatologic examination is performed after the physical examination. All areas of the skin should be carefully palpated and visually examined. A hand lens or other form of magnification is often helpful to identify lesions. The veterinarian's sense of smell may help identify diseased ears or other body odors associated with disease. The appearance of the pelage (hair coat), the ease of hair removal from follicles (epilation), and the pattern of lesions on the skin should be noted.

It is helpful to carefully record findings on a

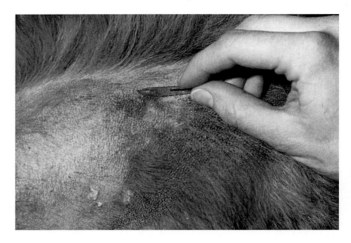

Figure 1–1
Skin scraping technique. Erythema at the site of the scraping indicates that the scraping has reached the proper depth.

special dermatologic examination form containing a silhouette of a dog or cat for recording the location of lesions. These drawings help the clinician monitor the disease and the efficacy of previous therapy at follow-up examinations. Photographs taken at regular intervals during the case management are also useful to monitor the disease.

Skin Scrapings

Skin scrapings should be done on all animals with dermatologic disease. They are primarily used to diagnose or rule out parasitic infections. Materials required for this procedure include a No. 10 scalpel blade, a glass slide, and mineral oil. The area to be scraped should be clipped or freed of hair so that the blade has access to the skin surface, where most parasites reside. The practitioner should remember to inform clients that small areas need to be clipped for scraping. The area to be scraped should be squeezed gently and released. This process is intended to extrude *Demodex* spp. mites from follicles. The blade is wiped in mineral oil, or oil is placed onto the skin, and the skin is scraped in one direction until it becomes reddened (capillary hemorrhage; Fig. 1–1). An appropriate size for each scraping is an area 2×2 cm. Multiple scrapings are recommended in most cases. The slides are examined microscopically.

Evaluation for Yeast Infections

Skin scrapings are also useful to identify yeast infections of the skin. The skin is scraped as described, except that mineral oil is not used. The scale collected during the scraping is pressed onto a glass slide, fixed with heat, and then stained with a modified Wright-Giemsa stain (Diff-Quik, Baxter Scientific Products).

The slide is examined with oil immersion objectives (50× or 100×) for the presence of yeast. Other stains may be used, depending on the preference of the clinician. Alternatively, a glass slide may be repeatedly pressed firmly against the involved area of skin. To prevent confusion when the slide is examined microscopically, the clinician should wear latex examination gloves to prevent fingerprints from accumulating on the slide.

Fungal Evaluation

Evaluation of a patient for fungal infections may involve several procedures, including Wood lamp examination, potassium hydroxide preparations, fungal culture and identification, and histopathology. Fungal culture followed by microscopic examination of the organism is the most reliable method to diagnose dermatophytosis. These procedures are discussed in Chapter 3.

Bacterial Culture and Susceptibility Testing

Cultures for bacteria are indicated for a patient that presents with recurring superficial pyoderma, acral lick dermatitis, deep pyodermas, cellulitis, fistulous tracts, or abscesses. The purpose of the procedure is to identify the pathogens involved and their pattern of susceptibility to antimicrobial agents. An intact pustule or erythematous papule is an ideal lesion for sampling. See Chapter 3 for information on the recommended technique for sample collection.

Cytology

The skin is ideally suited for cytologic evaluation because lesions are usually very accessible. Cytology provides useful information whenever pustules, papules, nodules, tumors, fistulous tracts, chronic ulcerations, or plaques are present. Supplies needed to perform cytologic evaluation of cutaneous lesions include cotton-tipped swabs, 3-mL syringes, 23-gauge needles, glass slides, a camel hair paint brush, an appropriate stain, and a microscope.

Several techniques are available to collect material from cutaneous lesions. *Fine-needle aspiration* is used to collect cells or fluid from nodules, tumors, pustules, and other lesions. *Impression smears* may be made of surface lesions or of cut surfaces of surgically removed lesions. Intact pustules or papules may be opened by lancing them with an injection needle or scalpel blade. Impression smears can then be made directly from the lesion. Although this technique is easily performed, material on the slide tends to clump and is often too thick for easy evaluation.

To maximize the usefulness of a cytologic

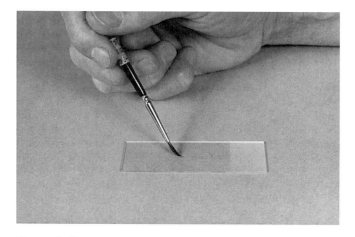

Figure 1–2
Use of a camel hair paintbrush for cytology. One can evenly distribute material over the slide by "painting" the sample onto the slide.

preparation, the material to be examined should be spread out on the glass slide to provide an adequate field for viewing. "Squash" preparations are made by placing the sample on one slide and then placing another slide on top of the sample. The top slide is then slid away, leaving the material distributed over the top slide. Alternatively, the material may be spread over the slide by using a camel hair paintbrush and gently "painting" the material over the slide (Fig. 1–2). This technique causes less distortion of the sample than the squash technique. The brush is cleaned after each use by rinsing with tap water.

The material on the slide is then fixed and stained. Several stains are suitable for routine cytologic examinations. Romanowsky stains, such as the Wright stain and modified Wright-Giemsa stains, are easily performed and provide excellent staining of cells and microorganisms. Supravital stains, such as new methylene blue, are also easy to use. Each clinician should select a stain for routine use and become accustomed to its qualities. In difficult or confusing cases, an extra (unstained) slide should be made and sent to a board-certified clinical pathologist for analysis. Slides made for interesting cases should be cleaned, and a permanent coverslip should be attached. These slides form an excellent reference slide set when matched with histopathologic or clinicopathologic results.

Skin Biopsy and Histopathology

Histopathologic examination of the skin is helpful in cases involving primary lesions such as pustules, papules, vesicles, bullae, tumors, and nodules. It is usually less helpful for secondary lesions, although it may still provide the key information to make the diagnosis in some cases.

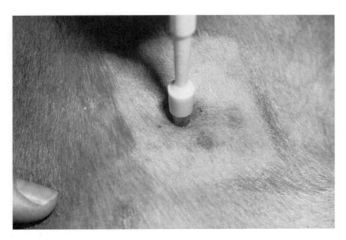

Figure 1–3
Use of a disposable biopsy instrument. The instrument is rotated in one direction with steady pressure until the skin is transected.

Supplies needed for sample collection include clippers, a local anesthetic, a suture pack (needle holder, hemostat, suture scissors, and surgical scissors), and 10% buffered formalin. The hair should gently be removed from each biopsy site with the clippers, taking care not to disturb or damage the lesion. Surgical scrubbing is not recommended, because it may damage the microscopic appearance of the lesion.

A local anesthetic should be infiltrated under the biopsy site, but the needle must not pass through the lesion to be removed. A general anesthetic is recommended if the biopsy is to be taken from the mucous membranes or mucocutaneous junctions, face, ears, extremities, or foot pads. Lesions may be removed with a disposable biopsy instrument or excised with a scalpel. Disposable biopsy punches are available in various sizes: the 6-mm size is recommended for most lesions, although the 4-mm size works well on the planum nasale and pinnae (Fig. 1–3). A biopsy punch is placed over the area to be sampled and rotated in one direction with moderate pressure until the biopsy instrument cuts through the skin. The edge of the skin plug is carefully grasped with forceps, with care taken not to traumatize the sample, and the sample is separated from the underlying fat or connective tissue. The biopsy site is sutured with the suture material of the clinician's choice, except on the planum or the skin over the pinnae, where the lesion is allowed to heal by secondary intention.

The keys to maximizing the benefits of this procedure are selection of the proper lesions for removal and careful handling of the samples to minimize artifact formation. Early lesions should be submitted for histopathologic evaluation whenever possible. It is also helpful to submit lesions from various stages of development. At least two skin samples should be submitted in each case, more if permitted by the pathology service or if the lesions vary in appearance. Both developing lesions and mature or chronic lesions should be sampled. It is good to include some "normal" skin with the biopsy, but the sample should consist mostly of affected skin so that a diagnostic lesion is certain to be present when the sample is processed by the pathologist. If there is any doubt, a variety of lesions should be submitted.

If an autoimmune disease is suspected and immunofluorescence staining is desired, the skin sample must be snap-frozen or fixed in Michel's fixative. The pathology service often can provide fixative for these special procedures.

Intradermal Skin Testing

Intradermal skin testing is indicated to confirm inhalant allergic diseases and to identify specific allergens for treatment. The procedure is described in Chapter 5.

In Vitro Allergy Tests

Three different laboratory techniques—the enzyme-linked immunosorbent assay, the radioallergosorbent test, and a liquid-phase immunoassay—are commercially available to measure antigen-specific immunoglobulin E in serum from allergic patients. The main advantage of these procedures over intradermal skin testing is the ability to perform the test on serum. This eliminates the need to clip the hair and the expense of purchasing antigens for testing. The main disadvantage is the tendency of these tests to give false-positive results.[20] These procedures are discussed in Chapter 5.

Routine Laboratory Evaluation

Clinical pathologic tests are often indicated because of the frequent associations between dermatologic diseases and systemic diseases. A complete blood count is helpful to identify changes consistent with inflammatory or infectious diseases, changes in the leukogram (e.g., eosinophilia) that may reflect allergic or parasitic disease, or evidence of systemic illness (e.g., anemia). Serum biochemistry analyses are helpful to identify underlying diseases (e.g., endocrine disorders) that may lead to recurring dermatologic problems such as pyoderma. Cats with recurring dermatologic signs should be evaluated for infection by the feline immunodeficiency virus and feline leukemia virus. Infection by either of these viruses may result in chronic or nonresponsive dermatologic disease. Urinalysis, although seemingly unimportant for dermatologic evaluation, may provide evidence of a systemic disease or urinary tract infection secondary to pyoderma.

Fecal Flotation

Fecal flotation is an inexpensive and important diagnostic procedure. Fecal flotation should be performed in all cases of pruritic skin disease to help confirm or rule out ectoparasitism or endoparasitism. Ectoparasites are often ingested as a result of biting (pruritus) and are passed in the feces. The presence of large amounts of hair in the stool may be the only evidence of pruritus in the cat. Gastrointestinal parasitic hypersensitivity can cause pruritus in dogs or cats.

Endocrine Evaluation

Endocrine disorders commonly associated with dermatologic changes include hypothyroidism, hyperadrenocorticism, and sex hormone imbalances of gonadal or adrenal origin. Growth hormone–responsive alopecia has also been described in the dog. Evaluation of the endocrine status of a patient is indicated if symmetrical alopecia is present, if the patient has recurring pyoderma, or if systemic signs of endocrine imbalance are present. Functional studies (stimulation or suppression tests) are preferred over the measurement of resting hormone levels. Results of endocrine studies must always be carefully interpreted in light of previous therapy, such as glucocorticoid therapy, that may have influenced endocrine function[21] (see Chap. 6).

Empiric Treatment

For many reasons, clients may not permit or be able to afford all diagnostic procedures deemed appropriate by the clinician. Therefore, empiric treatment is often prescribed by the veterinarian. Whenever treatment is administered or prescribed without a clear diagnosis, the treatment should be considered a diagnostic procedure. Medications that are appropriate for use in this manner include acaricides to rule out scabies in a pruritic patient, glucocorticoids in anti-inflammatory doses to help rule out allergies, antimicrobials to rule out or reduce bacterial dermatitis, and hypoallergenic (elimination) diets to identify adverse reactions to food. The key to the use of empiric treatments is to recheck the patient after an appropriate time has been allowed for an adequate response.

References

1. Yager JA. The skin as an immune organ. In: Ihrke PJ, Mason IS, White SD, eds. Advances in Veterinary Dermatology, vol 2. Oxford, Permagon Press, 1993:3–31.
2. Baker BB, Maibach HI, Park RD, et al. Epidermal cell renewal in the dog. Am J Vet Res 1973;34:93–94.
3. Kwochka KW, Rademaker AM. Cell proliferation of epidermis, hair follicles, and sebaceous glands of beagles and cocker spaniels with healthy skin. Am J Vet Res 1989;50:587–591.
4. Muller GH, Kirk RW, Scott DW. Small Animal Dermatology. Philadelphia, WB Saunders, 1989:1–48.
5. Morrison WB. The clinical relevance of APUD cells. Compen Contin Educ Pract Vet 1984;6:884–889.
6. Holbrook KA, Wolff K. The structure and development of skin. In: Fitzpatrick TB, Eisen AZ, Wolff K, et al., eds. Dermatology in General Medicine, 3rd ed. New York, McGraw-Hill, 1987:93–131.
7. Gunaratnam P, Wilkinson GT. A study of normal hair growth in the dog. J Small Anim Pract 1983;24:445–453.
8. Thomsett LR. Structure of canine skin. Br Vet J 1986;142:116–123.
9. Muller GH, Kirk RW, Scott DW. Small Animal Dermatology. Philadelphia, WB Saunders, 1989:42–45.
10. Caughey GH. Tryptase and chymase in dog mast cells. In: Schwartz LB, ed. Monographs in Allergy: Neutral Proteases of Mast Cells. Basel, Karger, 1990:67–89.
11. Rothe MJ, Nowak M, Kerdel FA. The mast cell in health and disease. J Am Acad Dermatol 1990;23:615–624.
12. Miller WH. Symmetrical truncal hair loss in cats. Compen Contin Educ Pract Vet 1990;12:461–470.
13. Merchant SA. Diagnosis of feline skin disease based on cutaneous reaction patterns. Compen Contin Educ Pract Vet 1994;16:163–171.
14. Scott DW. Feline dermatology 1983–1985: "The secret sits." J Am Anim Hosp Assoc 1987;23:255–274.
15. Scott DW. Feline dermatology 1986 to 1988: Looking to the 1990s through the eyes of many counsellors. J Am Anim Hosp Assoc 1990;26:515–537.
16. Gross TL, Kwochka KW, Kunkle GA. Correlation of histologic and immunologic findings in cats with miliary dermatitis. J Am Vet Med Assoc 1986;189:1322–1325.
17. McDougal BJ. Allergy testing and hyposensitization for three common feline dermatoses. Mod Vet Pract 1986;67:629–633.
18. Reedy LM. Feline miliary dermatitis with emphasis on dermatomycosis. Compen Contin Educ Pract Vet 1980;2:833–838.
19. Muller GH, Kirk RW, Scott DW. Small Animal Dermatology. Philadelphia, WB Saunders, 1989:97–99.
20. Codner EC, Lessard P. Comparison of intradermal allergy test and enzyme-linked assay in dogs with allergic skin disease. J Am Vet Med Assoc 1993;202:739–743.
21. Noxon JO. The effects of glucocorticoids on diagnostic procedures used in dermatology. In: Kirk RW, Bonagura JR, eds. Current Veterinary Therapy 11. Philadelphia, WB Saunders, 1992:498–502.

Parasitic Diseases of the Skin

James O. Noxon

Parasitic diseases are common in small animals. They can cause severe, painful skin disorders in companion animals and, in many cases, can cause disease in humans in contact with infested animals. Some parasites spend their entire life cycle on the animal, whereas others are only visitors, pausing long enough to feed or inflict damage to the skin. Parasites of the skin belong to several etiologic groups, including protozoans, nematodes, and several types of arthropods.

Cutaneous parasites cause damage to the host by several mechanisms, including direct irritation of the skin, induction of hypersensitivity reactions, transmission of infectious agents, and creation of metabolic disturbances such as anemia.

Problem Identification

Pruritus

Pruritus is the most common clinical sign associated with ectoparasitic infestations. The pruritus may result from local irritation produced by a bite by a parasite or from a hypersensitivity reaction induced by a parasite. Pruritus associated with hypersensitivity reactions tends to be intense and debilitating. Physical and dermatologic examination, multiple skin scrapings, careful combing with a fine-toothed comb, and fecal flotation can often isolate a parasite from an infested patient. If the historical or physical evidence is consistent with scabies (e.g., multiple animals affected, humans in the household with lesions, characteristic crusted lesions on the ears and elbows), the diagnosis may be confirmed by the response of the patient to appropriate therapy. If fleas are present, they should be suspected as the cause of pruritus, and aggressive flea control efforts should be instituted to eliminate fleas from the environment. The administration of glucocorticoids in anti-inflammatory doses (e.g., 1.1 mg/kg per day of prednisone) relieves much of the discomfort associated with ectoparasitic infestations, but it may not completely resolve the pruritus. See Chapter 1 for a complete discussion of pruritus.

Alopecia

The alopecia that occurs in conjunction with ectoparasitic infections is usually caused by the removal of hair by biting or chewing by the animal in response to pruritus. Some parasitic infections (e.g., demodicosis) cause follicular or perifollicular inflammation, which can induce hair follicles to shift into the telogen growth phase. Hairs are more easily epilated during this phase of the growth cycle. See Chapter 1 for a complete discussion of alopecia.

Scaling

Hyperkeratosis of the skin may occur in ectoparasitic infections as a response of the skin to irritation. In addition, some parasites (e.g., lice, *Cheyletiella* spp.) resemble scale or crusts on the skin and may cause the scaling to appear more severe than it actually is. Evaluation, as described for pruritus, often leads to a diagnosis (see Chapter 1).

Diagnostic Procedures

Direct Examination

Direct examination of the skin, ears, and hair may allow visualization of some ectoparasites, such as lice, ticks, and fleas. A 5× to 10× magnifying lens is useful to facilitate the examination. The entire surface of the patient, including the external ear canals, should be examined.

Skin Scrapings

Skin scrapings are part of the minimum database recommended for dermatologic cases. Because some parasites are difficult to isolate, multiple scrapings should be performed if an ectoparasitic infestation is suspected. Scrapings should be repeated each time a pruritic patient is presented to the veterinarian if the disease has not been clearly diagnosed or if the patient has not responded to therapy.

Fecal Flotation

Fecal flotation may identify ectoparasites ingested during the process of biting or chewing by pruritic animals. *Demodex, Sarcoptes,* and *Cheyletiella* mites are frequently isolated from the feces of animals infested by those parasites.

Flea Combing and Scale Digestion

Surface scale may be collected, digested with 10% potassium hydroxide for 15 to 30 minutes, and then examined according to a standard fecal flotation technique. The procedure has been shown to be more effective in isolating *Cheyletiella* mites from infested patients than are skin scrapings or acetate tape preparations.[1]

Empiric Treatment

Response to empiric treatment may also be used to rule out an ectoparasitic infestation, most reliably scabies and cheyletiellosis. Ivermectin is given orally once a week, at a dose of 0.3 mg/kg, for three to four doses. Pruritus usually abates within 7 to 10 days after the first treatment. This is an extralabel use of iver-mectin and should not be used in collies, Shetland sheepdogs, or other herding-breed dogs. Topical acar-icidal agents may also be used for this purpose. If topical antiparasitic drugs are recommended and are to be applied by the pet owner, the owner should be instructed to apply the medication in a well-ventilated area and to wear protective apparel (e.g., gloves, eye protection) in order to avoid direct contact with these toxic compounds.

Dermatologic Disease Caused by Mites

Demodicosis

Demodicosis (demodectic mange, red mange, follicular mange) is a parasitic infection of the skin by *Demodex* mites, most commonly *Demodex canis* in the dog and *Demodex cati* in the cat. The mite is considered a commensal organism of the skin in all mammalian species, although it is not easy to isolate a mite from normal skin of a dog or cat. The mite spends its entire life cycle on the host, residing within the hair follicle and feeding on cellular debris and sebum. An un-named species of *Demodex,* which is much shorter than the common canine and feline demodectic mite, appears to inhabit only the stratum corneum. It is uncommon in both dogs and cats.

Pathophysiology

Demodex mites are transmitted from the mother to the neonate during the first few days of life.[2] Puppies and kittens probably acquire the mite during nursing. Except for this short time period, the mites are not considered to be contagious.

Much has been written about the immunosup-pression that accompanies demodicosis. Abnormal lymphocyte response to mitogens has been reported in dogs with generalized demodicosis, prompting the theory that a specific immunosuppressive factor is present in dogs with demodicosis and leads to prolif-eration of mites and development of secondary bacte-rial infections.[3, 4] More recently, lymphocyte suppres-sion has been determined to result from the pyoderma that frequently accompanies demodicosis.[5] The patho-genesis of the initial mite proliferation and that of the secondary infections, both bacterial and fungal, re-mains unclear. Genetic factors, nutritional status of the animal, and environmental stress may play a role.

Clinical Signs

Demodicosis is common in dogs and uncom-mon in cats. Many dog breeds have been reported to be predisposed to develop generalized demodicosis, al-though any breed may be affected.[6] There is no sex predilection.

There are two distinct clinical forms of demodi-cosis. The first is localized demodicosis, a condition usually seen in dogs younger than 1 year of age. By definition, the lesions are confined to one body area, usually the face or head. However, several small lesions may be present. Lesions consist of nonpruritic, patchy areas of alopecia. Animals are usually pre-sented to the veterinarian because the owners notice hair loss in the affected area.

Generalized demodicosis involves more than one area of the body and is usually associated with secondary bacterial skin infections. This form of demodicosis is also more common in the first year of life, but it may be seen at any age. Animals that are younger than 1 year of age and have no complicating factors such as pyoderma may undergo spontaneous remission of clinical signs. The patient should be closely monitored if the client chooses not to treat an uncomplicated case of generalized demodicosis, be-cause severe, secondary infections can appear sud-denly.

Alopecia is the predominant clinical sign early in generalized demodicosis. After secondary pyo-derma develops, the disease becomes more severe, with papulopustular lesions, erythema, scale, crusts, greasiness of the skin, and lichenification. Pruritus may be moderate to intense if pyoderma is present. Involve-ment of the feet, referred to as pododemodicosis, is considered a severe manifestation of the disease and is difficult to control. Peripheral lymph nodes are usually enlarged as a result of the inflammation and general-ized pyoderma. Cats with demodicosis may show only pruritus (short-bodied mite), alopecia, or miliary der-matitis.

Adult-onset demodicosis has been associated with several systemic diseases, including hyperad-renocorticism, hypothyroidism, neoplasia, diabetes mellitus, and immunosuppressive diseases, as well as with immunosuppressive drug therapy. An underly-ing cause may be found in 60% to 75% of infested animals older than 2 years of age with no history or previous evidence of demodicosis.[7]

Diagnostic Plan

This disease is diagnosed by observation of the parasite or any of the life stages of the parasite (e.g., larva, nymph, adult) in debris collected by skin scrapings. Although the parasite is an inhabitant of normal skin, the recovery of any mites from a clinically normal animal is rare. The presence of even one mite in skin scrapings from a patient with clinical signs consistent with demodicosis constitutes a positive diagnosis. Scrapings should be performed after the skin is squeezed to extrude mites from the follicles, and they should be deep enough to induce capillary hemorrhage.

Treatment

Localized Demodicosis

Treatment of localized demodicosis is not necessary, nor does it increase the speed of recovery. If empiric or symptomatic treatment is desired, topical applications of benzoyl peroxide (Pyoben Gel, OxyDex Gel) or amitraz (Mitaban) are recommended. Owners should be informed that the areas of alopecia initially enlarge after treatment, because the act of applying medication dislodges hairs surrounding the lesion. Localized demodicosis rarely becomes generalized unless other factors, such as immunosuppressive drug therapy, are introduced.

Generalized Demodicosis

The first step in the treatment of generalized demodicosis is management of complicating factors, specifically the pyoderma. The bacterium most often isolated from patients with demodicosis is *Staphylococcus intermedius*.[8] Antimicrobials effective against this organism should be administered for a minimum period of 3 weeks or for 2 weeks beyond clinical resolution of the pyoderma. Cephalexin is a consistently effective drug; however, other antimicrobial agents are also effective (see Chap. 3). Weekly application of a topical antimicrobial agent, such as benzoyl peroxide, ethyl lactate, or triclosan, may help reduce the severity of lesions.

Amitraz is the acaricidal agent recommended for generalized demodicosis. It may safely be applied as a rinse (dip), even in the presence of pyoderma and draining lesions. The product is available in 10.6-mL vials as a 19.9% weight/volume concentrate solution, which is diluted in 7.6 L of water for application. The product is labeled for application every 2 weeks; however, weekly treatments have been shown to provide maximal response to therapy.[8] Although not labeled for use in cats, the drug has been used successfully to treat *D. cati* infections.

A total body clip should be performed on all animals with a medium- or long-haired coat. Animals should be bathed with a keratolytic shampoo to remove surface crusts and debris and towel-dried before being rinsed with amitraz. Many of these products contain antibacterial agents, such as benzoyl peroxide or triclosan, that also help control the pyoderma. Owners may safely apply the medication, but they should be instructed to wear latex gloves to avoid unnecessary contact with the drug. The solution is volatile and should be applied in a well-ventilated area. The entire (diluted) contents of the vial are applied; the animal should be soaked for 10 to 15 minutes with the diluted solution before being allowed to dry and is not rinsed after each application. Contact with the eyes and ears should be avoided.

Treatment is monitored by performing skin scrapings after four treatments and after every two treatments thereafter. Treatment is discontinued when no mites are found on two consecutive scrapings. The infection clears within eight treatments in 50% to 70% of dogs with generalized demodicosis.

Veterinarians should be aware that application of amitraz every other week is the only protocol approved by the US Food and Drug Administration. All other protocols described are not approved and constitute extralabel use of the drug.

Amitraz-Resistant Demodicosis

If the patient remains infected after 8 to 12 treatments, the infection is considered to be resistant to amitraz, and other therapy is indicated. Milbemycin oxime (Interceptor) has been reported to cure up to 60% of amitraz-resistant cases of canine demodicosis.[9, 10] The drug is administered at 1.0 mg/kg, orally, once a day for 30 to 90 days. Because relapses may occur in animals successfully treated with this protocol, patients should be monitored for up to 1 year after cessation of treatment. This protocol for the treatment of generalized demodicosis is very expensive and should be reserved for infections that have failed to respond to amitraz therapy.

Aggressive treatment with concentrated amitraz (Taktic EC) has also been reported to clear the mites in 75% of resistant cases.[11] Dogs are treated with a 0.125% solution of amitraz (1.0 mL Taktic EC in 100 mL water) by application of the solution to one half of the body daily and allowing it to dry. Resolution is indicated by two negative skin scrapings 1 week apart. Side effects of this therapy may include depression, anorexia, irritation at the site of application, and bradycardia. Yohimbine (Yobine), given intravenously at 0.1 mg/kg, has been shown to reverse the side effects of intravenously administered amitraz and may be of value in dogs showing severe reactions after topical applications.[12]

Ivermectin (Ivomec) is not effective in the treatment of demodicosis when administered at doses commonly employed to treat ectoparasitic infestations.[13] However, a recent study showed successful clearing of the infestation when ivermectin was administered orally at a dose of 0.6 mg/kg per day.[14] The mean treatment period was 8 weeks. Side effects included mydriasis, ataxia, and weakness, which resolved after treatment was discontinued. The use of ivermectin in this manner constitutes extralabel use. Some anecdotal evidence suggests that the efficacy of amitraz rinses may be increased if ivermectin is administered concurrently (0.3 mg/kg every 7 days). Controlled studies are needed to confirm this effect. Ivermectin should not be administered to collies, Shetland sheepdogs, and other herding-breed dogs.

The short-bodied *Demodex* mites that are occasionally found on the surface of the skin of dogs and cats are susceptible to weekly rinses with 2% lime sulfur solution for 6 to 8 weeks and to other acaricidal drugs.

Glucocorticoids are absolutely contraindicated in all forms of demodicosis. The administration of topical, otic, ophthalmic, or systemic glucocorticoids may precipitate generalized demodicosis in patients with localized lesions and may increase the severity of the disease and exacerbate pyoderma in dogs with generalized disease.

The American Academy of Veterinary Dermatology has recommended that dogs with generalized demodicosis be neutered, because genetic factors are thought to play an important role in the pathogenesis of this disease.

Scabies

Scabies (sarcoptic mange) is a severely pruritic condition caused by the ectoparasite *Sarcoptes scabiei* var. *canis*. This parasite infests dogs as well as other canids and, transiently, humans. The life cycle of this parasite (e.g., larva, nymph, and adult) takes place entirely on the host and is completed in approximately 3 weeks. After mating on the surface of the skin, female mites burrow into the stratum corneum, leaving behind a trail of feces and eggs. The males reside on the surface. The key distinguishing features of *Sarcoptes* mites are the long, unsegmented pedicles (stalks) on the pretarsi and the posterior anus (Fig. 2–1). Transmission occurs by direct contact or through fomites. Adult scabies mites can live for up to 72 hours off the host and may transiently infest humans, creating small pruritic, erythematous papules (Fig. 2–2).

Pathophysiology

S. scabiei causes irritation as it burrows through the skin. However, the intense pruritus associated with this disease is probably the result of a hypersensitivity reaction. Elevations in the serum concentrations of immunoglobulins A, G, and M have been reported in dogs with scabies.[15] However, concentrations of immunoglobulin E have not been reported for dogs with scabies, and the mechanism of hypersensitivity remains unclear.

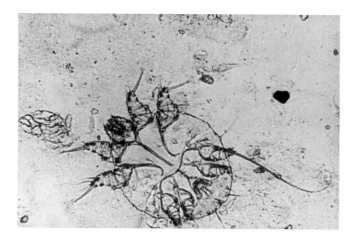

Figure 2–1
Adult *Sarcoptes canis* mite. A key identifying feature is the presence of long, unjointed stalks on the ends of the legs.

Clinical Signs

The disease is seen in animals of any age, although young dogs and those in crowded conditions are more likely to develop the disease. Intense pruritus is the hallmark of this disease. Infested animals scratch, chew, and rub almost continuously. Common secondary lesions include alopecia, erythema, heavy accumulations of crusts, lichenification, and excoriations. Peripheral lymph nodes are mildly to moderately enlarged, probably because of the inflammation and hypersensitivity caused by the infestation.

Lesions may be found on any area of the body but are most frequently noticed on the periocular areas, the ear margins, the elbows, and the lateral aspects of the extremities (Fig. 2–3). Alopecia with crust accumulation on the ear margin is the classic lesion for scabies.

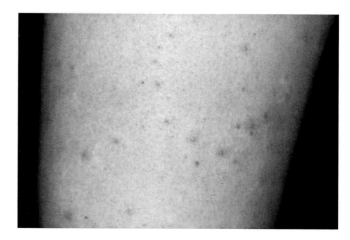

Figure 2–2
Erythematous papules and pustules on the leg of a human exposed to a dog with scabies.

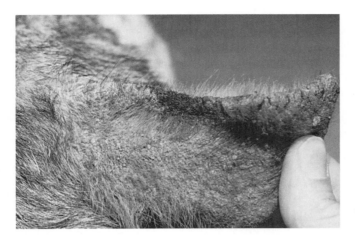

Figure 2-3
Alopecia, erythema, and crusting on the pinna of a dog with scabies.

Dogs often exhibit scratching movements when the pinnae are rubbed (ear-scratch or pinna-femoral reflex). Many dogs develop pyoderma as a result of the intense pruritus and self-mutilation.

Many dogs with scabies have been empirically treated with glucocorticoids for a presumed allergic disorder. The pruritus may be reduced for a short period or partially suppressed, but the response is usually unsatisfactory. This transient or incomplete response to previous glucocorticoid therapy provides an important diagnostic clue to this condition.

Diagnostic Plan

Scabies is difficult to diagnose early in the course of the condition. Differential diagnosis includes atopy, food allergy, dermatophytosis, pyoderma, *Malassezia* dermatitis, idiopathic seborrhea, and other ectoparasitic infestations.

The only definitive diagnostic procedure is identification of the mite in epidermal debris collected by skin scrapings. Multiple scrapings, up to 20, may be needed to find even a single mite or egg. The locations most likely to yield the parasite are the ear margins and the lateral aspects of the elbows. However, mites may be recovered from any affected area if the condition is generalized. Mites or eggs may also be recovered from feces by fecal flotation, so this procedure is strongly recommended in suspected cases. Other techniques that have been used to recover mites from the skin include potassium hydroxide digestion of scale or crust recovered from the patient and the use of a vacuum cleaner fitted with a filter to lift parasites from the surface of the skin.[16]

All patients with intense pruritus should be considered to have scabies until proven otherwise.

Response to acaricidal treatment is a reasonable diagnostic indicator if mites cannot be found.

Treatment

The topical application of acaricidal agents has been the standard therapy for scabies. Many agents, including lime sulfur, organophosphates, and amitraz, are effective against the mite.[17] The safest and most consistently effective topical agent is lime sulfur (LymDyp) diluted to a 2% solution. This and other topical preparations should be applied weekly for 6 to 8 weeks. Pet owners or other persons applying the medication should wear gloves and perform the rinses in a well-ventilated area. Before application, a total body clip of the patient is recommended to ensure adequate penetration and contact of the acaricide to the skin. Keratolytic shampoos applied before the acaricidal rinse help to remove the crust and scale.

Ivermectin also is an effective scabicidal agent when administered orally or subcutaneously once weekly at a dosage of 0.3 mg/kg for three or four treatments.[18] Oral administration of the drug is recommended, because subcutaneous injection may be painful to the patient. The drug may be diluted in propylene glycol to allow accurate measurement for smaller patients. This is an extralabel use of this drug. It should not be administered or prescribed to collies, Shetland sheepdogs, and other herding-breed dogs, because these dogs may have idiosyncratic reactions to the drug. Because ivermectin is a potent microfilaricide, treatment with the drug eliminates the usefulness of filter tests for heartworm diagnosis.

Prednisone or prednisolone (1.1 mg/kg per day for 5 days, then 1.1 mg/kg every other day for five doses) may be prescribed to suppress the pruritus accompanying this disease. As mentioned previously, prednisone does not completely eliminate the pruritus, but it does make the patient more comfortable. Pyoderma and other complications of scabies should be concurrently managed.

The environment should be treated to reduce reinfestation, although the mites live only a few days off the host. Bedding should be washed, and areas frequented by the animal should be vacuumed and the vacuum bag discarded. All dogs in the household should be treated. Humans with pruritic papules or pustules should contact their physicians for treatment.

Prognosis

The prognosis for this disease is excellent, and pet owners are uniformly grateful for an accurate diagnosis and successful treatment.

Cheyletiellosis

Cheyletiellosis ("walking dandruff") is the inflammatory skin disease resulting from infestation by *Cheyletiella* mites. Dogs are infested primarily by *Cheyletiella yasguri* and cats by *Cheyletiella blakei*, although there may be cross-infection by the various species. These mites are surface-dwelling parasites that are highly contagious and spread by direct contact or by fomites. They may transiently infest humans and cause erythematous, papular eruptions. The life stages of *Cheyletiella* mites include the egg, larva, nymph, and adult. The adult is characterized by the prominent palpal claws, often referred to as a "Viking helmet" (Fig. 2–4). Eggs are attached to hairs by fine fibrillar strands.[19] The cycle is completed in 3 to 4 weeks.

Pathophysiology

The mite induces disease by irritating the skin and probably by causing hypersensitivity reactions in the host.

Clinical Signs

Animals of any age may become infested by this mite. Pruritus and scaling are the two most prominent features of the infestation. Some animals appear to be asymptomatic carriers and exhibit little or no pruritus, whereas others become severely pruritic. Scaling may be mild to severe. Other lesions include erythematous papulopustular eruptions, crusts, and excoriations. The dorsal midline, from the rump to the neck, is the area most commonly affected. Multiple animals may be affected in a household, with some showing severe clinical signs and others minimal signs.

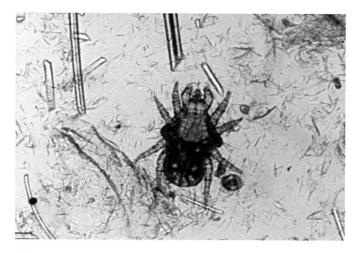

Figure 2–4
Adult *Cheyletiella* mite. Notice the large palpal hooks characteristic of this mite.

Diagnostic Plan

The infestation is confirmed by demonstration of the organism by one of several acceptable techniques: direct visualization, microscopic examination, flotation technique, vacuum technique, and fecal flotation.

Direct visualization of the mites, with or without magnification, is difficult and is not a sensitive diagnostic method in my experience. Microscopic examination of scale and hair collected by impressions with cellulose acetate tape may identify mites or eggs, but this method gives inconsistent results. Microscopic examination of material collected from skin scrapings is more reliable, if care is taken to collect as much scale from the hair and skin as possible. A flotation technique has been reported to be a simple and accurate diagnostic test. Hair and scale collected from the patient are digested with potassium hydroxide and then microscopically examined after flotation.[1] A vacuum technique is reported to recover mites from affected animals in many cases.[16] Mites may also be detected by fecal flotation.

Treatment

All infested animals and other animals that have been in contact with them should be treated for cheyletiellosis. Weekly topical application of acaricides controls the infestation in most cases. Effective agents include pyrethrin, pyrethroids (synthetic pyrethrin), organophosphates, carbaryl, and lime sulfur. Rinses (dips) and shampoos work best, but powders and sprays may also be effective. The common use of flea control products may be one reason the parasite is difficult to isolate in some cases. The mite population may be reduced by intermittent application of some insecticides. To be effective, topical acaricidal treatment should occur at regular intervals and should continue for a minimum of 4 weeks.

Ivermectin, administered orally or subcutaneously at a dose of 0.3 mg/kg, is also effective in eliminating the parasite.[1, 20] Two to three treatments, with the last treatment 4 weeks after the first, are recommended.

The environment should be disinfected by cleaning the animal's bedding and vacuuming exposed areas. Flea control products appear to work well for environmental control.

Dermatologic Disease Caused by Lice

The common lice of dogs include the biting lice, *Trichodectes canis* and *Heterodoxus spiniger*, and the sucking louse, *Linognathus setosus*. The only louse to infest the cat is *Felicola subrostratus*, a biting louse. Louse infestation is called pediculosis. Lice are host-specific, obligate parasites that are transmitted by direct contact or through fomites. The life cycle is completed in 17 to 21 days. Eggs (nits) are firmly attached to hairs and may be seen on the hair in some infected animals.

Pathophysiology

Lice cause disease in animals by irritation. If the animal is infected by large numbers of sucking lice, anemia may occur.

Clinical Signs

Pruritus is the main clinical sign, and lesions include scales and crusts (Fig. 2–5). Evidence of secondary bacterial infection may be present.

Diagnostic Plan

Diagnosis is confirmed by identification of the parasite by direct visualization or after removal from the skin with the use of skin scrapings, flea combs, or the vacuum technique.

Treatment

Lice are susceptible to most parasiticides, including pyrethrin, pyrethroids, organophosphates, amitraz, and 2% lime sulfur. In my experience, ivermectin is not effective against biting lice but may be effective against sucking lice. Antiparasitic agents should be applied topically once a week for 3 weeks. The use of organophosphates is not recommended in cats because of their sensitivity to these drugs. Clipping of the hair coat helps to remove all stages of the

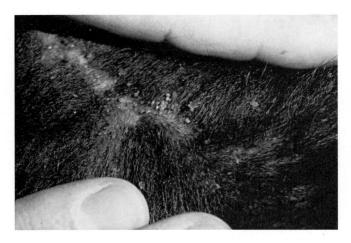

Figure 2–5
Pediculosis in a dog. Lice and scale are present on the skin and hair.

parasite but is usually not necessary to ensure complete eradication.

Dermatologic Disease Caused by Fleas

Fleas are the most common insect parasite of dogs and cats. The cat flea, *Ctenocephalides felis*, is the most common flea found on both dogs and cats, although *Ctenocephalides canis*, *Pulex irritans*, and *Echidnophaga gallinacea* (poultry sticktight flea) are also capable of parasitizing dogs and cats. Flea infestation is known as pulicosis. Cat fleas are not host specific, so almost any mammal can be infested. Raccoons, opossums, and other small mammal hosts may serve as reservoirs for the cat flea. Fleas are found in most parts of the world but are less prevalent at high altitudes (>1500 m) and in areas with low relative humidity.

Pathophysiology

An excellent review of the biology of the cat flea has recently been published and is recommended for review.[21] The life cycle is completed in as little as 12 to 14 days or as long as 180 days, depending on environmental conditions. The life stages of the flea include the egg, three larval stages, the cocoon (containing the pre-emergent adult), and the adult.

The egg is smooth, oval, white, and approximately 0.5 mm in diameter. Eggs are laid by the flea on the host but are easily dislodged into the environment. Humidity and temperature are key factors in determining the time until hatching, which is usually 1 to 10 days.

Larvae are free-living, are white on hatching, and feed on organic debris, including the feces of adult fleas. Larvae are negatively phototactic and positively geotropic; that is, they tend to move downward and away from light. This represents a survival characteristic of flea larvae. Larvae molt twice, becoming larger and darker as they ingest flea feces, and then develop into the pupal stage. The larval stage lasts from 5 to 11 days. Flea larvae are highly susceptible to destruction by heat or desiccation.

The cocoon spun by the last larval stage is approximately 0.5 cm in length. It is very sticky and quickly becomes coated with environmental debris, which acts as camouflage. The pre-emergent adult may survive for up to 140 days in the cocoon, emerging when properly stimulated by temperature, physical pressure, vibration, carbon dioxide concentration, or light.[22] Emergence of the cat flea from the cocoon takes only a few seconds, and the newly emerged adult immediately seeks a host. Because emergence is delayed until proper stimuli are present, it is possible for a family and pets to be absent from their home for several weeks and still return to find a hoard of fleas seeking a host.

The newly emerged adults move to the surface of the carpet or vegetation to better position themselves to find a suitable host. Survival time of a newly emerged flea depends on the ambient temperature and humidity and may extend past 2 months. The adult female flea feeds frequently: 72 females could cause a loss of 1 mL of blood daily.[21] Eggs are copiously produced by the female flea, with up to 1348 eggs produced within 50 days, and females have been reported to produce eggs for more than 100 days.[23]

Fleas cause disease in animals in several ways: they cause irritation by biting the host; they induce an allergic reaction, which is followed by severe pruritus; they serve as vectors of infectious agents and parasites such as the bacterium *Yersinia pestis* and the tapeworm *Dipylidium caninum*; and finally, they cause anemia in young or debilitated animals. Fleas cause dermatologic disease by irritating the skin and by eliciting hypersensitivity reactions[24] (see Chap. 5). Blood loss may be significant in young or debilitated animals that are unable to groom themselves to remove fleas.

Clinical Signs

Flea-induced dermatitis is a year-round problem in warm and tropical climates but is more seasonal in temperate climates with moderate to severe winters. Fleas may survive year-round indoors, even during severe winters, although the low humidity seen in many colder climates seems to reduce the population. Nevertheless, fleas are available to cause disease in any season, regardless of the climate.

Two separate clinical syndromes follow flea infestation: flea bite dermatitis and flea allergy dermatitis (FAD, also called flea bite hypersensitivity). Flea bite dermatitis causes pruritus, excoriations, crusts, and scaling; clinical signs of FAD include, in addition, erythema and self-induced alopecia. Papules, pustules, and epidermal collarettes, clinical signs of secondary bacterial infection, are also often present. Lesions may occur anywhere on the body but are pronounced over the dorsal lumbar area and base of the tail in patients with allergic reactions (Fig. 2–6). The most common clinical manifestation of flea bite dermatitis and FAD in cats is miliary dermatitis, which consists of multiple crusted papules over the trunk and head. Cats may also show signs similar to those described in dogs.

Diagnostic Plan

The diagnosis of flea infestation is made by finding fleas or flea dirt (flea feces) on the host or in the environment. The diagnosis of FAD does not require

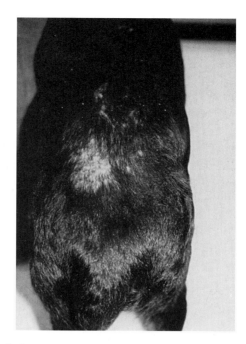

Figure 2–6
Characteristic pattern of alopecia and crusts in a dog with flea allergy dermatitis.

finding fleas on the animal, although that would be helpful. The diagnosis may be based on the clinical features and history of flea infestation. Fleas may not be seen on a patient at the time of examination if the flea population is low. To complicate the diagnosis, many owners unwittingly remove the fleas (and evidence of flea infection) by bathing their pets before presenting them to the veterinarian. The diagnosis is more acceptable to the client if fleas or flea dirt is present on the patient.

FAD can be confirmed in some patients by intradermal skin testing with a whole flea extract (Chap. 5). This procedure should not be overly promoted by the veterinarian, because flea allergy has many mechanisms of action, and the intradermal test evaluates only for an immediate-type hypersensitivity.

Because the flea is an intermediate host for *D. caninum*, flea-infested animals should be screened for tapeworm infestation by close examination of the perineal region for tapeworm segments and by a fecal flotation test.

Treatment

Treatment of flea-induced dermatologic disease has two components. The first is management of secondary problems, primarily the allergic component and secondary bacterial infections. The allergic reaction and pruritus are well controlled by administration of prednisone at anti-inflammatory doses (1.1 mg/kg per day for 7 days, then 1.1 mg/kg on alternate days as needed) until the flea infestation is controlled. In some cases, it is not possible to eradicate the flea population, and long-term glucocorticoid therapy is required. The pyoderma usually responds well to the administration of antibiotics for 2 to 3 weeks (see Chap. 3).

The second component of treatment is flea control and eradication (Table 2–1). The key to successful flea control is understanding the life cycle of the flea. There are three steps necessary in order to eliminate or control the flea population on the pet (and all pets in the household) and in the environment.[25]

Treatment of the Pet

The first step in flea eradication, treatment of the pet, is aimed at removal of fleas from the animal. Physical removal of fleas can be accomplished by careful combing with a fine-toothed comb (12.5 teeth per centimeter), although it is unlikely that all fleas will be removed by this method. Chemical removal may be accomplished by the use of a variety of insecticides delivered to the pet in a variety of manners. Effective insecticides include citric acid extracts, pyrethrin, pyrethroids, organophosphates, and carbamates. These agents may be applied to the pet in shampoos, powders, sprays, rinses (dips), topical ("pour-on") solu-

tions, and oral solutions. A list of delivery methods and their advantages and disadvantages is found in Table 2–2. A few of the commonly used flea control agents or delivery systems merit additional discussion.

Pyrethrin is the most commonly used insecticidal agent. It provides excellent knock-down (rapid kill) of exposed fleas but has poor residual action unless specially packaged. Pyrethrin is derived from the chrysanthemum and therefore may suit the need of clients who desire a "natural" flea-control agent. Pyrethrins are usually packaged with piperonyl butoxide, a chemical that prevents pyrethrin breakdown by microsomal enzymes of the flea. Pyrethrins are effective when applied as shampoos, sprays, or powders. They are rapidly inactivated by ultraviolet light and therefore do not make good premises insecticides.

Permethrin is another commonly used insecticide. This is a synthetic pyrethrin (pyrethroid) that has poor knock-down ability but good residual action. Permethrin is used in sprays, shampoos, creme rinses, and topical solutions for application on the pet. It is also used in foggers and premises sprays because it has good residual action and a low rate of breakdown by ultraviolet radiation.

Chlorpyrifos is the most commonly used organophosphate insecticide. It is available for topical use on dogs only; this organophosphate is very toxic to

---

Table 2–1
Recommended Flea Control Program

Step 1. Treatment of the Pet
1. Bathe or rinse the pet weekly.
2. Spray with pyrethrin spray (preferably containing an insect growth regulator) twice weekly or after the animal has been outdoors. Use flea foam on cats.
3. Flea comb the pet on each entry into the house.
4. Treat all dogs and cats in the household.

Step 2. Treatment of the Indoor Environment
1. Vacuum one to two times weekly.
2. Apply household spray containing an adulticide and insect growth regulator every 2 weeks.
3. Treat all mats and throw rugs the same as carpets.
4. Remove or clean all animal bedding weekly.

Step 3. Treatment of the Outdoor Environment
1. Remove all loose organic material in areas available to the pet.
2. Spray adulticide-femoxycarb combination spray in sunlight-protected areas. This includes sheds, garages, under porches, crawl spaces, and under foliage.
3. Treat the dog house as an indoor environment.

Step 4. Treatment Options for Resistant Infestations
1. Apply a flea collar containing an IGR if the problem is long-standing or recurrent.
2. Use microencapsulated products on the pet and in the premises.
3. Apply topical (residual) or systemic insecticides: cythioate (Proban), fenthion (Spotton), permethrin (Defend)
4. Use a professional exterminator in conjunction with routine treatment of the pet.
5. Apply sodium polyborate to the premises (carpet, furniture).

Table 2–2
Advantages and Disadvantages of Various Insecticide Patient Delivery Systems

MECHANISM	ADVANTAGES	DISADVANTAGES
Shampoo	Usually contains conditioners and soothing agents	Not effective or available with all insecticides; requires patience to achieve adequate contact time; gloves should be worn
Rinse (dip)	Generally good residual action	Requires proper dilution; gloves should be worn; possible danger to humans if exposed
Powder	Excellent for supplemental use (between baths or rinses); easily applied to focal areas on the pet	Not effective or available with all insecticides; messy; forms a dust cloud when applied
Spray	Same as for powder	Not effective or available with all insecticides; spraying sound frightens some cats
Foam	Same as for powder	Not effective or available with all insecticides; gloves should be worn; messy
Topical solution	Generally good residual action	Not effective or available with all insecticides; gloves should be worn; possible danger to humans if exposed
Oral solution	Generally good residual action	Only organophosphates are delivered in this manner; precludes use of topical organophosphates because of toxicities

cats. Chlorpyrifos is commonly used in foggers and premises sprays and has excellent residual activity.

Several insecticides have recently been developed and will soon be released for use on the dog and cat. These compounds, which include imidacloprid (Advantage) and fipronil (Frontline), are adulticides with residual action of 30 days or longer.

Microencapsulation is a process by which chemicals are placed inside microspheres made of various materials. Insecticides delivered in these microcapsules are less sensitive to breakdown and less toxic to the pet. The process extends the effective life of the insecticide but reduces its knock-down capability. Pyrethrin, chlorpyrifos, and other insecticides are available as microencapsulated products.

Flea collars are not considered highly effective in controlling the flea population on a pet. They should not be the only component of a flea control program. Collars containing methoprene, an insect growth regulator (IGR), may reduce the numbers and viability of eggs produced by female fleas. Flea collars may help to prevent development of a flea problem but are less effective after a problem exists. Ultrasonic flea collars have been shown to be ineffective.[26]

Topical and oral insecticide solutions may be helpful in households in which the owners are unable to bathe or rinse their pet or as a preventive measure early in a flea season. These products work by producing blood or tissue levels of insecticide that are toxic for fleas but not for the host. Theoretically, a flea dies after ingestion of a blood meal containing the insecticide. However, these preparations do not pre- vent the flea from biting and therefore are of limited value in the patient with FAD. Fenthion (ProSpot) is very effective when applied in this manner, but it is a toxic organophosphate.[27] The use of topical or systemic products precludes the use of additional insecticides with similar mechanisms of action because of the risk of toxicosis.

A number of home remedies have been used for flea control. Thiamine has been shown to be ineffective, but Avon's Skin-So-Soft does have some repellent effects.[28, 29] The efficacy of home remedies should be critically considered before they are recommended by the veterinarian.

Indoor Flea Control

The second step in flea eradication is control of the flea population in the indoor environment. IGRs are chemicals that disrupt the growth cycle of the flea. These compounds are integral products in control of the infestation, both on the pet and in the environment. The two general categories of IGRs are juvenile hormone analogs and inhibitors of chitin synthesis.

Juvenile Hormone Analogs. The two juvenile hormone analogs that are commercially available are methoprene and fenoxycarb. Pyriproxifen is another, more potent, IGR that is not yet commercially available in the United States. These compounds disrupt the molting process of the flea by providing growth hormone to the various life stages. Flea larvae normally molt and mature into the next growth stage when natural growth hormone levels become depleted. Treatment with juvenile hormone analogs causes abnormal pupal development and death. IGRs are ovicidal, and contact with an egg-laying female flea reduces the number and viability of eggs that are laid. IGRs are not lethal to adult fleas and therefore should be combined with an adulticide when used in a flea-control program. Methoprene is extremely safe for mammals and is stable in the environment for several weeks. Fenoxycarb is more stable than methoprene when exposed to ultraviolet light and therefore had been recommended for outdoor use of an IGR. Unfortunately, fenoxycarb has been withdrawn from the market due to studies that suggest it may be carcinogenic.

Chitin Inhibitors. Chitin inhibitors are compounds that disrupt synthesis of chitin, the substance required for development of the cuticle or exoskeleton of an insect. These compounds may be applied topically or given orally to the animal and are ingested by the flea during a blood meal. Lufenuron (Program) is a chitin inhibitor available in tablet form and given orally once a month to dogs.[30] It is available in liquid form for cats. This product and other chitin inhibitors do not kill adult fleas, and therefore adulticide therapy is still indicated in infested animals and households. However, these agents show excellent promise for long-term flea control in a controlled environment. Cyromazine is another chitin inhibitor that has shown promise for flea control in Australia, but it is not currently available in the United States.[31]

Mechanical Methods of Control. Indoor survival of the flea depends on having a hospitable microenvironment in which it can develop. Carpeted areas represent the most favorable location for development, because the environment deep in the carpet provides adequate humidity and protection from chemicals.

Thorough vacuuming every 7 days is recommended to remove fleas, larvae, and eggs from the environment. The vacuum should be emptied or the vacuum bag discarded after each vacuuming. The vacuuming process should be extremely thorough and should include areas under furniture, especially beds, and any other areas frequented by the pet. Vacuuming may stimulate emergence of adult fleas from the cocoon, so insecticides should be applied to the carpet after vacuuming.

The household, especially all carpeted areas, should be treated with products containing both an adulticide and an IGR. Treatment should be repeated 2 and 4 weeks later to kill newly emerged adult fleas. Carpet mats, throw rugs, and doormats should also be treated by cleaning and spraying. Owners often neglect to treat a carpeted mat (e.g., outdoors by a water bowl) that could provide a hatching area for fleas.

The application of sodium polyborate (Flea-busters, Rx for Fleas) into the carpet and furniture is an effective way to minimize flea infestation indoors. Sodium polyborate acts as a desiccant to reduce the humidity in those areas that normally provide a microenvironment suitable for flea development.

Outdoor Flea Control

The third step in flea control is elimination of fleas from the outdoor environment. Areas in direct sunlight are not conducive to flea survival, but areas protected from sunlight by porches, trees, bushes, or organic ground cover should be treated. Ground cover that can be removed should be raked and discarded. A spray containing an adulticide and an IGR should then be applied to the area. Dog houses should be treated the same as the indoor environment.

Special Considerations

The treatment of puppies and kittens warrants special care and caution. The safest products for animals younger than 16 weeks of age are IGRs and citric acid extracts. Physical removal of fleas with a flea comb is recommended along with good premises control.

Dermatologic Disease Caused by Ticks

The most common ticks found on dogs and cats in North America are the brown dog tick, *Rhipicephalus sanguineus*, and the American dog tick, *Dermacentor variabilis*.

Pathophysiology

Ticks induce disease in animals by irritating the skin at the site of the bite, by inducing a hypersensitivity reaction in some animals, by serving as vectors of infectious disease (see Chap. 37), by causing blood loss, and by producing toxins (e.g., tick paralysis; see Chap. 28). Dermatologic problems caused by ticks are related to irritation and possible hypersensitivity reactions. However, tick infestation does not cause any apparent clinical problem in most patients, unless a secondary condition occurs (e.g., allergy, infection) or unless large numbers of ticks are present.

Clinical Signs

Ticks are more frequently found in the spring and fall seasons. Ticks can occur anywhere on the body of a dog or cat, but they are frequently found on the neck, in the ears, in the axillary regions, and between the digits. Ticks may induce a localized area of inflammation (erythema) at the site of attachment, but infestation in low numbers rarely causes enough discomfort in the patient to be noticed by an owner. These parasites are often found incidentally as an owner pets or grooms the animal.

Treatment

Ticks can be physically removed by grasping the head parts with forceps and applying gentle traction. Ticks collected from the animal should be placed in alcohol or another fixative until dead.

If large numbers of ticks are present on the animal, shampoos or rinses can be used to kill the parasites. Organophosphates (in dogs) or carbamates are effective. Pyrethrin and other mild insecticides are less effective. *R. sanguineus* may infest premises such as kennels, garages, and houses, so these areas must be treated aggressively with insecticides. Removal of excessive vegetation and population control of intermediate hosts, such as small mammals, are required if outdoor areas are infested. The infested areas may also be sprayed with 0.5% malathion or other insecticides to reduce tick numbers.

Prevention of pet infestation is largely ineffective, although some promise has been seen with a collar containing amitraz (Preventic).[32] Amitraz allegedly paralyzes the mouth parts of the tick, thereby preventing feeding and infestation.

Dermatologic Disease Caused by Flies

Flies from a number of genera are capable of causing cutaneous lesions. *Stomoxys* spp. (stable flies), Simuliidae (black flies), *Tabanus* spp. (horseflies), *Chrysops* spp. (deer flies), and various genera of obligatory myiasis-producing flies cause dermatologic lesions.

Pathophysiology

Flies cause dermatologic disease in small animals by direct irritation, by infection of fly bites, by facultative myiasis, and by obligatory myiasis. Facultative myiasis is infection of contaminated or traumatic wounds by fly larvae of various fly genera.[33] Debilitated, young, and old animals are predisposed. As larvae develop on the skin, they induce disease by irritation, by secretion of toxins, and by transportation of bacteria into tissues. A heavy undercoat may also predispose dogs to infestation by *Sarcophaga* spp.

Obligatory myiasis is a condition in which the fly larva, to complete its development, is dependent on an animal host during part of its life cycle. Cuterebriasis falls into this category.[34] The eggs of the *Cuterebra* fly are usually laid in the nests or burrows of preferred host species, including rabbits and rodents.

Dogs and cats are not preferred hosts but may become infested. First-stage larvae enter the host through natural body openings and develop in subcutaneous pockets, which open to the surface to form a breathing pore. The larvae leave the host after development to the third stage.

Clinical Signs

Fly dermatitis is usually seen as small, alopecic, crusted areas on the ear margins of dogs housed outdoors. Affected dogs shake their heads and rub their ears and may have secondary excoriations or infections. Patients with facultative myiasis usually present with draining wounds containing fly larvae (maggots). The larvae are often found in punched-out lesions (holes) in the skin or large pockets formed by coalescing lesions. Many patients are overtly depressed, either from an underlying debilitating disease or from toxicosis and secondary wound infection.

Cuterebra spp. infestation appears as a single subcutaneous nodule, usually with a central opening to the exterior. Serosanguineous to purulent exudate often drains from the opening, which may also be large enough to reveal the larva (Fig. 2–7). Several larvae may infest a patient.

Treatment

The affected areas should be cleaned, and antimicrobials should be prescribed if an infection is present. Prevention is difficult, but application of gels containing repellents or insecticides (Fly Repellent Ointment for Wounds and Sores) to the ears may reduce the frequency of fly bites. Treatment of facul-

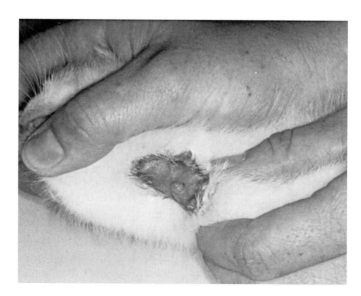

Figure 2–7
Typical appearance of *Cuterebra* infestation in a kitten. Notice the prominent breathing pore of the larva.

tative myiasis involves clipping the hair to facilitate physical removal of the larvae and application of insecticides in heavily infested animals to remove all the larvae. Heavily infested animals may require supportive care, including intravenous fluids and antimicrobial therapy.

Treatment of *Cuterebra* spp. infestation requires removal of the larvae and symptomatic treatment of the subcutaneous pocket. Larvae should be removed carefully in order to prevent retention of larval tissues.

Uncommon Ectoparasitic Diseases

Notoedres cati Infection

Infestation of cats by the mite *Notoedres cati* is often called head mange or feline scabies.[35] The parasite is endemic in some geographic areas and creates a disease in cats similar to scabies in the dog. Diagnosis and treatment of this condition is similar to diagnosis and treatment of scabies.

Fur Mite Infection

Infection by the cat fur mite, *Lynxacarus radovsky*, should be considered as a cause of feline pruritus in endemic areas, which include Florida, Puerto Rico, and Hawaii.[36] The diagnosis is based on identification of the parasite on skin scrapings, and treatment with oral ivermectin or weekly lime sulfur rinses is effective.

Chiggers Infection

Chiggers are parasitic larvae of harvest mites belonging to the family Trombiculidae. Infestation of dogs or cats causes pruritus and development of erythematous, crusted, papulopustular lesions on exposed skin.[37, 38] Diagnosis is made by identification of the larvae by skin scrapings. A single topical application of most insecticides (e.g., pyrethrin, organophosphate) is curative.

Hookworm Dermatitis

Hookworm dermatitis (cutaneous larval migrans) is a condition characterized by inflammation and irritation of the skin at the site of migration of infective larvae of the hookworms, *Ancylostoma* spp. and *Uncinaria stenocephala*.[39] Treatment includes symptomatic control of the pruritus, elimination of the hookworm infection, elimination of the migrating larvae, and environmental control of hookworm larvae. Ivermectin or fenbendazole (Panacur) eliminates the migrating larvae, and anti-inflammatory doses of

prednisone (1.1 mg/kg, orally) are recommended for 5 to 7 days after larvicidal treatment.

Rhabditic Mange

Rhabditic mange, or *Pelodera* dermatitis, is caused by cutaneous invasion by larvae of the free-living nematode, *Pelodera strongyloides*. These parasites have a predilection for moist straw or hay, and infection by any stage results in a papulopustular, pruritic dermatitis of exposed skin.[39] Topical acaricides or ivermectin eliminates the infestation. Anti-inflammatory doses of prednisone relieve the pruritus that accompanies the condition.

Dracunculus insignis Infection

Dracunculus insignis is a nematode parasite of dogs, raccoons, and wild carnivores in North America that may rarely infect dogs.[39] This parasite develops in a subcutaneous nodule that ulcerates to form an exit route for larvae. The nodule may become secondarily infected. Lesions are treated by physical removal of the parasite and symptomatic care of the ulcer.

References

1. Paradis M, Scott D, Villeneuve A. Efficacy of ivermectin against *Cheyletiella blakei* infestation in cats. J Am Anim Hosp Assoc 1990;26:125–128.
2. Greve JH, Gaafer SM. Natural transmission of *Demodex canis* in dogs. J Am Vet Med Assoc 1966;148:1043–1045.
3. Scott DW, Farrow BRH, Schultz RD. Studies on the therapeutic and immunologic aspects of generalized demodectic mange in the dog. J Am Anim Hosp Assoc 1974;10:233–244.
4. Scott DW, Schultz RD, Baker E. Further studies on the therapeutic and immunologic aspects of generalized demodectic mange in the dog. J Am Anim Hosp Assoc 1976;12:203–213.
5. Barta O, Waltman C, Oyekan PP, et al. Lymphocyte transformation suppression caused by pyoderma, failure to demonstrate it in uncomplicated demodectic mange. Comp Immunol Microbiol Infect Dis 1983;6:9–17.
6. Muller GH, Kirk RW, Scott DW. Small Animal Dermatology. Philadelphia, WB Saunders, 1989:381.
7. Duclos D. A retrospective study of canine adult-onset demodicosis. Proceedings of the Sixth Annual Members' Meeting, American Academy of Veterinary Dermatology and American College of Veterinary Dermatology, San Francisco, 1990:29–30.
8. Kwochka KW, Kunkle GA, Foil CO. The efficacy of amitraz for generalized demodicosis in dogs: A study of two concentrations and frequencies of application. Compen Contin Educ Pract Vet 1985;7:8–18.
9. Miller WH, Scott DW, Wellington JR, et al. Clinical efficacy of milbemycin oxime in the treatment of gener-

alized demodicosis in adult dogs. J Am Vet Med Assoc 1993;203:1426–1429.

10. Reedy LM, Garfield RA. Results of a clinical study with an oral antiparasitic agent in generalized demodicosis. Proceedings of the Seventh Annual Members' Meeting, American Academy of Veterinary Dermatology and American College of Veterinary Dermatology, Scottsdale, 1991:43.

11. Medleau L, Willemse T. Efficacy of amitraz therapy for generalized demodicosis in dogs: Two independent studies. Proceedings of the Seventh Annual Members' Meeting, American Academy of Veterinary Dermatology and American College of Veterinary Dermatology, Scottsdale, 1991:41.

12. Hsu WH, Hopper DL. Effect of yohimbine on amitraz-induced CNS depression and bradycardia in dogs. J Toxicol Environ Health 1986;18:423–429.

13. Scott DW, Walton DK. Experiences with the use of amitraz and ivermectin for the treatment of generalized demodicosis in dogs. J Am Anim Hosp Assoc 1985; 21:535.

14. Ristic Z. Ivermectin in the treatment of generalized demodicosis in the dog. Proceedings of the Ninth Annual Members' Meeting, American Academy of Veterinary Dermatology and American College of Veterinary Dermatology, San Diego, 1993:31.

15. Thoday KL. Serum immunoglobulin concentrations in canine scabies. In: Ihrke PJ, Mason IA, White SD, eds. Advances in Veterinary Dermatology, vol 2. Oxford, Permagon Press, 1993:211–227.

16. Klayman E, Schillhorn van Veen TW. Vacuum cleaner method of diagnosis of ectoparasitism. Mod Vet Pract 1981;62:767–771.

17. Folz SD, Kakuk TJ, Henke CL, et al. Clinical evaluation of amitraz for treatment of canine scabies. Mod Vet Pract 1984;65:597–600.

18. Scheidt VJ, Medleau L, Seward RL, et al. An evaluation of ivermectin in the treatment of sarcoptic mange in dogs. Am J Vet Res 1984;45:1201–1202.

19. Muller GH, Kirk RW, Scott DW. Small Animal Dermatology. Philadelphia, WB Saunders, 1989:369–376.

20. Paradis M, Villeneuve A. Efficacy of ivermectin against *Cheyletiella yasguri* infestation in dogs. Can Vet J 1988;29: 633–635.

21. Dryden MW. Biology of fleas of dogs and cats. Compen Contin Educ Pract Vet 1993;15:569–578.

22. Silverman J, Rust MK. Extended longevity of the pre-emergent adult cat flea (Siphonaptera:Pulicidae) and factors stimulating emergence from the pupal cocoon. Ann Entomol Soc Am 1985;78:763–768.

23. Dryden MW. Host association, on-host longevity, and egg production of *Ctenocephalides felis*. Vet Parasitol 1989;34:117–122.

24. Reedy LM. Common parasitic problems in small animal dermatology. J Am Vet Med Assoc 1986;188:362–364.

25. Dryden MW, Prestwood AK. Successful flea control. Compen Contin Educ Pract Vet 1993;15:821–830.

26. Dryden MW, Long GR, Gaafar SM. Effects of ultrasonic flea collars on *Ctenocephalides felis* on cats. J Am Vet Med Assoc 1989;195:1717–1718.

27. Mason KV, Ring J, Duggan J. Fenthion of flea control on dogs under field conditions: Dose response efficacy studies and effect on cholinesterase activity. J Am Anim Hosp Assoc 1984;20:591–595.

28. Halliwell REW. Ineffectiveness of thiamine (Vitamin B$_1$) as a flea repellent in dogs. J Am Anim Hosp Assoc 1982;18:423–426.

29. Fehrer SL, Halliwell REW. Effectiveness of Avon's Skin-So Soft® as a flea repellent on dogs. J Am Anim Hosp Assoc 1987;23:217–220.

30. Willemse T. The effect of insect growth regulator lufenuron on flea reproduction. In: Ihrke PJ, Mason IS, White SD, eds. Advances in Veterinary Dermatology, vol 2. Oxford, Pergamon Press, 1993:207–210.

31. Shipstone MA, Mason KV, Stone BF. A multi-centre field trial with DecaFlea, a cyromazine and diethylcarbamazine tablet for the control of fleas and the prevention of heartworm. Proceedings of the Tenth Annual Members' Meeting, American Academy of Veterinary Dermatology and American College of Veterinary Dermatology, Charleston, 1994:41–42.

32. Blagburn BL, Hendrix CM, Vaughan JL, et al. Efficacy of the Preventic (9% amitraz) collar for control of *Rhipicephalus sanguineous* and *Dermacentor variabilis* infestations on dogs. Proc North Am Vet Conf 1993:7;387–390.

33. Hendrix CM. Facultative myiasis in dogs and cats. Compen Contin Educ Pract Vet 1991;13:86–93.

34. Georgi JR. Parasitology for Veterinarians. Philadelphia, WB Saunders, 1985:22–23.

35. Muller GH, Kirk RW, Scott DW. Small Animal Dermatology. Philadelphia, WB Saunders, 1989:404–407.

36. Craig TM, Teel PD, Dubuisson LM, et al. *Lynxacarus radovskyi* infestation in a cat. J Am Vet Med Assoc 1993;202:613–614.

37. Fleming EJ, Chastain CB. Miliary dermatitis associated with *Eutrombicula* infestation in a cat. J Am Anim Hosp Assoc 1991;27:529–531.

38. Lowenstine LJ, Carpenter JL, O'Connor BM. Trombiculosis in a cat. J Am Vet Med Assoc 1979;175:289–292.

39. Muller GH, Kirk RW, Scott DW. Small Animal Dermatology. Philadelphia, WB Saunders, 1989:347–357.

Chapter 3

Bacterial and Fungal Diseases of the Skin

James O. Noxon

Bacterial Infections of the Skin

Problem Identification

Pyoderma

Pyoderma is defined as bacterial infection of the skin. Surface pyodermas are those infections that are restricted to the surface of the skin and do not extend into the follicle. Superficial pyodermas include infections that involve the hair follicle but do not extend into the dermis. Deep pyodermas are infections that extend into the dermis and underlying panniculus.

Pathophysiology

Staphylococcus intermedius is the primary pathogen of canine skin. It is a coagulase-positive, β-lactamase–producing staphylococcus.[1] The cell wall of this bacterium contains the substance protein A, which has many biologic effects, including activation of complement, induction of immediate and delayed hypersensitivity reactions, lymphocyte stimulation, and inhibition of phagocytosis.[2] Staphylococci also produce a variety of enzymes that may participate in pathologic processes.[3] Although coagulase-positive staphylococci are not considered part of the resident microflora of canine skin, they are consistently present on normal canine hair.[4, 5] Pyoderma is uncommon in the cat, but coagulase-positive staphylococci, including *Staphylococcus aureus* and *S. intermedius*, have been isolated from feline skin lesions.[6]

Pruritus is a constant feature of bacterial skin infections. The intensity varies from mild to severe, depending on the depth of the infection. The pruritus is induced by several factors, including exotoxins, proteolytic enzymes, and cell wall toxins of the bacteria. The proteolytic enzymes are thought to be responsible for much of the pruritus associated with bacterial skin infections. When the hair follicles are disrupted (furunculosis) by the infection, keratinized material (e.g., hair) is released into the dermis and induces a foreign body reaction, causing intense pruritus.

A number of factors may predispose an animal to a bacterial infection of the skin. Underlying diseases, such as atopy, adverse reactions to food, and ectoparasite infection, may result in secondary infections caused by self-induced trauma. Nonpruritic conditions associated with bacterial infections include specific immunoinsufficiency syndromes (e.g., immunoglobulin A deficiency in Chinese shar-peis or German shepherds), canine demodicosis, keratinization disorders, poor nutritional status, trauma, and endocrine disorders, especially hypothyroidism, hyperadrenocorticism, and sex hormone imbalances.[4, 7] These primary disease processes should be considered when-

ever a patient has recurring pyoderma or pyoderma that does not respond to the appropriate therapy.

Pyoderma has been classified according to the depth of infection, which correlates with the severity of infection and the intensity of the treatment required to clear the infection (Table 3–1). In general, more aggressive efforts are required to diagnose and treat infections that occur deep in the skin.

Clinical Signs

Bacterial skin infections are very common in dogs. Pyoderma should be suspected if the patient has a history of pruritus, especially if the pruritus has previously responded to antimicrobial therapy. Glucocorticoids reduce pruritus associated with pyoderma, but the lesions tend to persist. However, both the pruritus and the lesions regress with appropriate antimicrobial therapy. The presence of papules, pustules, and epidermal collarettes should create a high index of suspicion for pyoderma.

Papules and Pustules. Papules are solid, elevated lesions of the skin up to 1 cm in diameter. Pustules are elevated lesions containing inflammatory cells. Bacteria may be found within neutrophils or macrophages contained in these inflammatory lesions (see Chap. 1).

Epidermal Collarettes. Epidermal collarettes are circular scale-crust lesions that represent the end stage of pustules. These lesions are commonly found on animals with bacterial skin infections, but they are not specific for bacterial infections. Other causes of these lesions include pemphigus foliaceus, dermatophytosis, and drug eruptions. Epidermal collarettes are often mistaken for ringworm lesions (dermatophytosis) because of their characteristic circular shape (Fig. 3–1).

Diagnostic Plan

Patients with their first or only episode of surface or superficial pyoderma do not require an extensive diagnostic work-up. Skin scrapings are indicated in all cases to rule out ectoparasitic infections. Patients can be treated empirically with an antistaphylococcal agent after common predisposing factors such as demodicosis and atopy have been ruled out. Patients with recurring disease or disease that fails to respond to the empiric treatment should have a more extensive diagnostic evaluation. Fungal cultures, bacterial culture and sensitivity testing, cytology, skin biopsy, intradermal skin testing, hypoallergenic diet trial, and thyroid-stimulating hormone and adrenocorticotropic hormone response testing may be required to diagnose and properly manage the case.

Patients with deep pyoderma should be scrutinized more carefully. Bacterial cultures are indicated to identify the causative organism and to establish the

Table 3–1
Classification of Canine Pyoderma Based on Depth of Infection

CLASSIFICATION	EXAMPLES	TREATMENT DURATION
Surface pyoderma	Acute moist dermatitis Intertrigo	7–10 days
Superficial pyoderma	Folliculitis Impetigo	3–4 weeks
Deep pyoderma	Deep folliculitis Furunculosis	3–26 weeks
	Interdigital pyoderma Canine acne Nasal pyoderma Pressure point pyoderma Generalized deep pyoderma	
Cellulitis and abscess	Actinomycosis Nocardiosis Feline abscess and cellulitis	Weeks to months

susceptibility pattern for the organism. Histopathologic examination of the skin is recommended in cases that fail to respond to antimicrobial therapy or that recur.

Fistulous Tracts

Fistulous tracts are abnormal passages that communicate from deep in the skin or subcutaneous tissues to the exterior. Technically, they are considered a form of pyoderma if the cause is a bacterial infection.

Pathophysiology

These lesions represent an attempt by the host to extrude the offending substance from the skin. This material may be exogenous matter (e.g., a splinter) or keratinized structures of the skin (e.g., hair) trapped deep in the dermis or subcutis. Fistulous tracts often develop after furunculosis caused by bacterial infections of the follicle. If the infection extends deep into the dermis and involves the fascial planes, cellulitis occurs. The differential diagnosis for fistulous tracts includes sterile pyogranulomas, panniculitis, foreign body reactions, fungal infections (e.g., phaeohyphomycosis, coccidioidomycosis, cryptococcosis), atypical mycobacterial infections, and bacterial infections.

Clinical Signs

A fistulous tract appears as a draining, ulcerated lesion of the skin.

Diagnostic Plan

Cytology helps to determine whether an infectious agent is involved in the pathophysiology of the lesion. Bacterial and fungal cultures are indicated to identify infectious agents. Histopathologic evaluation of the affected skin may help to identify plant material or fungal agents. Occasionally, surgical exploration of the tract is necessary to determine the origin of the passage, which may be deep in the skin or in internal organs.

Diagnostic Procedures

Cytology

Cytology is a useful diagnostic procedure in patients with bacterial skin infections. If intact pustules are present, a slide should be prepared for cytologic evaluation (see Chap. 1). A Wright or Wright-Giemsa

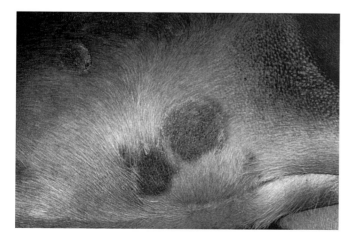

Figure 3–1
Circular scale-crust lesion (epidermal collarette) associated with bacterial dermatitis. The skin often becomes hyperpigmented as the lesions enlarge or heal.

Table 3–2

Antimicrobial Agents Effective Against _Staphylococcus intermedius_

ANTIMICROBIAL AGENT	DOSAGE	MECHANISM OF ACTION	MAJOR ADVERSE EFFECTS
Lincomycin	22 mg/kg PO, b.i.d.	Bacteriostatic*	Vomiting; colitis
Erythromycin	11 mg/kg PO, t.i.d.	Bacteriostatic	Vomiting
Trimethoprim-sulfonamide	30 mg/kg PO, s.i.d.	Bactericidal	Keratoconjunctivitis sicca; drug hypersensitivity; lameness in Doberman pinschers and other breeds
Ormetroprim-sulfadimethoxine	5 mg/kg† PO, s.i.d.	Bactericidal	Keratoconjunctivitis sicca; drug hypersensitivity
Amoxicillin–clavulanic acid	14-22 mg/kg PO, b.i.d.	Bactericidal	Vomiting; nephrotoxicosis
Oxacillin	22 mg/kg PO, t.i.d.‡	Bactericidal	Vomiting; nephrotoxicosis
Cefadroxil	22 mg/kg PO, b.i.d.	Bactericidal	Vomiting; nephrotoxicosis
Cephalexin	22 mg/kg PO, b.i.d.	Bactericidal	Vomiting; nephrotoxicosis

b.i.d., twice per day; PO, oral; s.i.d., once per day; t.i.d., three times per day.
*Shares cross-resistance with erythromycin.
†Dosage based on sulfadimethoxine content; twice this dose is administered on day 1 of treatment.
‡Do not give with food (interferes with absorption).

stain (Diff-Quik) is adequate. The clinician should look for the presence of infectious agents, usually coccoid bacteria, within inflammatory cells. If bacteria are not detected, histopathologic evaluation of the skin may be indicated to determine the cause of the pustular dermatitis.

Bacterial Culture and Susceptibility Testing

Bacterial culture and susceptibility testing is not necessary in all bacterial skin infections. The primary purpose is not to identify the causative organism, because _S. intermedius_ is known to be the inciting organism in most cases of pyoderma. The test is used to provide the clinician with the susceptibility pattern of the organism, so that the antimicrobial agent most likely to be effective against this organism can be prescribed[1] (Table 3–2). Bacterial cultures are indicated if the lesions do not clear after empiric antimicrobial therapy, if the bacterial infection recurs after cessation of therapy, in cases of deep pyoderma, or if fistulous tracts are present.

Intact pustules are the best lesion to culture. Pus or serosanguineous fluid should be collected, using aseptic techniques. Hair should be carefully clipped from the area around the lesion, taking care not to disturb or destroy the lesion. Most pustules are fragile and will not withstand a surgical scrub. Two or three gentle wipings of the lesion with alcohol help to reduce contamination. The lesion is then lanced with a sterile scalpel blade or 20-gauge needle, and the culture swab is carefully touched to the lesion. Material may also be collected for culture by aspiration of an intact pustule with a syringe and 20-gauge needle.

Therapeutic Procedures

Topical Antibacterial Therapy

Topical therapy with antimicrobial agents in gel, cream, or ointment preparations may be useful if a single, superficial lesion is present. Salicylic acid, benzoyl peroxide, and various antibiotics, including mupirocin (Bactoderm), have antibacterial properties. These products should be applied to the lesion two or three times per day until clinical remission has occurred. Topical antimicrobial agents are not useful or effective for generalized or multifocal disease.

A more effective method to deliver topical antimicrobial agents to the skin is by shampoos. Commercially available products containing benzoyl peroxide, salicylic acid, or triclosan may be used as the sole therapeutic agent in surface pyodermas or as an adjunct to systemic therapy in the treatment of surface and superficial pyodermas. Shampoos should be applied every 5 to 7 days and should contact the skin for 5 to 10 minutes at each application. Owners should be instructed to watch a timer while shampooing their pet to ensure adequate contact time.

Systemic Antibacterial Therapy

Systemic antimicrobial therapy is required to resolve the pyoderma in most cases. An appropriate antimicrobial drug should (1) be effective against β-lactamase–producing staphylococci, (2) be available as an oral preparation, because therapy may be prolonged, (3) have minimal side effects, and (4) be effective when administered one or two times per day, so that owners will be more likely to comply with instructions. Cost is also a factor when selecting an antimicrobial agent, because prolonged therapy is often necessary. It is important to know the mechanism of action of these drugs and to inform the client of possible adverse effects of drugs prescribed for the pet (see Table 3–2).

Penicillin, amoxicillin, ampicillin, and tetracycline are poor choices for the management of canine pyoderma, even if culture and susceptibility tests show the organism to be sensitive to these drugs. *S. intermedius* is frequently resistant to these drugs or develops resistance within several days of treatment. First-line drugs (i.e., those that are often effective for surface or mild superficial infections) include lincomycin, erythromycin, and the potentiated sulfonamides. Clavulanic acid–potentiated amoxicillin, penicillinase-resistant penicillins, and the cephalosporins are also very effective for these infections but should be reserved for deep pyodermas, subcutaneous infections, or systemic infections. Bactericidal antibiotics are recommended for deep pyodermas or if an immunosuppressive process is suspected.

The duration of therapy is important to ensure complete elimination of the infection. In general, the deeper the infection, the longer systemic therapy must be administered to clear the infection. Surface pyodermas may be managed by 5 to 7 days of antimicrobial therapy, superficial pyoderma may be managed by 21 to 28 days of therapy, and deep pyoderma may require 21 to 180 days of therapy. Antimicrobial therapy should continue for 7 days past clinical resolution of the lesions, except in the management of surface pyodermas. Clients should be cautioned not to adjust the dose without consent of the veterinarian, because alterations adversely affect the response of the animal to the medication.

Other antimicrobial agents that may be useful for resistant deep pyoderma include enrofloxacin, rifampin, and some of the aminoglycosides. These antibiotics are generally considered more useful for infections located in other organs systems.

Immunomodulating agents are occasionally indicated in recurring cases of pyoderma or if the response to antimicrobials is incomplete. Patients should be thoroughly evaluated for other disorders that may affect the response to antibacterial therapy. Predisposing diseases, such as demodicosis, hypothyroidism, or adverse reactions to food, should be ruled out before immunomodulators are administered.

Specific immunomodulators include autogenous bacterins, staphylococcal cell wall antigen toxoid, a bacteriophage-lysed preparation of *S. aureus* (Staphage Lysate), and a *Propionibacterium acnes* bacterin (ImmunoRegulin).[8, 9] In clinical trials involving dogs with superficial pyoderma, patients treated with a bacteriophage-lysed staphylococcal preparation had significant clinical improvement, compared with control dogs.[8] This product is my choice whenever immunomodulator therapy is indicated. A dose of 0.5 mL is administered subcutaneously twice weekly for a trial period of 10 weeks. If improvement is observed, injections are continued and the treatment intervals are gradually increased. Antimicrobials are usually given concurrently for the first few weeks.

Common Bacterial Diseases of the Skin

Surface Pyodermas

Surface pyoderma is defined as a bacterial infection limited to the surface of the skin. It does not extend deeper than the stratum corneum or into hair follicles.

Acute Moist Dermatitis

Acute moist dermatitis (hot spots, pyotraumatic dermatitis) is a common surface bacterial infection of the dog. The disease is seen more commonly in thick-coated breeds and in dogs that swim frequently.

Pathophysiology

These lesions develop secondary to precipitating factors that include self-induced trauma to the skin from pruritus, ectoparasitism, and alterations of the microenvironment of the skin. The microenvironmental change is exacerbated in long- or thick-coated breeds and in high relative humidity or heat and is compounded by some behaviors of animals, such as swimming. Bacterial proliferation on the skin and subsequent release of bacterial toxins and enzymes results in inflammation and pruritus. As the animal traumatizes the skin in response to the pruritus, the infection becomes more severe and a vicious circle of pyoderma and pruritus is established.

Clinical Signs

Lesions consist of moist, exudative areas of erythema and are generally well demarcated and severely pruritic. The lesions may develop and expand very rapidly, with animals showing severe, debilitating pruritus within a few hours. Alopecia results from self-induced trauma. These lesions are one of the few dermatologic diseases that constitute an emergency in the eyes of pet owners.

Diagnostic Plan

The diagnosis is made from the history and the findings on physical examination. Skin scrapings and fungal evaluation are recommended to rule out precipitating factors. If lesions fail to respond to treatment, bacterial culture and biopsy may be indicated. Two histologic forms of lesions have been identified.[10] The first pattern is an ulcerative, superficial inflammation of the skin. The second pattern is a deep, suppurative folliculitis and probably represents progression of the infection. If a patient has recurring lesions of acute moist dermatitis, active lesions should be treated and diagnostic testing should concentrate on identification of predisposing diseases.

Treatment

Treatment goals include control of the pruritus and pain and elimination of the infection. The lesions respond best to combination therapy with topical and systemic medications. First, the lesion should be cleaned and dried. Hair should be clipped from the lesion, although this may require an anesthetic because of the painful nature of some lesions. Astringents, such as aluminum acetate solution (Domeboro), may be applied to the lesion two to three times a day. Glucocorticoids help to reduce the inflammation, pain, and pruritus associated with these lesions. Oral prednisone (1.1 mg/kg per day for 5 days, then 1.1 mg/kg every other day for five doses) or a single injection of prednisone (e.g., Meticorten) at 1.1 mg/kg alleviates the pruritus. An appropriate antistaphylococcal antimicrobial agent should be administered for 5 to 7 days.

Prognosis

The prognosis is excellent if these recommendations are followed. The patient should be comfortable within 24 hours and the lesions healed within 7 days.

Intertrigo

Surface bacterial infections often develop in skin folds in some breeds and are referred to as intertrigo or intertriginous pyoderma (skin-fold pyoderma). The location, depth, and number of folds vary with the breed. Pyoderma may occur in the facial folds of brachycephalic breeds, such as English and French bulldogs and Boston terriers. Lip-fold pyoderma occurs in spaniel breeds, Irish setters, and other dogs with heavy jowls. Bacterial infection can develop in folds of skin around the vulva of female dogs, especially if the animal is obese. Animals with corkscrew tails may develop pyoderma in the folds around the tail. The Chinese shar-pei can develop skin-fold pyoderma in almost any area of the body.

Pathophysiology

Changes in the microenvironment of the skin surface permit proliferation of bacteria and other microorganisms. Secondary inflammation and necrosis induce pruritus and proliferative dermatologic changes. Obesity predisposes a female dog to develop vulvar-fold pyoderma.

Clinical Signs

The classic lesion is moist erythema in the affected area. Purulent exudate may collect in the affected area. There is often a foul odor emanating from the lesions, which are painful when severe. The level of pruritus is variable; if present, it is manifested as rubbing of the face, scratching, or scooting the perineal area on a carpet, depending on the area that is involved.

Diagnostic Plan

The diagnosis is based on the findings of the physical examination. Skin scrapings, fungal culture, cytology, and other tests may be necessary to identify predisposing factors. Animals with vulvar-fold pyoderma should be evaluated for ascending (secondary) urinary tract infections.

Treatment

Medical management of this condition is accomplished by cleaning and drying of the lesions and by treatment with appropriate antimicrobial medications. Owners should clean the affected areas daily with an antiseptic soap, such as chlorhexidine. Astringents (e.g., Domeboro solution) are useful to keep the areas dry. In severe cases, systemic antimicrobial agents should be prescribed for 7 to 10 days. Occasionally, surgical correction of a conformational problem is necessary to prevent recurrence of the inflammation. Episioplasty benefits some patients with vulvar-fold pyoderma; however, the condition may recur despite the surgical effort.

Prognosis

The prognosis is excellent, although the pyoderma may recur if the skin fold is not reduced by weight loss or surgical correction.

Superficial Pyodermas

Impetigo

Impetigo is a bacterial infection characterized by invasion of the stratum corneum and the development of subcorneal pustules. Impetigo is usually diagnosed in immature dogs.

Pathophysiology

Contributing pathologic factors may include specific immunodeficiency syndromes, inadequate nutrition, poor husbandry (e.g., crowding, inadequate housing), and stress. Staphylococci and streptococci are most frequently isolated from the lesions.

Clinical Signs

Lesions include papules and pustules in the ventral abdominal and inguinal areas. The pustules do not usually involve the follicles. If pruritus is present, it is usually mild.

Diagnostic Plan

The condition is easily diagnosed on physical examination. Skin scrapings and cytologic analysis of a pustule help to rule out predisposing factors and confirm the presence of a bacterial infection.

Treatment

Topical therapy is often sufficient to clear the infection after predisposing factors are controlled. Weekly baths with a benzoyl peroxide shampoo or a shampoo containing triclosan are effective. Systemic antibiotic therapy (10–14 days) is indicated in the rare cases that do not respond to topical therapy.

Prognosis

The prognosis is excellent, although some patients require topical treatment until they reach maturity.

Folliculitis

Folliculitis is defined as inflammation of the hair follicle. There are three diseases in which folliculitis is a common feature: demodicosis, dermatophytosis, and bacterial infections of the skin. Short-coated dogs seem predisposed to bacterial folliculitis, and the condition has been referred to as short-coated dog pyoderma.

Pathophysiology

Predisposing factors include breed (e.g., hair coat type), allergies, ectoparasitic infections, immunodeficiency syndromes, and endocrine imbalances. Two distinct forms of folliculitis are recognized. In superficial folliculitis, the inflammation is concentrated in the outer third of the follicle. In deep folliculitis, the inflammation occurs deep within the follicle. In both cases, the follicle growth cycle may shift to the telogen phase after inflammation occurs in and around the hair follicle. Hairs are then easily dislodged, resulting in diffuse or patchy alopecia.

The three most common causes of folliculitis are demodicosis, dermatophytosis, and bacterial infections. Folliculitis may also be seen in drug reactions, in autoimmune diseases, and in an idiopathic eosinophilic form.

Clinical Signs

Physical examination findings include patchy alopecia and the presence of many papules and pustules (Fig. 3–2). The large numbers of papules has led to the term lumpy-bumpy disease as a synonym for folliculitis. The clinician may notice that some hairs or tufts of hairs protrude from the rest of the hair coat and that hairs epilate easily. These findings are consistent with follicular disease.

Diagnostic Plan

The signalment of the patient (short-coated dogs) and the history provide the first evidence of folliculitis. Skin scrapings and fungal culture are indicated to rule out demodicosis and dermatophytosis, the other main causes of folliculitis. If pustules are present, cytology is recommended to search for infectious agents. Pustules or papules may be cultured for bacteria in order to determine the susceptibility of the organism to specific antibiotics. Histopathologic examination confirms the diagnosis, but other diagnostic tests are necessary to identify predisposing conditions.

Treatment

Bacterial folliculitis is treated with an appropriate antimicrobial agent for 21 to 28 days. The antimicrobial agent should be selected based on results of culture and sensitivity testing if the patient has had folliculitis previously or if the disease has not responded to empiric treatment. Topical antimicrobial shampoos are recommended as adjunctive treatment.

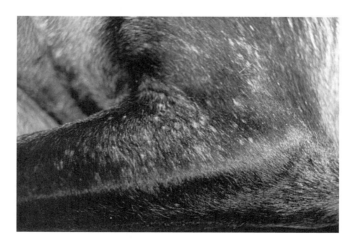

Figure 3–2
Papules, pustules, and patchy alopecia caused by bacterial folliculitis.

Benzoyl peroxide shampoos are administered weekly until the disease is in remission. Many owners find that administration of shampoos every 10 to 21 days keeps the disease in remission after completion of systemic antimicrobial therapy.

Prognosis

The prognosis is good for this condition, although patients may have recurring disease. If the patient has recurring disease and specific underlying conditions are ruled out, immunomodulator therapy is recommended.

Deep Pyodermas

Furunculosis

Furunculosis is defined as disruption of the hair follicle as a result of any underlying disease process. The condition may be seen in any breed predisposed to folliculitis.

Pathophysiology

Furunculosis is the end stage of untreated folliculitis. When furunculosis occurs, the infectious agent responsible for folliculitis and the keratinized structures of the follicle (e.g., hair) are released into the surrounding dermis. The result is a deep infection of the skin and a secondary foreign body reaction in the dermis. Draining tracts develop if large amounts of keratinized material are released into the dermis. Permanent hair loss occurs if the follicle is destroyed.

Clinical Signs

Furunculosis is clinically similar to folliculitis. Lesions include papules, pustules, and alopecia. However, as the lesions progress, draining tracts, nodules, ulcerations, and lichenification of the skin are seen. Clinicians are often able to express a serosanguineous, blood-tinged fluid from the skin in affected areas. The inflammation causes moderate to severe pruritus.

Furunculosis is often classified based on the location of the lesions. Canine acne is a form of folliculitis and furunculosis localized to the face and chin. Other examples include facial pyoderma, pressure point pyoderma, and interdigital pyoderma. A form of deep pyoderma and furunculosis has been recognized in German shepherds. The lesions are characterized by fistulization and ulceration, pustules, erythema, and crusts adherent to the hair[11, 12] (Fig. 3–3). The role of underlying immunodeficiencies in these patients is unclear.[13]

Diagnostic Plan

The diagnosis is based on the history and findings of the physical examination. Skin scrapings and fungal culture are always indicated to rule out

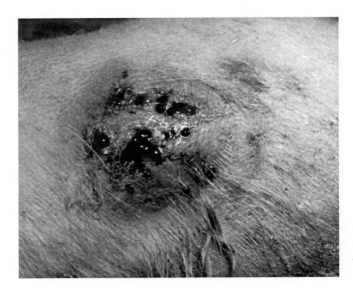

Figure 3–3
Ulcers and fistulous tracts associated with deep pyoderma in a German shepherd.

demodicosis and dermatophytosis. Cytologic evaluation of material collected from the draining lesions or from intact pustules helps to confirm the presence of bacteria. Bacterial culture should be performed to identify the causative organism and, more importantly, to assist in the selection of the most appropriate antimicrobial agent. Histopathologic examination may be indicated to rule out other causes of draining lesions and exudative dermatitis. Considerations in the differential diagnosis include foreign body reactions, mycobacterial infection, intermediate and deep fungal infections, sterile pyogranulomas, and neoplasia.

Treatment

The recommended treatment is long-term administration of an antimicrobial agent that has been selected based on culture and susceptibility testing. The duration of therapy is based on clinical response. Bacterial culture and sensitivity testing should be repeated if the clinical response seems to diminish after several days or weeks of treatment. Antimicrobial therapy is usually necessary for a minimum of 4 weeks; in some cases, treatment may be needed for several months.

Antimicrobial shampoos are helpful to clear surface crust and scale but are not of major therapeutic value in deep pyodermas. Whirlpool sessions reduce the pain and pruritus of the condition, enhance the drainage of lesions, and increase blood flow to the skin. Many clients find the purchase of a home whirlpool unit to be within their financial budget. Ultrasonic baths (HydroSound) have similar effects. Immunomodulator therapy is recommended if there is incomplete response to antimicrobial therapy or if the condition recurs.

Prognosis

The prognosis is fair to good; however, underlying disorders must be identified and managed. Hair will not regrow in areas where hair follicles have been destroyed. The prognosis is guarded in German shepherds with furunculosis, because response to antimicrobial therapy varies from patient to patient.[12]

Interdigital Pyoderma

Interdigital pyoderma is a form of folliculitis and furunculosis of the interdigital areas.

Pathophysiology

Interdigital pyoderma may be initiated by foreign material (e.g., plant awns), bacterial folliculitis, or trauma. Underlying conditions associated with interdigital pyoderma or pododermatitis (see Chap. 1) include atopy, adverse reactions to food, demodicosis, and contact dermatitis. The bacterial component of the pododermatitis may be a primary factor or an opportunistic infection. A hypersensitivity reaction to one or more bacterial cell wall components is suspected in some cases. A sterile pyogranulomatous condition involving the feet may present with similar lesions.

Clinical Signs

Erythema, papules, pustules, ulcerations, and fistulous tracts are found in the interdigital spaces on the dorsum of the foot and between the pads on the ventrum. In severe cases, the feet may become severely swollen, resulting in lameness. The prescapular and popliteal lymph nodes are usually enlarged.

Diagnostic Plan

An intensive diagnostic work-up of these patients is required to identify predisposing factors and diseases such as atopy, adverse reactions to food, or immunoinsufficiency syndromes. Skin scrapings, fungal cultures, cytologic evaluation of lesions, bacterial culture and sensitivity testing, and skin biopsies are recommended.

Treatment

Long-term administration of an appropriate antimicrobial agent is necessary to clear most infections. Antimicrobials are prescribed for a minimum of 3 to 4 weeks, and it may be necessary to continue treatment for 180 days or longer. Bacterial cultures are recommended every 30 to 60 days to determine whether bacteria are still present and to evaluate the susceptibility of the bacteria to the antimicrobial agent in use. Astringents are indicated in moist, exudative lesions. Whirlpool sessions are recommended to clean and dry the lesions and to improve blood flow to the affected areas. Foot soaks in antiseptic solutions may provide relief to some patients but are not as effective as active hydrotherapy.

If antimicrobial therapy does not control the problem, treatment with an immunomodulating drug is indicated. Improvement may be seen in up to 40% of patients after immunomodulator therapy. As previously stated, treatment with immunomodulators is not recommended until a thorough evaluation of the patient to identify predisposing conditions has been completed.

Glucocorticoid therapy is indicated in cases of interdigital pyoderma caused by sterile pyogranulomatous reactions.[13] These sterile lesions respond to aggressive glucocorticoid therapy (2.2 mg/kg per day). However, bacterial and other infectious causes of interdigital granulomas must be ruled out before immunosuppressive therapy is initiated. Two consecutive negative bacterial and fungal cultures and the absence of infectious agents on histologic evaluation of the skin are criteria used to recommend this therapy.

Cellulitis and Abscess

Cellulitis is defined as inflammation involving the deep subcutaneous tissues and fascial planes. An abscess is a localized collection of inflammatory cells.

Pathophysiology

These conditions are frequently caused by bacterial infections and are seen most commonly in cats with bite wounds. Organisms commonly identified in cat bite abscesses include *Pasteurella* spp., *Fusobacterium* spp., *Bacteroides* spp., streptococci, staphylococci, and other aerobic and anaerobic bacteria, including *Actinomyces* spp. and *Nocardia* spp.[6, 14, 15] Cats with recurring abscesses should be evaluated for the presence of the feline immunodeficiency virus and the feline leukemia virus. Other immunosuppressive disorders, such as the immunoglobulin A deficiency seen in shar-peis and German shepherds, should also be considered. Cellulitis and abscess formation may also accompany noninfectious dermatologic conditions, such as juvenile cellulitis (see Chap. 6) and panniculitis (see Chap. 5).

Clinical Signs

Cellulitis is characterized by swelling and pain over the affected area. Fistulous tracts, with draining serosanguineous or purulent material, are often present. An abscess is characterized by a localized, fluctuant swelling of soft tissue structures. Fever is common in animals with cellulitis or an abscess.

Diagnostic Plan

Diagnosis of a bacterial infection is easily confirmed by cytologic examination of material collected from the lesion. A 23-gauge needle and syringe may be used to perform a fine-needle aspiration to collect material for cytology or culture. Culture and sensitivity testing are not necessary unless the condition is recurrent or there is inadequate response to therapy.

Treatment

Treatment of cellulitis includes hot soaks of the affected area and antimicrobial therapy until the lesion is resolved. Appropriate treatment of an abscess includes surgical drainage.

Prognosis

The prognosis is excellent after drainage has been established.

Uncommon Bacterial Diseases of the Skin

Dermatophilus congolensis Infection

Dermatophilus congolensis infection has been reported in both dogs and cats. Infection by this actinomycete responds well to cleaning and drying of the skin and to appropriate antimicrobial therapy.

Nocardiosis and Actinomycosis

Cutaneous lesions may be associated with nocardiosis and actinomycosis in the dog or cat.[16, 17] Clinical findings include fever, anorexia, and depression, with ulcerative, fistulous lesions, erythema, and swelling of the affected areas.

Yersinia pestis Infection

Cellulitis and abscess formation may be seen with plague (*Yersinia pestis* infection), which is endemic in the western United States and carries strong public health risks to exposed humans.[18]

Mycobacterial Infection

Mycobacterial infections may result in nodules, ulcerations, and fistulous tracts in the skin of dogs and cats. *Mycobacterium leprosum* (leprosy), *Mycobacterium tuberculosis*, *Mycobacterium avium*, and mycobacteria classified as Runyon type IV (atypical mycobacteria) can cause lesions in both dogs and cats.[19–22]

Fungal Infections of the Skin

Problem Identification

Alopecia

Hair loss frequently accompanies dermatophyte infections of the skin. The alopecia is caused by structural damage of hairs by fungal organisms. These hairs are then easily broken and lost from the skin. Damage to hairs and alopecia also result from pruritus. The presence of broken hairs is a common feature of dermatophytosis. If broken hairs are present, they should be selected for potassium hydroxide (KOH) preparations and fungal culture.

The alopecia associated with fungal disease is often patchy, and animals looked disheveled. Cats often appear as though they have stopped grooming. Fungal culture for dermatophytes should be part of the minimum database for all patients with alopecia. See Chapter 1 for a complete discussion of alopecia.

Crusts

Serocellular crusts, accumulations of inflammatory cells and serum on the surface of the epidermis, are frequently seen in dermatophytosis. Crusts may also contain fungal hyphae. Because there is no specific appearance of a crust to suggest that it is associated with fungal disease, fungal evaluation is crucial whenever an animal presents with crusts. See Chapter 1 for a complete discussion of crusts.

Nodules

Fungal infections of the skin may produce severe localized swelling and accumulation of inflammatory cells, resulting in the formation of a nodule. Occasionally, these nodules are the result of deep invasion of the dermis by the fungal agent and form a kerion (dermatophytosis) or fungal pyogranuloma (systemic mycotic infections). Diagnosis is based on fungal culture, fine-needle aspiration, imprint cytology, or biopsy. See Chapter 7 for a complete discussion of nodules.

Diagnostic Procedures

Wood Lamp Examination

Wood lamp examination is a screening test for dermatophytes. Infected hairs and crusts exhibit an apple-green fluorescence on exposure to light from a Wood lamp, which has an ultraviolet light filtered through a nickel oxide filter. The longer the lesion is exposed to the light, the stronger the fluorescence. False fluorescence may be seen with scaling disorders or with some topical medications. Positive fluorescence should not be the sole basis for the diagnosis of dermatophytosis: of the common pathogens of the dog and cat, only *Microsporum canis* exhibits fluorescence, and even then only about half of samples fluoresce. Both positive and negative findings should be confirmed by fungal culture. The value of the test is early detection of some infections, because cultures may take weeks to develop.

Potassium Hydroxide Preparations

KOH digestion is another screening test used to confirm dermatophytosis. Hair samples or crusts are taken from patients suspected of having dermatophytosis. Hairs that fluoresce and those located at the periphery of a lesion are most likely to be infected. A few drops of 10% to 20% KOH are placed on a glass slide, a few hairs are added, and a coverslip is applied. After 5 to 30 minutes, the hairs are examined for spores or hyphae. To perform the procedure accurately requires experience. In most cases, positive or negative findings should be confirmed by fungal culture.

Fungal Culture

Fungal culture is the most definitive test to confirm the diagnosis of dermatophytosis. Hair or scale collected with mosquito forceps from the periphery and center of suspected fungal lesions should gently be placed on the culture medium. Hairs should not be clumped but should be separated as much as possible to reduce overgrowth from contaminants. Alternatively, samples of hair and scale may be collected by brushing the entire hair coat with a sterile toothbrush. The bristles are then shaken over the agar, embedded in agar, or trimmed over the culture medium. Sabouraud dextrose agar is an excellent growth medium, as are commercially available media that contain antimicrobial agents to reduce bacteria growth and pH indicators to aid in the identification of pathogenic fungi (Fungassay Dermatophyte Test Medium, Derm Duet). Samples should be incubated in a warm, humid environment for up to 28 days, and they should be examined every 2 to 3 days for evidence of growth.

Pathogenic fungi use protein in the culture medium as a substrate for growth and produce alkaline metabolites, causing a red color change on a dermatophyte test medium. Saprophytes use carbohydrate in the medium and do not produce the same color change. However, saprophytes eventually metabolize proteins and cause a color change in the medium. In addition, some saprophytes will cause a red color change during early stages of growth on a dermatophyte test medium. Therefore, microscopic confirmation of the identity of the fungus is required to avoid a false diagnosis of dermatophytosis.

A small amount of mycelial growth from a mature colony is easily teased onto a glass slide with forceps. Alternatively, a small strip of clear acetate tape can be pressed onto the surface of the mature colony to collect hyphae. The teased specimen or tape is placed onto a glass slide and stained with lactophenol cotton blue or new methylene blue stain for microscopic examination. The identification of a *Microsporum* spp. or *Trichophyton* spp. is easily made based on the characteristics of their hyphae and macroconidia.[23]

Skin Biopsy

Histopathologic examination of affected skin is a useful diagnostic procedure for dermatophytosis and for the intermediate and deep fungal infections. Special stains, such as silver stains or periodic acid–Schiff stain, are used by pathologists to help identify fungal elements in the microscopic section. However, dermatophytes may not be detected by histopathologic examination because of the relatively low numbers of infected hair follicles present on a patient at any given time. The procedure is useful if fungal elements are present, but fungal culture should be performed if the findings are negative for fungi.

Common Fungal Diseases of the Skin

Dermatophytosis

Dermatophytosis (ringworm) is the most common fungal infection of the skin. It is defined as infection of the keratinized structures of the skin by pathogenic fungi. The infection is seen more commonly in immunosuppressed animals, animals younger than 1 year of age, and older or debilitated animals. Dermatophytosis is a common problem in catteries and may be more prevalent in Persian cats.

Pathophysiology

Three microorganisms, *Microsporum canis*, *Microsporum gypseum*, and *Trichophyton mentagrophytes*, account for most infections. The prevalence of each of these agents varies with the geographic location: *M.*

canis is the most common isolate in some geographic regions, *T. mentagrophytes* in others. Factors that may predispose animals to infections include crowding, poor nutritional status, immunodeficiency syndromes, and debilitating diseases. Barring any of these factors, dermatophytosis is thought to be a self-limiting disease, with remission occurring in 1 to 3 months.

Dermatophytes invade only keratinized structures, including the stratum corneum of the skin, planum nasale, foot pads, hair, and claws. These fungal agents invade the nonliving portion of actively growing keratinized structures. They elicit an inflammatory response by the production of exotoxins and other fungal metabolites. The inflammatory response may result in control of the infection or may lead to secondary problems such as pruritus. Folliculitis is commonly seen in dermatophyte infections. If the lesions are severe, furunculosis may occur, resulting in the formation of nodules or fistulous tracts. Dermatophytes, usually *M. canis*, can rarely localize in granulomatous lesions in the dermis; the resulting ulcerated nodules are called pseudomycetomas.

Clinical Signs

Alopecia is the most common clinical finding associated with dermatophytosis. The alopecic areas may be circular or irregular, focal or generalized. They occur secondary to structurally damaged hairs, pruritus, and follicular inflammation. The presence of broken hairs is a key diagnostic feature. Erythema, crusts, and scale are also common findings (Fig. 3–4). The skin is often pigmented in chronically affected areas and areas undergoing healing. Pruritus is a common feature of dermatophytosis, although the intensity is variable.

Diagnostic Plan

Dermatophytosis should be suspected from the signalment, history, and clinical lesions. Fluorescence on Wood lamp examination helps to confirm the diagnosis. Fluorescing hairs should be selected for fungal culture for definitive diagnosis. Microscopic examination of hairs with or without digestion with KOH confirms the diagnosis if fungal elements or spores are visualized on the examination. Because this procedure requires some experience to avoid a false-positive diagnosis, it is not recommended as the sole diagnostic procedure.

Fungal culture remains the most definitive test to confirm the diagnosis of dermatophytosis.

Treatment

Not all animals with dermatophytosis require extensive therapy, because the disease is considered to be self-limited. However, these agents are a public health risk, and this fact must be considered when deciding whether systemic treatment is warranted. Most cases should be aggressively treated to avoid the risk of continued human exposure. Treatment of dermatophytosis has three components.

Decontamination of the Pet

The first component of therapy is decontamination of the infected animal. Topical antifungal preparations, used as the sole treatment, do not appear to significantly alter the course of experimentally induced dermatophyte infections in cats.[24] However, the use of these products may speed recovery of naturally infected animals and reduce infectivity to the humans in the household. Animals with diffuse or multifocal disease should have a total body clip performed to remove infected hairs. Application of antifungal shampoos containing lime sulfur, enilconazole, povidone-iodine, chlorhexidine, miconazole, or ketoconazole is recommended every 5 days. In a recent study using infected hairs, application of lime sulfur and enilconazole resulted in the most rapid negative culture results, but chlorhexidine and povidone-iodine were also effective.[25] Miconazole and ketoconazole were not included in that study. Topical antifungal agents, available as creams, ointments, and solutions, are also used to control localized or minor infections.

Systemic Antifungal Therapy

The implementation of systemic therapy is the second component of therapy. Systemic therapy with griseofulvin is recommended if the condition is generalized or recurrent. The drug is available in micro-sized or ultramicrosized formulations; particle size affects absorption of the drug. The drug is available in tablet form and as a pediatric suspension. Griseofulvin

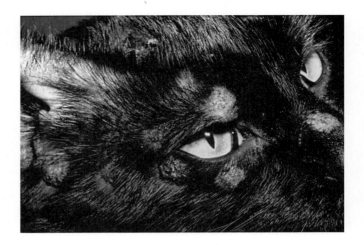

Figure 3–4
Microsporum canis infection in a cat with multiple, alopecic, scale-crust lesions.

Table 3–3
Control of Dermatophytosis in the Cattery

General Management

1. Screen all cats using the toothbrush technique for collection of samples (recommended if any cats show lesions).
2. Screen all new cats using the toothbrush technique before introducing into the cattery.
3. Keep new cats isolated until culture results are available.

Infected Animals

1. Isolate infected animals away from noninfected animals.
2. Clip and topically disinfect all infected animals.
3. Treat nonpregnant queens and cats older than 12 weeks of age with a systemic antifungal agent and with topical antifungal therapy every 5 to 7 days.
4. Treat pregnant queens and cats younger than 12 weeks of age with topical antifungal agents every 5 days.

Environment

1. Vacuum environment and discard vacuum bag every 2 to 3 days.
2. Clean all appropriate surfaces with a topical antifungal disinfectant (e.g., 1:30 dilution of sodium hypochlorite).
3. Clean and disinfect fans, air conditioning ducts, and other hardware in the cattery.
4. Clean and disinfect all grooming aids after each use.
5. Wash all carpets, bedding, and draperies every 7 to 10 days.
6. Replace furnace filters every 2 to 4 weeks.

is fungistatic, and absorption from the gastrointestinal tract is enhanced by reduction of particle size and by concurrent feeding of a fatty meal. Griseofulvin is teratogenic and may induce vomiting, diarrhea, and bone marrow suppression resulting in leukopenia. Bone marrow reactions appear to be idiosyncratic, although cats concurrently infected with the feline immunodeficiency virus appear to have an increased frequency of griseofulvin-associated neutropenia.[26, 27] Microsized formulations of griseofulvin are administered at 25 to 100 mg/kg per day, whereas ultramicrosized griseofulvin is administered at 5 to 15 mg/kg per day. The treatment duration varies and should extend for 2 to 3 weeks beyond clinical recovery. Six to eight weeks of therapy is usually required to clear the infection, which may be evaluated by fungal culture of hair and scale collected by the toothbrush technique.

Ketoconazole (Nizoral) is an imidazole drug that is also effective against dermatophytes.[28, 29] The use of this drug is reserved for patients that have adverse reactions to griseofulvin. Side effects may include anorexia, vomiting, and elevated liver enzyme concentrations. Ketoconazole is administered at 10 mg/kg per day for 6 to 8 weeks. Itraconazole is another imidazole drug that has shown efficacy against dermatophytes. The recommended dose is 5 mg/kg per day. Side effects in cats may include anorexia and vomiting.

Disinfection of the Environment

This third component of antifungal therapy is necessary to reduce the risk of reinfection. Fungal spores may remain viable for several months in the environment. Sodium hypochlorite at a 1:10 dilution should be used to clean appropriate surfaces in affected households. The staining or bleaching qualities of this disinfectant should be considered when it is used in the home. Chlorhexidine or another topical antifungal agent may also be used, but the effectiveness of any topical disinfectant is questionable. In addition, bedding should be cleaned, and furnace filters and airways should be changed or cleaned. Carpets and furniture should be vacuumed to remove contaminated hairs and debris.

Management of Catteries

Catteries represent an especially difficult management problem for the veterinarian. *M. canis* is the most frequently isolated dermatophyte from the cattery environment. Aggressive management of the cattery is essential to control the infection (Table 3–3). Extra attention should be directed to decontamination required in catteries.[30]

Special Considerations

Dermatophytosis in kittens and puppies should be managed with topical antifungal agents until the animals are 12 weeks of age, at which time oral griseofulvin may be used. In some cases, griseofulvin may be necessary in animals 8 to 12 weeks of age.

Prevention

A vaccine labeled for dermatophytosis (Fel-O-Vax MC-K) has recently been released. Preliminary work with the vaccine in catteries has shown that the product may reduce the number and severity of lesions seen in cats infected by *M. canis*. However, at this time there are no published studies supporting claims that the vaccine actually prevents infection. The vaccine may be useful in catteries or in households with large numbers of infected animals as an aid to treatment. Animals should be monitored with fungal cultures by the brush technique to determine whether the infection has been eliminated.

Prognosis

The prognosis is good for individual animals, although reinfection can occur. Catteries represent a difficult and troublesome source of infected hairs and cellular debris, and the prognosis for clearance is guarded.

Malassezia Dermatitis

Infection of the skin by the yeast *Malassezia pachydermatis*, formerly called *Pityrosporum canis*, has been recently recognized as a common problem in dogs. The disease may be seen in any breed of dog, but dachshunds, boxers, West Highland white terriers, basset hounds, and American cocker spaniels appear to be at increased risk of developing the infection. The infection is uncommon in cats.

Pathophysiology

The organism may be found in low numbers on the skin of normal dogs.[31] Proliferation of this yeast may occur if the host's immune system is compromised or if the skin surface is modified to allow or enhance growth. Predisposing factors for yeast proliferation include the presence of seborrheic dermatitis, recent antibiotic therapy, and susceptible breed.[32] Allergic skin disease is commonly associated with *Malassezia* dermatitis.

Clinical Signs

Cutaneous signs associated with proliferation of *Malassezia* spp. yeasts include erythema, lichenification, hyperpigmentation, and scale-crust accumulation. Pruritus is a constant feature and is often very intense. The interdigital areas, muzzle, ventral neck, abdominal and inguinal area, and axillae are commonly affected (Fig. 3–5). Otitis externa with accumulation of a dark, waxy exudate is a common feature of this syndrome. However, some animals have extensive cutaneous lesions and clinically normal ears.

Diagnostic Plan

Diagnosis is confirmed by identification of the organism from lesional skin. Because low numbers of

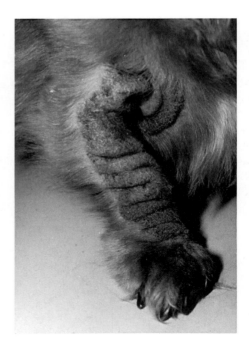

Figure 3–5
Erythema, hyperpigmentation, and lichenification commonly seen in *Malassezia* dermatitis.

yeast cells may be found on the skin of normal animals, it is useful to subjectively quantify the numbers found on samples (Table 3–4). Samples may be collected by dry skin scrapings, by vigorous rubbing of a cotton-tipped swab on the skin, by impression smears on glass slides, or by repeatedly pressing acetate tape onto the surface of the skin. The skin scraping technique is an excellent method to isolate yeast. In this procedure, a dull scalpel is used to scrape the surface of affected skin. Scale collected from the scraping is pressed onto a glass slide, which is then fixed with heat. Impression smears are made by repeatedly pressing a glass slide against lesions on the skin. A latex glove should be worn by the clinician to avoid leaving fingerprints or debris on the slide.

Table 3–4
Subjective Classification of Yeast Numbers on Cytologic Preparations

SCALE	INTERPRETATION
0	No yeast seen
1+	Yeast organisms present sporadically on the slide
2+	Organisms seen every 2 to 3 oil-immersion fields (1000×)
3+	One to two organisms seen every oil-immersion field
4+	More than two organisms per oil-immersion field

Microscopic examination of the slide is performed using a 50× to 100× objective lens. Yeasts appear as blue to purple, oval to budding (peanut-shaped) organisms on slides stained with a modified Wright-Giemsa stain (Diff-Quik) (Fig. 3–6). Histopathologic changes associated with *Malassezia* dermatitis include a superficial, perivascular dermatitis, acanthosis, and hyperkeratosis. Yeast organisms are difficult to visualize with routine stains but are easily identified in the stratum corneum or upper third of the follicle with fungal stains.

Other diagnostic procedures may be indicated to rule out ectoparasitic infections, allergies, endocrinopathies, and keratinization defects that may be predisposing factors.

Treatment

Ketoconazole (5–10 mg/kg orally, twice a day for 30 days) is the treatment of choice for *Malassezia* dermatitis. Shampoos containing selenium disulfide (Seleen Plus), miconazole (Dermazole), ketoconazole (Nizoral shampoo), or chlorhexidine are most effective when used as adjunctive treatment to systemic therapy. However, topical therapy may be effective as the sole form of treatment if the owner is willing to bathe the animal every day or every other day for 6 to 8 weeks.

The prognosis for response to treatment is good, but underlying conditions must be identified and controlled or the condition will recur.

Uncommon Fungal Diseases of the Skin

Subcutaneous (Intermediate) Mycoses

The subcutaneous mycoses represent a group of fungal infections that involve the skin and deeper subcutaneous tissues. The terminology of these conditions is often confusing, but this group of diseases includes pythiosis, phaeohyphomycosis, and sporotrichosis.[33] Clinical signs include nodules, fistulous tracts, ulcers, and varying degrees of swelling in affected areas. Diagnosis is made by histopathologic examination of the skin for fungal elements. Treatment of these conditions involves medical or surgical management, or both. Medical management is often unsuccessful, but treatment with amphotericin B or one of the imidazole drugs has been effective in some cases. Surgical excision of the lesion or amputation of a limb may be the only therapeutic option in some cases of intermediate mycotic infections. Some infections (e.g., sporotrichosis) represent a serious public health risk and must be managed with caution.[34]

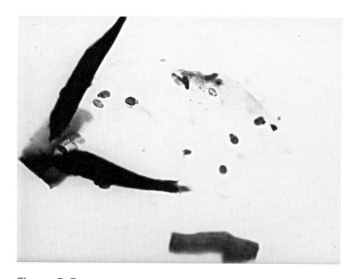

Figure 3–6
Classic peanut-shaped budding yeast, *Malassezia pachydermatis*. (Diff-Quik stain; ×1000)

Systemic (Deep) Mycoses

Cutaneous lesions may accompany infection by *Histoplasma capsulatum, Blastomyces dermatitis, Coccidioides immitis,* or *Cryptococcus neoformans.*[35–37] Lesions include alopecia, erythema, crusts, nodules, ulcerations, and fistulous tracts. Cutaneous changes may accompany systemic signs of fungal infection, such as respiratory distress, fever, diarrhea, and enlarged peripheral lymph nodes, although cutaneous lesions may be the only clinical sign early in the infection. Culture of material collected from lesions suspected to be caused by deep mycotic infection is not recommended because of the difficulty in growing these agents and the possible public health risk. Cytologic evaluation of material collected from cutaneous lesions may help identify the causative organism. Fungal agents may also be identified on histologic examination of the skin. Systemic therapy (see Chap. 39) is always necessary in deep mycotic infections with cutaneous lesions.

References

1. Medleau L, Long RE, Brown J, et al. Frequency and antimicrobial susceptibility of *Staphylococcus* species isolated from canine pyodermas. Am J Vet Res 1986;47:229–231.
2. Cox HU, Schmeer N, Newman SS. Protein A in *Staphylococcus intermedius* isolates from dogs and cats. Am J Vet Res 1986;47:1881–1884.
3. Sheagre JN. *Staphylococcus aureus*: The persistent pathogen. N Engl J Med 1984;310:1368–1373.
4. Ihrke PJ, Schwartzman RM, McGinley K, et al. Microbiology of normal and seborrheic canine skin. Am J Vet Res 1978;39:1487–1489.

5. White SD, Ihrke PJ, Stannard AA, et al. Occurrence of *Staphylococcus aureus* on the clinically normal canine hair coat. Am J Vet Res 1983;44:332–334.

6. Medleau L, Blue JL. Frequency and antimicrobial susceptibility of *Staphylococcus* spp. isolated from feline skin lesions. J Am Vet Med Assoc 1988;193:1080–1081.

7. Moroff SD, Hurvita AI, Peterson ME, et al. IgA deficiency in shar-pei dogs. Vet Immunol Immunopathol 1986;13:181–188.

8. DeBoer DJ, Moriello KA, Thomas CB, et al. Evaluation of a commercial staphylococcal bacterin for management of idiopathic recurrent superficial pyoderma in dogs. Am J Vet Res 1990;51:636–639.

9. Becker AM, Janik TA, Smith EK, et al. *Propionibacterium acnes* immunotherapy in chronic canine pyoderma. J Vet Intern Med 1989;3:26–30.

10. Reinke SI, Stannard AA, Ihrke PJ, et al. Histopathologic features of pyotraumatic dermatitis. J Am Vet Med Assoc 1987;190:57–60.

11. Krick SA, Scott DW. Bacterial folliculitis, furunculosis, and cellulitis in the German shepherd dog: A retrospective analysis of 17 cases. J Am Anim Hosp Assoc 1989;25:23–30.

12. Wisselink MA, Willemse A, Koeman JP. Deep pyoderma in the German shepherd dog. J Am Anim Hosp Assoc 1985;21:770–776.

13. Panich R, Scott DW, Miller WH. Canine cutaneous sterile pyogranuloma/granuloma syndrome: A retrospective analysis of 29 cases (1976 to 1988). J Am Anim Hosp Assoc 1991;27:519–528.

14. Scott DW. Feline dermatology 1983–1985: "The secret sits." J Am Anim Hosp Assoc 1987:23:255–274.

15. Greene CE. Feline abscesses. In: Greene CE, ed. Infectious Disease of the Dog and Cat, 2nd ed. Philadelphia, WB Saunders, 1990:595–598.

16. Muller GH, Kirk RW, Scott DW. Small Animal Dermatology. Philadelphia, WB Saunders, 1989:244–287.

17. Kirpenstein J, Fingland RB. Cutaneous actinomycosis and nocardiosis in dogs: 48 cases (1980–1990). J Am Vet Med Assoc 1992;201:917–920.

18. Edison M, Thilsted JP, Rollag OJ. Clinical, clinicopathologic, and pathologic features of plague in cats: 119 cases (1977–1988). J Am Vet Med Assoc 1991;199:1191–1197.

19. Monroe WE, August JR, Chickering WR, et al. Atypical mycobacterial infections in cats. Compen Contin Educ Pract Vet 1988;10:1044–1048.

20. McIntosh W. Feline leprosy: A review of forty-four cases from western Canada. Can Vet J 1982;23:291–295.

21. White SD, Ihrke PJ, Stannard AA, et al. Cutaneous atypical mycobacteriosis in cats. J Am Vet Med Assoc 1983;182:1218–1222.

22. Kunkle GA, Gulbas NK, Fadok V, et al. Rapidly growing mycobacteria as a cause of cutaneous granulomas: A report of five cases. J Am Anim Hosp Assoc 1983;19:513–521.

23. Rebell G, Taplin D. Dermatophytes: Their Recognition and Identification. Coral Gables, Florida, University of Miami Press, 1964.

24. DeBoer DJ, Moriello KA. Inability of topical treatment to influence the course of experimental feline dermatophytosis. Proceedings of the Tenth Annual Members' Meeting, American Academy of Veterinary Dermatology and American College of Veterinary Dermatology, Charleston, 1994:38–39.

25. White-Weithers N. Evaluation of topical therapies for the treatment of dermatophytosis in dogs and cats. Proceedings of the Ninth Annual Members' Meeting, American Academy of Veterinary Dermatology and American College of Veterinary Dermatology, San Diego, 1993:29.

26. Kunkle GA, Meyer DJ. Toxicity of high dose griseofulvin in cats. J Am Vet Med Assoc 1987;191:322–323.

27. Shelton GH, Grant CK, Linenberger ML, et al. Severe neutropenia associated with griseofulvin therapy in cats with feline immunodeficiency virus infection. J Vet Intern Med 1990;4:317–319.

28. Medleau L, Chalmers SA. Ketoconazole for treatment of dermatophytosis in cats. J Am Vet Med Am 1992;200:77–78.

29. De Keyser H, Van den Brande M. Ketoconazole in the treatment of dermatophytosis in cats and dogs. Vet Q 1983;5:142–144.

30. Moriello KA. Management of dermatophytes in catteries and multiple-cat households. Vet Clin North Am Small Anim Pract 1990;20:1457–1474.

31. Kennis RA. Quantitation and topographical analysis of *Malassezia* organisms on normal canine skin. Proceedings of the Ninth Annual Members' Meeting, American Academy of Veterinary Dermatology and American College of Veterinary Dermatology, San Diego, 1993:23–24.

32. Plant JD, Rosencrantz WS, Griffen CE. Factors associated with and prevalence of high *Malassezia pachydermatis* numbers on dog skin. J Am Vet Med Assoc 1992;201:879–882.

33. Muller GH, Kirk RW, Scott DW. Small Animal Dermatology. Philadelphia, WB Saunders, 1989:319–344.

34. Dunstan RW, Reimann KA, Langham RF. Feline sporotrichosis. J Am Vet Med Assoc 1986;189:880–883.

35. Noxon JO, Monroe WE, Chinn DR. Ketoconazole therapy in canine and feline cryptococcosis. J Am Anim Hosp Assoc 1986;22:179–183.

36. Legendre AM, Walker M, Buyukmihci N, et al. Canine blastomycosis: A review of 47 clinical cases. J Am Vet Med Assoc 1981;178:1163–1168.

37. Barsanti JA, Jeffery KL. Coccidioidomycosis. In: Greene CE, ed. Infectious Diseases of the Dog and Cat, 2nd ed. Philadelphia, WB Saunders, 1990:696–706.

Chapter 4

Otitis Externa

James O. Noxon

Anatomy

Pinna

The pinna, or auricle, is the outer part of the ear. It is shaped like a funnel to help direct sound into the ear canal. The pinna derives its shape from the auricular cartilage and its movement from a set of auricular muscles attached to the skull. The pinna is covered with skin, which can develop cutaneous lesions identical to those on skin located elsewhere on the body.[1]

External Ear Canal

The external ear canal, or external auditory meatus, extends from the point at which the auricular cartilage forms a tube to the tympanum. The structure of the external canal is provided by the annular cartilage, which is lined with skin that contains sebaceous glands, apocrine sweat glands, and variable numbers of hair follicles. The sebaceous and apocrine sweat gland secretions combine to form an emulsion known as cerumen. The external ear canal has a vertical (descending) component and a horizontal component that extends to the tympanum. The external canal may have several folds or wrinkles, and it varies in length in different breeds.

Tympanum

The tympanum (tympanic membrane, eardrum) is the membrane that separates the external ear canal from the middle ear. It is semitransparent, allowing the handle of the malleus to be seen during an otoscopic examination. The tympanum has a tense and a flaccid part (Fig 4–1). The tense part is stretched across the ear canal and is semitransparent in the normal ear. The smaller flaccid part, opaque white with blood vessels on the surface, extends downward from the roof of the canal. The flaccid part of the tympanum moves with respiration in some animals because of pressure changes occurring in the middle ear during respiration.

Experimental studies have shown that a dog may undergo moderate damage to the tympanum with only a moderate degree of hearing loss.[2] These studies showed that healing of the tympanum, in an otherwise healthy ear, occurs within 35 days after trauma.

Problem Identification

Pinnal Dermatitis

The skin over the pinna may develop the same lesions or problems as skin elsewhere on the body. Any disease causing lesions on this part of the ear can cause discomfort and clinical changes.

Pathophysiology

Pinnal dermatitis may be caused by any of the pathogenic factors that influence the skin elsewhere on the body (Table 4–1). Although dermatologic changes of the pinna may be the only signs of dermatologic disease, they most often accompany otitis externa and have a similar pathophysiology. Diseases of the pinna and external ear canal may be the only dermatologic problems of a patient, but they are almost always part of a more extensive dermatologic problem.

In response to disease, the skin of the external canal develops gross and microscopic changes similar to those seen in skin elsewhere on the body. For example, *Demodex* mites may inhabit follicles of the external canal and induce folliculitis and furunculosis, the same lesions seen in skin on other locations. Diseases affecting the pinna may extend to the external ear canal to induce changes within the ear canal.

Clinical Signs

Alopecia, scaling, papules, pustules, scale, crusts, hyperpigmentation, ulcers, vesicles, bullae, erythema, and lichenification may be present on the medial or lateral aspect of the pinna, depending on the disease process. Pruritus is often present.

Diagnostic Plan

Lesions on the pinna should be evaluated in the same manner as any cutaneous lesions. Skin scrapings, evaluation for fungal infection (Wood lamp examination, potassium hydroxide preparation, and fungal culture), and histopathologic evaluation of the skin are often indicated. In addition, the external ear canal should be examined thoroughly whenever dermatitis is present on the pinna.

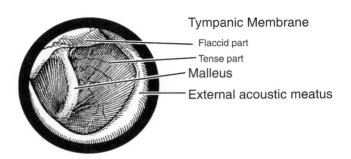

Figure 4–1
Otoscopic view of the tympanic membrane. (Modified from de Lahunta A, Habel RE. Applied Veterinary Anatomy. Philadelphia, WB Saunders, 1986.)

Table 4–1

Dermatologic Diseases Affecting the Pinna

Parasitic Diseases
Scabies
Notoedric mange
Otodectic mange
Fly-bite dermatitis
Tick infestation

Scaling Disorders
Idiopathic primary seborrhea
Sebaceous adenitis
Ear margin seborrhea
Zinc-responsive dermatosis
Hypothyroidism

Allergic Diseases
Atopy
Food allergy (hypersensitivity)

Autoimmune Diseases
Pemphigus foliaceus
Pemphigus erythematosus
Pemphigus vulgaris
Bullous pemphigoid
Systemic lupus erythematosus
Vasculitis
Cold-agglutinin disease

Environmental Diseases
Frostbite
Actinic dermatitis (solar-induced)

Neoplasia
Squamous cell carcinoma

Miscellaneous Diseases
Juvenile cellulitis
Pattern baldness (dachshunds)

Otitis Externa

Otitis externa is the clinical condition caused by inflammation of the external ear canal (auditory meatus).

Pathophysiology

Understanding of the pathologic mechanisms of otitis externa is the key to successful diagnosis and treatment. Factors affecting the development and maintenance of otitis externa are logically divided into three categories: predisposing factors, primary factors, and perpetuating factors.[3]

The external ear canal progresses through several pathologic stages as disease persists in the area. Some of the changes seen in the skin lining the external ear canal include hyperplasia of apocrine sweat glands, edema, inflammation, fibrosis, and hyperplasia resulting in stenosis of the ear canal, and calcification of the cartilage lining the external ear canal.

Predisposing Factors

Predisposing factors create an environment in the external canal that facilitates the establishment of primary or perpetuating factors.

The conformation of the canal is a predisposing factor. Dogs with long, tortuous external ear canals readily retain foreign material in the external canals. Dogs that swim frequently or live or work in wet areas may retain water in the horizontal external ear canals because of the shape of the canal. The moisture then facilitates overgrowth by some microorganisms. The Chinese shar-pei has a stenotic ear canal and a small pinna that is bent forward, covering the external opening. Some dog breeds have copious amounts of hair in the canals; this does not induce otitis externa but may impair ventilation and increase the retention of fluids in the external canal. There seems to be no clear evidence that the type of pinnae (pendulous versus upright) alters the risk of developing otitis externa. However, after otitis externa is present, ears with pendulous pinnae may be more difficult to medicate and to keep dry.

Environmental factors may predispose animals to otitis externa by altering the microclimate of the external ear canal. These factors include high humidity, warm temperatures, and rainfall.[4] As mentioned previously, moisture retained in the external ear after swimming or bathing can facilitate a change in the microflora and the subsequent development of inflammation.

Inappropriate care of the external ear during grooming may irritate or damage the skin lining the canal and predispose it to secondary invasion by microorganisms. Hair should not routinely be removed from the external canal by plucking unless inflammation is present and the purpose of hair removal is to allow for better penetration of medication.

Immunodeficiency syndromes, known to occur in some breeds of dogs, may permit recurrent ear infections or interfere with normal immune clearance of organisms.

Primary Factors

Primary factors are those conditions that induce inflammation in the external canal. In some cases, the inflammation may originate in the pinna and then move into the external ear canal. In other cases, the inflammation begins within the canal.

Ectoparasites, especially the ear mite *Otodectes cynotis*, are a common cause of otitis in dogs and the most common cause in cats.

The spinous ear tick, *Otobius megnini*, may be found in the external ear of dogs and cats in the southern United States. Other ectoparasitic infections, such as scabies, notoedric mange, and cheyletiellosis, may induce severe dermatitis on the pinna, and inflammation may extend down into the external ear canal.

Foreign bodies, including plant awns, gravel, and household items, are frequently responsible for the initial inflammatory reaction in otitis externa.

Hypersensitivity reactions are the most common cause of otitis externa in the dog and are also common in the cat. Inflammation of the pinna and external ear canal, especially in the area immediately surrounding the opening of the ear canal, is a common feature of atopy in the dog. Inflammation of the pinna and the external canal is a common feature of adverse reactions to food in both dogs and cats. Otitis externa may also be associated with allergic contact dermatitis (ACD), which may develop after application of otic medications. Most otic medications are combination products, and they often contain antibiotics, glucocorticoids, and topical anesthetics, common sensitizers of ACD. The diagnosis of ACD is made by observing a regression in clinical signs after all medications have been discontinued.

Scaling disorders frequently involve the pinnae. The external ear canal may be directly affected by these diseases or may become involved by extension of the pinnal lesions, resulting in secondary inflammation and irritation. Primary idiopathic seborrhea is the most common of these disorders. It is frequently seen in the American cocker spaniel, English springer spaniel, basset hound, German shepherd, and other breeds.[5] Patients with other scaling disorders may also have otitis externa secondary to the generalized cutaneous changes (see Chap. 6).

Perpetuating Factors

Perpetuating factors are those conditions responsible for the maintenance of the inflammatory process within the external ear canal. These factors are often the most obvious ongoing problems in the patient with otitis externa and must be controlled to alleviate the clinical signs.

Bacterial infections are common perpetuating factors. Normal bacterial flora of the external ear canal of dogs includes coagulase-positive and coagulase-negative staphylococci and micrococci. These and other bacteria are present in low numbers in healthy ears.[6, 7] The bacteria most commonly isolated in inflamed ears are *Staphylococcus intermedius*, *Pseudomonas aeruginosa*, β-hemolytic streptococci, *Proteus* spp., *Escherichia coli*, and *Corynebacterium* spp.[6–8]

Fungal infections may also perpetuate otitis externa. The most common fungal organism isolated from inflamed ears is *Malassezia pachydermatis*. This organism is readily identified on stained smears of exudate and can be cultured on Sabouraud dextrose agar or 5% blood agar.

Chronic inflammatory changes of the external ear canal perpetuate otitis externa by occluding the canal, favoring changes in the microclimate and flora of the external ear canal, and by increasing the activity of sebaceous and apocrine glands. These changes are reflected in severe lichenification at the opening of the external canal and throughout the vertical and horizontal canals. Inflammatory polyps may develop, further obstructing the canal. Glucocorticoids should be given topically and systemically in anti-inflammatory doses to reduce the swelling of the skin lining the canal and the opening of the canal. Lateral ear canal resection provides some relief in patients with changes that are long-standing and severe.[9]

Otitis media, or inflammation of the middle ear, may result from extension of an inflammatory process that begins in the external ear, from spread through the eustachian tube, or from hematogenous spread from another focus in the body. Regardless of the source of the infection, the middle ear may provide a nidus of resistance to medical therapy and is often an important factor in resistant or recurring otitis externa. Otitis media is often present when the tympanum is ruptured. Radiography of the tympanic bullae shows thickened osseus bullae and proliferative bony changes in chronic infections. Aspiration of purulent or caseous material through the tympanum helps to identify the causative infectious agent. Bulla osteotomy is required in most cases of otitis media to resolve the infection.[10, 11]

Aural hematomas develop after cartilage damage and blood vessel rupture in the pinna, secondary to severe inflammation and pruritus. There are many satisfactory methods available to treat the lesions. If the hematoma is not treated properly, severe scarring of the pinna can result, leading to additional conformational changes conducive for the development of otitis externa.

Clinical Signs

Pruritus is the clinical problem most commonly associated with otitis externa. Pruritus of the external ear canal is manifested as shaking of the head, scratching at the pinnae, rubbing the ears on the carpet or floor, and whining or crying.

The most common dermatologic lesions associated with otitis externa are erythema, scaling, crusts, and lichenification. Secondary changes, such as hyperpigmentation, develop as the disease becomes chronic. Lichenification occurs secondary to chronic rubbing and inflammation. It may be severe enough to obstruct

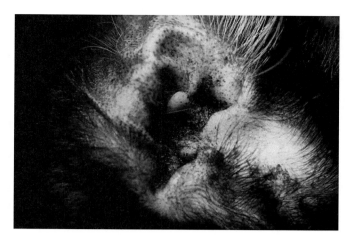

Figure 4-2
Characteristic dark, granular exudate associated with ear mite infestation in a cat.

Table 4–2
Diagnostic Plan for Otitis Externa

1. Perform cytologic examination of unstained exudate for parasites *and* stained slides for evidence of perpetuating factors (bacteria, yeast).
2. Perform bacterial culture if indicated (see text).
3. Control perpetuating factors.
   a. Clean the ears.
   b. Dry the ears.
   c. Apply specific therapy (systemic and topical anti-microbial agents).
   d. Perform surgical correction of hyperplastic changes.
4. Identify primary factors.
   a. Perform otoscopic examination for foreign bodies.
   b. Perform intradermal or in vitro allergy testing.
   c. Perform elimination dietary trial.
   d. Perform skin biopsy.
5. Correct predisposing factors.

the external ear canal and act as a perpetuating factor of the otitis. Intense pruritus affecting the head or ears is the key clinical feature of ear mite infestation. A dark, granular exudate accumulates in the external canal, especially at the infundibulum of the external canal (Fig. 4–2). Secondary excoriations, erythema, and crusts are often present on the skin of the head and pinnae. Alopecia and crusted papules may be seen in the periauricular area or on other infested areas of the body.

Malodor is also a common owner complaint of animals with otitis externa. In many cases, the owners are not sure of the origin of the bad odor because many patients with otitis externa also have severe generalized dermatitis.

Diagnostic Plan

The diagnostic approach includes a few key procedures that should be performed in a consistent order (Table 4–2). Routine diagnostic procedures in cases of otitis externa include a thorough history, a complete physical examination, otoscopic examination of the external ear canal, and cytologic evaluation of the ear canal.

There are several key elements in the history. First, the duration of the disease may help to define the primary disease process. An acute onset is most likely associated with a foreign body response or trauma, whereas chronic, intermittent otitis externa is more likely a feature of an allergic disease. Second, any seasonal predisposition would suggest an underlying allergic disease. Third, the presence of other animals with ear problems in the household is consistent with a parasitic cause of otitis.

The physical examination must be complete to identify other medical or dermatologic problems. For

example, atopy should be the primary differential diagnosis in a patient with otitis if the patient also licks its feet and rubs its face on the carpet. The otoscopic examination is a key diagnostic test to identify foreign bodies, parasites, obstructive disease, and the integrity of the tympanum.

Because otitis externa is usually only one manifestation of a more extensive dermatologic or systemic disease, diagnostic procedures should include tests to rule out common primary factors of otitis externa. Virtually any of the diagnostic procedures used to identify the cause of generalized dermatologic problems may be indicated in some patients presenting with otitis externa.

Diagnostic Procedures

Otoscopic Examination

Every patient with otitis externa should have a complete examination of the ear canal with an otoscope to visualize the entire ear canal and the tympanum. However, the ears of patients with otitis externa are often so painful that a thorough otoscopic examination is difficult to perform. In such patients, three options are available. First, the patient can be anesthetized. A general anesthetic agent is recommended, because most analgesics do not provide enough restraint. Second, the ear canal can be anesthetized by application of 4 to 5 drops of a topical anesthetic intended for ophthalmic use (e.g., 0.5% proparacaine hydrochloride). Third, if the disease is bilateral and a foreign body is not suspected, the ears can be treated empirically with any combination product containing a glucocorticoid and antimicrobial agents for 5 to 7 days. At that time, the animal should be re-examined to determine the integrity of the tympanum.

When performing an otoscopic examination, the clinician should gently grasp the pinna and pull the external canal upward and outward to introduce the otoscope into the external canal. Manipulation of the pinna helps to facilitate movement of the otoscope cone down the canal. The cone should never be advanced unless the examiner has a clear field of vision. The clinician must exercise caution when performing an otoscopic examination and take care not to damage the tympanum, because it is structurally weakened in the presence of inflammation.

The tympanum should be examined for structural integrity, the presence of exudate behind the membrane (a fluid line), and swelling. Edema of the flaccid part of the tympanum is commonly seen in atopic patients.

Cytology

Cytology is recommended in all cases of otitis externa and should be done early in the diagnostic process. Material that accumulates on the otoscope cone during otoscopic examination or material collected on a cotton-tipped swab manipulated into the horizontal canal should be rolled onto a glass slide for staining. A Wright-Giemsa stain (Diff-Quik) is recommended for routine use, because it is easy to apply and has excellent staining qualities. The slide is microscopically examined for inflammatory cells, bacteria, yeast, or parasites such as *Demodex* mites. If the exudate is dry or ear mite infection is suspected, some exudate should be mixed with mineral oil and examined for *O. cynotis* mites or ova.

Bacterial Culture

Bacterial culture of the external canal is rarely necessary, because most bacterial infections are secondary (perpetuating) factors of otitis and respond to empiric treatment with topical broad-spectrum antibiotics. However, culture of the external canal is indicated in nonresponsive or recurring bacterial infections. Both external ear canals should be cultured, because the infectious agent may be different in the two ears. Material is collected for culture by passing a sterile swab down into the horizontal section of the external ear canal, taking care not to touch the hair or skin at the opening of the canal.

Treatment of Otitis Externa

Therapeutic Plan

The first step in management of a patient with otitis externa is control and removal of the perpetuating factors, which are associated with discomfort and pain of the ears. After these factors are controlled, the predisposing and primary factors (e.g., foreign bodies, ear mites) must be identified and resolved. Management of only the perpetuating factors (e.g., bacterial or yeast infections) ultimately leads to frustration in the veterinarian and the client and a patient with progressive disease.

Symptomatic Management

Two aspects of therapy are important in all cases of otitis externa: cleaning the external ear canal and drying the external canal. A large number of pharmaceutical agents are available for cleaning and drying the ears, for removing wax from the canals, and as antimicrobial agents.[12] Each veterinarian should become familiar with the actions, side effects, and efficacy of one or two drugs in each category for use in patients with otitis externa.

Cleaning the External Ear Canal

The external ear canal should be thoroughly cleaned in all cases of otitis externa (Table 4–3). If the disease is mild, the ears can be satisfactorily cleaned with commercially available ear cleansers (Table 4–4). In addition, a povidone-iodine solution may be diluted in a 1:10 ratio with water and used as a cleansing solution. An otoscopic examination should be performed after cleaning to ensure complete removal of exudate and debris.

Ceruminolytic agents, including dioctyl sodium sulfosuccinate and carbamide peroxide, may be applied to loosen exudate in impacted ears. Ceruminolytic agents are contraindicated if the tympanum is known to be perforated.

If the otitis is chronic or severe, or the animal refuses to allow adequate cleaning, a general anesthetic is recommended to facilitate proper cleaning. The ear should be cleaned by infusion of a cleansing solution during observation through the otoscope. This permits direct infusion of the solution to all areas with exudate. The solution and exudate should then be aspirated through a soft rubber catheter attached to a bulb syringe or suction apparatus. The catheter or feeding tube should be visually guided to moist areas of the ear canal. The cycle should be repeated until the ear is clean. Saline is an effective debriding and cleansing agent and is the only cleansing solution recommended if the tympanum is known or suspected to be perforated.

Drying the External Ear Canal

After the ear is cleaned, a drying agent should be applied to reduce the moisture level in the canal.

Table 4–3
Ear Cleaning Technique for a Nonanesthetized Dog or Cat

Necessary Supplies
Ear cleansing solution
Cotton balls
3.0-mL injection syringe or bulb syringe

Process
1. The pinna is gently held in an upright position, and the cleansing solution is infused (with the injection syringe, bulb syringe, or applicator bottle) into the ear until the external canal is full.
2. A cotton ball is placed in the opening of the canal.
3. The external canal is gently massaged, using an upward and outward motion.
4. The cotton ball is removed and the process (infusion and massage) is repeated several times or until no exudate adheres to the cotton ball.
5. After the ear appears clean, the ear is massaged with a dry cotton ball in place to remove any excess solution.
6. Cotton-tipped applicators may be used to swab and dry the vertical canal.
7. The ear should be otoscopically examined, and the cleansing process should be repeated if exudate remains in the canal.

Table 4–4
Commercially Available Ear Cleansing and Drying Solutions*

TYPE OF AGENT	PRODUCT	COMPANY	ACTIVE INGREDIENTS†
Cleansing agents	Oti-Clens	SmithKline Beecham	Propylene glycol; malic acid; benzoic acid
	Epi-Otic Cleanser	Allerderm/Virbac	Lactic acid; salicylic acid; propylene glycol; docusate sodium
	OtiCalm	DVM Pharmaceuticals	Propylene glycol; benzoic acid; malic acid; salicylic acid; oil of eucalyptus
	Solvaprep	Solvay Animal Health	Propylene glycol; isopropyl alcohol
	Novasan Otic	Fort Dodge Laboratories	Propylene glycol; isopropyl alcohol
	Clear$_x$ Cleansing Solution	DVM Pharmaceuticals	Diocytyl sodium sulfosuccinate; urea peroxide
Drying agents	Panodry	Solvay Animal Health	Boric acid; isopropyl alcohol
	HB101	Maurry Biological	Hydrocortisone; Burow solution
	Clear$_x$ Ear Treatment Drying Solution	DVM Pharmaceuticals	Acetic acid; sulfur; hydrocortisone

*This table is not intended to list all available products; other ear cleansing and drying solutions are available.
†Antiseptics, drying agents, keratolytics, and humectants. Many products contain proprietary solvents and surfactants.

Bacteria and yeast thrive in areas of high humidity, and drying of the canal helps to control these infectious agents. Several agents are available in commercial products designed for this purpose.

Surgical Management

Surgery is indicated to correct perpetuating and predisposing factors (e.g., hyperplastic changes of the ear canal), to remove inflammatory polyps, and to facilitate drainage if otitis media is present. Lateral ear canal resection and bulla osteotomy are the surgical procedures most commonly performed on animals with otitis externa. These procedures are reported to reduce or eliminate the clinical signs of otitis externa in 50% to 95% of surgically managed cases.[9–11] The most successful procedure is total ear canal ablation combined with bulla osteotomy.[10, 11] However, potentially severe postoperative complications are associated with this procedure, including facial paralysis. In my experience, surgery rarely cures otitis externa, although it may help the patient by providing drainage and facilitating treatment with topical medications. There is often only marginal improvement of clinical signs after surgery in patients with atopy or adverse reactions to food, diseases that are common primary factors of otitis externa.

Diseases Causing Otitis Externa

Ear Mite Infestation

O. cynotis infestation (otodectic mange, otoacariasis) is the most common cause of otitis externa in cats. This parasite also infects dogs, and cross-infection between the two species occurs commonly. Like other ectoparasites of companion animals, this parasite may transiently infest humans.[13] The mite is an obligate parasite and completes its life cycle in approximately 3 weeks. Stages of the life cycle include the egg, larva, protonymph, deutonymph, and adult. Parasites in any or all of these stages may be found on an infested animal. The mites generally reside within the external ear canal, usually near the opening of the external ear, although they may be found on the skin of the pinna, head, or body. Ear mites feed on lymph and other cellular fluids on the surface of the skin and induce a pronounced hypersensitivity reaction.[14]

Pathophysiology

Mites are highly contagious and are transmitted by direct contact. They cause disease by direct irritation and by induction of a hypersensitivity reaction.[15]

Clinical Signs

Otoacariasis is associated with severe pruritus and pain affecting the head and ears. Scratching is common and often results in secondary excoriations around the ears. The characteristic discharge associated with ear mite infestation is a dark, dry, granular exudate (see Fig. 4–2).

Diagnostic Plan

Ear mite infestation is often suspected if multiple animals in a household have clinical signs of otitis externa or if a patient has recently been acquired from a pet store, an animal shelter, or a household with a large population of animals. Diagnosis of ectoparasitic infection is by direct identification of the parasite on otoscopic examination or on microscopic examination of exudate collected from the canal or skin of the pinnae. The otoscope should be introduced into the ear canal and then held still in one location to observe the exudate for movement. Mites appear as white, rapidly moving specks on the dark background of exudate. Cytology for ear mites is performed by collecting exudate from the external canal with a cotton-tipped swab, adding a few drops of mineral oil and a cover-slip, and examining the slide under scanning objectives. Mites are very active and will be seen rapidly moving across the slide.

Treatment

Thorough cleaning of the external ear canal is recommended before acaricidal therapy. Several acaricides, including sulfur, rotenone, pyrethrin, and thiabendazole, are effective topically against *O. cynotis*. Commercial preparations often contain a topical anesthetic or glucocorticoid to reduce the inflammation and pain associated with this infestation. Topical acaricides should be applied in the external canal daily or every other day for a minimum duration of 3 weeks. In addition, an insecticide should be applied weekly to the remainder of the body, because the mites may reside outside the ear canal. Most flea control products (e.g., powders, sprays) are effective acaricides against *O. cynotis*.

Ivermectin (0.3 mg/kg) is effective against this parasite if it is administered subcutaneously and again 2 to 3 weeks later.[16, 17] One study using cats in animal shelters showed that an average of 4.2 weekly treatments were required to eliminate mites from infested cats when ivermectin was administered subcutaneously, and 5.4 applications were required when ivermectin (0.5 mg/kg) was applied topically in the ear.[18] In most cases, two to three treatments with ivermectin (0.3 mg/kg, orally or subcutaneously) serve to eliminate the infestation.

Regardless of the specific treatment protocol used, all animals in the household should be treated, even those without obvious clinical signs. The environment should be cleaned and disinfected. Spontaneous remission of clinical signs may occur in some patients.

Bacterial Infection

Bacterial infections are very common in dogs and are common in cats. *S. intermedius*, *P. aeruginosa*, β-hemolytic streptococci, *Proteus* spp., and *E. coli* are the bacteria most commonly isolated from inflamed ears.[6–8]

Pathophysiology

As previously discussed, bacterial infections of the external ear canal are considered perpetuating factors of otitis externa. The external ear canal becomes an excellent incubator for bacteria once inflammation is initiated by primary factors.

Clinical Signs

Erythema, pain, and swelling of the epithelial lining of the external ear canal accompany bacterial infection. Ulceration may occur if the disease is severe or chronic. *Pseudomonas* spp. infections seem to be associated with ulcers more often than other bacterial infections. Many patients develop a purulent exudate within the external ear canal that causes the animal to shake the head in an attempt to clear fluid from the canal.

Diagnostic Plan

Otoscopic examination of the external ear canal should be attempted to examine for the presence of ulcers and to evaluate the integrity of the tympanum. However, pain, a common feature of bacterial infections, may be intense and may preclude a thorough examination unless an anesthetic is administered. Cytology provides key information about diagnosis and management. Clinicians should examine slides to determine what types of bacteria are present (gram-positive versus gram-negative), whether one type of bacterium or a mixed infection is present, and whether neutrophils are present (Fig. 4–3). Cultures are indicated if the infection is recurrent or has been nonresponsive to routine antimicrobial treatment.

Treatment

Bacterial infections can usually be managed with one of several excellent combination products containing antibacterial, antifungal, and anti-inflammatory medications. Topical antimicrobial-glucocorticoid combination products containing neomycin, chloramphenicol, or gentamicin are effective in most cases. Glucocorticoids are helpful in managing bacterial infections by reducing inflammation and swelling of the external canal. However, glucocorticoids are not recommended in ulcerated ears.

More aggressive or specific treatment is necessary if otitis is recurrent or resistant to previous therapy, if rod-shaped bacteria are detected on cytologic examination of exudate, or if indicated by culture and susceptibility results. Resistant cases of bacterial otitis can be managed with various antibacterial preparations that are available for ophthalmic use or with broad-spectrum antibacterial products (Table 4–5). Medications should be applied in large enough volume to ensure delivery deep into the horizontal canal. It may be necessary to recommend that the entire external ear canal be filled with medication to ensure adequate penetration and coverage by topical preparations. One to two drops is not an adequate amount for each application.

Resistant gram-negative bacterial infections may be controlled with a topical buffered solution of ethylenediaminetetraacetate (EDTA), referred to as Wooley's solution. This solution can be used alone or in combination with several different antimicrobial agents to treat resistant bacterial infections.[19]

Systemic antimicrobial agents are recommended if neutrophils are detected during cytologic examination of exudate, if the external canal is so swollen that topical medications are unable to penetrate into the canal, or if the patient is showing signs of systemic disease (e.g., fever). The selection of an antibacterial agent should be based on the culture and susceptibility pattern.

Malassezia Infection

M. pachydermatis is a common inhabitant of the external ear canal. Estimates of the prevalence of this yeast in normal canine ears range from 36% to 80%.[7, 8, 20, 21] The organism has a characteristic oval to budding (peanut) shape, stains a pale to dark blue color with modified Wright stain, and is gram positive. Although it may be the only infectious agent identified on cytologic examination of exudate taken from inflamed ears, it is usually found in conjunction with bacteria (see Fig. 4–3).

Clinical Signs

Malassezia infection may be associated with all the classic signs of otitis externa, such as pruritus, shaking of the head, pain, erythema, and swelling of soft tissue structures of the ear. In addition, a cream to dark waxy exudate is typical in yeast infections. The exudate often has a sweet smell.

Diagnostic Plan

Cytologic examination of a smear made of the exudate stained with Wright stain reveals the organisms. The yeast also grows on blood agar and may be cultured.

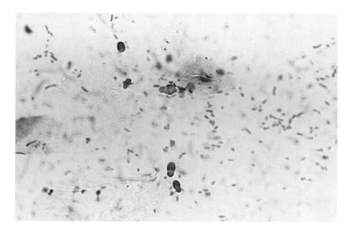

Figure 4–3
Cytology of the ear showing mixed bacterial and yeast infection. (Diff-Quik stain; ×1000)

Table 4–5
Topical Antimicrobial and Anti-inflammatory Agents Useful in the Treatment of Infectious Otitis Externa

TYPE OF AGENT	ACTIVE INGREDIENT	PRODUCT EXAMPLE	GLUCOCORTICOID	COMMENTS*
Antibacterials	Neomycin	Tresaderm (MSD-Agvet)	Dexamethasone	a, c
	Chloramphenicol	Liquichlor (Evsco)	Triamcinolone	a
	Neomycin/thiostrepton	Panolog (Solvay)	Triamcinolone	j
	Gentamicin	Gentocin Otic (Schering)	Betamethasone	b
	Gentamicin	Otomax (Schering)	Betamethasone	b, i
	Tobramycin	Tobrex (Alcan)	None	d
	Silver sulfadiazine	SSD cream (Boots)	None	b, f
	TRIS-EDTA	—	None	g, h
Antifungals	Nystatin	Panolog (Solvay)	Triamcinolone	f
	Clotrimazole	Lotrimin (Schering)	None	c
	Clotrimazole	Otomax (Schering)	Betamethasone	f
	Miconazole	Conofite (Pitman-Moore)	None	e
Anti-inflammatory agents	Dimethyl sulfoxide	Synotic (Syntex)	Fluocinolone	h
	Burow solution	HB101 (Maurry Biological)	Hydrocortisone	—
	—	EpiOtic HC (Allerderm)	Hydrocortisone	—

*Comments:
a = Excellent first choice for routine bacterial otitis ("first-line" product).
b = Excellent choice for resistant bacterial infections ("second-line" product).
c = Also contains an effective antifungal agent (thiabendazole).
d = Marketed for ophthalmologic application.
e = Marketed for cutaneous application.
f = Broad spectrum of antimicrobial activity.
g = Thick consistency; mix 1:1 with propylene glycol for application.
h = Activity may be enhanced when combined with some antibacterial agents.
i = Also contains an effective antifungal agent (clotrimazole).
j = Also contains an effective antifungal agent (nystatin).

Treatment

Treatment of the yeast infection is accomplished by cleaning and drying the external ear canal, controlling other perpetuating factors such as bacterial infections, and, if necessary, applying antifungal medications into the external ear canal. Miconazole, clotrimazole, cuprimyxin, thiabendazole, and silver sulfadiazine are effective agents against yeast. Ketoconazole (Nizoral) may be administered orally (5–10 mg/kg, twice daily) to patients with severe otitis externa associated with *M. pachydermatis*.

References

1. Angarano DW. Diseases of the pinna. Vet Clin North Am Small Anim Pract 1988;18:869–884.
2. Steiss JE, Boosinger TR, Wright JC, et al. Healing of experimentally perforated tympanic membranes demonstrated by electrodiagnostic testing and histopathology. J Am Anim Hosp Assoc 1992;28:307–310.
3. August JR. Otitis externa: A disease of multifactorial etiology. Vet Clin North Am Small Anim Pract 1988;18:731–742.
4. Hayes HM, Pickle LW, Wilson GP. Effects of ear type and weather on the hospital prevalence of canine otitis externa. Res Vet Sci 1987;42:294–298.
5. Kwochka KW. Primary keratinization disorders of dogs. In: Griffen CE, Kwochka KW, MacDonald JM, eds. Current Veterinary Dermatology: The Science and Art of Therapy. St Louis, Mosby–Year Book, 1993:176–190.
6. Dickson DB, Love DN. Bacteriology of the horizontal ear canal of dogs. J Small Anim Pract 1983;24:413–421.
7. McCarthy G, Kelly WR. Microbial species associated with the canine ear and their antibacterial sensitivity patterns. Ir Vet J 1982;36:53–56.
8. Kowalski JJ. The microbial environment of the ear canal in health and disease. Vet Clin North Am Small Anim Pract 1988;18:743–754.
9. Gregory CR, Vasseur PB. Clinical results of lateral ear resection in dogs. J Am Vet Med Assoc 1983;182:1087–1090.
10. Beckman SL, Henry WB, Cechner P. Total ear canal ablation combining bulla osteotomy and curettage in dogs with chronic otitis externa and media. J Am Vet Med Assoc 1990;196:84–90.
11. Matthiesen DT, Scavelli T. Total ear canal ablation and lateral bulla osteotomy in 38 dogs. J Am Anim Hosp Assoc 1990;26:257–267.
12. Wilcke JR. Otopharmacology. Vet Clin North Am Small Anim Pract 1988;18:783–797.

13. Lopez RA. Of mites and man. J Am Vet Med Assoc 1993;203:606–607 (letter).

14. Powell MB, Weisbroth SH, Roth L, et al. Reaginic hypersensitivity in *Otodectes cynotis* infestation of cats and mode of mite feeding. Am J Vet Res 1980;41:877–882.

15. Weisbroth SH, Powell MB, Roth L, et al. Immunopathology of naturally occurring otodectic otoacariasis in the domestic cat. J Am Vet Med Assoc 1974;165:1088–1093.

16. Song MD. Using ivermectin to treat feline dermatoses caused by external parasites. Vet Med 1991;86:498–502.

17. Foreyt WJ. Safety and efficacy of ivermectin against ear mites (*Otodectes cynotis*) in ranch foxes. J Am Vet Med Assoc 1991;198:96–98.

18. Gram D. Treatment of ear mites (*Otodectes cynotis*) in cats: Comparison of subcutaneous and topical ivermectin. Proceedings of the Seventh Annual Members' Meeting, American Academy of Veterinary Dermatology and American College of Veterinary Dermatology, Scottsdale, 1991:26–27.

19. Greene CE, Ferguson DC. Antibacterial chemotherapy. In: Greene CE, ed. Infectious Disease of the Dog and Cat, 2nd ed. Philadelphia, WB Saunders, 1990:461–493.

20. Merchant A. Quantitative and qualitative analysis of bacteria and yeast from normal canine ears. Proceedings of the Fourth Annual Members' Meeting, American Academy of Veterinary Dermatology and American College of Veterinary Dermatology, Washington, 1988:12.

21. Trettien AL. The prevalence of *Malassezia pachydermatis* in the external ear canal of normal dogs. Proceedings of the Third Annual Members' Meeting, American Academy of Veterinary Dermatology and American College of Veterinary Dermatology, Phoenix, 1987:26–27.

Chapter 5

Immune-Mediated Skin Diseases

James O. Noxon

Allergic Skin Diseases

Problem Identification

Pruritus

Pruritus is the unpleasant sensation that provokes the desire to scratch (see Chap. 1).

Pathophysiology

Several pathophysiologic mechanisms associated with allergy cause pruritus. The most common mechanisms are type I (immediate) hypersensitivity and type IV (delayed-type) hypersensitivity reactions. Type I hypersensitivity reactions result from production of high levels of immunoglobulin E (IgE) in animals that are genetically determined to produce that antibody. The IgE molecules bind to mast cells in the skin, and with repeated exposure to an allergen, cross-linking of the IgE molecules and mast cell degranulation occur. Pruritus associated with type I hypersensitivity disorders (e.g., atopy) results from the release of preformed inflammatory mediators, such as proteases, histamine, and serotonin, and generation of inflammatory mediators, such as prostaglandins and leukotrienes, from mast cells. These mediators and the inflammation caused by them irritate nerve endings in the superficial dermis, resulting in the sensation of pruritus.

Type IV hypersensitivity reactions are involved in some allergic diseases, especially food allergies and contact allergies. In this reaction, sensitized lymphocytes secrete lymphokines, which attract other lymphocytes and macrophages over a period of 24 to 72 hours.

Clinical Signs

Pruritus is the hallmark of allergic skin disease. The pruritus varies from mild to intense, depending on the cause and the presence of complicating factors. Each patient should be examined carefully for evidence of pruritus, such as licking, scratching, chewing, or rubbing. This is especially important in cats that present with dermatologic problems. Owners frequently misinterpret their pets' licking as normal grooming, not realizing that licking may be a reaction to a pruritic stimulus.

Excoriations are self-induced lesions, reflecting removal of the superficial layers of the epidermis. They are often linear scratches or crusted lesions and are secondary to pruritus.

Diagnostic Plan

Evidence that supports the diagnosis of pruritus includes excoriations, secondary bacterial infections, broken hairs, and increased hair in the feces.

Pruritus associated with allergies may be either a seasonal or a year-round problem, depending on the allergic disease that is present. The season of occurrence may help identify the inciting allergen by incriminating seasonal exacerbations of parasitic problems (e.g., flea infestation) or seasonal availability of plants (e.g., atopy or contact allergy).

Identification of the precise hypersensitivity mechanism and inciting substance is not necessary to properly manage most patients with allergic skin disease. However, if the patient fails to respond to empiric treatment, if there is recurring disease, or if the patient shows signs of systemic illness, diagnostic procedures should be performed to confirm the diagnosis. Intradermal skin testing and serologic tests are available to aid in the diagnosis of atopy. Other procedures used to diagnose allergic skin disease include elimination dietary trials (food allergy), patch testing (contact allergy), and isolation of the pet from the home environment. Atopy should be considered in a pruritic patient whenever the problem is seasonal and when seasonal ectoparasites (e.g., fleas) have been eliminated as the cause of the pruritus. An adverse reaction to food (i.e., food allergy) should be considered if the problem is nonseasonal and poorly responsive to anti-inflammatory doses of glucocorticoids.

Pustules, Papules, and Epidermal Collarettes

Pustules, papules, and epidermal collarettes are classic lesions of pyoderma, which is a common secondary finding in allergic skin diseases of the dog and cat (see Chap. 1).

Plaques

A plaque is a flat, elevated lesion of the skin. The lesion results from edema and infiltration of the skin by inflammatory cells.

Pathophysiology

This lesion is one manifestation of the eosinophilic granuloma complex, a cutaneous reaction pattern of feline skin. Eosinophilic plaques may be associated with atopy, food allergy, or flea allergy dermatitis (FAD) in the cat.

Clinical Signs

Plaques are elevated, flat leasons. They are usually hairless, and in eosinophilic diseases of the cat they are frequently an orange-yellow color. Plaques range in size from a few millimeters to several centimeters in diameter.

Diagnostic Plan

Histopathologic examination of the plaque is the best method to determine the cause of the lesion. The differential diagnosis of a plaque includes eosinophilic plaque, bacterial infection, fungal infection, and neoplasia, especially squamous cell carcinoma.

Wheals

A wheal is a flat, circumscribed elevation of the skin caused by edema.

Pathophysiology

Wheals are associated with type I hypersensitivity reactions. They are formed by edema resulting from increased permeability of small capillaries of the dermis, secondary to endothelial damage. Wheals are most frequently associated with type I hypersensitivity reactions caused by atopy, insect bites, and adverse reactions to food or medications.

Clinical Signs

Wheals may be singular or multiple and may appear in the skin over any area of the body. They may be palpated more easily than seen in animals with medium- to long-haired coats.

Diagnostic Plan

Wheals are flat lesions caused by edema. Papules are elevated lesions, not necessarily flat, caused by infiltration of the dermis by inflammatory cells or other cells. Confirmation of the lesion type may be made by histopathologic examination of the skin. Diagnostic procedures indicated in patients with recurrent wheals include intradermal skin tests or serologic tests for atopy and elimination dietary trials.

Diagnostic Procedures

Intradermal Skin Testing

The purpose of the intradermal skin test is to confirm the diagnosis of a type I hypersensitivity reaction and to provide information that will help the clinician formulate a therapeutic plan. Advantages of intradermal allergy testing include the reliability of the test and the familiarity that most dermatologists have with the procedure. Disadvantages include the need to clip the hair for testing, the need to sedate some patients for the injections, the experience required to read and interpret the reactions, and occasional false-negative results. Several excellent references describe this procedure in detail.[1, 2]

The intradermal skin test is an in vivo allergy test in which allergens are injected intradermally in predetermined amounts and concentrations.[2, 3] If antigen-specific IgE is present and bound to tissue (skin) mast cells, the addition of the antigen by injection results in mast cell degranulation and the development of a wheal and flare cutaneous reaction.

Antigens are available from several commercial sources. They are provided in vials as highly concentrated solutions that must be diluted to testing strength before use. Testing-strength antigens are available from most suppliers, but the antigens are not as stable in that concentration. Selection of antigens to be used in a testing panel is a crucial step in the skin testing process. The geographic region is the most crucial factor to consider, because many environmental allergens, such as grasses, weeds, trees, and molds, vary in importance from area to area. Antigen suppliers provide lists of important allergenic plants found in each geographic area. When beginning intradermal testing in a practice, it is useful to consult a local human-medicine allergist. The allergist can provide a list of the most common or significant allergens in the area. Indoor allergens tend to be fairly consistent from region to region.

Results of intradermal skin testing are influenced by previous medications, stress on the patient during the procedure, and anesthetics used for restraint during the test. Anti-inflammatory medications must be withheld from patients before allergy testing (Table 5–1). Medications that do not interfere with the testing may be used to control pruritus during the withdrawal period (Table 5–2).

In most cases, sedation is not necessary to perform this test. However, sedation reduces the anxiety of the patient and speeds up the procedure in apprehensive patients, which usually include all patients weighing less than 10 kg. Xylazine is a reliable

Table 5–1
Medication Withdrawal Times Recommended Before Allergy Testing

DRUG	RECOMMENDED WITHDRAWAL TIME (DAYS)
Glucocorticoids	
Oral alternate-day prednisone*	21–28
Daily prednisone	28
Injectable methylprednisolone	28–56
Injectable betamethasone	180
Topical glucocorticoids	14–28
Otic glucocorticoids	14–28
Ophthalmic glucocorticoids	14–28
Antihistamines (systemic or topical)	7–14
Fatty acid supplements	7–14

*Includes prednisone, prednisolone, and methylprednisolone.

Table 5–2

Medications Recommended to Control Pruritus While Preparing Patients for Allergy Testing

1. Place the patient on an antistaphylococcal antibiotic. Discontinue 2 to 3 days before intradermal testing.
2. If glucocorticoids have been administered, place the patient on antihistamines until 2 weeks before testing is scheduled.
3. Bathe the patient with colloidal oatmeal shampoos, oatmeal-antihistamine shampoos, oatmeal-topical anesthetic shampoos, or shampoos containing sulfur every 3 to 4 days. Discontinue shampoos containing antihistamines or glucocorticoids 7 days before testing.
4. Follow withdrawal times recommended in Table 5–1.

sedative for dogs when administered intravenously at 0.1 to 0.2 mg/kg. The patient's heart rate and rhythm should be monitored when this sedative is used. Atropine sulfate is given at 0.02 mg/kg intravenously to minimize any disturbances of the cardiac rate or rhythm. If necessary, yohimbine (Yobine) can be administered to the patient to reverse the effects of the xylazine. A combination product containing tiletamine and zolazepam (Telazol) has also been shown to provide adequate sedation without influencing intradermal test results.[4]

The hair is clipped over the lateral thoracic area, and the skin is gently wiped clean with cool water. Marks that correspond to the number of antigens to be tested are made on the skin with a permanent marking pen. The individual antigens are injected in a predetermined order, along with positive (histamine) and negative (diluent) control solutions. If mast cell degranulation occurs, a wheal and flare response appears within 10 to 15 minutes of the injection. The injection sites are observed for reactions on conclusion of the injections and again 15 minutes later. Reactions are read as 0 to 4+, with the wheal diameter of the negative

control assigned a value of 0 and the wheal diameter of the positive control assigned a value of 4+. Reactions 2+ or greater are considered significant (Fig. 5–1).

False-negative results may be seen if the patient has received anesthetic agents that interfere with the test, if outdated antigens are used, if endogenous or exogenous progesterone levels are high, if the skin has concurrent infections, or if the test is performed within several months after a seasonal allergy problem. Most of the drugs used to manage allergic skin diseases, including glucocorticoids, antihistamines, and essential fatty acid supplements, cause false-negative reactions. False-positive reactions can occur if the dilution is inadequate (important for some antigens), if there is contamination of the allergens, if poor technique results in trauma, or if dermographism is present. Despite the difficulties associated with intradermal skin testing, this procedure remains the most reliable method to diagnose atopy in the dog or cat.

In Vitro Allergy Testing

There are currently three techniques used in commercially available serum allergy tests for dogs: the radioallergosorbent test (RAST), the enzyme-linked immunosorbent assay (ELISA), and a liquid-phase immunoassay. ELISA and RAST are also available for cats. These tests attempt to measure IgE-specific antigen for allergens causing atopic disease. ELISA and RAST have been evaluated repeatedly, but the sensitivity and specificity of the liquid-phase immunoassay remain unknown. Poor correlation has been reported between intradermal skin test results and results of ELISA.[5, 6] Comparisons of intradermal skin tests and ELISA in allergic dogs suggest that false-positive reactions are common with in vitro tests.[7] Studies in cats have shown a poor correlation between intradermal and in vitro test results, but there have been good results from hyposensitization of cats with allergic disease based on in vitro test findings.[8]

These findings suggest that there is a place for

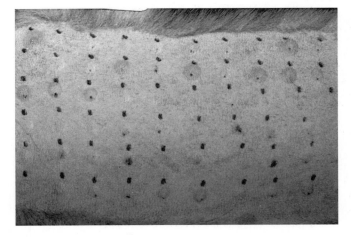

Figure 5–1
Positive reactions on the intradermal skin test are reflected as erythematous wheals.

in vitro testing in veterinary dermatology. The intradermal skin test is still considered the gold standard of allergy testing by veterinary dermatologists, but in vitro testing is an option for veterinarians isolated from referral centers and for practitioners who do not have a sufficient allergy caseload to justify the time and expense of developing in-clinic allergy testing. Their main disadvantage is the tendency to give false-positive results, which reduces the specificity of the test.[8]

Hypoallergenic (Elimination) Dietary Trial

The best procedure to identify an adverse reaction to food is a dietary trial with food containing limited dietary antigens. It is impossible to feed a diet that completely eliminates all antigenic material. All of the dietary ingredients of homemade and commercial diets are potential food allergens, but most food antigens are proteins. Therefore, the goal in an elimination dietary trial is to feed the patient a protein source that is novel or unknown to the patient. It is unlikely that a patient would be allergic to a dietary ingredient that it has never been fed.

Both commercially prepared diets and homemade diets can be used as hypoallergenic diets. A meal of lamb and rice is the most popular homemade diet for this purpose among veterinary dermatologists. This diet has become the gold standard to identify food-related dermatologic problems, but it is not a nutri-tionally balanced diet. In addition, it may be difficult or expensive to provide lamb in some geographic areas. Several substitute diets are available (Table 5–3). Formulas for homemade balanced hypoallergenic diets are also available.[9, 10] One example of a balanced homemade diet for the cat is provided in Table 5–4.[10] This diet was computer-analyzed and found to be balanced but has not yet been evaluated with feeding trials. Commercial diets are also available for this purpose and may be more acceptable to owners of large dogs. However, the name of the diet does not necessarily reflect all ingredients of that diet. The list of ingredients should be examined carefully before a commercial diet is recommended for an elimination trial.

The diet selected should be provided as the sole dietary source for 8 to 12 weeks.[11] No flavored vitamins, flavored medications (e.g., heartworm preventative), dog or cat treats, or table food should be given to the patient during the trial. Improvement in the clinical signs is seen in 75% of patients within 6 weeks if an adverse reaction to food is present. Secondary dermatologic problems, especially bacterial infections, should be treated and controlled during the early weeks of the dietary trial. If the purity of the water is in question, distilled water should be used during the trial.

A positive result of a dietary trial is determined by observing a 50% or greater reduction in pruritus during the feeding trial.

Table 5–3

Hypoallergenic Diets for the Dog and Cat

TYPE OF DIET	SPECIES	INGREDIENTS	PRODUCT
Homemade*	Dog/cat	Lamb and rice	
	Dog/cat	Tofu and rice	
	Dog	Fish and rice	
	Dog	Pinto beans and rice	
Commercial dry†	Dog	Whole egg and rice	Prescription Diet d/d
	Dog	Barley, carrots, rice	Nature's Recipe Vegetarian diet
	Dog	Fish and potato	Eukanuba Response Formula FP
	Cat	Lamb and rice	KenVet Nutritional Care, Specialized Protein
Commercial canned†	Dog	Lamb and rice	Prescription Diet d/d
	Dog	Duck and potato	Innovative Veterinary Diets
	Dog	Venison and potato	Innovative Veterinary Diets
	Dog	Rabbit and potato	Innovative Veterinary Diets
	Cat	Lamb and rice	Prescription Diet d/d
	Cat	Venison and potato	Innovative Veterinary Diets
	Cat	Rabbit and potato	Innovative Veterinary Diets

*Homemade diets are generally not nutritionally balanced diets. See Table 5–4 for a nutritionally balanced lamb and rice diet for the cat.

†Other commercial diets may be acceptable. Read the list of ingredients to determine the nature of the diet.

Table 5–4
Nutritionally Balanced Homemade Diet for Cats

9 jars (900 g) of lamb baby food, strained
5 cups (900 g) of cooked white rice
2 tsp of light salt
4.7 g of calcium carbonate (1880 mg calcium)
1 tsp dicalcium phosphate OR 3.6 g of bone meal (1180 mg calcium)
1 Tbs of safflower oil
350 mg taurine in a nonflavored, additive-free multivitamin supplement

Directions: Cook white rice according to package directions and add light salt to the water. Pulverize the calcium carbonate, the dicalcium phosphate or bone meal, and the taurine and vitamin supplement. Mix the oil, minerals, and supplements with the rice and then add to the lamb baby food. Mix well, cover, and refrigerate. Feed 66 g/kg per day, or 5.3 oz (150 g) for a 5-lb cat. Palatability will be increased if the daily portion is heated to body temperature. Makes enough to feed a 10-lb cat for 6 days.

Modified from Roudebush P. Homemade elimination diets. Derm Dialogue, Spring/Summer 1993:7.

Common Allergic Skin Diseases

Atopy

Atopy (allergic inhalant dermatitis) is an immediate-type hypersensitivity reaction seen in animals that are genetically predisposed to produce high quantities of IgE. Estimates of the incidence of atopy in dogs range up to 10%, but this figure seems low considering the number of atopic patients seen in practice. There is no sex predilection. Atopy is known to occur more frequently in some breeds, such as golden retrievers, Dalmatians, English bulldogs, Chinese shar-peis, and terrier breeds (Table 5–5).[12–14] Signs of atopy initially appear between 1 and 3 years of age and are often seasonal for the first year or two of the disease. The age of onset may be earlier, particularly in some breeds, such as the Chinese shar-pei. Atopy is the most common allergic disease of dogs and is a significant problem in cats.

Pathophysiology

Atopy is an immediate-type hypersensitivity reaction mediated by IgE and, in some cases, by immunoglobulin G_d (IgG_d).[15] Genetic influences are thought to play a major role in the development of this disease. Some animals are genetically predetermined to respond to exposure to some antigens by producing high levels of IgE.

Antigens that cause allergic reactions are called allergens. Not all allergens are complete antigens. Some are haptens, incomplete antigens that require bonding with another substance, usually a polypeptide, to form a complete antigen. All true allergic diseases require that the patient become sensitized to the antigen. During this sensitization period, the allergen stimulates the production of IgE (or IgG_d), which then circulates and binds to tissue mast cells.

Degranulation of mast cells follows subsequent exposures to the antigen and bridging of antigen-specific IgE on the surface of cutaneous mast cells. Inflammation resulting from mast cell degranulation and activation irritates nerve endings in the superficial dermis and initiates the sensation of pruritus. Allergens are classically thought to gain access to the host through the respiratory tract, but evidence suggests that percutaneous absorption of antigens also occurs.[16, 17] An allergic disease can be thought of as an exaggerated protective response of the immune system.

Sensitization of genetically predisposed patients usually occurs within the first 1 to 2 years of life, which accounts for the typical age of onset of clinical

Table 5–5
Dog Breeds Predisposed to Atopy

Akita
Boston terrier
Boxer
Chow chow
Chinese shar-pei
Dalmatian
English bulldog
English setter
Golden retriever
Irish setter
Labrador retriever
Lhasa apso
Miniature schnauzer
Poodle
Pug
Terriers

    Cairn terrier
    Scottish terrier
    West Highland white terrier
    Wirehaired fox terrier

signs in atopic patients. As atopic animals are exposed to more allergens with each successive year, they may become sensitized to additional allergens, and the clinical signs may continue year-round.

Atopic patients have also been shown to have abnormalities of the immune system, including altered lymphocyte function and increased adherence of bacteria to corneocytes.[18] These immunologic abnormalities help explain the frequent occurrence of secondary bacterial infections in atopic patients.

Clinical Signs

Pruritus is the hallmark of atopy. It is the initial clinical feature and is manifested as otitis externa, rubbing of the face, licking and chewing of the feet, scratching, and licking or rubbing of the skin of the ventral abdomen or perineum. Varying degrees of erythema, scale, crusts, papulopustular eruptions, lichenification, and alopecia may be seen (Fig. 5–2). Excessive licking of the feet or any body area results in salivary staining of the hair, which appears as a brownish-red discoloration of light-colored hair. Chewing or biting may result in broken hairs. Patients with atopy may show all or any combination of these signs. For example, unilateral or bilateral otitis externa may be the only clinical problem in an atopic patient.

Pyoderma is a common finding in atopic patients. Lesions include papules, pustules, erythema, crusts, scaling, and epidermal collarettes. Bacterial skin infections also induce pruritus and are frequently the cause of (apparent) glucocorticoid resistance in atopic patients. Secondary infection by *Malassezia pachydermatis*, a commensal yeast organism, is also common in atopic patients.

Cats with atopy develop a variety of clinical signs, including the common feline reaction patterns,

such as miliary dermatitis or lesions of the eosinophilic granuloma complex. Alopecia, caused by excessive licking (e.g., grooming), is also a common finding in cats. It is often difficult for a cat owner to recognize licking as abnormal behavior, because normal cats spend a large amount of time each day grooming.

Clinical signs are often seasonal for the first few years of the disease, when animals develop a hypersensitivity reaction to allergens that are more prevalent during specific seasons (Table 5–6). These signs often progress to a year-round problem as the patient develops reactions to increasing numbers of allergens. However, atopy can be a year-round problem from the initial demonstration of clinical signs, depending on the patient and the allergens involved.

Diagnostic Plan

A tentative diagnosis of atopy is made from the history and physical findings. Confirmation of the diagnosis is indicated if the clinical signs are not classic, if the client wants confirmation of the disease process, if alternative treatments to symptomatic management are desired, or if empiric treatment with glucocorticoids has not resulted in adequate control of clinical signs.

Secondary or coexisting skin diseases should be controlled before allergy testing is initiated. The most common concurrent dermatologic problems are bacterial infections, *Malassezia* dermatitis, and flea infestation or allergy. After these conditions are controlled, the patient is re-examined to confirm the presence of signs consistent with atopy.

Intradermal Skin Testing

Intradermal skin testing remains the diagnostic procedure most widely accepted for the diagnosis of atopy. However, intradermal skin testing is not necessary to confirm the diagnosis in most atopy patients. The history of the problem, physical findings, and results of the dermatologic database (e.g., skin scraping, fungal culture) provide sufficient information to make a presumptive diagnosis and begin medical management in most cases.

If testing is indicated, the patient should be prepared for intradermal skin testing by treatment of secondary infections and withdrawal of all medications that may interfere with the testing procedure (see Table 5–1). As mentioned previously, sedation is useful in most cases to expedite the procedure.

In Vitro Allergy Testing

The indications for in vitro testing are the same as for intradermal skin testing. As with intradermal skin testing, results of these procedures should be

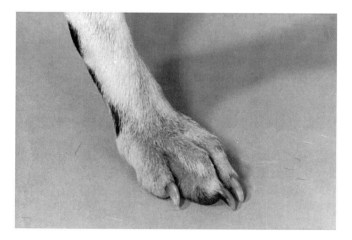

Figure 5–2
Erythema and alopecia in a patient with pododermatitis caused by atopy.

Table 5–6
Seasonality of Various Allergens*

ALLERGEN	SPRING	SUMMER	AUTUMN	WINTER	YEAR-ROUND
Grasses	—	X	—	—	—
Weeds	—	X	X	—	—
Trees	X	—	—	X†	—
Molds (fungi)	—	X‡	X	X§	X‖
Miscellaneous					
House dust mite	—	—	—	—	X
House dust	—	—	—	—	X
Tobacco smoke	—	—	—	—	X
Epidermals (wool, feathers, cat dander)	—	—	—	—	X
Arthropods	—	—	—	—	X¶
Cotton linters#	—	—	—	—	X
Kapok**	—	—	—	—	X

*Specific seasons of importance and distribution of allergens vary with the geographic region and climate.
†Includes some cedars and junipers.
‡*Alternaria* spp. and *Cladosporium* spp. during hot, breezy periods.
§Indoor fungi, such as *Penicillium* spp., *Aspergillus* spp., *Fusarium* spp.
‖Molds are found in areas of high humidity, including shower stalls, refrigerator drip trays, window moldings, cool basements, and air conditioning units.
¶Includes house fly, cockroach, mayfly, grasshoppers, and others. Season varies with occurrence of the specific arthropod.
#Degenerative cotton fibers, derived from cotton garments.
**Seed hair from kapok trees, used to stuff pillows, mattresses, cushions.

carefully interpreted by considering the season of occurrence and the known allergens in the geographic region.

Treatment

Most atopic patients require a combination of treatment modalities to adequately control their clinical signs. Topical therapy is used to provide temporary and symptomatic relief from pruritus. Medical management is directed at symptomatic relief of the pruritus, and immunotherapy is directed at altering the host response to the allergens.

Secondary infections, caused by bacteria or yeast, should be controlled before any specific treatment is prescribed for the atopy. In most cases, control of these secondary problems reduces the pruritus by 50% or more.

Topical Therapy

Many topical products are available to help manage the patient with atopy. Products include moisturizers and humectants, medicated ointments and creams, and medicated shampoos. Because dehydration of the stratum corneum increases pruritus, moisturizers and humectants can reduce pruritus in some patients by hydrating the stratum corneum. These products contain various combinations of oils, fatty acids, lactic acid, urea, amino acids, phospholip-ids, and glycerin. Oil-based products are occlusive and increase the water content of the skin when applied after a bath. Topical glucocorticoids formulated as creams or ointments are not recommended for use in atopic patients, because they are not well suited for treating extensive areas and animals often remove the medication by licking.

Some shampoos contain specific antipruritic medications such as colloidal oatmeal, antihistamines, glucocorticoids, and topical anesthetics. Shampoos containing colloidal oatmeal usually reduce the pruritus in atopic patients for 24 to 48 hours. A shampoo containing diphenhydramine hydrochloride and colloidal oatmeal (Histacalm) provides relief for 24 to 72 hours in many patients. Shampoos containing glucocorticoids (Cortisoothe, FS Shampoo) are also commercially available. These products seem to provide slightly longer relief than other shampoos, but they rarely are sufficient to control the pruritus if used as the sole form of antipruritic therapy. Although topically applied glucocorticoid products can suppress the hypothalamic-pituitary-adrenal axis, one study reported that application of one shampoo (FS Shampoo) twice weekly for 6 months did not do so significantly.[19]

These topical products rarely are effective when used alone to treat atopic patients. However, they are useful for adjunctive treatment of atopic animals and during seasonal exacerbations of clinical signs.

Medical Management

Antihistamines. Although antihistamines are commonly used to control signs of allergies in humans, histamine appears to be less significant as a mediator of inflammation in dogs. The percentage of canine patients that respond to antihistamine therapy is generally low, although the response is quite variable. For example, hydroxyzine hydrochloride may dramatically reduce pruritus in one patient yet provide no relief in another patient with similar clinical signs.

Antihistamines are best suited for use in mild cases of atopy or in combination with glucocorticoids or fatty acid supplements. They may be used to provide relief from pruritus on the nontreatment day of alternate-day glucocorticoid therapy, or they may be helpful during the most severe season for seasonally atopic patients. In general, these drugs provide some relief in 25% to 40% of atopic patients.

If antihistamine therapy is considered, several different products are prescribed for trial use in each patient. The owner is asked to give each drug for 7 to 10 days and to monitor the pet carefully for signs of pruritus. The pet is then re-examined, and a written log kept by the owner is reviewed to determine the best antihistamine, if any, for use in that patient. A list of antihistamines, their doses, and their side effects is provided in Table 5–7.

Chlorpheniramine maleate has been shown to be an effective antihistamine to control nonspecific pruritus in cats. In one clinical study, 2 mg given orally every 12 hours completely eliminated the pruritus in 73% of the cats studied.[20]

Fatty Acids. Fatty acid supplements have also been shown to have benefit in the treatment of atopy. Most products contain high levels of ω-3 fatty acids (e.g., eicosapentaenoic acid) or ω-6 fatty acids (e.g., γ-linolenic acid). High doses of these fatty acids are thought to modulate the arachidonic acid pathway by overwhelming some enzyme-limited pathways and promoting the formation of noninflammatory prostaglandins over proinflammatory prostaglandins and leukotrienes. The most effective combination of the various fatty acids has not yet been determined, but studies with various formulations of commercially available supplements and evening primrose oil (high in γ-linolenic acid) have demonstrated benefit in approximately 30% to 35% of atopic patients. One study evaluated the use of eicosapentaenoic acid (8.2 mg/kg, once daily) for 6 weeks and found that approximately one half of the atopic dogs on the protocol had better than 75% improvement in clinical signs.[21] Because beneficial effects may not be noticed until several weeks of therapy have been completed, these products are best used in combination with glucocorticoids or antihistamines.

Glucocorticoids. Glucocorticoid therapy remains the most consistently reliable medical treatment for atopy. Glucocorticoids decrease inflammation and pruritus by inhibiting the release of some inflammatory mediators, by inhibiting chemotaxis of inflammatory cells, and by reducing the effects (e.g., vasodilation, edema) of many of the inflammatory mediators released from mast cells. Glucocorticoids have many adverse effects, including polydipsia, polyuria, polyphagia, and personality changes. Gastrointestinal ulceration, pancreatitis, and hepatomegaly may occur with prolonged or high-dose therapy. In addition, all

Table 5–7
Antihistamines Used to Manage Canine Atopy*

COMPOUND	TRADE NAME	DOSAGE (mg/kg)	NO. DOSES PER DAY
Hydroxyzine hydrochloride†	Atarax	2.2	3
Diphenhydramine hydrochloride†	Benadryl	2.2	3
Chlorpheniramine†	Chlor-Trimeton	0.2–0.5	2–3
Terfenadine	Seldane	30–60 mg per dog	2
Doxepin hydrochloride†,‡	Sinequan	0.5–1.0	2
Astemizole	Hismanal	1.0	1–2
Trimeprazine	Temaril	0.12	2–3
Clemastine	Tavist	0.05	2

*Some antihistamines have antianxiety, sedative, or analgesic effects.
†Available as a generic compound.
‡Classified as a tricyclic antidepressant with antihistaminic properties.

Table 5–8
Prednisone Schedule for Treatment of Canine Atopy*

1. Administer 1.1 mg/kg once daily for 7 to 14 days, then
2. Administer 1.1 mg/kg every other day for 7 to 10 doses, then
3. Administer decreasing doses of 0.5 to 1.1 mg/kg every other day, until maintenance

*Oral doses.

glucocorticoids suppress the hypothalamic-pituitary-adrenal axis. These adverse effects are minimized by administering short-acting glucocorticoids and by using alternate-day therapy for treatment periods exceeding 1 week. Because of their short half-life, prednisone, prednisolone, and methylprednisolone are the only oral products acceptable for alternate-day administration.

Prednisone and prednisolone are the glucocorticoids of choice for atopy. They are administered orally each day until clinical signs remit and then on alternate days (Table 5–8). Eventually, the dose is decreased to the lowest alternate-day dose that controls the clinical signs. Complicated schedules of administration for these products are not necessary and confuse clients. Clients should be reminded to give the drugs only every other day unless otherwise directed. Injectable glucocorticoids provide no benefit over orally administered products. Depot formulations of glucocorticoids are not indicated to control atopy: the risks and side effects are not worth the benefits.

A low percentage of atopy patients cannot tolerate prednisone even at low doses and have severe side effects, such as polydipsia, polyuria, or panting. Oral dexamethasone or triamcinolone may be effective in those patients; however, the dose should be given as infrequently as possible (e.g., every third day) to prevent development of iatrogenic hyperadrenocorticism.

If the pruritus cannot be controlled with alternate-day prednisone, the patient should be evaluated for secondary infections or concurrent problems. Some patients benefit from the addition of an antihistamine, a fatty acid supplement, or topical therapy to the treatment plan. If the patient is still pruritic, the diagnosis should be reconsidered.

Immunotherapy

Hyposensitization is an excellent treatment option after the inciting allergens have been identified. Hyposensitization is not necessary in seasonally pruritic patients or in patients with signs that are well controlled with low doses of glucocorticoids, antihistamines, or fatty acid supplements. Hyposensitization

Table 5–9
Hyposensitization Schedule for Canine Atopy

TREATMENT DAY	200-pnu/ml VIAL	2000-pnu/ml VIAL	20,000-pnu/ml VIAL
1	0.2	—	—
3	0.4	—	—
5	0.8	—	—
7	1.0	—	—
9	—	0.2	—
11	—	0.4	—
13	—	0.8	—
15	—	1.0	—
17	—	—	0.2
19	—	—	0.4
21	—	—	0.6
23	—	—	0.8
25	—	—	1.0
32	—	—	1.0
39	—	—	1.0
46	—	—	1.0
52	—	—	1.0*

pnu, protein nitrogen unit.
*Dose is administered weekly until maximum beneficial effect is achieved, then dosing frequency is decreased as possible.

is recommended if the patient is pruritic for most of the year, if the condition is not well controlled with medical management, or if the patient develops unacceptable side effects from medication.

The mechanism of action for hyposensitization is not completely understood, but it may include the development of so-called blocking IgG antibodies. Other mechanisms may include stimulation of suppressor T cells to inhibit IgE production or alteration of receptors on mast cells. Hyposensitization is effective in reducing the clinical signs of atopy in 65% to 75% of patients treated.[1, 22] Results are affected by the accuracy of allergy testing, the involvement of allergens not included in the test battery of antigens, the schedule used for hyposensitization, and concurrent dermatologic problems of the patient.

A hyposensitization solution, commonly referred to as a vaccine, is prepared in various concentrations. Owners are taught to administer the solution subcutaneously. The patient receives increasing amounts and concentrations of solution over a period of several days to weeks (Table 5–9). Although most patients improve within a few weeks, injections should be continued for 6 to 12 months before a decision is made to discontinue the therapy because of lack of response. Most patients reach a point at which maximum benefit occurs with weekly to biweekly injections of a maintenance-strength solution. Several effective protocols are used by veterinary allergists.[13, 22]

Possible adverse effects of hyposensitization include increased pruritus at the time of injection, urticaria or angioedema after injection, and anaphylaxis. The increase in pruritus is usually transient and is managed by adding a systemic glucocorticoid or antihistamine to the treatment schedule for a few weeks. The other two reactions are serious but rare. Urticaria and angioedema may be controlled by decreasing the frequency, amount, or strength of the solution. However, they may also be a prologue to anaphylaxis, which is a life-threatening systemic reaction requiring immediate treatment with epinephrine. The initial sign of anaphylaxis in dogs is usually vomiting; in cats, the initial sign is respiratory distress. Life-threatening reactions to hyposensitization are rare, but the owners must be informed of the possibility of these reactions. Adverse reactions may develop at any time in the hyposensitization schedule, and owners should be instructed to observe the animal for 30 minutes after each injection.

Oral glucocorticoids or antihistamines are often prescribed for use during the first 30 days of hyposensitization, in order to increase the comfort level of the patient.

Client Education

Client education is an important aspect of management of the atopic dog or cat. Owners must understand the results to expect from the drugs prescribed for their pet and the side effects that may accompany the use of each drug. In addition, owners must be made aware that secondary bacterial or yeast infections may still occur in their pet and produce recurrence of the clinical signs. Re-examinations are encouraged on a regular basis, preferably every 6 months, to check on drug doses and secondary complications of atopy or treatment.

Prognosis

The prognosis for control of clinical signs of seasonal allergies is excellent. However, these patients may develop nonseasonal (year-round) signs through development of allergic responses to additional allergens. Patients with nonseasonal pruritus have a good prognosis and usually can be managed very well with the treatment options described here.

Atopic patients are prone to secondary bacterial and yeast infections. Clients should be warned that the pet may appear to have a relapse of the allergy and become less responsive to therapy. If an allergic patient ceases to respond to routine management, the patient should be re-examined by a veterinarian for secondary infections or other pruritic skin diseases.

Adverse Reactions to Food

Adverse reactions to food are those abnormal clinical conditions caused by ingestion of foods or food additives. The term food allergy is often used to describe all cutaneous reactions resulting from an adverse reaction to food, because it is difficult to clinically distinguish reactions caused by the various pathogenic mechanisms. However, the term adverse reaction to food is preferred to describe clinical conditions in which the pathogenic mechanism is unknown.

The prevalence of adverse reactions to food is unknown, but these conditions probably account for fewer than 15% of allergic skin disorders. There appears to be no age, breed, or sex predilection. Animals may show clinical signs initially at a very young age (<6 months) or at any age throughout life. Food allergy usually occurs after an animal has been on the same diet for months or years, a concept difficult for many clients to understand.

Pathophysiology

The terminology used to describe the various pathogenic mechanisms of food-related problems is confusing. Adverse reactions to food in the dog and cat may be immunologically mediated (food allergy) or nonimmunologically mediated (food intolerance, food idiosyncrasy).

True food allergy is thought to result from type I and type III hypersensitivity reactions, although type IV and type II mechanisms have also been proposed. The allergic phenomenon results from absorption of dietary antigens or haptens, which are usually derived from proteins in the diet. Factors that may influence the antigenicity of a food include the amount of antigen (protein) in the diet, the digestibility and thus the availability of antigen in the diet, and the source of the antigen (protein source).[23] As has been mentioned, other pathogenic mechanisms may be responsible for adverse food reactions in dogs and cats. For example, the histamine content of food (especially fish-based feline diets) may affect the patient's response to some foods.[24] The diagnostic and therapeutic techniques recommended for these problems are effective for both immunologically and nonimmunologically mediated disease.

Clinical Signs

Clinical features of adverse reactions to food are variable. Nonseasonal pruritus is the most common complaint. In dogs, the pruritus is poorly responsive to glucocorticoid therapy.[11] Cats with adverse reactions to food tend to be more responsive to glucocorticoids, especially if high doses are administered.

The clinical signs associated with adverse reactions to food are similar to those associated with atopy. Facial pruritus, perianal pruritus, pododermatitis (and foot licking), and otitis externa are common features of this disease. As in atopy, otitis externa, either unilateral or bilateral, may be the only clinical sign. Facial and head pruritus is a common manifestation of food reactions in cats.[25] Specific lesions include erythema, hyperpigmentation, papules, pustules, alopecia, scale accumulation, crusts, and epidermal collarettes. Recurrent superficial pyoderma and *Malassezia* dermatitis are also common in patients with adverse food reactions.

Signs localized to the gastrointestinal tract, such as vomiting, diarrhea, hematochezia, or anorexia, may occur with adverse reactions to food. However, their prevalence in this condition is unknown. The percentage reported has varied from less than 2% to 15%, depending on the perspective of the clinician (i.e., dermatologist or gastroenterologist). Reports of clinical signs (e.g., seizures) in other organ systems are rare and largely anecdotal.

Diagnostic Plan

Diagnosis of an adverse reaction to food is made by feeding the animal a hypoallergenic diet in an elimination dietary trial. Twenty-five percent of dogs with food allergies have remission of clinical signs within 3 weeks after beginning the diet, and another 49% within 6 weeks.[11] However, the trial should extend for 10 to 12 weeks if positive results are not seen earlier. Intradermal skin testing and in vitro allergy testing have been used to identify food allergens, but the accuracy of these procedures is questionable.[26] The application of food extracts through an endoscope onto the gastric mucosa has recently been described as a diagnostic procedure for food allergy.[27] The mucosa is evaluated for swelling and erythema. This procedure appears promising, but additional studies are needed to determine its clinical value.

Identification of the specific antigen may be accomplished by provocative exposure, a process that involves feeding a new protein source every 7 to 10 days while observing for recurrence of clinical signs. The goal of this procedure is to identify the offending food allergens in order to find a commercial diet that is tolerated by the patient.

Treatment

An adverse reaction to food is managed by avoiding the offending allergen. Patients with adverse reactions to food may develop clinical signs while on the treatment diet, requiring repetition of the elimination dietary trial and identification of a different maintenance diet that is acceptable to the animal.

Prognosis

The prognosis is excellent once the offending dietary substance has been identified. However, some patients develop an adverse reaction to an ingredient of the hypoallergenic or replacement diet. The incidence of this reaction is unknown but appears to be low.

Contact Dermatitis

Contact dermatitis may be divided into two syndromes: irritant contact dermatitis (ICD) and allergic contact dermatitis (ACD). ICD is produced by physical or chemical irritation of the skin, and ACD is a type IV allergic reaction. These conditions can occur in animals of any age, breed, or sex.

Pathophysiology

ICD results from contact of the skin by irritating substances; the damage may be caused by caustic reactions, temperature variations, or chemical reactions. ACD is a delayed-type hypersensitivity reaction that occurs after haptens contact the skin, are absorbed, and combine with cutaneous proteins to form a hapten-protein complex. The Langerhans cell modifies and transports the complex to a regional lymph node, where T-lymphocyte stimulation occurs. Sensitized T lymphocytes migrate to the site of exposure, and on subsequent exposure to the sensitizing allergen, the lymphocytes release cytokines that induce vascular changes and recruit inflammatory cells into the area.

Clinical Signs

ACD may be induced in dogs and cats after exposure to various substances, including plants, carpet deodorizers, chemicals, antibiotics, topical anesthetic agents, and cosmetics.[28–30] Lesions are confined to areas of contact between the antigen (or hapten) and the skin, with glabrous (hairless) skin most commonly affected. Lesions are often found on the chin, ventral neck, ventral thorax and abdomen, perineum, scrotum, and interdigital areas. The ears are often involved if the allergen is present in medication. Erythema, vesicles, or pustules may be seen early in the course of the reaction; scaling, crusts, hyperpigmentation, and lichenification develop with prolonged or repeated exposure. Pruritus may be mild or severe, and excoriations may be present. The lesions may be painful, especially with ICD.

Diagnostic Plan

ACD should be considered based on the history and physical findings. The differential diagnosis includes atopy, ectoparasitic infections, food allergy, pyoderma, *Malassezia* dermatitis, and other immunologically mediated diseases. Histopathologic examination of skin from affected areas may show spongiosis of the epidermis with perivascular dermatitis, intraepidermal spongiotic vesicles containing lymphocytes and eosinophils, and serocellular crusts on the epidermal surface. The most definitive test to confirm ACD is the patch test, which may be performed by using material suspected in the allergic reaction or by using purified allergens that are commercially available.[28,30] If ACD is suspected to be caused by a substance in the home, isolation (boarding) in a veterinary hospital helps to alleviate the clinical signs and can be used as both a diagnostic and a therapeutic procedure. However, many atopic dogs also improve with this environmental isolation, so other diagnostic tests may be necessary to confirm the cause of the response.

Treatment

Avoidance of the offending substance is the best treatment for ICD or ACD. Symptomatic management of the affected areas is necessary. Astringents (Domeboro) help to dry moist exudative lesions, and antimicrobial agents are indicated if secondary infections are present. Anti-inflammatory doses of prednisone reduce the inflammation and pruritus associated with ACD but provide minimal relief in ICD.

Prognosis

The prognosis is good if the offending substance is removed from contact with the patient. However, lesions may intermittently develop if the substance is not identified. Patient response to glucocorticoid therapy is variable, from poor to excellent.

Flea Allergy Dermatitis

FAD, also known as flea bite hypersensitivity, is the clinical disease resulting from a hypersensitivity to flea bites. Clinical signs may be seen in dogs or cats as young as 6 months of age, or the onset may also be delayed until the patient is older than 6 or 7 years of age. There is no age, breed, or sex predilection.

Pathophysiology

Haptens in flea saliva are introduced into the animal during feeding by the flea. These haptens combine with dermal proteins (collagen) to induce an allergic reaction. Allergic mechanisms that have been identified or suspected in animals with FAD include type I hypersensitivity reactions, delayed-type hypersensitivity reactions, cutaneous basophilic hypersensitivity reactions, and late-phase, IgE-mediated reactions.[31]

The net result of these hypersensitivity reactions is intense pruritus. The patient does not have to be exposed to large numbers of fleas to become severely affected, because the mechanism of the pruritus is allergic. Only a few fleas are required to induce the intense, debilitating pruritus associated with FAD.

Clinical Signs

The predominant clinical sign in dogs is intense pruritus affecting the base of the tail. Generalized pruritus may also be seen. The pruritus may be less localized in cats, although tail pruritus is also common. Clinical signs associated with FAD may be seasonal in some patients because of the seasonal nature of flea populations in some geographic areas. Lesions include erythema, alopecia, crusts, scale, excoriations, hyperpigmentation, and lichenification. Secondary changes include excoriations, alopecia from self-trauma, and pyoderma. Miliary dermatitis is a common reaction pattern in cats with FAD.

Diagnostic Plan

Differential diagnosis includes other ectoparasitic infections (e.g., scabies), pyoderma, atopy, food allergy, and seborrheic disorders. A tentative diagnosis can be based on the clinical features, even if fleas are not present at the time of the examination. The distribution of lesions and the severity of the pruritus are sufficient criteria to permit the initial diagnosis. Confirmation of FAD is difficult, although intradermal skin testing with flea antigen shows a positive wheal and flare response in those animals with a type I hypersensitivity reaction. Up to 90% of animals with FAD are reported to exhibit a positive reaction to the intradermal injection of flea antigen.[32] Clinicians should be cautious in promoting this diagnostic tool to the client, however, because FAD may be present with a negative intradermal test. Most in vitro allergy tests contain flea antigen in the test battery, but they also reflect only a type I hypersensitivity.

Treatment

Initial treatment of FAD includes symptomatic control of the pruritus and treatment of secondary changes created by the intense pruritus. Sulfur–salicylic acid or colloidal oatmeal shampoos help to remove crusts and reduce pruritus. Systemic antimicrobial agents are indicated if pyoderma is present. They may be used concurrently with glucocorticoids or other medications to control pruritus. Antihistamines provide relief from pruritus in some patients, but the response is often incomplete or transient. Glucocorticoids are the most effective medication for controlling the pruritus of FAD. Prednisone is administered with the use of the same protocol as for atopy (see Table 5–8). Clinical studies have shown no significant clinical improvement in either dogs or cats after hyposensitization with commercial flea extracts.[33-35]

Ultimately, successful management of FAD depends on adequate flea control. Because exposure to one flea may induce a severe response in the allergic patient, flea control efforts are paramount (see Chap. 2).

Autoimmune Skin Diseases

Problem Identification

Pustules

Pustules are circumscribed elevations of the epidermis containing inflammatory cells. Autoimmune diseases associated with the presence of pustules include pemphigus (all forms), bullous pemphigoid, systemic lupus erythematosus (SLE), and drug eruptions. Pustules developing secondary to autoimmune disease are clinically indistinguishable from those caused by infectious agents. Cytologic analysis is necessary to identify infectious agents or acantholytic cells, which are diagnostic of pemphigus. (See Chapter 1 for a complete discussion of pustules.)

Vesicles and Bullae

Vesicles and bullae are elevated lesions of the epidermis containing clear fluid.

Pathophysiology

These lesions are associated with urticarial reactions, bullous pemphigoid, irritant reactions, and drug eruptions. The lesions contain filtrate of blood or lymph, which escapes vessels after vascular damage.

Clinical Signs

Vesicles are small lesions less than 1 cm in diameter, and bullae are larger lesions; both are included in the lay term "blister." Vesicles and bullae are easily damaged, resulting in formation of an erosion or ulcer. Therefore, if a vesicle is present, the lesion should be resected for histopathology (if indicated) as soon as possible.

Diagnostic Plan

Histopathologic evaluation of the skin confirms the type of lesion. Cytology may be useful to differentiate the lesion from a pustule. Culture may be warranted if inflammatory cells are seen on cytologic examination.

Prognosis

The prognosis is excellent if flea control is successful. If fleas are eliminated from the patient's environment and no further contact occurs, medical therapy is not necessary. However, relapse can occur acutely when the patient is exposed to fleas.

Pathophysiology of Autoimmune Diseases

Autoimmune disease can arise from failure in immunoregulation due to overstimulation of B lymphocytes, defects in suppressor T-lymphocyte function, circumvention of normal suppressor T-cell control by helper T lymphocytes, and the presence of cross-reacting antigens. Immunologic damage to the host takes place through types II, III, and IV hypersensitivity reactions. In some cases, autoantibody production may be the result of a disease process, rather than the cause.

Diagnostic Procedures

Routine Laboratory Evaluation

Systemic signs of illness often accompany autoimmune diseases. Therefore, complete evaluation of the patient for hematologic abnormalities or serum biochemical alterations is indicated. These tests also help determine the functional status of various organ systems, which is important because treatment of these disorders involves the use of drugs that are metabolized or excreted by internal organs. A complete blood count and platelet count should be performed to rule out anemia or thrombocytopenia, features of SLE. Several biochemical parameters should be determined, including concentrations of serum creatinine and urea nitrogen, serum alkaline phosphatase, and alanine aminotransferase. A complete urinalysis is recommended to help rule out any pre-existing renal disease.

Cytology

Cytology is a useful diagnostic tool if pustules are present. The autoimmune disease most commonly associated with pustules is pemphigus foliaceus (PF). Neutrophils are the most common inflammatory cell seen on cytologic examination, and eosinophils and macrophages may also be present. Infectious agents are not present in pustules caused by autoimmune disease.

Histopathology

Histopathologic examination of the skin is the definitive procedure for identification of the specific autoimmune disease (see Chap. 1). Multiple skin biopsies should be collected and submitted to a dermatopathologist for evaluation. Special procedures, such as direct immunofluorescence and immunoperoxidase staining, may be useful on skin samples to identify the presence and location of antibody in the skin. Direct immunofluorescence is the standard test for localization of antibody, but the procedure requires that the skin biopsy specimen be frozen in liquid nitrogen or stored in Michel's fixative. Immunoperoxidase techniques may be performed on formalin-fixed tissues, but they are extremely sensitive and may give false-positive findings in inflamed skin.[36]

Common Autoimmune Skin Diseases

Pemphigus Foliaceus

PF is the most common form of pemphigus, a group of autoimmune skin diseases affecting the epidermis. Other forms of pemphigus include pemphigus vulgaris, pemphigus vegetans, and pemphigus erythematosus, a form with characteristics of both PF and SLE.[37] PF is commonly seen in dogs and cats, as well as in other animals and humans. Some breeds, such as Akitas, bearded collies, chow chows, Newfoundlands, and schipperkes, have been reported to be at increased risk.[38–40] Most dogs are young adults at the time of diagnosis, but dogs younger than 1 year of age can develop the disease.

Pathophysiology

The immunologic damage in PF is caused by a type II hypersensitivity reaction. Autoantibodies are directed at adhesion molecules that are part of desmosomes, the intercellular attachments of epithelial cells.[41] The hypersensitivity reaction induces a cascade of inflammatory events, culminating in the destruction of epidermal cellular attachments. The breakdown of epidermal cohesion is called acantholysis, and it is the key pathogenic mechanism in pemphigus. In PF, acantholytic epidermal cells and inflammatory cells form vesicles and pustules at or underneath the stratum corneum (subcorneal lesions). The precipitating cause of autoantibody formation is not known, although genetic factors are likely.

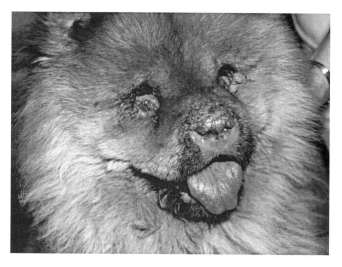

Figure 5–3
Depigmentation, crusting, and erythema involving the eyelids, bridge of the nose, and planum nasale in a chow chow with pemphigus foliaceus.

Clinical Signs

Pustular dermatitis is the characteristic change associated with PF. Although pustules are the classic lesion, they are fragile and may not be present at the time of examination. Crusts, scales, papules, and epidermal collarettes are commonly present. Mild to moderate pruritus may be reported by the owner, and alopecia may result from the inflammation and pruritus. Lesions are most commonly seen on the planum nasale, bridge of the nose, periocular skin, pinnae, and foot pads (Fig. 5–3). Oral ulcers are rare in this autoimmune skin disease. Lesions on the planum nasale often start as depigmenting areas, with subsequent development of crusts and erosions. Affected foot pads are hyperkeratotic and crusted, and they may develop fissures to the extent that lameness is reported by the owners. Paronychia may be seen in some animals.

Diagnostic Plan

Differential diagnosis includes demodicosis, dermatophytosis, discoid lupus erythematosus (DLE), SLE, pemphigus erythematosus, zinc-responsive dermatosis, superficial necrolytic dermatosis, and pyoderma. If pustules are present, material should be collected for cytologic examination. The presence of inflammatory cells and acantholytic epithelial cells and the absence of infectious agents are suggestive of PF. Histopathologic examination of an intact pustule is the definitive diagnostic procedure. If pustules are not present, crusts removed from the planum nasale, skin, or foot pad may be submitted for examination. It may be worthwhile to hospitalize the patient for 1 to 2 days and frequently examine the animal for pustules, because these lesions appear and regress rapidly. Routine histopathologic evaluation shows acantholytic cells within subcorneal pustules or crusts. These findings are usually sufficient to confirm the diagnosis of PF. However, in some cases, direct immunofluorescence or immunoperoxidase staining may be useful to demonstrate the presence of intercellular antibody.

Treatment

Immunosuppressive therapy is initiated to prevent formation of autoantibodies. Immunosuppressive doses of prednisone (2.2 mg/kg per day in the dog, 4.4 mg/kg per day in the cat) are given until remission of clinical signs. Some clinicians also concurrently administer azathioprine (2.2 mg/kg, once daily) in the dog, because fewer than 50% of dogs with PF respond to prednisone alone.[40] After remission has been achieved, the doses of drugs are slowly decreased over several weeks. Aurothioglucose, a gold salt, is also a useful immunosuppressive agent. It may be used concurrently with glucocorticoids in dogs or cats and is recommended if response to other immunosuppressive drugs is incomplete. Test doses of 0.25 mg/kg and 0.5 mg/kg are given intramuscularly on weeks 1 and 2, respectively. If adverse effects are not observed, the drug is administered in doses of 1.0 mg/kg intramuscularly every 7 days until remission of clinical signs occurs. The frequency of administration is then slowly decreased over several weeks to months. Combination therapy with tetracycline and niacinamide (the amide salt of the B vitamin nicotinic acid) has also been useful to treat PF in some cases[42] (see Discoid Lupus Erythematosus). All of the above-mentioned drugs are potent immunosuppressive agents, and patients should be carefully monitored for evidence of bacterial or viral infections, internal parasitic infections, and adverse effects of these agents (Table 5–10).

Prognosis

The prognosis varies from good to poor. Subjectively, it seems to vary from breed to breed, with some (e.g., chow chow, Akita) having a worse prognosis. Relapses may occur in any case if the animal is withdrawn from immunosuppressive therapy or if doses are decreased too rapidly. Therefore, careful monitoring is recommended.

Discoid Lupus Erythematosus

DLE is a common, cutaneous autoimmune disease with no systemic involvement. Female dogs are predisposed to develop DLE, and some breeds, such as

Table 5–10
Adverse Reactions of Common Immunosuppressive Drugs

DRUG	ADVERSE EFFECTS
Glucocorticoids	Polydipsia and polyuria
	Panting
	Polyphagia and weight gain
	Gastric ulcers and vomiting
	Secondary infections
Azathioprine	Bone marrow suppression
	Vomiting
	Secondary infections
	Pancreatitis
	Peripheral neuropathy (cats)
Cyclophosphamide	Bone marrow suppression
	Hemorrhagic cystitis
	Vomiting
	Secondary infections
Aurothioglucose	Thrombocytopenia
	Cutaneous drug eruptions (toxic epidermal necrolysis, erythema multiforme)
	Secondary infections

the collie, Shetland sheepdog, German shepherd, and Akita, also appear predisposed to develop the disease. DLE is rare in cats.

Pathophysiology

The cause of DLE is unclear, but it probably involves contributing factors such as exposure to ultraviolet irradiation, similar to those recognized for SLE. DLE is often considered a benign variant of SLE.[37]

Clinical Signs

Clinical signs associated with DLE in dogs include depigmentation, crusting, and ulceration of the planum nasale, margins of the eyelids, periocular skin, lips, pinnae, foot pads, or skin. The planum nasale is the most common site of involvement (Fig. 5–4). Lesions progress from hypopigmentation to ulceration of the skin and erosion of cartilage, which can be disfiguring. Severe ulceration may occasionally result in hemorrhage as arteries are damaged.

Diagnostic Plan

Diagnosis of DLE is based on histopathologic examination of the skin and the lack of systemic signs associated with SLE. Patients with DLE rarely have a significant titer of antinuclear antibodies. Samples for histopathologic examination should be obtained from affected areas and should include lesional and perilesional skin. Crusts, recently depigmented areas, and skin from the margins of ulcerated lesions may be selected for submission. A general anesthetic is required, because the most common location of lesions is the planum nasale or pinna.

Classic histopathologic findings include thickening of the basement membrane, hydropic degeneration of basal epithelial cells, and the presence of colloid (Civatte) bodies in the basal cell layer of the epidermis. Vacuolar changes in the basement membrane zone and the presence of an interface dermatitis are also frequently seen. Pigmentary incontinence, another common histopathologic finding, reflects the loss of epidermal pigment from the damaged basal cell layer into the underlying dermis. Immunoperoxidase or immunofluorescence staining of the skin, the so-called lupus band test, may identify immunoglobulins or complement along the dermal-epidermal junction.

Treatment

Many treatment options are available for DLE. Because ultraviolet radiation can exacerbate the clinical signs, avoidance of direct sunlight is recommended. Sunscreens may also help reduce the severity of lesions, but they tend to be of limited value because most dogs do not tolerate application of lotions to the planum nasale. Topical glucocorticoids may also reduce the inflammation associated with DLE, but they have the same limitations as topical sunscreens.

Vitamin E (400–800 IU given twice per day) has been reported to alleviate clinical signs in some dogs, but the response is unpredictable and is not dramatic in severe cases. Combination therapy with tetracycline and niacinamide has been shown to induce remission or reduce the severity of clinical lesions in some patients with DLE.[42] For patients weighing less than 10 kg, tetracycline is given orally at a dose of 250 mg three

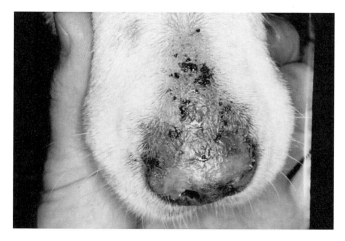

Figure 5-4
Depigmentation and crusting of the planum nasale in a dog with discoid lupus erythematosus.

times per day, along with niacinamide at the same dose and rate, for an 8-week trial period. Patients weighing more than 10 kg receive oral doses of 500 mg of each drug three times per day. A satisfactory level of response is seen in approximately half of patients treated with this protocol. If the response is good, the doses may be decreased to twice daily, or in some cases, once daily.

If the lesions are unresponsive to these medications, immunosuppressive therapy with prednisone (2.2 mg/kg per day orally) is recommended. Remission occurs in most cases within 14 days; however, higher doses of prednisone (up to 2.2 mg/kg twice daily) may be needed. Azathioprine (Imuran) is added to the treatment program at 1.0 to 2.0 mg/kg per day if prednisone alone fails to induce remission. After existing lesions have resolved and no new lesions have developed, doses of both prednisone and azathioprine are reduced by switching to alternate-day administration and then by tapering the doses over several weeks. Low doses of prednisone are usually required for long-term control of signs. A complete blood count should be performed every 3 to 4 weeks if azathioprine is included in the protocol, because the drug can be toxic to the bone marrow. As always, adverse effects of therapeutic agents should be explained to pet owners.

Prognosis

The prognosis for DLE is good, although some patients require aggressive immunosuppressive therapy for many months.

Uncommon Immune-Mediated Skin Diseases

Erythema Multiforme and Toxic Epidermal Necrolysis

Erythema multiforme (EM) and toxic epidermal necrolysis (TEN) are cutaneous reactions with an immune-mediated basis, although the precise mechanisms are not clear. These two entities probably represent a spectrum of the same disease, with EM considered a milder reaction than TEN.

These reactions have been reported after administration of various drugs or biologic agents, including trimethoprim-sulfadiazine, cephalexin, aurothioglucose, gentamicin, and levamisole.[43-45] With the ever-expanding list of drugs reportedly associated with this condition, it seems safe to assume that any drug may be responsible for EM or TEN. The history of lesion development in relation to drug administration should be investigated carefully in each case, and either cutaneous disorder should be considered an adverse drug reaction until proven otherwise. These reactions may also be associated with systemic illnesses, including neoplasia, systemic infections, and heat stroke.

Lesions include erythematous papules and macules, annular erythematous patches, epidermal collarettes, vesicles, bullae, and ulcerations. Common sites of involvement include the glabrous skin, mucocutaneous junctions, oral mucosa, ears, axillae, and trunk. TEN is often associated with signs of systemic illness, such as fever, depression, lethargy, and intense cutaneous pain.

Diagnosis of these reactions is confirmed by histopathologic examination of the skin. EM is characterized by single to multiple epidermal cell necrosis and interface dermatitis, and the differential diagnosis includes SLE, DLE, cutaneous neoplasia, burns, pyoderma, superficial necrolytic dermatitis, and drug eruption. Histologic changes seen in TEN are more severe and include full- or split-thickness coagulation necrosis of the epidermis.

Treatment for both conditions is supportive and symptomatic, with removal of the initiating factor being of paramount importance. Antimicrobial agents (not any previously administered) are indicated if ulcers are present. The use of glucocorticoids for these conditions is controversial because of their immunosuppressive effects. However, administration of glucocorticoid in anti-inflammatory doses early in the disease seems to reduce morbidity. The prognosis is guarded until the initiating factor can be identified and removed.

Familial Canine Dermatomyositis

Dermatomyositis is a familial, immune-mediated disease of collies and Shetland sheepdogs that appears to be inherited as an autosomal dominant trait with variable expressivity.[46] The disease is usually seen initially in dogs younger than 6 months of age, although an adult-onset form may also be seen.[47, 48] Both skeletal muscle and skin are affected. Dermatologic lesions include alopecia, erythema, crusts, and development of a fine scale on the face, tips of the pinnae, tip of the tail, foot pads, and skin over bony prominences (Fig. 5–5). Ulceration and depigmentation of the planum nasale occur in many cases. Diagnosis is confirmed by electromyography and histopathologic examination of skin and muscle. Treatment is variably effective and includes the use of anti-inflammatory and immunosuppressive drugs.[48] The prognosis is guarded. The disease waxes and wanes, and recurrence of clinical signs is common.

Systemic Lupus Erythematosus

SLE is a rare, multisystem, autoimmune disease seen uncommonly in the dog and cat. Genetic influences, environmental factors, infectious agents, and

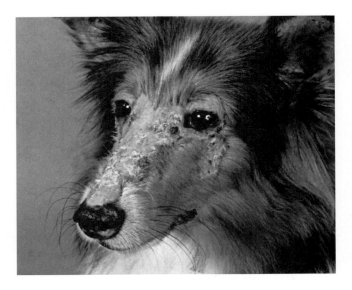

Figure 5–5
Dermatomyositis in an 8-month-old Shetland sheepdog. Notice the alopecia, crusts, and depigmentation of the planum nasale.

hormonal interactions may contribute to the pathogenesis of this syndrome. Clinical manifestations of SLE include autoimmune hemolytic anemia, immune-mediated thrombocytopenia, nonerosive polysynovitis, glomerulonephritis, polymyositis, and dermatitis. The cutaneous lesions include erythema, crusts, and erosions of thin-skinned areas such as the periocular skin, axillae, and ventral abdomen. Ulcers may develop in skin of the mucocutaneous junctions and mucosa of the oral cavity. Diagnosis is confirmed by histopathologic examination of affected organs, especially skin, and by the presence of specific laboratory findings, such as significantly high antinuclear antibody titers. Treatment usually involves administration of immunosuppressive agents such as glucocorticoids, azathioprine, and cyclophosphamide. The prognosis is guarded and depends on the extent of damage to internal organs such as the kidneys.

Pemphigus Vulgaris, Erythematosus, and Vegetans

PF is the most common form of pemphigus in the dog and cat. Other forms of pemphigus reported in dogs and cats include pemphigus vulgaris, pemphigus vegetans, and pemphigus erythematosus.[39] In pemphigus vulgaris, a rare form of pemphigus,[38, 39] the autoantibodies are directed at antigens deep in the epidermis, and the acantholysis and resulting lesions are suprabasilar (i.e., they develop immediately above the stratum basale). The disease is characterized by oral, cutaneous, and mucocutaneous vesicles, bullae, pustules, erosions, and ulcers. The clinical signs of pemphigus erythematosus include alopecia, crust formation, and pustules of the planum nasale and bridge of the nose. Pemphigus vegetans is a proliferative form of pemphigus that manifests as heavy crust formation. All of these conditions are diagnosed and treated as for PF. Immunosuppressive therapy is indicated to control the lesions.

Bullous Pemphigoid

Bullous pemphigoid is an uncommon autoimmune disease of the dog and cat with the antibody directed against antigens located in the basement membrane zone.[38, 39] Lesions include oral and cutaneous vesicles and bullae, erosions, and ulcerations. The condition is easily controlled with immunosuppressive therapy.

Adverse Drug Reactions

Adverse drug reactions may be idiopathic, or they may result from altered biochemical pathways that change the host's reaction to the drug or from a hypersensitivity reaction in a sensitized individual. Fixed drug eruptions are cutaneous reactions that occur in the same location of the body on each exposure to the drug.[49] Other clinical forms of adverse drug reactions include urticaria, angioedema, erythematous maculopapular reactions, and vesiculobullous reactions.[50] Sulfonamides and penicillins are most commonly incriminated as the cause of drug eruptions.[50, 51] Diagnosis of drug reactions is based on the perspective obtained from a history of lesion development after drug administration and on histopathologic findings of the skin. Treatment includes removal of the drug from the patient (if possible) and symptomatic management of the cutaneous lesions.

Vasculitis

Vasculitis is a syndrome characterized by inflammation of blood vessels that results in vascular damage and occlusion. The most common causes of vasculitis in humans are drug reactions, infectious diseases, secondary reactions to systemic inflammatory diseases, and malignancy.[52] Vasculitis has been described in dogs and cats in association with the same diseases.[53, 54] Several histopathologic forms of vasculitis occur in the dog and cat, reflecting different pathologic mechanisms.[55] A form of lymphocytic vasculitis secondary to vaccination may result in alopecia at the site of injection. Poodles seem to be predisposed to this reaction after rabies vaccination.[56]

Clinical signs of vasculitis include erythematous macules, petechiae, ecchymoses, ulcerations, alopecia, and crusts, which are most commonly found on the pinnae, distal extremities, and tip of the tail. Edema, which is caused by fluid leakage from small vessels, is another common sign of vasculitis. Erythematous macules and petechiae are differentiated from cutaneous hemorrhage by a procedure known as diascopy, performed by pressing a glass slide against the lesion. If the lesion blanches, the erythema is caused by vascular dilation, a common finding in vasculitis. Treatment includes removal of the initiating factor and immunosuppressive therapy.[53]

Vogt-Koyanagi-Harada–like Syndrome

The Vogt-Koyanagi-Harada (VKH) syndrome in humans is associated with uveitis, chorioretinitis, poliosis (whitening of hair), and meningitis. The disease is thought to be an autoimmune disease in which the target cell is the melanocyte. A similar disease occurs in dogs; clinical signs include progressive loss of pigment from the planum nasale, the pigmented mucous membranes, the hair (poliosis), and the skin around the lips and eyelids.[57, 58] Uveitis is a consistent feature of the disease in the dog.

Although the VKH-like syndrome has been described in several breeds, the condition is seen most commonly in Akitas and Samoyeds. Histologic changes in the uvea and skin include granulomatous inflammation with a lichenoid, interface dermatitis. Treatment has been most successful with immunosuppressive agents, both systemically and topically on the eyes. The prognosis is guarded: long-term therapy is needed, and recurrence is often seen in affected patients.

Panniculitis

Panniculitis is defined as inflammation of the subcutaneous fat, or panniculus. The inflammation is presumed to be immune-mediated based on response to therapy and the lack of infectious agents isolated from affected patients. The classic clinical lesion is an ulcerated nodule or fistulous tract, draining a serosanguineous fluid.[59] Firm to fluctuant subcutaneous masses are often present and may be painful. These lesions eventually fistulate. Solitary or multiple lesions may be present. Diagnosis is made by histopathologic evaluation of the subcutaneous lesion. The lesions respond to surgical removal (if solitary) or to immunosuppressive doses of prednisone.

References

1. Reedy LM, Miller WH. Allergic Skin Diseases of Dogs and Cats. Philadelphia, WB Saunders, 1989:81–109.
2. Halliwell REW, Gorman NT. Veterinary Clinical Immunology. Philadelphia, WB Saunders, 1989:238–242.
3. August JR. The reaction of canine skin to the intradermal

injection of allergenic extracts. J Am Anim Hosp Assoc 1982;18:157–163.

4. Codner EC, Lessard P, McGrath CJ. Effect of tiletamine/zolazepam sedation on intradermal allergy testing in atopic dogs. J Am Vet Med Assoc 1992;201:1857–1860.

5. Kleinbeck ML, Hites MJ, Loker JL, et al. Enzyme-linked immunosorbent assay for measurement of allergen-specific IgE in canine serum. Am J Vet Res 1989;50:1831–1839.

6. Miller WH, Scott DW, Wellington JR, et al. Evaluation of the performance of a serologic allergy system in atopic dogs. J Am Anim Hosp Assoc 1993;29:545–550.

7. Codner EC, Lessard P. Comparison of intradermal allergy test and enzyme-linked assay in dogs with allergic skin disease. J Am Vet Med Assoc 1993;202:739–743.

8. Halliwell REW. In-vitro allergy testing. Proceedings of the 11th Annual Congress of the European Society of Veterinary Dermatology, Bordeaux, June 1994.

9. Roudebush P. Nutritional management of the allergic patient. In: August JR, ed. Consultations in Feline Internal Medicine 2. Philadelphia, WB Saunders, 1994.

10. Roudebush P. Homemade elimination diets. Derm Dialogue, Spring/Summer 1993:7.

11. Rosser EJ. Diagnosis of food allergy in dogs. J Am Vet Med Assoc 1993;203:259–262.

12. Schick RO, Fadok VA. Responses of atopic dogs to regional allergens: 268 cases (1981–1984). J Am Vet Med Assoc 1986;189:1493–1494.

13. Muller GD, Kirk RW, Scott DW. Small Animal Dermatology. Philadelphia, WB Saunders, 1989:450–464.

14. Griffen CE. Canine atopic disease. In: Griffen CE, Kwochka KW, MacDonald JM, eds. Current Veterinary Dermatology. St Louis, Mosby–Year Book, 1993:99–120.

15. Willemse A, Noordzij A, Rutten PMG, et al. Induction of non-IgE anaphylactic antibodies in dogs. Clin Exp Immunol 1985;59:351–358.

16. Halliwell REW, Gorman NT: Atopic diseases. In: Halliwell REW, Gorman NT, eds. Veterinary Clinical Immunology. Philadelphia, WB Saunders, 1989:232.

17. Bruynzeel-Koomen C, van Wichen DF, Toonstra J, et al. The presence of IgE molecules on epidermal Langerhans cells in patients with atopic dermatitis. Arch Dermatol Res 1986:278;199-205.

18. McEwan NA. Bacterial adherence to canine corneocytes. In: von Tscharner C, Halliwell REW, eds. Advances in Veterinary Dermatology, vol 1. London, Balliere Tindall, 1990:454.

19. Beal KM, Kunkle GA, Keisling K. A study of long-term administration of F shampoo in dogs. Proceedings of the Ninth Annual Members' Meeting, American Academy of Veterinary Dermatology and American College of Veterinary Dermatology, San Diego, 1993:36.

20. Miller WH, Scott DW. Efficacy of chlorpheniramine maleate for management of pruritus in cats. J Am Vet Med Assoc 1990;197:67–70.

21. Logas D. Double blind crossover study with high-dose eicosapentaenoic acid supplementation for the treatment of canine allergic pruritus. Proceedings of the Ninth Annual Members' Meeting, American Academy of Veterinary Dermatology and American College of Veterinary Dermatology, San Diego, 1993:37.

22. Scott KV, White SD, Rosychuk RAW. A retrospective study of hyposensitization in atopic dogs in a flea-scarce environment. In: Ihrke PJ, Mason IS, White SD, eds. Advances in Veterinary Dermatology. Oxford, Pergamon Press, 1993:79–87.

23. Roudebush P, Gross KL, Lowry SR. Protein digestibility of commercial canine and feline hypoallergenic diets. Proceedings of the Ninth Annual Members' Meeting, American Academy of Veterinary Dermatology and American College of Veterinary Dermatology, San Diego, 1993:8–9.

24. Roudebush P, Guilford WG. A preliminary study of histamine in pet foods and pet food ingredients. Proceedings of the Seventh Annual Members' Meeting, American Academy of Veterinary Dermatology and American College of Veterinary Dermatology, Scottsdale, 1991:53.

25. White SD, Sequoia D. Food hypersensitivity in cats: 14 cases (1982–1987). J Am Vet Med Assoc 1989;194:692–695.

26. Kunkle GA, Horner S. Validity of skin testing for diagnosis of food allergy in dogs. J Am Vet Med Assoc 1992;200:677–680.

27. Guilford WG, Strombeck DE, Rogers Q, et al. Development of gastroscopic food sensitivity testing in dogs. J Am Coll Vet Intern Med 1994:414–422.

28. Olivry T, Prélaud P, Héripret D, et al. Allergic contact dermatitis in the dog. Vet Clin North Am Small Anim Pract 1990;20:1443–1456.

29. White PD. Contact dermatitis in the dog and cat. Semin Vet Med Surg (Small Anim) 1991;6:303–315.

30. Lewis TP. Adverse reactions to contactants. J Vet Allerg Clin Immunol 1993;2:21–24.

31. Halliwell REW, Gorman NT. Nonatopic allergic skin diseases. In: Halliwell REW, Gorman NT, eds. Veterinary Clinical Immunology. Philadelphia, WB Saunders, 1989:261–268.

32. MacDonald JM. Flea allergy dermatitis and flea control. In: Griffen CE, Kwochka KA, MacDonald JM, eds. Current Veterinary Dermatology. St Louis, Mosby–Year Book, 1993:57–71.

33. Schemmer KR, Halliwell REW. Efficacy of alum-precipitated flea antigen for hyposensitization of flea-allergic dogs. Semin Vet Med Surg (Small Anim) 1987;2:195–198.

34. Kunkle GA, Milcarsky J. Double-blind flea hyposensitization trial in cats. J Am Vet Med Assoc 1985;186:677–680.

35. Halliwell REW. Clinical and immunological response to alum-precipitated flea antigen in immunotherapy of flea-allergic dogs: Results of a double blind study. In: Ihrke PJ, Mason IA, White SD, eds. Advances in Veterinary Dermatology. Oxford: Pergamon Press, 1993:41–50.

36. Moore FM, White SD, Carpenter JL, et al. Localization of immunoglobulins and complement by the peroxidase antiperoxidase method in autoimmune and non-autoimmune canine dermatopathies. Vet Immunol Immunopathol 1987;14:1–9.

37. Muller GH, Kirk RW, Scott DW. Small Animal Dermatology. Philadelphia, WB Saunders, 1989:498–530.

38. Ackerman LJ. Canine and feline pemphigus and pemphigoid: II. Pemphigoid. Compen Contin Educ Pract Vet 1985;7:281–286.

39. Griffen CE. Diagnosis and management of primary autoimmune skin diseases: A review. Semin Vet Med Surg (Small Anim) 1987;2:173–185.

40. Ihrke PJ, Stannard AA, Ardans AA, et al. Pemphigus foliaceus in dogs: A review of 37 cases. J Am Vet Med Assoc 1985;186:59–66.

41. Suter MM, Ziegra CJ, Cayatte SM, et al. Identification of canine pemphigus antigens. In: Ihrke PJ, Mason IS, White SD, eds. Advances in Veterinary Dermatology. Oxford, Pergamon Press, 1993:367–380.

42. White SD, Rosychuk RAW, Reinke SI, et al. Use of tetracycline and niacinamide for treatment of autoimmune disease in 31 dogs. J Am Vet Med Assoc 1992;200: 1497–1500.

43. van Hees J, Mason KV, Gross TL, et al. Levamisole-induced drug eruptions in the dog. J Am Anim Hosp Assoc 1985;21:255–260.

44. Scott DW, Miller WH, Goldschmidt MH. Erythema multiforme in the dog. J Am Anim Hosp Assoc 1983;19: 453–459.

45. Rachofsky MA, Chester DK, Read WK. Toxic epidermal necrolysis. Compen Contin Educ Pract Vet 1989;11: 840–845.

46. Haupt KH, Prieur DJ, Moore MP, et al. Familial canine dermatomyositis: Clinical, electrodiagnostic, and genetic studies. Am J Vet Res 1985;46:1861–1869.

47. Hargis AM, Haupt KH, Prieur DJ, et al. A skin disorder in three Shetland sheepdogs: Comparison with familial canine dermatomyositis of collies. Compen Contin Educ Pract Vet 1985;7:306–315.

48. Hargis AM, Mundell AC. Familial canine dermatomyositis. Compen Contin Educ Pract Vet 1992;14:855–871.

49. Korkij W, Soltani K. Fixed drug eruption. Arch Dermatol 1984;120:520–524.

50. Rosencrantz WS. Cutaneous drug reactions. In: Griffen CE, Kwochka KA, MacDonald JM. Current Veterinary Dermatology. St Louis, Mosby–Year Book, 1993:154–164.

51. Cribb AE. Idiosyncratic reactions to sulfonamides in dogs. J Am Vet Med Assoc 1989;195:1612–1614.

52. Gibson LE. Cutaneous vasculitis: Approach to diagnosis and systemic associations. Mayo Clin Proc 1990;65: 221–229.

53. Crawford MA, Foil CS. Vasculitis: Clinical syndromes in small animals. Compen Contin Educ Pract Vet 1989;11: 400–415.

54. Randell MG, Hurvitz AI. Immune-mediated vasculitis in five dogs. J Am Vet Med Assoc 1983;183:207–211.

55. Gross TL, Ihrke PJ, Walder EJ. Veterinary Dermatopathology. St Louis, Mosby–Year Book, 1992:138–139.

56. Wilcock BP, Yager JA. Focal cutaneous vasculitis and alopecia at sites of rabies vaccination in dogs. J Am Vet Med Assoc 1986;188:1174–1177.

57. Kern TJ, Walton DK, Riis RC, et al. Uveitis associated with poliosis and vitiligo in six dogs. J Am Vet Med Assoc 1985;187:408–414.

58. Morgan RV. Vogt-Koyanagi-Harada syndrome in humans and dogs. Compen Contin Educ Pract Vet 1989;11: 1211–1218.

59. Scott DW, Anderson WI. Panniculitis in dogs and cats: A retrospective analysis of 78 cases. J Am Anim Hosp Assoc 1988;24:551–559.

Chapter 6

Miscellaneous Diseases of the Skin

James O. Noxon

Problem Identification

Scale

Scale is a loose collection of epidermal cells derived from the stratum corneum. (The lay term for scale is dandruff.) Scale may be dry or greasy to the touch. Scaling disorders are a group of diseases that appear clinically as excessive scale accumulation on the skin.

Pathophysiology

Excessive accumulation of scale may be caused by a primary keratinization disorder, or it may be secondary to various underlying dermatoses (Table 6–1). Scale accumulation occurs in primary keratinization disorders if there is an abnormality of epidermopoiesis, keratinization, apocrine or sebaceous gland function, intercellular lipid formation, epidermal cell cohesion, or cellular desquamation.[1] Scaling may also occur secondary to pruritus, from irritation of the skin by parasites or infectious agents, or as a result of environmental influences.

Clinical Signs

Scale accumulation appears as flaky, white to yellow debris on the surface of the skin or hair. The scale tends to fall off as the animal is handled. Patients with scaling disorders often leave copious amounts of scale on the examination table after the examination is concluded. Scale accumulation does not necessarily imply that the skin is dry. Scale is present in many greasy dermatologic disorders. Dehydration of the skin also results in scale formation. Pruritus may be present, especially if the skin is dehydrated.

Diagnostic Plan

Differential diagnosis of a scaling disorder includes parasite infestation (especially scabies and infestations due to *Cheyletiella* mites and fleas), dermatophytosis, primary idiopathic seborrhea, sebaceous adenitis, and a variety of keratinization disorders of the skin. Skin scrapings are indicated to rule out parasitism. Fungal culture is required to rule out dermatophytosis. Histopathologic evaluation of the skin helps to identify primary idiopathic seborrhea, sebaceous adenitis, or other scaling disorders. A complete blood count, serum biochemistry panel, urinalysis, and tests to evaluate the thyroid and adrenal gland function may be necessary to identify secondary causes of scaling.

Hyperkeratosis

Hyperkeratosis is an increased thickness of the stratum corneum that often produces excessive collection of keratinocytes on the surface of the skin.

Pathophysiology

Hyperkeratosis may result from increased epidermal proliferation or from reduced removal of keratinocytes from the surface of the skin. The changes may affect any of the keratinized structures of the skin, including hair, claws, planum nasale, and foot pads.

Clinical Signs

The classic sign of hyperkeratosis is lichenification of the skin or other affected structures. Hyperkeratosis of the foot pad is manifested as a thick, hard pad (Fig. 6–1). The planum nasale appears thick and has a cobblestone appearance when hyperkeratosis is present. Cracks or fissures may appear in affected areas.

Diagnostic Plan

The differential diagnosis of hyperkeratosis includes many of the scaling disorders, such as seborrhea, sebaceous adenitis, nasodigital hyperkeratosis, zinc-responsive dermatosis, and vitamin A–responsive dermatosis. In addition, it may be a feature of hormonal imbalances (e.g., hypothyroidism) or chronic inflammatory skin disease. Hyperkeratosis is a histopathologic finding and is therefore confirmed by histopathologic examination of the affected structure.

Diagnostic Procedures

Histopathologic examination of the skin is helpful to confirm the type of lesion and to identify specific disease processes (see Chap. 1).

Common Scaling (Keratinization) Diseases

Primary Idiopathic Seborrhea

Primary idiopathic seborrhea is the most common keratinization disorder of the dog. Commonly affected breeds include the American cocker spaniel, Irish setter, West Highland white terrier, English springer spaniel, Chinese shar-pei, basset hound, German shepherd, and Doberman pinscher. Clinical signs are usually noticed before 2 years of age.

Pathophysiology

The pathogenesis has been studied most extensively in the American cocker spaniel. In that breed, the epidermal turnover time is reduced from the normal 22 days to 8 days, resulting in excessive accumulation of scale on the skin.[2] Epidermal turnover in Irish setters with clinical signs of seborrhea has also been shown to

Table 6-1
Classification of Scaling Diseases

Keratinization Disorders
Primary idiopathic seborrhea
Epidermal dysplasia of West Highland white terriers
Sebaceous adenitis
Ear margin seborrhea
Zinc-responsive dermatosis
Follicular dysplasia or dystrophy
Ichthyosis
Fatty acid deficiency

Secondary Scaling Disorders
Ectoparasitism
  Scabies
  Cheyletiellosis
  Flea infestation or allergy
Allergies
  Atopy
  Food hypersensitivity
Endocrine imbalances
  Hyperadrenocorticism
  Hypothyroidism
  Sex hormone imbalance
  Growth hormone–responsive alopecia
Infectious dermatosis
  Pyoderma
  Dermatophytosis
Autoimmune disorders
  Pemphigus foliaceus
Neoplasia
  Mycosis fungoides

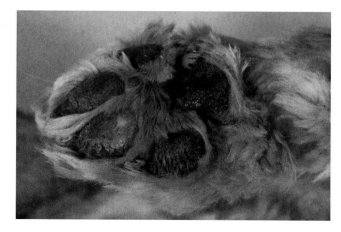

Figure 6-1
Hyperkeratosis of a foot pad in a dog with primary idiopathic seborrhea.

Clinical Signs

Primary seborrhea of the dog is often divided into three categories. This classification system is somewhat arbitrary and merely represents clinical variations in the disease. The first category is seborrhea sicca, which is characterized by the heavy accumulation of scales and a dry, dull hair coat. This condition is seen in Irish setters, German shepherds, and Doberman pinschers. The second category, seborrhea oleosa, is characterized by scaling and excessive lipid accumulation on the skin and is common in American cocker spaniels, basset hounds, English springer spaniels, and Chinese shar-peis. The third category of seborrhea is seborrheic dermatitis. This is an inflammatory condition, characterized by scale accumulation, occasionally by excessive lipid accumulation, and by lesions typical of pyoderma. Papules, pustules, and epidermal collarettes are commonly present.

Pruritus is the most consistent clinical feature of primary idiopathic seborrhea. It is often intense and may result in excoriations and secondary bacterial infections. Scale accumulation is the hallmark lesion of the disease. Excessive scale also accumulates within the hair follicle, and the scale is often packed around the hairs as they grow out of the follicle, forming a follicular cast (Fig. 6-2). Alopecia, crusts, comedones, malodor, and ceruminous otitis externa are also common signs. Peripheral lymph nodes are typically mildly to moderately enlarged.

Lesions are pronounced around the muzzle, ears, trunk, perineum, and ventral abdomen. Muzzle lesions usually consist of erythema and crusts. The ceruminous otitis externa is accompanied by erythema and lichenification of the external ear canal and the skin over the medial aspect of the pinnae. These hyper-

be reduced from 22 to 6 days.[3] Studies of cutaneous lipids in various seborrheic breeds have shown some changes in the relative amounts of fatty acids and diester waxes, but no differences in ω-3, ω-6, or ω-9 fatty acid levels were detected when seborrheic cocker spaniels were compared with normal dogs.[4, 5] These studies indicate that the metabolic defect associated with seborrhea involves epidermal cell proliferation. Alterations of the surface lipid layer may also occur as a result of abnormalities of lipid production or metabolism.

This disease is typically accompanied by bacterial overgrowth and clinical signs of pyoderma. *Staphylococcus intermedius* is frequently isolated from the skin and lesions of patients with primary idiopathic seborrhea. The bacterial infection exacerbates and potentiates the pruritus and therefore acts as a perpetuating factor of seborrhea. *Malassezia pachydermatis* is also frequently isolated from seborrheic lesions.

plastic changes may be so severe that the diameter of the external ear canal is greatly reduced. Seborrheic plaques, consisting of erythematous patches with scale, crust, or epidermal collarettes, are found on skin over the trunk. Crusts and centrally pigmented epidermal collarettes, representing secondary pyoderma, are commonly found on the ventral abdominal skin. The nipples are frequently hyperkeratotic and are surrounded by scale and crusts. Foot pads are typically hyperkeratotic and may have fissures.

Otitis externa is a common feature of this disease, with copious amounts of ceruminous material accumulating in the external ear canal (Fig. 6–3). Erythema, lichenification, and edema of the pinnae and opening of the external ear canal are common findings. The ears are often painful or tender to the touch.

Diagnostic Plan

The differential diagnosis includes atopy, adverse reactions to food, scabies, flea allergy dermatitis, primary pyoderma, *Malassezia* dermatitis, and other primary keratinization disorders.

The signalment, history, and physical findings provide sufficient information to make a tentative diagnosis of primary idiopathic seborrhea. Histopathologic examination of the skin shows a superficial perivascular dermatitis, with epidermal hyperplasia. Follicular and epidermal hyperkeratosis is a classic feature, and focal accumulations of parakeratotic crusts may be present at the infundibulum of hair follicles.[6] Practitioners are encouraged to send biopsies to an experienced veterinary dermatopathologist, because diagnostic lesions associated with this condition may be subtle. Other diagnostic procedures are directed at ruling out other scaling disorders and concurrent diseases, such as atopy, adverse reactions to food, and endocrinopathies.

Treatment

Management of Perpetuating Factors

It is essential to control the pyoderma that is uniformly present in these patients. Pyoderma is responsible for a major portion of the pruritus that accompanies this disease (see Chap. 3). A systemic antimicrobial agent that is effective against *S. intermedius* should be administered for 21 to 28 days. If *M. pachydermatis* is present on the skin, the patient should be treated with systemic and topical antifungal agents.

Treatment of Otitis Externa

The ears should be meticulously cleaned every 3 to 7 days with an appropriate cleansing solution. They should be kept dry to reduce secondary infections (see Chap. 4). Yeast infections may be controlled with antifungal agents used alone (Lotrimin) or in combination with other therapeutic agents (Tresaderm). Bacterial infections are adequately controlled with topical antimicrobial agents, unless ulcers are present in the external ear canal or inflammatory cells are seen on cytologic examination of exudate; a systemic antibiotic is indicated in those cases. Glucocorticoid therapy, both topical and systemic, has an integral role in the management of seborrheic otitis externa, but glucocorticoids should not be used until all diagnostic procedures are completed, to avoid interference with the tests. Failure to control the progression of the ceruminous otitis externa is the most common reason that owners elect to euthanize a pet with this disease.

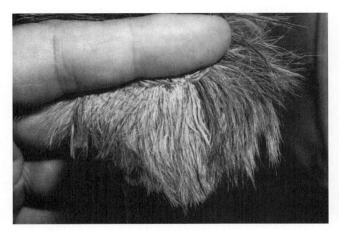

Figure 6–2
Follicular casts (keratinized debris packed around the base of hair) in a dog with primary idiopathic seborrhea.

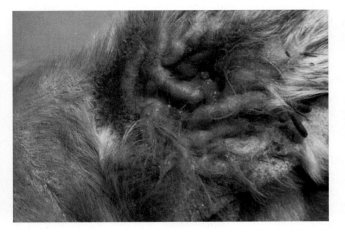

Figure 6–3
Ceruminous otitis externa in a cocker spaniel with idiopathic seborrhea.

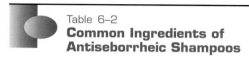

Table 6–2
Common Ingredients of Antiseborrheic Shampoos

INGREDIENT	ACTIONS	EXAMPLES OF COMMERCIAL PRODUCTS
Coal tar*	Keratolytic Keratoplastic Antipruritic	NuSal-T Allerseb-T
Sulfur	Keratoplastic Keratolytic*† Antipruritic*† Antiparasitic Antibacterial Antifungal	NuSal-T Allerseb-T SebaLyt Sulfoxydex Sebbafon Sebolux
Salicylic acid	Antibacterial Keratoplastic Keratolytic*†	
Selenium disulfide	Degreasing*† Antifungal	Seleen Plus
Benzoyl peroxide	Antibacterial*† Keratolytic Astringent Degreasing*† Follicular flushing action	Pyoben OxyDex Suf-OxyDex

*Tar shampoos should not be used on cats.
†Key or most useful function/ingredient.

Shampoo Therapy

Shampoos are the most effective carriers of topical medications. The functions of antiseborrheic shampoos include removal of scale and crusts from the skin surface, control of pyoderma, reduction of pruritus, and rehydration of the skin. Active components of antiseborrheic shampoos include coal tar derivatives, sulfur, salicylic acid, selenium disulfide, and benzoyl peroxide. Each of these substances has multiple therapeutic effects (Table 6–2). Keratolytic agents damage the keratinocyte and increase the moisture content of these cells, thus facilitating softening and removal of the scale. Keratoplastic agents alter the epidermal cell kinetics to "normalize" keratinization. The degree that each keratoplastic agent affects the cornification process varies. Some ingredients are potent degreasing agents and effectively remove the surface lipid layer. Excessive removal of surface lipids results in dehydration of the skin, which facilitates bacterial infections and pruritus.

Emollients, emulsifiers, and humectants are used to rehydrate and soften the skin. Emollients are lipids that are applied to replace lost surface lipids. They include many oils, such as olive oil, cottonseed oil, peanut oil, coconut oil, sesame seed oil, lanolin, and hydrocarbons. Humectants, such as propylene glycol, lactic acid, urea, and glycerin, are natural moisturizers that rehydrate the skin by increasing transepidermal movement of water. Moisturizers are beneficial in scaling disorders and should be applied after aggressive antiseborrheic shampoo therapy.

There are many commercial antiseborrheic shampoos available for use. The specific shampoos for each patient are selected by considering the clinical signs of the patient. If pyoderma is present, benzoyl peroxide is an excellent choice for initial shampoo therapy. Medications with antipruritic effects, such as sulfur, salicylic acid, and tar, are indicated if the patient is pruritic. Patients with greasy or oily dermatitis can receive benefit from treatment with degreasing shampoos containing benzoyl peroxide or selenium disulfide.

Patients are initially bathed twice weekly, with alternating use of the two shampoos considered most appropriate for that patient. After 3 weeks, the client is allowed to decrease the frequency of shampooing to once weekly. At that time, the client may introduce a third shampoo to compare the effects in the pet. Shampoos containing various combinations of active ingredients, such as sulfur and salicylic acid, tar and sulfur, and benzoyl peroxide, should be tried with each patient. Clients are encouraged to develop their own shampoo schedule based on the needs of their pet and the results of therapy. In most cases, shampoos are necessary every 10 to 14 days to control the scale, oil production, pruritus, and odor associated with seborrhea. Patients should be reexamined regularly to evaluate the efficacy of the therapy.

Retinoid Therapy

The retinoids are a group of naturally occurring and synthetic vitamin A derivatives. These compounds have many biologic effects, including promotion of growth, differentiation and maintenance of epithelial tissues, and maintenance of visual functions. Retinoids are available for topical application or systemic administration. Two synthetic retinoids, isotretinoin (Accutane) and etretinate (Tegison), have been used to manage primary idiopathic seborrhea.[7, 8] The most effective drug, etretinate, is administered at a dose of 0.75 to 2.0 mg/kg, daily by mouth.[8] Side effects of systemic retinoid therapy in the dog may include keratoconjunctivitis sicca, vomiting, increased liver enzyme activity, elevated serum triglyceride levels, and reluctance to eat hard food because of tenderness in the mouth. The synthetic retinoids are considered extremely teratogenic. Clients should be warned of the side effects and the dangers of accidental human ingestion of these drugs. Clinical improvement is reflected by the development of fewer seborrheic plaques, reduction of scale and crust formation, and decreased pruritus. Etretinate does not have a significant beneficial effect on the otitis externa that usually accompanies this condition, and the drug is prohibitively expensive for most clients.

One form of canine seborrhea has been found to be responsive to high doses of vitamin A.[9] This disease is characterized by heavy scale accumulation and specific histologic features, including prominent hyperkeratosis and dilatation of the follicles.

Treatment Summary

Effective management of the seborrheic patient begins with client education. Clients must understand that a cure is not available for this condition and that the primary goal of treatment is to improve the patient's quality of life and make it a functional pet. Combination therapy using all of the treatments described here provides the best clinical results.

Prognosis

The prognosis for this condition is guarded. Many animals respond well to treatment and become functional pets with minimal discomfort. However, some dogs do not respond significantly to treatment, and the condition persists. Many dogs with this disease are euthanized because of the difficulty in controlling the ceruminous otitis externa.

Feline Acne

Feline acne is a keratinization disorder affecting the skin over the chin and around the lips of cats. The condition may be seen in any breed of cat and is usually seen in adult cats of any age.

Pathophysiology

The cause of this condition is unclear, but it appears to be similar to acne in humans. Keratinized debris from the normal epidermal turnover process collects in the hair follicle, which may become obstructed and form a comedo (i.e., blackhead). Secondary bacterial infection leads to folliculitis.

Clinical Signs

Lesions include comedones, papules, and pustules in severe cases. The lesions are distributed on the ventral chin and may extend around the commissures of the lips and on the skin of the upper lip (Fig. 6–4). Bacterial involvement may lead to bacterial folliculitis, furunculosis, and cellulitis. The lesions are usually not pruritic unless secondary infections are present.

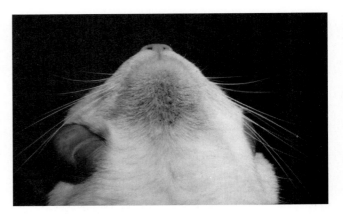

Figure 6–4
Comedones on the chin of a cat with feline acne.

Diagnostic Plan

The differential diagnosis for these lesions includes demodicosis and dermatophytosis. The diagnosis is based on the clinical signs. Infectious diseases and parasites should be ruled out with skin scrapings and fungal cultures. In some severe cases, histopathologic evaluation of the skin helps to rule out other dermatologic conditions.

Treatment

The affected areas should be cleaned to remove the comedones and prevent folliculitis. Warm soaks help to loosen the follicular plugs. Benzoyl peroxide gel can be applied to the affected areas to help remove the follicular debris, although this product irritates the skin of some cats. Antibiotics are indicated if bacterial involvement is present. Clindamycin (Antirobe) is a good choice for therapy and reduces the severity of lesions in many patients, possibly as a result of nonspecific anti-inflammatory properties.

Prognosis

The prognosis is good to excellent, although the condition often persists to some degree despite treatment.

Sebaceous Adenitis

Sebaceous adenitis is an inflammatory skin disease reported in standard poodles, miniature poodles, toy poodles, Akitas, chow chows, collies, dachshunds, Dalmatians, German shepherds, golden retrievers, Irish setters, Lhasa apsos, Old English sheepdogs, Pomeranians, Samoyeds, Scottish terriers, English springer spaniels, Saint Bernards, vizslas, weimaraners, and undoubtedly other breeds. It seems to be an autosomally recessive trait in the standard poodle, and clinical signs may appear between 6 months and 9 years of age.

Pathophysiology

Sebaceous adenitis is an immune-mediated disease with inflammation directed at the sebaceous glands of the skin. Histologic findings suggest that more than one form of the disease may exist.[10] The pathogenesis may include a primary follicular keratinization defect with obstruction of the follicle and sebaceous ducts, an abnormality in lipid production and metabolism of sebaceous secretions, and an immune-mediated destruction of the sebaceous glands.

Clinical Signs

Clinical features of sebaceous adenitis include scaling, alopecia, thickened skin, and secondary bacterial infections.[11] There seems to be two distinct clinical forms of the disease. The first is seen in standard poodles, Akitas, and other long-haired dogs. In these patients, there is heavy accumulation of white to silver-white scale on the skin. Often, scale is tightly adhered to hairs, forming follicular casts. Alopecia and a dry, brittle hair coat are commonly seen. Lesions are commonly found on the face, pinnae, trunk, and extremities.

The second form of this disease is seen in the vizsla and other short-coated dogs and consists primarily of erythema, alopecia, and scaling. The alopecia often spreads across the body in circular or serpiginous patterns (Fig. 6–5). The tail is commonly affected and develops the classic "rat tail" appearance often associated with endocrine disease. The ears have varying amounts of dry scale on the pinnae and extending down into the external ear canals. Pruritus may be present, but it varies in intensity.

Diagnostic Plan

The differential diagnosis includes seborrhea, dermatophytosis, ectoparasitism, *Malassezia* dermatitis, hypothyroidism, and other endocrinopathies. Diagnostic procedures are directed at ruling out these possible causes of scaling and identifying the classic lesions of sebaceous adenitis. Histopathologic examination of the skin is the definitive test for this condition. Biopsies may be obtained from any affected area, but they are most diagnostic if they reflect the entire spectrum of lesions on the patient. Early in the disease, histologic changes include mild perifollicular and periadenexal pyogranulomatous to granulomatous inflammation focused around the sebaceous glands. The glands may be completely obliterated by the inflammatory process. Later in the

disease, there is a complete absence (destruction) of the sebaceous glands, with perifollicular fibrosis. The severity of the histologic changes does not necessarily correlate with clinical signs. The sebaceous glands may be severely damaged before any clinical signs of the disease are detectable. Histopathologic examination is considered a useful screening test to detect carrier or subclinical animals, and screening of standard poodles for this disease is currently recommended. The skin biopsy for this screening procedure is obtained from the area between the scapulae.

Treatment

Treatment goals are to eliminate the scaling and return the coat to normal density and luster. Many breeders of predisposed dogs recommend that affected dogs have baby oil applied to the entire body for several minutes each day, followed by shampoos with dishwashing detergent (Palmolive) to remove the oil. Topical application of 50% propylene glycol to half of the body each day also reduces the severity of lesions in many patients. Both of these treatment protocols are messy, but the clinical response may be excellent. Dietary fatty acid supplements containing ω-3 and ω-6 fatty acids subjectively help many affected animals, although clinical studies have not confirmed their

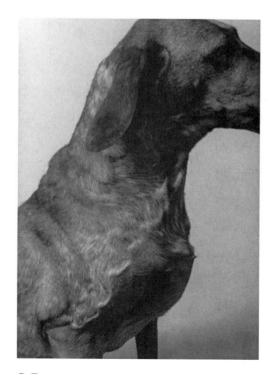

Figure 6–5
Serpiginous pattern of hair loss in a vizsla with sebaceous adenitis.

efficacy. These supplements are generally recommended and used in conjunction with other therapeutic options.

Systemic therapy has focused on the systemic use of retinoid compounds. Etretinate may be effective in some long-haired dogs. Likewise, isotretinoin may be effective in some cases, especially in the short-haired breeds. This drug is initially given daily at a dosage of 1.0 mg/kg, by mouth. Possible side effects of this therapy include keratoconjunctivitis sicca, vomiting and diarrhea, conjunctivitis, increased thirst, and elevated liver enzymes. Histopathologic examination of skin reveals significant inflammation and fibrosis around the sebaceous glands, even in dogs showing excellent clinical response to this therapy. Treatment is necessary for the life of the patient. The prognosis is fair to good for reduction of scale and regrowth of hair.

Other treatments that may be effective in some cases include immunosuppressive doses of glucocorticoids early in the course of disease and of cyclosporine (Sandimmune) in refractory cases.

Prognosis

The prognosis is good for short-haired dogs with this disease, but it is guarded for long-haired dogs. Clinical signs may diminish, but the patient usually requires long-term therapy.

Uncommon Scaling Diseases

Schnauzer Comedo Syndrome (Schnauzer Bumps)

The schnauzer comedo syndrome is a seborrheic disorder of the miniature schnauzer.[12] It is characterized by the presence of papules and comedones over the dorsal midline of the trunk and lumbar area. Occasionally, the condition progresses into bacterial folliculitis and furunculosis. Histologic examination of the skin shows orthokeratotic hyperkeratosis of the skin and hair follicle, with dilation and obstruction of the superficial third of the follicle. Diagnosis is based on the characteristic clinical signs and histopathologic examination of the skin. Treatment with antimicrobial agents is indicated if secondary pyoderma is present. Keratolytic shampoos containing benzoyl peroxide, with its follicular flushing action, control the severity of disease in most cases. Isotretinoin may help control the disease in severe cases.

Nasodigital Hyperkeratosis

Nasodigital hyperkeratosis is a condition characterized by scale and crust accumulation on the planum nasale, on foot pads, or on both areas.[12, 13] It may be seen in any breed but is most frequently recognized in American cocker spaniels, English springer spaniels, and English bulldogs. The differential diagnosis includes dermatophytosis, ectoparasitism, zinc-responsive dermatosis, canine distemper, and several autoimmune skin diseases. Diagnosis is based on ruling out of these other possibilities, clinical signs, and histologic evaluation of the skin. The affected areas are treated by hot soaks and daily applications of a gel containing salicylic acid, lactic acid, and urea (KeraSolv Gel).

Epidermal Dysplasia of West Highland White Terriers

A severe keratinization defect occurs in the West Highland white terrier.[12, 13] The condition is characterized by a progressive, severely pruritic dermatitis with alopecia, extensive lichenification, hyperpigmentation, scale and crust accumulation, ceruminous otitis externa, malodor, and generalized lymphadenopathy. Differential diagnosis in this breed includes demodicosis, dermatophytosis, atopy, adverse reactions to food, *Malassezia* dermatitis, and primary idiopathic seborrhea. Diagnosis is based on clinical signs and histopathologic evaluation of the skin. Treatment of the primary process is unrewarding, although many of these patients can be greatly improved by treatment and control of secondary yeast and bacterial infections or other underlying conditions. The long-term prognosis is guarded to poor.

Color Dilution Alopecia

Color dilution alopecia, also known as color mutant alopecia or the blue Doberman syndrome, is a hereditary tardive condition characterized by follicular dystrophy and dysplasia. The condition may be associated with blue, fawn, red, or other coat colors of the Doberman pinscher, Great Dane, whippet, dachshund, Irish setter, and other breeds.[14, 15] Clinical changes are manifested within the first 3 years of life, usually within the first year, and include alopecia, scaling, papules, pustules, and a dry and brittle hair coat. The differential diagnosis includes demodicosis, dermatophytosis, bacterial folliculitis, hypothyroidism, and idiopathic seborrhea. The diagnosis is based on the signalment, clinical signs, histopathologic evaluation of the skin, and ruling out of infectious and parasitic diseases. The condition is controlled with antiseborrheic shampoos followed by applications of moisturizers and humectants. Antibiotics are indicated if secondary pyoderma is present. There is some anecdotal evidence to suggest that retinoids may be effective therapeutic agents for this condition.

Zinc-Responsive Dermatosis

Zinc-responsive dermatosis is a diet-related condition characterized by scale and crust accumulation on the skin of the face and over various pressure points.[12, 13] The condition is seen most frequently in Siberian huskies and Alaskan malamutes, although other breeds may be affected.[16] The condition does not reflect a true zinc deficiency but may involve a genetic defect involving zinc absorption or dietary binding of available zinc in the diet. The lesions may be quite pruritic, and secondary bacterial infections may be present. Oral zinc supplementation with zinc sulfate (10 mg/kg, daily by mouth) or zinc methionine (2 mg/kg, daily by mouth) is effective, although the sulfate salt occasionally causes gastrointestinal upsets. Prednisone (1.1 mg/kg, daily by mouth) may be necessary in some cases to control the pruritus and facilitate resolution of the lesions. Zinc absorption from the diet may be facilitated by the use of a commercial dietary enzyme (Prozyme), although this therapy has not been evaluated as a treatment for zinc-responsive dermatosis.[17]

Miscellaneous Feline Dermatologic Diseases

Historically, the indolent ulcer, eosinophilic plaque, and collagenolytic (linear) granuloma have been considered to be components of the eosinophilic granuloma complex. The "complex" is a group of clinical reaction patterns in the cat[18]; they are best considered as clinical signs, not as definitive diagnoses. Other common feline reaction patterns are miliary dermatitis and symmetrical alopecia.

Feline Indolent Ulcer

The indolent ulcer is one of the lesions of the feline eosinophilic granuloma complex. It has been described in cats of all ages and is reported to occur more frequently in female cats.

Pathophysiology

The cause of the indolent ulcer is unknown. Pathogenic factors considered include genetics; infections by bacterial, viral, and fungal agents; insect bites; parasitic infestations; and allergic diseases. Adverse reactions to food and atopy are commonly associated with these lesions.

Clinical Signs

Indolent ulcers are well-circumscribed, ulcerated lesions that develop on the upper lip. The lesions are also thought to occur in skin elsewhere on the body.

They are not painful or pruritic. Lesions may be unilateral or bilateral, and if not controlled, they may erode into the planum nasale.

Diagnostic Plan

The differential diagnosis for an ulcer of the lip includes bacterial and fungal infections, squamous cell carcinoma, and other neoplasms (rare). The diagnosis is based on histopathologic examination of the skin, which reveals an inflammatory reaction containing neutrophils, macrophages, plasma cells, and eosinophils in varying numbers. Additional diagnostic procedures, such as an elimination dietary trial and intradermal skin testing, are useful to identify the underlying cause of the lesion.

Treatment

Treatment is directed at removal or control of the underlying disease process. If that is not possible, the lesions do respond to glucocorticoid therapy. Prednisone (2.2 mg/kg, daily by mouth) is given for 7 to 14 days, or methylprednisolone acetate (Depo-Medrol) is administered subcutaneously at a dose of 20 mg. The injections are repeated every 14 days until remission is achieved. Adverse effects of glucocorticoid therapy include increased appetite, polydipsia, polyuria, behavioral changes, weight gain, secondary infections, and diabetes mellitus. Cats are more resistant to the development of severe side effects than are dogs, but treatment must be monitored and the dose reduced as quickly as possible.

Megestrol acetate (Ovaban) has also been shown to be an effective treatment.[19] However, it has potent progestational and glucocorticoid effects, and its use is associated with many serious side effects, including polyphagia, weight gain, fibroadenomatous hyperplasia of mammary glands, pyometra, mammary adenocarcinoma, diabetes mellitus, and adrenocortical atrophy. Because of the frequency and severity of adverse reactions, this drug is not recommended for the management of dermatologic problems in the cat.

Prognosis

The prognosis is guarded for this condition. The lesion usually responds to treatment, but it may recur unless the underlying disease is identified and controlled.

Eosinophilic Plaque

The eosinophilic plaque is one of the lesions of the feline eosinophilic granuloma complex. It is most commonly associated with allergic diseases in the cat. The lesion may occur in cats of all ages, although it is seen most frequently in young adult cats. There is no breed or sex predilection.

Pathophysiology

Eosinophilic plaques are strongly associated with allergic diseases, such as atopy, flea allergy dermatitis, and adverse reactions to food. These lesions represent a clinical reaction pattern, similar to indolent ulcers and collagenolytic granulomas.

Clinical Signs

These lesions are single or multiple elevated plaques and may be located on the head, extremities, or trunk or in the oral cavity. The lesions are intensely pruritic and occasionally painful. Eosinophilia is a common finding in cats with these lesions.

Diagnostic Plan

The differential diagnosis of the lesion includes bacterial dermatitis, fungal infection, trauma, and neoplasia. Increased numbers of eosinophils are usually present on a hemogram. Histopathologic examination confirms the identity of the lesion. Skin scrapings, fungal cultures, intradermal skin testing, serologic tests for allergies, and elimination dietary trials may be necessary to identify the underlying cause.

Treatment

Treatment should be directed at removing the underlying disease process. Symptomatic treatment of these lesions is the same as described for the indolent ulcer.

Prognosis

The prognosis for control of the lesion is good. However, the lesions often recur unless the primary disease process is identified and controlled.

Collagenolytic (Linear) Granuloma

The collagenolytic granuloma (linear granuloma) is also one of the manifestations of the feline eosinophilic granuloma complex. The lesions may occur at any age but are frequently seen in cats younger than 1 year of age. No breed predilection has been observed, but females are more likely to develop this condition than males.

Pathophysiology

The cause of linear granuloma is unknown, although these lesions are commonly associated with atopy, flea allergy dermatitis, and adverse reactions to food. In addition, the lesions have been shown to develop at the sites of insect bites, suggesting an etiologic role for insect hypersensitivity.

Clinical Signs

This condition is characterized by well-circumscribed, raised plaques with a linear or arciform configuration. These lesions may be found at any location on the body or in the oral cavity, but they are classically located along the caudal aspects of the rear legs. They are the lesion responsible for the swollen chin seen in many cats. The lesions may appear as papules or nodules on the head, pinnae, planum nasale, or foot pads. The lesions are usually not pruritic.

Diagnostic Plan

The lesion is confirmed by histopathologic examination of the skin. Histologically, the lesions consist of degenerative collagen (collagenolysis) contained within foci of granulomatous inflammation. Eosinophils and multinucleated giant cells surround the area of collagenolysis. Eosinophilia may be present in some cases.

Treatment

The preferred mechanism of treatment is identification and removal of the underlying cause. If this is not possible, the lesions usually respond to symptomatic treatment as described for eosinophilic plaques.

Prognosis

The recurrence rate is high unless an underlying cause is identified and controlled.

Miscellaneous Canine Dermatologic Diseases

Acral Lick Dermatitis

Acral lick dermatitis (acral pruritic nodule, lick granuloma) is a common dermatologic lesion of the dog. The disease is seen most frequently in large-breed dogs, including the Doberman pinscher, golden retriever, Labrador retriever, Great Dane, and Irish setter.[20]

Pathophysiology

Acral lick dermatitis is reported to be a disease caused by psychogenic factors.[20] Boredom is frequently cited as a major pathogenic factor in development of this lesion. Further evaluation of these lesions provides evidence that the lesion is caused by bacterial infection. *S. intermedius* can be isolated from deep cultures in 93% of the lesions, although other bacteria may also occasionally be isolated. Histologic changes include folliculitis and furunculosis, lesions commonly associated with bacterial infections.[21] Atopy is a common concurrent disease and may be the initiating factor of the pruritus that leads to the development of the lesion. Excessive licking may lead to localized bacterial folliculitis and furunculosis, which serves to potentiate and intensify the pruritus. Boredom, also a factor in allergy, probably increases the tendency to lick. A primary behavioral disorder may be responsible for the development of lesions in some breeds, such as the Doberman pinscher, in which the lesions are more refractory to treatment.

Clinical Signs

The classic lesion of acral lick dermatitis is an elevated, erythematous, alopecic nodule, which is often ulcerated. Lesions range in size from less than 1 cm to several centimeters in length. Single lesions are usually present, but up to 30% of the cases have multiple lesions. Lesions are most frequently located on the dorsal aspect of the carpus or antebrachium but may also be found on the dorsolateral aspect of the tarsus. As lesions persist, they become fibrotic and hard.

Pruritus is the hallmark of acral lick dermatitis. Dogs typically spend many hours each day licking at the lesions.

Diagnostic Plan

Differential diagnosis should include dermatophytosis, folliculitis, foreign body reaction, and neoplasia. Bacterial culture and susceptibility testing should be performed on exudate collected from deep in the lesion. Histopathologic changes include superficial perivascular dermatitis, folliculitis, furunculosis, marked epithelial hyperplasia, apocrine gland dilatation and adenitis, and vertical alignment of collagen fibrils (fibrosis) in the superficial dermis.[21]

Treatment

Many treatments have been recommended for this condition, including physical restraint, behavioral modification (environmental, chemical, and surgical), surgical excision, cryosurgery, radiation therapy, ultrasound, topical therapy, acupuncture, cobra venom injections, injectable glucocorticoid, nonsteroidal anti-inflammatory agents (e.g., orgotein), naltrexone (a narcotic antagonist), and fluoxetine (Prozac).[20, 22–24] Most of these treatments are associated with success rates of approximately 50%.

In most cases, treatment of the bacterial infection is the key to initial management of acral lick dermatitis. The infection must be controlled, and predisposing diseases identified and treated. The selection of an antibiotic should be based on culture and susceptibility testing. If antibiotic treatment is begun before the development of extensive fibrosis, the pruritus usually decreases within 7 days, and the lesion regresses. Antibiotic therapy is necessary for 3 to 6 weeks in most cases. Severely fibrotic lesions may require several months of antibacterial therapy before the maximum benefit is noticed. Because lesions may recur after cessation of therapy, underlying diseases should be controlled. The topical application of a 2:1 mixture of Bitter Apple and Heet applied two to three times daily often results in regression of lesions less than 3 cm in diameter. This treatment in combination with appropriate systemic antimicrobial therapy reduces the size of most lesions and dramatically reduces the associated pruritus.

Nevertheless, the key to long-term management of these lesions is identification and control of underlying diseases. Because allergic skin diseases, such as atopy and adverse reactions to food, are common underlying diseases, allergy testing and dietary trials should be performed.

In some patients, these treatments are not successful and underlying diseases cannot be identified. The Doberman pinscher is one breed that is commonly affected with these lesions and seems to have a poor response to treatment. Behavioral (psychogenic) factors should be considered in such patients, and they should be treated with behavioral modification and training, by altering the environment if appropriate, or with behavior-modifying drugs. Fluoxetine has been used for this purpose at a dose of 1 mg/kg per day and may result in dramatic reduction of pruritus in some patients; the rate of success is not clear at this time. This drug is not approved by the US Food and Drug Administration for use in the dog; side effects may include lethargy, excitation, and urticaria.

Prognosis

The prognosis varies from poor to good, depending on the degree of fibrosis present in the lesion and the ability to identify the underlying cause of the lesion.

Juvenile Cellulitis

Juvenile cellulitis (puppy strangles, moist juvenile pyoderma) is an inflammatory disease of unknown cause that occurs in young dogs. It has historically been classified as a form of pyoderma, but clinical and microbiologic findings do not support this classification. Juvenile cellulitis is seen in golden retrievers, Labrador retrievers, miniature dachshunds,

Siberian huskies, and other breeds.[25] Multiple animals of the same litter may be involved, supporting a hereditary basis for the disease. The disease is usually seen in dogs younger than 4 months of age.

Pathophysiology

Bacterial hypersensitivity and autoimmune mechanisms have been proposed as possible pathogenic mechanisms, but these have not been confirmed. The disease is characterized by severe inflammation that destroys hair follicles and results in permanent scarring and alopecia if the disease is not properly treated.

Clinical Signs

Specific dermatologic lesions include severe edema, erythema, pustules and fistulous tracts, papules, crusts, and ulcers. Otitis externa, fever, depression, lethargy, and anorexia often accompany the disorder. The lesions initially develop on the muzzle and chin and then spread to involve the periocular skin, chin, ears, extremities, and truncal skin (Fig. 6–6). Mandibular and other peripheral lymph nodes are routinely enlarged, and cytologic evaluation shows lymphadenitis.

Diagnostic Plan

The development of classic lesions in dogs younger than 4 months of age is highly suggestive of juvenile cellulitis. The differential diagnosis includes demodicosis, dermatophytosis, pemphigus foliaceus, systemic and discoid lupus erythematosus, and drug eruption. Skin scrapings must be obtained to rule out demodicosis. Fungal culture and histopathologic examination of the skin may be necessary to rule out other diseases. Bacterial culture and susceptibility testing should be performed in these cases to identify any bacterial component, since the pathogenesis is unclear. Histopathologic examination reveals nodular to diffuse, granulomatous to pyogranulomatous dermatitis and panniculitis.

Treatment

Prednisone should be administered (2.0 mg/kg, daily by mouth) until lesions resolve. The dosage is then reduced and tapered over several days. Most patients require treatment with glucocorticoids for 2 to 4 weeks to prevent a relapse of clinical signs. Antimicrobial agents should be given based on results of culture and susceptibility testing. Hot soaks or astringents applied topically to affected areas help resolve the lesions.

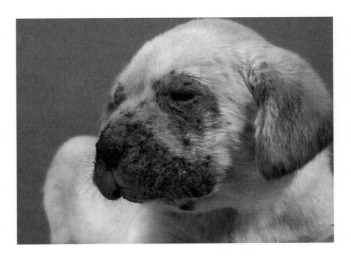

Figure 6–6
Juvenile cellulitis in a puppy. Notice the severe edema and crusting of the chin, lips, and eyelids.

Prognosis

The prognosis is excellent for complete recovery if the condition is recognized early and treated appropriately. The most critical component of treatment is the administration of a glucocorticoid. The lesions do not resolve adequately without glucocorticoid therapy, and permanent scarring with alopecia results from delay of treatment with these anti-inflammatory drugs.

Anal Sacculitis

Inflammation and infection of the anal sacs is a common problem in dogs, although the incidence is unknown.

Pathophysiology

Inflammation of these specialized tubuloalveolar, apocrine glands may be a primary process or a secondary process associated with dermatologic disease.[26] Anal sac inflammation may be associated with otitis externa, pyotraumatic dermatitis, recurrent pyoderma, perianal fistula, atopy, an adverse reaction to food, or contact dermatitis.

Clinical Signs

The most common clinical sign associated with anal sac disease is pruritus, manifested as licking at the perineum or scooting and dragging the perineal area on a carpeted area. Occasionally animals suddenly turn around to bite at the perineum as though they were in pain. The skin around the anus is frequently erythematous and may be lichenified if the area is chronically rubbed.

Diagnostic Plan

The clinical signs are highly suggestive of an anal sac disorder. Careful palpation of the anal sacs often reveals distended sacs. A fistulous tract indicates rupture of an anal sac. Cytologic analysis of the anal sac secretion may help to determine whether an active infection is present or whether the irritation is secondary to another dermatologic condition. Normal anal sac secretions contain bacteria and *Malassezia* spp. yeast. It is important to consider underlying causes of anal sacculitis, especially atopy, and to perform the diagnostic procedures necessary to rule out those conditions.

Treatment

Infusion of antibacterial or anti-inflammatory agents, systemic antimicrobial agents, topical warm soaks, and surgical drainage may be required to control infections. Underlying diseases must be identified and controlled if the patient has recurring problems. Surgical removal of the anal sacs should not be considered a panacea for anal sac disorders. Pruritus and inflammation continue if the underlying disease is present. Surgical removal of the sacs is recommended if there are recurring infections.

Prognosis

Anal sacculitis often recurs, especially if the underlying problem is not identified and treated. Perianal irritation may continue even after the anal sacs are surgically removed.

Cutaneous Manifestations and Markers of Systemic Disease

Cutaneous Manifestations of Internal Disease

Skin lesions and signs associated with internal disease are usually nonspecific. The skin may be structurally or functionally altered (e.g., hyperkeratosis), or it may merely reflect internal metabolic changes (e.g., jaundice). Lesions associated with internal disorders are often identical to those seen with diseases limited to the skin, such as pruritus, erythema, alopecia, scaling, or hyperpigmentation. Bacterial skin infections (papules, pustules, and epidermal collarettes), alterations in the hair cycle (alopecia), keratinization defects and seborrhea (scaling), and pigmentary changes (depigmentation and hyperpigmentation) are common cutaneous manifestations. Most cutaneous manifestations of internal disease are nonspecific, although some skin changes may be suggestive of certain types of internal disease (Table 6–3). Examples include pallor associated with cardiovascular and hematologic disease, icterus associated with hemolytic or biliary disease, purpura associated with coagulopathies, and bilaterally symmetrical alopecia associated with endocrinopathies. Cutaneous manifestations may be a marker of a pathologic process but not a specific disease.

Cutaneous Markers of Internal Disease

Cutaneous lesions that are highly specific and diagnostic for a specific systemic disorder are consid-

Table 6–3
Cutaneous Manifestations of Internal Disease

ORGAN SYSTEM	DERMATOLOGIC LESIONS
Hematologic disease	Pallor, cyanosis, jaundice, ulcers, purpura
Endocrine disease	Alopecia, atrophy, increased skin thickness, vascular fragility, impaired wound healing, secondary infections (bacterial and fungal), hirsutism, calcinosis cutis, seborrhea, phlebectasia, xanthoma, pigmentary changes
Infectious disease	Ulcers, vasculitis, erythema multiforme, toxic epidermal necrolysis
Parasitic infection	Pruritus, draining tracts, erythema, nodules
Immune-mediated disease	Pruritus, erythema, urticaria angioedema, vesicles, pustules, bullae, ulcers and erosions, erythema multiforme, toxic epidermal necrolysis, purpura, jaundice, vitiligo
Malignancy	Nodules, tumors, erythema, seborrhea, erythema multiforme
Hereditary or congenital disease	Alopecia, changes in skin tone, mucinosis, hair color pattern changes, pigmentary abnormalities
Nutritional imbalance	Alopecia, infections, parakeratosis, ulcers, seborrhea, poor wound healing
Toxicity	Hyperkeratosis, ulceration, secondary infections, alopecia, erythema, abnormal keratinization
Renal disease	Ulcers, alopecia, scaling, edema

ered to be cutaneous markers of that internal disease. The cutaneous changes may be caused by the same etiologic agent or process, which can be identified by examination and evaluation of the skin.

Diseases that often have both skin and internal organ involvement are infectious, neoplastic, and autoimmune diseases. Infectious diseases affecting both the skin and the internal organs are very common. Causative agents include viruses (e.g., poxvirus), bacteria, protozoa (e.g., *Leishmania* spp.), and fungi (e.g., *Blastomyces* spp.). Not all systemic infections caused by these and other agents have cutaneous changes, but if present, the skin lesions may provide rapid access to diagnostic material.

Malignancies of internal organs may have concurrent involvement of the skin or cutaneous metastatic lesions, although the incidence of cutaneous metastasis of internal malignancies appears to be low. Histopathologic examination of the skin may not always give the origin of the tumor, but the pathologic process and general tumor type are usually determined. Approximately 20% of skin tumors are malignant and may metastasize to internal organs.

Autoimmune disease may be multisystemic and involve the skin. Examples include systemic lupus erythematosus, familial dermatomyositis of collies and Shetland sheepdogs, and a variety of less well defined immunologic diseases. Histologic and immunodiagnostic evaluation of the skin can be diagnostic.

Endocrine Diseases With Cutaneous Manifestations

Endocrine imbalances are frequently associated with cutaneous changes. Lesions are usually nonspecific, and they include alopecia, scaling, crusting,

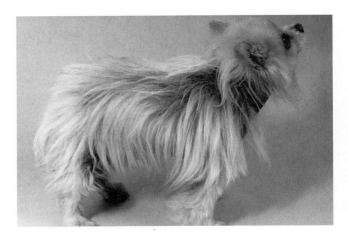

Figure 6-7
Bilaterally symmetrical alopecia of the neck and trunk in a Pomeranian with an adrenal sex hormone imbalance.

lichenification, pigmentation changes, and cutaneous atrophy. Occasionally, lesions that are more specific may be present, such as calcinosis cutis (hyperadrenocorticism), myxedema (hypothyroidism), and xanthomas (diabetes mellitus).

Hormones regulate physiologic processes in the body. Excesses or deficiencies produce quantitative changes in morphology or function. Cutaneous changes resulting from endocrine imbalance may occur through several different mechanisms. First, the skin may respond as a target organ, with different hormones having effects on specific areas of the skin. The target areas include all elements of the skin, including the epidermis, melanocytes, pilosebaceous units, dermal elements, adipose tissue, cutaneous immune system, and endothelial cells.[27] For example, growth hormone deficiency results in decreased amounts of dermal elastin, decreased thyroid hormone levels lead to pilosebaceous atrophy, and excessive glucocorticoid levels result in epidermal and dermal atrophy.

Table 6-4
Dermatologic Manifestations of Endocrine Disease

ENDOCRINE DISEASE	CUTANEOUS CHANGES*
Hypothyroidism	Bilaterally symmetrical alopecia
	Pyoderma
	Hyperpigmentation
	Thickened skin, lichenification
	Myxedema
Hyperadrenocorticism	Bilaterally symmetrical alopecia
	Pyoderma
	Cutaneous atrophy
	Calcinosis cutis
	Phlebectasia
	Loss of elasticity
	Bruising
Sex hormone imbalances	Bilaterally symmetrical alopecia
	Pyoderma
	Hyperpigmentation
	Purpura or bruising (hyperestrogenism)
	Perianal adenoma
Growth hormone-responsive alopecia	Bilaterally symmetrical alopecia
	Hyperpigmentation
Hypercalcemia of malignancy, hypervitaminosis D	Calcinosis cutis
Diabetes mellitus	Xanthoma

*Only major cutaneous changes are listed. Other common lesions include scaling and lichenification.

Second, hormonal excesses or deficiencies may affect various metabolic functions, which may indirectly influence the structure and function of the skin. Pinnal erythema may be associated with increased blood flow in hyperthyroid cats, xanthomas with dyslipoproteinemias, and calcinosis cutis with hyperadrenocorticism or hypervitaminosis D. Immunologic effects of hormonal disturbances are also responsible for many cutaneous lesions. Secondary infections are common in patients with decreased thyroid function or hyperadrenocorticism.

Bilaterally symmetrical alopecia is the classic dermatologic lesion of endocrine disease. It is associated with hypothyroidism, hyperadrenocorticism, adrenal and gonadal sex hormone imbalances, and growth hormone–responsive alopecia (Fig. 6–7). Other cutaneous lesions are associated with specific endocrinopathies (Table 6–4). Pyoderma is the most common dermatologic manifestation of endocrine imbalance, and endocrine disease should always be in the differential diagnosis for the patient with recurrent or nonresponsive pyoderma.

References

1. Kwochka KW. Overview of normal keratinization and cutaneous scaling disorders of dogs. In: Griffen CE, Kwochka KW, MacDonald JM, eds. Current Veterinary Dermatology. St Louis, Mosby–Year Book, 1993:167–175.
2. Kwochka KW, Rademaker AM. Cell proliferation kinetics of epidermis, hair follicles, and sebaceous glands of cocker spaniels with idiopathic seborrhea. Am J Vet Res 1989;50:1918–1922.
3. Baker BB, Maibach HI. Epidermal cell renewal in seborrheic skin of dogs. Am J Vet Res 1987;48:726–728.
4. Horwitz LN, Ihrke PJ. Canine seborrhea. In: Kirk RW, ed., Current Veterinary Therapy VI. Philadelphia, WB Saunders, 1977:519.
5. White PD. Evaluation of serum and cutaneous essential fatty acid profiles in normal, atopic, and seborrheic dogs. Proceedings of the Sixth Annual Members' Meeting, American Academy of Veterinary Dermatology and American College of Veterinary Dermatology, San Francisco, 1990:37–38.
6. Gross TL, Ihrke PJ, Walder EJ. Veterinary Dermatopathology. St Louis, Mosby–Year Book, 1992:88–92.
7. Fadok VA. Treatment of canine idiopathic seborrhea with isotretinoin. J Am Vet Med Assoc 1986;47:1730–1733.
8. Power HT, Ihrke PJ, Stannard AA, et al. Use of etretinate for treatment of primary keratinization disorders (idiopathic seborrhea) in cocker spaniels, West Highland white terriers, and basset hounds. J Am Vet Med Assoc 1992;201:419–429.
9. Ihrke PJ, Goldschmidt MH. Vitamin A–responsive dermatosis in the dog. J Am Vet Med Assoc 1983;182:687–690.
10. Gross TL, Ihrke PJ, Walder EJ. Veterinary Dermatopathology. St Louis, Mosby–Year Book, 1992:247–249.
11. Rosser EJ, Dunstan RW, Breen PT, et al. Sebaceous adenitis with hyperkeratosis in the standard poodle. J Am Anim Hosp Assoc 1987;23:341–345.
12. Muller GH, Kirk RW, Scott DW. Small Animal Dermatology. Philadelphia, WB Saunders, 1989:726–748.
13. Kwochka KW. Primary keratinization disorders of dogs. In: Griffen CE, Kwochka KW, MacDonald JM, eds. Current Veterinary Dermatology. St Louis, Mosby–Year Book, 1993:176–190.
14. O'Neill CS. Hereditary skin disease in the dog and cat. Compen Contin Educ Pract Vet 1981;3:791–798.
15. Miller WH. Alopecia associated with coat color dilution in two Yorkshire terriers, one saluki, and one mix-breed dog. J Am Anim Hosp Assoc 1991;27:39–43.
16. Van den Brock AHM, Thoday KL. Skin disease in dogs associated with zinc deficiency: A report of five cases. J Small Anim Pract 1986;27:313–323.
17. Ackerman L. Effect of an enzyme supplement (Prozyme) on selected nutrient levels in dogs. J Vet Allerg Clin Immunol 1993;1:25–29.
18. Merchant SR. Diagnosis of feline skin diseases based on cutaneous reaction patterns. Compen Contin Educ Pract Vet 1994;16:163–171.
19. Henik RA, Olson PN, Rosychuk RAW. Progestogen therapy in cats. Compen Contin Educ Pract Vet 1985;7:132–140.
20. Muller GH, Kirk RW, Scott DW. Small Animal Dermatology. Philadelphia, WB Saunders, 1989:750–757.
21. Gross TL, Ihrke PJ, Walder EJ. Veterinary Dermatopathology. St Louis, Mosby–Year Book, 1992:71–74.
22. White SD. Naltrexone for treatment of acral lick dermatitis in dogs. J Am Vet Med Assoc 1990;190:1073–1076.
23. Goldberger E, Rapoport JL. Canine acral lick dermatitis: Response to the antiobsessional drug clomipramine. J Am Anim Hosp Assoc 1991;27:179–182.
24. Shoulberg N. The efficacy of fluoxetine (Prozac) in the treatment of acral lick and allergic inhalant dermatitis in canines. Proceedings of the Sixth Annual Members' Meeting, American Academy of Veterinary Dermatology and American College of Veterinary Dermatology, San Francisco, 1990:31–32.
25. White SD, Rosychuk RAW, Stewart LJ, et al. Juvenile cellulitis: 15 cases (1979–1988). J Am Vet Med Assoc 1989;195:1609–1611.
26. Anderson RK. Anal sac disease and its related dermatoses. Compen Contin Educ Pract Vet 1984;6:829–837.
27. Scott DW. Histopathologic findings in endocrine skin disorders. J Am Anim Hosp Assoc 1982;18:173–183.

Chapter 7

Tumors of the Skin and Subcutis

James O. Noxon
Wallace B. Morrison

Problem Identification

Tumor

There is always considerable confusion over the most appropriate terminology to use when discussing tumors. In its narrowest definition, the word tumor is used to describe swelling, one of the cardinal signs of inflammation. However, in vernacular use the word is usually a synonym for the term cancer, although cancer is usually taken to mean a malignant tumor. The term neoplasia is usually applied to an abnormal growth of tissue, especially if uncontrolled and progressive. The term neoplasm is another synonym for tumor. Unless otherwise indicated, the term tumor in this chapter is used to mean a neoplastic mass or swelling.

Skin tumors develop from the epidermis and sebaceous glands, sweat glands, and connective tissue components of the dermis and subcutis. Tumors of the skin and subcutis account for about 30% of all canine and 15% to 20% of all feline tumors. In dogs, approximately 20% of these tumors are malignant; in cats, approximately 65% are malignant.[1]

Pathophysiology

Tumors can be categorized as benign or malignant based on histologic criteria that are well established. However, to divide tumors into benign and malignant categories is to oversimplify the behavioral differences among tumors in terms of local invasiveness and metastatic potential. There is a tendency to restrict the term malignant to describe only tumors with metastatic behavior. Clinically, however, malignant behavior includes local invasiveness as well as metastasis. Benign tumors lack these behavior characteristics. The suffix *-oma*, when applied to a tumor, is usually an indication of benign behavior.

The simple division of tumors into two categories (i.e., benign or malignant) makes the classification of some tumors with unpredictable or variable clinical behavior difficult. For example, mast cell tumors can be histologically graded based on established criteria as well-differentiated, differentiated, or poorly differentiated. Each histologic grade of mast cell tumor is associated with a different predicted clinical behavior. Variations in clinical behavior of mast cell tumors make the terms benign and malignant harder to apply with certainty.

Tumors are usually identified as originating in epithelial, mesenchymal (connective tissue), or neural crest tissue. Carcinomas are malignant epithelial neoplasms. Sarcomas are malignant mesenchymal tissue tumors that are usually categorized according to the tissue phenotype that they most resemble.

Until recently, the classic interpretation of tumor development was a two-step model involving an initial mutation followed by tumor promotion, during which mutated cells grew in number without restriction or inhibition. Tumor development is now known to be much more complicated. It is characterized by a multistep process resulting in cumulative changes in DNA that cause the transformation of a normal cell into a cell that is recognizable as a tumor cell. This multistep model of tumor development relies on a combination of changes in gene regulation, such as activation of one or more proto-oncogenes or inactivation of one or more tumor suppressor genes or antimetastasis genes. These changes alter the signal transduction pathways in affected cells, and a malignant phenotype is expressed.

The cause of skin tumors in domestic animals is usually unknown. However, there are some well-recognized environmental causes of cutaneous tumor development. Animals lacking protective pigments in their skin may develop tumors in areas that receive excessive exposure to ultraviolet (UV) radiation. The best-known example of a UV-induced skin tumor is squamous cell carcinoma in the white-haired regions of cats and dogs. These tumors may begin as an inflammatory dermatitis, called actinic or solar keratosis, which is exacerbated by exposure to direct sunlight. The prevalence of solar-induced skin tumors is higher in cats than in dogs.[2]

There are also some well-recognized viral causes of tumors that affect the skin and subcutis. The feline leukemia virus (FeLV) and the feline sarcoma virus (FeSV) are clinically the two most important viruses associated with tumors of the skin and subcutis in small animals. FeLV contains an enzyme known as reverse transcriptase (RNA-dependent DNA polymerase) that can copy viral RNA into the normal double-stranded DNA of an infected cell so that it becomes integrated into that cell's genome. This non-native DNA contains one or more transforming genes that induce normal cellular oncogenes to mediate malignant transformation. FeSV is the cause of multicentric fibrosarcoma in young cats when it is associated with FeLV as a helper virus. FeLV is not the cause of the solitary fibrosarcomas that occur more often in older cats, and it does not appear to be involved with the fibrosarcomas in cats that are associated with vaccine injection sites.[2, 3]

Clinical Signs

Solitary or multiple tumors may be present, depending on the cell line involved. Often, the presence of a mass is the only clinical sign. Tumors of the skin often outgrow their blood supply, become necrotic, and ulcerate. Tissues surrounding the tumor may become distorted or nonfunctional, depending on the size and invasiveness of the tumor.

Diagnostic Plan

Cytologic examination of material collected by fine-needle aspiration or imprinting may provide useful information about tumor type.[4] Ultimately, histopathologic examination of the tumor is needed to confirm the type of tumor and the behavioral characteristics of the neoplasm. If malignancy is identified, the extent of metastasis and the presence of concurrent disease need to be evaluated with a complete blood count, biochemical profile, urinalysis, thoracic radiography, and fine-needle aspiration of regional lymph nodes. Other specific tests may be indicated based on tumor type.

Nodule

A nodule is a solid enlargement of the skin that is more than 1 cm in diameter.

Pathophysiology

A nodule is formed by infiltration of the skin by inflammatory (bacterial or fungal) or neoplastic cells. A nodule may be a tumor, but the latter term is more encompassing.

Clinical Signs

A nodule is a small, solid enlargement of the skin. It may be covered by hair or be alopecic. It may be solid or have a fluctuant center, and it may become ulcerated.

Diagnostic Plan

Cytologic examination of material collected by imprinting with a glass slide or by fine-needle aspiration usually provides useful information to help identify the cause of the nodule. However, histopathologic evaluation of the lesion is required in most cases to provide a definitive diagnosis of the lesion. If malignancy is identified, further evaluation is indicated, as described for tumor.

Diagnostic Procedures

Physical Examination

In general, skin tumors are discovered by owners during petting or grooming activities. Skin tumors may also be discovered by veterinarians during the course of routine physical examinations, or during physical examinations performed as part of the evaluation of an unrelated problem. After a skin tumor is diagnosed, a complete medical history should be taken to identify medical problems associated with the skin tumor. The extent of the diagnostic procedures to be done in patients with skin tumors varies with the tentative diagnosis and the expected clinical behavior of the tumor type.

Routine Laboratory Evaluation

The need for clinical laboratory evaluation of a patient with a tumor of the skin also varies with the nature of the lesion. Treatment decisions may be highly influenced by the presence or absence of concurrent disorders. The clinical laboratory findings are therefore important, and evaluation of blood and urine should be routine in most cases.

Imaging Techniques

In cases of tumors with known metastatic potential, it is useful to include thoracic and abdominal radiography in the diagnostic plan to assess for metastasis. For the thoracic study, it is best to take right and left lateral projections in addition to the ventral-dorsal projection. The right and left lateral projections allow for better expansion of the lung on the up side, providing better contrast and making visualization of small metastases easier. Abdominal radiographs may help detect enlargement of external iliac (sublumbar) lymph nodes, malignant effusion, or masses. The absence of radiographic evidence of metastasis in tumors with a tendency toward hematogenous or lymphatic spread should be viewed with caution, because small lesions below the limits of resolution cannot be detected by this method.

Survey radiographs of the area of a skin tumor are usually not helpful because conventional radiography provides poor contrast discrimination between normal and tumorous tissue. Invasiveness and tissue architecture cannot be assessed with conventional radiographs, and soft tissue structures in contact with one another cannot be differentiated as separate entities if they have the same physical density.

Ultrasonography is usually not useful in evaluation of the invasiveness of a tumor of the skin or subcutis. Sharp definitions of the far margins of the tumor are limited by the heterogeneity of the echoic and anechoic signals from the many composite structures in the beam.

Computed tomography is much better at contrast discrimination among different tissue types. The physical density of a tumor may be compared with that of surrounding normal tissue to provide better information regarding size and invasiveness than is

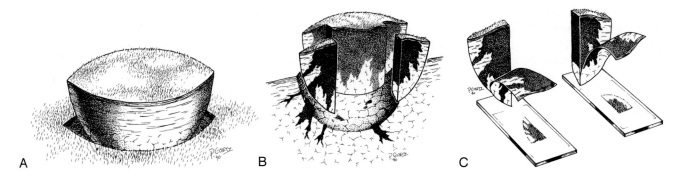

Figure 7-1
(A) A representation of a portion of skin containing an invasive neoplasm after surgical excision. **(B)** The same neoplasm *(shaded area)* after formalin fixation and initial trimming. **(C)** Only a 5- to 6-μm slice of a portion of a tumor is mounted and examined. If tissue from the right side of the specimen is examined, the excision appears complete. However, examination of the left side of the specimen reveals tumor cells extending to the biopsy margin. The choice of which portion of a tumor to consider representative is subjective and may lead to erroneous conclusions about the completeness of the excision. (From Morrison WB, Hamilton TA, Hahn KA, et al. Diagnosis of neoplasia. In: Slatter DS, ed. Textbook of Small Animal Surgery, 2nd ed. Philadelphia, WB Saunders, 1993:2043.)

possible with ultrasonography or conventional radiography.[5]

Cytology and Histopathology

Cytologic and histopathologic evaluations of a lesion are used to diagnose skin tumors. These techniques of cell evaluation often complement one another. Each method has advantages and disadvantages, and each is highly dependent on the interpretive skills of the pathologist. Cytology allows for a better assessment of cytoplasmic and nuclear detail than is possible with histopathology. For example, some poorly differentiated, discrete cell tumors (e.g., mast cell tumors with poorly staining granules, histiocytomas, melanocytic tumors containing little pigment) may resemble poorly differentiated carcinomas histologically, especially if inflammation is present. In such instances, cytologic analysis can be useful to assess cytoplasmic and nuclear detail and assist the pathologist in deriving an accurate diagnosis. However, histopathology is far superior to cytology in assessment of the structural and architectural relations (e.g., tissue invasion) of a tissue. In most situations, histopathology is the standard against which cytologic interpretation is compared, yet in some cases each of the two modalities contributes different but important information toward a diagnosis.

Interpretation of the Biopsy Report

The biopsy report should contain information that provides the clinician with some prognostic information. If that information is absent, it is important to ask more of the pathologist than simply the final diagnosis.

Microscopic examination of the cut margins of a tumor is a common way to try to determine the completeness of a surgical excision. The presence or absence of tumor cells extending to the margin of a surgical excision can influence decisions about the need for additional surgery or adjunctive treatment with irradiation or chemotherapy. If tumor cells are observed at the cut margin, the assumption is that tumor tissue was left behind and recurrence can be expected. If the biopsy report indicates that no tumor cells are observed at the cut margin, the clinician often assumes the excision to be complete. However, the report of clean surgical margins can be misleading with respect to the completeness of a surgical excision. Pathologists routinely trim a submitted sample to a small size that will fit into a special cassette used for automated processing. After the biopsy specimen has been embedded in paraffin, a 5- to 6-μm slice of tissue is mounted on a glass slide and evaluated. To conclude that all margins of an excised tumor are free of infiltrating cells based on the evaluation of a thin slice of a small portion of excised tissue can lead to an erroneous interpretation (Fig. 7–1). Knowledge of a tumor's usual biologic behavior (invasiveness and metastatic potential) is in many ways more important than histopathologic evaluation of tissue margins.[2]

Whenever there is doubt about the accuracy of a biopsy report, it is wise to talk directly with the pathologist and review the clinical and biopsy information. There are times when the clinician should request a tissue review by an additional qualified pathologist. At large laboratories, difficult or atypical specimens are often automatically reviewed internally by other pathologists. At small laboratories, there may only be one pathologist to evaluate the tissue and only one point of view applied toward the final diagnosis. In most cases, pathologists are very cooperative with requests for tissue reviews.

Many tumor types have well-established histologic criteria for the application of a numeric score or grade of malignancy. Tumor grading can provide the clinician with extremely valuable information relating to prognosis. Among tumors that affect the skin and subcutis, the mast cell tumor provides the best-known example of the prognostic value of the histologic grade of a tumor. Mast cell tumors can be graded as poorly differentiated, differentiated, or well-differentiated. The more differentiated the mast cell tumor, the better the prognosis after treatment with surgery alone or radiation therapy alone.

If the tumor is so undifferentiated that it is difficult to classify, a good pathologist uses special stains to bring out one or more of the structural components to clarify the diagnosis. A poorly differentiated tumor that has been assessed only with standard hematoxylin and eosin stain should prompt a discussion with the pathologist of the value of special stains in resolving basic tumor identification.

Immunohistochemistry, using monoclonal or polyclonal antibodies, can be very helpful to identify an anaplastic or undifferentiated tumor if the origin of the tumor cannot be determined with special stains. Various characteristic cytoplasmic markers that are found in normal tissue, when identified in undifferentiated tumor tissue, help to determine identity. The presence or absence of intermediate filaments is one of the more important classes of tumor markers that is used in veterinary medicine to help identify poorly differentiated tumor tissue.[6]

Non-neoplastic Masses of the Skin and Subcutis

Follicular Cysts

Follicular cysts (epidermal inclusion cysts, epidermoid cysts) are non-neoplastic, sac-like structures lined with epithelium. These cysts are usually found as round to oval, firm to fluctuant, smooth, well-delineated structures within the skin. They may be hairless or covered with hair. There is no age, breed, or sex predilection for these lesions.

Pathophysiology

The stimuli that promote formation of these cysts is unknown, although some investigators suspect trauma to the hair follicle. The cysts appear to develop from buried epidermal remnants or hair follicles, and different histologic forms of these lesions arise from different levels of the follicle. The cyst enlarges as a result of accumulation of keratinized debris formed by the epithelial lining of the cyst. This keratinized debris is white to pale yellow and caseous or doughy in consistency.

Clinical Signs

Follicular cysts appear as round papules or nodules in the skin. They may occur anywhere on the body as single or multiple masses. Follicular cysts have a fluctuant or soft center that is detectable on careful palpation. If the lesion ruptures, the keratinized material contained within the cyst is released into the dermis, where it causes a pronounced foreign body reaction. If the cyst is aspirated or lanced with a needle, caseous, white to pale yellow material can usually be expressed.

Diagnostic Plan

Cytologic evaluation of the contents of the cyst reveals blue-staining keratin debris (i.e., epidermal cells) with varying numbers of inflammatory cells. Often, the cytologic preparations of these lesions appear as a smear of acellular debris. Other skin tumors, such as intracutaneous cornifying epitheliomas and keratoacanthomas, may also contain similar debris. Histopathologic examination of the lesion provides a definitive diagnosis.

Treatment

Surgical removal of the lesion is the treatment of choice. The synthetic retinoids, etretinate and isotretinoin, have also been used to induce regression of the mass and decrease the likelihood of recurrence after the lesion has been removed.[7] Etretinate or isotretinoin may be administered in doses of 1 to 2 mg/kg per day; this treatment is recommended if the patient has multiple lesions or if new lesions develop frequently and rapidly enlarge. Symptomatic treatment with hot soaks of the affected area helps resolve the inflammation and encourages drainage of the lesion after the lesion has ruptured. Antimicrobial therapy is indicated if a secondary bacterial infection is present. Surgical removal of those lesions should take place after the acute swelling has resolved.

Prognosis

The prognosis is excellent if the lesion is removed. However, new lesions may develop in predisposed animals.

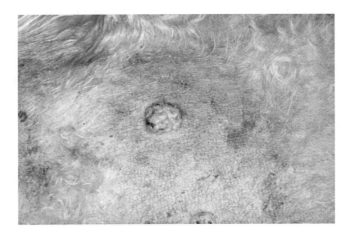

Figure 7-2
Typical lobulated lesion of nodular sebaceous hyperplasia.

Nodular Sebaceous Hyperplasia

The term nodular sebaceous hyperplasia is given to the small, papillated papules and nodules found frequently on the skin of older dogs. These are hyperplastic lesions of sebaceous glands. Poodles, American cocker spaniels, and other small breeds of dog appear to be predisposed to develop these lesions.[8, 9]

Pathophysiology

Nodular sebaceous hyperplasia is a hyperplastic lesion of the sebaceous gland. The exact cause and stimuli for this developmental change are unclear.

Clinical Signs

Nodular sebaceous hyperplasia appears as single to multiple, white or pale yellow, papillated (cauliflower-like) papules or nodules of the skin (Fig. 7-2). These common lesions of the dog grow slowly and are not of clinical significance until they become large enough to be traumatized during grooming. Some dogs bite at the lesions, although they do not appear to be pruritic.

Diagnostic Plan

A tentative diagnosis is based on the clinical appearance of the lesions, although histopathologic examination is required for a definitive diagnosis. In nodular sebaceous gland hyperplasia, the normal histopathologic orientation of sebaceous glands to ductal structures and the follicle is maintained.[10]

Treatment

Surgical removal of the lesion is the treatment of choice if the lesion is large enough to cause morbidity.

Prognosis

The prognosis is excellent if the lesions are surgically removed. New lesions frequently develop in predisposed animals.

Common Tumors of the Skin and Subcutis

Histiocytoma

Histiocytomas are common, benign tumors of the epidermis. Boxers, dachshunds, American cocker spaniels, Great Danes, Shetland sheepdogs, and many other breeds are reportedly predisposed to develop this tumor, but it may be seen in any breed of dog.[1, 8, 11] Young dogs are more likely to develop these tumors.

Pathophysiology

These benign tumors are derived from the Langerhans cell, the epidermal component of the macrophage-monocyte system. Some histiocytomas regress spontaneously.

Clinical Signs

Histiocytomas usually appear as solitary, 1- to 2-cm, circular, dome-shaped, hairless masses (Fig. 7-3). The lesions are frequently referred to as "button tumors" because of their characteristic appearance. The tumors may ulcerate and develop a crater-like appearance. Multiple histiocytomas have been reported but are uncommon.

Diagnostic Plan

The lesions have a characteristic dome shape, which, when combined with the young age of onset,

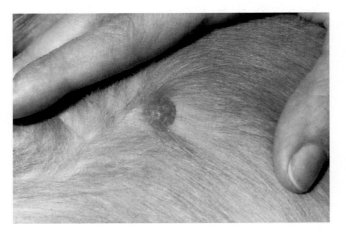

Figure 7-3
Characteristic appearance of a histiocytoma, one of the "button" or "round cell" tumors of the skin.

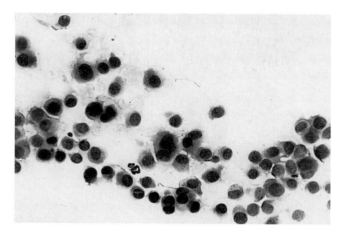

Figure 7-4
Cytologic examination of a histiocytoma reveals characteristic cells with large round nuclei and prominent nucleoli.

helps to increase the index of suspicion for this lesion. The differential diagnosis includes granuloma, lymphosarcoma, transmissible venereal tumor, and mast cell tumor. The cytologic appearance of a histiocytoma is unique. Cytologic preparations are moderately cellular, with the predominant cell being a round cell with moderate granularity and a large nucleus containing a single nucleolus (Fig. 7–4). Histiocytomas and other tumors (mast cell tumors, lymphosarcomas, transmissible venereal tumors) are often classified as round cell tumors based on the cytologic appearance of round cells, which are easily exfoliated as single cells rather than clumps and have distinct cell membranes.[4] The cytologic results, when combined with the age of the patient and clinical signs, provide ample evidence of the diagnosis in most cases. Histologically, histiocytomas have a high mitotic index, a feature that is usually associated with malignancy, but they are benign in their clinical behavior.

Treatment

Surgical removal is the treatment of choice, although injection of the tumor with a glucocorticoid induces remission in some cases. The prognosis is excellent.

Squamous Cell Carcinoma

Squamous cell carcinoma is a malignant tumor of epidermal cell origin that affects dogs and cats. In both species, it most frequently develops in skin on the nonpigmented or white-haired regions of the body, especially the planum nasale and the pinnae. In one study, the incidence rate for squamous cell carcinoma on sun-exposed sites of the skin in cats was estimated to be 26.9 cases per 100,000 cats, and the risk for white

cats was 13.4 times greater than the risk for nonwhite cats.[12] Dalmatians, beagles, whippets, and English bull terriers may be at increased risk to develop squamous cell carcinoma on white skin and hair coat areas of the body.

Pathophysiology

Squamous cell carcinomas are known to develop secondary to exposure to ultraviolet radiation. The site of these tumors reflects the influence of the radiation. They are highly invasive but are usually slow to develop metastasis. Subungual squamous cell carcinomas are locally invasive and early to metastasize.

Clinical Signs

Squamous cell carcinomas most commonly involve lightly pigmented or unpigmented skin. The lesions may be proliferative or erosive, and ulcers, necrosis, and secondary infection may be present.

Lesions on the cat are common on the pinnae, planum nasale, lips, and eyelids (Figure 7–5). Premalignant lesions (actinic keratosis) appears as erythematous plaques, often accompanied by fine scale and alopecia. As the tumor develops, it becomes erythematous, crusted, or ulcerated.

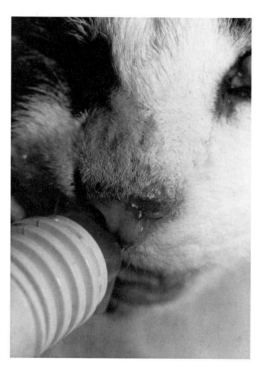

Figure 7-5
Squamous cell carcinoma on the planum nasale. This is a typical early, crusted, ulcerative lesion.

Subungual Squamous Cell Carcinoma

Squamous cell carcinoma may involve the nail-bed of dogs and cats. These tumors present as a nonresponding paronychia that develops into ulcerated or proliferative lesions. Squamous cell carcinoma of multiple digits has been described in large breeds of dogs (especially Labrador retrievers, giant schnauzers, and standard poodles) with black skin and hair coats. These tumors have a reputation for being especially prone to invade bone under their primary subungual location, and early metastasis to regional lymph nodes is common.[13]

Multicentric Squamous Cell Carcinoma In Situ

Multicentric squamous cell carcinoma in situ has been reported by several investigators.[14, 15] Typical lesions begin as pigmented areas that ulcerate in the center and then form an overlying crust. Lesions expand peripherally, so that some become larger than 4 cm in diameter. Several lesions may be present. Hair in the affected area is easily epilated and often has crusty debris clinging to the hair shafts. Histologically, the neoplastic cells are confined to the epidermis and do not penetrate the basement membrane into the surrounding dermis. In contrast to the more common forms of squamous cell carcinoma that usually affect cats, multicentric squamous cell carcinoma in situ occurs in areas that are heavily pigmented, or in nonpigmented sites that have limited solar exposure. This form of squamous cell carcinoma appears to affect predominantly older, mixed breed cats.

Diagnostic Plan

The tumor type is confirmed by histopathologic evaluation of the lesion. Biopsies are best obtained from the margin of the lesion, especially if the lesion is ulcerated. Because squamous cell carcinoma is locally invasive and may be metastatic in its clinical behavior, complete clinical laboratory and radiographic evaluation is advised to determine the full extent of the disease before treatment is initiated.

Treatment

Small lesions, especially those on the planum nasale and the pinnae, may be cured with surgery that allows adequate margins to ensure complete excision.[16] Cryosurgical techniques may also be used. In general, the smaller the initial lesion at the time of diagnosis, the better the overall prognosis. Because bone invasion is expected with subungual squamous cell carcinoma, these tumors are often treated by digital amputation and frequent monitoring to assess for the development of metastasis.

Nonresectable tumors may respond to radiation therapy, especially if they are located on the head.[17]

Systemic chemotherapy with doxorubicin or cisplatin (cisplatin cannot be used in cats) may be useful as adjunctive therapy. Retinoids can inhibit carcinogenesis and suppress the growth and expression of transformed phenotypes in certain cell lines in the laboratory. Retinoid therapy has been reported to be of use in the treatment of preneoplastic squamous cell carcinoma in dogs, but studies of the treatment of actinic dermatoses of the cat have not shown significant preventive benefit from retinoid therapy.[18, 19]

Prognosis

The prognosis for small, solitary lesions is fair to good if the tumor is in an area conducive to proper surgical removal. However, the invasive and malignant nature of tumors on the digits allows only a guarded prognosis in those cases.

Basal Cell Tumors

Basal cell tumors are benign tumors that develop from the basal epithelial cell layer of the epidermis. They are uncommon in dogs but common in cats older than 6 years of age. These tumors comprise 10% to 28% of feline skin tumors and 3% to 6% of feline neoplasms.[20]

Pathophysiology

These tumors generally exhibit benign behavior.

Clinical Signs

Basal cell tumors appear as firm, hairless, often pigmented, dome-shaped nodules in the skin that are freely movable over the underlying structures. Their cut surface is often white or gray. These lesions often appear as cystic, fluid-filled dermal masses.

Diagnostic Plan

Cytologic examination of cells collected by fine-needle aspiration shows single cells or clumps of small epithelial cells with a nucleus-to-cytoplasm ratio of approximately one (1:1). Spindle-shaped melanocytes and free melanin pigment are occasionally present on the cytologic preparation.[4] Histopathologic confirmation of any excised tissue is always necessary.

Treatment

Surgical removal of the tumor is the recommended treatment.

Prognosis

The prognosis is excellent after surgical excision.

Mast Cell Tumors

Mast cell tumors are common, comprising 7% to 21% of cutaneous tumors in dogs and 15% in cats.[11, 21, 22] They may involve other organs (e.g., liver, spleen, bone marrow, lymph nodes), but they are most commonly encountered as primary tumors of the skin or subcutis.

Pathophysiology

Mast cells have a variable number of cytoplasmic granules that contain histamine, heparin, serotonin, proteolytic enzymes, and other vasoactive substances. Histamine can be released in large amounts from these tumors and results in local inflammation and edema around the tumor, severe gastrointestinal irritation from stimulation of H_2 (histamine) receptors in the stomach and production of excess acid, and delayed wound healing from stimulation of macrophages to elaborate a fibroblast suppressor factor.

The biologic behavior of mast cell tumors is highly variable and difficult to predict with consistent accuracy. The biologic behavior of the tumor is most closely related to histologic tumor classification: well-differentiated, differentiated, or poorly differentiated. Differentiated and poorly differentiated tumors have a much higher metastatic potential that can result in systemic dissemination. Metastasis to regional lymph nodes is common and occasionally occurs in other sites such as the liver or spleen. Mast cell tumors in dogs rarely metastasize to the lungs.

Clinical Signs

Mast cell tumors in dogs usually present as single papules or nodules, although multiple tumors may be present. The tumors may be firm or fluctuant, alopecic or haired, and are most commonly found over the trunk and perineal area or on the extremities. They range in size from a few millimeters to several centimeters in diameter, although they are most frequently less than 2 cm in diameter. Manipulation of the tumor may stimulate degranulation of the cells, resulting in edema, erythema, and wheal formation, a phenomenon referred to as Darier's sign.

Mast cell tumors in cats usually present as solitary or multiple cutaneous lesions, or as a primary visceral form that involves the spleen or liver (or both) and occasionally the bone marrow. Some cats have both a cutaneous and a visceral component to their disease. Most cats with visceral mast cell disease show signs of systemic illness such as vomiting, weight loss, and anorexia. Large spleens, reflecting mast cell tumor localization there, can often be palpated, and occasionally circulating mast cells, eosinophilia, and basophilia may be observed in a hemogram.

Cutaneous mast cell tumors in cats usually present as multiple dermal masses that are found primarily on the head and neck. Histologically, cutaneous mast cell tumors in cats can be classified as mast cell–type or histiocytic-type. Mast cell–type tumors usually occur in cats older than 4 years of age as a solitary dermal mass. Histiocytic-type tumors usually occur in Siamese cats younger than 4 years of age as multiple, small masses that may be characterized by benign behavior.

Diagnostic Plan

Cytologic examination of material collected by fine-needle aspiration shows numerous mast cells, although the granularity of the cells varies from tumor to tumor (Fig. 7–6). Eosinophils are also found on cytologic preparations and on histopathologic examination of tumors. Care should be taken to avoid excessive manipulation of the tumor during the aspiration or biopsy process, to prevent degranulation of the tumor.

All mast cell tumors should be regarded as potentially life-threatening, and a complete medical and radiographic evaluation is advised before starting any treatment, especially in cases with suspected metastasis or if multiple cutaneous sites are apparent at initial diagnosis. In addition to routine procedures, a bone marrow aspiration biopsy and a buffy coat smear should be examined as an indication of systemic dissemination. If metastasis or circulating mast cells are detected, systemic chemotherapy should be considered as a primary treatment modality or as an adjunct to surgery or radiation therapy.

Treatment

Mast cell tumors in dogs are among the most difficult tumors to treat. Well-differentiated tumors are

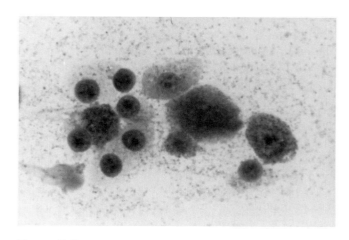

Figure 7–6
Typical appearance of mast cells obtained by fine-needle aspiration from a cutaneous tumor (Diff-Quik stain, ×1000).

associated with a good prognosis after complete surgical removal, and differentiated and poorly differentiated tumors have a progressively poorer prognosis after surgery alone.[23]

Higher-grade mast cell tumors (differentiated and poorly differentiated) may be treated with surgery, chemotherapy, radiation therapy, or combinations of these modalities. Solitary lesions may be treated with surgery, radiation therapy, or combinations of the two. For solitary differentiated or poorly differentiated tumors, surgery plus radiation therapy may be the optimal treatment.[24] Mast cell tumors can be highly invasive, so extensive margins should be taken on all sides of the tumor. If mast cell tumors occur in anatomic sites that make complete excision unlikely, aggressive surgery (amputation if located on an extremity) or radiation therapy should be considered. If solitary differentiated or poorly differentiated lesions exist on the body wall, full-thickness removal and reconstruction of the abdominal or thoracic wall should be considered as initial treatment, rather than as a salvage procedure after the tumor has grown or recurred.

Mast cell tumors that are too extensive for surgery or radiation therapy, or that have evidence of systemic dissemination, should be treated with some form of chemotherapy. However, the evidence for chemotherapeutic treatment of these tumors is largely anecdotal, and such treatment is generally thought to be unrewarding. They are variably and transiently responsive to prednisone alone; combinations of prednisone, vincristine, and cyclophosphamide; and vinblastine, L-asparaginase, and triamcinolone. Although several specific chemotherapy protocols have been described,[25] no published protocol has clear superiority over another. Prednisone administered orally at 1 mg/kg per day was shown to reduce tumor volume in approximately 20% of the patients in one study.[26] However, the ideal dose and specific indications for prednisone therapy have not been established. Triamcinolone has been injected intralesionally (1 mg triamcinolone for every centimeter of diameter, administered every 2 weeks) to reduce tumor size before surgical removal, but the efficacy and benefits of this practice are not clear.

Vomiting and gastroduodenal ulceration, caused by histamine release from mast cell tumors, is a serious complication that may occur if the tumor burden is large or as a result of histamine release after chemotherapy, radiation therapy, or surgical manipulation. During the initial stages of treatment, especially in cases in which the tumor burden is large, concurrent treatment with H_2 blocking agents (e.g., cimetidine) and synthetic polymers (e.g., sucralfate) should be considered. Gastroduodenal ulcers from histamine excess often contribute directly to the death of the patient.

Most cutaneous mast cell tumors in cats do not have the aggressive behavior that is shown by similar tumors in dogs. Surgical removal of the tumor is the recommended treatment. Surgery is indicated in cats with visceral involvement. Splenectomy and intestinal resection as needed, followed by chemotherapy with prednisone or a combination protocol, has been suggested to provide survival times of approximately 1 year.

Prognosis

The prognosis for a canine mast cell tumor treated with surgery, radiation therapy, or chemotherapy varies directly with the histologic classification and clinical stage. The better differentiated a mast cell tumor is, the better the prognosis is likely to be. Small, solitary, well-differentiated mast cell tumors can have an excellent prognosis.

Melanocytic Tumors

Tumors derived from melanocytes are common in dogs but rare in cats.[8] These tumors can be either benign or malignant, and they may occur on any part of the body. Dogs with pigmented skin, such as Scottish terriers, are predisposed to develop these tumors.[27]

Pathophysiology

Approximately 60% of melanomas that appear on hair-bearing skin are benign. Malignant melanomas of the oral cavity or distal extremities may be locally invasive into underlying bone.

Clinical Signs

Melanocytic tumors present as well-circumscribed, dome-shaped papules or nodules, ranging from 0.5 to 2.0 cm in diameter. Benign melanomas are usually well defined and heavily pigmented, although varying degrees of pigmentation may be present. Melanomas may be found anywhere on the body, including the oral cavity and distal extremities.

Diagnostic Plan

Cells are usually easily collected by fine-needle aspiration for cytologic evaluation. Microscopic examination of melanocytic tumors reveals melanocytes, melanophages (macrophages containing phagocytized pigment granules), and free melanin pigment.[4] Histopathologic evaluation of the lesion confirms the tumor type and the behavior (benign or malignant) of the tumor. Regional lymph nodes should be cytologically evaluated for evidence of metastasis. Radiography of the thorax should be performed on patients with malignant melanocytic tumors.

Treatment

The treatment and prognosis for melanomas vary with the location, size, and histologic appearance. Benign tumors respond well to surgical treatment and have an excellent prognosis. Malignant melanomas require aggressive surgical treatment as well as adjuvant treatment to address the metastatic nature of the tumor.

Prognosis

The prognosis for benign tumors is excellent after surgical resection, but it is guarded for malignant tumors.

Sebaceous Adenoma

Sebaceous adenomas are benign tumors derived from sebaceous glands or ducts. These lesions are common in dogs, accounting for approximately 6% of canine cutaneous tumors. They are also seen occasionally in cats. These tumors are seen more frequently in poodles, American cocker spaniels, dachshunds, and Boston terriers.[8, 9]

Pathophysiology

The lesions are not clinically significant unless they are pruritic, bleed after laceration, or are aesthetically unpleasing to the owner.

Clinical Signs

Sebaceous adenomas present as solitary or multiple, papillated lesions. Tumors are most frequently found on the head but may be found in any location.[27] They are usually white, tan, or pale yellow, have a shiny surface, and vary in size from a few millimeters to a few centimeters in diameter. Occasionally, dogs lick or chew at the lesions, although they are usually not pruritic. Patients are often presented after lesions are nicked or lacerated while the animal is being groomed.

Diagnostic Plan

The lesions are grossly indistinguishable from nodular sebaceous hyperplasia, and there is no practical advantage in differentiating a hyperplastic lesion from an adenoma. Histopathologic evaluation is required to confirm the identity of the lesion.

Treatment

Surgical removal of the lesion is the recommended treatment.

Prognosis

The prognosis is excellent, although new lesions often develop in predisposed patients.

Fibrosarcoma

Fibrosarcoma is a malignant connective tissue tumor that occurs in dogs and cats.

Pathophysiology

All fibrosarcomas have the potential to metastasize, but metastasis usually occurs late in the course of the disease. Fibrosarcomas affecting the skin and subcutis are usually poorly circumscribed and highly invasive. A pseudocapsule may form as rapidly growing tumor cells compress surrounding tissue into a thick band, but tumor cells invariably penetrate and extend through the pseudocapsule.

Recent reports indicate that fibrosarcoma and other sarcomas can develop in cats at sites routinely used by veterinarians for vaccinations as an adverse reaction.[3, 28] Many of these tumors are surrounded by a characteristic inflammatory infiltrate resembling that of previously recognized vaccine-induced inflammatory nodules. Foreign material identified as aluminum has been seen in macrophages associated with many of these sarcomas. Because aluminum hydroxide and aluminum phosphate are used as adjuvants in some feline vaccines, some investigators have suggested that inflammation associated with aluminum at injection sites may predispose cats to events that lead to malignant transformation of connective tissue. Whether the aluminum is oncogenic or just a marker of the injection site reaction is unclear.

Clinical Signs

Fibrosarcomas often appear as firm, smooth or lobulated masses within or under the skin. Tumors associated with vaccines are frequently located at sites of vaccination, such as the dorsal thoracic region.

Diagnostic Plan

Histopathologic evaluation of the tumor is necessary to confirm the tumor type. Fine-needle aspiration of the mass usually gives a poor yield of cells for cytologic evaluation because of the fibrotic nature of this tumor. Because fibrosarcomas have the potential for metastasis, a complete medical and radiographic evaluation is indicated before treatment.

Treatment

Surgical removal with generous surgical margins is indicated if it is possible. Radiation therapy may be helpful to control nonresectable tumors or tumors that have been incompletely removed. Treatment with doxorubicin may be of benefit in cases of nonresectable tumors or if metastasis is present.

Prognosis

The prognosis for fibrosarcoma in dogs varies with the size of the tumor and the presence or absence of metastasis. In general, the smaller the tumor at the time of diagnosis, the better the prognosis.

Hemangiopericytoma

Hemangiopericytomas are highly invasive tumors that develop from cells (pericytes) that surround small blood vessels in the dermis and subcutis. Hemangiopericytomas usually occur in middle-aged and older, large (>29 kg) dogs.

Pathophysiology

Although hemangiopericytomas are often classified as benign in behavior, up to 5% of them do metastasize, and all of them are highly invasive.

Clinical Signs

Hemangiopericytomas usually appear as firm, slow-growing, solitary to lobulated masses that are often firmly attached to underlying tissues. The surface of the tumor may be alopecic, erythematous, or ulcerated. Tumor size ranges from less than 1 cm to several centimeters in diameter. The tumors are located most frequently on the extremities.

Diagnostic Plan

Because these tumors have the potential to metastasize, a full medical evaluation, including clinical laboratory evaluation and thoracic radiographs, is indicated. Abdominal radiographs are appropriate if the primary lesion is located on the caudal portion of the body, in an area likely to have lymphatic drainage through abdominal structures.

Hemangiopericytomas can tentatively be diagnosed with cytology based on their typical appearance. Despite the mesenchymal nature of the tumor, cells are easily recovered by fine-needle aspiration of the firm areas of the tumor. The spindle-shaped cells have uniform, round nuclei with scant cytoplasm. They also have a distinct histologic appearance that should make a biopsy diagnosis unequivocal.

Treatment

Surgical resection of the tumor is the treatment of choice. However, these tumors often have pseudopods ("fingers") that extend and infiltrate for several centimeters away from the primary tumor mass. Therefore, surgical resection must be aggressive, with wide surgical margins. Amputation of the affected limb may be the best option in recurring or locally extensive tumors.

There is a high recurrence rate after surgery alone. Nonresectable tumors may be treated with radiation therapy after surgical debulking or chemotherapy, but the response to these treatments is variable. Hemangiopericytomas are usually resistant to treatment with radiation therapy alone.[29]

Prognosis

The prognosis after surgical resection of tumors is guarded. Metastatic lesions are usually slow-growing, and metastasis alone does not necessarily give the patient a poor prognosis.[29] The mitotic index has been shown to be of prognostic significance in soft tissue sarcomas in dogs, including hemangiopericytomas. In one study of sarcomas in dogs, tumors with nine or more mitotic figures per field when viewed at a magnification of 400× had a median survival time of 49 weeks and a recurrence rate of 62%, compared with 118 weeks and 25% for tumors with fewer than nine mitotic figures per field.[30]

Perianal Gland Tumors

Perianal gland tumors (circumanal gland tumors) are common in dogs, accounting for 10% to 20% of cutaneous tumors. The tumors are found in older animals. Adenomas are more prevalent in intact male dogs than in neutered males or female dogs; neutered female dogs are at greater risk than intact female dogs. There appears to be no sex predilection for adenocarcinomas.

Pathophysiology

Perianal gland tumors arise from perianal glands (hepatoid glands), which may be found around the anal area, the area lateral to the prepuce, the thighs, the dorsal midline, and the skin along the ventral midline. The tumors may represent hyperplastic lesions or benign or malignant tumors. Tumors in male dogs are several times more likely to be benign than malignant, but malignant and benign tumors appear with similar frequency in female dogs.

Hyperplastic lesions and adenomas are under hormonal influence, as suggested by the predisposition in intact male dogs to develop these tumors.

Clinical Signs

Perianal gland tumors appear as single to multiple, solid papules to nodules in the skin around the anus. The tumors are often well circumscribed and frequently ulcerate. The tumors may also be found in other areas where hepatoid glands may be found, such as the proximal third of the tail, the dorsal lumbar area, the area lateral to the prepuce, and the skin along the ventral midline.[9–11]

Perianal adenocarcinomas tend to grow faster than adenomas and ulcerate more easily. Adenocarcinomas are locally invasive and may have widespread metastasis.

Diagnostic Plan

Cytologic examination of material collected by fine-needle aspiration reveals typical hepatoid cells, cells with a large, round nucleus and abundant cytoplasm that appears foamy at higher magnification (Fig. 7–7). Because hyperplasia cannot be differentiated from adenoma, histopathologic evaluation of the lesion is needed to confirm the tumor type and behavior.

Treatment

Hyperplastic lesions may regress in male dogs after castration. Surgical resection or cryosurgery is the recommended treatment for most adenomas and all adenocarcinomas. Radiation therapy may also be used to treat adenocarcinomas and may slow progression of the disease. However, it is rarely curative. Adjuvant chemotherapy of adenocarcinomas with doxorubicin or cisplatin may result in short-term or partial remission of the tumor.

Hormonal therapy of hyperplastic lesions or benign tumors with diethylstilbestrol or estradiol may result in tumor regression within a few weeks of the initiation of treatment. However, estrogen therapy is not recommended because of unacceptable side effects, including bone marrow suppression.

Lipoma

Lipomas are benign tumors of fat. They are very common in the subcutaneous tissue of middle-aged and older dogs.

Pathophysiology

Lipomas are not considered to be aggressive tumors, and they present problems to the patient only if they interfere with function or are aesthetically unpleasing to the owner. Some lipomas behave entirely differently from most lipomas; these tumors, called infiltrative lipomas, are characterized by aggressive infiltration of histologically normal fat into surrounding muscle and connective tissue. Affected dogs and cats have a diffuse enlargement of the affected area. Although these tumors are not likely to metastasize, they should be regarded as malignant because of their aggressive invasive behavior.

Clinical Signs

Lipomas usually present as soft, fluctuant, subcutaneous masses. They may be solitary tumors, although most patients tend to develop multiple tumors over time. Lipomas are usually well encapsulated and are freely moveable beneath the skin.

Diagnostic Plan

Lipomas are frequently diagnosed by cytology. Material aspirated from a lipoma appears as glistening droplets of fat when placed on a glass slide. A smear of fat that is stained and examined microscopically appears acellular because alcohol, commonly found in commercial fixatives and stains, dissolves the fat cells off the slide during the staining process.

Treatment

Lipomas usually do not require treatment unless because of their size or location they interfere with limb function or cosmetic appearance. Surgical removal is the treatment of choice.

Prognosis

The prognosis for lipomas is excellent after surgical removal. However, there is a high local recurrence rate (up to 42%) after resection of infiltrative lipomas. Subsequent surgeries are frequently characterized by an even more vigorous local invasiveness than existed before the initial surgery.[31] Therefore, infiltrative lipomas have a guarded prognosis.

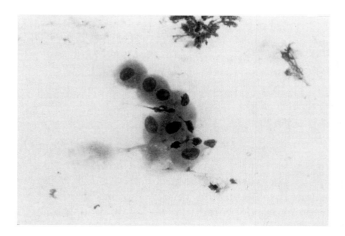

Figure 7–7
Cytologic preparation of a perianal adenoma. Notice the clumped hepatoid cells (Diff-Quik stain, ×1000).

Uncommon Tumors of the Skin and Subcutis

Hair Follicle Tumors

Hair follicle tumors are termed trichoepitheliomas if they arise from hair follicle sheaths and pilomatricomas if they arise from hair matrix. Poodles and Kerry blue terriers are reported to be predisposed to develop these types of tumors.[1, 8]

Trichoepitheliomas

Trichoepitheliomas account for 2% to 3% of all skin tumors in dogs and 1.5% to 4% of all skin tumors in cats.[10] They may occur anywhere on the body, but they are most common on the back. They appear as solitary, well-circumscribed, round to oval, intradermal masses. Diagnosis is confirmed by histopathologic evaluation of the tumor. Surgical removal is the treatment of choice, and the prognosis is good.

Pilomatricomas

Pilomatricomas are uncommon tumors of the skin that appear as firm, well-circumscribed, freely movable subcutaneous masses arising from the hair bulb. The skin over them is frequently hairless. Rarely, this tumor may be malignant. The diagnosis is confirmed by histopathologic evaluation of the tumor, and surgical removal is the recommended treatment. The prognosis after removal is good.

Intracutaneous Cornifying Epithelioma

Intracutaneous cornifying epitheliomas (infundibular keratinizing acanthomas) are uncommon tumors of the hair follicle that appear clinically similar to follicular cysts and other follicular tumors. They are more prevalent in the Norwegian elkhound. These tumors present as single or multiple, haired or alopecic nodules that often contain an opening from the lesion to the exterior. Keratinized cellular debris and hair can often be expressed from the lesion (Fig. 7–8). Surgical removal of the lesions is the recommended treatment, although there have been limited reports of regression of tumor after retinoid therapy.[7] The prognosis is good, although predisposed animals frequently develop additional tumors, which then require removal or medical management.

Lymphosarcoma

Nonepitheliotropic Cutaneous Lymphosarcoma

Nonepitheliotropic cutaneous lymphosarcoma usually appears as a solitary, erythmatous, hairy or hairless nodule or tumor. The diagnosis is confirmed

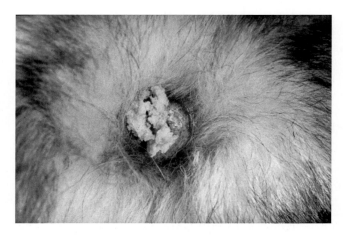

Figure 7–8
Caseous material, typical of the material found within follicular cysts and follicular tumors, expressed from an intracutaneous cornifying epithelioma in a Norwegian elkhound.

by cytologic and histopathologic evaluation. Treatment options for cutaneous lymphosarcoma are usually limited to surgery or irradiation for solitary lesions and systemic chemotherapy for disseminated disease. Surgical excision of solitary tumor is usually curative, and nonresectable tumors may be radiosensitive. Nonresectable lesions may be treated with chemotherapy using standard protocols with vincristine, cyclophosphamide, and prednisone. The prognosis is excellent if the tumor can be completely removed. However, dissemination to regional lymph nodes and internal organs is common.

Epitheliotropic Cutaneous Lymphosarcoma

Epitheliotropic lymphosarcoma (mycosis fungoides) is a malignant tumor that is believed to be of T-lymphocyte origin.[32, 33] Erythema is the most common clinical sign associated with this tumor. Pruritus, alopecia, and scaling are also common, and multiple plaque-like lesions, raised annular lesions, or nodules may be present. The epidermis may be intact, or it may show extensive ulceration, necrosis, and secondary infection. Involvement of the oral cavity is common.[32]

The clinical evaluation of dogs and cats with cutaneous lymphosarcoma should be as complete as possible because lymphosarcoma is usually a multicentric disease at the time of initial presentation. Recommended procedures for evaluation include a complete blood count, serum biochemical analysis, urinalysis, thoracic and abdominal radiography, bone marrow biopsy, ophthalmic examination, tissue biopsy of a representative lesion, and FeLV test (cats). Evidence of neoplastic involvement of the lymph nodes is seen in approximately one third of dogs with epitheliotropic cutaneous lymphosarcoma.

This form of cutaneous lymphosarcoma is histologically characterized by epitheliotropism of malignant lymphocytes and the presence of aggregations of malignant lymphocytes, referred to as Pautrier's microabscesses, within the epidermis and adnexa. Metastasis is to internal organs, including the liver and spleen. Therapy with the retinoids, isotretinoin and etretinate, has been shown to induce regression of the tumor, but the effects are largely palliative. Other treatment modalities, such as radiation therapy and chemotherapy, have generally been ineffective.

Ceruminous Gland Adenocarcinoma

These tumors, which develop from apocrine glands found in the external ear canal, are the most common malignant tumor of the ear of both dogs and cats. They most commonly occur in the horizontal ear canal, are pedunculated, and can extend into the middle ear. Clinical signs are usually indistinguishable from those of chronic otitis externa. A diagnosis is dependent on observation of a mass in the ear canal and histologic evaluation of the tumor. Radiography may be helpful to identify involvement of the middle ear or bones of the skull. The clinical behavior of these tumors is variable. They should be regarded as aggressive tumors with the potential for both local invasion of soft tissue and bone and distant metastasis. Surgical removal with total ear ablation is the recommended therapy.[34, 35] Radiation therapy may be an effective treatment if the tumor has not been completely resected.[36]

References

1. Susaneck SJ, Withrow SJ. Tumors of the skin and subcutaneous tissues. In: Withrow SJ, MacEwen EG, eds. Clinical Veterinary Oncology, 2nd ed. Philadelphia, WB Saunders, 1989;139–155.

2. Morrison WB, Hamilton TA, Hahn KA, et al. Diagnosis of neoplasia. In: Slatter DS, ed. Textbook of Small Animal Surgery, 2nd ed. Philadelphia, WB Saunders, 1993:2036–2048.

3. Esplin DG, McGill LD, Meiniger AC, Wilson SR. Postvaccination sarcomas in cats. J Am Vet Med Assoc 1993;202:1245–1247.

4. Barton CL. Cytologic diagnosis of cutaneous neoplasia: An algorithmic approach. Compen Contin Educ Pract Vet 1987;9:20–33.

5. Hahn KH, Lantz GC, Salisbury SK, et al. Comparison of survey radiography with ultrasonography and x-ray computed tomography for the clinical staging of subcutaneous neoplasms in dogs. J Am Vet Med Assoc 1990;196:1795–1798.

6. Sandusky GE, Carlton WW, Wrightman KA. Diagnostic immunohistochemistry of canine round cell tumors. Vet Pathol 1987;24:495–499.

7. White SD, Rosychuk RAW, Scott KV, et al. Use of isotretinoin and etretinate for the treatment of benign cutaneous neoplasia and cutaneous lymphoma in dogs. J Am Vet Med Assoc 1993;202:387–391.

8. Conroy JD. Canine skin tumors. J Am Anim Hosp Assoc 1983;19:91–114.

9. Bevier DE, Goldschmidt MH. Skin tumors in dogs: Part I. Epithelial tumors and tumorlike lesions. Compen Contin Educ Pract Vet 1981;3:389–398.

10. Gross TL, Ihrke PJ, Walder EJ. Veterinary Dermatopathology. St Louis, Mosby–Year Book, 1992:374–385.

11. Priester WA, Mantel N. Skin tumors of domestic animals. Data from 12 United States and Canadian colleges of veterinary medicine. J Natl Cancer Inst 1973;50:457–466.

12. Dorn CR, Taylor D, Schneider R. Sunlight exposure and the risk of developing cutaneous and oral squamous cell carcinoma in white cats. J Natl Cancer Inst 1971;46:1073–1078.

13. O'Brien MG, Berg RJ, Engler SJ. A retrospective study of 21 dogs with subungual squamous cell carcinoma treated by digital amputation. Proceedings of the Veterinary Cancer Society 10th Annual Conference, Auburn, Alabama, 1990:54–55.

14. Turrel JM, Gross TL. Multicentric squamous cell carcinoma in situ (Bowens disease) of cats. Proceedings of the Veterinary Cancer Society 11th Annual Conference, Minneapolis, Minnesota, 1991:84.

15. Baer KE, Rhodes KH. Feline epidermal squamous cell carcinoma in situ. Proceedings of Ninth Annual Members' Meeting, American Academy of Veterinary Dermatology and American College of Veterinary Dermatology, San Diego, 1993:100.

16. Withrow SJ, Straw RC. Resection of the nasal planum in nine cats and five dogs. J Am Anim Hosp Assoc 1990;26:219–222.

17. Madewell BR, Theilen GH. Tumors and Tumor-like Conditions of Epithelial Origin. In: Madewell BR, Theilen GH, eds. Veterinary Cancer Medicine, 2nd ed. Philadelphia, Lea & Febiger, 1987:240–281.

18. Marks SL, Song MD, Stannard AA, Power HT. Clinical evaluation of etretinate (Tegison) for the treatment of preneoplastic and neoplastic squamous cell carcinoma in 10 dogs. Proceedings of the Veterinary Cancer Society 10th Annual Conference, Auburn, Alabama, 1990:43–44.

19. Evans AG, Madewell BR, Stannard AA. A trial of 13-cis-retinoic acid for treatment of squamous cell carcinoma and preneoplastic lesions of the head in cats. Am J Vet Res 1985;46:2553–2557.

20. Diters RW, Walsh KM. Feline basal cell tumors: A review of 124 cases. Vet Pathol 1984;21:51–56.

21. Macy DW, Reynolds HA. The incidence, characteristics, and clinical management of skin tumors of cats. J Am Anim Hosp Assoc 1981;17:1026–1033.

22. Macy DW, MacEwen EG. Mast cell tumors. In: Withrow SJ, MacEwen EG, eds. Clinical Veterinary Oncology, 2nd ed, Philadelphia, WB Saunders, 1989:156–165.

23. Patniak AK, Ehler WJ, MacEwen EG. Canine cutaneous

mast cell tumors: Morphologic grading and survival in 83 dogs. Vet Pathol 1984;21:469–474.

24. Turrel JM, Kitchell BE, Miller LM, Theon A. Prognostic factors for radiation treatment of mast cell tumors in 85 dogs. J Am Vet Med Assoc 1988;193:936–940.

25. Couto GC. Selected canine and feline neoplasms. In: Nelson RW, Couto GC, eds. Essentials of Small Animal Medicine, St Louis, Mosby–Year Book, 1992:879–892.

26. McCaw DL, Miller MA, Olgilvie GK, et al. Response of canine mast cell tumors to treatment with oral prednisone. J Vet Intern Med 1994;8:406–408.

27. Bostock DE. Neoplasms of the skin and subcutaneous tissues in dogs and cats. Br Vet J 1986;142:1–19.

28. Hendrick MJ, Goldschmidt MH, Shofer FS, et al. Postvaccinal sarcomas in the cat: Epidemiology and electron probe microanalytical identification of aluminum. Cancer Res 1992;52:5391–5394.

29. Postorino NC, Berg RJ, Powers BE, et al. Prognostic variables for canine hemangiopericytoma: 50 cases (1979–1984). J Am Anim Hosp Assoc 1988;24:501–509.

30. Bostock DE, Dye MT. Prognosis after surgical excision of canine fibrous connective tissue sarcomas. Vet Pathol 1980;17:581–588.

31. Bergman PJ, Withrow SJ, Straw RC, Powers BE. Canine infiltrative lipoma: 11 cases (1981–1990). Proceedings of the Veterinary Cancer Society 11th Annual Conference, Minneapolis, Minnesota, 1991:39.

32. Beale KM, Bolon B. Canine cutaneous lymphosarcoma, epitheliotropic and non-epitheliotropic: A retrospective study. In: Ihrke PJ, Mason IS, White SD, eds. Advances in Veterinary Dermatology, vol 2. Oxford, Pergamon Press, 1993:273–284.

33. DeBoer DJ, Turrell JM, Moore PF. Mycosis fungoides in a dog: Demonstration of T-cell specificity and response to radiotherapy. J Am Anim Hosp Assoc 1990;26:566–572.

34. Marino DJ, MacDonald JM, Matthiesen DT, et al. Results of surgery in cats with ceruminous gland adenocarcinoma. J Am Anim Hosp Assoc 1994;30:54–58.

35. Williams JM, White RAS. Total ear ablation combined with lateral bulla osteotomy in the cat. J Small Anim Pract 1992;33:225–227.

36. Thoen AP, Barthea PY, Madewell BR, et al. Radiation therapy of ceruminous gland carcinomas in dogs and cats. J Am Vet Med Assoc 1994;205:566–569.

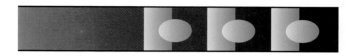

Cardiovascular Diseases

Chapter 8

Anatomy and Physiology of the Heart

Betsy R. Bond

In the recent past, all that was required to adequately treat heart disease was to hear a heart murmur in an elderly coughing poodle and dispense the two cardiac drugs that were available (digoxin and furosemide). Our current understanding of heart failure has made that approach obsolete. We can no longer be satisfied with simply relieving symptoms when we can help our patients live longer and feel better. The newer drugs that alter neurohormonal regulation represent a shift in the way heart failure is perceived and could be a harbinger of other changes. Because of an enlarging body of knowledge concerning cardiac disease and pathophysiology, it is increasingly important to maintain a working knowledge of the anatomy and physiology of the heart and circulatory system. Misdiagnoses and therapeutic errors occur if normal anatomy, physiology, and circulation through the heart and lungs are not considered in light of symptoms, physical findings, radiographic abnormalities, and electrocardiographic changes.

Anatomy

Gross Anatomy

The mammalian heart is a four-chamber pump, the right ventricle being the low-pressure side pumping blood to the lungs and the left ventricle the high-pressure side delivering blood to the circulation (Fig. 8–1). Blood returns from the systemic circulation into the right atrium through the cranial and caudal venae cavae. It then traverses the tricuspid valve into the right ventricle, which pumps blood through the pulmonary valve and pulmonary artery into the lungs for oxygenation. This intimate link of the lungs with the right side of the heart explains the cardiomegaly in pulmonary disease (e.g., heartworm disease, chronic obstructive pulmonary disease) that is often mistaken for left-sided heart problems such as mitral valve disease.

After circulating through the lungs, the blood returns to the left atrium through the pulmonary veins, then flows through the mitral valves into the left ventricle to be pumped to the systemic circulation. Therefore, left-sided heart failure (e.g., mitral regurgitation) causes pulmonary edema, whereas right-sided heart disease causes ascites (in the dog) and pleural effusion (in the cat). Cats may also exhibit pleural effusion with left-sided heart failure.

Cellular Anatomy

Ventricular myocytes are made up of cross-banded strands or bundles called myofibrils, which are composed of sarcomeres (Fig. 8–2). Actin (thin filaments of a two-stranded double helix) and myosin (thick filaments) are proteins that overlap with one another to form the sarcomeres. Myosin has cross-bridges that attach to actin during contraction[1](Fig. 8–3).When activated, the cross-bridges attach to actin and move, pulling the filaments along one another to generate force and shortening. Tropomyosin and troponin are regulatory proteins that control contraction and relaxation with the help of calcium. Tropomyosin is a strand of protein that lies slightly off the groove between actin chains (Fig. 8–4). Troponin is a complex of three components that lie at intervals along the tropomyosin: troponin C is a calcium-sensitizing factor that binds calcium ions; troponin I is the inhibitory factor of contraction; troponin T is necessary for function of the entire complex and allows attachment of tropomyosin to actin and myosin.[1]

Physiology

Current studies of heart failure have emphasized the underlying mechanisms of both systolic and diastolic

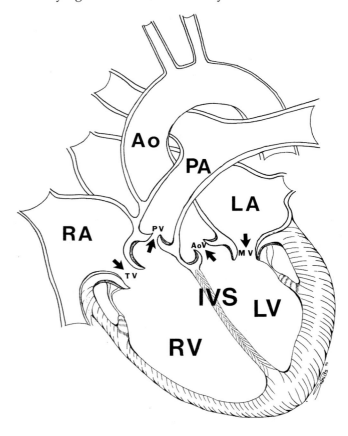

Figure 8–1
Structure of the mammalian heart. Arrows show direction of blood flow through the cardiac valves. Ao, aorta; AoV, aortic valve; IVS, interventricular septum; LA, left atrium; LV, left ventricle; MV, mitral valve; PA, pulmonary artery; PV, pulmonary valve; RA, right atrium; RV, right ventricle; TV, tricuspid valve.

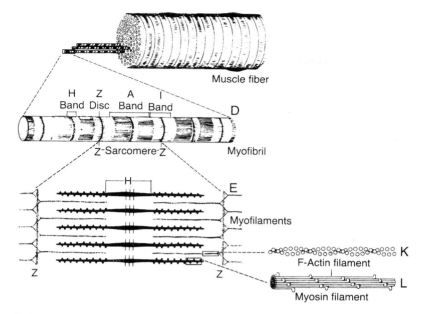

Figure 8–2
Sarcomeres are the major components of the ventricular myocytes. (Modified from Fawcett-Bloom and Fawcett: A Textbook of Histology. New York, Chapman & Hall, 1994. Drawing by Sylvia Colard Keene.)

dysfunction. To fully appreciate the varied mechanisms of heart failure, the clinician should thoroughly understand cellular processes.

Cellular Mechanisms of Contraction

The components of contraction include calcium (Ca^{++}); the contractile proteins actin, myosin, tropomyosin, and troponin; magnesium (Mg^{++}); and adenosine triphosphate (ATP). Only actin, myosin, Mg^{++}, and ATP are really needed for contraction to occur, but Ca^{++} interacts with the contractile proteins to regulate contraction, relaxation, and contractility.[1]

Contraction and Relaxation by Contractile Proteins

During relaxation, troponin I is bound to actin and inhibits cross-bridge formation of actin with myosin. Contraction occurs after Ca^{++} enters the cell and is bound to troponin C, which prevents binding of troponin I to actin. This allows a conformational change in tropomyosin so that tropomyosin can enhance cross-bridging of actin to myosin (see Fig. 8–3). The cross-bridging facilitates a relative change in the positions of actin and myosin with one another, similar to oars rowing a boat in water, and muscle shortening occurs[1] (Fig. 8–5).

Role of Calcium

A small amount of extracellular Ca^{++} enters the cell through either the slow Ca^{++} channels or the sodium-calcium (Na^{+}-Ca^{++}) exchange mechanism during the plateau phase of depolarization (Fig. 8-6). This Ca^{++} is not the trigger for contraction, but it causes release of larger stores of Ca^{++} from the cisternae of the sarcoplasmic reticulum. The Ca^{++} released from the sarcoplasmic reticulum is bound to troponin C and causes contraction. Relaxation occurs by reuptake of Ca^{++} into a temporary store, after which the Ca^{++} gradually returns to the sarcoplasmic reticulum to await another stimulus. It is the amount of Ca^{++} in the sarcoplasmic reticulum that determines the contractile state of the myocardium.[1] However, too much intracellular Ca^{++} impairs relaxation of the ventricular cells and can lead to diastolic dysfunction as a cause of heart failure.[2] Relaxation is not simply a passive process, but one that requires energy.

The process of contraction can be described as follows. At first, the cell is in a relaxed state. Troponin I has inhibited cross-bridging of actin and myosin. Calcium that has entered the cell during the plateau phase of depolarization triggers the release of a larger store of Ca^{++} from the sarcoplasmic reticulum. This Ca^{++} combines with troponin C to inhibit troponin I and allow cross-bridges of actin and myosin to form. The myosin head attaches to actin and flexes to slide

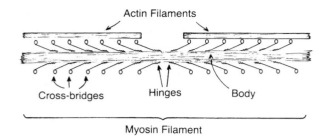

Figure 8–3
Many myosin molecules combine to form a myosin filament. Also shown are the cross-bridges and their proximity to adjacent actin filaments. (From Guyton AC. Textbook of Medical Physiology, 8th ed. Philadelphia, WB
Saunders, 1991:70.)

the actin and myosin filaments alongside one another.
This attaching and flexing of the myosin head occurs
several times in rapid succession until calcium is
depleted. At this point, full contraction has occurred
and the muscle is ready to relax. Relaxation occurs
as calcium is taken up into storage and then gradually into the sarcoplasmic reticulum to await the next
contraction.

The Autonomic Nervous System

The autonomic nervous system is the critical
regulator of heart rate, contractility, and vascular tone
and therefore has moment-to-moment control of cardiac output, blood flow distribution, and arterial
pressure. Neural control and cardiovascular reflexes
together ensure that heart function meets the physiologic demands of the peripheral circulation and the
body.

Neural control of the heart and blood vessels is
regulated primarily by the medullary cardiovascular
centers, which may be influenced by higher centers in
the cerebral cortex. Efferent impulses are sent from the
central nervous system to the sympathetic and parasympathetic preganglionic cells, and from there they

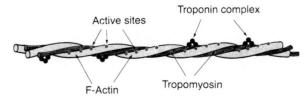

Figure 8–4
The actin filament is composed of two helical strands of
actin and tropomyosin molecules that fit loosely in the
grooves between the actin strands. Attached to one end
of each tropomyosin molecule is a troponin complex that
initiates contraction. (From Guyton AC. Textbook of
Medical Physiology, 8th ed. Philadelphia, WB Saunders,
1991:71.)

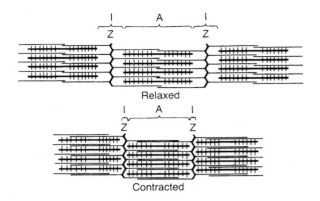

Figure 8–5
The relaxed and contracted states of a myofibril, showing
the actin filaments sliding into the spaces between the
myosin filaments. (From Guyton AC. Textbook of Medical
Physiology, 8th ed. Philadelphia, WB Saunders, 1991:70.)

travel to the heart, blood vessels, and adrenal medulla.
Most areas of the heart receive both sympathetic and
parasympathetic innervation, but different areas have
a predominance of one or the other. For instance,
sympathetic nerve endings primarily serve the myocardium and are interposed between muscle bundles
of the atria and ventricles, but they also innervate the
sinoatrial (SA) and atrioventricular (A-V) nodes. Parasympathetic efferent nerves richly supply the SA and

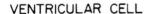
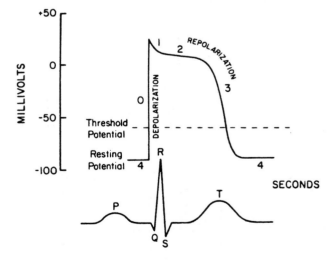

Figure 8–6
Diagram of the action potential of a Purkinje cell. Phase 0
represents the initial depolarization of the cell. Phase 2
is the plateau phase, in which calcium enters the cell for
contraction. In phase 3 (repolarization), the cell returns toward its resting state (phase 4). (From Tilley LP. Essentials of Canine and Feline Electrocardiography, 3rd ed.
Philadelphia, Lea & Febiger, 1992:4.)

A-V nodes but only sparsely innervate the ventricular myocardium[1] (Fig. 8–7).

The main neurotransmitter for the adrenergic nervous system is norepinephrine. Norepinephrine is released into the circulation and also acts at the nerve endings in the heart. Epinephrine is released by the adrenal medulla and circulates in the blood stream to stimulate adrenoceptors. Acetylcholine is the neurotransmitter for the parasympathetic nervous system, and it has effects on the heart opposite those of norepinephrine (i.e., it slows heart rate and mildly decreases cardiac contractility).[1]

Cardiac adrenoceptors are divided into two subtypes, α and β. β-Receptors can be divided further into β_1-receptors, which include the majority of myocardial receptors, and β_2-receptors, which cause relaxation of vascular and bronchial smooth muscle. The β_1-adrenergic myocardial receptors are primarily (although not exclusively) stimulated by norepinephrine. The β_2- and α-receptors mainly respond to circulating epinephrine and control dilation and constriction of blood vessels, respectively.[3] Epinephrine and norepinephrine together can increase both the force and the rate of contraction. Myocardial α-receptors also help modulate cardiac contractility, but they are more important in stimulating vasoconstriction.[1]

The mechanism by which the adrenergic nervous system affects the heart is as follows. Sympathomimetic amines react with β-receptors on cardiac sarcolemma to activate adenyl cyclase. Adenyl cyclase catalyzes the production of cyclic adenosine monophosphate (AMP) from ATP in the presence of Ca^{++}. Cyclic AMP allows Ca^{++} to enter the cell to enhance cardiac contraction. The sympathetic nervous system also enhances Ca^{++} uptake by the sarcoplasmic reticulum, facilitating relaxation.[1] Therefore, β-adrenergic stimulation can augment both contractility and relaxation.

Contraction in the Intact Heart

Definitions

A brief review of definitions will help ensure full comprehension of the mechanisms discussed. *Cardiac output* is the volume of blood being pumped out of the heart in liters per minute. Every time the heart beats, it pumps out a volume of blood called the *stroke volume.* The stroke volume is affected by preload, afterload, and contractility. *Stress* is the force put on each square centimeter of cross-sectional area of myocardium.[1] It is important for two reasons: (1) it is a major determinant of myocardial oxygen consumption, and (2) a chronic increase in wall stress over time probably causes irreversible myocardial damage. *Laplace's law* states that wall stress is directly related to the product of intraventricular pressure and the ventricle's internal radius and is inversely proportional to wall thickness.[1] In other words, as the ventricle dilates or as ventricular pressure increases, so does wall stress. Conversely, ventricular hypertrophy relieves wall stress.

Oxygen consumption or *oxygen demand* is the amount of oxygen extracted by the myocardium. Its three major determinants are wall stress, contractility, and heart rate. *Stroke work,* the amount of work performed by the pumping heart every time it beats, correlates directly with oxygen consumption and equals the stroke volume times the mean arterial pressure. Because the systemic pressure is higher than the pulmonary artery pressure, the left ventricle does seven times more stroke work than the right ventricle.[3] *Stiffness* describes the ability of the muscle to change in size with application of pressure. The stiffer a ventricular wall, the more pressure required to stretch the muscle. *Compliance* is the opposite of stiffness, so that a more compliant ventricle stretches more easily as pressure and volume are applied to it.[1] The terms *inotropic* and *chronotropic* refer to the force and rate of contraction, respectively; *lusitropic* refers to relaxation ability.

Starling's Law

One of the main mechanisms of contraction, the Frank-Starling phenomenon, explains the change in contractility that occurs on a beat-to-beat basis. It comes from the relation of sarcomere length to both the force of contraction and the extent of fiber shortening. The more the heart is filled in diastole, the more the

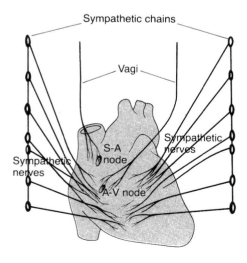

Figure 8–7

Diagram showing sympathetic innervation to the S-A node, A-V node, and myocardium. (From Guyton AC. Textbook of Medical Physiology, 8th ed. Philadelphia, WB Saunders, 1991:107.)

Table 8–1
Factors That Control Preload

Venous return
Total blood volume
Distribution of blood volume
    Body position
    Intrathoracic pressure
    Intrapericardial pressure
    Venous tone
Atrial contraction

myocardium is stretched and the more blood the heart is able to pump into the aorta.[3] There is an optimum length of sarcomere for the greatest force of myocardial contraction; above or below this optimum, the heart muscle loses force.[1]

The normal, unstressed diastolic sarcomere length is too short for maximum tension development. There is an optimal sarcomere length that is brought about by ventricular dilation. As left ventricular filling pressures increase, resting sarcomeres are stretched to provide increased force of contraction and enhanced left ventricular emptying. Mid-wall sarcomeres tend to be longer than those in the subendocardium and subepicardium and are stretched first. As filling pressures increase further, these "outer" and "inner" sarcomeres are recruited, providing a functional reserve of the Frank-Starling mechanism.[1]

Preload

Ventricular preload is end-diastolic wall stress, and it arises from either pressure or volume loading on the ventricle. The concept of preload reserve states that volume loading (increasing preload) increases stroke volume (Frank-Starling mechanism). There is a limit to preload reserve, and it diminishes as the ventricle progressively dilates. Atrial contraction is another means by which ventricular filling is enhanced. It assists ventricular filling in left ventricular hypertrophy and other types of decreased ventricular compliance.[1]

Control of preload is determined primarily by venous return, total blood volume, and distribution of blood volume (Table 8–1). Preload is increased by conditions that lower peripheral vascular resistance and increase venous return, such as fever, pregnancy, thyrotoxicosis, A-V fistulae, and anemia. If total blood volume is reduced, as in severe dehydration or blood loss, preload also drops.[1]

Distribution of blood between the intrathoracic and extrathoracic compartments is determined by intrathoracic pressure, intrapericardial pressure, and venous tone. Animals are affected by intrathoracic

pressure changes during respiration: the pressure becomes more negative during inspiration, normally drawing blood into the right ventricle and increasing preload and venous return. Elevation of intrathoracic pressure from conditions such as severe coughing can diminish venous return and cardiac output to the point that animals may faint (so-called cough drop). Elevated pericardial pressure (e.g., pericardial effusions, pericarditis) also interferes with cardiac filling. This is why diuretics (acting as preload reducers) are contraindicated for pericardial effusions. Venous tone by itself can enhance venous return, and it is increased by exercise, anxiety, deep respiration, or marked hypotension. Sympathomimetic drugs cause vasoconstriction, whereas sympatholytic drugs or drugs such as nitroglycerin do the opposite.[1]

Afterload

Afterload is the force or stress applied to the ventricular wall after the onset of shortening (Table 8–2). It greatly determines the amount of blood ejected by the ventricle, and it can decrease wall shortening and stroke volume. Elevated afterload is more important in the heart that is pressure- or volume-overloaded (or both) in which there is no preload reserve, and any increase in afterload has an adverse effect. This is especially true if contractility is depressed. Conversely, some clinical conditions, such as mitral regurgitation, patent ductus arteriosus, and ventricular septal defects, can lower impedance (decrease afterload) to left ventricular ejection and increase the extent of fiber shortening.[1] This frequently occurs with mitral regurgitation in small animals.

In most normal hearts, an increase in afterload often leads to a corresponding elevation in preload because of incomplete emptying and a larger end-diastolic diameter. Myocardial contractility is enhanced through the Frank-Starling mechanism, but the higher preload increases tension (afterload) even more, which in turn reduces myocardial fiber shortening. The dilated ventricle of a normal heart requires less shortening to deliver an equivalent stroke volume, so cardiac output can be maintained even in the presence of a higher afterload. However, in the failing heart, there is less preload reserve to help maintain stroke volume, and cardiac output falls with even small

Table 8–2
Factors That Control Afterload

Peripheral vascular resistance
Physical characteristics of the vascular tree
Volume of blood at onset of ejection
Outflow obstruction

Table 8–3
Pressure–Volume Relations

Myocardial fiber shortening is affected by
  More preload (*increases* shortening)
  More contractility (*increases* shortening)
  More afterload (*decreases* shortening)
Afterload is increased by
  More dilated left ventricle
  Increased arterial pressure
Stroke volume is increased by
  More dilated left ventricle
  Increased myocardial fiber shortening
Arterial pressure is increased by
  Increased peripheral resistance
  Increased cardiac output

increases in afterload.[1] Administration of a balanced vasodilator in this situation decreases systemic vascular resistance and shifts blood volume away from the central to the peripheral vascular space. The peripheral blood vessels hold more volume, and the heart empties more easily. Ventricular volume falls, which reduces left ventricular end-diastolic pressure and systolic wall stress. This reduction in afterload allows an increase in stroke volume and cardiac output.[1]

The interaction of arterial pressure, myocardial fiber shortening, and loading conditions of the ventricle profoundly affects the failing heart. Table 8–3 shows the interrelations of myocardial loading with peripheral pressure. Myocardial fiber shortening, a main determinant of stroke volume, is increased by both preload and contractility but is decreased by afterload. Arterial pressure is determined by the product of cardiac output and systemic vascular resistance. Arterial pressure rises if more volume is put into the system (increased cardiac output) or if vessels resist dilation (increased systemic vascular resistance). Arterial pressure directly affects afterload (as does left ventricular size). Therefore, if vasoconstriction raises arterial pressure, afterload is increased and myocardial fiber shortening is reduced. Stroke volume and cardiac output fall, and arterial pressure returns to normal.[1] These interactions are complex, and whether stroke volume and cardiac output are maintained to overcome an increased afterload, as has been described, or drop to re-establish a normal arterial blood pressure depends on the immediate needs of the animal and its ability to respond.

If ventricular function is impaired, afterload becomes an even more critical determinant of cardiac performance. In most instances of heart failure, neurohumoral influences raise afterload as a consequence of vasoconstriction. Cardiac output drops, and a failing myocardium is unable to respond. In this case, pharmacologic interventions can help restore cardiac output.[1]

Contractility

Contractility (inotropic state) refers to the strength and speed of contraction of the heart muscle. The cellular mechanism involves increasing Ca^{++} availability to the myofilaments or altering myofilament Ca^{++} sensitivity.[1] The measure of contractility is $\frac{dP}{dT}$, or the rate of change of ventricular pressure over time.[3] Contractility is analogous to the ability to lift weights; it refers to the heart's ability to "lift" heavier weights with more speed. The greater the contractility of the ventricles, the faster the contraction occurs and the more afterload (weight) the heart can comfortably handle.

Contractility and inotropic state are equivalent terms that are often used erroneously as synonyms for ventricular performance. Ventricular performance refers to global cardiac function, which is affected by mechanisms such as preload, afterload, heart rate, and contractility; contractility is only one part of cardiac performance. Performance and contractility are related in that, given constant loading conditions, an improved contractility augments cardiac performance (a positive inotropic effect), and a depressed contractility lowers cardiac performance (a negative inotropic effect).[1]

Factors that modify contractility (Table 8–4) do so at any amount of preload; that is, they act independently of Starling's law. The greatest determinant for contractility is the amount of norepinephrine released by sympathetic nerve endings in the heart, which serves to stimulate cardiac β-adrenergic receptors. Norepinephrine release is decreased by a negative feedback mechanism whereby prejunctional α-adrenergic receptors are stimulated by norepinephrine. The prejunctional α-adrenergic receptors then turn off norepinephrine release. Therefore, the effects of α-adrenergic blockade are similar to those of exercise-induced norepinephrine stimulation. Epinephrine released from the adrenal medulla and carried by the

Table 8–4
Factors That Control Contractility

Sympathetic nervous system activity
Circulating catecholamines
Force-frequency relation
Exogenous inotropic agents
Physiologic and pharmacologic depressants
Loss of contractile mass
Intrinsic myocardial depression

blood stream to the myocardium also augments contractility through stimulation of β-receptors.[1]

Another physiologic mechanism for increasing contractility in the intact ventricle is the interval-strength relation. This refers to the increased contractility manifested in the interval after a premature depolarization. The premature depolarization itself diminishes ventricular contraction, but the beat that follows the pause is more forceful than normal, a phenomenon called "postextrasystolic potentiation."[1] Contractility is also increased, within limits, as the heart rate is increased. This response is called the force-frequency relation, and it arises because an increased frequency of depolarization allows more intracellular Ca^{++} to be available to contractile proteins.[1]

Exogenous inotropic agents include the cardiac glycosides, sympathomimetic agents, caffeine, theophylline, amrinone, and their derivatives. Changes in the level of ionized calcium in the blood also affects contractility. Physiologic and pharmacologic depressants of contractility include anoxia, ischemia, acidosis, local anesthetics, most barbiturates, and general anesthesia. Loss of contractile mass, as occurs in people with ischemic heart disease, can reduce the overall performance of the myocardium. Lastly, congestive heart failure leads to a depression of contractility through an unknown mechanism.[1]

Heart Rate

Heart rate is a major determinant of cardiac output, especially during exercise, but an elevated heart rate can have detrimental effects in heart failure and during tachyarrhythmias. In exercise-induced tachycardia, the speed of ventricular contraction and relaxation are markedly augmented, atrial contraction is enhanced, and venous return is increased in spite of shortened diastolic filling time. These factors combine to increase cardiac output in exercise. With tachyarrhythmias, diastole is shortened and there is interference with ventricular filling, thereby lowering cardiac output. Chronically elevated heart rates in heart failure put a double strain on the heart: myocardial oxygen demand increases, and diastolic filling time shortens, decreasing coronary blood flow to the myocardium.[1]

Abnormalities in Relaxation

Abnormalities in relaxation, or diastolic dysfunction, are being increasingly recognized as important mechanisms of congestive heart failure. Systolic function is normal, but a stiff, noncompliant ventricle, caused by hypertrophy, fibrosis, or pericardial restraint, is not able to relax and fill properly. End-diastolic pressures rise, and backward failure ensues.[2, 4]

Neural Control of Cardiac Function

In the basal state, sympathetic activity is low and parasympathetic restraint predominates. This is why β-adrenergic blockade has little effect on SA automaticity or A-V nodal conduction at rest but atropine increases heart rate and accelerates A-V nodal conduction.[1] Alternatively, β-blockers can limit the amount of tachycardia during exercise without affecting the heart at rest. Increasing the heart rate by stimulation of cardiac adrenoceptors provides the most rapid control of the heart and blood vessels to accommodate the elevated metabolic needs during exercise. This is similar to the response seen in heart failure. But what is a good adaptive change in an exercising animal is detrimental to the heart on a chronic basis.

Pathophysiology of Heart Failure

Traditionally, congestive heart failure was considered to be a disorder in which the heart was unable to adequately pump blood to meet the needs of the body. Treatment regimens were aimed at assisting myocardial function with digitalis and removing excess fluid with diuretics. Symptoms were relieved, but nothing was done to slow progression of the primary heart problem or to protect the heart from further damage. It is now known that disorders of the neurohumoral system play as important a role as specific myocardial abnormalities, and they may have a greater influence on the progression of heart failure than damage to the heart muscle does. Compensatory mechanisms such as vasoconstriction and sodium and water retention, which support the heart in the early stages of cardiac disease, exert adverse effects when the myocardium fails.[5–7]

It is important to differentiate between heart failure and myocardial failure. *Heart failure,* a general term, denotes any abnormality in tissue perfusion or fluid buildup that results from any heart problem. It may involve the muscle, valves, or pericardium and endocardium. *Myocardial failure,* a more specific term, describes systolic failure of one or both ventricles, which occurs as a result of primary myocardial disease or secondary to a chronic overload that has damaged the ventricular muscle. Because myocardial failure progresses in a downward spiral to death, the goal of therapy is to stave off myocardial failure as long as possible, not just to relieve symptoms of heart failure.

Recent research has centered on the effect of the neurohumoral system and how compensatory mechanisms in later stages of cardiac disease actually accelerate heart failure and death. What starts as support for the heart and circulation turns into a system that places increasingly heavy burdens on an

Table 8-5
Causes of Heart Failure

Volume overload
  Mitral or tricuspid regurgitation
  Patent ductus arteriosus
  Ventricular septal defect
  Hyperthryoidism
Pressure overload
  Subaortic stenosis
  Hypertrophic obstructive cardiomyopathy
  Pulmonic stenosis
  Hypertension
  Heartworm disease
Restricted filling
  Hypertrophic cardiomyopathy (nonobstructed)
  Restrictive cardiomyopathy
  Pericardial effusion
Decreased myocardial contractility
  Dilated cardiomyopathy
Loss of muscle
  Myocardial infarction

already weakened and failing myocardium.[5–9] Clinicians should be familiar with the circulatory abnormalities known to occur in heart failure, so that they can select the best drugs to control abnormal humoral mechanisms and take advantage of new therapies as they are developed.

A number of conditions contribute to heart failure (Table 8–5). Because most cardiac abnormalities in small animals occur secondary to volume overload with or without myocardial failure, this condition is used as the model for discussion of the pathophysiology of congestive heart failure. Other conditions are covered in their respective chapters.

Compensatory Mechanisms

Volume overload of the ventricles activates both hemodynamic and neurohormonal mechanisms to enhance cardiac performance. First, the heart responds to increased volume (preload) by increasing contractility (Frank-Starling law). This maintains cardiac output for awhile, even in the presence of low-pressure run-off (e.g., mitral regurgitation). Then, after the regurgitant fraction becomes so high that aortic flow is reduced, baroreceptors (pressure receptors) in the aortic arch and carotid sinus stimulate the sympathetic nervous system. In turn, β-adrenergic receptors in the myocardium increase both the force and the rate of contraction in order to overcome loss of outflow through the mitral valve. The ventricular dilatation and peripheral vascular constriction (elevated afterload) thus produced increase internal wall stress in

diastole. The heart expends more energy, especially if the sympathetic nervous system also causes a resting tachycardia.[5, 7]

Several reactions regulate the ventricular response and sympathetic activation. The increase in wall stress induces ventricular hypertrophy by triggering synthesis of myofibrillar proteins. According to the law of Laplace, this hypertrophy should relieve wall stress, thereby reducing oxygen consumption. In addition, high atrial end-diastolic pressure increases atrial wall stress. Atrial stretch receptors that inhibit sympathetic flow and cause secretion of atrial natriuretic peptide are activated. Atrial natriuretic peptide inhibits the release of norepinephrine and exerts direct vasodilating and natriuretic effects, both of which reduce the hemodynamic load on the heart.[5, 7]

Loss of Compensatory Mechanisms

In the presence of severe, chronic overloads, compensatory mechanisms are unable to offset the effects of a stretched myocardium and an excessive blood volume. Prolonged ventricular dilation causes microscopic intramural myocardial infarcts, which limit the heart's ability to undergo hypertrophy in response to stress. Atrial distention damages atrial receptor endings, reducing their ability to inhibit sympathetic outflow. Atrial dilatation also depletes atrial natriuretic peptide. With these losses, ventricular dilatation progresses, and the sympathetic nervous system persistently overreacts.[5]

Loss of Contractility

After chronic volume overload causes maximally elevated preload, the failing heart loses its ability to contract adequately. Sarcomeres have become stretched to their limits, and preload reserve is nonexistent. Also, the heart no longer responds to the positive inotropic effects of catecholamines through downregulation (lowering the number of receptors) and uncoupling (interference with attachment of catecholamines to receptors) of β-receptors in the myocardium. The heart becomes unable to overcome increases in peripheral resistance (afterload) from higher sympathetic output and α-adrenergic stimuli in peripheral vessels. Systolic function cannot be maintained, and cardiac output declines further. With loss of systolic function, filling pressures also decrease more, and a vicious circle is in place.

Neurohumoral Activation

The main contributors to neurohumoral activation are listed in Table 8–6. Early in heart failure, compensatory mechanisms support cardiac performance;

Table 8–6
Neurohumoral Contributors to Congestive Heart Failure

Renin-angiotensin-aldosterone system
Sympathetic nervous system
Atrial natriuretic peptide
Arginine vasopressin

later, the focus is on maintaining perfusion. If cardiac output falls, perfusion pressure is maintained by vasoconstriction and sodium retention. Sympathetic stimulation occurs early in heart failure; the other two main mechanisms, renin-angiotensin-aldosterone system and vasopressin, are triggered later.[10] The renin-angiotensin-aldosterone system is usually activated by the time clinical signs develop; it leads to production of both circulating and local angiotensin II. Angiotensin II not only acts as a powerful vasoconstrictor but also increases sodium and water retention, both directly and by stimulation of aldosterone production. Vasopressin (antidiuretic hormone) is released primarily in the terminal stages of heart failure and causes even more sodium and water retention, along with vasoconstriction. Current research has revealed additional local vasoconstrictors (e.g., endothelin) and their antagonists (e.g., endothelium-derived relaxing factor), produced by the vascular endothelium, that may play a role in this process. However, in heart failure the actions of circulating and locally acting vasodilators are attenuated. Vasoconstriction keeps increasing from angiotensin II, which enhances the release of norepinephrine, which in turn stimulates the renin-angiotensin-aldosterone system so that more angiotensin II is released, and so on.[5]

Retention of sodium and water occurs by different mechanisms and has several adverse effects. Angiotensin II causes sodium resorption in the proximal renal tubules through aldosterone release. Water intake increases from stimulation of thirst centers (angiotensin), and water excretion decreases from the effects of vasopressin on the kidneys. Salt retention and edema thicken vascular walls and cause pressure on vessels by perivascular swelling, exacerbating vasoconstriction.[5]

End-Stage Heart Failure

Many cardiac therapies in veterinary medicine (e.g., digitalis, diuretics) do not correct the underlying problem but only attempt to relieve symptoms. Consequently, myocardial cells gradually undergo necrosis, and ventricular function continues to deteriorate.

Unabated increases in wall stress cause irreversible structural remodeling, augmented energy expenditure, and decreased coronary perfusion. Furthermore, high concentrations of norepinephrine and angiotensin II probably exert direct toxic effects on myocardial cells.[5] Death ensues when therapy can no longer control heart failure, when there is failure of other organs such as the kidneys, or suddenly as a result of a fatal arrhythmia.

Types of Heart Failure

Volume overload can occur with a number of heart disorders. There are several ways to interpret the heart's response to specific diseases. Understanding these responses provides a broadened concept of heart disease and aids selection of appropriate treatment. It also helps in understanding and anticipating the development of heart problems from specific diseases.

Forward Versus Backward Failure

Although these terms seem to differentiate two kinds of heart failure, they represent two sides of the same coin. Forward failure denotes a decrease in cardiac output, usually with myocardial failure and increased afterload. The primary symptoms, such as muscle weakness, come from diminished tissue perfusion rather than from hypoxia secondary to pulmonary edema and congestion. The animal may even be dyspneic but lacks radiographic signs of congestion. In backward failure, an overloaded ventricle backs up blood into the atrium, which cannot handle the load. Fluid backs up farther into the lungs or the abdominal cavity. In reality, both types of failure usually coexist in most cases of chronic heart failure.[4] Dilated cardiomyopathy is one disorder that causes both forward and backward failure.

Right-Sided Versus Left-Sided Failure

The question of right-sided versus left-sided failure pertains to the symptoms that occur when one side of the heart fails. Most heart diseases in dogs cause left-sided heart failure first; if they persist long enough, fluid can back up through the lungs to affect the right side of the heart as well. Some diseases affect both cardiac chambers (e.g., cardiomyopathy); others affect only the right ventricle (e.g., heartworm disease). Also, neurohumoral activity in response to failure of one ventricle influences the other. In addition, the chambers connect in their function through a common structure, the interventricular septum, so that what happens to one ventricle affects the other.[4]

Low-Output Versus High-Output Failure

Low cardiac output characterizes most types of cardiac disease and leads to neurohumoral stimulation. Low-output failure is almost synonymous with forward failure, but it can also cause backward failure. If a weak ventricle (i.e., dilated cardiomyopathy) is unable to pump blood forward, the blood backs up as fluid into the lungs and abdomen. In high-output heart disease, cardiac output (forward flow) is maintained, but there are varying degrees of backward failure and congestive symptoms. This is because high-output heart disease results from noncardiac conditions that increase total body fluid volume and metabolism. The heart at maximum function cannot adequately pump forward all of the blood that is delivered to it. Thyrotoxicosis and anemia are two diseases that cause high-output failure.[4]

Systolic Versus Diastolic Failure

The most common perception is that heart failure is synonymous with systolic failure. But it is commonly recognized now that diastolic abnormalities occur early in heart failure,[2] whereas systolic dysfunction is more of an end-stage event. These two types of heart failure are easily differentiated on echocardiography. Systolic failure is identified as a low shortening fraction (diminished contractility) with M-mode echocardiography, but animals with diastolic failure have a normal shortening fraction while exhibiting congestive heart failure.[2, 4] The paradigm for systolic failure is

dilated cardiomyopathy, whereas diastolic dysfunction is seen with hypertrophic cardiomyopathy.

References

1. Braunwald E, Sonnenblick EH, Ross J. Mechanisms of cardiac contraction and relaxation. In: Braunwald E, ed. Heart Disease. Philadelphia, WB Saunders, 1992:351–392.
2. Bonow RO, Udelson JE. Left ventricular diastolic dysfunction as a cause of congestive heart failure. Ann Intern Med 1992;117:502–510.
3. Guyton AC. Textbook of Medical Physiology, 8th ed. Philadelphia, WB Saunders, 1991.
4. Braunwald E, Grossman W. Clinical aspects of heart failure. In: Braunwald E, ed. Heart Disease. Philadelphia, WB Saunders, 1992:444–463.
5. Packer M. Pathophysiology of chronic heart failure. Lancet 1992;340:88–92.
6. Packer M. How should physicians view heart failure? The philosophical and physiological evolution of three conceptual models of the disease. Am J Cardiol 1993;71: 3C–11C.
7. Mancia G. Neurohumoral activation in congestive heart failure. Am Heart J 1990;120:1532–1537.
8. Francis G. Heart failure in 1991. Cardiology 1991; 78:81–94.
9. Parmley WW. Pathophysiology of congestive heart failure. Clin Cardiol 1992;15(Suppl. I):I5–I12.
10. Knowlen GG, Kittleson MD, Nachreiner RF, Eyster GE. Comparison of plasma aldosterone concentrations among clinical status groups of dogs with chronic heart failure. J Am Vet Med Assoc 1983;183:991–996.

Chapter 9

Clinical Approach to Heart Disease

Betsy R. Bond

With all the equipment available to veterinarians, especially on a referral basis, it is easy to rely on technology rather than on the most important diagnostic tools available: the history and physical examination. Good listening skills, auscultation, palpation, and observation are becoming lost arts. A diagnosis can frequently be made in the examination room. Radiography, electrocardiography (ECG), and echocardiography should be used to confirm or refute a suspected diagnosis, monitor progression of disease, and guide therapy. This chapter emphasizes parts of the history and physical examination that are important in diagnosing heart disease. The six most important problems are discussed first.

Problem Identification

Cough

A cough is an explosive expiration of air that clears the air passages of secretions and foreign material.[1] It is the most common cardiac symptom in dogs but a rare one in cats, in which it usually indicates respiratory disease. A cardiac cough results from backup of blood from the left atrium into the pulmonary veins or the alveoli (pulmonary edema). An enlarged heart that compresses the mainstem bronchi also causes coughing.

Pathophysiology

Pulmonary edema is divided into cardiogenic and noncardiogenic causes[2, 3] (Table 9–1). Noncardiogenic edema originates from injury to the alveolar-capillary membrane between the vessels and the pulmonary interstitium and alveoli. Because the permeability defect allows both water and solutes to escape vessels, noncardiogenic edema is more like plasma than what is found in cardiogenic edema.[3] Most edema is cardiogenic, caused by increased pulmonary capillary hydrostatic pressure secondary to increased left atrial pressure.[3, 4] Elevated pulmonary venous pressure can occur with or without left ventricle failure. Edema in early mitral regurgitation, mitral stenosis, and hypertrophic and restrictive cardiomyopathies are usually formed with normal left ventricular systolic function. In dilated cardiomyopathy or chronic heart failure, left ventricular failure contributes to the edema.

There are three stages of edema, representing the location of fluid accumulation in the lungs. There is normally a small amount of liquid and colloid that moves from the vessels to the interstitial space, where it is picked up by lymphatics and pumped into systemic veins. In stage 1, an increased amount of liquid and colloid is transferred through the interstitium to the lymphatics. Lymphatic flow is increased so that there is very little accumulation of fluid. The only symptom is mild exertional dyspnea.[2] In stage 2, edema fluid accumulates in the interstitium around the bronchi and alveoli, and there is a loss of radiographic definition of pulmonary vascular markings. There may also be reflex bronchoconstriction. Animals become tachypneic and cough, both of which augment the pumping action of the lymphatics. Stage 3 represents alveolar flooding, which shows the typical air bronchogram on radiographs.[2] Dogs and cats are usually moderately dyspneic and require emergency therapy.

Clinical Signs

A cough is the most common cardiac and respiratory symptom in dogs. Because small-breed dogs are prone to both mitral regurgitation and collapsing tra-

Table 9–1
Classification of Causes of Pulmonary Edema

Imbalance of Starling Forces
  Increased pulmonary venous pressure (left-sided heart failure)
  Decreased plasma oncotic pressure (hypoalbuminemia)
  Increased negativity of interstitial pressure
    Rapid removal of large pleural effusion or pneumothorax
    Large negative pleural pressures resulting from acute airway obstruction

Altered Alveolar-Capillary Membrane Permeability
  Infectious pneumonia
  Inhaled toxins (e.g., smoke)
  Circulating foreign substances (e.g., snake venom, bacterial endotoxins)
  Aspiration of acidic gastric contents
  Endogenous vasoactive substances (e.g., kinins)
  Disseminated intravascular coagulopathy
  Immunologic or hypersensitivity pneumonitis, drugs
  Acute hemorrhagic pancreatitis

Lymphatic Insufficiency
  Lymphangitic carcinomatosis

Unknown or Incompletely Understood Causes
  High-altitude pulmonary edema
  Neurogenic pulmonary edema
  Narcotic overdose
  Pulmonary embolism
  Eclampsia
  Postcardioversion
  Postanesthesia

From Ingram RH, Braunwald E. Pulmonary edema: Cardiogenic and noncardiogenic. In: Braunwald E, ed. Heart Disease. Philadelphia, WB Saunders, 1992:556.

Table 9–2
Differential Cough History Between Heart and Pulmonary Disease

ITEM	HEART DISEASE	PULMONARY DISEASE
Duration	Weeks to months	Months to years
Progression	Progresses rapidly	Relatively stable
Exercise intolerance	Present	Absent
Body type	Normal to thin	Obese
Type of cough	Moist	Dry, hacking

cheas or chronic obstructive pulmonary disease, determining the current cause of a cough is often difficult. Questioning the owner about the duration of the cough and its quality, progression, and response to medication is extremely helpful (Table 9–2).

One consideration in the history is the duration of the cough. A cough associated with a cardiac problem that goes untreated for more than a few weeks usually ends in death, whereas a cough of pulmonary origin can last for years. Coughing caused by pulmonary disease, although it may wax and wane, tends to be relatively consistent over time, but a cough from cardiac disease progressively worsens. However, a new cardiac cough may be superimposed over a long-standing pulmonary problem. The fact that a dog has had tracheal collapse for years does not eliminate heart failure as a current cause of the cough.

Response to medication also gives a clue to the underlying problem. Because small-breed dogs can have concomitant pulmonary and heart disease, and because both conditions cause cardiomegaly, veterinarians often treat coughing dogs with a diuretic or other cardiac medication, presuming that heart failure is present. A dog that has been treated for heart failure for more than a few weeks with no improvement of symptoms probably has respiratory disease. However, the converse is not necessarily true. Dogs with chronic obstructive pulmonary disease and collapsing tracheas respond poorly to medications, even if appropriate, and dogs with respiratory disease occasionally have a good short-term response to diuretics. This positive response possibly occurs because of edema caused by marked negative intrathoracic pressure.[5]

The character of the cough is also important. A dry, hacking, "honking" cough is usually heard with collapsing tracheas. Although cardiac disease may also cause a dry cough, especially early in disease progression, it more commonly causes a moist cough from pulmonary edema. A moist cough may also result from other respiratory problems, such as pneumonia.

A nocturnal cough may be heard in the early stages of heart failure. As a dog lies down to sleep, venous pooling causes pulmonary congestion that is absent when the dog is sitting up or walking. The owner may report that the dog wakes up in the middle of the night and paces and coughs before it is able to go back to sleep.

Symptoms such as lethargy and anorexia frequently accompany heart problems, whereas normal activity and appetite usually occur with chronic obstructive pulmonary disease and collapsing tracheas. Exercise initiates symptoms with both cardiac and pulmonary abnormalities, but drinking of water usually causes a cough only in dogs with collapsing tracheas.

Auscultation should reveal a murmur in dogs with heart failure unless the crackles are so loud they obscure it. Cats usually have a murmur or a gallop, but they can have significant heart disease without either sign. Most dogs and cats in left-sided heart failure have strong pulses unless they have dilated cardiomyopathy or myocardial failure from long-standing disease. Palpation of the chest may reveal a more prominent apex beat, indicating hypertrophy.

Lung sounds are similar in cardiac disease and respiratory disease,[4] although the location of crackles is occasionally significant. Dogs in heart failure may have dorsal and caudal crackles, or popping sounds, whereas dogs with respiratory disease can have crackles anywhere. In severe heart failure, crackles are heard in all lung fields. Listening over the trachea during a coughing fit may reveal the snap of a collapsing trachea.

Diagnostic Plan

Even with a suspected diagnosis based on history (i.e., presence or absence of heart murmur, length and severity of cough), a thoracic radiograph is the clinician's most important diagnostic tool. Location of infiltrates is a key to the cause of cough in dogs, because cardiogenic edema is usually located in the hilar region rather than in the ventral lung fields. Pulmonary edema in cats can be located anywhere, and it can even be diffuse and patchy. An enlarged left atrium is usually present in dogs and cats with heart disease. Right ventricular enlargement with an interstitial pattern is usually present in dogs with respiratory disease, whereas cats have a bronchial pattern and no cardiac enlargement. If caught at the appropriate part of the respiratory cycle, a collapsing trachea may be seen on thoracic radiography, although fluoroscopy may be necessary for definitive diagnosis. Dogs and cats coughing from heartworm disease have enlarged pulmonary arteries, and dogs can have an enlarged right ventricle. Pulmonary neoplasia causes an interstitial rather than an alveolar pattern.

ECGs in patients without cardiac disease should be normal, whereas arrhythmias and evidence of chamber enlargement are present in dogs and cats with cardiac disease. Echocardiograms reveal thickened valves, dilated atria and ventricles, and sometimes dilated aortas and pulmonary arteries in animals with heart disease.

A complete blood count is helpful in diagnosing animals with a cough caused by infection (leukocytosis), heartworm disease (eosinophilia and basophilia), or asthma (eosinophilia). Knott's test or immunologic tests for *Dirofilaria immitis* (or both) should be performed in all dogs with coughing of unknown cause. A tracheal aspirate may also be helpful if the cause of an infiltrate is not obvious.

Dyspnea

Dyspnea is an increase in the work required for respiration.[6] Owners describe dyspnea as "trouble breathing," "breathing with the abdomen," and "pumping of the chest." It is the second most common symptom of heart disease in dogs and is one of the most common symptoms (along with anorexia and lethargy) in cats.

Pathophysiology

Dyspnea usually results from pulmonary edema or pleural effusion but may be associated with upper airway obstruction (see Chaps. 52, 53, and 54). Pulmonary edema is associated with left-sided heart failure in both dogs and cats. Pleural effusion is caused by right-sided heart disease in dogs but is a less common sign than ascites. Pleural effusion in cats is caused by right- or left-sided heart failure and is much more common than ascites, which is rare.

The vital capacity of the lungs is reduced because of replacement of air by fluid or because of lung compression from pleural effusion. Pulmonary edema also severely impairs lung compliance, so that higher intrapleural pressure is required to expand the lungs. Engorgement of blood vessels also puts pressure on the smaller airways, increasing airway resistance.[4, 6]

Clinical Signs

Dyspnea is the most common symptom of heart failure in cats, and it is usually accompanied by lethargy and anorexia. Occasionally, a dog in heart failure presents with dyspnea alone, but it is usually accompanied by coughing. Heavy breathing along with coughing means a higher likelihood of cardiac problems as opposed to respiratory disease, for which coughing is usually the only symptom. Dyspnea may be nocturnal, and as edema worsens the dog may not be able to lie down comfortably at all (orthopnea).[4]

Dyspneic animals appear in obvious distress and frequently have the elbows abducted and the head and neck extended. Mucous membranes are cyanotic, and if the dyspnea is caused by edema there may be pink, frothy fluid dripping from the nostrils. Dyspneic cats prefer sternal recumbence, whereas dogs will sit or stand. Neither animal is comfortable in lateral recumbence.[4] Cats should be observed for dyspnea in the carrier before they are examined. Some cats develop open-mouth breathing from the stress of the hospital visit, and owners should be asked whether this is the respiratory pattern seen at home or a new development.

Auscultation of animals that are dyspneic because of pulmonary edema reveals crackles, wheezes, and increased bronchovesicular sounds primarily in the dorsal lung fields, although severe edema is generalized. Crackles are popping sounds that resemble the wadding of stiff plastic wrap. Wheezes are high-pitched sounds that occur during prolonged expiration and result from air being pushed out through compromised small airways. Increased bronchovesicular sounds are louder than normal lung sounds. Animals that are dyspneic from pleural effusion have decreased heart and lung sounds, especially ventrally. The fluid level can often be found by careful auscultation or percussion.

Dogs that are dyspneic secondary to pleural effusion from right-sided heart failure should have a murmur that is loudest over the tricuspid valve area. The murmur in dogs with left-sided heart failure and pulmonary edema is on the left, over the mitral valve area. The murmur in cats is ventral, but a murmur may not be auscultated in some cats with heart disease.

Diagnostic Plan

Often, diagnostic tests must be postponed because of the stress they represent to a dyspneic animal. However, thoracentesis in a dyspneic animal withpleural effusion is both diagnostic and therapeutic. As much fluid as possible should be withdrawn, and a sample should be submitted for cytologic analysis unless the diagnosis is already known. Both sides of the chest should be aspirated. Some fractious or anxious animals require sedation for successful thoracentesis. Although tranquilization carries some risk, it is less risky than tapping the chest of a moving animal (see Chap. 53). Thoracentesis of dyspneic animals with crackles is not recommended because of the high risk of pneumothorax. A balance needs to be maintained between tapping every dyspneic animal and never tapping. A good, quick auscultation should differentiate those animals that need thoracentesis from those that need oxygen and medical therapy.

Chest radiographs should be taken as soon as the animal is stable and examined for an enlarged cardiac silhouette, pleural fluid, or masses. Animals with pleural effusion should undergo echocardiography before thoracentesis, if possible, because fluid is a more compatible medium for ultrasound waves than is air, and it allows better visualization of the heart and other intrathoracic structures.

ECGs may be normal, even in animals with pleural effusion secondary to heart disease. Dogs in right-sided heart failure may have an axis deviation or arrhythmias, but cats can have pleural effusion caused by both right- and left-sided heart failure, so the ECG is more variable.

Echocardiography is superior to radiography in animals with pleural effusions. It reveals masses and other intrathoracic abnormalities hidden on radiographs. Echocardiography can also show right ventricular enlargement in dogs and cats with right-sided heart failure secondary to tricuspid regurgitation.

A complete blood count should be performed for the same reasons as in animals with cough. A biochemical profile and urinalysis reveal any metabolic abnormalities that may be related to heart failure, such as prerenal azotemia.

Exercise Intolerance

Exercise intolerance (fatigue, weakness) is usually reported along with other symptoms of heart failure and consists of an inability to complete a walk or perform normal activities. Animals may prefer recumbence, be reluctant to rise and walk, or simply stop in the middle of a walk or play to rest. They may or may not exhibit dyspnea.

Pathophysiology

Weakness and exercise intolerance can result from cardiac, orthopedic, neurologic, or metabolic abnormalities (Table 9–3). Animals with congestive heart failure may become fatigued for two reasons. The first is that with backward heart failure (see Chap. 8), pulmonary edema decreases the lung's ability to oxygenate, and exercise is shortened by hypoxemia. Pleural effusion decreases vital capacity of the lungs, again making it harder for oxygenation to occur. Dogs

Table 9–3
Common Categories of Causes of Weakness in Small Animals

Anemia
Ascites
Cardiovascular signs
Chronic inflammation and infection
   Tick-borne diseases
   Feline leukemia virus
   Feline immunodeficiency virus
Chronic wasting diseases
   Neoplasia
   Hyperthyroidism
Drug-related weakness
   Vasodilators
   Digoxin
Electrolyte disorders
   Hypokalemia
Endocrine disturbances
   Hypothyroidism
   Apathetic hyperthyroidism
   Diabetes mellitus
   Hyperadrenocorticism
   Hypoadrenocorticism
Fever
Metabolic dysfunction states
   Chronic renal failure
   Liver disease
   Hypoglycemia
Neoplasia
Neurologic disorders
   Diseases of the spinal cord
   Brain tumors
Neuromuscular diseases and polyneuropathies
Nutritional disorders
Overactivity
Psychological factors
Pulmonary diseases

Modified from Ettinger SJ. Weakness and syncope. In: Ettinger SJ, ed. Textbook of Veterinary Internal Medicine, 3rd ed. Philadelphia, WB Saunders, 1989:47.

usually develop pulmonary edema in left-sided heart failure; cats develop both pleural effusion and pulmonary edema. The second reason for weakness in congestive heart failure is poor perfusion of skeletal muscles,[6] which is caused by poor myocardial function, persistent tachyarrhythmias or bradyarrhythmias, outflow obstructions, pericardial effusions, or hypotension. In forward failure (see Chap. 8), cardiac output is so low that needed oxygen cannot be delivered to the muscles.

Poor myocardial function, or systolic failure, occurs in dilated cardiomyopathy of dogs and cats and in cases of long-standing volume overload to the left ventricle. The heart fails to deliver oxygen because of pump failure.

Arrhythmias cause low cardiac output by either decreasing stroke volume (tachyarrhythmias) or slowing heart rate. Bradyarrhythmias cause the heart to fill normally, but it does not pump a sufficient number of beats per minute. Tachyarrhythmias shorten diastole, so there is inadequate ventricular filling for normal stroke volume. Dogs generally require a heart rate of about 60 to 180 beats per minute, and cats a heart rate of 100 to 240 beats per minute, to maintain cardiac output at rest. Factors that affect the decreased cardiac output in arrhythmias include the ventricular rate, the duration of the abnormal rate, the relation of ventricular filling to atrial contraction, the sequence of ventricular activation, the status of the myocardium, the amount of rhythm irregularity, and associated cardiac drug therapies.[7]

Outflow obstructions, such as aortic or pulmonary stenosis or hypertrophic obstructive cardiomyopathy, block blood flow out of the heart and do not allow enough increase in stroke volume during exercise or stress to maintain cardiac output.

Pericardial effusions block venous return, which decreases ventricular filling so that there is insufficient volume to maintain stroke volume.

Hypotension also decreases venous return and filling pressures, so that cardiac output is difficult to preserve. A common cause of hypotension is overzealous use of diuretics and vasodilators.[6]

Clinical Signs

The owner usually reports that the dog or cat wants to sleep more, is reluctant to move around, or asks to be carried back from its walk. Strength in the front legs with stiffness or weakness in the rear usually indicates a neurologic or orthopedic problem, whereas generalized weakness is caused by metabolic, cardiac, and some neurologic conditions. Dogs with arthritis usually walk more easily as they warm up, whereas dogs with heart failure have greater fatigue as they exercise.

Weight loss, especially with abdominal distention (ascites), is common in right-sided heart failure in dogs and may accompany weakness. Severe weight loss from a heart problem is known as cardiac cachexia. It represents an end stage of heart disease and is seen with the most severe forms (e.g., canine dilated cardiomyopathy and long-standing atrioventricular [A-V] valvular disease). Cats with hyperthyroidism may have severe weight loss, and they can be weak from an "apathetic" form of hyperthyroidism.[8]

Murmurs, gallops, and tachycardia or severe bradycardia should also be present in weak animals with heart disease. These animals may be dyspneic and have crackles from pulmonary edema or muffled lung sounds from pleural effusion. Pulses are normal in early mitral regurgitation but become weaker with advanced disease or myocardial failure. Animals weak from myocardial failure have low body temperature, pallor, poor capillary refill time, weak pulses, and a weak apex beat.

Diagnostic Plan

Many of the conditions listed in Table 9–3 can be identified on physical examination—for example, ascites and neoplasia by abdominal palpation, cardiovascular disease by the presence of murmur or gallop, and a fever by rectal temperature. Some diseases are eliminated by simple tests such as a determination of packed cell volume for anemia. The history clarifies the presence of drug-related weakness, nutritional disorders, overactivity, or psychological factors. A complete blood count, biochemical profile, and urinalysis can identify electrolyte abnormalities, metabolic diseases, and inflammation. Titers for Rocky Mountain spotted fever, *Ehrlichia canis*, or Lyme disease are helpful in dogs with chronic inflammation. Specialized endocrine tests (i.e., thyroid-stimulating hormone, adrenocorticotropic hormone) help diagnose endocrine abnormalities.

Thoracic radiography helps differentiate pulmonary from cardiac disease and may be the only test to reveal neoplasia. Abdominal radiography can reveal a mass that was not palpated, and abdominal ultrasound may detect a mass not seen on radiographs. If an arrhythmia is causing the weakness, it should easily be found on a routine ECG. If no arrhythmias are found and other tests are normal, use of a 24-hour Holter monitor may be necessary (see Syncope). Patients without these findings should have a complete neurologic examination. Abnormalities of the cranial nerves, postural reactions, segmental reflexes, or gait indicate neuromuscular disease and should be pursued.

Syncope

Syncope is loss of consciousness as a result of deprivation of oxygen to the brain. In cardiac patients, it is related to cessation of blood flow to the cerebrum. It is often difficult to distinguish between syncope, seizures, and episodic weakness.[9]

Pathophysiology

Cardiac syncope usually results from arrhythmias, myocardial dysfunction, or obstruction to blood flow,[9] although it can occur in animals that are in left-sided heart failure during excitement or exercise. Tachyarrhythmias, bradyarrhythmias, or loss of atrial contraction can decrease cardiac output enough to cause syncope. Tachyarrhythmias and bradyarrhythmias are usually episodic, whereas persistent atrial arrhythmias and heart failure cause syncope related to exercise intolerance.

Obstruction to blood flow from the heart is caused by outflow obstructions, ball thrombi, and pericardial disease. Outflow obstructions may be fixed or dynamic. During exercise, more oxygen is needed and systemic resistance drops, but the obstruction prevents cardiac output from meeting the demand. Perfusion is decreased because of low systemic resistance, and syncope occurs.[9] Aortic stenosis and pulmonary stenosis are examples of fixed outflow obstructions. In aortic stenosis, a fibrous ring keeps the outflow tract the same size, so the obstruction remains the same throughout systole. A dynamic outflow obstruction occurs in hypertrophic cardiomyopathy, in which the mitral valve is either pulled or pushed into the left ventricular outflow tract in systole. Obstruction increases throughout systole, with the maximum occurring after midsystole.[10, 11]

A ball thrombus in the atrium acts as a pop-off valve in the mitral annulus. Flow to the ventricle is suddenly stopped, and cardiac output drops to zero. Pericardial disease impedes diastolic filling, which decreases cardiac output and causes syncope with stress or excitement.[9] Animals with pulmonary edema become hypoxic and faint secondary to hypoxemia. They may take longer to recover than animals with arrhythmia-induced syncope.

Other related dysfunctions also cause syncope (Table 9–4). "Cough drop," not related to heart failure, is common and occurs when strenuous coughing precedes syncope. Several mechanisms are involved, including acute reduction in cardiac output and increased intracranial pressure transmitted from the thorax through the cerebrospinal fluid. Vasovagal syncope is more commonly recognized in humans than in animals, but it probably does occur. It is associated with fear or excitement and results from a high level of sympathetic activity followed by paradoxical hypotension and, occasionally, bradycardia.

Clinical Signs

Syncope is a confusing symptom of heart disease, because it is easily mistaken for other problems. Seizures are particularly difficult to differentiate from cardiac syncope, but certain points of the history are helpful. Cardiac syncope is a sudden event that is over quickly and leaves no residual effects. Seizures usually have premonitory symptoms and leave the animal dazed for a period of time (postictal period). Autonomic release (urinating and defecating) is usually seen with seizures but occurs uncommonly with syncope. Paddling, frothing at the mouth, and opis-

Table 9–4
Common Causes of Cardiovascular and Cardiopulmonary Syncope

Peripheral vascular or neurologic dysfunction with normal heart
  Vasovagal
Cardiovascular dysfunction
  Intracardiac obstruction to blood flow
    Aortic stenosis
    Pulmonic stenosis
    Ball thrombus
    Hypertrophic obstructive cardiomyopathy
  Extracardiac obstruction to blood flow
    Cardiac tamponade
    Constrictive pericarditis
    Dirofilariasis
  Arrhythmias
    Tachycardias
    Bradycardias
    Bradycardia-tachycardia (sick sinus) syndrome
    Atrioventricular block (high-grade second-degree, third-degree)
Cardiopulmonary dysfunction
Cough (tussive) syncope
Right-to-left shunt (congenital heart disease)
Pulmonary hypertension
Pulmonary embolism

Modified from Lush RH, Ettinger SJ. Cardiovascular syncope. In: Fox PR, ed. Canine and Feline Cardiology. New York, Churchill Livingstone, 1988:336.

thotonus are common with seizures but not with syncope. If pulmonary edema causes syncope, dogs usually have other symptoms (e.g., cough, dyspnea), and the syncope is initiated by either coughing or excitement. Rarely, however, a dog may faint as the first and only sign of congestive heart failure.

Collapse is similar to syncope, but the animal falls, or almost falls, without losing consciousness. This may occur with arrhythmias, pericardial effusions, neuromuscular disorders, metabolic derangements, anemia, or certain neoplasias (e.g., hemangiosarcoma).[9]

Diagnostic Plan

Outflow obstructions occur in dogs and cats with loud murmurs, usually at the left cranial thorax. Outflow obstructions usually occur in young dogs because of congenital aortic or pulmonary stenosis, and they are confirmed by radiographic and ECG evidence of left- or right-sided heart enlargement, respectively. Pulses are weak in dogs with aortic stenosis but are normal in dogs with pulmonary stenosis. Doppler echocardiography or angiography is required for definitive diagnosis (see Chap. 14).

Outflow obstructions in cats are caused by hypertrophic cardiomyopathy (see Chap. 12). Radiography is nonspecific and is not helpful except to confirm cardiomegaly. Echocardiography is necessary to diagnose hypertrophic obstructive cardiomyopathy. Changes present include a thick ventricle, especially at the base of the septum, and systolic anterior motion of the mitral valve.

Pulmonary edema is diagnosed on thoracic radiography by location of an alveolar infiltrate in the hilar area, which may extend to the dorsocaudal lung lobes. Ball thrombi are seen in cats with severe left atrial enlargement and are easily diagnosed by echocardiography.

Pericardial effusion causing inflow obstruction may often be suspected by detection of muffled heart sounds and may be diagnosed by thoracic radiography; however, echocardiography may be required, because dilated cardiomyopathy also causes cardiomegaly. Dogs with cardiomyopathy should have a murmur, although it is sometimes very soft and may not be auscultated. Dogs with an arrhythmia are more likely to have cardiomyopathy, and poor pulses are present in dogs with cardiomyopathy and pericardial effusion.

D. immitis infection is suspected in dogs that have a cough with right ventricular enlargement and dilated pulmonary arteries. These dogs may also have pulmonary infiltrates on thoracic radiography. A definitive diagnosis is made by a positive Knott's test or enzyme-linked immunosorbent assay (see Chap. 13). Vasovagal syncope is a diagnosis made in sick animals after all other causes have been excluded.

Most arrhythmias are discovered by routine ECG on a lead II rhythm strip. The chances of discovering an arrhythmia causing syncope are increased if the rhythm strip is at least 2 minutes long. If an arrhythmia is not discovered, a 24-hour Holter monitor may be used. The owners should record any syncopal events that they witness, so that these observations can be matched with the Holter results to see whether they correspond to an arrhythmia. It is also important to note the times during which the animal is sleeping, because it is not unusual for the heart rate to drop to 40 beats per minute or less during sleep.

A thorough neurologic examination should be performed if all other tests are inconclusive. Dogs and cats may also be admitted for observation if the episodes occur often.

Murmurs

A murmur is a series of auditory vibrations and may be classified according to intensity (loudness), timing in the cardiac cycle, configuration (shape), and location. The three basic categories of murmurs are systolic, diastolic, and continuous. A systolic murmur occurs after the first heart sound (S_1) and before the second heart sound (S_2). A diastolic murmur begins with or after S_2 and ends before S_1. A continuous murmur begins in systole and continues through all or part of diastole.[12]

Pathophysiology

Murmurs arise because of turbulence of blood, which in turn arises from high blood flow through a small orifice.[13] The most commonly used category, intensity, is based on a six-grade system (Table 9–5). The intensity of a murmur is determined by the quantity and velocity of blood flow across the defect, the distance of the defect from the stethoscope, and the ability of the tissue between the murmur and the stethoscope to transmit sound. Murmurs are louder in thin animals and are diminished in obese animals and in animals with pulmonary disease or with pleural or pericardial fluid. Hyperdynamic hearts accentuate murmurs, whereas murmurs are softer in hearts with myocardial failure.[13] In general, the loudness of the murmur does not indicate the seriousness of the underlying condition, but there are exceptions. For example, because ventricular septal defects cause higher flow rates and therefore more turbulence, a small ventricular septal defect sounds louder than a larger one and carries a more favorable prognosis. A second exception

Table 9–5
Classification of Heart Murmurs

Grade I	Softest murmur, heard only in a quiet room.
Grade II	Soft murmur, heard when the stethoscope is placed on the chest wall; does not radiate.
Grade III	Moderate murmur, easily heard with stethoscope placed on the chest wall; radiates somewhat. Most clinically significant murmurs are at least grade III.
Grade IV	Moderate murmur, radiates over a larger area than grade III.
Grade V	Loud murmur, easily heard over a large area; thrill can be palpated through the chest wall.
Grade VI	Loudest murmur, heard even when the stethoscope is slightly removed from the chest wall.

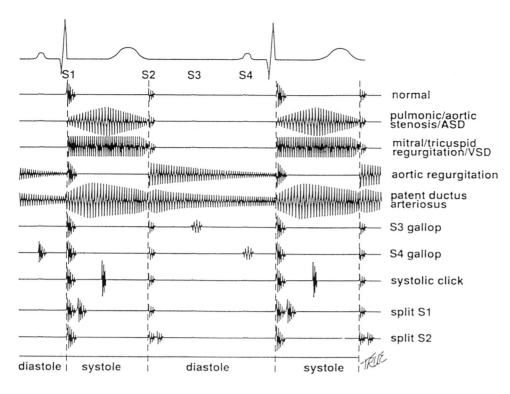

Figure 9–1

Cardiac cycle with electrocardiogram and phonocardiogram schematized. Both normal and abnormal sounds are included. ASD, atrial septal defect; VSD, ventricular septal defect. (From Atkins, CE. Abnormal heart sounds. In: Allen DG, ed. Small Animal Medicine. Philadelphia, JB Lippincott, 1991:198.)

occurs in cats with hypertrophic obstructive cardiomyopathy, because the murmur decreases or disappears as the obstruction decreases with medication.

The timing of a murmur refers to its occurrence in the cardiac cycle (i.e., systolic or diastolic). It is further characterized as holosystolic (i.e., lasting throughout systole) or as an early-, middle-, or late-systolic murmur (Fig. 9–1). Commonly used but confusing terms are regurgitant murmur and systolic ejection murmur. Regurgitant murmur was a term originally applied to murmurs that occurred throughout systole, but the term regurgitation can be applied to systolic murmurs that occur in early, middle, or late systole. The term systolic ejection murmur was originally applied to murmurs that occur in midsystole and included pulmonary stenosis and aortic stenosis. However, midsystolic murmurs do not necessarily occur during ventricular ejection,[12] and there is great variability in murmurs that occur during systole.

Systolic murmurs are the most common type heard in companion animals. Mitral and tricuspid regurgitation, ventricular septal defects, and pulmonary and aortic stenoses all cause systolic murmurs (see Fig. 9–1). Soft mitral and tricuspid murmurs are heard in dilated cardiomyopathy because of stretching of the valve annulus.[14] Loud systolic murmurs may be heard in cats with hypertrophic cardiomyopathy because of abnormal mitral valve motion leading to dynamic outflow obstruction and mitral regurgitation.[10, 15, 16]

Diastolic murmurs are rare in dogs and cats. If they are heard, they are usually a result of aortic regurgitation secondary to bacterial endocarditis. Continuous (machinery) murmurs are caused by patent ductus arteriosus and are produced by continuous flow from the aorta through the ductus to the pulmonary artery[16] (see Fig. 9–1).

The configuration of a murmur describes the appearance of the murmur on a phonocardiogram. A holosystolic murmur has the same loudness throughout systole and has a plateau configuration. It occurs most commonly with ventricular septal defects and with mitral and tricuspid regurgitation. A crescendo-decrescendo murmur starts and ends softly and builds to its loudest point in midsystole. Aortic and pulmonary stenoses cause crescendo-decrescendo murmurs[16] (see Fig. 9–1).

The location of a murmur is important in diagnosing the cause. Murmurs that are loudest at the base of the heart on the left side are caused by lesions of or around the aortic and pulmonary valves. Pulmonary stenosis, aortic stenosis, and patent ductus arteriosus are examples of murmurs in those locations. The murmur of mitral regurgitation is heard best over the left apex, and a tricuspid regurgitation is heard best from the right ventral thorax. Ventricular septal defects are heard on both sides but are louder on the right than on the left because of the pattern of radiation. Radiation is also responsible for the murmur heard over the carotid arteries in aortic stenosis.[17]

Although certain types of heart disease do not cause a murmur (e.g., right-to-left shunts, pericardial effusions, arrhythmias), others, such as mitral regurgitation, should not be diagnosed without auscultation of a murmur. However, not all murmurs are indicative of disease. Functional murmurs are low- to moderate-grade physiologic murmurs caused by high-output conditions such as anemia, fever, and hyperthyroidism. Puppies can have soft, innocent murmurs not caused by cardiac pathology that disappear by 4 to 9 months of age.[16]

Clinical Signs

Murmurs in puppies and kittens are usually caused by congenital heart defects, whereas murmurs in animals older than 1 year of age are usually caused by acquired problems. Congenital heart defects are discussed in Chapter 14, and acquired valvular disease is discussed in Chapter 11. Most murmurs are heard for the first time during routine examination, although a murmur may be auscultated initially when the animal is examined for symptoms of heart failure. Clinical signs associated with murmurs are coughing, dyspnea, exercise intolerance, and syncope.

Diagnostic Plan

Thoracic radiography, ECG, and echocardiography should be performed on all animals with murmurs. Congenital heart disease is suspected in puppies and kittens with heart murmurs, especially with murmurs of grade III/VI or greater. Echocardiography is the most important diagnostic test to perform in animals with suspected congenital heart disease.

Middle-aged and older small-breed dogs with holosystolic murmurs over the left apex usually have acquired mitral valve disease. Tricuspid valve degeneration is less common than mitral valve disease, and it may be associated with the latter or occur alone.

Young to middle-aged giant breeds (e.g., Great Danes, Saint Bernards), Doberman pinschers, boxers, and American and English cocker spaniels develop murmurs secondary to cardiomyopathy. Cardiomyopathy also occurs in cats and is the most common cause of a murmur in a mature cat (see Chap. 12).

Pulse Abnormalities

Pulses are pressure waves that are derived from cardiac contractions and travel down the artery or vein to points at which they are superficial enough to be seen or palpated. They are normal findings in the arterial system, but pulses do not normally occur in veins.

Pathophysiology

The pathophysiology of abnormal pulses depends on whether they are venous or arterial pulses. Persistent distention of the jugular vein more than one third of the way up the neck or strong jugular pulses indicate abnormally high central venous pressure and are usually seen with right-sided heart failure, cranial mediastinal masses, pericardial disease, or thrombosis of the jugular vein or cranial vena cava.[16] Occasionally, the hair must be clipped or wetted to see the jugular vein.

A waves are the normal, small pulses that arise from right atrial contraction and precede the apex beat. They are usually detected only by intravenous monitoring (i.e., central venous pressure) or in quiet animals in lateral recumbence. *Giant a waves* are jugular pulses that occur with decreased right ventricular compliance (right ventricular hypertrophy). They occur because of right atrial contraction against a stiff ventricle. Causes include pulmonary stenosis, pulmonary hypertension or severe chronic obstructive pulmonary disease, and heartworm disease. *Cannon a waves* are intermittent giant a waves that result from right atrial contraction against a closed A-V valve, as in third-degree A-V block.[17, 18] The hepatojugular reflex is elicited by compressing the cranial abdomen for 30 seconds. This increases venous return from a congested liver, and a jugular pulse arises because of the volume overload on the failing right ventricle. A simultaneous gallop may be auscultated.[18]

Pulse deficits arise from arrhythmias, especially atrial fibrillation, and occur because there are a higher number of apex contractions than there are pulses. The heart is beating so rapidly and irregularly that the left ventricle cannot fill adequately with every beat to produce a pulse.

Weak pulses are caused by a decreased stroke volume from conditions such as left ventricular failure, hypovolemia, pericardial disease or effusions, and aortic stenosis. An absence of femoral pulses in a cat with acute posterior paresis, cold hind limbs, and cyanotic nail beds is diagnostic of aortic thromboembolism (see Chap. 12). There are varying degrees of severity, the worst being total absence of arterial flow bilaterally. Mild involvement is characterized by a weak pulse unilaterally or bilaterally. Often, both hind legs are affected but to different degrees.[15]

Patent ductus arteriosus causes a bounding pulse because of rapid run-off from the aorta into the pulmonary artery in diastole. The hyperdynamic pulse comes from a higher systolic pressure and a wider pulse pressure.[17] A bounding pulse may also occur with severe aortic regurgitation, but this is an uncommon condition among small animals. Regular pulses of varying intensity are called pulsus alternans and come from severe left ventricular failure. Pulsus paradoxus is a pulse that paradoxically decreases with inspiration; it is caused by pericardial effusions.[18]

Clinical Signs

Palpation of arterial pulses for rate, quality, and pulse deficits should be performed at the same time as thoracic palpation or auscultation. Because abnormal pulses are secondary abnormalities and are insignificant without concomitant cardiac pathology, their importance is in correlating them with other physical findings. In other words, abnormal pulses add to the information about the cardiac status that is already known but do not have significance of their own.

Diagnostic Plan

Jugular pulses usually indicate right-sided heart failure, pericardial effusion, or thoracic masses. These are best evaluated by thoracic radiography and echocardiography. Pericardial effusions cause an enlarged, rounded cardiac silhouette; right-sided heart failure is usually related to right ventricular enlargement; and thoracic masses are water-tissue densities in the cranial thorax.

If weak arterial pulses are caused by cardiac disease, thoracic radiography should reveal an enlarged cardiac silhouette, although echocardiography may be necessary to differentiate cardiomyopathy from pericardial effusion. The heart should also be enlarged radiographically if pulses are bounding from heart disease. A packed cell volume reveals anemia, which can mimic heart disease because of the enlarged heart and bounding pulses.

History

A good history helps the clinician to make a correct diagnosis and, along with the physical examination, guides the clinician in ordering the most appropriate diagnostic tests. The history also assists the clinician in choosing proper therapy. A functional classification of heart failure in dogs according to activity that initiates symptoms has been modified from a similar classification for humans (Table 9–6). Dogs are classified as being asymptomatic, having mild to moderate heart failure, or having advanced heart failure. Dogs that are asymptomatic may have a cardiac murmur, arrhythmia, or cardiac enlargement detected by radiography or echocardiography but are not affected by the disease. Dogs with mild to moderate heart failure are symptomatic at rest or with mild exercise and exhibit typical radiographic changes. Dogs with advanced heart failure have immediately obvious clinical signs of

Table 9–6
Functional Classification of Heart Failure

Asymptomatic Heart Disease
Heart disease is detected by the presence of a heart murmur, arrhythmia, or radiographic evidence of cardiac chamber. Signs of compensation such as ventricular dilation or hypertrophy may or may not be present. The need for treatment may or may not be justified.

Mild to Moderate Heart Failure
Clinical signs of heart failure are evident at rest or with mild exercise and adversely affect the quality of life. Typical signs include cough, exercise intolerance, dyspnea, tachypnea, and mild to moderate ascites. Treatment is indicated.

Advanced Heart Failure
Symptoms of congestive heart failure are immediately obvious even when the animal is at rest. With any physical activity, discomfort is increased. Cardiogenic shock is present in severe cases. Many dogs can be treated at home, but severe cases must be hospitalized. Death is likely without some kind of therapy.

Modified from Kittleson MD. The pathophysiology and treatment of mitral regurgitation in the dog. In: The 18th Annual Waltham/OSU Symposium for the Treatment of Small Animal Diseases. Vernon, Calilfornia: Waltham USA, Inc, 1994;33–43.

congestive heart failure (e.g., cough, marked dyspnea, or exercise intolerance).[18a]

Signalment

The age, breed, and sex of the animal are the initial components of the history. Young animals are more likely to have congenital cardiac disorders, and older animals are more likely to have acquired problems. Hyperthyroidism is usually seen in older cats (average age, 12–13 years),[8] and older small-breed dogs often have acquired A-V valve disease. Cardiomyopathy may occur in cats of any age, although such patients tend to be middle-aged or older.[15]

Some congenital defects are specific to certain breeds, although other breeds may also be affected.[17] Dilated cardiomyopathy is more prevalent among large breeds of dogs, and other types of cardiomyopathy have been recognized in Doberman pinschers, English cocker spaniels, and boxers.[14] German shepherds have an inherited problem with ventricular arrhythmias and sudden cardiac death.[19] The sex of the animal seems to play a minor role in disease prevalence, but patent ductus arteriosus occurs more commonly in females,[17, 20] and cardiomyopathy in dogs is seen more commonly in males.[14, 21]

Previous Medications

The effect of previous medications is an important aspect of the history. If the animal is suspected to have pulmonary edema and is being treated with diuretics and other cardiac medications, obvious clinical improvement should occur, or the pulmonary infiltrate is probably not cardiogenic edema. One exception to this is ruptured chordae tendineae causing acute severe pulmonary edema, which responds poorly to even the most intensive therapy. Most dogs with this problem deteriorate rapidly and die because the lungs are overwhelmed by the sudden fluid overload. A history of response to medications is also an important guide to future therapy. Failure at a lower dose indicates that a higher dose may be required or additional medications may be needed.

Environmental History

Finding out an animal's travel history helps determine the probability of exposure to heartworms or systemic fungal diseases. A history of previous heartworm tests and compliance with heartworm preventative measures is also valuable information. It is worthwhile to get a good dietary history. Taurine-deficiency dilated cardiomyopathy of cats is now rare, but it is still periodically diagnosed in cats fed unusual diets. Also, many pets in heart failure are fed commercially prepared diets high in sodium and should be switched to low-sodium home-cooked or prescription diets.

Previous Illnesses

Any previous illnesses should be discussed, especially if they have a bearing on heart disease. For instance, hyperthyroidism, hypertension, and chronic renal failure may cause heart disease or exacerbate existing heart problems. Dogs with a recent history of surgery for a bleeding splenic tumor may develop pericardial effusion secondary to a right atrial hemangiosarcoma.

Physical Examination

A good physical examination is as important as the history in helping to determine which additional tests to pursue. The best tools for diagnosis are available in the examination room: the eyes, the hands, and the ears.

Visual Examination

The physical examination should begin as the dog walks into the examination room or as the cat is sitting in the carrier. Does the dog rise slowly and walk with effort? Is there a swollen abdomen or severe weight loss? How does the effort of walking affect respiration? What is the animal's demeanor, and how does the dog or cat respond to external stimuli? The animal should be observed for weakness, dyspnea, and general body condition before the hands-on examination is begun.

General Physical Examination

A good physical examination follows the same routine regardless of symptoms, history, or physical appearance. In this manner, unanticipated problems that may change the diagnosis or the therapeutic approach are not overlooked. I usually start with the head and work caudad.

Head and Neck

Mucous membranes should be examined for pallor or cyanosis. Cyanosis in young dogs indicates a congenital right-to-left shunt, such as tetralogy of Fallot, and is caused by unoxygenated blood's being shunted away from the lungs to the systemic circulation.[17] In older dogs and cats, it is seen with severe pulmonary disease or advanced congestive heart failure. Gums should be examined for gingivitis associated with dental disease, which can be a source of bacterial infection in cases of endocarditis, especially in dogs with chronic A-V valvular fibrosis. Pallor with a slow capillary refill time is caused by low-output heart disease.[16] Brachycephalic breeds of dogs often have upper respiratory abnormalities that may cause bradyarrhythmias, such as sinus bradycardia or second-degree heart block. These arrhythmias in brachycephalic breeds are "normal" unless the animal is symptomatic. Upper respiratory sounds are often heard without a stethoscope, and careful auscultation should be performed over the trachea as well as the lungs to determine the source of loudest noise in a dyspneic animal. Palpation of the trachea elicits a honking cough in dogs with collapsing tracheas and should not be performed until the end of the examination, so that coughing does not obscure auscultation of the heart and lungs.

The cervical region should be examined for jugular pulses or persistent jugular distention and, in cats, for a thyroid nodule. Thyroid nodules in cats are palpated by extending the head and neck and sliding the thumb and index finger from the larynx down the trachea. Some tumors are more distal and must be manipulated up from the thoracic inlet. A fundic examination in older cats suspected of having hyperthyroidism or chronic renal disease may reveal retinal detachment or hemorrhage caused by hypertension.[18]

Thorax

Next, the ventral thorax should be palpated to locate the apex beat, or point of maximal thrust by the ventricle, and to detect thrills. An apical beat more intense than normal may be caused by left ventricular hypertrophy, especially if the apex beat is caudally displaced. This usually occurs in cats with primary hypertrophic cardiomyopathy or hyperthyroidism. A weaker beat is associated with myocardial failure, pericardial or pleural effusions, obesity, pneumothorax, or thoracic masses. Thoracic masses, pleural fluid, and collapsed lung lobes may shift the point of maximal intensity to the right, whereas anterior mediastinal masses usually cause caudal displacement. Anterior mediastinal masses also cause a noncompressible cranial thorax. A dyspneic cat should have the thorax compressed carefully,[16] because thoracic compression further compromises breathing.

Abdomen

The clinician should palpate for ascites, hepatomegaly, and masses. Hepatomegaly and ascites are seen with right-sided heart failure. An enlarged liver may be a result of Cushing disease, which can also cause dyspnea because of chronic obstructive pulmonary disease and pulmonary thromboembolism. If ascites is severe, it may exacerbate or cause dyspnea.[16]

Auscultation

Auscultation of the heart and lungs is one of the main parts of the cardiovascular examination and deserves much attention. Optimum auscultation is performed in a quiet room without distractions. Dogs should be standing; cats should be sternal or standing. A nervous, active, or aggressive animal is difficult to examine, but with time and patience adequate auscultation can often be accomplished. Even purring and panting do not have to be major hindrances. A dog's mouth can be held shut by the veterinarian or the owner, but purring cats represent more of a problem. My favorite way to stop purring is to hold my index finger over both nostrils of the cat while listening. Some cats object, but most stop purring long enough for thorough auscultation. Shivering, movement, and breathing mimic murmurs, and it takes great care to listen "through" these sounds.

Both the bell and the diaphragm of the stethoscope should be used for listening, and all areas of the heart should be auscultated for heart sounds and murmurs (Fig. 9–2). Most murmurs in cats are auscultated ventrally, just to the right or the left of the sternum. The diaphragm of the stethoscope is best for high-frequency murmurs and for S_1 and S_2 sounds. The bell picks up lower-frequency sounds, such as gallops and

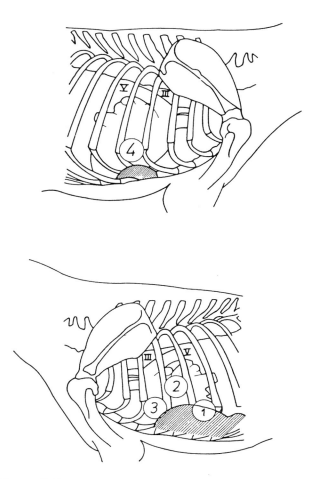

Figure 9–2
Principal areas of cardiac auscultation in the dog. The valve relations are the same in the cat, except that most murmurs are heard ventrally near the sternum. 1, mitral valve area; 2, aortic valve area; 3, pulmonary valve area; 4, tricuspid valve area. Mitral, aortic, and pulmonary valves are auscultated on the left hemithorax. The tricuspid valve is auscultated on the right. The shaded area is the area of cardiac dullness. (From Detweiler D. Heart sounds of the dog. Ann N Y Acad Sci 1965;127:323–324.)

some murmurs. It should be used with light pressure, because pressing against the chest tightens the skin and causes the bell to perform like the diaphragm.[16, 22] Light pressure is also important in cats, because murmurs can be created by squeezing both sides of the thorax while auscultating the heart.

Systematic auscultation should include listening for and identifying S_1 and S_2, the points of maximal intensity of murmurs and heart sounds, and the radiation, pitch, duration, quality, and timing of murmurs. The effects of respiration on the heart rate or on murmurs and the synchronization of heartbeats with pulses should also be noted. The clinician should also listen carefully for split heart sounds, clicks, gallops, and arrhythmias. Loudness of heart sounds and murmurs is decreased by the same conditions that affect thoracic palpation; that is, by obesity, pleural and pericardial effusions, pneumothorax, masses, diaphragmatic hernias, and systolic dysfunction.[16, 22] Systolic dysfunction can cause decreased heart sounds and is often omitted from a differential diagnosis.

Heart Sounds

S_1 is produced by closure of the mitral and tricuspid valves and is best heard at the ventricular apex (see Fig. 9–2). The peripheral pulse occurs just after S_1 and helps to differentiate S_1 from S_2. There is also a longer pause between S_2 and S_1, because diastole is longer than systole. The tricuspid component of S_1 is heard best over the tricuspid valve on the right side of the thorax[22] (see Fig. 9–2). A split S_1, caused by asynchronous closure of the A-V valves, is rare in dogs and cats but is occasionally heard in giant breeds of dogs. It must be differentiated from an S_4 gallop, an S_1 ejection sound, and a systolic click.[22]

S_2 is best heard at the heart base and results from closure of the aortic and pulmonary valves (see Fig. 9–2) at the end of systole. There is a physiologic splitting of S_2 that is not heard in normal dogs and cats. A split S_2 almost always results from either pulmonary hypertension (right-to-left shunts or heartworm disease) or a right bundle branch block.[16, 22]

Gallops are extra heart sounds caused by a loud third (S_3) or fourth (S_4) heart sound. An S_3 gallop occurs in diastole during the rapid ventricular filling phase of the cardiac cycle. Most S_3 gallops are associated with rapid filling of a severely dilated ventricle; they are heard in cats and dogs with dilated cardiomyopathy or severe chronic mitral regurgitation. An S_4 gallop follows atrial systole and usually results from atrial contraction into a noncompliant ventricle. Most S_4 gallops occur in cats with hypertrophic heart disease.[15] Both S_3 and S_4 gallops are best heard with the bell portion of the stethoscope and may be accentuated with exercise.[16, 22]

Heart sounds may differ in intensity from beat to beat. Causes include atrial fibrillation, extrasystoles, pericardial effusions, and third-degree A-V block. Differing intensity results from changes in ventricular filling. A premature contraction that occurs before the ventricle is adequately filled causes a softer beat. In pericardial effusion, the difference occurs because of the swinging of the heart toward or away from the area of auscultation.[16]

Lung Sounds

Inspiratory dyspnea is associated with upper respiratory problems and expiratory dyspnea with lower respiratory disease. Dogs in heart failure usually exhibit an expiratory dyspnea. The locations of crackles, wheezes, bronchovesicular sounds, and friction rubs should be noted. Crackles are snapping sounds of very short duration that are caused by fluid accumulation or by the popping open of airways plugged with mucous. Bronchovesicular sounds are harsh, blowing sounds normally heard over the trachea and anterior thorax. Their presence in the peripheral lung regions indicates pulmonary disease. Wheezes are high-pitched breath sounds that occur more frequently during expiration and indicate narrow airways. Friction rubs are described as creaky-leather sounds and are produced by diseased pleural surfaces rubbing against one another.[23]

Crackles in heart failure should be heard mainly dorsally and caudally, but dogs with severe heart failure may have generalized crackles. Crackles and wheezes also occur with chronic obstructive pulmonary disease, so their presence alone does not always equate with cardiogenic edema. In fact, if a murmur is not present in dogs, cardiac disease should probably not be diagnosed. A mistake that is often made is to diagnose edema on auscultation alone. Unless the animal is too dyspneic to undergo the stress associated with radiography, a chest radiograph should be taken before the administration of any medications. There are, however, three exceptions to the "no heart murmur, no cardiac edema" rule: (1) dogs whose crackles are so loud they obscure the murmur; (2) dogs with dilated cardiomyopathy that have low-grade murmurs that are easily missed; and (3) cats, which can have severe cardiac disease without a murmur or a gallop.

Decreased heart and lung sounds are caused by pleural effusions, masses, and pericardial effusions. Pleural effusions (see Chap. 53) obscure heart and lung sounds ventrally. Frequently, the level of the fluid in the chest can be ascertained by determining the horizontal line along which lung sounds are heard. Pneumothorax can cause decreased lung sounds.

Diagnostic Procedures

If the history and physical examination suggest a possible heart abnormality, the additional diagnostic tests that should be performed include chest radiography, a 6- or 10-lead ECG, echocardiography, and routine blood tests.

Radiography

Of all the diagnostic tests available, the most important in dogs is the chest radiograph. No older coughing dog should be administered medication without evaluation of a thoracic radiograph unless the owner refuses it. In many cases of suspected heart failure, radiography reveals neoplasia, pneumonia, or

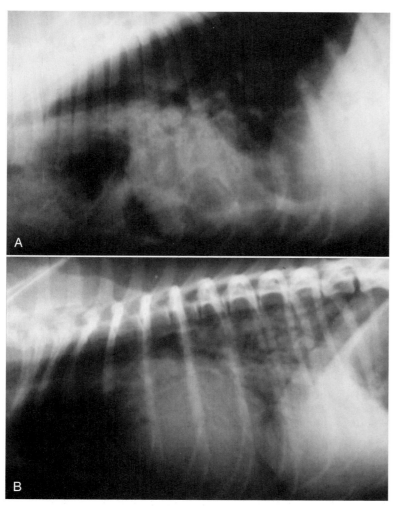

Figure 9–3
Lateral radiographs of two dogs illustrating different patterns of distribution of pneumonia and heart failure. **(A)** Four-year-old dog with pneumonia. The alveolar infiltrate is patchy and ventral. **(B)** Ten-year-old cavalier King Charles spaniel with mitral regurgitation and congestive heart failure. The alveolar infiltrate is hilar and exends to the dorsal and caudal lung lobes.

chronic obstructive pulmonary disease instead. The presence of a murmur in an older, small-breed dog does not eliminate the possibility of respiratory disease.

A chest radiograph helps to differentiate pulmonary from cardiac disease, to judge the severity of edema or pleural effusions, and to evaluate response to therapy. Both heart failure and pneumonia cause alveolar infiltrates, but the location of the infiltrate often helps to differentiate them. In dogs, edema associated with heart failure is more hilar, dorsal-caudal, and bilaterally symmetrical, whereas pneumonia is more anterior and cranial-ventral and is often more severe on one side[24] (Fig. 9–3). Pulmonary edema in cats is patchy and diffuse and is harder to diagnose by location (Fig. 9–4).

Radiographic signs of pleural effusions include rounding of the lung lobes and prominent fissure lines between lung lobes. A severe effusion obscures the cardiac silhouette and makes the diagnosis of cardiac disease more difficult. Echocardiography allows evalu-ation in patients with effusions, because fluid is a good medium to carry ultrasound waves, and hidden masses are easily seen.

The size and shape of the heart on the radiograph should be considered. Careful positioning and good radiographic technique are important but are more difficult in dyspneic patients. Some animals may require sedation to obtain good radiographs; poor positioning can cause one area of the heart to appear enlarged and abnormal bulges to be obscured. Both a lateral and a ventrodorsal radiograph should be made. The cardiac silhouette on the ventrodorsal film can be examined for chamber or vessel enlargements as if the heart were the face of a clock (Fig. 9–5). Pericardial effusions appear as a severely rounded, globoid cardiac silhouette (Fig. 9–6). However, echocardiography is usually necessary to identify the cause of the pericardial effusion. Pneumo-pericardiography can also define masses, but it is not often performed because of the wide availability of echocardiography.

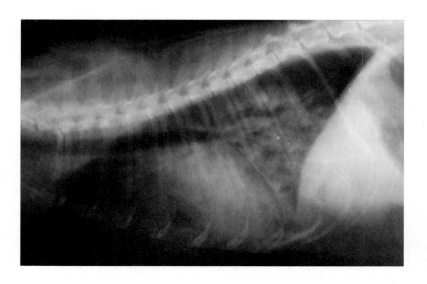

Figure 9–4
Pulmonary edema in a cat. Notice the generalized, patchy appearance, which is more ventral than it is dorsal and caudal. The heart is enlarged, and the pulmonary vessels are congested.

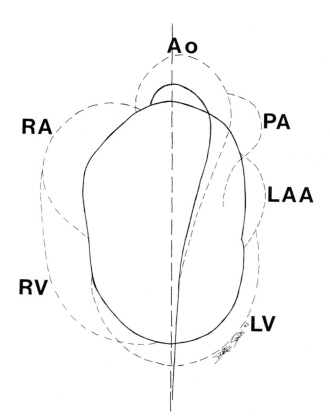

Figure 9–5
Anatomy of the heart from the perspective of a ventrodorsal radiograph. The enlargements are read as if looking at the face of a clock. The main body of the left atrium is in the lower middle section of the heart. Ao, aorta (12 o'clock); PA, main pulmonary artery (1–2 o'clock); LAA, left atrial appendage (3 o'clock); LV, left ventricle (4–6 o'clock); RV, right ventricle (6–9 o'clock); and RA, right atrium (9–11 o'clock).

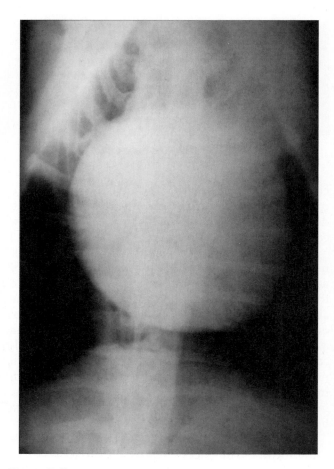

Figure 9–6
Pericardial effusion in a 9-year-old golden retriever. The cardiac silhouette is enlarged and rounded.

Electrocardiography

The next most valuable aid for a complete cardiac evaluation is an ECG. Although rhythm disturbances are the primary reason for running an ECG, other useful information can be obtained. Height and width of P waves and QRS complexes can reveal chamber enlargements. Abnormal QRS configuration can show electrolyte imbalances such as hyperkalemia in hypoadrenocorticism and urethral obstructions. Other types of aberrancy (abnormal conduction) are related to specific cardiac abnormalities; for example, left anterior fascicular block is closely associated with hypertrophic cardiomyopathy.[15] Specific arrhythmias are covered more completely in Chapter 10.

Echocardiography

If the chest radiograph is the most important diagnostic test for dogs, echocardiography is the most important one for cats. Echocardiography is simply ultrasonography of the heart and related structures, but many clients think echocardiography and sonography are two different procedures. Echocardiographic images are produced when electricity strikes a piezo-electric ("pressure-electric") crystal and an ultrasound wave is emitted that penetrates body tissues and is reflected back to the transducer. Each time the sound wave hits a different interface, it is seen as different tissue. The heart is visualized by two-dimensional and M-mode echocardiography because the object being scanned (e.g., the wall of a cardiac chamber) is perpendicular to the transducer. A special gel is required to facilitate contact of the transducer with the skin, because air hinders travel of ultrasound waves.[25, 26] Doppler echocardiography (both color flow Doppler and spectral Doppler) measures the direction and velocity of blood flow. It is optimized when the transducer beam is parallel to blood flow, because this configuration allows the beam to be perpendicular to the moving mass of red blood cells.[27]

Many veterinarians are presently learning echocardiography either for their own practice or to provide a service for other veterinarians. It is difficult to learn quickly, and many hours should be spent performing echocardiograms on normal dogs and cats, reading the literature,[25–31] and receiving instruction from an experienced sonographer. Basics may be picked up in a few weeks, but to do a professional job requires more than an echocardiograph machine and good intentions. Cost may run from $20,000 for a machine that does only two-dimensional and M-mode echocardiography to $250,000 for one that also has color flow and spectral Doppler capabilities. Any machine should have at least a 7.5-mHz transducer and a 5.0-mHz transducer. A 3.25-mHz transducer also is required to examine large dogs.

Echocardiography has revolutionized the practice of cardiology. Pleural effusions have become aids to diagnosis rather than hindrances, because fluid carries sound waves easily and enhances visualization of masses rather than obscuring them. Pericardial effusions can be examined for right atrial or heart base tumors. Cardiac chamber size, wall thickness, valve motion, and myocardial function are visualized in a noninvasive format. The diversity of feline heart disease is becoming more apparent, and therapy can be tailored to the individual patient. Most congenital defects are now easily diagnosed without cardiac catheterization. Echocardiography can also help to diagnose radiographic cardiomegaly in dogs that are coughing and dyspneic as a result of pulmonary disease, because pulmonary hypertension in these dogs dilates the right ventricle and pulmonary artery. Heartworms may be seen in the right ventricle and pulmonary artery, and severity of heartworm disease may be judged.[31] However, as good a tool as it is, echocardiography should be considered a part of the work-up and not used as a substitute for the physical examination, ECG, and chest radiograph.

Laboratory Evaluation

Blood tests are necessary to assess metabolic status and guide treatment with cardiac medications. For example, a dog with elevated blood urea nitrogen and creatinine requires a lower dose of digoxin than a dog with normal kidney function. Dogs treated with both furosemide and enalapril are more likely to develop azotemia than dogs receiving only enalapril. However, if the blood urea nitrogen and creatinine results of dogs treated with angiotensin-converting enzyme inhibitors rise less than 30% and the animal suffers no ill effects, there is no need to change therapy. If a greater change occurs, it is more important to lower the amount of diuretic rather than the amount of enalapril. It is also important to evaluate electrolytes, because low potassium can exacerbate digoxin toxicity, and low sodium (<135 mEq/L) is an indication of severe heart failure.

A complete white blood cell count can help differentiate pneumonia and pulmonary edema. Leukocytosis, especially with a left shift, indicates infection more than edema. Polycythemia is seen in dogs with right-to-left shunts. Heartworm tests should be performed routinely; they are discussed in detail in Chapter 13.

References

1. Braunwald E. The history. In: Braunwald E, ed. Heart Disease. Philadelphia, WB Saunders, 1992:1–12.

2. Ingram RH, Braunwald E. Pulmonary edema: Cardiogenic and noncardiogenic. In: Braunwald E, ed. Heart Disease. Philadelphia, WB Saunders, 1992:551–568.

3. Sibbald WJ, Cunningham DR, Chin DN. Non-cardiac or cardiac pulmonary edema? A practical approach to clinical differentiation in critically ill patients. Chest 1983;84:452–461.

4. Ware WA, Bonagura JD. Pulmonary edema. In: Fox PR, ed. Canine and Feline Cardiology. New York, Churchill Livingstone, 1988:205–217.

5. Kerr LY. Pulmonary edema secondary to upper airway obstruction in the dog: A review of nine cases. J Am Anim Hosp Assoc 1989;25:207–212.

6. Braunwald E, Grossman W. Clinical aspects of heart failure. In: Braunwald E, ed. Heart Disease. Philadelphia, WB Saunders, 1992:444–463.

7. Ettinger SJ. Weakness and syncope. In: Ettinger SJ, ed. Textbook of Veterinary Internal Medicine, 3rd ed. Philadelphia, WB Saunders, 1989:46–53.

8. Peterson ME, Kintzer PP, Cavanagh PG, et al. Feline hyperthyroidism: Pretreatment and clinical and laboratory evaluation of 131 cases. J Am Vet Med Assoc 1983;183:103–110.

9. Lusk RH, Ettinger SF. Cardiovascular syncope. In: Fox PR, ed. Canine and Feline Cardiology. New York, Churchill Livingstone, 1988:335–339.

10. Wigle ED. Hypertrophic cardiomyopathy: A 1987 viewpoint. Circulation 1987;75:311–322.

11. Sisson D. Fixed and dynamic subvalvular aortic outflow stenosis in dogs. In: Kirk RW, Bonagura JD, eds. Current Veterinary Therapy XI. Philadelphia, WB Saunders, 1992:760–766.

12. Perloff JK. Heart sounds and murmurs: Physiologic mechanisms. In: Braunwald E, ed. Heart Disease. Philadelphia, WB Saunders, 1992:43–63.

13. Braunwald E. The physical examination. In: Braunwald E, ed. Heart Disease. Philadelphia, WB Saunders, 1992: 13–42.

14. Fox PR. Canine myocardial disease. In: Fox PR, ed. Canine and Feline Cardiology. New York, Churchill Livingstone, 1988:467–493.

15. Fox PR. Feline myocardial disease. In: Fox PR, ed. Canine and Feline Cardiology. New York, Churchill Livingstone, 1988:435–466.

16. Gompf RE. The clinical approach to heart disease: History and physical examination. In: Fox PR, ed. Canine and Feline Cardiology. New York, Churchill Livingstone, 1988:29–42.

17. Olivier NB. Congenital heart disease in dogs. In: Fox PR, ed. Canine and Feline Cardiology. New York, Churchill Livingstone, 1988:357–389.

18. Ross JN. The no equipment cardiology examination. Proc North Am Vet Conf, 1993:12–18.

18a. Kittleson MD. The pathophysiology and treatment of mitral regurgitation in the dog. In: The 18th Annual Waltham/OSU Symposium for the Treatment of Small Animal Diseases. Vernon, California: Waltham USA, Inc., 1994:33–43.

19. Moise NS, Gilmour RF. Inherited sudden cardiac death in German shepherds. In: Kirk RW, Bonagura JD, eds. Current Veterinary Therapy XI. Philadelphia, WB Saunders, 1992:749–751.

20. Bonagura JD. Congenital heart disease. In: Bonagura JD, ed. Cardiology. New York, Churchill Livingstone, 1987: 1–19.

21. Thomas WP. Myocardial diseases of the dog. In: Bonagura JD, ed. Cardiology. New York, Churchill Livingstone, 1987:117–155.

22. Smith FWK. Rapid Interpretation of Heart Sounds, Murmurs, and Arrhythmias. Philadelphia, Lea & Febiger, 1992.

23. Schaer M, Ackerman N, King RR. Clinical approach to the patient with respiratory disease. In: Ettinger SJ, ed. Textbook of Veterinary Internal Medicine. Philadelphia, WB Saunders, 1989:747–767.

24. Hawkins EC. Diseases of the lower respiratory tract (lung) and pulmonary edema. In: Ettinger SJ, ed. Textbook of Veterinary Internal Medicine. Philadelphia, WB Saunders, 1989:816–866.

25. Feigenbaum H. Echocardiography, 4th ed. Philadelphia, Lea & Febiger, 1986:1–49.

26. Kaplan PM. Instrumentation, principles, and pitfalls of ultrasonography. Problems in Veterinary Medicine: Ultrasound. 1991;3:457–478.

27. Gaber C. Doppler echocardiography. In: Kaplan PM, ed. Problems in Veterinary Medicine: Ultrasound. Philadelphia, JB Lippincott, 1991;3:479–499.

28. Thomas WP. Two-dimensional, real-time echocardiography in the dog: Technique and anatomic validation. Vet Radiol 1986;27:34–49.

29. Moise NS. Echocardiography. In: Fox PR, ed. Canine and Feline Cardiology. New York, Churchill Livingstone, 1988:113–156.

30. Thomas WP, Gaber CE, Jacobs GJ, et al. Recommendations for standards in transthoracic two-dimensional echocardiography in the dog and cat. J Vet Intern Med 1993;7:247–252.

31. Bonagura JD. Echocardiography. J Am Vet Med Assoc 1994;204:516–522.

Electrocardiography

Betsy R. Bond

The electrocardiogram (ECG) is one of the simplest and most widely used of the diagnostic tools available to evaluate heart disease. Problems arise if it is asked to do too much (e.g., to recognize heart abnormalities in every case) or if it is never used because it is an insensitive measure of disease. Many veterinarians also have an aversion to ECG interpretation because they assume that ECGs are hard to understand. This antipathy can be dispelled by reviewing the basic anatomy of the conduction system, by understanding how electrical impulses are formed and conducted, and by developing a systematic method of evaluation of the ECG.

Of primary importance is recording a high-quality ECG and following certain standards of recording. This means laying the animal in right lateral recumbence, with the legs perpendicular to the animal's body. The leads are attached to the point of the elbow and the stifle. Contact between leads and skin is facilitated by use of an alcohol swab. I have also found it to helpful to bend down or flatten the teeth of the clips so that their application is less traumatic to the animal. The first ECG run on an animal should consist of six leads and a long lead II rhythm strip. The six leads include the standard limb leads (leads I, II, and III) and the augmented limb leads (leads aVR, aVL, and aVF).[1] A 10-lead ECG (standard leads plus augmented limb leads plus chest leads) should be obtained in all cases in which there is a possibility of subtle axis deviation, as in suspected right-sided heart failure or congenital heart defects. If an ECG is being repeated to follow progression of an arrhythmia, a standing or sitting lead II rhythm strip is acceptable.

Paper speed for the first six leads can be either 25 mm/sec or 50 mm/sec. All rhythm strips should be run at 50 mm/sec. The rhythm strip should be long enough to catch the occasional extrasystole. This sometimes requires running a strip at 25 mm/sec (to conserve paper) for several minutes. Standard calibration is 1 cm = 1 mV. This can be altered to half-sensitivity if the complexes are so tall or deep that they run off the page.[1] Alternatively, some animals have ECG complexes so small they are difficult to interpret, and the calibration can be switched to twice-sensitivity. This is common in normal cats, and a general rule of thumb for cats is that if the complexes are so small they are unrecognizable, they are probably normal.

A small investment in a caliper is helpful in measuring ECGs. The height and width of P waves and QRS complexes are measured with the caliper and compared with the small boxes of the ECG paper. At a paper speed of 50 mm/sec, every small box is equal to 0.02 sec, and at a calibration of 1 cm = 1 mV, every small box is 0.1 mV. If a caliper is not available, a card or stiff piece of paper can be used to mark off distances

between the beginning and ending points of complexes.[1]

There are two ways to obtain heart rate from an ECG. One is to count the number of R waves in a 3-sec interval and multiply by 20. Most ECG paper has marks every 1.5 sec at the top of the paper when paper speed is 50 mm/sec. A standard BIC pen can also be used because its length is equal to a 3-sec interval. The pen is laid on the ECG, and the number of R waves that appear along its length is multiplied by 20. If the paper speed is 25 mm/sec, the marks occur every 3 sec, and the number of R waves is multiplied by 10. The second way to estimate heart rate is to count the number of small boxes between two R waves at a paper speed of 50 mm/sec and divide that number into 3000. For this method to be accurate, the rhythm must be regular or many measurements must be taken and averaged.[1]

There are also two methods for calculating the axis. The first method requires finding the isoelectric lead, or the lead that is equal above and below the baseline. This is usually the lead with the smallest QRS deflections. Next, the lead perpendicular to the isoelectric lead is located. This is the lead that is the electrical axis, and it is examined to see whether it is primarily positive or primarily negative in deflection. On an axis wheel, all leads have a positive and a negative end (Fig. 10–1). This positivity and negativity

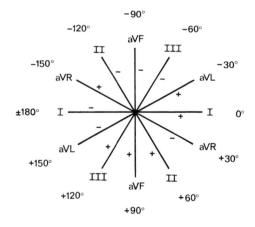

Figure 10–1

Bailey six-axis reference system. The diagram represents the combination of the standard limb leads (I, II, and III) and augmented limb leads (aVR, aVL, and aVF) after being redrawn through the center of the body in the frontal plane. The lead axes are marked in 30° increments from 0° to +180° at the bottom and from 0° to −180° at the top. Each of the six leads is marked with a "+" at the positive end (the electrode toward which the electrical forces flow) and a "−" at the negative end. Notice that the positive electrode for leads I, II, III, and aVF are all in the positive direction, whereas leads aVR and aVL are positive at the positions of −150° and −30°, respectively. (Modified from Ettinger SJ, Suter PF. Canine Cardiology. Philadelphia, WB Saunders, 1970:119.)

has been assigned by the ECG machine. For instance, the positive end of lead I is to the far right, and the negative end is to the far left. The positive end of aVF is down toward the feet, and the negative end is up toward the head. Once it has been determined whether the lead of the electrical axis is positive or negative, the axis wheel is analyzed to see which way positive or negative is for that lead. The wheel is divided into two 180° arcs, both of which start at the right (0°, the positive end of lead I) and curve around, meeting at the far left (the negative end of lead I). The bottom arc is +1° to +180°, and the top arc is −1° to −180°. If the electrical axis is formed by lead II and lead II is negative, the axis is −120°.[1] The second method for calculating the axis is to find the lead with the largest deflection, either positive or negative, and call that the electrical axis. The procedure after that is the same as in the first method.[1]

Anatomy and Physiology

Anatomy

The conduction system of the heart consists of the sinoatrial (SA) node, specialized conducting fibers in the atrial myocardium, the atrioventricular (A-V) node, the bundle of His, right and left bundle branches, anterior and posterior fascicles of the left bundle branch, and the Purkinje cells (Fig. 10–2). The normal impulse begins in the SA node (located in the right atrium near the cranial vena cava) and travels through the atrial myocardium to the A-V node (near the A-V junction next to the interventricular septum). The impulse then goes through the bundle of His and bundle branches to the Purkinje cells in the ventricular myocardium so that the right and left ventricles contract simultaneously. The SA node in the dog covers a larger anatomic area than it does in other species; this allows dogs to have a varying configuration of the P wave (wandering sinus pacemaker). The right bundle branch goes down the right side of the interventricular septum and divides into small fibers radiating over the right ventricular wall. The left bundle branch divides into anterior and posterior fascicles just past the upper one third of the septum.[1]

Normal Physiology

The ECG shows the sum of electrical forces that travel through the heart muscle, causing the heart to contract (Fig. 10–3). Most muscle cells are unable to spontaneously generate electrical activity unless damaged, but there are specialized cells called pacemaking cells throughout the heart that are capable of initiating these events. The SA node usually has control of heart rate and rhythm because it has a faster intrinsic rate than subsidiary pacemakers, but if it fails to fire, other pacemakers are ready to take over.

Action potentials from nonpacemaking and pacemaking cells differ (Fig. 10–4). The nonpacemaking cell is stimulated to threshold by an electrical impulse that causes influxes and effluxes of ionic charges across the cell membrane. These ionic charges are carried primarily by sodium, potassium, and calcium. Different phases of contraction result from the flow of electrolytes. Phase 0 (depolarization) occurs when one cell is stimulated by an adjacent cell and depends on a rapid inflow of sodium. Phase 0 of ventricular myocardial cells corresponds to the QRS of the ECG. Phases 1 through 3 are the stages of repolarization, or restoration of the myocardium to readiness for the next impulse. Phase 2 (plateau phase) results from a slow inward calcium current and is the phase affected by calcium channel blockers.[1]

Pacemaking cells differ from nonpacemaking cells in that they spontaneously depolarize in phase 4. During this phase, while nonpacemaking cells rest, pacemakers are activated by an inward slow leak of sodium. The upstroke of phase 0 is also slower in pacemaking cells, and the current in the SA and A-V nodes is carried more by calcium than by sodium.[2] The main pacemaking cells in the heart are found in the SA node. If the SA node fails to fire, subsidiary pacemaking cells in other locations take over to prevent asystole and cardiac arrest, resulting in an escape rhythm. Subsidiary pacemaking cells reside in the distal region of the A-V node, the bundle branches, and the Purkinje network.[1]

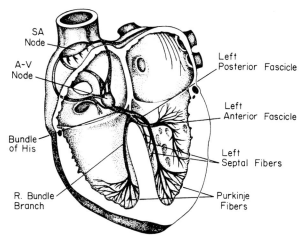

Figure 10–2
The labeled areas form the conduction system of the heart. (From Tilley LP. Feline cardiac arrhythmias. Vet Clin North Am 1977;7:274.)

Pathophysiology of Arrhythmias

Arrhythmias occur because of abnormalities in impulse formation, impulse conduction, or both.[2–4]

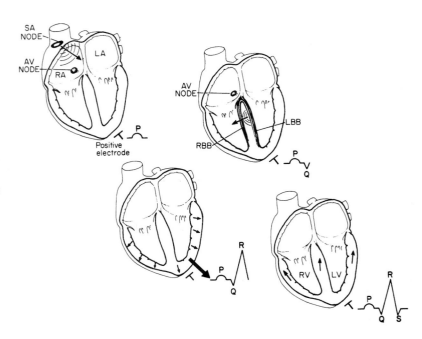

Figure 10–3
These four diagrams depict the electrocardiogram in connection with the cardiac conduction system as an electrical impulse travels from the sinoatrial node to the Purkinje network. The positive electrode of lead II is located over the left ventricle. (From Tilley LP. Feline cardiology. Proc Am Anim Hosp Assoc 1976;43:84.)

Disorders of impulse formation are caused by abnormal automaticity or by triggered arrhythmias. One form of abnormal automaticity occurs when normal pacemakers in the SA node fire too slowly or too rapidly, causing a bradyarrhythmia or tachyarrhythmia. Another type of automaticity, increased automaticity, occurs from the discharge of latent pacemakers because of disease in surrounding muscle (e.g., ischemia) or because of drugs or neurohormones that lower threshold (e.g, epinephrine). The increased automaticity causes latent pacemakers to fire faster than the SA node and take control of the heart rhythm.[2]

Triggered arrhythmias come from afterdepolarizations, which may or may not reach threshold and fire another beat. Early afterdepolarizations arise during phases 2 and 3 of the cardiac action potential, whereas delayed afterdepolarizations occur after completion of repolarization (Fig. 10–5). Early afterdepolarizations are thought to be the mechanism underlying proarrhythmia caused by antiarrhythmic drugs and arrhythmias caused by adrenergic stimulation. In proarrhythmia, antiarrhythmic drugs paradoxically increase, rather than decrease, the number of extrasystoles.[5] Delayed afterdepolarizations are probably responsible for arrhythmias secondary to cellular calcium overload and digitalis toxicity.[2]

Disorders of impulse conduction include heart blocks and re-entry. Heart blocks that arise in the SA and A-V nodes cause slow heart rates, whereas bundle branch blocks cause a bizarre configuration of the QRS

Figure 10–4
The diagrammed action potential of a nonpacemaking cell (on the left) correlates with the electrocardiogram beneath it. Compare this with the action potential of a pacemaking cell illustrated on the right. (From Tilley LP. Essentials of Canine and Feline Electrocardiography, 3rd ed. Philadelphia, Lea & Febiger, 1992:4.)

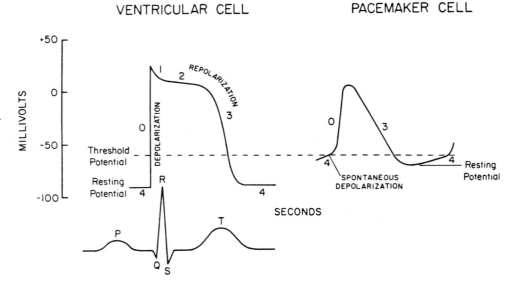

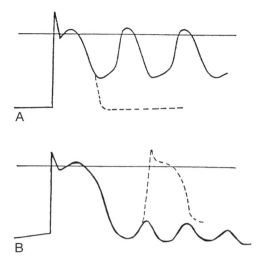

Figure 10–5

(A) If a fiber fails to repolarize completely, repetitive depolarizations can originate at a low level of membrane potential. These are called early afterdepolarizations. **(B)** A fiber can completely repolarize and then develop one or more small depolarizations. These are called delayed afterdepolarizations. (From Boyden PA. Cellular electrophysiologic basis of cardiac arrhythmias. In: Tilley LP. Essentials of Canine and Feline Electrocardiography, 3rd ed. Philadelphia, Lea & Febiger, 1992:279.)

complex but no change in heart rate. Re-entry is thought to be the most common mechanism behind supraventricular tachyarrhythmias. There are various types of re-entry, but common to all are two connecting pathways of fibers with different refractory periods, one slow and one fast. Slow conduction in one pathway is caused by unidirectional block (Fig. 10–6). When an impulse traveling down the slow pathway reaches the area of unidirectional block, it slows down. When the impulse reaches the other, fast pathway, it stimulates cells that were refractory milliseconds earlier but have had time to recover. By the time the fast pathway conducts the impulse back to its origin, the cells in the slow pathway are ready to discharge again. So starts a circus movement that can be a self-perpetuating tachycardia. A re-entry circuit uses either dual pathways in the A-V node or an accessory pathway and the A-V node to travel between the atrium and ventricles. Re-entry can also utilize a microscopic area of atrial or ventricular myocardium.[6]

Interpretation of Electrocardiograms

Principles of Interpretation

Application of a few principles of ECG interpretation can change ECG reading from a dreaded chore to an enjoyable experience.

1. Remember that all supraventricular depolarizations start above the A-V node and follow the same pathway through the ventricle, causing their QRS complexes to look alike, whether they are sinus, junctional, or atrial.

2. Interpret ECGs systematically.

   a. Note the heart rate: is it fast (tachycardia) or slow (bradycardia)?

   b. Note whether there is a P wave for every QRS and a QRS for every P wave.

   c. Note changes in the configuration of the QRS complex or uniformity of complexes.

   d. Measure the height and width of *all* deflections and of *all* intervals and compare with normal values.

   e. Look for miscellaneous changes (e.g., S-T slurring, tall peaked T wave).

   f. Note pauses and the events that precede or follow them. Is there an early complex before the pause? If so, the pause represents compensation for a premature complex. Is the pause greater than two R-R intervals? If so, it is a sinus arrest.

3. If the normal sinus pacemaker fails or there is a block in the A-V node such that the heart rate is seriously slowed, subsidiary pacemakers farther down in the conduction

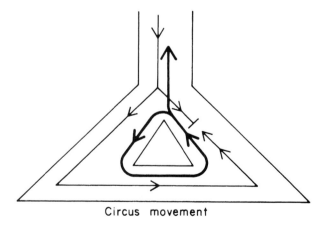

Circus movement

Figure 10–6

A diagram of re-entry by circus movement shows the initial impulse conduction *(fine lines)*. This initial impulse is stopped at a region of unidirectional block *(small perpendicular line)*. Heavier lines and arrows indicate regions of slow or delayed impulses, which are conducted in a retrograde direction by circus movement that perpetuates the tachyarrhythmia. (From Edwards NJ. Bolton's Handbook of Canine and Feline Electrocardiography, 2nd ed. Philadelphia, WB Saunders, 1987:64.)

Figure 10–7
Normal electrocardiogram from a cat who was shivering. Notice the sharp deflections *(arrows)* that are characteristic for shivering artifact. The QRS complexes (identified by the R wave) are almost too small to see.

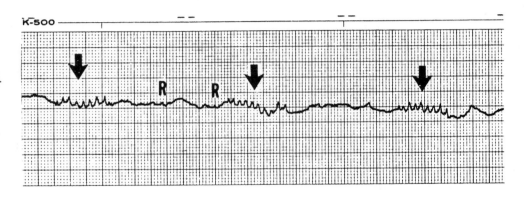

system take over control of the heart's rhythm. They produce escape rhythms, which are recognized by a pause before the QRS complex. Escape rhythms are slower than the normal sinus rhythm; the farther down the conduction system they originate, the slower they are. The ventricular escape rhythm in complete heart block for a dog is about 40 to 60 beats per minute (bpm); for a cat, it is about 100 bpm. Junctional rhythms are slightly faster for both species.

4. If the rhythm is irregular, is it a regularly irregular rhythm, occurring with respirations (sinus arrhythmia), or an irregularly irregular rhythm, sounding like tennis shoes in a washing machine (atrial fibrillation)? Or is it simply irregular (atrial premature complexes, ventricular premature complexes, sinus arrest, A-V nodal blocks)? Are there accompanying pulse deficits, indicating atrial fibrillation or extrasystoles?

5. Don't miss the forest for the trees. Look at the ECG from a distance to pick out pat-

terns that may be overlooked by observing too closely.

Pitfalls in Interpretation

The following common errors should be guarded against:

1. Making something out of every movement in the baseline ("I *think* it's a P wave, but I see only one.") Shivering often causes configurations that mimic P waves (Fig. 10–7).

2. Calling a bizarre-looking complex a ventricular premature complex (VPC) when it occurs after a pause and is actually a ventricular escape beat, or mistaking artifact for a ventricular premature complex (Fig. 10–8). Ventricular premature complexes usually break the rhythm and always have a T wave opposite in direction from the QRS.

3. Labeling a wave as a "deep" (negative) R wave or a "tall" (positive) S wave. By definition, R waves are always positive and S waves are always negative.

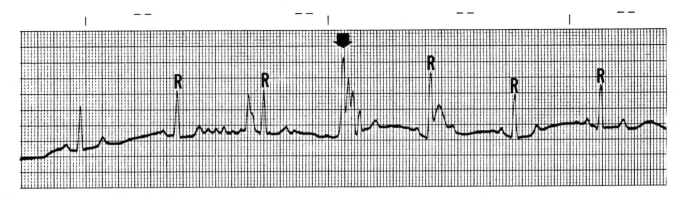

Figure 10–8
Electrocardiogram from a normal dog with movement artifact *(arrow)*. Careful measurement of the R-R intervals reveals that there is very little change in the rhythm, signifying that the "abnormality" did not disrupt the rhythm. There is a positive, wide deflection but no corresponding negative T wave, indicating artifact rather than ventricular premature complex.

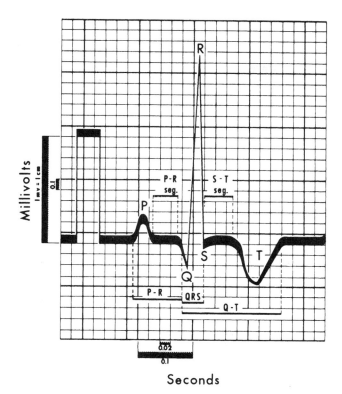

Figure 10–9

Diagram of the parts of the QRS. The P-R interval is from the beginning of the P wave to the beginning of the QRS, whereas the P-R segment is between the P wave and the QRS. The Q wave is the first negative deflection of the QRS, the R wave is the first positive deflection of the QRS, and the S wave is the first negative deflection after the R wave. The S-T segment is between the S wave and the T wave and should be even with the baseline. The Q-T interval is measured from the beginning of the QRS complex to the end of the T wave. (From Edwards NJ. Bolton's Handbook of Canine and Feline Electrocardiography, 2nd ed. Philadelphia, WB Saunders, 1987:42.)

P-QRS-T Deflections

Many abnormalities on the ECG are missed because the examiner does not take the few extra seconds required to measure height and width of P waves, P-R intervals, R-R intervals, P-P intervals, and QRS complexes (Fig. 10–9). Also often forgotten is which parts of the ECG reflect depolarization of various parts of the heart.

Normal Deflections

P waves represent depolarization of the atrial muscle, and their size and shape change depending on the location of the origin of the impulse and the size of the atria. An atrial premature complex should have a P wave that differs in configuration from that of a sinus beat; however, the QRS should look like that that of a sinus complex because conduction from the A-V node down is the same as in a sinus complex. The segment between the P wave and the QRS represents travel of the impulse through the A-V node, and because there is no large muscle to carry the charge, the surface ECG looks like a flat line. The QRS is the summation of all the electrical forces of both ventricles. Because most muscle mass is in the left ventricle, the mean electrical axis of the QRS "points" to the left ventricle (see Fig. 10–3).

Chamber Enlargements

ECG changes indicating chamber enlargements are listed in Tables 10–1 and 10–2.[7, 8] Although the published normal value for the height of the R wave in cats is 0.9 mV, that is probably too tall.[8a] A tall P wave is called P pulmonale, and it arises from *right atrial enlargement* (Fig. 10–10). The reference of the name to the lungs indicates the association of tall P waves with respiratory diseases such as a collapsing trachea and chronic obstructive pulmonary disease. P pulmonale is also caused by congenital or acquired diseases that lead to right atrial dilation (i.e., congenital or acquired tricuspid regurgitation).[1]

A wide P wave is caused by *left atrial enlargement* and is called P mitrale (Fig. 10–11). Again, the name relates to the associated structure, the mitral valve. P mitrale in dogs is usually seen with conditions that cause left atrial stretching, either from primary mitral valve disease (e.g., acquired mitral regurgitation) or from diseases that cause left ventricular dilation and secondary stretching of the mitral valve annulus (e.g., patent ductus arteriosus, dilated cardiomyopathy). P

Table 10–1 **Chamber Enlargements in Cats**	
CHAMBER ENLARGED	**CONFIGURATION**
Right atrium	P wave >0.2 mV tall (P pulmonale)
Left atrium	P wave >0.04 sec wide (P mitrale)
Left ventricle	R wave taller than 0.9 mV
	QRS wider than 0.04 sec
	Axis less than ±0°
Right ventricle	S waves in leads I, II, III, aVF
	Mean electrical axis in the frontal plane >+160°
	Deep S waves in leads CV_6LL and CV_6LU (usually >0.7 mV)

Data from Tilley LP. Essentials of Canine and Feline Electrocardiography, 3rd ed. Philadelphia, Lea & Febiger, 1992:440; and Edwards NJ. Bolton's Handbook of Canine and Feline Electrocardiography, 2nd ed. Philadelphia, WB Saunders, 1987:52.

Table 10–2
Chamber Enlargements in Dogs

CHAMBER ENLARGED	CONFIGURATION
Right atrium	P wave >0.4 mV tall (P pulmonale)
Left atrium	P wave >0.04 sec wide (P mitrale)
Left ventricle	R wave >3.0 mV in leads II and aVF in dogs younger than 2 years of age with narrow chests
	R wave >2.5 mV in leads II, III, and aVF
	R wave >3.0 mV in lead CV_6LU or CV_6LL
	QRS duration >0.05 sec in small and medium breeds or >0.06 sec in large breeds
	S-T segment slurring
	T wave more than 25% taller than R wave
	Mean electrical axis less than +40°
Right ventricle (any three criteria)	S wave in lead CV_6LL >0.08 sec
	Mean electrical axis in the frontal plane greater than +103°
	S wave in lead CV_6LU >0.7 mV
	S wave in lead I >0.05 mV
	R/S ratio in CV_6LU <0.87 mV
	S wave in lead II >0.35 mV
	S waves in leads I, II, III, and aVF
	Positive T wave in lead 10 (except in Chihuahuas)
	W-shaped QRS in lead 10

From Tilley LP. Essentials of Canine and Feline Electrocardiography, 3rd ed. Philadelphia, Lea & Febiger, 1992:438.

mitrale in cats is usually caused by hypertrophic or restrictive cardiomyopathy, but it can also be caused by mitral regurgitation and other diseases that produce left atrial dilation.[1]

Increased left ventricular muscle mass from either hypertrophy or dilation (*left ventricular enlarge-ment*) adds more voltage to the QRS and causes a taller QRS (Fig. 10–12). If the left ventricular dilation is severe, the QRS may also be wide and indistinguishable from that seen with a left bundle branch block. Common associated conditions include dilated cardiomyopathy, aortic stenosis, hypertrophic cardiomyopathy, and feline hyperthyroidism.[1]

Right ventricular enlargement adds muscle mass to the right ventricle, shifting the axis rightward (Fig. 10–13). Severe right ventricular hypertrophy usually occurs secondary to pulmonary stenosis and tetralogy of Fallot. Other conditions that may cause a right axis deviation are severe heartworm disease, other congenital right-to-left shunts, severe pulmonary disease, and tricuspid dysplasia.[1]

Intervals, Segments, and Miscellaneous Measurements

The P-R interval is measured from the beginning of the P wave to the beginning of the QRS and therefore includes the P wave. It represents all of atrial depolarization plus conduction across the A-V node and down the bundle of His. The time between the P wave and the QRS is relatively quiescent because no muscle mass is being depolarized to reveal itself on the surface ECG. The primary change in the P-R interval that may be seen is a prolongation of the interval because of first-degree heart block (see Conduction Disturbances). A changing of the P-R interval with changes in the heart rate may be insignificant, but more often it reflects an abnormality.[1]

The S-T segment is the time between the end of the QRS and the beginning of the T wave. Slurring into the T wave is abnormal, and so is depression of the S-T segment more than 0.2 mV or elevation more than 0.15 mV from the baseline (Fig. 10–14). S-T segment depression is associated with myocardial ischemia or infarction, hyperkalemia, hypokalemia, digitalis toxicity, or trauma to the myocardium. S-T segment el-

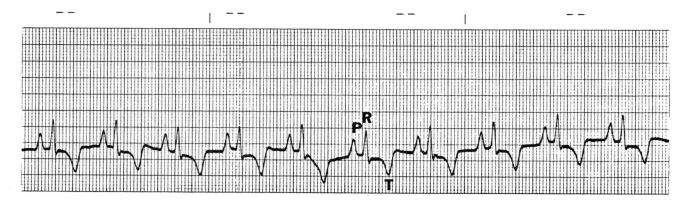

Figure 10–10
P pulmonale (tall P waves) in a dog with chronic bronchitis. The P waves are 0.5 mV high. Notice also the large, negative T waves.

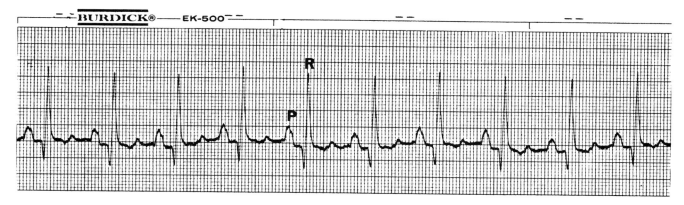

Figure 10-11
P mitrale (wide P waves) in a dog with chronic mitral regurgitation. The P waves measure 0.05 sec in width and are notched.

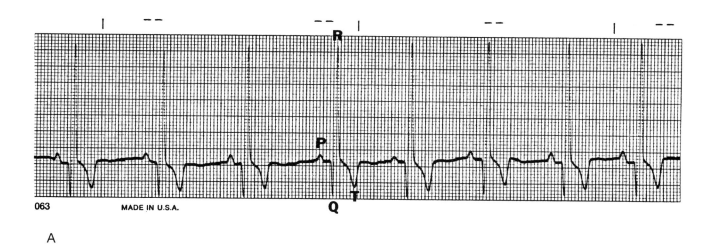

A

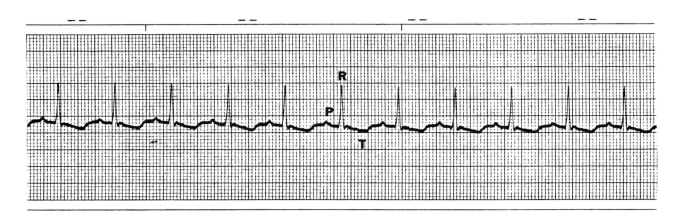

B

Figure 10-12
(A) Left ventricular enlargement in a puppy with a patent ductus arteriosus, indicated by R waves that are 3.6 mV high. The Q waves are deep (1.0 mV) and there is S-T segment slurring. **(B)** Left ventricular enlargement (tall R waves) in a cat with hypertrophic cardiomyopathy. The R waves are 1.2 mV tall but normal in width.

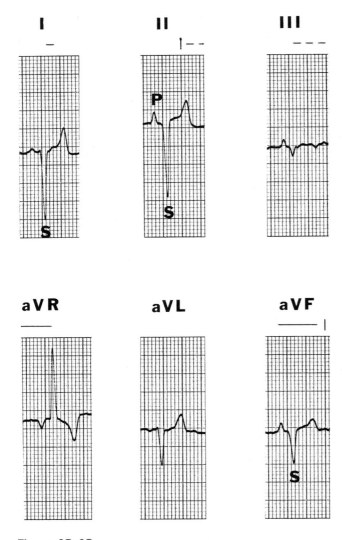

Figure 10-13
Right-axis deviation in a puppy caused by right ventricular hypertrophy secondary to pulmonary stenosis. The S waves are deep in leads I, II, III, and aVF. The axis is −150°.

evation is seen in myocardial infarction or ischemia and in pericarditis. S-T segment changes also occur secondary to changes in the QRS (e.g., hypertrophy, bundle branch blocks).[1]

The Q-T interval is measured from the beginning of the QRS to the end of the T wave and represents the whole of ventricular depolarization and repolarization. Heart rate affects the Q-T interval, with faster heart rates causing shorter Q-T intervals. Abnormalities of the Q-T interval alone are not often seen and do not have the clinical significance that other changes do. A prolonged Q-T interval occurs with hypocalcemia, hypokalemia, quinidine therapy or toxicity, prolonged QRS, ethylene glycol poisoning, strenuous exercise, or hypothermia. A shortened Q-T interval is seen with hypercalcemia, digitalis treatment, and hyperkalemia.[1]

T waves represent repolarization of the ventricle and should not be any higher than 25% of the amplitude of the R wave. T waves may be asymmetrical but should not be sharply pointed or notched. They may be positive, negative, or biphasic but should not change polarity in the same strip. T waves are expected to look abnormal if the QRS has an abnormal depolarization wave (e.g., bundle branch block). Causes of T wave enlargement include myocardial hypoxia and electrolyte imbalances. T waves can also change with other metabolic disorders, such as anemia, shock, uremia, ketoacidosis, hypoglycemia, and fever, and with drug toxicity (e.g., digitalis, quinidine, procainamide).[1]

Small QRS complexes with electrical alternans (alternating amplitudes of R waves) are often found in animals with a pericardial effusion (Fig. 10–15). Although they strongly suggest pericardial effusion, not all animals with the disorder have these changes.[1]

Most texts on arrhythmias arrange them by source or location (e.g., supraventricular versus ventricular arrhythmias). The arrangement in this chapter is problem-oriented and describes all bradycardias in one section, tachycardias in another, and conduction disturbances last of all. In all arrhythmias, the name is descriptive of the location of the origin of the complex (i.e., sinus, atrial, or junctional) and the type of activity (i.e., tachycardia, bradycardia, or escape).

Bradyarrhythmias

Bradycardias are slow heart rates (<60 bpm for giant breeds of dogs, <70 for other dogs, and <120 for cats).[1] They arise either because the sinus node fails to fire when it should or because the impulse is blocked at the A-V node so that it cannot depolarize the ventricles. The reasons for SA and A-V nodal blocks may be pathologic, metabolic, or drug-related (Table 10-3).

Clinical Signs

Many bradyarrhythmias are first discovered on auscultation in asymptomatic dogs and cats. Pulses are usually synchronous and are weak or strong depending on myocardial function and the condition of the animal. Animals with decreased myocardial function, obesity, or shivering have weaker pulses or pulses that are harder to palpate. Symptomatic animals are either lethargic or syncopal, depending on the severity, frequency, and type of arrhythmia. Syncopal dogs resemble animals with seizure, except that there is no aura or postictal period. They collapse for a few seconds, then quickly recover as if nothing had happened.

Diagnostic Plan

All bradycardic dogs and cats should have an ECG as the first diagnostic step, and most also need a

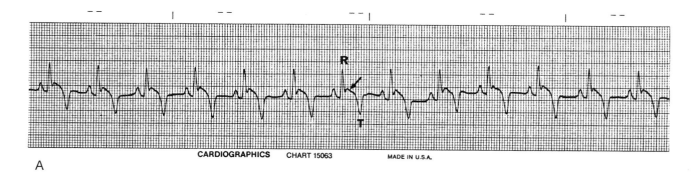

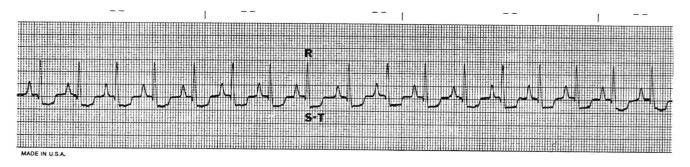

Figure 10–14
(A) S-T segment elevation *(arrow)* and large T waves in a dog with pericardial effusion.
(B) S-T segment depression in a dog with digoxin toxicity.

chest radiograph, depending on the ECG findings. For instance, an asymptomatic Pekingese with SA arrest associated with breathing does not need a chest radiograph, but a cat with third-degree A-V block does. Radiographs show the size and shape of the heart, the state of the pulmonary vasculature and pulmonary tissue, and the presence of intrathoracic masses. An echocardiogram should be done in all animals that have cardiomegaly, have a murmur, or may need to have a pacemaker implanted. Echocardiography may reveal an intracardiac reason for the arrhythmia, and it may show that a pacemaker is not indicated because of myocardial failure.

Types

Descriptions of common bradyarrhythmias follow.

Sinus Arrest

In sinus arrest, or SA nodal block, a long pause follows a sinus complex. The pause is greater than twice the distance between two normal beats, and no P waves are visible. A junctional or ventricular escape beat usually follows the pause and prevents asystole (Fig 10–16 and 10–17). The heart rate varies with the length and frequency of sinus arrest. Sinus arrest is

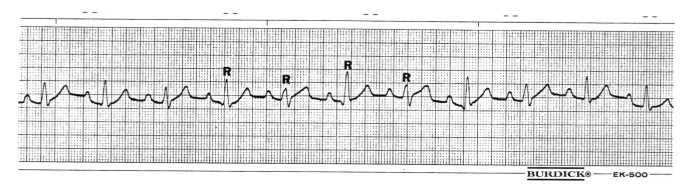

Figure 10–15
Electrical alternans in a dog with a large pericardial effusion. Notice that the R and S waves change in size with alternating beats, but the P and T waves remain the same.

Table 10–3
Conditions and Drugs That Cause Sinoatrial and Atrioventricular Nodal Blocks

High vagal tone
Degenerative diseases
Drugs
    Digitalis glycosides
    Calcium channel blockers
    β-blockers
    Antiarrhythmic drugs
      Quinidine
      Procainamide
Metabolic conditions
    Hyperkalemia
    Hypokalemia

of increased vagal tone in small animals, and SA arrest is often normal in brachycephalic breeds of dogs. Other causes of SA arrest include dilation or fibrosis of the atrium, cardiomyopathy, drug toxicity, electrolyte imbalances, and neoplasias of the head or neck that damage the vagus nerve.[1]

Sinus Bradycardia

Sinus bradycardia is similar to sinus arrest but is more regular, producing less variation in the R-R interval (Fig. 10–18). The heart rate falls below 70 bpm in dogs and 120 bpm in cats.[1] Both sinus arrest and sinus bradycardia are affected by diseases that increase vagal tone.

Sick Sinus Syndrome

Sick sinus syndrome is a severe form of SA block that is usually caused by disease in the SA node rather than by high parasympathetic tone (see Fig. 10–17). It has often been reported in female miniature schnauzers[9] but also occurs in other breeds of dogs. Sick sinus syndrome may be accompanied by a paroxysmal tachycardia that alternates with the sinus arrest, which has led to the other name for the syndrome, "brady-

usually caused by high parasympathetic tone.[1] The body systems that can cause increased vagal tone—the respiratory, gastrointestinal, and neurologic systems—should be examined for abnormalities if sinus arrest is present. Respiratory disease is the most common cause

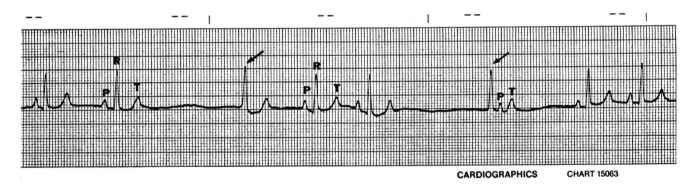

Figure 10–16
Sinus arrest with junctional escape beats (arrows) in a dog. The second escape beat has a P wave between it and the T wave.

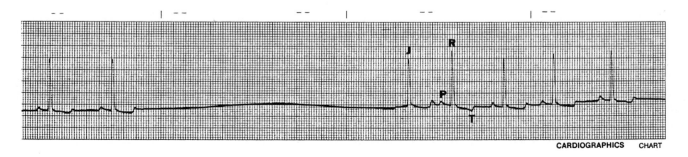

Figure 10–17
Severe sinus arrest (sick sinus syndrome) with a junctional escape beat (J) in a 13-year-old female schnauzer.

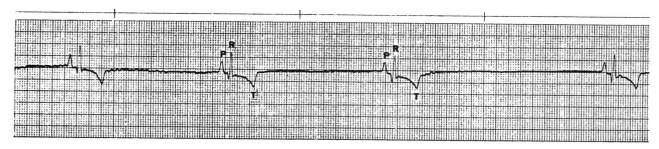

Figure 10–18
Sinus bradycardia in a 7-year-old female schnauzer with sick sinus syndrome.

cardia-tachycardia syndrome." The tachycardia in sick sinus syndrome inhibits the SA node more than normal through a mechanism called overdrive suppression and causes a longer-than-expected pause after cessation of the tachycardia. Sick sinus syndrome does not respond well to drug therapy, and the animal usually requires a pacemaker.[1]

A-V Nodal Blocks

A-V nodal blocks occur when the electrical impulse is stopped or slowed at the A-V node. There are different degrees or severity of block. The mildest form is first-degree A-V block. This is a conduction disturbance that does not alter the heart rate and is discussed later this chapter (see Conduction Disturbances).

In second-degree A-V block, there are P waves with and without conducted QRS complexes. The severity of the condition varies greatly (Figs. 10–19 and 10–20), depending on the number of P waves that eventuate in a QRS complex.[1] There may be only an occasional dropped QRS, or most of them may be dropped, in which case the condition resembles third-degree A-V block (see Fig. 10–19C).

Second-degree heart block is also divided into Mobitz I (Wenckebach phenomenon) and Mobitz II. In Mobitz I, the P-R interval progressively lengthens until there is a dropped QRS complex, or else the P-R interval may be prolonged only before the last conducted P wave.[1] Mobitz I second-degree A-V block is often a normal finding and usually requires no therapy. The P-R intervals in Mobitz II block are all the same, and the QRS is abruptly dropped. If the QRS is abnormal in configuration, indicating a block farther down in the bundle of His close to the bundle branches, it usually indicates a poorer prognosis. There is often a pattern to the block, such as 3:2 (three P waves for every two QRS complexes) or 2:1 (two P waves for every QRS). A number of conditions and drugs can cause SA and A-V nodal blocks (see Table 10–3). In pugs, type II A-V block can occur because of hereditary

stenosis of the bundle of His. A-V nodal blocks can also occur normally after atrial premature complexes or during atrial tachyarrhythmias. If the atrial premature complex comes while the A-V node is still refractory, the P wave is seen without a corresponding QRS.[1] Most second-degree heart blocks do not require therapy. Symptomatic second-degree heart blocks may respond to adrenergic or vagolytic drugs (Table 10–4), but if those drugs are unsuccessful, a pacemaker is required.

In third-degree (complete) A-V block, there is no association between P waves and QRSs, and the rhythm is usually a slow ventricular escape rhythm (Fig. 10–21). The rate is about 40 bpm for a dog and 100 bpm for a cat. Most dogs with third-degree heart block are either lethargic or exhibit collapsing episodes, whereas most cats can comfortably tolerate complete heart block because of their faster escape rhythm. Causes of third-degree A-V block (see Table 10–3) include congenital aortic stenosis or ventricular septal defect, infiltrative cardiomyopathy, myocardial fibrosis, hypertrophic cardiomyopathy, bacterial endocarditis, and Lyme disease. Drug therapies are usually ineffective, and an artificial pacemaker is frequently required.[1]

Persistent Atrial Standstill

An uncommon problem, persistent atrial standstill occurs when the atrial muscle is so fibrotic that it can no longer conduct impulses, and the heart must depend on ventricular escape beats (Fig. 10–22). Persistent atrial standstill is important because it looks like atrial standstill secondary to hyperkalemia in hypoadrenocorticism. It is thought to be congenital in English springer spaniels, although it has been reported in other breeds. Long-standing mitral regurgitation can also cause enough atrial damage to lead to this condition.[1, 10, 11] A pacemaker is required for these dogs, assuming ventricular function is normal.

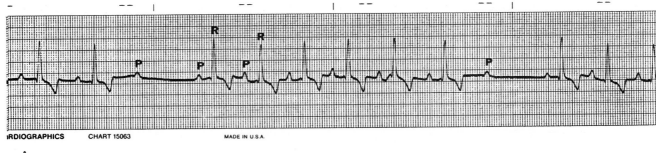

IRDIOGRAPHICS   CHART 15063   MADE IN U.S.A.

A

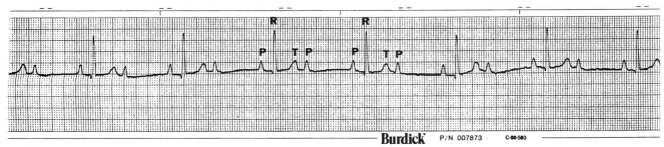

Burdick P/N 007873   C-00-503

B

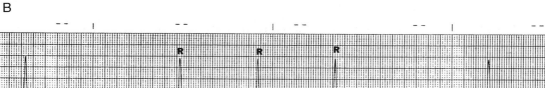

S   CHART 15063   MADE IN U.S.A.

C

Figure 10–19
(A) Mild second-degree A-V block (Mobitz II) in an asymptomatic dog. The P-R interval is a consistent length, and there are occasional P waves without corresponding QRS complexes. **(B)** 2:1 second-degree A-V block. There are two P waves for every QRS complex. This dog was mildly symptomatic and responsive to atropine. **(C)** Severe second-degree A-V block (many P waves without QRS complexes) in a dog that was responsive to atropine. A first-degree A-V block (prolongation of the P-R interval) is also present.

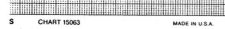

Ventricular Asystole

Ventricular asystole, an end-stage event, should be treated as cardiopulmonary arrest. It is usually seen after repeated attempts at cardiopulmonary resuscitation, although it may be seen prior to arrest. There are long periods of no electrical activity, occasionally broken by ventricular complexes with bizarre configurations (Fig. 10–23). It is a harbinger of imminent death in those dogs who are resuscitated to normal sinus rhythm only to revert to asystole. As the myocardium weakens, periods of sinus rhythm become shorter, periods of asystole become longer, and even rigorous therapy cannot maintain the heart in normal rhythm.

Treatment

Bradyarrhythmias in dogs and cats do not require therapy unless they cause lethargy or syncope. There are three ways to treat: parasympatholytic drugs, sympathomimetic agents, or a pacemaker. The drugs that are available for acute and chronic therapy are listed in (Table 10–4. Atropine sulfate is a good drug to start. Try isoproterenol if atropine is unsuccessful. If drugs fail, a permanent pacemaker is required.[12–15] Symptomatic second degree A-V block in a dog has also been successfully treated with terbutaline.[16] Occasionally, a symptomatic bradycardia is temporary and needs to be treated for only a few

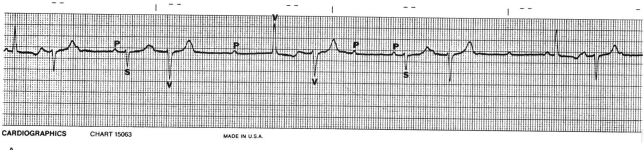

CARDIOGRAPHICS   CHART 15063   MADE IN U.S.A.

A

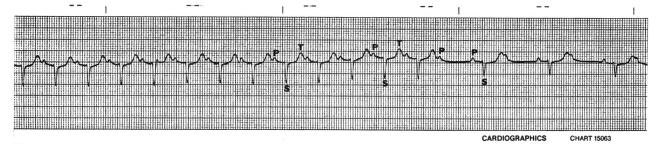

CARDIOGRAPHICS   CHART 15063

B

Figure 10–20

(A) Severe second-degree A-V block (P waves that do not always conduct across the A-V node) in a 2-year-old feline leukemia virus–positive cat. There are multiform ventricular escape beats (V). Sinus beats are the negative deflections (S wave) that follow P waves at a constant P-R interval. **(B)** Same cat as in **A**, after administration of intravenous atropine. There is 1:1 conduction on the left, which goes to 2:1 on the right-hand side of the strip.

weeks. Dogs should be rechecked no longer than 1 month after beginning therapy. If the heart rate is normal and the dog is asymptomatic, the drug can be discontinued gradually. If symptoms recur, the medication should be reinstituted. Some animals may require therapy for life.

Tachyarrhythmias

Tachycardias are fast heart rates (>140 bpm for giant breeds of dogs, >180 bpm for toy breeds, and >240 bpm for cats) that originate above the A-V node (supraventricular) or below the A-V node (ventricular). Technically, supraventricular tachycardias include any tachy-

Table 10–4
Drug Therapies for Symptomatic Bradyarrhythmias

DRUG	ACTION	DOSAGE*
Atropine sulfate (Atropine)	Parasympatholytic	0.01–0.04 mg/kg IV, IM 0.02–0.04 mg/kg SC
Isoproterenol (Isuprel)	Sympathomimetic	0.04–0.08 µg/kg/min IV, titrating to effect 0.1–0.2 mg q4-6 hr IM, SC
Glycopyrrolate (Robinul V)	Parasympatholytic	0.005–0.01 mg/kg IV, IM 0.01–0.02 mg/kg SC
Probantheline bromide (Pro-Banthine)	Parasympatholytic	Small dogs, 7.5 mg PO, t.i.d. Medium dogs, 15 mg PO, t.i.d. Large dogs, 30 mg PO, t.i.d. Cats, 7.5 mg PO, t.i.d.
Terbutaline (Brethine)	Sympathomimetic	Dogs, 0.2 mg/kg PO, b.i.d. to t.i.d. Cats, 0.625 mg PO b.i.d.

IV, intravenous; IM, intramuscular; SC, subcutaneous; PO, by mouth; b.i.d., twice per day; t.i.d., three times per day.
*All dosages the same for dogs and cats unless otherwise stated.

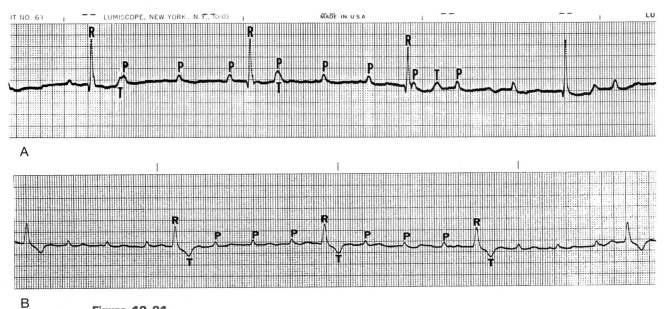

A

B

Figure 10–21
Complete (third-degree) A-V block **(A)** in a 12-year-old poodle and **(B)** in a 16-year-old cat. In third-degree A-V block, no P waves are conducted across the A-V node and the rhythm is a ventricular escape rhythm.

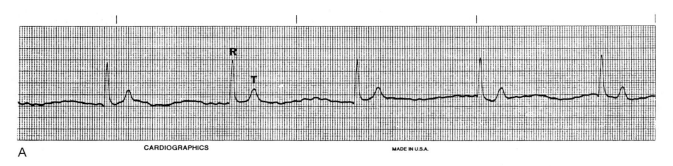

A

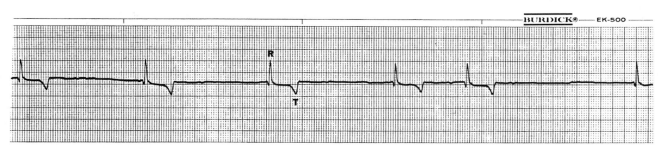

B

Figure 10–22
Atrial standstill in two dogs. **(A)** Persistent atrial standstill in an 11-year-old German shepherd with severe chronic mitral and tricuspid regurgitation. The atrium is so damaged that it cannot conduct electrical impulses. The rhythm is a ventricular escape rhythm. This electrocardiogram could also be interpreted as showing atrial fibrillation with third-degree heart block, but on postmortem examination the left atrium was found to be thin, dilated, and fibrotic. No atrial muscle was left. 1 mV = 0.5 cm.
(B) Atrial standstill secondary to hyperkalemia in a dog with an acute addisonian crisis. The heart rate is only 40 bpm and there are no P waves. The dog responded well to therapy. Paper speed = 25 mm/sec.

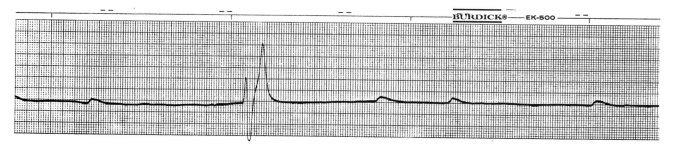

Figure 10–23
Ventricular asystole in a dog with mitral regurgitation and severe congestive heart failure during cardiopulmonary resuscitation for cardiac arrest.

cardia that occurs above the A-V node: sinus tachycardia, atrial tachycardia, junctional tachycardia, atrial flutter, or atrial fibrillation. However, the term supraventricular tachycardia is usually reserved for atrial or junctional tachycardia.[17] The following discussion includes atrial and junctional premature complexes, even though they do not usually cause a tachycardia.

Pathophysiology

The pathophysiology differs depending on the location of the tachycardia and is discussed separately for each type of arrhythmia.

Clinical Signs

Dogs and cats with tachycardias may be asymptomatic, but if the arrhythmia is fast enough, the animal may experience acute collapse. The tachycardia itself, if rapid enough, can cause pulmonary edema because of shortened diastole and incomplete ventricular emptying that backs up into the lungs. The tachycardia may also be caused by heart failure.[18] Signs of forward failure or cardiogenic shock (i.e., pallor, slow refill time, weakness, and hypothermia) are present in some animals. Pulses are weak in these animals, and pulse deficits may be present. Harsh lung sounds and a murmur may be auscultated if the tachycardia is associated with heart failure.

Diagnostic Plan

An ECG should be run first to define the type of tachycardia. Treatment can be instituted immediately if the type of arrhythmia is readily diagnosed. Some wide-complex tachycardias are difficult to differentiate as ventricular or supraventricular,[19–22] making the choice of correct therapy difficult. Supraventricular arrhythmias can safely be treated with ventricular antiarrhythmic drugs such as lidocaine, but it is dangerous to treat ventricular arrhythmias with supraventricular antiarrhythmic drugs, especially cal-

cium channel blockers.[20, 21] β-blockers, however, can safely be used in both supraventricular and ventricular arrhythmias. Ocular or carotid sinus pressure is also safe and may be used to see whether the rate slows.[18] Atrial tachycardias are broken suddenly if ocular or carotid pressure is successful; sinus tachycardias slow temporarily, then resume their pace after the stimulus is discontinued. If the rate does not slow, however, it does not mean the rhythm is ventricular. Intravenous lidocaine, procainamide, and propranolol should be used in wide-complex tachycardia if there is confusion about the origin of the rhythm.

If the animal is stable or the arrhythmia is not severe, routine chest radiographs should be taken and a complete blood count and serum chemistry analysis should be performed. If the rhythm is ventricular, dogs should also have tests for immune disease (e.g., systemic lupus erythematosus) and for Lyme disease, and cats should be tested for feline leukemia and feline immunodeficiency viruses. An echocardiogram should also be done to see whether the heart function is normal and whether there are any obvious myocardial abnormalities.

Types

Supraventricular Tachyarrhythmias

Atrial Premature Complexes

Atrial premature complexes are single supraventricular complexes that originate in the atrial muscle rather than in the sinus node. They are characterized by three things: prematurity, a QRS of similar configuration to those that originate from the SA node, and a P' wave that looks different from the sinus P wave (Fig. 10–24). These complexes are usually caused by diseases of the atrium, especially primary myocardial disease or mitral regurgitation, which causes atrial stretching. They may also be caused by drugs such as digitalis and catecholamines. Atrial premature complexes usually require no treatment,

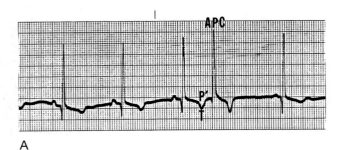

A

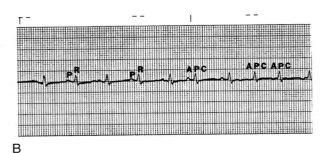

B

Figure 10-24
(A) Atrial premature complex (APC) in a poodle with mitral regurgitation. The QRS is early and has a similar configuration to the QRS complexes of sinus origin. The P' wave looks different from sinus P waves and has changed the configuration of the T wave of the preceding complex. (B) Atrial premature complexes in a cat with intergrade cardiomyopathy. Atrial premature complexes in cats are often subtle and can be found only by measuring R-R intervals.

because they do not cause problems and are indicators of other conditions.[18] Treatment should be aimed at the underlying disease.

Junctional Premature Complexes

Junctional premature complexes are similar to atrial premature complexes in that they arise above the A-V node and therefore have normal-appearing QRS complexes. They come early and may or may not have a P' wave preceding them. Often, the P' wave is negative. Junctional premature complexes can occur anywhere along the junction; they can be equidistant from the atria and ventricles or be closer to one or the other. The location of the focus determines whether the P' and QRS occur simultaneously or whether the P' occurs before or after the QRS. Junctional premature complexes are caused by the same conditions that cause atrial premature complexes, especially digoxin toxicity.

Sinus Tachycardia

Sinus tachycardia (Fig 10–25) is caused by sympathetic stimulation of the SA node and is a normal physiologic response to fever, pain, excitement, or other causes of adrenergic release. It also occurs with

drugs that block the parasympathetic nervous system. Sinus tachycardia requires no treatment unless the tachycardia is sustained, extremely rapid, or related to other disease processes that take time to control, such as hyperthyroidism. β-Blockers may be required in hyperthyroidism until other treatment stabilizes the underlying disease. Sinus tachycardia is recognized by its rapid rate, the normal size and shape of the P waves, the association of P waves with normal QRS complexes, and the presence of any condition of the animal that elevates sympathetic tone. Vagal maneuvers only temporarily slow the heart rate in sinus tachycardia, rather than abolish the arrhythmia; this is an important distinction between sinus and supraventricular tachycardia.[1]

Atrial and Junctional Tachycardias

Atrial and junctional tachycardias are often considered together because they are so difficult to differentiate. Sinus tachycardia is also frequently confused with atrial or junctional tachycardia (Fig. 10–26). However, atrial and junctional tachyarrhythmias are caused by diseased cardiac tissue, whereas sinus tachycardia is physiologic. If the exact location of the tachycardia cannot be discerned, it is called a supraventricular tachycardia. This category is used for atrial and junctional tachycardias more than for sinus tachycardia, because sinus tachycardia is usually recognized on clinical examination. Pathologic supraventricular tachycardias are caused by stretch, hypoxia, infection, and digitalis toxicity. The most common mechanism in humans is re-entry in the A-V node or in a bypass tract (extraconduction tissue that connects the atria with the ventricles and allows impulses to "bypass" the A-V node). The mechanism is unknown in dogs, although dogs do have bypass tracts and dual tracts in the A-V node. Vagal maneuvers such as ocular pressure or carotid sinus massage may break supraventricular tachycardias,[1, 3] but they only temporarily slow down a sinus tachycardia. The reason is that the re-entry circuit requires a delicate balance to continue, which is annulled by increased vagal tone. However, sinus tachycardia is caused by high sympathetic tone and is "turned off" only as long as the competing parasympathetic nervous system is stimulated.[17]

Supraventricular tachycardia should be treated if it is sustained, if there is a history of collapse or weakness, or if there is structural heart disease that would be compromised by a tachyarrhythmia. Vagal maneuvers such as ocular or carotid pressure should be attempted first, and if they are unsuccessful, a series of intravenous antiarrhythmic drugs should be tried[3] (Table 10–5). To use ocular pressure to stimulate vagal tone, the veterinarian applies strong and steady pressure to the eyes, pushing them firmly into the sockets.

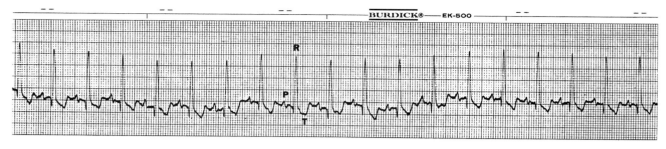

Figure 10-25
Sinus tachycardia in a nervous dog without heart disease. The heart rate is 220 bpm.

Carotid sinus pressure is increased by pressing deep into the neck just lateral to the trachea. This puts enough pressure on the carotid artery to stimulate baroreceptors and increase parasympathetic tone. If one drug trial proves unsuccessful, vagal stimulation should be repeated before going to the next drug, because the effects of drug and parasympathetic stimulation are often additive.[17] There are differing opinions about the best order in which to administer intravenous drugs, but I recommend digitalis first, followed by a β-blocker, then diltiazem. Verapamil has been used, but it must be administered with extreme care.[23] Most of the time, chronic oral therapy is required to prevent recurrence of the supraventricular tachycardia. The exception is supraventricular tachycardia caused by noncardiac disease, such as seizures or electric cord bites.

Atrial Flutter

Atrial flutter is an uncommon arrhythmia with an extremely rapid atrial rate. The rate and rhythm of the ventricular response depend on the state of the A-V node (Fig. 10-27). The atrial rate is frequently faster than 300 bpm; if the ventricular response approaches 1:1 conduction, it should be treated as soon as possible. Again, vagal stimulation is tried first. If that fails,

intravenous digitalis, β-blockers, or calcium channel blockers (see Table 10-5) may be given.[17] Some animals spontaneously convert without drugs.[1]

Atrial Fibrillation

Atrial fibrillation is one of the most common arrhythmias seen in veterinary medicine. It is found, in order of frequency, in dogs with dilated cardiomyopathy; in dogs with severe, chronic, mitral regurgitation[24]; and in dogs with congenital defects that cause severe atrial dilation. An idiopathic form occurs in large breeds of dogs with a normal left ventricle. Atrial fibrillation is characterized by a usually rapid, irregularly irregular rhythm; an absence of P waves; and fibrillation waves in the baseline (Fig. 10-28). Cats can also have atrial fibrillation (Fig. 10-29), usually in association with restrictive cardiomyopathy.[1, 17]

Because most atrial fibrillation in small animals is associated with left ventricular dysfunction, oral digoxin should be used first to slow the heart rate. Most of the time, however, digoxin alone does not slow an extremely rapid ventricular rate, and another drug is required. Both calcium channel blockers and β-blockers have been recommended for atrial fibrillation,[25] but they are negative inotropic drugs and can exacerbate heart failure.[10] Both drugs have side effects

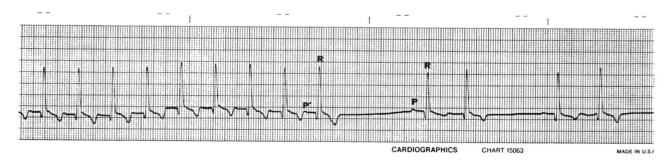

Figure 10-26
Supraventricular (atrial) tachycardia in a 13-year-old poodle with cardiac disease and collapsing episodes. The fast heart rate (220 bpm) makes it difficult to distinguish P waves. The sudden break from tachycardia to sinus rhythm confirms the diagnosis of atrial tachycardia.

Table 10–5
Classes of Antiarrhythmic Drugs

DRUG	DOSAGE*
Class 1A	
Quinidine sulfate, oral	10–20 mg/kg t.i.d. (cats)
Quinidine sulfate, injectable (Quinidex)	5–15 mg/kg PO, IM, q.i.d.
Quinidine gluconate (Quinaglute Dura-Tabs)	5–15 mg/kg PO with SR, q.i.d.
Quinidine polygalacturonate (Cardioquin)	5–15 mg/kg PO, t.i.d.
Procainamide (Procan SR)	5–15 mg/kg IM, PO, q.i.d. (SR-t.i.d.)
Procainamide (Pronestyl)	10–20 mg/kg PO, t.i.d. (cats)
	2 mg/kg IV over 3–5 min (total dose 5–10 mg/kg); 20–50 µg/kg/min CRI
Class 1B	
Lidocaine (Xylocaine)	2–8 mg/kg total dose slowly in boluses of 2 mg/kg; 50–75 mg/kg/min CRI
	Cats, 0.25–0.75 mg/kg slowly over 5 min
Mexiletene (Mexitil)	5–10 mg/kg PO, b.i.d. to t.i.d.
Tocainide (Tonocard)	10–20 mg/kg PO, b.i.d. to t.i.d.
Class 1C (not used in veterinary medicine)	
Class 2	
Propranolol (Inderal)	0.2–1.0 mg/kg PO, t.i.d.; 0.1–0.3 mg/kg IV over 5–10 min
	Cats, 2.5–10 mg PO, b.i.d. to t.i.d.; 0.04–0.06 mg/kg IV over 5–10 min
Atenolol (Tenormin)	0.25–1.0 mg/kg PO, s.i.d. to b.i.d.
	Cats, 6.25–12.5 mg PO, s.i.d. to b.i.d.
Class 3	
Sotalol (Betapace)	40–80 mg total dose, b.i.d.
Class 4 (not recommended for ventricular arrhythmias)	
Verapamil (Calan, Isoptin)	0.05–0.20 mg/kg IV slowly in boluses of 0.05 mg/kg at 10–30 min intervals
Diltiazem (Cardizem)	0.5–1.5 mg/kg PO, t.i.d. (to effect); 0.25 mg/kg IV slowly over 5–10 min (used by author)
Nifedipine (Procardia)	0.66 mg/kg PO, b.i.d.

*All dosages are for dogs unless stated otherwise.
IV, intravenous; IM, intramuscular; PO, by mouth; s.i.d., once a day; b.i.d., twice per day; t.i.d., three times per day; q.i.d., four times per day; CRI, constant-rate infusion; SR, sustained release.
Data from Muir WM III, Sams RA. Pharmacology and pharmacokinetics of antiarrhythmic drugs. In: Fox PR. Canine and Feline Cardiology. New York, Churchill Livingstone, 1988:309–333.

Figure 10–27
Atrial flutter in a young dog with a normal heart. The dog had had a seizure and developed pulmonary edema. The heart rate on presentation was more than 300 bpm. This strip was taken just before the dog's heart rate was converted with intravenous diltiazem. Notice the rapid, irregular rate and the sawtooth appearance to the P waves. The rhythm was not recognizable as atrial flutter until the ventricular response was slowed with the diltiazem, enabling the flutter waves (F) to be seen. The heart rate is 180 bpm. Paper speed = 25 mm/sec; there is no calibration, because the strip was taken from a monitor.

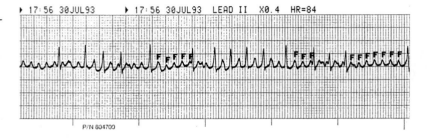

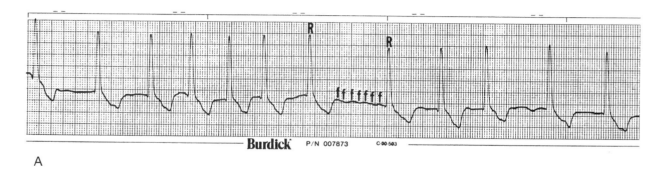

A

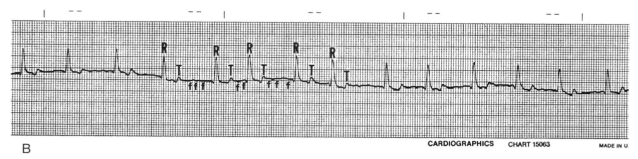

B

Figure 10-28

(A) Atrial fibrillation in a 12-year-old mixed breed dog with chronic mitral regurgitation being treated with digoxin. There are no recognizable P waves, and the baseline has fine fibrillation waves (f). The rhythm is irregularly irregular. The heart rate in atrial fibrillation is often too fast to confirm the absence of P waves, but a longer strip usually provides at least one area in which the irregular rhythm breaks enough to show the fibrillation waves instead of P waves. **(B)** Idiopathic atrial fibrillation in a Great Dane with a normal echocardiogram. T waves are often confused with P waves, but they can be differentiated by measuring the Q-T interval and the P-R interval. If the Q-T intervals are constant, it is a T wave. If the P-R intervals are constant, it is a P wave. f = fibrillation waves.

such as weakness, anorexia, and diarrhea. Dogs with idiopathic atrial fibrillation and normal cardiac function may respond to conversion with quinidine or electrical cardioversion, especially if the arrhythmia is caused by a noncardiac condition.[17] Idiopathic atrial fibrillation is not common, and most dogs need to have their therapy continued for life.

It is usually advisable to give a dog with atrial fibrillation secondary to cardiac disease digoxin for 3 to 5 days, then to add either a β-blocker or calcium channel blocker. If the heart rate is so rapid that there is low cardiac output, then the second drug may be started simultaneously with digoxin. The dog should be hospitalized during the attempt to slow the

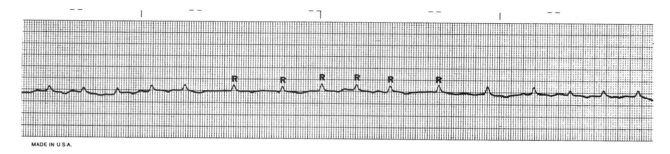

Figure 10-29

Atrial fibrillation in a cat with restrictive cardiomyopathy and severe left atrial dilation. Notice the irregularly irregular rhythm and the absence of P waves. Fibrillation waves in cats are often too small to be seen.

heart rate, then rechecked 1 week after discharge to monitor heart rate and possible drug reactions. If the rate is still high despite maximum dosages of either calcium channel blockers or β-blockers in addition to digoxin and if adequate time has passed for all the drugs to have full effect, both a β-blocker and a calcium channel blocker can be used together, but they should be used in lower doses and with extreme caution.

Ventricular Tachyarrhythmias

Ventricular tachyarrhythmias are the most common ECG abnormalities seen in veterinary medicine.[1] Causes vary greatly (Table 10–6). Discussion of both ventricular tachycardia and VPCs follows.

Table 10–6
Causes of Ventricular Arrhythmias

Cardiac Causes
Congenital heart disease
Cardiomyopathy
Chronic valvular disease
Pericarditis
Cardiac tumor
Myocarditis
Ischemia
Heartworm disease
Cardiac trauma

Drug Causes
Digitalis
Sympathomimetic agents
All anesthetic agents*
Phenothiazine tranquilizers
Atropine
Antiarrhythmic drugs

Noncardiac Causes
Hypoxia
Acidosis
Alkalosis
Electrolyte abnormalities (low potassium and
　magnesium)†
High sympathetic tone
Pheochromocytoma
Thyrotoxicosis
Sepsis and toxemia
Central nervous system disease
Gastric dilatation or volvulus
Pulmonary disease
Renal failure
Hypothermia
Splenic disease

*See Musselman[36] and Hubbell et al.[37]
†See Hollifield,[38] Podrid et al.,[39] and Gettes.[40]
Data from Bonagura JD. Therapy of cardiac arrhythmias. In: Kirk FW, ed. Current Veterinary Therapy VIII. Philadelphia, WB Saunders, 1983:360–376.

Ventricular Premature Complexes

Ventricular premature complexes (VPCs) are early ventricular beats. They are wide and bizarre and do not have an associated P wave preceding them unless the association is coincidental (Figs. 10–30 and 10–31). VPCs may be in pairs (two in a row), in runs (three in a row), or in a bigeminy (see Fig. 10–31A) or trigeminy (see Fig. 10–31B). If there are four or more VPCs in a row, it is called ventricular tachycardia. The QRS in VPCs may be positive or negative, indicating a right ventricular or left ventricular focus, respectively. Isolated, occasional VPCs do not need treatment and point to another disease.[1, 17] Sometimes an underlying cause is not determined. In that case, the animal should be referred to a cardiologist for an endomyocardial biopsy or simply re-evaluated regularly to make sure the arrhythmia does not worsen.

Ventricular Tachycardia

Ventricular tachycardia can be either monomorphic (uniform in configuration; see Fig. 10–31C) or polymorphic (multiform; see Fig. 10–31D). Monomorphic ventricular tachycardia is much more benign than polymorphic ventricular tachycardia and does not need to be treated unless the heart rate is very high or the tachycardia is causing hemodynamic compromise. Polymorphic ventricular tachycardia, on the other hand, is an unstable rhythm that should be treated with intravenous antiarrhythmic drugs (see Table 10–5). Lidocaine is the drug of first choice. If it is ineffective, procainamide should be tried next. If both fail to convert the rhythm, I recommend a combination of a constant-rate infusion of lidocaine with intramuscular quinidine or procainamide. A quick method for figuring the number of milligrams needed for a constant-rate infusion follows (note the change in units from μg to mg):

$$\text{constant-rate infusion} =$$
$$\text{animal's weight (kg)} \times \text{dose (μg/kg/min)} \times 0.36 =$$
$$\text{mg needed over a 6-hour period}$$

Example: $40 \text{ kg} \times 50 \text{ μg of lidocaine} \times 0.36 = 720 \text{ mg}$

The required amount of drug is added to a 6-hour dose of fluids and dripped at a constant rate. Infusion pumps are available for reasonable cost and should be used in this situation.

If the combination of lidocaine plus quinidine or procainamide does not work, I suggest antiarrhythmic drugs from different classifications, such as β-adrenergic blockers (see Table 10–5). Occasionally, even an oral antiarrhythmic drug such as sotalol is effective where injectable drugs are not.[26] A slow intravenous injection of propranolol (0.25 to 0.5 mg total dose over 3 to 5 min) can be used in cats with

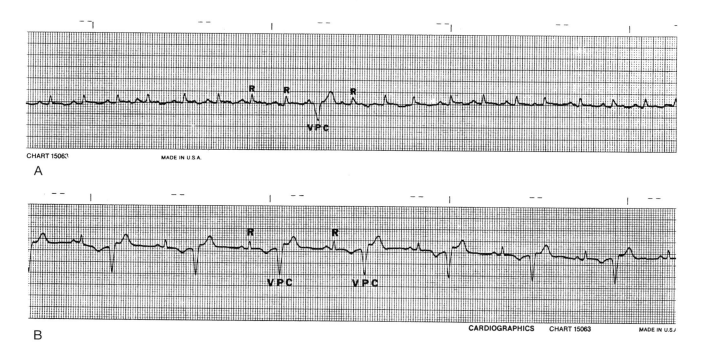

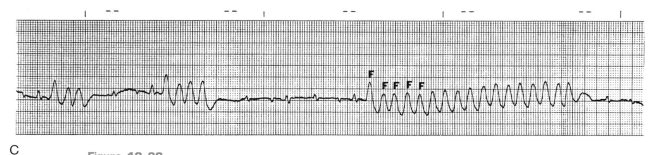

C

Figure 10–30

(A) Ventricular premature complex (VPC) in a cat with severe hypertrophic cardiomyopathy. The VPC is early and is followed by a pause, it is bizarre in configuration, and it has a T wave opposite in direction from the QRS. **(B)** Ventricular bigeminy (alternating VPCs with sinus beats) in an 8-month-old cat with left ventricular hypertrophy. **(C)** Ventricular flutter in a cat with hypertrophic cardiomyopathy and fainting episodes. The cat responded poorly to β-blocker therapy and died suddenly soon after this. These three ECGs represent increasing severity of ventricular arrhythmias. The first does not need therapy, the second may depending on the cat's clinical signs, and the third absolutely must be treated. F = ventricular flutter waves.

ventricular tachycardia. Injectable lidocaine (0.5–1.0 mg/kg bolus over 5 minutes, followed by constant-rate infusion at 10–20 μg/kg per minute) and procainamide (7.5–15 mg/kg intramuscularly) have also been used in cats. Oral procainamide (10–20 mg/kg three times per day [t.i.d.]), quinidine sulfate (10–20 mg/kg t.i.d.), and propranolol (2.5–10 mg/kg t.i.d.) all have been used in cats.[18]

After the rhythm has been controlled for 24 to 48 hours on injectable medications, the dog or cat can be switched to oral medications. The pet should be monitored another 24 hours to ensure a successful transition from injectable to oral medications. The first recheck should be in 1 to 2 weeks, then in 1 month, then every 6 months. If the cause of the underlying arrhythmia is cardiac and is not expected to resolve, antiarrhythmic drugs are continued for the life of the animal unless adverse reactions occur (e.g., proarrhythmia, untenable side effects such as vomiting). If the cause is underlying gastric dilatation or volvulus, most dogs do not even need to be sent home with antiarrhythmic therapy.[27, 28]

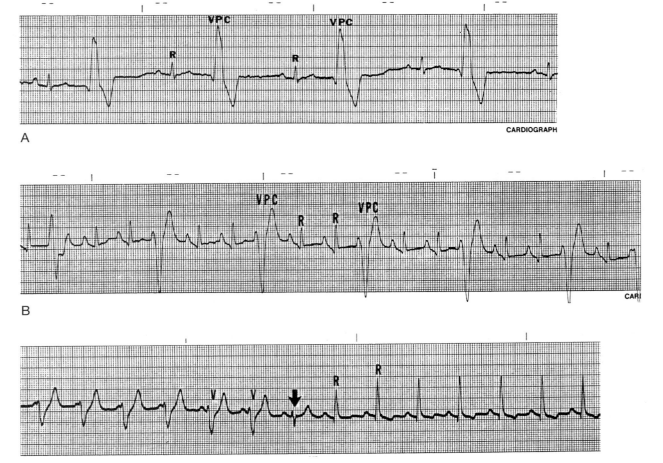

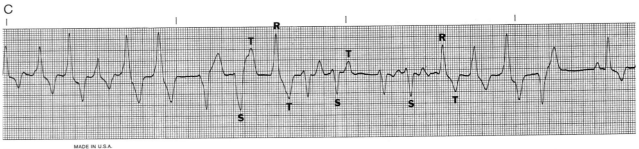

Figure 10–31
(A) Ventricular bigeminy in a dog. Ventricular premature complexes (VPCs) alternate with sinus beats. 1 mV = 0.5 cm. **(B)** Ventricular trigeminy (two sinus beats for every VPC) in a dog with congestive heart failure. **(C)** Uniform ventricular tachycardia in a dog. The seventh complex from the left is a fusion beat *(arrow)*. The dog was recovering from gastric dilatation-volvulus and was asymptomatic for the arrhythmia. 1 mV = 0.5 cm; V = ventricular complexes. **(D)** Polymorphic ventricular tachycardia in a dog with a bleeding liver tumor. Antiarrhythmic therapy was initially successful, but the arrhythmia became refractory and the dog died 6 hours after admission to the hospital. 1 mV = 0.5 cm.

Ventricular Flutter

Ventricular flutter is the step just before ventricular fibrillation, and as such it poses an emergency. It is extremely fast, bizarre, and unstable (see Fig. 10–30C). Intravenous drugs such as lidocaine or procainamide should be used as soon as the abnormal rhythm is recognized.

Ventricular Fibrillation

Ventricular fibrillation is an uncoordinated, chaotic rhythm synonymous with cardiac arrest (Fig 10–32). It does not cause cardiac arrest as commonly in animals (especially in cats) as was previously thought: most cardiac-related deaths in animals occur from asystole or electromechanical dissociation.[29] However, it is important to be able to recognize ventricular fibrillation early, because prompt treatment with direct-current countershock can reverse it.

If defibrillation equipment is unavailable, an intracardiac dose of epinephrine should be given, and the dog should be thumped. This is a procedure whereby the veterinarian hits the chest of the fibrillating animal with a closed fist, using enough force to cause a mechanical defibrillation. The thump must be delivered with more force than most are comfortable with, but one must not be timid in delivering it. Chemical defibrillation may also be attempted with 1 mEq/kg of potassium chloride (intracardiac) followed by 0.2 mL of 10% calcium chloride per kilogram, intracardiac.[30] Unfortunately, the chance of defibrillating the heart chemically or mechanically and then successfully resuscitating it is low.

As in any emergency situation, there is no time to refer to a textbook on cardiopulmonary resuscitation. Therefore, doses of emergency drugs for cardiopulmonary resuscitation should be memorized and constantly reviewed. Several excellent reviews covering cardiopulmonary resuscitation in animals may be referred to for details.[31–34]

Electromechanical Dissociation

Electromechanical dissociation occurs whenever there is continued electrical activity and a recognizable QRS complex but no mechanical heartbeat. This also poses an emergency, and it is probably one of the few emergencies in which calcium should be given. Calcium gluconate 10% can be given at a dose of 5 to 10 mg/kg intravenously.[31] Otherwise, the protocol is the same as for cardiac arrest with atrial fibrillation or asystole.

Conduction Disturbances

Conduction disturbances occur whenever the normal electrical circuit through the heart is interrupted or altered. Disturbances include slowing of conduction through the A-V node (first-degree heart block); partial to complete block through the A-V node (second- and third-degree heart block); disruption of normal conduction through the bundle branches, fascicles, and ventricular myocardium; and use of a pathway other than the A-V node. Second- and third-degree A-V blocks have been discussed (see Bradyarrhythmias), so only first-degree A-V block is covered here.

First-Degree A-V Block

First-degree A-V block occurs when slowing of conduction through the A-V node prolongs the P-R interval but every impulse reaches the ventricles (Fig. 10–33). The heart rate is normal, and there is a P wave for every QRS complex. A longer P-R interval in older dogs is common. Possible reasons for first-degree heart block (see Table 10–3) are the same as for second- and third-degree A-V block. If digitalis causes first-degree block, it can be a digitalis effect rather than toxicity as long as other symptoms of toxicity are absent, and it does not require therapy or a change of dosage.[1]

Right Bundle Branch Block

Right bundle branch blocks are probably more common in dogs and cats than realized. In general, they are benign conduction abnormalities, not usually related to cardiac disease in dogs. In cats, they may be caused by an underlying disease but in themselves are not harmful. Treatment of right bundle branch block is not necessary. Pathologic conditions causing right bundle branch block include congenital defects, myocardial disease, cardiac neoplasia, trauma, postcardiac arrest, and chronic valvular disease. It is important to differentiate bundle branch blocks from ventricular tachycardia, which they resemble. Right bundle branch blocks, unlike ventricular tachycardia, always have an associated P wave unless they are part of a complex arrhythmia (e.g., atrial fibrillation with right bundle branch block). ECG features of right bundle branch block (Figs. 10–34 and 10–35) include the following[1]:

1. QRS duration >0.08 sec in dogs (>0.06 sec in cats)

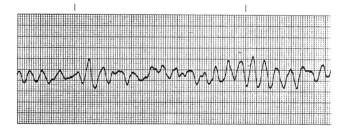

Figure 10–32
Ventricular fibrillation in a dog with severe congestive heart failure. Cardiopulmonary resuscitation was unsuccessful. 1 mV = 0.5 cm.

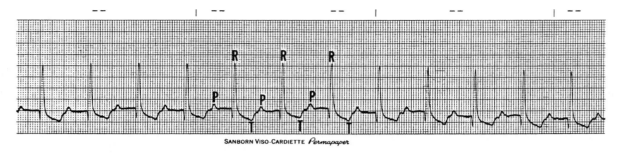

SANBORN VISO-CARDIETTE *Permapaper*

Figure 10–33
First-degree A-V block (prolonged P-R interval) in a mixed breed dog with mitral regurgitation and digitalis toxicity. The P-R interval is 0.18 sec long; normal is 0.13 sec.

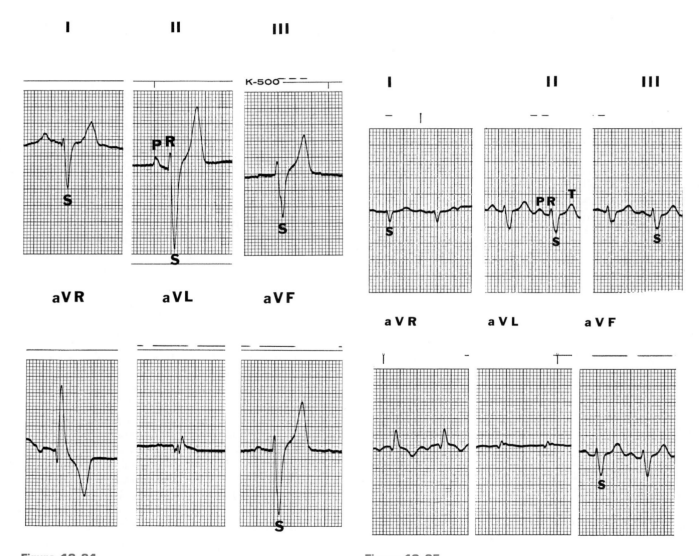

Figure 10–34
Right bundle branch block in a 14-year-old West Highland white terrier with a heart murmur but no other abnormal findings. The QRS is 0.08 sec wide, and the axis is −120°. There are deep S waves in leads I, II, III, and aVF.

Figure 10–35
Right bundle branch block in a 3-month-old kitten with a ventricular septal defect. The QRS is 0.06 sec wide, and the axis is −120°. There are deep S waves in leads I, II, III, and aVF.

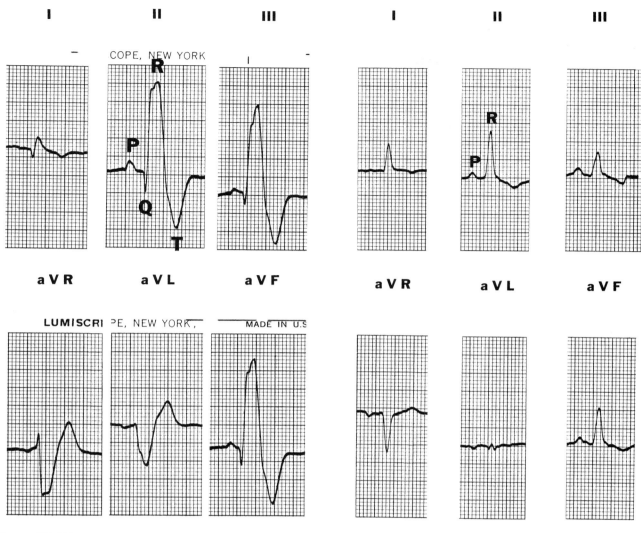

Figure 10–36
Left bundle branch block in a 4-year-old mixed breed dog with a patent ductus arteriosus. The QRS is 0.12 sec wide, and the axis is +90°. There is also P mitrale and S-T segment slurring. 1 mV = 0.5 cm.

Figure 10–37
Left bundle branch block in a cat with severe left ventricular hypertrophy. The QRS is 0.06 sec wide, and the axis is +60°.

2. Right axis deviation
3. Positive QRS in aVR, aVL, and CV_5RL leads, with a wide RSR' or rsR in CV_5RL
4. Large, wide S waves in leads I, II, III, aVF, CV_6LL, and CV_6LU

Left Bundle Branch Block

Unlike right bundle branch blocks, left bundle branch blocks are usually associated with severe underlying disease in both dogs and cats. The two most common diseases are primary myocardial disease (e.g., dilated cardiomyopathy in dogs, restrictive cardiomyopathy in cats) and long-standing mitral regur-

gitation in dogs. The complexes are wide and bizarre, but the axis is normal and there are associated P waves (Figs. 10–36 and 10–37). Like right bundle branch block, it is the underlying heart disease, rather than the left bundle branch block, that requires treatment.[1]

Left Anterior Fascicular Block

Left anterior fascicular block is rare in dogs but relatively common in cats. It is seen with hypertrophic and restrictive cardiomyopathy, other causes of left ventricular hypertrophy, and hyperkalemia. Left anterior fascicular block (Fig. 10–38) is recognized by the following features:

I   II   III

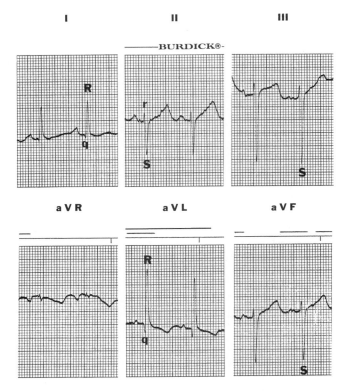

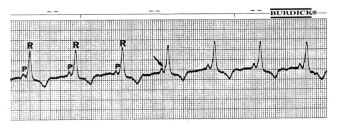

Figure 10-39
Wolff-Parkinson-White (pre-excitation) in an otherwise normal Irish setter. Notice the short P-R interval (0.04 sec) and the slurring (delta wave) in the upstroke of the QRS *(arrow)*.

Figure 10-38
Left anterior fascicular block in a cat with hypertrophic cardiomyopathy. There is a qR in leads I and aVL, there are deep S waves in leads II, III, and aVF, and there is a left axis deviation of −60°.

1. Normal to mildly prolonged QRS complex duration
2. Marked left axis deviation
3. Small q and tall R waves in leads I and aVL
4. Deep S waves in leads II, III, and aVF.

These changes should be rather marked to be called left anterior fascicular block. That is, the S waves should be significantly deep and not just present. Once again, the conduction abnormality does not require treatment; the underlying disease does.

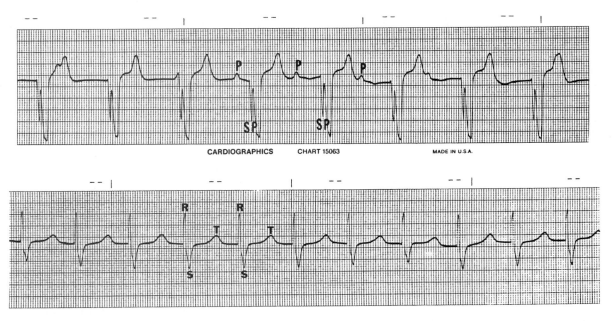

Figure 10-40
(A) Permanent transdiaphragmatic pacemaker in the left ventricle of a dog with third-degree heart block. P waves are unassociated with QRS complexes. There is a large pacemaking spike (SP) in front of every QRS. **(B)** Permanent transvenous pacemaker in the right ventricle of a cat with third-degree heart block. The pacemaking spike is too small to be seen.

Pre-excitation (Wolff-Parkinson-White) Syndrome

Pre-excitation syndrome is an uncommon conduction abnormality in which an extra tract bypasses the A-V node, allowing the depolarization wave to go from the atrium to the ventricle at a faster rate. If this impulse then restimulates the atrium, a re-entry circuit begins that can lead to a symptomatic supraventricular tachycardia called Wolff-Parkinson-White syndrome.[35] Pre-excitation syndrome is recognized by the short P-R interval, the slurred upstroke of the R wave (delta wave), and the slightly widened QRS complex[1] (Fig. 10-39).

Pacemaker

With more pacemakers being placed in dogs and cats, the veterinarian should be able to recognize the ECG tracing from a pacemaker. First, it is extremely regular unless the battery is failing. Second, there is a short, sharp spike in front of the QRS, representing the electrical discharge from the pacemaker that stimulates cardiac contraction (Fig. 10-40). Most pacemakers are demand pacemakers and do not fire unless the heart rate drops below a specified level.[1]

References

1. Tilley LP. Essentials of Canine and Feline Electrocardiography, 3rd ed. Philadelphia, Lea & Febiger, 1992.
2. Zipes DP. Genesis of cardiac arrhythmias: Electrophysiological considerations. In: Braunwald E, ed. Heart Disease, 4th ed. Philadelphia, WB Saunders, 1992: 588–627.
3. Manolis AS, Estes NAM. Supraventricular tachycardia: Mechanisms and therapy. Arch Intern Med 1987;147: 1706–1716.
4. Dangman KH, Boyden PE. Cellular mechanism of cardiac arrhythmias. In: Fox PR, ed. Canine and Feline Cardiology. New York, Churchill Livingstone, 1988: 269–287.
5. Zipes DP. Proarrhythmic effects of antiarrhythmic drugs. Am J Cardiol 1987;59:26E–31E.
6. Boyden PA. Cellular electrophysiologic basis of cardiac arrhythmias. In: Tilley LP. Essentials of Canine and Feline Electrocardiography, 3rd ed. Philadelphia, Lea & Febiger, 1992:274–286.
7. Gompf RE, Tilley LP. Comparison of lateral and sternal recumbent positions for electrocardiography of the cat. Am J Vet Res 1979;40:1483–1486.
8. Calvert CA, Coulter DB. Electrocardiographic values for anesthetized cats in lateral and sternal recumbencies. Am J Vet Res 1981;42:1453–1455.
8a. Schrope DP, Fox PR, Hahn AW. Effects of electrocardiograph frequency filters on P-QRS-T amplitudes of the feline electrocardiogram. Am J Vet Res 1995;56:1534–1540.
9. Hamlin RL, Smetzer DL, Breznock EM. Sinoatrial syncope in miniature schnauzers. J Am Vet Med Assoc 1972;161:1022–1028.
10. Miller MS, Tilley LP, Atkins CE. Persistent atrial standstill. In: Kirk RW, Bonagura JD, eds. Current Veterinary Therapy XI. Philadelphia, WB Saunders, 1992: 786–791.
11. Lombard CW, Tilley LP, Yoshioka M. Pacemaker implantation in the dog: Survey and literature review. J Am Anim Hosp Assoc 1981;17:751–758.
12. Yoshioka MM, Tilley LP, Harvey HJ, et al. Permanent pacemaker implantation in the dog. J Am Anim Hosp Assoc 1981;17:746–750.
13. Darke PGG, McAreavey D, Been M. Transvenous cardiac pacing in 19 dogs and one cat. J Small Anim Pract 1989;30:491–499.
14. Fox PR, Moise NS, Woodfield JA, et al. Techniques and complications of pacemaker implantation in four cats. J Am Vet Med Assoc 1991;199:1742–1753.
15. Sisson D, Thomas WP, Woodfield J, et al. Permanent transvenous pacemaker implantation in forty dogs. J Vet Intern Med 1991;5:322–331.
16. Sellon RD, Atkins CE, Hardie EM. Variable rate pacing and terbutaline in the treatment of syncope associated with second-degree atrioventricular block in a dog. J Am Anim Hosp Assoc 1992:28:311–317.
17. Sisson DD. The clinical management of cardiac arrhythmias in the dog and cat. In: Fox PR. Canine and Feline Cardiology. New York, Churchill Livingstone, 1988; 289–308.
18. Harpster NK. Feline arrhythmias: Diagnosis and management. In: Kirk RW, Bonagura JD, eds. Current Veterinary Therapy XI. Philadelphia, WB Saunders, 1992:732–744.
19. Litwin SE, Fenster PE. Diagnosis of wide QRS complex tachycardias. Choices in Cardiology 1989;3:342–344.
20. Stewart RB, Bardy GH, Greene HL. Wide complex tachycardia: Misdiagnosis and outcome after emergency therapy. Ann Intern Med 1986;104:766–771.
21. Akhtar M, Shenasa M, Jazayeri M, et al. Wide QRS complex tachycardia. Reappraisal of a common clinical problem. Ann Intern Med 1988;109:905–912.
22. Hamlin RL. Therapy of supraventricular tachycardia and atrial fibrillation. In: Kirk RW, Bonagura JD. Current Veterinary Therapy XI. Philadelphia, WB Saunders, 1992; 745–749.
23. Kittleson M, Keene B, Pion P, et al. Verapamil administration for acute termination of supraventricular tachycardia in dogs. J Am Vet Med Assoc 1988;193:1525–1529.
24. Bonagura JD, Ware WA. Atrial fibrillation in the dog: Clinical findings in 81 cases. J Am Anim Hosp Assoc 1986;25:111–120.
25. Prichett ELC. Management of atrial fibrillation. N Engl J Med 1992;326:1264–1271.
26. Lunney J, Ettinger SJ. Mexiletine administration for management of ventricular arrhythmia in 22 dogs. J Am Anim Hosp Assoc 1991;27:597–600.
27. Muir WW, Lipowitz AJ. Cardiac dysrhythmias associated with gastric dilatation–volvulus in the dog. J Am Vet Med Assoc 1978;172;683–689.
28. Muir WW. Gastric dilatation–volvulus in the dog, with

emphasis on cardiac dysrhythmias. J Am Vet Med Assoc 1982;180:739–742.

29. Rush JE, Wingfield WE. Recognition and frequency of dysrhythmias during cardiopulmonary arrest. J Am Vet Med Assoc 1992;200:1932–1944.

30. Haskins SC. Cardiopulmonary resuscitation. In: Kirk RW, ed. Current Veterinary Therapy X. Philadelphia, WB Saunders, 1989:330–336.

31. Robello CD, Crowe DT. Cardiopulmonary resuscitation: Current recommendations. Vet Clin North Am Small Anim Pract 1989;19:1127–1149.

32. Henik RA. Basic life support and external cardiac compression in dogs and cats. J Am Vet Med Assoc 1992;200:1925–1931.

33. Van Pelt DR, Wingfield WE. Controversial issues in drug treatment during cardiopulmonary resuscitation. J Am Vet Med Assoc 1992;200:1938–1944.

34. Wingfield WE, Van Pelt DR. Respiratory and cardiopul-monary arrest in dogs and cats: 265 cases (1986–1991). J Am Vet Med Assoc 1992;200:1993–1996.

35. Hill BL, Tilley LP. Ventricular preexcitation in seven dogs and nine cats. J Am Vet Med Assoc 1985;187:1026–1031.

36. Musselman EE. Arrhythmogenic properties of thiamylal sodium in the dog. J Am Vet Med Assoc 1976;168:145–148.

37. Hubbell JAE, Muir WW, Bendarski RM, et al. Change of inhalation anesthetic agents for management of ventricular premature depolarizations in anesthetized dogs and cats. J Am Vet Med Assoc 1984;185:643–646.

38. Hollifield JW. Magnesium depletion, diuretics, and arrhythmias. Am J Med 1987;82(Suppl 3A):30–37.

39. Podrid PJ, Fogel RI, Fuchs TT. Ventricular arrhythmia in congestive heart failure. Am J Cardiol 1992;69:82G–96G.

40. Gettes LS. Electrolyte abnormalities underlying lethal and ventricular arrhythmias. Circulation 1992;85(Suppl I):70–76.

Valvular Diseases

Betsy R. Bond

Valvular disease is caused by degeneration, infection, or damage to the mitral, tricuspid, aortic, or pulmonary valve. Chronic mitral valve disease in small breeds of dogs, the most common cardiac problem seen in small animal veterinary medicine, is discussed in the most detail. In addition to acquired mitral valve disease, this chapter covers acquired tricuspid valve disease and bacterial endocarditis. Acquired valvular disease in cats is rare as a primary entity.

Anatomy and Physiology

Semilunar and Atrioventricular Valves

There are four sets of cardiac valves that permit blood flow in one direction through the heart. The mitral and tricuspid, or atrioventricular (A-V), valves are open in diastole, allowing blood to flow from the atria to the ventricles. They should completely close in systole while blood is being ejected from the ventricles. Damage to these valves causes regurgitation into the left and right atria. Incomplete opening of the A-V valves in diastole (mitral or tricuspid stenosis) is rare in dogs and cats.

The aortic and pulmonary (semilunar) valves should open in systole and close in diastole. Blood is pumped from the right ventricle through the pulmonary artery into the lungs and from the left ventricle through the aorta to the rest of the body. Pulmonary and aortic stenoses create turbulence (murmurs) in systole; these conditions are discussed in Chapter 14.

Pulmonary and aortic insufficiencies occur in diastole and are usually associated with congenital aortic and pulmonary stenosis. Acquired aortic regurgitation usually occurs secondary to bacterial endocarditis, but a small aortic regurgitation may be seen on Doppler echocardiography as a result of systemic hypertension. Clinical disease is a rare cause of pulmonary insufficiency, but pulmonary insufficiency may be caused by pulmonary hypertension. However, a trivial pulmonary insufficiency is often visualized in normal animals during Doppler examinations, and this finding must be differentiated from diseased valves. Severe insufficiencies cause a diastolic murmur and a volume overload of the affected ventricle.[1]

Mitral Valve Apparatus

More has been written about the mitral valve than about the other valves, because it is usually the one affected in acquired valvular disease. Mitral regurgitation is caused by degeneration of the mitral valve leaflets, but it may also be caused by structural alteration of one or more regions of the mitral valve complex.[2] The mitral valve complex consists of four parts: mitral valve annulus, leaflets, chordae tendineae, and papillary muscle.[2, 3]

The mitral valve is not truly a bicuspid valve, although it has two main cusps, the aortic (anterior) and the mural (posterior). The anterior and posterior mitral valve cusps are unequal in length, but the free edges are level with one another and facilitate optimum coaptation. The purpose of the mitral valves is to prevent regurgitation of blood into the left atrium during systole. They are assisted in this by the papillary muscles, projections of the left ventricular myocardium that are connected to the mitral valves by chordae tendineae. As the normal left ventricle contracts in systole, the papillary muscles also contract and pull the mitral valves together, preventing insufficiency. The mitral valve annulus is the circular opening to which the mitral valves are attached; it separates the atria from the ventricles.[3]

The normal microscopic anatomy of the mitral valve consists of three layers, the first being a continuation of atrial muscle into the mitral valve. The atrial muscle is gradually replaced by collagen fibers (fibrosa), which become a mesh of loose collagen fibers (spongiosa) embedded in a mucopolysaccharide protein ground substance. There is a single unit of fibrous tissue that extends from the annulus through the collagen fibers of the leaflet to the collagen core of the chordae tendineae and papillary muscle. These collagen fibers divide into many small branches of chordae tendineae, which increase the surface area of the chordae and dissipate stress over the entire valve annulus.[2] The chordae must be the optimum size: too long, and they permit inversion or prolapse into the left atrium; too short, and they prevent coaptation.[3]

Problem Identification

Acquired Cardiac Murmurs

An acquired heart murmur is an abnormal vibration that is heard on auscultation in dogs older than 1 year of age, although it is very unusual to hear an acquired murmur in a small-breed dog younger than 3 years of age. Most murmurs are auscultated for the first time in dogs that are 7 years of age or older, although some dogs, such as cavalier King Charles spaniels, may have murmurs at as young as 2 years of age.[4] Systolic murmurs are extremely common in companion animals, especially small breeds of dogs.

Pathophysiology

Murmurs are caused by turbulent blood flow and may reflect damage to one or more of the heart valves (see Chap. 9). The turbulence arises because a valve is thickened and unable to fully close (coapt), or because stenosis prevents it from fully opening. Most murmurs caused by acquired valvular disease are systolic murmurs of the mitral or tricuspid valve. Murmurs associated with bacterial endocarditis are caused by vegetations on the valves, most commonly the aortic and mitral valves. The major consequence of most acquired valvular disease is a volume overload to the side of the heart that is affected. Mitral valve disease causes fluid retention in the lungs (pulmonary edema), whereas tricuspid valve disease causes fluid in the chest (pleural effusion) or abdomen (ascites).

Clinical Signs

Although murmurs of acquired valvular disease are usually heard during a routine physical examination, they often occur with symptoms of heart failure (i.e., crackles, dyspnea, coughing, ascites, arrhythmias). The age and breed of dog help determine the underlying cause. For example, disease of the mitral or tricuspid valve occurs in older, small breeds of dogs,[5-7] and dilated cardiomyopathy is found in middle-aged giant breeds (e.g., Great Danes, Saint Bernards), Doberman pinschers, boxers, and English cocker spaniels (see Chap. 12). Cavalier King Charles spaniels have a particularly virulent form of mitral regurgitation, and they develop signs earlier than other breeds.[4, 8] Murmurs from bacterial endocarditis occur in middle-aged large breeds of dogs (e.g., German shepherds); these murmurs are usually accompanied by a fever, lameness, lethargy, and other signs of systemic illness, and they are usually louder than those caused by cardiomyopathy.

The murmur of mitral valve disease is usually a grade III/VI or louder (see Chap. 9), although it may be softer when it is first heard. The loudness of the murmur frequently does not correlate well with clinical signs; that is, it cannot be assumed that a grade V/VI murmur is caused by worse mitral regurgitation than is a III/VI murmur.[9, 10] However, there is a general trend of worsening heart disease with increasing loudness of murmurs in cavalier King Charles spaniels.[8] Most murmurs of mitral regurgitation are loudest on the left at the ventricular apex (low on the thorax at the fifth to sixth intercostal space) and are holosystolic (i.e., occur throughout systole and often obliterate the first and second heart sounds). Tricuspid valve murmurs are auscultated best at the fifth to sixth intercostal space low on the right, although murmurs of mitral regurgitation are often loud enough to radiate to the right and mimic murmurs of tricuspid regurgitation. Diastolic decrescendo murmurs are usually caused by aortic insufficiency from bacterial endocarditis[5, 10] and radiate from the aortic valve to the left ventricle.

Diagnostic Plan

All dogs and cats in which murmurs have been auscultated should have an electrocardiogram (ECG), a chest radiograph, and an echocardiogram. Older dogs and cats should also have routine blood tests; dogs should be tested for heartworm disease, and cats should be screened for hyperthyroidism. Most diagnoses may be made by considering the age and breed of the dog, the history, and the clinical signs. Dogs with mitral valve disease and tricuspid valve disease are older, small breeds of dogs.[9] Approximately half of dogs with valvular disease have a normal ECG; if abnormalities are present, they include wide P waves, tall and wide QRS complexes, atrial arrhythmias, and occasionally, ventricular arrhythmias. Thoracic radiography is the most helpful of the tests available to veterinarians. Mitral regurgitation causes generalized cardiomegaly and left atrial enlargement. Right atrial enlargement may or may not be present, but the right ventricle usually appears enlarged even if only the mitral valves are involved. Echocardiography is not necessary for diagnosis, but it can indicate the severity of valvular thickening, chamber enlargement, and the presence of myocardial failure.

Bacterial endocarditis as a cause of heart murmur is often difficult to diagnose. A heart murmur in the presence of fever and leukocytosis is a strong indicator of endocarditis, especially if the ECG reveals arrhythmias or tall and wide QRS complexes and thoracic radiography shows cardiomegaly and pulmonary congestion or edema. Murmurs caused by bacterial endocarditis are systolic murmurs located over the mitral valve or decrescendo diastolic murmurs over the aortic valve and left ventricle. Echocardiography should be performed to look for thickened aortic or mitral valves with mitral or aortic regurgitation. A complete blood count (CBC) should be performed to look for leukocytosis, a serum biochemistry profile to see whether damage has occurred to the liver or kidneys, and a urinalysis to look for white cells, red cells, and casts. Blood culture and sensitivity, urine culture, and culture of joint fluid may reveal a source of infection.

Acquired valvular disease in the cat is rare. See Chapter 12 for a discussion of acquired heart murmurs in cats and of murmurs in dogs related to cardiomyopathy.

Fever

Dogs with chronic fever unresponsive to antibiotics may have bacterial endocarditis. A murmur of recent onset or changing intensity, or a ventricular arrhythmia, should accompany these fevers. Other signs supporting endocarditis include episodic lameness, anorexia, weight loss, lethargy, and coughing. A

CBC, serum chemistries, urinalysis, ECG, chest radiograph, echocardiogram, and multiple cultures of blood, urine, or joints should be performed. Leukocytosis, septic polyarthritis, urinary tract infection, left-sided heart failure, and thickened mitral or aortic valves are supportive of the diagnosis of bacterial endocarditis, and a positive blood culture is diagnostic (see Chap. 35 for a further discussion of fever).

Cough

A cough is a forceful expiration of fluid or foreign material from the lungs. The presence of a mitral regurgitation murmur in an older, small-breed dog with cough strongly indicates that the cough is caused by left-sided heart failure. Other symptoms that support a diagnosis of heart failure include dyspnea, lethargy, and anorexia. Crackles, dyspnea, cyanosis, and a heart murmur are usually auscultated. A cough in the absence of a murmur is not usually caused by heart failure, and a cough is not caused by tricuspid regurgitation. Radiographic changes consistent with mitral regurgitation include cardiomegaly, left atrial enlargement, and pulmonary venous congestion and edema.

A cough may also be caused by compression of the trachea and bronchi by a severely enlarged left atrium, in which case the lungs are clear of fluid but the enlarged left atrium and tracheal compression are visualized on the lateral radiograph. These dogs are not lethargic, but they have a harsh, dry cough that is similar to the cough caused by collapsing trachea (see Chaps. 9 and 54 for a further discussion of cough).

Ascites

Ascites is fluid accumulation within the abdomen. It is caused by isolated tricuspid regurgitation or by long-standing mitral regurgitation that has led to right-sided heart failure in older, small-breed dogs. Ascites is often present in dogs with atrial fibrillation. These dogs have murmurs of mitral or tricuspid insufficiency. Other symptoms include severe weight loss (cardiac cachexia), hepatomegaly, and jugular pulses. Radiography reveals cardiomegaly, but right atrial and ventricular enlargement are best visualized on echocardiography. Cytologic characteristics of ascites caused by right-sided heart failure are consistent with a modified transudate (see Chap. 34 for a further discussion of ascites).

Syncope

Syncope is an uncommon sign of acquired valvular disease, but it occurs often enough in small-breed dogs to be considered a symptom of heart failure. It may occur in dogs with bacterial endocarditis because of arrhythmias, or with left-sided heart failure because of pulmonary edema and hypoxia. Dogs that have syncope and endocarditis are usually large-breed male dogs with fever, lethargy, and an arrhythmia on auscultation. Other clinical signs in dogs with left-sided heart failure causing syncope include dyspnea, coughing, and lethargy, although none of these signs must be present. A murmur, however, is present in dogs with syncope secondary to heart failure. Radiography reveals cardiomegaly and pulmonary edema (see Chap. 9 for a further discussion of syncope).

Arrhythmias

Arrhythmias in dogs with bacterial endocarditis are usually ventricular in origin and are associated with fever, lethargy, and weight loss. Mitral and tricuspid regurgitation usually cause atrial arrhythmias (i.e., atrial tachycardia or atrial fibrillation) because of stretching of the atrial muscle,[11] although ventricular arrhythmias may occur. Atrial tachycardia is characterized by tachycardia (heart rate >160 beats per minute [bpm]), QRS complexes that are normal in configuration, and P waves that differ from sinus complexes. Atrial tachycardia causing syncope is usually paroxysmal and has a rate faster than 200 bpm. Atrial fibrillation is an irregularly irregular rhythm with an absence of P waves and fibrillation waves in the baseline. Clinical signs that should be present with heart disease include coughing, dyspnea, exercise intolerance, and weight loss (especially with atrial fibrillation). A heart murmur with or without crackles (pulmonary edema) or muffled heart and lung sounds (pleural effusion) should be auscultated in dogs with arrhythmias caused by mitral or tricuspid regurgitation (see Chap. 10 for a further discussion of arrhythmias).

Canine Mitral Valve Disease

Canine mitral valve disease is the most common heart disease seen in small animal medicine, affecting from 17% to 40% of all dogs.[1, 5, 7, 9, 10, 12, 13] It is an acquired condition whereby the mitral valve becomes thick and fails to close in systole, causing regurgitation of blood into the left atrium. It primarily occurs in geriatric, small breeds of dogs and rarely affects cats.[10] The mitral valve alone is affected in most cases; degeneration of both mitral and tricuspid valves together or of the tricuspid valve alone is less common.[5, 13] Acquired abnormalities of the aortic and pulmonary valves are rarely seen.[13]

Pathophysiology

The terms endocardiosis and myxomatous degeneration of the mitral valve have been used to

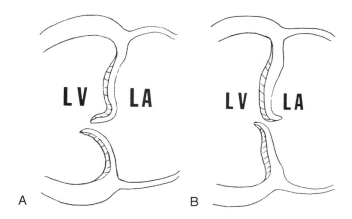

Figure 11-1

Abnormalities of mitral valve coaptation, as seen from a right parasternal long-axis echocardiogram. **(A)** Mild mitral valve prolapse. The body of the mitral valve protrudes into the left atrium. **(B)** In flail tip of the mitral valve, the tip of the mitral valve flips into the left atrium. LA, left atrium; LV, left ventricle.

describe a condition in which normal tissue is replaced by defective or degenerative collagen or glycosaminoglycans, or both, resulting in a nodular, thickened valve that does not close properly during systole.[1, 10, 13] The underlying cause is elusive, but it may be genetic.[10] The hallmark is myxomatous degeneration and mucopolysaccharide infiltration of the valve leaflet, which causes the valves to become voluminous, ballooning into the left atrium.[14, 15]

Abnormal coaptation (closure) of the valves causes regurgitation into the atrium and volume overload of the atrium and ventricle.[1] The severity of mitral regurgitation is related to several factors, such as the size of the mitral valve orifice in systole, the pressure gradient between the left ventricle and the left atrium,[1, 16, 17] the presence and severity of mitral valve prolapse or flail tip of the mitral valve, rupture of chordae tendineae, and left ventricular dilation.[1, 18]

Terms related to mitral valve dysfunction are helpful to describe echocardiographic abnormalities. Prolapse of the mitral valve is a bulging of the body of the mitral valve into the left atrium with regurgitation; it is often seen on echocardiography (Figs. 11–1A and 11–2A). A flail tip of the mitral valve occurs when the tip of the mitral valve flips into the left atrium (Figs. 11–1B and 11–2B).[14]

Rupture of the chordae tendineae is a special condition that causes more severe heart failure than does slowly developing mitral regurgitation. With chronic mitral regurgitation, the left atrium gradually stretches and holds a greater volume of blood than a left atrium that is suddenly overloaded by acute chordal rupture. The blood in acute mitral regurgitation is forced into the lungs, causing severe pulmonary

edema. There is evidence from studies in humans that animals with mitral valve prolapse may have a greater probability of rupture of the chordae tendineae because of increased tension on the valve and degeneration of collagen within the core of the chordae.[1, 19]

Left ventricular dilation also adversely affects mitral regurgitation.[20] First, as the left ventricle dilates, so does the mitral valve annulus,[18] and as the annulus dilates, so does the mitral valve orifice. Second, left ventricular dilation distorts normal left ventricular shape. Instead of being elliptic, it becomes more spheric, which affects the position of the papillary muscles. The papillary muscles move laterally and actually pull the mitral valves open in systole, instead of assisting closure during contraction.[21, 22]

Mitral regurgitation can be divided into acute, chronic compensated, and chronic decompensated mitral regurgitation.[23] Mitral regurgitation causes a volume overload to the left ventricle, which eventually leads to congestive heart failure (fluid retention) and myocardial failure (decreased contractility). The two main pathophysiologic mechanisms in heart failure are wall stress from left ventricular dilation and stimulation of neurohormones. Diuretics, vasodilators, and positive inotropic agents help relieve wall stress, but they may increase sympathetic tone or stimulate the renin-angiotensin-aldosterone system, thereby doing harm.[24]

Acute mitral regurgitation is usually caused by ruptured chordae tendineae. The regurgitant volume is added to pulmonary venous return,[23] so that a large amount of blood is delivered to a normal left atrium. The left atrium is unable to stretch acutely to accommodate the extra load, and blood backs up into the lungs, causing pulmonary edema. The left ventricle is also overwhelmed, and left-sided heart failure ensues.[25] Because contractility is normal, the shortening fraction on echocardiography is increased because of low pressure in the left atrium, compared with the systemic circulation. However, forward flow is severely compromised because of left atrial run-off.[23]

In chronic compensated mitral regurgitation, the heart has dilated and undergone eccentric hypertrophy (Fig. 11–3).[5, 20, 26, 27] Increased total left ventricular volume increases stroke volume and maintains cardiac output. Left ventricular and left atrial compliance are increased (less stiffness), so that there is a lower filling pressure even with an increased volume, and pulmonary venous congestion decreases.[1, 23]

The change from compensated mitral regurgitation to decompensated mitral regurgitation could be caused by rupture of the chordae tendineae or by worsening mitral regurgitation.[28] The left ventricle is more dilated, but the eccentric hypertrophy is inadequate to meet the needs of the ventricle, and wall stress is increased. There is maximum preload but

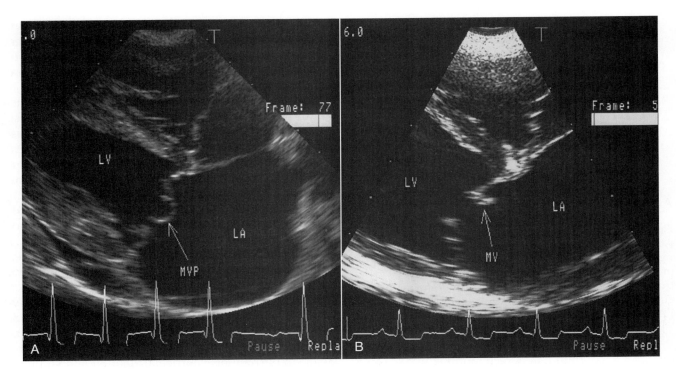

Figure 11–2
(A) Two-dimensional echocardiogram of a Chihuahua with mitral valve regurgitation and mild mitral valve prolapse. The middle portion of the mitral valve moves farther into the left atrium than it should *(arrow)*. The left atrium is severely dilated. LA, left atrium; LV, left ventricle; MVP, mitral valve prolapse. **(B)** Two-dimensional echocardiogram of a cavalier King Charles spaniel with mitral regurgitation and flail tip of the anterior mitral valve leaflet *(arrow)*. This abnormal coaptation allows regurgitation into the left atrium. LA, left atrium; LV, left ventricle; MV, mitral valve.

decreased cardiac output. The ventricle is weaker but must empty a higher load (larger volume), hastening the decline of ventricular function. As contractility decreases, the ventricle dilates more, putting more stress on the failing myocardium. Left ventricular dilation also dilates the mitral valve annulus, worsening the mitral regurgitation.[20, 23, 26, 27] Chamber stiffness also increases in animals with mitral regurgitation and myocardial failure,[21] decreasing ventricular filling.

In addition to cardiac changes in chronic compensated and decompensated mitral regurgitation, neurohumoral mechanisms exacerbate heart failure and put more stress on the myocardium.[20] The two most important systems are the sympathetic nervous system and the renin-angiotensin-aldosterone system (see Chap. 8). An important point is that the renin-angiotensin-aldosterone system is not stimulated in early heart failure until diuretics are administered; therefore, diuretics should not be prescribed until needed to treat fluid retention. In addition, the effectiveness of diuretics may become attenuated over time.[24, 29, 30]

Clinical Signs

Asymptomatic Heart Disease

A murmur is often heard for the first time when a dog is examined by a veterinarian for other problems or for a routine checkup.[1, 5] These dogs have a normal apex beat, normal pulses, and normal lung sounds.[30a] Many dogs have a murmur for years without clinical symptoms,[1] and although mitral regurgitation is a progressive disease, it is impossible to know how quickly an individual animal will deteriorate.[10]

Mild to Moderate Heart Failure

The most common symptom of heart failure caused by mitral regurgitation is a cough,[1, 5] usually of short duration (i.e., a few days to 2 months), and it can start suddenly. The cough in mild heart failure may be heard more at night or early in the morning, and it is exacerbated by exercise or excitement. Some owners report that their dog wakes up restless at night, coughing, and then goes back to sleep for a few hours (nocturnal dyspnea). As pulmonary congestion wors-

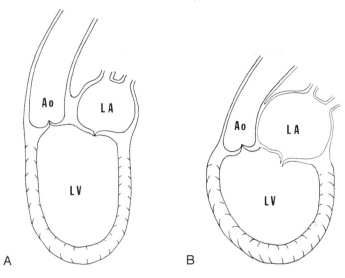

Figure 11-3
Diagram of **(A)** a normal heart compared with **(B)** a heart that has undergone eccentric hypertrophy. The ventricle is dilated, and the hypertrophy is a response to the dilation. Because most hypertrophy is inadequate to meet the needs of the dilated ventricle, the hypertrophy is not obvious. The ventricle also becomes more rounded than normal as heart failure progresses. Ao, aorta; LA, left atrium; LV, left ventricle.

ens, the cough becomes more persistent, and it is usually accompanied by dyspnea, tachypnea, and exercise intolerance (moderate heart failure).[1, 5, 10, 30a] However, not all geriatric dogs with a cough have mitral valve disease; many older dogs with or without mitral regurgitation cough from pulmonary disease.[9]

Advanced Heart Failure

Symptoms of congestive heart failure are immediately obvious even when the animal is at rest. With any physical activity, discomfort is increased. Cardiogenic shock is present in severe cases. Many dogs can be treated at home, but dogs with severe cases must be hospitalized. Death is likely without some kind of therapy.[30a]

Other symptoms of heart failure include exercise intolerance and syncope.[1, 5, 9] Because of the mitral regurgitation, blood is unable to perfuse muscle tissues and the brain, and animals become weak or they faint with exercise. Another mechanism for weakness is hypoxemia from pulmonary edema. Arrhythmias can also cause a sudden drop in cardiac output, leading to syncope. Generalized muscle weakness with exercise intolerance is usually not seen until there is myocardial failure from advanced disease.[10]

Physical findings other than a murmur depend on the class of heart failure and which valve is affected. Dogs with mitral regurgitation in asymptomatic or

mild heart failure usually have lungs that appear normal on auscultation, whereas dyspnea, crackles, and cyanosis are found in dogs with moderate or advanced heart failure. Weight loss is not a common finding except in chronic, severe mitral valve disease or tricuspid valve disease. The presence of a gallop—the third heart sound—in chronic advanced heart failure may indicate left ventricular dilation and impaired left ventricular function.[5, 31] A sinus tachycardia is usually present, and an arrhythmia caused by atrial or ventricular premature contractions may also be auscultated.[1, 9, 10] Atrial fibrillation in small dogs that is caused by severe left atrial dilation is a poor prognostic sign. Most of these dogs are also thin or cachectic.

Pulses in early mitral regurgitation are usually strong and synchronous with the heartbeat unless an arrhythmia is present. In later stages of heart failure, contractility decreases and pulses become weaker. Pulse deficits can be palpated in dogs with atrial and ventricular premature beats, because the beat is auscultated but ventricular filling is inadequate to generate a pulse. Atrial fibrillation causes pulses that may equal only half the number of beats auscultated.

End-Stage Complications

End-stage complications of mitral valve disease can be divided into those conditions that usually cause acute death (ruptured chordae or left atrial tear) and those that are more chronic but have very serious effects (atrial fibrillation and renal disease).

Dogs with ruptured chordae tendineae present in acute heart failure,[32] often with pink, frothy fluid dripping from their nostrils. They constitute the most immediate of emergencies, and many of them die within hours after presentation, even with intensive treatment. In addition to the therapies listed under acute heart failure, if the dog arrests and requires intubation, positive pressure ventilation may be helpful, as may suction through the tracheal tube to remove fluid. I have even turned some dogs so their heads are down for a few seconds to let edema fluid run out of the tube while waiting for suction to be set up. Unfortunately, most of these efforts are futile.[10]

Left atrial tears are also devastating complications of mitral valve disease.[6, 10] Dogs with left atrial tears experience acute collapse secondary to cardiac tamponade. Heart sounds are mildly muffled but not as much as in other kinds of pericardial effusion. The effusion develops so quickly that even small amounts of fluid produce severe symptoms. The cardiac silhouette is somewhat round, but not as much as is expected with pericardial effusions that develop more slowly and stretch the pericardial sac. Echocardiography is diagnostic of pericardial effusion, and a clot is often visualized in the pericardial fluid.[10] Pericardiocentesis yields clotting blood, and surgery, pericardiocentesis, or medical treatment (cage rest and oxygen) has not been successful, in my experience.

Atrial fibrillation is a late event in dogs with severely enlarged left atria. After atrial fibrillation develops, there is usually a slowly progressing, downward course until death. Most dogs live only 6 to 8 months after the development of atrial fibrillation. In addition, they begin to develop cardiac cachexia and ascites, and abdominocentesis often must be performed every 2 to 4 weeks.

Renal failure is a common condition in dogs with heart failure. The combination of heart disease, old age, and high levels of diuretics and vasodilators eventually takes its toll on the kidneys. This is an extremely difficult situation to manage, because the treatment for heart disease is detrimental to the kidneys, and vice versa. If owners elect to proceed with treatment, one half to three fourths of the calculated maintenance intravenous (IV) fluids (one-half strength lactated Ringer's solution with 2.5% dextrose) and decreased dosages of cardiac drugs may be helpful. Central venous pressure is monitored during fluid treatment, and if it rises above 15 cm H_2O or more than 10 cm H_2O above baseline measurement, the next fluid treatment is not administered. Central venous pressure is, however, an insensitive measurement of left atrial pressure. Worsening heart failure is monitored carefully by auscultation and thoracic radiography.

Serum chemistry determinations are repeated every 48 hours to check for worsening azotemia, and fluids and heart medications are adjusted according to the results of these tests. If renal function deteriorates, the dosage of furosemide should be decreased before the dosage of the angiotensin-converting enzyme (ACE) inhibitor is reduced. Changes in treatment are made gradually, if possible, unless acute heart failure develops. Digoxin is either discontinued or decreased by 50%. Dobutamine or dopamine may be administered by constant-rate infusion to give inotropic support to the heart. Dopamine has the added advantage of increasing renal blood flow. Some dogs respond favorably and may be sent home for a period of time, but treatment of heart failure complicated by renal disease is often unsuccessful and dogs must be euthanatized.

Diagnostic Plan

A thoracic radiograph should be taken on all dogs with a heart murmur except those that are too critical to undergo the test and that require immediate medical treatment and oxygen. There are several reasons to take a radiograph. One is to check for heart enlargement and pulmonary congestion or edema, which helps determine prognosis and the therapeutic plan.[9, 10] Another reason is to be certain of the diagnosis. Not all dogs with a heart murmur and crackles have pulmonary edema. Some have pneumonia or severe chronic obstructive pulmonary disease (Fig. 11–4), and the crackles from chronic obstructive pulmonary disease are not distinguishable from the crackles of pulmonary edema. Finally, radiography is important to monitor the success of treatment and the progression of disease. A baseline radiograph is helpful to observe changes with time.

The most common radiographic finding in dogs with mitral regurgitation is an enlarged left atrium.[5] The left atrium on the lateral view causes loss of the caudal waist and elevates and splits the mainstem bronchus (Fig. 11–5). It is important to differentiate the enlarged left atrium from hilar pulmonary edema. The left atrium has a distinct outline, whereas pulmonary edema causes a loss of the edge of the left atrium, looks indistinct, and is accompanied by engorged pulmonary vessels (Fig. 11–6).[33] On the ventrodorsal film, the left atrial appendage is seen as a bulge at the 3 o'clock position. The body of the left atrium is an increased density in the middle of the cardiac silhouette that separates the left and right mainstem bronchi (see Fig. 11–5).

As heart failure progresses, the left ventricle also enlarges,[34] resembling generalized cardiomegaly on thoracic radiography.[1] The right ventricle may even appear enlarged (see Fig. 11–6). As a general rule, contractility declines as the left ventricle becomes more dilated radiographically.[10] Dogs with moderate to severe heart failure have varying degrees of pulmonary congestion (enlarged pulmonary veins) and pulmonary edema (see Fig. 11–6). Interstitial edema causes loss of vascular detail, whereas alveolar edema has a mottled, "fluffy" appearance with indistinct edges.[33, 34]

The simplest cardiac diagnostic test to run is an ECG. However, the absence of an arrhythmia or ECG changes indicative of chamber enlargement does not rule out heart failure. A high percentage of dogs with severe mitral regurgitation have a normal ECG, although they may have sinus tachycardia,[5] wide P waves (left atrial enlargement), tall and wide QRS complexes[1] (left ventricular enlargement; Fig. 11–7), S-T segment slurring (hypoxia and left atrial enlargement), and atrial and ventricular arrhythmias[12] (Fig. 11–8).

Atrial arrhythmias in particular are caused by atrial stretching and strongly indicate the presence of mitral valve disease and left atrial dilation.[5, 11] Because high sympathetic tone causing sinus tachycardia is expected in heart failure, a normal to slow heart rate with a sinus arrhythmia may be indicative of pulmonary disease.[5]

Echocardiography is the best test to visualize

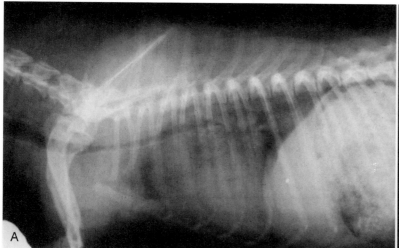

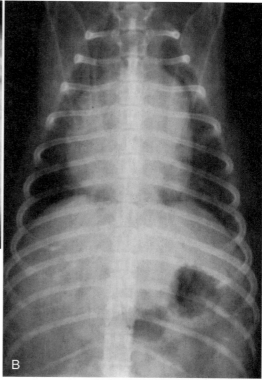

Figure 11–4
(A) Lateral and **(B)** ventrodorsal radiographs of a dog with chronic obstructive pulmonary disease and a collapsing trachea. Notice the narrowed trachea and interstitial lung pattern on the lateral radiograph. Right ventricular enlargement is easily visualized on the ventrodorsal radiograph.

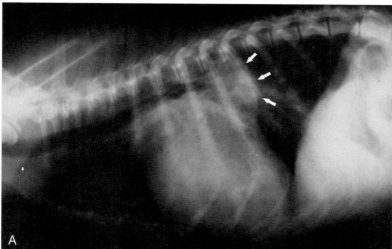

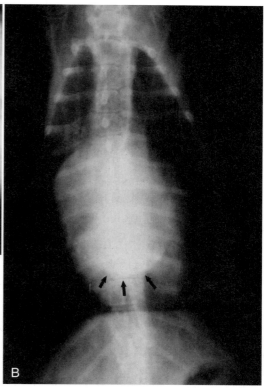

Figure 11–5
(A) Lateral and **(B)** ventrodorsal radiographs of a dog with mitral regurgitation and severe left atrial enlargement. A common error is to mistake the density of the enlarged left atrium on the lateral radiograph *(arrows)* for pulmonary edema. The left atrium in dogs with pulmonary edema has indistinct borders, whereas the caudal edge of the left atrium is clearly visible in dogs without pulmonary edema. The body of the left atrium can be seen in the middle of the heart on the ventrodorsal radiograph *(arrows)*; the left atrial appendage appears at the 3 o'clock postion.

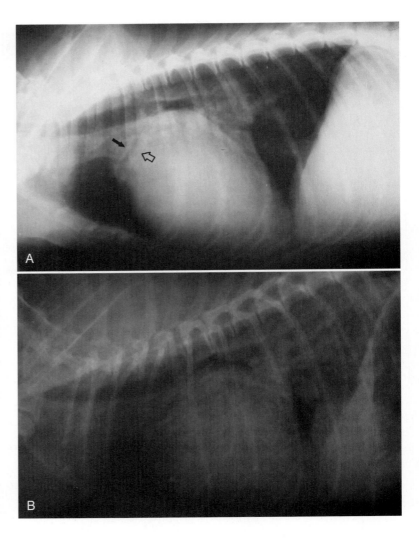

Figure 11-6
Lateral radiographs of two dogs with mitral regurgitation and congestive heart failure. **(A)** The cranial pulmonary vein *(open arrow)* is larger than the corresponding artery *(closed arrow)*, indicating venous congestion. **(B)** The pulmonary vessels are not visualized in the caudal-dorsal lung fields because of pulmonary edema, which appears as a fluffy density in the lungs.

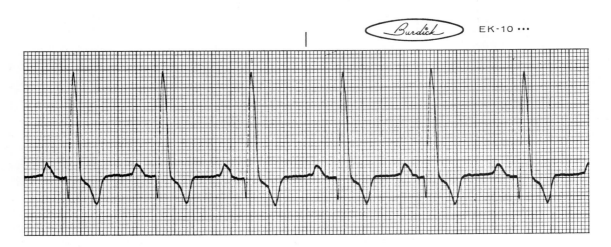

Figure 11-7
Electrocardiogram of a dog with mitral regurgitation. The P waves are wide (P mitrale), indicating left atrial dilation. The QRS is wide secondary to left ventricular dilation.

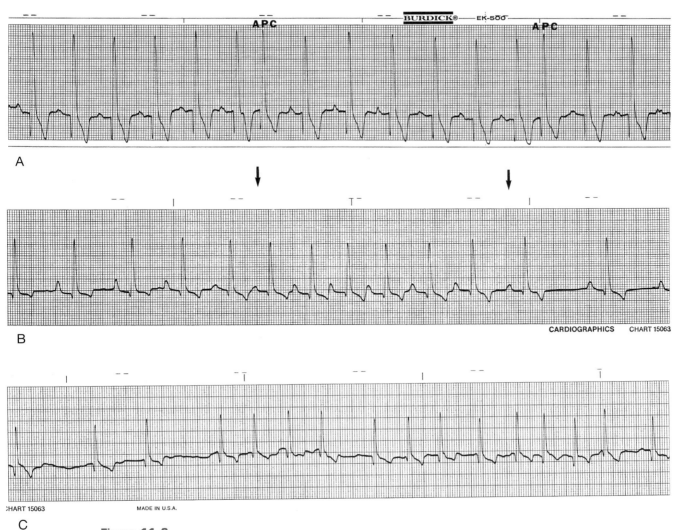

Figure 11–8

Examples of atrial arrhythmias in dogs caused by mitral regurgitation. **(A)** Atrial premature complexes (APC) in a cocker spaniel. **(B)** Paroxysmal atrial tachycardia in a poodle. The heart rate suddenly increases *(first arrow)*, then spontaneously breaks and converts to a sinus rhythm *(second arrow)*. **(C)** Atrial fibrillation in a poodle. Atrial fibrillation is characterized by an irregularly irregular rhythm, an absence of P waves, and fibrillation waves in the baseline.

the heart and see valve thickness, chamber size, and myocardial function. Most dogs with early mitral regurgitation retain good contractility, even if they are symptomatic and have a large regurgitant volume[35] (Fig. 11–9). The mitral valves, especially the anterior leaflet, are thick and may exhibit prolapse or flail tip. The left atrium is dilated to varying degrees, as is the left ventricle[34, 36] (Fig. 11–10). As with radiography, the larger the left ventricle on echocardiography, the poorer the systolic function. Contractility looks better than it actually is because of low impedance in the left atrium. Large excursions of the septum and free wall occur even with marginal myocardial strength.[5, 35] Mitral regurgitant volume is difficult to quantitate,

although left atrial and left ventricular diameters are approximate indicators of severity.[37]

Routine blood tests should also be performed on all animals in heart failure. A CBC helps differentiate infection from anemia,[1] although pneumonia can be present concurrently with heart failure. It is also less likely that bacterial endocarditis is present if the CBC is normal. Even with a leukocytosis and thick mitral valves, bacterial endocarditis is less likely in small breeds than is mitral valve disease without endocarditis. Serum chemistry analyses should be done to reveal abnormalities involving the kidneys, liver, electrolytes, and proteins.[1] Concurrent cardiac and renal disease presents a special therapeutic dilemma, because inten-

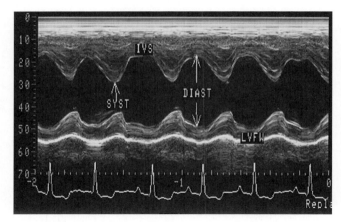

Figure 11-9
M-mode echocardiogram of a Chihuahua with mitral re-gurgitaion and heart failure. Notice the vigorous excursions of both the free wall of the left ventricle (LVFW) and the interventricular septum (IVS). DIAST, diastole; SYST, systole.

sive treatment of one exacerbates failure of the other. Low serum sodium occurs in severe heart failure and is an indicator of poor prognosis in heart disease.[26, 38] Low potassium can occur with high doses of loop diuretics; it increases sensitivity to digitalis toxicity and increases the likelihood of arrhythmias.[24, 29] Certain drugs, such as enalapril (Vasotec, Enacard), require hepatic biotransformation into their active forms (enalaprilat),[39] and low serum proteins can indicate dilution by free water retention.

Treatment

Treatment varies depending on the acuteness of presenting symptoms, severity of heart enlargement, myocardial function, presence and severity of edema, and response to previous medications (Table 11–1). Because the primary defect of myxomatous mitral valve degeneration cannot be repaired, cardiac drugs are used to control symptoms, improve quality of life, and prevent progression of disease. Clients should be told that treatment represents a means of control, not a cure. Once started, medications should be continued for the life of the animal. Routine follow-up visits should be scheduled to monitor symptoms, kidney function, electrolytes, heart rhythm, and adverse effects of medications.

Acute Heart Failure

Acute heart failure is usually caused by ruptured chordae tendineae. Signs are sudden and severe, and aggressive treatment must be instituted quickly.[10] Diagnostic tests should be withheld until the dog is stable. Cage rest and oxygen are two basic treatments that are often underappreciated, but oxygen should

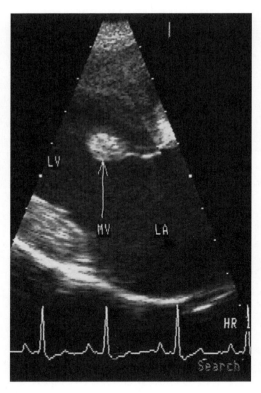

Figure 11-10
Two-dimensional echocardiogram of a poodle with mitral regurgitaion. Notice the thick anterior mitral valve leaflet (arrow). LA, left atrium; LV, left ventricle; MV, mitral valve.

never be substituted for emergency medical treatment (diuretics and vasodilators). The oxygen cage should be set at 40% to 50% oxygen. If an oxygen cage is not available, nasal oxygen can be used. A 1.6- to 2.6-mm (5- to 8-Fr) red rubber catheter is placed in the nostril and sutured in place. The oxygen should be humidified by bubbling it through water. If nasal oxygen is used, it should be set at a flow rate of 50 to 100 mL/kg per minute.[40]

Animals should be closely monitored, with checks of respiratory rate, pulse rate and quality, and capillary refill time every 1 to 2 hours. Intermittent or constant ECG may also be employed. Central venous pressure recordings are not always helpful in left-sided congestive heart failure, and they require the placement of a jugular catheter.[40] However, a peripheral catheter should be placed as soon as possible for ease of administration of IV drugs and for venous access in the event of cardiac arrest.

Diuretics

Diuretics such as furosemide (Lasix) are administered immediately at an IV dosage of 2 to 4 mg/kg[41] and are continued as often as every 2[40] to 4 hours. IV furosemide is thought to have hemodynamic effects on pulmonary vasculature that help remove edema before the onset of its diuretic effect.[42, 43] Another reason to give furosemide IV to animals in heart failure is the prolonged absorption of oral diuretics in patients with decompensated heart failure. Because IV furosemide does not need to be absorbed from the gastrointestinal tract and is therefore not affected by heart failure, the IV route allows a more effective amount to be delivered to the kidney.[29] After the initial doses, furosemide is continued at a dosage of 1 to 2 mg/kg, with IV, intramuscular, or subcutaneous administration, twice (b.i.d.) or three times (t.i.d.) per day, depending on response.

Afterload Reducers

One of the most important classes of drugs for acute heart failure is vasodilators, especially afterload reducers.[44] Afterload reducers are effective in mitral regurgitation because of their ability to lower aortic impedance, which reduces left atrial pressure, decreases pulmonary edema,[17, 41, 45] and lowers wall stress.[44, 46] Hydralazine (Apresoline), 1 to 2 mg/kg by mouth, b.i.d., is a powerful direct-acting arterial dilator that is often effective in cases of acute or chronic clinical mitral regurgitation in dogs.[28, 40, 42, 44, 45, 47, 48] It is more effective than ACE inhibitors in the early stage of severe heart failure because it is a stronger afterload reducer.[46] Its vasodilating effect begins within 1 hour, peaks in 5 hours, and has a duration of effect of about 12 hours.[44, 49] Hydralazine does not, however, affect filling pressures or contractility.[17, 44, 49] The major side effect is hypotension, which leads to tachycardia and diminished glomerular filtration rate. Tachycardia increases myocardial oxygen demand, and decreased glomerular filtration rate can cause azotemia.

Preload Reducers

A preload reducer is any compound or maneuver (e.g., phlebotomy) that lowers end-diastolic ventricular volume and concomitantly decreases ventricular filling pressures. The most commonly used preload reducer is furosemide, but there are specific vasodilators that may benefit dogs in acute heart failure.[48, 41] Nitrates are direct-acting venodilators that increase venous capacitance, thereby decreasing ventricular filling pressures.[46, 50] If the peripheral veins hold more blood, fluid is shifted away from the thoracic compartment to the periphery, and pulmonary edema is indirectly reduced.[40, 46, 48] The most commonly used nitrate is 2% nitroglycerin ointment (Nitro-Bid, Nitrol Ointment). It is applied to the pinna of the ear every 4 to 6 hours at a dosage of 0.625 cm for cats and small dogs and 1.25 cm for medium dogs.[10, 40] Because of rapid development of tolerance, nitroglycerin probably loses effectiveness after the first 24 hours.[51]

Positive Inotropic Support

Rarely, dogs with chronic mitral valve disease have myocardial failure as well as congestive heart failure and require positive inotropic support. The best positive inotropic drug to use in the acute situation is dobutamine (Dobutrex),[40, 42, 52] a synthetic sympathomimetic catecholamine that stimulates β_1-, β_2-, and α-adrenoceptors.[40] Dopamine (Inotropin, 2.5–15 µg/kg per minute) is another catecholamine that can be used, especially if renal failure is present.[42, 52] However, dobutamine is more effective than dopamine in heart failure; it has been shown in human studies to lower filling pressures while having little effect on heart rate or myocardial excitability.[52–54] Dopamine, on the other hand, increases filling pressures and ventricular ectopic activity, especially at higher dosages.[54, 55] The dosage of dobutamine in dogs is 5 to 20 µg/kg per minute by constant-rate infusion, although it is probably not necessary to go above 10 µg/kg per minute.[40] It is usually administered for 48 to 72 hours, but residual benefits that last beyond the treatment period may occur.[47, 52, 53] Because dobutamine increases the speed of A-V nodal conduction and can therefore speed up the ventricular response in animals with atrial fibrillation, it should be used cautiously in these patients.[47, 52]

Table 11–1
Drugs Commonly Used for Treatment of Heart Disease in Dogs

DRUG	AVERAGE DOSAGE
Digitalis Glycosides	
Digoxin	0.022 mg/kg PO, divided b.i.d. based on lean body weight
Digitoxin	0.033 mg/kg PO, b.i.d. (large dogs); t.i.d. (small dogs)
Vasodilators	
Enalapril	0.5 mg/kg PO, s.i.d. to b.i.d.
Lisinopril	0.5 mg/kg PO, s.i.d.
Hydralazine	1–2 mg/kg PO, b.i.d.
Isosorbide dinitrate	0.5–2 mg/kg PO, t.i.d.
Nitroglycerin ointment	0.6–2.5 cm inside ear pinna, q.i.d.
Diuretics	
Furosemide	1–4 mg/kg PO, IV, IM, b.i.d. or t.i.d.
Hydrochlorothiazide	2–4 mg/kg PO, b.i.d.
Spironolactone	2 mg/kg, b.i.d.
Nonglycoside Positive Inotropes	
Dobutamine	5–10 µg/kg/min IV

IV, intravenous; IM, imtramuscular; PO, by mouth; s.i.d., once per day; b.i.d., twice per day; t.i.d., three times per day; q.i.d., four times per day.

Antiarrhythmic Treatment

Antiarrhythmic treatment should be administered only if the resting heart rate is extremely rapid or the ventricular arrhythmia seems life-threatening, because antiarrhythmic drugs, except digoxin (Lanoxin), have negative inotropic activity and proarrhythmic effects.[27, 56] Ventricular arrhythmias may result from congestive heart failure, and treating the heart failure sometimes abolishes the arrhythmia. Treatment of ventricular premature beats is unnecessary except in the presence of rapid ventricular tachycardia (>160 bpm) that causes syncope, but significant ventricular tachycardia is rare in dogs with mitral valve disease and is not discussed further here.[42]

Atrial premature beats should be considered a marker of atrial disease rather than something dangerous that requires treatment. Rapid atrial tachycardia, on the other hand, increases myocardial oxygen demand and decreases cardiac output and should be controlled. Treatment is the same as for atrial fibrillation.

Atrial fibrillation at rates faster than 200 bpm should be treated because of the negative effect of tachycardia on cardiac output. Dogs treated with β-adrenergic blockers or calcium channel blockers should be monitored carefully, because both types of drugs have been reported to cause a worsening of heart failure.[24, 57, 58] The most commonly used calcium channel blocker in veterinary medicine today is diltiazem (Cardizem). The recommended dosage is 0.5 to 1.5 mg/kg, t.i.d.[59] The β-adrenergic blockers propranolol (Inderal) and atenolol (Tenormin), 0.25 to 1.0 mg/kg administered by mouth, once per day (s.i.d.) or b.i.d., have also been used. The dose of propranolol may be as high as 1.0 mg/kg by mouth, t.i.d., but it should be titrated upward slowly from a beginning dosage of 0.1 mg/kg.[60]

The therapies described (cage rest, oxygen, IV furosemide, hydralazine, and nitroglycerin ointment) may cause enough clinical improvement in 24 hours to abolish acute heart failure and allow further diagnostic tests to be performed.[41] However, many dogs in acute heart failure die because of the severity of regurgitation.[32] Those that do survive should have repeat blood tests for kidney function and electrolytes 24 to 48 hours after institution of drug treatment, because overzealous administration of diuretics and vasodilators can lower cardiac output and cause azotemia and symptoms of low-output heart failure.[43]

Mild to Moderate Heart Failure

Mild to moderate heart failure occurs more gradually but may still have a history of only a few days. Some dogs have remarkably mild signs for the amount of pulmonary edema and cardiomegaly that is shown to be present on chest radiography. Many are already on cardiac medications and require alterations of dosages or additions of new drugs. Absolute recommendations are difficult to make, because there are many cardiac medications, and only general guidelines can be suggested. Each dog must be treated as an individual. However, general guidelines may be presented.

Diuretics

All dogs that are in left-sided heart failure (pulmonary edema) secondary to mitral regurgitation should be treated with diuretics and vasodilators. Diuretics should be used in conjunction with ACE inhibitors, because one side effect of diuretic treatment is stimulation of the renin-angiotensin-aldosterone system.[20, 24, 29, 43, 57] The dosage of diuretic varies depending on the severity of edema and previous response to medications. The loop diuretic furosemide is the most commonly used diuretic in dogs and cats. It is a preload reducer as well as a diuretic,[43] because preload is lowered by removal of fluid from the vascular space. Furosemide acts at the thick ascending loop of Henle to inhibit sodium and chloride reabsorption.[29, 43] Natriuresis occurs even in the presence of decreased glomerular filtration rate and decreased renal blood flow.[43]

The most common side effects of diuretics are dehydration, hypotension, and electrolyte imbalance. As a powerful diuretic, furosemide can cause volume contraction, which in turn leads to decreased cardiac output and decreased stroke volume,[43] even though cardiac output is already low in heart failure. One of the most common side effects of diuretic administration in people is hypokalemia, but this is rare in dogs,[43] except if furosemide is combined with another diuretic such as hydrochlorothiazide (HydroDIURIL, 2–4 mg/kg, b.i.d.).[29] Diuretics are contraindicated if there is already decreased ventricular compliance,[43] because preload is needed in these conditions to help maintain pumping action through the Frank-Starling mechanism. If the ventricle is noncompliant and filling pressures fall even a little, cardiac output is dangerously reduced. Chronic obstructive pulmonary disease is the most common disease in which this happens. Diuretics should be avoided in pulmonary disease because they dry airway secretions that are necessary for normal pulmonary function.[43]

I begin treatment for all dogs with first-time heart failure with 1.0 mg/kg of furosemide given b.i.d. This is a smaller dosage than has been recommended,[10] but I rely more on ACE inhibitors than on diuretics. The ACE inhibitor should be started first at regular dosages (0.5 mg/kg, s.i.d.), with the diuretic dosage being adjusted up or down according to signs. Should side effects such as weakness, anorexia, or gastrointestinal signs occur with the combination of high-dose diuretics and ACE inhibitors, the diuretic should be lowered before the ACE inhibitor is reduced.[38]

Vasodilators

Vasodilators used in veterinary medicine include ACE inhibitors, hydralazine, and nitroglycerin. The ACE inhibitor used most frequently is enalapril, a long-acting, balanced vasodilator that replaced an earlier ACE inhibitor, captopril (Capoten). The advantages of enalapril over captopril include s.i.d. versus b.i.d. dosing and fewer side effects (e.g., anorexia, weakness, lethargy). Enalapril is hydrolyzed in the liver to the active form, enalaprilat. Its onset of action is slow, with the peak occurring at 4 to 6 hours.[39, 46] The recommended dosage is 0.5 mg/kg, s.i.d., but some animals must be given a lower dosage because of side effects (e.g., weakness, anorexia). As heart failure progresses, the dosage can be increased by giving the same amount b.i.d. Enalapril has been shown to prolong survival in humans and in dogs with severe congestive heart failure being treated with digitalis and diuretics.[57, 61–67]

ACE inhibitors are effective primarily where angiotensin II is active. Angiotensin II is the end product of the renin-angiotensin system. It is a powerful vasoconstrictor and helps maintain perfusion in early heart failure, but it is detrimental as heart failure progresses. Angiotensin II also stimulates release of aldosterone, antidiuretic hormone (i.e., vasopressin), and norepinephrine, and it preserves glomerular filtration rate in the presence of decreased renal blood flow by constricting the efferent or exiting glomerular arteriole.[46] By blocking angiotensin II, ACE inhibitors lower blood pressure, inhibit sodium and water retention (thereby diminishing potassium loss), and lower circulating norepinephrine. Some veterinarians fear the effects of ACE inhibitors on the kidneys, but azotemia is likely to occur only in cases of severely decreased renal blood flow, in which glomerular filtration depends on the efferent arteriole. If azotemia occurs, renal function can often be restored by decreasing the dosage of diuretic.[29] Mild increases in creatinine (i.e., 10%–15% over baseline) are usually insignificant.[68] Only rarely is fluid replacement required.

Problems with ACE inhibitors can be avoided if some guidelines are followed. First, renal function should be monitored, beginning 3 to 5 days after starting the ACE inhibitor, then 2 to 3 weeks later, then on follow-up visits. Second, if heart failure is severe and there is hyponatremia, plasma volume depletion, dehydration, or recent history of intensive diuretic therapy, a dosage lower than 0.5 mg/kg should be given and the dosage adjusted upward every 2 to 3 weeks. Finally, prostaglandin inhibitors such as aspirin, which can prevent prostaglandin-induced renal vasodilation, should be avoided.[46]

Combinations of vasodilators, such as hydralazine and isosorbide dinitrate (Isordil), have also been shown to be beneficial in heart failure.[66, 69–71] Hydralazine should not be used as a sole vasodilator because it stimulates the neurohumoral system by lowering blood pressure, thereby increasing the heart rate and enhancing retention of sodium and water.[41, 45] Prazosin is no longer recommended because it is no better than placebo in lowering mortality.[69]

Positive Inotropic Drugs

The digitalis glycosides, especially digoxin, are currently the only oral positive inotropic drugs available.[72, 73] Digoxin is administered primarily to slow the heart rate in supraventricular tachyarrhythmias such as atrial fibrillation and to increase contractility in animals with myocardial failure.[52, 74–76] Its use in heart failure with normal sinus rhythm is controversial.[75, 77] However, digoxin treatment in humans improves exercise tolerance and lowers the number of hospitalizations.[57, 72, 73] In addition, withdrawal of some patients from digoxin treatment results in clinical deterioration.[73, 78] Therefore, unless future studies indicate increased mortality with digoxin, it seems to be a worthwhile drug in animals with left ventricular dysfunction, atrial tachyarrhythmias, or resting sinus tachycardia.

Digoxin exerts its positive inotropic effect by binding to the sodium-potassium adenosine triphosphatase pump where potassium normally attaches. Pump activity stops, and sodium that would normally be extruded from the cell accumulates intracellularly. This sodium is then available to exchange with calcium, so that intracellular calcium rises and is available for contraction.[25, 75, 76] The mechanism for toxicity also involves accumulation of excess intracellular calcium, which causes delayed afterpotentials that can lead to arrhythmias.[75, 79]

The negative chronotropic effects of digoxin are caused by increased parasympathetic tone to the sinoatrial and A-V nodes. This helps break an atrial tachycardia or slow the ventricular response rate in atrial fibrillation.[56, 74–76, 79] Because digoxin works primarily through the parasympathetic nervous system, its beneficial effects are offset by sympathetic stimulation and administration of atropine.[52, 75, 76] Only at high levels, which are frequently toxic, does digoxin act directly on the A-V node.[52, 74, 75] Therefore, digoxin usually must be combined with either a β-blocker or a calcium channel blocker in atrial fibrillation,[80] and it should not be used as a first-line drug for idiopathic atrial fibrillation (atrial fibrillation with normal myocardial function).[52, 56, 75, 76]

A recently discovered effect of digoxin is the

restoration of baroreceptor sensitivity. The ability to slow the heart rate through baroreceptor stimulation is lost in heart failure,[20, 27, 81] and the resulting increased sympathetic drive causes a higher resting heart rate. Digoxin restores lost baroreceptor tone, and it has been shown to lower norepinephrine levels in humans with heart failure.[24, 76, 82–84] Its effectiveness is probably related to the dosage of digoxin, the species of animal being treated, and the degree of baroreceptor malfunction.[82]

Oral digoxin is well absorbed from the gastrointestinal tract, with about 60% of the tablet and 75% of the elixir being absorbed. The serum halflife of oral digoxin in dogs is 23 to 39 hours. Although it is supposed to take five halflives to reach therapeutic serum concentrations, it actually takes only 2 to 4.5 days with maintenance doses.[76, 79] Therefore, there is no reason to use rapid oral digitalization except in emergency situations of extremely fast atrial fibrillation.[52, 79] Most digoxin is excreted through the kidneys, necessitating a lowering of the dosage in renal disease. Digitoxin may also be used in place of digoxin in renal failure, because digitoxin is excreted primarily by the liver.[74, 75, 79] Other conditions that can raise serum concentrations of digoxin are listed in Table 11–2.

To optimize treatment, serum digoxin levels should be measured 1 week after treatment is started and periodically after that. Samples should be drawn 8 to 12 hours after the last dose of digoxin. The therapeutic range is between 1.0 and 2.5 ng/mL.[79]

Toxicity usually is manifested as gastrointestinal disturbances before arrhythmias occur. Anorexia and vomiting are probably caused by a direct effect of digoxin on the chemoreceptor trigger zone in the medulla, not from the effect of the drug on the gastrointestinal tract.[75, 76] If digoxin is stopped as soon as symptoms appear, the more serious arrhythmogenic effects are usually avoided. Almost every known rhythm disturbance can be caused by digoxin toxicity, but the most common arrhythmias seen are extrasystoles from delayed afterdepolarizations and A-V nodal blocks. The first treatment for toxicity is to stop the drug. Next, fluid and electrolyte abnormalities, especially hypokalemia, must be corrected. Serious ventricular arrhythmias are treated with IV lidocaine (Xylocaine), 50 to 75 µg/kg per minute. High-degree (i.e., second-degree with bradycardia and third-degree) A-V nodal blocks are treated with atropine, 0.02 to 0.04 mg/kg, subcutaneously, every 4 to 6 hours.[76, 79]

In severe kidney failure, digitoxin (Foxalin or Crystodigin, 0.02–0.03 mg/kg, t.i.d.) may be administered, because it is excreted primarily by the liver. Its halflife is only 8 to 12 hours, and therapeutic serum concentrations may be achieved more rapidly than with digoxin.[79]

Summary

A summary can now be made concerning the treatment of heart failure:

Asymptomatic heart disease—Dogs that are asymptomatic should be treated only with a low-salt diet, although that is not always necessary. Most dogs do not need drug treatment at this point but should have a follow-up examination with thoracic radiograph every 6 to 12 months.

Mild heart failure—Dogs with mild heart failure should be treated with a low-salt diet. If cardiomegaly is present on thoracic radiography or echocardiography, an ACE inhibitor should be administered. Low dosages of diuretics are also indicated if there is pulmonary congestion or edema, because they are more potent natriuretics than are ACE inhibitors.[29] Diuretics should not be administered alone, because they stimulate the renin-angiotensin-aldosterone system,[24, 29] although some veterinarians prefer diuretics over vasodilators as a first-line drug in mild heart failure.[5] Some dogs improve clinically with a bronchodilator such as aminophylline (10 mg/kg by mouth, t.i.d.), theophylline (Theo-Dur, 20 mg/kg by mouth, b.i.d.), or oxtriphylline (Choledyl Pediatric Elixir, 47 mg/kg by mouth, t.i.d.) instead of an ACE inhibitor or diuretic.[1] Exercise should be limited; there should be no strenuous activity, and stairs should be avoided.

Table 11–2
Conditions That Elevate Serum Digoxin Concentrations

Renal disease
Hypokalemia
Hypercalcemia
Hypernatremia
Hyperthyroidism
Hypothyroidism
Myocardial failure
Hypoxemia
Other drugs
   Quinidine
   Verapamil
   Tetracycline
   Chloramphenicol (possible)

Data from Kittleson MD. Management of heart failure: Concepts, therapeutic strategies, and drug pharmacology. In: Fox PR, ed. Canine and Feline Cardiology. Philadelphia, WB Saunders, 1988:189–191.

Moderate to severe heart failure—These dogs usually require an ACE inhibitor and a diuretic[67] in addition to salt and exercise restriction. Thinking has recently changed concerning the relative importance of diuretics and ACE inhibitors. Clinicians previously depended primarily on diuretics, titrating the ACE inhibitor upward until symptoms were controlled or side effects occurred. Now the recommendation is to administer the ACE inhibitor as the first-line drug and adjust the diuretic as needed for control of edema and symptomatic relief.[24, 29] Dogs with persistently high heart rates or low shortening fractions on echocardiography should also be treated with digoxin. Arrhythmias such as atrial fibrillation or ventricular premature contractions should be treated with appropriate antiarrhythmic treatment.

Severe chronic heart failure—Dogs in severe heart failure require higher amounts of diuretics and may even need more than one vasodilator and diuretic.[29, 85] After the maximum dosages of an ACE inhibitor (enalapril, 0.5 mg/kg, b.i.d.) and a diuretic (furosemide, 2–4 mg/kg, t.i.d.) are being administered, a low dosage of hydralazine (0.5–1.0 mg/kg, s.i.d. or b.i.d.) may be added. Dogs on this regimen must be watched carefully for signs of hypotension (e.g., lethargy, anorexia).[1, 41] Finally, diuretics such as hydrochlorothiazide (2–4 mg/kg, b.i.d.) or spironolactone (Aldactone, 2 mg/kg, b.i.d.) may be added.[5] The risks of hypokalemia and dehydration greatly increase if furosemide and hydrochlorothiazide are used together.[29, 30] The combination of an ACE inhibitor with spironolactone can increase serum potassium.[86] β-Adrenergic blockers or calcium channel blockers may be required in addition to digoxin to control tachycardias associated with atrial fibrillation.[80] Some dogs in severe heart failure also require periodic hospitalization for cage rest, oxygen, injectable diuretics, and, occasionally, dobutamine infusion.

Client Communications

Most clients must be told that salt, not cholesterol, is the problem in their dog. A handout describing the various medications and their potential side effects is very helpful. Clients should be told to skip the next treatment and call if they notice any adverse signs (i.e., anorexia, vomiting, lethargy, or diarrhea). They must also be warned about acute exacerbations of heart failure and urged to return their pet to the hospital as an emergency if they notice a sudden increase in coughing accompanied by heavy breathing. Clients must understand that cardiac drugs will not cure their dog but only control symptoms and that medications must be continued for life even if the animal is doing well.

Prognosis

Prognosis is extremely variable, but it is rare for dogs to live longer than 2 years after clinical signs develop. On the other hand, a heart murmur may be auscultated in a dog years before heart failure occurs. In general, however, the larger the heart, the poorer the prognosis. Dogs with severe left atrial enlargement usually do not live more than 1 year after diagnosis. Atrial fibrillation is also a very poor prognostic sign in dogs with acquired valvular disease, and dogs with mitral regurgitation and atrial fibrillation are unlikely to live longer than 6 to 8 months after the onset of the arrhythmia. It is impossible to predict which dogs will suddenly die from left atrial tear, rupture of the chordae tendineae and left-sided heart failure, or an acute arrhythmia.

Tricuspid Valve Disease

Tricuspid valve degeneration as an isolated problem is rare; it is usually seen as a sequela of or coincident with mitral valve disease.[1, 10, 13] The signalment is the same as for mitral valve disease. Both forward failure and backward failure occur, so symptoms of tricuspid valve disease include weakness, syncope, ascites, anorexia, diarrhea, and weight loss. Occasionally dogs also have pleural effusion. A harsh murmur and jugular pulses are common findings on the physical examination. Jugular venous distention may be more obvious when the abdomen is compressed.[10]

For pathophysiology, see Canine Mitral Valve Disease.

Clinical Signs

The history is often the same as for dogs with mitral valve disease: a murmur is auscultated on a routine physical examination. Dogs may also be brought in for lethargy, weight loss, anorexia, and ascites. Coughing is uncommon in isolated tricuspid valve disease. A heart murmur of at least grade III/VI intensity is auscultated, primarily at the right fourth intercostal space. Pulses are normal, and dogs are usually eupneic unless moderate or severe pleural effusion is present.

Diagnostic Plan

ECG may reveal tall P waves but often shows only evidence of left ventricular enlargement if mitral valve disease is also present. Right ventricular and right atrial enlargement are seen on thoracic radiographs, although generalized cardiomegaly is often present and may be difficult to differentiate from cardiomegaly caused by isolated mitral valve disease. An enlarged vena cava, hepatomegaly, and ascites may also be visualized on thoracic radiographs.[10] Echocardiography provides the best tool for documenting tricuspid valve disease. The right ventricle and right atrium are dilated, and the volume overload in the right ventricle may flatten or displace the septum toward the left ventricle in diastole.[10] The tricuspid valves may appear thickened and can prolapse in a manner similar to that of mitral valve prolapse.

Ascites from tricuspid valve disease must be differentiated from that caused by pericardial disease, obstruction of the caudal vena cava, liver disease, hypoproteinemia, abdominal neoplasia, or other causes of right-sided heart failure such as heartworm disease (see Chap. 13). ECG, radiography, echocardiography, routine blood tests, and heartworm tests should be performed on all patients with suspected tricuspid valve disease.

Abdominal sonography is especially helpful, because fluid analysis of many conditions causing ascites produces a modified transudate, as does right-sided heart failure. Ultrasonography in heart failure reveals enlarged vessels in the liver from hepatic congestion. Pericardial disease or obstruction of the caudal vena cava also produces hepatic congestion, but without enlargement of the right ventricle. Liver disease may be diagnosed as abnormal liver parenchyma, and liver biopsy may be required for final diagnosis. Pericardial disease or masses obstructing the caudal vena cava should be seen on ultrasonography of the heart or abdomen.

Treatment

Treatment for tricuspid valve disease is similar to treatment of mitral valve disease except that it must be more intensive. Digoxin is used in all cases unless cor pulmonale is suspected because of evidence such as dilated pulmonary arteries on echocardiography and dilated, tortuous vessels on thoracic radiography. Combinations of two or more diuretics and vasodilators are the rule rather than the exception. Preload reducers such as isosorbide dinitrate combined with ACE inhibitors are more important in isolated tricuspid valve disease than are afterload reducers. Periodic abdominocentesis is usually required,[10] and the long-term prognosis is poor.

Bacterial Endocarditis

Bacterial endocarditis is bacterial destruction and proliferation of the endocardium involving the valves (valvular bacterial endocarditis) or endocardial wall (mural bacterial endocarditis).[87] Its incidence is very low,[7] and it is usually seen in large-breed dogs older than 4 years of age. German shepherds and boxers are affected more often than other breeds, and males more commonly than females.[88–93]

Pathophysiology

Several factors combine to create an environment in which bacterial endocarditis can occur. Certain bacteria have an ability to adhere to the valve surface, especially if the valve is damaged.[91, 94] A second factor is bacteremia from an active infection at a distant site.[91] This can originate from dental procedures (although dental work is not as much of a culprit as many claim),[89] endoscopy, bronchoscopy, poor IV catheter placement, or any localized infection.[86, 88, 89, 91, 92, 94] The most common bacteria isolated are *Staphylococcus aureus, Pseudomonas aeruginosa, Corynebacterium* spp., *Erysipelothrix rhusiopathiae, Escherichia coli, Aerobacter aerogenes*,[1, 91] and *Streptococcus* spp.[86, 92, 94] However, overuse of antibiotics may select for other, more resistant bacteria.

A third factor is the presence of previous damage to the valve.[86, 91, 92] Bacterial endocarditis is rarely seen in older, small-breed dogs with mitral valve disease, even though the mitral valve is one of the valves most commonly affected in companion animals.[91, 92] There is a higher incidence of bacterial endocarditis in dogs with subaortic stenosis, possibly because the high-velocity jet damages the aortic valves.[90] Vegetations are then deposited on the low-pressure side of the valve (i.e., the ventricular side for aortic regurgitation and the atrial side for mitral regurgitation).[94] Another factor is the formation of a platelet-fibrin thrombus because of exposed collagen from the valve. Bacteria colonize inside the thrombus and are protected against antibodies and antibiotics.[86, 91, 94] A fifth factor is the use of immunosuppressive drugs or the presence of conditions that suppress an animal's immune system, such as neoplasia.[86, 90, 94]

Septic emboli can be carried to almost any organ of the body, with the kidney and spleen most commonly affected.[88, 91, 94, 95] Symptoms depend on the organ systems involved. Congestive heart failure may occur secondary to volume overload from aortic or mitral regurgitation.[91] Death usually results from heart failure, arrhythmias, infarction, sepsis, or renal failure.[90] Heart failure and renal failure significantly worsen the prognosis.[88, 91, 94]

Clinical Signs

Bacterial endocarditis is known as the "great imitator" because of its ability to mimic so many diseases. Lethargy, weight loss, anorexia, and lameness (polyarthritis) are the most frequent symptoms.[1, 86, 89–94] Other symptoms include epistaxis, hemoptysis, dyspnea,[93] abdominal pain,[95] syncope,[91] hematuria, cough, convulsions, and paralysis.[86, 90, 92] Symptoms probably occur because of sepsis, embolization, or disseminated intravascular coagulation.

An unexplained, recurrent fever and a murmur that is new or has recently changed are strong indicators of bacterial endocarditis. The murmur is usually systolic, although it may be diastolic as a result of aortic regurgitation. If moderate or severe aortic regurgitation is present, the pulses feel bounding because of a widened pulse pressure. Arrhythmias may also occur, as well as a gallop, the third heart sound.[86, 88, 90–94] Dyspnea is present with congestive heart failure, and abdominal pain is present if the kidneys have been infarcted.[86, 95]

Diagnostic Plan

Radiography of the chest frequently shows cardiomegaly if significant aortic or mitral regurgitation is present,[88, 90, 91, 93, 94] and there may be pulmonary edema with congestive heart failure. Arrhythmias seen on ECGs are usually ventricular,[88] but A-V nodal blocks, atrial arrhythmias, and bundle branch blocks may also be present.[86, 90, 92, 94] Echocardiography is one of the most specific tests for diagnosis of bacterial endocarditis, but lesions must be at least 2 mm thick to be seen. In addition to thickened valves (the most specific finding), left ventricular dilation, flail leaflets, ruptured chordae tendineae, or diastolic mitral valve flutter (from aortic regurgitation) may be present[90–94] (Figs. 11–11 and 11–12). Abdominal sonography may reveal a source of the infection and should also be performed.

Blood tests and urinalysis may show several abnormalities. Liver enzymes and kidney function tests are abnormal if septic embolization of organs has occurred. Renal infarction causes hypoalbuminemia and proteinuria.[95] If pyelonephritis is the source of the infection, pyuria and hematuria are also present. Dogs usually have a normocytic normochromic anemia and a leukocytosis with a left shift.[86, 88, 90, 91, 93, 94] Some dogs even have positive antinuclear antibodies and positive results on Coombs testing and on testing for rheumatoid factor.[88, 91] This occurs because of nonspecific immune stimulation and should not be confused with immune-mediated disease. Treatment should still be aggressively aimed at the bacteremia.

Blood cultures are critical. A positive blood

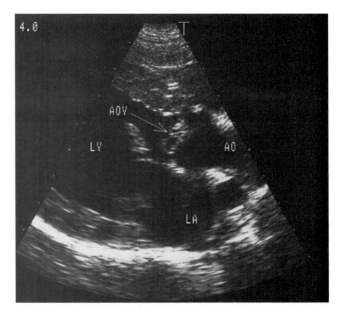

Figure 11–11
Two-dimensional echocardiogram of a dog with bacterial endocarditis. Notice the thickened, hyperechoic aortic valve *(arrow)*. The dog had high systolic aortic flows and aortic regurgitation on Doppler echocardiography. AO, aorta; AOV, aortic valve; LA, left atrium; LV, left ventricle.

culture combined with suggestive clinical signs is proof of bacterial endocarditis, although a diagnosis can be made on clinical and laboratory evidence of heart involvement (new or progressive murmur, anemia, leukocytosis, echocardiographic changes, embolism).[91, 92] Reasons for a negative culture in bacterial endocarditis include recent antibiotic use, uremia, chronic endocarditis, and noninfectious endocarditis. In general, cultures are positive in 75% of cases of bacterial endocarditis.[91] More than one culture should be obtained, because the chance of getting a positive culture is directly related to the number of cultures. At least two or three samples should be taken, at least 1 hour apart, within a 24-hour period. It is not critical to obtain the samples during a fever spike, because the bacteremia is constant. Samples should be at least 10 mL, because a greater volume of blood correlates with a better chance of obtaining a positive result. Both aerobic and anaerobic cultures should be obtained and tested for bacterial identification and antimicrobial sensitivity. In addition, mean inhibitory concentration should be determined.[88, 91, 92, 94]

Cultures in addition to blood cultures are often helpful. Urine, joint fluid, and abdominal or pleural effusions may produce positive cultures.

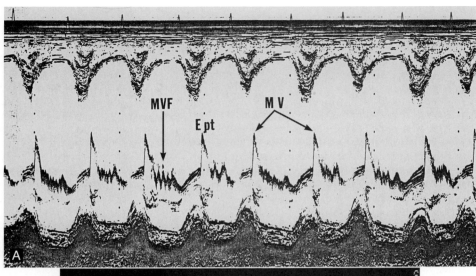

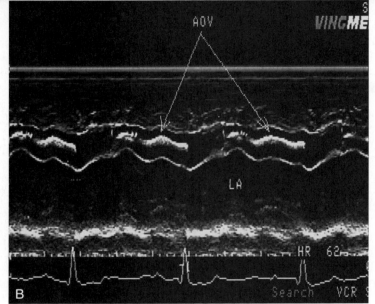

Figure 11–12
M-mode echocardiograms of two dogs with bacterial endocarditis. **(A)** Notice the poor contractility and the large separation of the E point of the mitral valve (rapid ventricular filling phase of diastole) from the septum, denoting left ventricular dilation. Aortic regurgitation has also caused flutter of the anterior mitral valve leaflet, characterized by high frequency vibration of the leaflet. E pt, E point; MV, mitral valve; MVF, mitral valve flutter. **(B)** The aortic valve can clearly be seen as a thick line during diastole. AOV, aortic valve; LA, left atrium.

Treatment

Treatment must be intensive and aggressive. Ideally, IV antibiotics should be administered for 4 to 6 weeks, but this usually is not practical in veterinary medicine. At the very least, a course of antibiotics based on blood cultures should be administered intravenously for 7 to 14 days and continued orally for 4 to 6 weeks. Antibiotics should be bactericidal and used in dosages that result in high serum concentrations. Therapy should be instituted before culture results are available. Antibiotics that are most effective include combinations of an aminoglycoside with penicillin, ampicillin, or a cephalosporin.[88, 92] If the source of the bacteremia is known, it should be treated medically or surgically. Arrhythmias should be treated if they are causing hemodynamic compromise, and congestive heart failure should be treated with vasodilators, diuretics, and possibly digoxin.[88, 91, 94] Blood cultures should be repeated at 1 and 2 months after initiation of treatment, and dogs should be examined every 1 to 2 weeks to monitor arrhythmias and heart failure.

Prognosis

The prognosis for dogs with bacterial endocarditis is extremely poor, especially in the presence of renal failure, heart failure, or aortic valve endocarditis with regurgitation. Most dogs die or are euthanatized within 6 months after diagnosis, although some live as long as 2 years.[92, 94]

References

1. Reed JR. Acquired valvular heart disease in the dog. In: Kirk RW, ed. Current Veterinary Therapy X. Philadelphia, WB Saunders, 1989:231–240.
2. Fenoglio JJ, Tuan DP, Wit AL, et al. Canine mitral valve complex. Circ Res 1972;31:417–430.
3. Frater RWM, Ellis FH. The anatomy of the canine mitral valve. J Surg Res 1961;1:171–178.
4. Beardow AW, Buchanan JW. Chronic mitral valve disease in cavalier King Charles spaniels: 95 cases (1987–1991). J Am Vet Med Assoc 1993;203:1023–1029.
5. Keene BW, Bonagura JB. Valvular heart disease. In: Kirk RW, ed. Current Veterinary Therapy VIII. Philadelphia, WB Saunders, 1983:311–320.
6. Ettinger SJ. Valvular heart disease. In: Ettinger SJ, ed. Textbook of Veterinary Small Animal Medicine. Philadelphia, WB Saunders, 1989:1031–1050.
7. Buchanan JW. Causes and prevalence of cardiovascular disease. In: Kirk RW, Bonagura JD. Current Veterinary Therapy XI. Philadelphia: WB Saunders, 1992:647–654.
8. Kvart C, Häggström. Chronic valvular disease in cavalier King Charles spaniels. Proc Am Coll Vet Intern Med Forum 1994;12:298–300.
9. Keene BW. Chronic valvular disease in the dog. In: Fox PR, ed. Canine and Feline Cardiology. New York, Churchill Livingstone, 1988:409–418.
10. Sisson D. Acquired valvular heart disease in dogs and cats. In: Bonagura JD, ed. Contemporary Issues in Small Animal Practice: Cardiology. New York, Churchill Livingstone, 1987;7:59–116.
11. Boyden PA, Tilley LP, Pham TD, et al. Effects of left atrial enlargement on atrial transmembrane potentials and structure in dogs with mitral valve fibrosis. Am J Cardiol 1982;49:1896–1908.
12. Das KM, Patnaik AK, Liu S-K, et al. Cardiovascular pathology of the dog and cat: A case study of 1000 consecutive cases. J Am Vet Med Assoc 1965;147:1648–1649.
13. Buchanan JW. Chronic valvular disease (endocardiosis) in dogs. Adv Vet Sci Comp Med 1977;21:75–106.
14. Virmani R, Atkinson JB, Forman MB, et al. Mitral valve prolapse. Hum Pathol 1987;18:596–602.
15. King BD, Clark MA, Baba N, et al. Myxomatous mitral valves: Collagen dissolution as the primary defect. Circulation 1982;66:288–296.
16. Pierpont GL, Talley RC. Pathophysiology of valvular heart disease: The dynamic nature of mitral valve regurgitation. Arch Intern Med 1982;142:998–1001.
17. Yoran C, Yellin EL, Becker RM, et al. Mechanism of reduction of mitral regurgitation with vasodilator therapy. Am J Cardiol 1979;43:773–777.
18. Braunwald E. Valvular heart disease. In: Braunwald E, ed. Heart Disease. Philadelphia, WB Saunders, 1992: 1007–1077.
19. Jeresaty RM, Edwards JE, Surendra KC. Mitral valve prolapse and ruptured chordae tendineae. Am J Cardiol 1985;55:138–142.
20. Packer M. Pathophysiology of chronic heart failure. Lancet 1992;340:88–92.
21. Corin WJ, Murakami T, Monrad ES, et al. Left ventricular passive diastolic properties in chronic mitral regurgitation. Circulation 1991;83:797–807.
22. Kono T, Sabbah HN, Stein PD, et al. Left ventricular shape as a determinant of functional mitral regurgitation in patients with severe heart failure secondary to either coronary artery disease or idiopathic dilated cardiomyopathy. Am J Cardiol 1991;68:355–359.
23. Carabello BA. Mitral regurgitation: Basic pathophysiologic principles. Mod Concepts Cardiovasc Dis 1988;57: 53–58.
24. Packer M. Treatment of chronic heart failure. Lancet 1992;340:92–95.
25. DePace NL, Nestico PF, Morganroth J. Acute severe mitral regurgitation: Pathophysiology, clinical recognition, and management. Am J Med 1985;78:293–306.
26. Weber KT, Janicki JS, Campbell C, et al. Pathophysiology of acute and chronic cardiac failure. Am J Cardiol 1987;60:3C–9C.
27. Francis G. Heart failure in 1991. Cardiology 1991;78:81–94.
28. Cody RJ. Management of refractory congestive heart failure. Am J Cardiol 1992;69:141G–149G.
29. Cody RJ. Clinical trials of diuretic therapy in heart failure: Research directions and clinical considerations. J Am Coll Cardiol 1993;22(Suppl A):165A–171A.
30. Pitt B. Use of converting enzyme inhibitors in patients with asymptomatic left ventricular dysfunction. J Am Coll Cardiol 1993;22(Suppl A):158A–161A.
30a. Kittleson MD. The pathophysiology and treatment of mitral regurgitation in the dog. In: The 18th Annual Waltham/OSU Symposium for the Treatment of Small Animal Diseases. Vernon, California: Waltham USA, Inc, 1994;33–43.
31. Braunwald E. The physical examination. In: Braunwald E, ed. Heart Disease. Philadelphia, WB Saunders, 1992: 13–42.
32. Ettinger S, Buergelt CD. Ruptured chordae tendineae in the dog. J Am Vet Med Assoc 1969;155:535–546.
33. Hawkins EC. Diseases of the lower respiratory tract (lung) and pulmonary edema. In: Ettinger SJ, ed. Textbook of Veterinary Internal Medicine. Philadelphia, WB Saunders,1989:816–866.
34. Lombard CW, Spencer CP. Correlation of radiographic, echocardiographic, and electrocardiographic signs of left heart enlargement in dogs with mitral regurgitation. Vet Radiol 1985;26:89–97.
35. Kittleson MD, Eyster GE, Knowlen GG, et al. Myocardial function in small dogs with chronic mitral regurgitation and severe congestive heart failure. J Am Vet Med Assoc 1984;184:455–459.
36. Pipers FS, Bonagura JD, Hamlin RL, et al. Echocardiographic abnormalities of the mitral valve associated with left-sided heart disease in the dog. J Am Vet Med Assoc 1981;179:580–586.
37. Burwash IG, Blackmore GL, Koilpillai CJ. Usefulness of left atrial and left ventricular chamber sizes as predictors of the severity of mitral regurgitation. Am J Cardiol 1992;70:774–779.
38. Dietz RD, Nagel F, Osterziel KJ. Angiotensin-converting

enzyme inhibitors and renal function in heart failure. Am J Cardiol 1992;70:119C–125C.

39. Allen TA, Wilke WL, Fettman MJ. Captopril and enalapril: Angiotensin-converting enzyme inhibitors. J Am Vet Med Assoc 1987;190:94–96.

40. Rush JE. Emergency therapy and monitoring of heart failure. In: Kirk RW, Bonagura JD. Current Veterinary Therapy XI. Philadelphia, WB Saunders, 1992:713–721.

41. Bonagura JD, Muir W. Vasodilator therapy. In: Kirk RW, ed. Current Veterinary Therapy IX. Philadelphia, WB Saunders, 1986:329–333.

42. Keene BW. Cardiovascular drugs. In: Bonagura JD, ed. Contemporary Issues in Small Animal Practice: Cardiology. New York, Churchill Livingstone, 1987;7:21–57.

43. Fox PR. Current uses and hazards of diuretic therapy. In: Kirk RW, Bonagura JD. Current Veterinary Therapy XI. Philadelphia, WB Saunders, 1992:668–676.

44. Sisson D. Evidence for or against the efficacy of afterload reducers for management of heart failure in dogs. Efficacy of cardiac therapy. Vet Clin North Am Small Anim Pract 1991;21:945–955.

45. Kittleson MD, Eyster GE, Olivier NB, et al. Oral hydralazine therapy for chronic mitral regurgitation in the dog. J Am Vet Med Assoc 1983;182:1205–1209.

46. DeLellis LA, Kittleson MD. Current uses and hazards of vasodilator therapy in heart failure. In: Kirk RW, Bonagura JD. Current Veterinary Therapy XI. Philadelphia, WB Saunders, 1992:700–708.

47. Kittleson MD. Dobutamine. J Am Vet Med Assoc 1980;177:642–643.

48. Hamlin RL. Evidence for or against clinical efficacy of preload reducers. Efficacy of cardiac therapy. Vet Clin North Am Small Anim Pract 1991;21:931–944.

49. Kittleson MD, Hamlin RL. Hydralazine pharmacodynamics in the dog. Am J Vet Res 1983;44:1501–1505.

50. Cohn JN. Mechanisms of action and efficacy of nitrates in heart failure. Am J Cardiol 1992;70:88B–92B.

51. Elkayam U, Roth A, Mehra A, et al. Randomized study to evaluate the relation between oral isosorbide dinitrate dosing interval and the development of early tolerance to its effect on left ventricular filling pressure in patients with chronic heart failure. Circulation 1991;84:2040–2048.

52. Knight DH. Efficacy of inotropic support of the failing heart. Vet Clin North Am Small Anim Pract 1991;21:879–904.

53. Kittleson MD, Knowlen GG. Positive inotropic drugs in heart failure. In: Kirk RW, ed. Current Veterinary Therapy IX. Philadelphia: WB Saunders, 1986:323–328.

54. Smith TW, Braunwald E, Kelly RA. The management of heart failure. In: Braunwald E, ed. Heart Disease. Philadelphia, WB Saunders, 1992:464–519.

55. Hosgood G. Pharmacologic features and physiologic effects of dopamine. J Am Vet Med Assoc 1990;197:1209–1211.

56. Sarter BH, Marchlinski FE. Redefining the role of digoxin in the treatment of atrial fibrillation. Am J Cardiol 1992;69:71G–81G.

57. Packer M. Therapeutic options in the management of chronic heart failure: Is there a drug of first choice? Circulation 1989;79:198–204.

58. Ware WA. Current uses and hazards of beta-blockers. In: Kirk RW, Bonagura JD. Current Veterinary Therapy XI. Philadelphia, WB Saunders, 1992:676–684.

59. Pion PD. Current uses and hazards of calcium channel blocking agents. In: Kirk RW, Bonagura JD. Current Veterinary Therapy XI. Philadelphia, WB Saunders, 1992:684–693.

60. Hamlin RL. Therapy of supraventricular tachycardia and atrial fibrillation. Current Veterinary Therapy XI. Philadelphia, WB Saunders, 1992:745–749.

61. The CONSENSUS Trial Study Group. Effects of enalapril on mortality in severe congestive heart failure. N Engl J Med 1987;316:1429–1435.

62. The SOLVD Investigators. Effect of enalapril on survival in patients with reduced left ventricular ejection fractions and congestive heart failure. N Engl J Med 1991;325:293–302.

63. Ettinger S, Lusk R, Brayley K, et al. Evaluation of enalapril therapy in dogs with heart failure in a large multicenter study: Cooperative veterinary enalapril (COVE) study group. Proc Am Coll Vet Intern Med Forum 1992;10:584–585.

64. Hamlin RL, Benitz AM, Ericsson GF. Clinical testing of angiotensin converting enzyme inhibitors for treatment of heart failure in dogs. Proc Am Coll Vet Intern Med Forum 1992;10:581–583.

65. Sisson DD. Hemodynamic, echocardiographic, radiographic, and clinical effects of enalapril in dogs with chronic heart failure. Proc Am Coll Vet Intern Med Forum 1992;10:589–591.

66. Cohn JN. Efficacy of vasodilators in the treatment of heart failure. J Am Coll Cardiol 1993;22(Suppl A):135A–138A.

67. Hood WB Jr. Role of converting enzyme inhibitors in the treatment of heart failure. J Am Coll Cardiol 1993;22(Suppl A):154A–157A.

68. Ljungman S, Kjekshus J, Swedberg K. Renal function in severe congestive heart failure during treatment with enalapril (the Cooperative North Scandinavian Enalapril Survival Study [CONSENSUS] Trial). Am J Cardiol 1992;70:479–487.

69. Cohn JN, Archibald DG, Francis GS, et al. Veterans administration cooperative study on vasodilator therapy of heart failure: Influence of prerandomization variables on the reduction of mortality by treatment with hydralazine and isosorbide dinitrate. Circulation 1987;75(Suppl IV):49–54.

70. Cohn JN, Johnson G, Ziesche S, et al. A comparison of enalapril with hydralazine-isosorbide dinitrate in the treatment of chronic congestive heart failure. N Engl J Med 1991;325:303–310.

71. Cohn JN. Nitrates versus angiotensin converting enzyme inhibitors for congestive heart failure. Am J Cardiol 1993;72:21C–26C.

72. Gheorghiade M, Zarowitz BJ. Review of randomized trials of digoxin therapy in patients with chronic heart failure. Am J Cardiol 1992;69:48G–63G.

73. Kelly RA, Smith TW. Digoxin in heart failure: implications of recent trials. J Am Coll Cardiol 1993;22(Suppl A):107A–112A.

74. Kaufman GM, Weirich WE. Oral glycoside therapy in the dog. Compen Contin Educ Pract Vet 1983;5:753–760.

75. Smith TW. Digitalis. Mechanisms of action and clinical use. N Engl J Med 1988;318:358–364.

76. Snyder PS, Atkins CE. Current uses and hazards of the digitalis glycosides. In: Kirk RW, Bonagura JD. Current Veterinary Therapy XI. Philadelphia, WB Saunders, 1992:689–693.

77. Bright JM. Controversies in veterinary medicine: Is the long-term use of digitalis for treatment of low output heart failure unwarranted? J Am Anim Hosp Assoc 1983;19:233–236.

78. Packer M, Gheorghiade M, Young JB, et al. Withdrawal of digoxin from patients with chronic heart failure treated with angiotensin-converting-enzyme inhibitors. N Engl J Med 1993;329:1–7.

79. Kittleson MD. Management of heart failure: Concepts, therapeutic strategies, and drug pharmacology. In: Fox PR, ed. Canine and Feline Cardiology. New York, Churchill Livingstone, 1988:171–204.

80. Klein HO, Kaplinsky E. Verapamil and digoxin: Their respective effects on atrial fibrillation and their interaction. Am J Cardiol 1982;50:894–902.

81. Parmley WW. Pathophysiology of congestive heart failure. Clin Cardiol 1992;15(Suppl I):I5–I12.

82. Gheorghiade M, Ferguson D. Digoxin: A neurohormonal modulator in heart failure? Circulation 1991;84:2181–2186.

83. Ferguson DW. Digitalis and neurohormonal abnormalities in heart failure and implications for therapy. Am J Cardiol 1992;69:24G–33G.

84. Packer M. The development of positive inotropic agents for chronic heart failure: How have we gone astray? J Am Coll Cardiol 1993;22(Suppl A):119A–126A.

85. Dahlstrom U, Karlsson E. Captopril and spironolactone therapy for refractory congestive heart failure. Am J Cardiol 1993;71:29A–33A.

86. Zannad F. Angiotensin-converting enzyme inhibitor and spironolactone combination therapy: New objectives in congestive heart failure treatment. Am J Cardiol 1993;71:34A–39A.

87. Drazner FH. Bacterial endocarditis in the dog. Comp Contin Educ Pract Vet 1979;1:918–924.

88. Calvert CA. Valvular endocarditis in the dog. J Am Vet Med Assoc 1982;180:1080–1084.

89. Anderson CA, Dubielzig RR. Vegetative endocarditis in dogs. J Am Anim Hosp Assoc 1984;20:149–152.

90. Sisson D, Thomas WP. Endocarditis of the aortic valve in the dog. J Am Vet Med Assoc 1984;184:570–577.

91. Sisson D, Thomas WP. Bacterial endocarditis. In: Kirk RW, ed. Current Veterinary Therapy IX. Philadelphia, WB Saunders, 1986:402–406.

92. Thomas WP. Update: Infective endocarditis. In: Kirk RW, Bonagura JD. Current Veterinary Therapy XI. Philadelphia, WB Saunders, 1992:752–755.

93. Elwood CM, Cobb MA, Stepien RL. Clinical and echocardiographic findings in 10 dogs with vegetative bacterial endocarditis. J Small Anim Pract 1993;34:420–427.

94. Woodfield JA, Sisson D. Infective endocarditis. In: Ettinger SJ, ed. Textbook of Veterinary Small Animal Medicine. Philadelphia, WB Saunders, 1989:1151–1162.

95. Taboada J, Palmer GH. Renal failure associated with bacterial endocarditis in the dog. J Am Anim Hosp Assoc 1989;25:243–251.

Chapter 12

Myocardial Diseases

Betsy R. Bond

Cardiomyopathy is a disorder of myocardial structure or function that is not the result of ischemic, congenital, valvular, or pericardial disease.[1-8] It is a diagnosis of exclusion of other forms of heart disease.[6] Cardiomyopathies are classified as primary or secondary (Table 12–1). Primary cardiomyopathy has no known cause and is usually further defined as dilated (congestive) cardiomyopathy, hypertrophic cardiomyopathy, or restrictive cardiomyopathy (Fig. 12–1).[5, 6, 8] Dilated cardiomyopathy is the most common type seen in dogs, and hypertrophic cardiomyopathy is most common in cats. Also, cardiomyopathy in cats is more complex than it is in dogs. Two types have been described that fall out of normal categories: excessive left ventricular moderator bands[9] and intermediate (intergrade) cardiomyopathy.[2] Distinct clinical forms of cardiomyopathy in dogs are found in giant breeds, Doberman pinschers, boxers, and English and American cocker spaniels, although many of the characteristics overlap.[10-13]

Secondary cardiomyopathy often mimics primary cardiomyopathy in its clinical presentation and course, but the cause is known (see Table 12–1) and must be treated in addition to treatment of existing heart failure. Two common secondary cardiomyopathies in cats are thyrotoxicosis and hypertensive heart disease.[2, 4]

Table 12–1
Classification of Heart Muscle Disease in Dogs and Cats

Primary (Idiopathic) Cardiomyopathy
Dilated/Congestive (dogs)*
Hypertrophic (cats)*
Restrictive (cats)*
Intermediate/Intergrade (cats)*
Excessive left ventricular moderator bands (cats)

Secondary Cardiomyopathy
Infective
  Bacterial
  Protozoal
  Fungal
  Viral
Metabolic
  Nutritional (taurine—cats)
  Endocrine
    Thyrotoxicosis (cats)*
    Acromegaly (cats)
    Hyperadrenocorticism (dogs)
  Uremic
Toxic
  Doxorubicin (Adriamycin)
Infiltrative
  Neoplasia
Physical agent
  Hyperpyrexia
  Hypothermia
Ischemic (dogs)
  Pancreatitis
  Gastric dilatation-volvulus*
  Shock
  Central nervous system trauma

*Common causes.
Modified from Fox PR. Feline myocardial disease. In: Fox PR, ed. Canine and Feline Cardiology. Philadelphia, WB Saunders, 1988:436; and Fox PR. Canine myocardial disease. In: Fox PR, ed. Canine and Feline Cardiology. Philadelphia, WB Saunders, 1988:468.

Problem Identification

Cough

Pathophysiology

A cough develops in animals with heart disease when pulmonary edema fluid irritates the air passages.

Clinical Signs

A cough is one of the most common signs in dogs with dilated cardiomyopathy, but it is rare in cats with heart disease. Therefore, this section pertains only to dogs. Owners often describe a cough as choking or gagging, not recognizing it as coughing,[13] and it usually accompanies dyspnea and tachypnea. Lethargy, anorexia, weakness, and abdominal swelling are often present as well.

Auscultation should reveal a murmur or gallop in dogs with dilated cardiomyopathy. Diffuse crackles indicative of pulmonary edema should also be present. Arrhythmias, weak pulses with pulse deficits (if an arrhythmia is present), pallor, hypothermia, and slow capillary refill time are also found in dogs with dilated cardiomyopathy.

Diagnostic Plan

Preliminary diagnosis of myocardial disease is often made after a murmur, arrhythmia, or crackles are auscultated in a breed that is predisposed to cardiomyopathy. A murmur should be present in dogs with cardiomyopathy. The differential diagnosis of cough includes pulmonary disease (e.g., bronchitis, pneumonia), heartworm disease, and pulmonary neoplasia.

Radiography should be performed in dogs that are stable and can withstand the stress of the procedure. Cardiomegaly is usually present in dogs with cardiomyopathy, although Doberman pinschers with cardiomyopathy often have a normal cardiac silhouette. Pulmonary edema causes the cough in heart failure, and it is associated with an alveolar infiltrate located primarily in the hilar area that extends to the dorsal and caudal lung lobes in dogs, although it can be present in all lung lobes in Doberman pinschers.

Heartworm disease causes right ventricular enlargement, dilation of the pulmonary arteries, and an interstitial as well as alveolar infiltrate around the lobar arteries. The heart is normal in pneumonia, and the alveolar infiltrate is usually located ventrally. Bronchitis causes a peribronchial infiltrate that is associated with a normal heart.

An electrocardiogram (ECG) is often helpful, revealing atrial and ventricular arrhythmias and chamber enlargements. The ECG should be normal in animals without heart disease, but a normal ECG does not indicate the absence of cardiomyopathy. Echocardiography is diagnostic of dilated cardiomyopathy in dogs (see Echocardiography). Blood tests, including a heartworm test, should be done. See Chapter 9 for a complete discussion of coughing caused by cardiac disease and Chapter 54 for a discussion of respiratory disease.

Dyspnea

Pathophysiology

Dyspnea in animals with cardiomyopathy is caused by either pulmonary edema or pleural effusion. Alveolar pulmonary edema interferes with normal gas exchange in the lungs and causes hypoxemia. In addition, interstitial pulmonary edema increases pulmonary stiffness, which makes it harder to breathe. Pleural effusion takes up space in the thoracic cavity into which lungs normally expand. Therefore, the lungs cannot fill with normal respirations, and the work of breathing is again increased.

Clinical Signs

Dyspnea is the most common sign of heart failure in cardiomyopathic cats, and it is common in dogs as well. It is usually accompanied by lethargy and anorexia in cats, and dogs usually cough. Dyspnea may be nocturnal, and as edema worsens, dogs may not be able to lie down comfortably (orthopnea).[14]

Auscultation of animals that are dyspneic because of pulmonary edema reveals crackles, wheezes, and increased bronchovesicular sounds, primarily in the dorsal lung fields, although severe edema is generalized. Animals that are dyspneic because of

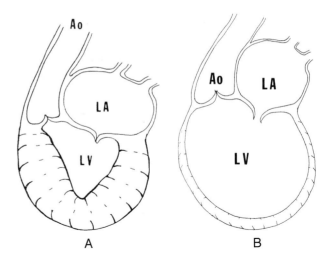

Figure 12–1
Diagram of **(A)** hypertrophic and **(B)** dilated cardiomyopathy. Hypertrophic cardiomyopathy is characterized by a thick wall and a normal to small ventricular chamber. It is primarily a diastolic dysfunction of the left ventricle. Dilated cardiomyopathy is characterized by a dilated, flabby ventricle. It is primarily a systolic dysfunction of the left ventricle. Ao, aorta; LA, left atrium; LV, left ventricle.

pleural effusion have decreased ventral lung sounds, and the extent of pleural effusion can often be determined by careful auscultation. Lung sounds are muffled ventrally, but as the stethoscope is moved dorsally lung sounds become more clear. The area at which the lung sounds are again clearly auscultated is the line of fluid within the chest. A murmur or gallop should be present in dogs and cats with cardiomyopathy, although some cats with cardiomyopathy will have neither.

Diagnostic Plan

Diagnostic tests may have to be postponed because of the stress they may cause a dyspneic animal. The exception is thoracentesis in a dyspneic animal with pleural effusion,[2] which is both diagnostic and therapeutic. This procedure may be life-saving in cats with severe pleural effusion, and it should not be delayed except to allow the cat to calm down from a car ride or stressful examination. The maximum amount of fluid should be withdrawn and submitted for cytologic analysis, although cytology is unnecessary if fluid has been analyzed previously and the diagnosis is known. Most cats with pleural effusion from right-sided heart failure have a modified transudate, but chylous effusions are caused by heart failure as well.[15] Other common causes of pleural effusion are neoplasia and pyothorax. Septic pleural effusions should have large numbers of white cells with bacteria. Neoplastic pleural effusions may contain cells diagnostic of the particular tumor causing the effusion. Lymphosarcoma usually causes an effusion with a high percentage of mature and immature lymphocytes.

Both sides of the chest should be aspirated, optimally with the animal in sternal recumbence. I prefer using a 21-gauge butterfly needle with a 12-mL syringe for thoracentesis in cats. I do not use a three-way stopcock to aspirate fluid, because the fluid in the tubing prevents a pneumothorax, and the stopcock is something additional to maneuver. I also prefer tapping cranial to the heart at about the second intercostal space, because there is less opportunity to run into the heart and because I think the thorax is more completely drained from this position than caudally. The disadvantage is that this location is less accessible than a caudal approach in cats that do not allow their forelimbs to be pulled forward. A location caudal to the heart is often easier to tap, because cats can rest comfortably and the forelimb does not hinder aspiration.

Although some veterinarians allow others to withdraw fluid while they maneuver the needle to different pockets of fluid within the thorax, it is safer to aspirate with one hand and hold the needle with the other. This way, the veterinarian is more aware of increasing negative intrathoracic pressure, which signals the end of thoracentesis. At this stage, aspiration of the syringe with strong pressure could draw lung tissue into the tip of the needle and cause a pneumothorax. Some fractious or anxious animals require sedation for successful thoracentesis. Although tranquilization involves some risk, it is less than the risk of tapping the chest of a moving animal. Dogs usually require a larger needle (i.e., 20-gauge) and an extension tube with a 12- or 35-mL syringe.

Thoracentesis of dyspneic animals with crackles is not recommended, because crackles usually indicate pulmonary edema, and there is a high risk of causing pneumothorax in these animals. Error can occur on both ends of the spectrum of tapping: some veterinarians tap every dyspneic animal, and some do not tap any. A good, quick auscultation should differentiate those animals that need thoracentesis from those that need cage rest, oxygen, and medical treatment.

Thoracic radiographs should be taken as soon as the animal is stable. ECG, echocardiography, and blood tests should be performed next. If possible, echocardiography should be performed before thoracentesis in animals with pleural effusion, because echocardiography can reveal masses and other intrathoracic abnormalities that are hidden on radiographs. See Cough for a complete discussion of the diagnostic plan, and see Chapter 53 for a discussion of pleural effusion.

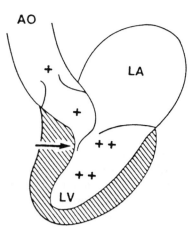

Figure 12–2
Diagram of a heart with the obstructive form of hypertrophic cardiomyopathy. The mitral valve is pulled or pushed anteriorly into the left ventricular outflow tract in systole *(arrow),* causing an outflow tract obstruction and mitral regurgitation. The plus signs indicate relative pressures within the left ventricle and aorta. AO, aorta; LA, left atrium. (From Wigle ED. Hypertrophic cardiomyopathy in 1988. Mod Concepts Cardiovasc Dis 1988;57:1–6. Reproduced with permission. Modern Concepts in Cardiovascular Disease. Copyright 1988 American Heart Association.)

Murmur

Pathophysiology

A murmur is often present in cats with hypertrophic cardiomyopathy. The murmur may be caused by outflow obstruction, mitral regurgitation, or both. Outflow obstruction is caused by abnormal mitral valve motion, commonly referred to as systolic anterior motion of the mitral valve. The most likely mechanism of outflow obstruction is a severely thickened septum that causes high-velocity blood flow (obstruction) through the left ventricular outflow tract during systole, although obstruction without septal hypertrophy can occur in cats with redundant mitral valves. This high-velocity blood flow in turn creates negative forces (i.e., Venturi forces) distal to the obstruction that either pull or push the mitral valve anteriorly. Mitral regurgitation is created when the mitral valve is displaced anteriorly in systole and contributes to the murmur (Fig. 12–2).[16] However, mitral regurgitation without systolic anterior motion of the mitral valve can occur in cats with restrictive cardiomyopathy.

In dogs and cats with dilated cardiomyopathy, a soft murmur of mitral regurgitation is caused by left ventricular dilation that stretches the mitral valve annulus and distorts left ventricular geometry, preventing mitral valve coaptation. Dogs with dilated cardiomyopathy may have concurrent mitral valve degeneration contributing to the mitral regurgitation.[6]

Clinical Signs

Murmurs in animals with dilated cardiomyopathy are usually low-grade (i.e., I/VI to II/VI), whereas murmurs in cats with the obstructive form of hypertrophic cardiomyopathy are higher-grade (i.e., III/VI to IV/VI). Other types of cardiomyopathy in cats can produce murmurs of any intensity. Many cats with murmurs are asymptomatic, but they may also have signs of heart failure on examination (e.g., acute dyspnea, lethargy, anorexia, posterior paresis). Dogs with heart murmurs may exhibit coughing, dyspnea, lethargy, syncope, weight loss, or ascites. A gallop, crackles, or muffled heart and lung sounds may be auscultated in dogs and cats. Arrhythmias are common in dogs and cats with cardiomyopathy.

Diagnostic Plan

Thoracic radiography, ECG, echocardiography, and routine blood tests should be performed in all animals with heart murmurs to elucidate a specific cause and determine severity of disease. Serum thyroxine (T_4) concentrations should be measured in all cats 7 years of age or older. The diagnostic plan is the same as for cough. See Chapter 9 for a complete discussion of heart murmurs.

Gallop

Pathophysiology

Although often referred to as a "gallop rhythm," a gallop is actually an extra heart sound caused by a loud third (S_3) or fourth (S_4) heart sound. An S_3 occurs in diastole during the rapid ventricular filling phase of the cardiac cycle. Most S_3 gallops are associated with rapid filling of a severely dilated ventricle and are found in cats and dogs with dilated cardiomyopathy. An S_4 gallop follows atrial systole and usually results from atrial contraction into a noncompliant ventricle. Most S_4 gallops occur in cats with hypertrophic or restrictive heart disease.[2]

Clinical Signs

Gallops are heard more commonly in cats than in dogs, and they are usually a sign of underlying heart disease, although gallops can occur in healthy cats. Occasionally, they are heard in cats that have received an overload of intravenous fluids, in which case they disappear after the fluid rate is decreased. The best single test for these cats is an echocardiogram. A gallop in a dog usually indicates severe cardiac disease, such as dilated cardiomyopathy. Radiography in dogs and cats with heart disease reveals cardiomegaly. Pulmonary edema and a pleural effusion may or may not be present. See Chapter 9 for a complete discussion of gallops.

Lethargy and Weakness

Pathophysiology

Exercise intolerance, lethargy, and weakness are common signs in dogs with dilated cardiomyopathy and in cats with all types of cardiomyopathy. Animals with cardiomyopathy become weak and exercise intolerant because of either backward or forward failure. Backward failure may be left-sided or right-sided. In left-sided heart failure, pulmonary edema decreases the lungs' ability to oxygenate, and exercise is hindered by hypoxemia. Pleural effusion caused by right-sided heart failure decreases vital capacity of the lungs, which also decreases oxygenation. Dogs and cats with cardiomyopathy develop both pleural effusion and pulmonary edema, although specific diseases are more likely to cause one or the other.[2, 6]

Forward failure, or low-output heart failure,[17] is caused by myocardial or systolic failure or tachyarrhythmias. Myocardial failure is the primary hemodynamic abnormality in dogs and cats with dilated cardiomyopathy. Because of poor contractility, the heart fails to deliver oxygen to tissues. Arrhythmias also cause low cardiac output. Several factors are involved, including the ventricular rate, the duration of the abnormal rate, the relation of ventricular filling to atrial contraction, the sequence of ventricular activation, the status of the myocardium, the amount of rhythm irregularity, and associated administration of cardiac drugs.[18] Tachyarrhythmias shorten diastole, leading to inadequate ventricular filling for normal stroke volume. Atrial contraction enhances ventricular filling at end-diastole, increasing cardiac output by as much as 20%. Loss of this effect because of atrial fibrillation is a significant loss in an animal that already has poor myocardial function.

Outflow obstructions can also cause lethargy and exercise intolerance. Although outflow obstructions are not thought to cause a decrease in cardiac output at rest, they can prevent the increase in stroke volume required during exercise or stress to maintain cardiac output. Stroke volume can also be reduced in cats with a ball thrombus in the left atrium that lodges in the mitral annulus and obstructs left ventricular filling. The thrombus may acutely cut off inflow to the left ventricle from the mitral valve, and with no ventricular filling there can be no outflow. In addition, cats with hypertrophic cardiomyopathy that have no signs of failure but are lethargic and anorexic may be experiencing chest pain. Angina pectoris is a common sign in humans with hypertrophic cardiomyopathy,[8] and it is possible that cats may also feel discomfort.

These cats often regain normal activity after treatment with a β-blocker.

Clinical Signs

The owner usually reports that the dog or cat wants to sleep more, is reluctant to move around, or has trouble walking even short distances. Murmurs, gallops, or arrhythmias should be present in weak animals with heart disease. Dyspnea, crackles, and muf fled heart and lung sounds on auscultation are common findings. The dyspnea may arise from pulmonary edema or pleural effusion. Decreased heart sounds may result from a hypocontractile ventricle or from pleural effusion, whereas muffling of both heart and lung sounds is usually caused by pleural effusion. Animals with dilated cardiomyopathy have low body temperature, pallor, poor capillary refill time, diminished pulses, and a weak apex beat. Cats with hypertrophic cardiomyopathy may have a hyperkinetic left apex beat.

Diagnostic procedures are the same as for animals with a heart murmur. See Chapter 9 for a complete discussion of lethargy and weakness.

Posterior Paresis or Lameness in Cats

Posterior paresis is the inability to move the hind limbs; in cats with cardiomyopathy, it is caused by thromboembolism of the distal aorta at the trifurcation (saddle thrombus). Thromboembolism occurs acutely, and it may be the first sign observed in cats with any form of cardiomyopathy.

Pathophysiology

Thromboemboli are thought to originate in the left ventricle or left atrium and to travel from there to a peripheral artery, where they cause lower motor neuron neuropathy and ischemic neuromyopathy.[2, 3, 19–21] Three factors associated with thrombus formation are local vessel or tissue injury, blood stasis, and altered blood coagulability.[2, 3, 19, 21] Tissue injury may be caused by atrial stretch or by damage to the outflow tract in cats with obstructive hypertrophic cardiomyopathy. Severe stretching of the left atrium, which occurs with hypertrophic cardiomyopathy and restrictive cardiomyopathy, exposes the subendocardium to platelets and creates a reservoir for stagnant blood. Stasis is also caused by an irregular ventricular chamber in some cats with restrictive cardiomyopathy or excessive numbers of moderator bands. Finally, altered blood coagulability is caused by hyperaggregable platelets in some myopathic cats[22] and by a chronic form of disseminated intravascular coagulopathy that

is found in 75% of cats with thromboembolism.[2]

The importance of the effect of substances that cause vasoconstriction distal to the clot is shown by the fact that ligation of the distal aorta does not cause the same clinical signs as does naturally occurring thromboembolism. Collateral circulation forms rapidly, but this too is impaired in cats with thromboembolism.[19, 21, 23] Serotonin and prostaglandins have been implicated as the vasoactive substances causing the damage in thromboembolism.[23]

Clinical Signs

Lameness or posterior paresis occurs acutely[19, 21, 23]; often, affected cats cry out in pain and then suddenly begin to drag their hind limbs. Cats may also develop heart failure as a result of the stress of the thromboembolism. Although any organ or limb may be affected, the caudal abdominal aorta is the most common site for emboli to lodge.[2, 19–21] If the embolus travels to a forelimb, the cat appears to be lame. Emboli to the renal, mesenteric, or pulmonary arteries are particularly devastating.[2]

Cats with thromboembolism of the distal aorta have different degrees of posterior paresis, which usually lateralizes to one side or the other. Pulses are severely diminished or absent, nail beds are cyanotic, and the distal limbs are cool to the touch. Immediately after the thromboembolic event, the muscles are soft, but within 12 to 18 hours they become hard and painful. The muscles below the stifle are affected most, with the cranial tibial muscles being firmer and more painful than the gastrocnemius muscles.[2, 3, 19, 21]

Signs of cardiac disease (i.e., murmur, gallop, and arrhythmias) are present in many cats with thromboembolism. Cats in decompensated heart failure may be dyspneic from pleural effusion, pulmonary edema, or both.[2, 3, 21]

Diagnostic Plan

Thromboembolism can be confused with tumors of the spinal cord or trauma (see Chap. 27). However, the clinical signs of cold extremities, absent pulses, and cyanotic nail beds are so distinct that misdiagnosis is rare. Because thromboembolism is associated with heart disease, a full cardiac work-up (i.e., ECG, thoracic radiographs, echocardiogram) should be performed. Abnormalities depend on the specific type of heart disease present. Serum biochemical analysis performed several hours after the event reveals extremely high alanine aminotransferase and aspartate aminotransferase as well as lactate dehydrogenase and creatine phosphokinase.[2, 3, 19–21] The cause of liver enzyme elevation is unknown, but it may arise from microthrombi to the liver or from generalized hypoxia. Nonselective angiography provides a definitive method of diagnosing thromboembolism,[2, 3, 19, 21] but this procedure is risky in cats with decompensated cardiac disease and is usually not necessary to reach a conclusive diagnosis.

Syncope

Pathophysiology

Some animals with heart failure faint during excitement or exercise because of an inability of the heart to deliver oxygenated blood to the brain. If pulmonary edema is present, blood is hypoxemic and animals faint even with adequate blood flow. Dogs and cats with forward failure may be able to oxygenate properly but because of poor cardiac output may not be able to deliver oxygen to the brain. Syncope usually results from a bradyarrhythmia or obstruction of blood flow,[24] although a tachyarrhythmia or loss of atrial contraction can also decrease cardiac output enough to cause syncope. Syncope secondary to tachyarrhythmias and bradyarrhythmias is usually episodic and unrelated to any activity, whereas persistent atrial arrhythmias cause syncope related to exercise intolerance because of increased oxygen demand during exercise.

Obstruction of blood flow from the heart is caused by a dynamic outflow obstruction in cats with hypertrophic cardiomyopathy or by a ball thrombus in the left atrium. Dynamic outflow obstruction in cats with hypertrophic cardiomyopathy is caused by abnormal mitral valve motion. The anterior leaflet is either pulled or pushed into the left ventricular outflow tract in systole, with maximum obstruction occurring after midsystole.[25] A ball thrombus in the atrium acts as a pop-off valve in the mitral annulus. Flow is suddenly stopped to the ventricle, and cardiac output drops to nothing.

Clinical Signs

Syncope of cardiac origin can often be differentiated from seizures on the basis of history and clinical signs. Cardiac syncope is a sudden event that has no premonitory signs and is over quickly. Dogs with syncope secondary to an arrhythmia have an irregular cardiac rhythm on auscultation as well as a cardiac murmur, congestive heart failure, and possibly marked weight loss. Cats with myocardial disease should have a murmur or gallop, and they may or may not have an arrhythmia. Animals with seizures, on the other hand, do not have any other signs of cardiac disease (e.g., murmur, gallop, arrhythmia) and may have abnormalities on a neurologic examination. They should also

have an aura and a postictal period, which are not seen in dogs with cardiac syncope.

Diagnostic Plan

The differential diagnosis includes any kind of neurologic or neuromuscular disorder and many metabolic problems. An ECG should be performed on all animals that have a history of syncope. Both bradycardias and tachycardias can cause syncope, although usually a heart rate slower than 40 beats per minute (bpm) in the dog (<80 in the cat) or faster than 180 bpm in the dog (>250 in the cat) is required to cause syncope. These heart rates are guidelines and not absolute numbers that always cause syncope. If cardiomyopathy is causing the syncope, radiographs should reveal cardiomegaly with or without heart failure (i.e., pulmonary edema or pleural effusion). A thorough neurologic examination should be performed in addition to thoracic radiographs, ECG, and routine blood tests. Animals may also need to be observed in the hospital for several days. In addition, a 24- or 48-hour Holter monitor may be necessary to detect occult arrhythmias.

See Chapter 9 for a complete discussion of cardiovascular syncope and Chapter 24 for a discussion of seizures.

Diagnostic Procedures

Electrocardiography

Approximately one half to two thirds of cats with cardiomyopathy have ECG abnormalities such as arrhythmias, conduction disturbances, or evidence of chamber enlargement.[2, 3, 20] In general, there are no distinguishing ECG abnormalities in cats with cardiomyopathy that definitively diagnose a particular form of cardiomyopathy. The one exception is a left anterior fascicular block pattern, which has a high association with hypertrophic cardiomyopathy.[3] I have also noticed an association of atrioventricular (A-V) nodal blocks with restrictive cardiomyopathy. Other abnormalities include tall and wide QRS complexes, wide P waves, atrial and ventricular arrhythmias, conduction disturbances such as first-degree A-V nodal block, and bradycardia.[1-3, 7, 20] A wide QRS complex may be slightly more common in cats with dilated cardiomyopathy than in those with other types of cardiomyopathy.[20]

In dogs, an arrhythmia is often the first sign of dilated cardiomyopathy.[6] Atrial fibrillation is usually auscultated in giant breeds,[26] whereas ventricular arrhythmias are more common in Doberman pinschers and boxers.[10, 27] Atrial fibrillation may also be present in Doberman pinschers,[26] but it is less common than ventricular arrhythmias.[10] Tall, wide QRS complexes with slurring S-T segments may also be present in giant breeds. English cocker spaniels rarely display arrhythmias, but they have deep Q waves, tall and wide QRS complexes, and right axis deviations.[28–30]

Radiography

Radiographs, like ECGs, show very few distinguishing characteristics that elucidate a particular type of heart disease in cats, although some general statements can be made. The left atrium in cats with hypertrophic or restrictive cardiomyopathy is more prominent than in cats with other cardiomyopathies, and the left ventricular apex in cats with dilated cardiomyopathy is more rounded (globoid).[1–3] Pulmonary edema is usually seen in cats with hypertrophic or restrictive cardiomyopathy, whereas pleural effusion is more common in cats with dilated cardiomyopathy. Pleural effusion in cats with hypertrophic or restrictive cardiomyopathy is usually mild. Cats with nonspecific types of heart disease can have pleural effusion or pulmonary edema.[1–3, 7, 31]

Giant breeds of dogs with dilated cardiomyopathy usually have generalized cardiomegaly with various degrees of left- and right-sided heart failure (pulmonary edema and pleural effusion).[11] In Doberman pinschers, the left ventricle may appear normal in size radiographically, even in the presence of severe heart failure, although the left atrium may be enlarged.[10–13] Boxers with ventricular arrhythmias as their only sign may also display a normal cardiac silhouette.[27] Boxers in heart failure usually have left atrial enlargement and hilar pulmonary edema.[6, 10–13] Radiographic abnormalities in English and American cocker spaniels include biventricular enlargement and pulmonary edema.[28–30]

Echocardiography

The best single method for elucidating the type and severity of cardiomyopathy is echocardiography.[32, 33] Its major advantages are safety, specificity, and ease of technique for the experienced echocardiographer. Disadvantages include expense of equipment and difficulty for the inexperienced echocardiographer. However, the services of experienced sonographers are becoming more widely available.

Knowledge of heart disease is expanding, and feline cardiomyopathy, in particular, constitutes a wider spectrum of disease than was previously recognized. Although earlier classifications of hypertrophic cardiomyopathy, dilated cardiomyopathy, and restrictive cardiomyopathy are still useful, there is also great overlap between types, and even echocardiography is often unable to identify a specific type of cardiomyopathy on the basis of structure or function of the heart.[2, 3] The term "intergrade cardiomyopathy" was introduced to give a name to the large number of cardiac abnormalities in cats that do not easily fit into any category. Even without naming the disease, echocardiography is necessary to determine wall thickness, measure systolic function, decide whether positive inotropic agents are required, and visualize clots in cats that develop thromboembolism. Categories of myocardial fibrosis and myocardial failure are also being included in the wider spectrum of heart disease in cats.

Dilated cardiomyopathy in dogs can usually be diagnosed by the breed, clinical signs, physical findings, and changes on ECG and radiography. Echocardiography is useful to estimate the severity of myocardial dysfunction in dogs prone to dilated cardiomyopathy and to determine whether myocardial dysfunction is present in boxers and English and American cocker spaniels. In addition, Doberman pinschers may have less systolic dysfunction and more mitral valve degeneration than other breeds.[6]

Routine Laboratory Evaluation

Routine serum biochemical analyses and complete blood counts should be performed on all dogs and cats with suspected cardiomyopathy. Many exhibit prerenal azotemia, which could worsen with overzealous use of diuretics and vasodilators. Some animals also have mild anemia. Muscle enzyme levels in cats with thromboembolism are extremely high, and some cats are hyperkalemic. Hyperthyroidism causes secondary hypertrophic cardiomyopathy, which may be mistaken for primary hypertrophic cardiomyopathy and inadequately treated. In addition, elevated liver enzymes may be found.[2, 3, 34–43]

Nonselective Angiography

Nonselective angiography has been advocated as a relatively safe method of identifying the distinct forms of cardiomyopathy in cats.[1, 20] With the widespread availability of echocardiography, it no longer seems advisable to sedate a cat and inject a dye that could induce cardiac arrest. However, in practices in which echocardiography is not routinely performed, it is still a reasonable procedure to complete the diagnosis. The technique has been well described and is not discussed further here.[20, 44, 45] Nonselective angiography is impractical in most dogs because of their size.

Blood Pressure

Routine blood pressure measurement in cats with renal disease, cardiac disease, or hyperthyroidism is not yet widely practiced, but it may become more available in the future. Recent reports indicate that a high proportion of cats with hyperthyroidism or renal disease also have hypertension. Because hypertension can cause left ventricular hypertrophy, cats with hypertrophic cardiomyopathy should be screened for hypertension.[46–48]

Common Myocardial Diseases

Hypertrophic Cardiomyopathy in Cats

Hypertrophic cardiomyopathy is the most common type of cardiomyopathy in cats.[2, 3, 20, 31] It is defined as inappropriate left ventricular hypertrophy, often accompanied by asymmetrical hypertrophy of the septum and preserved or enhanced myocardial function.[49, 50] The primary pathophysiologic abnormality is diastolic dysfunction because of increased stiffness and abnormal relaxation of the left ventricle. The discovery that hypertrophic cardiomyopathy in cats closely resembles the same syndrome in humans[5, 7, 51, 52a] has enhanced our understanding of the disease because of the large numbers of studies performed on humans with hypertrophic cardiomyopathy.

Prevalence of hypertrophic cardiomyopathy in cats varies from 1% of a hospital population based on echocardiography[53] to 5% based on necropsy findings.[31] The prevalence may even be higher, because sudden death is a result of hypertrophic cardiomyopathy in cats.[3] Many cats are asymptomatic until they are examined in acute heart failure or with an aortic thromboembolism.[2, 3, 20, 52a]

The typical cat with hypertrophic cardiomyopathy is a middle-aged (5–6.5 years old), male domestic shorthair cat; however, cats from less than 1 to 16 years of age can be affected.[1–3, 5, 7, 20, 53] Persian cats have been reported to have a higher prevalence of hypertrophic cardiomyopathy,[5, 54] and it has been found in a family of Maine coon cats.[55]

Pathophysiology

The cause of hypertrophic cardiomyopathy is unknown, although high concentrations of growth hormone have been reported in cats with hypertrophic cardiomyopathy.[56] The hallmark of hypertrophic cardiomyopathy is pathologic hypertrophy of the left ventricle that leads to diastolic dysfunction of the left ventricle. Left ventricular diastolic failure causes high left ventricular filling pressure. The left atrium is unable to empty into a stiff ventricle, and left atrial pressure rises. The left atrium stretches to accommodate high pressure, but as left atrial pressure rises, so does pulmonary venous pressure. Eventually, pulmonary edema ensues.[8, 49, 50, 52a]

The diastolic abnormalities of hypertrophic cardiomyopathy arise from two different mechanisms: left ventricular stiffness and impaired relaxation. Increased myocardial stiffness is associated with a greatly thickened left ventricular wall and with increased deposition of collagen in the myocardium. Left ventricular relaxation, an energy-dependent process, is also impaired in cats with hypertrophic cardiomyopathy.[8, 25, 49]

Hypertrophic cardiomyopathy has been divided into obstructive and nonobstructive forms, depending on the gradient between the left ventricle and aorta.[8, 25, 49, 50, 52a] Several conditions are known to increase outflow obstruction. Increasing contractility, dramatically decreasing preload, and decreasing afterload all increase the gradient. Therefore, drugs that should be avoided in cats with obstructive hypertrophic cardiomyopathy include positive inotropic agents such as digitalis, dopamine, dobutamine, or isoproterenol; overzealously used diuretics plus nitroglycerin, which decrease preload; and strong afterload reducers such as hydralazine (Apresoline).[8]

It is thought that the obstruction starts from a pronounced thickening of the basilar interventricular septum, which causes a progressive narrowing of the left ventricular outflow tract during systole. This narrowing either sucks or pushes the mitral valve into the outflow tract and causes systolic anterior motion of the mitral valve, which in turn increases apposition of the mitral valve against the septum and causes outflow tract obstruction[25, 49, 52a] (see Fig. 12–2). This type of obstruction is dynamic, meaning that it is not the same throughout systole but increases in severity during systole, with the worst obstruction occurring at the end.[52a] It is also labile and varies from day to day depending on hemodynamic conditions.[25, 49, 57]

Mitral regurgitation also occurs in cats with hypertrophic cardiomyopathy because of the abnormal motion of the mitral valve,[49, 52a, 57] and its severity is related to the degree of systolic anterior motion of the mitral valve.[16] The murmur in cats with hypertrophic cardiomyopathy is caused by the turbulence from left ventricular outflow obstruction and by mitral regurgitation.[49] There is also a direct correlation between the severity of outflow obstruction and the amount of mitral regurgitation, which in turn further elevates left atrial pressure.[58] Therefore, it seems imprudent to disregard high aortic outflow, and treatment that is effective in reducing the gradient should be chosen.

Pathologic alterations on postmortem examination are similar in cats and dogs with hypertrophic cardiomyopathy.[5, 51, 52, 59, 60] The primary abnormality is thickening of the interventricular septum and segments of the left ventricular wall. There is asymmetrical hypertrophy, defined as a ratio of septal wall to free wall greater than 1:1; disorganized cardiac muscle cells are also found on necropsy examination in many cats with hypertrophic cardiomyopathy.[5, 7, 51, 52a, 61]

Clinical Signs

Cats with hypertrophic cardiomyopathy are usually examined because of acute dyspnea from pulmonary edema, although anorexia, vomiting, lethargy, and posterior paresis from thromboembolism are also common signs.[1–3, 20, 50, 52a] Cats with pulmonary edema rarely cough, and a cat with acute dyspnea, a cough, and crackles is more likely to have asthma or bronchitis than heart failure.

A murmur is often present in cats with hypertrophic cardiomyopathy, even before other signs develop. Dyspnea, tachypnea, crackles, a murmur, and occasionally an arrhythmia are common in cats with heart failure.[52a] The only ECG abnormality specific for hypertrophic cardiomyopathy is a left anterior fascicular block pattern (Fig. 12–3), but this is not seen in every cat with hypertrophic cardiomyopathy. Radiographs reveal an enlarged heart, often with marked left atrial enlargement, and patchy pulmonary edema (Fig. 12–4). Cats with early hypertrophic cardiomyopathy and without heart failure may display minimal evidence of cardiomegaly on thoracic radiographs.[1–3, 20, 50]

Diagnostic Plan

Echocardiography is the best tool to diagnose hypertrophic cardiomyopathy, because ECG and radiographic changes are not specific.[50, 52a] The most definitive abnormality is thickening of the septum or left ventricular free wall. Hypertrophic cardiomyopathy is probably overdiagnosed, because some veterinarians performing echocardiograms diagnose as hypertrophy any amount of wall thickening. The wall thickness should be at least 5.5 mm for the average-sized cat, and other causes of left ventricular hypertrophy (i.e., hypertension and hyperthyroidism) should be excluded.

Systolic anterior motion of the mitral valve may also be visualized during M-mode or two-dimensional echocardiography in cats with the obstructive form of hypertrophic cardiomyopathy[50, 52a] (Figs. 12–5 and 12–6). Doppler echocardiography definitively diagnoses obstructive hypertrophic cardiomyopathy by revealing high-velocity left ventricular outflow[52a] (see Fig. 12–6C). There is a broad range of severity of hypertrophy; it may be symmetrical and concentric, or it may involve only segments of the left ventricle, which appears hyperdynamic.[49, 50, 52a] Mild to severe left atrial dilation is also commonly found. Because hyperthyroidism mimics primary hypertrophic cardiomyopathy, serum T_4 concentrations should be determined in all cats with hypertrophic cardiomyopathy.[46]

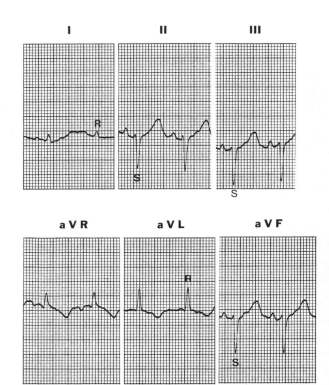

Figure 12–3

Left anterior fascicular block pattern in a cat with hypertrophic cardiomyopathy. There is a predominant R wave in leads I and aVL, deep S waves in leads II, III, and aVF, and a left axis deviation.

Treatment

The aims of treating hypertrophic cardiomyopathy in cats include resolving edema, slowing the heart rate to decrease myocardial oxygen demand and relieve ischemia, alleviating or lessening left ventricular outflow tract obstruction, and facilitating left ventricular relaxation.[8, 25] Diuretics such as furosemide should be used with caution in cats because of their propensity to cause dehydration.[8] An intravenous dose of 1 mg/kg twice (b.i.d.) or three times (t.i.d.) per day is usually adequate to control acute pulmonary edema. A preload reducer such as nitroglycerin ointment (0.3–0.6 cm in the ear pinna) may also be used to move fluid from the chest to the periphery, but it should be discontinued as soon as possible. Administration of oxygen and cage rest are absolute necessities for cats in heart failure. Digitalis glycosides should be avoided except in cases of severe, right-sided heart failure. Any kind of fluid therapy should also be avoided in cats that are in fulminant left-sided heart failure, because it increases edema.[1–3, 20] The most promising therapy in cats with refractory pulmonary edema unresponsive to furosemide is a single 15-mg oral dose of diltiazem (Cardizem).

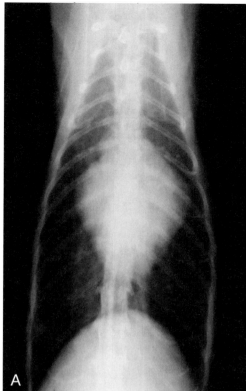

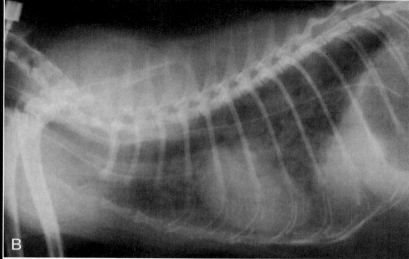

Figure 12-4

(A) Ventrodorsal radiograph of a cat with hypertrophic cardiomyopathy. Both atria are large, causing the heart to appear wide at the base. The left ventricle is long. **(B)** Lateral radiograph of a cat with left-sided heart failure and pulmonary edema. Notice the diffuse nature of the edema. The radiopaque lines are a nasoesophageal tube and a jugular catheter.

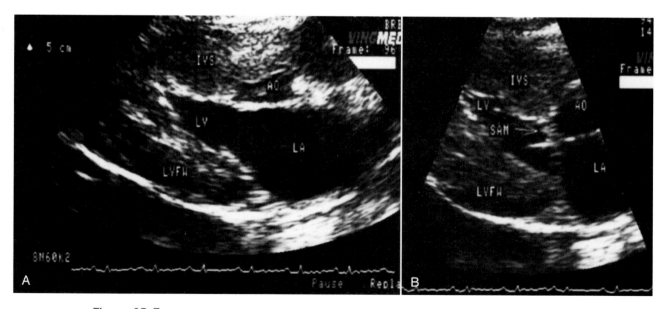

Figure 12-5

Two-dimensional echocardiogram of a cat with hypertrophic cardiomyopathy in **(A)** diastole and **(B)** systole. In **A,** the septum and free wall of the heart are thick, and the left ventricle is not dilated. In **B,** systolic anterior motion of the mitral valve (SAM) is present. AO, aorta; IVS, interventricular septum; LA, left atrium; LV, left ventricle; LVFW, left ventricular free wall.

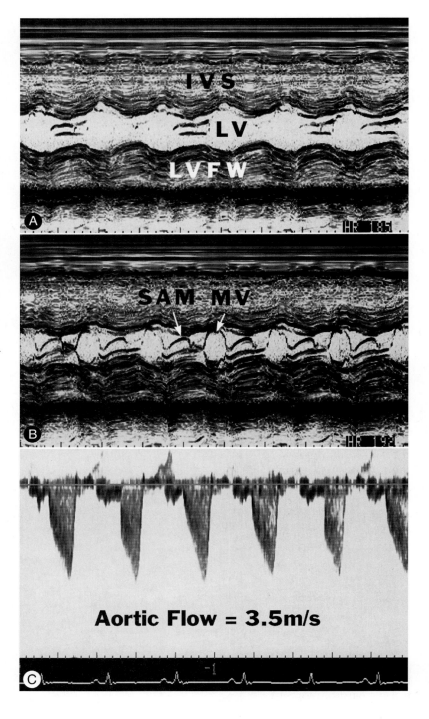

Figure 12-6
(A) M-mode echocardiogram of the left ventricle of a cat with hypertrophic cardiomyopathy. The septum and free wall of the left ventricle are thick, and the left ventricular cavity is small. **(B)** M-mode echocardiogram of the mitral valve of a cat with hypertrophic cardiomyopathy. The mitral valve moves anteriorly in systole (SAM), touching the septum and causing an outflow tract obstruction. **(C)** Doppler echocardiogram of a cat with hypertrophic cardiomyopathy. Notice the "ski slope" shape of the envelope that is characteristic of dynamic outflow obstructions. The highest velocities are reached after midsystole. Velocity of aortic flow in this cat is 3.5 m/sec. Normal aortic flow should be approximately 1 m/sec. IVS, interventricular septum; LV, left ventricular cavity; LVFW, left ventricular free wall; MV, mitral valve; SAM, systolic anterior motion of the mitral valve.

The two main classes of drugs appropriate for long-term treatment of hypertrophic cardiomyopathy are β-adrenergic blocking agents[62] and calcium channel blockers.[63] Although β-blockers have been the mainstay of therapy in the past, calcium channel blockers are now the drugs of choice in human medicine.[8, 25, 64, 65] There is controversy in veterinary medicine over which class of drugs is more efficacious in cats,[50, 62, 63, 66] and further studies are needed to clarify this issue. Both classes act to slow the heart rate,

which both decreases myocardial oxygen consumption[67] and enhances ventricular filling by allowing more time for diastole. The calcium channel blockers are the only drugs that actually facilitate relaxation by their action on intracellular calcium.[65]

The biggest problem with some therapies may be lack of owner compliance in administering the proper dosage. For this reason, the sustained-release or long-acting drugs are preferable in cats. My β-blocker of choice is atenolol (Tenormin), a β$_1$-selective adrenergic blocker.[67] The dosage in cats is 6.25 to 12.5 mg by mouth, once per day (s.i.d.) or b.i.d. The dosage is adjusted upward until the heart rate drops to 170 bpm or less. When the heart rate slows on auscultation, the murmur also becomes softer, and left ventricular outflow velocity decreases on repeat echocardiographic evaluations. Problems such as increased mortality, which were reported with propranolol (Inderal),[68] have not been encountered with atenolol, and β-blockers are probably as good or better in reducing heart rate and decreasing obstruction than calcium blocking agents in cats with obstructive hypertrophic cardiomyopathy. However, calcium channel blockers are preferable in cats with severe hypertrophic cardiomyopathy and small left ventricular cavities. Diltiazem, the calcium channel blocker used most commonly in cats with hypertrophic cardiomyopathy, must be administered b.i.d. or t.i.d. in the usual dosage of 7.5 to 15 mg. The difficulty with frequent administration of diltiazem can be eliminated by administering a long-acting form at a dosage of 10 mg/kg every 24 hours.[69] A new form of diltiazem comes with 60-mg timed-release caplets that are combined in an extended-release capsule of 120 mg (Dilacor XR). The capsule may be broken open and the caplets administered individually. Care must be taken to administer the caplets without breaking them.

Side effects of calcium channel blockers relate to their effect on the A-V node (slow conduction) and on the cardiac muscle (negative inotropic activity), which can cause heart rates to become too low. Both calcium channel blockers and β-blockers can exacerbate heart failure,[67, 70–72] and both can cause diarrhea,[67] although diarrhea is uncommon in cats in my experience. Animals that react adversely to these drugs appear weak.

Prognosis

Prognosis is better than expected for most cats with hypertrophic cardiomyopathy, although cats with aortic thrombi, severe left ventricular hypertrophy, or posterior walls that are thicker than the septum have a much poorer prognosis than other cats with hypertrophic cardiomyopathy.[52a, 53]

Restrictive Cardiomyopathy in Cats

The term "restrictive" refers to a restriction of ventricular filling. Therefore, restrictive cardiomyopathy, like hypertrophic cardiomyopathy, produces diastolic dysfunction, but to a greater degree than hypertrophic cardiomyopathy does. The underlying cause is unknown; the end result is myocardial or endomyocardial fibrosis. Restrictive cardiomyopathy has been considered a relatively rare form of cardiomyopathy,

but it is probably more common than was previously recognized. Many cats formerly designated with intermediate or intergrade cardiomyopathy probably had restrictive cardiomyopathy.[4, 72a, 73] Signalment is the same as for other forms of cardiomyopathy.[1–3, 7, 31]

Pathophysiology

Restrictive cardiomyopathy causes severe left ventricular diastolic dysfunction. There is rapid completion of ventricular filling in early diastole, with little or no further filling during middle to late diastole. High end-diastolic pressures prevent normal left atrial emptying, producing the typical severely dilated left atrium.[4] This explains the S_4 gallop (atrial contraction against a noncompliant ventricle) that is auscultated in some cats with restrictive cardiomyopathy. There is also overlap between hypertrophic cardiomyopathy and restrictive cardiomyopathy in cats, but it is preferable to reserve the term "restrictive" for those cats with obvious fibrosis on necropsy or echocardiographic examination, or evidence of restrictive filling (e.g., severe left atrial enlargement without severe mitral regurgitation[4] or Doppler echocardiographic indices of restrictive physiology).[72a]

Clinical Signs

Clinical signs are similar to those in cats with hypertrophic cardiomyopathy; dyspnea is the most common sign, but lethargy and anorexia are also characteristic. A murmur or S_4 gallop is often heard, and muffled heart sounds (indicating pleural effusion) or crackles (indicating pulmonary edema) may be auscultated.[1–3, 7, 31, 72a] An aortic clot may be the first sign of restrictive cardiomyopathy.[72a]

Diagnostic Plan

Echocardiography is the best method of diagnosing restrictive cardiomyopathy. The most characteristic finding is a severely dilated left atrium. Shortening, as measured on the M-mode echocardiogram, is either normal or only slightly decreased (usually >25%), and areas of marked wall dysfunction are seen. The left ventricular diameter is usually slightly dilated, and discrete areas of thinning caused by infarction, atrophy, or scarring may be imaged. Cats with a hyperechoic, thick endocardium or hyperechoic areas within the myocardium probably have restrictive cardiomyopathy[4, 72a, 73] (Fig. 12–7).

Nonselective angiography may be employed in practices in which echocardiography is not available, but echocardiography is much preferred as a diagnostic tool.[2] Angiography reveals filling defects in the left ventricular cavity if the restriction is caused by endomyocardial fibrosis. There may be a higher number of

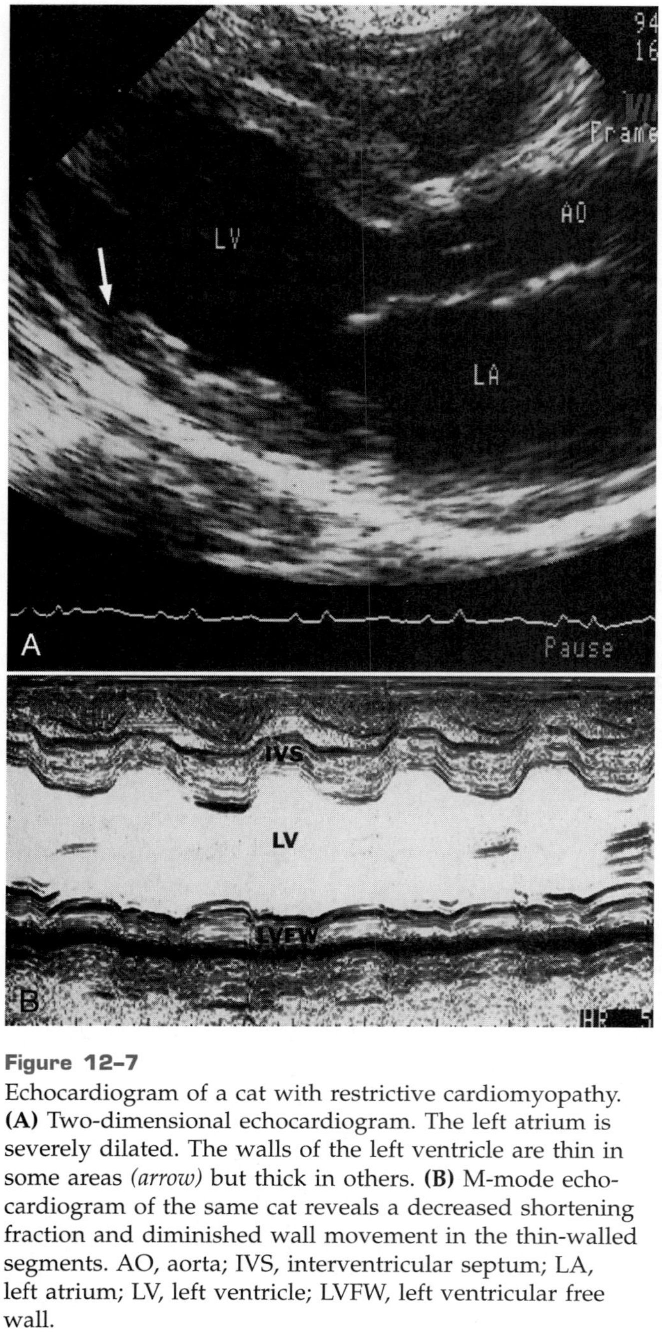

Figure 12–7
Echocardiogram of a cat with restrictive cardiomyopathy.
(A) Two-dimensional echocardiogram. The left atrium is
severely dilated. The walls of the left ventricle are thin in
some areas *(arrow)* but thick in others. **(B)** M-mode echocardiogram of the same cat reveals a decreased shortening
fraction and diminished wall movement in the thin-walled
segments. AO, aorta; IVS, interventricular septum; LA,
left atrium; LV, left ventricle; LVFW, left ventricular free
wall.

cats with A-V nodal blocks, atrial and ventricular premature complexes, atrial fibrillation, or wide P waves
on ECG (Fig. 12–8) than with other types of cardiomyopathy, but this is an insensitive diagnostic test for
restrictive cardiomyopathy. Thoracic radiography likewise is not specific for restrictive cardiomyopathy, although moderate to severe left atrial enlargement with
pulmonary edema is a characteristic finding.[73] Pleural
effusion is also occasionally seen on radiographs (Fig.
12–9).[1–3, 7, 31]

Treatment

Treatment is aimed at relieving signs of heart
failure or thromboembolism, because the fibrosis is
nonreversible. Most cats have pulmonary edema, but
some have pleural effusion as a major problem. The
most important immediate treatment for cats with
pleural effusion on examination is thoracentesis. This
is much more efficacious in improving clinical status
than administration of any drug or oxygen. Occasionally, light sedation (0.05 mL ketamine plus 0.05 mL
diazepam [Valium] intravenously for the average cat)
is required, and it should be administered to fractious
cats. Cats should be observed carefully for paradoxical
worsening of dyspnea after thoracentesis as a result of
pneumothorax or pulmonary edema. Pneumothorax
may occur because of puncture of a lung lobe or
because of the inability of the lungs to expand with
removal of a large amount (>200 mL) of pleural fluid.
Pleural fibrosis in cats with chronic pleural effusion
prevents normal expansion of the lung lobes, causing
their collapse and more severe dyspnea after thoracentesis. Repeated thoracentesis may resolve the problem, or placement of a chest tube may be required.
Pulmonary edema may also occur secondary to thoracentesis because of the negative pressure required to
drain fluid from the chest cavity.

Pulmonary edema is treated initially with furosemide (Lasix), nitroglycerin ointment, and oxygen.
Care must be taken with injectable furosemide in cats
because of their tendency to become dehydrated with
seemingly appropriate dosages: 1 mg/kg, b.i.d. or
t.i.d., intravenously or intramuscularly, is usually adequate, even for cats in acute pulmonary edema.[1–3, 7, 31]

Furosemide at a dosage adequate to control
signs is continued as one of the mainstays of long-term
treatment. Vasodilators, especially angiotensin-converting enzyme (ACE) inhibitors such as enalapril
(Vasotec or Enacard, 0.25–0.5 mg/kg by mouth every
24–48 hours), are important drugs to use not only
because of their vasodilating capabilities but also
because of their ability to block sodium and water
retention and decrease stimulation of the sympathetic
nervous system. Digoxin may be instituted if the
fibrosis does not appear to be severe or widespread
and if there is concurrent systolic dysfunction, but
digoxin does not improve contractility of a myocardium that is largely fibrous tissue.

Prognosis

Prognosis for cats with restrictive cardiomyopathy is extremely variable, depending on the amount of
myocardium that is fibrotic and the degree of diastolic
dysfunction. It is not known whether the presence of
atrial fibrillation or ventricular arrhythmias worsens
the prognosis. Longevity is variable; some cats die

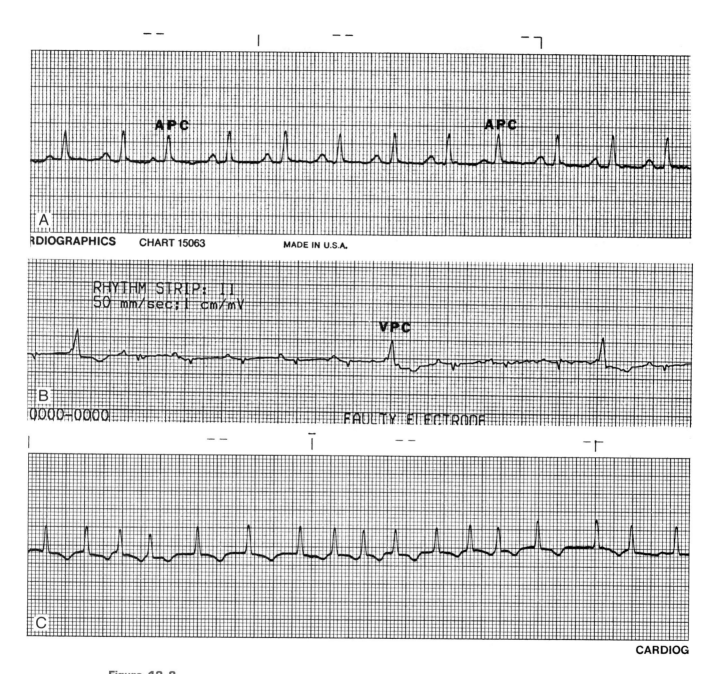

Figure 12-8

Electrocardiograms of cats with cardiomyopathy. **(A)** Atrial premature complexes (APC). The complexes are similar in configuration to the sinus complexes, occur early, and are followed by a pause. **(B)** Ventricular premature complexes (VPC). The complexes occur early, are followed by a pause, and differ in configuration from the sinus complexes. **(C)** Atrial fibrillation. The rhythm is irregularly irregular, P waves are absent, and fine fibrillation waves are present in the baseline.

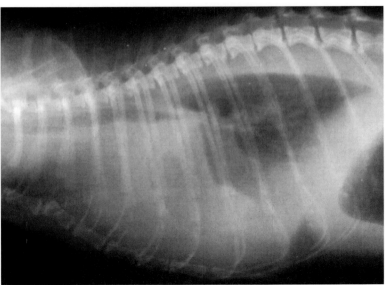

Figure 12–9
Severe pleural effusion in a cat with restrictive cardiomyopathy. The fluid obscures the heart and causes separation of the lungs from the thoracic wall. The lung borders have a leafy appearance.

within a few weeks after diagnosis, and others live for years.

Intergrade Cardiomyopathy in Cats

Intergrade or intermediate cardiomyopathy is a term that has been devised to describe heart disease in cats that does not fit into any category of myocardial disease.[2, 20] These patients exhibit a broad range of systolic and diastolic dysfunction, left ventricular hypertrophy, and left and right ventricular dilation, and many may actually have restrictive cardiomyopathy.[73] This category can also be divided into myocardial failure and restrictive cardiomyopathy.[4] Excessive left ventricular moderator bands constitutes a subgroup of heart disease in cats that should probably be included in the category of restrictive cardiomyopathy when the moderator bands obliterate the left ventricle, but the pathophysiology and hemodynamic abnormalities of this form of cardiomyopathy in cats are unknown. For the purpose of this chapter, excessive moderator bands is included in the category of intergrade cardiomyopathy.[9] The incidence of intergrade cardiomyopathy is unknown. Signalment is similar to that for other kinds of cardiomyopathy; that is, it is found in cats of any age, breed, or sex.

Pathophysiology

The pathophysiology varies and is probably similar to that of other cardiomyopathies. The veterinarian should become familiar with the pathophysiology of hypertrophic cardiomyopathy and restrictive cardiomyopathy and be able to recognize indicators of systolic and diastolic dysfunction.

Clinical Signs

Clinical signs and physical examination findings are the same as with other types of cardiomyopathy: lethargy, anorexia, or dyspnea of short duration; a murmur, gallop, or arrhythmia revealed by auscultation of the heart; and crackles (pulmonary edema) or diminished lung sounds (pleural effusion) revealed by thoracic auscultation.

Diagnostic Plan

Diagnosis is reached by exclusion of other types of cardiomyopathy by echocardiography. For instance, if a cat's heart is hypertrophied but too dilated for a diagnosis of hypertrophic cardiomyopathy, it is said to exhibit intergrade cardiomyopathy. This is an example of the principle that it is more important in cats with heart disease to determine the type and severity of hemodynamic abnormalities (systolic or diastolic) than to classify the condition with a name.

Treatment

Treatment is similar to that for other types of heart disease: oxygen, cage rest, and nitroglycerin ointment for cats with pulmonary edema; and thoracentesis for cats with marked pleural effusion. Once the type of failure has been recognized (systolic, diastolic, or volume overload), treatment may be individualized for each cat. Systolic dysfunction should be treated with digoxin (Lanoxin), the only known positive inotropic drug available for oral administration in cats.[74] Administration is usually started immediately, even if dobutamine is being infused. Although the elixir has the advantages of ease of measuring and better absorption,[75, 76] the tablet form is used most frequently because some cats salivate excessively when given the elixir. The dosage is 0.01 mg/kg every 48 hours,[74, 77] or one quarter of a 0.125-mg tablet every 2 or 3 days for a cat weighing 1.9 to 3.2 kg; one quarter of a 0.125-mg tablet s.i.d. or every 48 hours for a cat weighing 3.3 to 6.9 kg; and one quarter of a 0.125-mg tablet s.i.d. for a cat weighing more than 6 kg.[2] Digoxin should not be administered with food, because this decreases absorption.[75] Steady state is reached 10 days after initiation of treatment, and serum digoxin concentrations should be obtained 8 hours after the last pill has been administered. Cats that are concurrently being given low-sodium diets, furosemide, and aspirin may be more sensitive to the effects of digoxin than other cats and should be monitored more closely.[74, 77]

The therapeutic range of digoxin concentrations in cats has been reported to be 1 to 2 ng/mL.[74, 77] The dosage should be lowered to 0.007 mg/kg every 48 hours if cats are concurrently being fed a low-salt diet and are being treated with furosemide and aspirin. Early signs of toxicity include vomiting accompanied by hypersalivation, anorexia, and lethargy.[76] Digoxin has a cumulative effect, so seemingly well-regulated cats may eventually require a lower dosage.[75, 78]

Furosemide is administered at a dosage of 1 to 2 mg/kg, s.i.d. or b.i.d. The dehydrating effects of furosemide in cats must be remembered, and the drug should be given cautiously to cats with azotemia or dehydration. The lowest dosage possible should be prescribed, and it should then be adjusted according to need (e.g., recurrence of pleural effusion or pulmonary edema).[2, 11]

Dobutamine (Dobutrex) should be considered if severe systolic dysfunction is present. Dopamine may also be considered, but dobutamine is preferable because it is less arrhythmogenic, causes less vasoconstriction, and is superior in increasing cardiac output to dopamine. The dosage of dobutamine is 2 to 3 µg/kg per minute by constant-rate infusion for 48 to 72 hours. Higher dosages have been known to cause seizures in cats, although we have recently used dosages as high as 7 µg/kg per minute without adverse effects.[2]

Heart failure is treated with an ACE inhibitor such as enalapril. ACE inhibitors benefit cats in heart failure by causing vasodilation and by reducing sodium and water retention, thereby decreasing pleural effusion. The dosage in cats is 0.25 to 0.5 mg/kg, s.i.d. or b.i.d. Enalapril must be administered with caution in cats that are receiving high dosages of furosemide, because azotemia is more likely to occur with the combination of diuretics and ACE inhibitors than when either drug is used alone. It is preferable to stabilize a cat with diuretics and digoxin for several days to a week, then add enalapril.

Follow-up radiography is important in cats with recurrent pleural effusion, because many cats do not become symptomatic until the pleural effusion is very severe (>150 mL of fluid). Even moderate amounts of pleural effusion may not cause muffling of heart and lung sounds. The lowest dose of diuretic required to control signs should be administered, because of the tendency for cats to become dehydrated with administration of diuretics.[1–3, 7, 31]

Prognosis

Prognosis is extremely variable and depends on the amount of hemodynamic derangement, the presence and severity of arrhythmias, the presence of metabolic abnormalities, and the presence or absence of a clot. Cats with thrombi in the left atrium or aortic trifurcation and cats with myocardial failure have a worse prognosis.

Thromboembolism

Thromboembolism in cats can occur as a sequela of any type of cardiomyopathy, and it often is the first sign of cardiac disease. A thrombus is a blockage of an artery by platelets and fibrin that begins at the site of the blockage. An embolus begins in another area of the body, usually the heart, and travels to the area of the blockage. The term "thromboembolus" is used if it is unclear whether the problem is a thrombus or embolus.

Clinical Signs

Common clinical signs and physical examination findings have been described (see Posterior Paresis). Thromboembolism may affect any limb or organ, including the heart, kidney, spinal cord, and liver. The diagnosis and pathophysiology have been described earlier in the chapter.[2, 3]

Treatment

Treatment of thromboembolism is controversial because no controlled studies have been done to indicate that one form of treatment is superior to another.[79] Heparin is administered acutely to prevent further thrombosis and to allow the body to decrease the size of the thromboembolus. It has no effect on an established thrombus. The initial dosage of heparin is 100 to 200 USP units/kg intravenously, followed by a dosage of 150 to 200 USP units/kg subcutaneously repeated every 8 hours and adjusted to maintain a prolonged activated clotting time of 1 to 1.5 times the baseline time. The use of acepromazine maleate (PromAce, 0.1–0.3 mg/kg subcutaneously, t.i.d.) or hydralazine (0.5–0.8 mg/kg by mouth, b.i.d.) has tentatively been advocated to improve collateral circulation, but their efficacy has not been established.[20] Propranolol should be avoided in cases of acute thromboembolism because of its tendency to cause vasoconstriction.[20]

Warfarin sodium (Coumadin, 0.5–1.0 mg total dose, s.i.d. or adjusted to maintain the prothrombin time at 15–20 seconds) has also been recommended.[20, 79a] However, warfarin has been shown to cause a hypercoagulable state for the first 3 to 4 days of administration, and it should be accompanied by heparin during that time.[79, 79a] Aspirin has been one of the mainstays of prevention of thromboembolism because it has been shown to decrease platelet aggregation and improve collateral blood flow in cats.[80–82] The recommended dosage is 25 mg/kg or one quarter of a 324-mg tablet every 2 or 3 days.[2, 3, 21] No studies have been conducted to ascertain the effectiveness of either aspirin[79] or warfarin in cats with thromboembolism compared with control cats. It is known that cats treated with aspirin or warfarin can have recurrences of thromboembolism.[2, 79, 79a]

Some cats with posterior paresis from thromboembolism regain full function of their hind limbs, but others continue to have loss of use of the distal portions of their limbs. These cats walk on the dorsum of their hind paws and must be bandaged to prevent abrasions. In addition, some cats have such severe thromboembolism that a limb or part must be amputated.[2, 3] This is usually a poor prognostic sign.

Prognosis

Prognosis for cats with aortic thromboembolism is poor. Even if the acute episode resolves and the cat is placed on long-term antiplatelet therapy, the recurrence rate is high.[2, 3, 83] If thrombi embolize to the kidneys, lungs, mesenteric artery, or more than three limbs, euthanasia should be recommended.

Hyperthyroidism in Cats

Hyperthyroidism is a relatively common disease of older cats that results from overproduction of thyroid hormone by benign tumors of the thyroid gland. It is usually seen in cats that are 12 years of age or older, although cats afflicted with the disease may be as young as 7 years of age. There is no age or sex predilection.[35–37, 41, 84, 85]

Pathophysiology

There are three major mechanisms of thyrotoxicosis. First, thyroid hormones act directly at the cellular level; second, they interact with the sympathetic nervous system; and third, they cause alterations in peripheral circulation and energy metabolism. At the cellular level, thyroid hormone stimulates hypertrophy of myocardial cells. Thyroid hormone also causes a hyperadrenergic state that increases heart rate, blood pressure, and contractility. Blood pressure may be only mildly elevated because of the third area of influence, energy metabolism. Hyperthyroidism causes increased tissue metabolism, which leads to vasodilation, increased blood volume, and augmented cardiac output. Heart failure secondary to hyperthyroidism is therefore known as high-output heart failure.[86, 87]

Clinical Signs

Cats are commonly brought in for weight loss in spite of a voracious appetite or for chronic vomiting or diarrhea, or a diagnosis is made when a routine serum T_4 concentration test is performed on an older cat with other disease. The typical cat is thin and hyperactive, with a heart murmur, tachycardia, and an increased left ventricular apex beat.[35–37, 41, 46, 85] Because veterinarians are more aware of hyperthyroidism in older cats than they were when the disease was first recognized, diagnosis is usually made before the disease has progressed to the point that cats become emaciated.[85] Other signs include bulky stools, polydipsia and polyuria, gallop rhythms, arrhythmias, and a thyroid nodule on cervical palpation.[35–37, 41, 46]

Hyperthyroidism can cause heart disease similar to hypertrophic cardiomyopathy,[38, 46] or it can exacerbate underlying cardiac abnormalities. Although hyperthyroidism may be associated with any ECG abnormalities, the most common findings are a tall R wave on lead II and sinus tachycardia.[42, 85] Other frequent ECG changes include atrial and ventricular arrhythmias and prolonged QRS duration.[42] Radiographically, an enlarged left ventricle and various degrees of pleural effusion or pulmonary edema may be present.[46] Liver enzyme levels are often high in cats with hyperthyroidism.[35, 37, 41, 85]

Cats with hyperthyroidism resemble cats with hypertrophic cardiomyopathy on echocardiography (i.e., they have a thick left ventricular free wall and septum and a dilated left atrium), except that the left ventricle is also mildly dilated. Shortening fraction, a measure of contractility, is high more often in cats with hyperthyroidism than in cats with hypertrophic cardiomyopathy.[34, 40] Blood pressure should be measured if possible, because hyperthyroidism in cats is known to cause hypertension.[47, 48]

Diagnostic Plan

Hyperthyroidism is suspected on the basis of the clinical signs listed. Definitive diagnosis is made on the basis of high resting serum T_4 concentrations. If hyperthyroidism is suspected but the T_4 is normal, other tests are necessary to confirm the diagnosis (see Chap. 47).[85]

Treatment

There are three possible treatment regimens for hyperthyroidism. Two, radioactive iodine (^{131}I) therapy and surgery,[88] are curative. The third, administration of an antithyroid drug,[41, 89, 90] only controls the disease, but this regimen is frequently chosen because treatment with ^{131}I and surgical thyroidectomy have special considerations that preclude their routine use[91] (see Chap. 47). Ancillary therapy includes a β-adrenergic blocking drug such as atenolol or propranolol to control the cardiovascular effects of hyperthyroidism. These drugs may not be necessary after the hyperthyroid state has been brought under control.

Prognosis

Prognosis is good with medical treatment, providing there are no adverse reactions to medications.[37, 46] Prognosis is also good with ^{131}I treatment and with surgery.

Hypertensive Heart Disease in Dogs and Cats

Systemic hypertension is an elevation of systolic and diastolic blood pressure above the normal range. It can be divided into essential (primary) hypertension and secondary hypertension (Table 12–2). The prevalence in all dogs is reported to be less than 1% or 2%; however, the reported prevalence in dogs with renal disease ranges from 50% to 93%.[92] Sixty-one percent of cats with chronic renal failure and 87% of hyperthyroid cats in one study were found to have high systolic or high diastolic blood pressure, or both.[47] Therefore, it is recommended that all cats with renal azotemia or high

Table 12–2
Causes of Hypertension in Dogs and Cats

Primary Hypertension

Secondary Hypertension
Renal*
Endocrine
    Pheochromocytoma
    Steroid excess (Cushing disease)*
    Acromegaly
    Hypothyroidism
    Thyrotoxicosis*
    Hyperparathyroidism
Neurogenic

*Common causes.
From Ross LA. Hypertension: Pathophysiology and management. Proc Am Anim Hosp Assoc 1987;54:350–353.

serum T_4 concentrations have their blood pressure measured.[93] In addition, cats with hypertrophic cardiomyopathy should be evaluated for hypertension, because hypertension can cause left ventricular hypertrophy.[94]

Because hypertension in cats is usually caused by chronic renal disease or hyperthyroidism, most cats with this condition are middle-aged or older (mean age, 13.8 years).[47] Dogs may be any age, consistent with the broader range of causes.[95, 96]

Pathophysiology

Arterial blood pressure is regulated by physical and physiologic means. The physical means are the total blood volume and the elasticity of the arterial wall. Physiologically, blood pressure is controlled by neural reflexes, primarily baroreceptors and the renin-angiotensin-aldosterone system. Baroreceptors, are located in the carotid sinus and aortic arch and are sensitive to changes in arterial blood pressure. If there is a drop in pressure, baroreceptors send a message to the vasomotor center in the brain to stimulate the sympathetic nervous system, which causes vasoconstriction and increased cardiac activity. Heightened blood pressure decreases sympathetic stimulation to restore pressure to normal.[96]

The renin-angiotensin-aldosterone system is the most important mechanism for regulating arterial blood pressure. Renin stored in the juxtaglomerular apparatus of the kidney is released in response to decreased pressure to the afferent glomerular artery or decreased sodium or chloride at the macula densa. Renin cleaves angiotensinogen to angiotensin I, which is converted to angiotensin II in the lung by ACE. Angiotensin II not only acts as a powerful vasoconstrictor, but stimulates aldosterone release from the adrenal cortex, which in turn facilitates retention of sodium and water by the kidney.[92, 96]

Consequences of systemic hypertension include left ventricular hypertrophy; retinal hemorrhage, exudates, and detachment leading to blindness; glomerulosclerosis and glomerular proliferation causing renal failure; and neurologic problems such as seizures, cerebrovascular accidents, and dementia.[92, 96]

Clinical Signs

Many dogs and cats show no signs of hypertension until they become acutely blind and are found to have retinal edema and detachment, retinal hemorrhage, and anterior chamber hemorrhage on ophthalmologic examination[97] (see Chap. 19). However, blood pressure should be measured in animals with those diseases that cause secondary hypertension, especially if retinal changes or left ventricular hypertrophy are discovered. An increasing number of cats with incidental hypertension are being discovered as more veterinarians refer patients with azotemia or hyperthyroidism for blood pressure evaluation.[93]

Diagnostic Plan

The diagnosis is made on the basis of direct or indirect measurement of systolic and diastolic blood pressure. Direct blood pressure measurement is not practical for practitioners.[96, 98] Indirect blood pressure is usually measured by the Doppler ultrasonic[47, 48, 93, 96, 99] or oscillometric techniques.[96] The oscillometric method depends on a cuff that blocks pulse pressure oscillations when inflated to suprasystemic pressures. Although the technique requires some practice, it is an attainable skill for most veterinarians, and equipment to measure blood pressure is becoming more available.

An occlusive cuff with an attached pressure gauge is placed around the distal hind limb or tail base. The width of the cuff should be 40% of the limb or tail circumference.[100] If a pulse is palpated, the sensing portion of the cuff is placed over the pulse. If not, the sensor is placed craniolaterally over the hock or just dorsal to the hock. Several measurements may have to be taken to obtain optimum readings. A pediatric or neonatal cuff is used for most dogs and cats. As pressure in the cuff is lowered, oscillations return. Systolic blood pressure is signaled at the point at which oscillations begin to increase in amplitude. Diastolic blood pressure is reached when the oscillations begin to decrease in amplitude.[101] A dinamap is an oscillometric blood pressure monitor widely used in veterinary medicine. Doppler measurements may also be made, but blood pressure machines that use Doppler are not widely available.

Serum biochemical analyses, measurement of serum T_4 concentration, echocardiography, and urinalysis should be performed on hypertensive animals. If a specific disease such as hyperadrenocorticism is suspected on the basis of clinical signs, biochemical abnormalities, or echocardiography, follow-up diagnostic tests should be performed.

Treatment

The goal of treatment is to lower systolic and diastolic blood pressure to normal. There is some disagreement as to what constitutes normal. Published normal values for dogs are 180/100 by two authors[95, 98] and 160/90 by another.[99] Normal values for cats are given as 141 to 160 systolic, and 100 to 108 diastolic.[48, 93] Although it is not clear how well hypertensive dogs respond to treatment, in my experience azotemic hypertensive cats respond poorly to medication, even to combinations. The hypertensive state in hyperthyroid cats often resolves along with a positive response to treatment for hyperthyroidism.[47]

Until the introduction of amlodipine (Norvasc–see later), a long-acting calcium channel blocker, single medications were unsuccessful, and combination drugs had to be tried. A low-salt diet may be implemented as first-line treatment.[92, 98] Feline or canine k/d or h/d (Prescription Diet) is a good diet. The owner may also cook a diet for the pet. The diet should be altered slowly over a period of 2 to 4 weeks in animals with renal failure because of the large amount of sodium that is excreted in the urine. Too-rapid introduction of a sodium-restricted diet may cause sodium and water depletion.[92, 95, 96]

Diuretics may be added to the regimen if dietary manipulations fail.[98] Diuretics must be used with caution, if at all, in animals whose hypertension is caused by renal disease. These animals are already volume-contracted, and further diuresis may exacerbate renal failure or hasten the change from compensated to decompensated renal failure.[92, 93, 96] Therefore, the use of diuretics in cats is not recommended, but they have been used in dogs with kidney disease with some success.[95, 98] A weak diuretic such as hydrochlorothiazide (HydroDIURIL, 2–4 mg/kg every 12 to 24 hours) should be attempted first. Dogs are treated for 2 to 4 weeks, after which the blood pressure is reassessed. Dogs with creatinine concentration higher than 4 mg/dL may not respond to thiazides. A loop diuretic such as furosemide (2–4 mg/kg, s.i.d. or b.i.d.) has been recommended, but complications such as hypokalemia and dehydration are common and are more likely to occur in the presence of strict dietary sodium restriction.[95] Even though diuretics have represented a first-line defense against hypertension, it is becoming more acceptable to initiate treatment with other drugs such as ACE inhibitors and calcium antagonists.[92, 102]

β-Adrenergic blockers are used in both dogs and cats with hypertension. The mechanism by which they lower blood pressure is complex and not completely understood. Proposed mechanisms include lowering of cardiac output, suppression of renin secretion, interference with sympathetic outflow, and blocking of presynaptic neurotransmitter release.[92, 95, 96] Propranolol (Inderal) is one of the most commonly used β-blockers. It is administered to dogs at a dosage of 5 to 20 mg every 8 to 12 hours in proportion to the patient's size, but the dosage may be titrated according to heart rate and blood pressure. The dosage in cats is 2.5 to 10 mg every 8 to 12 hours.[67] Atenolol, a $β_1$-selective β-blocker, can be substituted for propranolol.[93] The dosage in dogs is 0.25 to 1.0 mg/kg by mouth, s.i.d. or b.i.d., and in cats it is 6.25 to 12.5 mg by mouth, s.i.d.

or b.i.d. Side effects include weakness or diarrhea, bradycardia, and congestive heart failure. Propranolol may also cause bronchospasm in patients with pre-existing pulmonary disease.[67, 95]

Vasodilators, especially ACE inhibitors, are becoming more popular as treatment for hypertension.[98] They are often used in combination with diuretics or β-blockers. Captopril (Capoten, 0.5–2 mg/kg every 8–12 hours in dogs) was one of the first used, but it had many side effects (i.e., anorexia, vomiting, diarrhea, and azotemia).[103] Most veterinarians now prescribe enalapril, a longer-acting ACE inhibitor, in both dogs and cats. It seems to cause fewer side effects than captopril, although it can cause weakness, anorexia, and azotemia. Although there may be some concern about using enalapril in cats, the concern appears to be unwarranted, because actual worsening of renal failure in cats being given ACE inhibitors is very low. The dosage in dogs is 0.5 mg/kg by mouth, s.i.d. or b.i.d., and in cats it is 0.25 to 0.5 mg/kg by mouth, s.i.d. or b.i.d.[92, 103]

Calcium channel blockers may also be administered to animals with hypertension.[17] Diltiazem is the most common calcium channel blocker used (7.5–15 mg/kg, b.i.d. or t.i.d., in cats; 0.5–1.5 mg/kg, t.i.d., in dogs), although amlodipine (Norvasc, 0.625 mg, s.i.d.), a long-acting calcium channel blocker, has been used with some success in cats.[104] Although relatively new, amlodipine currently seems the most promising monotherapy to treat hypertension. If that fails, good results seem to be achieved by combining a calcium channel blocker with either a β-blocker or an ACE inhibitor in cats with chronic renal disease. In my experience, these patients are the most difficult to manage because they are often refractory to treatment.

Combinations of two and sometimes three drugs may be required to lower blood pressure to acceptable values,[98] and even this may not be completely successful. One study reported that combinations that included either a β-blocker or an ACE inhibitor were most helpful.[93] Animals treated for hypertension should be monitored every 2 weeks for azotemia and changes in blood pressure during the period of therapeutic trial and adjustment. After that, stable animals should be rechecked every 1 to 2 months.

Prognosis

Prognosis is variable, depending on the cause and severity of the disease causing the hypertension. One recent study concluded that control of hypertension in cats did not necessarily improve survival.[93] More research needs to elucidate the benefits of treatment in dogs and cats.

Cardiomyopathy in Dogs

Cardiomyopathy in dogs, like that in cats, may be classified as primary or secondary, although most dogs have primary disease. The term "dilated" cardiomyopathy is preferred to the earlier term, "congestive" cardiomyopathy, because dilation often precedes heart failure and is more descriptive of the actual condition of the myocardium: a dilated, poorly contracting ventricle that eventually causes congestive heart failure.[8]

Approximately 1% of all dogs are affected by cardiomyopathy,[105] and the disease is divided into specific types on the basis of breed. Dilated cardiomyopathy occurs in giant breeds of dog (e.g., German shepherd, Great Dane, Saint Bernard, and Irish wolfhound) and Doberman pinschers.[32] Dogs affected are primarily male and young to middle-aged (mean age, 6 years).[6, 106] Doberman pinschers acquire a particularly virulent form of dilated cardiomyopathy and have a higher mortality rate than other breeds. In boxers with cardiomyopathy the heart may not be dilated, but congestive heart failure and syncope induced by ventricular arrhythmias are typical. Cardiomyopathy in English and American cocker spaniels causes heart failure and arrhythmias. Although they are seemingly different, the common denominator in all types of cardiomyopathy is a heart muscle disorder that does not arise secondary to abnormalities of other cardiac structures such as valves or vessels.[106] This disorder eventually leads to congestive heart failure and death. Table 12–3 lists distinctive features of cardiomyopathy according to breed. Giant breeds represent the prototype and therefore are not included.

Pathophysiology

The hallmark of dilated cardiomyopathy is ventricular dilation with poor contractility and congestive heart failure[8]; this is systolic failure, not the diastolic failure seen in animals with hypertrophic or restrictive cardiomyopathy. The typical heart in animals with dilated cardiomyopathy is severely dilated in all four chambers, but the ventricles are more severely affected than the atria, and there is inadequate hypertrophy to compensate for the dilation.

Decreased systolic function leads to high ventricular filling pressures and congestion of both pulmonary and systemic veins. Poor contractility also causes low cardiac output and decreased perfusion of kidneys and body tissues (low-output heart failure). Signs arise from inability to oxygenate blood as well as inability to deliver oxygen to tissues (left-sided heart failure). Right-sided heart failure causes weight loss and retention of fluid in body cavities and tissues. Dilation causes a transformation from an elliptic shape of the left ventricle to one that is more globoid and less

Table 12–3
Distinctive Features of Cardiomyopathy in Dogs

Doberman Pinschers

Short survival time[11, 111]
Acute left-sided heart failure[12, 111]
Weight loss and syncope[6, 12, 111]
Radiographic changes
   Less cardiomegaly[6, 12, 13]
   Left atrial enlargement[5, 11]
   Diffuse pulmonary edema[11, 12]
Nodular degeneration of the mitral valve with regurgitation[6]
Ventricular arrhythmias common[6, 11, 12]
Ventricular arrhythmias an early sign[10]
Increased sensitivity to digoxin[11–13, 111]
Weight loss an early sign[111]
Atrial fibrillation poor prognostic sign[11]
Right side of heart not affected[6]
Sudden death from arrhythmias[6, 11, 12]
Rapid deterioration[12]
L-Carnitine deficiency[110]

Boxers

Ventricular arrhythmias only sign[6, 11, 27]
Syncope[6, 27]
Radiographic changes
   Normal left ventricle[6, 11]
   Left atrial dilation[6]
Myxomatous mitral valve[6]
Right side of heart not affected[6]
Sudden death from arrhythmias[6, 11]
Worst prognosis with combined heart failure and arrhythmias[11]
L-Carnitine deficiency[12, 109]

English Cocker Spaniels

Tall R and deep Q on lead II[28–30]
Dyspnea, cardiomegaly, pulmonary edema common[30]
Absence of murmur[30]

efficient. It also produces dilation of the mitral valve annulus and distortion of the geometry of the papillary muscles, both of which can aggravate or cause mitral regurgitation.[107]

Continued stretching of the left ventricle leads to arrhythmias and ventricular remodeling (i.e., changing from normal myocardium to scar tissue). Loss of myocardium through remodeling decreases systolic function even further, and cardiac performance rapidly declines to inevitable death. The cause of the original insult to the myocardium is unknown,[6, 8] so there is no known method of prevention. Most treatments help to resolve signs but do not reverse the process.

The neurohumoral system plays an important role in propagating and exacerbating dilated cardiomyopathy, especially the sympathetic nervous system and the renin-angiotensin-aldosterone system.[108] Concentrations of circulating catecholamines are high and lead to resting tachycardia and vasoconstriction. In addition, β-adrenergic receptors in the myocardium are reduced in number (downregulated), which has led to speculation that high concentrations of catecholamines are toxic or damaging to the heart muscle. Stimulation of the renin-angiotensin system increases angiotensin II, which in turn causes vasoconstriction and retention of sodium and water.

The cause of cardiomyopathy in dogs is unknown, but low myocardial concentrations of L-carnitine have been found by some investigators.[109, 110] It is likely that there are many different causes and that dilated cardiomyopathy represents an end stage of several types of myocardial injury.[11–13]

Clinical Signs

General statements about cardiomyopathy apply to all types; additional findings are particular to certain breeds. Clinical signs often occur acutely and consist of dyspnea, cough, syncope, exercise intolerance, and abdominal distention. Chronic signs include anorexia, weight loss, and lethargy. On physical examination, dogs may display weakness, dyspnea, crackles or muffled heart and lung sounds, a murmur, weak pulses, tachycardia, irregular rhythm, pallor, slow capillary refill time, and an S_3 gallop.[11, 106]

The most common signs in Doberman pinschers are sudden onset of a cough and weight loss,[10, 111] although weakness and syncope are also common.[6] Ventricular arrhythmias auscultated on routine physical examination are an early sign of cardiomyopathy in Dobermans and boxers, and they are more common in those breeds of dogs than in giant breeds.[6, 10, 111]

Boxers have been reported to have three different categories of disease: ventricular arrhythmias without signs, ventricular arrhythmias causing syncope, and left-sided heart failure.[10, 111]

Diagnostic Plan

Diagnosis is made on the basis of breed predilection, clinical signs, ECG abnormalities, radiographic changes, and echocardiography.[106] ECG changes consistent with cardiomyopathy in dogs include tall and wide QRS complexes with slurring (left ventricular enlargement or left bundle branch block), atrial fibrillation, ventricular arrhythmias, and wide P waves (Fig. 12–10). Supraventricular tachycardia other than atrial fibrillation may also be present.[6, 11] Deep Q waves and tall R waves with S-T segment slurring and right axis

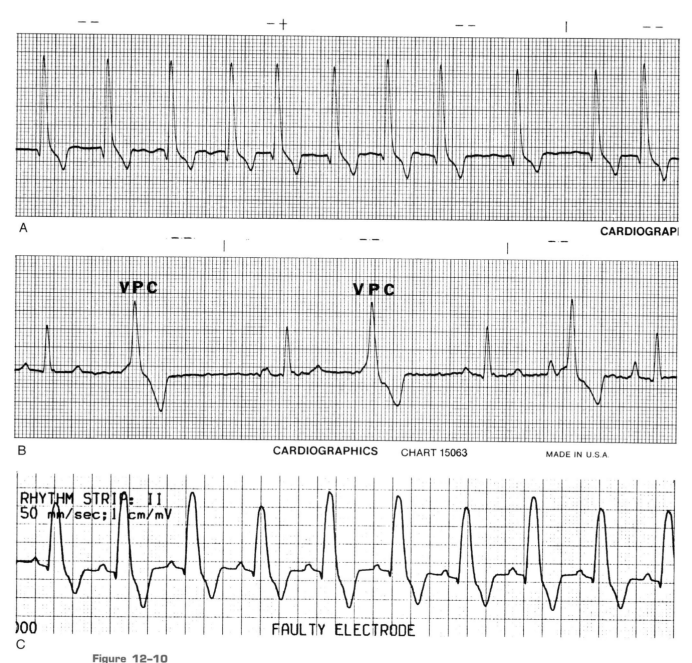

Figure 12–10

(A) Atrial fibrillation in a Great Dane with dilated cardiomyopathy. The rhythm is irregularly irregular, there is an absence of P waves, and there are fibrillation waves in the baseline. **(B)** Ventricular premature complexes (VPC) in a boxer with cardiomyopathy who was examined because of syncope. The complexes are early and differ in appearance from sinus beats. The QRS is positive in lead II, denoting a right ventricular origin. **(C)** Left bundle branch block pattern in a golden retriever with dilated cardiomyopathy. The axis is normal, but the QRS complex is more than 0.08 sec in width.

deviations are typical findings in English cocker spaniels.[28, 30] Ventricular arrhythmias (singles, pairs, runs, and ventricular tachycardia) are the most common findings in boxers[27] and may be the first sign of cardiomyopathy in Doberman pinschers.[10]

Radiography, in all breeds except Doberman pinschers, usually reveals cardiomegaly.[6, 10, 11, 106] Although left atrial enlargement is common in Dobermans, generalized cardiac enlargement is a less reliable finding.[10] Giant breeds of dogs may display various

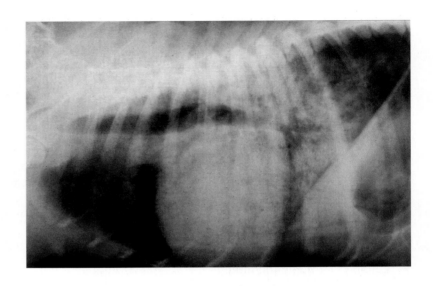

Figure 12–11
Lateral radiograph of a Doberman pinscher with dilated cardiomyopathy. Cardiomegaly and pulmonary edema are present.

degrees of right- and left-sided heart failure (i.e., pleural effusion and pulmonary edema), whereas Doberman pinschers usually have pulmonary edema, which may be severe and diffuse (Fig. 12–11).[6, 10, 11, 13] Radiographic changes in boxers are variable and nonspecific.[27, 106] English cocker spaniels display biventricular enlargement and pulmonary edema.[28, 30]

Echocardiographic findings of dilated cardiomyopathy are typical and diagnostic regardless of breed or even species. They include a severely dilated left ventricular cavity (Fig. 12–12) with very poor indices of contractility (e.g., shortening fraction <20%–25%).[6, 10, 11, 13, 32, 106] In addition, the right atrium and right ventricle are usually dilated, there is separation of E point to septum, and a decrease in septal and posterior wall thickening is present (Fig. 12–13). Myocardial function in English and American cocker spaniels is usually less depressed than in other breeds, although congestive heart failure frequently arises from progressive systolic dysfunction.[11] Boxers with ventricular arrhythmias may not develop myocardial failure.

Treatment

In addition to low-salt diets and exercise restriction, a large number of drugs are currently available to treat dogs with cardiomyopathy, including positive inotropic drugs, diuretics, vasodilators, and antiarrhythmic drugs. However, treatment is much more effective for relieving signs than for prolonging life.[63]

Positive Inotropic Drugs

Positive inotropic drugs should be prescribed to all dogs with dilated cardiomyopathy; they may be administered either intravenously or orally, depending on the severity of clinical signs.[63] The major drawback of intravenous administration is the need for constant-rate infusion of dobutamine. The dosage of dobutamine is 5 to 10 µg/kg per minute by constant-rate infusion for 48 to 72 hours. The infusion should be started at the low end of the dosage range and increased every 2 hours. If the heart rate increases by more than 20%, if tachyarrhythmias develop, or if the frequency of pre-existing arrhythmia increases, the dosage should be decreased.[12]

The digitalis glycosides remain the only positive inotropic drugs available for oral administration, and although there is controversy regarding their use in dogs with dilated cardiomyopathy, most cardiologists advocate their inclusion in the protocol.[6, 10–13, 63, 106, 112] Digitalis is given primarily to slow the heart rate in dogs with supraventricular tachyarrhythmias such as atrial fibrillation and to increase contractility in animals with myocardial failure.[113, 114] In addition, digoxin is known to restore baroreceptor tone, which is lost in humans with heart failure; this, in turn, allows high sympathetic tone to return to normal.[63, 107] Digoxin (Lanoxin) is the digitalis glycoside used most frequently in veterinary medicine. The dosage is lower per kilogram in large-breed dogs than in small-breed dogs. A good rule of thumb is that no dog should be prescribed more than 0.75 mg per day, divided b.i.d., and any dog weighing more than 20 kg should be given a dosage lower than the routine 0.01 to 0.02 mg/kg per day, divided b.i.d. In addition, Doberman pinschers are sensitive to digoxin and should not receive more than 0.375 mg/day, divided b.i.d. Most Doberman pinschers tolerate only 0.125 to 0.25 mg/day, divided b.i.d.[10–13, 112] Digoxin may also be administered intravenously at a dosage of 0.005 to 0.01 mg/kg every hour, for two to three doses or until the heart slows

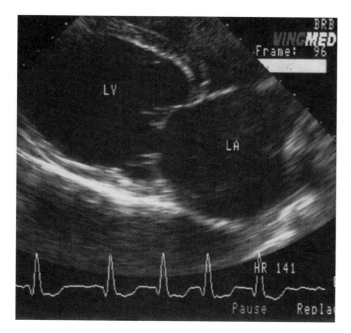

Figure 12–12
Two-dimensional echocardiogram of a Doberman pinscher with dilated cardiomyopathy. The left ventricle (LV) and left atrium (LA) are severely dilated.

or signs of toxicity (e.g., ventricular arrhythmias) appear.

Diuretics

Diuretics such as furosemide are one of the mainstays of treatment for congestive heart failure.[63, 107, 112] No other drugs are as efficient at removing excess fluid, but they are not without side effects. Dehydration, hypokalemia, and azotemia are potential adverse effects that should be anticipated and watched for with scheduled recheck examinations and follow-up blood tests. The most common diuretic is furosemide (Lasix, 1–4 mg/kg, b.i.d. or t.i.d., either by mouth, intramuscularly, or intravenously).[115] Furosemide should be administered intravenously to dogs in acute heart failure because of decreased absorption by the gastrointestinal tract.[63] Hydrochlorothiazide (HydroDIURIL, 2–4 mg/kg by mouth, b.i.d.) or spironolactone (Aldactone, 2–4 mg/kg per day, s.i.d. or b.i.d.) may be added to furosemide to enhance diuresis in dogs with refractory heart failure.[63] The risks of hypokalemia and dehydration greatly increase when furosemide and hydrochlorothiazide are used together,[115, 116] and the combination of an ACE inhibitor and spironolactone can cause potassium concentration to increase.[115, 117]

Vasodilators

Vasodilators are being administered with increasing frequency in humans and animals with dilated cardiomyopathy. Studies indicate that all animals with heart failure and left ventricular dysfunction should be treated with an ACE inhibitor, not only because of its vasodilating properties but also because of its ability to increase survival time in dogs and humans with severe congestive heart failure who are being given digitalis and diuretics.[63, 107, 118–120] There is also evidence that ACE inhibitors slow progression of left ventricular failure because they slow ventricular remodeling.[63, 107, 121] The ACE inhibitor that has been most extensively studied and therefore used most frequently in dogs is enalapril.[63, 119, 122] The recommended dosage is 0.5 mg/kg, s.i.d. or b.i.d., but some animals must be given a lower dosage because of side effects (primarily weakness and anorexia). Another long-acting ACE inhibitor, lisinopril (Zestril, 0.5 mg/kg by mouth, s.i.d.), is being used by some veterinarians because it seems to be as effective as enalapril but is less expensive.[63, 123]

The combination of hydralazine (0.5 mg/kg by mouth, b.i.d.) and isosorbide dinitrate (Isordil, 2.5–5 mg per dog by mouth, t.i.d) has also been shown to prolong life in humans with dilated cardiomyopathy and, in addition, to improve exercise tolerance.[8, 121, 124] These drugs may be added alone or together to the therapeutic regimen of dogs with refractory heart failure.[107] They are also useful in dogs that cannot tolerate any dosage of an ACE inhibitor.

Antiarrhythmic Drugs

Antiarrhythmic drugs may be needed to treat ventricular arrhythmias or to slow rapid atrial fibrillation. Boxers with syncope from ventricular arrhythmias require antiarrhythmic treatment, but attempting to suppress all ventricular arrhythmias in dogs with congestive heart failure and left ventricular dysfunction is not recommended. Although it may seem logical to attempt to eliminate ventricular arrhythmias, there is no evidence that decreasing ventricular arrhythmias prolongs life, and antiarrhythmic drugs may actually increase the severity of the arrhythmia (proarrhythmia) or exacerbate heart failure because of their negative inotropic effects.[8, 63, 107]

Boxers are the most likely breed to require intravenous administration of ventricular antiarrhythmic drugs because of syncope. Both lidocaine (Xylocaine, 50–80 μg/kg per minute) and procainamide (Pronestyl, 25–40 μg/kg per minute) may be effective in acutely suppressing ventricular arrhythmias, but lidocaine is preferable to procainamide because it causes less myocardial depression and has a shorter duration of action. Lidocaine is administered as an intravenous bolus of 2.2 mg/kg. The first may be followed by a second, similar intravenous bolus, and then the drug is administered slowly to effect or to a total dosage of 8.8 mg/kg. Toxic effects include central

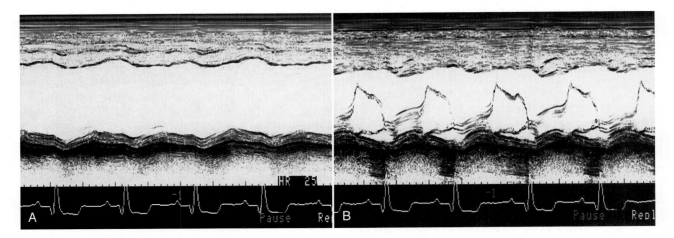

Figure 12-13
M-mode echocardiogram of a Great Dane with dilated cardiomyopathy. **(A)** The left ventricle is severely dilated, the walls are thin for the size of the heart, and the contractility is severely decreased. **(B)** There is E point–to–septal separation of the anterior mitral valve leaflet from the septum (EPSS). IVS, interventricular septum; LV, left ventricular cavity; LVFW, left ventricular free wall; MV, mitral valve.

nervous system depression and seizures, both of which disappear after the dosage of antiarrhythmic drug is lowered. Muscular twitching is a sign of an impending seizure, which can be averted by discontinuing the lidocaine. Seizures are easily controlled with one intravenous dose (2.5–5 mg) of diazepam (Valium).

After the arrhythmia is controlled, procainamide can be administered at a dosage of 8 to 20 mg/kg every 6 hours, intramuscularly.[27] Dogs controlled on this dosage for 24 hours may be switched to procainamide given orally (Procan SR, 20–50 mg/kg, t.i.d.). Refractory arrhythmias may require combinations such as procainamide given orally with a β-blocker such as propranolol (0.6–1.4 mg/kg, t.i.d.) or atenolol (0.25–1.0 mg/kg by mouth, s.i.d. or b.i.d.). Sotalol (Betapace, 40–80 mg per dose by mouth, b.i.d.), a class III antiarrhythmic drug with β-blocking properties, is being used as a monotherapy with success in boxers with symptomatic ventricular arrhythmias.

Atrial fibrillation at rates faster than 200 bpm should be treated because of the negative effect of tachycardia on cardiac output. Most dogs are already receiving digoxin, but digoxin alone is usually inadequate in slowing heart rate. Both β-blockers and calcium channel blockers are effective in slowing the ventricular response in dogs with atrial fibrillation because of their action on the A-V node.[63, 72] The most commonly used calcium channel blocker in veterinary medicine today is diltiazem (Cardizem); the recommended dosage is 0.5 to 1.5 mg/kg, t.i.d.[125] The β-adrenergic blockers propranolol (Inderal, up to 1.0 mg/kg by mouth, t.i.d.) and atenolol (Tenormin, 0.25–1.0 mg/kg by mouth, s.i.d. or b.i.d.) have also

been used.[67, 126] Calcium channel blockers and β-blockers should be started at the low end of the dosage range and carefully titrated until the heart rate falls below 170 bpm.[67]

Side effects of β-blockers and calcium channel blockers include weakness because of low blood pressure and gastrointestinal signs, especially with calcium channel blockers.[70] A more serious complication of the use of these drugs is exacerbation of heart failure because of their negative inotropic effects.[67, 71, 72, 127–129]

Despite their similarities, calcium channel blockers and β-blockers differ with regard to deleterious effects in animals with heart failure. Paradoxically, β-blockers have been advocated for people with dilated cardiomyopathy, and there has been evidence that their addition may improve survival.[63, 130] One of the major mechanisms for this effect is the lowering of sympathetic tone. Because catecholamines are toxic to the myocardium, decreasing their circulating concentrations is beneficial. β-blockers also indirectly decrease arterial and venous constriction, because there is less sympathetically induced elevation in plasma renin activity and angiotensin II. Myocardial β-adrenergic receptors that have been downregulated (i.e., decreased in number because of high resting sympathetic tone) may be increased by treatment with β-blockers, providing a method for the heart to be stimulated if necessary.[106, 130]

Calcium channel blockers, on the other hand, exacerbate heart failure with no benefit other than slowing heart rate. The sympathetic nervous system may even be stimulated by calcium channel blockers because they lower blood pressure and stimulate baroreceptors. One of the advantages of diltiazem over other calcium channel blockers is that it is one of the least potent negative inotropic drugs.[131]

L-Carnitine

L-Carnitine is a naturally occurring constituent of the body that is synthesized from lysine and methionine. Adequate myocardial concentrations are critical for myocardial fatty acid metabolism, and long-chain fatty acids are the most important energy-producing substrate of the myocardium. The current recommended dosage for Doberman pinschers, boxers, and giant breeds is 50 to 100 mg/kg administered with food, t.i.d.[106] The benefit for all dogs is uncertain, but it has been shown to benefit some Doberman pinschers and boxers. Positive clinical response (decreased lethargy and increased appetite) is seen by owners within 1 to 4 weeks after supplementation begins. Echocardiographic improvement in indices of contractility (i.e., shortening fraction) are seen after 2 to 3 months of supplementation, and a plateau is reached after 6 to 8 months of therapy. Dogs appear clinically well during this time but still have a markedly decreased shortening fraction.[63, 111]

Recent reports indicate that American cocker spaniels with dilated cardiomyopathy respond well to a combination of L-carnitine (50 mg/kg, t.i.d.) and taurine (250 mg by mouth, b.i.d.).[106] Most dogs that responded to this regimen had low plasma taurine levels but normal concentrations of L-carnitine.[132] However, biopsy samples of myocardium are the only way that L-carnitine can currently be accurately measured.[111] After 2 months of treatment, the end-diastolic diameter and shortening fraction had improved in most dogs, so that all drugs except taurine and L-carnitine were discontinued.[132]

In summary, diuretics decrease ventricular filling pressures through fluid removal. Positive inotropic drugs improve cardiac output and tissue perfusion. Vasodilators such as the ACE inhibitors and combinations of hydralazine and isosorbide dinitrate have been shown to improve exercise tolerance, relieve signs of heart failure, and improve survival in humans and dogs with dilated cardiomyopathy. ACE inhibitors have also been effective in slowing progression of ventricular remodeling.[107] Calcium channel blockers and β-blockers slow ventricular response in animals with atrial fibrillation, and β-adrenergic blocking agents may also reduce myocardial damage from circulating catecholamines and increase the number of β-receptors in the myocardium.[107] Ventricular antiarrhythmic drugs should be avoided except in dogs with symptomatic ventricular tachycardia because of their negative inotropic and proarrhythmic effects.

Prognosis

Prognosis in dogs with cardiomyopathy is extremely guarded, with a lifespan of 2 to 24 months after diagnosis. Survival time for Doberman pinschers with dilated cardiomyopathy averages 6 months. It is currently unknown whether ACE inhibitors or L-carnitine significantly improve long-term survival. Boxers have a fair prognosis unless congestive heart failure is a part of their cardiomyopathy.

Uncommon Disorders

Dilated Cardiomyopathy in Cats

Dilated cardiomyopathy used to be the scourge of heart disease in cats. Cats would appear to be perfectly healthy until they suddenly collapsed from cardiogenic shock, developed heart failure (usually manifested as pleural effusion), and died within days of the onset of clinical signs. However, since the discovery that taurine deficiency is a major cause of dilated cardiomyopathy,[133] the verification by follow-up studies,[134, 135] and the resolution of most cases of dilated cardiomyopathy by taurine supplementation,[136] dilated cardiomyopathy in cats has become an uncommon disorder. However, idiopathic myocardial failure (i.e., shortening fraction <26%) is still seen in 2.5% to 6% of cardiomyopathic cats that have echocardiograms performed for suspected heart disease.[4]

The disease is characterized by systolic dysfunction that involves both the left and right ventricles and causes severe dilation of all four cardiac chambers and poor contractility of the ventricles. Even though most pet food companies currently supplement cat foods with adequate concentrations of taurine to prevent dilated cardiomyopathy, some cats fed uncommon brands may develop this devastating disease. In addition to poor diet, some cats are thought to have a genetic tendency to develop dilated cardiomyopathy.[137] Cats with dilated cardiomyopathy may be any age, breed, or sex.

Pathophysiology

See the section on dilated cardiomyopathy in dogs for the pathophysiology.

Clinical Signs

Cats with dilated cardiomyopathy are usually examined because of acute onset of weakness, anorexia, vomiting, or lethargy. Signs are characteristic of low-output heart failure: hypothermia, dehydration, pallor, slow capillary refill time, and weak pulses. A gallop rhythm is auscultated more often than a murmur, and the intensity of heart sounds is usually decreased because of decreased contractility or pleural effusion, or both.

Diagnostic Plan

Although a presumptive diagnosis can be made on the basis of history, physical examination, and radiographic and ECG abnormalities, echocardiography is required for definitive diagnosis. Echocardiographic abnormalities include a dilated left ventricle with separation of E point to septum and severely depressed shortening fraction.[138] Cats with nontaurine myocardial failure may have only mild left ventricular dilation with segmental thinning or hypertrophy of the left ventricular free wall and septum.[4]

ECG abnormalities include arrhythmias and tall QRS complexes in lead II. Radiographic changes include generalized cardiomegaly, a rounded left ventricular apex, and various amounts of pleural effusion or pulmonary edema. Pleural effusion is more common than pulmonary edema (see Fig. 12–9). Mild prerenal azotemia is frequently present.[2]

Treatment

Cats with dilated cardiomyopathy should be treated like cats with intergrade cardiomyopathy and myocardial failure.

The most revolutionary treatment for dilated cardiomyopathy in cats is taurine, a sulfur-containing amino acid that is highly concentrated in the heart, retinas, central nervous system, skeletal muscle, and white blood cells and platelets. It is the most abundant free amino acid in the myocardium and retina.[134]

Early work with taurine demonstrated that it is essential for normal retinal function, but its importance for normal myocardial function was only recently recognized,[133–136] after cats fed low-taurine diets developed dilated cardiomyopathy as demonstrated by echocardiography (i.e., end-systolic diameter >12 mm and shortening fraction <35%).[133] Taurine supplementation produced echocardiographic improvement in 2 to 4 weeks and clinical improvement within 2 weeks, but it took at least 6 to 8 weeks for hearts to normalize.[133, 136]

Taurine in one study was administered at a dosage of 500 to 1000 mg, divided b.i.d., and cats that lived longer than 30 days remained clinically stable despite discontinuation of all drugs except taurine.[136] The current recommended dosage is 250 mg, s.i.d. or b.i.d.

Prognosis

Prognosis for cats with dilated cardiomyopathy is extremely poor. Cats with the comparatively mild form of taurine-deficient dilated cardiomyopathy should respond favorably to supplementation within 2 to 4 weeks. The most difficult aspect is helping cats survive long enough for taurine supplementation to reverse the dilated cardiomyopathy. If dilated cardiomyopathy is caused by taurine deficiency and the cat lives through the period of conventional treatment, prognosis is good and all cardiac drugs can be discontinued. Cats with nontaurine-related dilated cardiomyopathy usually survive only 2 to 3 weeks after diagnosis.

Canine Hypertrophic Cardiomyopathy

Unlike feline hypertrophic cardiomyopathy, hypertrophic cardiomyopathy in dogs is rare.[51, 52, 59, 60] The age range of affected dogs is 1 to 13 years, and males and German shepherds are overrepresented. Many are diagnosed on necropsy after sudden death.[51, 59, 60] The pathophysiology is the same as for feline hypertrophic cardiomyopathy.

If present, clinical signs of heart disease include pulmonary edema or syncope. Conduction disturbances[51, 59, 60] and evidence of left ventricular enlargement (tall QRS complexes on lead II) may be found on ECGs. Thoracic radiographs reveal cardiomegaly, pulmonary edema, pleural effusion, or ascites.[51, 59, 60]

The best tool to diagnose canine hypertrophic cardiomyopathy is echocardiography. Typical findings include left ventricular hypertrophy and left atrial dilation. Systolic anterior motion of the mitral valve and midsystolic closure of the aortic valve may be present in dogs with left ventricular outflow tract obstruction.

Treatment is directed toward removing fluid with diuretics and either increasing left ventricular filling with β-blockers (atenolol, 0.25–1.0 mg/kg by mouth, s.i.d. or b.i.d.) or using calcium channel blockers (diltiazem, 0.5–1.5 mg/kg, t.i.d.) to enhance left ventricular relaxation and filling. Dogs with third-degree A-V nodal blocks require a pacemaker, but owners should be aware of the risk of anesthetic death.[59] Prognosis seems to be guarded in dogs with untreated hypertrophic cardiomyopathy, although treatment studies are lacking. However, the prognosis is probably variable in dogs without heart block, with dogs with severe hypertrophy or arrhythmias having the worst prognosis.

Myocarditis

Bacterial, viral, fungal, and rickettsial causes of myocarditis are rare in dogs and cats.[3] A few years ago, parvovirus myocarditis caused acute death in puppies 4 to 6 weeks of age, but this is rare now, owing to widespread vaccination for parvovirus.[139–141] Trypanosomiasis (Chagas disease), caused by the protozoan *Trypanosoma cruzi*, is a common disorder in

Central and South America[6] and has been described in dogs in the southeastern United States.[142] Lyme myocarditis is caused by the spirochete *Borrelia burgdorferi*, which is vectored by the ticks *Ixodes dammini* and *Ixodes pacificus*.

Sudden death is often the first sign that myocarditis is present, especially in puppies with parvovirus.[139] Arrhythmias (i.e., ventricular extrasystoles) and congestive heart failure (i.e., pulmonary edema, ascites, and pleural effusion) are also signs of myocarditis.[142] Lyme disease has caused second- and third-degree A-V block in dogs.[143]

Final diagnosis of myocarditis is most often made on necropsy by examination of heart muscle. Lyme disease is usually diagnosed before necropsy examination because titers are readily available. Trypanosomiasis must be diagnosed on necropsy examination or myocardial biopsy.[142] Diagnosis is often made on the basis of clinical signs and associated abnormalities, such as arthropathy in dogs with Lyme disease. Myocarditis can cause acute dilated cardiomyopathy because of infiltration of the myocardium by the infectious agent, which causes active inflammation and necrosis of myocardial cells. If the A-V node is affected, conduction disturbances leading to heart block may occur. Irritative lesions may develop and cause ventricular extrasystoles.

Success of treatment depends on the cause of the myocarditis and the availability of drugs effective against the offending organism. Treatment is often ineffective in dogs with parvovirus and trypanosomiasis because of the rapid onset of clinical signs and death. Dogs and cats should also be treated for any signs of heart failure with diuretics, vasodilators, positive inotropic drugs, and antiarrhythmic drugs if needed. Dogs with Lyme disease are treated with tetracyclines. Prognosis is extremely guarded: most dogs die within hours to weeks after diagnosis.[139–142]

Doxorubicin Toxicity

Doxorubicin (Adriamycin) is an anthracycline antibiotic that is widely used in veterinary medicine as an antineoplastic agent. Its use is limited, however, because of cardiotoxicity. Cardiomyopathy caused by doxorubicin is dose-dependent and can occur immediately or develop several years after treatment has ended. ECG abnormalities in dogs are detectable in approximately 1 to 287 days after treatment, but development of congestive heart failure may take longer (42 to 287 days).[144]

In one study, the most common ECG abnormalities included ventricular arrhythmias and changes in R wave amplitude. Clinical signs were not always evident in dogs with arrhythmias, but dogs that eventually developed heart failure and died continued to receive doxorubicin after the appearance of ECG abnormalities. Echocardiograms performed in dogs with heart failure revealed left ventricular dilation and a greatly reduced fractional shortening.[144] It is recommended that doxorubicin be discontinued if the ejection fraction is less than 50%, if the left ventricular shortening fraction is less than 27%, or if there is a new onset of frequent or multiform ventricular premature complexes.[145] No therapy is recommended at this point unless signs of congestive heart failure (i.e., cough, dyspnea, exercise intolerance, ascites) are present.

Doxorubicin causes myocardiocytolysis, degeneration, and myocardial fibrillar vacuolation with fibrosis, which produces a condition similar to dilated cardiomyopathy in clinical appearance, signs, and outcome.[144, 145] Treatment is the same as for canine dilated cardiomyopathy (see earlier discussion). Prognosis is extremely guarded. Dogs may survive up to 90 days with treatment, but most die within 24 hours.[144]

References

1. Bond BR, Fox PR. Advances in feline cardiomyopathy. Vet Clin North Am Small Anim Pract 1984;14:1021–1038.
2. Fox PR. Feline myocardial disease. In: Fox PR, ed. Canine and Feline Cardiology. New York, Churchill Livingstone, 1988:435–466.
3. Fox PR. Feline myocardial diseases. In: Kirk RW, ed. Current Veterinary Therapy VIII. Philadelphia, WB Saunders, 1983:337–348.
4. Fox PR. Feline myocardial diseases. Waltham/OSU Symposium for the Treatment of Small Animal Diseases. Vernon, California, Waltham USA, Inc, 1994: 119–128.
5. Liu S-K, Tilley LP. Animal models of primary myocardial disease. Yale J Biol Med 1980;53:191–211.
6. Thomas WP. Myocardial diseases of the dog. In: Bonagura JD, ed. Contemporary Issues in Small Animal Practice: Cardiology. New York, Churchill Livingstone, 1987;7:117–155.
7. Tilley LP, Liu S-K, Gilbertson SR, et al. Primary myocardial disease in the cat: A model for human cardiomyopathy. Am J Pathol 1977;87:493–514.
8. Wynne J, Braunwald E. The cardiomyopathies and myocarditides: Toxic, chemical, and physical damage to the heart. In: Braunwald E, ed. Heart Disease, 4th ed. Philadelphia, WB Saunders, 1992:1394–1450.
9. Liu S-K, Fox PR, Tilley LP. Excessive moderator bands in the left ventricle of 21 cats. J Am Vet Med Assoc 1982;180:1215–1219.
10. Calvert CA. Dilated cardiomyopathy in Doberman pinschers. Compen Contin Educ Pract Vet 1986;8: 417–430.
11. Fox PR. Canine myocardial disease. In: Fox PR, ed. Canine and Feline Cardiology. New York, Churchill Livingstone, 1988:467–493.
12. Keene BW. Canine cardiomyopathy. In: Kirk RW,

Bonagura JD, eds. Current Veterinary Therapy X. Philadelphia, WB Saunders, 1989:240–251.

13. Ware WA, Bonagura JD. Canine myocardial diseases. In: Kirk RW, ed. Current Veterinary Therapy IX. Philadelphia, WB Saunders, 1986:370–380.

14. Ware WA, Bonagura JD. Pulmonary edema. In: Fox PR, ed. Canine and Feline Cardiology. New York, Churchill Livingstone, 1988:205–217.

15. Fossum TW, Miller MW, Rogers KS, et al. Chylothorax associated with right-sided heart failure in five cats. J Am Vet Med Assoc 1994;204:84–89.

16. Panza JA, Maron BJ. Simultaneous occurrence of mitral valve prolapse and systolic anterior motion in hypertrophic cardiomyopathy. Am J Cardiol 1991;67:404–410.

17. Braunwald E, Grossman W. Clinical aspects of heart failure. In: Braunwald E, ed. Heart Disease. Philadelphia, WB Saunders, 1992:444–463.

18. Ettinger SJ. Weakness and syncope. In: Ettinger SJ, ed. Textbook of Veterinary Internal Medicine, 3rd ed. Philadelphia, WB Saunders, 1989:46–53.

19. Fox PR. Feline thromboembolism associated with cardiomyopathy. Proc Am Coll Vet Intern Med Forum 1987;5:714–718.

20. Harpster NK. Feline myocardial diseases. In: Kirk RW, ed. Current Veterinary Therapy IX. Philadelphia, WB Saunders, 1986:380–398.

21. Pion PD, Kittleson MD. Therapy for feline aortic thromboembolism. In: Kirk RW, Bonagura JD, eds. Current Veterinary Therapy X. Philadelphia, WB Saunders, 1989:295–302.

22. Helenski CA, Ross JN Jr. Platelet aggregation in feline cardiomyopathy. J Vet Intern Med 1987;1:24–28.

23. Pion PD. Feline aortic thromboemboli and the potential utility of thrombolytic therapy with tissue plasminogen activator. Vet Clin North Am Small Anim Pract 1988;18:79–86.

24. Lusk RH, Ettinger SF. Cardiovascular syncope. In: Fox PR, ed. Canine and Feline Cardiology. New York, Churchill Livingstone, 1988:335–339.

25. Wigle ED. Hypertrophic cardiomyopathy in 1988. Mod Concepts Cardiovasc Dis 1988;57:1–6.

26. Bonagura JD, Ware WA. Atrial fibrillation in the dog: Clinical findings in 81 cases. J Am Anim Hosp Assoc 1986;22:111–120.

27. Harpster NK. Boxer cardiomyopathy. In: Kirk RW, ed. Current Veterinary Therapy VIII. Philadelphia, WB Saunders, 1983;329–337.

28. Gooding JP, Robinson WF, Wyburn S, et al. A cardiomyopathy in the English cocker spaniel: A clinicopathological investigation. J Sm Anim Pract 1982;23:133–149.

29. Gooding JP, Robinson WF, Mews GC. Echocardiographic characterization of dilatation cardiomyopathy in the English cocker spaniel. Am J Vet Res 1986;47:1978–1983.

30. Staaden RV. Cardiomyopathy of English cocker spaniels. J Am Vet Med Assoc 1981;178:1289–1292.

31. Tilley LP. Feline cardiology. Vet Clin North Am Small Anim Pract 1976;6:415–432.

32. Calvert CA, Brown J. Use of M-mode echocardiography in the diagnosis of congestive cardiomyopathy in

33. Soderberg SF, Boon JA, Wingfield WE et al. M-mode echocardiography as a diagnostic aid for feline cardiomyopathy. Vet Radiol 1983;24:66–73.

34. Bond BR, Fox PR, Peterson ME, et al. Echocardiographic findings in 103 cats with hyperthyroidism. J Am Vet Med Assoc 1988;192:1546–1549.

35. Bond BR. Hyperthyroid heart disease in cats. Current Veterinary Therapy IX. Philadelphia, WB Saunders, 1989;399–402.

36. Holzworth J, Theran P, Carpenter JL, et al. Hyperthyroidism in the cat: Ten cases. J Am Vet Med Assoc 1980;176:345–353.

37. Jacobs G, Hutson C, Dougherty J, et al. Congestive heart failure associated with hyperthyroidism in cats. J Am Vet Med Assoc 1986;188:52–56.

38. Liu S-K, Peterson ME, Fox PR. Hypertrophic cardiomyopathy and hyperthyroidism in the cat. J Am Med Assoc 1984;185:52–57.

39. Moise NS, Dietze AE, Mezza LE, et al. Echocardiography, electrocardiography, and radiography of cats with dilatation cardiomyopathy, hypertrophic cardiomyopathy, and hyperthyroidism. Am J Vet Res 1986;47:1476–1486.

40. Moise NS, Dietze AE, Mezza LE, et al. Echocardiography, electrocardiography, and radiographic cardiomegaly in hyperthyroid cats. Am J Vet Res 1986;47:1487–1494.

41. Peterson ME, Kintzer PP, Cavanagh PG, et al. Feline hyperthyroidism: Pretreatment and clinical and laboratory evaluation of 131 cases. J Am Vet Med Assoc 1983;183:103–110.

42. Peterson ME, Keene B, Ferguson DC, et al. Electrocardiographic findings in 45 cats with hyperthyroidism. J Am Vet Med Assoc 1982;180:934–937.

43. Peterson EN, Moise NS, Brown CA, et al. Heterogeneity of hypertrophy in feline hypertrophic heart disease. J Vet Intern Med 1993;7:183–189.

44. Fox PR, Bond BR. Nonselective and selective angiography. Vet Clin North Am Small Anim Pract 1983;13:259–272.

45. Owens JM, Twedt DC. Nonselective angiography in the cat. Vet Clin North Am Small Anim Pract 1977;7:309–321.

46. Jacobs G, Panciera D. Cardiovascular complications of feline hyperthyroidism. In: Kirk RW, Bonagura JD, eds. Current Veterinary Therapy XI. Philadelphia, WB Saunders, 1992:756–759.

47. Kobayashi DL, Peterson ME, Graves TK, et al. Hypertension in cats with chronic renal failure or hyperthyroidism. J Vet Intern Med 1990;4:58–62.

48. Lesser M, Fox PR, Bond BR. Assessment of hypertension in 40 cats with left ventricular hypertrophy by Doppler-shift sphygmomanometry. J Small Anim Pract 1992;33:55–58.

49. Maron BJ, Bonow RO, Cannon RO, et al. Hypertrophic cardiomyopathy: Interrelations of clinical manifestations, pathophysiology, and therapy. Part I. N Engl J Med 1987;316:780–789.

50. Thomas WP. Feline hypertrophic cardiomyopathy.

Waltham/OSU Symposium for the Treatment of Small Animal Diseases. Vernon, California, Waltham USA, Inc, 1994;112–118.

51. Liu S-K, Roberts WC, Maron BJ. Comparison of morphologic findings in spontaneously occurring hypertrophic cardiomyopathy in humans, cats, and dogs. Am J Cardiol 1993;72:944–951.

52. Maron BJ, Liu S-K, Tilley LP. Spontaneously-occurring hypertrophic cardiomyopathy in dogs and cats: A potential animal model of a human disease. In: Kaltenbach M, Epstein SE, eds. Hypertrophic Cardiomyopathy. Berlin: Springer-Verlag, 1982;73–87.

52a. Fox PR, Liu S-K, Maron BJ. Echocardiographic assessment of spontaneously occurring feline hypertrophic cardiomyopathy. An animal model of human disease. Circulation 1995;92:2645–2651.

53. Atkins CE, Gallo AM, Kurzman ID, et al. Risk factors, clinical signs, and survival in cats with a clinical diagnosis of idiopathic hypertrophic cardiomyopathy: 74 cases (1985–1989). J Am Vet Med Assoc 1992;201:613–618.

54. Martin L, VandeWoude S, Boon J, Brown D. Left ventricular hypertrophy in a closed colony of Persian cats (abstract). J Vet Intern Med 1994;8:143.

55. Kittleson MD. CVT update: Feline hypertrophic cardiomyopathy. In: Bonagura JD, ed. Current Veterinary Therapy XII. Philadelphia, WB Saunders, 1995:854–862.

56. Kittleson MD, Pion PD, DeLellis LA, et al. Increased serum growth hormone concentrations in feline hypertrophic cardiomyopathy. J Vet Intern Med 1992;6:320–324.

57. Maron BJ, Epstein SE. Clinical significance and therapeutic implications of the left ventricular outflow tract pressure gradient in hypertrophic cardiomyopathy. Am J Cardiol 1986;58:1093–1096.

58. Tunick PA, Lampert R, Perez JL, et al. Effect of mitral regurgitation on the left ventricular outflow pressure gradient in obstructive hypertrophic cardiomyopathy. Am J Cardiol 1990;66:1271–1273.

59. Liu S-K, Maron BJ, Tilley LP. Canine hypertrophic cardiomyopathy. J Am Vet Med Assoc 1979;708–713.

60. Liu S-K, Maron BJ, Tilley LP. Hypertrophic cardiomyopathy in the dog. Am J Pathol 1979;94:497–508.

61. Van Vleet JF, Ferrans VJ, Weirich WE. Pathologic alterations in hypertrophic and congestive cardiomyopathy of cats. Am J Vet Res 1980;41:2037–2048.

62. Fox PR. Evidence for or against efficacy of beta-blockers and aspirin for management of feline cardiomyopathies. Vet Clin North Am Small Anim Pract 1991;21:1011–1022.

63. Smith CA. Current concepts: Looking for consensus in treatment of cardiac disease. J Am Vet Med Assoc 1995;206:307–312.

64. Maron BJ, Bonow RO, Cannon RO, et al. Hypertrophic cardiomyopathy: Interrelations of clinical manifestations, pathophysiology, and therapy. N Engl J Med 1987;316:844–852.

65. Allert JA, Adams HR. New perspectives in cardiovascular medicine: The calcium channel blocking drugs. J Am Vet Med Assoc 1987;190:573–578.

66. Bright JM, Golder AL. Evidence for or against the efficacy of calcium channel blockers for management of hypertrophic cardiomyopathy in cats. Vet Clin North Am Small Anim Pract 1991;21:1023–1034.

67. Muir W. Beta-blocking therapy in dogs and cats. In: Kirk RW, ed. Current Veterinary Therapy IX. Philadelphia, WB Saunders, 1986;343–346.

68. Bright JM, Golden AL, Gompf RE, et al. Evaluation of the calcium channel-blocking agents diltiazem and verapamil for treatment of feline hypertrophic cardiomyopathy. J Vet Intern Med 1991;5:272–282.

69. Atkins C, Johnson L, Keene B, et al. Diltiazem pharmacokinetics and pharmacodynamics in cats (abstract). J Vet Intern Med 1994;8:144.

70. Baughman KL. Calcium channel blocking agents in congestive heart failure. Am J Med 1986;80(Suppl 2B):46–50.

71. Eichhorn EJ. The paradox of β-adrenergic blockade for the management of congestive heart failure. Am J Med 1992;92:527–538.

72. Keene BW, Hamlin RL. Calcium antagonists. In: Kirk RW, ed. Current Veterinary Therapy IX. Philadelphia, WB Saunders, 1986:340–342.

72a. Bonagura JD, Fox PR. Restrictive cardiomyopathy. Current Veterinary Therapy XII. Philadelphia: WB Saunders, 1995:863–867.

73. Bonagura JD. Feline restrictive cardiomyopathy. Proc Am Coll Vet Intern Med Forum 1994;12:205–209.

74. Atkins CE, Snyder PS, Keene BW, et al. Efficacy of digoxin for treatment of cats with dilated cardiomyopathy. J Am Vet Med Assoc 1990;196:1463–1469.

75. Erichsen DF, Harris SG, Upson DW. Plasma levels of digoxin in the cat: Some clinical applications. J Am Anim Hosp Assoc 1978;14:734–737.

76. Erichsen DF, Harris SG, Upson DW. Therapeutic and toxic plasma concentrations of digoxin in the cat. Am J Vet Res 1980;41:2049–2058.

77. Atkins CE, Snyder PS, Keene BW. Effect of aspirin, furosemide, and commercial low-salt diet on digoxin pharmacokinetic properties in clinically normal cats. J Am Vet Med Assoc 1988;193:1264–1268.

78. Bolton GR, Powell W. Plasma kinetics of digoxin in the cat. Am J Vet Res 1982;43:1994–1999.

79. Baty CJ. Warfarin prophylaxis in feline aortic thromboembolism. Proc Am Coll Vet Intern Med Forum 1993;11:519–520.

79a. Harpster NK, Baty CJ. Warfarin therapy of the cat at risk of thromboembolism. In: Kirk RW, Bonagura JD, eds. Current Veterinary Therapy XII. Philadelphia: WB Saunders, 1995:868–873.

80. Allen DG, Johnstone IB, Crane S. Effects of aspirin and propranolol alone and in combination on hemostatic determinants in the healthy cat. Am J Vet Res 1985;46:660–663.

81. Greene CE. Effects of aspirin and propranolol on feline platelet aggregation. Am J Vet Res 1985;46:1820–1823.

82. Schaub RG, Gates KA, Roberts RE. Effect of aspirin on collateral blood flow after experimental thrombosis of the feline aorta. Am J Vet Res 1982;43:1647–1650.

83. Bonagura JD. Feline hypertrophic cardiomyopathy. Proc North Am Vet Conf 1992;6:23–24.

84. Peterson ME. Treatment of feline hyperthyroidism. In:

Kirk RW, Bonagura JD, eds. Current Veterinary Therapy X. Philadelphia, WB Saunders, 1989:1002–1008.

85. Broussard JD, Peterson ME, Fox PR. Changes in clinical and laboratory findings in cats with hyperthyroidism from 1983 to 1993. J Am Vet Med Assoc 1995;206:302–305.

86. Klein I, Levey GS. New perspectives on thyroid hormone, catecholamines, and the heart. Am J Med 1984;76:167–172.

87. Polikar R, Burger AG, Scherrer U, et al. The thyroid and the heart. Circulation 1993;87:1435–1441.

88. Birchard SJ, Peterson ME, Jacobson A. Surgical treatment of feline hyperthyroidism: Results of 85 cases. J Am Anim Hosp Assoc 1984;20:705–709.

89. Peterson ME, Kintzer PP, Hurvitz AI. Methimazole treatment of 262 cats with hyperthyroidism. J Vet Intern Med 1988;2:150–157.

90. Thoday KL, Mooney CT. Medical management of feline hyperthyroidism. In: Kirk RW, Bonagura JD, eds. Current Veterinary Therapy XI. Philadelphia, WB Saunders, 1992:338–345.

91. Turrel JM, Feldman EC, Hays M, et al. Radioactive iodine therapy in cats with hyperthyroidism. J Am Vet Med Assoc 1984;184:554–559.

92. Ross LA. Hypertension and chronic renal failure. Semin Vet Med Surg (Small Anim) 1992;7:221–226.

93. Littman MP. Spontaneous hypertension in 24 cats. J Vet Intern Med 1994;8:79–86.

94. Frohlich ED, Apstein C, Chobanian AV, et al. The heart in hypertension. N Engl J Med 1992;327:998–1008.

95. Cowgill LD, Kallet AJ. Systemic hypertension. In: Kirk RW, Bonagura JD, eds. Current Veterinary Therapy IX. Philadelphia, WB Saunders, 1989:360–364.

96. Ross LA. Hypertension: Pathophysiology and management. Proc Am Anim Hosp Assoc 1987;54:350–353.

97. Morgan RV. Systemic hypertension in four cats: Ocular and medical findings. J Am Anim Hosp Assoc 1986;22:615–621.

98. Littman MP, Robertson JL, Bovee KC. Spontaneous systemic hypertension in dogs: Five cases (1981–1983). J Am Vet Med Assoc 1988;193:486–494.

99. Spangler WL, Gribble DH, Weiser MG. Canine hypertension: A review. J Am Vet Med Assoc 1977;170:995–998.

100. Snyder PS, Henik RA. Feline systemic hypertension. Proc Am Coll Vet Intern Med Forum 1994;12:126–128.

101. Snyder PS. Canine hypertensive disease. Compen Contin Educ Pract Vet 1991;13:1785–1793.

102. Zusman RM. Angiotensin-converting enzyme inhibitors: more different than alike? Focus on cardiac performance. Am J Cardiol 1993;72:25H–36H.

103. DeLellis LA, Kittleson MD. Current uses and hazards of vasodilator therapy in heart failure. In: Kirk RW, Bonagura JD, eds. Current Veterinary Therapy XI. Philadelphia, WB Saunders, 1992:700–708.

104. Henik RA, Snyder PS, Volk LM. Amlodipine besylate therapy in cats with systemic arterial hypertension secondary to chronic renal disease (abstract). Proc Am Coll Vet Intern Med Forum 1994;12:976.

105. Buchanan JW. Causes and prevalence of cardiovascular disease. In: Kirk RW, Bonagura JD, eds. Current Veterinary Therapy XI. Philadelphia, WB Saunders, 1992;647–655.

106. Keene BW. Dilated cardiomyopathy in dogs: Diagnosis and long-term management. Waltham/OSU Symposium for the Treatment of Small Animal Diseases. Vernon, California, Waltham USA, Inc, 1994:27–32.

107. Armstrong PW, Moe GW. Medical advances in the treatment of congestive heart failure. Circulation 1993;88:2941–2952.

108. Ware WA, Lund DD, Subieta AR, et al. Sympathetic activation in dogs with congestive heart failure caused by chronic mitral valve disease and dilated cardiomyopathy. J Am Vet Med Assoc 1990;197:1475–1481.

109. Keene BW, Panciera DP, Atkins CE, et al. Myocardial L-carnitine deficiency in a family of dogs with dilated cardiomyopathy. J Am Vet Med Assoc 1991;198:647–650.

110. Keene BW. L-Carnitine supplementation in the therapy of canine dilated cardiomyopathy. Vet Clin North Am Small Anim Pract 1991;21:1005–1009.

111. Calvert CA, Chapman WL, Toal RL. Congestive cardiomyopathy in Doberman pinscher dogs. J Am Vet Med Assoc 1982;181:598–602.

112. Calvert CA. Effect of medical therapy on survival of patients with dilated cardiomyopathy. Vet Clin North Am Small Anim Pract 1991;21:919–930.

113. Knight DH. Efficacy of inotropic support of the failing heart. In: Hamlin RL, ed. Efficacy of cardiac therapy. Vet Clin North Am Small Anim Pract 1991;21:879–904.

114. Snyder PS, Atkins CE. Current uses and hazards of the digitalis glycosides. In: Kirk RW, Bonagura JD, eds. Current Veterinary Therapy XI. Philadelphia, WB Saunders, 1992;689–693.

115. Fox PR. Current uses and hazards of diuretic therapy. In: Kirk RW, Bonagura JD, eds. Current Veterinary Therapy XI. Philadelphia, WB Saunders, 1992:668–676.

116. Cody RJ. Clinical trials of diuretic therapy in heart failure: Research directions and clinical considerations. J Am Coll Cardiol 1993;22(Suppl A):165A–171A.

117. Zannad F. Angiotensin-converting enzyme inhibitor and spironolactone combination therapy: New objectives in congestive heart failure treatment. Am J Cardiol 1993;71:34A–39A.

118. The CONSENSUS Trial Study Group. Effects of enalapril on mortality in severe congestive heart failure. N Engl J Med 1987;316:1429–1435.

119. Ettinger S, Lusk R, Brayley K, et al. Evaluation of enalapril therapy in dogs with heart failure in a large multicenter study: Cooperative veterinary enalapril (COVE) study group. Proc Am Coll Vet Intern Med Forum 1992;10:584–585.

120. The SOLVD Investigators. Effect of enalapril on survival in patients with reduced left ventricular ejection fractions and congestive heart failure. N Engl J Med 1991;325:293–302.

121. Cohn JN. Efficacy of vasodilators in the treatment of heart failure. J Am Coll Cardiol 1993;22(Suppl A):135A–138A.

122. Sisson DD. Hemodynamic, echocardiographic, radiographic, and clinical effects of enalapril in dogs with

chronic heart failure. Proc Am Coll Vet Intern Med Forum 1992;10:589–591.

123. Buoscio DA, Stepien RL. Limitations and complications of ACE inhibitors for treating heart failure in dogs. Proc Am Coll Vet Intern Med Forum 1994;12:348–352.

124. Cohn JN, Archibald DG, Francis GS, et al. Veterans administration cooperative study on vasodilator therapy of heart failure: Influence of prerandomization variables on the reduction of mortality by treatment with hydralazine and isosorbide dinitrate. Circulation 1987;75(Suppl IV):49–54.

125. Pion PD. Current uses and hazards of calcium channel blocking agents. In: Kirk RW, Bonagura JD, eds. Current Veterinary Therapy XI. Philadelphia, WB Saunders, 1992:684–693.

126. Hamlin RL. Therapy of supraventricular tachycardia and atrial fibrillation. In: Kirk RW, Bonagura JD, eds. Current Veterinary Therapy XI. Philadelphia, WB Saunders, 1992:745–749.

127. Packer M. Therapeutic options in the management of chronic heart failure: Is there a drug of first choice? Circulation 1989;79:198–204.

128. Packer M. Treatment of chronic heart failure. Lancet 1992;340:92–95.

129. Ware WA. Current uses and hazards of beta-blockers. In: Kirk RW, Bonagura JD, eds. Current Veterinary Therapy XI. Philadelphia, WB Saunders, 1992:676–684.

130. Shanes JG. β-Blockade: Rational or irrational therapy for congestive heart failure? Circulation 1987;76:971–973.

131. Colucci WS, Fifer MA, Lorell BH, et al. Calcium channel blockers in congestive heart failure: Theoretical considerations and clinical experience. Am J Med 1985;78 (Suppl 2B):9–17.

132. Kittleson MD. Results of the taurine/carnitine multicenter spaniel trial. 12th American College of Veterinary Internal Medicine Forum, June 4, 1994.

133. Pion PD, Kittleson MD, Rogers QR, et al. Myocardial failure in cats associated with low plasma taurine: A reversible cardiomyopathy. Science 1987;237:764–767.

134. Pion PD, Kittleson MD, Rogers QR. Cardiomyopathy in the cat and its relation to taurine deficiency. In: Kirk RW, Bonagura JD, eds. Current Veterinary Therapy X. Philadelphia, WB Saunders, 1989:251–262.

135. Pion PD, Kittleson MD, Thomas WP, et al. Clinical findings in cats with dilated cardiomyopathy and relationship of findings to taurine deficiency. J Am Vet Med Assoc 1992;201:267–284.

136. Pion PD, Kittleson MD, Thomas WP, et al. Response of cats with dilated cardiomyopathy to taurine supplementation. J Am Vet Med Assoc 1992;201:275–284.

137. Lawler DF, Templeton AJ, Monti KL. Evidence for genetic involvement in feline dilated cardiomyopathy. J Vet Intern Med 1993;7:383–387.

138. Sisson DD, Knight DH, Helinski C, et al. Plasma taurine concentrations and M-mode echocardiographic measures in healthy cats and in cats with dilated cardiomyopathy. J Vet Intern Med 1991;5:232–238.

139. Hayes MA, Russell RG, Babiuk LA. Sudden death in young dogs with myocarditis caused by parvovirus. J Am Vet Med Assoc 1979;174:1197–1203.

140. Jezyk PF, Haskins ME, Jones CL. Myocarditis of probable viral origin in pups of weaning age. J Am Vet Med Assoc 1979;174:1204–1207.

141. Mulvey JJ, Bech-Nielsen S, Haskins ME, et al. Myocarditis induced by parvoviral infection in weanling pups in the United States. J Am Vet Med Assoc 1980;177:695–698.

142. Williams GD, Adams LG, Yaeger RG, et al. Naturally occurring trypanosomiasis (Chagas' disease) in dogs. J Am Vet Med Assoc 1977;171:171–177.

143. Steere AC, Batsford WP, Weinberg M, et al. Lyme carditis: Cardiac abnormalities of Lyme disease. Ann Intern Med 1980;93:8–16.

144. Mauldin GE, Fox PR, Patnaik AK, et al. Doxorubicin-induced cardiotoxicosis: Clinical features in 32 dogs. J Vet Intern Med 1992;6:82–88.

145. Page RL; Keene BW. Doxorubicin cardiomyopathy. In: Kirk RW, Bonagura JD, eds. Current Veterinary Therapy XI. Philadelphia, WB Saunders, 1992;783–785.

Chapter 13

Heartworm Disease

Betsy R. Bond

Heartworm infection, caused by *Dirofilaria immitis,* is a widespread problem that affects both dogs and cats. Although prevalence is higher in some areas than in others, the disease has been diagnosed in almost every state.[1]

Heartworm *infection,* or the mere presence of heartworms in a dog or cat, should be differentiated from heartworm *disease,* which refers to the pathologic changes that result from heartworm infection. Dogs and cats that are heartworm-infected may or may not be symptomatic (i.e., have clinical disease), but signs are always present in dogs and cats with heartworm disease.[1]

The term occult heartworm infection refers to the presence of adult *D. immitis* worms without circulating microfilariae (microfilaria −/antigen +).[2] Table 13–1 lists possible causes of occult infection.

The prevalence of heartworm infection is increasing, probably because of the movement of infected dogs. Infection rates in endemic areas have been estimated to be from 45% to 100%,[1] with the prevalence of occult infection ranging from 10% to 67% of all heartworm-infected dogs.[3] In the United States, heartworm disease is endemic in the southeastern coastlands,[2] the Gulf Coast states,[3] and the Mississippi River valley. Cats are infected at a rate about 20% that of dogs.[1]

Large sporting breeds of dog are predisposed to heartworm disease,[4] and in both dogs and cats, males are infected more often than females.[1]

Problem Identification

Cough (Dogs and Cats)

Pathophysiology

Heartworm disease is associated with a cough reflex because it causes endothelial inflammation that extends to the alveoli and bronchioles. It is usually associated with moderate to severe pulmonary artery disease or pulmonary infiltrates with eosinophilia. Embolization after treatment with an adulticide also causes coughing.[2]

Clinical Signs

A cough is one of the earliest signs of heartworm disease, and it is detected in dogs before dyspnea or exercise intolerance. It is also a common sign in cats with heartworm disease. Crackles may be heard in the dorsal and caudal lung lobes, especially in dogs with advanced disease.[1, 2, 5]

Diagnostic Plan

Electrocardiography (ECG), radiography, echocardiography, routine blood tests, urinalysis, and Knott's test should be performed, although thoracic radiographs are the best diagnostic tool to differentiate heartworm disease from other causes of cough (see Radiography). See Chapters 9 and 54 for a complete discussion of cough. Common findings in dogs with heartworm disease include right ventricular enlargement, pulmonary artery enlargement with blunting, and alveolar or interstitial infiltrates (Fig. 13–1).

Other diseases can usually be easily differentiated from heartworm disease. Pneumonia causes an alveolar infiltrate but usually without cardiac enlargement. An alveolar infiltrate is also caused by left-sided heart failure, but the cardiac enlargement is left-sided rather than right-sided and characteristically causes left atrial enlargement. Chronic obstructive pulmonary disease results in cough and right ventricular enlargement, but the pulmonary arteries are not as dilated as they are in animals with heartworm disease. In addition, chronic obstructive pulmonary disease usually affects small breeds of dog, and affected dogs are characteristically old and obese and live primarily indoors. An interstitial pattern without cardiac enlargement is found in animals with pulmonary neoplasia.

Knott's test is definitive for heartworm infection and should be performed in all coughing dogs with characteristic findings on thoracic radiography. If the Knott's test is negative, serologic tests for adult heartworms may be diagnostic (see Table 13–1).

Transtracheal lavage may be useful in coughing dogs and cats with bronchial, alveolar, or interstitial pulmonary infiltrates, especially in animals with a fever or leukocytosis. Results are not specific for heartworm disease, but the procedure can reveal a high percentage of eosinophils and help to differentiate heartworm disease from pneumonia.[2] Eosinophilia, basophilia, anemia, and high levels of globulins are associated with heartworm disease. Their presence should increase suspicion that the cough is caused by heartworms.

Dyspnea (Dogs)

Pathophysiology

Dyspnea that results from heartworm disease is always associated with severe pulmonary artery disease, pulmonary thromboembolism, pulmonary infiltrates with eosinophilia, or caval syndrome. It indicates more severe disease than coughing and usually is detected before exercise intolerance.[2] Dyspnea is

Table 13-1

Interpretation of Knott's Test and Antigen Test Results for *Dirofilaria immitis*

Microfilaria +/Antigen +
Patent infection

Microfilaria +/Antigen −
False-positive Knott's test result (approximately 1% of all cases), no adult heartworms
Low worm burden
New infection (within past 6 months), heartworms present
Immune response removing antigen from circulation, heartworms present
Prenatal microfilariae (from bitch with microfilaremia), no heartworms
Dirofilaria reconditum or other microfilariae, no heartworms
Transfusion of contaminated blood
Ineffective microfilaricide treatment
Test performed before microfilaricide treatment
Adult worms dead of natural causes (microfilariae may survive for 2 years after the death of adult worms)

Microfilaria −/Antigen +
False-positive antigen test result, technical error, no heartworms
All female or all male adults (in approximately one third of all infected dogs), heartworms present
New infection (within past 6 months), heartworms present
Antibody against microfilariae prevents detection of microfilariae (in approximately one third of all dogs with occult
    infection), heartworms present
Treatment with microfilaricide, heartworms present
Seasonal changes in microfilariae number, heartworms present
Monthly preventative induced embryostasis, heartworms present

Microfilaria −/Antigen −
True negative, no adult heartworms
Low worm burden
All male or all female adults, low number of adult heartworms
Prepatent, immature infection (L_5 larvae reach heart by 100 days; therefore, results of both tests may be negative for
    first 180 days, heartworms present)
Immune-mediated occult plus spontaneous clearance of antigen, heartworms present

From Henry CJ, Dillon R. Heartworm disease in dogs. J Am Vet Med Assoc 1994; 204:1148–1151.

caused by impaired blood flow through the pulmonary arteries for oxygenation.

Clinical Signs

Dogs with dyspnea secondary to heartworm disease rarely have a murmur, but they may have crackles and rales indicative of pulmonary disease. Arterial pulses are normal, but abnormal jugular pulses indicating right-sided heart failure may be present.[1] A cough may also be present.

Diagnostic Plan

The diagnostic plan is the same as for coughing dogs, although radiographic changes are usually more severe in dyspneic than in coughing dogs. Pulmonary arteries are more dilated and blunted, and there is an increased severity of pulmonary infiltrates. See Chapters 9 and 52 for a complete description of dyspnea.

Exercise Intolerance (Dogs)

Pathophysiology

Exercise intolerance occurs in dogs with heartworm disease when pulmonary hypertension from thrombosis exerts such pressure on the right ventricle that it can no longer increase its output. In addition, damaged pulmonary arteries cannot allow normal intrapulmonary blood flow and oxygen exchange. The lungs are unable to increase intrapulmonary blood flow by dilation of collateral small pulmonary arteries and recruitment of unused or partially collapsed vessels. Exercise intolerance is usually associated with moderate to severe pulmonary artery disease and may be seen in dogs with right-sided heart failure.[2]

Clinical Signs

Clinical signs are the same as for dogs with dyspnea, although there is more likely to be a split second heart sound (S_2) in these dogs.

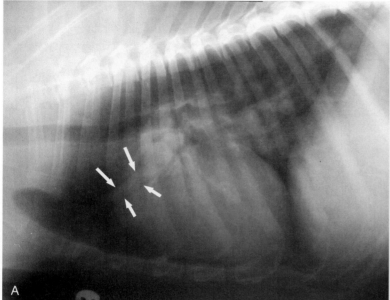
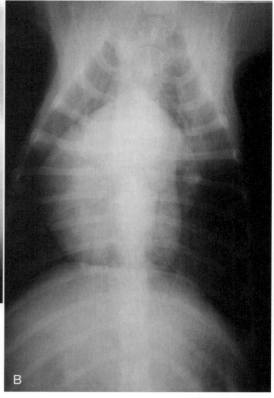

Figure 13-1
(**A**) Lateral and (**B**) ventrodorsal radiographs of a bull mastiff with severe heartworm disease after treatment with thiacetarsamide. In **A**, the cranial lobar artery (*arrows*) is extremely dilated. There are nodular densities in the caudal dorsal lung lobes. In **B**, the right ventricle is enlarged, and there is dilation of the main pulmonary artery, which can be seen at the 1 o'clock position.

Diagnostic Plan

The diagnostic plan is the same as for coughing dogs. See Chapter 9 for a complete description of exercise intolerance.

Ascites (Dogs)

Ascites is accumulation of fluid in the abdominal cavity.

Pathophysiology

Severe heartworm disease causes pulmonary hypertension that eventually leads to right-sided heart failure. Ascites, which is caused by backward failure of the right ventricle,[1] is a sign of the most severe form of pulmonary hypertension.[2, 6]

Clinical Signs

Dogs with abdominal distention caused by ascites secondary to heartworm disease also exhibit exercise intolerance, coughing, dyspnea, syncope, weight loss, and hemoptysis.[1, 2] A systolic murmur over the tricuspid valve is common, and a split S_2 may be auscultated.[6]

Diagnostic Plan

The diagnostic plan is the same as for coughing dogs. In most dogs with ascites, a right axis deviation and deep S waves in leads I, II, and III can be seen on ECG, indicating right ventricular hypertrophy. The right ventricle and pulmonary arteries are larger than normal on thoracic radiographs.[1, 2, 6] Echocardiography may be performed to determine the size of the right ventricle and gauge the severity of right ventricular failure. Heartworms are often seen in the pulmonary arteries. Any dog with ascites and right ventricular enlargement with pulmonary artery dilation seen on thoracic radiographs should be tested for *D. immitis*. See Chapter 34 for a complete description of ascites.

Vomiting (Cats)

Clinical Signs

Intermittent vomiting is one of the common signs associated with chronic heartworm disease in cats. Retching and severe paroxysmal vomiting are unusual, and concomitant respiratory signs are usually absent.[7]

Diagnostic Plan

Thoracic radiography should be done in vomiting outdoor cats that live in heartworm-endemic areas. If an abdominal radiograph is taken because of vomiting, abnormal pulmonary parenchyma may be seen in the part of the thorax that is included in the radiograph. Routine blood tests and an enzyme-linked immunosorbent assay (ELISA) for adult heartworm antigens should be performed if thoracic radiographs reveal signs of heartworm disease. A tracheal wash may be performed, but results are nonspecific for diagnosis of heartworms, because eosinophils are also present in cats with asthma. Heartworm disease should also be considered in cats with nonregenerative anemia, eosinophilia, and basophilia. Contrast radiography that reveals blunting of pulmonary arteries and filling defects indicating the heartworms themselves may be the most diagnostic test available.[7, 8] See Chapter 31 for a complete description of vomiting.

Hemoptysis

Hemoptysis, or coughing of blood, occurs secondary to severe heartworm disease and is caused by rupture of pulmonary arteries into alveoli. It may result from naturally occurring pulmonary embolism and is accompanied by other symptoms of severe heartworm disease (e.g., weight loss, ascites, heart murmur). Radiographic changes include right ventricular enlargement and dilated, tortuous, blunted pulmonary arteries. Alveolar pulmonary infiltrates are usually present. Hempotysis also occurs after treatment for adult dirofilariae. It is a severe prognostic sign, with mortality reaching almost 100%. See Chapters 9 and 54 for a complete discussion of hemoptysis.

Eosinophilia

Eosinophilia, or an absolute increase in circulating eosinophils, is seen in heartworm disease at any stage. Any dog or cat with elevated eosinophils should be tested for heartworm disease. Radiographic abnormalities may or may not accompany eosinophilia. See Chapter 42 for a complete discussion of eosinophilia.

Hemoglobinuria

Hemoglobinuria, or a reddish color to the urine caused by massive destruction of red blood cells, is present in dogs with caval syndrome because of trauma to red blood cells and increased red blood cell fragility. Hematuria or myoglobinuria can also cause reddish urine, and hemoglobinuria of suspected caval syndrome origin must be differentiated from other causes of red blood cell destruction, such as immune-mediated hemolytic anemia. Dogs with caval syndrome have signs of right-sided heart failure such as ascites, hepatomegaly, murmurs, and arrhythmias. Microscopic hematuria is not present. Echocardiography is diagnostic of caval syndrome, showing the mass of worms in the right atrium and ventricle. See Chapter 17 for a complete discussion of discolored urine.

Anemia

Anemia, or a deficiency of red blood cells, is seen in dogs with caval syndrome. It is associated with hemoglobinuria and has the same cause; it is also differentiated from other causes of anemia in the same way (see Chap. 41).

Icterus

Icterus, or a yellow tinge to the sclerae and mucous membranes caused by increased bilirubin, is seen in heartworm disease in caval syndrome or after treatment with thiacetarsamide. Hepatic dysfunction from passive congestion of the liver and hemolysis cause the icterus in heartworm disease. Icterus caused by heartworm disease must be differentiated from icterus resulting from other causes. See Chapter 34 for a complete discussion of icterus.

Heartworm Disease in Dogs

Pathophysiology

Life Cycle

See Table 13–2 for the life cycle of heartworm in dogs. Two points are significant. First, the L_3 larvae exist for only a short period (1 to 12 days), which is the

Table 13–2
Life Cycle of *Dirofilaria immitis*

EVENT	TIME
Mosquito ingests L_1	Day 0
L_1 moults to L_3	8 to 17 d
L_3 transmitted to host	
L_3 moults to L_4	1 to 12 d
L_4 moults to L_5	50 to 68 d after infection
L_5 enters vascular system and migrates	
L_5 matures and produces microfilariae	6 to 7 mo after infection

period of time that diethylcarbamazine is effective. Second, it takes about 6 months before microfilariae appear in the blood stream after the host is bitten by an infected mosquito.[1, 2]

Although young adults (L5 larvae) and adults generally reside in the right ventricle and pulmonary artery,[1] the number of worms determines their anatomic location. In an average 25-kg dog, 25 or fewer worms are found in the pulmonary artery. If there are more than 25 adult worms, they are found in the right ventricle as well, and dogs with more than 50 worms have some in the right atrium. Obstruction to the caudal vena cava may occur with 75 or more worms.[2]

Lungs

The severity of pulmonary artery disease depends on the number of adult worms, the duration of infection, and the interaction between host and parasite.[1] In experiments involving induced heartworm infection, exposure of pulmonary artery endothelium and platelet aggregation occurred within 3 days after transplantation of adult heartworms into the jugular vein.[5] Pulmonary hypertension is caused by endothelial damage by adult worms; this leads to villous myointimal proliferation and vascular reaction to worms rather than physical obstruction by worms.[1, 5, 9] Platelets adhere to the exposed subendothelium, and intimal smooth muscle cells proliferate. Large arteries dilate and become tortuous and blunted.[2, 5] Diseased pulmonary arteries are unable to dilate in response to the need for more oxygen, and the result is pressure overload to the right ventricle.[1, 5]

Pulmonary infiltrates with eosinophilia, or allergic pneumonitis, can cause severe clinical signs. Antibodies trap microfilariae within pulmonary arteries. Immune-mediated hypersensitization with infiltration of eosinophils occurs around the entrapped microfilariae, causing allergic pneumonitis. Microfilariae may eventually become engulfed in a granulomatous inflammatory response, a more severe form of allergic pneumonitis.[10] In general, immune-mediated occult heartworm disease causes more severe pulmonary artery disease and hypertension than does heartworm infection with microfilaremia.[1, 2, 3] Although there is usually a direct correlation between severity of pulmonary artery changes and clinical signs, some dogs with moderate to severe respiratory disease have only mildly enlarged pulmonary arteries because their pathologic response consists of an immune reaction against microfilariae within the pulmonary parenchyma.[2]

Treatment of dogs with heartworm disease causes extensive pulmonary changes associated with the death of adult heartworms. These changes are most severe during the first 3 to 6 weeks after treatment

begins. Whereas live heartworms possess mechanisms to protect themselves against the host's immune system, dead heartworms are susceptible to immune destruction, which leads to severe thrombosis and a granulomatous inflammatory response. The myointimal and villous proliferation that was produced by live worms is intensified, and there is increased focal loss of endothelium.[1, 2] Coagulation is initiated, and in animals with severe disease, fibrinolysis may initiate disseminated intravascular coagulation. Resolution of changes within the pulmonary arteries may begin 6 weeks after treatment, but pulmonary hypertension can take 6 months to resolve.[2]

Heart

Hypertrophy of the intima of the pulmonary arteries increases pulmonary artery resistance and pressure, leading to pressure overload of the right ventricle. If the pulmonary hypertension is long-standing, right-sided heart failure ensues.[1, 2, 5] Signs of right-sided heart failure include ascites, cachexia (if chronic), and exercise intolerance. The severity of hypertension and subsequent development of heart failure depend on the number of heartworms relative to the size of the dog, the amount the dog usually exercises, the duration of infection, and the host's response to the infection. The lungs cannot recruit collateral circulation, because blood flow to underperfused vessels is blocked in heartworm-infected dogs; therefore, pulmonary vascular resistance increases. Exercise increases pulmonary hypertension and causes volume overload of the right ventricle, which results in ascites and exercise intolerance. However, even dogs with severe heartworm disease have normal cardiac output at rest.[11]

Liver

The hepatic enzymes alanine aminotransferase and alkaline phosphatase are often abnormally high in dogs that are severely affected with heartworm disease and caval syndrome. Liver damage results from hepatic congestion and causes lower serum albumin and higher gamma globulin concentrations than normal. The inability of the liver to remove procoagulate may contribute to the initiation of disseminated intravascular coagulation.[11]

Kidneys

Antigen-antibody complexes can cause glomerulonephritis secondary to reaction against heartworm antigens. Proteinuria with hypoalbuminemia is seen on biochemical testing.[1] Prognosis for this complication of heartworm disease is extremely guarded. Caval syndrome, with acute increases in venous pressures, can cause the glomerular filtration rate to fall, the renal venous pressure to rise, and the proximal tubular sodium reabsorption rate to fall. High blood urea nitrogen (BUN) may also worsen hemolysis.[11]

Diagnostic Plan

In the past, infection with *D. immitis* was usually diagnosed during routine examination by recognition of the microfilariae on a direct smear or by results of a modified Knott's test. Tests against adult antigens are now available and widely used. These tests may be more accurate than tests for microfilariae, because the most commonly used preventative agents, the macrolides (i.e., ivermectin and milbemycin), reduce or eliminate microfilariae concentrations.[12] Ancillary tests such as radiography, ECG, echocardiography, and routine blood screening can also help, not only in diagnosis but also in determining the severity of disease, prognosis, and success of treatment.

Modified Knott's Test

The most definitive means of diagnosing heartworm infection in dogs used to be the identification of *D. immitis* microfilariae in the peripheral blood.[1] Although immunodiagnostic tests are rapidly replacing identification of microfilariae,[12] dogs older than 6 months of age that are not being treated with any macrolides and dogs that are being given diethylcarbamazine need to be tested for microfilariae.

A confusing situation has arisen with the widespread use of macrolides for prevention. Because the macrolides decrease or eliminate microfilariae in dogs with a patent infection and induce sterility in adult worms, a routine microfilaria test is inadequate to demonstrate the presence of heartworms in a dog that has been given ivermectin or milbemycin. An occult infection usually develops within 6 months after monthly macrolide treatment is initiated and continues for 6 months after discontinuation of administration.[3, 13] The diagnosis is especially difficult in a dog that has adult worms and then is given a macrolide. The adult worms continue to exert their influence on the lungs, but microfilariae no longer circulate, and a test for microfilariae to diagnose heartworm infection is no longer definitive.

However, testing for microfilariae plays an important role, because all the drugs available for prevention react with circulating microfilariae. Diethylcarbamazine (Filaribits) induces the greatest adverse effects, milbemycin is next in severity, and ivermectin causes the fewest adverse reactions in microfilaremic dogs.[13] Without testing for microfilariae, it cannot be assumed that they are not present. This is especially important in dogs from cold climates in whom treatment is suspended during the winter months.[12]

Table 13–3
Comparison of Microfilariae of *Dirofilaria immitis* and *Dirofilaria reconditum*

D. IMMITIS	D. RECONDITUM
279–324 µm long	213–270 µm long
Less active (move in place)	More active (move across slide)
6.1–7.2 µm wide	4.7–5.8 µm wide
Tapered head	Blunt head
Straight tail	Tail hook >180 degrees

Diagnosis is made by recognition of microfilariae on a direct blood smear, although concentration tests (i.e., the modified Knott's test) are more likely to pick up the L_1 larvae.[2] One advantage of the direct smear is the ability to see movement of microfilariae, an important distinction between *D. immitis* and *Dirofilaria reconditum*.[1] Table 13–3 lists differences between *D. immitis* and *D. reconditum*.[2] *D. reconditum* should always be considered if microfilariae are found in the blood, because one of the most common reasons for a false-positive heartworm result is technical errors in the identification of microfilariae.[13]

The number of microfilariae present is affected by the season, time of day, ambient temperature, stage of infection, host immune response, and drug therapy; therefore, there is no relation between the number of circulating microfilariae and the severity of cardiopulmonary disease or the number of adult worms in the heart. A positive diagnosis is more likely if the count of microfilariae is high, which is generally between 4 PM and 10 PM, during periods of warm weather, and when the mosquito population is high.[1, 2]

Screening of dogs younger than 6 months old for microfilariae is not warranted, because neither antigens nor microfilariae are detected in the blood until about 6 or 7 months after infection.[1, 3, 13] However, adult dogs in endemic areas should be tested yearly.[1, 13]

Immunodiagnostic Tests

ELISAs test for either heartworm antibody or heartworm antigen,[1] although antigen tests are used more commonly. Fewer than 1% of dogs with mature heartworms are free of circulating antigens, and most antigens are produced in the female reproductive tract.[14] An ELISA can be positive as early as 10 weeks after infection by an L_3 larva (i.e., during prepotency). Results of these tests should be interpreted cautiously, because the host immune response varies and the tests can cross-react with intestinal nematodes.[2] Tests for heartworm antigens work best in dogs with high worm burdens (i.e., more than five worms) and can be used after treatment to gauge efficacy of adulticide therapy.[3, 14] The ELISA remains positive for at least 12 weeks after successful adulticide therapy[1]; to be sure there are no false-positive results, an interval of at least 12 weeks is recommended before retesting.[12] Reasons for false-positive and false-negative results are listed in Table 13–1.

Titers of adult antigens peak about 4 weeks after thiacetarsamide administration and killing of adult heartworms. These titers should not be detectable after 6 months if all adults are eradicated.[2, 14] Cross-reactivity with ascarids and *D. reconditum* is common, giving a false-positive result.[2, 12, 14, 15] A negative result of an ELISA or indirect fluorescent antibody test almost eliminates the possibility of heartworm infection,[2, 14] but false-positive results can occur. The most common reason for a false-positive result is technical error in antigen detection procedures.[13]

The sensitivity and longevity of antigen-detecting tests can be a problem. For instance, results of ELISA can be positive as early as 70 days after infection, but the efficacy of thiacetarsamide that early is unknown. If the treatment is administered at day 110 after infection, it is possible that only 50% of male and 20% of female worms will be killed, because males are less resistant than females, and not all young worms will be killed. Because the infection is not eradicated, microfilaremia from remaining adults can be detected over the ensuing 5 to 6 months. Thiacetarsamide administered at that time would also probably be ineffective, because adult worms are not mature enough to be fully sensitive. If microfilariae are killed, the presence of infection can be documented only with repeat ELISA or indirect fluorescence antibody tests.[2] It must be remembered that antigens circulate for 3 months after adults are killed.[1]

Because of the problems associated with tests for microfilariae, antigen tests are replacing concentration tests for routine screening of microfilariae. The occurrence of macrolide-induced occult heartworm infections is very common, and most dogs with heartworm infection that are treated with ivermectin or milbemycin should not have circulating microfilariae.[12] The only way to be sure, however, is to run both tests.

Radiography

Radiography can be used to diagnose heartworm disease in the absence of microfilariae or positive serologic test results. Radiographs are also an effective method of assessing the severity of heartworm disease. However, young dogs without clinical signs are unlikely to display abnormalities. The right ventricle in severely affected dogs is abnormally large, and the main pulmonary arteries, especially the caudal lobar arteries, appear dilated, tortuous, and blunted (see Fig. 13–1).[1–3, 5] Extensions of endothelial inflammation produce focal areas of alveolar edema or consolidation, which surround the caudal lobar arteries.[5] The severity of radiographic abnormalities is related to the adult worm burden, the duration of infection, and the host-parasite interaction. Some dogs with severe pulmonary disease have a relatively low adult worm burden, demonstrating the importance of the host-parasite interaction.[2, 3, 16]

Another radiographic manifestation of heartworm disease is occult heartworm disease allergic pneumonitis (Fig. 13–2). This causes a mixed, linear, interstitial and alveolar pattern that frequently obscures the lobar pulmonary arteries. The pattern is most obvious in the caudal lung fields, and pulmonary arteries are not severely affected.[1, 2] A more severe form of pneumonitis is eosinophilic nodular pulmonary granulomatous disease, which causes interstitial nodular densities, bronchial lymphadenopathy, and occasionally, pleural effusion (Fig. 13–3).[1, 10]

Embolism of worms after administration of an adulticide causes characteristic radiographic signs. Focal areas of increased alveolar density and consolidation can be seen in the caudal and accessory lung lobes[5] and occasionally involve whole lung lobes (see Fig. 13–1). Radiographic and arteriographic changes caused by dead heartworms start resolving within 3 to 4 weeks after treatment,[1, 2, 5] but it may be months before they completely disappear.

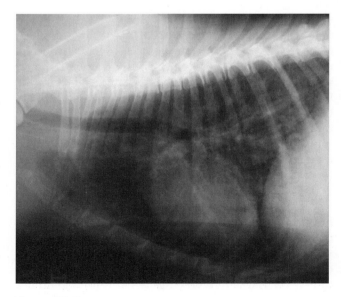

Figure 13–2

Radiograph of a 6-year-old rottweiler with eosinophilic pneumonitis. Diffuse alveolar and interstitial infiltrates and an enhanced bronchial pattern are present.

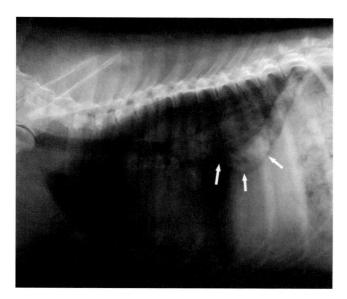

Figure 13–3
Lateral radiograph of a 6-year-old Doberman pinscher with eosinophilic granulomas in the caudal lung lobes secondary to heartworm disease.

Electrocardiography

ECG is an insensitive measure of the presence of heartworms, although the presence of three or more criteria of right ventricular hypertrophy usually indicates severe pulmonary arterial and right ventricular abnormalities and clinical right-sided heart failure.[2, 3, 5] Arrhythmias are uncommon in animals with heartworm disease.[1]

Routine Laboratory Evaluation

A complete blood count, serum biochemistry profile, and urinalysis should be performed in any dog with heartworm disease, even those without clinical signs. Underlying disorders might need to be corrected before treatment of heartworm disease can be instituted or might preclude adulticide therapy.[1] This is more true in dogs with renal failure than it is in dogs with high liver enzymes. The presence of high liver enzymes alone is not associated with adverse drug reactions and should not cause a delay in administration of thiacetarsamide.[3]

Most asymptomatic dogs have no important hematologic or biochemical abnormalities other than possible eosinophilia or basophilia. Anemia may occur in symptomatic dogs, with the degree of anemia corresponding to the severity of disease. Mildly symptomatic dogs display mild normocytic normochromic anemia because of fragility of red blood cells; more severely affected dogs are more anemic. Severe anemia is associated with disseminated intravascular coagulation.[6, 11] Caval syndrome causes macrocytic, regenerative anemia and hemoglobinuria. Target cells, spherocytes, spur cells, and poikilocytes may be present.[11]

Most dogs with severe pulmonary hypertension have corresponding leukocytosis, usually with a left shift and monocytosis. Eosinophilia is most common when young adult worms reach the heart and when the first microfilariae appear. Basophilia is usually associated with eosinophilia, and both conditions are more noticeable in dogs with occult, symptomatic infection.[2]

Liver enzymes are usually not high in asymptomatic dogs, and increases are not well correlated with either severity of disease or adverse reactions to thiacetarsamide.[2]

Proteinuria is common in symptomatic dogs and is caused by immune complex glomerulopathy.[1] Mild changes are of little clinical significance and resolve within several months after adulticide treatment.[2] However, severe proteinuria, especially with hypoalbuminemia, may indicate nephrotic syndrome, which carries an extremely guarded prognosis.[11] Such severe renal involvement is rare in dogs with heartworm disease.[2]

Eosinophilia, hyperglobulinemia, and basophilia are consistent findings in dogs with pneumonitis associated with occult heartworm disease. Serologic tests for adult and microfilaria antigens are positive, but a Knott's test is negative. Cytologic examination of a tracheal lavage specimen reveals eosinophils, nondegenerate neutrophils, and macrophages.[1, 2] However, this is not diagnostic of heartworm disease, because allergic pneumonitis can cause similar cytologic changes.

Echocardiography

Whereas echocardiography is unnecessary and insensitive in most animals,[1] it does reveal right ventricular dilation, right ventricular hypertrophy, and the presence of worms in the right ventricle and atrium in dogs with severe heartworm disease and caval syndrome.[3, 6, 17] In addition, results are obtained quickly in practices with echocardiographic equipment. Echocardiography can definitively diagnose some dogs even with mild disease before serologic results are available by enabling one to see worms in pulmonary arteries (Fig. 13–4).[1, 17]

Angiography

Nonselective or selective angiography of the pulmonary arteries reveals linear lucencies of adult heartworms in pulmonary arteries. Abrupt pruning of pulmonary arteries caused by thromboembolism is easier to see on an angiogram than on a plain radiograph.[2] Angiography may be especially helpful in cats,

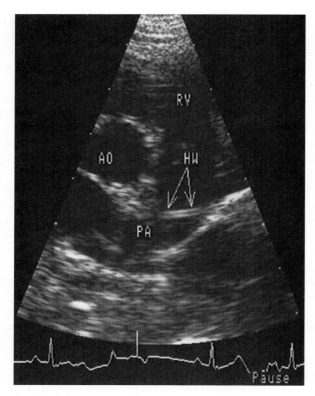

Figure 13-4
Echocardiogram of a dog with heartworm disease and heartworms (HW) in the pulmonary artery. Heartworms are seen as parallel lines in the pulmonary artery. AO, aorta; PA, pulmonary artery; RV, right ventricle.

because results of serodiagnostic tests in cats are unreliable.[7, 8]

Treatment

Adults

Although treatment should be administered to all dogs with confirmed heartworm infection, treatment causes pulmonary embolization in all dogs, even those that are asymptomatic.[9, 18] One must stress the likelihood of pulmonary embolization to clients. This should encourage owner compliance with instructions that the dog rest after treatment with adulticide and should allow a lower rate of post-treatment complications.

Until recently, thiacetarsamide was the only drug approved for the treatment of *D. immitis* infection.[12] It is considered to be effective, although not all adults are killed. However, pulmonary function improves even if there is incomplete kill. The treatment should be administered in four doses over a 2-day period at 8- to 16-hour intervals. The dosage is 2.2 mg/kg of 1% thiacetarsamide.[1–3, 10] Other regimens have been attempted (i.e., five or six doses over 3 days),

but none has proved superior. With a treatment period longer than 2 days, worms die faster and pulmonary embolism is more severe.[2, 3]

Melarsomine dihydrochloride (Immiticide) is a new drug for treating *D. immitis* that has the advantages of intramuscular versus intravenous administration, no sloughing of the injection site, no liver or kidney impairment, and a higher rate of kill than thiacetarsamide. Dogs with asymptomatic to moderate heartworm disease are given a dosage of 2.5 mg/kg twice, 24 hours apart, in the epaxial muscles in the third to fifth lumbar region. Dogs with severe heartworm disease receive 2.5 mg/kg once, with two doses of 2.5 mg/kg administered 24 hours apart 30 days after the first dose.

Dogs should be fed half an hour before each treatment[2] and monitored for anorexia, excessive vomiting, icterus, and gross bilirubinuria.[3] I prefer giving injections through a 23-gauge butterfly needle and following them with a saline flush.[1] The injection of saline helps prevent even a drop of thiacetarsamide from touching extravascular tissues as the needle is withdrawn. I also aspirate several times during the injection, which accomplishes two things. First, the injection is slower because I am stopping to aspirate. Second, I ensure that I am still in the vein by aspirating and seeing blood in the tubing. Consecutive injections should not be given in the same vein because of local vascular damage, and later injections should be administered more proximally than earlier ones. A different vein should be selected if there is any possibility of drug extravasation.[2]

Perivascular reactions from leakage of thiacetarsamide may not be evident immediately, but they appear as swelling and inflammation at the previous injection site. Known extravascular injection of thiacetarsamide and inflammatory reactions of injection sites should be treated with dimethyl sulfoxide topically three times per day (t.i.d.) or four times per day (q.i.d.).[3] Obvious perivascular injection at the time of treatment can be treated with local injection of saline and a corticosteroid such as dexamethasone.

Each dose of the recommended regimen is additive, and it is critical not to miss any doses.[2, 3] The interval between doses is 8 to 16 hours, but it is best if the second dose is given not more than 10 hours after the first. Efficacy is not 100%: young female adult worms are more likely to survive. If a repeat ELISA indicates that not all adults were killed by the first treatment regimen, a 20% higher dose can provide greater efficacy but also causes greater toxicity. This regimen should be used only after initial treatment fails.[3, 13] An alternative method is to wait for a year to repeat the dose, thereby allowing the worms to become more mature and therefore more susceptible to the drug.[16] Successful adulticide treatment results in a negative antigen test 10 to 12 weeks after treatment.[13]

Adult worms begin to die within a few days and continue to die over a 3-week period.[1, 2] Approximately 90% or more of adult male worms and 70% of adult females are killed by this protocol, with females younger than 4 to 12 months being the most difficult to kill. If the worm burden is primarily young females and evidence of adult worms is found after treatment, a second treatment is more effective if it is delayed for a year after the first.[2]

Treatment to kill adult worms is the same for all dogs with heartworm disease, but dogs with severe pulmonary hypertension, right-sided heart failure, or pneumonitis require special consideration because they are the dogs most likely to develop severe complications after administration of adulticide.[2] Dogs with severe pulmonary hypertension are at greater risk than dogs with ascites or chronic caval syndrome if the latter are without cor pulmonale or have only mild pulmonary hypertension.[11]

Treatment of dogs with pulmonary hypertension or right-sided heart failure consists of the following[1-3, 11]:

1. Allow cage rest for 1 to 2 weeks before and 4 weeks after administration of adulticide.

2. Give adulticide therapy not sooner than after 1 week of cage rest and after resolution of pulmonary parenchymal disease.

3. Administer judicious dosages of furosemide (Lasix) and a low-sodium diet for dogs with ascites.

4. Administer corticosteroid hormones (prednisone, 1 to 2 mg/kg per day, divided into two doses) where indicated (i.e., allergic pneumonitis or eosinophilic granulomatosis).[1, 2, 10]

5. Administer broad-spectrum antibiotics, such as amoxicillin (11–22 mg/kg by mouth, twice per day [b.i.d.]); amoxicillin plus clavulanate (12.5–25 mg/kg by mouth, b.i.d.); or trimethoprim plus sulfadiazine (15 mg/kg by mouth or intramuscularly [IM], b.i.d.) and aminophylline (10 mg/kg t.i.d., by mouth, IM, or intravenously [IV]).[1]

Right-sided heart failure requires special considerations. Cage rest seems to be one of the most important treatments for dogs with right-sided heart failure; it significantly increases survival rates in dogs receiving adulticide therapy.[19] Digoxin is not indicated, because it does not increase survival or right-sided cardiac output. Aspiration of fluid from the thorax or abdomen is performed only if the fluid is causing dyspnea or discomfort.[1, 12]

There is controversy about the use of aspirin in heartworm-infected dogs. Some clinicians recommend administration of aspirin before adulticide treatment in dogs with severe clinical signs and evidence of severe pulmonary artery disease on thoracic radiographs. Some studies have demonstrated that platelet adhesion, thromboembolism, and myointimal proliferation in response to endothelial damage are markedly reduced by aspirin, and aspirin would therefore decrease the size of pre-existing lesions.[2, 3, 20] However, recent controlled studies have shown that aspirin does not consistently benefit dogs with heartworm disease, either before or after treatment.[13, 21] Newer drugs such as the antiplatelet agent ticlopidine hydrochloride may be of benefit; however, these drugs need to be studied further.[13] Considering the side effects of aspirin (i.e., gastrointestinal ulceration, exacerbation of bleeding tendencies), it should not be administered to dogs with heartworm disease.

Corticosteroids have been shown to decrease arterial blood flow and increase intimal damage in dogs that are treated compared with untreated dogs.[20] Thrombosis and obstruction to pulmonary blood flow are more severe in corticosteroid-treated dogs, and therefore corticosteroids should be reserved for dogs that have allergic pneumonitis or eosinophilic granulomas.[1, 2, 10, 12] Radiographic evidence of pneumonitis should be largely cleared in about 1 week after administration of corticosteroids. Granulomas respond less favorably and may only partially resolve in 2 weeks.[1] Even dogs that respond initially relapse if the dosage of corticosteroids is reduced or even if the dosage is not altered.[10]

Administration of corticosteroids should also be considered in dogs that have a severe pulmonary reaction to adulticide treatment. Although corticosteroids given before or during the first week after adulticide administration may decrease the kill rate of young female heartworms,[2, 12] they should be considered in dogs with severe post-treatment alveolar and parenchymal reactions.[2]

It is sometimes necessary to stop treatment before the four doses of adulticide are given. Vomiting often occurs after the first or second injection, but it should not cause cessation of treatment if it consists of only one or two episodes.[1-3] The presence of anorexia with vomiting or of depression, icterus, or bilirubinuria is a reason to stop treatment before it is completed,[1-3] especially if persistent or numerous vomiting episodes occur.[3] High levels of liver enzymes are common, and this is not an indication to stop treatment.[1, 2] If treatment has been aborted, supportive care with IV fluids may be needed.[3] Retreatment with thiacetarsamide after 4 weeks is recommended. Owners should be reassured that repeat treatment is seldom associated with complications.[2, 3]

Treatment is not usually administered to azotemic animals, so it is unknown whether treatment of these animals is associated with a high number of adverse reactions. If the azotemia is prerenal, fluid therapy can help the BUN and creatinine return to normal. If the azotemia is renal and there is right ventricular enlargement (i.e., elevated preload), fluid therapy is contraindicated. Long-term prognosis is guarded if the azotemia is caused by renal disease.[2]

Echocardiographic evidence of a worm mass in the right atrium and inferior vena cava is a reason to physically remove worms before administration of thiacetarsamide.[11, 12] Use of alligator forceps has also been advocated in dogs with severe heartworm infection not obstructing the caudal vena cava. The forceps are introduced into the jugular vein and can be passed into the pulmonary arteries for worm retrieval.[22–24] Efficacy can approach 92% for an experienced operator. Lower removal rates occur in dogs with severe pulmonary artery enlargement, extensive embolization with dead worms, stricture of the pulmonary arteries, or immature worms in the distal pulmonary arteries.[22] Resolution of clinical signs can be expected within 4 weeks after worm removal.[25]

It must be emphasized to owners that treatment with an adulticide must be followed by strict rest, because almost all dogs have embolization of worms and worm fragments.[1, 12, 21] Dogs who die usually do so 10 to 14 days after administration of thiacetarsamide, when embolization is the greatest. Most of these dogs have signs and laboratory data consistent with disseminated intravascular coagulation. Thrombocytopenia is often seen 7 to 14 days after adulticide treatment, even in dogs without signs, and it may be severe.[2]

In general, prognosis is very poor in dogs with severe pulmonary hypertension, dogs older than 12 years, and dogs that develop disseminated intravascular coagulation. The presence of ascites does not seem to worsen the prognosis.[2]

Microfilariae

Microfilariae should be eliminated for two reasons. First, the dog remains infectious as long as it has circulating microfilariae. Second, accurate diagnosis of future infection is compromised by the presence of microfilariae, making it difficult to know whether the circulating microfilariae are new or have survived from a previous infection.[1] Although some think treatment of microfilariae before adults are treated ensures ease of thiacetarsamide therapy, there is no evidence to support this theory.[2, 3, 24]

Medication to kill microfilariae should be given approximately 4 weeks after the adulticide is administered.[2, 3] Because adult heartworms may live and produce microfilariae for 3 weeks after administration of thiacetarsamide, the microfilaricide should not be administered until 4 weeks after adulticide administration to ensure that all microfilariae are killed. Rarely, a dog that was positive before adulticide therapy may test negative for microfilariae without specific treatment.[2]

Levamisole, milbemycin, and ivermectin (Ivomec) are available for use as microfilaricides,[13] although ivermectin is the most widely used drug. One oral dose of ivermectin removes microfilariae in 1 to 3 weeks, usually within 1 week. The recommended dosage is 50 µg/kg for ivermectin[2, 3, 12, 13, 26] or 0.5 mg/kg for milbemycin, 4 weeks after treatment with an adulticide.[12, 13]

Ivermectin also kills L_3 and L_4 larvae up to 2 months after infection, so reinfection is prevented if ivermectin is administered within 2 months after treatment with thiacetarsamide. Ivermectin should be administered only orally, because there are more adverse reactions if the drug is administered by injection. It should not be given to collies, and possibly not to Shetland sheepdogs. It can be diluted 1:10 with propylene glycol and administered orally at a dosage of 1 mL of the mixture per 20 kg body weight. A Knott's test is performed 4 weeks after administration of a microfilaricide, and if that test is negative, the dog is started on preventative medication. Nine percent to 13% of dogs have a positive Knott's test 3 weeks after treatment with ivermectin[26] but a negative result after a second administration of ivermectin at the same dosage.[2, 3, 26]

Adverse reactions to ivermectin include lethargy, ataxia, vomiting, diarrhea, and shock. Most reactions are mild, although occasionally a dog requires administration of IV fluids and corticosteroids.[1, 3] Collies and related breeds may have an idiosyncratic reaction to ivermectin that is more severe than reactions in other breeds. Signs include salivation, tremors, confusion, ataxia, convulsions, coma, and, occasionally, death.[1] Dogs that are severely microfilaremic develop microgranulomas in the lungs, kidneys, and liver, indicating that treatment for microfilariae is not a benign procedure.[27]

It is difficult to determine whether persistent microfilaremia has resulted from incomplete elimination of adults or from microfilariae, especially if low numbers of adults are present. A second dose of microfilaricide should be administered, followed by thiacetarsamide or melarsomine if microfilariae are still present. If that regimen is ineffective, the best option is to wait 1 year and repeat the entire treatment. If it is suspected that persistent microfilaremia is a result of resistant female worms, once-monthly preventative treatment can still be administered.[2]

The most severe reaction to microfilaricide is circulatory collapse, which is caused by rapid death of large numbers of microfilariae in dogs that have severe microfilaremia.[13, 26] Therefore, dogs should be observed for 6 to 8 hours after administration of microfilaricide. Small dogs (<16 kg) with large numbers of microfilariae are more likely to experience adverse reactions. Treatment with fluids and rapid-acting glucocorticoids (prednisolone sodium succinate, Solu-Delta-Cortef, 20 mg/kg IV once) brings clinical improvement.[26] Because of the susceptibility of collies to adverse reactions to ivermectin, milbemycin (0.5 mg/kg once) has been recommended.[12] However, the preventative and microfilaricidal doses of ivermectin have been shown to be safe in collies.[13]

Prevention

Prevention should be the primary aim of the veterinarian, because it is much easier than treatment. Dogs without microfilariae that have been treated can and should be started on prevention as soon as treatment with adulticide is completed.[1] Diethylcarbamazine, ivermectin, milbemycin, and thiacetarsamide all are capable of killing the tissue-migrating larvae of *D. immitis*.[2] Although diethylcarbamazine has largely been replaced by ivermectin and milbemycin, it is still useful in dogs that cannot tolerate the other two drugs. The dosage of diethylcarbamazine is 5.0 to 7.0 mg/kg by mouth, once daily. Although it is efficacious when administered every other day, daily dosing is recommended[2, 3] because of the small window of efficacy. Because it only kills L_3 and early L_4 larvae, the window of opportunity may only be 1 or 2 days (see Table 13–2).[1] If diethylcarbamazine is discontinued for 2 to 3 days, protection is compromised.[10] The drug is started before mosquito season begins and is continued until 60 days after it ends; dogs in warmer climates should be given preventative year-round. Diethylcarbamazine must not be administered to dogs with circulating microfilariae because of the possibility of immune-mediated reactions[2, 3] (i.e., depression, ptyalism, vomiting, diarrhea, weak pulses, pale mucous membranes, prolonged capillary refill time, and bradycardia). Dogs become recumbent, weak, and tachycardic, and approximately 9% of these dogs die.[1]

Ivermectin (Heartguard, 6–12 μg/kg) and milbemycin oxime (Interceptor, 0.5–1.0 mg/kg) are the two most commonly used drugs for heartworm prophylaxis. Their greatest advantage is their once-a-month dosing schedule.[13] Because they kill L_4 larvae, they have a therapeutic window of approximately 6 weeks after an infective mosquito bites a dog (see Table 13–2).[1, 13] In addition, they may be administered to dogs who are microfilaremic, decreasing the possibility of reinfection between adulticide and microfilaricide treatments.[2] Although collies have been shown to have more adverse reactions to ivermectin than other breeds, milbemycin appears to be safe in this breed.[28] Also, recent studies have shown that dosages of ivermectin up to 60 μg/kg (10 times the recommended dosage for prevention) are safe even in sensitive collies.[29] Thiacetarsamide can also be administered at 6-month intervals to prevent heartworm infection,[2] but this is a poor alternative to ivermectin and milbemycin.

Puppies should be started on chemoprophylaxis when they are 6 to 8 weeks old.[12] They do not require testing at that time but should be checked by antigen testing 6 to 12 months later. At 8 weeks, they can have worms that are too immature to produce measurable antigen or too old (L_5) to be eliminated by once-a-month administration of preventative.[13]

There are several reasons why dogs remain heartworm-positive while receiving heartworm preventative: (1) the product has poor efficacy; (2) there is lack of owner compliance; (3) the product was not swallowed or metabolized by the dog; (4) the dog was infected with developing larvae that were too old for the product to eliminate when it was first administered; (5) the test outcome is a false-positive result.[13]

Adverse reactions to ivermectin are rare (<5%) and are usually mild. Most occur within 1 to 4 hours of administration of the drug and include vomiting, trembling, and lethargy. More severe reactions include tachycardia, hypotension, tachypnea, and collapse. Shock should be treated by administration of IV fluids and corticosteroids.[2]

Severe Adverse Effects of Treatment

Pulmonary Thromboembolism

Pulmonary thromboembolism is the most serious effect of treatment. Worms begin to die within a few days after treatment, and they continue to die over a 3-week period. All dogs experience some degree of thromboembolism, but dogs with radiographic evidence of moderate to severe pulmonary artery enlargement, alveolar disease, or parenchymal disease (e.g., granulomas) are at increased risk for thromboembolism. Fever, anorexia, lethargy, and coughing begin 7 to 14 days after treatment and peak at 10 to 14 days; this is when dogs usually die. High fever, dyspnea, and hemoptysis are associated with severe, pre-existing pulmonary disease. Treatment with corticosteroids reduces the fever and inflammation associated with mild reactions. However, corticosteroids should not be started until 1 week after completion of thiacetarsamide treatment,[2, 3] if possible, because they decrease the effectiveness of the drug.

Dogs with severe reactions should be hospitalized for cage confinement and administration of corticosteroids (prednisone, 1–2 mg/kg, divided b.i.d.), bronchodilators (aminophylline, 10 mg/kg, t.i.d.), antibiotics, and oxygen. Disseminated intravascular coagulation occurs in dogs with advanced disease. Thrombocytopenia is common and is seen 5 to 21 days after adulticide treatment, with the lowest count occurring at 10 to 14 days.[2, 3]

The best drugs for treatment of pulmonary thromboembolism include corticosteroids (prednisone, 1–2 mg/kg, divided b.i.d.) and oxygen. Administration of a large volume of fluids should be avoided because of the risk of promoting inflammatory lung damage, decreasing right ventricular free wall perfusion, and increasing right ventricular preload. Platelets are consumed during thromboembolism, and thus platelet numbers should be expected to be low.[13]

Disseminated Intravascular Coagulation

Disseminated intravascular coagulation is associated with caval syndrome, severe reaction to diethylcarbamazine, or pulmonary thromboembolism. It usually occurs 5 to 14 days after adulticide treatment and is diagnosed by the presence of a low platelet count and other coagulation abnormalities. Progression of disseminated intravascular coagulation is documented by a continuing decrease in platelets; an increase in prothrombin, thrombin, and partial thromboplastin times; and the appearance of fibrin degradation products. However, not all dogs with disseminated intravascular coagulation exhibit all coagulation abnormalities. Therefore, it is difficult to differentiate disseminated intravascular coagulation from other thrombocytopenic conditions.[30] Dogs with disseminated intravascular coagulation may have epistaxis, hemoptysis, petechial hemorrhages, and hemolytic serum.[2, 3]

The mortality rate for dogs with acute or severe disseminated intravascular coagulation is almost 100%.[2] Cage confinement, supportive care, and plasma transfusion to replace clotting factors constitute the treatment of choice, but most dogs die even with intensive therapy. See Chapter 44 for a complete discussion of the treatment of disseminated intravascular coagulation.

Caval Syndrome

Caval syndrome is a severe complication of heartworm disease associated with a heavy worm burden in the right atrium and caudal vena cava, although the reason some dogs develop caval syndrome and others do not is unclear.[1, 3] It is characterized by high mortality and causes hemoglobinemia, hemoglobinuria, anemia, and renal and hepatic dysfunction. The actual incidence of caval syndrome in dogs is unknown.[4] Prevalence is higher in early spring and early summer than in other seasons.[1, 11] It occurs most often in male dogs 3 to 5 years old. No breed predilection has been reported.[1, 11, 24]

Caval syndrome can be divided into acute, subacute, and chronic forms. The acute form is classic caval syndrome; the subacute form takes several days to develop but is still fatal without treatment; the chronic form may be indistinguishable from right-sided heart failure.[11]

Pathophysiology

As a general rule, the number of worms required to cause caval syndrome (<100) is higher than the number found in dogs with chronic forms of heartworm disease (50–60).[11] Other factors seem to be necessary, because dogs with caval syndrome can carry the same number of worms (80–85) as dogs that do not develop the syndrome. However, dogs with caval syndrome do have a high prevalence of pulmonary hypertension, making pulmonary hypertension a possible contributing factor.[4] Dogs with acute caval syndrome have worms concentrated in the right atrium, whereas dogs with the subacute form have a greater concentration of worms in the pulmonary arteries or right ventricle.[11]

Both forward and backward failure are present in dogs with caval syndrome. Poor perfusion of mucous membranes, weak pulses, and tachycardia indicate forward failure; jugular distention indicates backward failure. Because the right ventricle is consistently dilated in most dogs owing to increased preload, it is unlikely that worm obstruction causes reduced preload to the right side of the heart. Instead, the decreased cardiac output is probably caused by pulmonary hypertension combined with tricuspid regurgitation.[1, 4, 31] Arrhythmias and tricuspid regurgitation may further jeopardize right ventricular function.[1]

Trauma to red blood cells and red blood cell fragility in dogs with heartworm disease are the causes of anemia. Hepatorenal dysfunction probably results from passive congestion of the liver, impaired perfusion of abdominal organs, and hemolysis. Intravascular hemolysis, metabolic acidosis, and hepatic dysfunction with impaired removal of circulating procoagulants probably lead to disseminated coagulation.[1]

Clinical Signs

Signs of classic caval syndrome in dogs include sudden onset of pallor, weak pulses, dyspnea, abnormal jugular pulses and distention, murmurs, gallops, arrhythmias, and right ventricular hypertrophy. These signs occur in dogs without any previous sign of heartworm disease.[1, 3, 4, 11] The murmur is usually a systolic murmur of recent onset over the tricuspid valve. Arrhythmias are both atrial and ventricular but are not life-threatening.[4] Hepatosplenomegaly, split S_2, ascites, jaundice, and hemoptysis are also characteristic.[1]

Macrocytic, regenerative anemia and hemoglobinuria are hallmarks of caval syndrome.[1, 11] Other laboratory abnormalities include hemoglobinemia, high BUN, and high activity of liver enzymes.[1, 32] The poor cardiac output and backward failure usually cause more severe metabolic disease than severe pulmonary hypertension.[11] One of the worst complications of caval syndrome is disseminated intravascular coagulation.[1]

Diagnostic Plan

Caval syndrome should be highly suspected in dogs with acute collapse, anemia, and hemoglobinuria. Echocardiography is highly diagnostic. A large worm mass can be seen residing in a dilated right atrium and flowing into a dilated right ventricle during rapid ventricular filling.[1, 4] If echocardiography is not available, caval syndrome is diagnosed in dogs with hemoglobinemia and microfilaremia (both of these are present in 85% of dogs with caval syndrome). Thoracic radiography reveals cardiomegaly and pulmonary artery dilation and tortuosity.[1]

Treatment

A database should be compiled that consists of thoracic radiographs and the results of a complete blood count, a biochemical profile to define liver and kidney function, a urinalysis, and coagulation tests including fibrin degradation products. A jugular catheter is placed to monitor central venous pressure and administer IV fluids as needed. Fluids should be withheld if central venous pressure is 10 to 20 cm H_2O or if it rises more than 10 cm H_2O above baseline. Digitalis and sodium bicarbonate are not indicated.[1]

Surgical removal of worms should be attempted immediately with flexible alligator forceps introduced through the right jugular vein. Sedation is rarely necessary, and a local anesthetic is usually all that is needed. The area is prepared antiseptically and draped. An incision approximately 7.5 cm long is made over the jugular vein, and 5 cm of jugular vein are exposed by blunt dissection. A loop of suture is preplaced cranially and tied after an incision large enough to accommodate alligator forceps is made caudal to the ligature. The alligator forceps is gently inserted down the jugular vein into the right atrium. The jaws of the forceps are opened, the forceps advanced slightly, the jaws are closed, and the worms are removed. This procedure is repeated until five or six passes are completed without retrieving worms. The jugular vein is sacrificed and ligated caudal to the incision. The incision is closed with routine subcutaneous and skin sutures.[23, 33]

A dramatic (40%) drop in central venous pressure is expected after worm removal and is accompanied by a reduction in the heart murmur, jugular pulses, and clinical signs. Monitoring of central venous pressure is continued, because pulmonary vascular resistance does not change and fluid overloading can still occur. Routine administration of thiacetarsamide is withheld until the dog's clinical status improves, usually within 2 weeks. Evaluation of renal and hepatic tests should precede adulticide treatment, and additional fluid therapy administered as necessary.[1, 3, 22, 24, 32]

Prognosis

Prognosis is guarded for dogs with caval syndrome, although 15% to 40% of dogs from which worms are successfully removed survive.[3]

Heartworm Disease in Cats

Heartworm disease in cats is recognized with increasing frequency, especially in heartworm-endemic areas. The prevalence in cats approximately parallels that of dogs, but with fewer numbers numbers of cats affected. It is experimentally more difficult to infect cats with heartworms, and the percentage of larvae that develop into adult worms is significantly less in cats than in dogs. Larvae also seem to develop more slowly in cats than in dogs. Microfilaremia is uncommon and is transient when it is present. In summary, the cat is a susceptible but resistant host with a shorter time course of disease than the dog.[7, 34]

Pathophysiology

Adult heartworms in cats have a shorter lifespan than in dogs (2 years versus 5 years). Otherwise, the life cycle is the same.[7, 34]

Pathologic changes in the lungs and pulmonary arteries of cats are identical to those seen in dogs. Embolization is a major factor causing clinical signs.[7, 20] The large, muscular arteries associated with bronchi are most severely affected.[34] Right axis deviation on ECG, radiographic right-sided enlargement, and right-sided heart failure are uncommon.[7] If present, these changes are more indicative of heartworm disease than of other pulmonary diseases in cats.

The heart seems to be relatively untouched by feline heartworm disease, perhaps because most of the pathologic changes are in the lungs or because cats with heartworm disease severe enough to cause heart failure do not live long enough for heart failure to develop.[7]

Clinical Signs

Cats with heartworm disease may die acutely, exhibit chronic signs, or be asymptomatic. Sudden death is usually caused by circulatory collapse and acute pulmonary artery embolism and may occur without previous clinical signs. Severe pulmonary infarction, congestion, and edema may be present, with or without pulmonary emboli.[7, 35]

The most common clinical signs include coughing, dyspnea, vomiting, lethargy, anorexia, and weight loss, with vomiting or respiratory signs being the most common owner complaints. Vomiting is sporadic and can be related to eating. Paroxysmal coughing can be severe but is interspersed with periods of days without signs. Dyspnea, especially acute dyspnea, may represent emboli and may be accompanied by radiographic evidence of lung lobe consolidation in the caudal lung lobes. Harsh, dry lung sounds are the most common finding on auscultation. Murmurs and gallops are uncommon, and other signs (e.g., ascites, exercise intolerance, right-sided heart failure) are rare.[7]

Nonregenerative anemia is present in about one third of heartworm-infected cats. Eosinophilia, basophilia, and nucleated erythrocytes may also be present.[7, 34, 35] Severe thrombocytopenia has not been reported in the cat.[36] Hyperglobulinemia is not a consistent or reliable indicator of heartworm disease in cats.[7] Microfilariae are rare, and their presence should not be depended on for diagnosis. The best serologic test to diagnose heartworms in cats is the ELISA for the detection of adult antigen in circulation.[7, 34] However, cats with sexually immature worms or with a low worm burden test negative.[7]

Radiography is one of the best screening tests for heartworm disease in cats. Nonspecific pulmonary parenchymal changes include diffuse or coalescing infiltrates, perivascular densities, and lung atelectasis. The most distinctive radiographic abnormality is a large pulmonary artery with blurred edges (Fig. 13–5A, C).[7, 34, 35] Blunting and tortuosity of the pul-

monary arteries is less common than in dogs. Nonselective angiography may confirm a tentative diagnosis of heartworm disease: 4 to 6 mL of contrast material are injected by butterfly needle into a cephalic or jugular vein, and a radiograph is taken 5 to 6 seconds after the injection to provide good imaging of the right-sided outflow. Classic lesions include blunting of the vessels, and linear defects caused by the presence of the worms may be seen (Fig. 13–5B, D).[7, 8, 20]

Heartworms have been detected by echocardiography in cats with heartworm infection. As in dogs, a double-lined echodensity is seen in the main pulmonary artery, in one of its branches, or in the right ventricle.[12]

Heartworm disease in cats must be differentiated from lungworm infestation, asthma, or bronchitis. Although the pulmonary parenchymal changes may be similar for all these diseases, pulmonary arterial changes are unique[10] and can easily be seen on contrast radiographs.[7] In addition, ECG evidence of right ventricular enlargement, hyperglobulinemia, heart murmurs, or gallops is more commonly seen in cats with heartworm disease than in cats with asthma or lungworm infestation.[10]

Treatment

Adults

Cats with heartworm disease have been successfully treated with thiacetarsamide (2.2 mg/kg IV at 8- to 12-hour intervals for 2 days), although it is not routinely advocated.[8, 10, 12, 36] Active cats may need sedation with a tranquilizer, such as a combination of ketamine and diazepam (Valium), to ensure safe administration of thiacetarsamide.[36] Some authors report a high prevalence of adverse reactions, including death from fulminant pulmonary edema and respiratory failure,[37] but slow injection of thiacetarsamide (i.e., over 1–2 minutes) should eliminate this problem.[36]

Embolization is the most important complication of adulticide treatment in cats. It can induce severe pulmonary infarction, hemoptysis, and dyspnea, and it is most likely to occur in cats with a strongly positive antigen test and a large heartworm mass. Death can be rapid, and clients should be warned that complications are more severe in cats than in dogs. The risk of postadulticide complications may even be greater than those posed by the slow, spontaneous death of heartworms in the asymptomatic cat.[35, 36]

Aspirin is of no benefit to cats with heartworm disease.[20] Oxygen, cage rest, and administration of corticosteroids (2–4 mg/kg of prednisone, IM or by mouth) should be considered in cats that develop dyspnea or cyanosis from pulmonary edema or thromboembolism.[36]

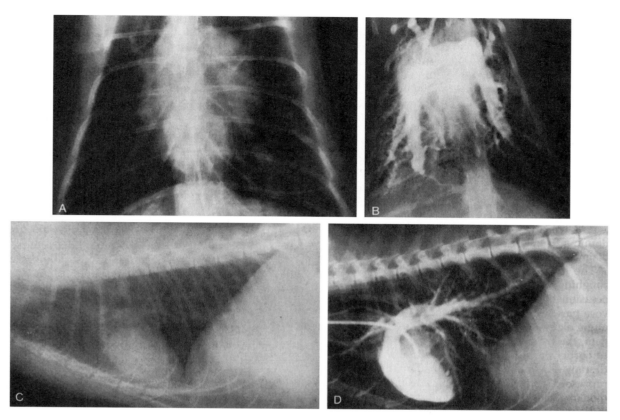

Figure 13-5
(A) Ventrodorsal radiograph of a cat infected with heartworms, showing marked prominence of the caudal pulmonary arteries. Severe radiographic changes are typical of the vascular lesions without cardiac changes. **(B)** Ventrodorsal radiograph taken 4 seconds after administration of contrast solution, illustrating the blunting of the pulmonary arteries. **(C)** Lateral radiograph of a cat with increased densities, especially in the caudal lung lobes. **(D)** Lateral radiograph taken 4 seconds after contrast administration, illustrating the blunting and embolization of the caudal arteries. Linear filling defects can be observed; these represent adult heartworms. (From Dillon R. Feline heartworm disease. In: Kirk RW, ed. Current Veterinary Therapy IX. Philadelphia, WB Saunders, 1986:422.)

Microfilariae

Because circulating microfilariae are rare in cats, they rarely require treatment.[12] However, cats that do have microfilariae have been successfully treated with levamisole hydrochloride, 4.4 mg/kg once by mouth.[36]

Prevention

Ivermectin has not yet been proven effective as a preventative in cats. Diethylcarbamazine has been safely administered to cats and can be used in susceptible cats in a highly endemic area. Routine prevention with diethylcarbamazine, however, is not currently recommended.[36]

References

1. Atkins CE. Heartworm disease. In: Allen DG, ed. Small Animal Medicine. Philadelphia, JB Lippincott, 1991: 341–363.
2. Calvert CA, Rawlings CA. Therapy of canine heartworm disease. In: Kirk RW, ed. Current Veterinary Therapy IX. Philadelphia, WB Saunders, 1986;406–419.
3. Hribernik TN. Canine and feline heartworm disease. In: Kirk RW, Bonagura JD, eds. Current Veterinary Therapy IX. Philadelphia, WB Saunders, 1989;263–270.
4. Atkins CE. Pathophysiology of heartworm caval syndrome: Recent advances. In: Otto GF, ed. Proceedings of the Heartworm Symposium. Washington, DC, The Heartworm Society, 1989;27–31.
5. Rawlings CA, McCall JW, Lewis RE. The response of the

canine's heart and lungs to *Dirofilaria immitis*. J Am Anim Hosp Assoc 1978;14:17–32.

6. Lombard CW, Buergelt CD. Echocardiographic and clinical findings in dogs with heartworm-induced cor pulmonale. Compen Contin Educ Pract Vet 1983; 1971–982.

7. Dillon R. Feline heartworm disease. In: Kirk RW, ed. Current Veterinary Therapy IX. Philadelphia, WB Saunders, 1986;420–424.

8. Green BJ, Lord PF, Grieve RB. Occult dirofilariasis confirmed by angiography and serology. J Am Anim Hosp Assoc 1983;19:847–854.

9. Rawlings CA. Cardiopulmonary function in the dog with *Dirofilaria immitis* infection: During infection and after treatment. Am J Vet Res 1980;41:319–325.

10. Calvert CA. Eosinophilic pulmonary granulomatosis. In: Kirk RW, Bonagura JD, eds. Current Veterinary Therapy XI. Philadelphia, WB Saunders, 1992;813–816.

11. Dillon R, Brawner B. Right-sided heart failure in heartworm dogs. In: Otto GF, ed. Proceedings of the Heartworm Symposium. Washington, DC, The Heartworm Society, 1989;173–177.

12. Atkins CE. Heartworm disease: An update on prevention, diagnosis, and management. Waltham/OSU Symposium for the Treatment of Small Animal Disease. Vernon, California, Waltham USA, Inc, 1994;97–106.

13. Henry CJ, Dillon R. Heartworm disease in dogs. J Am Vet Med Assoc 1994;204:1148–1151.

14. Courtney CH, Zeng Q-Y. Applications of heartworm immunodiagnostic tests. In: Otto GF, ed. Proceedings of the Heartworm Symposium. Washington, DC, The Heartworm Society, 1989;167–172.

15. Reference deleted.

16. Thrall DE, Badertscher RR, Lewis RE, et al. Radiographic changes associated with developing dirofilariasis in experimentally infected dogs. Am J Vet Res 1980;41:81–90.

17. Badertscher RR II, Losonsky JM, Paul AJ, et al. Two-dimensional echocardiography for diagnosis of dirofilariasis in nine dogs. J Am Vet Med Assoc 1988;193:843–846.

18. Keith JC, Rawlings CA, Schaub RG. Treatment of canine dirofilariasis: Pulmonary thromboembolism caused by thiacetarsamide. Microscopic changes. Am J Vet Res 1983;44:1272–1277.

19. Calvert CA, Thrall DE. Treatment of canine heartworm disease coexisting with right-sided heart failure. J Am Vet Med Assoc 1982;180:1201–1203.

20. Rawlings CA, Keith JC, Losonsky JM, et al. Aspirin and prednisolone modification of postadulticide pulmonary arterial disease in heartworm-infected dogs: Arteriographic study. Am J Vet Res 1983;44:821–827.

21. Luethy MW, Sisson DD, Kneiller SK, et al. Angiographic assessment of aspirin and heparin therapy for the prevention of pulmonary thromboembolism following adulticide therapy. In: Otto GF, ed. Proceedings of the Heartworm Symposium. Washington, DC, The Heartworm Society, 1989;53–57.

22. Ishihara K, Sasaki Y, Kitagawa H. Removal of canine heartworms using flexible alligator forceps: The con-struction and manipulation of the forceps, removal techniques and efficiency. In: Otto GF, ed. Proceedings of the Heartworm Symposium. Washington, DC, The Heartworm Society, 1989;33–43.

23. Jackson RF, Seymour WG, Growney PJ, et al. Surgical treatment of the caval syndrome of canine heartworm disease. J Am Vet Med Assoc 1977;171:1065–1069.

24. Jackson, RF. Treatment of heartworm disease. California Veterinarian: Proceedings of the Heartworm Symposium, Washington, DC, 1989;26–30.

25. Sasaki Y, Kitagawa H, Ishihara K. Clinical and pathological effects of heartworm removal from the pulmonary arteries using flexible alligator forceps. In: Otto GF, ed. Proceedings of the Heartworm Symposium. Washington, DC, The Heartworm Society, 1989;45–51.

26. Neer TM, Hoskins JD. Clinical experience with ivermectin used as a microfilaricide and for prophylaxis in the dog. In: Otto GF, ed. Proceedings of the Heartworm Symposium. Washington, DC, The Heartworm Society, 1989;95–97.

27. McManus ED, Pulliam JD. Histopathologic features of canine heartworm microfilarial infection after treatment with ivermectin. Am J Vet Res 1984;45:91–97.

28. Blagburn BL, Hendrix CM, Lindsay DS, et al. Milbemycin: efficacy and toxicity in beagle and collie dogs. In: Otto GF, ed. Proceedings of the Heartworm Symposium. Washington, DC: The Heartworm Society, 1989;109–113.

29. Fassler PE, Tranquilli WJ, Paul AJ, et al. Evaluation of the safety of ivermectin administered in a beef-based formulation to ivermectin-sensitive Collies. J Am Vet Med Assoc 1991;199:457–460.

30. Carr AP, Johnson GS. A review of hemostatic abnormalities in dogs and cats. J Am Anim Hosp Assoc 1994;30:475–482.

31. Atkins CE, Keene BW, McGuirk SM. Pathophysiologic mechanism of cardiac dysfunction in experimentally induced heartworm caval syndrome in dogs: An echocardiographic study. Am J Vet Res 1988;49:403–410.

32. Heartworm Society. Recommended procedures for the diagnosis and management of heartworm (*Dirofilaria immitis*) infection. In: Otto GF, ed. Proceedings of the Heartworm Symposium. Washington, DC, The Heartworm Society, 1989;229–232.

33. Rawlings CA, Calvert CA, Glaus TM, Jacobs GJ. Surgical removal of heartworms. Semin Vet Med Surg (Small Anim) 1994;9:200–205.

34. Wong MM, Petersen NC, Cullen J. Dirofilariasis in cats. J Am Anim Hosp Assoc 1983;19:855–864.

35. Calvert CA, Mandell CP. Diagnosis and management of feline heartworm disease. J Am Vet Med Assoc 1982;180:550–552.

36. Dillon R. Clinical management of feline heartworm disease. California Veterinarian: Proceedings of the Heartworm Symposium, Washington, DC, 1989;36–37.

37. Turner JL, Lees GE, Brown SA, et al. In: Otto GF, ed. Thiacetarsamide in normal cats: Pharmacokinetic, clinical and laboratory features. Proceedings of the Heartworm Symposium. Washington, DC, The Heartworm Society, 1989;135–141.

Congenital Heart Defects

Betsy R. Bond

Congenital heart disease is diagnosed in approximately 0.5% to 0.85% of all dogs examined by veterinarians, and this percentage seems to be increasing. The apparent increase in prevalence is probably a result of more-accurate diagnostic methods and more veterinary cardiologists.[1] Any young animal with a heart murmur should be suspected of having a congenital cardiac defect unless the murmur is a low-grade, innocent murmur. Innocent murmurs, which are heard in many young dogs, usually disappear by 16 weeks of age.[2]

Congenital heart defects are less common in cats than in dogs. Table 14–1 lists defects in cats in order of frequency. The defects in cats tend to be more complex and more difficult to diagnose. However, in general, simple heart defects are associated with the same pathophysiology as in dogs, and all that is said about dogs in that regard is applicable to cats. The other difference between cats and dogs is that cats experience fewer problems and live longer with congenital heart defects, probably because they are more likely to rest when they are tired and thus to preserve their myocardial reserve.

Knowledge of the pathophysiology and common cardiac abnormalities seen on physical examination, electrocardiography (ECG), and radiography can often lead the veterinarian to an accurate diagnosis without specialized tests, although echocardiography (especially with Doppler) is extremely helpful. The signalment can help guide the veterinarian to concentrate on the most common anomaly for a particular breed, although breed predisposition alone does not guarantee a diagnosis of a specific congenital defect.[3] For example, in a litter of Newfoundlands that I recently examined, two dogs had subaortic stenosis on echocardiography, but a third puppy in the same litter had pulmonary stenosis. Auscultation was similar in all three dogs. Also, complex defects or defects with unusual characteristics require echocardiography with color flow and spectral Doppler or selective angiography for diagnosis.[3]

Problem Identification

Murmur

A murmur is an abnormal sound that occurs between the first and second heart sounds (systolic murmur) or between the second and first heart sounds (diastolic murmur). It is the most common finding on physical examination in dogs and cats with congenital heart disease.

An innocent murmur is a soft (grade I/VI to II/VI), systolic murmur with greatest intensity in the area of the left cranial thorax. It may be confused with an early pulmonary or subvalvular aortic stenosis. A murmur that is grade III/VI to VI/VI, continuous, diastolic, or heard best over the right hemithorax or over the mitral valve is probably not an innocent murmur[2] (see Chap. 9).

Pathophysiology

Murmurs are caused by turbulent blood flow within the heart or near it. They result from stenotic (narrow) valves, dysplastic valves that do not close properly and lead to regurgitation, abnormal openings between the chambers of the heart (septal defects), or abnormal connections between vessels (patent ductus arteriosus). The defect determines the point of maximal intensity, timing, and radiation of the murmur. Congenital defects that are not associated with murmurs include some right-to-left shunts.[3]

Clinical Signs

History and clinical signs are also determined by the type and severity of the defect. Outflow obstructions such as pulmonary and aortic stenosis cause exercise intolerance or syncope, whereas volume overloads such as patent ductus arteriosus usually cause signs of left-sided heart failure (i.e., coughing and dyspnea). Right-to-left shunts can cause cyanosis and polycythemia (packed cell volume [PCV] <65%) before other signs develop.[3] Ascites is usually caused by right-sided defects such as tricuspid dysplasia and long-standing pulmonary stenosis.

Diagnostic Plan

The physical examination is the important first step in diagnosing a congenital heart problem in dogs and cats. After that, the minimum database needed

Table 14–1

Relative Incidence of the Most Common Feline Congenital Cardiovascular Anomalies

Atrioventricular valve malformation

  Mitral valve complex malformation
  Tricuspid valve complex dysplasia

Ventricular septal defect
Endocardial fibroelastosis
Patent ductus arteriosus
Vascular anomalies

  Persistent right aortic arch
  Venous anomalies

Aortic stenosis
Tetralogy of Fallot
Atrial septal defect
Common atrioventricular canal
Pulmonary stenosis

Table 14–2
Breed Predispositions for Congenital Cardiac Disorders

DISORDER	BREEDS PREDISPOSED
Patent ductus arteriosus	Poodle, Pomeranian, collie, Shetland sheepdog, English springer spaniel, cocker spaniel, Irish setter, German shepherd, Maltese, Yorkshire terrier
Pulmonary stenosis	English bulldog, cocker spaniel, terrier, miniature schnauzer, Chihuahua, beagle, Samoyed
Aortic stenosis	Newfoundland, golden retriever, German shepherd, rottweiler, boxer
Tetralogy of Fallot	Keeshond, English bulldog
Persistent right aortic arch	German shepherd, Irish setter
Mitral insufficiency	English bulldog, Chihuahua, Great Dane
Tricuspid insufficiency	Great Dane, weimaraner
Ventricular septal defect	English bulldog
Atrial septal defect	Samoyed

Data from Buchanan JW. Causes and prevalence of cardiovascular disease. In: Kirk RW, Bonagura JD, eds. Current Veterinary Therapy XI. Philadelphia, WB Saunders, 1992:647–655 and Gompf RE. The clinical approach to heart disease: history and physical examination. In: Fox PR, ed. Canine and Feline Cardiology. Philadelphia, WB Saunders, 1988:29–42.

includes thoracic radiographs, ECG, and echocardiogram, preferably with Doppler echocardiography. If a right-to-left shunt is suspected, PCV and arterial blood gases should also be determined.[3]

The type, loudness, and location of the heart murmur often lead to a presumptive diagnosis. Systolic murmurs located at the left base are usually caused by aortic stenosis, pulmonary stenosis,[3–5] or tetralogy of Fallot. These murmurs are crescendo-decrescendo murmurs; that is, they are softest at the beginning and end and loudest in midsystole. The murmur of aortic stenosis often radiates to the right cranial thorax or up the carotid arteries.[3, 4, 6] Pulmonary and aortic stenoses can often be differentiated by ECG: pulmonary stenosis causes a right axis deviation,[3–5, 7, 8] and in animals with aortic stenosis the ECG is either normal or indicative of left ventricular enlargement (tall and wide R waves).[9] Pulses are normal in dogs with pulmonary stenosis[3, 5] and mild aortic stenosis but are weak in dogs with moderate to severe aortic stenosis.[3, 4] Knowing breed predisposition is also helpful (Table 14–2).

Radiographic changes include right ventricular enlargement with a prominent main pulmonary artery bulge in pulmonary stenosis[3–5, 7, 8] and left ventricular enlargement in aortic stenosis. The aortic bulge is not always visualized in dogs with aortic stenosis.[3, 4, 6, 7] Pulmonary stenosis and tetralogy of Fallot cause similar ECG and radiographic changes and usually require other tests for differentiation.[4, 5, 7, 10] The simplest is a PCV, which is often elevated (>65%) in symptomatic dogs and cats with tetralogy of Fallot but normal in animals with pulmonary stenosis.[4, 10] Echocardiography with a bubble study (injection of 3 to 6 mL of agitated saline into a peripheral vein) is also helpful.

The murmur of a patent ductus arteriosus is distinct enough to lead to the diagnosis based on auscultation alone, but it is sometimes missed. A systolic murmur heard at the left apex could be associated with patent ductus arteriosus, ventricular septal defect, or mitral valve dysplasia. Because most routine auscultation procedures begin at the left ventricular apex, a murmur of mitral insufficiency is often the first murmur heard. The continuous murmur of patent ductus occasionally is auscultated only very cranially, and it is easily missed in dogs with faint diastolic murmurs.[3, 4, 11] Pulses are hyperdynamic in patent ductus arteriosus and normal in ventricular septal defect or mitral valve dysplasia. ECG is normal or indicates left ventricular or left atrial enlargement in all three defects.[3, 4, 11, 12]

Radiographic changes that are diagnostic for patent ductus arteriosus include three bulges on a ventrodorsal film: aortic, pulmonary, and left atrial. The left ventricle is also enlarged, and there is overcirculation of the lungs.[3, 4, 7, 11, 12] The murmur in dogs and cats with ventricular septal defect is holosystolic and is louder on the right thorax than on the left. Radiographs in animals with ventricular septal defect are usually normal, but if the defect is large they may reveal left ventricular enlargement.

Echocardiography is usually the best single test to diagnose congenital heart defects. In dogs and cats with pulmonary stenosis, the right ventricle is hypertrophied and often dilated. The pulmonary valve is thickened, and a poststenotic bulge is present.[4, 5, 8, 13] Aortic stenosis causes a hypertrophied left ventricle in severe cases. A fibrous ring is often seen just below the aortic valve leaflets.[4, 6, 14] In animals with ventricular septal defect, the defect itself is often seen on two-dimensional echocardiography.[13, 15, 16] The size of the ventricular septal defect determines the amount of left ventricular and left atrial enlargement, with a larger defect causing a more significant volume overload. The ductus in patent ductus arteriosus can be visualized by a skilled and experienced echocardiographer.[4, 7] In addition, the left atrium and ventricle are usually dilated in animals with patent ductus arteriosus, and the shortening fraction may be decreased.[4, 11, 13, 15] An injection of agitated saline into a peripheral vein during echocardiography reveals a right-to-left shunt (e.g., in tetralogy of Fallot).[4, 13, 17] Doppler echocardiography can be invaluable in some dogs and cats.

Nonselective angiography can also be used to diagnose congenital heart defects. Right-to-left shunts are diagnosed by visualizing the aorta before dye has circulated through the lungs, left atrium, and left ventricle. Right ventricular hypertrophy and a post-stenotic pulmonary artery bulge are seen in animals with pulmonary stenosis. A patent ductus arteriosus is seen after dye has circulated through the lungs and returned to the left side of the heart.[7]

Exercise Intolerance

Exercise intolerance is an inability to complete normal activities without resting. See Chapter 9 for a complete discussion of exercise intolerance.

Pathophysiology

Exercise intolerance in dogs and cats with congenital heart disease is usually caused by an outflow obstruction such as aortic or pulmonary stenosis,[3, 5, 6, 18] but it may also result from severe left-sided heart failure or right-to-left shunt.[4, 10] Exercise increases the body's need for oxygen, but the narrow outflow prevents normal circulation of blood to the lungs or to the peripheral tissues.

Clinical Signs

Exercise and play time are shorter compared with normal, and activity suddenly ceases so that the dog or cat can rest and pant before resuming play. If the exercise intolerance is caused by aortic or pulmonary stenosis, the main finding on physical examination is a heart murmur. In addition, aortic stenosis causes weak pulses that are directly correlated with severity of disease (i.e., the weaker the pulse, the more severe the stenosis). Dogs with left-sided heart failure should be dyspneic, and crackles should be auscultated along with the murmur.

Diagnostic Plan

Auscultation of a murmur in young dogs with exercise intolerance is reason to suspect congenital heart disease. The diagnostic plan is the same as for heart murmurs.

Syncope

Syncope is loss of consciousness caused by deprivation of oxygen to the brain because of cessation of blood flow to the cerebrum. It is often difficult to distinguish between syncope, seizures, and episodic weakness.[19] See Chapter 9 for a complete discussion of syncope.

Pathophysiology

Cardiac syncope is usually caused by a paroxysmal arrhythmia, a hypoxic event from a right-to-left shunt, or a ventricular outflow tract obstruction.[2–6, 10, 19] Left ventricular outflow tract obstruction, which can be either fixed or dynamic, is the most common cause of syncope in animals with congenital heart disease. In dogs with a fixed outflow obstruction, a fibrous ring keeps the outflow tract the same size throughout systole. A dynamic outflow obstruction is caused by abnormal mitral valve motion. The mitral valve is either pulled or pushed into the left ventricular outflow tract in systole, causing maximum obstruction after midsystole.[20] During exercise, more oxygen is needed and systemic resistance drops, but the obstruction prevents an increase in cardiac output. Perfusion is decreased because of low systemic resistance, and syncope occurs.[19]

Clinical Signs

Dogs with syncope secondary to an outflow obstruction are normal at rest, but they collapse with strenuous exercise. They usually have a harsh systolic murmur of at least grade III/VI intensity over the left base of the heart, consistent with pulmonary or aortic stenosis. Dogs with aortic stenosis also have weak or absent pulses, whereas dogs with pulmonary stenosis have normal pulses.[3, 5, 6]

Diagnostic Plan

The diagnostic plan is the same as for murmurs. Evidence of right ventricular enlargement (right axis deviation on the ECG and right ventricular enlargement with a pulmonary artery bulge on thoracic radiography) is present in dogs with pulmonary stenosis. Changes consistent with left ventricular enlargement (tall, wide QRS complexes on the ECG and left ventricular enlargement on thoracic radiography) are seen in dogs with aortic stenosis. Dogs with a right-to-left shunt are polycythemic and hypoxemic.[3, 4, 10]

Cough

Coughing is a forced expiration of material from the respiratory tract. In dogs with congenital heart disease, it is usually caused by pulmonary edema. The most common defect causing left-sided heart failure in dogs is patent ductus arteriosus, although a large ventricular septal defect can also cause left-sided heart failure.[4] See Chapters 9 and 54 for a complete discussion of cough.

Pathophysiology

Pulmonary edema in patent ductus arteriosus is caused by a volume overload to the lungs that eventually overwhelms the pulmonary vasculature and floods the alveoli. Patent ductus arteriosus is the most common congenital cause of pulmonary edema.

Clinical Signs

Dogs with patent ductus arteriosus and left-sided heart failure usually develop signs gradually over weeks to months. Exercise intolerance is often present. A loud continuous murmur of at least grade III/VI intensity is auscultated over the left base of the heart. Pulses are hyperdynamic unless myocardial failure or atrial fibrillation is present. An irregularly irregular rhythm with pulse deficits of atrial fibrillation occurs in dogs with severe or long-standing patent ductus arteriosus.[4]

Diagnostic Plan

The diagnostic plan is the same as for murmurs. A tall R wave with a normal axis is the most common ECG finding in dogs with patent ductus arteriosus, but atrial fibrillation may be present in dogs with long-standing disease. The classic ventrodorsal radiograph reveals three bulges—at the 12 o'clock, 2 o'clock, and 3 o'clock positions—representing the aorta, pulmonary artery, and left atrial appendage, respectively. Also, the heart appears long on the ventrodorsal film. Vessels appear prominent because of overcirculation of the lung fields.

Dyspnea

Dyspnea is an increase in the work required for respiration. It is the second most common sign of heart disease in dogs and is the most common sign (along with anorexia and lethargy) in cats. See Chapters 9 and 52 for a complete discussion of dyspnea.

Pathophysiology

Dyspnea is usually caused by congestive heart failure or cyanotic heart disease.[3] Pulmonary edema is associated with left-sided heart failure and is usually caused by patent ductus arteriosus. Pleural effusion is caused by right-sided heart disease in dogs but is less common than ascites. Pleural effusion in cats is caused by right- or left-sided heart failure. Cyanotic heart disease is usually caused by tetralogy of Fallot.[4, 10]

Clinical Signs

Dyspnea in cats is usually accompanied by lethargy and anorexia. Dogs in heart failure usually have dyspnea combined with coughing.

Diagnostic Plan

Diagnostic tests must often be postponed because of the stress they represent to a dyspneic animal. However, thoracentesis in a dyspneic animal with pleural effusion is both diagnostic and therapeutic.

Thoracic radiographs should be taken as soon as possible. ECGs, echocardiograms, and blood tests (PCV and blood gas determinations) should be performed next. A bubble study should be done during echocardiography if a right-to-left shunt is suspected.

Cyanosis

Cyanosis is a bluish tinge to the mucous membranes; it is caused by poorly oxygenated blood.

Pathophysiology

Cyanosis in animals with congenital heart disease is caused by a right-to-left shunt, congestive heart failure, or cyanotic lung disease. Two features must be present in animals with a right-to-left shunt in order for cyanosis to occur: a defect in the partitions of the heart or great vessels and an obstruction to pulmonary flow.[4] Right-to-left defects cause cyanosis because blood is shunted into the peripheral circulation before it circulates through the lungs for oxygenation. Congestive heart failure causes cyanosis because of pulmonary edema that hinders normal oxygenation.

Clinical Signs

Most dogs and cats are examined because of lethargy, weakness, and stunted growth. They may display exercise intolerance and dyspnea. Mucous membranes have a bluish tinge. A murmur caused by pulmonary stenosis is heard over the base of the heart on the left side if tetralogy of Fallot is present. A right-to-left shunt caused by a ventricular septal defect and patent ductus arteriosus is rare and is characterized by an absence of a heart murmur and occasionally a split second heart sound. A right-to-left shunt usually causes a right axis deviation on the ECG and right ventricular enlargement with a pulmonary artery bulge on thoracic radiographs.[7]

Diagnostic Plan

The diagnostic plan is the same as for murmur. A bubble study should be done during echocardiography; it is positive in animals with tetralogy of Fallot or right-to-left ventricular septal defects. It is difficult to see bubbles in animals with right-to-left patent ductus arteriosus because of the extracardiac location of the ductus (i.e., echolucent bubbles are seen flowing from the pulmonary artery directly into the aorta). Because bubbles should be cleared by the pulmonary capillaries, only those bubbles that flow directly from the right to the left side of the heart are visible.[17] If the bubble study is negative, nonselective or selective angiography may reveal the source of the shunt. A PCV often shows polycythemia.

Polycythemia

Polycythemia is an abnormally high number of circulating red blood cells.

Pathophysiology

Polycythemia in animals with congenital heart disease is often caused by hypoxia from a right-to-left shunt. Hypoxia stimulates erythropoietin production in the kidney, which causes increased production and release of red blood cells from the bone marrow. A PCV greater than 65% is likely to cause clinical signs because of increased blood viscosity and decreased oxygenation.[3, 4]

Clinical Signs

Symptomatic dogs display syncope or exercise intolerance. Cyanosis is usually seen on physical examination, and a murmur may be auscultated over the base of the left side of the heart.

Diagnostic Plan

After an elevated hematocrit is found, the diagnostic plan is the same as for murmur. Most dogs have ECG and radiographic signs of right ventricular enlargement. A bubble study should be done during echocardiography, and if it is negative, cardiac catheterization should be performed.

Abnormal Arterial Pulses

Hyperdynamic pulses are often palpated in animals with patent ductus arteriosus. There is a widened pulse pressure, caused by the run-off in diastole from the aorta to the pulmonary artery. Pulses are decreased in intensity in dogs with subaortic stenosis.[3] The severity of the stenosis is often correlated with the weakness of the pulse. See Chapter 9 for a complete discussion of abnormal pulses.

Patent Ductus Arteriosus

Patent ductus arteriosus is the most frequently diagnosed congenital cardiac defect in dogs.[1, 4, 11, 21] It has been reported in cats but is uncommon. Patent ductus arteriosus is usually an isolated defect (i.e., no other defects exist with it).[4] It also tends to occur in purebred female dogs,[2, 4, 12, 17] and it has been found to be inherited in poodles.[4] Table 14–2 lists breeds of dogs in which patent ductus arteriosus is commonly diagnosed.

Pathophysiology

Patent ductus arteriosus is a connection between the pulmonary artery and aorta at the level of the bifurcation of the pulmonary arteries. It is normal in fetal circulation and allows blood from the right ventricle to bypass the unexpanded lungs and go to the placenta, the fetal organ of oxygenation.[22] It should close within hours after birth[17] as a response to the sudden rise in arterial partial pressure of oxygen. Failure to close is related to a lack of oxygen at birth or, more likely in animals, to a primary anatomic defect of the elastic tissue within the wall of the ductus.[22]

In animals with patent ductus arteriosus, pulmonary vascular resistance is less than that of the systemic circulation in both systole and diastole. This hemodynamic situation encourages continuous flow of blood from the aorta through the pulmonary artery to the lungs (i.e., left-to-right shunt) (Fig. 14–1). Filling pressures are normal on the right side of the heart, but the filling pressures of the left side of the heart and pulmonary vessels are high because of a volume overload.[2, 4, 17]

Rarely, a right-to-left shunt develops in dogs with patent ductus arteriosus[17, 23] because of increased pulmonary artery pressure caused by high pulmonary artery flow. However, a pulmonary vascular defect probably coexists and predisposes animals to develop pulmonary hypertension and a right-to-left shunt. Dogs that do not have surgery usually die of left-sided congestive heart failure rather than have a change in the direction of their shunt.

Clinical Signs

Most dogs display normal growth and do not show clinical signs. Clinical signs, if present, include those of left-sided heart failure (coughing, dyspnea, and exercise intolerance). The murmur is usually discovered on routine examination when the puppy is vaccinated. The murmur of patent ductus arteriosus is the most characteristic of all congenital heart defects. It is a continuous murmur that is heard best high at the base of the heart under the left axilla.[2, 3, 4, 17] The diastolic portion of the murmur is localized in some

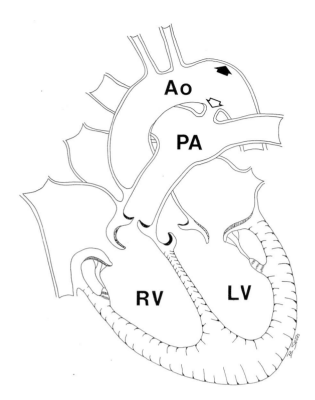

Figure 14-1
Diagram of a dog with patent ductus arteriosus. Bulges are present in the aorta *(solid arrow)* and the pulmonary artery because of turbulence through the patent ductus arteriosus *(open arrow)*. The left atrium and left ventricle are often dilated. Ao, aorta; LV, left ventricle; PA, pulmonary artery; RV, right ventricle.

dogs and is easily missed if thorough auscultation is not performed.[4] A murmur of mitral regurgitation can also be auscultated over the left ventricular apex.[2, 3, 4] Palpation over the anterior thorax usually reveals a thrill (vibration), and pulses are usually hyperdynamic.[2, 4, 17]

Diagnostic Plan

Diagnosis is usually made on the basis of signalment and physical examination. Any small-breed female dog with a murmur is considered to have a patent ductus arteriosus until proven otherwise. Ancillary tests that confirm the diagnosis and indicate the severity of the defect include ECG and radiography. Echocardiography and angiography may be helpful in dogs that do not display typical findings on physical examination or on diagnostic tests.

The ECG early in the course of disease or in dogs that are mildly affected is normal, but most dogs display a tall R wave (Fig. 14-2) and wide P waves in lead II.[2-4, 12, 17] Of all congenital heart defects, patent ductus arteriosus causes the most dramatically tall R

waves.[3] ECG abnormalities in dogs with severe or long-standing patent ductus arteriosus include atrial fibrillation,[3, 4, 17] sinus tachycardia, and ventricular premature complexes.[4]

Ventrodorsal radiographs in dogs with patent ductus arteriosus are diagnostic if they display the three characteristic bulges (aorta, pulmonary artery, and left atrium) with a long left ventricle (Fig. 14-3).[3] Other abnormalities include left ventricular and left atrial enlargement and overcirculated pulmonary arteries and veins.[2-4, 7, 12, 17] Pulmonary edema is present in dogs that have congestive heart failure.[3]

The ductus is not easily seen on an echocardiogram, but it may be found by an experienced echocardiographer.[4, 13, 15, 17] Doppler echocardiography is the best method to confirm patent ductus arteriosus. Continuous flow is seen in the pulmonary artery and can direct the echocardiographer to the ductus itself.[4, 13, 15, 16] Other common echocardiographic changes (e.g., left atrial and ventricular dilation)[13, 17] are not specific for patent ductus arteriosus.

Right-to-left shunting in animals with patent ductus arteriosus is rare[13, 15] and is not discussed in detail here. Dogs usually do not have a murmur on auscultation, but a split second heart sound may be present as a result of pulmonary hypertension.[4] ECG changes indicative of right ventricular hypertrophy include a right axis deviation with prominent S waves in leads I, II, II, and aVF and the right chest leads. Thoracic radiographs reveal evidence of pulmonary hypertension, such as right ventricular enlargement, pulmonary artery bulge, tortuous pulmonary vessels, and hypovascular lung fields.[3, 7] A bubble study does not reveal the ductus on an echocardiogram, because the ductus is too distal to be easily seen, but microbubbles may be detected in the abdominal aorta adjacent to the kidney.[13] The best diagnostic test is angiography, and even nonselective angiography demonstrates the ductus.[7]

Treatment

The treatment of choice is surgical ligation of the ductus in all dogs and cats with a left-to-right shunt,[4, 21, 24, 25] even if the animals are old.[12] Dogs who have congestive heart failure require rest, diuretics, and vasodilators before surgery. Dogs with supraventricular arrhythmias (e.g., atrial fibrillation) that increase the heart rate should also be treated with digoxin and either a β-blocker or a calcium channel blocker.[4] Surgery should not be attempted in animals with a right-to-left shunt.[17]

Prognosis

Prognosis is good if dogs are surgically treated before they are 1 year old,[4, 11] especially if the patent

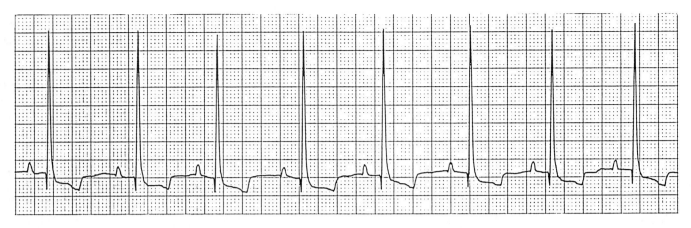

Figure 14-2
Lead II electrocardiogram in a 2.5-kg Maltese with patent ductus arteriosus. The R wave is almost 4 mV in height, which is extraordinarily tall for a dog this size.

ductus arteriosus is small.[17] The surgical death rate increases in dogs older than 2 years of age.[11] If dogs do not have surgery, 60% to 70% die within the first year or two of life,[4, 17, 21] and it is rare for a dog to live beyond 5 to 7 years with this condition.[23] In my experience, very small dogs (<2 kg) with congestive heart failure, dogs with severe myocardial failure, and dogs with atrial fibrillation have the poorest prognoses and may not survive surgery.

Subaortic (Aortic) Stenosis

Aortic stenosis used to be the third most common congenital defect in dogs after pulmonary stenosis, but it is now considered by many to be second in prevalence.[1] It may be supravalvular (rarely), valvular, or subvalvular.[4] The lesion in most dogs is characterized by an obstructive, fibromuscular band below the aortic valve in the left ventricular outflow tract[4, 6, 26]—hence the common term subvalvular stenosis or subaortic stenosis. It is inherited in Newfoundlands and is usually an isolated defect, although it may coexist with aortic insufficiency, pulmonary stenosis, or mitral regurgitation. The severity of subaortic stenosis ranges from mild, with only subvalvular fibrous nodules, to very severe, with a thick fibrous ring, aortic insufficiency, and mitral regurgitation.[2, 4, 6]

Pathophysiology

Subaortic stenosis causes a pressure overload to the left ventricle because of a fibrous ring located just below the aortic valve that narrows the left ventricular outflow tract (Fig. 14-4). The pressure overload causes left ventricular hypertrophy, which also causes narrowing of coronary arteries and decreased myocardial blood flow. The severity of the stenosis is directly related to the degree of hypertrophy: the more severe the stenosis, the thicker the left ventricle. If tachycardia occurs because of exercise or excitement, myocardial oxygen demand increases and the coronary arteries are not able to meet the demand (myocardial ischemia).

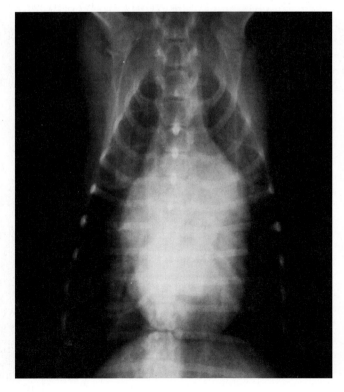

Figure 14-3
Ventrodorsal radiograph of a dog with patent ductus arteriosus. The aorta, pulmonary artery, and left atrium are seen as bulges at the 1 o'clock, 2 o'clock, and 3 o'clock positions, respectively. The left ventricle appears long.

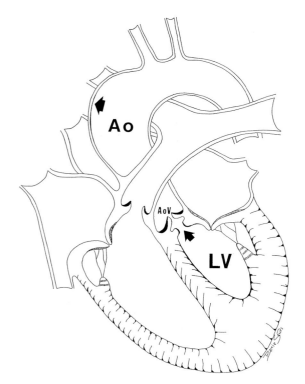

Figure 14–4
Diagram of aortic stenosis. There is a ring under the aortic valve *(arrow)* that causes high flow out of the aorta and a bulge in the ascending aorta *(thick arrow)*. The high pressure in the left ventricle causes left ventricular hypertrophy. Ao, aorta; AoV, aortic valve; LV, left ventricle.

If left ventricular pressure is high enough, left ventricular baroreceptors are stimulated, which causes reflex vasodilation, bradycardia,[4] and syncope. Myocardial ischemia also causes arrhythmias, decreased ventricular compliance, and decreased contractility.[2, 4, 26]

High-velocity systolic flow strikes the aortic valve and causes thickening of the valve, which then causes aortic insufficiency. If the aortic insufficiency is severe enough, the regurgitant blood flow causes diastolic fluttering of the mitral valve. Therefore, diastolic mitral valve fluttering on M-mode echocardiography is also suggestive of subaortic stenosis, even with a near-normal gradient.[2]

Clinical Signs

Aortic stenosis should be suspected in a dog of any commonly susceptible breed (see Table 14–2) with a crescendo-decrescendo murmur that is auscultated best at the left third to fourth intercostal space.[3, 4] The murmur may radiate up the carotid arteries and be auscultated in the cervical area,[3, 4, 6] or it may radiate to the ascending aorta, where it is auscultated at the right cranial thorax.[3] Dogs can be asymptomatic, or

they may be brought in for examination because of syncope or exercise intolerance.[3, 6] The left apex beat can be more prominent than is usual because of left ventricular hypertrophy, and pulses are slow-rising and attenuated.[3, 4] In general, the more severe the stenosis, the more attenuated the pulse and the louder the murmur.[2]

Diagnostic Plan

Tentative diagnosis is made on the basis of an auscultated murmur in a breed that is associated with subaortic stenosis (see Table 14–2). However, the absence of a murmur in a very young puppy does not guarantee that subaortic stenosis is not present, because dogs may not manifest a murmur for several weeks or months after birth.[4] In addition, breeds other than the common ones may develop subaortic stenosis.

ECG and radiography may or may not be helpful in diagnosing subaortic stenosis. Dogs that are mildly affected have a normal ECG, but severely affected dogs display a tall and wide QRS complex on lead II and S-T segment depression (Fig. 14–5). Ventricular premature complexes, ventricular tachycardia,[2, 9] and atrial fibrillation may also be present in dogs with severe subaortic stenosis. Radiographic changes, if present, include left ventricular enlargement and poststenotic aortic dilation (wide cranial mediastinum on the ventrodorsal film and loss of cranial waist on the lateral view) (Fig. 14–6).[2–4, 6, 7]

Echocardiography is the best tool for both diagnosis and prognosis, because the degree of left ventricular hypertrophy can be seen on an echocardiogram.[4, 6, 14] Other abnormalities consistent with subaortic stenosis include an echo-dense ridge or band just below the aortic valve (Fig. 14–7), poststenotic aortic bulge, narrow left ventricular outflow tract, partial aortic valve closure during systole, thick aortic valves, and mitral valve fluttering.[4, 13, 14] Doppler echocardiography is a noninvasive method for determining the severity of the stenosis; the gradient can be calculated from the velocity of blood flow through the stenotic area.[4, 13, 15, 16, 27, 28] Puppies with mild subaortic stenosis, especially giant-breed dogs, may worsen as they become adults.[6]

Cardiac catheterization and direct measurement of pressures can also determine the severity of the gradient, but anesthesia may cause the gradient to appear lower than it actually is.[4, 6] Cardiac catheterization is not usually performed unless aortic balloon dilation is done.

Treatment

Treatment is related to severity of stenosis and consists of medical control or surgical correction. Mild

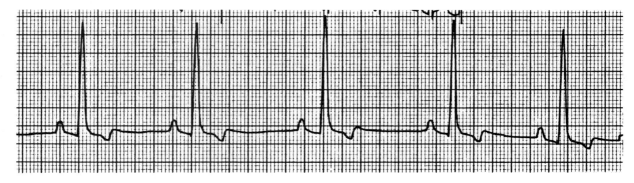

Figure 14–5
Lead II electrocardiogram of a golden retriever with subaortic stenosis. The QRS complexes are tall (3 mV in height) and wide (0.06 sec).

subaortic stenosis is not treated. Moderate subaortic stenosis with a gradient between 50 and 80 mm Hg is treated on an individual basis.[26] If a dog has syncope, exercise intolerance, or ventricular arrhythmias, β-blockers[29] or calcium channel blockers can be used. The effect of medical therapy on mortality is unknown,[4, 26] but in my experience some animals respond favorably (i.e., less syncope or exercise intolerance) to β-blockers.[2] Atenolol (Tenormin, 0.25–1.0 mg/kg by mouth, once or twice per day) is my preferred β-blocker.

Open heart surgery has been performed in some dogs with success. Balloon aortic valvuloplasty has also been attempted; it was reported to be immediately successful in 50% of the dogs undergoing the procedure,[2, 6] but long-term results are unknown. In my experience in a limited number of dogs, the fibrous ring is extremely hard to break down with a balloon, and the rate of recurrence is high. A conduit from the left ventricle to the aorta has been attempted[29] but is not widely recommended.[25]

Prognosis

Dogs with mild subaortic stenosis have a good prognosis for a long life without symptoms. Dogs with mild to moderate stenosis have a good to fair prognosis but tend to develop infective endocarditis and left-sided heart failure later in life (after 5 years of age). Dogs with severe subaortic stenosis have a poor prognosis; most die suddenly before 3 years of age or develop left-sided heart failure.[4, 6, 18]

Aortic Stenosis in Cats

Aortic stenosis in cats is relatively rare but has been reported. In general, it is associated with a poor prognosis, with most cats dying of congestive heart failure. As in dogs, it is also caused by a fibrous band beneath the aortic valve, which leads to left ventricular, left atrial, and aortic dilation. High aortic flow can be seen on a Doppler echocardiogram. Furosemide and nitroglycerin ointment are used in cats with acute pulmonary edema secondary to subaortic stenosis. The

Figure 14–6
Lateral radiograph of a 1-year-old Newfoundland with subaortic stenosis. The aorta bulges cranial to the heart (*arrow*).

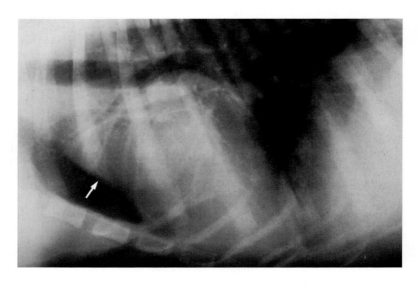

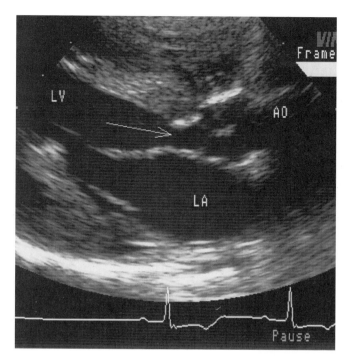

Figure 14–7
Echocardiogram of a 9-month-old mixed breed dog with subaortic stenosis from the right parasternal long-axis view. The arrow points to the narrowed subvalvular area. The hyperechoic area above the narrowing represents the fibrous tissue of subaortic stenosis. There is severe hypertrophy of the left ventricular free wall and septum. AO, aorta; LA, left atrium; LV, left ventricular cavity.

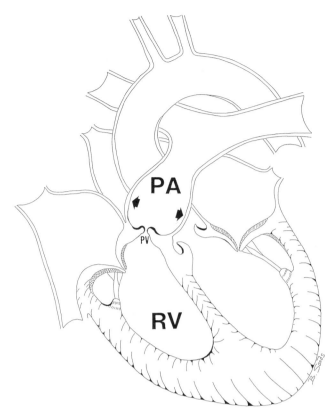

Figure 14–8
Diagram of pulmonary stenosis. The pulmonary valves (PV) are thickened, causing right ventricle hypertrophy and a pulmonary artery bulge distal to the stenosis *(arrows)*. PA, main pulmonary artery; RV, right ventricle.

effectiveness of β-blockers for long-term treatment is unproven.[30]

Pulmonary Stenosis

Pulmonary stenosis is a common defect in dogs.[1, 31] It usually occurs as an isolated defect, and it can be supravalvular (rare), valvular, or subvalvular (infundibular).[4, 5] Most dogs have dysplasia of the valves (i.e., thickening, fusion, and hypoplasia of the leaflets)[2, 5] that causes secondary subvalvular stenosis.[4, 5] An anomalous left main coronary artery that originates from a single right coronary artery has also been described in English bulldogs and boxers with pulmonary stenosis.[2, 31]

Pathophysiology

Pulmonary valve dysplasia causes narrowing at the level of the pulmonary valves (pulmonary stenosis). Pulmonary stenosis in turn increases systolic pressure to the right ventricle and causes right ventricular hypertrophy (Fig. 14–8). Subvalvular (infundibular) hypertrophy develops secondary to pulmonary stenosis, which worsens an already narrow right ventricular outflow tract. High right ventricular pressure inhibits right ventricular myocardial perfusion and causes ischemia and fibrosis. Ischemia and fibrosis, in turn, cause arrhythmias and impair right ventricular performance.[2, 4] Right-sided congestive heart failure is an end stage of pulmonary stenosis.[5]

Clinical Signs

In most dogs, pulmonary stenosis is diagnosed when a typical murmur is heard during a routine examination. The murmur is a crescendo-decrescendo murmur heard best at the second to third intercostal space low on the left thorax.[2–5] Symptomatic dogs have syncope, exercise intolerance, and right-sided congestive heart failure.[2, 3, 5] With severe pulmonary stenosis and right ventricular hypertrophy, a prominent beat is palpated on the right side near the right ventricular apex.[2–4] Arterial pulses are usually normal, but abnormal jugular pulses are evident in dogs with severe pulmonary stenosis.[3, 5]

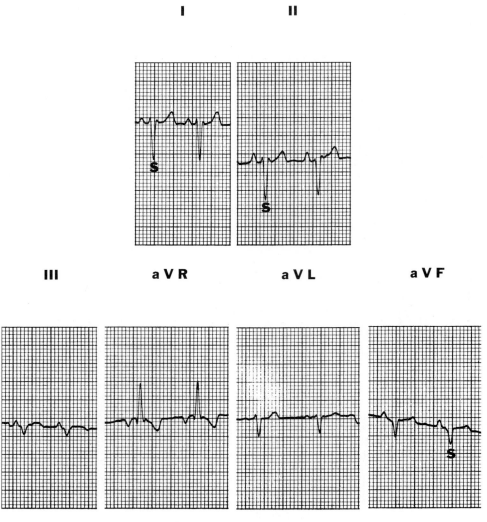

Figure 14-9
Right axis deviation in a puppy caused by right ventricular hypertrophy secondary to pulmonary stenosis. There are deep S waves in leads I, II, and aVF, and the axis is −150°.

Diagnostic Plan

Diagnosis of pulmonary stenosis is made on the basis of characteristic physical examination findings, especially in common breeds (see Table 14–2), along with findings on ECG, radiography, and echocardiography. The ECG is normal in dogs with mild cases of pulmonary stenosis, but a right axis deviation is found in dogs with more severe disease (Fig. 14–9). Radiographs usually reveal right ventricular enlargement and a pulmonary bulge at the 2 o'clock area on the ventrodorsal radiograph (Fig. 14–10).[2–5, 7, 8] Angiography reveals the stenosis, poststenotic dilation in the main pulmonary artery, and right ventricular hypertrophy (Fig. 14–11).[7]

Echocardiography is helpful both in diagnosing pulmonary stenosis and in estimating severity of disease. The most common echocardiographic abnormalities include right ventricular hypertrophy, thick and poorly movable pulmonary valve leaflets, and poststenotic dilation of the pulmonary artery (Fig. 14–12).[2, 4, 5, 8, 13] Doming of the pulmonary valve is also occasionally seen.[13, 32] The interventricular septum is often flattened in diastole because of the high right ventricular pressure.[2–4, 13] Doppler echocardiography can help estimate the pressure gradient from the velocity of blood flow distal to the stenosis.[2, 4, 13, 15, 16]

Treatment

Dogs that are asymptomatic and have a mild gradient (<50 mm Hg) need no treatment and usually live normally.[2, 4] Dogs with a gradient greater than

50 to 80 mm Hg according to Doppler echocardiography or catheterization, along with dogs that are symptomatic or have significant right ventricular hypertrophy, should undergo either surgical correction or balloon valvuloplasty. The techniques for surgical correction[33, 34] and balloon valvuloplasty[35] have been described. Both surgery and balloon valvuloplasty should be performed only by those experienced in the techniques. Ventricular arrhythmias, which are rare, require antiarrhythmic drugs.[4] Other medical therapy consists of administering drugs that slow the heart rate and preserve myocardial oxygenation, such as β-blockers.[4]

Prognosis

Dogs with mild pulmonary stenosis have a good prognosis for an asymptomatic, normal life span.[5] Dogs with severe pulmonary stenosis may do surprisingly well, even without surgical correction or balloon valvuloplasty. Prognosis with surgery or balloon valvuloplasty is variable. Balloon valvuloplasty is less invasive than surgery, but stenosis often recurs.[25] Balloon valvuloplasty produces better results in humans who have true pulmonary stenosis or valve

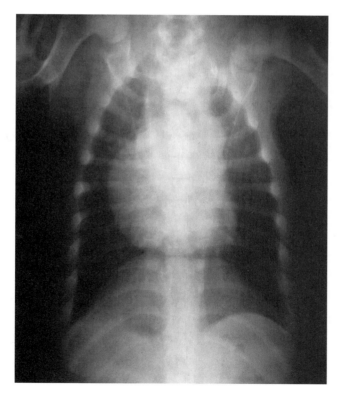

Figure 14–10
Ventrodorsal radiograph of a dog with pulmonary stenosis. The right ventricle is enlarged, and dilation of the main pulmonary artery is represented by a bulge at the 1 o'clock position.

fusion than in dogs that have pulmonary valve dysplasia.[36, 37]

Ventricular Septal Defect

Ventricular septal defects represent between 5% and 10% of all congenital heart defects in dogs. Most defects are between the ventricles only, although they may involve the atrioventricular valves and atrial septum. Ventricular septal defects usually occur in the membranous portion of the septum beneath the tricuspid valve, although they can also occur below the pulmonary valve (supracristal). Muscular ventricular septal defects are rare.[4]

Pathophysiology

Ventricular septal defects usually cause a volume overload to the left side of the heart. The amount of blood shunted depends on the size of the defect and the amount of pulmonary vascular resistance—the larger the defect and the lower the pulmonary artery pressure, the greater the flow. High shunt flows may also cause obstructive pulmonary vascular disease that decreases the amount of left-to-right shunting or even causes a right-to-left shunt.[3, 4]

Eisenmenger's syndrome is the term given to animals that have high pulmonary vascular resistance so that flow is right-to-left instead of left-to-right. It is more often associated with ventricular septal defects than with other defects.[38] The pulmonary hypertension causes unoxygenated blood to circulate and leads to polycythemia. If the PCV is high enough, animals can experience seizure or syncope during exercise because of hyperviscosity. A high PCV can also predispose an animal to thromboembolism.[3, 4]

Clinical Signs

Clinical signs depend on the size of the defect and whether there is a reverse shunt. Most dogs and cats remain asymptomatic, and some have spontaneous closure of the ventricular septal defect. Animals with large defects develop congestive heart failure because of a volume overload to the left side of the heart. Dogs that develop clinical signs (e.g., cough, exercise intolerance, lethargy) usually do so by 18 months of age.[4] Right-to-left shunts in dogs and cats with ventricular septal defects are rare.

Small ventricular septal defects are termed "restrictive," because there is restriction of flow from the left to the right ventricle.[15] These animals usually have loud, harsh, holosystolic murmurs that are heard best at the right cranial sternal border. Animals with very small ventricular septal defects may also have murmurs that are auscultated only in early systole

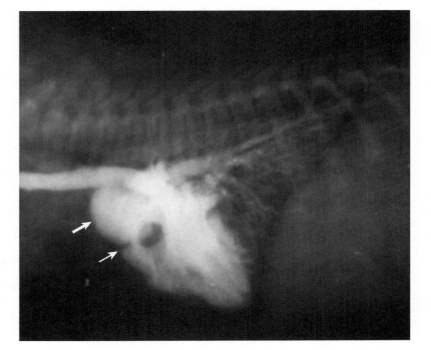

Figure 14–11
Nonselective angiogram of a dog with pulmonary stenosis. There is severe narrowing of the valvular area *(arrow)* and a bulge of the pulmonary artery above the stenosis *(thick arrow).*

because the defect closes during ventricular contraction. Large defects cause murmurs of variable intensity and may also cause a left basilar murmur because of high flow rates through the pulmonary valve. Arterial pulses vary.[2–4]

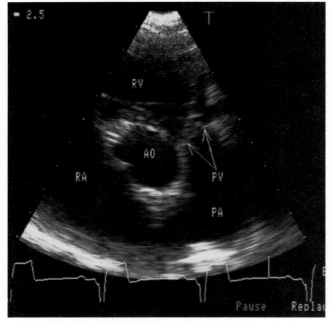

Figure 14–12
Echocardiogram of a dog with pulmonary stenosis from the right cranial short-axis view. There is malformation of the pulmonary valve *(arrows)* and dilation of the pulmonary artery below the valve (PA). AO, aorta; PV, pulmonary valve; RA, right atrium; RV, right ventricle.

Diagnostic Plan

Diagnosis is often made by echocardiography, especially if the defect is large enough to be seen. Doppler echocardiography reveals the turbulent flow in the right ventricle caused by small defects. However, cardiac catheterization and selective angiography may be required for diagnosis and to determine the severity of the shunt if Doppler is not available or the ventricular septal defect is not seen.[2, 4, 7]

ECG changes depend on the ventricle that is affected. A left-to-right shunt (i.e., volume overload of the left ventricle) causes left ventricular and left atrial enlargement (a tall R wave and a wide P wave in lead II), whereas a right-to-left ventricular septal defect causes right axis deviation. A right bundle branch block or ventricular arrhythmia may also be present.[3, 4] Radiographs usually reveal left ventricular and left atrial enlargement similar to but less severe than is seen in patent ductus arteriosus.[4, 7] Dogs with a right-to-left ventricular septal defect have right ventricular enlargement, pulmonary artery dilation, and hypovascularity of the lung fields. The heart does not appear as large as it does in dogs with pulmonary stenosis.[3]

Ventricular septal defects greater than 1 cm can often be directly seen on an echocardiogram as discontinuity between the interventricular septum and the anterior wall of the aorta (Fig. 14–13). Large shunts cause left ventricular enlargement and pulmonary artery dilation that is also easily identified on an echocardiogram. Color flow Doppler reveals turbulent flow on the right ventricular side of the septum.[13, 15, 16] Aortic regurgitation and mitral valve flutter may also

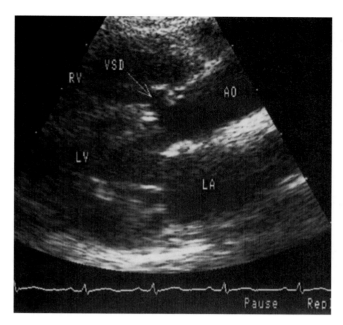

Figure 14-13
Echocardiogram of a dog with ventricular septal defect (VSD) from the left parasternal long-axis view. The ultrasound beam is angled to maximize visualization of the defect. AO, aorta; LA, left atrium; LV, left ventricle; RV, right ventricle.

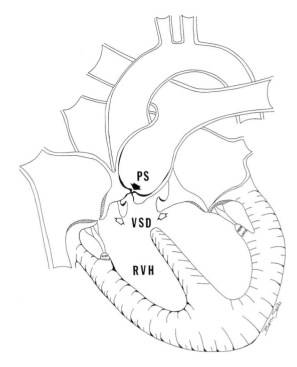

Figure 14-14
Diagram of tetralogy of Fallot. The four components of this defect are a ventricular septal defect (VSD), an aorta that is shifted to the right and receives blood from ventricles (*open arrows*), a pulmonary stenosis (PS, *solid arrow*), and right ventricular hypertrophy (RVH).

be seen if the septal cusp of the aortic valve is affected by flow through the defect.[4] A right-to-left shunt can be identified during a bubble study.[17]

Blood tests should be performed if a right-to-left shunt is suspected. The PCV is high, and measurement of arterial blood gases reveals hypoxemia.

Treatment

Treatment of small defects is not required, but large defects need primary repair by open heart surgery. Pulmonary artery banding has been attempted with some success, but it is not widely practiced.[4, 21] Dogs with a bidirectional or right-to-left shunt are not surgical candidates.[4] Dogs that develop left-sided congestive heart failure that cannot be surgically corrected can be treated with diuretics and vasodilators. Digoxin is administered to dogs in end-stage heart disease with myocardial failure.

Prognosis

Prognosis is excellent in dogs and cats with small ventricular septal defects and low shunt flows. It is variable in animals with larger defects or right-to-left shunts, although some animals can live years with the defect. Prolapse of the aortic valve into the defect causes concurrent aortic regurgitation. Significant regurgitation is related to a less favorable outcome.[2]

Tetralogy of Fallot

Tetralogy of Fallot is actually a combination of four cardiac abnormalities: ventricular septal defect, pulmonary stenosis, right ventricular hypertrophy, and dextroposition (overriding) of the aorta (Fig. 14–14). The two clinically important problems are a large ventricular septal defect and pulmonary stenosis, because these two defects encourage blood flow from the right ventricle to the aorta. Other defects may coexist with tetralogy of Fallot.[2, 4] Tetralogy of Fallot has also been reported in cats.[39]

Pathophysiology

The pathophysiology depends on the size of the ventricular septal defect and the pressure difference between pulmonary outflow and systemic vascular resistance. A large ventricular septal defect with minimal pulmonary stenosis causes volume overload similar to that caused by a left-to-right ventricular septal defect. In animals with worse pulmonary stenosis, less blood is shunted through the lungs, and the left-to-right shunting decreases. If resistance to pulmonary artery flow exceeds systemic vascular resistance, a right-to-left shunt is created.

This causes right ventricular pressure overload

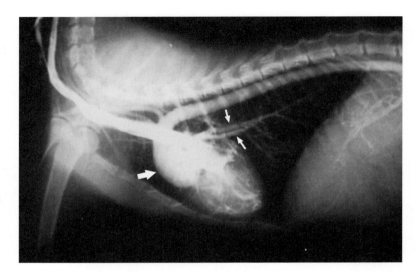

Figure 14–15
Nonselective angiogram of a cat with tetralogy of Fallot. Contrast material is filling the cranial vena cava, right ventricle, pulmonary arteries, and aorta without filling the left atrium or ventricle. Note the diminished pulmonary arteries (*small arrows*) and the pulmonary artery bulge (*large arrow*). The right ventricle is minimally filled with contrast material because of the right ventricular hypertrophy.

and right ventricular hypertrophy. During excitement, infundibular hypertrophy aggravates the pulmonary stenosis and intensifies shunting. Chronic hypoxemia from continuous right-to-left shunting causes polycythemia, which is the cause of death in most animals. Right-sided congestive heart failure is uncommon. If it occurs, it is exacerbated by pulmonary or tricuspid insufficiency.[4]

Clinical Signs

Animals usually become symptomatic by 1 year of age; however, animals with mild pulmonary stenosis with less shunting may remain asymptomatic.[4] Tachypnea, stunted growth, seizures, severe exercise intolerance, and syncope are signs associated with tetralogy of Fallot.[2, 4, 10] Arterial thromboembolism may occur in dogs with polycythemia (PCV >65%).[4]

Physical examination reveals a murmur of pulmonary stenosis (i.e., crescendo-decrescendo murmur heard best at the second to third intercostal space low on the left thorax)[4, 10] or ventricular septal defect (i.e., loud, harsh, holosystolic murmur that is loudest at the right cranial sternal border). Tetralogy of Fallot is the most common cause of cyanosis in animals with congenital heart disease. The right ventricular apex beat is usually more prominent because of right ventricular hypertrophy.[2, 4]

Diagnostic Plan

Diagnosis is usually evident from the results of the physical examination, thoracic radiography, ECG, hematology (i.e., polycythemia), and arterial blood gas determination (arterial desaturation).[10] Echocardiography is the best noninvasive method of making a definitive diagnosis, especially if a bubble study is included,[4] but nonselective angiography may also be used.[7]

A right axis shift indicative of right ventricular enlargement is present on the ECG. Thoracic radiography also reveals right ventricular enlargement, and pulmonary artery vessels appear smaller than normal.[4, 10] The size of the main pulmonary artery varies from normal to dilated.[4, 7]

The four characteristics of tetralogy of Fallot (i.e., ventricular septal defect, pulmonary stenosis, right ventricular hypertrophy, and overriding aorta) can usually be seen on an echocardiogram. However, proper technique is required, and misdiagnosis is possible. If there is any suspicion that tetralogy of Fallot is present, a bubble study should be performed.[4, 13, 17] Occasionally, cardiac catheterization is required to determine the size and severity of the defects.[7] In addition to the four characteristic findings, the right ventricular pressure during catheterization equals systemic pressure.[4, 10] Nonselective angiography also readily diagnoses tetralogy of Fallot by demonstrating simultaneous filling of the pulmonary artery and aorta without the appearance of contrast material in the left ventricle (Fig. 14–15).[7]

Treatment

Primary surgical repair is not usually possible because it requires open heart surgery. However, creation of a systemic-pulmonary artery shunt by connection of an artery to the main pulmonary artery may act as a palliative procedure.[4, 10, 25]

β-Adrenergic blocking drugs have been advocated to decrease myocardial oxygen demand by slowing the heart rate.[4, 10] It is also important to control polycythemia greater than 60% with periodic phlebotomy, because high blood viscosity increases the risk of thromboembolic disease and decreases cerebral perfusion.[2, 4] Phlebotomy should be performed cautiously, because a dramatically decreased systemic blood pressure and number of red blood cells serve to decrease oxygen transport.[10]

Prognosis

Prognosis is extremely guarded, although some dogs and cats live for years if polycythemia is controlled.[2] Signs usually occur by 1 year of age and progress until death by 2 years of age.[4]

References

1. Buchanan JW. Causes and prevalence of cardiovascular disease. In: Kirk RW, Bonagura JW, eds. Current Veterinary Therapy XI. Philadelphia, WB Saunders, 1992: 647–655.
2. Lehmkuhl LB, Bonagura JD. Congenital heart disease in the dog. Waltham/OSU Symposium for the Treatment of Small Animal Diseases. Vernon, California, Waltham USA, Inc, 1994:57–67.
3. Miller MW, Bonagura JD. Congenital heart disease. In: Kirk RW, Bonagura JW, eds. Current Veterinary Therapy X. Philadelphia, WB Saunders, 1989:224–231.
4. Olivier NB. Congenital heart disease in dogs. In: Fox PR, ed. Canine and Feline Cardiology. New York, Churchill Livingstone, 1988:357–389.
5. Fingland RB, Bonagura JD, Myer CW. Pulmonic stenosis in the dog: 29 cases (1975–1984). J Am Vet Med Assoc 1986;189:218–226.
6. Lehmkuhl LB, Bonagura JD. Congenital subaortic stenosis in the dog. Proc Am Coll Vet Intern Med Forum 1993;11:392–395.
7. Stickles L, Anderson LK. Diagnosis of common congenital heart anomalies in the dog using survey and nonselective contrast radiography. Vet Radiol 1987; 28:6–12.
8. Jacobs G, Mahaffey M, Rawlings CA. Valvular pulmonic stenosis in four Boykin spaniels. J Am Anim Hosp Assoc 1990;26:247–252.
9. Lehmkuhl LB, Bonagura JD. Results of Holter monitoring in dogs with congenital subaortic stenosis. Proc Am Coll Vet Intern Med Forum 1993;11:553–556.
10. Ringwald RJ, Bonagura JD. Tetralogy of Fallot in the dog: Clinical findings in 13 cases. J Am Anim Hosp Assoc 1988;24:33–43.
11. Birchard SJ, Bonagura JD, Fingland RB. Results of ligation of patent ductus arteriosus in dogs: 201 cases (1969–1988). J Am Vet Med Assoc 1990;196:2011–2013.
12. Goodwin J-K, Lombard CW. Patent ductus arteriosus in adult dogs: Clinical features of 14 cases. J Am Anim Hosp Assoc 1992;28:349–354.
13. Kaplan PM. Congenital heart disease. Probl Vet Med 1991;3:500–519.
14. Wingfield WE, Boon JA, Miller CW. Echocardiographic assessment of congenital aortic stenosis in dogs. J Am Vet Med Assoc 1983;183:673–676.
15. Moise NS. Doppler echocardiographic evaluation of congenital cardiac disease. J Vet Intern Med 1989;3: 195–207.
16. Reeder GS, Currie PJ, Hagler DJ, et al. Use of Doppler techniques (continuous-wave, pulsed-wave, and color flow imaging) in the noninvasive hemodynamic assessment of congenital heart disease). Mayo Clin Proc 1986; 61:725–744.
17. Bonagura JD, Pipers FS. Diagnosis of cardiac lesions by contrast echocardiography. J Am Vet Med Assoc 1983; 182:396–402.
18. Kienle RD, Thomas WP, Pion PD. The natural clinical history of canine congenital subaortic stenosis. J Vet Intern Med 1994;8:423–431.
19. Lusk RH, Ettinger SF. Cardiovascular syncope. In: Fox PR, ed. Canine and Feline Cardiology. New York, Churchill Livingstone, 1988:335–339.
20. Sisson D. Fixed and dynamic subvalvular aortic outflow stenosis in dogs. In: Kirk RW, Bonagura JD, eds. Current Veterinary Therapy XI. Philadelphia, WB Saunders, 1992:760–766.
21. Eyster GE, Eyster JT, Cords GB, et al. Patent ductus arteriosus in the dog: Characteristics of occurrence and results of surgery in one hundred consecutive cases. J Am Vet Med Assoc 1976;168:435–438.
22. Friedman WF. Congenital heart disease in infancy and childhood. In: Braunwald E, ed. Heart Disease. Philadelphia, WB Saunders, 1992:887–965.
23. Oswald GP, Orton EC. Patent ductus arteriosus and pulmonary hypertension in related Pembroke Welsh corgis. J Am Vet Med Assoc 1993;202:761–764.
24. Wolfe DA. Patent ductus arteriosus in dogs: A surgical review and simplified technique. J Am Anim Hosp Assoc 1979;15:323–328.
25. Hardie EM. Surgical management of selected congenital heart diseases. Proc Am Coll Vet Intern Med Forum 1992;10:177–179.
26. Levitt L, Fowler JD, Schuh JCL. Aortic stenosis in the dog: A review of 12 cases. J Am Anim Hosp Assoc 1989;25: 357–362.
27. Lehmkuhl LB, Bonagura JD. Comparing transducer placement for quantifying outflow gradients in subaortic stenosis. Proc Am Coll Vet Intern Med Forum 1993;11: 528–529.
28. Brown DJ. Evaluation of cardiac defects by echodoppler. Proc Am Coll Vet Intern Med Forum 1993;11: 396–399.
29. Breznock EM, Whiting P, Pendray D, et al. Valved apico-aortic conduit for relief of left ventricular hypertension caused by discrete subaortic stenosis in dogs. J Am Vet Med Assoc 1983;182:51:56.
30. Stepien RL, Bonagura JD. Aortic stenosis: clinical findings in six cats. J Small Anim Pract 1991;32:341–350.
31. Buchanan JW. Pulmonic stenosis caused by single coronary artery in dogs: Four cases (1965–1984). J Am Vet Med Assoc 1990;196:115–120.
32. Patterson DF, Haskins ME, Schnarr WR. Hereditary dysplasia of the pulmonary valve in beagle dogs: Pathologic and genetic studies. Am J Cardiol 1981;47: 631–641.
33. Shores A, Weirich WE. A modified pericardial patch graft technique for correction of pulmonic stenosis in the dog. J Am Anim Hosp Assoc 1985;21:809–812.
34. Breznock EM, Wood GL. A patch-graft technique for

correction of pulmonic stenosis in dogs. J Am Vet Med Assoc 1976;169:1090–1094.

35. Sisson DD, MacCoy DM. Treatment of congenital pulmonic stenosis in two dogs by balloon valvuloplasty. J Vet Intern Med 1988;2:92–99.

36. Kopecky SL, Gersh BJ, McGoon MD, et al. Long-term outcome of patients undergoing surgical repair of isolated pulmonary valve stenosis: Follow-up at 20–30 years. Circulation 1988;78:1150–1156.

37. McCrindle BW, Kan JS. Long-term results after balloon pulmonary valvuloplasty. Circulation 1991;83:1915–1922.

38. Grossman W, Braunwald E. Pulmonary hypertension. In: Braunwald E, ed. Heart Disease. Philadelphia, WB Saunders, 1992:790–816.

39. Fox PR. Congenital feline heart disease. In: Fox PR, ed. Canine and Feline Cardiology. New York, Churchill Livingstone, 1988:391–408.

Chapter 15

Pericardial Disease

Betsy R. Bond

Pericardial disease is caused by damage to or infiltration of the pericardial sac, the tissue that surrounds the heart. It is most simply divided into diseases causing pericardial effusion (i.e., excessive fluid accumulation within the pericardial cavity) and diseases causing constrictive pericarditis. Pericardial effusion is caused by damage to the pericardial sac or by disease that causes fluid buildup but does not affect the pericardium per se.[1] Congenital pericardial disease is usually caused by a defect in the diaphragm and pericardium that allows herniation of abdominal organs (i.e., the liver, small intestines, or stomach) through both the diaphragm and the pericardial sac into the thoracic cavity.[2]

Cardiac tamponade is a rapid accumulation of pericardial fluid that causes signs of cardiovascular shock.[2–4] Fluid that accumulates more slowly usually causes signs of right-sided heart failure (e.g., exercise intolerance, ascites).[4] Pericardial effusion without a known cause is referred to as idiopathic pericardial effusion.[1] Pericardial effusion in dogs can be caused by neoplasia (e.g., hemangiosarcoma of the right atrium, heart base tumor, mesothelioma), infectious pericarditis, renal failure, trauma, left atrial tear, right-sided heart failure, and metastatic neoplasia.[1, 2] The most common cause of pericardial effusion in cats is heart disease, with feline infectious peritonitis being the next most common cause. Other causes include renal failure, metastatic neoplasia, coagulopathies, and bacterial pericarditis. Idiopathic pericardial effusion has not been diagnosed in cats.[1, 5]

The prevalence of clinically significant pericardial disease in dogs is estimated at 1% of all cardiovascular disease.[6] The two most common types of pericardial effusion in dogs are idiopathic pericardial effusion and pericardial effusion caused by neoplasia.[2, 3] Constrictive pericarditis is rarely recognized.[1] Cats are rarely affected by pericardial effusion.[5]

Anatomy and Physiology

The pericardial sac is composed of a fibrous outer layer and an inner serous layer. The fibrous pericardium has both elastic and fibrous properties and is attached to the great vessels at the base of the heart. The serous pericardium adheres to the surface of the heart and becomes the epicardium. It then turns back on itself and adheres to the fibrous pericardium. Pericardial effusions develop in the space between the two layers of the serous pericardium.[1, 2]

The pericardial cavity normally contains a small amount (0.5–2.5 mL) of clear, serous fluid that lubricates the epicardial surface. The pericardial sac also protects the heart from infectious processes, prevents acute overfilling of the heart, and maintains equality of right and left ventricular stroke volumes.[1]

Problem Identification

Exercise Intolerance

Pathophysiology

The development of clinical signs is related to the distensibility of the pericardium and the rapidity with which fluid accumulates.[1–4, 6] As fluid develops within the pericardial space, the stretching capacity is exceeded and pressure in the pericardial sac is transmitted to the heart. As pericardial pressure exceeds cardiac filling pressures, diastolic filling is impaired. If pericardial pressures are high or pericardial effusion occurs rapidly, venous return is blocked, and the left side of the heart receives an inadequate supply of blood to maintain cardiac output. Signs of forward heart failure (e.g., exercise intolerance, syncope, weakness) result.[1–3, 6] In most dogs, cardiac contractility is unaffected by pericardial effusion.[6]

Clinical Signs

Dogs become extremely weak and cannot perform normal activities, preferring to lie down. Even mild exercise induces dyspnea. Other clinical signs include weight loss, ascites, syncope, and tachypnea. Physical examination reveals muffled heart sounds, weak arterial pulses, abnormal jugular venous distention, pallor, sinus tachycardia, and arrhythmias.[1, 3, 6]

Diagnostic Plan

Any dog with exercise intolerance and muffled heart sounds should have a thoracic radiograph taken. Radiographic appearance of a large, round cardiac silhouette (Fig. 15–1) and the presence of small QRS complexes with electrical alternans on the electrocardiogram (ECG) provide strong evidence of the presence of pericardial effusion[6] (Fig. 15–2). However, radiography is not always characteristic, and electrical alternans is not always present. The differential diagnosis for radiographic evidence of cardiomegaly includes primary myocardial disease, mitral insufficiency with biventricular enlargement, and congenital cardiac defect. Definitive diagnosis of pericardial effusion is made by echocardiography (Fig. 15–3).[1] Care should be taken to examine the right atrium and great vessels for hemangiosarcoma and heart base masses. See Chapter 9 for further discussion of exercise intolerance.

Syncope

Pathophysiology

The pathophysiology for syncope is the same as for exercise intolerance and weakness, but syncope usually indicates a more sudden onset of effusion.

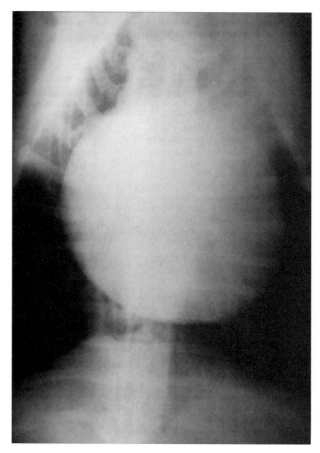

Figure 15-1
Pericardial effusion in a 9-year-old golden retriever. The cardiac silhouette is enlarged and rounded.

Clinical Signs

Dogs with syncope caused by pericardial effusion are usually weak and have episodes of sudden collapse. They may or may not lose consciousness. Other clinical signs are the same as those of exercise intolerance.[1, 6]

Diagnostic Plan

If radiography reveals an extremely large cardiac silhouette, tests to determine the cause of cardiomegaly should be performed. The diagnostic plan is the same as for exercise intolerance. See Chapter 9 for further discussion of syncope.

Dyspnea and Tachypnea

Pathophysiology

Occasionally, pleural effusion accompanies pericardial effusion. Pleural effusion causes compression of the lung lobes and their inability to expand normally. In addition, venous return to the heart is impaired, which decreases blood flow through the lungs for oxygenation.[4]

Clinical Signs

Animals display difficult or rapid, shallow breathing. Other clinical signs are the same as those of exercise intolerance.[1]

Diagnostic Plan

Thoracic radiographs should be taken in all animals with dyspnea and tachypnea. Pleural effusion can obscure the large, round cardiac silhouette that is characteristic of pericardial effusion. Severely dyspneic animals with pleural effusion should undergo thoracentesis for both therapeutic and diagnostic purposes. Thoracic effusions caused by pericardial disease are usually modified transudates. Repeat thoracic radiography can then be performed, al-

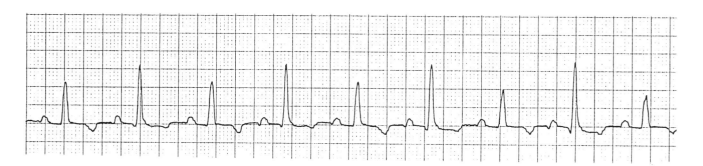

Figure 15-2
Lead II electrocardiogram of a 13-year-old German shepherd with a heart base mass and pericardial effusion The QRS complexes alternate in height as the heart swings in the percardial sac. As the heart moves toward the left chest wall in the percardial sac, the R waves become taller. When the heart moves away from the chest wall, the R waves shorten.

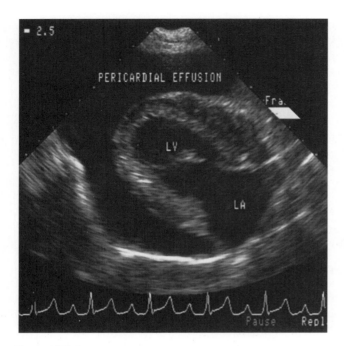

Figure 15–3
Two-dimensional echocardiogram of a pericardial effusion in a 9-year-old mixed breed dog with a right atrial mass. There is a large, echo-free space around the heart. The pericardium is represented by the hyperechoic line at the bottom of the echocardiogram. LA, left atrium; LV, left ventricle.

though echocardiography is more sensitive and specific for diagnosis of pericardial effusion and differentiation from right-sided congestive heart failure. See Chapters 9, 52, and 53 for further discussion of dyspnea.

Vomiting

Pathophysiology

Vomiting is common in animals with congenital peritoneopericardial diaphragmatic hernia. It is caused by compression or blockage of the portion of the gastrointestinal tract (i.e., stomach and small intestine) that has herniated into the pericardial sac.

Clinical Signs

Animals may have anorexia and diarrhea in addition to vomiting. Other clinical signs are the same as those of exercise intolerance.[1]

Diagnostic Plan

Abdominal radiography reveals loss of abdominal organs in the cranial abdomen, and thoracic radiographs reveal a large, round cardiac silhouette. A gaseous pattern may overlie the heart.[1] If the liver has herniated into the pericardial sac, it may be seen on echocardiography. Animals with vomiting caused by gastrointestinal disease should not have cardiomegaly. See Chapter 31 for further discussion of vomiting.

Ascites

Ascites is the accumulation of fluid within the abdominal cavity.

Pathophysiology

Ascites develops in animals with pericardial disease because pericardial pressure exceeds cardiac filling pressures, impairing diastolic filling. This causes increased venous pressures and right-sided congestive heart failure (e.g., ascites).[1, 4, 6] Ascites is usually associated with pericardial effusion that develops slowly.[4]

Clinical Signs

The abdomen is swollen, and a fluid wave and large liver may be palpable unless the ascites is severe. Other clinical signs are the same as those of exercise intolerance.[1]

Diagnostic Plan

If radiography reveals a large cardiac silhouette, echocardiography should be performed to determine the cause of cardiomegaly. The diagnostic plan is described in the section on exercise intolerance. In addition, abdominal fluid can be aspirated for analysis, which usually reveals a transudate or modified transudate that is compatible with right-sided heart failure. Bloody abdominal fluid may be a sign of abdominal neoplasia, in which case an ultrasound examination of the abdomen should be performed, because tumors such as hemangiosarcoma can cause both pericardial and abdominal effusions. See Chapter 34 for further discussion of ascites.

Muffled Heart Sounds

Heart sounds are considered muffled if the first and second heart sounds are softer than normal on auscultation.

Pathophysiology

Fluid in the pericardial sac or pleural cavity, excessive subcutaneous fat, or thoracic masses block normal heart sounds from being carried as well as usual to the thoracic wall.[3, 4]

Clinical Signs

Clinical signs are the same as those for exercise intolerance. Differentiation of pericardial from pleural effusion is often difficult from auscultation alone, because both conditions may cause dyspnea and muffled heart and lung sounds if both pleural and pericardial effusion are present. However, lung sounds are heard in animals with only pericardial effusion (i.e., no pleural effusion).

Diagnostic Plan

Other conditions that cause muffling of heart sounds include obesity, thoracic masses, pleural effusion, pneumothorax, and myocardial failure (decreased contractility). Radiography is usually sufficient to differentiate pericardial effusion from other causes of muffled heart sounds, because pericardial effusion is associated with a rounded appearance of the cardiac silhouette. Radiography is insufficient in animals that have both pericardial and pleural effusions. In animals with cardiomegaly secondary to myocardial disease or myocardial failure, the silhouette is not as rounded, and cardiac structures can be seen on radiographs. If the pericardial effusion is mild, the heart does not appear as rounded, and echocardiography is required to differentiate mild pericardial disease from severe myocardial disease. Echocardiography is diagnostic of pericardial effusion in animals that have cardiomegaly or pleural effusion not easily diagnosed by thoracic radiography.

Diagnostic Procedures

Radiography

In many animals, thoracic radiography alone is diagnostic of pericardial effusion. However, the size and shape of the cardiac silhouette on thoracic radiography changes depending on the underlying cause. Dogs with acute left atrial tear may exhibit near-normal cardiac size or cardiomegaly and left atrial enlargement, whereas long-standing pericardial disease causes stretching of the pericardial sac and the characteristic large, globoid cardiac silhouette with loss of cardiac chamber definition (see Fig. 15–1). Enlargement of the caudal vena cava is occasionally seen, and pleural effusion may interfere with evaluation of the cardiac silhouette. Dogs with heart base tumors may have a radiodense soft tissue mass effect at the heart base that displaces the trachea (Fig. 15–4).[1, 3, 4, 6] Differential diagnosis includes primary myocardial disease, mitral insufficiency with biventricular failure, and congenital defects.[1]

Pneumopericardiography (see Pericardiocentesis) can be performed if echocardiography is unavailable or if a tumor is suspected but not definitively seen on the echocardiogram. Pneumopericardiography accurately outlines most cardiac masses and usually differentiates idiopathic from neoplastic effusions.[6] Inadequate studies are caused by failure to remove all the pericardial fluid or to inject an adequate amount of air to distend the pericardial sac. The injection of carbon dioxide or room air should be equivalent to two thirds to three quarters of the fluid volume removed. Radiographs are immediately obtained with the animal in the right lateral, left lateral, dorsoventral, and ventrodorsal positions. Residual air may be removed after the radiographs are taken, but the air is absorbed quickly.[6]

Electrocardiography

Several ECG abnormalities have been reported in dogs and cats with pericardial effusion, including small QRS complexes (<1 mV in all leads), electrical alternans, and S-T segment elevation.[1–3, 6] Electrical alternans is the regular variation in QRS size or morphology every second or third complex; it is caused by swinging of the heart within the fluid-filled pericardial sac (see Fig. 15–2). It is not as common as low-amplitude QRS complexes in animals with pericardial effusion,[3] but its presence is highly suggestive of pericardial effusion.[1]

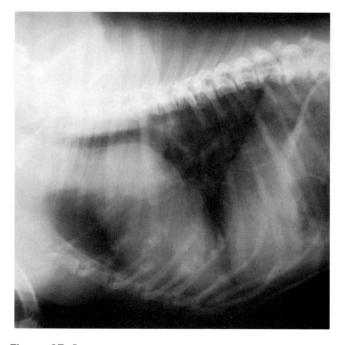

Figure 15–4
Radiograph of an 11-year-old boxer with a heart base tumor. There is a radiodense mass dorsal to the heart that also displaces the trachea dorsally.

Echocardiography

Echocardiography is the most sensitive and specific test for diagnosing pericardial effusion.[3] An echo-free space is present between the myocardium and pericardium, and the heart is observed to swing to and fro within the pericardial sac (see Fig. 15–3). Cardiac tamponade is characterized by right atrial and right ventricular diastolic collapse.[1, 4, 6–8]

The cause of pericardial effusion may also be evident on two-dimensional echocardiography. In dogs with neoplasia of the right atrium or heart base, the mass can be imaged directly.[3] The lack of an identifiable mass suggests idiopathic pericardial effusion, although some masses are not readily seen. Cats with pericardial effusion caused by heart failure have obvious cardiac chamber enlargement, and dogs with a left atrial tear have left atrial enlargement and thick mitral valves. A clot forming from the left atrium and extending into the pericardial effusion may also be seen in these dogs. In dogs and cats with a peritoneopericardial diaphragmatic hernia, the liver may be seen in the pericardial sac.[1]

Pericardiocentesis

Mild sedation of dogs is usually required to perform pericardiocentesis. Animals are placed in left lateral recumbence, and the right hemithorax is clipped and aseptically prepared between the third and eighth intercostal spaces from the sternum to an area above the costochondral junction.[1] I prefer to use a large-bore, long intravenous (IV) catheter for dogs and a butterfly needle with flexible tubing for cats. The patient is attached to a continuous ECG and monitored for ventricular arrhythmias.

Penetration into the pericardium is accomplished by attaching the needle from the IV catheter to a sterile 12-mL syringe and slowly advancing with mild suction until pericardial fluid is obtained. If the procedure is performed carefully, it is often possible to feel the needle "pop" through the pericardium. Major risks of pericardiocentesis are laceration of a coronary artery, ventricular arrhythmias, and exacerbation of active hemorrhage. The potential for coronary artery laceration is reduced if aspiration is performed from the right hemithorax. Ventricular arrhythmias are caused by contact of the needle with the ventricular myocardium; they are easily seen on the cardiac monitor. In addition, the heart can usually be felt as it beats against the needle. The needle should be retracted a short distance to continue the procedure.

After the needle enters the pericardium, a sample is withdrawn for fluid analysis and culture and sensitivity testing if indicated. The intravenous catheter with stylet is passed through the needle approximately one third of the length, and then the catheter is fully inserted over the stylet. A large syringe is then used to aspirate as much of the pericardial fluid as possible. A large catheter should be used, because most pericardial effusion is hemorrhagic and very viscous. Effusion that is withdrawn is periodically examined for clotting, which would indicate either that the fluid is from the heart or that there is active bleeding into the pericardial sac. Measurement of a packed cell volume usually differentiates pericardial effusion from blood; they should be significantly different except in animals with acute, recent hemorrhage.[6] However, differentiation of acute pericardial hemorrhage from cardiac puncture is difficult. If clotting blood is obtained, it is recommended that pericardiocentesis be attempted in a different area. If clotting blood is again obtained, the risk of continuing should be evaluated versus the benefit that may be gained from the pericardiocentesis.

Routine Laboratory Evaluation

Routine laboratory testing is usually not helpful in diagnosing pericardial disease, but it should be performed to assess the effects of the pericardial disease on other systems. Dogs with pericardial disease may have hypoproteinemia, anemia, or neutrophilic leukocytosis. Serum biochemical abnormalities include elevated liver enzymes and mild prerenal azotemia. Dogs with hemangiosarcoma are more likely to have anemia, circulating nucleated red blood cells,[1, 9] and schistocytes than dogs with pericardial effusion from other causes. Cats may have a high antibody titer for feline infectious peritonitis and may test positive for feline leukemia virus.[1]

Cytologic analysis of pericardial fluid is not helpful in differentiating idiopathic from neoplastic pericardial effusion. In both conditions, the fluid contains red blood cells, macrophages, and reactive mesothelial cells.[2, 10] Fluid from both of these conditions is thick and very hemorrhagic. However, fluid that is clear or only mildly hemorrhagic could come from congestive heart failure or an infection (e.g., bacterial or feline infectious peritonitis). Any fluid obtained from an animal with a concurrent pneumonia or septic process should be cultured.

Idiopathic Pericardial Effusion

Pericardial effusion without a known cause is referred to as idiopathic pericardial effusion. It is one of the most common causes of pericardial effusion in dogs.[1–3, 6, 11] Male dogs of medium and large breeds[11] with an age range of 1 to 14 years (average, 6 years) are most commonly affected. Golden retrievers, German shepherds, Great Danes, and Saint Bernards appear to be overrepresented.[1, 3, 6] It has not been reported in cats.[5] The cause is unknown, but thickening of the parietal pericardium and epicardium with fibrosis and mild inflammation are the predominant histologic features.[1, 11]

Pathophysiology

Pericardial effusion causes clinical signs if fluid collects within the pericardial space such that the elastic limit or stretching capacity is exceeded. The pressure in the pericardial sac rises and is transmitted to the structures within the pericardial cavity. As pericardial pressure exceeds cardiac filling pressure, diastolic filling is impaired, causing abnormally high venous pressure and right-sided congestive heart failure (e.g., ascites, hepatomegaly, jugular venous distention). Most dogs with idiopathic pericardial effusion have very large volumes, because fluid collects slowly, allowing for stretching of the pericardial sac. It is not unusual to aspirate 500 to 1000 mL of fluid from the pericardial sac.[1]

Signs of right-sided heart failure predominate in some dogs, because the right ventricular filling pressure is lower than that of the left ventricle and the right ventricle is affected earlier in the disease process. However, as pericardial pressure increases, venous return is blocked, the left side of the heart receives an inadequate supply of blood to maintain cardiac output, and signs of forward heart failure result (e.g., exercise intolerance, syncope, hypotension).[1, 6, 11]

Clinical Signs

Clinical signs of idiopathic pericardial effusion include lethargy, weakness, exercise intolerance, weight loss, ascites, syncope, muffled heart sounds, weak peripheral pulses, and tachypnea.[1, 3] Pericardial friction rubs and pulsus paradoxus (exaggerated decline of the pulse during inspiration), although reported,[2] are infrequently seen.[3]

Diagnostic Plan

Diagnosis is suspected on the basis of characteristic changes on thoracic radiography and ECG, but definitive diagnosis is made when pericardial effusion without a mass is seen on an echocardiogram in a medium- to large-breed dog.[1, 11]

Fluid from pericardiocentesis may be submitted for evaluation, although cytologic examination usually fails to differentiate among hemangiosarcoma, heart base tumor, and idiopathic pericardial effusion.[3, 9, 11] Reactive mesothelial cells are a finding in all three diseases (not just neoplasia), and the protein content, red blood cell count, and nucleated cell blood count are similar in all three diseases.[1]

Treatment

Pericardiocentesis is the initial treatment of choice for dogs with idiopathic pericardial effusion.[4, 6, 11] If active pericardial hemorrhage is suspected, the decision to perform pericardiocentesis is difficult. However, most dogs that would be harmed by pericardiocentesis because of continuous hemorrhage are small-breed dogs with murmurs of mitral regurgitation (e.g., left atrial tears). Because medium- to large-breed dogs are the ones characteristically affected by idiopathic pericardial effusion, these dogs should have pericardiocentesis performed as early as possible for relief of signs.

There is no medical treatment that provides relief from clinical signs caused by pericardial effusion. Treatment with diuretics is of no benefit, because the pericardial space has limited venous and lymphatic drainage, and inflammation further impedes fluid escape.[1, 6] In fact, treatment with diuretics is contraindicated in dogs and cats with pericardial effusion because venous return and cardiac output are already low as a result of the effusion. Administration of diuretics diminishes vascular volume and further diminishes venous return. Treatment with vasodilators, especially afterload reducers, is likewise contraindicated. These agents only worsen the hypotension that is usually already present.[1, 6] Digitalization is not indicated because myocardial function is normal. Repeat pericardiocentesis is the nonsurgical treatment of choice for recurrent pericardial effusion.[1]

Approximately 50% of dogs respond to one or two therapeutic pericardiocenteses. The remaining dogs have recurring pericardial effusion, usually within days to weeks after the initial pericardiocentesis. Administration of anti-inflammatory agents such as corticosteroids has been advocated to prevent recurrence, although no controlled studies have documented their benefit.[1]

Dogs with recurrent pericardial effusion should be considered candidates for surgical removal of the pericardium. Subtotal pericardiectomy is the procedure of choice, and most dogs become asymptomatic after surgery.[3, 11] Creation of a small pericardial window, rather than removal of a substantial portion of the pericardium, has proven unsuccessful. Although most dogs remain asymptomatic after pericardiectomy, a small percentage of dogs develop hemorrhagic pleural effusion and require repeat thoracentesis.[1, 12]

Prognosis

Dogs that respond favorably to pericardiocentesis and those that become asymptomatic after pericardiectomy have a good prognosis for normal life expectancy.[1]

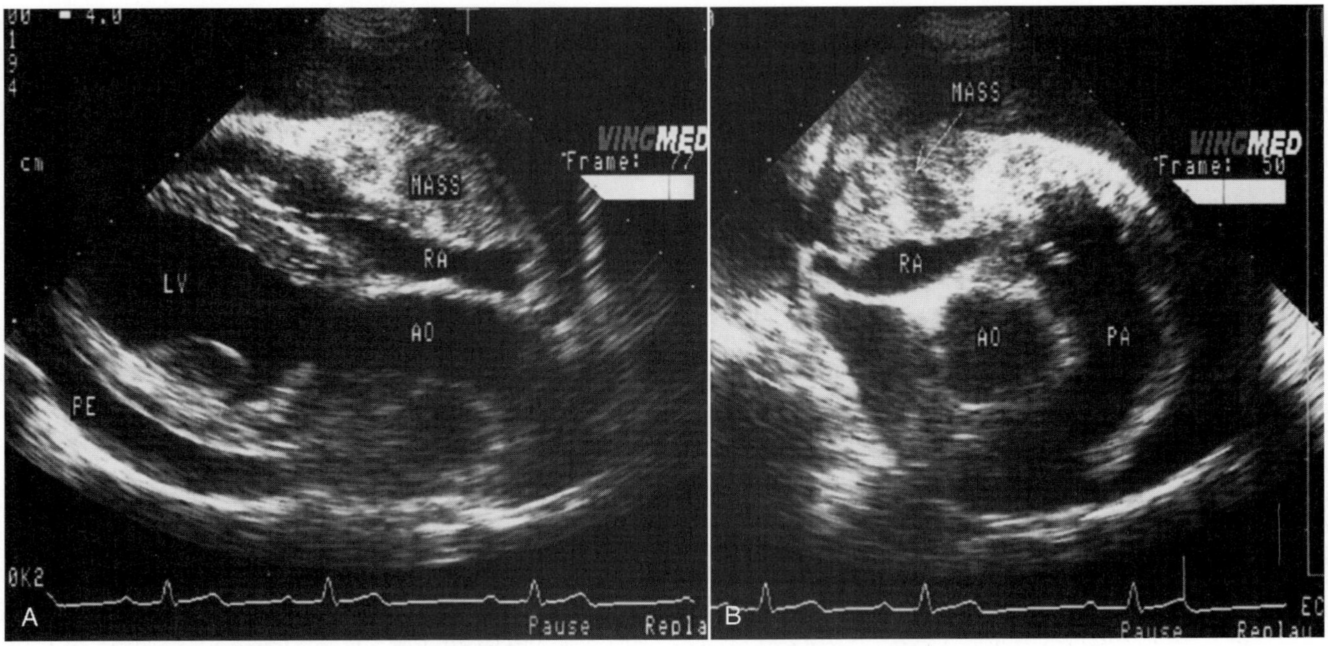

Figure 15-5
(A) Long-axis and (B) short-axis echocardiograms of a 10-year-old golden retriever with a mass in the right atrium. The mass is located primarily in the wall of the right atrium but also involves the wall of the right ventricle. AO, aorta; LV, left ventricle; PA, pulmonary artery; PE, pericardial effusion; RA, right atrium.

Neoplastic Pericardial Effusion

Neoplastic pericardial effusion is usually caused by a mass that is located in the wall of the right atrium (e.g., hemangiosarcoma) or arises from the aortic arch (e.g., chemodectoma).[6] Hemangiosarcoma of the right atrium is an uncommon form of hemangiosarcoma, comprising only 3% of cases of hemangiosarcoma.[13] German shepherds, golden retrievers, and poodles[9, 13, 14] are predisposed to right atrial hemangiosarcoma, whereas boxers, bulldogs, and Boston terriers are predisposed to heart base tumors.[1, 6] Chemodectomas are rare in cats, and hemangiosarcomas usually appear in the myocardium rather than in the right atrium.[15] Neoplasias such as mesotheliomas and metastatic carcinomas are uncommon in both dogs and cats.[5, 6, 15]

Pathophysiology

Pathophysiology is the same as for idiopathic pericardial effusion, although cardiac tamponade is more likely in dogs with neoplastic pericardial effusion. Therefore, collapse, syncope, and signs of low-output heart failure are more likely in dogs with neoplastic than with idiopathic pericardial effusion.[1, 6, 11]

Clinical Signs

Clinical signs of neoplastic pericardial effusion include lethargy, weakness, exercise intolerance, weight loss, ascites, syncope, muffled heart sounds, weak peripheral pulses, and tachypnea.[1, 6, 9] Dogs with bleeding tumors may also have a heart murmur and tachycardia.[9] Dogs with splenic masses often have arrhythmias.

Diagnostic Plan

Many neoplastic masses can easily be identified by echocardiography, but others are less obvious. It is important to view the heart and pericardium from as many different positions as possible, angling the probe to optimally visualize any suspicious areas (Fig. 15-5). It is also preferable to perform echocardiography if fluid is still present in the pericardium, because fluid helps to outline masses. Cytologic analysis is of limited diagnostic value in dogs with idiopathic or neoplastic effusions, but it can help in animals with septic pericarditis or cats with feline infectious peritonitis.[6, 10] Anemia, leukocytosis with neutrophilia and a left shift, and nucleated red blood cells are characteristic.[9]

Treatment

Pericardiocentesis is the treatment of choice for neoplastic pericardial effusion. If active pericardial hemorrhage is suspected, the decision to perform pericardiocentesis is difficult. However, dogs that are hemorrhaging because of a ruptured neoplasm usually have cardiac tamponade and require pericardiocentesis as an emergency treatment. Pericardiocentesis is performed with the understanding that further hemorrhage and exsanguination may occur because of tears in the pericardium. Prognosis in these dogs is extremely guarded regardless of treatment, and pericardiocentesis is often a temporary procedure that merely provides extra time for owners to prepare for their dogs' death. Cats with lymphosarcoma can be treated with chemotherapeutic agents, although a favorable response is not well documented.[1]

After initial pericardiocentesis, the most aggressive treatment is thoracotomy and removal of the mass and pericardial sac. In dogs with hemangiosarcoma, results of surgery are usually poor,[14] because the tumor has usually metastasized by the time surgery is performed.[6] Limited but better success has been achieved with removal of heart base tumors. A more conservative approach would be to remove the pericardial sac in the hope that the pleural cavity would absorb more fluid than the pericardial sac. Radiation therapy of heart base tumors has not been successful.[6]

Prognosis

Prognosis is variable but generally poor,[3] depending on the location, size, and type of tumor. Right atrial masses, which often metastasize,[14] carry an extremely guarded prognosis.[1, 6, 9, 14] Surgical removal is usually not helpful. Complications include atrial and ventricular arrhythmias, anemia, disseminated intravascular coagulation, and pneumonia. Mean survival is only 4 months (range, 2 days to 8 months) after surgical removal.[14]

Heart base tumors grow more slowly than right atrial tumors and are less likely to metastasize in dogs, but they are difficult or impossible to excise. Pericardiectomy may help relieve clinical signs in dogs. Heart base tumors in cats are rare, but they are extremely malignant.

Congenital Pericardial Disease

Congenital abnormalities of the pericardial sac in dogs and cats include partial or complete absence of the pericardial sac, pericardial cysts, and peritoneopericardial diaphragmatic hernia. Peritoneopericardial dia-

phragmatic hernia is the only common cause of clinical disease in dogs and cats[1, 2] and is the only disease discussed here. It is usually diagnosed in young animals, although some cats can reach middle age or older without displaying clinical signs. Weimaraners are thought to be predisposed to this disease.[1]

Pathophysiology

Pathophysiology is the same as for causes of pericardial effusion, although displacement of the lungs is usually caused by entrapped intestines or liver rather than fluid. Fluid accumulation is probably caused by pressure on the entrapped liver. Pathophysiology may also be related to entrapment of abdominal organs within the pericardial sac, which causes blockage or obstruction of the gastrointestinal tract.

Clinical Signs

Many animals remain asymptomatic, especially cats. Clinical signs are referable to the gastrointestinal, respiratory, or cardiovascular system, depending on the organs herniated, the amount of lung displaced by the herniated organs, and the amount of pressure exerted on the heart and great vessels. Signs include vomiting, anorexia, dyspnea, cough, weakness, and collapse. Physical examination reveals muffled or absent heart sounds, displaced apical beat, sternal deformity,[1, 2] and weak pulses.

Diagnostic Plan

Diagnosis is often made by thoracic radiography, especially if it is combined with physical examination. The cardiac silhouette is extremely large and round with loss of cardiac shape, with the caudal border of the heart overlapping the diaphragm. Abnormal gaseous densities may overlie the heart, and abdominal radiographs may demonstrate absence of cranial abdominal organs. An upper gastrointestinal barium series often reveals the stomach or intestines within the pericardial sac. Echocardiography is the preferred method of diagnosing liver entrapment within the pericardium.[1] Fluid aspirated from the pericardial sac is usually clear or only mildly serosanguineous.

Treatment

Surgical repair of the defect within the pericardium and diaphragm is the treatment of choice.[1]

Prognosis

Prognosis is excellent for young animals with uncomplicated peritoneopericardial diaphragmatic hernia after surgery.[1] Care must be taken with old cats (>10 years) who have lived with peritoneopericardial diaphragmatic hernia and adjusted to it, especially if the liver is involved.

Uncommon Causes of Pericardial Effusion

Constrictive Pericarditis

Constrictive pericarditis is rare in dogs and cats. If it does occur, it is in medium- to large-breed, middle-aged dogs. It is caused by thickening and fibrosis of the pericardial sac, which sometimes adheres to the epicardial surface and impairs late diastolic filling.[1, 6] Constrictive pericarditis causes right-sided heart failure (e.g., ascites). The cause of constrictive pericarditis is unknown, although it is usually a sequela of idiopathic or septic pericardial effusion.[16] Surgical removal is the treatment of choice, and it is most successful if only the parietal pericardium is involved. Fibrosis of the visceral pericardium requires epicardial stripping and can lead to complications such as myocardial hemorrhage. Prognosis is favorable in dogs that undergo successful surgical removal of the pericardium.[1, 16]

Left Atrial Tear

Left atrial tear is a serious cause of cardiac tamponade. It usually occurs in dogs with a history of mitral regurgitation and severe left atrial enlargement and leads to dramatic clinical signs of collapse, shock, or worsening heart failure. Signs occur with only a small volume of pericardial effusion (50–100 mL in the dog), because the elastic limit of the pericardium is quickly exceeded.[1, 2]

Septic Pericardial Effusion

Septic pericardial effusion is caused by viral (e.g., feline infectious peritonitis), bacterial, fungal (e.g., *Coccidioides immitis*), or protozoal (e.g., toxoplasmosis) infection of the pericardial sac. Diagnosis is made on the basis of culture or cytologic examination of the pericardial effusion. Both IV and intrapericardial administration of antibiotics may be required. Infectious pericarditis often results in fibrous tissue deposition and constrictive pericarditis. Prognosis is guarded to poor.[1]

Pericardial Mass Lesions

Pericardial mass lesions are caused by neoplasms, cysts,[17] abscesses, and granulomas. They cause pericardial effusions and are diagnosed by echocardiography or pneumopericardiography. Surgery to remove the affected pericardial sac and mass is the treatment of choice.[6] In cats, tumors found in the pericardial sac include mesothelioma, bronchoalveolar carcinoma, lymphosarcoma, mammary gland adenocarcinoma, pulmonary carcinoma, tonsillar carcinoma, and melanoma.[5, 15] Tumors in dogs include lymphosarcoma, thymoma, thyroid carcinoma, and mesothelioma.[2, 3]

References

1. Rush JE, Atkins CE. Pericardial disease. In: Allen DG, ed. Small Animal Medicine. Philadelphia, JB Lippincott, 1991:309–321.
2. Bouvy BM, Bjorling DE. Pericardial effusion in dogs and cats: Part I. Normal pericardium and causes and pathophysiology of pericardial effusion. Compen Contin Educ Pract Vet 1991;13:417–424.
3. Berg RJ. Pericardial effusion in the dog: A review of 42 cases. J Am Anim Hosp Assoc 1984;20:721–730.
4. Jones CL. Pericardial effusion in the dog. Compen Contin Educ Pract Vet 1979;1:680–686.
5. Rush JE, Keene BW, Fox PR. Pericardial disease in the cat: A retrospective evaluation of 66 cases. J Am Anim Hosp Assoc 1990;26:39–46.
6. Thomas WP, Reed JR. Pericardial disease. In: Kirk RW, ed. Current Veterinary Therapy IX. Philadelphia, WB Saunders, 1986:364–370.
7. Bonagura JD, Pipers FS. Echocardiographic features of pericardial effusion in dogs. J Am Vet Med Assoc 1981;179:49–55.
8. Chuttani K, Pandian NG, Mohanty PK, et al. Left ventricular diastolic collapse: An echocardiographic sign of regional cardiac tamponade. Circulation 1991;83:1999–2006.
9. Kleine LJ, Zook BC, Munson TO. Primary cardiac hemangiosarcoma in dogs. J Am Vet Med Assoc 1970;157:326–337.
10. Sisson D, Thomas WP, Ruehl WW, et al. Diagnostic value of pericardial fluid analysis in the dog. J Am Vet Med Assoc 1984;184:51–59.
11. Berg RJ, Wingfield WE, Hoopes PJ. Idiopathic hemorrhagic pericardial effusion in eight dogs. J Am Vet Med Assoc 1984;185:988–992.
12. Matthiesen DT, Lammerding J. Partial pericardiectomy for idiopathic hemorrhagic pericardial effusion in the dog. J Am Anim Hosp Assoc 1985;21:41–47.
13. Brown NO, Patnaik AK, MacEwen EG. Canine hemangiosarcoma: Retrospective analysis of 104 cases. J Am Vet Med Assoc 1985;186:56–58.
14. Aronsohn M. Cardiac hemangiosarcoma in the dog: A review of 38 cases. J Am Vet Med Assoc 1985;187:922–926.
15. Tilley LP, Bond B, Patnaik AK, et al. Cardiovascular tumors in the cat. J Am Anim Hosp Assoc 1981;17:1009–1021.
16. Thomas WP, Reed JR, Bauer TG, et al. Constrictive pericardial disease in the dog. J Am Vet Med Assoc 1984;184:546–553.
17. Sisson D, Thomas WP, Reed J, et al. Intrapericardial cysts in the dog. J Vet Intern Med 1993;7:364–369.

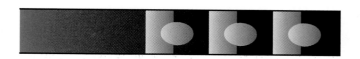

Urinary
Diseases

Chapter 16

Diseases of the Kidney and Ureter

S. Dru Forrester

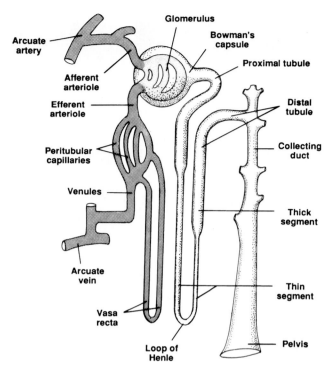

Figure 16-1
Segments that compose a nephron, the functional unit of
the kidney, including the blood supply. (Adapted from
Guyton AC. Textbook of Medical Physiology, 8th ed. Philadelphia, WB Saunders, 1991:289.)

Anatomy

Both kidneys in dogs and cats are located in the
retroperitoneal space, with the left kidney lying more
caudally. Each kidney consists of an outer layer, the
renal cortex, and an inner portion, the medulla. The
functional units of the kidney (nephrons) consist of a
glomerulus, Bowman's capsule, proximal tubule, loop
of Henle, distal tubule, and collecting duct (Fig. 16–1).
Each kidney is supplied by a renal artery, which
subdivides to eventually form the afferent arteriole
that supplies the glomerular capillary tuft. The efferent
arteriole exits the glomerulus to form an extensive
peritubular capillary network. Nephrons that originate
at the corticomedullary junction (i.e., juxtamedullary
nephrons) have efferent arterioles that give rise to vasa
recta, vessels that extend deep into the medulla. Vasa
recta run parallel to long loops of Henle and are
important in maintaining the hypertonic medullary
interstitium necessary for urinary concentration.

The glomerulus is a tuft of highly branched
capillaries that consist of endothelial cells, basement
membrane, epithelial cells, and mesangium (matrix
and cells).[1] The inner surface of capillary basement
membranes is lined by a thin layer of endothelium. The
glomerular basement membrane, composed of glyco-

protein and a collagen-like substance, acts as a filtration barrier, although it restricts passage only of large
proteins. Visceral epithelial cells cover the outer
surface of the basement membrane and have numerous extensions, called foot processes or podocytes, that
extend to the basement membrane. Spaces between
foot processes are slit pores through which glomerular
filtrate passes. Because of their size and associated
negative charge, the slit pores prevent passage of
proteins such as albumin into glomerular filtrate.
Located between capillaries are mesangial cells and
matrix (material similar to basement membrane),
which serve as support structures. Mesangial cells also
may have phagocytic activity.[1]

Physiology

The three basic functions of the kidneys are to excrete
waste products of metabolism; to regulate fluid, electrolyte, and acid-base balances; and to produce or
activate hormones necessary for hematopoiesis, regulation of blood pressure, and maintenance of calcium
balance. These functions are carried out by the processes of glomerular filtration, tubular absorption and
secretion, production of erythropoietin and renin, and
activation of vitamin D.

Glomerular Filtration

The kidneys excrete metabolic wastes such as
urea and creatinine primarily by filtering them through
the glomerulus and failing to reabsorb them; in
addition, some substances (e.g., potassium, hydrogen
ions) are actively secreted by renal tubular cells.
Glomerular filtration is a passive process that is
dependent on generation of adequate perfusion pressure by the heart. Changes in renal vascular resistance
maintain a constant perfusion pressure as long as
systolic blood pressure remains between 90 and 220
mm Hg.[2] If mean arterial pressure decreases below 70
to 80 mm Hg, glomerular filtration begins to decline.[3]
The glomerular filtrate that enters Bowman's capsule is
similar to plasma except that it contains no appreciable
amount of cells or proteins.

Tubular Function

Composition of glomerular filtrate is altered by
tubular reabsorption and secretion. Sodium, chloride,
water, glucose, potassium, phosphate, and amino acids
are reabsorbed in the proximal tubule. Reabsorption of
glucose and amino acids is complete, and these
substances are not normally present in urine; in
contrast, sodium, potassium, phosphate, and bicarbonate are reabsorbed or excreted, depending on the
body's needs. The kidney is the major organ for control

of serum phosphorus concentration, and most reabsorption of phosphate occurs in the proximal tubule.[4] Parathyroid hormone (PTH) inhibits reabsorption of phosphate, thus promoting urinary phosphate excretion. The kidney is a major source for elimination of potassium from the body, a process regulated in the distal tubule by aldosterone, which causes secretion of potassium and reabsorption of sodium. The kidneys also are important regulators of acid-base balance; bicarbonate is regenerated in the proximal tubule, and hydrogen ion is secreted by the distal tubule.

The kidneys play a critical role in maintaining extracellular fluid volume. Approximately 90% of water in glomerular filtrate is reabsorbed by the time it reaches the distal tubule and collecting duct.[4] In the absence of antidiuretic hormone (ADH), the collecting duct is impermeable to water, and dilute urine is produced. In contrast, states of decreased extracellular fluid volume or increased plasma osmolality cause release of ADH from the pituitary gland, which increases permeability of the collecting duct, enhancing reabsorption of water and facilitating excretion of concentrated urine. In addition to the action of ADH, a hypertonic medullary interstitium is necessary for the kidney to produce concentrated urine. This is maintained by the loops of Henle, which operate as countercurrent multipliers, and the vasa recta, which act as countercurrent exchangers (Fig. 16–2). Chloride is actively transported out of the thick portion of the ascending loop of Henle into the interstitium. In addition, passive diffusion of urea from the collecting duct and sodium and chloride from the thin limb of the loop of Henle contribute to medullary hypertonicity. The relatively slow flow of blood through the vasa recta minimizes removal of solutes from the interstitium, and the countercurrent exchanger system results in recirculation of solutes within the medulla.

Hormone Production

In addition to excretory and regulatory functions, the kidneys produce erythropoietin and renin and activate vitamin D. Erythropoietin is produced by peritubular endothelial cells in the renal cortex in response to anemia or hypoxia; it stimulates erythroid progenitor cells in the bone marrow to produce red blood cells.[5] Renin is produced by juxtaglomerular cells located in the wall of the afferent arterioles and is released in response to decreased extracellular fluid volume or blood pressure and increased sympathetic stimulation.[6] Renin release results in production of angiotensin II and aldosterone, which increase blood pressure and extracellular fluid volume. The kidneys also convert 25-hydroxyvitamin D_3 to 1,25-dihydroxyvitamin D_3 (calcitriol), a process facilitated by the renal tubular enzyme 1α-hydroxylase. The activity of this enzyme is increased by PTH and hypophosphatemia and is inhibited by hypercalcemia, hyperphosphatemia, and calcitriol.[7, 8]

Problem Identification

Polyuria and Polydipsia

Polyuria and polydipsia (PU/PD) are commonly reported problems in veterinary patients. Polyuria is production of more than 50 mL/kg per day of urine, whereas PD is consumption of more than 100 mL/kg per day of water. With few exceptions, these two problems usually occur together; primary PD

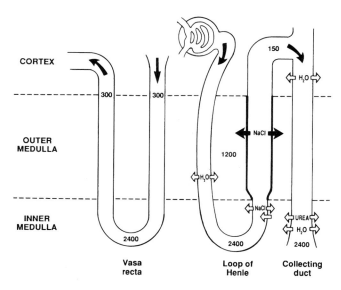

Figure 16–2

Drawing illustrating the countercurrent multiplier system, which is responsible for urine concentrating ability. Numbers represent osmolality in milliosmoles per liter (mOsm/L). Glomerular filtrate enters the descending loop of Henle, and solutes are concentrated as water (H_2O) moves passively *(open arrows)* into the hypertonic medullary interstitium. The thick ascending limb of Henle *(dark lines)* is impermeable to H_2O. In contrast, sodium chloride (NaCl) moves from the loop of Henle by passive transport *(open arrows)* into the inner medulla and by active transport *(shaded arrows)* into the outer medulla, resulting in dilute urine (150 mOsm/L) as it enters the distal tubule. In the presence of antidiuretic hormone, H_2O is passively reabsorbed *(open arrows)* into the hypertonic medullary interstitium, producing concentrated urine. The vasa recta help maintain medullary hypertonicity by recirculating solutes such as NaCl and urea and preventing their removal in excessive quantities. (Adapted from Guyton AC. Textbook of Medical Physiology, 8th ed. Philadelphia, WB Saunders, 1991:310; Finco D. Kidney function. In: Kaneko JJ, ed. Clinical Biochemistry of Domestic Animals, 4th ed. San Diego, Academic Press, 1989:506.)

Table 16-1
Causes of Polyuria and Polydipsia in Dogs and Cats

CAUSE	MECHANISM OF POLYURIA AND POLYDIPSIA
Drugs and Dietary Supplements	
Corticosteroids	Interfere with action of ADH on tubule
Anticonvulsants	Interfere with action of ADH on tubule
Phenobarbital	
Primidone	
Diuretics	Interfere with renal tubular function
Excessive thyroid hormone	Increased blood flow through vasa recta?
Salt supplementation	Compensatory polyuria due to increased water intake
Intravenous fluid therapy	Medullary solute washout
Vitamin D	Secondary to hypercalcemia
Endocrine Disorders	
Hyperadrenocorticism	Interferes with action of ADH
Diabetes mellitus	Osmotic diuresis due to glucosuria and ketonuria
Hyperthyroidism	Increased blood flow through vasa recta?
Hypoadrenocorticism	Renal sodium loss due to aldosterone deficiency
Central diabetes insipidus	Decreased production and release of ADH
Hypersomatotropism (acromegaly)	Usually occurs with diabetes mellitus
Renal Disorders	
Chronic renal disease/failure	Insufficient numbers of functional nephrons
Pyelonephritis	Increased medullary blood flow; renal tubular dysfunction
Primary renal glucosuria	Osmotic diuresis
Nephrogenic diabetes insipidus	Congenital lack of renal tubular ADH receptors; acquired ADH receptor dysfunction (e.g., pyometra, hypercalcemia, hypokalemia)
Hepatic Disorders	
Hepatic insufficiency	Decreased medullary tonicity from lack of urea
Portosystemic shunts	Compensatory polyuria due to increased water intake
Electrolyte Disorders	
Hypercalcemia	Interferes with action of ADH on renal tubule; increased medullary blood flow; reduced transport of sodium into interstitium; renal tubular mineralization
Hypokalemia	Increased thirst due to release of angiotensin II; decreased renal tubular response to ADH; decreased medullary tonicity
Miscellaneous	
Pyometra	Endotoxin-induced renal tubular damage; decreased tubular response to ADH
Psychogenic polydipsia	Compensatory polyuria due to increased water intake
Polycythemia	Mechanism unknown

ADH, antidiuretic hormone.

usually is accompanied by compensatory PU, and diseases that cause PU are associated with compensatory PD.

Pathophysiology

PU/PD may be a physiologic response to increased environmental temperature or increased water content of the diet, or they may indicate an underlying disease. The mechanism of PU/PD varies depending on the underlying cause (Table 16-1).

Clinical Signs

Owners of pets with PU/PD may notice that the pet drinks more frequently or appears to be consuming larger volumes of water, wakes the owner in the middle of the night to urinate (i.e., nocturia), or appears to no longer be housebroken. The history should elucidate any environmental changes (e.g., increased humidity or temperature) or treatment with drugs that may have caused increased water consumption (see Table 16-1). Other historical and abnormal physical examination findings depend on the cause of PU/PD. Diabetes mellitus, hyperthyroidism, and hyperadrenocorticism usually cause increased appetite, whereas chronic renal failure (CRF), hypercalcemia, and hepatic disease usually are associated with decreased appetite and weight loss. In addition, weight loss often occurs despite an increased appetite with diabetes mellitus and hyperthyroidism. Patients with hyperadrenocorticism often have bilaterally symmetrical alopecia, thinning and hyperpigmentation of skin, and abdominal enlargement. Cats with hyperthyroidism usually have a palpable thyroid nodule and also may have signs of cardiac disease (e.g., tachycardia, gallop rhythm, murmur). Kidneys may be small and irregular in CRF or enlarged and painful in pyelonephritis or acute renal failure (ARF). Patients with pyometra may have fever, purulent vaginal discharge, or an enlarged uterus. Lymphadenopathy, hepatosplenomegaly, or a perianal mass may be present in hypercalcemic patients.

Diagnostic Plan

The initial step in evaluating patients with suspected PU/PD is to confirm that these problems actually exist. Polyuria sometimes is confused with pollakiuria, which is characterized by increased frequency of urination but with only small amounts of urine passed. Careful questioning of the owner helps differentiate these two disorders. Patients with pollakiuria usually have lower urinary tract disease and other abnormal historical findings such as stranguria, dysuria, and discolored urine. The only definitive method for confirming the presence of PU/PD is to measure water consumption and urine output. This is best accomplished by having the owner measure the pet's water consumption for 2 to 3 days at home, because hospitalization tends to decrease consumption of water. As an initial screening test, a urinalysis should be performed. A urine specific gravity (USG) greater than 1.030 in an otherwise normal urine sample (i.e., no glucosuria or significant proteinuria) in a nondehydrated patient suggests that PU/PD is highly unlikely.[9] Some patients with psychogenic PD, however, may concentrate urine to a USG greater than 1.030.

After it has been established that PU/PD exists, routine laboratory tests are performed, including complete blood count (CBC), serum biochemical profile, and urinalysis, to screen for an underlying cause. CRF, hypercalcemia, hypokalemia, diabetes mellitus, polycythemia, and primary renal glucosuria can be excluded on the basis of these results. Normal values for serum sodium and potassium make hypoadrenocorticism unlikely. Increased activity of serum alkaline

phosphatase often occurs in patients with hyperadrenocorticism, but it also may indicate hepatic disease, especially if there are other abnormalities, such as low blood urea nitrogen (BUN) and hyperbilirubinemia. A regenerative left shift often occurs in patients with pyometra or acute pyelonephritis, whereas a stress leukogram may be present in patients with hyperadrenocorticism. Pyuria can occur with pyelonephritis, pyometra, hyperadrenocorticism, and diabetes mellitus, and its presence indicates need for bacterial urine culture. USG is an extremely useful test for evaluation of patients with PU/PD. Hyposthenuria (USG <1.008) most often occurs with hypercalcemia, hyperadrenocorticism, pyometra, diabetes insipidus, and primary polydipsia; its presence essentially rules out renal failure as a cause of PU/PD.[9] Renal disease is suspected if isosthenuria (USG 1.008–1.013) is identified, especially on repeated urinalyses. If the patient is not azotemic, a creatinine clearance determination may be considered to detect renal dysfunction. Again, if USG is greater than 1.030 in the absence of glucosuria and proteinuria, PU/PD is unlikely, except for the rare case of psychogenic PD.

Ancillary tests may be necessary to confirm a diagnosis of some diseases that cause PU/PD. Serum thyroid hormone concentration may be measured to rule out hyperthyroidism in cats. Abdominal radiography or ultrasonography is useful to evaluate the size of the liver and look for adrenal masses or an enlarged uterus. Hepatic function testing, such as sulphabromophthalein (BSP) retention and serum bile acid concentrations, is indicated in patients with suspected hepatic disease. Hyperadrenocorticism is ruled out by performing an adrenocorticotropic hormone (ACTH) response test or a low-dose dexamethasone suppression test. This should be done before a water deprivation test is performed, because hyperadrenocorticism is much more common than either diabetes insipidus or psychogenic PD. In addition, patients with hyperadrenocorticism have confusing results on water deprivation testing.

If no cause for PU/PD has been identified by this point in the diagnostic evaluation, the possibilities of central or nephrogenic diabetes insipidus or psychogenic PD should be considered. A modified water deprivation test (see Chap. 45) may be used to distinguish among these three uncommon causes of PU/PD.[10] A more convenient and less expensive alternative to water deprivation is to administer exogenous ADH, such as DDAVP (desmopressin), for 2 to 3 days and monitor changes in water intake and USG (see Chap. 45). If renal disease is suspected (i.e., persistent isosthenuria), measurement of creatinine clearance before performance of a water deprivation test is strongly recommended.

Inappetence, Vomiting, and Diarrhea

Inappetence, vomiting, and diarrhea are nonspecific signs that may result from systemic or primary gastrointestinal disorders. These problems occur often in dogs and cats with renal failure; therefore, determination of serum concentrations of urea nitrogen and creatinine are indicated. For a more detailed discussion of these problems, see Chapters 31 and 32.

Retinal Lesions

Retinal lesions, including tortuous vessels, hemorrhages, edema, and detachments, may be associated with primary ophthalmic disorders as well as systemic disorders. These lesions have been documented in dogs and cats secondary to hypertension associated with CRF; it appears that retinal lesions are more common in cats than dogs.[11-13] Diagnostic evaluation of patients, therefore, should include evaluation of renal function and measurement of blood pressure. For further discussion of these problems, see Chapter 19.

Hypertension

Hypertension is a sustained increase in systolic or diastolic blood pressure; it is infrequently recognized in veterinary patients because it is difficult to measure blood pressure accurately. Direct arterial puncture is the most accurate method for measuring blood pressure; however, it may artificially elevate blood pressure because of the patient's fear, pain, or excitement. Results of blood pressure measurements obtained by indirect methods (i.e., Doppler and oscillometric techniques) have correlated closely with direct measurements and are more practical in veterinary patients.[14-16] Systolic and diastolic blood pressures greater than 180 and 100 mm Hg, respectively, are generally consistent with a diagnosis of hypertension, although some hypertensive patients may have values slightly lower and others have pressures that are much greater.[11-13, 17, 18]

Pathophysiology

Hypertension may be a primary disorder (essential hypertension) or it may occur secondary to another disease. Essential hypertension is uncommon in veterinary patients; most dogs and cats have hypertension associated with renal or endocrine disease. The incidence of hypertension associated with CRF in dogs may be 60%, and up to 80% of dogs with glomerular disease may be hypertensive.[11, 19] Other disorders associated with hypertension include hyperadrenocorticism and hyperthyroidism.[11, 13, 18]

Clinical Signs

Dogs and cats with hypertension may have clinical signs caused by hypertension; however, it is not uncommon for patients to have only signs of the underlying disease. The organs or body systems most often affected by hypertension include the eyes, heart, nervous system, and kidneys. The most common clinical signs are blindness, retinal lesions (see Retinal Lesions), and cardiac murmurs.[12, 13, 18, 20] Neurologic signs (e.g., altered mentation, head tilt, seizures) and epistaxis occur less frequently.[20, 21]

Diagnostic Plan

If hypertension is suspected on the basis of clinical findings, blood pressure should be measured and appropriate tests performed to identify an underlying disease. A minimum database, including CBC, serum chemistries, and urinalysis, should be gathered initially. Depending on results of history, physical examination, and minimum database, additional tests (e.g., ACTH response, low-dose dexamethasone suppression, serum thyroxine concentration) may be indicated.

Oral Ulcerations

Ulcerations of oral mucous membranes occur in dogs and cats secondary to trauma, ingestion of toxic substances, infectious diseases, and systemic disorders. Careful evaluation of the history and physical examination findings should help to identify the cause of oral ulcerations. Patients with uremia secondary to either ARF or CRF may have oral ulcerations; therefore, measurement of serum chemistries and analysis of urine are indicated to evaluate renal function.

Pallor

Pale mucous membranes occur secondary to anemia or peripheral vasoconstriction. Physical examination of patients with decreased perfusion secondary to peripheral vasoconstriction usually reveals other abnormal findings, such as prolonged capillary refill time, tachycardia, and poor pulse quality. A CBC documents anemia. Pallor of mucous membranes often is noted in patients with CRF caused by nonregenerative anemia; therefore, evaluation of renal function may be indicated.

Abdominal Enlargement

Abdominal enlargement results from organomegaly, fluid accumulation (ascites), or weakness of

Table 16–2
Causes of Renomegaly in Dogs and Cats

Inflammation
Leptospirosis
Feline infectious peritonitis
Renal abscesses

Neoplasia
Lymphoma (primarily cats)
Renal cell carcinoma
Cystadenocarcinoma
Sarcomas
Nephroblastoma (Wilms tumor)

Obstruction
Hydronephrosis

Cysts
Polycystic kidney disease
Feline perirenal pseudocysts

Miscellaneous
Hematomas
Compensatory hypertrophy
Ethylene glycol toxicosis

the abdominal muscles (e.g., hyperadrenocorticism). The distinction between organomegaly and ascites usually can be made on physical examination, although abdominal radiography and ultrasonography also are helpful. Additional diagnostic tests are useful to determine the cause of abdominal fluid (see Chap. 34). Disorders of the kidneys and ureters that are most likely to cause abdominal accumulation of fluid include nephrotic syndrome and ruptured urinary tract. Results of serum chemistries and urinalysis reveal hypoalbuminemia and significant proteinuria in patients with nephrotic syndrome (see Nephrotic Syndrome). Ruptured urinary tract usually is suspected on the basis of history, physical examination, laboratory evaluation, and radiographic findings (see Chap. 17).

Renomegaly

Renomegaly is the finding of abnormally enlarged kidneys. Although kidney size can be subjectively determined by abdominal palpation, it is more objectively evaluated by abdominal radiography.

Pathophysiology

The kidneys may become enlarged secondary to inflammatory or infectious diseases, neoplastic infiltration, urinary tract obstruction, acute tubular necrosis (e.g., ethylene glycol toxicosis), or development of renal cysts or pseudocysts (Table 16–2).

Clinical Signs

Clinical findings in patients with renomegaly may include lethargy, depression, inappetence, vomiting, and weight loss; some owners may detect abdominal enlargement. Physical examination findings may include unilateral or bilateral renomegaly as well as abnormalities that result from the cause of renomegaly (e.g., fever and chorioretinitis with feline infectious peritonitis). Signs of renal failure, such as dehydration, pale mucous membranes, and oral ulcerations, also may be present.

Diagnostic Plan

If renomegaly is suspected on the basis of physical examination findings, it should be confirmed by abdominal radiography. In general, the length of the kidney on the ventrodorsal view should be 2.0 to 3.0 times the length of the second lumbar vertebra in cats, and 2.5 to 3.5 times in dogs.[22, 23] Determining whether there is unilateral or bilateral renomegaly may help in the initial evaluation of an underlying cause (Figs. 16–3 and 16–4). Disorders that cause unilateral renomegaly include primary renal neoplasms, compensatory hypertrophy, and renal abscesses or hematomas; bilateral renomegaly is most likely to result from feline infectious peritonitis (FIP), lymphoma, leptospirosis, ethylene glycol (antifreeze) toxicosis, and polycystic kidney disease. Perirenal pseudocysts, hydronephrosis, and some primary renal tumors may cause either unilateral or bilateral renomegaly.

Additional diagnostic tests are indicated to determine the cause of renomegaly. A CBC, serum chemistries, and urinalysis are performed to detect renal failure and signs of other organ system involvement (e.g., hyperglobulinemia with FIP, hepatic disease with leptospirosis). Thoracic radiographs reveal pulmonary metastases in patients with suspected renal neoplasia. Abdominal ultrasonography is useful for evaluation of renal architecture and detection of changes consistent with polycystic kidney disease, perirenal cysts, hydronephrosis, or renal neoplasia.[24–27] Excretory urography is indicated if an abdominal mass is suspected to be an enlarged kidney but is not confirmed by plain films or if urinary tract obstruction is suspected. After cystic lesions have been ruled out, the next step is to obtain a sample of renal tissue by fine-needle aspiration. Renal neoplasia, especially lymphoma, may readily be diagnosed by cytologic evaluation of renal aspirates; however, if results are inconclusive, a renal biopsy is indicated.

Peripheral Edema

Peripheral edema occurs secondary to increased hydrostatic pressure, decreased oncotic pressure

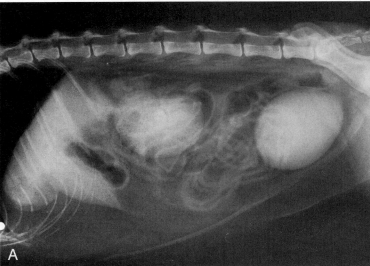

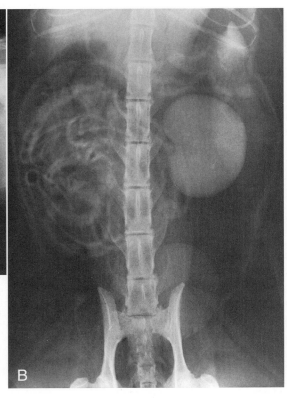

Figure 16–3
Lateral **(A)** and ventrodorsal **(B)** radiographs demonstrate unilateral renomegaly due to compensatory hypertrophy in a cat with chronic renal failure and unilateral renal agenesis.

caused by hypoalbuminemia, increased capillary membrane permeability caused by inflammation, and lymphatic dysfunction or obstruction. Patients with protein-losing glomerular diseases (e.g., amyloidosis, glomerulonephritis) may develop peripheral edema from decreased oncotic pressure. As with patients with ascites, results of laboratory evaluation can rule out hypoalbuminemia as the cause of edema.

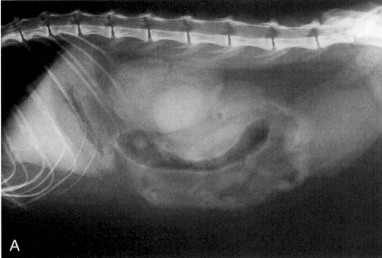

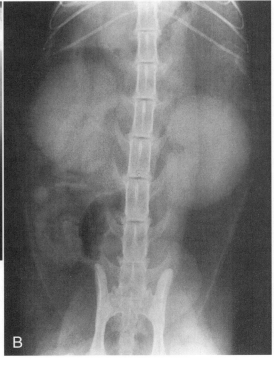

Figure 16–4
Lateral **(A)** and ventrodorsal **(B)** radiographs of a cat with bilateral renomegaly due to renal lymphoma.

Azotemia

Azotemia is the laboratory finding of increased concentrations of BUN and serum creatinine.

Pathophysiology

Increased concentrations of BUN or serum creatinine may result from increased rate of production, decreased rate of excretion, or both.[28] Increased production of urea may occur with catabolic states (e.g., treatment with corticosteroids), consumption of a high-protein diet, or gastrointestinal hemorrhage; with these conditions, azotemia usually is mild (BUN < 60–80 mg/dL, creatinine normal) and is not associated with decreased glomerular filtration rate (GFR). In other instances, azotemia is caused by decreased GFR, which may result from prerenal, renal, or postrenal disorders (Table 16–3). Prerenal azotemia results from any disorder that causes decreased renal perfusion; renal structure remains normal, and the kidneys are capable of normal function if the prerenal insult is corrected before permanent renal damage occurs. Renal azotemia (renal failure) occurs when 75% of nephrons are nonfunctional and may be caused by a variety of disorders that affect glomeruli, tubules, renal interstitium, or renal vasculature. Postrenal azotemia is caused by disorders that impair elimination of urine from the body, such as urinary tract obstruction or rupture. Sites most often involved are the urethra, the urinary bladder, and, less frequently, the ureters and kidneys. In order for upper urinary tract disease to cause postrenal azotemia, both kidneys or ureters must be affected, unless the patient has concomitant renal disease or failure. As with prerenal disorders, renal function in patients with postrenal azotemia is initially normal, and development of renal injury depends on the severity, duration, and nature of the disorder that impairs urine outflow (i.e., ureteral obstruction versus rupture).

Diagnostic Plan

The initial diagnostic step in evaluating patients with azotemia is to distinguish among prerenal, renal, and postrenal disorders. Patients with prerenal azotemia often have evidence of dehydration, hypovolemia, or cardiac disease; therefore, physical examination should include evaluation of capillary refill time, skin turgor, mucous membrane color, pulse rate and quality, and heart sounds. Patients with renal azotemia caused by CRF may have a history of polyuria, whereas patients with prerenal azotemia and ARF often have oliguria. Complete absence of urine production (anuria) is most often caused by lower urinary tract obstruction, although it also may occur in some cases of ARF caused by ethylene glycol toxicosis. If there is

Table 16–3
Disorders Associated With Azotemia

Prerenal Disorders
Normal glomerular filtration rate
High-protein diet
Gastrointestinal hemorrhage
Catabolic drugs
   Corticosteroids
   Tetracyclines
   Early dehydration
Decreased glomerular filtration rate
Hypovolemia
   Dehydration (vomiting, diarrhea, ascites)
   Hypoalbuminemia
   Hemorrhage
   Hypoadrenocorticism
Hypotension
   Inhalational anesthesia
   Vasodilator drugs
Decreased cardiac output
   Congestive heart failure
   Pericardial disease
   Cardiac arrhythmias

Renal Disorders
Glomerular
Glomerulonephritis
Amyloidosis
Tubular
Congenital disorders
Tubular necrosis
Nephrotoxicosis
Ischemia
Neoplasia
Interstitial
Nephritis (leptospirosis)
Pyelonephritis
Neoplasia
Vascular
Thrombosis
Embolic disease
Vasculitis

Postrenal Disorders
Urinary tract obstruction or rupture
Urolithiasis
Urethral plugs
Neoplasia
Herniated urinary bladder
Trauma
Blood clots
Iatrogenic
   Inadvertent surgical ligation (ureters)
   Traumatic urethral catheterization
   Manual compression of urinary bladder

any question regarding patency of the lower urinary tract, an attempt to pass a urinary catheter should be made. Other signs that suggest postrenal azotemia from lower urinary tract disease include stranguria, dysuria, pollakiuria, and discolored urine. Abdominal pain, ascites, renomegaly, a firm and painful urinary bladder, subcutaneous swelling or discoloration of the perineum, or palpable masses of the urethra, urinary bladder, or prostate gland suggests postrenal azotemia. Abdominal ultrasonography is helpful for detecting masses and accumulation of fluid if urinary tract obstruction or rupture is suspected. Abdominal fluid analysis in patients with uroabdomen reveals a modified transudate or exudate, characterized cytologically by neutrophils, macrophages, mesothelial cells, and occasionally bacteria, especially if there is urinary tract infection.[28, 29] Urea concentration in abdominal fluid often equals that of plasma, whereas creatinine concentration in the fluid usually equals or exceeds concurrent serum creatinine. Contrast urethrocystography is indicated if rupture or obstruction of the urethra or urinary bladder is likely; excretory urography is indicated if rupture of the upper urinary tract is suspected.

One of the most useful tests for distinguishing between prerenal and renal azotemia is analysis of urine obtained before any treatment. Azotemic patients with evidence of urinary concentration (i.e., USG >1.030 in dogs, >1.045 in cats) most likely have prerenal azotemia, although there are some exceptions. Hypoadrenocorticism, diabetes mellitus, hypercalcemia, and administration of drugs such as diuretics, corticosteroids, or fluids may be associated with prerenal azotemia and decreased USG, despite normal renal function. In fact, hypoadrenocorticism may easily be misdiagnosed as ARF, because these patients have similar clinical and laboratory findings.[30] Dogs and cats with renal azotemia usually have isosthenuria (USG 1.008–1.013) or minimally concentrated urine (USG <1.025).[31] Because cats with experimentally induced renal azotemia may produce concentrated urine, renal failure cannot definitively be excluded in azotemic cats with USG values greater than 1.045.[32] However, most cats with naturally occurring CRF have USG values lower than 1.035.[31, 33] USG analysis often is not helpful in patients with postrenal azotemia, because urinary tract obstruction may cause renal tubular dysfunction and interfere with urine concentrating ability.[28, 34]

Finally, response to treatment may help differentiate among prerenal, renal, and postrenal azotemia. Prerenal and postrenal azotemia usually resolve rapidly (within 1–3 days) after correction of the underlying cause, whereas azotemia from renal failure decreases more slowly or persists after appropriate treatment. Severe or prolonged prerenal or postrenal azotemia may cause renal injury, which eventually leads to renal failure. It also is possible for renal azotemia to exist concomitantly with either prerenal or postrenal disorders, and this should be suspected in patients that do not respond to treatment as expected.

Hypoalbuminemia

Decreased concentrations of serum albumin usually result from either decreased production (i.e., hepatic dysfunction) or increased loss, as in gastrointestinal, glomerular, or third-space disorders. Glomerular diseases, amyloidosis and glomerulonephritis, are the only diseases of the urinary tract that cause hypoalbuminemia. For further discussion of hypoalbuminemia, see Chapter 34.

Hyperphosphatemia

Hyperphosphatemia is the laboratory finding of increased serum concentration of phosphorus. Like potassium, most phosphorus in the body is found in the intracellular space; however, clinical signs of hyperphosphatemia usually correlate with serum phosphorus concentration.[35]

Pathophysiology

The consequences of hyperphosphatemia include precipitation of calcium phosphate in soft tissues, suppression of 1α-hydroxylase activity, and hypocalcemia. Soft tissue mineralization is most likely to occur when the product of serum phosphorus and calcium concentration exceeds 60.[36] Complications of soft tissue mineralization depend on the organ affected (e.g., lungs, heart, kidneys) but may include cardiac arrhythmias and renal failure. Hyperphosphatemia has a direct inhibitory effect on 1α-hydroxylase, which decreases renal production of active vitamin D.[7] This, in turn, decreases mobilization of calcium from bone and the intestines, which causes hypocalcemia. Hypocalcemia also may occur as a result of the mass-law effect or soft tissue deposition of calcium.

Hyperphosphatemia may be physiologic, or it may result from transcellular shifts, increased intake, or decreased excretion (Table 16–4). Mild hyperphosphatemia is considered normal in young, growing puppies, especially in giant breeds; however, it is not as evident in kittens.[36] Because serum phosphorus concentration may increase postprandially, blood samples should be collected after a 12- to 18-hour fast. Disorders that cause release of phosphorus from the intracellular space are potential causes of hyperphosphatemia, although this rarely occurs in veterinary patients.[37, 38] Use of phosphate-containing enemas in cats and small dogs may cause hyperphosphatemia from colonic absorption as well as hypocalcemia, hyperglycemia, and hypernatremia.[39–41] Iatrogenic hy-

Table 16–4
Causes of Hyperphosphatemia

Physiologic
Postprandial
Young, growing dogs
Healing fracture

Transcellular Shifts
Hemolysis
Tumor lysis syndrome
Soft tissue trauma
Rhabdomyolysis
Osteolysis

Increased Intake and Absorption
Phosphate enemas
Excessive IV phosphate administration
Vitamin D toxicosis

Decreased Excretion
Azotemia
 Prerenal
 Renal
 Postrenal
Primary hypoparathyroidism
Hyperthyroidism (cats)
Hypersomatotropism (acromegaly)

perphosphatemia may result from excessive intravenous (IV) administration of potassium phosphate to treat hypophosphatemia, which is most often associated with diabetic ketoacidosis in small animals.[42] Vitamin D rodenticide toxicosis in dogs and cats is associated with hyperphosphatemia, hypercalcemia from increased gastrointestinal absorption, and subsequent azotemia.[43, 44] Because most phosphorus is eliminated through the kidneys, decreased renal excretion is the most common cause of clinically important hyperphosphatemia in veterinary patients. Disorders that cause prerenal azotemia also may be associated with mild to moderate hyperphosphatemia, whereas renal failure usually causes moderate to severe hyperphosphatemia. Primary hypoparathyroidism, hyperthyroidism, and acromegaly also may cause decreased renal excretion of phosphorus and hyperphosphatemia, although this usually is not clinically important.[45–49] Rarely, hemolysis, rapid tumor cell lysis, and severe soft tissue trauma can lead to hyperphosphatemia in small animal patients.[37, 38]

Diagnostic Plan

The initial approach to patients depends on the severity of hyperphosphatemia and the presence of other laboratory abnormalities. Mild hyperphosphatemia in young, growing puppies, especially giant breeds, requires no further evaluation. Many causes of hyperphosphatemia can be excluded on the basis of history (e.g., patient not fasted, administration of phosphate enemas or parenteral phosphate). Patients with hypoparathyroidism show clinical signs (e.g., tetany) as a result of hypocalcemia and not hyperphosphatemia (see Chap. 49). If the patient has hyperphosphatemia and concurrent azotemia, it should be determined whether the cause is prerenal, renal, or postrenal (see Azotemia). If a patient has concurrent hyperphosphatemia and hypercalcemia, vitamin D toxicosis is a possibility; the owner should be asked about potential exposure to rodenticides containing cholecalciferol. Hypercalcemia occurs rarely along with hyperphosphatemia in some patients with CRF, particularly in young dogs.[50] In these cases, it may be difficult to determine whether renal failure is secondary to hypercalcemia or vice versa.[31, 50]

Anemia

Anemia is classified as either regenerative or nonregenerative on the basis of the number of reticulocytes present. Nonregenerative anemias result from decreased bone marrow production of red cells. A variety of toxic, neoplastic, infectious, inflammatory, and endocrine disorders can cause nonregenerative anemia. CRF is the most important disorder of the urinary system that causes nonregenerative anemia. For further discussion of anemia see Chapter 41.

Failure of Maximal Urine Concentrating Ability

Urine concentrating ability is most often measured by USG, and there is a wide range of normal values for dogs and cats. Many disorders can interfere with urine concentrating ability (see Polyuria and Polydipsia).

Proteinuria

Proteinuria is the laboratory finding of urine protein by urinalysis. Normal dogs and cats excrete less than 30 to 35 mg of protein per kilogram of body weight per day in their urine; amounts greater than these values are considered significant.[51–56] Such a finding often coincides with a protein value of 2+ or higher on routine urinalyses.

Pathophysiology

The glomerulus prevents entry of most plasma proteins into urine by acting as a charge- and size-selective barrier. Large proteins (e.g., albumin, immunoglobulins) usually are not present in urine, although a small amount of albumin does filter through the glomerulus in normal animals. Proteins such as myoglobin and immunoglobulin light chains (e.g., Bence

Jones proteins) are small enough to pass through the glomerulus. Although the size of hemoglobin allows hemoglobin to pass through the glomerulus, it usually does not appear in urine because it is bound to haptoglobin. However, if the binding capacity of haptoglobin is exceeded, as in acute intravascular hemolysis, hemoglobinuria occurs. In addition to size restriction, negative charges on glomerular capillary walls hinder passage of negatively charged molecules such as albumin. Proteins that do enter glomerular filtrate often are completely absorbed by renal tubular cells. Some proteins, such as mucoproteins and secretory immunoglobulins, are produced in the renal tubules and are found in urine. A small amount of protein may be detected in the urine of normal dogs and cats, especially in concentrated urine samples.

Causes of proteinuria may be prerenal, renal, or postrenal or, in some cases, a combination (Table 16–5). Hyperproteinemia may cause spilling of proteins into the urine, although inflammatory diseases associated with hyperproteinemia also may cause glomerulonephritis and subsequent proteinuria. Hemoglobinuria associated with intravascular hemolysis, and rarely, myoglobinuria associated with rhabdomyolysis, may cause prerenal proteinuria.[57] Excess production of immunoglobulins and Bence Jones proteinuria may occur in some dogs and cats with multiple myeloma.[58–61] Renal proteinuria may result from glomerular, tubular, or interstitial disease, although glomerular protein loss is more clinically significant. Postrenal proteinuria results from disorders of the urogenital system, most commonly from lower urinary tract inflammation.

Diagnostic Plan

The screening tests used most often to detect proteinuria are the dipstick and the sulfosalicylic acid (SSA) tests. The dipstick is a colorimetric test that primarily detects albumin.[62] Negative dipstick reactions may occur despite significant proteinuria if the urine sample is dilute or if the protein present is not albumin (e.g., Bence Jones proteins). An extremely alkaline urine (pH >9) may cause a false-positive protein reaction.[63] The SSA test (Bumintest Tabs) is a turbidimetric test that is most sensitive to albumin but also detects globulins and Bence Jones proteins. Therefore, patients with Bence Jones proteinuria may have a negative dipstick protein reaction but a positive SSA test.[64] Because the SSA test is more sensitive than a dipstick, it usually detects smaller amounts of protein. In contrast to the dipstick, the SSA test is not affected by urine pH. Both tests, however, must be interpreted in light of USG. A trace protein reaction with either the dipstick or the SSA test may be normal at any USG, and values of 1+ may be normal with USG greater than

1.030; however, a urine protein value of 2+ or higher at any USG should be considered abnormal, and the patient should be evaluated further.[51] It also is possible for patients with significant proteinuria to have a negative dipstick test; these patients, especially if hypoalbuminemic, may best be screened by determining the ratio of protein to creatinine in the urine.

The initial approach to patients with proteinuria identified by a screening test is to rule out prerenal and postrenal causes. Most patients with postrenal proteinuria have signs of lower urinary tract disease (e.g., stranguria, dysuria, pollakiuria) or urinary sediment abnormalities (e.g., pyuria, hematuria, cylindruria). Collection of urine by cystocentesis excludes the genital tract as a source of proteinuria. Results of CBC and serum chemistries are helpful for identification of

Table 16–5
Causes of Pathologic Proteinuria in Dogs and Cats

Prerenal
Hyperproteinemia
  Infectious and inflammatory disorders
  Plasma transfusion
Hemoglobinemia
Myoglobinemia
Bence Jones proteinuria
Congestive heart failure
Hypertension

Renal
Glomerular
  Glomerulonephritis
  Amyloidosis (dogs)
  Glomerulosclerosis
Tubular
  Tubular necrosis
    Ischemia
    Toxicosis
  Tubular dysfunction
    Fanconi's syndrome
Interstitial
  Pyelonephritis
  Leptospirosis
  Neoplasia

Postrenal
Urinary (Bladder and Urethra)
  Bacterial cystitis
  Urolithiasis
  Feline lower urinary tract disease
  Neoplasia
  Sterile hemorrhagic cystitis
Genital
  Vaginitis
  Prostatitis

Table 16–6
Mean Values of Diagnostic Test Results in Patients With Renal Disease and Proteinuria*

DISORDER	URINARY PROTEIN LOSS (mg/day)	URINARY PROTEIN LOSS (mg/kg body weight per day)	URINE PROTEIN/ CREATININE RATIO
Glomerulonephritis	2265.3 (245.5–17,520)	116 (7.5–526.1)	5.73 (0.47–43.4)
Amyloidosis	9059.8 (5742–14,400)	481.7 (350.8–533.7)	22.5 (11.17–46.65)
Chronic interstitial nephritis	536.5 (409.5–4074)	38.9 (17.6–138.1)	2.89 (1.51–10.52)
Normal dogs	36.0 (5.4–286.4)	1.5 (0.2–7.7)	0.05 (0.01–0.38)

*Numbers in parentheses represent range of reported values.
From Center SA, Wilkinson E, Smith CA, et al. 24-Hour urine protein/creatinine ratio in dogs with protein-losing nephropathies. J Am Vet Med Assoc 1985; 187:820–824.

potential causes of prerenal proteinuria such as hyperproteinemia and hemolysis. If a monoclonal hyperglobulinemia is identified by serum protein electrophoresis, urine immunoelectrophoresis should be done to detect Bence Jones proteins. If there is no evidence of hematuria (i.e., red cells on urinalysis) and the urine dipstick test is positive for occult blood, the possibility of hemoglobinuria or myoglobinuria is considered. Patients with hemoglobinuria have pink plasma and evidence of intravascular hemolysis; patients with myoglobinuria have clear plasma and evidence of severe muscle damage (e.g., painful muscles, increased activity of creatine kinase).

After prerenal and postrenal causes of proteinuria have been excluded, renal proteinuria should be considered. In general, glomerular disease is more likely to cause significant proteinuria than either renal tubular disease or interstitial disease. Patients with renal tubular or interstitial disease usually have other abnormal findings on physical examination or urinalysis (e.g., cylindruria, pyuria, hematuria, glucosuria). Therefore, a finding of proteinuria in an otherwise normal urinalysis suggests glomerular protein loss, especially if hypoalbuminemia exists. In order to determine the significance and severity of proteinuria, the ratio of urine protein to creatinine should be obtained next. This test has eliminated the need for 24-hour quantitation of urine output because it can be used to predict daily protein loss in dogs and cats and requires only one urine sample.[55, 56, 65–67] Urine protein/creatinine ratios are not affected by urine volume or concentration, so they are useful regardless of USG. However, postrenal proteinuria increases the protein/creatinine ratio despite absence of renal protein loss, and the ratio therefore should be interpreted in light of urine sediment findings.[68, 69] Most normal dogs and cats have a urine protein/creatinine ratio of less than 0.5.[55, 56, 65, 66] A ratio greater than 1 in dogs is consistent with urine protein loss in excess of

30 mg/kg per day and indicates significant proteinuria.[65, 67, 69] Dogs with glomerular disease often have ratios greater than 5.[67–69] Although amyloidosis is associated with more severe urinary protein loss and higher protein/creatinine ratios (>15) than are found in nonamyloid glomerular disease, there is considerable overlap, and the ratio cannot be used to reliably predict which disease exists. (Table 16–6).[67, 69, 70]

If a patient has persistently increased protein/creatinine ratios and normal urine sediment findings, further diagnostic tests are indicated. First, an attempt should be made to identify any disorders that may be associated with glomerular disease (Table 16–7).[34, 71–85] If an underlying disease cannot be found, renal biopsy should be considered (see Diagnostic Procedures). This allows for distinction among amyloidosis, glomerulonephritis, and interstitial nephritis, which have different prognoses and treatments.

Hematuria

Hematuria results from passage of red blood cells into urine; this may occur secondary to infection, inflammation, neoplasia, trauma, or bleeding disorders. Hematuria most often occurs secondary to diseases of the lower urinary tract and is accompanied by other signs, including pollakiuria, stranguria, and dysuria. Infrequently, hematuria results from disorders affecting the kidneys and ureters, such as urolithiasis, neoplasia, pyelonephritis, or idiopathic renal hematuria. These patients usually do not have signs of lower urinary tract disease. For a more complete discussion of hematuria, see Chapter 17.

Pyuria

Increased numbers of white blood cells in urine (pyuria) most often occurs secondary to infectious, inflammatory, or neoplastic disorders of the urinary tract. As with hematuria, signs of lower urinary tract

Table 16–7
Disorders Associated With Glomerular Diseases in Dogs and Cats

Inflammatory Disorders
Systemic lupus erythematosus
Polyarthritis
Chronic pancreatitis

Infectious Disorders
Bacterial
  Cholangiohepatitis
  Brucellosis
  Pyometra
  Chronic pyoderma
  Endocarditis
  Bacteremia
  Borreliosis
Viral
  Infectious canine hepatitis
  Feline leukemia virus
  Feline infectious peritonitis
Rickettsial
  Rocky Mountain spotted fever
  Ehrlichiosis
Parasitic
  Dirofilariasis
  Hepatozoonosis
  Leishmaniasis
  Trypanosomiasis

Neoplasia
Lymphoma
Leukemia (myeloid, lymphocytic)
Systemic mastocytosis
Primary erythrocytosis
Carcinoma

Familial Disorders
Beagle (amyloidosis)
Bernese mountain dog
Bull terrier
Chinese shar-pei (amyloidosis)
Doberman pinscher
Samoyed

Miscellaneous
Chronic hepatic disease
Hyperadrenocorticism
Diabetes mellitus
Chronic corticosteroid treatment

disease usually are present if the urinary bladder or urethra is affected. Upper urinary tract disorders that may cause pyuria include pyelonephritis, renal and ureteral neoplasms, and urolithiasis. For a more detailed discussion of pyuria, see Chapter 17.

Bacteriuria

A finding of bacteria on microscopic examination of sediment in urine collected by cystocentesis is abnormal in dogs and cats and suggests urinary tract infection. Not all patients with urinary tract infection, however, have bacteriuria apparent in urine sediment. If bacteriuria is identified, a sample of urine should be cultured to rule out infection. For a more detailed discussion of bacteriuria, see Chapter 17.

Diagnostic Procedures

Routine Laboratory Evaluation

Complete Blood Count and Serum Chemistries

Results of CBC and serum chemistries are helpful in evaluating patients with diseases of the kidneys and ureters. Changes in the hemogram (e.g., nonregenerative anemia) and leukogram (e.g., leukocytosis) are usually nonspecific. Evaluation of serum chemistries is necessary to identify abnormalities that occur in patients with renal disease or failure (e.g., azotemia, hyperphosphatemia, hyperkalemia) and to help differentiate these conditions from other disorders that cause azotemia, such as hypoadrenocorticism.

Urinalysis

Analysis of urine obtained before treatment is extremely helpful in the evaluation of patients with suspected renal disease. Cystocentesis is the preferred method for collecting urine, although a sample obtained by catheterization or during voiding may be appropriate in some cases. If a urinalysis cannot be done within 30 minutes of collection, the sample should be refrigerated until it can be evaluated, preferably within 12 hours.

Initial evaluation of urine includes determination of physical properties, such as color, transparency, and USG, and chemical properties, such as pH, protein, occult blood, and glucose. Normal urine should be yellow and clear. Concentrated samples tend to be darker, whereas dilute urine may appear colorless. Other substances such as bilirubin and hemoglobin also may affect urine color. USG is determined with a refractometer; if the sample is turbid, the supernatant should be used for measuring USG. USG is the only part of the urinalysis that helps evaluate renal function, and it is very useful for localizing azotemia. Chemical properties of urine are determined with the use of dipsticks that react by a change in color. Values for urinary pH vary in dogs and cats but usually are between 5.5 and 7.5. Urine pH values higher than 7.5 should prompt suspicion of urinary tract infection with urease-producing bacteria, especially if other signs of infection exist (e.g., dysuria, pollakiuria, pyuria). Proteinuria may be normal or abnormal, depending on USG and the amount of protein present. A positive occult blood reaction indicates the presence of blood, hemoglobin, or myoglobin in urine. Glucosuria is abnormal and occurs in patients with hyperglycemia (e.g., diabetes mellitus, hyperadrenocorticism) and, less often, with renal tubular dysfunction (e.g., Fanconi's syndrome, renal tubular necrosis).

Microscopic evaluation of urinary sediment provides valuable information, and it should be done in all cases.[86] A 5- to 10-mL sample of urine is centrifuged at 1000 to 3000 rotations per minute for 5 minutes. All but 0.5 mL of supernatant is removed, and the urine sediment is resuspended by agitation of the tube. One to two drops of resuspended urine sediment are transferred to a microscope slide, and a coverslip is placed over it. The slide is examined under low intensity with the 40× objective for white and red blood cells, epithelial cells, bacteria, and crystals; the 10× objective is used to look for casts.[87]

Interpretation of sediment findings must always be made with the method of collection in mind. Urine collected by cystocentesis from normal dogs and cats should contain no bacteria, fewer than 5 red or white blood cells per high-power field (40× lens), occasional epithelial cells, and fewer than two hyaline or granular casts per low-power field (10× lens). Absence of bacteria on urine sediment evaluation does not rule out urinary tract infection, because some bacteria, especially cocci, are difficult to identify unless they are present in large numbers. Cellular casts composed of red cells, white cells, or epithelial cells are always considered abnormal regardless of their number. Certain crystals, such as struvite, amorphous phosphate, bilirubin, and calcium oxalate, may be observed in urine of normal dogs and cats, whereas others, such as calcium phosphate or carbonate, ammonium biurate, and cystine, are considered abnormal.

Urine Culture

Culture of urine for bacteria is indicated if pyelonephritis is suspected on the basis of clinical findings, (fever, lumbar pain), laboratory results (leukocytosis, white blood cell casts, pyuria), or radiographic findings (dilated renal pelvis, hydronephrosis, or hydroureter). This is discussed in more detail in Chapter 17.

Evaluation of Glomerular Function

Blood Urea Nitrogen and Serum Creatinine

Once prerenal and postrenal factors have been excluded, BUN and serum creatinine concentrations serve as crude estimates of renal function in dogs and cats.[88] These factors increase as GFR decreases, although not in a linear fashion. The large changes in GFR that occur in early renal disease cause small changes in BUN and serum creatinine, whereas small changes in GFR in advanced renal failure may cause large changes in BUN and serum creatinine. Therefore, the magnitude of elevation in these factors cannot be used to distinguish among prerenal, renal, and postrenal disorders, to predict the reversibility of the underlying disease, or to differentiate ARF from CRF.[88] Finally, renal azotemia is not apparent until 75% of nephrons are nonfunctional; therefore, it is possible to have appreciable renal dysfunction in the absence of azotemia.

Measurement of Glomerular Filtration Rate

GFR is a more sensitive indicator of renal function than BUN or serum creatinine, and it should be measured if renal disease is suspected in nonazotemic patients. Creatinine clearance serves as a reliable estimate of GFR in dogs with normal renal function and in those with reduced renal mass.[89–91] Values for creatinine clearance appear to slightly underestimate GFR in cats.[32] For an endogenous creatinine clearance analysis, usually all urine produced during a 24-hour period is collected.[92] A period of time shorter than 24 hours may be used; however, it is important to accurately collect and measure all urine produced to lessen the chances of affecting the accuracy of calculated creatinine clearance. At the beginning of the collection period, the urinary bladder must be empty; either the patient should be allowed to urinate or a urinary catheter should be passed. Then all urine produced during the next 24 hours is collected with the use of a metabolic cage or intermittent catheterization. Samples of urine should be refrigerated until the end of the collection. At a point midway through the collection period, blood is collected for measurement of serum creatinine concentration. At the end of the collection period, the urinary bladder is again emptied, preferably by catheterization. The volume of urine produced is recorded, and the sample is thoroughly mixed before an aliquot is submitted for measurement of urine creatinine. Creatinine clearance is calculated using the formula

$$Cl = (U_{Cr} \times V) \div (S_{Cr} \times T \times BW)$$

where Cl is creatinine clearance (mL/min/kg), U_{Cr} is urine creatinine (mg/dL), V is urine volume (mL), S_{Cr} is serum creatinine (mg/dL), T is the collection period (min), and BW is body weight (kg). Normal values for endogenous creatinine clearance are 2.0 to 4.0 mL/min/kg in dogs and 1.6 to 3.8 mL/min/kg in cats.[92]

Radiography

Abdominal radiography is used to evaluate patients with suspected diseases of the kidneys and ureters. The right lateral recumbent view is recommended, because the outline of each individual kidney is more readily distinguishable. Plain films are helpful for evaluating kidney size, shape, and position and the presence of radiopaque uroliths. Kidney size is evaluated by comparing the length of the kidney on the ventrodorsal view with the length of the second lumbar vertebra. In normal dogs, the kidneys should be 2.5 to 3.5 times the length of the second lumbar vertebra; in cats, 2.0 to 3.0 times.[22, 23] Other findings on plain abdominal radiographs often are nonspecific. Patients with urinary tract trauma and rupture may have an increased density in the retroperitoneal space, which is consistent with accumulation of fluid.[93]

Excretory urography is useful in patients with upper urinary tract disorders, including pyelonephritis, upper urinary tract rupture or obstruction, and ectopic ureters.[94] In addition, the nephrogram phase of excretory urography may be used as a crude estimate of individual renal function, which is important if nephrectomy is being considered. Before excretory urography, the patient must be well prepared; food is withheld for 12 to 24 hours, and enemas are performed the night before and again no later than 2 hours before the procedure. An IV catheter is placed, and a bolus of water-soluble iodinated contrast medium (Conray) is administered at a dose of 180 mg of iodine per kilogram of body weight.[95] Patients with dilute urine as a result of decreased renal function or fluid therapy may require 360 mg/kg to enhance renal opacification. Ventrodorsal and lateral films should be taken immediately and at 5 to 10, 10 to 20, and 30 to 40 minutes after injection. Normal dogs experience decreased GFR for several days after excretory urography.[96] Although the risk of contrast-induced nephropathy appears to be minimal in dogs and cats, excretory urography should be performed only in hydrated patients.[94, 97, 98]

Ultrasonography

Ultrasonography is a noninvasive method for evaluating renal architecture and distinguishing between cystic and solid masses.[25, 27, 99] It may be used to confirm urinary tract obstruction (e.g., hydroureter, hydronephrosis), neoplasia, cystic renal disease, or uroliths.[24-27, 100] Ultrasonography of the kidneys is less useful for evaluation of diffuse renal parenchymal diseases such as glomerulonephritis and renal tubular necrosis; however, it may be used to guide renal biopsy in these cases.[26, 101]

Renal Biopsy

It is helpful to obtain samples of renal tissue for either cytologic or histologic examination in certain patients with renal disease. Fine-needle aspiration cytology may be used to diagnose renal neoplasia, especially lymphoma. Renal biopsy for histologic evaluation should be considered if findings are likely to result in improved patient management.[102] Patients with well-defined acute tubular necrosis do not require renal biopsy and are best evaluated by response to treatment.[34] However, if the patient does not respond as expected or if aggressive treatment such as dialysis is contemplated, renal biopsy should be considered. In such cases, histologic evaluation may help determine the reversibility of renal lesions.[103] In those cases in which it is difficult to differentiate between ARF and CRF (i.e., acutely decompensated CRF), renal histologic evaluation can provide important prognostic information. Renal biopsy also is indicated in patients with suspected glomerular disease to distinguish between glomerulonephritis and amyloidosis. Renal biopsy is contraindicated in patients with renal cysts, pyonephrosis, perirenal abscess, hydronephrosis, or coagulopathy,[23, 104] and it should be performed with caution in patients with a single kidney.

Renal biopsy should be performed only after careful patient evaluation, including coagulation studies (e.g., platelet count, bleeding time), measurement of hematocrit and total protein, plain film radiography, ultrasonography (if available), and, if indicated, contrast radiography. The laboratory should be contacted before renal biopsy to determine the appropriate solution in which to place specimens of renal tissue. Usually, samples of kidney for routine histologic evaluation, immunofluorescence, and electron microscopy are placed in formalin, Michel's solution, and glutaraldehyde, respectively.

Renal tissue may be obtained by several methods, including percutaneous (blind, keyhole, and ultrasound-guided) methods, at laparotomy, and by laparoscopy.[101, 102, 105] All techniques may be performed using a biopsy needle such as the Tru-Cut or Franklin-Silverman needle. General anesthesia or heavy sedation is recommended for all these procedures to provide analgesia and to minimize risks associated with renal biopsy. The keyhole approach is commonly used in dogs to obtain samples from the right kidney (Fig. 16–5).[104] The patient is placed in lateral recumbence with the vertebrae facing the surgeon. An oblique paralumbar incision 2 to 3 cm long is made through the skin (just caudal to the last rib and just below the ventral border of the lumbar muscles). The underlying tissue is bluntly dissected, with care being taken to avoid the intercostal artery located caudal to the last rib. The index finger is inserted into the abdominal cavity, and the kidney is palpated. At a separate site, a small skin incision is made, and the biopsy needle is introduced through the body wall. The index finger is used to guide the needle to the immobilized kidney. The long axis of the biopsy needle should not be directed toward the renal pelvis; instead, samples of renal cortex should be obtained by appropriate placement of the needle (Fig. 16–6). The biopsy

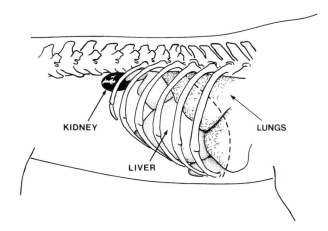

Figure 16-5
Drawing of landmarks for obtaining renal biopsy sample percutaneously by the keyhole technique.

needle is removed from the kidney, and digital pressure is applied to the site for several minutes. Before routine closure of the incision, the area is inspected for excessive hemorrhage.

The blind percutaneous technique is best suited for cats.[104] The kidney is localized and immobilized by digital palpation through the abdomen. A small skin incision is made over the proposed biopsy site. The remainder of the procedure is similar to that described for the keyhole approach.

If it is available, ultrasonography can be used to guide insertion of the biopsy needle into the kidney in both dogs and cats.[101] The technique is similar to that for the blind percutaneous method. Alternatively, samples of kidney may be obtained by laparoscopy, which also requires use of a biopsy needle.[105] If the clinician is unfamiliar with these techniques or a larger sample of kidney is needed, a wedge biopsy can be obtained by laparotomy.

Complications of renal biopsy include hematuria, hemorrhage, and hydronephrosis. Microscopic hematuria occurs in almost all patients and usually resolves within 3 days.[102, 105] The most serious complication of renal biopsy is severe hemorrhage, which in most cases is caused by faulty technique. Hydronephrosis caused by intrarenal blood clots occurs infrequently; IV administration of fluids to induce diuresis may prevent development of this complication.[102]

Common Diseases of the Kidney and Ureter

Acute Renal Failure

ARF is a syndrome characterized by an abrupt decline in renal function that occurs over a period of hours to days. The incidence of ARF is unknown; however, it does occur with some frequency, although less commonly than CRF. There seems to be no age, breed, or sex predisposition for development of ARF; however, older patients with pre-existing renal disease may be more likely to develop ARF, especially from ischemia. Free-roaming dogs and cats are more likely to develop ARF from ethylene glycol intoxication.

Pathophysiology

The clinical course of ARF consists of three phases: induction, maintenance, and recovery.[23, 106] The induction phase is the period of time from initial renal injury to development of azotemia and decreased urine concentrating ability. Intervention at this stage may prevent progression to the next phase, but most veterinary patients are presented for evaluation after the induction phase. The maintenance phase is characterized by irreversible renal injury; elimination of the underlying cause does not necessarily improve renal function. Urine volume may be characterized as either oliguria (<1.0 mL/kg per hour) or nonoliguria (>1.0 mL/kg per hour).[107] The maintenance phase usually lasts for several weeks, although most dogs and cats with ARF die or are euthanized during this phase unless supported by dialysis. Survival through the maintenance phase leads to the recovery phase, which may last several months. GFR may improve such that azotemia resolves during recovery; however, it still remains below normal.

Major pathophysiologic mechanisms proposed to cause ARF include (1) tubular obstruction from either intratubular casts or interstitial edema, (2) increased tubular permeability, such that glomerular

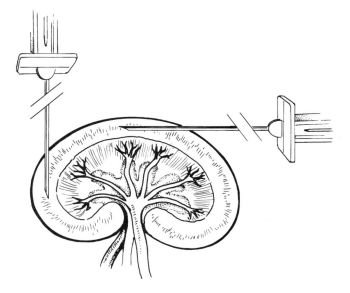

Figure 16-6
Drawing illustrating appropriate sites for renal biopsy using a Tru-Cut biopsy needle. Ideally, the needle should be guided through the cortex and should avoid the renal hilus, which contains the renal pelvis, artery, and vein.

filtrate passively leaks back into the renal interstitium, and (3) altered renal hemodynamics resulting in decreased GFR.[108] It is not known which of these is most important; it is possible that all play a role in the pathogenesis of ARF. Regardless of the mechanism, the end result appears to be preglomerular vasoconstriction with subsequent azotemia and, with some exceptions (e.g., aminoglycoside nephrotoxicosis), oliguria.

Many diseases and conditions are associated with ARF in small animal patients, and in some cases a cause is not identified. ARF occurs with disorders that cause either nephrosis (i.e., acute tubular necrosis) or nephritis. Acute tubular necrosis is by far the most common cause of ARF in dogs and cats, and it usually occurs secondary to nephrotoxicosis. However, renal ischemia may also be a cause of ARF, especially in those patients with conditions that predispose to such injury. Nephritis, although less common than nephrosis, may occur with some infectious diseases, such as leptospirosis. Unlike in humans, noninfectious causes of nephritis (e.g., immune-mediated) are not recognized as causes of ARF in veterinary patients.

Nephrotoxicosis

Clinically, the most important cause of ARF in small animal patients is nephrotoxicosis. Although many substances can potentially cause ARF, only a few occur with any frequency in veterinary patients (Table 16–8). With the exception of ethylene glycol, most substances that commonly cause ARF are therapeutic agents. Ethylene glycol toxicosis probably is the most common cause of ARF in dogs and cats.[23] Ethylene glycol becomes toxic only after hepatic conversion to its toxic metabolites (glyoxalate, oxalate), a reaction that is greatly accelerated by the enzyme alcohol dehydrogenase.[109] Metabolites of ethylene glycol inhibit important cellular enzymes and interfere with cellular respiration, which causes renal tubular necrosis. Tubular deposition of calcium oxalate crystals may contribute to renal injury but is not essential. All aminoglycosides are potentially nephrotoxic; however, gentamicin (Gentocin) often is responsible, probably because of its extensive use compared with other agents.[110] Aminoglycosides interfere with renal tubular respiration, causing tubular necrosis and decreased GFR. Decreased GFR leads to reduced elimination of gentamicin, which potentiates additional renal injury. The antifungal agent amphotericin B (Fungizone) is reported to be the third most common cause of ARF in veterinary patients.[23] Amphotericin B causes renal vasoconstriction, which reduces renal blood flow and GFR.[111]

Other agents infrequently cause nephrotoxic ARF in small animals. The antineoplastic agent cisplatin (Platinol) causes renal tubular necrosis and ARF; the severity of nephrotoxicosis is dose-dependent, and

Table 16–8
Potential Causes of Nephrotoxicosis in Dogs and Cats

Therapeutic Agents
Aminoglycosides
Amphotericin B
Tetracycline (IV)
Cisplatin
Thiacetarsamide

Endogenous Substances
Hypercalcemia
Hemoglobinuria
Myoglobinuria

Miscellaneous Substances
Ethylene glycol
Iodinated contrast agents
New methylene blue (hemoglobinuria)

most dogs with clinically normal renal function tolerate doses of 60 to 70 mg/m² if appropriate preventive measures are employed.[112] Hypercalcemia can cause ARF, especially if concurrent hyperphosphatemia exists.[23] IV administration of 30 mg/kg or more of oxytetracycline to dogs can cause ARF that may be fatal.[113] The severity appears to be dose-related. Trivalent arsenical compounds such as thiacetarsamide (Caparsolate), used to treat heartworm disease, have the potential to cause ARF.[114, 115] Toxicity can occur after as few as two doses; however, the severity of ARF and renal lesions may be directly proportional to the dose of arsenic.[114, 115] In general, doses used to treat heartworm disease are associated with only mild renal tubular lesions and no clinical or laboratory signs of renal failure. Hemoglobinuria secondary to intravascular hemolysis and myoglobinuruia associated with seizure-induced rhabdomyolysis rarely cause ARF in dogs.[57, 116, 117] Nephrotoxicosis appears to be most likely when either myoglobinuria or hemoglobinuria occur with disorders that cause decreased urinary pH and renal hypoperfusion, such as dehydration, hypovolemia, or acidosis.[118, 119] ARF associated with IV administration of a radiographic contrast medium occurs rarely in dogs.[98] From personal observations, it appears that inhalational anesthesia may enhance the occurrence of contrast-induced ARF in veterinary patients.

Renal Ischemia

Renal ischemia infrequently is recognized as a cause of ARF in small animal patients, but it may occur in clinical conditions associated with impaired renal perfusion[23, 116, 117, 120–128] (Table 16–9). Ischemia initially causes prerenal azotemia with no evidence of intrinsic renal injury. In the normal kidney, adequate perfusion is maintained by production of renal vasodilators, which balance the systemic vasoconstriction that occurs in response to decreased renal perfusion. However, if renal hypoperfusion persists, renal vasoconstriction may lead to ARF. In general, ischemic injury usually causes ARF in patients with pre-existing renal disease.[129] Conditions that favor hypoperfusion and subsequent ischemic injury include decreased circulating blood volume, thromboembolic disease, use of certain vasoactive pharmacologic agents, and changes in systemic vascular resistance.

Some pharmacologic agents such as nonsteroidal anti-inflammatory drugs (NSAIDs) and angiotensin-converting enzyme (ACE) inhibitors interfere with the kidney's normal ability to counteract systemic vasoconstriction, thereby allowing renal ischemic in-

jury to occur. Administration of NSAIDs to patients with conditions that are associated with systemic vasoconstriction, such as congestive heart failure, hypovolemia, general anesthesia, dehydration, or renal disease, can result in failure of compensatory mechanisms and subsequent renal ischemia.[129] ARF in dogs has been associated with administration of ibuprofen,[124, 125] naproxen,[126] phenylbutazone,[127] and flunixin meglumine.[128] As with NSAIDs, administration of ACE inhibitors (e.g., captopril, enalapril) to an individual whose renal autoregulatory abilities are compromised potentiates deleterious effects on renal perfusion and may lead to ARF.

Nephritis

Nephritis secondary to infectious disease is an infrequent cause of ARF in small animal patients; however, it should be considered if the physical examination or laboratory findings suggest systemic infection or inflammation.[130] Leptospirosis is clinically the most important cause of nephritis and ARF in dogs. In cats, clinical signs usually are inapparent, and renal failure does not occur.[131] Leptospirosis is caused by infection with several different serovars of *Leptospira interrogans; pomona* and *grippotyphosa* may be the most common.[132] Leptospires are acquired from the environment or directly from an infected animal. The organisms penetrate mucous membranes or abraded skin, multiply in the bloodstream, and then colonize renal tubular epithelial cells, where pathologic damage ensues.[131] Leptospires also produce a toxin that directly compromises capillary structure and function.[133] Patients with leptospirosis also may have concurrent hepatic involvement, although most dogs with leptospirosis have only signs of renal disease.[132] Acute pyelonephritis infrequently causes ARF in dogs and cats.[34] Rarely, other infectious diseases cause nephritis and ARF; these include Rocky Mountain spotted fever, ehrlichiosis, and bacterial endocarditis.[122–124, 130, 134]

Clinical Signs

Clinical findings are nonspecific and include lethargy, vomiting, diarrhea, dehydration, oral ulcers, and foul-smelling breath. These signs result from inability of the kidneys to adequately regulate fluid and electrolyte balance and excrete catabolic wastes. Other signs, such as fever, icterus, hepatosplenomegaly, and petechial hemorrhages, may also exist, depending on the underlying cause of ARF.

Diagnostic Plan

The goals of diagnostic evaluation of patients with suspected ARF are to identify life-threatening abnormalities, to establish a diagnosis of renal failure, to differentiate ARF from CRF, and to identify a cause so that specific treatment can be administered.

Table 16–9
Disorders Associated With Renal Hypoperfusion

Hypovolemia
Dehydration
Hypoalbuminemia
Hemorrhage
Hypoadrenocorticism

Decreased Cardiac Output
Congestive heart failure
Pericardial disease
Cardiac arrhythmias
Inhalational anesthesia

Renal Vasoconstriction
Myoglobinuria
Hemoglobinuria
Angiotensin-converting enzyme inhibitors
  Captopril
  Enalapril
Nonsteroidal anti-inflammatory drugs
  Phenylbutazone
  Ibuprofen
  Naproxen
  Flunixin meglumine
Amphotericin B

Renal Vascular Thrombosis
Bacterial endocarditis
Disseminated intravascular coagulation
Nephrotic syndrome
  Amyloidosis
  Glomerulonephritis

Systemic Vasodilation
Anaphylaxis
Inhalational anesthesia
Septic shock
Heatstroke
Drugs (arteriolar dilators)

Before extensive diagnostic evaluation is begun, patients are assessed for presence of life-threatening abnormalities, including severe dehydration, metabolic acidosis, and hyperkalemia. In some patients, treatment may be necessary before results of initial laboratory tests are available; however, samples of blood and urine should be collected before any treatment begins, if possible, to facilitate interpretation of results later. Early detection and correction of dehydration helps prevent additional renal injury from hypoperfusion. Patients with bradycardia or other cardiac arrhythmias may have hyperkalemia. Electrocardiographic (ECG) changes, including prolonged P-R intervals, spiked T waves, absent P waves, and widened QRS complexes, also suggest hyperkalemia (Fig. 16–7). Patients with cardiac arrhythmias or serum potassium concentrations higher than 8.0 mEq/L require immediate treatment to lower serum potassium. Severe metabolic acidosis (pH <7.2 or total carbon dioxide <12 mEq/L) also may have detrimental effects on the cardiovascular system; therefore, treatment to increase blood pH above 7.2 is indicated (see later section).

Renal failure is diagnosed by a finding of azotemia and concomitant isosthenuria or minimally concentrated urine with a specific gravity of 1.014 to 1.025. Other causes of azotemia should be excluded; however, some patients with renal failure also have prerenal and postrenal disorders that exist concurrently (see Azotemia).

After a diagnosis of renal failure has been established, it is important to distinguish between ARF and CRF, because ARF is potentially reversible with aggressive treatment and carries a better long-term prognosis. Although findings from the history and physical examination usually allow for distinction between these two syndromes, other tests (e.g., CBC, serum chemistries, radiography) are helpful (Table 16–10). Patients with ARF usually are healthy before the sudden onset of lethargy, depression, and vomiting in a period of less than 1 week. In contrast, the clinical signs in CRF (e.g., inappetence, weight loss, PU/PD) often occur over a period of weeks to months. Patients with an acute exacerbation of CRF present a diagnostic challenge, but careful questioning of the owners often establishes a more chronic history in these cases. Patients with ARF usually have a normal or increased hematocrit, although anemia may occur because of gastrointestinal hemorrhage, hemodilution from fluid therapy, or presence of a concurrent disease that causes anemia. CRF often is associated with nonregenerative anemia. In general, serum creatinine and BUN concentrations are stable in CRF, whereas these values progressively increase in ARF. Both hyperkalemia and oliguria (<1.0 mL urine/kg per hour) are most likely to occur with ARF; however, they may be observed in the terminal stages of CRF. Polyuria is characteristic of CRF, although some patients with ARF caused by aminoglycoside toxicosis have PU also.[135] Small, irregularly shaped kidneys indicate CRF, whereas normal to enlarged kidneys may occur with either ARF or CRF. Infrequently, patients with CRF demonstrate signs of renal osteodystrophy (e.g., rubber jaw); this does not occur in patients with ARF. If it still is not possible to adequately distinguish between ARF and CRF on the basis of these findings, a renal biopsy should be done.

If ARF has been diagnosed, an attempt should be made to determine the underlying cause. This allows for rendering of a more accurate prognosis and guides the need for specific treatment. Information obtained from the history, physical examination, laboratory evaluation, and ancillary diagnostic tests may be helpful, although many cases of ARF are idiopathic.

A　　　　　　　　　　　　　　　　　　　　**B**

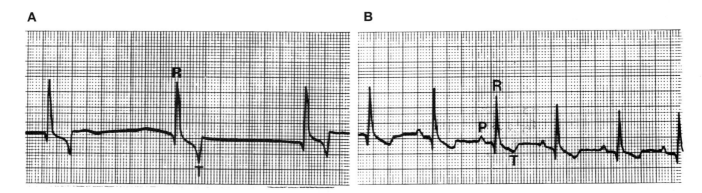

Figure 16–7
(A) Electrocardiographic tracing from dog with hyperkalemia. Notice bradycardia, absent P waves, and spiked T waves. **(B)** Tracing from same dog after treatment of hyperkalemia. Notice increased heart rate, return of P waves, and shortening of T waves.

Table 16–10
Distinguishing Characteristics of Acute and Chronic Renal Failure

PARAMETER	ACUTE RENAL FAILURE	CHRONIC RENAL FAILURE
History	Previously normal	Polyuria and polydipsia
		Weight loss or poor growth
Hematocrit	Normal or increased	Decreased
Serum urea nitrogen and creatinine	Previously normal	Previously increased
	Progressive increase	Typically stable
Hyperkalemia	May be present	Absent unless terminal
Urine volume	Oliguric, nonoliguric	Polyuric unless terminal
Renal size	Normal or increased	Normal or decreased or increased
Bone density	Normal	Often decreased (rubber jaw)

Ethylene Glycol Toxicosis

Ethylene glycol toxicosis should be considered a potential cause of ARF, especially if the patient lives outdoors or has a history of possible exposure. Clinical signs depend on the time between the ingestion of ethylene glycol and presentation to the veterinarian. Initial signs include ataxia, depression, and dehydration; some patients may have severe neurologic signs, including dementia, stupor, and seizures. Signs of renal failure usually occur 24 to 72 hours after ingestion in dogs and 12 to 24 hours after ingestion in cats.[109] Physical examination findings often are unremarkable; abdominal pain may occur from renal capsular swelling.[136] In addition to azotemia and hyperphosphatemia, serum chemistry abnormalities may include hypocalcemia, hyperglycemia, severe metabolic acidosis, and increased anion gap, often greater than 40.[136] Urinalysis findings include proteinuria, hematuria, normoglycemic glucosuria, and cellular or granular casts.[136] Calcium oxalate crystalluria supports a diagnosis of ethylene glycol toxicosis if other signs exist concurrently; however, they also may be observed in urine of normal dogs and cats.[109, 136] Calcium oxalate crystals are observed more often in dogs than cats with ethylene glycol toxicosis.[136]

Drug-Induced Nephrotoxicosis

Drug-induced ARF should be suspected in patients that have been receiving nephrotoxic drugs such as aminoglycosides, amphotericin B, and cisplatin (see Table 16–8). Renal failure associated with aminoglycosides may not occur until 3 to 5 days after the drug has been discontinued.[135] Aminoglycosides often cause nonoliguric ARF, so PU/PD may be noted. Serum chemistry abnormalities in patients with drug-induced ARF are typical of renal failure, and urinalysis findings are similar to those for ethylene glycol toxicosis.[135]

Leptospirosis

Leptospirosis should be suspected if ARF is diagnosed in a patient with signs of systemic infection or inflammation. Clinical signs of leptospirosis include anorexia, vomiting, fever, abdominal pain, reluctance to move, and, rarely, icterus.[132] In addition to findings of renal failure, laboratory abnormalities may include leukocytosis, thrombocytopenia, and increased activities of hepatic enzymes; urinalysis may show glucosuria, hematuria, pyuria, proteinuria, and granular casts.[132] A diagnosis of leptospirosis is confirmed by demonstration of a single titer higher than 1:3200 or a fourfold rise in titers from samples collected 2 to 4 weeks apart.[131, 132]

Pyelonephritis

Acute pyelonephritis is an uncommon cause of ARF in dogs and cats but should be suspected if findings such as fever, abdominal pain, leukocytosis, and pyuria exist. A sample of urine should be cultured to rule out urinary tract infection (see Pyelonephritis).

Miscellaneous Causes

If a readily identifiable cause of ARF cannot be identified, consideration should be given to disorders that are infrequently associated with ARF, such as ischemia, Rocky Mountain spotted fever, and ehrlichiosis. Owners should be asked about administration of over-the-counter preparations (e.g., aspirin, ibuprofen) or other drugs such as ACE inhibitors. Any recent episode such as prolonged dehydration, hypotensive anesthesia, or cardiac disease that may have caused renal hypoperfusion and ischemic-induced ARF should be determined. Disseminated intravascular coagulation (DIC) can be ruled out by a coagulation profile and platelet count, especially in patients with unexplained hemorrhage or disorders that predispose to DIC. If rickettsial disease is suspected, serum should be submitted for measurement of titers (see Chap. 37).

Treatment

The goals of treating patients with ARF are to minimize further renal injury, to promote diuresis if oliguria exists, to combat metabolic consequences of uremia, and to establish a prognosis for recovery.[34, 137] Additional renal injury can be avoided by discontinuation of potentially nephrotoxic drugs or appropriate modification of the dosage regimen, by correction of any prerenal or postrenal disorders (e.g., dehydration, decreased cardiac output, urinary obstruction), and by administration of specific treatment for the underlying cause of ARF, if one can be identified. Methods to stimulate urine production are indicated in oliguric patients. Although increased urine production does not indicate increased GFR, clinical management (e.g., control of hyperkalemia, acidosis) is facilitated in patients that are nonoliguric. Control of metabolic complications of ARF, such as hyperkalemia, metabolic acidosis, hyperphosphatemia, hypocalcemia, and vomiting, also contributes to improved patient care. Prognosis in patients with ARF often is guarded; however, institution of these measures may sustain the patient until adequate renal function returns.

Initial Patient Assessment

Before treatment is begun, the patient is assessed and baseline laboratory data are collected. Physical examination should include determination of body weight, hydration status (Table 16–11), pulse rate and quality, and capillary refill time.[107, 138] Body weight after rehydration should be used for comparisons. Baseline values for packed cell volume (PCV), total protein, BUN, serum creatinine, phosphorus, potassium, calcium, and total carbon dioxide also should be determined and recorded for future comparisons. An indwelling catheter should be aseptically placed, preferably in the jugular vein, for administration of fluids and other treatments. This also allows for measurement of central venous pressure, which is indicated in patients that are oliguric and susceptible to overhydration.[137] Patients that remain oliguric (<1.0 mL/kg per hour) after rehydration should have an indwelling urinary catheter placed and connected to a closed drainage system for at least 24 to 48 hours. This allows for accurate determination of urine volume and helps in adjusting fluid therapy as well as determining need for administration of drugs to stimulate diuresis.[137]

Measurement of urine volume may be accomplished by intermittent collection of all voided urine, by use of a metabolism cage, or by urethral catheterization (indwelling or intermittent). The first two

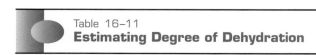

Table 16–11
Estimating Degree of Dehydration

PERCENT DEHYDRATION	CLINICAL FINDINGS
<5	History of vomiting, diarrhea No physical examination abnormalities
5	Possibly dry mucous membranes Slightly decreased skin turgor
6–8	Dry mucous membranes Mildly to moderately decreased skin turgor Slightly prolonged capillary refill time
10–12	Dry mucous membranes Markedly decreased skin turgor Weak and rapid pulse Prolonged capillary refill time Enophthalmos Moderate to marked mental depression

methods are helpful for quantitating urine volume in nonoliguric patients; however, they may not be accurate in patients with oliguria. Urinary catheterization is associated with increased risk of urinary tract infection, which is a problem in uremic patients that are already predisposed to infection.[139] If catheterization is deemed necessary, it should be done intermittently if possible. If an indwelling catheter is placed, it should remain in place for as short a time as possible. I usually reserve indwelling urinary catheterization for monitoring of oliguric patients that require treatment to stimulate urine production and for patients that may be difficult to intermittently catheterize (e.g., female dogs). Administration of antimicrobials should be avoided in patients with indwelling urinary catheters because this may predispose to infection with resistant bacteria.[139] Instead, the urine should be cultured when the catheter is removed and the patient treated with an appropriate antimicrobial agent, if indicated.

Fluid Therapy

The first goal of fluid therapy in patients with ARF is to correct hydration deficits. Degree of dehydration is estimated by physical examination findings (see Table 16–11). If a patient does not appear dehydrated, it is best to assume subclinical dehydration (<5%) and treat accordingly. It is better to slightly overhydrate a patient with ARF than to risk continued renal hypoperfusion associated with subclinical dehydration. The dehydration deficit in milliliters is equal to the percent dehydration times the body weight in kilograms times 1000. This deficit should be rapidly replaced (i.e., over 4–8 hours) unless there is concurrent cardiac dysfunction. Normal saline solution (0.9%) is an appropriate fluid for rehydration because it contains a relatively large amount of sodium and no potassium. Although lactated Ringer's solution may be used, it contains 4 mEq/L of potassium, which may be undesirable in patients with ARF.

After rehydration, fluid therapy is aimed at maintaining hydration by administration of fluids to meet daily needs and replace any ongoing losses (e.g., vomiting, diarrhea). Maintenance fluids (Normosol, Plasma-Lyte) should be used in patients with ARF instead of solutions that tend to cause hypernatremia, such as 0.9% saline or lactated Ringer's solution. Maintenance fluid requirements are 40 to 60 mL/kg per day, including both insensible losses (20 mL/kg per day) and sensible losses (20 to 40 mL/kg per day primarily urine volume). If oliguria exists, placement of an indwelling urinary catheter to accurately measure urine volume is strongly recommended.[107] After the patient is rehydrated, the volume of urine produced every 4 to 6 hours is recorded. The volume of fluids to be administered in each 4- to 6-hour interval is the sum of calculated insensible losses (20 mL/kg per day) and urine volume for the previous interval. Ongoing losses such as vomiting and diarrhea also must be estimated and added to the volume of fluids administered; it is usually safe to assume that patients with ARF become 3% to 5% dehydrated each day because of ongoing losses.

Strict monitoring of fluid therapy in nonoliguric patients is not as critical; however, urine output should be estimated so that appropriate fluid volumes, usually 1.5 to 3 times maintenance volume, are administered.[140] After dehydration has been corrected, periodic monitoring of body weight is an objective method for detecting changes in fluid balance.

Conversion of Oliguria to Nonoliguria

If patients remain oliguric after apparent rehydration or administration of a volume of fluids equal to 5% of body weight, additional measures are indicated to stimulate urine production (Table 16–12).[141–143] The nonoliguric state facilitates management of patients with ARF, because it is easier to correct metabolic abnormalities such as hyperkalemia and azotemia, and overhydration is less likely to occur. Conversion from oliguria to nonoliguria, however, does not necessarily indicate improved renal function (i.e., increased GFR), although it may indicate a better prognosis. Patients with ARF that are nonoliguric seem to have less severe renal injury and are more likely to respond to treatment than oliguric patients.[135, 144] Stimulating diuresis in patients that are nonoliguric by any means other than volume diuresis should be avoided because it increases risk

of fluid and electrolyte depletion, which could potentially worsen renal injury.

Agents such as diuretics and vasodilators, used to initiate a diuresis in oliguric patients, should not be administered until the patient has been rehydrated by appropriate fluid therapy. Administration of IV fluids (i.e., at rates 1.5–3 times maintenance) is not an effective method to stimulate diuresis in patients with ARF that remain oliguric after rehydration. These patients are not capable of excreting an excess water load, in part because of tubular dysfunction, and therefore are susceptible to overhydration.

Osmotic diuretics such as mannitol and hypertonic dextrose may be used initially to stimulate urine production. Because of their hypertonicity, osmotic diuretics should be administered through a central vein. Dextrose has the advantage of being relatively inexpensive, being easily measured in urine, and providing some calories. Beneficial effects of mannitol include increased GFR, scavenging of oxygen free radicals, inhibition of renin secretion, and increased tubular flow rates, which may prevent tubular obstruction with casts and debris.[145, 146] Mannitol exerts its effects along the entire nephron and may be more effective than dextrose for patients with renal tubular swelling (e.g., ischemic renal injury). Mannitol should not be used in overhydrated patients because it may precipitate or worsen pulmonary edema. Mannitol also probably should be avoided in patients with vasculitis (e.g., rickettsial diseases, DIC), because it may leak into extravascular spaces and cause peripheral edema.[146]

If an osmotic diuretic is contraindicated or has not been effective at stimulating urine production, furosemide or dopamine (or both) should be administered next (see Table 16–12). Both agents have been used alone to treat oliguric patients; however, they appear to be most effective when used together.[143] Furosemide should be avoided in patients with suspected aminoglycoside nephrotoxicosis because it may worsen renal injury.[147] Dopamine should not be diluted in alkaline solutions, because this inactivates the drug.[107] Side effects of dopamine include tachycardia, cardiac arrhythmias, and renal vasoconstriction; these are most likely to occur if dopamine is infused too rapidly. Ideally, ECG monitoring should be done during dopamine infusion. Heart rate should be measured every 15 minutes during the first hour and hourly thereafter. If heart rate increases suddenly (>180/min in dogs, >200/min in cats), the rate of infusion should be decreased.[107]

If oliguria persists after all of these measures have been attempted, prognosis for survival is grave. Fluid therapy should be restricted to match urine output and any ongoing losses, because these patients are very susceptible to overhydration. Dialysis, if available, is indicated to control metabolic complications of uremia.

Patient Monitoring

Monitoring of patients is important so that treatment can be adjusted and the patient's response and prognosis determined. A physical examination should be performed daily to assess hydration status (e.g., mental status, skin turgor, moistness of mucous membranes, capillary refill time, pulse quality, thoracic auscultation). Body weight is measured on the same scales every 6 to 8 hours during the first 48 hours of treatment and every 12 hours thereafter. Failure to gain weight during the first 24 hours indicates insufficient rehydration because of initial underestimation of dehydration or failure to adequately replace ongoing losses; unexpected weight gain above hydration deficits suggests overhydration. Patients lose approximately 0.5% to 1.0% of body weight per day from anorexia.[148]

Values for PCV and total protein (TP) should be determined twice daily for the first 48 hours and daily thereafter.[107] This helps to document rehydration (decreasing PCV and TP), overhydration (continually decreasing PCV and TP), dehydration (increasing PCV and TP), or hemorrhage (decreasing PCV and TP).[107] Central venous pressure is monitored to prevent overhydration in predisposed patients. Normal pressure is less than 5 cm H_2O; initial values greater than 10 to 12 cm H_2O or an increase of 2 cm H_2O or more in a 10-minute period indicates need for discontinuation or marked reduction in rate of fluid administration.[107, 137] Serum chemistries should be measured once daily to determine whether the patient is responding appropriately. Values for potassium and total carbon dioxide should be monitored more frequently if severe metabolic acidosis or hyperkalemia exist; this allows for administration of additional treatment if indicated.

Table 16–12
Methods to Stimulate Urine Production in Oliguric Patients[140–143]

I. Administer an osmotic diuretic
  A. Mannitol (20% or 25%)
    1. Administer 0.25–0.5 g/kg, IV over 5 min
    2. If urine flow increases, continue mannitol:
      a. At 0.25–0.5 g/kg, IV, every 6–8 h as needed
      or
      b. Administer 5%–10% solution (diluted in lactated Ringer's solution) IV at constant rate of 2–5 mL/min
    3. If urine flow does not increase within 30–60 min of initial administration, do not give additional osmotic diuretic; another method to stimulate urine production should be attempted
  B. Dextrose (20%)
    1. Administer 0.5–1 g/kg IV over 15–20 min (20% = 0.2 g dextrose per mL)
    2. If adequate diuresis occurs:
      a. Repeat dose every 8–12 h as needed (continue maintenance fluids between doses)
      or
      b. Administer a maintenance infusion of 10% dextrose for 12–24 h
    3. If adequate urine flow (1–2 mL/kg/h) is not observed within 60 minutes of the initial infusion, discontinue osmotic diuretic therapy and attempt to stimulate urine production by another method
II. If an osmotic diuretic is not effective, administer furosemide or dopamine, or both
  A. Furosemide
    1. Administer 2.2 mg/kg, IV
    2. If urine production increases, continue every 8 h
    3. If urine production does not increase within 30–60 min, administer 4.4 mg/kg, IV
    4. If still unsuccessful, administer 6.6 mg/kg, IV
    5. If unsuccessful after three doses of furosemide, attempt other therapy to stimulate urine production
  B. Dopamine
    1. Dilute 30 mg of dopamine in 500 mL of lactated Ringer's solution, 0.9% saline, or 5% dextrose to make a final dopamine concentration of 60 µg/mL
    2. Infuse at 1–3 µg/kg/min using an infusion pump or pediatric infusion set
    3. If urine production increases, continue dopamine for 12–24 h or until urine flow can be maintained by fluid therapy
  C. Dopamine/Furosemide combination
    1. Infuse dopamine continuously as specified above and administer furosemide, 1 mg/kg, IV every hour
    2. If there is no improvement within 6 h, additional treatment is unlikely to be successful

Data from Ross, 1989[140]; Finco and Low, 1980[141]; Cornelius, 1983[142]; and Lindner, 1979.[143]

Table 16–13
Addition of Potassium to Fluids for Treatment of Hypokalemia

SERUM POTASSIUM (mEq/L)	POTASSIUM IN FLUIDS (mEq/L)	MAXIMAL FLUID RATE (mL/kg/h)
3.5–4.0	20	25
3.0–3.4	30	17
2.5–2.9	40	12
2.0–2.4	60	8
<2.0	80	6

Managing Complications of Acute Renal Failure

Hyperkalemia. Hyperkalemia often occurs in patients with ARF, and treatment is indicated if serum potassium exceeds 8 mEq/L or signs of cardiac toxicity occur. Mild hyperkalemia (6–8 mEq/L) usually responds to fluid replacement with 0.9% saline and elimination of the underlying cause. If other treatment is necessary, then sodium bicarbonate (0.5–1.0 mEq/kg, IV over 15–20 minutes), 25% dextrose (2–4 mL/kg, IV), or dextrose added to IV fluids to make a 5% or 10% solution should be administered. Sodium bicarbonate usually is a good first choice in ARF patients because metabolic acidosis often exists concurrently; potassium-lowering effects persist for several hours. Alternatively, dextrose can be administered; it acts by stimulating endogenous insulin release, which causes potassium to shift intracellularly. Insulin and dextrose also may be administered; however, this rarely is needed and may cause iatrogenic hypoglycemia. Calcium gluconate directly antagonizes the cardiotoxic effects of hyperkalemia and should be administered to patients with life-threatening arrhythmias. In addition, 10% calcium gluconate (0.5–1.0 mL/kg, IV) should be administered slowly. ECG monitoring is employed, and the infusion is slowed or discontinued if signs of toxicosis (e.g., vomiting, bradycardia, shortening of the Q-T interval) occur. Because calcium gluconate is effective for only 10 to 15 minutes and does not lower serum potassium, concurrent treatment with either bicarbonate or dextrose is indicated to lower serum potassium.

Hypokalemia. Hypokalemia may occur during the maintenance or recovery phase of ARF and may require potassium supplementation. The amount of potassium added to IV fluids is based on serum potassium concentration (Table 16–13). In order to avoid iatrogenic hyperkalemia and its side effects, the rate of potassium infusion should not exceed 0.5 mEq/kg per hour. If the patient is not vomiting, potassium can be supplemented orally (see Chronic Renal Failure).

Metabolic Acidosis. Patients with mild to moderate acidosis usually respond to fluid therapy; however, if severe metabolic acidosis exists (i.e., blood pH <7.2 or total carbon dioxide <12–15 mEq/L), sodium bicarbonate should be administered. If blood gas data or total carbon dioxide data are available, the milliequivalents of bicarbonate needed can be calculated by multiplying 0.3 times the body weight in kilograms times either the base deficit or 20 minus the total carbon dioxide. One quarter to one half of the deficit is administered over 1 to 2 hours, and the remaining volume is added to the IV fluids and administered over 12 hours. Blood gas parameters are then reassessed to determine the need for additional bicarbonate therapy. Alternatively, if blood gas data are unavailable, bicarbonate is added at a dose of 1 to 5 mEq/kg, depending on estimated severity of acidosis, to calcium-free maintenance fluids (not lactated Ringer's solution) and administered over 12 to 24 hours.[107, 137]

Hyperphosphatemia. There is no specific treatment for hyperphosphatemia; however, measures directed at correcting prerenal factors and improving GFR result in lowering of serum phosphorus. If the patient is able to tolerate oral feeding, phosphate binders are indicated (see Chronic Renal Failure).

Hypocalcemia. Specific treatment of hypocalcemia should be given only in patients that have clinical signs associated with hypocalcemia, such as tremors, seizures, or weakness. Calcium must be administered cautiously, because concurrent hyperphosphatemia increases risk of soft tissue mineralization, which may worsen renal tubular injury. If indicated, calcium gluconate (10%) is administered slowly at a dosage of 0.5 to 1.5 mL/kg, IV. Bicarbonate should not be administered to hypocalcemic patients, because alkalinization lowers ionized calcium and may precipitate clinical signs of hypocalcemia.

Vomiting. Persistent vomiting and nausea are problems that require treatment in patients with ARF. Vomiting is thought to be mediated both centrally, by effects of uremic toxins on the chemoreceptor trigger zone, and locally, by gastrointestinal ulceration, which may result from decreased renal elimination of gastrin. Antiemetic agents that act centrally include trimethobenzamide (Tigan, 3 mg/kg every 8 hours, intramuscularly [IM] in dogs, or 100-mg rectal suppositories in dogs weighing more than 6.8 kg), chlorpromazine (Thorazine, 0.5–1.5 mg/kg every 6–8 hours, IM or IV), and metoclopramide (Reglan, 0.2–0.4 mg/kg, subcutaneously every 6–8 hours). Because metoclopramide is a dopamine antagonist, it should be avoided during the time patients are receiving dopamine. Chlorpromazine may cause hypotension and should not be used until the patient is well hydrated. Histamine$_2$-receptor antagonists are indicated to decrease gastric acid secretion. These include cimetidine (Tagamet, 5–10 mg/kg every, 12 hours, IV in dogs; 5 mg/kg every 12 hours, IV in cats) and ranitidine (Zantac, 2.2–4.4 mg/kg every 12 hours, by mouth in dogs; 2.2 mg/kg every 12 hours, by mouth in cats). The presence of oral ulcerations often contributes to anorexia, and treatment with viscous lidocaine (0.5–1 mL, topically before meals) may improve patient comfort.

Nutritional Support. If the patient survives the initial period of treatment (3–5 days) and does not begin to eat on its own, some form of nutritional support is indicated. Vomiting often precludes oral feeding initially; however, after azotemia and other complications are being managed, many patients that do not eat voluntarily can tolerate tube feeding. Pureed prescription diets such as Prescription Diet k/d may be used, or liquid diets such as Renal Care may be tried. Diets that are moderately restricted in protein and phosphorus are preferred because they help control clinical signs of uremia. Such diets should be continued until azotemia resolves. Dietary guidelines for long-term management of patients that recover from ARF and have resolution of azotemia have not been established.

Specific Treatment of Underlying Causes of Acute Renal Failure

Ethylene Glycol Toxicosis. Treatment of ethylene glycol toxicosis includes measures to prevent its absorption and metabolism and enhance its excretion. Gastric lavage should be done if the patient is presented within 6 to 12 hours of ingestion.[107] If it has been 24 hours or less since ingestion of ethylene glycol, ethanol or 4-methylpyrazole should be administered to prevent metabolism of ethylene glycol to its toxic metabolites (Table 16–14). Ethanol and 4-methylpyrazole are most effective if administered within 1 and 8 hours of ingestion, respectively.[109, 149] Most patients are presented several days after ingestion, after established renal failure exists. Although ethanol is readily available, it worsens central nervous system depression.[109] 4-Methylpyrazole is the treatment of choice for ethylene glycol toxicosis in dogs; it is not effective in cats.[150]

Infectious Diseases. In addition to general supportive measures, specific treatment is indicated for infectious diseases associated with ARF (see Chap. 37).[131] Some adjustments need to be made in patients with decreased renal function, and parenteral treatment usually is indicated because of the nature of the underlying disease (e.g., septicemia) or the presence of vomiting.

Leptospirosis is treated either with penicillin G

Table 16–14
Treatment of Ethylene Glycol Toxicosis

	Ethanol (20%)
Dogs	5.5 mL/kg IV every 4 h for 5 treatments, then every 6 hours for 4 additional treatments
Cats	5 mL/kg IV every 6 h for 5 treatments, then every 8 hours for 4 additional treatments
	4-Methylpyrazole (5%)
Dogs	0.4 mL/kg IV initially, then 0.3 mL/kg IV at 12 and 24 h, then 0.1 mL/kg IV at 36 h
Cats	Not currently recommended

(25,000–40,000 U/kg every 12 hours, IM or IV) or with ampicillin (10–20 mg/kg every 8–12 hours, IV, subcutaneously, or by mouth) for 2 weeks. Although penicillins are eliminated primarily by the kidneys, precise adjustments in the dosage regimen usually are unnecessary, and in general either the dose is halved or the dosing interval is doubled in patients with ARF.[34] After BUN and creatinine return to normal, dihydrostreptomycin (15 mg/kg every 12 hours, IM), if available, is administered, for 2 weeks to eliminate leptospires from the kidney and terminate the carrier state. Administration of doxycycline (Vibramycin, 5–10 mg/kg every 24 hours, IV or by mouth for 5–10 days) effectively terminates leptospiremia and leptospiruria in humans and therefore may be an effective alternative for veterinary patients with ARF and leptospirosis.[151]

Selection of antimicrobial drugs for treatment of pyelonephritis ideally is based on results of urine culture and susceptibility (see Chap. 17). However, if immediate treatment is necessary, as in suspected sepsis, empiric treatment with either ampicillin (25 mg/kg every 8 hours, IV) or enrofloxacin (Baytril, 2.5 mg/kg every 12 hours, IM or IV) may be used (see Pyelonephritis). Enrofloxacin has not been approved for IV administration; however, it has been used without any recognized complications. It should be diluted 1:1 with sterile saline and injected slowly.

Rickettsial infections in patients with ARF are probably best treated with doxycycline (5–10 mg/kg every 24 hours, IV or by mouth for 5 to 10 days) because it undergoes less renal elimination than tetracycline; in addition, tetracycline can cause renal tubular necrosis and ARF if it is administered IV.

Prevention of Acute Renal Failure

Because ARF requires intensive and expensive treatment and carries a guarded to grave prognosis in many cases, every effort should be made to prevent its occurrence. The first step is to recognize patients that are at risk for ARF (Table 16–15). Correction or

Table 16–15
Risk Factors for Acute Renal Failure

Dehydration
Advanced age
Renal disease (pre-existing or active)
Renal hypoperfusion
Electrolyte abnormalities
   Hyponatremia
   Hypocalcemia
   Hypokalemia
Metabolic acidosis
Concurrent nephrotoxic drugs
Other drugs (with nephrotoxic drug)
   Furosemide
   Cytotoxic drugs (e.g., chemotherapeutics)
   Nonsteroidal anti-inflammatory drugs
Fever
Sepsis

avoidance of these risk factors, if possible, is especially important in patients with pre-existing renal disease.

Nephrotoxic drugs should be avoided if possible. A quinolone antibiotic often can be used instead of aminoglycosides to treat gram-negative infections. If a nephrotoxic drug must be used, for example to treat a life-threatening infection with an organism that is resistant to all other antibiotics on the basis of culture and susceptibility, the patient must be monitored closely for signs of nephrotoxicosis. Dehydration, electrolyte, and acid-base abnormalities should be corrected before potentially nephrotoxic drugs are used. Furosemide should not be used in a patient that is receiving or has received gentamicin in the recent past (2–4 weeks). If there is any question about hydration status in a patient receiving aminoglycosides, it is probably best to administer maintenance IV fluids to ensure adequate hydration and renal perfusion.

Even after risk factors have been corrected, patients receiving aminoglycosides must still be closely monitored. Nephrotoxicosis is most likely to occur after prolonged treatment (>5–10 days); however, exceptions occur and are unpredictable.[135] Gentamicin should be used for as short a time as possible, and patients that are treated for longer than 5 days should be closely monitored. Laboratory evaluation, including serial urinalyses and BUN and serum creatinine concentrations, is probably the most readily available method for detecting gentamicin nephrotoxicosis in small animals. Baseline values should be obtained before treatment and monitored on alternate days during treatment with aminoglycosides. In general, changes in the urinalysis occur before azotemia is

observed. Increased numbers of casts, proteinuria, glucosuria, or azotemia is an indication to discontinue aminoglycosides. After cessation of treatment, monitoring should continue for a period of 7 days, because it is not uncommon for nephrotoxicosis to be detected several days after discontinuation of aminoglycosides.[135] Therapeutic drug monitoring should be considered in patients with concurrent risk factors or if treatment is prolonged.[152] Because of the great pharmacokinetic variations among patients receiving aminoglycosides, monitoring of serum concentrations helps to individualize the dosage regimen.[152, 153] Many veterinary schools and human hospitals have laboratories that can readily measure serum concentrations of aminoglycosides.

Measures must be taken to prevent ARF in patients requiring general anesthesia, especially older patients and those with renal disease.[152] Water should not be withheld before anesthesia, particularly in patients that are polyuric. Anesthetic agents and regimens that cause significant cardiovascular depression, including xylazine (Rompun), high doses of acepromazine (PromAce, >0.2 mg/kg or 4 mg total), and high concentrations of any inhalant anesthetic, should be avoided. Ketamine (Ketaset) should not be used in cats with renal disease because it is excreted predominately by the kidneys. To promote adequate renal perfusion in high-risk patients, a diuresis is induced before induction of anesthesia with a balanced electrolyte solution (5–10 mL/kg, IV over 30 minutes); urine output is maintained during the anesthetic episode by a relatively high rate of fluid administration (20 mL/kg per hour). Adequacy of renal perfusion is determined by monitoring of urine output, which should remain above 0.5 to 1.0 mL/kg per hour. The urinary bladder is palpated to grossly estimate urine volume or, in high-risk patients, an indwelling urinary catheter is placed. Urine production decreases as mean arterial blood pressure falls below 60 to 70 mm Hg; therefore, monitoring of blood pressure should be considered in critical patients or during prolonged procedures. If blood pressure monitoring is not available, at least strong peripheral pulses (e.g., dorsal pedal artery) should be preserved.

Prognosis

Although the long-term prognosis for patients with ARF is better than for those with CRF, many patients are euthanized before recovery. Prognostic indicators are important, because treatment of ARF is time-consuming and expensive. Patients with the best chance for recovery are those with moderate azotemia that are nonoliguric and have an acute renal insult that is reversible or transient.[137] Some examples include ARF associated with prerenal or postrenal insults such as dehydration or urinary obstruction or administration of NSAIDs, new methylene blue, or iodinated contrast agents. Patients with an acute exacerbation of CRF may survive through the acute crisis, although long-term prognosis is poor. ARF associated with gentamicin has a variable prognosis; oliguric patients have a poor chance for recovery, but those that are nonoliguric may have a favorable outcome after several weeks of intensive care.[135, 144] Patients with ARF caused by infectious diseases such as leptospirosis and pyelonephritis often recover if the underlying disease is treated aggressively. Most patients with ethylene glycol toxicosis are presented with established renal failure and have a grave prognosis. In general, poor prognostic signs include persistent oliguria despite attempts to induce diuresis, overhydration, intractable hyperkalemia, and severe metabolic acidosis.[107] If azotemia and clinical signs of uremia persist and improvement in clinical condition or laboratory parameters does not occur after 5 to 7 days of intensive treatment, euthanasia should be considered, unless dialysis is available.[107]

Chronic Renal Failure

CRF is a syndrome characterized by a slowly progressive deterioration in renal function that occurs over a period of months to years. Chronic renal failure occurs more often than ARF in dogs and cats and is probably the most common disorder affecting the kidneys. In general, CRF occurs most often in older dogs and cats, although congenital renal diseases should be suspected if CRF is diagnosed in young animals or in certain breeds of dogs and cats (Table 16–16).[34, 79, 80, 82–84, 154–163] Although most dogs with juvenile renal disease are younger than 2 years of age when presented for evaluation, some may be older.[81]

Pathophysiology

The consequences of CRF result from failure of the kidneys to adequately perform their normal excretory, regulatory, and synthetic functions. Loss of excretory function causes retention of nitrogenous wastes that are normally eliminated by glomerular filtration. This is characterized by increased concentrations of serum creatinine, BUN, and phosphorus. Inability to perform regulatory functions eventually leads to changes in fluid, electrolyte, and acid-base balance. The most common abnormalties are metabolic acidosis and hypokalemia. Failure to synthesize erythropoietin leads to nonregenerative anemia, whereas decreased conversion of vitamin D to its active metabolite impairs intestinal absorption of calcium and contributes to development of renal secondary hyperparathyroidism.

Many adaptive changes occur in patients with

Table 16–16
Breeds With Congenital or Familial Renal Disease

BREEDS	DISORDER
Canine	
Basenji	Renal tubular dysfunction
Beagle	Unilateral renal agenesis
	Renal amyloidosis
Bull terrier	Glomerulopathy
Cairn terrier	Polycystic kidney disease
Chinese shar-pei	Renal amyloidosis
Cocker spaniel	Tubulointerstitial fibrosis; renal cortical hypoplasia
Doberman pinscher	Glomerulosclerosis
Lhasa apso	Renal dysplasia
Norwegian elkhound	Tubulointerstitial fibrosis
Pembroke Welsh corgi	Renal telangiectasia
Samoyed	Glomerular atrophy
Shih tzu	Renal dysplasia
Soft-coated wheaten terrier	Renal dysplasia
Feline	
Abyssinian	Renal amyloidosis
Domestic longhair	Polycystic kidney disease
Persian	Polycystic kidney disease

CRF in an attempt to maintain homeostasis. As the number of functional nephrons decreases, the remaining nephrons filter a proportionately larger amount of the total glomerular filtrate per nephron. This increase in single-nephron GFR (i.e., glomerular hyperfiltration) initially helps blunt the overall decline in GFR, but, with time, it leads to progressive nephron injury and death. Serum concentrations of sodium and potassium are maintained because there is a compensatory increase in the amount excreted per nephron. Water balance also is maintained by a progressive increase in the amount of water excreted per nephron. The high rate of fluid that flows through remaining functional nephrons contributes to the PU that occurs in patients with CRF. There is a tendency toward metabolic acidosis because of decreased ability of the kidneys to excrete acids.

Perhaps one of the best-known compensatory mechanisms in CRF is renal secondary hyperparathyroidism. In CRF, production of 1α-hydroxylase, the renal tubular enzyme that converts vitamin D to its active form, calcitriol, is deficient. This prevents intestinal absorption of calcium and leads to a slight decrease in serum calcium. In addition, as GFR declines and serum phosphorus increases, serum calcium decreases as a result of the mass law effect. This slight decrease of serum ionized calcium stimulates release of PTH from the parathyroid glands. Increased PTH normalizes serum concentrations of calcium and phosphorus by causing release of calcium from bone and increasing renal phosphate excretion. Initially, this is a beneficial effect; however, it eventually leads to renal osteodystrophy, which is characteristic of CRF. In addition, hyperphosphatemia and increased serum concentrations of PTH may exacerbate clinical signs of uremia and contribute to further deterioration of renal function.[164, 165]

Most cases of CRF result from some acquired disorder that affects glomeruli, tubules, or renal interstitium. A variety of infectious and inflammatory diseases (e.g., glomerulonephritis, feline infectious peritonitis) and neoplastic diseases (e.g., lymphoma) can cause CRF also; however, in most cases, a specific cause cannot be identified. Regardless of the initial cause of renal injury, there tends to be a progressive loss of nephron function over time that eventually results in CRF.

Clinical Signs

The most common historical signs of CRF are lethargy, inappetence, vomiting, diarrhea, weight loss, and PU/PD. PU/PD and nocturia may be the earliest signs noted by owners of dogs with CRF; however, they may be less obvious in cats.[31, 34] Physical examination often reveals dehydration, emaciation, pale mucous membranes, and, less frequently, oral ulcerations and retinal lesions suggestive of hypertension (e.g., retinal detachments, tortuous vessels).[31, 34] Renal size varies depending on the cause of CRF. Classically, kidneys are small, firm, and irregularly shaped; however, some disorders that cause CRF may be associated with normal or enlarged kidneys (e.g., lymphoma, feline infectious peritonitis, polycystic kidney disease).[31, 33]

Diagnostic Plan

Results of laboratory evaluation, including CBC, serum chemistries, and urinalysis, are used to confirm a diagnosis of CRF. Normocytic, normochromic, nonregenerative anemia is the most common hemogram finding; this may not become apparent until after rehydration. Serum chemistry abnormalities include azotemia, hyperphosphatemia, and metabolic acidosis; hypokalemia, hypocalcemia, and, uncommonly, hypercalcemia also may occur. Urinalysis reveals minimally concentrated urine (USG 1.014–1.025) or isosthenuria in most cases; however, some cats with naturally occurring CRF may produce relatively concentrated urine (USG up to 1.035).[31, 33] The remainder of the urinalysis usually is unremarkable, although some patients may have proteinuria, especially if glomerular disease exists. If bacteriuria, pyuria, or hematuria is present, additional tests such as bacterial urine culture and, possibly, abdominal radiographs or ultrasonography are indicated.

It is important to distinguish between CRF and ARF because of differences in treatment and long-term prognosis (see Table 16–10 and Acute Renal Failure). In addition to historical findings, results of abdominal radiographs (small, irregularly shaped kidneys), ultrasonography (hyperechogenicity and small kidneys) and histologic evaluation of renal tissue may aid the diagnosis.

After a diagnosis of CRF is made, every attempt should be made to identify any potentially reversible disorders that may be contributing to renal dysfunction. These include pyelonephritis, urinary obstruction (e.g., uroliths, neoplasia), renal lymphoma, concurrent hypercalcemia and hyperphosphatemia, and systemic hypertension. Although correction of these disorders does not reverse CRF, it could potentially decrease the rate of progression of renal disease.

Treatment

Initial management of patients with CRF and clinical signs of uremia such as inappetence, vomiting, and dehyration is aimed at short-term support until the patient is eating and drinking sufficiently to maintain hydration and body weight (see Acute Renal Failure). Hydration deficits should be corrected rapidly (over 4–8 hours), and ongoing losses should be estimated and replaced as needed. If the patient is polyuric (>2.0 mL urine/kg per hour), fluids are administered at a rate 1.5 to 3 times maintenance in an attempt to enhance diuresis and decrease severity of azotemia and uremia to the point that the patient is stable (i.e., able to eat and drink without assistance). Antiemetics and histamine$_2$ receptor antagonists are administered as needed to control nausea and vomiting. Nutritional support is implemented as soon as the patient can tolerate it (see Acute Renal Failure).

After the patient is stable, treatment of CRF consists primarily of conservative medical management, which includes dietary alterations and administration of agents to control metabolic consequences of renal failure. The goals of treatment are to control the clinical signs of uremia; maintain adequate fluid, electrolyte, and acid-base balance; provide adequate nutrition; and minimize progression of CRF.[34]

Some general supportive measures should be considered in all patients. If an underlying cause can be identified, it should be treated as quickly as possible to prevent additional renal injury. Because of the detrimental effects of dehydration, animals with CRF should always have access to fresh, clean water. Any disorder that causes prerenal azotemia, such as vomiting or dehydration, should be treated promptly. Stressful situations, such as elective surgeries or boarding in a kennel, should be avoided. Nephrotoxic

Table 16-17
Homemade Diets for Dogs and Cats With Chronic Renal Failure

DOGS	CATS
¼ lb ground beef* 1 large egg, hard-boiled 2 cups cooked rice (no salt) 3 slices white bread, crumbled 1 tsp calcium carbonate	¼ lb liver 2 large eggs, hard-boiled 2 cups cooked rice (no salt) 1 T vegetable oil 1 tsp calcium carbonate
Brown meat and retain fat. Combine all ingredients and mix well. Can add some water to improve palatability. Makes 1¼ lbs (750 kcal/lb)	Dice and braise liver, retaining fat. Combine all ingredients and mix well. Can add some water to improve palatability. Yields 1¼ lbs (635 kcal/lb)

*Do not use lean ground round or chuck.
From Lewis LD, Morris ML, Hand MS. Small Animal Clinical Nutrition. Topeka, Mark Morris Associates, 1987:8-3-8-51.

drugs (e.g., aminoglycosides) should not be used in patients with renal disease because of the potential for additional renal injury and ARF.

Dietary Management

Dietary management has been the mainstay of medical treatment of CRF in veterinary patients. It is indicated to lessen severity of uremic signs (e.g., anorexia, vomiting) and possibly to prevent progression of CRF. Diets for patients with CRF, either commercially available (Prescription Diet k/d) or homemade, are restricted in protein, phosphorus, and sodium (Table 16–17).[166] Changes in diet should be made gradually over a period of 2 to 4 weeks to allow the kidneys adequate time to adapt to lower sodium intake and also to increase acceptability of the diet by patients. As a general rule, the daily ration should be divided into three or four meals. To increase palatability, the food can be warmed, or flavoring agents such as garlic powder, tuna or clam juice, or chicken broth can be added.[33]

The amount of dietary protein should be restricted, and it should be of high biologic value (80% or greater; Table 16–18).[167] As a general guideline, dogs should be fed 2.0 to 2.2 g/kg per day, and cats should be fed 3.3 to 3.5 g/kg per day.[34] A commercial diet (Prescription Diet k/d) based on recommended caloric requirements supplies approximately this amount of protein. Because of individual differences, however, each patient should be monitored periodically and the amount of protein adjusted to prevent protein malnu-

trition, which may be characterized by weight loss, hypoalbuminemia, and worsening anemia or azotemia. Diets that are severely restricted in protein (1.25 g/kg/day; for example, Prescription Diet u/d) should be used only in patients that are refractory to moderately restricted protein diets, and then with caution. The primary beneficial effect of dietary protein restriction is to control uremic signs. Dietary protein restriction reduces glomerular hyperfiltration and prevents progression of renal failure in rats; however, this has not been proven in dogs.[165]

Fluid, Electrolyte, and Acid-Base Balances

Most patients with CRF have an obligatory PU, and fluid balance is maintained by increased consumption of water; however, if water intake is not adequate to maintain hydration, as is the case with some cats, supplemental fluids should be administered. Owners can be instructed to administer these fluids subcutaneously at home.

Hypokalemia may occur in patients with CRF, especially cats.[31, 168] Hypokalemia results from decreased oral intake or increased renal loss of potassium. The primary clinical sign of hypokalemia is muscle weakness, which may be characterized by lethargy, ventroflexion of the neck (cats), and respiratory distress. In addition, hypokalemia may contribute to renal dysfunction in dogs and cats.[169, 170] Because of these consequences, hypokalemia should be corrected. If possible, it is best to administer potassium orally. Potassium gluconate, available as an elixir (Kaon) or powder (Tumil-K) is the drug of choice for cats. Potassium chloride should be avoided because it is unpalatable and may contribute to metabolic acidosis.[171] An initial dose of 2 to 6 mEq per cat is administered, depending on severity of hypokalemia

Table 16-18
Protein Biologic Value of Pet Food Ingredients

FOOD	BIOLOGIC VALUE (%)
Egg	100
Fish meal	92
Milk	92
Liver	79
Beef	78
Casein	78
Soybean meal	67
Meat and bone meal	50
Whole wheat	48
Whole corn	45

From Lewis LD, Morris ML, Hand MS. Small Animal Clinical Nutrition. Topeka, Mark Morris Associates, 1987:1-1-1-25.

and size of the cat. Serum potassium is monitored weekly to determine the appropriate maintenance dose. Most older cats require potassium supplementation for the remainder of their lives, whereas younger cats may not.[171] It may be prudent to supplement normokalemic cats with a low maintenance dose (2 mEq per cat) to prevent hypokalemia and worsening renal function; however, this remains to be evaluated in controlled studies.

If parenteral potassium is required (e.g., vomiting patient, severe hypokalemia), potassium chloride is added to IV fluids, not exceeding a rate of 0.5 mEq/kg per hour (see Table 16–13). Initially, patients may experience a decline of serum potassium when IV fluids are administered. To avoid this, all nonoliguric patients that are anorectic should receive supplemental potassium in IV fluids (20 mEq of potassium chloride per liter of fluids), even if serum potassium initially is normal. Rapid rates of fluid administration should be avoided, the fluids used should not contain glucose, and oral potassium supplementation should be started as soon as possible. In an emergency situation with severe hypokalemia (e.g., respiratory paralysis), administration of dopamine (0.5 µg/kg per hour) should be considered to shift potassium out of cells and into the extracellular space.[172]

Hyperkalemia is uncommon in CRF unless the patient is oliguric, which is most likely to occur terminally. If serum potassium is higher than 8 mEq/L or signs of cardiac toxicity exist, treatment is administered to lower serum potassium (see Acute Renal Failure).

Metabolic acidosis is the most common acid-base abnormality in CRF, and treatment is indicated if total carbon dioxide is less than 15 mEq/L. Sodium bicarbonate is administered at a dose of 8 to 12 mg/kg every 8 to 12 hours[34] (1 teaspoon baking soda equals 2000 mg bicarbonate). In order to avoid fluctuations in blood pH, it is best to start at the lower end of the dose range and administer it several times daily. Other alkalinizing agents, such as potassium citrate or calcium carbonate, should be considered in patients that are subject to volume overload (e.g., those with congestive heart failure). Total carbon dioxide is monitored and values are maintained at 18 to 24 mEq/L. Urinary acidifiers and diets that are intended to acidify urine (e.g., Prescription Diet Feline c/d) should not be used because they may worsen metabolic acidosis.

Hyperphosphatemia

Hyperphosphatemia exists in most patients with CRF and may contribute to progression of renal disease and worsening of clinical signs. Phosphate restriction has been shown to be beneficial in dogs and cats with experimentally induced CRF.[164, 173] The initial step is to feed a phosphate-restricted diet; most low-protein diets are also low in phosphate. The goal is to maintain serum phosphorus concentrations within reference ranges (3.5–5.5 mg/dL). Serum phosphorus concentration is monitored every 2 weeks, after a 12-hour fast. Dietary treatment alone is most effective in patients with early CRF that have mild to moderate hyperphosphatemia.

If normophosphatemia cannot be achieved by dietary phosphate restriction alone, phosphate binders may be used in combination with a low-phosphate diet. This is the most effective regimen for patients with advanced CRF. The phosphate binders most often used are aluminum hydroxide (Amphojel), calcium carbonate (Rolaids; Tums E-X, Cal Carb-HD), and calcium acetate (PhosLo, Phos-Ex). Liquid and gel formulations are more effective at binding phosphate than tablets; however, these products may be more difficult to administer long-term to veterinary patients.[174] Aluminum hydroxide and calcium carbonate should be administered at an initial dose of 100 mg/kg per day.[175] Calcium acetate binds more phosphorus per milligram of calcium, so a starting dose of 60 mg/kg per day is adequate. Phosphate binders are most effective when administered concurrently with a phosphate-restricted diet.[176] Also, it is important that the total daily dose be divided so that the agent is administered several times daily with meals. Potential side effects of calcium-containing phosphate binders include hypercalcemia and diarrhea. Because of the risk of soft tissue mineralization, it is probably best to administer aluminum hydroxide initially until the product of calcium times phosphorus is less than 70. Side effects of aluminum hydroxide include constipation and hypophosphatemia, which is unlikely in patients with CRF. Serum concentrations of phosphorus and calcium are monitored every 2 to 4 weeks initially, and the dose of phosphate binder is adjusted to maintain serum calcium and phosphorus within reference ranges. It may require several weeks to achieve normal phosphorus concentrations.

Hypocalcemia

Hypocalcemia occurs infrequently in patients with CRF, but if it is associated with clinical signs (e.g., weakness, inappetence, tremors, seizures), treatment is required. Calcium must be supplemented carefully in patients with CRF because of the risk of soft tissue mineralization and additional renal injury. Therefore, serum phosphorus should be normalized by phosphate-restricted diet and phosphate binders before calcium is administered. Calcium carbonate (100 mg/kg per day) may be preferred because of its alkalinizing properties.[34] Serum calcium and phosphorus are monitored every 2 to 4 weeks, and the dose is adjusted as needed.

Table 16–19
Dosages of Androgens Used to Treat Anemia of Chronic Renal Failure

DRUG	CANINE DOSAGE	FELINE DOSAGE
Stanozolol (Winstrol-V)	1–4 mg/dog, PO every 12 h	1 mg/cat, PO every 12 h
	25–50 mg/dog, IM weekly	25 mg/cat, IM weekly
Oxymetholone (Anadrol)	1–5 mg/kg, PO daily	1–5 mg/kg, PO daily
Nandrolone (Deca-Durabolin)	1–1.5 mg/kg, IM every 7–10 d	1 mg/kg, IM every 7–10 d

IM, intramuscularly; PO, by mouth.

Control of Serum Parathyroid Hormone Concentration

Normalization of serum phosphorus concentration does not cause maximal suppression of PTH, so additional treatment may be indicated to lower serum PTH. Administration of calcitriol (Rocaltrol) has been advocated to accomplish this.[177] Suppression of PTH could decrease severity of uremia as well as slow progression of CRF; however, results of long-term studies evaluating these effects in veterinary patients with CRF are not yet available. In addition, administration of vitamin D can cause hypercalcemia and potentially exacerbate renal disease secondary to nephrocalcinosis. Fortunately, the dose required to suppress PTH is lower than the dose that usually causes hypercalcemia.

Calcitriol should be administered only after the serum phosphorus concentration is lower than 6 mg/dL and the calcium-phosphorus product is less than 70.[178] An initial dose of 1.5 to 2.5 ng/kg is administered once daily by mouth. Calcitriol should be used in combination with a phosphate-restricted diet in order to cause maximal suppression of serum PTH.[179] Serum calcium and phosphorus are measured after 1 week and after 1 month of treatment, then monthly thereafter, to detect hypercalcemia and hyperphosphatemia.[178] If hyperphosphatemia develops, the dose of phosphate binders is increased to maintain serum phosphorus below 6 mg/dL. Hypercalcemia is most likely to occur in patients receiving calcium carbonate; if this occurs, another phosphate binder should be used. If hypercalcemia persists, the dose of calcitriol should be lowered. Serum PTH is measured at 1, 3, and 6 months to evaluate the efficacy of calcitriol treatment.[180] Serum PTH concentration normalizes within 1 to 2 months in most dogs; however, some patients may require a longer period of treatment.[179]

Anemia

Treatment of anemia in patients with CRF is indicated to improve quality of life and resolve the clinical signs associated with anemia. Options for treatment include administration of blood products, androgens, and recombinant human erythropoietin (Epogen). Administration of whole blood or packed cells is usually reserved for patients with clinical signs referable to severe anemia. If multiple transfusions are anticipated, as often occurs in CRF, a universal donor should be used, and a cross-match should be performed before each transfusion. Either whole blood or packed red cells are administered to raise the hematocrit above 25%.[34]

Androgens may be administered orally or parenterally in an attempt to increase hematocrit; other beneficial effects include increased appetite and weight gain (Table 16–19). In general, androgens must be administered for several months before a change in hematocrit is observed.[34] Parenterally administered androgens may be more effective; however, studies documenting efficacy of androgens for treatment of anemia in veterinary patients with CRF are lacking. Potential side effects of androgens include sodium and water retention, prostatomegaly, and hepatotoxicity, which may be more likely to occur with orally administered products.

Recombinant human erythropoietin has been used successfully to treat anemia of CRF in dogs and cats.[181] It should be considered if hematocrit decreases below 30% in dogs or 25% in cats.[181] Because treatment with erythropoietin may exacerbate hypertension, blood pressure should be measured before treatment begins. In addition, iron status, including serum iron, total iron-binding capacity (TIBC), and percent saturation (i.e., serum iron divided by TIBC), should be evaluated so that iron deficiency can be identified and corrected before beginning treatment with erythropoietin. The initial dose of 75 to 100 U/kg is administered subcutaneously three times weekly for 12 weeks, or until a target hematocrit is reached (i.e., 37%–45% for dogs and 30%–40% for cats).[181] Alternatively, a transfusion of either packed red cells or whole blood can be administered to raise the PCV before beginning treatment with erythropoietin; this may actually be more cost effective in larger patients. After the hematocrit reaches the lower end of the target range, the frequency of administration of erythropoietin is decreased to twice weekly. If the patient becomes anemic during twice-weekly treatment, erythropoietin is administered three times weekly again. Most patients can be maintained on a dose of 75 to 100 U/kg, two or three times weekly. Because of the potential for iron deficiency, it is probably best to administer ferrous sulfate orally to cats (50–100 mg/day) and dogs (100–300 mg/day) receiving erythropoietin. Oral administration of iron may cause gastric irritation and vomiting in some patients. Some ferrous sulfate products (Slow Fe) are less likely to cause vomiting, and they may be considered for veterinary patients that cannot tolerate other iron products.

Patients receiving erythropoietin should be monitored periodically to determine the efficacy of treatment and detect side effects such as iron deficiency, worsening hypertension, or development of erythropoietin antibodies. Hematocrit is measured weekly until it reaches the target range and remains stable for at least 4 weeks on a maintenance dosage. Thereafter, a CBC is taken every 1 or 2 months to monitor efficacy of treatment. Iron status is determined 4 weeks after beginning erythropoietin and every 2 to 3 months thereafter. Iron supplementation should be increased if serum iron is less than 84 μL/dL or percent saturation is less than 20%. Blood pressure is monitored monthly during initiation of treatment and every 1 to 2 months thereafter. Potential side effects of erythropoietin include exacerbation of hypertension, iron deficiency, and allergic reactions to the human serum albumin contained in the product. Up to 50% of dogs and cats may develop antibodies against erythropoietin (LD Cowgill, University of California at Davis, personal communication, 1992). Allergic reaction is characterized by a precipitous drop in hematocrit and is preceded by erythrocytic hypoplasia of the bone marrow; if this occurs, erythropoietin should be discontinued. Because antibodies also may form against endogenous erythropoietin, these patients usually are dependent on transfusions indefinitely.

Hypertension

The initial step in management of hypertensive patients is to restrict dietary sodium intake; diets containing 0.1% to 0.3% sodium on a dry matter basis should be used. Commercial (e.g., Prescription Diet k/d) or homemade diets are adequate.[166] Changes in dietary sodium intake should be made gradually over 2 to 4 weeks to allow the diseased kidneys sufficient time to adapt to a lower level of sodium. Diets that are severely sodium restricted (e.g., Prescription Diet h/d) should be avoided in patients with CRF because they may decrease renal perfusion and cause additional renal injury. Blood pressure is measured within 2 to 4 weeks to determine need for other treatment.

Most hypertensive veterinary patients require additional treatment in combination with dietary sodium restriction to control blood pressure. Diuretics are the first line of pharmacologic agents used. Furosemide (Lasix) is administered at 2 to 4 mg/kg every 12 to 24 hours, by mouth. If dietary sodium restriction and administration of a diuretic does not decrease blood pressure adequately, a β-blocker is added to the therapeutic regimen. Either propranolol (Inderal), at 0.2 to 1 mg/kg every 8 to 12 hours, by mouth, or atenolol (Tenormin) at 2 mg/kg every 24 hours, by mouth, may be used. Atenolol is a β_1-selective blocker and may be preferred over propranolol because it is more conveniently dosed and does not have the potential to cause bronchospasm from blocking of β_2-receptors. If additional control of blood pressure is needed, hydralazine (0.5–2 mg/kg every 12 hours, by mouth) is administered. Hydralazine causes direct arteriolar dilation, which helps lower blood pressure; however, it also causes reflex tachycardia and renin release and therefore should be administered with a β-blocker and a diuretic. If hypertension is still refractory to these measures, an ACE inhibitor may be substituted for hydralazine or used alone. Either captopril (Capoten at 0.5 to 1.0 mg/kg every 8 to 12 hours, by mouth), enalapril (Vasotec) at 0.5 mg/kg every 12 to 24 hours, by mouth), or lisinopril (Zestril at 0.5 mg/kg every 24 hours, by mouth) may be administered. Inhibition of ACE inhibitors causes efferent arteriolar dilation, which may decrease GFR and lead to ARF; this is most likely to occur in the presence of dehydration, hyponatremia, or pre-existing renal disease. Therefore, ACE inhibitors should be used cautiously in patients with CRF; renal function should be monitored every 2 to 4 weeks for the first 3 to 4 months, then every 2 to 6 months as needed.

Patient Monitoring

Patients with CRF should be monitored periodically so that treatment can be adjusted as needed. The frequency of evaluation depends on the occurrence and severity of metabolic disturbances. Patients that are stable (i.e., maintaining body weight and hydration status) should be evaluated every 2 to 4 months, and patients with persistent abnormalities such as hypokalemia, hyperphosphatemia, or metabolic acidosis need to monitored more frequently. A physical examination detects changes in body weight and hydration status. Laboratory tests, including CBC, serum chemistries, and urinalysis, are performed to evaluate renal function and the need for additional treatment or alteration of dosage. Parameters should be recorded in a flow chart so that trends can be more easily detected and adjustments in treatment made as needed.

Prognosis

Eventually, patients with CRF die because renal function continues to deteriorate; however, many patients can live a comfortable life for several years with careful medical management. Several factors should be considered when establishing a prognosis for animals with CRF, including severity of clinical signs, presence of a reversible disorder contributing to renal dysfunction, severity of renal functional impairment, and rate of progression of renal disease.[34] The short-term (weeks to months) prognosis is good for patients without clinical signs of uremia and those that respond to supportive treatment; patients with severe clinical signs (e.g., vomiting, anorexia, weight loss) that persist for longer than 2 to 4 days despite appropriate treatment have a guarded to poor prognosis. Identification and successful treatment of an underlying disorder that impairs renal function (e.g., prerenal or postrenal azotemia) is a favorable prognostic sign. A persistent decline in renal function, determined by serially increased values for serum creatinine and BUN, indicates a less favorable prognosis than does more stable renal function. In addition to laboratory parameters, the clinical condition of the patient also must be considered in determining prognosis.

Nephrotic Syndrome

Nephrotic syndrome is caused by glomerular disease and is characterized by proteinuria, hypoalbuminemia, hypercholesterolemia, and peripheral edema or ascites. Because many dogs and cats with glomerular disease do not have all these characteristics, a more practical definition in veterinary patients is proteinuria of sufficient magnitude to cause clinically important hypoalbuminemia. This definition of nephrotic syndrome is adequate considering that diagnostic evaluation of patients with hypoalbuminemia and proteinuria is the same whether or not edema or ascites exist.[34] The incidence of nephrotic syndrome in veterinary patients is unknown, although it seems to occur more often in dogs than cats. Although nephrotic syndrome may affect dogs and cats of all ages, most are older than 5 years of age, except for Abyssinian cats and Chinese shar-peis with amyloidosis.[79, 161] Some breeds have a familial tendency to develop glomerular diseases that cause nephrotic syndrome (see Table 16–7).[34, 71–85]

Pathophysiology

Nephrotic syndrome results from glomerular diseases, which are differentiated from other renal diseases because they primarily affect glomeruli, at least initially. Glomerulonephritis and amyloidosis are clinically the two most important glomerular diseases that cause nephrotic syndrome in dogs and cats.

Glomerulonephritis is an immune-mediated phenomenon that results from glomerular deposition of circulating immune complexes. Immune complexes form in the presence of moderate antigen excess, which may result from a variety of infectious, inflammatory, and neoplastic diseases (see Table 16–7). In some cases, an underlying disease is not identified, and the patient is said to have idiopathic glomerulonephritis. Glomerular deposition of immune complexes activates the complement cascade, which leads to an inflammatory response characterized by influx of neutrophils and other cells. Release of lysosomal enzymes causes glomerular injury. Damage to glomerular endothelium exposes collagen, which activates platelets, causing release of vasoactive and inflammatory substances (e.g., thromboxanes). Increased capillary membrane permeability occurs, potentiating additional immune complex deposition, which causes further glomerular injury.

Reactive systemic amyloidosis occurs in dogs and cats and is associated with hepatic production of an acute phase protein, serum amyloid A. Amyloidosis, like glomerulonephritis, may be associated with any infectious, inflammatory, or neoplastic disease; an underlying cause is identified in approximately 25% to 50% of cases.[120, 121] Although amyloid may affect many tissues, it often deposits in the kidneys. In dogs, it primarily affects glomeruli, causing a protein-losing nephropathy; in cats, CRF occurs secondary to medullary deposition of amyloid.

Regardless of the cause of glomerular injury (i.e., glomerulonephritis or amyloidosis), it eventually leads to glomerular sclerosis and replacement of the entire nephron segment with fibrous tissue. If enough nephrons become nonfunctional (i.e., 75%), CRF develops. Glomerular disease appears to be a common cause of CRF in dogs and cats.

Thrombosis of major vessels may be a complication of nephrotic syndrome in dogs and cats. Potential causes include urinary loss of antithrombin III and increased platelet aggregation.[182, 183] It seems to occur more often in patients with amyloidosis, probably because of the severity of urine protein loss and subsequent hypoalbuminemia.[120]

Clinical Signs

Clinical signs of glomerular disease may result from complications of urinary protein loss, renal failure, or an underlying infectious, inflammatory, or neoplastic disease. Historical findings often include anorexia, weight loss, vomiting, lethargy, PU/PD, and, rarely, signs of thromboembolic disease (e.g., severe dyspnea, posterior paresis). Physical examination findings include emaciation, dehydration, and, less often, edema and ascites.

Diagnostic Plan

Results of CBC, serum chemistries, and urinalysis vary depending on the severity and longevity of glomerular disease. If hypoalbuminemia and proteinuria occur together, glomerular disease should be strongly suspected, especially if urinary sediment examination is unremarkable and the patient has no signs of lower urinary tract disease. The magnitude of proteinuria tends to be more severe with amyloidosis, although patients with severe glomerulonephritis may lose similar amounts of urinary protein (see Table 16–6 and Proteinuria). Urine protein/creatinine ratios less than 13 usually are associated with nonamyloid glomerular disease, whereas ratios greater than 13 often result from either severe glomerulonephritis or amyloidosis.[69] Hypoalbuminemia exists in most patients that are presented with clinically important glomerular disease; however, total protein may be normal, especially in patients with hyperglobulinemia caused by underlying infectious, inflammatory, or neoplastic disorders. Hypercholesterolemia also exists in many patients and may be caused by increased hepatic synthesis of cholesterol or loss of some regulatory protein into the urine.[184] If CRF has developed, other laboratory findings include nonregenerative anemia, azotemia, hyperphosphatemia, and metabolic acidosis. In addition to proteinuria, other urinalysis findings may include decreased urine concentrating ability, presence of hyaline casts, and pyuria.

Underlying Diseases

If glomerular disease is suspected on the basis of clinical and laboratory findings, additional diagnostic evaluation should be done to identify potentially treatable underlying diseases (see Table 16–7). The evaluation should be guided by historical findings, physical examination, and laboratory findings (e.g., fever, joint pain, splenomegaly, lymphadenopathy, vaginal discharge, thrombocytopenia, hemolytic anemia). Diagnostic tests may include thoracic and abdominal radiography, abdominal ultrasonography, serologic evaluation (i.e., antinuclear antibodies, LE cell test, rickettsial/viral/fungal titers, occult heartworm test), adrenocorticotropic hormone response test, synovial fluid analysis, and cytologic evaluation of tissue aspirates, depending on other clinical findings. A suspected source of immune complex production is identified in 50% to 70% of patients with glomerular disease.[73, 121] Before recommending more invasive tests, such as renal biopsy, it may be worthwhile to treat the underlying disease and monitor the patient for response to treatment.

Renal Biopsy and Immunofluorescence

If there is lack of response to treatment of the suspected underlying cause, or if a predisposing cause cannot be identified, a renal biopsy should be done. Microscopic evaluation of renal tissue is the only definitive method to diagnose glomerular disease and distinguish between amyloidosis and glomerulonephritis. This is important clinically because of differences between these disorders regarding prognosis and treatment. Special stains such as Congo red often are necessary for definitive diagnosis of amyloidosis.

Additional studies, such as immunofluorescence, may be needed to diagnose glomerulonephritis. With immunofluorescent staining, glomerulonephritis is characterized by fluorescence of granular, discontinuous deposits on glomerular basement membranes. However, finding of fluorescent deposits in glomeruli indicates the presence of immunoglobulin, complement, or antigen but by itself is not diagnostic of glomerulonephritis.[185] Results must be interpreted with the clinical and laboratory findings in mind. It also is possible to have immune-mediated glomerular disease in the absence of fluorescence.

Treatment

Treatment of Underlying Disease

The initial step in managing patients with nephrotic syndrome and glomerular disease is to treat any underlying disease. Severity of proteinuria and hypoalbuminemia may decrease after treatment of these disorders, in particular with pyometra and heartworm disease.[34] In some cases, however, an associated infectious, inflammatory, or neoplastic condition cannot be identified, or it may not be amenable to treatment (e.g., metastatic neoplasia, FIP, feline leukemia virus).

Immunosuppressive agents such as corticosteroids, azathioprine, or cyclophosphamide have been used to treat glomerulonephritis in dogs and cats on the premise that they prevent formation of immune complexes and alter the inflammatory response; however, this practice now is considered questionable. It is not known whether patients with glomerulonephritis have a hyperactive immune system or a deficient immune response. In addition, corticosteroids can potentially cause adverse effects, including worsening of uremic signs in patients with CRF, increased proteinuria and glomerular injury, increased risk of secondary infections, and increased risk of thromboembolic disease.[34, 72] For these reasons, and because no controlled studies have documented the efficacy of administering immunosuppressive agents to dogs and cats with glomerulonephritis, their use should be avoided unless the underlying disease is amenable to such therapy (e.g., systemic lupus erythematosus, lymphoma).

Administration of drugs that prevent platelet activation and release of vasoactive substances such as thromboxane may be helpful for treatment of glomerulonephritis. Thromboxane synthetase inhibitors specifically inhibit production of thromboxane, a potent inducer of platelet aggregation. These substances have been shown to lessen the severity of proteinuria in dogs with experimentally induced and spontaneously occurring glomerulonephritis.[186, 187] Although not currently available on the market, these agents may prove useful in the future. At present, a low dose of aspirin (0.5–5 mg/kg every 12–24 hours, by mouth) can be administered to selectively inhibit cyclo-oxygenase without preventing formation of prostacyclin (renal vasodilatory prostaglandin and platelet aggregation antagonist).[71] All NSAIDs, including aspirin, should be used cautiously in patients with renal disease because of the potential for causing ARF.[125, 126]

There is no consistently reliable treatment for amyloidosis, although occasionally patients have responded to administration of dimethylsulfoxide (DMSO).[188, 189] For lack of any better treatment and because of few reported side effects, a therapeutic trial with DMSO probably is appropriate. Dosage regimens of DMSO that have been used are 125 mg/kg every 12 hours, by mouth and 80 mg/kg three times weekly, by subcutaneous administration.[188, 189]

*Supportive Treatment and
Management of Complications*

Dogs and cats with glomerular disease should be fed a diet that is moderately restricted in protein, phosphorus, and sodium, similar to diets recommended for patients with CRF (e.g., Prescription Diet k/d). Sodium restriction is indicated because of the high incidence of systemic hypertension and the potential for ascites and peripheral edema in patients with glomerular disease. At one time, it was believed that dietary protein should be supplemented to account for the amount of protein lost in urine; however, this is no longer recommended because of potential for worsening proteinuria and hypoalbuminemia.[190] Dogs and cats with glomerular disease should be fed a protein-restricted diet (see Chronic Renal Failure), and they should be monitored every 2 to 4 weeks initially to detect signs of protein malnutrition such as weight loss, decreased muscle mass, worsening hypoalbuminemia, increased proteinuria, and decreased PCV. If these signs occur, the diet is carefully supplemented with additional protein up to the amount lost daily in the urine. A boiled egg contains 6.5 to 7.0 g of protein of high biologic value and may be used for protein supplementation. If proteinuria or hypoalbuminemia worsen, however, protein supplementation should be discontinued because of the risk of additional renal injury.

Administration of ACE inhibitors lessens the severity of proteinuria in human and veterinary patients with glomerular disease.[191–194] These drugs cause efferent arteriolar dilation and lessen intraglomerular pressure, which may partially explain how ACE inhibitors decrease proteinuria. Because of the potential benefits of ACE inhibition, it may be worthwhile to administer an ACE inhibitor to dogs and cats with glomerular disease (see section on hypertension in CRF for dosage regimens). Because the efficacy of ACE inhibitors at reducing proteinuria is affected by dietary sodium intake, treatment should be combined with a sodium-restricted diet (e.g., Prescription Diet k/d).[195] Because of potential side effects of ACE inhibition (e.g., ARF), patients with renal disease should be monitored closely when these drugs are administered, especially if a diuretic is being administered concurrently.

Urine protein loss should be monitored carefully so that treatment can be adjusted as necessary. This can be accomplished by measuring urine protein/creatinine ratios every 2 to 4 weeks initially, then after any changes in treatment. A decrease in the ratio indicates decreased urine protein loss, which may occur as a result of successful treatment (e.g., dietary protein restriction, ACE inhibition). However, decreased proteinuria also may occur as renal function deteriorates and less protein is filtered through the glomerulus. In order to interpret the significance of declining proteinuria, serial measurements of BUN and serum creatinine also should be done.

Because of potential harmful effects of systemic hypertension on progression of renal disease, treatment to control blood pressure is indicated in hypertensive patients if blood pressure can be monitored (see Chronic Renal Failure). Because of the potential beneficial effects of ACE inhibitors in patients with glomerular disease, these drugs may be preferable to other antihypertensive agents.

The best treatment for edema or ascites is cage rest and dietary sodium restriction. Cage confinement for a few days often causes marked improvement in edematous patients. Administration of diuretics and paracentesis is reserved for patients that experience respiratory distress or clinically important abdominal discomfort. Furosemide may be administered (2–4 mg/kg every 6–24 hours, by mouth, subcutaneously, or IV) until edema resolves; the dose is gradually tapered and discontinued. Diuretics should be avoided because of the potential for electrolyte disturbances, dehydration, and renal hypoperfusion. Unless necessary, fluid is not removed from body cavities, because this potentiates volume depletion, protein loss, and further edema formation. Because edema results from decreased oncotic pressure as a result of hypoalbuminemia, the best long-term method for controlling edema is to reduce urine protein loss.

Because of the difficulty of successfully treating the uncommon complication of thromboembolism of major vessels, every effort should be made to prevent its occurrence. Methods to reduce urine protein loss are indicated, as are general measures to prevent thrombosis, including maintenance of hydration and avoidance of predisposing drugs such as corticosteroids (see Chap. 13 for treatment of pulmonary thrombosis).

Prognosis

Although it is generally agreed that glomerulonephritis often progresses to cause terminal CRF in dogs and cats, the prognosis for individual patients varies considerably. If an underlying disease such as pyometra or heartworm disease can be identified and successfully treated, glomerulonephritis often resolves. The prognosis for recovery remains guarded if an underlying cause either cannot be identified or does not respond to treatment (e.g., systemic lupus erythematosus). Spontaneous remissions may occur in idiopathic cases of glomerulonephritis, and it is not uncommon for dogs and cats with glomerulonephritis and proteinuria to live for 2 to 5 years.[196–199] Although dogs with severe proteinuria, weight loss, and ascites seem to have a poor prognosis, some cats with edema and ascites may experience resolution of clinical signs and survive for years.[34, 197, 199] However, if renal failure is present, the prognosis is grave, because these patients do not respond well to treatment.

In contrast to glomerulonephritis, amyloidosis invariably progresses to death as a result of terminal CRF. Also, complications of nephrotic syndrome (e.g., weight loss, thromboembolism, edema, and ascites) may be more likely to occur in patients with amyloidosis because of the large amount of urinary protein loss.

Pyelonephritis

Pyelonephritis is inflammation of the renal parenchyma and its pelvis; however, the term often is used to mean bacterial urinary tract infection that involves one or both kidneys.[34] Pyelonephritis is recognized less frequently than urethrocystitis, possibly because of the lack of clinical signs in patients with upper urinary tract infection and the difficulty of localizing infection to the upper urinary tract. Urinary tract infection is more common in dogs than in cats, and females appear to be more often affected than males.[200, 201] Although not documented, pyelonephritis may be more common in females as a result of ascending infections from the lower urinary tract.

Pathophysiology

Ascending infection from the urinary bladder is believed to cause most renal infections in dogs and cats. Altered host defense mechanisms (e.g., nephrolithiasis, ectopic ureters, vesicoureteral reflux) may predispose to pyelonephritis; however, some patients have no apparent cause. Although uncommon, microbial invasion may occur by the hematogenous route (e.g., septicemia). Organisms that cause pyelonephritis are similar to those that cause urethrocystitis; *Escherichia coli, Staphylococcus* spp., and *Proteus* spp. are the most common.

Clinical Signs

Clinical findings in patients with pyelonephritis depend on whether the disorder is acute or chronic. Problems in patients with acute pyelonephritis may include depression, lethargy, anorexia, vomiting, fever, and abdominal pain or discomfort. Owners may notice discolored or malodorous urine. PU/PD may occur with chronic pyelonephritis because of loss of urine-concentrating ability.[202] Patients with pyelonephritis may have concomitant signs of urethrocystitis, including pollakiuria, stranguria, and dysuria. Pyelonephritis should be suspected, especially if relapse of infection occurs in a patient treated for urethrocystitis. Some patients with acute pyelonephritis may have no clinical signs, although this is more common in patients with chronic pyelonephritis.

Diagnostic Plan

Although it may be difficult, an attempt should be made to distinguish between pyelonephritis and urethrocystitis. This is important because pyelonephritis may cause renal damage and requires a longer period of treatment. Fever and other signs of systemic illness are much more common with pyelonephritis than with simple cystitis. Laboratory findings may help support a diagnosis of pyelonephritis; however, they are rarely specific and often are normal. Serum chemistries often are unremarkable, although azotemia and hyperphosphatemia may occur as a result of dehydration or renal failure. Patients with acute pyelonephritis may have leukocytosis and a left shift. Urinalysis may reveal low USG, pyuria, and bacteriuria; isosthenuria usually is not present unless the disease is chronic.[202, 203] The presence of white blood cell casts is a reliable indicator of renal involvement; however, they are not observed in most patients with pyelonephritis. Quantitative urine culture should be done in patients with suspected urinary tract infection (see Chap. 17). Some patients with pyelonephritis, especially those with chronic disease, may have a negative urine culture. In addition, a positive urine culture does not localize disease to the kidneys.

Results of excretory urography or ultrasonography may support a diagnosis of pyelonephritis, although the findings are neither sensitive nor specific.[204, 205] Approximately 64% to 73% of dogs with experimentally induced pyelonephritis have abnormal findings on excretory urography.[204, 206] Radiographic findings include dilation of the renal pelvis and ureter and decreased opacity of contrast media in the collecting system.[204] Some dogs with pyelonephritis do not have any radiographic changes; however, radiography may help to identify disorders that predispose to pyelonephritis (e.g., nephroliths, vesicoureteral reflux on contrast cystography).[204] Ultrasonographic findings of pyelonephritis include renal pelvic dilatation, proximal ureteral dilatation, and generalized hyperechogenicity of the renal cortex.[206] Ability to detect changes consistent with acute pyelonephritis may be better with ultrasonography than with excretory urography.[206] In addition, ultrasonography is noninvasive, requires little patient preparation, and is not affected by poor renal function.[206]

Because the clinical findings of pyelonephritis often are nonspecific, clinicians must maintain a high index of suspicion. In many cases, a presumptive diagnosis is made on the basis of clinical findings and a positive urine culture. Radiographic and ultrasonographic findings also may be used to support the diagnosis. If there is any question about the diagnosis, it is probably best to assume that pyelonephritis exists and to treat accordingly.

Treatment

Treatment of pyelonephritis includes correction of impaired host defenses and administration of appropriate antimicrobials. Maintaining adequate serum concentrations of antimicrobial drugs may be more important in patients with pyelonephritis than in those with urethrocystitis, where urinary drug concentrations primarily determine efficacy of treatment. Animals with pyelonephritis or sepsis should be treated with parenteral antimicrobials until systemic signs such as fever and pain subside, usually within 48 to 72 hours. Ideally, selection of antimicrobial drugs should be based on results of culture and susceptibility testing, although most urinary pathogens have predictable susceptibility patterns (see Chap. 17). Antimicrobials should be administered for a minimum of 4 to 6 weeks. Ideally, a urine sample obtained by cystocentesis should be cultured 7 to 14 days after treatment begins to determine efficacy of the selected drug. Another urine culture should be done 5 to 7 days after cessation of treatment and every 4 to 8 weeks thereafter until three consecutive negative cultures are obtained. If the infection relapses, an appropriate antimicrobial should be administered for a longer period of time (i.e., 8–12 weeks). Some patients with persistent infections may benefit from low-dose antimicrobial treatment administered daily (see Chap. 17).

Some measures can be taken to lessen the likelihood of development of pyelonephritis. Because most renal infections are believed to result from ascending infections from the lower urinary tract, prompt recognition and treatment of urethrocystitis may prevent pyelonephritis. Also, manual compression of the urinary bladder should be avoided in patients with urinary tract infection because it causes vesicoureteral reflux (i.e., reflux of urine from the urinary bladder into the ureters and renal pelves), which may lead to renal infection.[34]

Prognosis

Adequate studies of dogs and cats with pyelonephritis are not available to accurately predict prognosis. Patients with acute pyelonephritis usually respond to supportive care and administration of parenteral antimicrobials. Patients with septicemia may have a more guarded prognosis. The long-term prognosis for patients with chronic pyelonephritis is unknown. It is possible that no sequelae may occur; however, destruction of enough nephrons may lead to CRF. Patients with chronic pyelonephritis also may be more susceptible to nephrotoxic substances such as aminoglycosides, and these agents should be avoided.[207]

Nephrolithiasis and Ureterolithiasis

Uroliths are polycrystalline concretions that are composed of organic or inorganic crystalloids (90%–95%) and a smaller amount of organic matrix (5%–10%).[208] Uroliths form in the urinary space within the excretory pathway, and they usually are classified according to their mineral composition. Uroliths rarely affect the upper urinary tract of dogs and cats.[209–212] Less than 6% of urinary tract uroliths are found in the kidneys; the majority are located in the urinary bladder or urethra.[209, 210] However, because nephroliths may not cause clinical signs, their true incidence in dogs and cats is unknown.

Breeds with a higher incidence of uroliths include miniature schnauzer, dachshund, Dalmatian, pug, bulldog, Welsh corgi, beagle, and basset hound.[209] Siamese cats were overrepresented in a study of feline nephroliths.[211] Certain uroliths occur most often in selected breeds of dogs, including urate (Dalmatian), cystine (dachshund, English bulldog), calcium oxalate (miniature schnauzer, miniature poodle, Yorkshire terrier, Lhasa apso, shih tzu), and silica (German shepherd).[213, 214] Uroliths that more often affect male dogs include calcium oxalate, xanthine, and silica.[213–215]

Pathophysiology

Uroliths may occur secondary to urinary tract infection, dietary factors, inborn errors of metabolism, portal vascular anomalies, or primary hyperparathyroidism; in some instances, the cause is unknown (see Chap. 17).

Clinical Signs

Clinical signs of renal and ureteral uroliths depend on the size, number, and location of stones; presence or absence of urinary obstruction; and whether urinary tract infection exists. Some patients may show evidence of sublumbar pain or abdominal discomfort. Discolored urine (hematuria) may be noted, and urine may be foul smelling if infection is present. Bilateral obstruction of renal pelves or ureters or unilateral obstruction with inadequate renal function in the contralateral kidney may cause signs of renal failure, including depression, inappetence, vomiting, and weight loss resulting from postrenal azotemia or uremia. Some patients may have a palpably enlarged kidney or kidneys. Despite these findings, some patients with nephroliths and ureteroliths have no clinical signs.

Diagnostic Plan

Uroliths of the upper urinary tract often are identified initially by abdominal radiography in patients with vague clinical signs or inadvertently in patients with other diseases. Patients with urinary bladder uroliths should always be evaluated for the presence of uroliths in the upper urinary tract. Excretory urography is indicated to detect radiolucent uroliths and to determine the presence and degree of urinary obstruction in patients with confirmed or suspected nephrolithiasis or ureterolithiasis. Abdominal ultrasonography also may help confirm presence and location of radiolucent uroliths and detect signs of urinary obstruction. A minimum database, including CBC, serum chemistries, urinalysis, and urine culture, is indicated in patients with uroliths, regardless of their location. Renal failure caused by urinary obstruction may be present in patients with bilateral nephroliths or ureteroliths. Results of the minimum database, together with radiographic findings, may provide clues to the type of urolith present, which guides initial medical treatment (see Chap. 17).

Treatment

Treatment for an individual patient with uroliths of the upper urinary tract depends on renal function, presence of urinary obstruction, and whether urinary tract infection exists. Nonobstructing, sterile nephroliths that do not increase in size, do not produce clinically important hematuria, or do not cause deterioration in renal function can be monitored without therapeutic intervention. If an underlying cause of urolithiasis can be identified (e.g., urinary tract infection, portosystemic shunt, primary hyperparathyroidism), it should be corrected. Medical treatment of urolithiasis should be considered, especially if the mineral composition of the urolith can be estimated with confidence. This primarily involves dietary changes, alteration of urine pH, and administration of agents to decrease urinary excretion of calculogenic substances (see Chap. 17).

Surgical removal of nephroliths or ureteroliths may be appropriate in several situations.[216] If uroliths are obstructing urine flow to any substantial degree, they should be surgically removed without delay. If renal function could deteriorate in the time required for medical dissolution, surgery also should be considered. Some uroliths (i.e., calcium oxalate, calcium phosphate, silica) are not amenable to medical dissolution; if treatment is indicated, surgical removal should be done. Surgery also should be considered for young animals, because the safety of low-protein and low-magnesium diets is unknown for growing animals. Also, males with uroliths at multiple sites that require abdominal surgery and cystotomy are candidates for surgical removal of uroliths affecting the upper urinary tract. Removal of bilateral nephroliths can be done during one surgical procedure if azotemia is not present and urine concentrating ability is adequate. It may be preferable to perform a more sensitive measurement of glomerular filtration, such as creatinine clearance, in these patients. If azotemia already exists and surgical excision is necessary, it is preferable to remove the urolith from only one kidney; surgery of the other kidney should be done later, only after careful evaluation of renal function.

Prognosis

The prognosis for patients with nephroliths or ureteroliths depends on whether urinary obstruction exists, the duration and degree of obstruction, the presence or absence of urinary infection, and whether one or both kidneys are affected.[34] Complete obstruction with infection can cause total renal destruction in a few days, but in the absence of infection, the kidneys have a remarkable capacity for recovery, even after long periods of obstruction.[34] After 7 days of complete unilateral ureteral obstruction in dogs, GFR returned to a maximal value that was 68% of baseline.[217] In addition, return of renal function after unilateral ureteral obstruction in dogs is directly proportional to duration of obstruction.[218]

Ectopic Ureters

Ureteral ectopia is a congenital disorder whereby either one or both ureters do not terminate normally in the trigone of the urinary bladder. In females, ectopic ureters terminate in the vagina most often, followed by urethra, neck of the urinary bladder, or uterus.[219] Ectopic ureters in males usually terminate in the pelvic urethra.

The incidence of ectopic ureters is unknown; however, it should be suspected in young patients that are presented for evaluation of urinary incontinence. Ectopic ureters usually are diagnosed in young animals and are 20 times more common in female dogs than males; cats are rarely affected.[219–224]

Pathophysiology

The cause of ectopic ureters is unknown, although a hereditary predisposition is suspected in some breeds of dogs (e.g., Siberian huskies).[222–224] Because of abnormal termination of ureters, these patients are susceptible to ascending urinary tract infection and development of pyelonephritis. Renal failure may be present in some patients. In addition, other urinary tract abnormalities such as urethral incompetence, hydroureter, and hydronephrosis often exist concurrently.[225]

Clinical Signs

Most dogs with ectopic ureters are presented for evaluation of urinary incontinence that is recognized soon after birth or at the time of weaning, although it has been reported in adult dogs up to 7 years of age.[224] Urinary incontinence may be continuous or intermittent. Animals with ectopic ureters often retain the ability to micturate normally, especially if unilateral disease exists. Clinical signs of urinary tract infection, such as foul-smelling urine, stranguria, and pollakiuria, often are present. Physical examination often is normal except for presence of a wet perineal area and possibly dermatitis caused by urine scalding. Animals with ectopic ureters should be carefully evaluated for other congenital abnormalities.

Diagnostic Plan

Ectopic ureters are most easily diagnosed by excretory urography; however, retrograde contrast urethrography, pneumocystography, or vaginography may help to localize the site of ureteral termination.[225] In addition to ectopic ureters, it is not uncommon for these patients to have other urinary system abnormalities, including hydroureter, hydronephrosis, pyelonephritis, and small urinary bladder.[219, 221–225] In addition to radiographic studies, other tests, including serum chemistries, urinalysis, and urine culture, should be done to detect renal failure and urinary tract infection.

Treatment

The treatment of choice for ectopic ureters is surgical correction. Ureterovesicular anastomosis is preferable in unilateral disease if the affected ureter appears normal; it also is indicated in patients with bilaterally ectopic ureters. If there is unilateral disease and the function of the affected ureter and the kidney is significantly compromised (e.g., severe hydroureter and hydronephrosis), ureteronephrectomy should be considered, provided that contralateral renal function is normal.

Administration of antimicrobial drugs is indicated in patients with urinary tract infection. Selection of antimicrobials should be based on results of culture and susceptibility. If pyelonephritis is suspected, antimicrobial drugs should be administered for at least 6 to 8 weeks. Because of compromised host defenses, many patients require long-term treatment (see Chap. 17).

Some patients also have urethral incompetence, which is characterized by incontinence despite successful correction of ectopic ureters. Administration of agents to increase urethral sphincter tone (e.g., phenylpropanolamine, diethylstilbestrol) may be helpful in these cases (see Chap. 17).

Prognosis

The response to surgical correction of ectopic ureters is variable; although some patients have complete resolution of clinical signs, others have persistent incontinence.[219, 222–224] Persistent urinary incontinence may be caused by other abnormalities, such as urethral incompetence or vestibulovaginal disorders, that often exist in these patients. The prognosis for resolution of signs appears to be better if the ectopic ureter terminates in the vagina or uterus instead of the urethra in females.[224] Also, patients that have marked hydroureter before surgery are less likely to respond than patients with mild to no ureteral dilation.[226] In contrast, the presence of hydroureter after surgery does not necessarily indicate a poor prognosis.[221, 226, 227] Other factors that worsen the prognosis include the presence of renal failure and persistent urinary tract infection.

Renal Neoplasia

Neoplasia affecting the kidneys may originate from renal tissue (i.e., primary tumors) or may secondarily affect the kidneys by metastasis. The most common primary renal tumors of dogs are epithelial in origin and include renal cell carcinoma and transitional cell carcinoma; mesenchymal tumors (e.g., sarcomas) also may affect the kidneys, but they occur less often.[228–230] Nephroblastoma is a congenital tumor of mixed-cell origin that also occurs infrequently in dogs.[229, 230] Renal neoplasia is uncommon in small animals, representing less than 1% of all canine neoplasms.[229] Primary renal tumors are more common in dogs than in cats, and males are more often affected than females.[228-231] Although nephroblastoma is usually considered a tumor of young dogs, it has been diagnosed in animals that are 8 years of age.[230] German shepherds have a disorder characterized by dermatofibrosis and bilateral renal cystadenocarcinoma.[230, 232] In cats, lymphoma is clinically the most important tumor that affects the kidneys, although it may infrequently occur in dogs as well.[233-235]

Pathophysiology

Approximately 90% of primary renal tumors behave malignantly, and they often metastasize to lungs, bone, liver, abdominal lymph nodes, and adrenal glands.[228-230] In contrast, nephroblastomas often behave benignly, although they have metastatic potential. Lymphoma in cats is caused by infection with feline leukemia virus, although only 50% of cats with renal lymphoma are viremic.[233]

Clinical Signs

Clinical signs of renal neoplasia often are vague and nonspecific and include lethargy, inappetence, weight loss, and fever.[228, 230, 235, 236] Discolored urine (hematuria) is infrequently observed; it is more likely to occur in patients with mesenchymal and transitional cell tumors.[230] Rarely, lameness may occur secondary to hypertrophic osteopathy. Clinical signs of CRF, such as vomiting, dehydration, and PU/PD, may be observed in some patients with renal neoplasia, especially cats with renal lymphoma.[234, 235] The most common physical examination finding with primary renal tumors is a palpable abdominal mass. Cats with renal lymphoma usually have bilateral renomegaly, although only one kidney may appear enlarged in some cases.[233-235]

Diagnostic Plan

Results of laboratory evaluation, including CBC, serum chemistries, and urinalysis, usually are nonspecific. Anemia and azotemia were the two most common findings in one study of dogs with renal neoplasia; rarely, polycythemia was observed.[230] Hematuria and proteinuria may be observed on urinalysis, although results of urinalysis often are normal. Neoplastic cells are rarely identified in urine from patients with renal tumors.

Radiography (including plain and contrast studies) and ultrasonography are helpful for confirming the presence of an abdominal mass.[24, 230] Plain films often do not allow identification of an abdominal mass as a kidney; in these cases, excretory urography or ultrasonography may be used.[230] In addition, thoracic radiographs should be taken in all patients with renal tumors to evaluate for metastasis. In one study of dogs with renal neoplasia, 34% of all dogs had

pulmonary metastases, whereas 48% of dogs with renal cell carcinoma had metastasis.[230]

A definitive diagnosis of renal neoplasia is made by either histologic or cytologic evaluation of renal tissue. Renal lymphoma in cats can easily be diagnosed by fine-needle aspiration cytology. Other malignant renal tumors also can be diagnosed by aspiration cytology; however, samples often are obtained at exploratory laparotomy and submitted for histologic evaluation. If available, ultrasonography may be used to guide renal biopsy (see Renal Biopsy).

Treatment

The treatment of choice for unilateral renal tumors is surgical excision of the affected kidney and its ureter. In addition, exploratory laparotomy allows for visual inspection of abdominal organs to detect metastases. There is no effective treatment for patients with bilateral involvement. Chemotherapy may be considered for patients with bilateral neoplasia, incompletely excised tumors, or evidence of metastasis.[236]

Renal lymphoma in cats is best treated by combination chemotherapy[233] (see Chap. 43). In one study of 28 cats with renal lymphoma, 17 responded completely to chemotherapy, 9 had a partial response, and only 2 showed no response.[233] The median survival time for cats that responded completely and were negative for feline leukemia virus was 256 days, whereas cats that were positive for feline leukemia virus had a median survival time of 131 days. In 40% of the cats with renal lymphoma, metastasis to the central nervous system occurred. It has been suggested that incorporation of cytosine arabinoside into the chemotherapy regimen may decrease this complication; however, this remains to be proven.[233]

Prognosis

Prognosis for patients with renal neoplasia depends somewhat on type of tumor, presence of other complicating factors (e.g., renal failure), and whether the disease is bilateral or unilateral. In general, the long-term prognosis for patients with malignant mesenchymal tumors and renal cell carcinoma is grave to guarded, whereas patients with nephroblastoma may have a favorable outcome. The median survival time after nephrectomy for dogs with renal cell carcinoma in one study was 8 months; however, some patients have lived for several years.[228, 230] For cats with renal lymphoma, the median survival time is longer if the animal is negative for feline leukemia virus. Although renal failure and azotemia have a negative effect on survival, some azotemic cats may have long survival times; therefore, the presence of renal failure should not exclude a recommendation of chemotherapy.

Uncommon Diseases of the Kidney and Ureter

Renal and Ureteral Trauma

Injury to the upper urinary tract (e.g., crush injury, ureteral avulsion) infrequently occurs in dogs and cats.[237] Renal and ureteral trauma should be suspected in patients with vague signs of abdominal discomfort, hematuria, or fractures of the caudal ribs, vertebrae, or pelvis.[93, 238–240] If there is any doubt about the integrity of the urinary tract, excretory urography should be performed. If the urinary tract remains intact, supportive care is all that is necessary; however, surgical correction is indicated if there is leakage of urine into the peritoneal or retroperitoneal spaces.

Renal Parasitic Infection

Renal infection with the giant kidney worm, *Dioctophyma renale,* occurs rarely in dogs.[241, 242] Dogs become infected by ingestion of the larvae directly or ingestion of a paratenic host, usually a fish, that contains the encysted larvae. Clinical signs include abdominal enlargement and hematuria. Diagnosis is made by finding double-operculated ova in urine sediment. Surgery is the treatment of choice, either a unilateral nephrectomy or nephrotomy to remove the parasite if both kidneys are affected.

Primary Renal Hematuria

Nontraumatic or idiopathic renal hematuria has been reported as a cause of massive hematuria in dogs.[243, 244] This disorder should be considered after more common causes of hematuria (e.g., lower urinary tract diseases, nephrolithiasis, pyelonephritis) have been excluded. The diagnosis is made by performing a cystotomy and catheterizing each ureter to obtain urine for urinalysis and bacterial culture. Surgical removal of the affected kidney and ureter causes resolution of clinical signs.

Polycystic Kidney Disease

Renal cysts are dilated nephron segments that contain fluid; they may be single or multiple (polycystic). The cause of cystic renal diseases is unknown; however, familial polycystic kidney disease occurs in cairn terriers, domestic longhair cats, and Persian cats.[156–159] Cysts also are present in the liver of cairn terriers.[157] The most common clinical finding is bilateral renomegaly. Ultrasonography is very useful for documenting the presence of multiple renal cysts. The disorder eventually progresses to cause renal failure. There is no specific treatment other than medical management of CRF.

Feline Perirenal Pseudocysts

Pseudocysts, accumulations of fluid that collect outside the renal parenchyma, occur rarely in cats.[245, 246] Most reported cases have been in male cats older than 8 years of age. The most common clinical finding is abdominal enlargement caused by nonpainful renomegaly. Ultrasonography reveals the presence of a cystic lesion associated with the kidney. Treatment of choice is surgical drainage and resection of the cyst wall.

Nephrogenic Diabetes Insipidus

Nephrogenic diabetes insipidus is characterized by renal tubular inability to respond to adequate amounts of ADH; it is a congenital disorder that affects young dogs.[247, 248] The most common clinical sign is extreme PU and PD. Other causes of PU/PD should be excluded before a water deprivation test is performed. Animals with nephrogenic diabetes insipidus cannot concentrate urine above a specific gravity of 1.008 after water deprivation and do not respond to exogenous administration of ADH. Patients may respond to treatment including dietary sodium restriction and administration of chlorthiazide (20–40 mg/kg by mouth every 12 hours).

Renal Tubular Acidosis

Proximal renal tubular acidosis (type II) is associated with bicarbonate wasting, whereas distal acidosis (type I) is characterized by inability of the distal tubule to secrete hydrogen ions and produce acid urine. Renal tubular acidosis may be acquired or congenital, and it is observed rarely in dogs and cats.[249, 250] Proximal disease usually is associated with other tubular disorders (e.g., Fanconi's syndrome, gentamicin nephrotoxicosis) that also cause glucosuria, aminoaciduria, and phosphaturia.[251, 252]

Fanconi's Syndrome

Fanconi's syndrome is a disorder characterized by proximal tubular dysfunction, which causes excessive urinary loss of many substances, including glucose, amino acids, phosphate, potassium, and bicarbonate. It is suspected to be an inherited disorder and has been observed in basenjis, Norwegian elkhounds, Shetland sheepdogs, and schnauzers.[251, 253, 254] Fanconi's syndrome also may be acquired and has been reported in a dog with gentamicin nephrotoxicosis.[252]

Renal Glucosuria

Renal glucosuria may occur without other signs of renal tubular dysfunction in Norwegian elkhounds, Scottish terriers, and mixed breed dogs.[255]

Ureteral Fibrosis

Ureteral fibrosis and secondary bilateral hydronephrosis has been reported in a Burmese cat.[256] Clinical signs primarily resulted from renal failure.

Ureteral Neoplasia

Primary ureteral tumors (e.g., leiomyosarcoma, leiomyoma) are uncommonly diagnosed; it is more common for tumors of the kidney, prostate gland, or urinary bladder to secondarily affect the ureters. Clinical signs often are not observed unless the urinary bladder, prostate, or urethra also are affected. Excretory urography may show ureteral obstruction; dilation of the ureter proximal to the obstruction and hydronephrosis often occur. Surgical excision is the treatment of choice for primary ureteral neoplasia.

References

1. Osborne CA, Vernier RL. Glomerulonephritis in the dog and cat: A comparative review. J Am Anim Hosp Assoc 1973;9:101–127.
2. Ganong WF. Renal function and micturition. In: Ganong WF, ed. Review of Medical Physiology, 13th ed. Norwalk, Appleton & Lange, 1987:581–606.
3. Rose BD. Clinical Physiology of Acid-Base and Electrolyte Disorders. New York, McGraw-Hill, 1984:66–67.
4. Finco DR. Kidney function. In: Kaneko JJ, ed. Clinical Biochemistry of Domestic Animals, 4th ed. San Diego, Academic Press, 1989:496–542.
5. Erslev AJ. Erythropoietin. N Engl J Med 1991;324:1339–1344.
6. Ganong WF. Review of Medical Physiology, 13th ed. Norwalk, Appleton & Lange, 1987:381–389.
7. Ganong WF. Hormonal control of calcium metabolism and the physiology of bone. In: Ganong WF, ed. Review of Medical Physiology, 13th ed. Norwalk, Appleton & Lange, 1987:321–332.
8. Allen TA, Weingand K. The vitamin D (calciferol) endocrine system. Compen Contin Educ Pract Vet 1985;7:482–491.
9. Bruyette DS, Nelson RW. How to approach the problems of polyuria and polydipsia. Vet Med 1986;81:112–128.
10. Feldman EC, Nelson RW. Diagnostic approach to polydipsia and polyuria. Vet Clin North Am Small Anim Pract 1989;19:327–341.
11. Cowgill LD, Kallet AJ. Recognition and management of hypertension in the dog. In: Kirk RW, ed. Current Veterinary Therapy VIII. Philadelphia, WB Saunders, 1983;1025–1028.
12. Morgan RV. Systemic hypertension in four cats: Ocular and medical findings. J Am Anim Hosp Assoc 1986;22:615–621.
13. Kobayashi DL, Peterson ME, Graves TK, et al. Hypertension in cats with chronic renal failure or hyperthyroidism. J Vet Intern Med 1990;4:58–62.
14. Garner HE, Hahn AW, Hartley JW, et al. Indirect blood pressure measurement in the dog. Lab Anim Sci 1975;25:197–202.
15. Hamlin RL, Kittleson MD, Rice D, et al. Non-invasive measurement of systemic arterial pressure in dogs with automatic sphygmomanometry. Am J Vet Res 1984;43:1271–1273.
16. Remillard RL, Ross JN, Eddy JB. Variance of indirect blood pressure measurements and prevalence of hypertension in clinically normal dogs. Am J Vet Res 1991;52:561–565.
17. Dukes J. Hypertension: a review of the mechanisms, manifestations and management. J Small Anim Pract 1992;33:119–129.
18. Littman MP, Robertson JL, Bovee KC. Spontaneous systemic hypertension in dogs: Five cases (1981–1983). J Am Vet Med Assoc 1988;193:486–494.
19. Spangler WL, Gribble DH, Weiser MG. Canine hypertension: A review. J Am Vet Med Assoc 1977;170:995–998.
20. Littman MP. Update: Treatment of hypertension in dogs and cats. In: Kirk RW, ed. Current Veterinary Therapy XI. Philadelphia, WB Saunders, 1992:838–841.
21. Snyder PS. Canine hypertensive disease. Compen Contin Educ Pract Vet 1991;13:1785–1793.
22. Finco DR, Stiles NS, Kneller SK, et al. Radiologic estimation of kidney size of the dog. J Am Vet Med Assoc 1971;159:995–1002.
23. Chew DJ, DiBartola SP. Diagnosis and pathophysiology of renal disease. In: Ettinger SJ, ed. Textbook of Veterinary Internal Medicine, 3rd ed. Philadelphia, WB Saunders, 1989:1893–1961.
24. Konde LJ, Wrigley RH, Park RD, et al. Sonographic appearance of renal neoplasia in the dog. Vet Radiol 1985;26:74–81.
25. Konde LJ, Park RD, Wrigley RH, et al. Comparison of radiography and ultrasonography in the evaluation of renal lesions in the dog. J Am Vet Med Assoc 1986;188:1420–1425.
26. Walter PA, Feeney DA, Johnston GR, et al. Ultrasonographic evaluation of renal parenchymal diseases in dogs: 32 cases (1981–1986). J Am Vet Med Assoc 1987;191:999–1007.
27. Walter PA, Johnston GR, Feeney DA, et al. Applications of ultrasonography in the diagnosis of parenchymal kidney disease in cats: 24 cases (1981–1986). J Am Vet Med Assoc 1988;192:92–98.
28. Osborne CA, Polzin DJ. Azotemia: A review of what's old and what's new. II. Localization. Compen Contin Educ Pract Vet 1983;5:561–577.
29. Burrows CF, Bovee KC. Metabolic changes due to experimentally induced rupture of the canine urinary bladder. Am J Vet Res 1974;35:1083–1088.
30. Willard MD, Schall WD, McCaw DE, et al. Canine hypoadrenocorticism: Report of 37 cases and review of 39 previously reported cases. J Am Vet Med Assoc 1982;180:59–62.
31. DiBartola SP, Rutgers HC, Zack PM, et al. Clinicopathologic findings associated with chronic renal disease in cats: 74 cases (1973–1984). J Am Vet Med Assoc 1987;190:1196–1202.

32. Ross LA, Finco DR. Relationship of selected clinical renal function tests to glomerular filtration rate and renal blood flow in cats. Am J Vet Res 1981;42:1704–1710.

33. Lulich JD, Osborne CA, O'Brien RD, et al. Feline renal failure: Questions, answers, questions. Compend Contin Educ Pract Vet 1992;14:127–153.

34. Polzin D, Osborne C, O'Brein T. Diseases of the kidneys and ureters. In: Ettinger SJ, ed. Textbook of Veterinary Internal Medicine, 3rd ed. Philadelphia, WB Saunders, 1989:1962–2046.

35. DiBartola SP. Disorders of phosphorus: Hypophosphatemia and hyperphosphatemia. In: DiBartola SP, ed. Fluid Therapy in Small Animal Practice. Philadelphia, WB Saunders, 1992:177–192.

36. Chew DJ, Meuten DJ. Disorders of calcium and phosphorus metabolism. Vet Clin North Am Small Anim Pract 1982;12:411–438.

37. Laing EJ, Carter RF. Acute tumor lysis syndrome following treatment of canine lymphoma. J Am Anim Hosp Assoc 1988;24:691–696.

38. Couto CG. Management of complications of cancer chemotherapy. Vet Clin North Am Small Anim Pract 1990;20:1037–1053.

39. Atkins CE, Tyler R, Greenlee P. Clinical, biochemical, acid-base, and electrolyte abnormalities in cats after hypertonic sodium phosphate enema administration. Am J Vet Res 1985;46:980–988.

40. Jorgensen LS, Center SA, Randolph JF, et al. Electrolyte abnormalities induced by hypertonic phosphate enemas in two cats. J Am Vet Med Assoc 1985;187:1367–1368.

41. Schaer M, Cavanaugh P, Hause W, et al. Iatrogenic hyperphosphatemia, hypocalcemia and hypernatremia in a cat. J Am Anim Hosp Assoc 1977;13:39–41.

42. Willard MD, Zerbe CA, Schall WD, et al. Severe hypophosphatemia associated with diabetes mellitus in six dogs and one cat. J Am Vet Med Assoc 1987;190:1007–1010.

43. Fooshee SK, Forrester SD. Hypercalcemia secondary to cholecalciferol rodenticide toxicosis in two dogs. J Am Vet Med Assoc 1990;196:1265–1268.

44. Gunther R, Felice LJ, Nelson RK, et al. Toxicity of vitamin D_3 rodenticide to dogs. J Am Vet Med Assoc 1988;193:211–214.

45. Peterson ME, Taylor RS, Greco DS, et al. Acromegaly in 14 cats. J Vet Intern Med 1990;4:192–201.

46. Peterson ME, Kinter PB, Cavanagh PG, et al. Feline hyperthyroidism: Pretreatment clinical and laboratory evaluation of 131 cases. J Am Vet Med Assoc 1983;183:103–110.

47. Bruyette DS, Feldman EC. Primary hypoparathyroidism in the dog. J Vet Intern Med 1988;2:7–14.

48. Sherding RG, Meuten DJ, Chew DJ, et al. Primary hypoparathyroidism in the dog. J Am Vet Med Assoc 1980;176:439–444.

49. Peterson ME, James KM, Wallace M, et al. Idiopathic hypoparathyroidism in five cats. J Vet Intern Med 1991;5:47–51.

50. Finco DR, Rowland GN. Hypercalcemia secondary to chronic renal failure in the dog: A report of four cases. J Am Vet Med Assoc 1978;173:990–994.

51. Barsanti JA, Finco DR. Protein concentration in urine of normal dogs. Am J Vet Res 1979;40:1583–1588.

52. Biewenga WJ. Urinary protein loss in the dog: Nephrological study of 29 dogs without signs of renal disease. Res Vet Sci 1982;33:366–374.

53. DiBartola SP, Chew DJ, Jacobs G. Quantitative urinalysis including 24-hour protein excretion in the dog. J Am Anim Hosp Assoc 1980;16:537–546.

54. Russo EA, Lees GE, Hightower D. Evaluation of renal function in cats, using quantitative urinalysis. Am J Vet Res 1986;47:1308–1312.

55. Monroe WE, Davenport DJ, Saunders GK. Twenty-four hour urinary protein loss in healthy cats and the urinary protein-creatinine ratio as an estimate. Am J Vet Res 1989;50:1906–1909.

56. Forrester SD, Lees GE, Russo EA. Urine protein-to-creatinine ratio determinations in healthy cats. J Vet Intern Med 1989;3:130.

57. Spangler WL, Muggli FM. Seizure-induced rhabdomyolysis accompanied by acute renal failure in a dog. J Am Vet Med Assoc 1978;172:1190–1194.

58. MacEwen EG, Hurvitz AI. Diagnosis and management of monoclonal gammopathies. Vet Clin North Am Small Anim Pract 1977;7:119–132.

59. Matus RE, Leifer CE, MacEwen EG, et al. Prognostic factors for multiple myeloma in the dog. J Am Vet Med Assoc 1986;188:1288–1292.

60. Hribernik TN, Barta O, Gaunt SD, et al. Serum hyperviscosity syndrome associated with IgG myeloma in a cat. J Am Vet Med Assoc 1982;181:169–170.

61. Forrester SD, Greco DS, Relford RL. Serum hyperviscosity syndrome associated with multiple myeloma in two cats. J Am Vet Med Assoc 1992;200:79–82.

62. Pesce AJ. Methods used for the analysis of proteins in urine. Nephron 1974;13:93–104.

63. Rennie IDB, Keen H. Evaluation of clinical methods for detecting proteinuria. Lancet 1967;2:489–492.

64. Abuelo JG. Proteinuria: Diagnostic principles and procedures. Ann Intern Med 1983;98:186–191.

65. Grauer GF, Thomas CB, Eicker SW. Estimation of quantitative proteinuria in the dog, using the urine protein-to-creatinine ratio from a random, voided sample. Am J Vet Res 1985;46:2116–2119.

66. White JV, Olivier NB, Reimann K, et al. Use of protein-to-creatinine ratio in a single urine specimen for quantitative estimation of canine proteinuria. J Am Vet Med Assoc 1984;185:882–885.

67. Center SA, Wilkinson E, Smith CA, et al. 24-Hour urine protein/creatinine ratio in dogs with proteinlosing nephropathies. J Am Vet Med Assoc 1985;187:820–824.

68. Bagley RS, Center SA, Lewis RM, et al. The effect of experimental cystitis and iatrogenic blood contamination on the urine protein/creatinine ratio in the dog. J Vet Intern Med 1991;5:66–70.

69. Lulich JP, Osborne CA. Interpretation of urine protein-creatinine ratio in dogs with glomerular and nonglomerular disorders. Compen Contin Educ Pract Vet 1990;12:59–73.

70. DiBartola SP, Spaulding GL, Chew DJ, et al. Urinary protein excretion and immunopathologic findings in

dogs with glomerular disease. J Am Vet Med Assoc 1980;177:73–77.

71. Grauer GF. Glomerulonephritis. Semin Vet Med Surg (Small Anim) 1992;7:187–197.

72. Center SA, Smith CA, Wilkinson E, et al. Clinicopathologic, renal immunofluorescent, and light microscopic features of glomerulonephritis in the dog: 41 cases (1975–1985). J Am Vet Med Assoc 1987;190:81–90.

73. Murray M, Wright NG. A morphologic study of canine glomerulonephritis. Lab Invest 1974;30:213–221.

74. Casey HW, Splitter GA. Membraneous glomerulonephritis in dogs infected with *Dirofilaria immitis*. Vet Pathol 1975;12:111–117.

75. Hottendorf GH, Nielsen SW. Pathologic report of 29 necropsies on dogs with mastocytoma. Vet Pathol 1968;5:102–121.

76. Grauer GF, Culham CA, Cooley AJ, et al. Clinicopathologic and histologic evaluation of *Dirofilaria immitis*-induced nephropathy in dogs. Am J Trop Med Hyg 1987;37:588–596.

77. Glick AD, Horn RG, Holscher M. Characterization of feline glomerulonephritis associated with viral-induced hematopoietic neoplasms. Am J Pathol 1978;92:321–332.

78. Hayashi T, Ishida T, Fujiwara K. Glomerulonephritis associated with feline infectious peritonitis. Jpn J Vet Sci 1982;44:909–916.

79. DiBartola SP, Tarr MJ, Webb DM, et al. Familial renal amyloidosis in Chinese shar pei dogs. J Am Vet Med Assoc 1990;197:483–487.

80. Bowles MH, Mosier DA. Renal amyloidosis in a family of beagles. J Am Vet Med Assoc 1992;201:569–574.

81. DiBartola SP, Davenport DJ, Chew DJ. Renal failure in young dogs. In: Kirk RW, ed. Current Veterinary Therapy X. Philadelphia, WB Saunders, 1989:1166–1169.

82. Bloedow AG. Familial renal disease in Samoyed dogs. Vet Rec 1981;108:167–168.

83. Wilcock BP, Patterson JM. Familial glomerulonephritis in Doberman pinscher dogs. Can Vet J 1979;20:244–249.

84. Chew DJ, DiBartola SP, Boyce JT, et al. Juvenile renal disease in Doberman pinscher dogs. J Am Vet Med Assoc 1983;182:481–485.

85. Reusch C, Liehs M, Brem G, et al. A new familial membrano-proliferative glomerulonephritis in Bernese mountain dogs. J Vet Intern Med 1992;6:120.

86. Barlough JE, Osborne CA, Stevens JB. Canine and feline urinalysis: Value of macroscopic and microscopic examinations. J Am Vet Med Assoc 1981;178:61–63.

87. Osborne CA, Stevens JB. Handbook of Canine and Feline Urinalysis. St. Louis, Ralston Purina Company, 1981:91–118.

88. Finco DR, Duncan JR. Evaluation of blood urea nitrogen and serum creatinine concentrations as indicators of renal dysfunction: A study of 111 cases and a review of related literature. J Am Vet Med Assoc 1976;168:593–601.

89. Finco DR, Coulter DB, Barsanti JA. Simple, accurate method for clinical estimation of glomerular filtration rate in the dog. Am J Vet Res 1981;42:1874–1877.

90. Bovee KC, Joyce T. Clinical evaluation of glomerular function: 24-hour creatinine clearance in dogs. J Am Vet Med Assoc 1979;174:488–491.

91. Finco DR, Brown SA, Crowell WA, et al. Exogenous creatinine clearance as a measure of glomerular filtration rate in dogs with reduced renal mass. Am J Vet Res 1991;52:1029–1032.

92. Ross LA. Assessment of renal function in the dog and cat. In: Kirk RW, ed. Current Veterinary Therapy IX. Philadelphia, WB Saunders, 1986:1103–1108.

93. Pechman RD. Urinary trauma in dogs and cats: a review. J Am Anim Hosp Assoc 1982;18:33–40.

94. Feeney DA, Barber DL, Johnston GR, et al. The excretory urogram: Part II. Interpretation of abnormal findings. Compen Contin Educ Pract Vet 1982;4:321–330.

95. Feeney DA, Johnston GR. Urogenital imaging: A practical update. Semin Vet Med Surg (Small Anim) 1986;1:144–164.

96. Feeney DA. Effect of multiple excretory urograms on glomerular filtration of normal dogs: A preliminary report. Am J Vet Res 1980;41:960–963.

97. Feeney DA, Barber DL, Osborne CA. Advances in canine excretory urography. Proceedings of the 30th Gaines Veterinary Symposium 1981:8–22.

98. Ihle SL, Kostolich M. Acute renal failure associated with contrast medium administration in a dog. J Am Vet Med Assoc 1991;199:899–901.

99. Konde LJ. Sonography of the kidney. Vet Clin North Am Small Anim Pract 1985;15:1149–1158.

100. Cartee RE, Selcer BA, Patton CS. Ultrasonographic diagnosis of renal disease in small animals. J Am Vet Med Assoc 1980;176:426–430.

101. Hager DA, Nyland TG, Fisher P. Ultrasound-guided biopsy of the canine liver, kidney, and prostate. Vet Radiol 1985;26:82–88.

102. Osborne CA. Clinical evaluation of needle biopsy of the kidney and its complications in the dog and cat. J Am Vet Med Assoc 1971;158:1213–1228.

103. Osborne CA, Low DG, Finco DR. Reversible versus irreversible renal disease in the dog. J Am Vet Med Assoc 1969;155:2062–2078.

104. Osborne C, Stevens J, Perman V. Kidney biopsy. Vet Clin North Am Small Anim Pract 1974;4:351–365.

105. Grauer GF, Twedt DC, Mero KN. Evaluation of laparoscopy for obtaining renal biopsy specimens from dogs and cats. J Am Vet Med Assoc 1983;183:677–679.

106. Finn WF. Postischemic acute renal failure. Initiation, maintenance, and recovery. Invest Urol 1980;17:427–431.

107. Chew DJ. Fluid therapy during intrinsic renal failure. In: DiBartola SP, ed. Fluid Therapy in Small Animal Practice. Philadelphia, WB Saunders, 1992:554–572.

108. Flamenbaum W. Pathophysiology of acute renal failure. Arch Intern Med 1973;131:911–928.

109. Grauer GF, Thrall MAF. Ethylene glycol (antifreeze) poisoning. In: Kirk RW, ed. Current Veterinary Therapy IX. Philadelphia, WB Saunders, 1986:206–212.

110. Brown SA, Barsanti JA. Gentamicin nephrotoxicosis in the dog. In: Kirk RW, ed. Current Veterinary Therapy IX. Philadelphia, WB Saunders, 1986:1146–1150.

111. Rubin SI. Nephrotoxicity of amphotericin B. In: Kirk RW, ed. Current Veterinary Therapy IX. Philadelphia, WB Saunders, 1986:1142–1146.

112. Ogilvie GK, Straw RC, Jameson VJ, et al. Prevalence of nephrotoxicosis associated with a four-hour saline

solution diuresis protocol for the administration of cisplatin to dogs with naturally developing neoplasms. J Am Vet Med Assoc 1993;202:1845–1848.

113. Stevenson S. Oxytetracycline nephrotoxicosis in two dogs. J Am Vet Med Assoc 1980;176:530–531.

114. Leib MS, Allen TA, Husted PW. Acute renal failure associated with thiacetarsamide sodium treatment for adult heartworms in a dog. J Am Anim Hosp Assoc 1984;20:973–978.

115. Tsukamoto H, Parker HR, Gribble DH, et al. Nephrotoxicity of sodium arsenate in dogs. Am J Vet Res 1983;44:2324–2330.

116. Krum SH, Osborne CA. Heatstroke in the dog: A polysystemic disorder. J Am Vet Med Assoc 1977;170:531–535.

117. Osuna DJ, Armstrong PJ, Duncan DE, et al. Acute renal failure after methylene blue infusion in a dog. J Am Anim Hosp Assoc 1990;26:410–412.

118. Flamenbaum W, Gehr M, Gross M, et al. Acute renal failure associated with myoglobinuria and hemoglobinuria. In: Brenner BM, Lazarus JM, ed. Acute Renal Failure. Philadelphia, WB Saunders, 1983:269–282.

119. Mandal AK, Davis JJ, Bell RD, et al. Myoglobinuria exacerbates ischemic renal damage in the dog. Nephron 1989;53:261–267.

120. Slauson DO, Gribble DH, Russell SW. A clinicopathologic study of renal amyloidosis in dogs. J Comp Pathol 1970;80:335–343.

121. DiBartola SP, Tarr MJ, Parker AT, et al. Clinicopathologic findings in dogs with renal amyloidosis: 59 cases (1976–1986). J Am Vet Med Assoc 1989;195:358–364.

122. Taboada J, Palmer GH. Renal failure associated with bacterial endocarditis in the dog. J Am Anim Hosp Assoc 1989;25:243–251.

123. Calvert CA. Valvular bacterial endocarditis in the dog. J Am Vet Med Assoc 1982;180:1080–1084.

124. Sisson D, Thomas WP. Endocarditis of the aortic valve in the dog. J Am Vet Med Assoc 1984;184:570–577.

125. Spyridakis LK, Bacia JJ, Barsanti JA, et al. Ibuprofen toxicosis in a dog. J Am Vet Med Assoc 1986;188:918–919.

126. Gilmour MA, Walshaw R. Naproxen-induced toxicosis in a dog. J Am Vet Med Assoc 1987;191:1431–1432.

127. Tandy J. A fatal syndrome in the dog following administration of phenylbutazone. Vet Rec 1967;81:398–399.

128. Elwood C, Boswood A, Simpson K, et al. Renal failure after flunixin meglumine administration. Vet Rec 1992;130:582–583. Letter.

129. Rubin SI. Nonsteroidal antiinflammatory drugs, prostaglandins, and the kidney. J Am Vet Med Assoc 1986;188:1065–1068.

130. Forrester SD, Lees GE. Acute renal failure associated with systemic infectious disease. In: Kirk RW, Bonagura JD, eds. Current Veterinary Therapy, vol XI. Philadelphia, WB Saunders, 1992:829–831.

131. Greene CE, Shotts EB. Leptospirosis. In: Greene CE, ed. Infectious Diseases of the Dog and Cat. Philadelphia, WB Saunders, 1990:498–507.

132. Rentko VT, Clark N, Ross LA, et al. Canine leptospirosis: A retrospective study of 17 cases. J Vet Intern Med 1992;6:235–244.

133. Greene CE. Leptospirosis. In: Greene CE, ed. Clinical Microbiology and Infectious Diseases of the Dog and Cat. Philadelphia, WB Saunders, 1984:588–598.

134. Greene CE, Breitschwerdt EB. Rocky mountain spotted fever and Q fever. In: Greene CE, ed. Infectious Diseases of the Dog and Cat. Philadelphia, WB Saunders, 1990:419–433.

135. Brown SA, Barsanti JA, Crowell WA. Gentamicin-associated acute renal failure in the dog. J Am Vet Med Assoc 1985;186:686–690.

136. Thrall MA, Grauer GF, Mero KN. Clinicopathologic findings in dogs and cats with ethylene glycol intoxication. J Am Vet Med Assoc 1984;184:37–41.

137. Lane IF, Grauer GF. Management of acute renal failure. Vet Med 1994;89:219–230.

138. Schaer M. General principles of fluid therapy in small animal medicine. Vet Clin North Am Small Anim Pract 1989;19:203–213.

139. Barsanti JA, Blue J, Edmunds J. Urinary tract infection due to indwelling bladder catheters in dogs and cats. J Am Vet Med Assoc 1985;187:384–388.

140. Ross LA. Fluid therapy for acute and chronic renal failure. Vet Clin North Am Small Anim Pract 1989;19:343–359.

141. Finco DR, Low DG. Intensive diuresis in polyuric renal failure. In: Kirk RW, ed. Current Veterinary Therapy VII. Philadelphia, WB Saunders, 1980;7:1091–1093.

142. Cornelius LM. Fluid therapy in the uremic patient. In: Kirk RW, ed. Current Veterinary Therapy VIII. Philadelphia, WB Saunders, 1983:989–994.

143. Lindner A. Synergism of dopamine plus furosemide in preventing acute renal failure in the dog. Kidney Int 1979;16:158–166.

144. Anderson RJ, Linas SL, Berns AS, et al. Nonoliguric acute renal failure. N Engl J Med 1977;296:1134–1138.

145. Levinsky NG, Bernard DB, Johnston PA. Mannitol and loop diuretics in acute renal failure. In: Brenner BM, Lazarus JM, ed. Acute Renal Failure. Philadelphia, WB Saunders, 1983:712–722.

146. Kirby R. Acute renal failure as a complication in the critically ill animal. Vet Clin North Am Small Anim Pract 1989;19:1189–1208.

147. Adelman RD, Spangler WL, Beason F, et al. Furosemide enhancement of experimental gentamicin nephrotoxicity: Comparison of functional and morphological changes with activities of urinary enzymes. J Infect Dis 1979;140:342–352.

148. English P. Acute renal failure in the dog and cat. Aust Vet J 1974;50:384–392.

149. Dial SM, Thrall MA, Hamar DW. 4-Methylpyrazole as treatment for naturally acquired ethylene glycol intoxication in dogs. J Am Vet Med Assoc 1989;195:73–76.

150. Dial SM, Thrall MAH, Hamar DW. Comparison of ethanol and 4-methylpyrazole as treatments for ethylene glycol intoxication in cats. Am J Vet Res 1994;55:1771–1782.

151. McClain BL, Ballou WR, Harrison SM, et al. Doxycycline therapy for leptospirosis. Ann Intern Med 1984;100:696–698.

152. Forrester SD, Jacobson JD, Fallin EA. Taking measures

to prevent acute renal failure. Vet Med 1994;89: 231–236.

153. Neff-Davis CA. Therapeutic drug monitoring in veterinary medicine. Vet Clin North Am Small Anim Pract 1988;18:1287–1307.

154. Eriksen K, Grondalen J. Familial renal disease in soft-coated wheaten terriers. J Small Anim Pract 1984; 25:489–500.

155. Nash AS, Kelly DF, Gaskell CJ. Progressive renal disease in soft-coated wheaten terriers: Possible familial nephropathy. J Small Anim Pract 1984;25:479–487.

156. Lulich JP, Osborne CA, Walter PA, et al. Feline idiopathic polycystic kidney disease. Compen Contin Educ Pract Vet 1988;10:1030–1041.

157. McKenna SC, Carpenter JL. Polycystic disease of the kidney and liver in the cairn terrier. Vet Pathol 1980;17: 436–442.

158. Biller DS, Chew DJ, DiBartola SP. Polycystic kidney disease in a family of Persian cats. J Am Vet Med Assoc 1990;196:1288–1290.

159. Crowell WA, Hubbell JJ, Riley JC. Polycystic renal in related cats. J Am Vet Med Assoc 1979;175:286–288.

160. Boyce JT, DiBartola SP, Chew DJ, et al. Familial renal amyloidosis in Abyssinian cats. Vet Pathol 1984;21: 33–38.

161. Chew DJ, DiBartola SP, Boyce JT, et al. Renal amyloidosis in related Abyssinian cats. J Am Vet Med Assoc 1982;181:139–142.

162. DiBartola SP, Chew DJ, Boyce JT. Juvenile renal disease in related standard poodles. J Am Vet Med Assoc 1983;183:693–696.

163. O'Brein TD, Osborne CA, Yano BL, et al. Clinicopathologic manifestations of progressive renal disease in Lhasa apso and shih tzu dogs. J Am Vet Med Assoc 1982;180:658–664.

164. Brown SA, Crowell WA, Barsanti JA, et al. Beneficial effects of dietary mineral restriction in dogs with marked reduction of functional renal mass. J Am Soc Nephrol 1991;1:1169–1179.

165. Finco DR, Brown SA, Crowell WA, et al. Effects of dietary phosphorus and protein in dogs with chronic renal failure. Am J Vet Res 1992;53:2264–2271.

166. Lewis LD, Morris ML, Hand MS. Small Animal Clinical Nutrition. Topeka, Mark Morris Associates, 1987:8-3– 8-51.

167. Lewis LD, Morris ML, Hand MS. Small Animal Clinical Nutrition. Topeka, Mark Morris Associates, 1987:1-1– 1-25.

168. Dow SW, Fettman MJ, LeCouteur RA, et al. Potassium depletion in cats: Renal and dietary influences. J Am Vet Med Assoc 1987;191:1569–1575.

169. Abbrecht PH. Effects of potassium deficiency on renal function in the dog. J Clin Invest 1969;48:432–442.

170. Dow SW, Fettman MJ, Smith KR, et al. Effect of dietary acidification and potassium depletion on acid-base balance, mineral metabolism, and renal function in adult cats. J Nutr 1990;120:569–578.

171. Dow SW, Fettman MJ. Renal disease in cats: The potassium connection. In: Kirk RW, Bonagura JD, eds. Kirk's Current Veterinary Therapy XI. Philadelphia, WB Saunders, 1992;11:820–822.

172. Dow SW, LeCouteur RA, Fettman MJ, et al. Potassium depletion in cats: Hypokalemia polymyopathy. J Am Vet Med Assoc 1987;191:1563–1568.

173. Ross LA, Finco DR, Crowell WA. Effect of dietary phosphorus restriction on the kidneys of cats with reduced renal mass. Am J Vet Res 1982;43: 1023–1026.

174. Balasa RW, Murray RL, Kondelis NP, et al. Phosphate-binding properties and electrolyte content of aluminum hydroxide antacids. Nephron 1987;45:16–21.

175. Chew DJ, DiBartola SP, Nagode LA, et al. Phosphorus restriction in the treatment of chronic renal failure. In: Kirk RW, Bonagura JD, eds. Kirk's Current Veterinary Therapy XI. Philadelphia, WB Saunders, 1992;11: 853–857.

176. Schiller LR, Santa Ana CA, Sheikh MS, et al. Effect of time of administration of calcium acetate on phosphorus binding. N Engl J Med 1989;320:1110–1113.

177. Nagode LA, Chew DJ. Nephrocalcinosis caused by hyperparathyroidism in progression of renal failure: Treatment with calcitriol. Semin Vet Med Surg (Small Anim) 1992;7:202–220.

178. Chew D, Nagode L. Calcitriol in the treatment of chronic renal failure. In: Kirk RW, Bonagura JD, eds. Kirk's Current Veterinary Therapy XI. Philadelphia, WB Saunders, 1992;11:857–860.

179. Brown S, Finco D. Efficacy of calcitriol in suppressing plasma parathyroid hormone (PTH) in dogs with renal disease. Proc Am Coll Vet Intern Med Forum 1993;11: 158–160.

180. Chew D, Nagode L, Carothers M, et al. Calcitriol treatment of renal secondary hyperparathyroidism in dogs and cats. Proc Am Coll Vet Intern Med Forum 1993;11:164–167.

181. Cowgill LD. Application of recombinant human erythropoietin in dogs and cats. In: Kirk RW, Bonagura JD, eds. Kirk's Current Veterinary Therapy XI. Philadelphia, WB Saunders, 1992:484–487.

182. Green RA, Russo EA. Hypoalbuminemia-related platelet hypersensitivity in two dogs with nephrotic syndrome. J Am Vet Med Assoc 1985;186:485–488.

183. Green RA, Kabel AL. Hypercoagulable state in three dogs with nephrotic syndrome: Role of acquired antithrombin III deficiency. J Am Vet Med Assoc 1982;181: 914–917.

184. Kaysen GA. Albumin synthesis, albuminuria and hyperlipemia in nephrotic patients. Kidney Int 1987;31: 1368–1376.

185. Robertson JL. Immunologic injury to the kidney and the renal response. In: Bovee KC, ed. Canine Nephrology. Media, PA, Harwal Publishing, 1984:439–460.

186. Grauer GF, Culham CA, Dubielzig RR, et al. Effects of a specific thromboxane synthetase inhibitor on development of experimental Dirofilaria immitis immune complex glomerulonephritis in the dog. J Vet Intern Med 1988;2:192–200.

187. Grauer GF, Frisbie DD, Longhofer SL, et al. Effects of a thromboxane synthetase inhibitor on established immune complex glomerulonephritis in dogs. Am J Vet Res 1992;53:808–813.

188. Cowgill LD. Diseases of the kidney. In: Ettinger SJ, ed.

Textbook of Veterinary Internal Medicine, 3rd ed. Philadelphia, WB Saunders, 1983:1793–1879.

189. Spyridakis L, Brown S, Barsanti J, et al. Amyloidosis in a dog: Treatment with dimethylsulfoxide. J Am Vet Med Assoc 1986;189:690–691.

190. Kaysen GA, Gambertoglio J, Jimenez I, et al. Effect of dietary protein intake on albumin homeostasis in nephrotic patients. Kidney Int 1986;29:572–577.

191. Heeg JE, De Jong Pe, van der Hem GK, et al. Reduction of proteinuria by angiotensin converting enzyme inhibition. Kidney Int 1987;32:78–83.

192. Keane WF, Anderson S, Aurell M, et al. Angiotensin converting enzymes inhibitors and progressive renal insufficiency. Ann Intern Med 1989;111:503–516.

193. Keane WF, Shapiro BE. Renal protective effects of angiotensin-converting enzyme inhibition. Am J Cardiol 1990;65:491–531.

194. Brown SA, Walton CL, Crawford P, et al. Long-term effects of antihypertensive regimens on renal hemodynamics and proteinuria. Kidney Int 1993;43:1210–1218.

195. Heeg J, de Jong PE, Gjalt K, et al. Efficacy and variability of the antiproteinuric effect of ACE inhibition by lisinopril. Kidney Int 1989;36:272–279.

196. Stuart BP, Phemister RD, Thomassen RW. Glomerular lesions associated with proteinuria in clinically healthy dogs. Vet Pathol 1975;12:125–144.

197. Arthur JE, Lucke VM, Newby TJ, et al. The long-term prognosis of feline idiopathic membranous glomerulonephropathy. J Am Anim Hosp Assoc 1986;22:731–737.

198. Nash AS, Wright NG, Spencer AJ, et al. Membranous nephropathy in the cat: A clinical and pathological study. Vet Rec 1979;105:71–77.

199. Lucke VM. Glomerulonephritis in the cat. Vet Annual 1982;22:270–278.

200. Kivisto AK, Vasenius H, Sandholm M. Canine bacteriuria. J Small Anim Pract 1977;18:707–712.

201. Osborne CA, Kruger JM, Johnston GR, et al. Feline lower urinary tract disorders. In: Ettinger SJ, ed. Textbook of Veterinary Internal Medicine, 3rd ed. Philadelphia, WB Saunders, 1989:2057–2082.

202. Finco DR, Barsanti JA. Bacterial pyelonephritis. Vet Clin North Am Small Anim Pract 1979;9:645–660.

203. Finco DR, Shotts EB, Crowell WA. Evaluation of methods for localization of urinary tract infection in the female dog. Am J Vet Res 1979;40:707–712.

204. Barber DL, Finco DR. Radiographic findings in induced bacterial pyelonephritis in dogs. J Am Vet Med Assoc 1979;175:1183–1190.

205. Lees GE, Rogers KS. Diagnosis and localization of urinary tract infection. In: Kirk RW, ed. Current Veterinary Therapy IX. Philadelphia, WB Saunders, 1986: 1118–1123.

206. Neuwirth L, Mahaffey M, Crowell W, et al. Comparison of excretory urography and ultrasonography for detection of experimentally induced pyelonephritis in dogs. Am J Vet Res 1993;54:660–669.

207. Beauchamp D, Poirier A, Bergeron MG. Increased nephrotoxicity of gentamicin in pyelonephritic rats. Kidney Int 1985;28:106–113.

208. Osborne CA, Polzin DJ, Johnston GR, et al. Canine urolithiasis. In: Ettinger SJ, ed. Textbook of Veterinary Internal Medicine, 3rd ed. Philadelphia, WB Saunders, 1989:2083–2107.

209. Brown NO, Parks JL, Greene RW. Canine urolithiasis: Retrospective analysis of 438 cases. J Am Vet Med Assoc 1977;170:414–418.

210. Osborne CA, Clinton CW, Bamman LK, et al. Prevalence of canine uroliths. Vet Clin North Am Small Anim Pract 1986;16:27–44.

211. Carter WO, Hawkins EC, Morrison WB. Feline nephrolithiasis: Eight cases (1984–1989). J Am Anim Hosp Assoc 1993;29:247–256.

212. Marretta SM, Pask AJ, Greene RW, et al. Urinary calculi associated with portosystemic shunts in six dogs. J Am Vet Med Assoc 1981;178:133–137.

213. Osborne CA, Clinton CW, Kim KM, et al. Etiopathogenesis, clinical manifestations, and management of canine silica urolithiasis. Vet Clin North Am Small Anim Pract 1986;16:185–207.

214. Lulich JP, Osborne CA, Parker ML, et al. Canine calcium oxalate urolithiasis. In: Kirk RW, ed. Current Veterinary Therapy X. Philadelphia, WB Saunders, 1989:1182–1188.

215. Bartges JW, Osborne CA, Felice LJ. Canine xanthine uroliths: Risk factor management. In: Kirk RW, Bonagura JD, eds. Kirk's Current Veterinary Therapy XI. Philadelphia, WB Saunders, 1992:900–905.

216. Dieringer TM, Lees GE. Nephroliths: Approach to therapy. In: Kirk RW, Bonagura JD, eds. Kirk's Current Veterinary Therapy XI. Philadelphia, WB Saunders, 1992:889–892.

217. Kerr WS. Effects of complete ureteral obstruction for one week on kidney function. J Appl Physiol 1954;6: 762–772.

218. Kerr WS. Effect of complete ureteral obstruction in dogs on kidney function. Am J Physiol 1956;184:521.

219. Owen RR. Canine ureteral ectopia: A review. 1: Embryology and aetiology. J Small Anim Pract 1973;14: 407–417.

220. Hayes HM. Breed associations of canine ectopic ureter: A study of 217 female cases. J Small Anim Pract 1984;25:501–504.

221. Holt PE, Gibbs C, Pearson H. Canine ectopic ureter: A review of twenty-nine cases. J Small Anim Pract 1982;23:195–208.

222. Stone EA, Mason LK. Surgery of ectopic ureters: Types, method of correction, and postoperative results. J Am Anim Hosp Assoc 1990;26:81–88.

223. Smith CW, Stowater JL, Kneller SK. Ectopic ureter in the dog: A review of cases. J Am Anim Hosp Assoc 1981;17:245–248.

224. Dean PW, Bojrab MJ, Constantinescu GM. Canine ectopic ureter. Compen Contin Educ Pract Vet 1988;10: 146–163.

225. Mason LK, Stone EA, Biery DN, et al. Surgery of ectopic ureters: Pre- and postoperative radiographic morphology. J Am Anim Hosp Assoc 1990;26:73–79.

226. Owen RR. Canine ureteral ectopia: A review. 2: Incidence, diagnosis and treatment. J Small Anim Pract 1973;14:419–427.

227. Ross LA, Lamb CR. Reduction of hydronephrosis and

hydroureter associated with ectopic ureters in two dogs after ureterovesical anastomosis. J Am Vet Med Assoc 1990;196:1497–1499.

228. Lucke VM, Kelly DF. Renal carcinoma in the dog. Vet Pathol 1976;13:264–276.

229. Baskin GB, De Paoli A. Primary renal neoplasms of the dog. Vet Pathol 1977;14:591–605.

230. Klein MK, Cockerell GL, Harris CK, et al. Canine primary renal neoplasms: A retrospective review of 54 cases. J Am Anim Hosp Assoc 1988;24:443–452.

231. Hayes HM, Fraumeni JF. Epidemiological features of canine renal neoplasms. Cancer Res 1977;37:2553–2556.

232. Suter M, Lott-Stolz G, Wild P. Generalized nodular dermatofibrosis in six Alsations. Vet Pathol 1983;20: 632–634.

233. Mooney SC, Hayes AA, Matus RE, et al. Renal lymphoma in cats: 28 cases (1977–1984). J Am Vet Med Assoc 1987;191:1473–1477.

234. Weller RE, Stann SE. Renal lymphosarcoma in the cat. J Am Anim Hosp Assoc 1983;19:363–367.

235. Osborne CA, Johnson KH, Kurtz HJ, et al. Renal lymphoma in the dog and cat. J Am Vet Med Assoc 1971;158:2058–2068.

236. Crow SE. Urinary tract neoplasms in dogs and cats. Compen Contin Educ Pract Vet 1985;7:607.

237. Kolata RJ. Motor vehicle accidents in urban dogs: A study of 600 cases. J Am Vet Med Assoc 1975;167: 938–941.

238. Bjorling DE. Traumatic injuries of the urogenital system. Vet Clin North Am Small Anim Pract 1984;14:61–75.

239. Kleine LJ, Thornton GW. Radiographic diagnosis of urinary tract trauma. J Am Anim Hosp Assoc 1971;7: 318–327.

240. Selcer BA. Urinary tract trauma associated with pelvic trauma. J Am Anim Hosp Assoc 1982;18:785–793.

241. Osborne CA, Stevens JB, Hanlon GF, et al. Dioctophyma renale in the dog. J Am Vet Med Assoc 1969;155:605–619.

242. Ehrenford FA, Snodgrass TB. Incidence of canine dioctophymiasis (giant kidney worm infection) with a summary of cases in North America. J Am Vet Med Assoc 1955;126:415–417.

243. Stone EA, DeNovo RC, Rawlings CA. Massive hematuria of nontraumatic renal origin in dogs. J Am Vet Med Assoc 1983;183:868–871.

244. Hitt ME, Straw RC, Lattimer JC, et al. Idiopathic hematuria of unilateral renal origin in a dog. J Am Vet Med Assoc 1985;187:1371–1373.

245. Abdinoor DJ. Perinephric pseudocysts in a cat. J Am Anim Hosp Assoc 1980;16:763–767.

246. Brace JJ. Perirenal cysts (pseudocysts) in the cat. In: Kirk RW, ed. Current Veterinary Therapy VIII. Philadelphia, WB Saunders, 1983:980–981.

247. Lage AL. Nephrogenic diabetes insipidus in a dog. J Am Vet Med Assoc 1973;163:251–254.

248. Breitschwerdt EB, Verlander JW, Hribernik TN. Nephrogenic diabetes insipidus in three dogs. J Am Vet Med Assoc 1986;179:235–238.

249. DiBartola SP, Leonard PO. Renal tubular acidosis in a dog. J Am Vet Med Assoc 1982;180:70–73.

250. Brown SA, Spyridakis LK, Crowell WA. Distal renal tubular acidosis and hepatic lipidosis in a cat. J Am Vet Med Assoc 1986;189:1350–1352.

251. Bovee KC, Joyce T, Blazer-Yost B, et al. Characterization of renal defects in dogs with a syndrome similar to the Fanconi syndrome in man. J Am Vet Med Assoc 1979;174:1094–1099.

252. Brown SA, Rakich PM, Barsanti JA, et al. Fanconi syndrome and acute renal failure associated with gentamicin therapy in a dog. J Am Anim Hosp Assoc 1986;22:635–640.

253. Easley JR, Breitschwerdt EB. Glucosuria associated with renal tubular dysfunction in three basenji dogs. J Am Vet Med Assoc 1976;168:938–942.

254. Brown SA. Fanconi's syndrome. Inherited and acquired. In: Kirk RW, ed. Current Veterinary Therapy X. Philadelphia, WB Saunders, 1989:1163–1165.

255. Bovee KC. Genetic and metabolic diseases of the kidney. In: Bovee KC, ed. Canine Nephrology. Media, Pennsylvania, Harwal Publishing, 1984:339–354.

256. Leib MS, Allen TA, Konde LJ, et al. Bilateral hydronephrosis attributable to bilateral ureteral fibrosis in a cat. J Am Vet Med Assoc 1988;192:795–797.

Chapter 17

Diseases of the Urinary Bladder and Urethra

S. Dru Forrester

Anatomy

The lower urinary tract (urinary bladder and urethra) functions primarily in storage and elimination of urine from the body. The urinary bladder is composed of smooth muscle, termed the detrusor muscle, and is divided into a neck, which empties into the urethra, and a body.[1] The trigone of the urinary bladder is a triangular area located internally between the urethral orifice and the ureteral openings. Ureters enter the urinary bladder by traversing the mucosa at an oblique angle; this forms vesicoureteral valves, which prevent reflux of urine from the urinary bladder to the kidneys. Smooth muscle of the urinary bladder is continuous with that of the urethra, forming the internal urethral sphincter. The urethra serves as a conduit for elimination of urine from the body. The urethra of male dogs is 10 to 35 cm long and is composed of prostatic, pelvic (membranous), and penile portions.[1] The urethra of female dogs is much shorter (7–10 cm) and empties into the vagina 4 to 5 cm cranial to the ventral commissure of the vulva.[1] The external urethral sphincter is composed of striated muscle and is located in the mid-urethral region of females and in the pelvic urethra of males.[2] The mucosal surface of the urinary bladder and the urethra are lined by transitional epithelium.

The lower urinary tract receives its innervation from somatic, sympathetic, and parasympathetic nervous systems. The pudendal nerve, derived from sacral spinal cord segments 1 to 3, supplies the external urethral sphincter. The hypogastric nerve, from lumbar spinal cord segments 1 to 4, provides sympathetic input to the detrusor muscle of the urinary bladder and the internal urethral sphincter. Parasympathetic input to the detrusor muscle is provided by the pelvic nerve, which is composed of fibers from sacral spinal cord segments 1 to 3.

Physiology

The micturition reflex consists of two phases: storage of urine and voiding of urine (urination).[2] The storage phase of micturition is maintained primarily by sympathetic activity, whereas the voiding phase is maintained by parasympathetic activity. As the urinary bladder fills with urine, sympathetic input causes relaxation of the detrusor muscle and contraction of the internal urethral sphincter. In addition, somatic input from the pudendal nerve causes contraction of the external urethral sphincter. The overall effect is to maintain urinary continence. When the urinary bladder becomes full, stimulation of stretch receptors sends impulses through the pelvic nerve to the spinal cord and higher centers, which are under voluntary control. If appropriate, voiding is initiated by parasympathetic stimulation of the detrusor muscle. At the same time, there is inhibition of sympathetic activity to the internal urethral sphincter and somatic input to the external urethral sphincter. Urethral relaxation and concomitant detrusor contraction produce sustained urine flow until the urinary bladder is almost empty.

Host defense mechanisms in normal animals prevent bacterial colonization of the urinary bladder and proximal urethra. Long urethral length and narrow diameter, especially in male dogs, reduce the potential for ascending infection. The urothelial surface of the urinary tract acts as a mechanical barrier against bacterial colonization. Periodic emptying of urine from the urinary bladder through the urethra physically removes bacteria. The distal urethra and lower genital tract are colonized by normal bacterial flora that compete with uropathogens for nutrients and attachment sites. Urine itself possesses antibacterial properties; the extremes of urine osmolality that occur in dogs and particularly in cats create an unfavorable environment for microbial growth.[3] Finally, local immunologic mechanisms (e.g., secretory immunoglobulins) probably serve an important role in preventing urinary tract infection (UTI).

Problem Identification

Stranguria, Dysuria, and Pollakiuria

Stranguria is slow and painful discharge of urine, characterized by straining, whereas dysuria is painful or difficult urination. Pollakiuria is frequent passage of small amounts of urine.

Pathophysiology

Dysuria and pollakiuria often occur concomitantly in patients with diseases of the urinary bladder and urethra (e.g., UTI, urolithiasis, neoplasia). Irritation secondary to inflammation initiates the detrusor reflex, and patients feel the need to void frequently. In addition, some disorders such as urolithiasis and neoplasia may cause partial or complete obstruction, which is most often associated with stranguria.

Clinical Signs

Most patients with stranguria, dysuria, or pollakiuria are presented because owners have noted urination in inappropriate places, discolored urine, increased frequency of attempts to urinate, or inability to pass urine after repeated attempts. If the patient has complete urethral obstruction and postrenal azotemia, other historical findings may include severe depression, inappetence, and vomiting. Physical examination findings may be normal; however, some patients may have dehydration, caudal abdominal mass, thickened urinary bladder, or enlarged or painful urinary bladder. Rectal examination may reveal prostatic disease in male dogs and masses affecting the caudal urinary bladder and urethra.

Diagnostic Plan

The initial step in evaluating patients with stranguria, dysuria, or pollakiuria is to determine whether a disorder of the lower urinary tract exists. Some patients that urinate in inappropriate places have behavioral problems; however, this is a diagnosis of exclusion. Urinary tract obstruction should be ruled out promptly on the basis of physical examination findings or an attempt to pass a urethral catheter, because obstruction can cause rapid deterioration of the patient's condition (see Urethral Obstruction). After urinary obstruction has been excluded, urinalysis and bacterial urine culture are indicated. Findings on urinalysis that support lower urinary tract disease include pyuria, hematuria, and bacteriuria. If urinalysis results on urine taken by cystocentesis are normal, the genital tract should be thoroughly examined. Most nonobstructed dogs with dysuria or pollakiuria have UTI.[4] If results of bacterial urine culture are negative or there is no response to antimicrobial treatment, abdominal radiographs should be taken to detect radiopaque uroliths or masses affecting the lower urinary tract. If results of plain radiographs are normal, other tests such as contrast studies (e.g., cystogram, urethrogram) and ultrasonography are indicated to detect radiolucent uroliths, space-occupying masses, or other abnormalities. Most nonobstructed cats with pollakiuria and dysuria have sterile cystitis, which is diagnosed by excluding other disorders. If bacterial urine culture is negative, a therapeutic trial should be considered before additional diagnostic tests are attempted (see Feline Lower Urinary Tract Disease). If clinical signs persist longer than 5 to 7 days or recur within 3 months, additional tests should be done as for dogs.

Urethral Obstruction

Urethral obstruction is blockage of the urethra such that urine cannot exit the body; it may be partial or complete.

Pathophysiology

Obstruction of the urethra may result from a mechanical (most commonly) or functional disorder. Mechanical obstruction is caused by a structural abnormality, which may be intraluminal (e.g., uroliths, amorphous plugs, urethral neoplasia) or extraluminal (e.g., prostatic disease). Functional obstruction results from inability of the urethra to dilate as the urinary bladder contracts. Neurologic dysfunction, most often caused by upper motor neuron lesions, and intramural lesions (e.g., neoplasia, fibrosis) of the urethra can cause functional obstruction.[4, 5]

Clinical Signs

Clinical findings in patients with urethral obstruction include dysuria, pollakiuria, and stranguria. The urinary bladder often is enlarged and painful; it is difficult for the veterinarian to express urine in animals with partial obstruction, and impossible with complete obstruction. Rectal examination may reveal mass lesions (e.g., uroliths, neoplasia) affecting the urinary bladder, urethra, or prostate gland. Uroliths also may be palpated in the external urethra of male dogs, particularly cranial to the os penis or in the tip of the penis. Patients with functional obstruction may have neurologic deficits such as posterior paresis.

Diagnostic Plan

If urethral obstruction is suspected on the basis of history and physical examination findings, it should be determined whether the blockage is functional or mechanical. Inability to pass a urinary catheter indicates mechanical obstruction, whereas ability to catheterize the patient suggests functional obstruction. Patients with apparent functional obstruction should be evaluated for neurologic disease by neurologic examination; if results are normal, the diagnostic evaluation is continued as for mechanical obstruction. Serum chemistries and electrolytes should be measured in patients with urethral obstruction to detect metabolic disturbances such as uremia, hyperkalemia, and metabolic acidosis. In some instances, these problems may be life-threatening and require immediate treatment. Urine should be collected for urinalysis and bacterial urine culture, preferably by cystocentesis. Findings on urinalysis such as crystalluria, urine pH, hematuria, pyuria, bacteriuria, and, infrequently, neoplastic cells may help determine the underlying cause of obstruction. Additional tests such as plain and contrast radiography and ultrasonography may be needed to identify intraluminal, extraluminal, and intramural disorders such as strictures, neoplasia, and uroliths. In some cases, samples of tissue may need to be obtained for cytologic or histologic evaluation so that a definitive diagnosis can be made.

Urinary Incontinence

Urinary incontinence is lack of voluntary control over flow of urine from the body. It may result from neurogenic or urinary disorders. The most common urinary disorders that cause incontinence are ectopic ureters, urethral incompetence, partial urethral obstruction, UTI, and acquired structural abnormalities that interfere with urinary bladder or urethral function (e.g., neoplasia, urolithiasis, stenosis). After neurogenic disorders have been excluded, the lower urinary system should be evaluated by physical examination and laboratory tests (i.e., urinalysis and urine culture). Depending on these findings, additional tests such as radiography (plain and contrast studies) or ultrasonography may be indicated, as previously described for dysuria and urethral obstruction. For a complete discussion of urinary incontinence see Chapter 27.

Discolored Urine

Normal urine is yellow to amber; any variation from this is considered discolored urine. Red, brown, reddish-brown, and orange-yellow are the most common abnormal urine colors of clinical importance in dogs and cats.

Pathophysiology

Discolored urine results from the presence of abnormal amounts of pigmented substances such as red blood cells (i.e., hematuria), bilirubin, hemoglobin, or myoglobin. Although exceptions occur, hematuria usually is associated with urogenital disorders, whereas bilirubinuria, hemoglobinuria, and myoglobinuria usually result from systemic disorders. Deep yellowish-orange or brown urine may occur with bilirubinuria, which results from increased serum concentrations of conjugated bilirubin. Causes of increased serum bilirubin include hemolysis, hepatic disease, and posthepatic biliary obstruction. Red, brown, or reddish-brown urine results most often from either hematuria or hemoglobinuria and, rarely, from myoglobinuria. Hematuria results from hemorrhage into the urogenital tract and may be caused by a variety of disorders (Table 17–1). Hemoglobin can enter urine either by filtration through the glomerulus or by release of hemoglobin from lysis of red blood cells that are present in urine. Hemoglobin in plasma does not pass through glomeruli because it is bound to haptoglobin; however, if the amount of hemoglobin exceeds the haptoglobin-binding capacity, free hemoglobin spills into the urine. Causes of hemoglobinuria in dogs and cats include intravascular hemolysis associated with parasitic or immune-mediated disease, splenic torsion, postcaval syndrome, and heatstroke. Myoglobin released from muscle after severe injury does not bind to plasma proteins and therefore readily crosses glomeruli to enter urine. Myoglobinuria occurs rarely in dogs with severe muscle injury such as rhabdomyolysis.[6]

Table 17–1
Causes of Hematuria in Dogs and Cats

Renal Causes
Acute pyelonephritis
Neoplasia
Trauma
Nephrolithiasis
Cystic disease
Infarction
Idiopathic hematuria
Parasitic infection

Lower Urinary Tract Causes
Urinary tract infection
Urolithiasis
Feline lower urinary tract disease
Neoplasia
Trauma
Hemorrhagic cystitis (cyclophosphamide)
Polypoid cystitis

Genital Tract Causes
Prostate
  Hypertrophy
  Infection
  Neoplasia
  Cysts
Uterus
  Subinvolution of placental sites
  Proestrus
Vagina and penis
  Trauma
  Transmissible venereal tumor

Clotting Disorders
Platelet disorder
  Thrombocytopenia
  von Willebrand's disease
Coagulation factor deficiency
  Vitamin K rodenticide toxicosis
  Hemophilia

Clinical Signs

Clinical findings in patients with discolored urine depend on the underlying cause. Patients with bilirubinuria may have weakness, depression, inappetence, and weight loss associated with hemolysis or hepatic dysfunction; physical examination may reveal dehydration, icterus, or pallor. Hemoglobinuria associated with intravascular hemolysis also may be associated with weakness, depression, and pale mucous membranes. Clinical signs in patients with hematuria usually are limited to the urogenital system (i.e., stranguria, dysuria, pollakiuria), although other findings suggestive of systemic coagulation disorders (e.g., petechiae, ecchymoses, hematomas) may exist. Physical examination of patients with hematuria may be normal or may reveal urolithiasis, prostatomegaly, renomegaly, or masses affecting the urogenital tract.

Diagnostic Plan

The first step in evaluating patients with discolored urine is to perform urinalysis on a voided sample of urine collected during midstream. Bilirubinuria is easily diagnosed by finding increased urine bilirubin (any amount in cats; >2+ in dogs); the remainder of urinalysis often is normal. A positive occult blood test indicates presence of red blood cells, hemoglobin, or myoglobin. If urine sediment examination reveals red blood cells, hematuria exists. If red blood cells are not present, hemoglobinuria and myoglobinuria should be considered. Patients with hemoglobinuria also have hemoglobinemia, which is associated with pink plasma. In contrast, patients with myoglobinuria have clear plasma. Additional tests may be indicated (e.g., complete blood count [CBC], platelet count, reticulocyte count, serum chemistries, creatine kinase activity) to determine the cause of bilirubinuria, hemoglobinuria, or myoglobinuria.

If hematuria is suspected, additional diagnostic evaluation is indicated to determine the source of hemorrhage. Most patients with hematuria have a urogenital disorder; an exception is hematuria that occurs secondary to systemic bleeding disorders such as thrombocytopenia. A finding of stranguria, dysuria, or pollakiuria localizes disease to the urinary bladder, urethra, vagina, or prostate, whereas hematuria in the absence of clinical signs is suggestive of renal hematuria.[7] Owners should be questioned to determine the stage of urination at which hematuria occurs (i.e., beginning, throughout, or at end of urination) and whether the patient is receiving medications such as cyclophosphamide. Hematuria at the beginning of urination suggests disease of the prostate, urethra, penis, uterus, or vagina; hematuria at the end of urination is typical of prostatic or urinary bladder disorders. Hematuria that persists for the duration of urination suggests disease of kidneys, ureters, urinary bladder, or prostate gland. If the owner is not certain of the pet's urinary habits, it is important to observe the patient urinating.

Owners should be asked about trauma, which may explain hematuria. Physical examination should include careful palpation of kidneys, urinary bladder, urethra, and prostate. External genitalia are examined for traumatic lesions or masses; it is important to completely extrude the penis of male dogs so that no proximal mass or lesion is overlooked. If a systemic coagulation disorder is suspected, a coagulation profile, including platelet count, activated partial thromboplastin time, and one-stage prothrombin time, should be done. Any abnormalities should be evaluated further before pursuing diagnostic tests of the urogenital system (see Chap. 44).

Repeating the urinalysis on urine collected by cystocentesis may be helpful for determining the source of hemorrhage. If hematuria is identified from a voided sample but is absent in urine collected by cystocentesis, hemorrhage from the urethra or genital tract is likely. Prostatic hemorrhage cannot be excluded, because prostatic fluid refluxes into the urinary bladder. Presence of red blood cell casts indicates that the kidneys are a source of hemorrhage. Urine collected by cystocentesis should be cultured to identify urinary tract infection, especially in patients with pyuria or bacteriuria.

After initial evaluation, additional tests often are necessary to determine the cause of hematuria. Plain abdominal radiographs and ultrasonography, if available, are helpful for detecting radiopaque uroliths, some masses of the urinary bladder or urethra, abnormalities in renal size or shape, and prostatomegaly. If results are normal, contrast radiography should be done next to identify radiolucent uroliths and space-occupying masses. Lower urinary tract disease should be ruled out first by contrast cystogram and urethrogram. If a lower urinary tract disorder cannot be identified, the kidneys and ureters should be evaluated next by excretory urography. Some patients may require an exploratory laparotomy to determine the source or cause of hematuria. Ideally, the source of hemorrhage should be determined before surgery to increase the likelihood of finding the cause. If renal hematuria is suspected, a cystotomy should be performed, and each ureter should be catheterized to determine which kidney is affected.[8] During surgery, samples of kidney, urinary bladder, and prostate are collected for histologic evaluation and culture, even if these organs appear grossly normal.

Pyuria

Pyuria is abnormally increased numbers of white blood cells (WBCs) on urine sediment examination. Urine obtained by cystocentesis from normal dogs and cats should have 0 to 3 WBCs, catheterized samples should have 0 to 5 WBCs, and voided samples collected during midstream should have 0 to 7 WBCs per high-power field; voided samples from male dogs usually contain more WBCs.[4]

Pathophysiology

Pyuria can result from inflammation of any part of the urogenital tract. Disorders that cause pyuria are similar to those that cause hematuria (see Table 17–1).

Clinical Signs

Patients with pyuria caused by lower urinary tract disease often have dysuria, stranguria, pollakiuria, or hematuria; these signs usually are absent in pyuria associated with disorders of the kidneys and ureters. Hyperadrenocorticism and exogenous administration of corticosteroids also can cause UTI and pyuria in the absence of clinical signs.[9, 10]

Diagnostic Plan

The diagnostic plan for patients with pyuria is similar to that described for patients with stranguria, dysuria, pollakiuria, or hematuria. If pyuria is identified in urine obtained by either catheterization or free catch of a voided sample, analysis of urine obtained by cystocentesis should be done to rule out the genital tract as the source of inflammation. Because prostatic fluid refluxes into the urinary bladder, a finding of increased numbers of WBCs in urine collected by cystocentesis does not exclude prostatic disease in male dogs. If pyuria exists in urine collected by cystocentesis, urine is submitted for bacterial culture; although other infections are less common, urine also may be cultured for *Mycoplasma* spp. and fungal organisms.[11, 12] If urine culture is negative, other causes of urinary tract inflammation should be evaluated. If the patient has signs of dysuria, stranguria, or pollakiuria, diagnostic tests should focus on the lower urinary tract (see previous section). Plain abdominal radiographs are performed first, followed by contrast cystography or urethrography. If lower urinary tract abnormalities are not identified, evaluation of the kidneys and ureters by CBC, serum chemistries, and excretory urogram or abdominal ultrasound is indicated (see Chap. 16).

Bacteriuria

Bacteriuria is presence of bacteria in urine detected by microscopic examination of urine sediment. Significant bacteriuria indicates colonization of the urinary tract with bacterial organisms.

Pathophysiology

The significance of bacteriuria depends on the method of urine collection. Urine in the bladder normally is sterile; therefore, bacteriuria in a sample collected by cystocentesis is abnormal and suggests bacterial UTI. Most organisms reach the urinary bladder by ascending from the lower urinary and genital tracts. Bacteria in urine collected by catheterization or free catch may not be abnormal, because the distal urethra and genital tract contain a resident population of bacteria.

Clinical Signs

Patients with bacteriuria often have signs consistent with UTI such as dysuria and pollakiuria; however, some patients (e.g., those with chronic pyelonephritis or hyperadrenocorticism) may have no clinical signs. Physical examination often is unremarkable unless the patient has a disorder that compromises host defenses and predisposes to UTI (e.g., urolithiasis, prostatic disease, urinary bladder tumor).

Diagnostic Plan

If bacteriuria is identified in urine collected by catheterization or free catch, cystocentesis should be done to rule out contamination from the lower urinary and genital tracts. Also, if other signs of UTI (e.g., pyuria, hematuria) are not present, it is likely that the bacteriuria was caused by contamination. If bacteria are identified in urine collected by cystocentesis, UTI is likely and urine culture should be done. Not all dogs and cats with UTI have microscopically apparent bacteriuria because at least 10^4 rods/mL and 10^5 cocci/mL must be present to be readily identified on sediment examination.[4] The prostate gland also should be evaluated in male dogs with bacteriuria by rectal examination and possibly by obtaining a sample of prostatic fluid from ejaculate or from prostatic washing, because the prostate often is involved when there is UTI (see Chap. 18).

Diagnostic Procedures

Routine Laboratory Evaluation

Urinalysis

Analysis of a fresh urine specimen, preferably obtained by cystocentesis, is extremely useful for evaluating diseases of the urinary bladder. For a complete discussion of urinalysis see Chapter 16.

Urine Culture

Bacterial culture of urine is indicated to diagnose UTI. Quantitative culture (i.e., determining number of bacterial organisms per milliliter of urine) helps determine the significance of bacterial growth in urine. Growth of any bacterial organisms from urine collected by cystocentesis is abnormal; however, the significance of bacterial growth in urine collected by catheterization or free catch depends on the number of organisms

Table 17–2
Identifying Characteristics of Common Uropathogens in Dogs and Cats

ORGANISM	GRAM STAIN	BLOOD AGAR	MacCONKEY AGAR
Escherichia coli	Negative rods	Smooth, gray colonies; may be hemolytic	Pink colonies
Proteus spp.	Negative rods	Swarming colonies	Colorless colonies
Staphylococcus spp.	Positive cocci	Small, white colonies; often hemolytic	No growth
Streptococcus spp.	Positive cocci	Tiny, pinpoint colonies; partial hemolysis	No growth
Klebsiella spp.	Negative rods	Mucoid, gray-white colonies	Pink colonies
Pseudomonas spp.	Negative rods	Gray or greenish colonies; fruity or ammonia odor; often hemolytic	Colorless colonies
Enterobacter spp.	Negative rods	Smooth, gray colonies	Pink colonies

From Ling GV, Biberstein EL, Hirsh DC. Bacterial pathogens associated with urinary tract infections. Vet Clin North Am Small Anim Pract 1979; 9:617–630.

cultured. In dogs, growth of more than 100,000 organisms/mL in urine obtained by catheterization is consistent with UTI, whereas growth of the same number of organisms in voided urine may indicate infection or contamination.[13, 14] In cats, growth of more than 1000 organisms/mL in urine collected by catheterization suggests infection; more than 10,000 organisms/mL in voided urine is consistent with infection, although it may result from contamination in some cats.[15] Because proper collection of urine by cystocentesis eliminates the possibility of contamination from the lower urogenital tract and does not cause iatrogenic infection, it is the method of choice for collection of urine samples for bacterial culture.

Samples must be handled appropriately after collection to obtain accurate results. If the sample cannot be processed immediately, it may be stored in a refrigerator for 2 to 6 hours without affecting culture results.[16] Quantitative urine cultures can be done in-house; required equipment includes an incubator, blood and MacConkey agar plates, calibrated bacteriologic loops (0.01 mL and 0.001 mL), and a flame source to sterilize the loops.[17] For each culture, one blood agar plate and one MacConkey agar plate are used; the agar plates are divided in half by drawing a line across the bottom on the outside of the plate. Immediately before inoculation, each bacteriologic loop is sterilized in the flame source; then the loop is placed into a well-mixed urine sample to obtain the calibrated amount. Half of each agar plate is streaked with 0.01 mL of urine and the other half with 0.001 mL. The agar plates are inverted and incubated at 37° C; most urinary pathogens grow within 12 to 24 hours. The presence of 100 or more colonies on the half-plate inoculated with 0.001 mL of urine indicates a bacterial count higher than 100,000 organisms/mL.[17] Growth characteristics of any colonies can be used to identify common uropathogens (Table 17–2).[18] Determination of antimicrobial susceptibility is easily accomplished by transferring one or two colonies of the organism to a culture swab and sending it to a commercial laboratory.[18, 19] Alternatively, urine samples can be sent to a commercial laboratory for quantitative culture and determination of antimicrobial susceptibility. If samples are mailed to an outside laboratory, urine must be packaged so that it remains at 4° C. Placing the sample in a tube containing a preservative (B-D Urine Culture Kit) ensures accurate results as long as the sample arrives and is processed within 72 hours of collection.[20]

Radiography

Although plain abdominal radiographs may demonstrate some abnormalities of the lower urinary system (e.g., radiopaque uroliths), most disorders require contrast procedures (Fig. 17–1). Indications for performing cystography include persistent dysuria or hematuria, incontinence, recurrent UTI, caudal abdominal masses, and suspected urinary bladder rupture, herniation, neoplasia, or radiolucent uroliths. If the location of the urinary bladder is unknown (e.g., suspected herniation) or if rupture is suspected, a positive-contrast cystogram is indicated. For evaluation of other disorders, both a positive-contrast cystogram and a double-contrast cystogram (i.e., positive and negative contrast concomitantly) are helpful. If space-occupying masses are identified at the urinary bladder trigone, excretory urography is indicated to determine the presence and extent of ureteral involvement.

Before contrast procedures of the urinary bladder are performed, the patient should be fasted for 12 to 24 hours. Cleansing enemas should be done no sooner than 2 hours before the procedure to remove

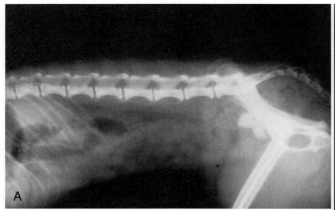

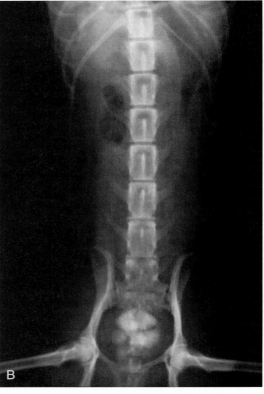

Figure 17–1
(A) Lateral abdominal radiograph of a dog presented for evaluation of stranguria and pollakiuria. Note several radiopaque uroliths in the urinary bladder, which were diagnosed as struvite. It is important to perform an enema prior to radiography because the presence of feces could make identification of uroliths more difficult. **(B)** Ventrodorsal abdominal radiograph of the same dog showing multiple radiopaque uroliths in the urinary bladder.

fecal material that could obscure radiographic changes. Survey abdominal radiographs are taken to determine whether the patient is adequately prepared and to detect obvious abnormalities, such as radiopaque uroliths, that would obviate the need for a contrast procedure. Although sedation is not required, it is very helpful, especially for patients that may be difficult to catheterize. A urinary catheter should be passed using sterile technique; Foley catheters are best for female dogs, and flexible urethral catheters can be used for male dogs. Both male and female cats can be catheterized using 3.5 Fr open-ended polypropylene catheters (Sovereign Tom-Cat Catheter). After catheterization, all urine is removed from the urinary bladder, and the catheter is connected to a three-way stopcock.

A positive-contrast cystogram is performed by injection of an organic iodide solution, such as meglumine iothalamate (Conray), that has been diluted with either sterile water or saline to a final concentration of 20% iodide.[21] The volume of contrast agent needed varies, although a general rule is 10 mL/kg of body weight.[21] To avoid complications such as urinary

bladder rupture, the injection should be discontinued if the urinary bladder feels adequately distended by abdominal palpation, if there is reflux around the catheter, or if back-pressure is felt on the plunger of the syringe.[21] Lateral and ventrodorsal views of the caudal abdomen are taken; ventrodorsal oblique views also may be necessary to avoid superimposition of the urinary bladder and spine.

If a double-contrast procedure is necessary, all but a small amount (2–10 mL) of positive-contrast agent is removed, and the bladder is distended with either room air or carbon dioxide. Radiographic views of the abdomen are obtained as described for positive-contrast cystography. Because of the risk of air embolization, the use of negative contrast material is avoided in patients with ulcerative cystitis or severe hematuria.

Contrast urethrography helps identify luminal filling defects, strictures, and urethral rupture; it also is indicated in patients with signs of lower urinary tract disease, especially if stranguria exists. Because of the relatively longer urethral length in males, urethrography is most often done in male dogs and cats; however, it may provide useful information in female dogs and cats. Fasting of patients is not necessary unless cystography is to be performed also; however, enemas should be given to remove fecal material from the distal colon. Survey radiographs should be done initially; the rear limbs of male dogs should be pulled forward so that the urethra can be more easily visualized. Sedation is helpful for urinary catheterization and urethrography. In male dogs, a Foley catheter (2 mm or smaller) is passed to a level so that the cuff is just proximal to the os penis. In female dogs, a Foley catheter is passed to the level of the urinary bladder and then slowly withdrawn until the cuff is just inside the external urethral orifice. Before the injection of contrast agent, the cuff is partially inflated. In cats, an open-ended polypropylene catheter can be used. After placement of the catheter, a three-way stopcock is attached. A small amount (2–5 mL) of 2% lidocaine without epinephrine can be injected initially to reduce urethral spasm. Organic iodide contrast agent is diluted as for cystography, and a bolus of 10 to 15 mL for male dogs or 5 to 10 mL for female dogs or cats is injected.[22] Radiographic exposures should be made during injection of the last 2 or 3 mL of contrast medium.[22] A lateral and a ventrodorsal oblique view should be taken, with a separate injection for each view.

Ultrasonography

If it is available, ultrasonography can be used to evaluate certain disorders of the lower urogenital tract. Some uroliths can be detected by ultrasonography (Fig. 17–2). Masses affecting the urinary bladder and urethra also can be identified readily by ultrasonographic evaluation. In addition, ultrasound-guided biopsy can be used to obtain samples for cytologic and histologic evaluation.

Cytologic and Histologic Evaluation

Many disorders of the urinary bladder and urethra require cytologic or histologic evaluation to make a definitive diagnosis. Tissue samples for these tests can be obtained by transabdominal fine-needle aspiration, urinary bladder wash, or surgical excision. Every effort should be made to obtain a diagnosis by the least invasive means possible.

Fine-needle aspiration of urinary bladder and urethral masses is easily accomplished with minimal patient discomfort. The only equipment needed is a 22- to 25-gauge needle attached to a 12-mL syringe; a 3.8- to 6.3-cm spinal needle with stylet removed can be used in larger dogs. Although it is not required, a device that stabilizes the syringe and needle (Aspir-Gun) is very helpful. Most patients do not require sedation; however, fractious patients probably should be sedated. The skin over the area to be aspirated should be clipped and scrubbed with an antiseptic solution. The mass to be aspirated should be localized by an assistant or with the free hand of the operator. Alternatively, the mass can be localized and aspirated with ultrasound guidance. The needle is introduced into the mass, and suction is applied to the syringe three or four times without moving the needle. All suction is released, and the needle is withdrawn from the mass. The needle is removed from the syringe, and air is aspirated into the syringe to force the contents in the hub of the needle onto glass slides. A pull-apart smear is made, and the slides are allowed to air dry before fixing and staining (Diff-Quik).[23] If slides are to be sent to a commercial laboratory for evaluation, inquiry should be made as

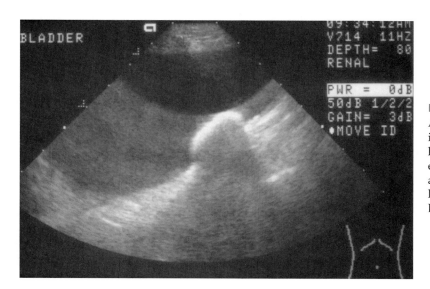

Figure 17–2
Abdominal ultrasonography revealed a urolith in the urinary bladder of this dog. Note the hypoechoic area dorsally (urine) and increased echogenicity ventrally (urolith). There also is acoustic shadowing, which is typical of uroliths. (Courtesy of Martha L. Moon, DVM, MS, Blacksburg, Virginia.)

to whether the clinical pathologist prefers stained or unstained slides.

Samples for cytologic and histologic evaluation also can be obtained with the help of a urinary catheter. Either a flexible urethral catheter or a ureteral catheter with openings on the sides at the proximal end is used; the diameter should be large enough so that the catheter can be passed atraumatically yet maximize the quantity of sample obtained.[24] Ideally, the mass or lesion to be evaluated should be localized by physical examination, ultrasonography, or contrast radiography. Sedation of the patient may facilitate the procedure but is not necessary. The catheter is passed with sterile technique through the urethra to the level of the lesion so that the side openings are adjacent to the lesion. Concomitant rectal or vaginal palpation or radiography (of radiopaque catheter) can be used to ensure proper positioning. A 12-mL syringe containing 3 to 10 mL of sterile saline is attached to the catheter and all but 1 mL is injected into the urinary tract. The plunger of the syringe is pulled back to create negative pressure, and the catheter is moved back and forth for a short distance; the goal is to aspirate part of the mass or lesion into one of the side holes in the catheter. The negative pressure is released slowly, and the catheter is removed from the urinary tract. Any tissue specimens are removed from the catheter by injection of sterile saline solution, forcing the contents of the catheter into a container. Large pieces of tissue may be placed in formalin and submitted for histologic evaluation. The remaining liquid can be centrifuged and the sediment resuspended and evaluated cytologically.

An alternative method for obtaining cytologic specimens from the urinary bladder is to perform a bladder wash. The urinary bladder is catheterized and emptied of all urine. Then 50 to 100 mL of sterile saline solution is instilled. The urinary bladder is massaged through the abdomen, and the saline is then aspirated. The retrieved fluid can be evaluated by making a direct smear or by examining resuspended sediment from a centrifuged sample.

If noninvasive methods fail to yield a diagnosis, samples for histologic evaluation should be obtained at surgery. Although it is preferable to obtain a diagnosis before surgical intervention, this may not be possible in some cases.

Common Diseases of the Urinary Bladder and Urethra

Urinary Tract Infection

UTI is microbial colonization of any part of the urinary tract that is normally sterile.[25] Bacterial infection of the urinary tract affects approximately 14% of dogs during their lifetime.[18] The incidence in cats is unknown, but it is much lower than in dogs.

There are no reported breed predispositions for development of UTI; however, it is known that female dogs have a two to four times higher incidence of UTI than male dogs.[26, 27] UTI is thought to be less common in cats as a primary disorder; it most often occurs as a complication of other urinary abnormalities.[28] Fewer than 3% of cats with clinical signs of lower urinary tract disease have bacterial UTI.[29]

Pathophysiology

Most UTI in dogs and cats results from colonization of the urinary tract with aerobic bacteria. Organisms most often isolated from dogs with UTI are (in order of decreasing frequency) *Escherichia coli*, *Staphylococcus* spp., *Proteus*, *Streptococcus*, *Klebsiella*, *Pseudomonas* spp., and *Enterobacter* spp.[17] Organisms most often identified in cats with UTI are *E. coli*, *Pasteurella* spp., *Proteus* spp., *Staphylococcus* spp., and *Streptococcus* spp.[30] Most cases of UTI are caused by colonization by a single organism; however, up to 18% of infections involve multiple organisms.[31]

Establishment of UTI requires that the organism gain access to and colonize the urinary tract. Most infections are caused by ascending colonization of the urinary tract from more distant sites such as the distal urethra. In normal animals, anatomic, physical, microbiologic, chemical, and immunologic barriers prevent colonization of the urinary tract (see Physiology).[32, 33] In order for an organism to colonize the urinary tract, there must be some compromise in these host defenses. Conditions that may alter host defenses and predispose to UTI include any disorder of the urinary tract (e.g., urolithiasis, urinary obstruction, neoplasia, perineal urethrostomy, neurogenic disorders of micturition, anatomic abnormalities such as urachal diverticula in dogs), urinary catheterization, immunosuppressive drug therapy, prolonged intervals between voiding episodes, and decreased urine osmolality (e.g., diuresis or polyuria).[32–40] In some patients, primarily female dogs with acute urethrocystitis, a predisposing cause cannot be identified and antimicrobial treatment produces a lasting cure. It is presumed that there is a temporary compromise in host defenses in these patients; however, an exact cause cannot be identified.

Clinical Signs

The most common clinical signs associated with lower UTI are stranguria, dysuria, pollakiuria, discolored urine, and urination in inappropriate places; however, some patients may show no clinical signs. Long-term administration of corticosteroids for treatment of dermatologic disease was associated with an increased frequency of UTI in one report; many of these dogs had no clinical or urinalysis findings suggestive of UTI.[10] Subclinical UTI also may occur in dogs with spontaneous hyperadrenocorticism or diabetes mellitus.[9, 41]

Diagnostic Plan

UTI may be suspected on the basis of findings from urinalysis. Gross examination of urine may reveal a foul odor and cloudy or discolored urine. Dipstick analysis often reveals proteinuria and positive occult blood reaction; urine pH may be increased, especially if there is infection with urea-splitting bacteria. Urine sediment changes include hematuria, pyuria, and bacteriuria. With the exception of bacteriuria, these urinalysis findings are not specific for UTI. Also, some patients may have UTI with normal results of urinalysis.

If UTI is suspected on the basis of clinical or laboratory findings or if the patient has a disorder that predisposes to UTI, bacterial culture of urine is indicated. Although cases of acute, simple urethrocystitis in female dogs can be treated empirically, it is preferable to perform urine culture to tentatively identify the infecting organism or organisms.[42] Urine culture should be done on all patients with recurrent, chronic, or complicated infections. Quantitative urine culture is preferred (see Diagnostic Procedures); determining the number of bacteria per milliliter of urine helps in evaluating significance of bacteriuria, especially in samples collected by any method other than cystocentesis. Identification of the organism allows for appropriate selection of antimicrobial agents for treatment. Antimicrobial susceptibility testing is not necessary in all patients; however, it should be done if UTI is chronic or recurrent or if the patient has received antimicrobial treatment for any reason.

Table 17–3
In Vivo Susceptibilities of Common Canine Uropathogens to Selected Antimicrobial Agents

ORGANISM	SUSCEPTIBILITY	
	Approaching 100%	Approaching 80%
Escherichia	—	Trimethoprim-sulfonamide
Proteus	—	Ampicillin
Staphylococcus	Ampicillin	—
Streptococcus	Ampicillin	—
Klebsiella	—	Cephalexin
Pseudomonas	—	Tetracycline
Enterobacter	—	Trimethoprim-sulfonamide

From Lees GE, Forrester SD. Update: Bacterial urinary tract infections. In: Kirk RW, Bonagura JD, eds. Kirk's Current Veterinary Therapy XI. Philadelphia, WB Saunders, 1992:909–914.

Treatment

Selection of Antimicrobial Agents

Antimicrobial drugs for treatment of UTI ideally are selected with knowledge of the infecting organism. If the infecting organism has been identified, an effective antimicrobial agent can be selected in most cases without determining susceptibility. This treatment is indicated primarily for dogs with single episodes of UTI or for multiple episodes that occur several months apart.[42] On the basis of previous studies in dogs, susceptibilities of common urinary pathogens to various antimicrobial drugs have been determined (Table 17–3).[18, 42, 43–49] These drugs at recommended dosages have been used effectively to treat most patients with UTI (Table 17–4).

Table 17–4
Guidelines for Oral Antimicrobial Treatment of Urinary Tract Infections

DRUG	SUGGESTED MINIMUM INHIBITORY CONCENTRATION CUTOFF FOR SUSCEPTIBILITY	DOSAGE	FREQUENCY
Ampicillin	≤64 µg/mL	25 mg/kg	Every 8 h
Amoxicillin	≤64 µg/mL	12 mg/kg	Every 8 h
Trimethoprim-sulfonamide	≤16 µg/mL	15 mg/kg	Every 12 h
Cephalexin	≤32 µg/mL	18 mg/kg	Every 8 h
Tetracycline	≤32 µg/mL	18 mg/kg	Every 8 h
Amoxicillin with clavulanic acid	≤32 µg/mL	16.5 mg/kg	Every 8 h
Enrofloxacin	≤8 µg/mL	2.5 mg/kg	Every 12 h

From Lees GE, Forrester SD. Update: Bacterial urinary tract infections. In: Kirk RW, Bonagura JD, eds. Kirk's Current Veterinary Therapy XI. Philadelphia, WB Saunders, 1992:909–914.

If susceptibility testing is done, antimicrobial agents should be selected with knowledge of minimum inhibitory concentration (MIC), or the minimum concentration of antimicrobial drug that will completely inhibit growth of an organism. Disc diffusion tests (e.g., Kirby-Bauer) are not appropriate for determining antimicrobial susceptibility to urinary pathogens because they are based on serum and not urine concentrations of drug. Because urine concentrations of drug often are 100 times greater than serum concentrations, an antimicrobial drug to which an organism is resistant on the basis of a disc diffusion test may actually be very effective at eliminating the organism from the urinary tract. This explains why UTI caused by a gram-negative organism such as *Proteus* can be treated effectively by penicillin, a drug not routinely used to treat gram-negative infections. In general, an antimicrobial drug whose mean urine concentration is at least four times the MIC for the infecting organism should be selected. Urine concentrations have been determined for many antimicrobial agents in dogs, and this information can be used to determine the MIC cutoff for susceptibility, or the value of MIC below which the antimicrobial should be effective (see Table 17–4).[18, 25]

Two new classes of drugs have become available for treatment of patients with UTI.[50–53] A combination of clavulanate potassium with amoxicillin (Clavamox) is very effective against UTI caused by *E. coli* and may be used instead of trimethoprim-sulfonamide.[52] Amoxicillin-clavulanate also may be effective against other urinary pathogens, including *Staphylococcus* and *Klebsiella*.[52] Another class of drugs, the fluoroquinolones, are effective for treatment of most uropathogens, especially gram-negative organisms.[51, 53–55] These drugs are bactericidal and achieve high concentrations in urine. Enrofloxacin (Baytril), norfloxacin (Noroxin), and ciprofloxacin (Cipro) are available for oral administration.

For treatment of UTI in male dogs, it is important to consider how readily the drug penetrates the blood-prostate barrier, because the prostate gland often is involved in male dogs with UTI. Drugs that penetrate the prostate gland include chloramphenicol, trimethoprim-sulfonamide, enrofloxacin, norfloxacin, and ciprofloxacin.[51, 53, 56]

Selection of antimicrobial agents for polymicrobic infections is somewhat different than for infections caused by a single organism. Ideally, an antimicrobial drug that is effective against all the infecting organisms is selected; however, this is not always possible. If multiple organisms with different susceptibilities are encountered, it usually is best to treat each organism sequentially instead of administering a combination of antimicrobial agents.[42]

Duration of Treatment

Duration of treatment with antimicrobial drugs depends on the presence of clinical signs, time-course of infection (acute or chronic), anatomic extent of infection (urinary bladder versus kidneys), and presence of concurrent urinary tract abnormalities. Animals with acute, simple urethrocystitis and subclinical UTI should receive antimicrobial treatment for 2 weeks. Because of presumed prostatic involvement, all intact male dogs should receive antimicrobial drugs for a minimum of 4 weeks. If pyelonephritis is suspected, treatment for at least 6 to 8 weeks is recommended. If a urinary disorder that predisposes to UTI is identified (e.g., urolithiasis), antimicrobials should be administered until the disorder is corrected and then for an additional 1 to 2 weeks.

Monitoring Success of Treatment

Efficacy of treatment is best determined by periodic urine cultures, especially in patients with recurrent, chronic, or complicated UTI. Ideally, urine cultures should be done 3 to 5 days after treatment begins and 7 to 14 days after completion of treatment.[57] If results of the first culture are negative, antimicrobial treatment is continued; however, if there is bacterial growth, another antimicrobial agent should be selected. Absence of bacterial growth 7 to 14 days after completion of treatment indicates that UTI has been eradicated, whereas growth of the same organism indicates relapse and the need for a longer course of treatment. It is important to determine MIC again, because the organism may have developed resistance to the initial antimicrobial. If a different organism is detected, reinfection is likely and the patient should be evaluated for disorders that predispose to UTI. For patients with acute, uncomplicated urethrocystitis (especially female dogs), therapeutic success may be monitored adequately by resolution of clinical signs or microscopic analysis of urinary sediment.

Management of Recurrent Urinary Tract Infection

Any disorders that predispose to development of UTI (see Pathophysiology) should be identified and corrected. Patients that develop frequent reinfections can be managed by treating each episode individually or by administering long-term treatment.[57] If more than three infections occur in a 1-year period, long-term treatment with low doses of antimicrobial drugs is indicated.[18] After eradication of bacteriuria (i.e., negative urine culture) by treatment at full dose for 2 to 3 weeks, approximately one third of the daily dose is administered once daily at bedtime. Urine is collected by cystocentesis for culture monthly, and low-dose antimicrobial treatment is continued for 6 months as long as urine cultures are negative. If a positive culture is obtained, the regular antimicrobial regimen is administered for 2 to 3 weeks to eradicate bacteriuria, and then low-dose treatment is reinstituted. Drugs used most often for low-dose treatment are penicillin, trimethoprim-sulfonamide, and cephalexin (Keflex).[42] Because of the potential for development of drug resistance, selection of antimicrobial agents should always be made on the basis of culture results and MIC.

Urinary Tract Infection Associated With Urinary Catheterization

Unless systemic infection such as sepsis or pyelonephritis is suspected, antimicrobials are avoided in patients with indwelling urinary catheters. Catheterized patients are at increased risk for development of UTI, and antimicrobial treatment during catheterization selects for organisms that often are resistant to many antimicrobial agents.[36, 37, 58, 59] In order to minimize risk of catheter-induced infection, urinary catheters should be used only when absolutely necessary, a closed collection system should be maintained, and the catheter should be removed as soon as possible. Just before the catheter is removed, a sample of urine is obtained for culture; this is most easily accomplished by inserting a needle through the catheter into its lumen and aspirating 1 to 2 mL of urine. Alternatively, urine can be collected by cystocentesis after the patient is urinating normally (i.e., 1 to 2 days after the catheter has been removed). Antimicrobials are administered for 10 to 14 days if urine culture reveals bacterial growth. In contrast to those with indwelling catheterization, patients that have a single episode of catheterization, especially female dogs, may benefit from short-term prophylactic antimicrobial treatment.[60] The goal is to sterilize urine before bacteria are able to establish infection. Administration of ampicillin (75 mg/kg by mouth) or amoxicillin (36 mg/kg by mouth) as a single high dose immediately after catheterization or at a regular dose for 24 hours (see Table 17–4) may prevent establishment of an infection.

Prognosis

Prognosis for patients with UTI depends on time-course of infection, presence of correctable disorders that predispose to UTI, and whether infection involves the kidneys or prostate gland. Patients with acute urethrocystitis often are cured by antimicrobial treatment, whereas patients with chronic, deep-seated infections (e.g., pyelonephritis, chronic prostatitis) are more difficult to treat and have a more guarded prognosis. Prognosis is guarded if pyelonephritis results in chronic renal failure, because this condition is irreversible. If a disorder that predisposes to UTI (e.g., urolithiasis, urinary catheterization) can be identified and eliminated, the prognosis for complete recovery is good; however, if the underlying cause cannot be effectively treated (e.g., urinary bladder neoplasia), the prognosis is guarded.

Canine Urolithiasis

Uroliths are polycrystalline concretions composed of 90% to 95% organic or inorganic crystalloids and 5% to 10% organic matrix that form within the urinary space.[61] Uroliths are classified according to their mineral content; although most uroliths are composed primarily of one mineral, some may be compound.

Reported incidence of urolithiasis in dogs ranges from 0.4% to 2.8%.[62, 63] Magnesium ammonium phosphate (struvite) is the most common urolith that affects dogs; other uroliths that occur less frequently include calcium oxalate, calcium phosphate, uric acid or urate, cystine, silica, and xanthine.[61, 64] Although uroliths may affect any part of the urinary tract, they most often are identified in the urinary bladder.[62–64]

Several breeds of dogs appear to have a higher incidence of uroliths, including miniature schnauzer, miniature poodle, dachshund, Dalmatian, bulldog, Scottish terrier, Yorkshire terrier, Pekingese, pug, basset hound, Welsh corgi, shih tzu, and cocker spaniel.[62–64] Not only are some breeds more likely to develop uroliths, but certain types of uroliths occur with greater frequency in certain breeds Table 17–5).[64–74] In general, uroliths primarily occur in middle-aged dogs; young dogs (<1 year) almost always have struvite uroliths.[64, 75] Struvite is the most common urolith of females, whereas metabolic stones such as calcium oxalate, cystine, urate, silica, and xanthine occur predominantly in males.[64]

Pathophysiology

The initial step in formation of uroliths is development of a crystal nidus, a process dependent on supersaturation of urine with calculogenic crystalloids. Supersaturation may be caused by increased renal excretion of crystalloids, altered urine pH, or decreased amounts of crystallization inhibitors in urine.[76] Growth of the crystal nidus depends on its ability to remain in the urinary tract, the degree and duration of supersaturation of urine with crystalloids, and the physical characteristics of the nidus.[76]

Struvite

In order for struvite uroliths to form, urine must be supersaturated with magnesium ammonium phos-

Table 17–5
**Breed and Sex Associations
for Canine Uroliths**

UROLITH	BREED	SEX
Struvite	Miniature schnauzer	>80% Female
Calcium oxalate	Miniature schnauzer	>70% Male
	Miniature poodle	
	Shih tzu	
	Lhasa apso	
	Yorkshire terrier	
Urate/Uric acid	Dalmatian	>85% Male
	Bulldog	
Cystine	Dachshund	>90% Male
	Bulldog	
	Chihuahua	
	Mastiff	
	Australian cattle dog	
Silica	German shepherd	>90% Male
Xanthine	Dalmatian	>80% Male

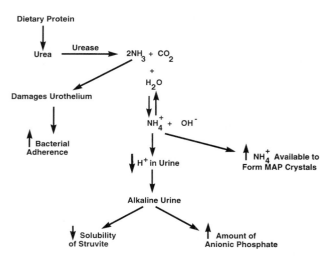

Figure 17–3
Pathogenesis of infection-induced struvite uroliths in dogs. Excess dietary protein is excreted into urine as urea. In the presence of urinary tract infection with a urease-producing microbe such as *Staphyloccocus aureus* or *Proteus* spp., urea is hydrolyzed to form two molecules of ammonia (NH_3) and a molecule of carbon dioxide (CO_2). Ammonia damages the urothelium, which increases bacterial adherence. In addition, ammonia reacts with water (H_2O) to form ammonium ion (NH_4^+) and hydroxyl ion (OH^-). Production of NH_4^+ increases its availability to form magnesium ammonium phosphate (MAP) (i.e., struvite) crystals. In addition, production of NH_4^+ consumes hydrogen ion (H^+) in urine, resulting in alkaline urine. Increased urine pH increases the amount of anionic phosphate available for formation of struvite crystals and also decreases the solubility of struvite. All these factors contribute to an environment that favors formation of struvite uroliths.

phate. Conditions that may cause this include UTI, alkaline urine, genetic predisposition, and diet.[77] The most common cause of struvite uroliths in dogs is UTI with urease-producing bacteria such as *Staphylococcus aureus* and *Proteus* (Fig. 17–3). Urea is derived from dietary protein and is excreted in urine. Urease acts on urea, resulting in formation of ammonia. Ammonia reacts with water to form ammonium, which increases its availability to form struvite crystals. Production of ammonium also decreases hydrogen ion concentration in urine, resulting in alkaline urine. Solubility of struvite is decreased and the amount of available anionic phosphate is increased in alkaline urine. All these factors create an environment that favors formation of struvite uroliths.[77] However, not all patients with struvite uroliths have UTI; unknown dietary or metabolic factors may be involved in formation of sterile struvite uroliths.[77]

Urate

Potential factors that predispose to development of urate uroliths in dogs include increased urinary concentrations of uric acid and ammonia and low urine pH.[61] In Dalmatians, the breed most often recognized as having urate uroliths, urinary excretion of urate is greatly increased because hepatic conversion of uric acid to allantoin is decreased.[61] In addition, reduced renal tubular reabsorption and increased distal tubular secretion of uric acid contribute to increased urinary excretion of urate.[78] Although all Dalmatians excrete increased concentrations of urate, not all Dalmatians develop uroliths; therefore, other factors probably play a role in development of urate uroliths. In non-Dalmatian breeds, the most common disorder that predisposes to formation of urate uroliths

is severe hepatic dysfunction, such as portosystemic shunts or cirrhosis.[79, 80] Presumably, there is inadequate conversion of urate and ammonia to allantoin and urea, respectively, such that urine concentrations of urate and ammonia are increased.[61, 80]

Calcium Oxalate

The most important predisposing factor to development of calcium oxalate uroliths in dogs is hypercalciuria.[72, 81] The mechanism by which hypercalciuria occurs is unknown; potential causes may include increased intestinal absorption of calcium and decreased renal tubular reabsorption of calcium. Most dogs with calcium oxalate uroliths have normal serum calcium concentrations. Calcium oxalate uroliths occur infrequently in dogs with hypercalcemia caused by primary hyperparathyroidism.[82]

Cystine

Cystine uroliths occur in dogs because of an inborn error of metabolism that prevents renal tubular reabsorption of the amino acid cystine.[61, 83, 84] Not all dogs with cystinuria develop uroliths; therefore, other factors probably are involved. Cystine uroliths are most likely to develop in urine with an acid pH.

Silica

Silica uroliths presumably develop in dogs as a result of increased dietary intake of silicates; diets containing corn gluten or soybean hulls have been incriminated.[61, 70] Silica is more soluble in alkaline urine; however, dogs with silica uroliths often have acid urine.[70]

Calcium Phosphate (Apatite)

Calcium phosphate uroliths may occur when urine concentrations of calcium and phosphate are increased. Disorders that have been associated with calcium phosphate uroliths in dogs include primary hyperparathyroidism, renal tubular acidosis, and excessive intake of calcium and phosphorus.[61, 74, 82, 85, 86] With few exceptions, calcium phosphate is more insoluble and more likely to form uroliths in alkaline urine.

Xanthine

Xanthine uroliths may develop in dogs receiving allopurinol for treatment of urate uroliths.[67, 68, 80, 87] Allopurinol inhibits activity of xanthine oxidase, an enzyme that facilitates conversion of purine metabolites, hypoxanthine and xanthine, to uric acid. Therefore, administration of allopurinol, especially at high doses, increases the amount of xanthine excreted into urine, predisposing to development of xanthine uroliths.[67, 80] Xanthine uroliths should be suspected in dogs with urate uroliths that initially respond to treatment with allopurinol but then become refractory to treatment.

Clinical Signs

Clinical signs of urolithiasis are similar to those for other lower urinary tract disorders and include dysuria, stranguria, pollakiuria, and discolored urine (hematuria). Findings consistent with urethral obstruction may occur, especially in male dogs. Depending on size and location of uroliths, physical examination may be normal or may reveal palpable masses in the urinary bladder; sometimes grating can be heard and felt as uroliths rub against one another during abdominal palpation. Uroliths also may be palpated in the pelvic urethra during rectal examination or, in males, in the external urethra or at the tip of the penis. The urinary bladder may be small and thickened from chronic inflammation, or it may be large and distended in dogs with urethral obstruction.

Diagnostic Plan

Routine Laboratory Evaluation

Urinalysis and urine culture are indicated in all dogs with suspected uroliths. Urinalysis findings in patients with urolithiasis may include discolored urine, abnormal urine pH, positive occult blood, proteinuria, hematuria, pyuria, and bacteriuria. Crystalluria indicates that the patient is at increased risk for uroliths; however, its presence is not diagnostic of urolithiasis.[61] Urine culture should be done, because UTI may predispose to struvite uroliths, and UTI can occur secondary to other uroliths.

Radiography and Ultrasonography

Radiographic and ultrasonographic evaluations are indicated to detect uroliths and determine their location, size, and radiodensity.[61] Most uroliths in dogs are radiopaque, although the degree of radiopacity varies.[88] Calcium oxalate, calcium phosphate, struvite, and silica uroliths are the most radiodense, and urate and cystine are the least radiodense; some urate and cystine uroliths may be radiolucent (Fig. 17–4).[88] If uroliths are identified in the urinary bladder, uroliths should be looked for in other parts of the urinary tract as well.

Urolith Analysis

If a urolith is obtained (by voiding, catheter retrieval, or surgical removal), it should be saved, preferably in a sterile container, and submitted to a commercial laboratory for quantitative stone analysis; this allows for definitive determination of mineral composition and helps in planning appropriate treatment (Table 17–6). Xanthine uroliths appear similar to urate uroliths by qualitative analysis, so quantitative analysis should be used for all uroliths.[67] Because uroliths may contain bacteria that are different from those on the urolith surface or in urine, bacterial culture of the center of uroliths should be done by the laboratory that performs quantitative analysis. Bacteria found within the urolith probably were present when the urolith formed; therefore, appropriate antimicrobial treatment may help with dissolution of the urolith.

Treatment

Urethral obstruction should be treated immediately, especially in patients with metabolic complications such as vomiting, dehydration, azotemia, and hyperkalemia. Urohydropropulsion may be used to flush uroliths back into the urinary bladder. A sterile, flexible catheter is passed into the urethra. An assistant places an index finger into the rectum and occludes the pelvic urethra while 35- to 60-mL aliquots of sterile

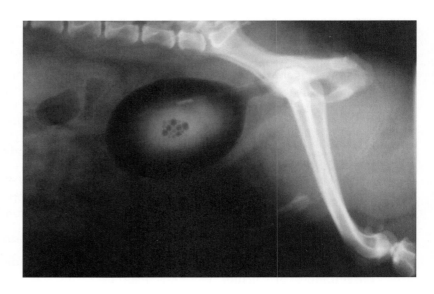

Figure 17–4
Double-contrast cystogram of a dog with stranguria and normal findings on plain abdominal radiographs. Note the presence of multiple, small radiolucent urinary calculi surrounded by positive contrast. (Courtesy of Martha L. Moon, DVM, MS, Blacksburg, Virginia.)

saline solution are injected through the catheter. As saline is injected, the penile urethra should be occluded by compression of the distal penis around the catheter. After the pelvic urethra is distended, pressure around the distal penis is quickly released. If uroliths are small enough, they should move toward the distal urethra; it may require several flushing attempts to accomplish their removal. If uroliths are too large to pass through the area of the os penis, occlusion of the distal penis is maintained during and after flushing with saline solution, and pressure is released on the pelvic urethra;

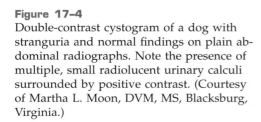

Table 17–6
Laboratories That Perform Urolith Analysis

Minnesota Urolith Center
College of Veterinary Medicine
University of Minnesota
St. Paul, MN 55108
(612) 625-4221

Urolithiasis Laboratory
Baylor College of Medicine
P.O. Box 25375
Houston, TX 77265-5375
(800) 235-4846

Urinary Stone Analysis Laboratory
Rm 3106 Medical Sciences Building
Department of Medicine
University of California, Davis
Davis, CA 95616
(916) 625-4221

Herring Laboratories
P.O. Box 2191
Orlando, FL 32802
(305) 841-6770

this facilitates movement of uroliths into the urinary bladder. After urethral obstruction is relieved, additional treatment is necessary for any remaining uroliths.

Before formulating a treatment plan, it is necessary to make an educated guess about the type of urolith present. This usually can be done by using information from signalment and results of laboratory, radiographic, and ultrasonographic evaluation (Table 17–7; see Table 17–5). If uroliths are available for quantitative analysis, these results can help select more definitive treatment. Small uroliths may be retrieved through a catheter for analysis. With the dog in lateral recumbence, a soft catheter is passed to just inside the bladder. If the bladder is not distended with urine, it is moderately distended with 0.9% NaCl solution. An assistant then vigorously moves the abdomen up and down while urine or saline (and small calculi) are aspirated through the catheter with a 60-mL syringe.[76]

Depending on urolith type, treatment consists of surgical removal or medical therapy (or both) to dissolve uroliths and prevent their recurrence. Uroliths that can be dissolved by medical treatment include struvite, urate, and cystine types; uroliths composed of calcium oxalate, calcium phosphate, or silica must be surgically removed. Uroliths that are composed of more than one mineral type may respond initially to medical treatment but later require surgical intervention.

Indications for surgical management include urinary obstruction that cannot be relieved by nonsurgical means, uroliths that do not respond to medical treatment, patient intolerance of severe dietary protein restriction (e.g., puppies, dogs with renal failure), surgically correctable anatomic defects that predispose to urolithiasis, and situations in which owners are unable to comply with recommendations for medical

Table 17–7
Characteristics of Most Common Canine Uroliths

UROLITH TYPE	RADIOPACITY	URINE pH
Struvite	++ to ++++	Alkaline
Urate	– to ++	Acid
Calcium oxalate	++++	Variable
Cystine	– to ++	Acid
Silica	++ to ++++	Variable
Calcium phosphate	+++	Alkaline

– not radiopaque
+ slightly radiopaque
++ moderately radiopaque
+++ moderately to markedly radiopaque
++++ markedly radiopaque

dissolution.[89] Advantages of surgical treatment are that it results in rapid removal of uroliths and it allows for definitive diagnosis of urolith type, correction of any anatomic defects such as urachal diverticula, and collection of urinary bladder tissue specimens for bacterial culture. Potential disadvantages of surgery include the need for anesthesia in older patients, incomplete removal of all uroliths from the urinary tract, and inability to correct the underlying cause of some uroliths (i.e., urate, cystine, calcium oxalate, silica, and xanthine uroliths). If uroliths are removed surgically, methods should be instituted to prevent recurrence of uroliths.

General goals for medical treatment of uroliths are to prevent further urolith growth and promote urolith dissolution. This is accomplished by increasing the solubility of crystalloids in urine, increasing the volume of urine in which crystalloids are contained, and decreasing the amount of calculogenic substances in urine.[61] Methods for medical dissolution of uroliths include administering drugs to change urine pH, inducing diuresis to increase urine volume, and altering diet to decrease the quantity of calculogenic substances in urine. Depending on mineral composition of uroliths, an individual therapeutic regimen should be established for each patient.

Struvite

Treatment of struvite uroliths consists of feeding a calculolytic diet (e.g., Prescription Diet s/d) and treating UTI when it exists. Calculolytic diets are restricted in dietary protein, phosphorus, and magnesium. In addition, these diets are supplemented with sodium chloride to stimulate diuresis and increased urine volume and with DL-methionine to decrease urine pH. To be effective, owners must feed the calculolytic diet exclusively; treats, table scraps, and other foods should not be fed. In addition to dietary management, eradication of UTI is necessary to effectively treat and prevent struvite urolithiasis. Antimicrobial agents should be selected on the basis of urine culture results and susceptibility testing.

Patients should be evaluated monthly to determine effectiveness of treatment. A urinalysis is helpful for detecting struvite crystals, which should be absent in patients treated appropriately. Urine culture and susceptibility should be done to guide antimicrobial treatment. Radiography is indicated to determine urolith size, number, and location. Because uroliths may pass into the urethra and cause obstruction, especially in male dogs, owners should be informed about signs of urinary obstruction. A continual decrease in size of uroliths at each re-evaluation indicates effective treatment. The time required to dissolve infection-induced struvite uroliths ranges from 2 to 5 months, whereas sterile struvite uroliths dissolve after approximately 4 to 6 weeks.[90, 91] The calculolytic diet and antimicrobial treatment should be continued 1 month beyond radiographic resolution of uroliths.

If uroliths remain the same size or become larger after 2 months of medical treatment, other management should be considered. First, the owner must be complying with all treatment recommendations, including feeding the calculolytic diet exclusively. Serum concentrations of urea nitrogen, albumin, and phosphorus should be decreased in dogs that are fed a calculolytic diet exclusively.[90] It also is important to make sure that bacteriuria has been eradicated and urine pH is no longer alkaline. Dogs with persistent bacteriuria may require additional treatment to lower urine pH and control signs of lower UTI. Acetohydroxamic acid (12.5 mg/kg by mouth every 12 hours), a urease inhibitor, may be helpful in such patients. Higher doses of acetohydroxamic acid are not recommended because they may cause hemolytic anemia.[92] In addition, the drug should not be administered to pregnant dogs because of its teratogenic effects.[92]

Methods to prevent recurrence of struvite urolithiasis include control of UTI, if present; a diet with reduced concentrations of protein, magnesium, and phosphorus; and maintenance of acid urine pH. Patients with recurrent UTI may benefit from prophylactic antimicrobial treatment (see Urinary Tract Infection). Results of studies documenting efficacy of dietary management for prevention of struvite uroliths are not yet available; however, such diets are often used and are probably beneficial. Commercial diets (Prescription Diets c/d and w/d) that are used to prevent struvite uroliths are mildly to moderately restricted in protein, magnesium, phosphorus, and sodium; DL-methionine is included in these diets as a urinary acidifier. Addition of sodium to the food (500 mg sodium chloride per day) may be necessary to increase urine volume.[93]

Urate and Uric Acid

Treatment of urate uroliths in dogs without hepatic dysfunction consists of feeding a calculolytic diet, administering allopurinol, alkalinizing urine, and treating any UTI. Prescription Diet u/d is recommended because it is purine-restricted and contains potassium citrate, a urinary alkalinizer. Allopurinol (Zyloprim) should be administered at a dose of 15 mg/kg by mouth every 12 hours. High doses of allopurinol may lead to development of xanthine uroliths, requiring adjustment in allopurinol dosage. If available, urine urate/creatinine ratios can be monitored; dosage of allopurinol should be adjusted to maintain a urine urate/creatinine ratio that is at least 50% of that obtained before treatment.[80] If dietary therapy does not cause formation of urine with pH of 7 to 7.5, a urinary alkalinizer is administered, either potassium citrate (Urocit-K, Polycitra syrup) at 75 mg/kg by mouth every 12 hours or sodium bicarbonate (1/4 tsp baking soda per 5 kg body weight, with food every 8 hours).[76, 80] If UTI is diagnosed, an appropriate antimicrobial agent should be administered until 1 month after radiographic disappearance of uroliths.

If urate uroliths occur in dogs with hepatic disease or portosystemic shunts, underlying hepatic dysfunction should be corrected if possible (e.g., by ligation of portosystemic shunts). In some cases, urate uroliths may dissolve without additional treatment in these patients. Uroliths also can be removed if abdominal surgery is performed to correct a portosystemic shunt. Diets that are severely protein-restricted (e.g., Prescription Diets u/d and s/d) are not recommended for patients with hepatic disease; therefore, an alternative diet such as Prescription Diet k/d should be fed. Urate uroliths may spontaneously resolve when dogs with portosystemic shunts are fed a diet that is moderately restricted in protein and sodium (i.e., Prescription Diet k/d).

Patients with urate uroliths should be monitored at monthly intervals to evaluate the effectiveness of medical treatment. Urine should be collected in the morning after the first meal for determination of pH, examination for ammonium urate crystals, and measurement of urate/creatinine ratio.[80] Radiographs are indicated to determine size, number, and location of uroliths; contrast cystography is necessary if uroliths are radiolucent. An antimicrobial agent should be administered at the time of catheterization to prevent UTI (see Urinary Tract Infection). Medical treatment should be continued 1 month beyond radiographic resolution of uroliths. If no dissolution of stones has occurred after 8 weeks of treatment and owner compliance is not a problem, surgical treatment should be considered.

After urate uroliths have been effectively treated, measures should be instituted to prevent recurrence. A diet restricted in purines that promotes formation of alkaline urine (Prescription Diet Canine u/d) should be fed. If urate crystalluria persists, urine pH is monitored and an alkalinizing agent is administered. If additional treatment is needed, allopurinol (10–20 mg/kg per day) should be administered.[76]

Calcium Oxalate

Medical treatment does not effectively dissolve calcium oxalate uroliths, so surgical removal is indicated. Measures can be attempted to prevent recurrence of uroliths after surgical removal. If hypercalcemia exists, the underlying cause should be treated. A diet that is moderately restricted in protein, calcium, oxalate, and sodium (e.g., Prescription Diets u/d and w/d) should be fed. The patient is re-evaluated by urinalysis and BUN measurement after 2 to 4 weeks of dietary therapy.[76] If aciduria or calcium oxalate crystalluria persists, potassium citrate (Urocit-K tablets, Polycitra syrup), 75 mg/kg by mouth every 12 hours, is administered. If, after 2 to 4 weeks, calcium oxalate crystalluria persists, vitamin B_6 (2–4 mg/kg by mouth every 24–48 hours) is administered to potentially decrease urinary oxalic acid excretion. The patient is re-evaluated in another 2 to 4 weeks to determine efficacy of treatment. If owner compliance is not a problem and calcium oxalate crystalluria is still present, hydrochlorothiazide (2 mg/kg by mouth every 12 hours) should be considered. Thiazide diuretics may decrease urinary calcium excretion; however, patients should be monitored for side effects of these drugs, including dehydration, hypokalemia, and hypercalcemia.[76] Patients are monitored every 3 to 6 months by urinalysis, BUN (which should be reduced), and abdominal radiographs to confirm dietary compliance and resolution of crystalluria and to detect recurrent uroliths.

Cystine

Medical treatment to dissolve cystine uroliths includes administration of a protein-restricted, alkalinizing diet (Prescription Diet u/d) and a thiol-containing drug such as N-2-mercaptopropionyl-glycine (MPG) (Thiola) or D-penicillamine (Cuprimine) to bind cystine and increase its solubility in urine.[61, 94] Because side effects (e.g., vomiting, fever, lymphadenopathy, and glomerulonephritis) are more likely to occur with D-penicillamine, MPG (15 mg/kg by mouth every 12 hours) is preferred for treatment of patients with cystine uroliths.[61, 76] If necessary, potassium citrate (75 mg/kg by mouth every 12 hours) is administered to maintain urine pH around 7.5. Patients are re-evaluated monthly by urinalysis and abdominal radiography. Contrast cystourethrography is necessary to detect radiolucent uroliths; an antimicrobial agent is administered at the time of urethral catheterization to prevent UTI (see Urinary Tract Infection). Medical treatment is continued 1 month beyond radiographic resolution of uroliths.

Measures to prevent cystine urolith recurrence include continued dietary management and administration of urinary alkalinizers. If cystine crystalluria persists or if uroliths begin to form, administration of either D-penicillamine or MPG is indicated.

Silica

Surgical removal is the treatment of choice for silica uroliths. Measures to prevent recurrence include avoidance of diets with increased plant proteins, especially soybean hulls and corn gluten; addition of water and salt to the diet to increase urine volume; and avoidance of efforts to acidify urine.[61]

Xanthine

Treatment and prevention of xanthine uroliths involves titration of the dose of allopurinol to prevent excessive urinary excretion of xanthine (see section on urate uroliths) and feeding of a diet (e.g., Prescription Diet u/d) that has decreased amounts of purine precursors. Foods such as organ meats, seafood, spinach, beans, lentils, and peas contain large amounts of purines and should be avoided.[87]

Prognosis

Prognosis for patients with uroliths depends in part on whether an underlying cause can be identified and eliminated. Patients with calcium oxalate, urate, and cystine uroliths have persistent metabolic defects that predispose to continued development of uroliths. Sterile struvite uroliths also have a tendency to recur because of an unidentified underlying defect. Infection-induced struvite uroliths have a good prognosis as long as UTI is treated appropriately; an exception is in miniature schnauzers, who have a familial tendency to develop recurrent UTI and struvite uroliths.[71, 73]

Feline Lower Urinary Tract Diseases

Feline lower urinary tract diseases include idiopathic lower urinary tract disease, also called idiopathic feline urologic syndrome (FUS); urolithiasis; and urethral plugs. FUS is characterized by hematuria, dysuria, or urethral obstruction; however, an underlying cause cannot be identified, and it is said to be idiopathic. Uroliths are polycrystalline concretions that consist mostly of minerals and a small quantity of matrix, whereas urethral plugs may be composed of

matrix with some minerals, aggregates of crystalline minerals, or tissue debris.[95] Some clinicians consider urethral plugs to be a part of idiopathic FUS, and others consider them a separate disorder.

Although the incidence of hematuria, dysuria, and urethral obstruction in cats ranges from 0.5% to 1.0% per year, 1% to 6% of cats with these signs are presented for veterinary evaluation.[96–98] In cats with naturally occurring signs of lower urinary tract disease, a cause cannot be found in 55%, urethral plugs are identified in 21%, and uroliths are found in 21%.[29] The most common urolith in cats is struvite, occurring in approximately 62% to 88% of cases.[95, 99–102] In contrast to dogs, most struvite uroliths in cats are not associated with UTI; an exception is immature cats (<1 year of age), who usually develop struvite uroliths secondary to UTI.[95] Uroliths that occur less frequently include (in order of decreasing frequency) calcium oxalate, urate, and calcium phosphate.[95, 99] Occurrence of sterile struvite uroliths has steadily decreased over the past 10 years, whereas urate and calcium uroliths have increased in frequency.[100, 102]

Idiopathic FUS and urolithiasis are recognized most often in middle-aged cats (2–6 years of age) that are neutered; males and females are affected equally.[95, 96] Although urethral plugs occur in cats of both sexes, they are most often diagnosed in castrated males. Also, urethral obstruction is most often observed in males.

Pathophysiology

Causes of uroliths in cats are similar to those described for dogs. Factors that predispose to development of sterile struvite uroliths include increased urinary concentrations of magnesium and increased urine pH. Pathogenesis of infection-induced struvite uroliths is similar to that for dogs; these uroliths contain a greater quantity of matrix, tend to grow more rapidly, and reach a larger size than sterile struvite uroliths.[95] Little is known about pathogenesis of urate, calcium oxalate, and calcium phosphate uroliths in cats. Increased dietary sodium and urinary acidifiers are associated with increased urinary excretion of calcium in some species. In addition, magnesium is an inhibitor of calcium oxalate crystal formation.[103] Therefore, diets with increased sodium, decreased magnesium, and urinary acidifiers (e.g., Prescription Diet Feline s/d) may predispose to development of calcium oxalate uroliths; however, this remains to be proven.

It is possible that urethral plugs and uroliths are caused by similar mechanisms; however, urethral plugs differ from uroliths in that they have the consistency of toothpaste and are composed of a larger amount of matrix. More than 90% of urethral plugs in cats are composed of struvite.[95] Urethral plugs appear to be the most common cause of urethral obstruction in cats.[95]

Pathogenesis of idiopathic FUS probably involves multiple factors that may or may not be related. Risk factors that may predispose to development of idiopathic FUS include neutering, obesity, decreased physical activity, consumption of dry food, and decreased water intake.[96] Viruses have been investigated as potential causes of idiopathic FUS; however, additional studies are required before definitive conclusions can be made.[104, 105] Most studies have focused on the role of dietary magnesium in development of idiopathic FUS; however, it appears that other factors are involved.[106, 107] Urine pH appears to play a role in development of struvite crystalluria; struvite crystals precipitate in alkaline urine. Although cats with signs of lower urinary tract disease often have struvite crystalluria, it is not known whether struvite crystals actually cause idiopathic FUS. Consequently, there is much that remains unknown regarding pathogenesis of idiopathic FUS.

Clinical Signs

Clinical signs of idiopathic FUS, urolithiasis, and urethral plugs are similar and include dysuria, hematuria, pollakiuria, and stranguria. If urethral obstruction occurs, stranguria may be the predominant sign, along with a palpably large, firm urinary bladder. Signs of postrenal uremia, such as lethargy, anorexia, vomiting, bradycardia, and stupor, may be present, depending on presence and duration of urethral obstruction.

Diagnostic Plan

Idiopathic FUS is diagnosed by ruling out all other disorders that can affect the feline lower urinary tract, including uroliths, urethral plugs, urinary bladder neoplasia, and UTI. Urinalysis and urine culture are performed initially or if there is no response to medical treatment in unobstructed cats. Additional evaluation, including abdominal radiographs and contrast cystourethrography, should be done if clinical signs persist longer than 5 to 7 days or recur within 3 months despite appropriate treatment. Serum chemistries and electrolytes should be measured in cats with systemic signs such as dehydration, vomiting, and weight loss and if urethral obstruction exists. Laboratory abnormalities in cats with urethral obstruction include azotemia, hyperphosphatemia, hyperkalemia, and metabolic acidosis.[108] Urinalysis may reveal hematuria, proteinuria, and crystalluria. Although urine culture is indicated to definitively exclude UTI, results often are negative, especially in cats presented for initial evaluation of signs. In one study of cats, plain abdominal radiographs were more likely to be helpful than urine culture; 20% of cats had radiopaque uroliths.[29]

Treatment

Urolithiasis

Medical treatment to dissolve struvite uroliths includes feeding a diet restricted in magnesium and maintaining urine pH at 6.0 or lower.[95] In contrast to dogs, dietary protein should not be restricted in cats. Feline calculolytic diets (e.g., Prescription Diet Feline s/d) also contain sodium chloride to increase urine volume and DL-methionine to acidify urine. If urine pH measured 4 to 8 hours after meals cannot be maintained at 6.0 or lower after 2 to 4 weeks of dietary treatment, urinary acidifiers should be administered cautiously; either DL-methionine (Methio-Tabs, (1000 mg/cat per day) or ammonium chloride (Uroeze, 800–1000 mg/cat per day) may be used.[109] Ideally, the total daily dose should be divided and given with meals because the goal is to lower postprandial urine pH. Acidifying diets or drugs should be avoided in immature cats and cats with disorders that cause metabolic acidosis (e.g., renal failure, postrenal azotemia).

Patients with struvite uroliths should be monitored every 2 to 4 weeks during medical treatment. Urinalysis is indicated to evaluate urine pH, preferably 4 to 8 hours postprandially, and to detect struvite crystalluria, which should not be present if treatment is successful. Radiographs should be done monthly to evaluate urolith size, number, and location. Medical treatment should be continued 1 month beyond radiographic resolution of uroliths. If UTI exists, antimicrobials also should be administered for this length of time. The average time required for dissolution of sterile struvite uroliths after beginning medical treatment is 36 days (range, 14–141 days), whereas infection-induced uroliths require an average of 79 days (range, 64–92 days) to dissolve.[110] If uroliths do not decrease in size after 4 to 8 weeks of medical treatment and owner compliance is not a problem, surgical removal of uroliths is indicated.

After struvite uroliths have been dissolved or removed surgically, measures to prevent their recurrence include maintaining urine pH at less than 6.5 and feeding a diet that is restricted in magnesium content. Diets should contain no more than 0.1% magnesium on a dry-matter basis, and ash content should be less than 3% of the diet.[109] Several commercial diets meet these criteria (Prescription Diet c/d, Feline Urological Diet, Iams Cat Food). If acid urine pH cannot be maintained by diet alone, urinary acidifiers should be administered.

Calcium oxalate, calcium phosphate, and urate

uroliths do not consistently respond to medical treatment and should be removed surgically if they are associated with clinical signs. Little is known about methods to prevent recurrence of these uroliths after surgical removal, although some guidelines may be useful pending results of controlled studies. Cats with calcium oxalate uroliths should be fed a nonacidifying diet that is moderately restricted in protein and sodium (Prescription Diet k/d); an alternative diet is Feline Prescription Diet w/d, especially if hypercalcemia exists.[100, 111] Potassium citrate (50–75 mg/kg by mouth every 12 hours) can be administered to alkalinize urine, which increases solubility of calcium oxalate.[111] If dietary treatment and urinary alkalinization are not effective, concurrent administration of vitamin B_6 (2 mg/kg by mouth every 24–48 hours) may be helpful.[111] Diets that cause excretion of acid urine or that contain increased purine precursors (e.g., liver) should be avoided in patients with urate uroliths.[100] Avoiding excessive dietary intake of protein and sodium may minimize hypercalciuria and calcium phosphate uroliths.[100]

Urethral Obstruction

Initial treatment of urethral obstruction is aimed at re-establishing urethral patency. Chemical restraint is unnecessary in severely depressed cats but facilitates urethral catheterization in other instances. Depending on the cat's physical condition, inhalational anesthesia with halothane or isofluorane, or injectable anesthesia with a combination of ketamine (2 Ketaset, 2–4 mg/kg IV to effect) and diazepam (Valium, 0.2 mg/kg IV to effect) can be used. After sedation, the penis is extruded, the distal urethra is massaged, and the urinary bladder is manually compressed in an attempt to dislodge a urethral plug. If unsuccessful, the next step is either to decompress the urinary bladder by performing cystocentesis or to pass a urethral catheter, according to personal choice. Advantages of cystocentesis are that it allows for collection of urine for culture and urinalysis before the urine is altered by a flushing solution and that it may facilitate repulsion of a urethral plug or urolith into the urinary bladder.[95] Disadvantages of cystocentesis are that it may cause extravasation of urine into the peritoneal cavity and injure the urinary bladder wall, but these complications are unlikely if proper technique is used and if the urinary bladder wall is not devitalized.[95] A 35- or 60-mL syringe connected to a 2.5- or 3.8-cm 22-gauge needle may be used to partially empty the urinary bladder.[112]

For urethral catheterization a sterile, open-ended, 1.15-mm catheter (Sovereign Tomcat catheter) or Minnesota olive-tipped urethral catheter can be used in an attempt to dislodge urethral plugs or uroliths. First, the penis and prepuce are cleaned with warm water, and the tip of the catheter is coated with sterile lubricant. The penis is extended dorsally so that it is parallel to the vertebral column.[95] The catheter is inserted through the urethral orifice and passed to the site of obstruction. A 35- or 60-mL syringe containing sterile saline or lactated Ringer's solution is attached to the urethral catheter, and the solution is flushed while an attempt is made to advance the catheter; several flushes, using a total of several hundred milliliters of solution, may be necessary. The goal is to soften urethral plugs so that they become dislodged and are flushed out around the catheter. If this procedure is unsuccessful, an attempt is made to repulse the plug or urolith back into the urinary bladder by occluding the distal end of the urethra around the catheter before flushing. If these procedures are unsuccessful at relieving urethral obstruction, a disorder other than a urethral plug or urolith (e.g., stricture, urethral mass) is likely, and contrast urethrography is indicated.

If, after relief of obstruction, urine contains a large amount of debris that may predispose to reobstruction, the urinary bladder should be flushed several times to remove excess debris. An indwelling urinary catheter should be placed if severe hematuria or crystalluria exists, if obstruction was difficult to relieve, if the urine stream remains small or weak, or if the urinary bladder was overdistended long enough to cause atony.[113] A flexible red rubber catheter (1.15- or 1.65-mm) is less traumatic and should be used instead of a polypropylene catheter.[113, 114] The catheter should be connected to a closed collection system, and it should be left in place for as short a time as possible (e.g., 24–48 hours) to lessen chances of causing UTI. Antimicrobials should not be administered to patients with indwelling urinary catheters, because UTI with resistant organisms may develop.[36, 37] Instead, urine is cultured immediately before removal of the catheter or a few days after removal, and antimicrobial drugs are administered if urine culture reveals bacterial growth. As many as 50% or more of cats previously catheterized for urethral obstruction may get iatrogenic UTI.[28] After removal of the urinary catheter, the patient is observed for 12 to 24 hours to detect signs of reobstruction.

Disorders of micturition (e.g., reflex dyssynergia, atony) may require treatment after relief of urethral obstruction. Reflex dyssynergia is characterized by inability to urinate because of concomitant urethral and detrusor contraction; the urinary bladder becomes distended because of functional outflow obstruction. Clinical findings of reflex dyssynergia are very similar to those of urethral obstruction; after the animal is positioned to urinate, an initial stream abruptly stops. In contrast to cats with urethral obstruction, a urinary catheter can be easily passed in cats with reflex dyssynergia. Urinary bladder atony occurs because of prolonged overdistention and is characterized by a flaccid urinary bladder and production of an adequate urine stream by manual expression. These cats also often position to urinate but produce a poor stream or only a few drops of urine. Phenoxybenzamine (Dibenzyline) is indicated to relax internal urethral sphincter tone in cats with reflex dyssynergia; an initial dose of 2.5 mg, by mouth every 24 hours can gradually be increased to 7.5 mg every 24 hours if needed. Diazepam also can be administered (2.5–5.0 mg per cat, by mouth every 8 hours) to decrease external urethral sphincter tone.[115] Urinary bladder atony usually responds if the urinary bladder is periodically emptied so that integrity of disrupted tight junctions can return. Emptying of the urinary bladder is most easily accomplished by placing an indwelling urinary catheter for 2 to 7 days and administering bethanechol (Urecholine). Treatment with bethanechol administered at a dose of 1.25 to 5 mg, by mouth every 8 hours for 7 to 10 days stimulates detrusor contraction. Because bethanechol stimulates urethral sphincter contraction, phenoxybenzamine should be given concomitantly.[116, 117]

Treatment of metabolic complications (e.g., dehydration, hyperkalemia, azotemia, metabolic acidosis) associated with urethral obstruction also is indicated after urethral obstruction has been relieved. An exception is emergency treatment of life-threatening hyperkalemia (e.g., cardiac arrhythmias), which should be done before relieving urethral obstruction or at the same time, if possible. Because results of serum potassium are not available at initial presentation, electrocardiographic changes (i.e., prolonged P-R interval, absent P waves, peaked T waves, widened QRS complexes) can be used to determine the need for treatment. Dehydration should be corrected rapidly (over 6–8 hours) by intravenous administration of 0.9% saline solution to prevent additional renal injury; lactated Ringer's solution is adequate if severe hyperkalemia does not exist. Maintenance fluid volume should be administered in addition to amounts necessary to replace ongoing losses from vomiting and postobstructive diuresis, which usually lasts less than 24 hours.[113] Potassium supplementation may be necessary for cats that develop hypokalemia after relief of urethral obstruction during diuresis. See Chapter 16 for a complete discussion of treatment of hyperkalemia, hypokalemia, metabolic acidosis, and fluid deficits.

Perineal urethrostomy should be considered in cats with repeated episodes of obstruction (e.g., within 6–12 months of each other) despite preventative medical treatment. It also may be indicated in male cats that cannot be closely observed by owners (e.g., outside cats). A retrograde cystourethrogram should be done before surgery to evaluate the proximal urethra and urinary bladder for strictures, uroliths, and neopla-

sia.[118] Owners should be informed that perineal urethrostomy prevents signs of obstruction but does not affect other signs of idiopathic FUS, such as dysuria and hematuria. In addition, perineal urethrostomy compromises host defenses and is associated with UTI in approximately 25% of cats.[38, 40, 119] Cats that develop UTI after surgery may not show clinical signs; therefore, urine cultures should be done periodically (e.g., every 6 months).[38, 120]

Idiopathic Feline Urologic Syndrome

Treatment of cats with nonobstructed idiopathic FUS includes feeding a diet that contains decreased magnesium and maintaining acidic urine (see section on prevention of struvite urolithiasis in cats for specific guidelines). Increased water intake and urine volume may help prevent recurrence of clinical signs. Adding water to the cat's food or stimulating thirst by adding salt or bouillon to the food may accomplish this. Obesity should be avoided, because increased consumption of food is likely to cause increased magnesium intake.

Because UTI is extremely uncommon in cats that have not been catheterized previously for urethral obstruction, routine administration of antimicrobials to cats with signs of idiopathic FUS is not indicated. Some veterinarians believe that cats with idiopathic FUS respond to antimicrobial treatment; however, it is not uncommon for cats with idiopathic FUS to have spontaneous resolution of clinical signs, whether antimicrobials are used or not.[104] Indiscriminate use of antimicrobial drugs may predispose to development of resistant strains of bacteria. If UTI is identified on the basis of urine culture, however, an appropriate antimicrobial agent should be administered (see Urinary Tract Infection).

Because the cause of FUS is unknown, symptomatic treatment of clinical signs is sometimes attempted. Urge incontinence, characterized by frequent detrusor contraction, often accompanies idiopathic FUS, and drugs that decrease detrusor contraction, such as propantheline (Pro-banthine, 7.5 mg by mouth every 72 hours), may be used, although response has been limited.[104] Administration of anti-inflammatory doses of corticosteroids (0.5–1 mg/kg per day) may relieve clinical signs in cats with idiopathic FUS. Ideally, corticosteroids should be used only after all other causes of lower urinary tract disease have been ruled out. Corticosteroids are contraindicated in cats with renal failure, postrenal azotemia, bacterial UTI, or indwelling urinary catheters.[59] As a last resort, dimethylsulfoxide (DMSO) has been used to treat cats with chronic idiopathic FUS that have persistent clinical signs.[109] All causes of lower urinary tract disease should be excluded before this procedure is done. A urinary catheter is placed with the cat under general anesthesia, and the urinary bladder is emptied. Approximately 10 to 20 mL of DMSO (10%) is instilled into the urinary bladder and allowed to remain for 10 minutes before it is removed. If necessary, this treatment can be repeated once in 2 weeks.

Prognosis

Prognosis for many disorders of the feline lower urinary tract is guarded because the underlying cause often is unknown. Patients with idiopathic FUS often have multiple recurrences of clinical signs. Because the causes of calcium oxalate, calcium phosphate, and urate uroliths are unknown, they may recur even though preventative measures are used. Struvite uroliths can be dissolved by medical treatment, and treatments are available to prevent their recurrence; only 7% of cats had recurrent struvite uroliths in one study.[110] Prognosis for patients with urethral obstruction depends on the cause and duration of obstruction. Urethral plugs usually can be removed; however, they have a tendency to recur, causing repeated episodes of obstruction in up to 37% of cats.[121] If urethral obstruction persists longer than 24 hours, azotemia, hyperkalemia, and severe metabolic acidosis develop, and death may result from severe dehydration, renal failure, or cardiac arrhythmias secondary to hyperkalemia.[108]

Neoplasia

Neoplasms of the lower urinary tract are progressive and uncontrolled growths of abnormal tissue in the urinary bladder or urethra. Urinary bladder neoplasms are uncommon in dogs and cats, representing 0.5% to 1% of all canine tumors and 0.07% to 0.38% of feline tumors.[32, 122–126] Urethral tumors occur less frequently than urinary bladder tumors in dogs and are rare in cats.[32, 126–129] Epithelial tumors of urinary bladder and urethra occur primarily in older dogs and cats; reported mean ages range from 9.1 to 11.6 years.[122, 124, 125, 127, 128, 130] Embryonal rhabdomyosarcoma is a tumor of mesenchymal origin that most often affects young dogs (<2 years).[131–135] Urinary bladder and urethral tumors occur more often in larger dogs (>10 kg) than in small breeds.[127, 131–135] Lower urinary tract tumors in dogs appear to be more common in females than in males; less is known about sex predilection in cats.[123, 127–129,136]

Pathophysiology

The cause of lower urinary tract neoplasia in dogs and cats is unknown. Chronic inflammation, urinary retention, and excretion of carcinogenic substances such as aromatic amines in urine have been suggested as potential causes of urinary bladder neoplasia.[122] Transitional cell carcinoma of the urinary bladder has been reported in dogs receiving cyclophosphamide; it is possible that either chronic inflammation or immunosuppression secondary to such treatment predisposes to development of neoplasia.[137, 138] Experimentally induced urinary bladder neoplasia occurs in dogs because of urinary excretion of carcinogenic substances such as aromatic amines or tryptophan.[139, 140] Cats may be less susceptible to lower urinary tract neoplasia because their urine contains virtually no tryptophan metabolites.[141] There seems to be no association between urinary bladder neoplasia in cats and feline leukemia virus infection.[130]

Most lower urinary tract tumors arise directly from tissues of urinary bladder and urethra, although some tumors result from secondary invasion (e.g., prostate gland) or metastasis from elsewhere. Some tumors of the lower urinary tract are benign; however, 80% in cats and 93% to 100% in dogs are malignant.[124, 127, 128, 130] Malignant epithelial neoplasms, including transitional cell carcinoma, squamous cell carcinoma, and adenocarcinoma, are most common. Rhabdomyosarcoma, leiomyosarcoma, and fibrosarcoma are the most common malignant mesenchymal tumors. Most malignant tumors of the lower urinary tract are locally invasive, and they frequently metastasize to lymph nodes in the abdomen; distant metastases (e.g., lungs) occur less often. Benign tumors of the lower urinary tract are rare but include fibroma, leiomyoma, papilloma, adenoma, and others.[124, 130, 136, 142]

Clinical Signs

Clinical signs of lower urinary tract neoplasia are nonspecific and include dysuria, stranguria, pollakiuria, and hematuria; of these, hematuria is most common.[127, 130, 142] Signs of uremia, such as inappetence, vomiting, weight loss, and dehydration, may occur secondary to postrenal azotemia and uremia, which may result from either urethral or ureteral obstruction. Lameness is observed infrequently in dogs with hypertrophic osteopathy, which has been reported in association with transitional cell carcinoma, rhabdomyosarcoma, and neurofibrosarcoma of the urinary bladder.[127, 135, 143–145]

Diagnostic Plan

Tests that are helpful for confirming a diagnosis of lower urinary tract neoplasia include urinalysis, radiography, and cytologic or histologic evaluation of tissue specimens. Urinalysis often reveals proteinuria, pyuria, hematuria, and sometimes bacteriuria resulting from secondary UTI.[127, 130] Lower urinary tract tumors are diagnosed by a finding of neoplastic cells on urine sediment examination in 30% to 70% of dogs

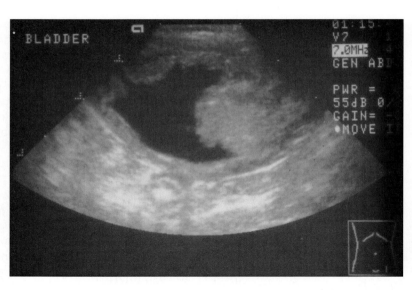

Figure 17-5
Abdominal ultrasonogram of a dog with chronic hematuria. Note the hyperechoic area on the right, consistent with a mass in the urinary bladder trigone. A transitional cell carcinoma was diagnosed by aspiration cytology. (Courtesy of Martha L. Moon, DVM, MS, Blacksburg, Virginia.)

and 13% of cats.[124, 127, 130] Caution is indicated when interpreting cytologic results because inflammation itself can cause dysplastic changes in epithelial cells that resemble neoplasia. Urine sediment examination and bladder washes should be done before contrast radiography because hypertonic contrast media distort cellular morphology. Plain abdominal radiographs are abnormal in only 30% of dogs with urinary bladder tumors; however, contrast cystography (see Diagnostic Procedures) reveals space-occupying masses in almost all cases.[124, 127, 130] Ultrasonography also is very useful for identifying masses in the urinary bladder (Fig. 17-5). Excretory urography (see Chap. 16) should be done to determine the presence and extent of ureteral involvement, especially with tumors located at the trigone. Thoracic radiographs also are indicated to detect distant metastasis before aggressive treatment is instituted. Fine-needle aspiration of urinary bladder and urethral masses, with ultrasound guidance when available, often allows for the making of a diagnosis.[127] Aspiration also may be performed without ultrasonography if the mass can be palpated through the abdominal wall.

It is preferable to obtain a diagnosis of lower urinary tract neoplasia before surgical intervention; however, if this is not possible, the surgeon should be prepared to obtain specimens for intraoperative cytologic or histologic evaluation and then to proceed with appropriate surgical treatment.[146] If a clinician is not prepared to do this, it is better to refer the case to a specialist before surgical biopsy for definitive diagnosis and treatment.[147] One reason for this is that the first surgery offers the best chance for complete tumor excision. Also, multiple surgeries may increase the potential for seeding of the abdominal cavity and incision with tumor cells.[148]

Treatment

By the time of diagnosis in most malignant tumors, local invasiveness, especially involving the urinary bladder trigone, and metastasis of tumor prevent curative treatment. Therefore, most treatments for urinary bladder and urethral tumors are palliative. Goals of treatment are to control local disease (e.g., dysuria, hematuria, urinary obstruction, incontinence) and to prevent or delay metastasis.[149] Options for treatment of lower urinary tract neoplasia include surgery, radiotherapy, and chemotherapy. At this time, ideal treatment of lower urinary tract tumors is unknown; most dogs are treated with a combination of modalities. Even less is known about treatment of lower urinary tract neoplasia in cats; most have been treated by surgical excision.[130, 150]

Surgical excision of benign urinary bladder tumors often is curative; however, malignant tumors frequently cannot be excised completely because of their invasive nature or location.[142, 147, 151] Median survival times after surgical excision of malignant tumors range from 86 to 365 days.[127, 152] Completeness of surgical excision influences survival times; dogs with excision of all visible tumor in one study had a median survival time of 365 days, whereas those with only partial excision had survival times of 75 to 120 days.[127] Radical excision (e.g., cystectomy) of many malignant tumors requires urinary diversion such as ureterocolonic anastomosis, and these procedures often are associated with postoperative complications and decreased quality of life.[151] Although debulking surgery may temporarily relieve clinical signs, regrowth of tumor usually occurs rapidly. Surgical reduction of tumor mass may help if it is used in conjunction with radiotherapy.[153]

Radiotherapy has been successful for prolonging survival times in patients with urinary bladder neoplasia.[153,154] Median survival time of 15 months was reported when urinary bladder neoplasia was treated with a combination of intraoperative radiotherapy and surgical reduction.[154] Potential complications of radiotherapy include urinary incontinence, urinary bladder fibrosis characterized by pollakiuria, and ureteral fibrosis and stenosis with secondary hydroureter, although hydronephrosis does not appear to cause clinically important renal disease and is not a common cause for euthanasia.[155] However, because of limited availability, costs, potential complications, and inability to cure patients with radiotherapy, most clients choose other modes of treatment.

Several chemotherapeutic agents have been used to treat urinary bladder and urethral neoplasia; however, measurable responses have occurred in only a few patients.[131, 132, 152, 156–158] A median survival time of 180 days was reported in one study of 12 dogs with transitional cell carcinoma treated with cisplatin alone.[156]

I administer cisplatin (Platinol) at a dose of 60 to 70 mg/m^2 intravenously every 3 weeks; depending on response of the tumor and renal function, a total of 2 to 6 treatments is given. However, in order to determine the efficacy of chemotherapy, it is recommended that a baseline contrast cystogram or ultrasonogram be done to determine tumor size. Before chemotherapy, laboratory evaluation including CBC, platelet count, serum chemistries, and urinalysis should be done. Chemotherapy should be postponed if neutropenia (<5000 neutrophils/µL), thrombocytopenia (<100,000 platelets/µL), or azotemia is identified. If renal failure exists (azotemia and urine specific gravity <1.030), carboplatin should be used instead of cisplatin.

After initial evaluation, the owners should be instructed to bring the dog to the hospital in the morning when the clinic opens; most dogs can be treated as outpatients if laboratory evaluation is done 1 or 2 days before chemotherapy or if results are available the same day. An indwelling IV catheter is placed and 0.9% saline is administered at 25 mL/kg per hour for 1 hour; an infusion pump is very helpful to accurately administer this large volume of fluids, especially to large patients (>40 kg). Because cisplatin causes emesis in virtually every patient, an antiemetic such as butorphanol (Torbugesic) (0.2–0.4 mg/kg SC) should be given 4 hours and then 1 hour before cisplatin, and 4 hours after cisplatin. The calculated dose of cisplatin is mixed in 8 mL/kg of 0.9% saline and infused at 25 mL/kg per hour over a 20-minute period. Saline diuresis is continued at the same rate for another hour after infusion of cisplatin. Hospital personnel and owners should be instructed to avoid contact with the animal's urine for the next 24 hours because most cisplatin is eliminated by the kidneys.

The patient should return every 3 weeks for evaluation prior to administration of cisplatin. Ideally, a contrast cystogram or ultrasonogram should be done between the second and third treatments to determine efficacy of cisplatin. Patients that have stable disease (no enlargement of tumor) or regression of tumor are given additional treatments as long as there is clinical improvement and no signs of nephrotoxicosis. Some dogs show clinical improvement (i.e., resolution of hematuria, dysuria, pollakiuria) even if the tumor does not regress; chemotherapy should be continued in these cases.

Partial responses have been seen in dogs with urinary bladder transitional cell carcinoma treated with carboplatin (DW Knapp, Purdue University, Personal Communication, 1994); a dose of 300 mg/m^2 IV every 3 to 4 weeks until there is no response is recommended.[159] Carboplatin is preferred for patients with renal disease because it is not nephrotoxic; however, myelosuppression does occur, and it usually peaks at about 14 days after treatment.[160] In another study of dogs with transitional cell carcinoma, median survival time of 259 days was reported with the use of a combination of doxorubicin (Adriamcyin, 30 mg/m^2 IV every 3 weeks) and cyclophosphamide (Cytoxan, 50–100 mg/m^2 by mouth once daily on days 3 through 6 after doxorubicin).

Prior to treatment with doxorubicin, thorough patient evaluation including CBC, platelet count, and echocardiogram should be done. The most common side effects of doxorubicin are hypersensitivity reactions (e.g., hives, urticaria) and myelosuppression. Chemotherapy should be postponed for 1 week if neutropenia (<5000 neutrophils/µL) or thrombocytopenia (<100,000 platelets/µL) exist, and then the patient should be re-evaluated by another CBC and platelet count. The most severe complication of treatment with doxorubicin, irreversible cardiomyopathy, is most likely to occur with cumulative doses >180 mg/m^2. A baseline echocardiogram is indicated to assess cardiac contractility, especially in breeds that are prone to cardiomyopathy.

Administration of doxorubicin can be done as an outpatient procedure. An indwelling IV catheter is placed and the dog is given diphenhydramine (Benadryl) at a dose of 0.5 mg/kg IV, 30 minutes before infusion of doxorubicin. Because doxorubicin causes severe tissue necrosis if given extravascularly, it is extremely important that the catheter be placed appropriately during the first attempt. If there is any question regarding catheter patency, it is best to replace the catheter in another vein. The calculated dose (30 mg/m^2) of doxorubicin is mixed in 50 to 150 mL of 0.9%

saline and infused over a 15-minute period. Because doxorubicin may be inactivated by light, the infusion bag and IV line should be covered with aluminum foil. Signs of hypersensitivity may occur during infusion; however, they usually subside if the infusion is stopped briefly and do not recur once infusion is continued. If they persist, another dose of diphenhydramine can be administered. The patient should be observed for 1 to 2 hours after treatment and then sent home.

The dog should return every 3 weeks for evaluation, including physical examination, CBC, and platelet count. If results are normal, doxorubicin is administered as described, for a total of 6 treatments. To assess cardiac contractility, another echocardiogram should be done between the third and fourth treatments. Also, evaluation of tumor response should be done, as described for cisplatin.

Treatment with piroxicam (Feldene), a non-steroidal anti-inflammatory drug, has been associated with partial and complete remissions in some dogs with urinary bladder transitional cell carcinoma, but the mechanism of action of piroxicam is unknown.[161, 162] Median survival time of 34 dogs was 181 days; however, some dogs lived longer than 720 days.[162] Dogs without evidence of remission appeared to benefit from treatment and had improved quality of life as judged by their owners. The recommended dose of piroxicam is 0.3 mg/kg by mouth once daily. Potential side effects include gastrointestinal ulceration and renal papillary necrosis. Concurrent administration of misoprostol (Cytotec, 3–5 μg/kg every 8 hours) may help prevent gastrointestinal complications.

Prognosis

Prognosis for patients with lower urinary tract tumors depends on histologic type and location of tumor. Benign tumors that can be surgically excised are associated with a good prognosis.[142] Malignant tumors carry a grave prognosis because no treatment has been curative; however, if surgical resection is successful at removing all visible tumor, prognosis is somewhat improved.[127] Tumors located in the trigone of the urinary bladder are difficult to completely excise, and chances for cure are less likely than for tumors located elsewhere in the urinary bladder. Presence of obstructive hydroureter, hydronephrosis, or abdominal lymphadenopathy also are poor prognostic findings.[32] Finally, dogs that have tumors located in either the urinary bladder or the urethra have a better prognosis than when both urinary bladder and urethra are affected.[127]

Urethral Incompetence

Urethral incompetence is decreased function of the internal urethral sphincter. Incidence of urethral incompetence in this country is unknown; however, 20% of 412 female dogs in a German study became incontinent after neutering, presumably because of urethral incompetence.[163] Urethral incompetence is diagnosed primarily in neutered female dogs, although male dogs and intact females may be affected.[163–165] Although incontinence caused by urethral incompetence may occur any time, most female dogs develop incontinence within 2 to 3 years of neutering.[163,165] Most dogs with urethral incompetence are of medium to large breeds (>20 kg body weight).[163, 165] Little is known about occurrence of urethral incompetence in cats.

Pathophysiology

The exact cause of urethral incompetence is unknown; it is likely that multiple factors are involved. It once was thought that deficiency of either estrogen or testosterone in neutered dogs was responsible; recent evidence suggests that this is not so.[164] The fact that neutered dogs may not respond to hormone replacement and that some intact dogs develop incontinence also suggests that other mechanisms are responsible for urethral incompetence. Results of a study in dogs suggest that incontinence may result in part from decreased effectiveness of adrenergic innervation to the urethra.[166] Other factors that may contribute to incontinence are a caudally located urinary bladder in the pelvic canal and decreased urethral length.[165]

Clinical Signs

Intermittent urinary incontinence during periods of rest is the most common clinical sign of urethral incompetence; in some cases incontinence occurs continuously.[165] Most dogs are able to initiate and maintain urination normally with complete emptying of the urinary bladder.

Diagnostic Plan

In most instances, urethral incompetence is tentatively diagnosed on the basis of history, physical and neurologic examination findings, and response to treatment. Urinalysis and urine culture should be done in all patients with incontinence. UTI occurs in 38% of dogs with urethral incompetence, sometimes in the absence of clinical signs of infection.[165] Persistent hyposthenuria (i.e., specific gravity <1.008 on several occasions) should prompt suspicion of polyuria and polydipsia. Any condition that causes polyuria and polydipsia may exacerbate clinical signs of incontinence. Additional testing (see Chap. 16), including CBC and serum chemistries, may be indicated to screen for systemic disorders such as renal disease, renal failure, or hyperadrenocorticism. Special diagnostic procedures such as urethral pressure profilometry are

Table 17–8
Drugs Used to Treat Urethral Incompetence

DRUG	DOSAGE REGIMEN
Phenylpropanolamine	Dogs and cats, 1.5 mg/kg PO every 8–12 h
Ephedrine	Dogs, 12.5–50 mg per dog PO every 8–12 h Cats, 2–4 mg/kg PO every 8–12 h
Diethylstilbestrol	Dogs, 0.1–1 mg PO per dog every 24 h for 3–5 d, then same dose PO once weekly not to exceed 1 mg/wk
Testosterone propionate	Dogs, 2.2 mg/kg IM 2 to 3 times weekly
Testosterone cypionate	Dogs, 2.2 mg/kg IM once monthly

PO, by mouth; IM, intramuscularly.

the most objective method for confirming urethral incompetence; however, these tests are not routinely available. For complete discussion of diagnostic evaluation of patients with urinary incontinence, see Chapter 27.

Treatment

Most dogs with urethral incompetence are treated by administering drugs that increase urethral tone (Table 17–8). α-Adrenergic agonists such as phenylpropanolamine (Propagest) and ephedrine may be used to increase urethral sphincter tone. Side effects of these drugs include anxious behavior, tremors, dizziness, cardiac arrhythmias, hypertension, and urinary retention.[117] Phenylpropanolamine may be preferable because it has fewer side effects and tends to be effective for a longer period of time.[117] Alternatively, diethylstilbestrol (DES) or testosterone can be administered to female and male dogs, respectively. The most serious complication of DES is bone marrow suppression; however, it is unlikely to occur at recommended doses. Still, it is best to inform owners of potential for this problem and monitor with a CBC every 1 to 2 months. Testosterone proprionate (Androlan) or testosterone cypionate (Depo-testosterone) can be administered to male dogs with incontinence caused by urethral incompetence.[167] If incontinence persists in female dogs after treatment with either an α-adrenergic agonist or DES, concurrent administration of both drugs may resolve clinical signs.[167]

For dogs that do not respond to medical treatment, other options can be considered. In 33 incontinent dogs that failed to respond to medical treatment, colposuspension (i.e., pulling the vagina cranially and anchoring it to the prepubic tendon)

resulted in complete resolution of incontinence in half of the dogs, and the majority of the remaining dogs were markedly improved.[168] In another study, incontinence was controlled in 19 of 22 dogs by one or two endoscopic injections of Teflon into the urethral submucosa.[169]

Prognosis

Most dogs with urethral incompetence appear to respond to medical treatment, although periodic adjustments of dosages or drugs may be needed. The majority of female dogs respond favorably to treatment with either estrogen or ephedrine.[163]

Lower Urinary Tract Trauma

Trauma of the lower urinary tract is injury to either the urinary bladder or the urethra. Incidence of lower urinary tract trauma is unknown; however, it was reported in 1.7% of dogs involved in motor vehicle accidents and 32% of dogs with pelvic fractures.[170, 171] Although some studies show that male dogs are more likely to experience urinary trauma, others show no difference between males and females.[170–173] However, urethral rupture occurs almost exclusively in male dogs.[171] Little is known about feline urinary tract trauma; it appears that cats are affected less often than dogs.

Pathophysiology

Most cases of lower urinary tract trauma occur secondary to vehicular accidents, although any type of blunt or penetrating trauma may injure the urinary bladder or urethra. Trauma may cause only soft tissue bruising and hemorrhage, or it may be associated with a ruptured urinary tract.[171] Other causes of urinary tract injury include traumatic catheterization and overzealous urinary bladder palpation, especially if bladder tissue is devitalized. Spontaneous rupture of the urinary bladder may occur secondary to urolithiasis, neoplasia, and atony resulting from prolonged overdistention.[32, 156] Urethral rupture occurs most frequently near the junction with the urinary bladder, and it causes retroperitoneal, perineal, or abdominal accumulation of urine, which may not be apparent for up to 72 hours after injury.[32] Leakage of urine from a ruptured urethra may cause periurethral inflammation, which leads to obstruction.

Clinical Signs

Clinical findings in patients with lower urinary tract trauma include depression, dehydration, vomiting, abdominal fluid or pain, perineal swelling, hematuria, dysuria, and anuria. However, not all dogs with urinary tract injury have clinical signs of urinary tract disease. Of dogs with pelvic fractures and

Figure 17–6
Positive-contrast cystogram of a dog that was hit by a car 5 days prior. After surgical treatment of pelvic fractures, the dog became depressed and inappetent, and azotemia and abdominal effusion were noted. Note leakage of contrast from the cranioventral surface of the urinary bladder. An exploratory laparotomy was done, and a rent in the cranial urinary bladder was identified and repaired.

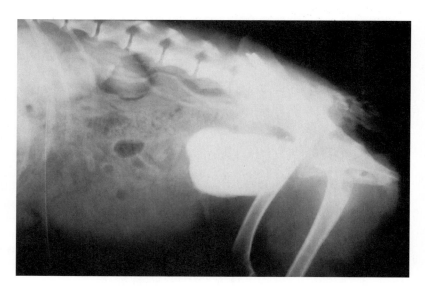

urinary tract injuries, 33% may have no clinical signs of urinary tract disease; this is especially true for females.[171] Dogs with ruptured urinary bladders may not show clinical signs for 1 to 3 days after a traumatic incident. Also, ability to urinate normally does not exclude urinary bladder rupture.[173]

Diagnostic Plan

Urinary tract trauma and rupture should be suspected in any patient with abdominal trauma, especially if pelvic fractures exist, whether clinical signs of urinary tract disease are present or not. Diagnostic tests, including serum chemistries, urinalysis, and analysis of abdominal fluid, if present, are indicated initially. Patients with experimentally ruptured urinary bladders developed increased packed cell volumes, azotemia, hyperphosphatemia, hypochloremia, and hyponatremia within 45 hours of urinary tract rupture; hyperkalemia occurred after 53 hours.[173] Analysis of abdominal fluid, if present, shows an exudate characterized cytologically by neutrophils, macrophages, and mesothelial cells; if UTI exists, bacteria also may be observed.[173] Although both urea nitrogen and creatinine concentrations are increased in abdominal fluid, creatinine may be a better indicator of urinary tract rupture, especially if rupture has been present for longer than a day. Finding an abdominal fluid creatinine concentration that is greater than concomitant serum creatinine is diagnostic of urinary tract rupture.[173]

Radiography is indicated in patients with suspected urinary tract rupture; rents of the urinary tract are most easily confirmed by positive-contrast procedures (Fig. 17–6).[171, 173, 174] Plain abdominal radiographs may show decreased contrast because of accumulation of fluid and inability to visualize the urinary bladder.[171] Positive-contrast cystography and retrograde cystourethrography (see Diagnostic Procedures) are indicated to diagnose urinary bladder and urethral rupture, respectively. It is important to fully distend the urinary bladder with contrast material; otherwise, small rents may be overlooked. If a urethral catheter cannot be passed, excretory urography can be performed instead; this is often sufficient for diagnosis of ruptured urinary bladder in female dogs.[171] It is important to confirm the location of urinary tract rupture before surgical correction.

Treatment

Patients with urinary tract bruising often respond to supportive care, including maintenance of hydration and elimination and treatment of skeletal fractures, but patients with a ruptured urinary tract also require surgical correction. Small urethral tears may heal over a catheter that is left in place for 7 to 21 days. Pelvic urethral tears require surgical exploration.[32] If urinary tract rupture is diagnosed, the patient should first be stabilized by administration of fluids to correct azotemia, hyperphosphatemia, hyponatremia, and hyperkalemia (see Chap. 16). A catheter should be placed into the urinary bladder and connected to a closed system so that urine can be drained from the abdominal cavity. If this is unsuccessful at draining the abdomen, an indwelling dialysis catheter or sterile rubber feeding tube with multiple holes can be inserted into the abdomen using a local anesthetic.[175] Antimicrobial treatment is indicated if there is UTI, septic abdominal effusion, or devitalized tissue.[32] After fluid, electrolyte, and serum chemistry abnormalities have been treated and the patient is stable, which may

require several days, surgical correction of the ruptured urinary tract can be done. Surgical correction
should not be done before correction of metabolic
abnormalities unless life-threatening hemorrhage or
urinary obstruction exists.

Prognosis

Prognosis for patients with urinary tract trauma
depends on the severity of injury and the time between
injury and diagnosis. Patients with minor injuries such
as bruising and hemorrhage have a better prognosis
than those with urinary tract rupture.[171] In one study,
mortality associated with urinary bladder rupture was
42%.[173] In another study of 16 dogs that required surgical treatment for ruptured urinary tract, 56% were
euthanized or died during surgery.[171] If diagnosis is
delayed, metabolic abnormalities develop and complicate management of patients with urinary tract rupture.

Uncommon Diseases of the Urinary Bladder and Urethra

Fungal Urinary Tract Infection

Fungal UTI is very uncommon and usually
affects patients that have compromised host defense
mechanisms.[12] It is diagnosed by identification of
budding yeasts or elongated hyphae on urine sediment
examination or by culture of urine in special media.
Treatment includes correction of predisposing causes
and administration of antifungal agents such as flucytosine.

Sterile Hemorrhagic Cystitis

Treatment with cyclophosphamide may cause
sterile, hemorrhagic cystitis. Most cases occur in dogs
after prolonged oral administration of the drug, usually longer than 18 weeks; however, it may occur after a
single intravenous dose.[176, 177] The disorder is diagnosed by excluding all other causes of lower urinary tract disease. Treatment includes discontinuation
of cyclophosphamide; intravesicular instillation of
DMSO may be helpful in patients with persistent clinical signs.[178]

Polypoid Cystitis

Polypoid cystitis is characterized by numerous
polyp-like lesions that protrude from the urinary
bladder mucosa in dogs.[179] Patients often have dysuria, hematuria, and secondary bacteriuria. Contrast
radiographic findings appear similar to those of
neoplasia; however, histologic evaluation reveals benign polyps. Surgical removal is the treatment of
choice.

Parasitic Infection

Urinary bladder infection with *Capillaria plica* or
Capillaria feliscati occurs infrequently in dogs and cats,
respectively.[180, 181] Clinical findings may include dysuria, pollakiuria, hematuria, and secondary bacterial
UTI. Urinary bladder capillariasis is diagnosed by
finding double-operculated ova, approximately 25 μm
wide by 50 μm long, on urine sediment examination.
Fenbendazole (Panacur) at 50 mg/kg by mouth every
24 hours in dogs and 25 mg/kg by mouth every 12
hours in cats for 10 days has been an effective
treatment. Albendazole (Valbazen) at 50 mg/kg by
mouth every 12 hours for 10 to 14 days can be used in
dogs; however, anorexia may occur at this dose.[180]
Dogs also may be treated with a single dose of
ivermectin (200–400 μg/kg by mouth).

Urethral Prolapse

Prolapse of the urethral mucosa may cause
dysuria and hemorrhage from the tip of the penis in
dogs; English bulldogs may be predisposed.[182, 183]
Diagnosis is made by observing the prolapsed urethra,
which appears as a red mass at the end of the penis.
Surgical resection of the urethral mucosa is the
treatment of choice.

References

1. Christensen GC. The urogenital apparatus. In: Evans
   HE, Christensen GC, ed. Miller's Anatomy of the Dog,
   Philadelphia, WB Saunders, 1979:544–601.
2. Moreau PM, Lees GE. Incontinence, enuresis, and
   nocturia. In: Ettinger SJ, ed. Textbook of Veterinary
   Internal Medicine, 3rd ed. Philadelphia, WB Saunders,
   1989:148–154.
3. Lees GE, Osborne CA, Stevens JB. Antibacterial properties of urine: Studies of feline urine specific gravity,
   osmolality, and pH. J Am Anim Hosp Assoc 1979;15:
   135–141.
4. Lees GE, Willard MD, Green RA. Urinary disorders. In:
   Willard MD, Tvedten H, Turnwald GH, eds. Small
   Animal Clinical Diagnosis by Laboratory Methods,
   Philadelphia, WB Saunders, 1994:115–146.
5. Moreau PM, Lees GE. Urinary obstruction and atony. In:
   Ettinger SJ, ed. Textbook of Veterinary Internal Medicine, 3rd ed. Philadelphia, WB Saunders, 1989:155–159.
6. Gannon JR. Exertional rhabdomyolysis (myoglobinuria) in the racing greyhound. In: Kirk RW, ed. Current
   Veterinary Therapy VII. Philadelphia, WB Saunders,
   1980:783–787.
7. Lage AL. Diagnostic approach to canine and feline

hematuria. In: Kirk RW, ed. Current Veterinary Therapy X. Philadelphia, WB Saunders, 1989:1117–1123.

8. Stone EA, DeNovo RC, Rawlings CA. Massive hematuria of nontraumatic renal origin in dogs. J Am Vet Med Assoc 1983;183:868–871.

9. Ling GV, Stabenfeldt GH, Comer KM, et al. Canine hyperadrenocorticism: Pretreatment clinical and laboratory evaluation of 17 cases. J Am Vet Med Assoc 1979;174:1211–1215.

10. Ihrke PJ, Norton AL, Ling GV, et al. Urinary tract infection associated with long-term corticosteroid administration in dogs with chronic skin diseases. J Am Vet Med Assoc 1985;186:43–46.

11. Jang SS, Ling GV, Yamamoto R. Mycoplasma as a cause of canine urinary tract infection. J Am Vet Med Assoc 1984;185:45–47.

12. Lulich JP, Osborne CA. Fungal urinary tract infections. In: Kirk RW, Bonagura JD, eds. Kirk's Current Veterinary Therapy XI. Philadelphia, WB Saunders, 1992:914–919.

13. Carter JM, Klausner JS, Osborne CA, et al. Comparison of collection techniques for quantitative urine culture in dogs. J Am Vet Med Assoc 1978;173:296–298.

14. Barsanti JA, Finco DR. Laboratory findings in urinary tract infections. Vet Clin North Am Small Anim Pract 1979;9:729–748.

15. Lees GE, Simpson RB, Green RA. Results of analyses and bacterial cultures of urine specimens obtained from clinically normal cats by three methods. J Am Vet Med Assoc 1984;184:449–454.

16. Padilla J, Osborne CA, Ward GE. Effects of storage time and temperature on quantitative culture of canine urine. J Am Vet Med Assoc 1981;178:1077–1081.

17. Ling GV, Biberstein EL, Hirsh DC. Bacterial pathogens associated with urinary tract infections. Vet Clin North Am Small Anim Pract 1979;9:617–630.

18. Ling GV. Therapeutic strategies involving antimicrobial treatment of the canine urinary tract. J Am Vet Med Assoc 1984;185:1162–1164.

19. Lees GE, Rogers KS. Diagnosis and localization of urinary tract infection. In: Kirk RW, ed. Current Veterinary Therapy IX. Philadelphia, WB Saunders, 1986:1118–1123.

20. Allen TA, Jones RL, Purvance J. Microbiologic evaluation of canine urine: Direct microscopic examination and preservation of specimen quality for culture. J Am Vet Med Assoc 1987;190:1289–1291.

21. Park RD. The urinary bladder. In: Thrall DE, ed. Textbook of Veterinary Diagnostic Radiology. Philadelphia, WB Saunders, 1994:459–474.

22. Pechman RD. The urethra. In: Thrall DE, ed. Textbook of Veterinary Diagnostic Radiology. Philadelphia, WB Saunders, 1994:475–478.

23. Tvedten H. Cytology of neoplastic and inflammatory masses. In: Willard MD, Tvedten H, Turnwald GH, eds. Small Animal Clinical Diagnosis by Laboratory Methods, 2nd ed. Philadelphia, WB Saunders, 1994:321–341.

24. Melhoff T, Osborne CA. Catheter biopsy of the urethra, urinary bladder, and prostate gland. In: Kirk RW, ed. Current Veterinary Therapy VII. Philadelphia, WB Saunders, 1977:1173–1175.

25. Lees GE, Forrester SD. Update: Bacterial urinary tract infections. In: Kirk RW, Bonagura JD, eds. Kirk's Current Veterinary Therapy XI. Philadelphia, WB Saunders, 1992:909–914.

26. Kivisto AK, Vasenius H, Sandholm M. Canine bacteriuria. J Small Anim Pract 1977;18:707–712.

27. Bush BM. A review of the etiology and consequences of urinary tract infections in the dog. Br Vet J 1976;132:632–641.

28. Lees GE. Epidemiology of naturally occurring feline bacterial urinary tract infections. Vet Clin North Am Small Anim Pract 1984;14:471–479.

29. Kruger JM, Osborne CA, Goyal SM, et al. Clinical evaluation of cats with lower urinary tract disease. J Am Vet Med Assoc 1991;199:211–216.

30. Wooley RE, Blue JL. Quantitative and bacteriological studies of urine specimens from canine and feline urinary tract infections. J Clin Microbiol 1976;4:326–329.

31. Ling GV. Treatment of urinary tract infections. Vet Clin North Am Small Anim Pract 1979;9:795–804.

32. Brown SA, Barsanti JA. Diseases of the bladder and urethra. In: Ettinger SJ, ed. Textbook of Veterinary Internal Medicine, 3rd ed. Philadelphia, WB Saunders, 1989:2108–2141.

33. Osborne CA, Klausner JS, Lees GE. Urinary tract infections: Normal and abnormal host defense mechanisms. Vet Clin North Am Small Anim Pract 1979;9:587–609.

34. Lees GE, Osborne CA. Antibacterial properties of urine: A comparative review. J Am Anim Hosp Assoc 1979;15:125–132.

35. Biertuempfel PH, Ling GV, Ling GA. Urinary tract infection resulting from catheterization in healthy adult dogs. J Am Vet Med Assoc 1981;178:989–991.

36. Barsanti JA, Blue J, Edmunds J. Urinary tract infection due to indwelling bladder catheters in dogs and cats. J Am Vet Med Assoc 1985;187:384–388.

37. Lees GE, Osborne CA. Adverse effects of open indwelling urethral catheterization in clinically normal male cats. Am J Vet Res 1981;42:825–833.

38. Gregory CR, Vasseur PB. Long-term examination of cats with perineal urethrostomy. Vet Surg 1983;12:210–212.

39. Klausner JS, Osborne CA. Urinary tract infection and urolithiasis. Vet Clin North Am Small Anim Pract 1979;9:701–711.

40. Smith CW, Schiller AG. Perineal urethrostomy in the cat: A retrospective study of complications. J Am Anim Hosp Assoc 1978;14:225–228.

41. Lorenz MD. Diagnosis and medical management of canine Cushing's syndrome: A study of 57 consecutive cases. J Am Anim Hosp Assoc 1982;18:707–716.

42. Ling GV. Management of urinary tract infections. In: Kirk RW, ed. Current Veterinary Therapy IX. Philadelphia, WB Saunders, 1986:1174–1177.

43. Ling GV, Gilmore CJ. Penicillin G or ampicillin for oral treatment of canine urinary tract infections. J Am Vet Med Assoc 1977;171:358–361.

44. Ling GV, Ruby AL. Chloramphenicol for oral treatment of canine urinary tract infections. J Am Vet Med Assoc 1978;172:914–916.

45. Ling GV, Ruby AL. Trimethoprim in combination with

a sulfonamide for oral treatment of canine urinary tract infections. J Am Vet Med Assoc 1979;174:1003–1005.

46. Ling GV, Creighton SR, Ruby AL. Tetracycline for oral treatment of canine urinary tract infection caused by *Pseudomonas aeruginosa*. J Am Vet Med Assoc 1981;179: 578–579.

47. Ling GV, Ruby AL. Cephalexin for oral treatment of canine urinary tract infection caused by *Klebsiella pneumoniae*. J Am Vet Med Assoc 1983;182:1346–1347.

48. Ling GV, Rohrich PJ, Ruby AL, et al. Canine urinary tract infections: A comparison of in vitro antimicrobial susceptibility test results and response to oral therapy with ampicillin or with trimethoprim-sulfa. J Am Vet Med Assoc 1984;185:277–281.

49. Rohrich PJ, Ling GV, Ruby AL, et al. In vitro susceptibilities of canine urinary bacteria to selected antimicrobial agents. J Am Vet Med Assoc 1983;183:863–867.

50. Kilgore WR. β-Lactamase inhibition: A new approach in overcoming bacterial resistance. Compen Contin Educ Pract Vet 1986;8:325–331.

51. Neer TM. Clinical pharmacologic features of fluoroquinolone antimicrobial drugs. J Am Vet Med Assoc 1988;193:577–580.

52. Senior DF, Gaskin JM, Buergelt CD, et al. Amoxycillin and clavulanic acid combination in the treatment of experimentally induced bacterial cystitis in cats. Res Vet Sci 1985;39:42–46.

53. Budsberg SC, Walker RD, Slusser P, et al. Norfloxacin therapy in infections of the canine urogenital tract caused by multiresistant bacteria. J Am Anim Hosp Assoc 1989;25:713–716.

54. Childs SJ, Goldstein EJC. Ciprofloxacin as treatment for genitourinary tract infection. J Urol 1989;141:1–5.

55. Hooper DC, Wolfson JS. Fluoroquinolone antimicrobial agents. N Engl J Med 1991;324 384–394.

56. Barsanti JA, Finco DR. Canine prostatic diseases. In: Ettinger SJ, ed. Textbook of Veterinary Internal Medicine, 3rd ed. Philadelphia, WB Saunders, 1989:1859–1880.

57. Rogers KS, Lees GE. Management of urinary tract infections. In: Kirk RW, ed. Current Veterinary Therapy X. Philadelphia, WB Saunders, 1989:1204–1209.

58. Lees GE, Osborne CA. Use and misuse of indwelling urinary catheters in cats. Vet Clin North Am Small Anim Pract 1984;14:599–608.

59. Barsanti JA, Shotts EB, Crowell WA, et al. Effect of therapy on susceptibility to urinary tract infection in male cats with indwelling urethral catheters. J Vet Intern Med 1992;6:64–70.

60. Lees GE, Osborne CA. Urinary tract infections associated with the use and misuse of urinary catheters. Vet Clin North Am Small Anim Pract 1979;9:713–727.

61. Osborne CA, Polzin DJ, Johnston GR, et al. Canine urolithiasis. In: Ettinger SJ, ed. Textbook of Veterinary Internal Medicine, 3rd ed. Philadelphia, WB Saunders, 1989:2083–2107.

62. Finco DR, Rosen E, Johnson KH. Canine urolithiasis: A review of 133 clinical and 23 necropsy cases. J Am Vet Med Assoc 1970;157:1225–1228.

63. Brown NO, Parks JL, Greene RW. Canine urolithiasis:

Retrospective analysis of 438 cases. J Am Vet Med Assoc 1977;170:414–418.

64. Osborne CA, Clinton CW, Bamman LK, et al. Prevalence of canine uroliths. Vet Clin North Am Small Anim Pract 1986;16:27–44.

65. Case LC, Ling GV, Franti CE, et al. Cystine-containing urinary calculi in dogs: 102 cases (1981–1989). J Am Vet Med Assoc 1992;201:129–133.

66. Bartges JW, Osborne CA, Lulich JP, et al. Prevalence of cystine and urate uroliths in bulldogs and urate uroliths in Dalmatians. J Am Vet Med Assoc 1994; 204:1914–1918.

67. Ling GV, Ruby AL, Harrold DR, et al. Xanthine-containing urinary calculi in dogs given allopurinol. J Am Vet Med Assoc 1991;198:1935–1940.

68. Case LC, Ling GV, Ruby AL, et al. Urolithiasis in Dalmatians: 275 cases (1981–1990). J Am Vet Med Assoc 1993;203:96–100.

69. Cornelius CE, Bishop JA, Schaffer MH. A quantitative study of amino aciduria in dachshunds with a history of cystine urolithiasis. Cornell Vet 1967;57:177–183.

70. Osborne CA, Clinton CW, Kim KM, et al. Etiopathogenesis, clinical manifestations, and management of canine silica urolithiasis. Vet Clin North Am Small Anim Pract 1986;16:185–207.

71. Lulich JP, Osborne CA, Unger LK, et al. Prevalence of calcium oxalate uroliths in miniature schnauzers. Am J Vet Res 1991;52:1579–1582.

72. Lulich JP, Osborne CA, Parker ML, et al. Canine calcium oxalate urolithiasis. In: Kirk RW, ed. Current Veterinary Therapy X. Philadelphia, WB Saunders, 1989:1182–1188.

73. Klausner JS, Osborne CA, O'Leary TP, et al. Struvite urolithiasis in a litter of miniature schnauzer dogs. Am J Vet Res 1980;41:712–719.

74. Klausner JS, Osborne CA, Clinton CW, et al. Mineral composition of urinary calculi from miniature schnauzer dogs. J Am Vet Med Assoc 1981;178:1082–1083.

75. Hardy RM, Osborne CA, Cassidy FC, et al. Urolithiasis in immature dogs. Vet Med Small Anim Clin 1972;67: 1205–1211.

76. Lulich JP, Osborne CA, Bartges JW, et al. Canine lower urinary tract disorders. In: Ettinger SJ, Feldman EC, eds. Textbook of Veterinary Internal Medicine, 4th ed. Philadelphia, WB Saunders, 1995:1833–1861.

77. Osborne CA, Klausner JS, Polzin DJ, et al. Etiopathogenesis of canine struvite urolithiasis. Vet Clin North Am Small Anim Pract 1986;16:67–86.

78. Foreman JW. Renal handling of urate and other organic acids. In: Bovee KC, ed. Canine Nephrology. Media, PA. Harwal Publishing, 1984:135–151.

79. Marretta SM, Pask AJ, Greene RW, et al. Urinary calculi associated with portosystemic shunts in six dogs. J Am Vet Med Assoc 1981;178:133–137.

80. Senior DF. Medical management of urate uroliths. In: Kirk RW, ed. Current Veterinary Therapy X. Philadelphia, WB Saunders, 1989:1178–1181.

81. Lulich JP, Osborne CA, Nagode LA, et al. Evaluation of urine and serum metabolites in miniature schnauzers with calcium oxalate urolithiasis. Am J Vet Res 1991;52: 1583–1590.

82. Klausner JS, O'Leary TP, Osborne CA. Calcium uro-

lithiasis in two dogs with parathyroid adenomas. J Am Vet Med Assoc 1987;191:1423–1426.

83. Bovee KC, Thier SO, Rea C, et al. Renal clearance of amino acids in canine cystinuria. Metabolism 1974;23: 51–58.

84. Bovee KC. Canine cystine urolithiasis. Vet Clin North Am Small Anim Pract 1986;16:211–215.

85. Klausner JS, Osborne CA. Canine calcium phosphate uroliths. Vet Clin North Am Small Anim Pract 1986;16: 171–184.

86. Polzin DJ, Osborne CA, Bell FW. Canine distal renal tubular acidosis and urolithiasis. Vet Clin North Am Small Anim Pract 1986;16:241–250.

87. Bartges JW, Osborne CA, Felice LJ. Canine xanthine uroliths: Risk factor management. In: Kirk RW, Bonagura JD, eds. Kirk's Current Veterinary Therapy XI. Philadelphia, WB Saunders, 1992:900–905.

88. Osborne CA, Klausner JS, Clinton CW. Analysis of canine and feline uroliths. In: Kirk RW, ed. Current Veterinary Therapy VIII. Philadelphia, WB Saunders, 1983:1061–1066.

89. Caywood DD, Osborne CA. Surgical removal of canine uroliths. Vet Clin North Am Small Anim Pract 1986;16: 389–407.

90. Osborne CA, Polzin DJ, Kruger JM, et al. Medical dissolution and prevention of canine struvite uroliths. In: Kirk RW, ed. Current Veterinary Therapy IX. Philadelphia, WB Saunders, 1986:1177–1187.

91. Abdullahi SU, Osborne CA, Lenninger JL, et al. Evaluation of a calculolytic diet in female dogs with induced struvite urolithiasis. Am J Vet Res 1984;45:459–469.

92. Bailie NC, Osborne CA, Leininger JR, et al. Teratogenic effect of acetohydroxamic acid in clinically normal beagles. Am J Vet Res 1986;47:2604–2611.

93. Grauer GF. Canine urolithiasis. In: Nelson RW, Couto CG, ed. Essentials of Small Animal Internal Medicine, St Louis, Mosby–Year Book, 1992:501–508.

94. Frimpter GW, Thouin P, Ewalds BH. Penicillamine in canine cystinuria. J Am Vet Med Assoc 1967;151:1084–1086.

95. Osborne CA, Kruger JM, Johnston GR, et al. Feline lower urinary tract disorders. In: Ettinger SJ, ed. Textbook of Veterinary Internal Medicine, 3rd ed. Philadelphia, WB Saunders, 1989:2057–2082.

96. Willeberg P. Epidemiology of naturally occurring feline urologic syndrome. Vet Clin North Am Small Anim Pract 1984;14:455–469.

97. Lawler DF, Sjolin DW, Collins JE. Incidence rates of feline lower urinary tract disease in the United States. Fel Pract 1985;15:13–16.

98. Walker AD, Weaver AD, Anderson RS, et al. An epidemiological survey of feline urological syndrome. J Small Anim Pract 1977;18:283–301.

99. Ling GV, Franti CE, Ruby AL, et al. Epizootiologic evaluation and quantitative analysis of urinary calculi from 150 cats. J Am Vet Med Assoc 1990;196:1459–1462.

100. Osborne CA, Lulich JP, Bartges JW, et al. Feline metabolic uroliths: Risk factor management. In: Kirk RW, Bonagura JD, eds. Kirk's Current Veterinary Therapy XI. Philadelphia, WB Saunders, 1992:905–909.

101. Hesse A, Sanders G. A survey of urolithiasis in cats. J Small Anim Pract 1985;26:465–476.

102. Osborne CA, Kruger JM, Lulich JP, et al. Feline lower urinary tract diseases: State of the science. Waltham/OSU Symposium for the Treatment of Small Animal Diseases 1992;16:89–98.

103. Osborne CA, Poffenbarger EM, Klausner JS, et al. Etiopathogenesis, clinical manifestations, and management of canine calcium oxalate urolithiasis. Vet Clin North Am Small Anim Pract 1986;16:133–170.

104. Barsanti JA, Finco DR, Shotts EB, et al. Feline urologic syndrome: Further investigation into etiology. J Am Anim Hosp Assoc 1982;18:391–395.

105. Kruger JM, Osborne CA. The role of viruses in feline lower urinary tract disease. J Vet Intern Med 1990;4: 71–78.

106. Finco DR, Barsanti JA, Crowell WA. Characterization of magnesium-induced urinary disease in the cat and comparison with feline urologic syndrome. Am J Vet Res 1985;46:391–400.

107. Finco DR, Barsanti JA. Diet-induced feline urethral obstruction. Vet Clin North Am Small Anim Pract 1984;14:529–536.

108. Burrows CF, Bovee KC. Characterization and treatment of acid-base and renal defects due to urethral obstruction in cats. J Am Vet Med Assoc 1978;172:801–805.

109. Ross LA. Treating FUS in unobstructed cats and preventing its recurrence. Vet Med 1990;85:1218–1222.

110. Osborne CA, Lulich JP, Kruger JM, et al. Medical dissolution of feline struvite urocystoliths. J Am Vet Med Assoc 1990;196:1053–1063.

111. Osborne CA, Kruger JM, Lulich JP, et al. Feline lower urinary tract disorders. In: Ettinger SJ, Feldman EC, eds. Textbook of Veterinary Internal Medicine, 4th ed. Philadelphia, WB Saunders, 1995:1805–1832.

112. Osborne CA, Lees GE, Polzin DJ, et al. Immediate relief of feline urethral obstruction. Vet Clin North Am Small Anim Pract 1984;14:585–597.

113. Ross LA. The protocol for treating cats with urethral obstructions. Vet Med 1990;85:1206–1214.

114. Lees GE, Osborne CA, Stevens JB, et al. Adverse effects caused by polypropylene and polyvinyl feline urinary catheters. Am J Vet Res 1980;41:1836–1840.

115. Lees GE, Moreau PM. Management of hypotonic and atonic urinary bladders in cats. Vet Clin North Am Small Anim Pract 1984;14:641–547.

116. Barsanti JA, Finco DR, Brown SA. Feline urethral obstruction: Medical management. In: Kirk RW, Bonagura JD, eds. Kirk's Current Veterinary Therapy XI. Philadelphia, WB Saunders, 1992:883–885.

117. Moreau PM, Lappin MR. Pharmacologic management of urinary incontinence. In: Kirk RW, ed. Current Veterinary Therapy X. Philadelphia, WB Saunders, 1989:1214–1222.

118. Stone EA, Barsanti JA. Urologic Surgery of the Dog and Cat. Philadelphia, Lea & Febiger, 1992:135–139.

119. Osborne CA, Caywood DD, Johnston GR, et al. Feline perineal urethrostomy. A potential cause of hematuria, dysuria, and urethral obstruction. In: Kirk RW, ed. Current Veterinary Therapy X. Philadelphia, WB Saunders, 1989:1209–1213.

120. Stone EA, Barsanti JA. Urologic Surgery of the Dog and Cat. Philadelphia, Lea & Febiger, 1992:140–142.

121. Bovee KC, Reif JS, Maguire TG, et al. Recurrence of feline urethral obstruction. J Am Vet Med Assoc 1979;174:93–96.

122. Osborne CA, Low DG, Perman V, et al. Neoplasms of the canine and feline urinary bladder: Incidence, etiologic factors, occurrence, and pathologic features. Am J Vet Res 1968;29:2041–2055.

123. Hayes HM. Canine bladder cancer: Epidemiologic features. Am J Epidemiol 1976;104:673–677.

124. Burnie AG, Weaver AD. Urinary bladder neoplasia in the dog: A review of seventy cases. J Small Anim Pract 1983;24:129–143.

125. Wimberly HC, Lewis RM. Transitional cell carcinoma in the domestic cat. Vet Pathol 1979;16:223–228.

126. Engle GC, Brodey RS. A retrospective study of 395 feline neoplasms. J Am Anim Hosp Assoc 1969;5:21–31.

127. Norris AM, Laing EJ, Vallie VEO, et al. Canine bladder and urethral tumors: A retrospective study of 115 cases (1980–1985). J Vet Intern Med 1992;6:145–153.

128. Tarvin G, Patnaik A, Greene R. Primary urethral tumors in dogs. J Am Vet Med Assoc 1978;172:931–933.

129. Wilson GP, Hayes HH, Casey HW. Canine urethral cancer. J Am Anim Hosp Assoc 1979;15:741–744.

130. Schwarz PD, Greene RW, Patnaik AK. Urinary bladder tumors in the cat: A review of 27 cases. J Am Anim Hosp Assoc 1985;21:237–245.

131. Van Vechten M, Goldschmidt MH, Wortman JA. Embryonal rhabdomyocarcoma of the urinary bladder in dogs. Compen Contin Educ Pract Vet 1990;12:783–793.

132. Senior DF, Lawrence DT, Gunson C, et al. Successful treatment of botryoid rhabdomyosarcoma in the bladder of a dog. Compen Contin Educ Pract Vet 1993;29:386–390.

133. Roszel JF. Cytology of urine from dogs with botryoid sarcoma of the bladder. Acta Cytologica 1972;16:443–446.

134. Kelly DF. Rhabdomyosarcoma of the urinary bladder in dogs. Vet Pathol 1973;10:375–384.

135. Halliwell WH, Ackerman N. Botryoid rhabdomyosarcoma of the urinary bladder and hypertrophic osteoarthropathy in a young dog. J Am Vet Med Assoc 1974;165:911–913.

136. Strafuss AC, Dean MJ. Neoplasms of the canine urinary bladder. J Am Vet Med Assoc 1975;166:1161–1163.

137. Weller RE, Wolf AM, Oyejide A. Transitional cell carcinoma of the bladder associated with cyclophosphamide therapy in a dog. J Am Anim Hosp Assoc 1979;15:733–736.

138. Macy DW, Withrow SJ, Hoopes J. Transitional cell carcinoma of the bladder associated with cyclophosphamide. J Am Anim Hosp Assoc 1983;19:965–969.

139. Hueper WC, Wiley FH, Wofle HD. Experimental production of bladder tumors in dogs by administration of beta-naphthylamine. J Indus Hyg Toxicol 1938;20:46–84.

140. Radomski JL, Glass EM, Diechmann WB. Transitional cell hyperplasia in the bladders of dogs fed DL-tryptophan. Cancer Res 1971;31:1690–1692.

141. Brown RR, Price JM. Quantitative studies on metabo-

lites of tryptophan in the urine of the dog, cat, and man. J Biol Chem 1956;219:985–997.

142. Esplin DG. Urinary bladder fibromas in dogs: 51 cases (1981–1985). J Am Vet Med Assoc 1987;190:440–444.

143. Mandel M. Hypertrophic osteoarthropathy secondary to neurofibrosarcoma of the urinary bladder in a Cocker Spaniel. Vet Med Small Anim Clin 1975;70:1307–1308.

144. Brodey RS, Riser WH, Allen H. Hypertrophic pulmonary osteoarthropathy in a dog with carcinoma of the urinary bladder. J Am Vet Med Assoc 1973;162:474–478.

145. Brodey RS. Hypertrophic osteoarthropathy in the dog: A clinicopathologic survey of 60 cases. J Am Vet Med Assoc 1971;159:1242–1256.

146. Gilson SD. Diagnosis and medical therapy of urinary tract neoplasia. In: Stone EA, Barsanti JA, eds. Urologic Surgery of the Dog and Cat, Philadelphia, Lea & Febiger, 1992:237–243.

147. Gilson SD. Surgical therapy for urinary tract neoplasia. In: Stone EA, Barsanti JA, eds. Urologic Surgery of the Dog and Cat, Philadelphia, Lea & Febiger, 1992:244–251.

148. Gilson SD, Stone EA. Surgically induced tumor seeding in eight dogs and two cats. J Am Vet Med Assoc 1990;196:1811–1815.

149. Crow SE. Urinary tract neoplasms in dogs and cats. Compen Contin Educ Pract Vet 1985;7:607–618.

150. Brearley MJ, Thatcher C, Cooper JE. Three cases of transitional cell carcinoma in the cat and a review of the literature. Vet Rec 1986;118:91–94.

151. Stone EA, Withrow SJ, Page RL, et al. Ureterocolonic anastomosis in ten dogs with transitional cell carcinoma. Vet Surg 1988;17:147–153.

152. Helfand SC, Hamilton TA, Hungerfor LL, et al. Comparison of three treatments for transitional cell carcinoma of the bladder in the dog. J Am Anim Hosp Assoc 1994;30:270–275.

153. Withrow SJ, Gillette EL, Hoopes PJ, et al. Intraoperative irradiation of 16 spontaneously occurring canine neoplasms. Vet Surg 1989;18:7–11.

154. Walker M, Breider M. Intraoperative radiotherapy of canine bladder cancer. Vet Radiol 1987;28:200–204.

155. Rogers KS, Walker MA. Therapy of transitional cell carcinoma of the canine bladder. In: Kirk RW, Bonagura JD, eds. Kirk's Current Veterinary Therapy XI. Philadelphia, WB Saunders, 1992:919–922.

156. Moore AS, Cardona A, Shapiro W, et al. Cisplatin cis-diamminedichloroplatinum) for treatment of transitional cell carcinoma of the urinary bladder and urethra. J Vet Intern Med 1990;4:148–152.

157. Shapiro W, Kitchell BE, Fossum TW, et al. Cisplatin for treatment of transitional cell and squamous cell carcinomas in dogs. J Am Vet Med Assoc 1988;193:1530–1533.

158. Knapp DW, Richardson RC, Bonney PL, et al. Cisplatin therapy in 41 dogs with malignant tumors. J Vet Intern Med 1988;2:41–46.

159. Hutson CA, Degen LA, Rackear DG. Preliminary results of carboplatin toxicity and efficacy in 12 canines and 4 felines. Proc Vet Cancer Soc Annual Meeting 1990;87–88.

160. Kraegel SA, Page RL. Advances in platinum compound chemotherapy. In: Kirk RW, Bonagura JD, eds. Kirk's Current Veterinary Therapy XI. Philadelphia, WB Saunders, 1992:395–399.

161. Knapp DW, Richardson RC, Bottoms GD, et al. Phase I trial of piroxicam in 62 dogs bearing naturally occurring tumors. Cancer Chemother Pharmacol 1992;29:214–218.

162. Knapp DW, Richardson RC, Chan TCK, et al. Piroxicam therapy in 34 dogs with transitional cell carcinoma of the urinary bladder. J Vet Intern Med 1994;8:273–278.

163. Arnold S, Arnold P, Hubler M, et al. Incontinentia urinae bei der kastrierten huendin: haeufigkeit und rassedisposition. Schweiz Arch Tierheilkd 1989;131:259–263.

164. Richter KP, Ling GV. Clinical response and urethral pressure profile changes after phenylpropanolamine in dogs with primary sphincter incompetence. J Am Vet Med Assoc 1985;187:605–611.

165. Holt PE. Urinary incontinence in the bitch due to sphincter mechanism incompetence: Prevalence in referred dogs and retrospective analysis of sixty cases. J Small Anim Pract 1985;26:181–190.

166. Creed KE. Effect of hormones on urethral sensitivity to phenylephrine in normal and incontinent dogs. Res Vet Sci 1983;34:177–181.

167. Chew DJ, DiBartola SP, Fenner WR. Pharmacologic manipulation of urination. In: Kirk RW, ed. Current Veterinary Therapy IX. Philadelphia, WB Saunders, 1986:1207–1212.

168. Holt PE. Urinary incontinence in the bitch due to sphincter mechanism incompetence: Surgical treatment. J Small Anim Pract 1985;26:237–246.

169. Arnold S, Jaeger P, DiBartola SP, et al. Treatment of urinary incontinence in dogs by endoscopic injection of Teflon. J Am Vet Med Assoc 1989;195:1369–1374.

170. Kolata RJ, Johnston DE. Motor vehicle accidents in urban dogs: A study of 600 cases. J Am Vet Med Assoc 1975;167:938–941.

171. Selcer BA. Urinary tract trauma associated with pelvic trauma. J Am Anim Hosp Assoc 1982;18:785–793.

172. Meynard JA. Traumatic rupture of the bladder in the dog. A clinical sutdy of nine cases. J Small Anim Pract 1961;2:131–134.

173. Burrows CF, Bovee KC. Metabolic changes due to experimentally induced rupture of the canine urinary bladder. Am J Vet Res 1974;35:1083–1088.

174. Kleine LJ, Thornton GW. Radiographic diagnosis of urinary tract trauma. J Am Anim Hosp Assoc 1971;7:318–327.

175. Stone EA, Barsanti JA. Urologic Surgery of the Dog and Cat. Philadelphia, Lea & Febiger, 1992:185–188.

176. Crow SE, Thielen GH, Madewell BR, et al. Cyclophosphamide-induced cystitis in the dog and cat. J Am Vet Med Assoc 1977;171:259–262.

177. Peterson JL, Couto CG, Hammer AS. Acute sterile hemorrhagic cystitis after a single intravenous administration of cyclophosphamide in three dogs. J Am Vet Med Assoc 1992;201:1572–1574.

178. Laing EJ, Miller CW, Cochrane SM. Treatment of cyclophosphamide-induced hemorrhagic cystitis in five dogs. J Am Vet Med Assoc 1988;193:233–236.

179. Johnston SD, Osborne CA, Stevens JB. Canine polypoid cystitis. J Am Vet Med Assoc 1975;166:1155–1160.

180. Senior DF, Solomon GB, Goldschmidt MH, et al. *Capillaria plica* infection in dogs. J Am Vet Med Assoc 1980;176:901–905.

181. Wilson-Hanson S, Prescott CW. *Capillaria* in the bladder of the domestic cat. Aust Vet J 1982;59:190–191.

182. Sinibaldi KR, Green RW. Surgical correction of prolapse of the male urethra in three English bulldogs. J Am Anim Hosp Assoc 1973;9:450–453.

183. Firestone WM. Prolapse of the male urethra. J Am Vet Med Assoc 1941;99:135.

Chapter 18

Diseases of the Prostate

S. Dru Forrester
Beverly J. Purswell

Anatomy and Physiology

The prostate gland is the only accessory sex gland in male dogs; it is a bilobed organ with a medial septum on its dorsal surface.[1] The prostate gland is located predominately in the retroperitoneal space, just caudal to the urinary bladder. With age, the gland enlarges and is located in the caudal abdominal cavity. The prostate gland encircles the proximal urethra, and its ducts enter the urethra throughout its circumference. Histologically, the prostate gland is composed of epithelial and stromal or connective tissue cells; after sexual maturity, epithelial cells predominate.

The primary function of the prostate gland is production of prostatic fluid, which serves as a transport medium for sperm during ejaculation. A small amount of fluid is released from the prostate gland constantly; this fluid enters the urinary bladder (prostatic fluid reflux) if neither ejaculation nor urination occurs.

The prostate gland of normal dogs increases in weight with aging.[2] In order to grow and maintain its size, the prostate gland requires testosterone. Prostatic growth is inhibited in dogs that are castrated before sexual maturity.[3] If adult dogs are castrated, the prostate gland decreases to 20% of its normal adult size.[4]

Problem Identification

Stranguria and Dysuria

Stranguria and dysuria occur with diseases of the lower urogenital tract. Prostatic diseases that cause moderate to marked prostatomegaly and partial urethral obstruction, such as abscesses, paraprostatic cysts, or neoplasia, may cause stranguria or dysuria. Benign prostatic hyperplasia (BPH) usually does not cause dysuria because the canine prostate enlarges outwardly, away from the urethral lumen.[1] For a complete discussion of stranguria and dysuria, see Chapter 17.

Discolored Urine

Discolored urine may occur secondary to many disorders of the urogenital tract. Dogs with prostatic disease may have discolored urine, which is most often red or reddish-brown as a result of prostatic hemorrhage. For a complete discussion of discolored urine, see Chapter 17.

Urinary Incontinence

Urinary incontinence may result from neurogenic or non-neurogenic disorders. Partial urethral obstruction from disorders that cause prostatomegaly

Table 18–1
Causes of Urethral Discharge in Dogs

Prostatic Disorders
Benign hyperplasia
Acute prostatitis
Chronic prostatitis
Abscessation
Neoplasia
Cysts
Abacterial hemorrhage

Urethral Disorders
Trauma
Neoplasia
Urolithiasis
Foreign bodies
Urethral prolapse

Systemic Disorders
Thrombocytopenia
von Willebrand's disease

may lead to dysfunction of the detrusor muscle and urethral sphincter and subsequent urinary incontinence. Dogs with prostatic disease may have urodynamic abnormalities (e.g., decreased urethral pressures), even in the absence of urinary incontinence.[5] For a complete discussion of urinary incontinence, see Chapter 27.

Urethral Discharge

Urethral discharge is abnormal drainage of blood, purulent exudate, serous fluid, or urine from the urethral orifice.

Pathophysiology

Any disorder of the distal urethra or prostate gland may cause urethral discharge (Table 18–1).[6] Infectious, neoplastic, and traumatic disorders are most common. Infrequently, systemic coagulopathies such as platelet abnormalities may cause hemorrhagic urethral discharge.

Clinical Signs

Patients may have a history of either intermittent or persistent urethral discharge. Depending on the underlying cause, other historical findings may include tenesmus, dysuria, stranguria, discolored urine, and abdominal distention. Urinalysis results may be normal or may reveal hematuria, pyuria, or bacteriuria. Patients with hemorrhagic urethral discharge caused by coagulopathies may have hemorrhage elsewhere (e.g., mucosal petechiae, ecchymoses).

Diagnostic Plan

The initial step is to perform a physical examination, which should include thorough evaluation of the prepuce and the entire penis for evidence of urethral prolapse, trauma, or neoplastic masses. Abdominal palpation may reveal a caudal abdominal mass with moderate to marked prostatomegaly, especially with paraprostatic cysts. Rectal examination is indicated to identify prostatic abnormalities (e.g., enlargement, pain, asymmetry). Next, it is important to determine whether the discharge is hemorrhagic, purulent, or serous; in addition to gross characteristics, cytologic evaluation of the discharge is necessary. Urethral trauma, uroliths, prolapse, neoplasia, and most prostatic diseases usually cause hemorrhagic discharge. Purulent urethral discharge most often results from prostatic infection, abscess, or neoplasia, although inflammatory urethral disorders (e.g., urolithiasis, neoplasia) also may be a cause. Serous urethral discharge most often occurs with prostatic cysts. At times, it may be difficult to distinguish between urethral discharge and urinary incontinence on the basis of history. Urine collected by cystocentesis should be evaluated in all patients with urethral discharge. Comparison of the results of analysis of the urethral discharge with results of urinalysis may help determine the source of discharge (e.g., urethra versus urinary bladder or prostate gland). Analysis of urine collected by cystocentesis often is normal in patients with urethral disease alone, whereas patients with prostatic or urinary bladder diseases often have abnormal findings such as hematuria, pyuria, bacteriuria, or crystalluria.

Additional diagnostic tests may be indicated depending on results of history and physical examination. Patients with urethral diseases usually have other abnormal findings such as dysuria and stranguria. In these cases, evaluation should include plain and contrast radiographs (e.g., cystourethrography) to rule out fractured os penis, uroliths, and neoplasia (see Chap. 17 for technique). The most common cause of hemorrhagic urethral discharge in the absence of other clinical findings is BPH. Additional diagnostic tests are indicated in dogs with suspected prostatic disease (see Prostatomegaly and Diagnostic Procedures).

Tenesmus

Tenesmus usually occurs as a result of large bowel diseases; however, rectal compression resulting from prostatomegaly from any cause also may be associated with tenesmus. In some dogs with prostatic hyperplasia, tenesmus is the only abnormal clinical finding.[1] For a complete discussion of this problem, see Chapter 32.

Abdominal Distention

Abdominal distention or enlargement results from organomegaly, abdominal fluid accumulation, abdominal fat, or abdominal muscle weakness. Marked prostatomegaly, especially because of paraprostatic cysts, may cause caudal abdominal distention. For a complete discussion of abdominal distention, see Chapter 34.

Prostatomegaly

Prostatomegaly is abnormal enlargement of the prostate gland.

Pathophysiology

Prostatomegaly may result from changes in prostatic epithelium (i.e., hyperplasia, hypertrophy, or metaplasia), infectious disorders (e.g., abscess), neoplasia, or cystic disease (e.g., cystic hyperplasia, paraprostatic cysts).[7] With aging, the canine prostate gland is subject to hyperplasia and enlargement, which may occur secondary to increased sensitivity of the gland to testosterone.[2] By 9 years of age, more than 95% of dogs may have prostatic hyperplasia.[8] Squamous metaplasia of the prostate occurs secondary to hyperestrogenism, either from endogenous sources such as testicular Sertoli cell tumors or from exogenous administration of estrogen. Prostatic infection may occur secondary to bacteria ascending from the urethra, spread of bacteria from infected urine, or hematogenous spread of bacteria. Although acute and chronic bacterial prostatitis often do not cause prostatomegaly, they may lead to development of prostatic abscesses, which do cause prostatic enlargement.[7] Neoplasia of prostatic epithelium (e.g., adenocarcinoma) and extension of tumors from the urethra or urinary bladder (e.g., transitional cell carcinoma) also cause prostatomegaly.

Clinical Signs

Historical and clinical findings in patients with prostatomegaly may include hemorrhagic, purulent, or serous urethral discharge, tenesmus, discolored urine, abdominal distention, stranguria, or dysuria.[9–11] Patients with prostatitis, abscesses, or neoplasia may have systemic signs such as lethargy, depression, inappetence, weight loss, abnormal gait, and fever.[9, 10, 12]

Diagnostic Plan

Initial evaluation of patients with prostatomegaly depends on signalment and the presence of clinical signs. Rectal examination is indicated to evaluate prostatic size, symmetry, consistency, moveability, and presence of pain; other structures, such as caudal abdominal lymph nodes, also should be evaluated for enlargement. After the prostate gland is located abdominally, palpation is facilitated by placing a hand on the abdomen and using it to move the prostate gland caudally so that it can be evaluated during rectal examination. Diseases associated with severe prostatomegaly include paraprostatic cysts, abscess, and neoplasia, whereas diseases associated with mild to moderate prostatomegaly include benign hyperplasia and squamous metaplasia.[13] Dogs with prostatitis usually do not have prostatomegaly, although acute prostatitis often causes pain on palpation. Symmetrical prostatic enlargement occurs with BPH and squamous metaplasia, whereas asymmetrical prostatomegaly with areas of variable consistency occurs with neoplasia, paraprostatic cysts, and abscess.[1] Older, intact male dogs often have mild prostatomegaly caused by benign hyperplasia with no other clinical signs, and additional diagnostic evaluation is not necessary; however, the owner should be informed of the potential for development of other prostatic disorders.

If clinical signs other than prostatomegaly exist (e.g., urethral discharge, dysuria, stranguria, discolored urine), or if prostatomegaly is detected in a castrated dog, further diagnostic tests are indicated to determine the underlying cause. Results of complete blood count (CBC) and serum chemistries should be determined in patients with systemic signs such as depression, dehydration, vomiting, and fever. Dogs with BPH and chronic bacterial prostatitis often have normal results of CBC and serum chemistries.[1] Patients with prostatic abscess, acute prostatitis, paraprostatic cysts, and, less commonly, prostatic neoplasia may have leukocytosis, with or without a left shift.[1, 11, 14–17] Azotemia caused by dehydration or ureteral obstruction may occur in dogs with paraprostatic cysts, acute prostatitis, prostatic abscess, or prostatic neoplasia.[14–18] Increased hepatic enzyme activities may occur in dogs with acute prostatitis, prostatic abscess, or prostatic neoplasia; in addition, dogs with acute prostatitis or abscess may have hyperbilirubinemia.[14–16, 18] Urinalysis and culture of urine collected by cystocentesis are indicated in all patients with suspected prostatic disease. Hematuria may occur with all prostatic diseases; however, it is most common with BPH and prostatic neoplasia and least common with paraprostatic cysts.[1, 11, 16] Pyuria, proteinuria, and bacteriuria occur in patients with acute and chronic prostatitis, prostatic abscess, and prostatic neoplasia.[1, 14–16, 18] Urine culture may be positive in more than 80% of dogs with chronic prostatitis; other prostatic disorders are less often associated with UTI.[11]

Cytologic evaluation and culture of prostatic fluid collected by ejaculation or prostatic massage is indicated for patients with clinical signs of prostatic disease (see Diagnostic Procedures). Results of prostatic fluid evaluation are used to help localize the site of origin of hemorrhage, inflammation, or infection to the prostate gland.[1] Prostatic fluid evaluation is most likely to provide useful information in patients with chronic bacterial prostatitis; other disorders such as paraprostatic cysts, acute prostatitis, prostatic abscess, and prostatic neoplasia usually can be diagnosed by other tests. Evaluation of prostatic fluid obtained by ejaculation is preferred; prostatic massage is reserved for patients from which an ejaculate cannot be obtained or for which a diagnosis cannot be made by other tests. The most common finding in dogs with BPH is hemorrhagic prostatic fluid, whereas dogs with chronic prostatitis and prostatic abscess have purulent prostatic fluid, sometimes with phagocytized bacteria.[1] Bacterial cultures of prostatic fluid obtained by ejaculation often reveal significant bacterial growth in dogs with prostatic infection or abscess. Epithelial cells with malignant characteristics may be seen on prostatic fluid evaluation in dogs with prostatic neoplasia. These cells also may occur secondary to inflammation; therefore, a diagnosis of neoplasia should be confirmed by aspiration cytology or biopsy of the prostate gland.[19]

Plain abdominal radiographs may help confirm the presence of prostatomegaly, especially if the prostate gland is located in the abdomen, making rectal palpation of the prostate gland difficult (Fig. 18–1). Ultrasonography of the prostate gland is most useful for detecting changes consistent with benign hyperplasia, cysts, abscesses, and neoplasia. Disorders most likely to cause marked, asymmetrical prostatomegaly with poor contrast of caudal abdominal structures include neoplasia, abscess, and paraprostatic cysts.[13, 20] Multifocal, irregularly shaped mineral densities within the prostate gland most often result from neoplasia but also may occur with chronic prostatitis.[13, 16] Periosteal proliferation or osteolysis of the pelvis or lumbar vertebral bodies may occur in patients with prostatic or urethral neoplasia.[13, 16] Sublumbar lymphadenopathy may occur secondary to metastasis in patients with prostatic neoplasia but also has been reported with prostatitis.[13]

Positive-contrast retrograde cystourethrography is indicated to evaluate the position of the urethra relative to an enlarged prostate gland and the involvement of the urinary bladder, especially in patients with dysuria and hematuria. It also is indicated to determine the location of the urinary bladder (e.g., in patients with suspected paraprostatic cysts).[21] Narrowing of the prostatic urethra may occur in patients with prostatic abscess, paraprostatic cysts, or neoplasia.[13] An undulant appearance of the prostatic urethral surface may occur secondary to inflammatory or neoplastic disorders; a markedly irregular surface with luminal disruption or distortion is highly suggestive of

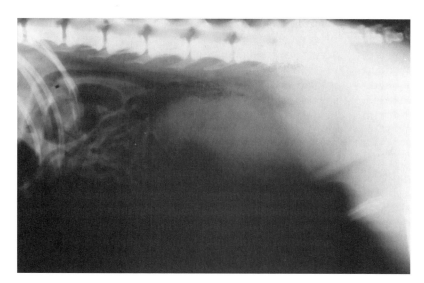

Figure 18-1
Lateral abdominal radiograph of an intact male dog with severe prostatomegaly that was bilaterally symmetrical and nonpainful on palpation. Note the soft tissue density in the caudal abdomen and dorsal displacement of the colon due to the enlarged prostate. Diagnostic evaluation revealed benign prostatic hypertrophy. (Courtesy of Martha L. Moon, DVM, MS, Blacksburg, Virginia.)

neoplasia.[13] Urethroprostatic reflux of contrast material is common with many prostatic diseases, although massive reflux usually occurs only with abscess or neoplasia.[13] Urethroprostatic reflux with neoplasia usually is characterized by an irregular, ragged appearance of urethral mucosa.[13]

Thoracic radiographs should be made to evaluate for distant metastases in dogs with suspected prostatic neoplasia. Pulmonary metastases are detected in 44% of dogs with prostatic adenocarcinoma.[16] Excretory urography should be done in patients with marked prostatomegaly, especially if renal dysfunction is suspected or azotemia exists, to determine the presence and degree of ureteral involvement.[1]

Definitive diagnosis may require collection of prostatic tissue by fine-needle aspiration or biopsy for cytologic or histologic evaluation. Results of cytologic evaluation of prostatic aspirates correlate with results of other diagnostic tests (e.g., histologic evaluation) in more than 95% of dogs.[19] Cytologic evaluation in dogs with BPH reveals normal prostatic cells, whereas neutrophils and sometimes bacteria are seen in dogs with prostatic inflammation.[19] Prostatic neoplasia is more likely to be diagnosed if samples are obtained by aspiration than by prostatic massage. Malignant epithelial cells often are identified, although their absence does not exclude a diagnosis of neoplasia.[19]

Diagnostic Procedures

Routine Laboratory Evaluation

Urinalysis and urine culture are indicated in all dogs with signs of prostatic disease; CBC and serum chemistry analyses should be performed if there are systemic signs of illness, such as lethargy, depression, inappetence, or fever. For complete discussion of urinalysis and urine culture, see Chapters 16 and 17.

Radiography

Survey radiography may be used to help identify location of the prostate gland; however, changes usually are not specific for any particular disease. Prostatomegaly displaces the urinary bladder cranially and the colon dorsally (see Diagnostic Plan).[21]

Positive-contrast retrograde cystourethrography aids in evaluating the position of the urethra relative to an enlarged prostate gland and the location of the urinary bladder; changes often are nonspecific, however.[21] Excretory urography is indicated to detect ureteral involvement in patients with prostatomegaly, especially if prostatic enlargement is marked or appears to affect the caudal urinary bladder or if postrenal azotemia is suspected (see Chaps. 16 and 17).

Ultrasonography

Ultrasonography is a noninvasive method for assessing the prostate gland. Intraparenchymal architecture can readily be evaluated, allowing for differentiation between cystic and solid lesions.[22] Paraprostatic cysts and caudal abdominal masses are easily identified by ultrasonography. Evidence of metastasis, such as sublumbar lymphadenopathy, also can be identified. Finally, ultrasonography can be used to guide fine-needle aspiration or biopsy of the prostate gland and to monitor response to treatment.[23, 24]

Prostatic Fluid Evaluation

Evaluation of an ejaculate provides useful information because the majority of semen is prostatic fluid. For a complete discussion on the method for collection of an ejaculate, see Chapter 21. Approximately 2 or 3 mL of the third fraction of an ejaculate should be collected in a sterile container; this represents prostatic fluid, which is normally clear. If the entire ejaculate appears abnormal, it cannot be divided into fractions, so the entire sample is analyzed. Evaluation should include cytologic examination and quantitative bacterial culture. Normal values for cytologic evaluation of canine prostatic fluid have not been determined; however, it has been suggested that normal prostatic fluid contains occasional red and white blood cells (probably less than 5 white blood cells/high-power field), squamous cells, and some contaminating bacteria.[1, 14] Increased numbers of white blood cells indicate inflammation, whereas large numbers of red blood cells occur with hemorrhage. A finding of bacteria phagocytized within white blood cells or macrophages suggests infection. Bacteria can be cultured from normal ejaculates because of contamination from the distal urethra; however, contaminating bacteria usually number less than 100,000/mL and are gram positive.[1] Culturing of multiple organisms also suggests contamination. Finding more than 100,000 gram-negative organisms/mL of ejaculate suggests infection, especially if cytologic evaluation reveals increased white blood cells. Dogs with prostatitis may have as few as 100 bacteria/mL of prostatic fluid; therefore, results of prostatic fluid culture must be interpreted together with findings from history, physical examination, urine culture, and prostatic fluid cytologic evaluation.[25] Culturing of 100 bacteria/mL of prostatic fluid in a patient with no other signs of prostatic disease probably indicates contamination, but this number of bacteria in a dog with clinical signs of prostatic disease, positive urine culture, or purulent prostatic fluid probably indicates infection.

Collection of an ejaculate is not possible in all dogs, especially those with acute prostatitis, prostatic abscessation, and prostatic neoplasia; therefore, another method of obtaining a sample of prostatic fluid or cells, such as prostatic massage, can be used.[12, 14, 25] The dog is allowed to empty the urinary bladder, and then a urinary catheter is passed with the use of aseptic technique. Any remaining urine is removed, and the bladder is flushed two or three times with 5 to 10 mL of sterile saline solution; the last flush should be saved as the premassage sample. The catheter is retracted so that the tip is just distal to the prostate gland, as determined by rectal palpation. The prostate is then vigorously massaged for 1 to 2 minutes through the rectum or, if the prostate is markedly enlarged, through the abdomen. Then another 5 to 10 mL of sterile saline solution is injected while the distal urethral orifice is occluded to prevent reflux of fluid. Continuous suction

is applied to the catheter while it is advanced into the urinary bladder. The remaining fluid is aspirated and serves as the postmassage sample.

The results from quantitative culture and cytologic evaluation of the premassage and postmassage samples are compared to determine abnormalities caused by prostatic disease. In normal dogs, the postmassage sample should be clear and should contain only a few red and white blood cells, squamous cells, and transitional epithelial cells.[1] Bacterial cultures of premassage and postmassage samples usually are negative or contain fewer than 100 organisms/mL in normal dogs.[25, 26] Prostatic disease is diagnosed by finding more severe abnormalities in the postmassage sample than in the premassage sample. If the number of bacteria cultured from the postmassage sample is greater than in the premassage sample, prostatic infection is likely. However, if concurrent UTI exists, both samples may contain more than 10^5 bacteria/mL, and it is not possible to determine whether prostatic infection exists.[11, 25] For this reason, it is important to obtain urine by cystocentesis for urinalysis and quantitative bacterial culture before performing prostatic massage. If UTI exists, obtaining prostatic fluid by ejaculation is preferable to prostatic massage.

Potential complications of prostatic massage include peritonitis from ruptured abscess, septicemia secondary to entry of bacteria into the blood stream from an infected prostate gland, and dissemination of neoplastic cells. These complications apparently are uncommon in dogs with prostatic disease.

Fine-Needle Aspiration

Prostatic aspiration is indicated if less invasive tests fail to yield a definitive diagnosis. Because of the potential for causing localized peritonitis, aspiration should be avoided in patients with signs of prostatic abscess, such as fever, leukocytosis, and asymmetrical, painful prostatomegaly.[14] If the prostate can be palpated and localized in the abdominal cavity, a transabdominal approach can be used; if it is available, ultrasonography may be used to guide aspiration. Sedation may or may not be necessary, depending on the patient's disposition. The area over the site to be aspirated should be prepared aseptically. A 22- to 25-gauge needle attached to a 12-mL syringe is inserted into the abdominal cavity and prostate gland. After several aspirations, the negative pressure is released and the needle is removed from the abdomen. Aspirated material can be used for bacterial cultures and cytologic evaluation.[27] If the prostate cannot be palpated in the abdomen, the perirectal approach can be used; mild sedation often is helpful with this technique. A 9-cm 22-gauge spinal needle attached to a 12-mL syringe is inserted lateral to the anus and passed through the perineal area to the prostate gland. At the same time, a finger is placed in the rectum to stabilize the prostate gland and guide insertion of the needle. Aspirates are then obtained as described for the transabdominal approach.[27]

Prostatic Biopsy

Samples of prostatic tissue should be obtained for histologic evaluation if less invasive tests do not yield a diagnosis, if treatment of the suspected underlying disease is not effective, or if the disorder is potentially serious and would require immediate and extensive treatment (e.g., neoplasia).[1] Specimens may be obtained percutaneously, by either the transabdominal or the perirectal approach. In general, prostatic biopsy is contraindicated in acute, septic inflammation of the prostate gland, particularly abscesses, because of the possibility of causing septicemia or peritonitis.[1] If prostatic aspiration is done in a patient with an abscess, surgical drainage of the abscess should be done as soon as possible. Sedation with local anesthesia is preferred for the transabdominal approach; general anesthesia may be required for the perirectal approach. Ultrasonography is very useful for guiding biopsy in the transabdominal approach.[23] If the prostate gland cannot be palpated in the abdominal cavity, the perirectal approach may be used. A biopsy needle (e.g., Tru-Cut) is inserted as previously described for perirectal aspiration. The needle is directed away from the center of the gland to avoid the urethra.[14] After biopsy samples are obtained, the patient is observed for several hours to detect signs of hemorrhage. The most common complication of prostatic biopsy is hematuria, which usually is mild and self-limited.[28]

Samples of prostate also may be obtained by direct visualization of the gland at exploratory laparotomy, using either a biopsy needle or wedge resection. An advantage of surgery is that it allows for collection of lymph node specimens, which help to more accurately stage prostatic neoplasia.

Common Diseases of the Prostate

Benign Prostatic Hyperplasia

BPH is an increase in prostatic epithelial cell size and number. The disorder affects nearly every sexually intact male dog, although not all dogs show clinical signs.[8, 29] Only intact male dogs are affected by BPH. The disorder is most common in older dogs; mean age at time of diagnosis is about 8 years.[10]

Pathophysiology

BPH is thought to be hormonally mediated. Apparently, there is increased responsiveness of the prostate gland to testosterone and an altered androgen/estrogen ratio.[30] Testosterone serves as a prohormone for formation of dihydrotestosterone, an active metabolite that mediates intracellular processes of androgen action.[31] Accumulation of dihydrotestosterone within the prostate gland appears to be the hormonal mediator for BPH in dogs.[31] In addition, hyperplasia is facilitated by estrogens, which may enhance androgen receptors. After 4 years of age, prostatic hyperplasia is accompanied by development of intraparenchymal cysts.[8, 29]

Clinical Signs

Most dogs with BPH have no clinical signs, but some have tenesmus, serous or hemorrhagic urethral discharge, or hematuria. Systemic signs of illness usually are not present, and dysuria and stranguria occur infrequently. Physical examination reveals mild to moderate, symmetrical, and nonpainful prostatomegaly.

Diagnostic Plan

Results of routine laboratory tests usually are normal except urinalysis, which may reveal hematuria. Results of analysis of semen or prostatic massage specimens may be normal or reveal hemorrhage. Cytologic evaluation of prostatic aspirates reveals normal epithelium.[19] Radiography reveals symmetrical prostatomegaly and sometimes compression of the colon dorsally and urinary bladder cranially. Retrograde urethrocystography may reveal urethroprostatic reflux and narrowing of the prostatic urethra.[13] Ultrasonography reveals symmetrical prostatomegaly with diffusely increased echogenicity and, in some cases, small intraparenchymal cysts (Fig. 18–2).[22, 24] Although definitive diagnosis requires prostatic biopsy, a clinical diagnosis can be made in most cases on the basis of history and physical examination findings. Response to castration also can be used to support a diagnosis of BPH.[1]

Treatment

Treatment generally is indicated only for patients that have clinical signs of prostatic disease. Treatment of choice for BPH is castration, which causes a 70% decrease in prostatic size.[4, 28] A decrease in prostatic size can be palpated within 7 to 10 days, and clinical signs usually resolve within 1 to 4 weeks.[26, 32]

If castration is not possible in a dog with clinical signs, (e.g., if the dog is used for breeding), medical

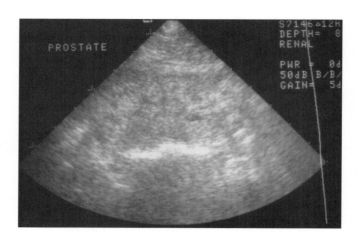

Figure 18–2
Ultrasonogram of a dog with prostatomegaly due to benign prostatiac hypertrophy. Note the presence of increased echogenicity throughout the prostate gland. Some dogs with BPH have small cysts characterized by hypoechoic areas within the prostate gland. (Courtesy of Martha L. Moon, DVM, MS, Blacksburg, Virginia.)

treatment can be attempted. Progestin compounds have antiandrogenic properties and have been used successfully to treat small numbers of dogs with BPH.[26, 33, 34] Administration of megestrol acetate (Ovaban; Megace) at a dosage of 0.55 mg/kg per day for 4 weeks caused resolution of clinical signs and decreased prostatic size in dogs with BPH; decreased numbers of spermatozoa did not occur.[26] Even though megestrol acetate may be effective, it is not approved for use in male dogs and should not be used for longer than 32 days.[26]

Another progestin, medroxyprogesterone acetate (Depo-Provera), also causes resolution of clinical signs in dogs with BPH.[33, 34] This drug appears to have no detrimental effects on semen quality. Medroxyprogesterone acetate is administered at 3 mg/kg subcutaneously; a minimal dose of 50 mg is recommended.[34] When this regimen is used, about 85% of dogs with BPH have resolution of clinical signs 4 to 6 weeks after treatment, and approximately 70% remain free of clinical signs for at least 10 months after a single treatment.[34] A decrease in prostatic size occurs in slightly more than half of dogs; however, clinical improvement may be noted even if prostatic size is not altered. Most dogs have relapses 10 to 24 months after treatment; additional treatment with medroxyprogesterone acetate causes resolution of signs in about half of dogs for at least another 7 months. It may be necessary to treat dogs at 8- to 10-month intervals; however, results of long-term studies are needed before such recommendations can be made.[34] Medroxyprogesterone acetate has not been approved for use in dogs. Potential complications of progestin compounds include increased appetite, weight gain, and diabetes mellitus.

Estrogens also have been used to treat BPH because they decrease secretion of gonadotropin from the pituitary gland, which subsequently depresses androgen secretion and causes prostatic atrophy. Although effective doses of estrogens have not been determined, diethylstilbestrol administered at a rate of 0.2 to 1 mg orally every 2 to 3 days for 3 to 4 weeks has been recommended.[35] Adverse effects of estrogen must be considered when selecting medical treatment for BPH. Bone marrow suppression may occur; it is characterized initially by leukocytosis and a left shift, followed by anemia, leukopenia, and thrombocytopenia. However, administration of DES at 1 mg/kg per day for 9 weeks is not associated with any side effects in dogs.[36] Although the higher doses used for prolonged duration are more likely to cause bone marrow hypoplasia, it also may occur as an idiosyncratic reaction at recommended doses.[28] In addition, repeated use of estrogen and excessive doses may cause prostatic enlargement from squamous metaplasia and predispose to development of cyst formation, bacterial infection, and abscessation.[4, 28, 37]

The antiandrogen drug flutamide (Eulexin) blocks dihydrotestosterone activity in the prostate gland with few effects on testicular function.[38] Administration of 5 mg/kg per day orally to dogs causes a decrease in prostatic size after 6 weeks.[39] Advantages of the drug are that it does not affect libido, production of sperm, or apparent fertility.[39] A decrease in prostatic size as detected by ultrasonography occurs after 10 days of treatment in dogs.[40] At present the drug is not approved for use in dogs.[1]

Prognosis

Prognosis for recovery is good in dogs treated by castration. Although dogs may respond favorably to medical treatment of BPH, prognosis is more guarded because less is known about the efficacy and safety of such treatment.

Paraprostatic Cysts

Paraprostatic cysts are fluid-filled structures located adjacent to the prostate gland.[17, 41] They differ from the intraparenchymal cysts that occur with BPH.

Incidence of paraprostatic cysts is low; approximately 5% of dogs with prostatic disease have paraprostatic cysts.[17] Paraprostatic cysts may be more common in older (>8 years), medium- to large-breed dogs; there appear to be no breed predispositions.[17] Intact males may be affected more than castrated males.[41]

Pathophysiology

The cause of paraprostatic cysts is unknown. It has been suggested that these cysts originate from embryologic structures such as remnants of müllerian ducts or uterus masculinus; however, this has not been confirmed by histologic evaluation.[17]

Clinical Signs

Clinical signs of paraprostatic cysts include dysuria; hemorrhagic, serosanguineous, or yellow urethral discharge; tenesmus; and urinary incontinence.[17, 41] Systemic signs usually are not present. Physical examination usually reveals a caudal abdominal mass that can be palpated on rectal examination. If the cyst extends caudally, it may cause perineal swelling.

Diagnostic Plan

Results of CBC, serum chemistries, and urinalysis may be normal or may reveal neutrophilic leukocytosis, azotemia, or hematuria.[17] Survey radiography often reveals a soft tissue density in the caudal abdomen; in some cases, it may appear as if there are two urinary bladders (Fig. 18–3). Contrast urethrocystography may reveal asymmetrical enlargement of the prostate gland and narrowed urethral lumen; urethroprostatic reflux may be increased, although there is no communication with the cyst.[13, 17] In addition, contrast cystography helps to differentiate the urinary bladder from a suspected paraprostatic cyst. Ultrasonography is the most useful test for confirming the diagnosis; a smoothly marginated anechoic structure resembling the urinary bladder and extending from the area of the prostate gland is visualized.[24] Results of ultrasonography of the prostate gland itself usually are normal.[24]

Analysis of cyst fluid aspirated with ultrasound guidance is helpful. Cyst fluid may be clear, serosanguineous, or dark brown and often contains low numbers of white blood cells.[1, 17] Cultures for aerobic and anaerobic bacteria usually are negative but may be positive if the cyst is secondarily infected.

Definitive diagnosis is made by confirming the presence of a paraprostatic cyst at surgery. Fluid should be obtained for cytologic evaluation and bacterial culture, and a sample of the cyst wall should be submitted for histologic evaluation.

Treatment

The recommended treatment for paraprostatic cysts is surgical drainage with either excision of the cyst or marsupialization.[41, 42] Castration should be done concomitantly.

Prognosis

Prognosis for recovery after surgical treatment of paraprostatic cysts is guarded. In one study, only 3 of 12 dogs had a favorable outcome; however, some dogs had complications not directly related to prostatic

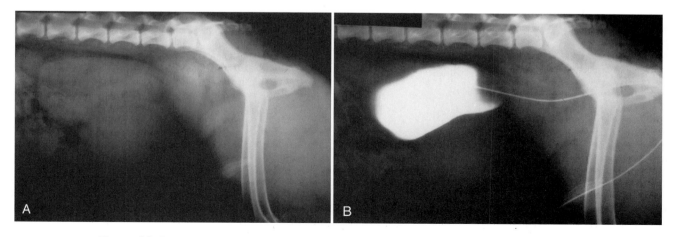

Figure 18–3
(A) Lateral abdominal radiograph of a dog with a palpable mass in the caudal abdomen. Note the two distinct areas of soft tissue density. **(B)** A positive-contrast cystogram reveals that the dorsal mass is the urinary bladder. The ventral mass was determined to be a paraprostatic cyst at surgery. (Courtesy of Gregory C. Troy, DVM, Blacksburg, Virginia.)

disease.[17] Surgical excision of cysts is difficult because of extensive attachments to the prostate gland and urinary bladder.[17] Potential complications of surgical treatment include chronic UTI and prostatic abscessation.[18]

Acute Bacterial Prostatitis

Acute bacterial prostatitis is sudden inflammation of the prostate gland from bacterial infection. Acute prostatitis occurs much less frequently than chronic prostatitis.[1, 10] Sexually intact male dogs older than 9 years of age are most often affected; there is no known breed predisposition.[1, 9]

Pathophysiology

Infecting organisms most often reach the prostate gland by ascending through the urethra, although infection also may result from hematogenous spread or infection of urine or semen. Normally, the prostate gland is sterile because of inherent host defenses that prevent infection, similar to those that prevent UTI. Any disorder of the urethra (e.g., urolithiasis, neoplasia) or prostate gland (e.g., BPH, cysts, neoplasia, squamous metaplasia) may predispose to development of prostatitis. In addition, UTI almost always is associated with concomitant infection of the prostate gland.[9, 11, 43] Organisms that usually cause prostatitis are similar to those that cause UTI. *Escherichia coli* is the most common infecting organism, but infection also may be caused by *Staphylococcus* spp., *Streptococcus* spp., *Klebsiella* spp., *Proteus* spp., *Pseudomonas* spp., and *Enterobacter* spp.[10, 14, 43] Although *Brucella canis* usually causes orchitis and scrotal dermatitis, it also may cause prostatitis.[44] Prostatitis caused by infection with *Blastomyces* spp. infrequently occurs in dogs with blastomycosis.[10] Mycoplasmas have been cultured from prostatic fluid of dogs with signs of prostatitis; however, their role is uncertain because these organisms may be cultured from ejaculates of clinically normal dogs.[26, 43]

Clinical Signs

Systemic signs such as lethargy, depression, vomiting, dehydration, and weight loss often are present in dogs with acute prostatitis; persistent urethral discharge also may be noted.[9] A few dogs have signs of altered locomotion such as a stiff, stilted gait, sometimes with an arched back. Physical examination findings often include depression, dehydration, and caudal abdominal pain. The prostate gland often is painful on palpation; however, usually it is not enlarged unless there is concurrent prostatic disease such as BPH or prostatic abscess.

Diagnostic Plan

A clinical diagnosis usually is made on the basis of history, physical examination findings, routine laboratory evaluation, and response to treatment. The CBC may show neutrophilic leukocytosis with or without a left shift. Urinalysis often reveals hematuria, pyuria, bacteriuria, and proteinuria.[14] Urine collected by cystocentesis should be cultured quantitatively, and antimicrobial susceptibility testing should be done. Serum chemistries may be normal, or azotemia may be present in dogs with dehydration or renal insufficiency. Signs of hepatic disease, including increased serum activities of alkaline phosphatase and alanine aminotransferase, hyperbilirubinemia, and prolonged excretion of sulphobromophthalein, occur in some dogs with acute prostatitis or prostatic abscessation. These abnormalities usually resolve within 1 month of treatment.[18] It is possible that hepatic disease occurs secondary to septicemia.[45] Culture of prostatic fluid is helpful but often is not possible because of difficulty in obtaining an ejaculate from a dog in pain. Results of prostatic massage can be difficult to interpret because UTI usually exists concomitantly (see Diagnostic Procedures).[11, 25] Also, there is a potential for causing septicemia secondary to prostatic massage.[14] Analysis of prostatic fluid is not necessary in most cases of acute prostatitis.

Treatment

An antimicrobial agent should be administered for 4 to 6 weeks to treat dogs with acute prostatitis. If clinical signs are severe (e.g., dehydration, vomiting), parenteral antimicrobial drugs should be administered for the first 48 to 72 hours. Intravenous fluids may be necessary to correct hydration deficits and provide maintenance needs during this time. If the dog's condition is stable (i.e., it is eating and drinking sufficiently to maintain hydration), oral antimicrobial treatment is indicated. Antimicrobial drugs should be selected on the basis of results of urine culture or, if it is available, prostatic fluid culture. Pending results of culture, a broad-spectrum antimicrobial agent that penetrates the blood-prostate barrier, such as trimethoprim-sulfonamide or chloramphenicol, may be used. Because acute inflammation compromises the blood-prostate barrier, most antimicrobials may be effective initially; however, for long-term oral treatment a drug with prostatic penetrance is preferred (see Chronic Bacterial Prostatitis).[1]

To determine effectiveness of treatment, reevaluation (including physical examination, culture of urine and prostatic fluid, and cytologic evaluation of prostatic fluid) should be done 3 to 7 days after cessation of antimicrobial treatment.[1] If persistent infection is identified, antimicrobial treatment should be administered for an additional 4 to 6 weeks. Castration may improve efficacy of treatment and should be considered, especially in dogs with recurrent signs of prostatitis.

Prognosis

Most dogs appear to respond rapidly to antimicrobial treatment; however, long-term prognosis is unknown. Some dogs may develop chronic prostatitis, which is difficult to eradicate. Other dogs may develop prostatic abscess as a consequence of acute prostatitis. Although it is not proven, castration may lessen chances of developing chronic prostatitis.

Chronic Bacterial Prostatitis

Chronic bacterial prostatitis is prolonged bacterial infection of the prostate gland. True incidence of chronic prostatitis is unknown; however, it may be the most common clinically apparent prostatic disease of dogs.[10] Although sexually intact males are most often affected, neutered dogs also may have prostatitis.[10] Mean age at time of diagnosis is about 8 years.[10]

Pathophysiology

The causes and pathogenesis of chronic prostatitis are similar to those described for acute prostatic infection.

Clinical Signs

Clinical signs of chronic bacterial prostatitis include recurrent hematuria, dysuria, or urethral discharge; some manifestations of chronic prostatitis may be subclinical. Except for lethargy, systemic signs usually are absent.[10] Chronic prostatitis also should be suspected in male dogs with recurrent UTI or infertility.[1, 10] Physical examination often is unremarkable. The prostate is nonpainful on palpation and usually is not enlarged unless there is concomitant disease such as BPH. Chronic inflammation may cause fibrosis and variable prostatic symmetry and consistency.[1]

Diagnostic Plan

Clinical diagnosis is based on results of history, physical examination, routine laboratory evaluation, and prostatic fluid evaluation. Results of CBC and serum chemistries usually are unremarkable. Urinalysis may reveal hematuria, pyuria, bacteriuria, or proteinuria. Urine should be collected by cystocentesis for quantitative culture to identify UTI. Cytologic examination and quantitative culture of prostatic fluid obtained by ejaculation or prostatic massage is essen-

tial in dogs with suspected chronic prostatitis (see Diagnostic Procedures).[1] Increased numbers of white blood cells and culture of more than 100,000 organisms/mL of prostatic fluid obtained by ejaculation indicate prostatic infection.[1] However, as few as 100 bacteria/mL may occur with infection. Results of culture must be interpreted together with clinical findings and results of urinalysis, urine culture, and prostatic fluid cytology.[25] Cultures of prostatic massage samples are not as helpful for diagnosing prostatitis, particularly if concomitant UTI exists.[25] For complete discussion of interpretation of prostatic fluid evaluation see Diagnostic Procedures.

Treatment

Administration of antimicrobial drugs that penetrate the blood-prostate barrier and achieve adequate concentrations in the prostate gland is necessary for management of chronic prostatitis. Antimicrobials should be selected on the basis of culture and susceptibility results. Drugs that diffuse into prostatic fluid include chloramphenicol, trimethoprim, quinolones (e.g., ciprofloxacin, norfloxacin, enrofloxacin), erythromycin, and clindamycin. Of the quinolones, enrofloxacin appears to achieve higher prostatic concentrations in dogs than ciprofloxacin or norfloxacin.[1, 46] Cephalosporins, tetracyclines, aminoglycosides, and penicillins, except for carbenicillin and hetacillin, do not penetrate the blood-prostate barrier very well. Antimicrobial agents should be administered for a minimum of 6 weeks (Table 18–2).[1] Ideally, urine and

Table 18–2
Dosage Regimens of Antimicrobial Agents Used to Treat Bacterial Prostatitis in Dogs

DRUG	DOSE (mg/kg)	FREQUENCY	ROUTE
Carbenicillin	15–20	Every 8 h	IV, SC
	20–30	Every 8 h	PO
Chloramphenicol	25	Every 8 h	PO, IV
Ciprofloxacin	2	Every 12 h	PO, IV
Clindamycin	2.5	Every 12 h	PO, IV
Enrofloxacin	2.5	Every 12 h	PO, IV*
Erythromycin	10	Every 8 h	PO
Hetacillin	20	Every 8 h	PO
Norfloxacin	4	Every 12 h	PO
Trimethoprim-sulfonamide	15	Every 12 h	PO, SC

IV, intravenous; PO, by mouth; SC, subcutaneous.
*Not approved for IV use but has been used safely by authors by diluting 1:1 with sterile saline and infusing slowly (i.e., over 5 min) IV.

prostatic fluid should be cultured within 3 to 7 days of beginning treatment and at least 1 month after completion of antimicrobial treatment to detect persistent or recurrent infection.[28] If relapsing infection is detected, a longer course of antimicrobial therapy (i.e., 3–6 months) is indicated.

Because long-term treatment of chronic prostatitis is necessary, patients should be monitored for potential complications of antimicrobial agents. Trimethoprim-sulfonamide products may cause keratoconjunctivitis sicca, folate deficiency anemia, hepatic disease, bone marrow dysfunction, and a lupus-like syndrome characterized by polyarthritis, ocular lesions, and proteinuria.[47–50] The drug should be discontinued if any of these disorders are suspected. Folic acid can be administered orally (5 mg/day) to dogs receiving trimethoprim-sulfonamide products longer than 6 weeks to lessen chances of anemia.

Castration probably is beneficial for management of chronic prostatitis, especially if antimicrobial treatment alone is unsuccessful. Castration performed 2 weeks after experimental induction of bacterial prostatitis in dogs reduced the duration of infection and resulted in fewer bacterial organisms/mL of urine.[51]

If castration and antimicrobial treatment are unsuccessful, low-dose antimicrobial treatment can be attempted to suppress infection and control clinical signs of chronic prostatitis.[1] Trimethoprim-sulfonamide (15 mg/kg by mouth) can be administered as a single daily dose at night.

Prognosis

Without castration, prognosis for dogs with chronic prostatitis is guarded, because it is difficult to completely eradicate infection, and relapses are common.

Prostatic Abscess

Prostatic abscess is an advanced form of chronic prostatitis characterized by one or more areas of septic, purulent exudate within the prostate gland.[1] Prostatic abscesses are relatively uncommon compared with other prostatic diseases; probably less than 5% of dogs with prostatic disease have prostatic abscess.[10] Sexually intact male dogs are most often affected by prostatic abscess; 87% of dogs in one study were intact, and an additional 6% had been neutered within a year of diagnosis.[15] Although older dogs usually are affected, young to middle-aged dogs also may develop prostatic abscess.[15, 18, 52] The average age of dogs with prostatic abscesses is about 11 years.[15]

Pathophysiology

The cause and pathogenesis of prostatic abscess are similar to those described for prostatitis. Appar-

ently, abscess is the end result of uncontrolled chronic prostatitis. Organisms most often isolated from prostatic abscesses are similar to those from dogs with prostatitis or UTI. E. coli is isolated from more than 80% of prostatic abscesses in dogs; other organisms that are isolated less frequently include Klebsiella spp., Staphylococcus spp., Streptococcus spp., Proteus spp., and Enterobacter spp.[15]

Clinical Signs

Clinical signs of prostatic abscess may include depression, lethargy, fever, inappetence, vomiting, stranguria, dysuria, hematuria, tenesmus, abdominal pain, and purulent or hemorrhagic urethral discharge.[15, 18, 52] Icterus and edema of the prepuce, scrotum, and rear legs occur less frequently.[15, 18] Signs of shock, such as pale mucous membranes, tachycardia, prolonged capillary refill time, and weak pulse quality, may be observed in patients presented with peritonitis or septicemia caused by ruptured prostatic abscess.[15, 52] Prostatomegaly and caudal abdominal mass and pain are detected in most dogs.[15] The prostate may be asymmetrically enlarged and contain one or more fluctuant areas.

Diagnostic Plan

Results of laboratory evaluation are helpful in patients with prostatic abscess. Laboratory findings often include neutrophilic leukocytosis with or without a left shift.[11, 15] Results of serum chemistries may show hypoglycemia, azotemia, hyperproteinemia, hyperbilirubinemia, and increased hepatic enzyme activities.[15] Hypoglycemia occurs in 40% of dogs, presumably secondary to sepsis.[15] Azotemia may be caused by prerenal disorders (e.g., dehydration), renal disorders (e.g., renal failure), or postrenal disorders (e.g., ureteral obstruction). Increased hepatic enzyme activities and hyperbilirubinemia are presumed to result from sepsis-induced hepatic disease; these abnormalities usually resolve after treatment of prostatic abscess.[18] Urinalysis usually reveals hematuria, pyuria, proteinuria, and bacteriuria. Prostatic fluid analysis often reveals septic, purulent inflammation that may be hemorrhagic; however, collection of prostatic fluid often is difficult and usually is not needed because other findings are used to make a diagnosis of prostatic abscess.

Radiographs may show sublumbar lymphadenopathy and decreased contrast of the caudal abdomen as a result of peritonitis. Results of contrast urethrography are not specific for prostatic abscess but may reveal reflux of contrast into the prostate gland, especially if the abscess communicates with the urethra. There also may be periurethral asymmetry, narrowing of the prostatic urethra, and undulation of the urethral lumen.[13] Ultrasonography reveals increased

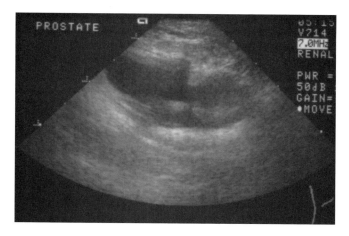

Figure 18–4
Ultrasonogram of a dog with fever, abdominal pain, and an asymetrically enlarged prostate gland. Further diagnostic tests revealed a large cystic area within the prostate gland, which was confirmed to be a prostatic abscess at surgery. (Courtesy of Gregory C. Troy, DVM, Blacksburg, Virginia.)

parenchymal echogenicity and focal areas of decreased echogenicity that may be very large (Fig. 18–4).[22]

A presumptive diagnosis is made on the basis of findings from the history, physical examination, laboratory evaluation, radiography, and ultrasonography. Diagnosis is confirmed either by aspiration of the suspected abscess for cytologic evaluation and culture or by exploratory laparotomy with collection of samples for culture at surgery. Aspiration carries the risk of rupture of the abscess and subsequent peritonitis; therefore, the clinician should be prepared to perform laparotomy immediately if purulent exudate is obtained. Because surgical drainage is the treatment of choice, an exploratory laparotomy usually should be done to confirm the diagnosis.

Treatment

The treatment of choice for prostatic abscess is surgical drainage of abscesses and concomitant castration. Several techniques have been described for establishing drainage; placement of multiple drains currently is recommended.[15, 53] Drains are removed after discharge subsides, usually 5 to 7 days after surgery. These patients require intensive care and treatment of potential postoperative complications such as peritonitis and septicemia. Urinary incontinence may occur in 25% of cases treated surgically; although incontinence resolves in some cases, it tends to persist in most.[15] Other complications, which occur in fewer than 20% of cases, include formation of prostatic urethrocutaneous fistulas, prostatic reabscess, and recurrent UTI.[15]

In addition to surgery, antimicrobial treatment is indicated in all dogs with prostatic abscess. Patients with severe systemic signs or suspected sepsis should receive intravenous antimicrobial drugs initially (for 48–72 hours) until the dog can tolerate oral medication (see Table 18–2). If septicemia exists, it is important to select an antimicrobial agent that is effective against gram-negative organisms, even if it does not penetrate the blood-prostate barrier as well as other agents.

Antimicrobial treatment may have to be modified after results of susceptibility become available. Antimicrobial treatment should be continued for a minimum of 6 weeks, as in patients with chronic prostatitis.

Patients with septicemia also should receive vigorous fluid therapy. Fluids such as lactated Ringer's solution and 0.9% sodium chloride often are sufficient initially. The rate of fluid administration should be based on cardiovascular status and clinical response; dogs with severe cardiovascular collapse may require up to 90 mL/kg per hour initially. Intravenous fluids containing 5% dextrose should be administered to patients with hypoglycemia. Potassium supplementation also is needed in patients with hypokalemia (see Chap. 16).

Prognosis

Prognosis for recovery in patients with prostatic abscess is guarded.[15, 18, 52] Approximately 21% of 92 dogs in one study died or were euthanized within 2 weeks of surgery, primarily as a result of peritonitis, sepsis, and shock; another 10% were euthanized later because of recurrent UTI or urinary incontinence.[15] Approximately 18% of dogs had prostatic reabscess, which required a second surgery in most cases.[15] Dogs that recover from surgery and survive for at least 2 weeks have a better prognosis. Fifty-eight percent of dogs that are alive 2 weeks after surgery have good to excellent results, and another 26% have fair results.[15]

Prostatic Neoplasia

Prostatic neoplasia is uncontrolled and disorganized proliferation of prostatic tissue, most often of epithelial cells. On the basis of necropsy studies, prevalence of prostatic neoplasia ranges from 0.29% to 0.6% in male dogs, although prostatic neoplasia accounts for 3.5% to 15% of dogs with prostatic disease.[10, 32, 54–57] In contrast to other prostatic disorders, prostatic neoplasia affects both sexually intact and neutered dogs.[16, 56, 58–60] It appears that neoplasia is the most common cause of prostatic disease in neutered dogs.[10] Older dogs are more often affected; mean age at time of diagnosis is 8 to 10 years.[9, 10, 16, 56, 59, 60] There are no breed predilections, although most dogs with prostatic neoplasia are of medium to large breeds.[16, 56, 59]

Pathophysiology

The cause of prostatic neoplasia is unknown; although it may be hormonally related, it does not appear to exclusively involve testicular hormones.[60] Prostatic neoplasms are virtually always malignant; adenocarcinoma is most common.[58] Transitional cell carcinoma is the second most common prostatic tumor; however, it occurs infrequently compared with adenocarcinoma. Prostatic tumors are locally invasive and may cause ureteral or urethral obstruction.[56, 59] Invasion through the prostatic capsule into surrounding pelvic musculature may occur.[59] Prostatic tumors frequently metastasize to pelvic lymph nodes, vertebrae, pelvic bones, and lungs.[16, 57, 59]

Clinical Signs

Clinical signs in dogs with prostatic neoplasia include tenesmus, constipation, dysuria, hematuria, stranguria, hemorrhagic urethral discharge, and rear limb weakness, lameness, or pain.[9, 10, 16, 56, 57] Compared with some prostatic disorders, systemic signs such as inappetence, weight loss, and fever are relatively common in dogs with prostatic neoplasia. Dogs with metastases to bone have significantly greater occurrence of weight loss, emaciation, and lumbar pain.[57] Rectal examination usually reveals asymmetrical prostatomegaly with areas of increased firmness. Neutered dogs should have a palpably small prostate gland; a finding of even mild prostatic enlargement in a neutered dog should prompt suspicion of neoplasia. In some dogs with prostatic neoplasia, the prostate gland may be attached to surrounding tissues.

Diagnostic Plan

A tentative diagnosis is based on findings from signalment, history, physical examination, radiography, and ultrasonography. Results of laboratory evaluation may provide evidence for the presence of prostatic disease; however, they rarely are diagnostic. Hemogram may reveal nonregenerative anemia, neutrophilic leukocytosis with or without a left shift, or monocytosis.[16] Serum chemistries may show increased activities of hepatic enzymes, especially alkaline phosphatase and hypoalbuminemia; hypocalcemia or hypercalcemia rarely is observed.[16] Some dogs have azotemia, which may result from bilateral ureteral obstruction. Hematuria and pyuria are the most

common findings on urinalysis; UTI may be identified in some cases.[16] Atypical cells suggestive of neoplasia are observed rarely in urine sediment.[16]

Radiography and ultrasonography are helpful for detecting abnormalities consistent with prostatic neoplasia and determining the extent of disease. Prostatomegaly and intraprostatic mineralization are the most common survey radiographic findings.[16] Other abnormalities may include sublumbar lymphadenopathy and proliferative or lytic lesions of pelvic bones or caudal lumbar vertebrae. Virtually any bone can be affected by metastatic lesions, including the scapulae, ribs, and digits.[57] The most common findings on retrograde urethrocystography are increased urethroprostatic reflux and narrowing, distortion, or destruction of the prostatic urethra.[13, 16] Thoracic radiographs are indicated to detect signs of distant metastases; about 45% of dogs with prostatic adenocarcinoma have pulmonary metastases.[16] Ultrasonography is useful for evaluating prostatic size, detecting prostatic masses and sublumbar lymphadenopathy, and guiding aspiration of the prostate gland.

Definitive diagnosis of prostatic neoplasia is made by identifying malignant prostatic cells. Analysis of prostatic fluid often is not possible because the difficulty of obtaining an ejaculate specimen from dogs with prostatic neoplasia. Neoplastic cells can be identified in prostatic massage samples (see Diagnostic Procedures); however, results sometimes are difficult to interpret, especially if concomitant inflammation exists.[19] Cytologic evaluation of prostatic aspirates (see Diagnostic Procedures) is very helpful for confirming prostatic neoplasia; ultrasound guidance may improve the ability to obtain diagnostic specimens. Histologic evaluation of biopsy specimens may be needed to confirm a diagnosis if cytologic findings are equivocal. If exploratory laparotomy is done to obtain prostatic tissue, samples of pelvic lymph nodes also should be collected to help determine extent of disease.

Treatment

Because of the biologic behavior of prostatic neoplasia in dogs, cure is unlikely and the goal of treatment is to control the tumor and make the patient more comfortable. Before treatment, patients should be thoroughly evaluated to determine the extent of disease. This evaluation should include thoracic and abdominal radiographs and retrograde cystourethrography; if they are available, ultrasonography and bone scan also may help detect metastatic disease. Excretory urography should be done to detect ureteral involvement if postrenal azotemia exists or if the tumor is large. Patients with localized tumor are better candidates for treatment than those with metastatic disease. Some dogs have responded to radiotherapy.[16, 61]

Median and mean survival times were 114 days and 196 days, respectively, in one study; dogs without evidence of metastasis lived longer and had a mean survival time of 8 months.[61] Prostatectomy may be considered for dogs with localized disease; however, owners should be informed that most dogs are incontinent after surgery.[18]

Prognosis

Prognosis for dogs with prostatic neoplasia is grave; most die or are euthanized shortly after diagnosis.[16] Patients with no evidence of metastasis may have longer survival times. It is likely that metastasis has already occurred at the time of initial diagnosis, even though it may not be detected by diagnostic tests.[16]

Uncommon Diseases of the Prostate

Squamous Metaplasia

Squamous metaplasia of prostatic epithelium occurs secondary to hyperestrogenism, either from exogenous administration or from increased endogenous release of estrogen from a testicular Sertoli cell tumor.[4, 37, 62] Mild to moderate symmetrical prostatomegaly may exist. Cytologic or histologic evaluation of prostatic tissue reveals squamous changes of prostatic epithelium. The treatment of choice is removal of exogenous sources of estrogen and castration if testicular neoplasia is identified.

Abacterial Prostatic Hemorrhage

Abacterial prostatic hemorrhage is a disorder characterized by hemorrhage from the prostate gland.[27] It may be more common in dogs exposed to chronic sexual excitement. Bacterial culture of prostatic fluid shows no growth, and cytologic evaluation shows primarily red blood cells with occasional inflammatory cells. The treatment of choice is castration. In breeding dogs, frequent ejaculation (i.e., every other day until prostatic hemorrhage diminishes) may be effective.

References

1. Barsanti JA, Finco DR. Prostatic diseases. In: Ettinger SJ, Feldman EC, eds. Textbook of Veterinary Internal Medicine, 4th ed. Philadelphia, WB Saunders, 1995:1662–1685.
2. Berry SJ, Coffey DS, Ewing LL. Effects of aging on prostate growth in beagles. Am J Physiol 1986;250:R1039–R1046.
3. Issacs JT. Common characteristics of human and canine benign prostatic hyperplasia. Prog Clin Biol Res 1984;145:217–234.
4. Huggins C, Clark PJ. Quantitative studies of prostatic secretion II: The effect of castration and of estrogen injection on the normal and on the hyperplastic prostate glands of dogs. J Exp Med 1940;72:747–761.
5. Basinger RR, Rawlings CA, Barsanti JA, et al. Urodynamic alterations associated with clinical prostatic diseases and prostatic surgery in 23 dogs. J Am Anim Hosp Assoc 1989;25:385–392.
6. Barsanti JA. Vaginal and preputial discharges. In: Lorenz MD, Cornelius LM, eds. Small Animal Medical Diagnosis. Philadelphia, JB Lippincott, 1993:357–363.
7. Stone EA, Barsanti JA. Urologic Surgery of the Dog and Cat. Philadelphia, Lea & Febiger, 1992:30–33.
8. Berry SJ, Strandberg JD, Saunders WJ, et al. Development of canine benign prostatic hyperplasia with age. Prostate 1986;9:363–373.
9. Hornbuckle WE, MacCoy DM, Allan GS, et al. Prostatic disease in the dog. Cornell Vet 1978;68:284–305.
10. Krawiec DR, Heflin D. Study of prostatic disease in dogs: 177 cases (1981–1986). J Am Vet Med Assoc 1992;200:1119–1122.
11. Barsanti JA, Finco DR. Evaluation of techniques for diagnosis of canine prostatic diseases. J Am Vet Med Assoc 1984;185:198–200.
12. Kay ND, Ling GV, Nyland TG, et al. Cytological diagnosis of canine prostatic disease using a urethral brush technique. J Am Anim Hosp Assoc 1989;25:517–526.
13. Feeney DA, Johnston GR, Klausner JS, et al. Canine prostatic disease: Comparison of radiographic appearance with morphologic and microbiologic findings, 30 cases (1981–1985). J Am Vet Med Assoc 1987;190:1018–1026.
14. Barsanti JA, Finco DR. Canine bacterial prostatitis. Vet Clin North Am Small Anim Pract 1979;9:679–700.
15. Mullen HS, Matthiesen DT, Scavelli TD. Results of surgery and postoperative complications in 92 dogs treated for prostatic abscessation by a multiple penrose drain technique. J Am Anim Hosp Assoc 1990;26:369–379.
16. Bell FW, Klausner JS, Hayden DW, et al. Clinical and pathologic features of prostatic adenocarcinoma in sexually intact and castrated dogs: 31 cases (1970–1987). J Am Vet Med Assoc 1991;199:1623–1630.
17. Weaver AD. Discrete prostatic (paraprostatic) cysts in the dog. Vet Rec 1978;102:435–440.
18. Hardie EM, Barsanti JA, Rawlings CA. Complications of prostatic surgery. J Am Anim Hosp Assoc 1984;20:50–56.
19. Thrall MA, Olson PN, Freemyer FG. Cytologic diagnosis of canine prostatic disease. J Am Anim Hosp Assoc 1985;21:95–102.
20. Stone EA, Thrall DE, Barber DL. Radiographic interpretation of prostatic disease in the dog. J Am Anim Hosp Assoc 1978;14:115–118.
21. Lattimer JC. The prostate gland. In: Thrall DE, ed. Textbook of Veterinary Diagnostic Radiology, 2nd ed. Philadelphia, WB Saunders, 1994:479–493.
22. Feeney DA, Johnston GR, Klausner JS, et al. Canine prostatic disease. Comparison of ultrasonographic appearance with morphologic and microbiologic findings, 30 cases (1981–1985). J Am Vet Med Assoc 1987;190:1027–1034.
23. Hager DA, Nyland TG, Fisher P. Ultrasound-guided

biopsy of the canine liver, kidney, and prostate. Vet Radiol 1985;26:82–88.

24. Feeney DA, Johnston GR, Klausner JS, et al. Canine prostatic ultrasonography: 1989. Semin Vet Med Surg (Small Anim) 1989;4:44–57.

25. Barsanti JA, Prasse KW, Crowell WA, et al. Evaluation of various techniques for diagnosis of chronic bacterial prostatis in the dog. J Am Vet Med Assoc 1983;183:219–224.

26. Olson PN. Disorders of the canine prostate gland: Pathogenesis, diagnosis, and medical therapy. Compen Contin Educ Pract Vet 1987;9:613–624.

27. Rogers KS, Wantschek L, Lees GE. Diagnostic evaluation of the canine prostate. Compen Contin Educ Pract Vet 1986;8:799–811.

28. Barsanti JA, Finco DR. Canine prostatic diseases. In: Ettinger SJ, ed. Textbook of Veterinary Internal Medicine, 3rd ed. Philadelphia, WB Saunders, 1989:1859–1880.

29. Lowseth LA, Gerlach RF, Gillett NA, et al. Age-related changes in the prostate and testes of the beagle. Vet Pathol 1990;27:347–353.

30. Lloyd JW, Thomas JA, Mawhinney MG. Androgens and estrogens in the plasma and prostatic tissue of normal dogs and dogs with benign prostatic hypertrophy. Invest Urol 1975;13:220–222.

31. Wilson JD. The pathogenesis of benign prostatic hyperplasia. Am J Med 1980;68:745–756.

32. Borthwick R, Mackenzie CP. The signs and results of treatment of prostatic disease in dogs. Vet Rec 1971;89:374–384.

33. Schubert BG, Weiger G. Zur therapie der prostatahypertrophie des hundes mit medroxyprogesteron. Kleintierpraxis 1978;23:331–332.

34. Bamberg-Thalen B, Linde-Forsberg C. Treatment of canine benign prostatic hyperplasia with medroxyprogesterone acetate. J Am Anim Hosp Assoc 1993;29:221–226.

35. Johnston DI. The prostate. In: Slatter DH, ed. Textbook of Small Animal Surgery, Philadelphia, WB Saunders, 1985:1635–1649.

36. Tyslowitz R, Dingemanse E. Effect of large doses of estrogens on the blood picture of dogs. Endocrinology 1941;29:817–827.

37. Berg OA. Effect of stilbestrol on the prostate gland in normal puppies and adult dogs. Acta Endocrinol (Copenh) 1958;27:155–169.

38. Geller J. Overview of benign prostatic hyperplasia. Urology 1989;34(4 Suppl):57–63.

39. Neri RO, Monahan M. Effects of a novel nonsteroidal antiandrogen on canine prostatic hyperplasia. Invest Urol 1972;10:123–130.

40. Cartee RE, Rumph PF, Kenter DC, et al. Evaluation of drug-induced prostatic involution in dogs by transabdominal B-mode ultrasonography. Am J Vet Res 1990;51:1773–1778.

41. White R, Herrtage ME, Dennis R. The diagnosis and management of paraprostatic and prostatic retention cysts in the dog. J Small Anim Pract 1987;28:551–574.

42. Basinger RR, Rawlings CA. Surgical management of prostatic disease. Compen Contin Educ Pract Vet 1987;9:993–1000.

43. Ling GV, Branam JE, Ruby RL, et al. Canine prostatic fluid: Techniques of collection, quantitative bacterial culture, and interpretation of results. J Am Vet Med Assoc 1983;183:201–206.

44. Greene CE, George LW. Canine brucellosis. In: Greene CE, ed. Clinical Microbiology and Infectious Diseases of the Dog and Cat. Philadelphia, WB Saunders, 1984:646–662.

45. Taboada J, Meyer DJ. Cholestasis associated with extrahepatic bacterial infection in five dogs. J Vet Intern Med 1989;3:216–221.

46. Dorfman M, Barsanti J, Budsberg S. Enrofloxacin concentrations in the normal prostate gland and in chronic bacterial prostatitis in the dog. J Vet Intern Med 1993;7:122.

47. Cribb AE. Idiosyncratic reactions to sulfonamides in dogs. J Am Vet Med Assoc 1989;195:1612–1613.

48. Rowland PH, Center SA, Dougherty SA. Presumptive trimethoprim-sulfadiazine–related hepatotoxicosis in a dog. J Am Vet Med Assoc 1992;200:348–350.

49. Giger U, Werner LL, Millichamp NJ, et al. Sulfadiazine-induced allergy in six Doberman pinschers. J Am Vet Med Assoc 1985;186:479–484.

50. Medleau L, Shanley KJ, Rakich PM, et al. Trimethoprim-sulfonamide–associated drug eruptions in dogs. J Am Anim Hosp Assoc 1990;26:305–311.

51. Cowan LA, Barsanti JA, Crowell W, et al. Effects of castration on chronic bacterial prostatitis in dogs. J Am Vet Med Assoc 1991;199:346–350.

52. Bauer MS. Prostatic abscess rupture in three dogs. J Am Vet Med Assoc 1986;188:735–737.

53. Zolton GM, Greiner TP. Prostatic abscesses: A surgical approach. J Am Anim Hosp Assoc 1978;14:698–702.

54. Krook LA. A statistical investigation or carcinoma in the dog. Acta Pathol Microbiol Scand 1954;35:407–422.

55. Schlotthauer CF, Millar JAS. Carcinoma of the prostate gland in dogs: A report of three cases. J Am Vet Med Assoc 1941;99:239–241.

56. Weaver AD. Fifteen cases of prostatic carcinoma in the dog. Vet Rec 1981;109:71–75.

57. Durham SK, Dietze AE. Prostatic adenocarcinoma with and without metastasis to bone in dogs. J Am Vet Med Assoc 1986;188:1432–1436.

58. O'Shea JP. Studies on the canine prostate gland II: Prostatic neoplasms. J Comp Pathol 1963;73:244–252.

59. Leav I, Ling GV. Adenocarcinoma of the canine prostate gland. Cancer 1968;22:1329–1345.

60. Obradovich J, Walshaw R, Goullaud E. The influence of castration on the development of prostatic carcinoma in the dog: 43 cases (1978–1985). J Vet Intern Med 1987;1:183–187.

61. Turrel JM. Intraoperative radiotherapy of carcinoma of the prostate gland in ten dogs. J Am Vet Med Assoc 1987;190:48–52.

62. Sherding RG, Wilson GP, Kociba GJ. Bone marrow hypoplasia in eight dogs with Sertoli cell tumor. J Am Vet Med Assoc 1981;178:497–500.

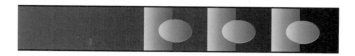

Ophthalmic
Diseases

Chapter 19

Ophthalmic Manifestations of Systemic Diseases

J. Phillip Pickett
Erin S. Champagne

It has been said that the eye is the window to the soul, and any ophthalmologist knows that there is some truth in this statement. Many systemic diseases commonly seen by the practicing veterinarian have ocular signs in addition to their systemic signs; in many cases, the ocular signs are the first clinical signs noticed by the owner and are the primary complaint for presentation of the animal to the veterinarian. It is not the purpose of this chapter to educate the veterinary practitioner in the diagnosis, pathophysiology, and treatment of every disease entity of the eye and adnexa. Rather, the purpose is to enlighten the practicing veterinarian to those systemic diseases that commonly have ophthalmic signs. With this information in mind, a thorough ophthalmic examination can become an integral part of every veterinary practitioner's diagnostic work-up.

Anatomy and Physiology

There are many excellent references in veterinary ophthalmology textbooks concerning basic and applied anatomy and physiology of the eye and adnexa.[1-4] These features are discussed here only in relation to ophthalmic manifestations of systemic disease.

The eye rests in the orbit, a complex structure made up of bone, periosteum, cartilage, ligaments, tendons, and muscles. In addition to the globe itself, extraocular muscles, fat, vascular structures, cranial nerves, and the lacrimal and zygomatic glands lie within the orbit. Structures immediately adjacent to the orbit include sinus cavities, tooth roots, and the soft palate.

Cranial nerves II through VIII, cranial nerve X, and the parasympathetic and sympathetic branches of the autonomic nervous system are involved either directly or indirectly with the innervation of the eye and adnexa. An understanding of the innervation to the eye and adnexa may be useful in the localization of more centrally located nervous system disorders (see Chap. 26).

The conjunctiva is the mucous membrane that lines the inside of the eyelid, the third eyelid, and the visible portions of the sclera. The conjunctivae are often concurrently affected by disease, along with the mucous membranes of the mouth, pharynx, and sinuses, especially with upper respiratory infection. Because the conjunctiva is highly vascular (and these vessels can be directly observed), disorders of the vasculature, anemia, bleeding disorders, and hepatic dysfunction may first be seen as conjunctival hyperemia, pallor, hemorrhages, or jaundiced discoloration, respectively.

The cornea is the clear "window" through which light rays pass into the eye on their way to stimulate the retina and begin the process of vision (Fig. 19–1). Corneal nourishment comes from the aqueous humor and the precorneal tear film. The cornea is involved with few systemic diseases, although there are some rather significant corneal disorders that may represent clinical signs of underlying systemic disease.

The crystalline lens normally resides behind the iris and cranial to the anterior vitreous face. Because the lens is without a direct vascular supply, nutrients for the metabolically active lens epithelial cells must come from the aqueous humor. Changes in aqueous humor composition may result in altered lens metabolism, usually resulting in cataract formation.

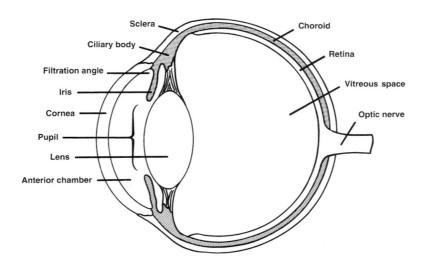

Figure 19–1
Line drawing of general anatomic features of the eye.

The uvea is the vessel-rich portion of the eye. Made up of the iris, ciliary body, and choroid, the uvea functions to provide nutrition to and remove metabolic waste products from the avascular structures of the eye (cornea and lens). The anterior uvea produces aqueous humor and the fluid component of the vitreous. The choroid, in conjunction with the true retinal vessels, provides nourishment to the neural retina. Like other well vascularized structures of the body (e.g., kidneys, lungs, choroid plexus of the brain), the uvea is made up of a rather complex system of arterioles, venules, and capillary beds with selective permeabilities to various ions, proteins, and other cellular and subcellular elements. Vascular endothelial cell tight junctions (in the iris stroma and the true retinal vessels) and overlying epithelial cell barriers (in the case of the nonpigmented ciliary body epithelium and the retinal epithelium overlying the choroid) are responsible for maintaining clear ocular media. The blood-ocular barrier (BOB) is made up of these tight junctions and epithelial cell barriers. Disruption of the BOB allows blood components (e.g., protein, red blood cells, white blood cells) to enter the aqueous humor, vitreous, retina, and subretinal spaces (see Uveitis).

The ocular fundus is one of the few places in the body in which blood vessels and nervous tissue may be noninvasively viewed by the veterinarian. True retinal vessels may be observed for signs of hemorrhage, perivasculitis, lipemia, engorgement, and excessive tortuosity. The neural retina and the optic papilla are direct extensions of the central nervous system and may be examined for signs of infectious, toxic, or neoplastic disorders of the central nervous system. Signs of hematogenous dissemination of infectious agents or neoplastic cells may be noted during a complete fundic examination.

Problem Identification

Exophthalmos

Exophthalmos is an abnormal protrusion of a normal-sized eyeball.

Pathophysiology

Exophthalmos is caused by abnormal fluid or abnormal tissue within the orbit pushing the globe outward. This could be in the form of purulent debris in a retrobulbar abscess; swelling of the extraocular muscles or masticatory muscles; or inflammation or neoplasia of any of the structures immediately adjacent to the orbit (i.e., tooth roots, sinuses, lacrimal or salivary glands).

Exophthalmos may be caused by apparent immune-mediated inflammation of, rarely, the extraocular muscles[5] or, more commonly, of the masticatory muscles[6-8] that make up the medial and ventral walls of the orbit. Exophthalmos may be caused by orbital cellulitis or abscess,[9-10] primary orbital or metastatic neoplasia,[11-15] or cystic diseases (zygomatic mucocele).[16]

Clinical Signs

Exophthalmos must be differentiated from buphthalmos or megalaglobus (enlargement of the globe caused by chronic glaucoma) before the diagnostic work-up is continued. With exophthalmos, the third eyelid is usually (but not always) prominent, the corneal diameter is usually the same as in the contralateral normal eye, exposure keratitis caused by lagophthalmos may or not be present, and intraocular pressure is usually within normal limits. Attempts to retropulse the globe into the orbit are usually met with resistance from some space-occupying mass or fluid deep to the globe. In the case of buphthalmos caused by chronic glaucoma, corneal diameter is usually greater and the corneal curvature flatter than in the contralateral normal eye; the third eyelid is usually not prominent, and retropulsion is usually not met with as much orbital resistance as in true exophthalmos. It must be remembered that brachiocephalic breeds of dogs have shallow, tight-fitting orbits, so the ability to retropulse the globe is naturally less than in a breed with a more normal eye-orbit conformation.

Important historical and physical examination findings may include unilateral or bilateral involvement; a history of sudden onset or progressive worsening; painful or nonpainful disease; axial displacement of the globe or dorsal, ventral, medial, or lateral strabismus; and other clinical and physical examination findings such as pyrexia, lymphadenopathy, anorexia, and ocular, oral, or nasal discharge.

Diagnostic Plan

Based on the initial history and physical examination findings, certain general conclusions may be reached that can narrow the diagnostic possibilities. Unilateral exophthalmos usually indicates a localized inflammatory disease of the orbit or its contents, orbital abscess, neoplasia, or cystic orbital structures (zygomatic sialocele).[9, 10, 15, 16] Bilateral exophthalmos usually (but not always) involves inflammation of the extraocular muscles or masticatory muscles.[5-8] Bilateral orbital neoplasia is seldom seen in cats and dogs.[12-14] Painful exophthalmos is most likely caused by inflammatory processes such as orbital cellulitis or abscess,[9-13, 17, 18] trauma, fracture, or masticatory muscle myositis.[6-8, 12] Nonpainful exophthalmos is most likely caused by orbital neoplasia,[9-13, 15] cystic orbital structures,[16] or extraocular muscle myositis.[5] Sudden onset of exophthalmos is more likely to involve inflammatory myositis disorders, cellulitis, or abscess; slowly progressive exophthalmos is more likely a result of neoplasia or cystic orbital disease. Fetid drool or purulent or sanguineous discharge from the caudal oral cavity may indicate orbital abscess or cellulitis, necrotic neoplasia, or an abscessed tooth root. Ipsilateral nasal discharge may indicate sinus neoplasia or infectious sinusitis. Localized lymphadenopathy may indicate orbital cellulitis or abscess caused by bacteria or fungi[12, 13, 17, 18]; generalized lymphadenopathy may indicate generalized fungal infection[17, 18] or lymphosarcoma.[12, 13]

Besides a thorough general physical examination and examination of the orbital, head, and oral cavity regions, the diagnostic work-up for unilateral exophthalmos may include a complete blood count (CBC) and serum biochemistry panel. An elevated white blood cell count with neutrophilia is consistent with retrobulbar abscess or cellulitis or necrosis of a localized neoplasm. Neoplasia (lymphosarcoma) may result in hypercalcemia.

Plain skull radiography under anesthesia may identify fractures, sinus disorders, or tooth root abscesses. Contrast orbitography[19] may help to localize an intraorbital mass better than plain films alone. Fine-needle aspiration and cytologic evaluation and cultures may contribute to the final diagnosis in cases of neoplasia or infectious causes of exophthalmos. Relative position of the globe may be helpful in the determination of the areas to be aspirated (e.g., lateral strabismus would indicate that fine-needle aspiration of the medial orbit should be performed). Probing of the oral cavity behind the last upper molar tooth on the ipsilateral side may be helpful in differentiating a true orbital abscess from cellulitis.[12] Orbital B-scan ultrasonography may be helpful in identifying fluid density versus solid tissue density in the retrobulbar space.[20, 21] Orbital exploratory surgery[22, 23] may be used to diagnose or treat orbital neoplasia and foreign bodies.

With bilateral exophthalmos, attempts to open the mouth may differentiate extraocular muscle myositis from masticatory myositis. Compared with extraocular muscle myositis, masticatory myositis may be met with more resistance because of swollen muscles or muscle fibrosis and pain. Masticatory myositis is typically seen in adult, larger breeds of dogs, although it may occasionally be seen in medium-sized and smaller dogs. Biopsy of swollen temporalis muscles for histopathologic evaluation, submission of serum samples for determination of type 2M muscle fiber antibodies, and evaluation of serum creatinine kinase may also contribute to a diagnosis of masticatory myositis.[6–8] Peripheral eosinophilia also may indicate masticatory myositis, although not all dogs with masticatory myositis have the condition, and

dogs may have it for other reasons. Extraocular muscle myositis is usually seen in prepubescent, large-breed dogs.[5]

Treatment

Specific therapy for exophthalmos depends on the cause. Because exposure keratoconjunctivitis secondary to lagophthalmos may lead to corneal ulceration, protection of the corneal surface with a temporary tarsorrhaphy is indicated if central corneal drying or ulceration occurs. Excessive, acute extraocular muscle inflammation or retrobulbar hemorrhage, abscess, or cellulitis may put pressure on the optic nerve and posterior globe, resulting in blindness secondary to optic nerve necrosis or retinal detachment. Resolution of pressure on these structures should be achieved as soon as possible. This may be accomplished through the use of antimicrobial therapy (for infectious orbital cellulitis or abscess), steroids (for masticatory or extraocular muscle myositis; see Chap. 28), nonsteroidal anti-inflammatory drugs (for inflammation caused by potentially infectious disease), drainage (for orbital abscess), or a combination of these treatments.[11] Orbital neoplasia always carries a poor prognosis; many of these tumors are malignant, and local infiltration is usually such that recurrence is likely even after aggressive excision followed by chemotherapy and radiation therapy.[15]

Enophthalmos

Enophthalmos is an abnormal retraction or sinking of a normal-sized globe into the orbit.

Pathophysiology

Enophthalmos occurs as either an active or a passive disorder. Active enophthalmos occurs when the retractor bulbi muscles retract the globe deep into the socket. This retraction may be a reflex that occurs secondary to ocular irritation or pain, or it may be caused by tetanic extraocular muscle contractions. Passive enophthalmos occurs when there is reduction of orbital contents that allows the globe to sink back into the orbit because of lack of support. In addition, the globe may be forced caudally into the orbit by space-occupying masses of the cranial orbit. Two neurologic disorders that can cause apparent passive enophthalmos are Horner's syndrome[24–29] (seen in all animals and in humans) and bilateral third eyelid protrusion[13] or haws syndrome in cats. Horner's syndrome usually occurs unilaterally, although there are rare cases of bilateral involvement, and is caused by a deficit of sympathetic innervation to the iris dilator muscles, the Müller's muscle of the upper eyelid, the conjunctival and retrobulbar vasculature, and the extraocular muscles. Haws syndrome is attributed to decreased sympathetic tone to the orbital vasculature and smooth muscles.

Active enophthalmos is usually caused by surface ocular irritation (e.g., conjunctivitis, keratitis) or intraocular irritation (e.g., uveitis, glaucoma). It may be bilateral or unilateral. Bilateral active enophthalmos also is a manifestation of tetanus. Passive enophthalmos may be caused by loss of orbital mass (e.g., dehydration, cachexia, atrophy of orbital contents as a result of previous inflammation), Horner's syndrome, haws syndrome in cats, or abnormal cranial orbital structures retropulsing the globe (i.e., inflammatory or neoplastic swelling of the lids, third eyelid, or conjunctiva).

Clinical Signs

Clinical signs include third eyelid protrusion, possible drooping of the upper eyelid (ptosis) from lack of support by the globe, and the appearance that the globe is sitting deeper in the eye socket than is normal. Less of the sclera and cornea are seen in an enophthalmic eye because of the altered eyeball positioning.

Enophthalmos must be differentiated from microphthalmos and phthisis bulbi before additional diagnostic testing is pursued. Microphthalmos refers to a globe of smaller than normal size; it is a congenital condition. Additional defects, such as corneal size and shape abnormalities, anterior uveal abnormalities, lens abnormalities, and globe position or motion abnormalities, may accompany microphthalmos. Physiologic enophthalmos or pseudomicrophthalmos may be seen in dolichocephalic breeds such as collies and Doberman pinschers, in whom the deep eye socket gives the appearance of the globe's being smaller than normal. Phthisis bulbi is a scarred, contracted, usually blind eye that, because of its contracted size, has the appearance of enophthalmos. Previous history of ocular inflammation or injury, a cloudy and misshapen cornea, and internal ocular anomalies such as synechia, iris bombe, and cataract formation are all consistent with phthisis bulbi.

Diagnostic Plan

A thorough ophthalmic examination, sometimes with the aid of a topical or general anesthetic agent, may be needed to rule out surface or intraocular irritation as a cause of active enophthalmos. Tetanus can also cause bilateral active enophthalmos because of the tetanic contractions of extraocular muscles. Other musculoskeletal signs are usually seen with tetanus, although rapid, intermittent, spastic third eyelid protrusion caused by globe retraction may be one of the first clinical signs of tetanus noted by an owner.

Bilateral, passive enophthalmos secondary to chronic masticatory myositis[6, 8] in dogs usually shows other signs of masticatory muscle wasting. Acute masticatory myositis results in pain on attempt at opening the mouth; in chronic cases, there is no pain, but the mouth may not be able to be opened because of the muscle fibrosis. Bilateral passive enophthalmos caused by dehydration (especially seen in cats) or by cachexia is usually obvious based on the rest of the physical examination. Old dogs occasionally have bilateral enophthalmos because of age-related periorbital muscle atrophy. This is usually seen in conjunction with loss of muscle tone in the rest of the body.

Haws syndrome in cats is seen as a bilateral enophthalmos and passive protrusion of the third eyelids with no other ophthalmic signs. It is important to rule out conjunctivitis, keratitis, and anterior uveitis as a source of pain and cause of active enophthalmos. Many cats historically have clinical signs of upper respiratory or gastrointestinal disease (diarrhea) before the onset of the third eyelid protrusion. Because cats have smooth muscle fibers in the third eyelid that are innervated by the sympathetic nervous system,[2, 4] it may be that a virus or other infectious agent is responsible for a generalized sympathetic nervous system disorder leading to both the diarrhea and the third eyelid protrusion.

The classic clinical signs for Horner's syndrome include miosis (especially noticeable after dark adaptation), ptosis, mild conjunctival hyperemia, enophthalmos, and third eyelid protrusion. Horner's syndrome must be differentiated from anterior uveitis (which also shows aqueous flare, corneal edema, episcleral injection, and decreased intraocular pressure) before additional testing is instituted. Because there are a number of disorders of the sympathetic nervous system that may lead to the clinical signs of Horner's syndrome, pharmacologic testing to localize the lesion causing the Horner's syndrome[29] may be helpful in the diagnostic work-up (see Chap. 26).

Most cases of enophthalmos caused by neoplasia of the lids, conjunctiva, third eyelid, or cranial orbital structures are obvious on ophthalmic and physical examination.

Treatment

Treatment of the underlying disease (i.e., keratitis, conjunctivitis, uveitis, glaucoma, or tetanus) usually resolves cases of active enophthalmos. Most patients of haws syndrome recover without medical therapy within 2 to 4 weeks with no apparent long-term ill effects. One of us (JPP) has seen a number of haws syndrome cats with giardiasis in whom the third eyelid protrusion has responded favorably to oral therapy with metronidazole (see Chap. 32). Treatment of Horner's syndrome depends on the cause. Most cases of idiopathic postganglionic Horner's syndrome resolve with no therapy within a few weeks to a few months. Appropriate treatment of specific lesions causing Horner's syndrome (otitis or orbital inflammation in the case of postganglionic lesions, or cervical or cranial thoracic disease in preganglionic lesions) hastens the resolution of the clinical signs of Horner's syndrome. If the third eyelid protrusion hinders vision, symptomatic therapy in the form of topical application of 1% to 10% phenylephrine drops, two or three times a day as needed to the affected eye, may be helpful until the problem resolves. Topical phenylephrine is irritating, however, and clients should be advised of this before therapy.

Depending on the type of neoplasm retropulsing the globe, appropriate surgical removal, radiation therapy, chemotherapy, or some combination of these treatments may be beneficial. However, the long-term prognosis is poor.[15, 30] All adnexal and orbital neoplasias in cats carry a poor long-term prognosis.[31] In dogs, with the exception of primary third eyelid adenocarcinoma and meibomian adenomas, all adnexal neoplasia carries a poor to guarded prognosis as well.[30, 32]

Conjunctivitis

Conjunctivitis is inflammation of the mucous membrane that covers the bulbar surface of the eyelids, the third eyelid, and the visible portion of the sclera.

Pathophysiology

Conjunctivitis has many causes; infection, irritants, immune-mediated disease, and exposure are the major broad categories. There are numerous primary ocular causes for conjunctivitis in animals, and systemic diseases may also cause conjunctivitis. Allergic conjunctivitis (to molds, pollens, or dust), rickettsial diseases (Rocky Mountain spotted fever,[33, 34] ehrlichiosis[35]), and specific upper respiratory diseases (distemper virus in the dog[35–38] and herpes virus,[35, 36, 38–42] chlamydia,[35, 36, 38, 39, 43] and calicivirus virus[35, 36, 38, 39] infections in cats) are all systemic diseases usually associated with conjunctivitis.

Clinical Signs

Clinical signs of conjunctivitis include vascular engorgement or hyperemia, swelling or chemosis, excessive ocular discharge ranging from serous to mucoid to mucopurulent, and varying degrees of pain as noted by blepharospasm and self-trauma to the eyelids and adjacent structures.

Diagnostic Plan

It is beyond the scope of this chapter to describe the diagnostic plan for all causes of conjunctivitis in small animals. Instead, the purpose of this section is to cover the major clinical signs and diagnostic procedures for those systemic diseases that commonly cause conjunctivitis in dogs and cats.

Systemic disease–associated conjunctivitis in the dog is a bilateral disorder. A thorough ophthalmic examination should rule out primary ocular disease (i.e., lash, eyelid, or nasolacrimal duct anomalies, foreign bodies, sicca, primary bacterial infection, and exposure) as the cause of conjunctivitis. Allergic conjunctivitis is a bilateral, chronic disorder that is diagnosed by ruling out other primary causes of blepharoconjunctivitis. Most dogs with allergic conjunctivitis have a mucoid rather than purulent ocular discharge, they usually have other clinical signs of atopy (see Chap. 5), and the ocular signs usually respond to systemic therapy for atopy. Cytologic evaluation of conjunctival scrapings in these dogs usually reveals conjunctival epithelial cells and lymphocytes, but the eosinophils or mast cells commonly seen in humans with allergic conjunctivitis are rarely observed.

Rocky Mountain spotted fever[33, 34] and ehrlichiosis[35] occasionally produce conjunctivitis as one of many clinical signs. Ehrlichiosis is more likely to cause anterior uveitis and intraocular hemorrhage than is Rocky Mountain spotted fever, but both can cause these ocular signs along with conjunctivitis. Definitive diagnosis of these two diseases is based on additional clinical signs, hematologic findings, and serology (see Chap. 37).

Canine distemper virus–associated conjunctivitis is usually seen in conjunction with the classic acute catarrhal form of distemper. A bilateral, mucopurulent ocular discharge is usually noted along with conjunctival hyperemia. Distemper virus–associated adenitis of the lacrimal gland may cause decreased aqueous tear production, which can be measured with Schirmer tear test (STT) strips. Conjunctival scrapings and cytology may be helpful in diagnosing distemper in the early stages of the disease. Early inflammatory cell types tend to be more lymphocytic, progressing to neutrophilic as the disease progresses. Within the first 5 to 20 days after inoculation, multinucleate giant cells and intracytoplasmic inclusions may be seen; however, these characteristic inclusions may not be seen later in the course of the disease.[35–37] Indirect immunofluorescent antibody techniques may detect distemper virus in the acute states but are usually noncontributory late in the acute disease or with chronic cases.[38]

In contrast to dogs, cats seldom have conjunctivitis that is not associated with systemic disease. Primary sicca; lash, lid, and nasolacrimal duct anomalies; allergies; and primary bacterial conjunctival infections are uncommon causes of conjunctivitis in the cat. Upper respiratory diseases in the cat are very commonly associated with conjunctivitis. Feline herpes virus type 1 (FHV-1), *Chlamydia psittaci*, and feline calicivirus infection are the three most common causes of acute conjunctivitis in cats.[13] Reovirus infection and *Mycoplasma felis* are less common causes of feline conjunctivitis. Chronic conjunctivitis in cats is usually secondary to latent infections with FHV-1 or chlamydia, although this is difficult to definitively diagnose with routine diagnostic testing.[39]

The typical syndrome of FHV-1 infection is an acute, conjunctival-respiratory infection in neonatal or adolescent cats (see Chap. 51). The conjunctivitis is bilateral, with conjunctival hyperemia and serous ocular discharge that becomes mucopurulent as the disease progresses. The initial FHV-1 infection usually runs its course over a 2-week period,[13, 40, 41] and most cats do not experience long-term disease. Of the infectious diseases causing conjunctivitis in cats, FHV-1 is the only agent that produces keratitis (see Keratitis). Symblepharon formation (covering of the corneal surface with an adherent conjunctival membrane or ablation of the conjunctival cul-de-sacs from conjunctival adhesions) may be seen in cats after neonatal herpetic keratoconjunctivitis, but most cats recover with no long-term sequelae. FHV-1 may also cause recurrent episodes of conjunctivitis in adult cats that have presumably been exposed to, and have recovered from, the viral infection earlier in life. Adult FHV-1 infection may be unilateral, and clinical signs (conjunctival hyperemia, intermittent blepharospasm, and mild serous ocular discharge) are nondiagnostic in themselves. Recurrent bouts of conjunctivitis in the adult form of FHV-1 may be associated with periods of stress, corticosteroid usage,[42] or immunosuppressive diseases (feline leukemia virus [FeLV] and feline immunodeficiency virus [FIV]).[39] In the acute disease, a tentative diagnosis of FHV-1 can be made based on classic clinical signs. Fluorescein antibody testing of conjunctival scrapings may be helpful in definitively diagnosing acute cases of FHV-1 infection. Serologic testing has been reported to be helpful in identifying FHV-1 carriers,[41] but laboratory testing to determine an underlying cause for chronic recurrent conjunctivitis in older cats is diagnostic less than half the time.[39]

Chlamydia psittaci infections typically involve conjunctivitis and rarely cause a primary respiratory infection.[13] Unilateral conjunctivitis that becomes bilateral, marked conjunctival chemosis with hyperemia and occasional conjunctival lymphoid follicular hyperplasia, and serous ocular discharge that becomes mucopurulent are typical clinical signs. Intracytoplasmic inclusions are readily seen within conjunctival epithelial cells between days 7 and 14 of the infection but may not be seen in the case of chronic disease. Fluorescent antibody techniques can detect chlamydial antigen in the acute disease state.[13, 43] Chlamydial infections may be a cause of chronic conjunctivitis in cats, but this has been difficult to prove with routine

diagnostic techniques.[39] Calicivirus infections may produce mild serous ocular discharge and mild conjunctival hyperemia during the acute respiratory disease state. Except for the occasional production of keratitis in FHV-1, the clinical signs of calicivirus infection may not be distinguishable from those of acute FHV-1 infection.[35, 36, 38]

Treatment

Allergic conjunctivitis in dogs usually responds well to topical or systemic corticosteroids. A therapeutic trial of corticosteroids with alleviation of clinical signs may be one indirect method of confirming the tentative diagnosis in this difficult-to-diagnose disorder. Allergy testing and desensitization for atopy (see Chap. 5) improves the conjunctivitis if there is a positive response to the desensitization in general.

Treatment for canine distemper virus–induced conjunctivitis is supportive: cleansing the conjunctival surfaces with sterile collyria, topical broad-spectrum antibiotics (triple antibiotic, chloramphenicol, or gentamicin) to restrict secondary bacterial overgrowth, and topical tear supplementation if sicca is a problem. If decreased tear production leads to corneal ulceration, supportive surgical therapy (e.g., temporary tarsorrhaphy, third eyelid flaps, conjunctival flaps) is indicated.

Therapy for the acute form of calicivirus and FHV-1 conjunctivitis is supportive and consists of cleansing of exudates from the eyes and nose and broad-spectrum systemic and topical antibiotics to prevent secondary bacterial infections. Because corticosteroid therapy can prolong the clinical course of FHV-1 infection and may lead to stromal keratitis[41] or formation of corneal sequestra in herpes-infected cats,[41] topical and systemic steroids are contraindicated. Topical antiviral therapy for acute conjunctivitis induced by FHV-1 is usually not necessary,[44] and in recurrent cases of conjunctivitis caused by FHV-1 it is usually of minor benefit.[39]

Medical therapy for chlamydial conjunctivitis is in the form of topical tetracycline (Terramycin with polymixin B sulfate ophthalmic ointment) or systemic tetracycline. Because topical therapy must be performed four times per day, it may be easier to treat adult cats with oral tetracycline instead of topical tetracycline. Oral tetracycline causes discoloration of the enamel in those animals that do not have permanent dentition. In multiple-cat households, all cats should be treated at the same time in an attempt to eradicate the organism from the population.

Keratoconjunctivitis Sicca

Keratoconjunctivitis sicca (KCS), or "dry eye," is inflammation of the cornea and conjunctiva secondary to decreased tear production. Normal values for aqueous tear production in dogs and cats have been reported.[45, 46] A good clinical rule of thumb for tear production in the dog is that an STT value higher than 15 mm/minute is normal, between 10 and 15 mm/minute is questionable for sicca, and less than 10 mm/minute definitely indicates hyposecretion of aqueous tear. STT values alone are not adequate to diagnose decreased tear production in cats. Although STT values of more than 10 mm/minute are considered normal for cats, many cats have STT values of less than that amount when they are stressed or excited. Without the additional clinical signs of KCS, feline STT values of less than 10 mm/minute of themselves are not diagnostic of chronic decreased aqueous tear production.

Pathophysiology

Decreased aqueous tear production leads to increased production of the mucus component of the tear, exposure and drying of the corneal and conjunctival surfaces, and poor surface ocular health. Overgrowth of normal bacterial flora may cause secondary bacterial conjunctivitis or keratitis, or both.

Causes of decreased aqueous tear production include decreased parasympathetic stimulation to the lacrimal gland (through nerve damage or drug administration),[47, 48] iatrogenic removal of tear secretory tissue,[49] drug toxicities,[50–54] active inflammation of the lacrimal gland, and chronic inflammation of the lacrimal glands with scarring.[39, 41, 55–58]

Clinical Signs

Clinical signs of KCS include signs of ocular pain (blepharospasm and self-trauma); dried crusts on the eyelids or mucoid to mucopurulent ocular discharge; conjunctival hyperemia with thickening or hyperpigmentation (or both); lackluster corneal and conjunctival surfaces; recurrent history of corneal ulcerations or rapidly deteriorating corneal ulcers; corneal neovascularization, pigmentation, or hyperkeratosis; and potentially thick, crusty discharge from the ipsilateral nares. Clinical KCS is more commonly seen in dogs but can also be seen in cats. Because so many mechanisms for decreased tear production may involve systemic diseases or the treatment of systemic diseases, a review of some of the causes of KCS is presented here.

Diagnostic Plan

After the STT has established that there is decreased aqueous tear production, additional historical consideration, ocular examination, and physical examination findings should be addressed. If the animal is being treated with a topical or systemic parasympatholytic agent (e.g., atropine) or has undergone general anesthesia or sedation within the previous 24 to 48 hours, aqueous tear production should return to normal levels within 2 to 7 days after discontinuation of drug therapy.[47, 48] Systemic drug therapy with parasympatholytic agents, anesthetic agents, or sulfonamides[50–54] usually results in bilateral reduction of aqueous tear production.

If the sicca is unilateral, a history of injury to the ipsilateral ear or zygomatic arch region, a history of ipsilateral orbital disease, or current otitis media or otitis interna could indicate damage to the parasympathetic innervation to the lacrimal gland and the third eyelid gland (neurogenic sicca).[59] Previous amputation or other surgical manipulation of the gland of the third eyelid could cause decreased aqueous tear production.[49]

If purulent ocular discharge is present, indicating bacterial conjunctivitis, or if there are general clinical signs of distemper virus infection, conjunctival scrapings and cytology, scrapings and fluorescein antibody testing for distemper virus, and bacterial cultures may be helpful in diagnosing the primary cause or a contributing cause of the sicca. If the animal does not have a history or physical examination findings consistent with previous distemper virus infection[58] (or previous or chronic FHV-1 infection in a cat[39, 41]), then chronic, immune-mediated lacrimal adenitis (previously termed "idiopathic KCS") may be the cause of the sicca.[55–57] This is the most common disorder that causes KCS in the dog. This type of KCS seems to have a high degree of breed predisposition similar to that seen for other immune-mediated diseases such as atopy (e.g., American cocker spaniels, English bulldogs, Boston terriers, shih tzus, Lhasa apsos, miniature schnauzers, West Highland white terriers).

Treatment

Therapy for KCS depends on the cause. Removal of causative agents (topical atropine, general anesthetic agents, or sulfonamide therapy) usually results in return of normal tear production within 2 to 7 days. However, chronic sulfonamide therapy may totally destroy the functional tissue of the lacrimal glands because of its toxic effect, and restoration of tear production after discontinuation of therapy may not occur (this is especially true in those animals whose STT values are 0–3 mm/minute while on systemic sulfonamide therapy). Neurogenic KCS may respond to topical pilocarpine drops (0.125% to 0.25% concentrations two or three times per day) or systemic pilocarpine (1–2 drops of 2% solution in food, twice a day) if total atrophy of the lacrimal gland has not occurred.[59, 60] Supportive care with frequent (every 2–4 hours) artificial tear drops, lubricant ointment, and appropriate topical antibiotic therapy (depending on culture and sensitivity results) is indicated in all cases of KCS. With the discovery that topical application of cyclosporine reduces immune-mediated lacrimal adenitis with resultant return of aqueous tear production in dogs,[61, 62] the treatment of KCS in dogs has become much easier for client, veterinarian, and patient.[62–64] Commercially available cyclosporine 0.2% ointment for topical ophthalmic use (Optimmune) is now available in the United States. Animals that do not respond to topical antibiotic therapy (in 1–2 weeks), oral or topical parasympathomimetics (within 1 week), or topical cyclosporine (within 8 weeks) may require chronic maintenance therapy in the form of topical artificial tear supplementation or surgical therapy such as canthal closure or parotid duct transposition.[59, 60]

Keratitis and Keratopathy

Keratitis is defined as inflammation of the cornea; keratopathy is defined as noninflammatory disease of the cornea. Although many diseases involving inflammation or noninflammatory lesions of the cornea are primary diseases of the eye, there are some significant disorders of the cornea that are associated with systemic diseases. Furthermore, the corneal disease may be the first or most obvious clinical sign to the owner or veterinarian.

Pathophysiology

The three keratitis or keratopathy syndromes associated with systemic diseases that are discussed here are endotheliitis or uveitis caused by canine adenovirus type 1 (CAV-1),[65–68] ulcerative keratitis and stromal keratitis caused by FHV-1,[35, 36, 39–42, 44, 69] and stromal lipid degeneration or deposition in dogs as a result of metabolic diseases.[70–73]

CAV-1 infection in the dog causes the clinical disease infectious canine hepatitis (see Chap. 38). In the eye, this disease may cause noticeable keratitis with severe corneal edema ("blue eye") and signs of anterior uveitis. When CAV-1 replicates in the corneal endothelial cells, antiviral antibody deposition on the endothelial cell membranes with activation of the complement cascade (type III immune-complex deposition hypersensitivity, or Arthus reaction) leads to massive destruction of corneal endothelial cells.[65–68] Inflammation or necrosis of endothelial cells (which are responsible for maintaining corneal deturgescence) leads to marked corneal edema. This reaction may be unilateral or bilateral, and other signs of anterior uveitis may be noticed (see Uveitis). Severe corneal disease occurs in approximately 20% of the dogs with infectious canine hepatitis.[74] It was also seen in approximately 0.4% of dogs vaccinated with the older CAV-1 modified live virus vaccines (postvaccinational blue eye)[74]; this

reaction is almost nonexistent with the newer CAV-2 vaccines. However, there have been anecdotal reports of cases of apparent postvaccinational blue eye after vaccination with combination distemper virus, CAV-2, parainfluenza, leptospirosis, and parvovirus vaccine.[74] Because of the multiple antigens present in these types of vaccines, it is impossible to incriminate the CAV-2 component as being the cause of the uveitis and keratitis.

FHV-1 is the only conjunctivitis-causing systemic disorder that causes primary corneal disease in cats. Two types of keratitis may be seen with FHV-1: ulcerative keratitis (dendritic ulcers) and stromal keratitis. With the acute infection in young cats, corneal ulceration may be seen along with the typical signs of upper respiratory disease and conjunctivitis (see Conjunctivitis). Viral replication in the corneal epithelial cells causes fine, branching irregularities of the epithelium that may not be readily noticed with fluorescein stain. These dendritic ulcers (so called because of their characteristic branching pattern) may be better appreciated with topical application of the vital stain rose bengal (which stains the necrotic epithelial cells red). In the acute viral infection, these ulcerative lesions heal as the conjunctivitis and respiratory disease resolve. Older cats may have recurrent episodes of unilateral or bilateral ulcerative keratitis and conjunctivitis as a result of FHV-1 recrudescence associated with stress or immune-compromising disease (e.g., FIV, FeLV).

The stromal keratitis induced by FHV-1 is a deeper, more severe form of herpetic keratitis that may be seen in cases of acute herpetic infection that are inappropriately treated with corticosteroids[41, 44] or in older cats with recurrent or chronic herpetic keratitis. Endogenous stress (e.g., other concurrent disease, travel, boarding, surgery, new housing, new animal brought into the environment) or exogenous corticosteroid administration (either topically or systemically) are usual historical findings in older cats with any type of recurrent ocular herpetic disease. It is believed that herpetic stromal keratitis is due to an overzealous immune response to stromal depth viral antigen and may not be caused by active viral replication, as is the case with acute herpetic keratitis or conjunctivitis.

In dogs, deposition of abnormal fats, cholesterol, triglycerides, or mineralized lipid materials may be seen secondary to systemic diseases such as hypothyroidism, hyperparathyroidism, hyperadrenocorticism, diabetes mellitus, and hyperlipoproteinemia.[70–73] These corneal degenerative disorders or keratopathies may or may not cause a foreign body–like inflammatory response and may involve the peripheral or central cornea. Ophthalmic examination alone usually does not differentiate between inherited canine corneal dystrophy and these keratopathies associated with systemic disease.

Clinical Signs

Dogs with CAV-1–induced blue eye typically have rapid onset (within 24 hours) of severe corneal edema that may be unilateral or bilateral. Other clinical signs of infectious canine hepatitis (see Chap. 38) are also seen in dogs with street virus infections. Dogs with postvaccinational blue eye have a history of immunization with a vaccine containing live CAV (usually CAV-1), usually 4 to 7 days before the appearance of corneal edema. Episcleral injection, pain, and other signs of anterior uveitis (see Uveitis) are usually seen as well.

Young cats with FHV-1–induced ulcerative keratitis usually have all of the other clinical signs of FHV-1 infection (see Chap. 51). As mentioned previously, fluorescein staining may not be as definitive for the dendritic ulcers as is staining with rose bengal stain.

Clinical signs of stromal keratitis include blepharospasm, serous to mucopurulent discharge, deep (stromal depth) corneal neovascularization, cellular infiltration of the corneal stroma, and generalized corneal edema and collagen fibrillar damage that gives the appearance of a cloudy cornea. If ulceration is present (in most instances it is not), it may be in the form of a broader branching pattern (geographic ulcer) than is seen with dendritic ulcers.[40, 41] Corneal sequestra (dark, usually raised plaques of the axial cornea) may be seen in conjunction with stromal keratitis (especially in those cases treated inappropriately with topical corticosteroids).[41]

Lipid keratopathy is seen clinically as a white, usually nonpainful or uninflamed discoloration of the cornea. Inherited lipid degenerations are usually axial in location and are horizontally oval. Lipid keratopathy induced by metabolic disease may be axial in location, may be diffuse throughout the cornea, or may involve the limbal portion of the cornea.

Diagnostic Plan

Because uveitis and corneal edema have so many different causes (see Uveitis), a good physical examination and work-up for systemic disease should be considered if CAV-induced keratitis and uveitis are suspected. Probably the most important clinical signs leading to a diagnosis of CAV-1 blue eye are corneal edema and uveitis in a dog with other supporting clinical signs of infectious canine hepatitis or in an otherwise healthy dog with a history of immunization with live CAV within 1 week of onset of clinical signs.

Concerning FHV-1 ulcerative keratitis, any cat with bilateral conjunctivitis, upper respiratory disease, and corneal ulcers should be considered to have FHV-1–associated disease. Dendritic ulcers are considered pathognomonic for FHV-1 keratitis. Corneal and conjunctival scrapings in these acute cases usually show virus particles with fluorescein antibody testing.

A definitive diagnosis of FHV-1–associated stromal keratitis is much more difficult to obtain than is the case with acute keratoconjunctivitis caused by FHV-1.[39] Serologic testing for FHV-1[41] may be contributory, but the combination of clinical signs of unilateral or bilateral stromal keratitis with a history of previous acute signs of FHV-1 infection or presence of immune suppression by exogenous topical or systemic corticosteroids, stress, or immunosuppressive diseases makes for a diagnosis of FHV-1–induced stromal keratitis.

A serum biochemistry panel, a serum lipid profile, and thyroid and adrenal function testing are necessary to make a definitive diagnosis of metabolic disease–induced lipid keratopathy in the dog (see Chaps. 46, 47, and 50).

Treatment

Therapy for CAV-1–induced keratitis or keratouveitis is debatable. Some ophthalmologists do not treat the disorder, for fear that immunosuppressive drugs will prolong the natural recovery from the disease: most animals recover from the ocular disease within 21 days after natural infection if they do not die of other systemic disorders associated with infectious canine hepatitis. However, because the keratitis is immune-mediated and because other intraocular inflammations (e.g., iridocyclitis) may lead to worse disease (e.g., synechia formation, secondary glaucoma, phthisis bulbi), we believe that symptomatic medical therapy (see Uveitis) for the keratouveitis is necessary to retain a functional eye.

Therapy for acute FHV-1–associated ulcerative keratitis is usually symptomatic (see Conjunctivitis).[40, 41] Cats with ulcerative keratitis need antiviral therapy to speed the resolution of the keratitis, although antiviral therapy seldom leads to permanent resolution of recurrent or chronic ocular disease. Medical therapy for FHV-1–induced dendritic ulcers includes administration of a topical antiviral agent for 3 to 5 weeks, along with other supportive care. Agents that may be used include trifluorothymidine (Viroptic, five or six times per day), idoxuridine (Herplex, five or six times per day up to every 2 hours), and adenine arabinoside (Vira-A, four times per day).[69] Studies have shown trifluorothymidine to be the most effective antiviral agent for treatment of laboratory FHV-1 infection, but because the ointment form of adenine arabinoside can be used less frequently than liquid forms of antiviral agents, client compliance may be greater with this form. Because these agents are virostatic and resolution of clinical signs is dependent on the cat's own immune competency, testing for immunosuppressive viruses (FIV and FeLV) should be part of a diagnostic work-up in cases of recurrent ocular herpes disease in older cats.

Treatment of the underlying disease may help reduce the clinical signs of lipid keratopathy in some cases, but lipid deposition in some cases of metabolic disease–induced lipid keratopathy may be permanent despite successful treatment of the underlying disease. Symptomatic therapy in the form of topical corticosteroids may be necessary to treat active nonulcerative keratitis, although with some degenerative corneal disorders, such as those caused by hyperadrenocorticism, topical steroid administration may exacerbate the condition. Superficial keratectomy to remove abnormal tissue is seldom necessary or indicated, but it may be helpful if the lesion is superficial and painful and continues to worsen despite treatment of the underlying disorder (e.g., in dystrophic calcification of the cornea as a result of hyperadrenocorticism or hyperparathyroidism). Specific ocular medical or surgical therapy for lipid degeneration in hypothyroidism, diabetes mellitus, and hyperlipoproteinemia is rarely necessary.

Cataract

A cataract is an opacity of the lens capsule or of the lens cells and fibers and their proteins. Dislocation of the crystalline lens from its normal anatomic position between the anterior vitreous and the posterior iris is defined as a luxated lens.

Pathophysiology

In the dog, cataracts are commonly caused by inherited local metabolic defects of the lens epithelial cells and fibers.[75] Many breeds of dogs are genetically predisposed to the development of cataracts at a young age (juvenile cataracts), and all animals may develop lens opacification because of protein changes within the lens associated with aging (this is most commonly seen in humans and in the dog). With the exception of cataracts induced by diabetes mellitus and chronic uveitis, there are few systemic diseases that cause cataracts that are of clinical importance in the dog or cat. Certain toxic substances (naphthalene, dinitrophenol, and dimethyl sulfoxide), heavy metals (thallium, cobalt, and selenium), megavoltage irradiation, microwaves, electric shock, and dietary deficiencies in orphaned wolf pups, dog pups, and kittens have been implicated in the formation of cataracts.[75–82]

Diabetes mellitus is the only metabolic disorder leading to cataract formation.[75] Diabetic cataracts are inevitably seen in diabetic dogs but are only occasionally seen in diabetic cats. With diabetes mellitus, elevated aqueous humor glucose concentrations overload the typical pathway of glucose metabolism. With overload of the hexokinase enzyme pathway, an alternate pathway of glucose metabolism occurs, involving the enzyme aldose reductase with production of the alcohol sorbitol. Sorbitol acts as an osmotic substance to increase influx of fluid into the lens. Early on, this influx of fluid may be seen as fracture lines (intercellular clefts), particularly in the equatorial lens cortex. Eventually, increasing intracellular fluid leads to rupture of lens cells and lens opacification (diabetic cataract).[83, 84] Diabetic cataracts may be rapid in development from first onset of equatorial clefts to total cataract (days to weeks). Cataract formation may take many weeks or months to occur in the insulin-treated, regulated diabetic dog. Cataracts may be the first clinical sign of diabetes mellitus noticed by the owner.

Chronic uveitis alters the quality of the aqueous humor formed. Abnormal aqueous humor eventually disrupts the metabolism of the lens cells, resulting in lens cell death and opacification (i.e., cataract formation). Because of the chronic nature of uveitis induced by FeLV, FIV, or toxoplasmosis and of idiopathic uveitis in older cats, cataract formation is many times the first sign of uveitis in older cats. In contrast, uveitis is quite noticeable in dogs, followed by secondary cataract formation. Chronic uveitis may also cause lens capsular and zonular changes that lead to breakdown of the lens zonules that hold the lens in its normal anatomic position. Breakdown of zonular attachments or of the zonules themselves leads to lens luxation.

Clinical Signs

Diabetic cataracts may appear swollen or intumescent because of imbibition of fluid into the lens, the anterior chamber may be quite shallow, and there is a classic accentuation of the Y-suture pattern of the lens.[75, 83, 84] Anterior uveitis caused by leakage of lens proteins through the lens capsule is common with diabetes mellitus–induced cataracts, and many times this uveitis can be quite severe.

Because most dogs with uveitis have clinical signs that are noticed by the owner well before cataract formation occurs, most uveitis-induced cataracts in dogs are noted after a protracted period of dealing with the original uveitis state. In cats, however, the owner may notice either blindness or the color change of the cataractous lens before noting that the cat has chronic uveitis. Aside from a cataractous lens or a lens luxated into the anterior chamber, other signs of uveitis-induced lens changes in cats include signs of pain (blepharospasm, tearing), an edematous cornea, keratic precipitates, and posterior synechia (see Uveitis).

Diagnostic Plan

Any mature dog with a rapid onset of bilateral cataracts with or without other clinical signs consistent with diabetes mellitus (e.g., polyphagia, polydipsia, polyuria, lethargy, weight loss) should have a blood glucose level determination to rule out diabetes mellitus.

Older cats with luxated lenses or cataracts should have a thorough work-up for infectious causes of uveitis (see Uveitis).

Treatment

There is no medical treatment for cataracts, and surgical removal of the cataractous lens remains the only effective treatment.[75] Studies into the prevention of diabetic cataracts using aldose reductase inhibitor drugs (including aspirin) have been promising, and specific potent aldose reductase inhibitors may be commercially developed in the future for prevention of diabetic cataracts.[85–87]

Older cats with uveitis-induced cataracts or luxated lenses have a poor prognosis for restoration of vision after lens removal. Chronic uveitis, secondary glaucoma, retinal detachment, and/or degeneration are all common sequelae in these cats. Medical therapy for the uveitis (see Uveitis) may be attempted if the eye is painful. Enucleation may also be indicated for painful, medically unresponsive, blind eyes.

Uveitis

Uveitis is inflammation of the vascular structures of the eye (i.e., iris, ciliary body, and choroid). Terms that are commonly used to differentiate the portion of the eye and uveal tract involved include iridocyclitis or anterior uveitis (iris and ciliary body together inflamed); chorioretinitis or posterior uveitis (inflammation of the choroid in conjunction with the adjacent retina); panuveitis (inflammation of all three of the ocular vascular tunic components); endophthalmitis (inflammation within the anterior and posterior chambers and vitreous space as well as the uvea); and panophthalmitis (inflammation of all of the ocular structures together—uvea, retina, cornea, and sclera—and extension to the extraocular muscles, to the conjunctiva, and potentially to the orbital structures). In many instances, it is clinically impossible to differentiate anterior uveitis from panuveitis, but with specific disease states the inflammatory process may classically involve one particular area of the eye more than another.

Pathophysiology

In the review of applied anatomy and physiology at the beginning of this chapter, four barriers to the passage of whole blood into the ocular tissues (the BOB) were mentioned. The iris vessel endothelial tight junctions and ciliary body epithelium comprise the blood-aqueous barrier (BAB), and the retinal vessel endothelial cell tight junctions and retinal pigment epithelium make up the blood-retinal barrier (BRB).

When inflammatory mediators (e.g., prostaglandins, leukotrienes, interleukins) disrupt these vascular beds, leading to breakdown of the vascular and epithelial cell integrity (the BOB), increased protein levels as well as abnormal cellular elements and other inflammatory debris may be seen in the aqueous humor, the vitreous space, and the subretinal space—as aqueous flare and cells, vitreous debris, and subretinal fluid with detachment of the neural retina, respectively. Because the uvea has a large capillary bed with a rather high blood flow, hematogenously spread infectious organisms, antigen-antibody complexes, and neoplastic cells may be disseminated from other body parts, with resultant secondary eye disease. Many times, the ocular inflammation (or even blindness) noted by the owner is one of the first clinical signs of an underlying systemic disease.

When ocular inflammation breaks down the BAB, blood cellular elements, inflammatory cells, and large protein molecules are seen in the normally clear aqueous humor; this is termed hyphema (red cells), hypopyon (white cells), or aqueous flare. When inflammation breaks down the BRB, retinal perivascular exudates, intraretinal edema, subretinal edema, or subretinal exudates and retinal detachments may be seen.

A cause of BAB breakdown that is seen with canine distemper virus keratoconjunctivitis and FHV-1 keratitis (but is seldom seen with other systemic diseases) involves the reflex arc between ocular surface irritation and reflex ciliary muscle and iris sphincter muscle spasm; cranial nerve V is the afferent receptor and cranial nerve III is the efferent transmitter nerve in this arc.

Uveitis that is more likely to be associated with systemic disease involves chemical mediators of inflammation. Histamine, arachidonic acid derivatives produced by cyclo-oxygenase metabolism (prostaglandins, thromboxane, prostacyclin) and lipoxygenase metabolism (leukotrienes, hydroxyeicosatetraenoic acids), reactive oxygen metabolites, and angiotensin-converting enzymes are all major chemical mediators of intraocular inflammation.[74, 88–95] Because the uveal tract is highly vascular and has a high rate of blood flow, transport of these inflammatory mediators from other parts of the body to the eye may cause breakdown of the BOB with clinical signs of uveitis despite the fact that the eye is not the primary focus of inflammation. Intraocular production of these inflammatory mediators by intraocular microbes, neutrophils, lymphocytes, and other inflammatory cells can also cause uveitis. Infectious organisms are brought to the eye by hematogenous or neurologic routes; their active intraocular growth and their destruction of intraocular tissue are common causes of uveitis associated with certain infectious diseases. Depending on the organism and its route of spread to the eye, clinical signs may range from a primary anterior uveitis or a primary chorioretinitis to a much more severe endophthalmitis or panophthalmitis.

Immunologic mechanisms are important in the pathophysiology of uveitis. The eye supports four types of immune responses: type II (cytotoxic response), mediated by antibody; type III (immune-complex response), mediated by immune complex deposition and complement activation; type IV (cell-mediated response), mediated by T lymphocytes; and type V, which is characterized by production of autoantibodies for certain target organs.[74] With uveitis induced by systemic disease, antibody or antigen-antibody complex deposition may occur in the capillary beds of the uvea or in intraocular fluids and result in immune-mediated damage to the eye, in much the same manner that antigen-antibody complex deposition causes glomerulonephritis in the kidney. This is the mechanism for the anterior uveitis seen in conjunction with the blue eye keratitis of infectious canine hepatitis.

Although uveitis in dogs and cats may be caused by primary ocular trauma, primary ocular diseases, and hematogenously spread inflammatory mediators from unlimited nonspecific systemic disease states, certain specific systemic diseases have traditionally been associated with uveitis. In the cat, specific infectious diseases associated with uveitis include the viral-induced diseases (feline infectious peritonitis [FIP],[13, 35, 36, 96–101] FeLV complex,[13, 35, 36, 96–102] and FIV complex[13, 96, 100, 103]), toxoplasmosis,[13, 35, 36, 96, 99–101, 104–106] and the systemic mycoses (histoplasmosis,[13, 35, 36, 107–111] blastomycosis,[13, 35, 36, 111–117] cryptococcosis,[13, 35, 36, 118–122] and coccidioidomycosis[13, 35, 36, 123]). Infectious diseases associated with uveitis in the dog include the viral diseases (infectious canine hepatitis[65–68, 74, 101] and canine distemper virus,[35, 36, 101, 124–127]), specific bacterial diseases (canine brucellosis,[35, 36, 101, 128–130] Lyme borreliosis,[131] and leptospirosis[35, 36, 74, 101]), rickettsial diseases (ehrlichiosis[35, 36, 101, 132–134] and Rocky Mountain spotted fever,[33–36, 101]), the systemic mycoses (histoplasmosis,[35, 36, 74, 101, 135, 136] blastomycosis,[35, 36, 74, 101, 137–140] cryptococcosis,[35, 36, 74, 101, 141–143] and coccidioidomycosis[35, 36, 74, 101, 144, 145]), and protothecosis.[74, 146–151] Disseminated neoplasia[35, 36, 74, 101, 152–159] (especially lymphosarcoma[35, 74, 101, 160–162]) and autoimmune diseases[74, 101, 163–169] may also cause uveitis in the dog.

Clinical Signs

Clinical signs of uveitis are many, and their intensity may vary from subtle to fulminant. Early diagnosis and treatment of an underlying systemic

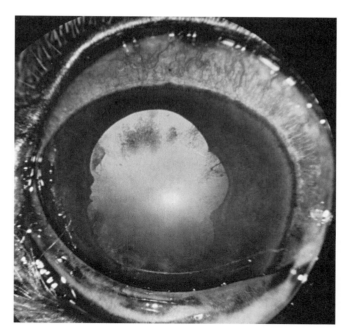

Figure 19–2

Injected episcleral vessels in a young dog recovering from anterior uveitis. The dog had been symptomatically treated with topical prednisolone acetate and atropine for 1 week before this photograph was taken. Notice the dyscoria caused by posterior synechia of the iris to the lens. Foci of iridal pigment ("pigment rests") are also noted on the anterior lens capsule.

disease that presents as a nonspecific uveitis may make the difference between retention and loss of ocular function (vision). More importantly, early detection and treatment of an underlying systemic disease may mean the difference between life and death of the patient. Client complaints that may be indicative of uveitis include signs of apparent pain with or without accompanying changes of behavior and attitude, ocular discharge, a red eye, a cloudy eye, or apparent vision loss. However, none of these complaints is specific for uveitis as opposed to other ocular diseases.

Blepharospasm, photophobia, and serous to mucoid ocular discharge are all clinical signs of ocular or periocular pain that may be caused by uveitis or other ocular disease. A red eye is a classic clinical sign of uveitis, but other external and internal ocular diseases may also cause a red eye. Typically, the red eye of uveitis involves engorgement of the deep, tortuous, somewhat individual vessels of the episclera (Fig. 19–2) instead of the generalized red discoloration of hyperemic conjunctiva seen with more superficial ocular disease. Episcleral injection may be first noted or most notable immediately adjacent to the corneoscleral limbus. Deep corneal neovascularization is seen as a red ring of short, straight vessels extending inward from the limbus; it is commonly seen with uveitis. Likewise, episcleral vessel injection may also be

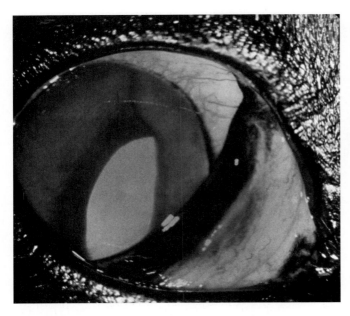

Figure 19-3
Swollen iris of an aged cat with anterior uveitis. The cat had disseminated lymphosarcoma that also involved the uveal tract of both eyes.

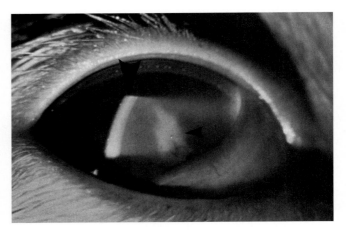

Figure 19-4
Granulomatous anterior uveitis in a young cat with ocular feline infectious peritonitis. The white line on the cornea *(large arrowhead)* is the slit beam of light as it passes obliquely through the edematous cornea. The beam of light can be seen in the anterior chamber as a result of the elevated protein levels in the aqueous humor ("aqueous flare"). A large "mutton fat" keratic precipitate on the corneal endothelial surface *(small arrowhead)* can be seen to the right of the slit beam of light.

secondary to deep corneal disease (deep microbial-induced ulcerative keratitis) or glaucoma as well as uveitis. Cats do not seem to have as marked an episcleral vessel injection or corneal neovascularization response as do dogs with apparently the same amount of intraocular inflammation. Generalized corneal edema may also be a sign of uveitis.

Iris changes are quite notable with uveitis and include miosis, changes in texture, and changes in color. In cases of subtle anterior uveitis, the miosis may not be readily apparent until the animal has been dark adapted and it is observed that the pupil does not dilate with dim light adaptation. When acutely inflamed, the iris "swells" and loses its normal lacy texture (Fig. 19–3). With chronic iritis, localized inflammatory cell accumulations (sometimes histologically seen as accumulations of lymphocytes and plasma cells) may give the iris stroma a nodular appearance. This is especially noticeable in cats with chronic uveitis. Chronic iritis may also cause degenerative changes seen as iris atrophy or thinning of the iris. In most animals, the iris color darkens with chronic inflammation, and ocular color change may be a presenting complaint. This hyperpigmentation is usually caused by the combination of inflammatory cells within the iris stroma and hypertrophy of iris melanocytes. With chronic iritis, a fibrovascular membrane (rubeosis irides) may grow across the iris surface and contribute a red or pink tint to the base iris color.

Decreased intraocular pressure or ocular hypotony is typical of uncomplicated uveitis. This de-creased intraocular pressure is caused by a combination of decreased active production of aqueous humor at the level of the ciliary body epithelium and increased outflow of aqueous humor through the uveoscleral outflow tract.[92, 94, 95, 170–173]

If the BAB in the iris and ciliary body is disrupted, the normally clear aqueous humor becomes turbid because of the increased level of protein or cells. This increased level of protein is best appreciated by shining a fine, bright, focused beam of light obliquely across the anterior chamber. As the light beam passes through the turbid aqueous humor, the protein molecules disperse the light beam, which makes the beam visible (Tyndall effect). Elevated aqueous humor protein that is seen clinically is termed aqueous flare (Fig. 19–4). With magnification, individual or clumped cells may also be seen suspended or settled within the aqueous humor.

Keratic precipitates are accumulations of inflammatory cells, pigment, and protein on the endothelial surface of the cornea. Typically, these precipitates are seen inferiorly because of the combined effects of gravity and the normal general circulation pattern of the aqueous humor in the anterior chamber. Large, waxy-yellow to tan accumulations are termed "mutton-fat" keratic precipitates and classically have been associated with granulomatous inflammatory processes (see Fig. 19–4). Elevated aqueous humor protein levels in conjunction with miosis may cause the posterior surface of the iris to become adherent to the anterior lens capsule. This adhesion (posterior synechia) inhibits mydriasis and can lead to a misshapen pupillary aperture (dyscoria; see Fig. 19–2) and an eccentric pupil (corectopia). If the pupillary margin is totally adherent to the lens, aqueous humor may not be able to circulate from the posterior chamber into the anterior chamber, which may cause the iris to bulge forward (iris bombe). This type of pupillary occlusion is a common cause of decreased aqueous outflow and glaucoma secondary to uveitis. Excessive accumulation of inflammatory cells and protein in the filtration angle may also inhibit outflow of aqueous humor with subsequent secondary glaucoma.

Because the lens receives its nourishment from the aqueous humor, chronic uveitis states may result in cataract formation because of less than optimal lens nourishment. It is important to determine, if possible, whether the cataract caused the uveitis (e.g., hypermature cataractous lenses seen with some inherited juvenile cataracts and with diabetic cataracts) or the uveitis led to the cataract formation. The history and other ocular and physical findings should be helpful in determining whether the uveitis or the cataract came first. Pigmented anterior lens capsule opacities may be seen where foci of posterior synechia have pulled loose, leaving behind uveal pigment on the lens capsule. These so-called pigment rests are indicative of previous anterior uveitis (see Fig. 19–2).

With inflammation of the choroid or retina, the most common owner complaint is vision deficit. Inflammatory debris in the vitreous space, retinal edema, inflammatory cell infiltration, or separation (detachment) can cause decreased vision or total vision loss. Posterior uveitis tends not to be as painful as is anterior uveitis (there is no painful ciliary muscle spasming associated with posterior uveitis), and clinical signs may go unnoticed until vision deficit is severe. Active chorioretinitis lesions appear "fuzzy" and poorly demarcated because of edema fluid or inflammatory cells within the retina or between the neural retina and the underlying reflective tapetum or pigmented nontapetal zone of the fundus. Vitreal debris and retinal detachment caused by inflammation may also obscure the normally sharp features of the tapetum and nontapetal zones. With active posterior uveitis, perivascular hemorrhage, fibrin, or exudates may make retinal blood vessels indistinct. Inflammation of the optic nerve may make the nerve head appear swollen, the edges indistinct, and the vessels overlying or adjacent to the nerve head indistinct. Subretinal inflammatory debris that has organized into the equivalent of a subretinal abscess has been termed "granulomatous chorioretinitis" (Figs. 19–5 and 19–6).

Areas of previously active chorioretinitis that have subsequently healed produce a sharply demarcated pattern, like scar tissue elsewhere in the body. Previous sites of chorioretinitis in the tapetal area of the

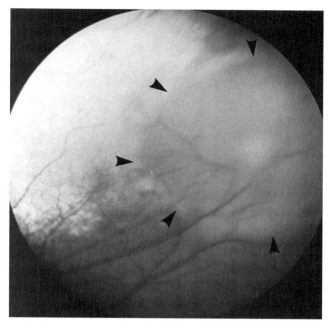

Figure 19–5

Granulomatous chorioretinitis in a dog with blastomycosis. Notice the dull, indistinct area to the right in the photograph, outlined by arrowheads. Retinal vessel and tapetal detail are lost in this area because of choroidal and intraretinal exudate.

ocular fundus may appear as sharply demarcated areas of tapetal hyperreflectivity because of the death of the overlying neural retina. Hyperpigmentation within this area of hyperreflectivity (Fig. 19–7) may represent hypertrophy and hyperpigmentation of the normally nonpigmented retinal pigment epithelial cells that overlie the tapetum. Vascular attenuation is commonly seen in areas of retinal death and degeneration from previous chorioretinitis.

Inactive (healed) optic neuritis may be seen as a loss of myelination, shrinkage of the optic nerve, vascular attenuation of the nerve head vessels, or sharply delineated peripapillary hyperreflectivity, depigmentation, or hyperpigmentation. In the nontapetal region of the fundus, sharply demarcated areas of depigmentation or hyperpigmentation are usually indicative of chorioretinal scarring from previous inflammation (Fig. 19–8). The amount of vision lost from previous chorioretinitis depends on the amount and specific area of retina death, how complete the destruction of the retinal layers (photoreceptors, bipolar cells, ganglion cells) has been, and the integrity of the optic nerve.

Diagnostic Plan

The diagnostic work-up for the underlying cause of uveitis is always a challenge to the generalist

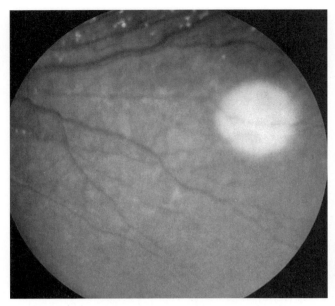

Figure 19–6
Granulomatous chorioretinitis in a dog with cryptococcosis. Notice the dull, indistinct gray area against the dark nontapetal area (to the right in the photograph). Notice the deviation of the retinal vessel, which results from retinal elevation caused by subretinal inflammatory debris.

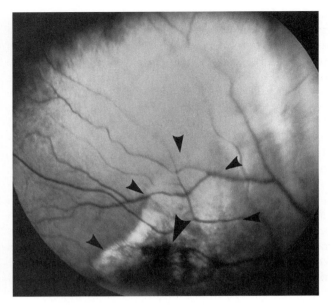

Figure 19–7
Area of retinal scarring and retinal pigment epithelium hypertrophy in the fundus of a dog that had recovered from blastomycosis. Notice the well-demarcated area of tapetal hyper-reflectivity *(small arrowheads)* in the inferior portion of the photograph and the hyperpigmented area *(large arrowhead)* within the zone of hyperreflectivity.

and the veterinary ophthalmologist alike. The clinical ocular signs (e.g., anterior uveitis, posterior uveitis, or panuveitis; unilateral versus bilateral involvement; granulomatous versus nongranulomatous uveitis), the history (e.g., duration of signs, progression, vaccination history, housing, area of the country involved, travel, other animals in the household that may or may not have physical problems), and the general physical examination findings (e.g., pyrexia; skin, lymphatic, pulmonary, gastrointestinal, or locomotor system abnormalities) all can contribute to the final definitive diagnosis.

Among cats younger than 1 year of age, more than half of the animals with bilateral anterior uveitis have FIP. Disease associated with FeLV or FIV complex or toxoplasmosis is also seen in these young cats, especially in outdoor cats and cats with a history of exposure to outdoor cats. In cases of unilateral anterior uveitis, primary ocular disease (e.g., trauma) should be ruled out, if possible, by ophthalmic examination. Although less commonly associated with anterior uveitis, other nonspecific systemic diseases (e.g., abscess, pneumonia, pyometra) should be ruled out by general physical examination. In young adult and middle-aged cats with anterior uveitis that are in endemic areas or have history of exposure, a diagnosis of systemic fungal disease may be considered (e.g., histoplasmosis, blastomycosis, coccidioidomycosis), although these diseases are rare in cats. In cases of

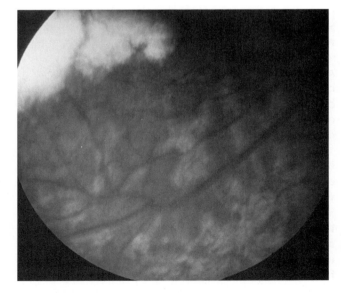

Figure 19–8
Multifocal areas of sharply demarcated, depigmented foci in the nontapetal zone of the ocular fundus of a dog that had recovered from canine distemper. These depigmented areas represent retinal thinning and retinal pigment epithelium depigmentation as a result of scarring of the retina and choroid after distemper virus infection.

unilateral or bilateral chronic anterior uveitis, posterior synechia, cataract formation, glaucoma, or lens luxation in middle-aged or older cats, FeLV complex, FIV complex, and toxoplasmosis should be considered as underlying systemic diseases. Granulomatous chorioretinitis and retinal detachments may be seen with FIP, toxoplasmosis, and lymphosarcoma caused by FeLV complex. Cats with granulomatous chorioretinitis and retinal detachments are more likely to have systemic fungal diseases than are cats with anterior uveitis alone.

The routine laboratory work-up on cats with uveitis should include a CBC and serum biochemistry panel. Increased total protein (especially globulins) may be indicative of FIP. Anemia, thrombocytopenia, or leukopenia may be indicative of FeLV or FIV complex. Presence of neoplastic lymphocytes is indicative of FeLV-associated lymphosarcoma. Elevation of hepatic enzymes may be consistent with toxoplasmosis or FIP. Thoracic and abdominal radiographs may be useful in locating multifocal pulmonary granulomas (i.e., fungal diseases), signs of pleuritis or peritonitis (FIP), and lymphadenopathy or organomegaly (FeLV-associated lymphosarcoma, systemic mycotic diseases, toxoplasmosis).

Infectious disease serology (especially for FeLV, FIV, toxoplasmosis, and cryptococcosis) may help identify the underlying cause of uveitis in cats (see Chaps. 38–40). In those animals that cannot be definitively diagnosed by physical examination, routine laboratory evaluation, radiology, and serology, ocular aspiration with cytology and culture may be helpful. Subretinal aspirates from animals with detached retinas may be especially helpful in the rare cases of systemic fungal infection. Aqueous humor centesis and evaluation in cases of anterior uveitis alone seldom contribute to the definitive diagnosis. Enucleation of a blind, painful eye and evaluation by a competent ophthalmic pathologist may be helpful in the definitive diagnosis of an underlying systemic disease.

Because uveitis is more common in the dog than in the cat, and because there are more systemic disease causes of uveitis in dogs than cats, a diagnostic work-up for uveitis in a dog tends to be more involved. Signalment and general history, ophthalmic examination, a thorough physical examination, general laboratory tests (CBC, serum biochemistry panel, and urinalysis), radiology, infectious disease serology, tests for immune-mediated disorders, and other tests such as impression smears and fine-needle aspirates of tissues with accompanying cytologic evaluation and culturing may all be necessary to come up with a definitive diagnosis for an underlying disease that is the cause of uveitis. Even with fairly exhaustive diagnostic work-ups, as many as one fourth to one half of uveitis cases remain idiopathic.

Pampered house dogs have a lower incidence of uveitis secondary to infectious disease than outside dogs that have exposure to other dogs and wildlife. Sexually intact dogs that are allowed to roam may have a higher incidence of uveitis caused by brucellosis. Dogs exposed to ticks have a higher potential for tick-borne diseases (i.e., Rocky Mountain spotted fever, ehrlichiosis, and Lyme borreliosis). Dogs with a questionable vaccination history may have an increased incidence of chorioretinitis resulting from distemper virus infection or blue eye from infectious canine hepatitis; likewise, a puppy with the history of having just had immunizations may be more likely to have vaccination-induced blue eye. Dogs that eat raw meat or rodents may be at risk for toxoplasmosis or leptospirosis. Hunting dogs and dogs that dig in the dirt may be at higher risk for uveitis induced by systemic fungal disease (especially coccidioidomycosis in the desert southwestern United States, blastomycosis in the American Midwest, especially in the Mississippi and Ohio River valleys, and histoplasmosis in the central United States). History of travel to an endemic area for an infectious disease that is not endemic in the home area is important in the work-up of a case of uveitis. Older dogs have a higher incidence of uveitis caused by disseminated neoplasia.

Very few clinical ophthalmic signs are pathognomonic for a specific disease in the dog. Many factors are responsible for what is seen on ophthalmic examination, including the stage at which the eye is examined (early or late in the disease course), how well the dog's immune system is handling the disease, whether the dog being treated effectively for the underlying disorder, and what kind of supportive therapy is being used. Nevertheless, some general guidelines concerning findings of the ophthalmic examination may be useful to the veterinary practitioner in the work-up to diagnose the underlying cause of the dog's uveitis.

It would seem logical that a systemic disease would lead to bilateral ocular involvement, but this is not necessarily the case. Early in the course of the disease, only one eye may be afflicted. Hematogenous spread of an infectious organism directly to the eye may be unilateral (this is especially true with systemic fungal infections). The typically nongranulomatous, mild anterior uveitis caused by release of systemic inflammatory mediators from localized nonocular infections (e.g., pyometras, bacterial pneumonias, localized abscesses, anal sac abscesses, prostatitis) and from some particular systemic infectious diseases (leptospirosis, Lyme borreliosis, and Rocky Mountain spotted fever) is usually bilateral in its presentation, as is the granulomatous or nongranulomatous uveitis caused by certain autoimmune disorders. The chorioretinitis of canine distemper virus infection is typically bilateral, as is the associated conjunctivitis and decreased tear production. Uveitis induced by ehrlichiosis or canine brucellosis may begin as a unilateral problem but usually becomes bilateral. Toxoplasmal uveitis may also begin unilaterally and eventually become bilateral. Uveitis caused by disseminated lymphosarcoma is typically bilateral, but other types of disseminated neoplasia (e.g., mammary, renal, and prostatic adenocarcinomas, hemangiosarcomas, melanomas, pulmonary and squamous cell carcinomas) are evenly distributed with regard to unilateral versus bilateral ocular metastasis and secondary uveitis.

The severity of episcleral injection that is seen depends on the stage of the disease at examination. As a whole, cases of endophthalmitis (caused by systemic fungal diseases such as blastomycosis and coccidioidomycosis, ehrlichiosis, brucellosis, and hematogenously disseminated nonspecific bacterial infections) tend to have the worst episcleral injection. Uveitis caused by release of inflammatory mediators from nonocular tissues tends not to cause as severe an episcleral injection. Autoimmune phenomena (especially uveodermatologic syndrome or Vogt-Koyanagi-Harada–like syndrome) and disseminated lymphosarcoma may cause severe episcleral injection. Uveitis from any cause with secondary glaucoma usually results in pronounced episcleral injection.

Severe corneal edema is commonly seen with adenoviral infections (e.g., infectious canine hepatitis). Endophthalmitis tends to cause severe corneal edema, as does glaucoma secondary to uveitis. Mild corneal edema is a nonspecific sign of anterior uveitis from any cause.

Early in the course of the disease, mild anterior uveitis (mild episcleral injection, minimal corneal edema, aqueous flare, and miosis) may be seen in conjunction with any underlying disease. Severe granulomatous anterior uveitis (with hypopyon, keratic precipitates, high anterior chamber cell counts, posterior synechia, and iris bombe) is most typically seen with coccidioidomycosis and blastomycosis, ehrlichiosis, brucellosis, septicemias that have hematogenously been spread to the eyes, uveodermatologic syndrome, and ocular lymphosarcoma.

Anterior chamber hemorrhage accompanying uveitis is seen most commonly with rickettsial infections (Rocky Mountain spotted fever and ehrlichiosis) and ocular lymphosarcoma (see later section on intraocular hemorrhage).

Autoimmune phenomena (uveal dermatologic syndrome and autoimmune chorioretinitis), cryptococcosis, histoplasmosis, distemper virus, protothecosis, and disseminated lymphosarcoma may cause chorioretinitis or retinal detachments (or both) alone or with minimal anterior segment inflammation. The systemic fungal or algal infections tend to cause more of a

granulomatous chorioretinitis (see Figs. 19–5 and 19–6), whereas autoimmune chorioretinitis may cause a clear, subretinal fluid with detachment or retinal edema. Active distemper virus retinochoroiditis appears as multifocal, serous areas of chorioretinitis. Old, healed lesions of distemper virus retinochoroiditis appear as well-delineated, multifocal scars (tapetal hyperreflectivity or "gold medallions" in the tapetal zone of the fundus and depigmented foci in the nontapetal fundus; see Figs. 19–7 and 19–8). Blastomycosis and coccidioidomycosis may cause granulomatous chorioretinitis and retinal detachments without severe anterior uveitis (especially early in the disease state). Optic neuritis may be seen with cryptococcal infections. Chorioretinitis with retinal hemorrhages is most commonly seen with rickettsial infections and disseminated lymphosarcoma but may be seen with almost any cause of chorioretinitis (see later section on posterior segment hemorrhage).

Nonspecific physical examination findings such as fever, depression, anorexia, and weight loss may or may not contribute significantly to a uveitis diagnostic work-up. Dogs with uveitis caused by immune-mediated diseases or disseminated neoplasia often are not febrile. Fever is an inconsistent finding with infectious disease–induced uveitis and depends on the state of disease and what other body systems may be involved in addition to the eyes. If the uveitis state is causing severe pain or blindness, nonspecific signs such as depression, anorexia, and weight loss may be present even if no other body systems are involved.

Granulomatous skin lesions may be caused by systemic fungal diseases (especially blastomycosis), and subcutaneous nodular skin lesions may be a sign of lymphosarcoma. Facial dermatitis (especially of the dorsal nose and around the eyelids) with depigmentation of the hair and skin (poliosis and vitiligo, respectively) in conjunction with bilateral granulomatous panuveitis may be indicative of uveodermatologic syndrome. Lymphadenopathy can be caused by a number of diseases. Systemic fungal diseases, rickettsial diseases (especially ehrlichiosis), brucellosis, and lymphosarcoma are common causes of uveitis with lymphadenopathy and should be ruled out in the uveitis work-up.

Dogs with active retinochoroiditis and seizures may have acute canine distemper virus (and dogs with old chorioretinal scars and neurologic abnormalities may have chronic distemper as an underlying cause). Stuporous or demented dogs and dogs with other cranial nerve disorders with accompanying optic neuritis, blindness, or granulomatous chorioretinitis should be evaluated for cryptococcosis, granulomatous meningoencephalitis, and central nervous system neoplasia. Respiratory system abnormalities (e.g., nasal discharge, coughing, dyspnea) associated with uveitis indicate canine distemper virus or systemic fungal disease.

Musculoskeletal abnormalities may be localizing or differentiating clinical findings in a uveitis work-up. Bone pain may indicate osteomyelitis caused by fungal disease (especially blastomycosis). Joint inflammation may be seen with Lyme borreliosis or autoimmune disorders. Myositis may be seen with toxoplasmosis. Back pain and neurologic disorders localized to spinal disease may be associated with brucellosis or discospondylitis from other infectious causes.

Splenomegaly and hepatomegaly may be important physical examination findings in a uveitis work-up. Splenomegaly may be seen with rickettsial diseases, chronic systemic infections (e.g., bacterial septicemias, discospondylitis), autoimmune phenomena, and specific neoplasia (especially hemangiosarcoma and lymphosarcoma) with ocular metastasis. Hepatomegaly may indicate toxoplasmosis, infectious canine hepatitis, and organ-specific or disseminated neoplasia. Both splenomegaly and hepatomegaly may be seen with systemic fungal infections. Urogenital abnormalities may also be important in a uveitis work-up. Abnormal urination with or without lumbar pain, fever, and weight loss may be seen with leptospirosis or pyelonephritis of any cause. A history of abortion or orchitis may be consistent with brucella infection. Orchitis may also be seen with systemic fungal infections (especially blastomycosis).

Gastrointestinal abnormalities such as vomiting and diarrhea may be important clinical signs in the work-up of a uveitis case. Chronic diarrhea with weight loss can be seen with histoplasmosis, acute vomiting and diarrhea may be seen with canine distemper, and chronic hemorrhagic diarrhea associated with granulomatous chorioretinitis may be seen with prototheccosis. Vomiting and diarrhea with or without icterus may be seen in animals with anterior uveitis who have infectious canine hepatitis or leptospirosis.

Thoracic and abdominal radiography are important diagnostic tests to be included in a uveitis work-up. Thoracic radiography may uncover subclinical pneumonia from a number of possible causes. Pulmonary granulomas and hilar lymphadenopathy may be seen with systemic fungal infections. Metastatic neoplasia may be detected with routine thoracic radiography. Abdominal radiographs may pick up liver, spleen, or kidney enlargement or irregularities. Enlarged abdominal lymph nodes that could not be palpated on physical examination may be detected. Peritonitis and vertebral abnormalities (e.g., discospondylitis) may be detected on routine abdominal radiography.

A CBC, serum biochemistry panel, and urinalysis are always indicated in a complete uveitis work-up.

Anemia or platelet deficiencies may indicate rickettsial diseases, chronic infection, autoimmune phenomena, or lymphosarcoma. Inflammatory leukograms may be indicative of an infectious disease as an underlying cause of the uveitis, although some animals with infectious disease–induced uveitis may not have an inflammatory leukogram. As was the case with clinical ocular signs and fever, the white blood cell count and differential are very much affected by the stage of the disease, the involvement of body systems other than the eyes, how the dog's immune system is handling the disease, the specific therapy, and supportive ocular or systemic therapies. A urinalysis may help in the diagnosis of pyelonephritis or cystitis as an underlying cause of uveitis; it may reveal glomerulonephritis secondary to infectious or immune-mediated disease, and it may contribute to the evaluation of the dog's renal function. A serum biochemistry panel can help localize other organ involvement (e.g., hepatic disorders) and may identify electrolyte abnormalities (e.g., hypercalcemia associated with lymphosarcoma); it is, therefore, useful in the diagnostic work-up of any uveitis case.

Serology for infectious diseases is often helpful, but the diagnostic tests run must be based on knowledge of potential findings based on the species and breed, clinical signs seen, area of the world in which the animal lives or has traveled, and potential exposures (see Chaps. 36–40). Tests for autoimmune diseases (e.g., antinuclear antibody, rheumatoid factor) may be indicated if clinical signs point to an immune-mediated disorder (see Chap. 55).

If applicable, fine-needle aspiration and cytology of lymph nodes, bone marrow, and draining skin wounds or cutaneous masses; transtracheal aspiration for cytology or culture; and urine culture may be helpful in making a definitive diagnosis. Although not always helpful or indicated, ocular aspiration for cytologic evaluation or culture may be of some benefit. Anterior chamber centesis is seldom helpful in the isolation of microbes causing anterior uveitis. Aqueous centesis of hypopyon in cases of lymphosarcoma may yield a diagnosis, but lymph node, splenic, and bone marrow aspirates are usually easier to obtain and have a higher diagnostic yield. Vitreal or subretinal aspirates (in animals with detached retina) may be especially helpful in reaching a diagnosis in cases of granulomatous endophthalmitis associated with mycotic, bacterial, or algal infections. The potential risk for causing more harm to the eye (i.e., worsening uveitis, hyphema, or detached retina) must be weighed against the potential for gaining useful information. Likewise, enucleation of a painful, irreparably blind eye and a subsequent histopathologic evaluation performed by an experienced ocular pathologist may be invaluable in the final determination of the uveitis.

Treatment

Definitive therapy for uveitis involves treatment of the underlying systemic disease. However, up to half of the cases of uveitis in veterinary medicine remain idiopathic despite thorough diagnostic workups. Symptomatic therapy for uveitis is, therefore, necessary to reduce ocular inflammation and to salvage ocular function (vision), if possible, while waiting for specific therapy to take effect. Supportive care of the eye only helps to alleviate the clinical signs, however, and systemic corticosteroids alone may inhibit resolution of a systemic infectious disease (with potential fatal consequences).

There are three major classifications of drugs that are used for treatment of intraocular inflammation: cycloplegic agents, corticosteroid agents, and nonsteroidal anti-inflammatory drugs. Cycloplegic agents are parasympatholytic drugs that block the effects of the parasympathetic nervous system on the iris and ciliary body smooth muscle. Paralysis of these smooth muscles stabilizes BAB integrity and blocks parasympatholytically stimulated neurotransmitters that mediate uveal inflammation.[174, 175] Paralysis of the ciliary and iris sphincter muscles diminishes the pain associated with anterior uveitis. Mydriasis also decreases the frequency of posterior synechia. A 1% atropine ophthalmic solution or ointment is recommended one to four times per day, depending on the severity of the inflammation and the clinical response to treatment. Although ciliary spasm may still be present with a maximally dilated pupil, pupillary dilation is a relatively reliable indicator of drug efficacy. After the pupil is fully dilated, frequency of atropine use may be decreased to a point at which a dilated pupil is maintained for most of the 24-hour period. Other factors, such as the presence of prostaglandins and other inflammatory mediators, play a part in miosis, and lack of immediate total mydriasis does not necessarily indicate a need for increased frequency of drug application. Adverse reactions to atropine use include decreased aqueous tear production, tachycardia, decreased gastrointestinal motility, and potential precipitation of acute glaucoma in those canine breeds predisposed to narrow filtration angles.[47, 74] Passage of atropine through the nasolacrimal duct system to the nares and licking of the drug from the nose may cause excessive salivation and even vomiting from the drug's bitter taste. This response is more common in cats, and use of atropine ointment instead of solution may prevent it.

Corticosteroids are the primary therapy of choice for uveitis. Despite the fact that there is some systemic absorption with topical application,[176–178] topical corticosteroids may be used to treat all cases of anterior uveitis except when ulcerative keratitis or uncontrolled ocular infectious disease is present. Although there is some debate over the use of topical steroids to treat uveitis in those cases that are caused by systemic infectious disease, the benefits of topical steroids to control intraocular inflammation and maintain vision outweigh the potential problems of minor local (or systemic) immunosuppression. Topical corticosteroids are of use in the treatment of anterior uveitis cases only. Chorioretinitis cannot successfully be treated with topical drugs because of the inability of the drug to reach the posterior segment. Posterior segment inflammation must be treated with systemic administration of corticosteroids if a beneficial effect is to be seen.

Concentration and penetrability of the drug are important factors to consider when choosing a topical corticosteroid. Topical 1% prednisolone acetate suspension produces the best anti-inflammatory effect with an intact cornea, followed by 0.1% dexamethasone alcohol suspension, 0.1% prednisolone phosphate solution, and 0.05% dexamethasone phosphate ointment.[179] Some advocate subconjunctival injection of repository corticosteroid suspensions (triamcinolone acetonide, methylprednisolone acetate, or betamethasone), but this form of administration results in increased systemic absorption of the drug over topical application alone[180] and may occasionally result in subconjunctival granuloma formation.[181] Subconjunctival corticosteroids should never be used alone, but they should be used to augment topical application of corticosteroids if client ability to treat topically is limited. We seldom use subconjunctival steroids in small animal patients.

Intensity of inflammation and contact time of the drug used dictate the frequency of topical drug administration. Initial therapy with solutions or suspensions may require application as often as four to six times per day, whereas corticosteroid-containing ointments may be used three to four times per day with the same efficacy. Because there is some systemic absorption of topically applied corticosteroids with an effect on the pituitary-adrenal axis,[176–178] a slow weaning of drug is necessary after long-term use.

Systemic corticosteroids may be used to treat both anterior and posterior uveitis, but they should be used with extreme caution in uveitis cases with potential or proven systemic bacterial or fungal origin. The dosage of systemic corticosteroid varies depending on the intensity of the inflammatory process and the cause of the disorder. Dosages may range from 0.22 to 1.1 mg/kg per day of oral prednisolone, for uveitis induced by mild, nonspecific, noninfectious disease, to 2.2 to 4.4 mg/kg per day of oral prednisolone for immune-mediated uveitis. If systemic steroids are to be used in an attempt to maintain vision in the presence of infectious disease, the dosages should be the lower anti-inflammatory levels, not the higher immunosuppressive levels. Systemic steroids must be used with extreme caution in cases of systemic infection or diabetes mellitus. Systemic corticosteroids can be used judiciously in cases of uveitis with superficial corneal ulceration, but they should not be used for deep ulcerative keratitis or herpetic keratitis.

Nonsteroidal anti-inflammatory drugs may be used topically and systemically in conjunction with or instead of corticosteroids to treat uveitis.[91–95, 182, 183] Because these drugs do not suppress the animal's natural immune system, they may be used more safely than corticosteroids to treat uveitis cases involving infectious systemic diseases. Flurbiprofen 0.03% solution (Ocufen) and suprofen 1% solution (Profenal) are topical medications marketed for use in humans to inhibit prostaglandin-induced intraoperative miosis during cataract surgery. Their ability to decrease intraocular inflammation is not as great as that of the previously recommended topical corticosteroids. Neither drug significantly inhibits corneal stromal healing, nor do they enhance collagenase activity as the topically applied corticosteroids do, so they may be used instead of topical steroids to treat patients with uveitis and ulcerative keratitis. They should not be used for viral keratitis, and they may potentiate intraocular or conjunctival hemorrhage.

Commonly used systemic nonsteroidal anti-inflammatory drugs include aspirin, phenylbutazone, and flunixin meglumine. Dosage of aspirin for the treatment of anterior uveitis in the dog is 15 to 25 mg/kg two to three times per day. Flunixin meglumine has not been approved by the US Food and Drug Administration for use in companion animals, but intravenous dosages of 0.25 to 1.0 mg/kg once, 0.25 mg/kg daily for 5 days, or 0.5 mg/kg daily for 3 days have been reported as acceptable.[74] Because gastrointestinal hemorrhage, gastric ulceration, and acute renal failure are adverse side effects occasionally seen after use of systemic nonsteroidal anti-inflammatory drugs, patients should be monitored for vomiting, diarrhea, melena, and urine output. We do not use these drugs in feline uveitis patients.

Lipemic Aqueous Humor

Lipemic aqueous humor is a milky, hazy-gray discoloration of the anterior chamber fluid caused by the presence of lipid material derived from the blood stream.

Pathophysiology

Lipemic aqueous humor occurs when lipoproteins in the systemic circulation gain entrance into the aqueous humor after what is usually a minor breakdown in the BAB. Although most animals with lipemic aqueous humor have minimal uveitis, marked uveitis with secondary glaucoma has been reported.[127, 184, 185]

Although some sort of breakdown of the BAB is necessary to have lipemic aqueous humor, finding the cause of the usually low-grade anterior uveitis is seldom as important as finding the cause of the underlying lipemia. Metabolic disorders that may cause lipemia and subsequent lipemic aqueous include hypothyroidism,[184] pancreatitis, diabetes mellitus, and hepatic dysfunction. A high-fat diet may also be an underlying cause of lipemia.

Clinical Signs

Lipemic aqueous humor is usually an acute disorder. Because of the marked ocular discoloration, it is usually soon noticed by the owner. The intensity of the white discoloration may wax and wane over a period of hours to days. Although the cornea is clear, the aqueous humor is milky white and may obstruct visualization of the iris and deeper ocular structures. The disorder may be bilateral, but unilateral involvement is more common. Subtle clinical signs of anterior uveitis (e.g., episcleral injection, ocular hypotension, miosis, photophobia) may be present, but most dogs have very minimal signs of anterior uveitis.

Diagnostic Plan

A work-up for lipemia should include a serum biochemistry panel, thyroid testing, tests for adrenal function, diet evaluation, and possibly tests for liver function.

Treatment

Specific therapy is geared toward reduction of lipemia. Supportive therapy for the mild anterior uveitis may include topical cycloplegic agents, topical corticosteroids, or systemic nonsteroidal anti-inflammatory drugs (see previous section).

Intraocular Hemorrhage

Free blood in the anterior chamber (or blood that has settled inferiorly because of gravitational forces as a fluid line) is termed hyphema. Blood suspended in the vitreous space is termed vitreous hemorrhage. Localization of blood as preretinal, intraretinal, or subretinal has little importance in the diagnosis of the underlying cause or treatment of fundic hemorrhage, and no attempt is made here to differentiate these three types of fundic hemorrhage.

Pathophysiology

Although primary ocular diseases such as ocular trauma, embryonal vascular anomalies, uveitis, chronic glaucoma, and retinal detachment may be a cause of hyphema or vitreal hemorrhage, many systemic disorders involving the coagulation system or the integrity of the vasculature may first manifest themselves as intraocular hemorrhage.

Many causes of uveitis (especially if chronic) can cause intraocular hemorrhage, but specific causes of uveitis with intraocular hemorrhage include immune-mediated vasculitis,[186] rickettsial diseases,[33–35, 132–134] and disseminated neoplasia[152–162] (especially lymphosarcoma). Disorders involving the coagulation system, such as dicoumarin toxicity, hepatic diseases, and disseminated intravascular coagulation, may produce signs of subconjunctival hemorrhage, hyphema, vitreal hemorrhage, and fundic hemorrhage. Platelet disorders (platelet function abnormalities such as von Willebrand's disease and thrombocytopenia) may also cause intraocular hemorrhage.[74, 187] Polycythemia[74, 185] and hyperviscosity syndromes[74, 185, 188–194] may cause retinal vessel engorgement and tortuosity, retinal hemorrhages, and subretinal hemorrhage or fluid with detached retinas. Anemia in cats has been reported as a cause of retinal hemorrhages.[195] Systemic hypertension may cause hyphema, but it is more likely to cause vitreous hemorrhage, retinal hemorrhage, or subretinal fluid or hemorrhage with retinal detachment[185, 196–199] (see next section).

Clinical Signs

An acute "red eye" may be the only history in some cases of hyphema. Signs of ocular pain (e.g., blepharospasm, photophobia, epiphora) may also be noted with hyphema, depending on the underlying cause. The anterior chamber may be totally filled with blood, so that the iris and deeper intraocular structures cannot be seen. The free red blood cells may be pooled inferiorly with formation of a fluid line (which may change with position and ocular or head movements), or there may be clotted blood and fibrin in the anterior chamber. Blindness may be a presenting clinical sign with bilateral vitreal or fundic hemorrhage. The lack of a tapetal reflection or a red or dark-brown pupil may also be noted with vitreal or subretinal hemorrhage. Perivascular hemorrhage of the retinal vessels, subretinal hemorrhage with partial or complete retinal detachment, and multifocal retinal hemorrhages may be incidental findings on ophthalmic examination in animals with no other clinical abnormalities.

Diagnostic Plan

Our diagnostic protocol for intraocular hemorrhage usually begins with a thorough physical examination. We look for other signs of hemorrhage, petechiae, and extravasations that may indicate a systemic problem rather than a strictly ocular problem; for lymphadenopathy that may indicate rickettsial diseases or lymphosarcoma; for cardiac abnormalities on auscultation that may indicate an underlying cardiovascular disorder; and for splenomegaly or other organomegaly on palpation, which may indicate rickettsial diseases, immune-mediated platelet disorders, hyperthyroidism, or disseminated neoplasia. A CBC, platelet count, and serum biochemistry panel are useful for revealing underlying anemias, polycythemias, and hepatic or renal disorders, and for determining whether platelet numbers are a problem. Activated clotting time, prothrombin time, and partial thromboplastin time are all clotting tests that may help in localizing the source of the disorder in the coagulation system. A blood pressure measurement may help determine whether fundic hemorrhages are caused by systemic hypertension.[196–198, 200-203] If intraocular structures cannot be visualized adequately, ocular B-scan ultrasonography may be performed to rule out intraocular tumors or retinal detachments.[204] Depending on the results of the initial work-up, further diagnostic testing may include serology for infectious diseases (Rocky Mountain spotted fever and ehrlichiosis), additional coagulation studies, a cardiac work-up (electrocardiography, radiography, and echocardiography), thyroid function testing, and bone marrow evaluation.

Treatment

Specific therapy for intraocular hemorrhage depends on the underlying disease. Symptomatic therapy for hyphema involves the use of drugs to reduce the intraocular inflammation and clot formation that may cause iridal adhesions and secondary glaucoma, to enhance the outflow of blood from the anterior chamber, and to reduce the incidence of repeated intraocular hemorrhage. Topical corticosteroids help reduce intraocular inflammation. Topical and systemic nonsteroidal anti-inflammatory drugs probably should not be used for fear of inducing additional hemorrhage. Although miotic agents (pilocarpine) theoretically enhance red blood cell outflow from the anterior chamber and increase anterior chamber fibrinolysin activity, miotic drugs cause ciliary body muscle and iris sphincter muscle spasm and may cause additional hemorrhage, worsen uveitis, and potentiate posterior synechia, iris bombe, and secondary glaucoma. Topical atropine causes paralysis of the ciliary musculature and the iris sphincter musculature, thereby decreasing the incidence of spasm of these muscles and the incidence of repeated intraocular hemorrhage. We usually treat hyphema with topical corticosteroids (prednisolone acetate suspension or dexamethasone alcohol solution, three to four times per day) and topical atropine (1% ophthalmic solution, one to three times per day to effect).

Blindness Associated With Retinal Disease

Blindness is a common presenting complaint to the veterinary practitioner. Dysfunction at any level in the eye (i.e., cornea, anterior chamber, lens, vitreous space, or retina) can lead to vision impairment or blindness. Rarely is a client able to discern whether the animal has vision loss in only one eye. Most animals presented for blindness have relatively severe disease bilaterally.

Diseases of the neural retina that may lead to blindness are retinal degeneration and retinal detachment. Retinal degeneration is death of the neurons that make up the retina. Retinal detachment is separation of the neural retina from the underlying retinal pigment epithelium and choroid.

Pathophysiology

Retinal degeneration occurs when the retinal cells die for whatever reason. There are many inherited retinal metabolism disorders seen in the dog that involve the eye alone and have no association with any other systemic diseases or disorders. These inherited retinal degenerations (or retinal atrophies) are progressive, and the dog progressively loses vision to and ends with total blindness. Loosely termed progressive retinal atrophy, these disorders may also rarely be seen in cats. Retinal degeneration may also be seen secondary to infectious diseases involving the retina (canine distemper virus, toxoplasmosis), infectious disease–associated chorioretinitis (fungal diseases, rickettsial diseases, brucellosis, Lyme borreliosis, protothecosis), nutritional deficits (feline central retinal degeneration [FCRD] or taurine deficiency retinopathy), vascular disorders (systemic hypertension associated retinopathy), and idiopathic acute retinal cell death (sudden acquired retinal degeneration syndrome [SARDS] of the dog).

Retinal detachment has been discussed in conjunction with systemic disease–induced uveitis (see Uveitis). If the inflammatory process can be halted before total retinal cell death occurs, then some vision may be restored. The most common infectious disease causing uveitis-induced retinal detachment in the cat is FIP. In addition to chorioretinitis, cryptococcosis, toxoplasmosis, FeLV complex, and FIV complex may also cause uveitis-induced retinal detachments. In the dog, blastomycosis and coccidioidomycosis in their endemic areas, cryptococcus, and ehrlichiosis are the most common infectious diseases causing chorioretinitis and secondary retinal detachment. Immune-mediated panuveitis or chorioretinitis and dissemi-

nated neoplasia are the most common noninfectious causes of chorioretinitis-related retinal detachments in the dog.

Retinopathy associated with systemic hypertension has been reported in the cat[196, 197, 199] and in the dog,[198, 200–202, 204] but we have found the disorder to be much more common in feline patients. With systemic hypertension, vascular changes in the choroid, choriocapillaris, and retinal vessels ultimately lead to vessel leakage of transudates and even whole blood (hemorrhage), which may cause partial or total retinal detachment. Intermittent, partial detachment and subretinal fluid may lead to slowly progressive vision loss. Massive subretinal edema or total subretinal hemorrhages may cause acute total retinal detachment with acute vision loss.

FCRD is a nutritional deficit–induced retinopathy caused by inadequate intake of the amino acid taurine.[205, 206] Restoration of an adequate diet stops the progression of retinal cell death, but there is no regenerative capability for cells that have already died.

SARDS is a disorder in dogs that is characterized by acute (sometimes within 24 hours), total, and irreversible blindness associated with no obvious ocular abnormality.[207–212] The disease appears to be an acute, total death of the photoreceptor cells (rods and cones) of the retina.[210] Although there have been studies and case reports linking the disorder to endocrinopathies, hepatopathies, pancreatic disease, and other systemic disorders, the cause of this disorder remains unknown.[207–212]

Causes for uveitis-induced retinal detachments and conditions to be ruled out have been covered in the section on uveitis. Other causes of intraocular hemorrhage in cats and dogs should be ruled out (see Intraocular Hemorrhage). Systemic hypertension in cats is usually associated with chronic renal failure and hyperthyroidism,[196, 199] but systemic hypertension may be a primary disorder, and it may be diet induced.[197, 198] Taurine deficiency retinopathy or FCRD is associated with feeding cats diets based on plant proteins. Cats fed dry dog food have been documented as having FCRD.[206] Since the publication of the report on taurine deficiency–induced cardiomyopathy[213] and the increase in taurine content in certain brands of cat foods, FCRD and taurine-induced congestive cardiomyopathy have become uncommon,[214] but clients who feed dog food or homemade vegetarian diets could cause this disorder in their cats. Because of the fairly classic bilateral distribution of the FCRD lesions and the slowly progressive nature of the disease, there are few other fundic disorders in the cat that even vaguely mimic FCRD.

With the exception of bilateral optic neuritis (or some other disruption of the optic nerves such as focal neoplasia), no other disorder besides SARDS causes acute blindness in a dog with no obvious ocular abnormalities. It is important in the ophthalmic examination to document poor pupillary light responses (normal pupillary light responses with blindness could indicate a brain lesion) and a normal fundus.

Clinical Signs

Pets with acute retinal detachments caused by chorioretinitis usually have a history of apparently normal vision followed by acute vision loss. Maze testings and menace responses are usually absent if the retinal detachments are total, but pupillary light responses may be intact if the retina is still functional. Other clinical signs of anterior, posterior, or panuveitis may be noted on ophthalmic examination (see Uveitis). With retinopathy induced by systemic hypertension, progressive vision loss (especially in cats) or acute vision loss may be the initial complaint. Depending on the extent of the disease at examination, results from menace testing, maze testing, and pupillary light response testing may range from almost normal to totally absent. With the exception of rare anterior chamber hyphema, the anterior chamber of the eye is normal. A red or dark brown pupil discoloration with a total lack of tapetal reflection may indicate hemorrhage filling the vitreal space or a total subretinal hemorrhage and detachment. Ophthalmic signs in animals that are not totally blind may include intraretinal or subretinal hemorrhages, large areas of gray discolored intraretinal or subretinal edema seen most easily in that area of the retina overlying the tapetum (Fig. 19–9), multifocal hyperpigmented foci of scarring in the tapetal zone, and partial retinal detachments. Retinal vascular engorgement and tortuosity are much more commonly seen in canine hypertension than in feline cases. Systemic hypertension–associated retinopathy is usually a disease of older animals. Most cats have general physical examination findings consistent with the underlying systemic disease (described in the following paragraphs), including weight loss, poor hair coat, tachycardia, small irregular kidneys, and possibly thyroid enlargement.

Cats with FCRD may present with histories of progressive vision loss or acute blindness. Because this disorder is a slowly progressive disease, supposed acute blindness may be seen if the animal has been taken to a new environment and the vision deficit becomes acutely evident to the owner. With the exception of the fundus, ophthalmic examination is unremarkable. Funduscopically, lesions are bilaterally symmetrical and begin in the area centralis (that retinal vessel–poor area dorsotemporal to the optic nerve). These typically are areas of tapetal hyperreflectivity. This zone of degeneration may extend horizontally above the optic disc to become a band of hyperreflec-

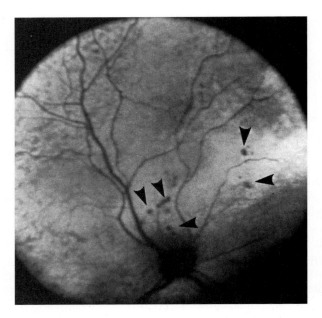

Figure 19–9
Multifocal retinal hemorrhages and subretinal and intraretinal edema in an aged cat with systemic hypertension. The punctate intraretinal hemorrhages are seen as dark spots against the tapetal background *(arrowheads)*. The less distinct, mottled gray discoloration of the dorsal tapetal zone in this photograph represents intraretinal and subretinal edema.

tivity, and with continued taurine deficiency in the diet, the entire retina degenerates, leaving behind the total tapetal hyperreflectivity and retinal vascular attenuation seen with generalized retinal degeneration. Cats on long-term taurine-deficient diets may have clinical signs of congestive cardiomyopathy.[213]

Common historical signs with SARDS-afflicted dogs include polyuria, polydipsia, polyphagia, and recent weight gain. Sometimes rather marked obesity, alopecia, hepatomegaly, pot-bellied appearance, and other clinical signs suggestive of hyperadrenocorticism are also seen. In addition, the condition may occur after severe episodes of vomiting and diarrhea. SARDS-afflicted dogs are typically middle-aged or older and small, pampered breeds (house dogs), but larger dogs and sporting dogs may also be affected. Most dogs have apparent total blindness within hours or days, although some observant owners have noted progressive vision loss over a week or more. Menace and maze responses and pupillary light reflexes are usually absent, but some animals have very slow and incomplete pupillary light reflexes early on. Both eyes are normal on ophthalmic examination; however, with the passage of time (months), classic signs of retinal degeneration are seen (i.e., tapetal hyperreflectivity and retinal vascular attenuation).

Diagnostic Plan

The diagnostic work-up depends on the retinal lesions present on ophthalmic examination. Work-up for fundic hemorrhage or retinal detachment from possible systemic hypertension should include tests for coagulopathies (see Intraocular Hemorrhage), and a CBC, serum biochemistry panel, and urinalysis are important to identify chronic renal failure as a cause of hypertension. Thyroid function testing is important in cats, and a cardiac work-up (thoracic radiography, electrocardiography, and cardiac ultrasonography) is useful for diagnosis and follow-up in response to therapy. The definitive diagnosis for hypertensive retinopathy is documentation of systemic hypertension by measurement of blood pressure (see Chaps. 12 and 16).

A history of poor diet and classic funduscopic signs are enough for a diagnosis of FCRD resulting from taurine deficiency. If the cat is still eating the defective diet, plasma taurine levels may be determined to document the deficient state.

Electroretinography is the definitive diagnostic test for blindness caused by SARDS. Animals with SARDS have a flat tracing, indicating no photoreceptor cell function. Dogs with optic neuritis or nonocular disease (e.g., cortical blindness) have a normal tracing. Because of the incidence of hyperadrenocorticism associated with SARDS, a work-up for Cushing's syndrome should be undertaken; this includes CBC, serum biochemistry panel, urinalysis, and testing with adrenocorticotropic stimulation or dexamethasone suppression. Dogs with SARDS typically have elevations in serum alkaline phosphatase and cortisol, with occasional mild elevations of other hepatocellular enzymes. It should not be immediately assumed that these dogs have Cushing's syndrome. Some dogs with SARDS have hyperadrenocorticism, but in most cases the biochemical and adrenal function abnormalities are transient and are thought to be caused by stress associated with acute blindness.

Treatment

There is no specific ocular therapy for systemic hypertension–induced retinopathy. Specific therapy for the hypertension may help reduce subretinal edema and reduce the incidence of continued retinal or choroidal hemorrhage. Animals with chronic end-stage retinal changes such as retinal degeneration regain little or no vision even with medical therapy for the hypertension. Animals with active retinal or sub-retinal hemorrhage may recover some vision with resolution of these active lesions. There is no specific ocular therapy for FCRD or SARDS. Once the retinal cells have degenerated, there is no regenerative capability and no hope for return of function.

References

1. Martin CL, Anderson BG. Ocular anatomy. In: Gelatt KN, ed. Textbook of Veterinary Ophthalmology. Philadelphia, Lea & Febiger, 1981:12–121.
2. Samuelson DA. Ophthalmic embryology and anatomy. In: Gelatt KN, ed. Veterinary Ophthalmology, 2nd ed. Philadelphia, Lea & Febiger, 1991:3–123.
3. Schmidt GM, Coulter DB. Physiology of the eye. In: Gelatt KN, ed. Textbook of Veterinary Ophthalmology. Philadelphia, Lea & Febiger, 1981:129–159.
4. Gum GG. Physiology of the eye. In: Gelatt KN, ed. Veterinary Ophthalmology, 2nd ed. Philadelphia, Lea & Febiger, 1991:124–161.
5. Carpenter JL, Schmidt GM, Moore FM, et al. Canine bilateral extraocular polymyositis. Vet Pathol 1989;26:510–512.
6. Gilmour MA, Morgan RV, Moore FM. Masticatory myopathy in the dog: A retrospective study of 18 cases. J Am Anim Hosp Assoc 1992;28:300–306.
7. Brogden JD, Brightman AH, McLaughlin SA. Diagnosing and treating masticatory myositis. Vet Med 1991;86:1164–1170.
8. Shelton GD, Cardinet GH. Canine masticatory muscle disorders. In: Kirk RW, ed. Current Veterinary Therapy X. Philadelphia, WB Saunders, 1989:816–819.
9. Koch SA. The differential diagnosis of exophthalmos in the dog. J Am Anim Hosp Assoc 1969;5:229–237.
10. McCalla TL, Moore CP. Exophthalmos in dogs and cats: Part I. Anatomic and diagnostic considerations. Compen Contin Educ Pract Vet 1989;11:784–792.
11. McCalla TL, Moore CP. Exophthalmos in dogs and cats: Part II. Compen Contin Educ Pract Vet 1989;11:911–925.
12. Kern TJ. The canine orbit. In: Gelatt KN, ed. Veterinary Ophthalmology, 2nd ed. Philadelphia, Lea & Febiger, 1991:239–255.
13. Nasisse MP: Feline ophthalmology. In: Gelatt KN, ed. Veterinary Ophthalmology, 2nd ed. Philadelphia, Lea & Febiger, 1991:529–575.
14. Lewis GT, Blanchard GL, Trapp AL, et al. Ophthalmoplegia caused by thyroid adenocarcinoma invasion of the cavernous sinuses in the dog. J Am Anim Hosp Assoc 1984;20:805–812.
15. Kern TJ. Orbital neoplasia in 23 dogs. J Am Vet Med Assoc 1985;186:489–491.
16. Martin CL, Kaswan RL, Doran CC. Cystic lesions of the periorbital region. Compen Contin Educ Pract Vet 1987;9:1022–1030.
17. Angell JA, Meredith R. Ocular lesions associated with coccidioidomycosis in dogs: 35 cases (1980–1985). J Am Vet Med Assoc 1987;190:1319–1322.
18. Buyukmichi N. Ocular lesions in blastomycosis in the dog. J Am Vet Med Assoc 1982;180:426–431.
19. Munger RJ, Ackerman N. Retrobulbar injections in the dog: A comparison of three techniques. J Am Anim Hosp Assoc 1978;14:490–498.
20. Cottrill NB, Banks WJ, Pechman RD. Ultrasonographic and biometric evaluation of the eye and orbit in dogs. Am J Vet Res 1989;50:898–903.
21. Dziezyc J, Hager DA, Millichamp MJ. Two-dimensional

real-time ocular ultrasonography in the diagnosis of ocular lesions in dogs. J Am Anim Hosp Assoc 1987;23: 501–508.

22. Slatter DH, Abdelbaki YZ. Lateral orbitotomy by zygomatic resection in the dog. J Am Vet Med Assoc 1979;175:1179–1182.

23. Bistner SI, Aguirre G, Batik G. Atlas of Veterinary Ophthalmic Surgery. Philadelphia, WB Saunders, 1977: 258–260.

24. Neer TM. Horner's syndrome: Anatomy, diagnosis, and causes. Compen Contin Educ Pract Vet 1984;6:740–745.

25. Wowk BJ, Olsen GA. Oculosympathetic paralysis (Horner's syndrome) in the dog. Vet Med Small Anim Clin 1979;74:521–527.

26. Morgan RV, Zanotti SW. Horner's syndrome in dogs and cats: 49 cases (1980–1986). J Am Vet Med Assoc 1989;194:1096–1099.

27. Kern TJ, Aromando MC, Erb HN. Horner's syndrome in dogs and cats: cases (1975–1985). J Am Vet Med Assoc 1989;195:369–373.

28. Scagliotti RH. Current concepts in veterinary neuro-ophthalmology. Vet Clin North Am Small Anim Pract 1980;10:431–434.

29. Scagliotti RH. Neuro-ophthalmology. In: Gelatt KN, ed. Veterinary Ophthalmology, 2nd ed. Philadelphia, Lea & Febiger. 1991:706–743.

30. Gwin RM, Gelatt KN, Williams LW. Ophthalmic neoplasms in the dog. J Am Anim Hosp Assoc 1982;18: 853–866.

31. Gilger BC, McLaughlin SA, Whitley RW, et. al. Orbital neoplasms in cats: 21 cases (1974–1990). J Am Vet Med Assoc 1992;201:1083–1086.

32. Wilcock B, Peiffer RL. Adenocarcinoma of the gland of the third eyelid in 7 dogs. J Am Vet Med Assoc 1988;193:1549–1550.

33. Breitschwerdt EB, Menten DJ, Walker DH, et al. Canine Rocky Mountain spotted fever: A kennel epizootic. Am J Vet Res 1985;46:2124–2128.

34. Davidson, MG, Breitschwerdt EB, Nasisse MP, et al. Ocular manifestations of Rocky Mountain spotted fever in dogs. J Am Vet Med Assoc 1989;194:777–781.

35. Martin CL. Ocular signs of systemic diseases: Part I. Mod Vet Pract 1982;63:689–694.

36. Peiffer RL. Ocular manifestations of systemic disease: Part I. Dog and cat. In: Gelatt KN, ed. Textbook of Veterinary Ophthalmology. Philadelphia, Lea & Febiger, 1981:699–723.

37. Brooks DE. Canine conjunctiva and nictitating membrane. In: Gelatt KN, ed. Veterinary Ophthalmology, 2nd ed. Philadelphia, Lea & Febiger, 1991:290–306.

38. Gaskin JM. Microbiology of the canine and feline eye. Vet Clin North Am Small Anim Pract 1980;10: 303–316.

39. Nasisse MP, Guy JS, Stevens JB, et al. Clinical and laboratory findings in chronic conjunctivitis in cats: 91 cases (1983–1991). J Am Vet Med Assoc 1993;203: 834–837.

40. Nasisse MP. Manifestations, diagnosis, and treatment of ocular herpes virus infection in the cat. Compen Contin Educ Pract Vet 1982;4:962–971.

41. Nasisse MP, Guy JS, Davidson, MG, et al. Experimental ocular herpes virus infection in the cat: Sites of virus replication, clinical features, and effects of corticosteroid administration. Invest Ophthalmol Vis Sci 1989;30: 1758–1768.

42. Gaskell RN, Povey RC. Re-excretion of feline viral rhinotracheitis virus following corticosteroid treatment. Vet Rec 1973;93:204–207.

43. Dorin SE, Miller WW, Goodwin J. Diagnosing and treating chlamydial conjunctivitis in cats. Vet Med 1993;88:322–330.

44. Nasisse MP, English RV, Tompkins MB, et al. Immunologic, histologic, and virologic features of herpes-virus induced stromal keratitis in cats. Am J Vet Res 1995;56: 51–55.

45. Gelatt KN, Peiffer RL, Erickson JL, et al. Evaluation of tear formation in the dog, using a modification of the Schirmer tear test. J Am Vet Med Assoc 1975;166: 368–370.

46. Veith LA, Cure TH, Gelatt KN. The Schirmer tear test in cats. Mod Vet Pract 1970;51:48–49.

47. Hollingsworth SR, Canton DD, Buyukmihci N, et al. Effect of topically administered atropine on tear production in dogs. J Am Vet Med Assoc 1992;200:1481–1484.

48. Vestre WA, Brightman AH, Helper LC, et al. Decreased tear production associated with general anesthesia in the dog. J Am Vet Med Assoc 1979;174:1006–1007.

49. Morgan RV, Duddy JM, McClurg K. Prolapse of the gland of the third eyelid in dogs: A retrospective study of 84 cases (1980–1990). J Am Anim Hosp Assoc 1993;29:56–62.

50. Slatter DH, Blogg JR. Keratoconjunctivitis sicca in dogs associated with sulfonamide administration. Aust Vet J 1978;54:444–446.

51. Slatter DH. KCS in the dog produced by oral phenazopyridine hydrochloride. J Small Anim Pract 1973;14:749–771.

52. Bryan GM, Slatter DH. Keratoconjunctivitis sicca induced by phenazopyridine in dogs. Arch Ophthalmol 1973;90:310–311.

53. Morgan RV, Bachrach A. Keratoconjunctivitis sicca associated with sulfonamide therapy in dogs. J Am Vet Med Assoc 1982;180:432–434.

54. Collins BK, Moore CP, Hagee JH. Sulfonamide-induced keratoconjunctivitis sicca and corneal ulceration in a dysuric dog. J Am Vet Med Assoc 1986;189:924–926.

55. Kaswan RL, Martin CL, Dawe DL. Rheumatoid factor determination in 50 dogs with keratoconjunctivitis sicca. J Am Vet Med Assoc 1983;183:1073–1075.

56. Kaswan RL, Martin CL, Dawe DL. Keratoconjunctivitis sicca: Immunological evaluation of 62 canine cases. Am J Vet Res 1985;46:376–383.

57. Sansom J, Barnett KC. Keratoconjunctivitis sicca in the dog: A review of 200 cases. J Small Anim Pract 1985;26:121–131.

58. Martin CL, Kaswan RL. Distemper-associated keratoconjunctivitis sicca. J Am Anim Hosp Assoc 1985;21: 355–361.

59. Gelatt KN. Canine lacrimal and nasolacrimal diseases. In: Gelatt KN, ed. Veterinary Ophthalmology, 2nd ed. Philadelphia, Lea & Febiger, 1991:276–289.

60. Whitley RD, McLaughlin SA, Gilger BC, et al. The treatment for keratoconjunctivitis sicca. Vet Med 1991; 86:1076–1093.

61. Kaswan RL, Salisbury MA. A new prospective on canine keratoconjunctivitis sicca. Treatment with ophthalmic cyclosporine. Vet Clin North Am Small Anim Pract 1990;20:583–613.

62. Salisbury MA, Kaswan RL, Ward DA, et al. Topical application of cyclosporine in the management of keratoconjunctivitis sicca in dogs. J Am Anim Hosp Assoc 1990;26:269–264.

63. Morgan RV, Abrams KL. Topical administration of cyclosporine for treatment of keratoconjunctivitis sicca in dogs. J Am Vet Med Assoc 1991;199:1043–1046.

64. Olivero DK, Davidson MG, English RV, et al. Clinical evaluation of 1% cyclosporine for topical treatment of keratoconjunctivitis sicca in dogs. J Am Vet Med Assoc 1991;199:1039–1042.

65. Carmicheal LE. The pathogenesis of ocular lesions of infectious canine hepatitis: I. Pathology and virological observation. Pathol Vet 1964;1:73–95.

66. Carmicheal LE. The pathogenesis of the ocular lesions of infectious canine hepatitis: II. Experimental ocular hypersensitivity produced by the virus. Pathol Vet 1965;2:344–359.

67. Aguirre G, Carmicheal LE, Bistner S. Corneal endothelium in viral induced anterior uveitis. Ultrastructural changes following canine adenovirus type-I infection. Arch Ophthalmol 1974;93:219–224.

68. Carmicheal LE, Medic BLS, Bistner SI, et al. Viral-antibody complexes in canine adenovirus type-I ocular lesion: Leukocyte chemotaxis and enzyme release. Cornell Vet 1975;65:331–351.

69. Nasisse MP, Guy JS, Davidson MG, et al. In vitro susceptibility of feline herpes virus-1 to vidarabine, idoxuridine, trifluridine, acyclovir, and bromobinyl-deoxyuridine. Am J Vet Res 1989;50:158–160.

70. Crispin SM, Barnett KC. Arcus lipoides corneae secondary to hypothyroidism in the Alsatian. J Small Anim Pract 1978;19:127–142.

71. Crispin SM, Barnett KC. Dystrophy, degeneration, and infiltration of the canine cornea. J Small Anim Pract 1983;24:63–83.

72. Ward DA, Martin CL, Weiser I. Band keratopathy associated with hyperadrenocorticism in the dog. J Am Anim Hosp Assoc 1989;25:583–586.

73. Whitley RD. Canine cornea. In: Gelatt KN, ed. Veterinary Ophthalmology, 2nd ed. Philadelphia, Lea & Febiger, 1991:307–356.

74. Collins BK, Moore CP. Canine anterior uvea. In: Gelatt KN, ed. Veterinary Ophthalmology, 2nd ed. Philadelphia, Lea & Febiger, 1991:357–395.

75. Gelatt KN. The canine lens. In: Gelatt KN, ed. Veterinary Ophthalmology, 2nd ed. Philadelphia, Lea & Febiger, 1991:429–460.

76. Roberts SM, Lavach JD, Severin GA, et al. Ophthalmic complications following megavoltage radiation of the nasal and perinasal cavities in dogs. J Am Vet Med Assoc 1987;190:43–47.

77. Brightman AH, Brogden JD, Helper LC, et al. Electric

78. Vainisi SJ, Edelhauser HF, Wolf ED, et al. Nutritional cataracts in timber wolves. J Am Vet Med Assoc 1982;179:1175–1180.

79. Martin CL, Chambreau T. Cataract production in experimentally orphaned puppies fed a commercial replacement for bitch's milk. J Am Anim Hosp Assoc 1982;18:115–119.

80. Glaze MB, Blanchard GL. Nutritional cataracts in a Samoyed litter. J Am Anim Hosp Assoc 1983;19:951–954.

81. Remillard RL, Pickett JP, Thatcher CD, et al. Comparison of kittens fed queen's milk with those fed milk replacers. Am J Vet Res 1993;54:901–907.

82. Rubin LF, Mattis PA. Dimethyl sulfoxide: Lens changes in dogs during oral administration. Science 1966;153:83–89.

83. Peiffer RL, Gelatt KN, Gwin RM. Diabetic cataracts in the dog. Canine Pract 1977;4:18–23.

84. Wyman M, Sato S, Akagi Y, et al. The dog as a model for ocular manifestations of high concentrations of blood sugars. J Am Vet Med Assoc 1988;193:1153–1156.

85. Kador P. Overview of the current attempts towards medical treatment of cataract. Ophthalmology 1983;90:352–364.

86. Cotlier E, Sharma YR, Niven T, et al. Distribution of salicylate in lens and intraocular fluids and its effect on cataract formation: Aspirin Symposium, June 1983. Am J Med 1983;74:83–90.

87. Ao S, Kikuchi C, Ono T, et al. Affect of installation of aldose reductase inhibitor FR74366 on diabetic cataract. Invest Ophthalmol Vis Sci 1991;32:3078–3083.

88. Peiffer, RL. Ocular immunology and mechanisms of ocular inflammation. Vet Clin North Am Small Anim Pract 1980;10:281–302.

89. Wilkie, DA. Control of ocular inflammation. Vet Clin North Am Small Anim Pract 1990;20:693–714.

90. Yoshitomi T, Ito Y. Effects of indomethacin and prostaglandins on the dog's iris sphincter and dilator muscles. Invest Ophthalmol Vis Sci 1988;29:127–132.

91. Regnier A, Whitley RD, Benard P, et. al. Effect of flunixin meglumine on breakdown of the blood-aqueous barrier following paracentesis of the canine eye. J Ocul Pharmacol 1986;2:165–170.

92. Millichamp NJ, Dziezyc J, Rohde BH, et al. Acute effects of anti-inflammatory drugs on neodymium:yttrium aluminum garnet laser–induced uveitis in dogs. Am J Vet Res 1991;52:1279–1284.

93. Spiess BM, Mathis GA, Franson KL, et. al. Kinetics of uptake and effects of topical indomethacin application on protein concentration in the aqueous humor of dogs. Am J Vet Res 1991;52:1159–1163.

94. Millichamp NJ, Dziezyc J. Comparison of flunixin meglumine and flurbiprofen for control of ocular irritative response in dogs. Am J Vet Res 1991;52:1452–1455.

95. Dziezyc J, Millichamp NJ, Rohde BH, et al. Comparison of prednisolone and RMI-1068 in the ocular irritative response in dogs. Invest Ophthalmol Vis Sci 1992;33:460–465.

96. Davidson MG, Nasisse MP, English RV, et al. Feline

anterior uveitis: A study of 53 cases. J Am Anim Hosp Assoc 1991;27:77–83.

97. Doherty M. Ocular manifestations of feline infectious peritonitis. J Am Vet Med Assoc 1971;159:417–424.

98. Slauson D, Finn J. Meningoencephalitis and panophthalmitis in feline infectious peritonitis. J Am Vet Med Assoc 1972;160:729–734.

99. Peiffer RL, Wilcock BP. Histopathologic study of uveitis in cats: 139 cases (1978–1988). J Am Vet Med Assoc 1991;198:135–138.

100. Lappin MR, Marks A, Greene CE, et al. Serology prevalence of selected infectious diseases in cats with uveitis. J Am Vet Med Assoc 1992;201:1005–1007.

101. Häkanson N, Forrester SD. Uveitis in the dog and cat. Vet Clin North Am Small Anim Pract 1990;20:715–735.

102. Brightman AH, Ogilvie GK, Tompkins M. Ocular disease in FeLV-positive cats: 11 cases (1981–1986). J Am Vet Med Assoc 1991;198:1049–1051.

103. English R, Davidson M, Nasisse M, et al. Intraocular disease associated with feline immunodeficiency virus infection in cats. J Am Vet Med Assoc 1990;197:1116–1119.

104. Vainisi SJ, Campbell LH. Ocular toxoplasmosis in cats. J Am Vet Med Assoc 1969;154:141–152.

105. Piper RC, Cole CR, Shadduck JA. Natural and experimental ocular toxoplasmosis in animals. Am J Ophthalmol 1970;69:662–668.

106. Dubey JP, Carpenter JL. Histologically-confirmed clinical toxoplasmosis in cats: 100 cases (1952–1990). J Am Vet Med Assoc 1993;203:1556–1566.

107. Clinkenbeard K, Cowell R, Tyler R. Disseminated histoplasmosis in cats: Twelve cases (1981–1986). J Am Vet Med Assoc 1987;190:1445–1448.

108. Mahaffey E, Gabbert N, Johnson D, et al. Disseminated histoplasmosis in three cats. J Am Anim Hosp Assoc 1977;13:46–50.

109. Wolf A, Belden M. Feline histoplasmosis: A literature review and retrospective study of 20 new cases. J Am Anim Hosp Assoc 1984;20:995–998.

110. Peiffer RL, Belkin PV. Ocular manifestations of disseminated histoplasmosis in a cat. Feline Pract 1979;9:24–29.

111. Whitley RD, Hamilton HL, Weigand CM. Glaucoma and disorders of the uvea, lens, and retina in cats. Vet Med 1993;88:1164–1173.

112. Jasmin AM, Carrol JA, Bancom JN, et al. Systemic blastomycosis in Siamese cats. Vet Med Small Anim Clin 1969;64:33–37.

113. Hatkin JM, Phillips WE, Utroska WR. Two cases of feline blastomycosis. J Am Anim Hosp Assoc 1979;15, 217–220.

114. Alden CL, Mokan R. Ocular blastomycosis in a cat. J Am Vet Med Assoc 1974;164, 527–528.

115. Easton KL. Cutaneous North American blastomycosis in a Siamese cat. Can Vet J 1961;2:350–351.

116. Nasisse MP, vanEe RF, Wright B. Ocular changes in a cat with disseminated blastomycosis. J Am Vet Med Assoc 1985;187, 629–631.

117. Miller PE, Miller LM, Schoster JV. Feline blastomycosis: A report of three cases and a literature review (1961–1968). J Am Anim Hosp Assoc 1990;26:417–424.

118. Rosenthal JJ, Heibgerd J, Peiffer RL. Ocular and sys-

temic cryptococcosis in a cat. J Am Anim Hosp Assoc 1991;11:307–310.

119. Fischer CA. Intraocular cryptococcosis in two cats. J Am Vet Med Assoc 1971;158:191–198.

120. Wilkinson GT. Feline cryptococcosis: A review and seven case reports. J Small Anim Pract 1979;20:749–768.

121. Gwin RM, Gelatt KN, Hardy R, et al. Ocular cryptococcosis in a cat. J Am Anim Hosp Assoc 1977;13:680–684.

122. Blouin P, Cello R. Experimental ocular cryptococcosis: Preliminary studies in cats and mice. Invest Ophthalmol Vis Sci 1980;19, 21–30.

123. Angell JA, Shively JN, Merideth RE, et al. Ocular coccidioidomycosis in a cat. J Am Vet Med Assoc 1985;187, 167–169.

124. Parry H. Degeneration of the dog retina: IV. Retinopathies associated with distemper-complex virus infections. Br J Ophthalmol 1954;38:295–309.

125. Jubb K, Saunders LZ, Coates H. The intraocular lesions of canine distemper. J Comp Pathol 1957;67:21–29.

126. Fischer C. Retinal and retinochoroidal lesions in early neuropathic canine distemper. J Am Vet Med Assoc 1971;158:740–752.

127. Aguirre GD, Gross SL. Ocular manifestations of selected systemic diseases. Compen Contin Educ Pract Vet 1980;2:144–153.

128. Rieke JA, Rhoades HE. *Brucella canis* isolated from the eye of a dog. J Am Vet Med Assoc 1975;166:583–584.

129. Saegusa J, Veda K, Goto Y, et. al. Ocular lesions in experimental canine brucellosis. Jpn J Vet Sci 1977;39:181–185.

130. Gwin RM, Kolwalski JJ, Wyman M, et. al. Ocular lesions associated with *Brucella canis* infection in a dog. J Am Anim Hosp Assoc 1980;16:607–610.

131. Munger RJ. Uveitis as a manifestation of *Borrelia burgdorferi* infection in dogs. J Am Vet Med Assoc 1990;197:811. Letter.

132. Glaze MB, Gaunt SD. Uveitis associated with *Ehrlichia platys* infection in a dog. J Am Vet Med Assoc 1986;188:916–917.

133. Ellett EW, Playtor RF, Pierce KR. Retinal lesions associated with induced canine ehrlichiosis: A preliminary report. J Am Anim Hosp Assoc 1979;9:214–218.

134. Troy GC, Vulgamott JC, Turnwald GH. Canine ehrlichiosis: A retrospective study of 30 natural occurring cases. J Am Anim Hosp Assoc 1980;16:181–187.

135. Salfelder K, Schwarz J, Akbarian M. Experimental ocular histoplasmosis in dogs. Am J Ophthalmol 1965;59:290–294.

136. Gwin RM, Makley T, Wyman M, et al. Multifocal ocular histoplasmosis in a dog and cat. J Am Vet Med Assoc 1980;176:638–642.

137. Albert RA, Whitley RD, Crawley RR. Ocular blastomycosis in the dog. Compen Contin Educ Pract Vet 1981;3:303–314.

138. Legendre AM, Walker M, Buyukmihci N, et. al. Canine blastomycosis: A review of 47 clinical cases. J Am Vet Med Assoc 1981;178:1163–1168.

139. Brooks DE, Legendre AM, Gum GG, et al. The treatment of canine ocular blastomycosis with systemically administered itraconazole. Prog Vet Comp Ophthalmol 1991;1:263–268.

140. Buyukmihci NC, Moore BF. Microscopic lesions of spontaneous ocular blastomycosis in dogs. J Comp Pathol 1987;97:321–328.

141. Jergens AE, Wheeler CA, Collier LL. Cryptococcosis involving the eye and central nervous system of a dog. J Am Vet Med Assoc 1986;189:302–304.

142. Panciera DL, Bevier D. Management of cryptococcosis and toxic epidermal necrolysis in a dog. J Am Vet Med Assoc 1987;191:1125–1127.

143. Stampley AR, Barsanti JA. Disseminated cryptococcosis in a dog. J Am Anim Hosp Assoc 1988;24:17–21.

144. Shively JN, Whiteman CE. Ocular lesions in disseminated coccidioidomycosis in 2 dogs. Pathol Vet 1970;7:1–6.

145. Angell JA, Merideth RE, Shively JN, et al. Ocular lesions associated with coccidioidomycosis in dogs: 35 cases. J Am Vet Med Assoc 1987;190:1319–1322.

146. Rakich PM, Latimer KS. Altered immune function in a dog with disseminated prototothecosis. J Am Vet Med Assoc 1984;185:681–683.

147. Gaunt SD, McGrath RK, Cox HU. Disseminated prototothecosis in a dog. J Am Vet Med Assoc 1984;185:906–907.

148. Font RL, Hook SR. Metastatic prototothecal retinitis in a dog: Electron microscopic observations. Vet Pathol 1984;21:61–66.

149. Tyler DE, Lorenz MD, Blue JL, et al. Disseminated prototothecosis with central nervous system involvement in a dog. J Am Vet Med Assoc 1980;176:987–993.

150. Cook JR, Tyler DE, Coulter DB, et al. Disseminated prototothecosis causing acute blindness and deafness in a dog. J Am Vet Med Assoc 1984;184:1266–1272.

151. Moore FM, Schmidt GM, Desai D, et al. Unsuccessful treatment of disseminated prototothecosis in a dog. J Am Vet Med Assoc 1985;186: 705–708.

152. Morgan G. Ocular tumors in animals. J Small Anim Pract 1969;10:563–570.

153. Peiffer RL. Secondary intraocular tumors in the dogs: Part II. Mod Vet Pract 1979;60:450–462.

154. Moore CP, Jones BD, Jensen H. Hyphema: Presenting sign of metastatic disease. A clinicopathologic case report. J Am Anim Hosp Assoc 1980;16:589–594.

155. Lavach JD. Disseminated neoplasia presenting with ocular signs: A report of two cases. J Am Anim Hosp Assoc 1984;20:459–462.

156. Whitley RD, Jensen HE, Andrews JJ. Renal adenocarcinoma with ocular metastasis in a dog. J Am Anim Hosp Assoc 1980;16:949–953.

157. Ladds PW, Gelatt KN, Strafuss AC. Canine ocular adenocarcinoma of mammary origin. J Am Anim Hosp Assoc 1970;156:63–65.

158. Szymanski CM. Bilateral metastatic intraocular hemangiosarcoma in a dog. J Am Anim Hosp Assoc 1972;17:803–805.

159. Fulton LM, Bromberg NM, Goldschmidt M. Soft-tissue fibrosarcoma with intraocular metastasis in a cat. Prog Vet Comp Ophthalmol 1991;1:129–132.

160. Saunders L, Barron C. Intraocular tumors in animals: IV. Lymphosarcoma. Br Vet J 1964;120:25–35.

161. Cello RM, Hutcherson B. Ocular changes in malignant lymphoma of dogs. Cornell Vet 1962;54:492–523.

162. Krohne SG, Vestre WA, Richardson RC, et al. Ocular involvement in canine lymphosarcoma: A retrospective study of 94 cases. Trans Am Coll Vet Ophthalmol 1987;18:68–89.

163. Asakura S, Takahashi K, Onishi T. Vogt–Koyanagi–Harada syndrome (uveitis diffusa acuta) in the dog. Jpn J Vet Med 1977;673:445–455.

164. Bussanich MN, Rootman J, Dolman CL. Granulomatous panuveitis and dermal depigmentation in dogs. J Am Anim Hosp Assoc 1982;18:131–138.

165. Halliwell RE. Autoimmune diseases in domestic animals. J Am Vet Med Assoc 1982;181:1088–1096.

166. Kern TJ, Walton DK, Riis RC, et al. Uveitis associated with poliosis and vitiligo in six dogs. J Am Vet Med Assoc 1985;187:409–414.

167. Romatowski J. A uveodermatological syndrome in an Akita dog. J Am Anim Hosp Assoc 1985;21:777–780.

168. Campbell KL, McLaughlin SA, Reynolds HA. Generalized leukoderma and poliosis following uveitis in the dog. J Am Anim Hosp Assoc 1986;22:121–124.

169. Morgan RV. Vogt–Koyanagi–Harada syndrome in humans and dogs. Compen Contin Educ Pract Vet 1989;11:1211–1218,1249.

170. Toris C, Pederson J. Aqueous humor dynamics in experimental iridocyclitis. Invest Ophthalmol Vis Sci 1987;28:477–481.

171. Kaufman PL, Crawford K, Gabelt BT. The effects of prostaglandins on aqueous humor dynamics. Ophthalmol Clin North Am 1989;2:141–150.

172. Gabelt BT, Kaufman PL. Prostaglandin F2a increases uveoscleral outflow in the cynomolgus monkey. Exp Eye Res 1989;49:389–402.

173. Millichamp NJ, Dziezyc J, Olsen JW. Effects of flurbiprofen of facility of aqueous outflow in eyes of dogs. Am J Vet Res 1991;52:1448–1451.

174. Mori M, Makoto A, Masahiko S, et al. Effects of pilocarpine and tropicamide on blood-aqueous barrier permeability in man. Invest Ophthalmol Vis Sci 1992;33:416–423.

175. O'Conner RG. Factors related to the initiation and recurrence of uveitis. Am J Ophthalmol 1983;95:577–583.

176. Roberts SM, Lavach JD, Macy DW, et al. Effect of ophthalmic prednisolone acetate on the canine adrenal gland and hepatic function. Am J Vet Res 1984;45:1711–1714.

177. Glaze MB, Crawford MA, Nachreiner RF, et al. Ophthalmic corticosteroid therapy: Systemic effects in the dog. J Am Vet Med Assoc 1988;192:73–75.

178. Eichenbaum JD, Macy DW, Severin GA, et al. Effect in large dogs of ophthalmic prednisolone acetate on adrenal gland and hepatic function. J Am Anim Hosp Assoc 1988;24:705–709.

179. Leibowitz HM, Kupferman A. Anti-inflammatory effectiveness in the cornea of topically administered prednisolone. Invest Ophthalmol Vis Sci 1974;13: 757–763.

180. Regnier A, Toutain PL, Alvinerie M, et al. Adrenocortical function and plasma biochemical values in dogs after subconjunctival treatment with methylprednisolone acetate. Res Vet Sci 1982;32:306–310.

181. Fischer CA. Granuloma formation associated with

subconjunctival injection of a corticosteroid in dogs. J Am Vet Med Assoc 1979;174:1086–1088.

182. Brightman AH, Helper LC, Hoffman WE. Effect of aspirin on aqueous protein values in the dog. J Am Vet Med Assoc 1981;178:572–573.

183. Krohne SD, Vestre WA. Ocular use of antiinflammatory drugs in companion animals. Compen Contin Educ Pract Vet 1987;9:1085–1097.

184. Kern TJ, Riis RC. Ocular manifestations of secondary hyperlipidemia associated with hypothyroidism and uveitis in a dog. J Am Anim Hosp Assoc 1980;16: 907–914.

185. Lane IF, Roberts SM, Lappin MR. Ocular manifestations of vascular disease: Hypertension, hyperviscosity, and hyperlipidemia. J Am Anim Hosp Assoc 1993;29:28–36.

186. Randell MG, Hurvitz AI. Immune-mediated vasculitis in five dogs. J Am Vet Med Assoc 1983;183:207–211.

187. Carter JD, Prasse KW, Baker GG. Ocular and clinical features of canine thrombocytic purpura. Vet Med Small Anim Clin 1971;125–128.

188. Szymanski CM. Multiple myeloma with hyperviscosity syndrome in a dog. Proc Am Coll Vet Ophthalmol 1976;5:143–145.

189. Center SA, Smith JF. Ocular lesions in a dog with serum hyperviscosity secondary to IgA myeloma. J Am Vet Med Assoc 1982;181:811–813.

190. Kirschner SE, Niyo Y, Hill BL, et al. Blindness in a dog with IgA-forming myeloma. J Am Vet Med Assoc 1988;193:349–350.

191. Shull RM, Osborne CA, Barrett RE, et al. Serum hyperviscosity syndrome associated with IgA multiple myeloma in dogs. J Am Anim Hosp Assoc 1978;14: 58–70.

192. MacEwen EG, Hurvitz AI, Hayes A. Hyperviscosity syndrome associated with lymphocytic leukemia in three dogs. J Am Vet Med Assoc 1977;170:1309–1312.

193. Hoenig M. Multiple myelomas associated with the heavy chains of IgA in the dog. J Am Vet Med Assoc 1987;190:1191–1192.

194. Hribernik TN, Barta O, Gaunt SD, et al. Serum hyperviscosity syndrome associated with IgG myeloma in a cat. J Am Vet Med Assoc 1982;181:169–170.

195. Fischer CA. Retinopathy in anemic cats. J Am Vet Med Assoc 1970;156:1415–1419.

196. Kobayashi D, Peterson M, Graves T, et al. Hypertension in cats with chronic renal failure or hyperthyroidism. J Vet Intern Med 1990;4:58–62.

197. Turner L, Brogden JD, Lees G. Idiopathic hypertension in a cat with secondary hypertensive retinopathy associated with a high salt diet. J Am Anim Hosp Assoc 1990;26:647–651.

198. Paulsen M, Allen T, Jaenke R, et al. Arterial hypertension in two canine siblings: Ocular and systemic manifestations. J Am Anim Hosp Assoc 1989;25:287–295.

199. Morgan R. Systemic hypertension in four cats: Ocular and medical findings. J Am Anim Hosp Assoc 1986;22: 615–621.

200. Gwin RM, Gelatt KN, Terrell TG, et al. Hypertensive retinopathy associated with hypothyroidism, hypercholesterolemia, and renal failure in a dog. J Am Anim Hosp Assoc 1978;14:200–209.

201. Bovee KC, Littman MP, Crabtree BJ, et al. Essential hypertension in a dog. J Am Vet Med Assoc 1989;195: 81–86.

202. Manning P. Thyroid gland and ocular lesions of beagles with familial hypothyroidism and hyperlipoproteinemia. Am J Vet Res 1979;40:820–828.

203. Littman MP, Robertson JL, Bovee KC. Spontaneous systemic hypertension in dogs: 5 cases. J Am Vet Med Assoc 1988;193:486–494.

204. Nelms SR, Nasisse MP, Davidson MB, et al. Hyphema associated with retinal disease in dogs: 17 cases (1986–1991). J Am Vet Med Assoc 1993;202:1289–1292.

205. Hayes K, Carey R, Schmidt S. Retinal degeneration associated with taurine deficiency in the cat. Science 1975;188:949–951.

206. Aguirre G. Retinal degeneration associated with the feeding of dog foods to cats. J Am Vet Med Assoc 1978;172:791–796.

207. Vainisi SJ, Schmidt GM, West CS, et al. Metabolic toxic retinopathy preliminary report. Trans Am Coll Vet Ophthalmol 1983;14:76–81.

208. Acland GM, Irby NL, Aguirre GD, et al. Sudden acquired retinal degeneration in the dog: Clinical and morphologic characterization of the "silent retina" syndrome. Trans Am Coll Vet Ophthalmol 1984;15: 86–104.

209. Vainisi SJ, Fond RL, Anderson R, et al. Idiopathic photoreceptor cell degeneration in dogs. Invest Ophthalmol Vis Sci 1985;26:129.

210. Acland GM, Aguirre GD. Sudden acquired retinal degeneration: clinical signs and diagnosis. Trans Am Coll Vet Ophthalmol 1986;17:58–63.

211. vanderWoerdt A, Nasisse MP, Davidson MG. Sudden acquired retinal degeneration syndrome in the dog: Clinical and laboratory findings in 36 cases. Prog Vet Comp Ophthalmol 1991;1:11–18.

212. Mattson A, Roberts SM, Isherwood JME. Clinical features suggesting hyperadrenocorticism in association with sudden acquired retinal degeneration syndrome in a dog. J Am Anim Hosp Assoc 1992;28: 199–202.

213. Pion P, Kittleson M, Rogers Q, et al. Myocardial failure in cats associated with low plasma taurine: A reversible cardiomyopathy. Science 1987;237:764–768.

214. Riis RC. Feline central retinal degeneration—going—going—gone? Proc Am Coll Vet Ophthalmol 1990;21: 116–125.

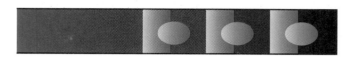

Reproductive
Diseases

Chapter 20

Diseases of the Uterus

Beverly J. Purswell

Anatomy

The uterus has a short body that originates at the internal os of the cervix and divides into two long, straight horns.[1] These two uterine horns diverge at an acute angle and end immediately caudal to the kidneys, where they join the ovaries and uterine tubes.

The cervix is a muscular, tubular sphincter between the vagina and uterus. In the bitch, the cervix is located in the abdomen anterior to a relatively long vagina. The cervix extends diagonally across the uterovaginal junction. The internal os faces almost directly dorsally, whereas the external os faces toward the vaginal floor.[2] Owing to the abdominal location of the cervix and the dorsoventral angle of the cervical lumen, the canine cervix is difficult or impossible to catheterize except during the periparturient period. In the queen, the cervix is located in the pelvis. The vagina in the queen is very narrow and does not accommodate catheterization except during the periparturient period.

The uterine diameter is uniform in the normal nonpregnant state. The uterine lumen is lined with glandular endometrium surrounded by the myometrium. The myometrium consists of an inner circular and an outer longitudinal layer of smooth muscle. The outer serosal layer of the uterus is the thin layer of peritoneum covering the entire uterus. When the uterus is under the influence of estrogen, increased blood flow and edema make the uterus more round. When it is under the influence of progesterone, the uterus has a gross appearance of being coiled. This is a result of the bulging of the myometrium between subserosal blood vessels. During anestrus, the uterus is rather flattened and atonic.[2]

Physiology

The endometrium of the uterus undergoes dramatic changes under the influence of the gonadal hormones, estrogen and progesterone. The endometrium may have transverse dark bands indicating implantation sites from previous pregnancies. Under the influence of estrogen, marked edema of the uterus occurs. Histologically, the endometrium undergoes marked hypertrophy and some hyperplasia of the glandular cells. There is differentiation of the glandular epithelium into mucus-secreting cells.

In the bitch, extensive extravasation of red blood cells occurs into the superficial part of the endometrium and into the uterine lumen by diapedesis. This luminal blood is discharged through the vulva, accounting for the characteristic vulvar bleeding seen during proestrus and estrus. In the queen, during proestrus and estrus the endometrial glands dilate but remain straight. In the luteal phase, which is dominated by progesterone, the endometrial glands grow rapidly and exhibit increased coiling and branching. Regressive changes begin to occur in the endometrium after the progesterone levels begin to fall at about the third week after estrus in the nonpregnant female.[2]

In both species, the luteal phase is prolonged, mimicking the pregnant state. Pseudopregnancy in the bitch is a normal phenomenon that follows every estrous period. The queen undergoes a luteal phase only if she is stimulated to release luteinizing hormone during estrus by copulation or mechanical stimulation of the vulva and vestibule. There is now evidence that the queen can be induced to ovulate by external stimuli such as contact with human handlers. This was documented in confined queens with no contact with male cats; the queens developed pyometra and were found to have progesterone levels indicative of ovulation.[3]

Problem Identification

Infertility

A bitch or queen is considered infertile if she has been bred to a fertile male at the correct time during estrus and has not become pregnant. Correct breeding management (see Chap. 23) and male fertility (see Chap. 21) are critical to successful reproduction. A variety of factors influence fertility, but uterine health plays a significant role in successful reproduction.

Pathophysiology

Cystic endometrial hyperplasia, with or without bacterial involvement, significantly interferes with a developing pregnancy at the local endometrial level; infertility usually represents embryonic death rather than conception failure. Segmental aplasia of the uterus prevents the passage of semen through the affected horns altogether. Infectious diseases, such as *Brucella canis*, must be considered as a potential cause of infertility. *B. canis* colonizes the placental epithelial cells, resulting in placentitis and loss of the pregnancy.[4] Systemic disease, such as hypothyroidism, causes infertility through poorly understood mechanisms. There may be no other clinical signs associated with uterine disease except for infertility.

Clinical Signs

Typically, one or more attempts have been made to breed the bitch to a fertile male, following good breeding management practices, with no puppies being born. There may be no abnormal physical examination findings. Uterine abnormalities may or may not be palpable abdominally.

Diagnostic Plan

All external factors for infertility must be considered and ruled out before invasive procedures are attempted. Breeding management, timing of breeding, and male dog infertility must be ruled out as the causative agents. Serology for *B. canis* is indicated. Thyroid-stimulating hormone stimulation tests may be done to evaluate thyroid function. Hypothyroidism may be clinically inapparent except for its affect on reproductive processes, and this condition is prevalent in a number of breeds of dogs. Vaginal cytology and vaginoscopy may reveal inflammation not evident by external signs such as vulvar discharges. Ultrasonography may be helpful in identifying abnormal uterine morphology or contents. Exploratory laparotomy may be necessary for examination or biopsy of the uterus.

Uterine Enlargement

Uterine enlargement refers to a thickening of the walls of the uterus or an accumulation of uterine contents, or both. Uterine enlargement may be caused by cystic endometrial hyperplasia, pyometra, hydrometra or mucometra, metritis, uterine neoplasia, or pregnancy. Uterine enlargement must be assessed in light of the stage of the estrous cycle and size of the animal. The slight enlargement of the uterus during estrus that is caused by increased circulation and edema should be accompanied by overt signs of proestrus and estrus. The uterus has slightly more tone during diestrus than during anestrus but is not enlarged. Prepubertal and anestrous uteri are small, atonic, and more difficult to identify by abdominal palpation.

Pathophysiology

Increases in uterine wall thickness may be caused by inflammation or cystic endometrial hyperplasia. Under the influence of progesterone, proliferation of the endometrium normally occurs. Degenerative cystic changes that occur within the endometrium are aggravated with each subsequent luteal phase. With the presence of bacteria in the uterus, this endometrial proliferation is compounded by inflammation, leading to gross uterine enlargement. Because of the closed cervix characteristic of the luteal phase, uterine contents are allowed to accumulate, thus contributing to uterine enlargement. With no bacteria present, mucus may accumulate in the uterine lumen during the luteal phase. In the bitch, both uterine disease and pregnancy occur during the 2 months after estrus, when the uterus is dominated by progesterone; therefore, pregnancy must be differentiated from other forms of uterine enlargement. In queens, spontaneous

luteinization of follicles or ovulation has been documented,[3] and breeding may or may not have occurred.

Clinical Signs

The affected animal must be intact. In the bitch, there is usually a history of a recent estrus (within 60–90 days). In the queen, there may or may not be a history of breeding. Mild to moderate uterine enlargement is detectable by abdominal palpation. Severe uterine enlargement, usually resulting from large amounts of uterine contents, may be difficult to distinguish from other abdominal contents. Uterine enlargement may be extensive enough to cause abdominal distention, more commonly in queens.[5] A vulvar discharge may be evident if the cervix relaxes sufficiently to allow drainage from the uterus. Systemic signs such as fever, depression, lethargy, and anorexia may be evident in cases of pyometra or metritis.

Diagnostic Plan

The enlarged uterus may be visualized by either radiography or ultrasonography. Radiography is not able to distinguish between pregnancy and pyometra until the fetal skeletons are calcified sufficiently to be radiopaque. Ultrasonographic examination of the abdomen allows visualization of the uterus and its contents, and pregnancies can be distinguished from abnormal uterine contents such as pyometra (Fig. 20–1). Actual measurements of uterine diameter and uterine wall thickness may be made by ultrasonography.

A serum progesterone determination is indicated to determine whether the animal is under the influence of progesterone. With incomplete histories, cycle information may not be accurate or available. If progesterone levels are higher than 1 ng/mL, luteal phase conditions such as uterine disease and pregnancy are more likely. Thickening of the uterine wall without luminal contents may indicate cystic endometrial hyperplasia, uterine inflammation, or uterine tumors (Fig. 20–2). Exploratory laparotomy may be necessary to differentiate these conditions.

Vulvar Discharge

Vulvar discharges should be evaluated cytologically to determined the nature of the discharge. If the discharge is purulent and the bitch is within 60 to 90 days of her last estrus, pyometra is strongly suggested. Any purulent vulvar discharge in the intact queen is strongly suggestive of pyometra. If the bitch or queen is in the immediate postpartum period and has a purulent vulvar discharge, metritis is likely. If the animal is older, is intact, and has a palpable abdominal mass or abdominal enlargement,

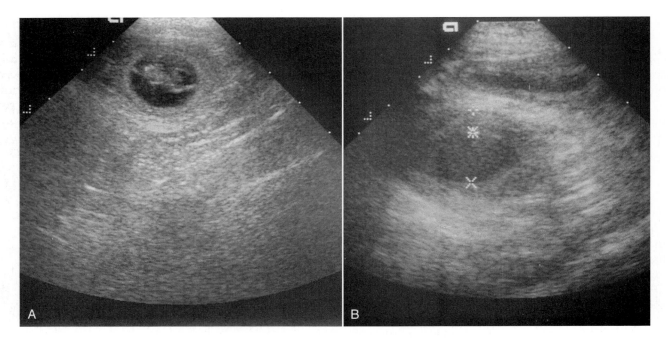

Figure 20-1
Ultrasonography of the canine uterus. (A) Early canine pregnancy showing the amnionic vesicle and a fetus within, approximately 28 days after luteinizing hormone peak. (B) Pyometra. The uterine lumen is approximately 1.3 cm in diameter (between the two Xs); the uterine wall is approximately 0.7 cm thick (between the two cross-hatches).

neoplasia of the uterus or vagina should be considered. The vulvar discharges with neoplasia are usually hemorrhagic but may have an inflammatory component (see Chap. 22).

Depression

The affected animal may be lethargic and anorexic. These signs are compatible with uterine inflammation and the absorption of inflammatory byproducts from the uterus. These signs may also indicate dehydration and azotemia, common metabolic problems seen as complications of uterine disease. Pyometra should be suspected in any intact bitch or queen with depression, particularly if there is a history of estrus within the last 60 to 90 days. In the queen, there may be no history of breeding. An enlarged uterus, purulent vulvar discharge, and a serum progesterone level higher than 1 ng/mL increase the suspicion of pyometra.

Polyuria and Polydipsia

Increased urination and increased thirst is referred to as polyuria with polydipsia. The endotoxin produced by *Escherichia coli* bacteria, the most common opportunistic pathogen isolated from canine and feline pyometras,[6, 7] has been shown to cause reduction in renal concentrating ability.[8] The resulting polyuria causes a compensatory polydipsia, which is consid-

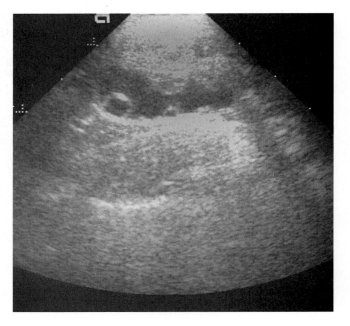

Figure 20-2
Ultrasonography of a canine uterus showing uterine luminal fluid. The fluid appears slightly hyperechoic, indicating mucopurulent uterine contents, which was confirmed by cytologic examination of the vulvar discharge. Within the uterine lumen are multiple cystic structures, indicative of cystic endometrial hyperplasia, which was confirmed at surgery.

ered a functional abnormality that resolves on resolution of the endotoxemia.[6] This condition is present in 28% of canine pyometras and 9% of the feline pyometras.[9–11] Pyometra should be suspected in any intact bitch or queen with polyuria and polydipsia, particularly if there is a history of estrus within the last 60 to 90 days. In the queen, there may be no history of breeding. An enlarged uterus, purulent vulvar discharge, and a serum progesterone level higher than 1 ng/mL increase the suspicion of pyometra (see Chap. 16).

Diagnostic Procedures

Routine Laboratory Evaluation

A complete blood count helps to detect systemic signs associated with uterine disease. The most common finding with metritis and pyometra is a leukocytosis with a regenerative left shift.[12] Biochemical profiles help to detect metabolic abnormalities such as azotemia and dehydration and to assess the health of other organ systems. Urinalysis, combined with the biochemical profile, may be used to evaluate renal function and screen for the presence of a concurrent urinary tract infection.

Abdominal Palpation

Abdominal palpation should allow for assessment of the size, consistency, and tone of the uterus. During abdominal palpation of the uterus, the colon is the most obvious landmark. Coming from below the animal, the clinician places the hands flat on each side of the abdomen. The fingertips are gently brought together immediately ventral to the lumbar vertebrae and dorsal to the colon. The colon is allowed to slip through the opposing fingers, after which the uterus should be the next palpable structure running lengthwise through the abdomen. Care must be taken when palpating a greatly enlarged uterus because it tends to be thin walled.

Vaginal Cytology

Vaginal cytology is indicated whenever reproductive disease is suspected. Estrus and inflammation or infection are two conditions easily detected with vaginal cytology (see Chap. 22).

Vaginoscopy

Vaginoscopy is indicated whenever vulvar discharges are present to determine the origin of these discharges. Vaginoscopy allows visualization of the vagina and discharges from the cervix that may not be evident as vulvar discharges (see Chap. 22).

Serum Progesterone Assays

Progesterone levels can easily be measured from serum with enzyme-linked immunosorbent assay (ELISA) kits available commercially or through laboratories that offer radioimmunoassay. If progesterone is present at levels higher than 1 ng/mL, luteal tissue is present on the ovaries. Because uterine disease is most prevalent during the luteal phase, progesterone levels are helpful in determining whether the animal is at risk. Serum should be separated promptly after the blood has clotted. If the progesterone assay cannot be run immediately, the serum sample should be frozen.

Vaginal Cultures

Bacterial cultures are indicated if purulent discharges are observed. Vaginal cultures should be obtained with a guarded culture instrument or carefully through a speculum. The distal part of the reproductive tract normally has higher numbers of bacteria and should be avoided. For interpretation, see Chapter 22.

Ultrasonography and Radiography

An enlarged uterus can readily be identified with either ultrasonography or radiography. Radiographically, the presence of a homogeneous, tubular, soft tissue density mass in the posterior abdomen is characteristic of uterine enlargement[13] (Fig. 20–3). Normal uterine enlargement is radiographically evident during the later stages of pregnancy and in the immediate postpartum period. Normal nongravid uteri cannot be visualized on radiographs or by ultrasonography. Ultrasonography offers the advantage of measurement of the uterine diameter and uterine wall thickness and assessment of uterine contents (see Fig. 20–1B). This is particularly helpful to distinguish between the normal uterine enlargement of pregnancy and uterine disease.

Uterine Biopsy

Uterine health can be evaluated definitively by a full-thickness biopsy obtained by means of a laparotomy. An exploratory laparotomy allows direct observation of the reproductive tract. Endometritis and cystic endometrial hyperplasia are easily seen histologically. Biopsies may be taken of any lesions found by excision or incision. Uterine biopsies should be taken from the antimesenteric border of the uterus. The biopsy should include both myometrium and endometrium for histologic examination.

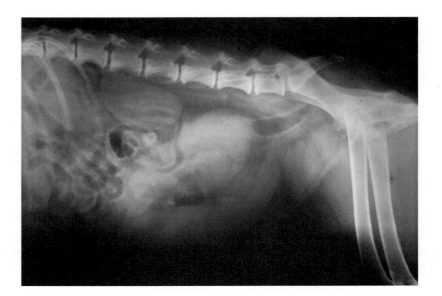

Figure 20-3
Lateral abdominal radiograph showing uterine enlargement consistent with canine pyometra. Note the tubular mass ventral to colon.

Brucella canis Serology

Screening for *B. canis* should be part of any reproductive tract examination. This organism is not common but has profound effects on reproduction if contracted (see Chap. 23).

Common Diseases of the Uterus

Pyometra and Cystic Endometrial Hyperplasia

Pyometra is the accumulation of purulent material within the lumen of the uterus. Pyometras are classified as open-cervix or closed-cervix pyometras, according to the presence or absence of a vulvar discharge. Pyometra almost exclusively occurs when the uterus is under the influence of progesterone. The progesterone-dominated luteal phase occurs 2 months after estrus in the bitch and pregnant queen or 40 to 45 days after ovulation in the nonpregnant queen. Spontaneous luteinization or ovulation in the queen has been documented; therefore, a history of breeding may not be present.[3] Clinically inapparent pyometras may become apparent after the progesterone levels have fallen. At that time, the cervix relaxes and the uterine contents begin to drain, producing a vulvar discharge. The incidence of pyometra increases with the age of the animal.[9] Older nulliparous animals may be in a higher risk category than animals that have had litters.[14]

Pathophysiology

Uterine infections occur only when the uterus is under the influence of progesterone or during the immediate postpartum period. Cystic endometrial hyperplasia can occur when the uterus is under the influence of progesterone and has responded in an exaggerated or abnormal manner. Cystic endometrial hyperplasia tends to occur more frequently in aged animals that have undergone numerous hormonal cycles throughout their lifetimes, and it may persist after the progesterone influence has been removed. Exogenous progesterone has been shown to cause cystic endometrial hyperplasia and is the experimental model for pyometra.[14]

The vulnerablility of the uterus to bacterial infections while under the influence of progesterone is poorly understood but widely accepted.[15] Once in the uterus, bacterial growth is relatively uninhibited. The uterine motility is decreased by progesterone, and uterine glands become more numerous, complex, and secretory. The cervix is typically closed during the luteal phase, which allows accumulation of bacteria and bacterial byproducts in the uterus. Bacterial toxins, especially endotoxins associated with *E. coli*, may be absorbed from the uterus and cause systemic signs of endotoxemia. Seepage of these uterine contents through the cervix may occur and may present as vulvar discharge. Neutrophils in vulvar discharges are present in high numbers when uterine infection is present.

Cystic endometrial hyperplasia is considered to predispose the uterus to pyometra.[14] Cystic endometrial hyperplasia develops over time, with age, and after multiple reproductive cycles and can be induced by exogenous progesterone administration. Cystic hyperplasia–pyometra complex has been described in progressive categories. Type I is uncomplicated cystic hyperplasia with mucoid vulvar discharge and can occur at any time during the estrous cycle. Type II is cystic hyperplasia with lymphoid infiltration and vulvar discharge, occurring 40 to 70 days after estrus, with slight leukocytosis. With type III, acute endometritis superimposed on cystic hyperplasia, the animal is clinically ill to a variable degree, depending on the degree of uterine distention; the complex occurs 20 to 40 days after estrus and produces moderate to severe leukocytosis. Finally, type IV, chronic endometritis, produces a degree of illness that varies inversely with the patency of cervix, occurs 55 to 90 days after estrus, and produces moderate to severe leukocytosis.[14] The majority of pyometra cases culture positive for *E. coli* in both bitches and queens.[16] Bacteria are considered opportunistic pathogens superimposed on the cystic hyperplasia–pyometra complex.

Clinical Signs

The clinical signs seen with pyometras vary with the severity of the condition. Any time that a purulent vulvar discharge is noted in an intact bitch or queen, pyometra must be considered. Clinically inapparent pyometras occur and may be identified only at the end of diestrus, when a purulent vulvar discharge is noted. Pyometra must be considered if depression, lethargy, anorexia, and polyuria with polydipsia occur in the intact bitch or queen, particularly if there is a history of estrus within the last 60 to 90 days.

Open-cervix pyometras present with a purulent vulvar discharge with variable systemic signs and account for approximately 85% of pyometras in the bitch[9] and 68% of pyometras in the queen.[10] Animals are often afebrile with a regenerative leukocytosis. Clinical signs of open-cervix pyometras range from a vulvar discharge and mildly enlarged uterus only to severe systemic signs of depression, anorexia, vomiting, and other signs indicative of septicemia or toxemia. Animals with closed-cervix pyometras tend to have more systemic signs of disease. Polyuria with polydipsia is observed in approximately 30% to 50% of bitches with pyometra.[9] This is considered to be an effect of *E. coli* endotoxins on renal tubules[8] or of reduction in the glomerular filtration rate.[6] Concurrent urinary tract infections are found in 22% of animals with pyometra (38% in animals older than 7 years of age).[6]

Diagnostic Plan

Diagnosis of pyometra begins with the signalment of an intact queen or bitch. The history usually includes a recent estrous episode (<70 days ago). Progesterone levels are typically higher than 1 ng/mL. A purulent vulvar discharge is diagnostic, particularly if it is shown to be originating from the cervix by vaginoscopy. Palpation, radiography, or ultrasonography can demonstrate uterine enlargement (see Figs. 20–1*B* and 20–2). Ultrasonography is preferable because of the ability to visualize uterine contents and rule out other causes of uterine enlargement.

Treatment

The treatment of choice for pyometra is ovariohysterectomy. Clinical improvement is rapid and permanent after removal of the uterus and appropriate supportive therapy such as intravenous (IV) fluids and antibiotics in all but the most critically ill patients. Ampicillin (10–25 mg/kg IV or by mouth three or four times per day) is a good first choice but should be substantiated by culture and sensitivity results of the bacteria involved. Medical management of pyometra can be considered if the client desires to keep the animal as breeding stock. Open-cervix pyometras respond the best to medical management. Closed-cervix pyometras are treated medically only with caution. Animals with closed-cervix pyometras tend to be more systemically ill, and the uterus is much more compromised. Vaginoscopy, in the absence of a vulvar discharge, may determine the presence of purulent discharge within the vagina, indicating an open cervix.

Medical management of pyometras involves the use of prostaglandin F_{2a} (PGF). PGF causes smooth muscle contraction and, with multiple small doses, lysing of the corpus luteum, thus removing the progesterone influence on the uterus.[17] Dinoprost tromethamine (Lutalyse) is the recommended product because of the wealth of information available on dosages, effects, side effects, and safety. PGF is not approved for use in the dog or cat but has been shown to be safe if used properly. Care must be taken in calculating the dose for each animal; the median lethal dose (LD_{50}) for PGF in the dog is 5 mg/kg.[18] Side effects, including lethal side effects, from PGF are dose related, and therefore the lowest effective dose should be used. Initially, subcutaneous doses of 0.05 to 0.1 mg/kg per day are used in the dog[19] (0.25–0.5 mg/kg per day in the cat), which causes adequate contraction of the myometrium to allow expression of uterine contents. After uterine evacuation has begun, the initial treatment can be expanded to twice daily without any untoward effects. Monitoring of the serum levels of progesterone demonstrates the luteolytic activity of PGF.

The side effects seen with PGF are panting, hypersalivation, restlessness, vomiting, and defecation or diarrhea. All side effects are transient, disappearing in 30 to 40 minutes after drug administration. Metabolism of PGF occurs rapidly in the lungs. Because side effects tend to diminish over the treatment period with each injection, they are most pronounced after the first injection. Systemic antibiotics are administered concurrently to protect against the possibility of bacteremia. Again, ampicillin (10–25 mg/kg three to four times per day) is a good first choice, because *E. coli* is the most common species found. Culture and sensitivity of the actual bacterium substantiate the choice of antibiotics. Treatment with PGF must continue until all clinical signs of pyometra have disappeared. Monitoring should include the animal's general attitude, vulvar discharge, vaginal cytology, complete blood count, and uterine size by abdominal palpation and ultrasonography. Most pyometras respond and resolve in 5 to 10 days.

Prognosis

Prognosis for pyometra treated surgically is excellent if the animal survives the perioperative period. Prognosis for medical treatment of pyometra depends on the extent of uterine disease and length of treatment necessary for the resolution of clinical signs. Breeding during the next estrus after treatment is recommended. Pyometra is reported to recur within 2 years in more than 70% of bitches successfully treated with PGF.[20] The underlying pathologic changes of cystic endometrial hyperplasia are apparently unaffected by PGF therapy and continue to place the animal at risk to develop pyometra with each luteal phase. Prognosis appears worse if PGF therapy of longer than 5 days' duration is necessary for clinical resolution.

Metritis

Metritis is defined as an inflammatory process involving the entire uterus—endometrium and myometrium. Metritis is most often seen in the postpartum period[21] but can be a consequence of the cystic endometrial hyperplasia–pyometra complex.

Pathophysiology

Postpartum metritis is a result of delayed uterine involution complicated by bacterial involvement.[21] Delayed uterine involution may be caused by uterine trauma or by underlying metabolic abnormalities, such as hypocalcemia or hypoglycemia, that interfere with normal uterine motility. Dystocia, abortion, obstetric manipulations, retained placentas or fetuses, contaminated whelping or queening environments, bacterial endometritis (pyometra) concurrent with pregnancy, and pre-existing cystic endometrial hyperplasia all may lead to metritis in the postpartum period. The relaxed and open cervix present at parturition allows the possibility of ascending bacterial invasion of the uterus. Delayed uterine involution allows ascending infections to proliferate and colonize the uterus.

Clinical Signs

Purulent vulvar discharges are usually evident. Animals with metritis show acute systemic signs of

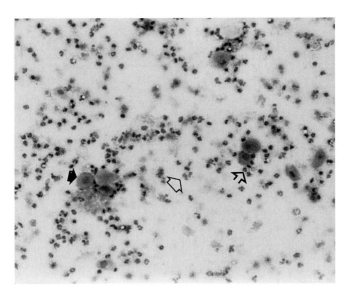

Figure 20–4
Vaginal cytology preparation from a bitch with pyometra. Notice the high ratio of neutrophils to epithelial cells and the presence of degenerate *(large open arrow)* and nondegenerate *(small open arrow)* neutrophils. Solid arrow indicates noncornified epithelial cell.

illness, including fever, anorexia, malaise, and dehydration. Rapid progression of clinical signs makes immediate intervention necessary. Dams lose interest in mothering activities.

Diagnostic Plan

Abdominal palpation reveals an enlarged, firm uterus. Leukocytosis with or without a left shift is usually present. Degenerative left shifts may be found in the more clinically ill patients. Other metabolic abnormalities, such as azotemia, may be present as a consequence of the dehydration and endotoxemia. Vaginal cytology shows a high ratio of neutrophils to epithelial cells, usually 10:1 or higher (Fig. 20–4). The enlarged uterus is easily identifiable with ultrasonography and radiography. With ultrasonography, the uterine walls are seen to be thickened, and a varying amount of luminal fluid is present.

Treatment

Treatment decisions are made based on the future breeding potential of the animal and the severity of the illness. Broad-spectrum antibiotics (ampicillin, 10–25 mg/kg three or four times per day) are administered, immediately preceded by anterior vaginal culture with sensitivities. Choice of antibiotics can be altered, if necessary, after the results of the vaginal culture and sensitivity determinations are known. Ovariohysterectomy may be the treatment of choice.

PGF may be used to treat metritis before ovariohysterectomy in order to reduce uterine contamination before surgery. PGF therapy promotes uterine evacuation and should be used to effect. Cessation of PGF therapy should be based on the animal's general attitude, vulvar discharge, vaginal cytology, complete blood count, and size of uterus as determined by abdominal palpation or ultrasonography. It should be kept in mind that antibiotics will be passed through the milk to the suckling neonates. Neonates should be monitored for the desired daily weight gain and normal feces.

Prognosis

With prompt and appropriate therapy, the prognosis for resolution of metritis is good. The prognosis for future reproduction varies depending on the underlying cause of the metritis and the degree of damage to the uterus.

Neoplasia

Neoplasia infrequently involves the uterus of the dog or cat. Neoplastic conditions may arise from the endometrium in the form of adenocarcinomas, but the most frequent tumor found in the uterus is leiomyoma.[2, 22, 23] Tumors of the uterus can arise from uterine remnants left behind from an ovariohysterectomy, but typically they are found in older intact bitches and queens that are 8 to 10 years of age or older. One study[24] reported the incidence of uterine tumors to be 0.033% among bitches examined over a 14-year period.

Pathophysiology

The cause of uterine tumors is unknown. Circumstantial evidence points to a hormonal dependency of some tumors, but this relationship has not been statistically documented.[22]

Clinical Signs

No specific clinical signs are associated with uterine neoplasia other than the detection of an abdominal mass or uterine enlargement by palpation, radiography, or ultrasonography. A vulvar discharge may be present, but it can vary from mucoid or mucopurulent to hemorrhagic.

Diagnostic Plan

An abdominal mass in the area of the uterus may be palpated or seen on radiography. Ultrasonography may help to delineate the mass and determine its connection to the uterus. Diagnosis is made conclusively at surgery. Thoracic radiographs should be taken to evaluate for metastasis.

Treatment

Treatment consists of surgical removal of the affected uterus. Removal of the tumor is possible, but it is not recommended in the aged patient.

Prognosis

Prognosis is good with the benign uterine tumors, such as leiomyomata, after surgical removal of the uterus. Adenocarcinomas may already have spread by local invasion or metastasis through blood or lymphatic vessels, which makes the prognosis poor.[23] If local invasion is not evident at surgery, area lymph nodes may be biopsied and thoracic radiographs taken to assess metastasis.

Uncommon Diseases of the Uterus

Hydrometra and Mucometra

The terms hydrometra and mucometra refer to the accumulation of watery to mucoid contents in the uterus without an inflammatory component. The incidence is unknown, and the condition is usually an incidental finding at ovariohysterectomy. This accumulation of a noninflammatory uterine content is most often seen during the luteal phase of the estrous cycle but may occur during estrogen stimulation as well.

Pathophysiology

Fluid accumulates in the uterus because of stimulation of the endometrium by the gonadal hormones. This accumulation of fluid is most pronounced during diestrus and may be associated with cystic endometrial hyperplasia.[2] Excessive estrogenic stimulation also induces hyperplasia of the endometrium and accumulation of fluid in the uterus. Endogenous sources of estrogen may include follicular cysts and granulosa cell tumors.

Clinical Signs

The only clinical sign that may be noticed is a mucoid vulvar discharge. In most cases, no clinical signs are recognized. Bitches may lick the vulvar area frequently, and they often attract male dogs. These signs are most often noticed at the end of diestrus, when signs of pseudopregnancy are at their maximum (approximately 2 months after estrus). Vaginal cytology is helpful in differentiating these conditions from pyometra by the absence of abundant inflammatory cells. Diagnosis can be made by ultrasonographic examination of the uterus, which reveals uterine luminal fluid that is generally hypoechoic. Only in cases of uterine or cervical hypoplasia or aplasia[2] is the accumulation of fluid great enough to be detected by abdominal palpation or radiography.

Treatment

Treatment of mucometra or hydrometra, if the bitch or queen is to be retained as a breeding animal, consists of PGF therapy for at least 5 consecutive days, until the uterus is completely evacuated. Ultrasonography is necessary to know when complete uterine evacuation has been obtained. Ovariohysterectomy may be performed if the animal will no longer be used for breeding or if the condition is secondary to anatomic defects such as segmental aplasia or cervical aplasia.

Prognosis

Prognosis for future fertility is variable. Most anatomic defects render the animal permanently sterile. Many animals successfully carry litters after PGF therapy for mucometra or hydrometra. The recommendation should be made to breed at the next estrus if possible. Because of the relation of cystic endometrial hyperplasia to mucometra or hydrometra, recurrence is likely, and the condition may progress to pyometra in subsequent estrous cycles. Ovariohysterectomy is the ultimate recommendation; it should be performed as soon as possible or when suitable to the client.

Congenital Abnormalities

Congenital uterine abnormalities usually involve aplasia, segmental aplasia, or hypoplasia of some portion of the uterus or cervix. Many times, the ipsilateral ovary and uterine tube are not involved.[2] These conditions are often incidental findings at surgery. There are no specific clinical signs associated with these abnormalities. Infertility or subfertility (small litter size) may be seen in these patients, depending on the extent of the involvement. Diagnosis of these conditions is confirmed by surgical exploration of the abdomen. There are no treatment options; therefore, ovariohysterectomy is advised. Prognosis for future fertility is dictated by the extent and degree of involvement of the abnormality. After ovariohysterectomy is performed, no other problems should arise from these congenital abnormalities.

References

1. Roberts SJ. Veterinary Obstetrics and Genital Diseases: Theriogenology. North Pomfret, Vermont, David and Charles, 1986:6–11.

2. McEntee K. Reproductive Pathology of Domestic Mammals. San Diego, Academic Press, 1990:110–115.

3. Lawler DF, Evans RH, Reimers TJ, et al. Histopathologic features, environmental factors, and serum estrogen, progesterone, and prolactin values associated with ovarian phases and inflammatory uterine disease in cats. Am J Vet Res 1991;52:1747–1753.

4. Johnson CA, Walker RD. Clinical signs and diagnosis of *Brucella canis* infection. Compen Contin Educ Pract Vet 1992;14:763–773.

5. Potter AK, Hancock DH, Gallina AM. Clinical and pathologic features of endometrial hyperplasia, pyometra, and endometritis in cats: 79 cases (1980–1985). J Am Vet Med Assoc 1991;198:1427–1431.

6. Stone EA, Littman MP, Robertson JL, et al. Renal dysfunction in dogs with pyometra. J Am Vet Med Assoc 1988;193:457–464.

7. Sandholm M, Vasenius H, Kivisto A-K. Pathogenesis of canine pyometra. J Am Vet Med Assoc 1975;167:1006–1010.

8. Asheim A. Pathogenesis of renal damage and polydipsia in dogs with pyometra. J Am Vet Med Assoc 1965;147:736–745.

9. Nelson RW, Feldman EC. Pyometra. Vet Clin North Am Small Anim Pract 1986;16:561–576.

10. Kenney KJ, Matthiesen DT, Brown NO, et al. Pyometra in cats: 183 cases (1979–1984). J Am Vet Med Assoc 1987;191:1130–1132.

11. Davidson AP, Feldman EC, Nelson RW. Treatment of pyometra in cats, using prostaglandin F_{2a}: 21 cases (1982-1990). J Am Vet Med Assoc 1992; 200:825-828.

12. Nelson RW, Feldman EC. Pyometra in the bitch. In: Morrow DA, ed. Current Therapy in Theriogenology, 2nd ed. Philadelphia, WB Saunders, 1986:484–489.

13. Hardy RM. Cystic endometrial hyperplasia-pyometra complex. In: Morrow DA, ed. Current Therapy in Theriogenology. Philadelphia, WB Saunders, 1980:624–631.

14. Dow C. The cystic hyperplasia-pyometra complex in the bitch. Vet Rec 1957;69:1409–1415.

15. Hawk HW, Turner GD, Sykes JF. The effect of ovarian hormones on the uterine defense mechanism during the early stages of induced infection. Am J Vet Res 1960;21:644–648.

16. Johnson CA. Cystic endometrial hyperplasia, pyometra, and infertility. In: Ettinger SJ, Feldman EC, eds. Textbook of Veterinary Internal Medicine, 4th ed, vol 2. Philadelphia, WB Saunders, 1995:1636–1642.

17. Lein DH. Prostaglandin therapy in small animal reproduction. In: Kirk RW, ed. Current Veterinary Therapy IX. Philadelphia, WB Saunders, 1986:1233–1235.

18. Sokolowski JH, Geng S. Effect of prostaglandin F_{2a}-THAM in the bitch. J Am Vet Med Assoc 1977;170:536-537.

19. Wheaton LG, Barbee DD. Comparison of two dosages of prostaglandin F_{2a} on canine uterine motility. Theriogenology 1993;40:111–120.

20. Meyers-Wallen VN, Goldschmidt MH, Flickinger GL. Prostaglandin F_{2a} treatment of canine pyometra. J Am Vet Med Assoc 1986;189:1557–1561.

21. Magne ML. Acute metritis in the bitch. In: Morrow DA, ed. Current Therapy in Theriogenology, 2nd ed. Philadelphia, WB Saunders, 1986:505–506.

22. Herron MA. Tumors of the canine genital system. J Am Anim Hosp Assoc 1983;19:981–994.

23. Crow SE. Neoplasms of the reproductive organs and mammary glands of the dog. In: Morrow DA, ed. Current Therapy in Theriogenology. Philadelphia, WB Saunders, 1980:640–646.

24. Brodey RS, Roszel JF. Neoplasms of the canine uterus, vagina, and vulva: A clinicopathologic survey of 90 cases. J Am Vet Med Assoc 1967;151:1294–1307.

Chapter 21

Diseases of the Gonads

Beverly J. Purswell
Nikola A. Parker

Anatomy

Male

The testes are paired, oval, laterally compressed organs with a smooth, regular surface and are located within the scrotal sac in the male. The size of the testes varies with the breed and age of the animal. Each organ is suspended from the ventral abdominal wall by the spermatic cord, which passes through the inguinal canal. The spermatic cord is composed of striated cremaster muscle, a ductus deferens, a spermatic artery, and a network of spermatic veins that form the pampiniform plexus. Each testis is closely associated with the epididymis along its dorsal border (in the dog) or its dorsocranial border (in the cat).

Microscopically, each testis consists of a connective tissue capsule, the tunica albuginea, surrounding testicular parenchyma. The parenchyma consists of seminiferous tubules and interstitial cells (Leydig cells) and is divided into lobules by connective tissue septa extending from the overlying capsule. These septa converge centrally, forming the mediastinum testis. Blood vessels, nerves, and lymphatics course within these septa. The seminiferous tubules are composed of layers of spermatogenic cells at different stages of development. The basal layer consists of spermatogonia and Sertoli cells. Sertoli cells are large, pleomorphic cells that extend throughout the width of the tubule and constitute a large part of the blood-testis barrier. The Sertoli cell functions in nutrition and maturation of spermatids.

Female

The ovaries are paired, flattened, firm, ellipsoid organs that lie caudal to the kidney in the female. The surface is smooth during the prepubertal period and during anestrus. During estrus and diestrus, the surface becomes irregular owing to the presence of follicles or corpora lutea. There is a tendency for the surface of the ovary to become wrinkled with age and multiple estrous cycles. The size of the ovary varies with the size of the animal. It should measure approximately $15 \times 7 \times 5$ mm in an 11.5-kg bitch.[1] Each ovary is suspended within a bursa formed from fusion of portions of the broad ligament. In the dog, this bursa contains much adipose tissue and totally surrounds the ovary. Each ovary is associated caudolaterally with the oviduct (uterine tube).

Histologically, the ovary consists of germinal epithelium surrounding ovarian stroma. Stroma consists mainly of developing follicles, luteal tissue, blood vessels, lymphatics, and cords of germinal epithelium from which follicles develop. Follicles are composed of multiple layers of granulosa cells surrounding an oocyte, which is enveloped by cumulus cells. Luteal tissue may be corpora hemorrhagica, corpora lutea, or corpora albicans, depending on the stage of the cycle. Corpora hemorrhagica are developing corpora lutea shortly after ovulation; on cross section, they are dark red. Corpora lutea (yellow bodies) are the mature functional structures producing progesterone during diestrus; they are yellow on cross section. Corpora albicans, the residual scar tissue left after the corpora lutea regress, are white on cross section.

Physiology

Male

The testes function primarily in the production of spermatozoa and steroid hormones. The principal steroid, testosterone, is produced by the Leydig (or interstitial) cells. Spermatogenesis and steroidogenesis are under the control of the hypothalamus and pituitary. Gonadotropin-releasing hormone (GnRH) from the hypothalamus stimulates the release of pituitary follicle-stimulating hormone (FSH) and luteinizing hormone (LH). LH acts on interstitial cells, which respond by producing testosterone, estradiol, progesterone, and other androgens. FSH regulates Sertoli cells to secrete androgen-binding protein and inhibin. Androgen-binding protein regulates testosterone concentrations within the seminiferous tubules.[2] Inhibin is thought to suppress FSH secretion from the pituitary.

FSH also stimulates spermatogenesis, which is the series of mitotic and meiotic divisions within the germinal epithelium of the seminiferous tubules that results in the production of sperm. Spermatogonia divide mitotically to form primary spermatocytes, which then divide meiotically to form spermatids. The latter give rise to spermatozoa. The duration of spermatogenesis is about 62 days in the dog.[3] The process is greatly influenced by temperature. Spermatogenesis cannot occur at normal body temperatures. Thermoregulation is maintained by numerous factors. These factors include the extra-abdominal or scrotal location of the testes, the action of the cremaster muscle and tunica dartos (smooth muscle within the wall of the scrotum), and the vascular arrangement of the testicular artery and pampiniform plexus. The cremaster muscle and tunica dartos are sensitive to temperature changes and act to bring the testes closer to the body in colder temperatures. The testicular artery is surrounded by the pampiniform plexus of veins, which cools arterial blood entering the testes.

The epididymis is the location of final spermatozoan maturation and sperm storage. Spermatozoa move from the seminiferous tubules to the rete testis, which is centrally located within the testicle. From the rete testis, the spermatozoa are moved through the

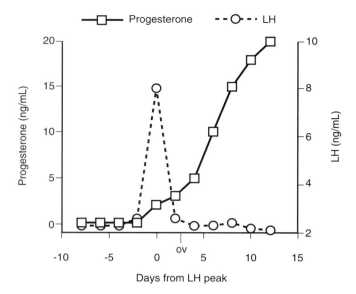

Figure 21-1
Graph showing the relationship between the ovulatory luteinizing hormone (LH) peak and the rise in progesterone levels before, during, and after ovulation (ov).

efferent ducts to the head of the epididymis. Spermatozoa move through the head and body of the epididymis to collect in the tail of the epididymis. The tail of the epididymis is a major storage area for spermatozoa before ejaculation or elimination through urination. The cytoplasmic droplet of the spermatozoa translocates from the proximal midpiece to the distal midpiece as the cell is transported through the epididymis. As the final stage of maturation takes place in the tail of the epididymis, the cytoplasmic droplet falls off the spermatozoa. These detached droplets may be seen floating free in the seminal fluid.

Female

The ovaries produce ova and steroid hormones. Under hypothalamic (GnRH) control, the pituitary releases LH and FSH. These act on the ovaries to stimulate follicular development; some of the follicles dominate, mature, and ovulate. Granulosa cells within these follicles produce estrogen and inhibin, both of which negatively feed back to the hypothalamus and pituitary to suppress hormonal secretion. Estrogen causes changes in the entire reproductive tract (increased blood supply, cornification of the vagina, edema) and elicits a preovulatory LH surge from the pituitary. Luteinization of follicular cells, followed by ovulation, occurs as a result of this LH surge (Fig. 21-1). The resulting structure is a corpus luteum. The corpus luteum produces progesterone and persists for approximately 2 months in the pregnant or nonpregnant bitch.[4] The queen is an induced ovulator and ovulates in response to copulation or stimulation of the

vulva or vestibule. After ovulation, the queen has a luteal phase lasting approximately 63 to 65 days if pregnant or 40 to 45 days if pseudopregnant.[5]

The estrous cycle is divided into proestrus, estrus, diestrus, postestrus, and anestrus. Cycle length varies dramatically among individual bitches. Interestrous periods (from the beginning of one estrus to the beginning of the next estrus) of 4 to 12 months are considered normal in dogs. In the bitch, the average duration of proestrus and estrus is 9 days, both having a range of 2 to 21 days. During proestrus, the period of follicular development, FSH and LH are low and estrogen levels are elevated. At the beginning of estrus (standing behavior), there is a preovulatory rise in FSH and LH. After this rise of gonadotropins, progesterone levels increase and estrogens begin to fall. It is the combination of estrogen and progesterone that elicits standing behavior in the bitch. Ovulation occurs between 24 and 72 hours after the LH peak[6] (see Fig. 21-1).

Diestrus, or the luteal phase, lasts in dogs for 65 days if pregnant or 60 to 90 days if pseudopregnant. In cats, diestrus lasts 63-65 days in the pregnant queen or 40 to 45 days in the pseudopregnant queen. Although progesterone levels are high during diestrus, FSH, LH, and estrogen are at basal levels. There is evidence that prolactin is luteotropic in both species during the last half of diestrus. The queen is seasonally polyestrous and cycles every 2 to 3 weeks during the season of long daylight hours.[7]

The queen, if not induced to ovulate, enters a postestrus period by regression of the previous set of follicles. This period is dominated by neither estrogen nor progesterone. The postestrus period ends with the recruitment of the next set of follicles. Both species exhibit anestrus. After diestrus, the bitch undergoes an anestrus period of variable duration until the next proestrus. The queen undergoes a seasonal anestrus in response to short daylight hours.

Problem Identification (Males)

Orchitis and Epididymitis

Orchitis is inflammation of the testicle and is characterized by a painful, hard swelling of the testicle. Epididymitis is a painful, hard swelling of the epididymis. Orchitis and epididymitis may or may not occur concurrently.

Pathophysiology

Inflammation may be caused by infectious or noninfectious processes. Trauma to the testicle; testicular torsion; infectious agents such as *Brucella canis* or *Blastomyces* spp., which have a tendency to localize in or around the testicle; cellulitis; and abscess from punctures in the scrotum all may result in orchitis. Insults to the testicle cause increased blood flow and polymorphonuclear cell activity within the testis. Localized swelling, hyperemia, and hyperthermia result. Disruption of thermoregulation to the testicle inhibits spermatogenesis and may result in irreversible damage to the seminiferous tubules in the affected testicle. Testicular degeneration is the usual sequela to orchitis. Testicular degeneration may be followed by testicular atrophy or testicular fibrosis. Testicular degeneration is characterized by a softening of the testicular parenchyma. If the testicle recovers from the inflammatory process, the testicular degeneration resolves and the testicle returns to normal.

Similar changes occur with inflammation to the epididymitis. Trauma, blunt or penetrating, may cause epididymitis. Some organisms, such as *B. canis* and *Blastomyces* spp., have a predilection for the epididymitis as a site of localization. Because of scarring, blockage of the epididymis is often the long-term result of epididymitis.

Clinical Signs

Orchitis or epididymitis may be either acute or chronic in onset. Beagles are particularly susceptible to lymphocytic orchitis,[8] indicating a possible hereditary component to certain kinds of orchitis. Orchitis and epididymitis are usually associated with subfertility or infertility. The clinical signs associated with orchitis or epididymitis vary with the extent and duration of the problem. The inflammation in the scrotal area may cause the male to lick the genital area more frequently than normal. Gait abnormalities may be seen because of pain in the inguinal area. In acute cases, the animal may show depression, inappetence, elevated body temperature, a painful and swollen testicle or epididymis, and a reluctance to move. Unilateral involvement is more common than bilateral involvement. Scrotal dermatitis may be present if the animal has been licking the area. Animals with chronic cases usually do not show clinical signs. Physical examination findings are usually localized to the affected area. Swelling, redness, heat, and pain may be found with palpation if the condition is acute. Atrophy or fibrosis of the testicle may be found if orchitis is a chronic condition. Lymphadenopathy may be present in the regional lymph nodes. The animal may be febrile and may show systemic signs of infection.

Diagnostic Plan

Cytologic evaluation of semen may reveal the presence of inflammatory cells. Evaluation of the sperm cell may reveal abnormal sperm morphology and the presence of spermatozoa precursors, suggesting tubular damage. Bacterial culture of the semen sample may help to identify any infectious agents present. In acute cases of orchitis or epididymitis, fine-needle aspiration of the epididymis or testicle for culture or cytology may be necessary to identify the offending organism. *B. canis* serology should be obtained on all dogs with orchitis or epididymitis. Ultrasound is useful to differentiate testicular swelling from neoplasia. In chronic cases, fine-needle, punch, or incisional biopsies may be taken to obtain a definitive diagnosis. A prostatic examination should be done, because ascending or descending spread of disease is possible. Castration is the best option if the animal is not to be used for breeding.

Testicular Degeneration, Fibrosis, and Atrophy

Testicular degeneration is characterized by the loss of functional testicular tissue, which results in a softening of the testicular parenchyma and a reduction in the size of the testicle. Testicular atrophy is the end result of irreversible testicular degeneration. In testicular atrophy, the testicular parenchyma shrinks until the epididymis may be the only palpable structure remaining. Testicular parenchyma may be replaced over time by connective tissue; this constitutes testicular fibrosis.

Pathophysiology

Testicular degeneration, fibrosis, or atrophy may result from inflammatory, age-related, nutritional, or hormone-induced processes. In a high percentage of cases, the cause is unknown and may be related to a genetically controlled early loss of fertility. Irreversible damage and complete loss of testicular tissue may result from trauma, infectious organisms such as *B. canis* or *Blastomyces* spp., testicular torsion, cellulitis, or abscess. Other bacterial agents may ascend from infections in the prostate gland.

Inflammation may cause only temporary dysfunction of the testicle because of the increase in temperature associated with the inflammatory process itself (disruption of thermoregulation). This less-damaging form of inflammation may be caused by scrotal skin inflammation, overheating in hot summer months, or trauma to the surrounding pelvic, inguinal, or perineal area. These less-damaging disruptions in testicular function are reflected in temporary testicular degeneration that resolves over time. If the testicular damage is reversible, recovery is slow, requiring 3 to 6 months in most cases. The slow recovery time is influenced by the length of the spermatogenic cycle. Inflammation that causes direct damage to the testicular tissue itself leads to irreversible changes within the testicle. Irreversible testicular degeneration progresses to testicular fibrosis, atrophy, or, more uncommonly, dystrophic calcification.

Testicular degeneration may be seen with increasing age. This type of testicular degeneration is typically irreversible. A decrease in libido may accompany testicular degeneration because of a reduction in Leydig cells, which are responsible for testosterone production. Reduction in the normal levels of testosterone may also result in shrinkage of the prostate gland, penis, and prepuce. Any severe nutritional deficiency has the potential to cause testicular degeneration, but this cause is uncommon because commercial diets are well balanced. Lack or excess of endogenous or exogenous steroid hormones or thyroxine (T_4) over time causes testicular degeneration that may or may not be reversible.

Clinical Signs

Male animals may first be presented because of problems with infertility with or without decreased libido. The animal may have a history of recurrent prostatitis or prior trauma. History of oligospermia or azoospermia may be present. These conditions are often found on physical examination without prior history of a problem or inciting cause. On testicular palpation, small, soft to firm testes are noted. Testicular degeneration causes a softening of the testicle and a concurrent loss of resiliency. Testicular fibrosis results in an increased firmness in the consistency of the testis, with a loss of testicular resiliency. The consistency of the affected organ varies with the amount of fibrosis. These conditions are often bilateral.

Diagnostic Plan

A breeding soundness examination that includes evaluation of semen can determine the extent of testicular damage. Evaluation of the ejaculate determines the presence of sperm, numbers of sperm cells ejaculated, motility of the sperm cells, and sperm morphology. Earlier forms of testicular degeneration are indicated by presence of a high percentage of abnormal spermatozoa within the ejaculate. More chronic forms are indicated by oligospermia or azoospermia. *B. canis* serology is indicated in all reproductive examinations. T_4 levels should be determined to rule out hypothyroidism. Testicular biopsy determines the extent of tubular degenerative changes and fibrosis. However, because of the invasive nature of the procedure and the possible complications (e.g., complete testicular atrophy), testicular biopsy is performed only with discretion.

Oligospermia and Azoospermia

Oligospermia is the production or ejaculation of sperm in numbers that are below what is considered normal. Azoospermia is the total lack of sperm in the ejaculate.

Pathophysiology

Oligospermia or azoospermia can result from any process that decreases or inhibits spermatogenesis or the transport of spermatozoa from the testis, including duct occlusion. These conditions may occur with epididymitis, orchitis, tubular ischemia, testicular degeneration, testicular neoplasia, hormonal disturbances (hypothyroidism, hyperadrenocorticism), and systemic diseases (any febrile or debilitating episode).

Clinical Signs

Depending on the use of the male for breeding, subfertility or infertility may be noted; this could be congenital or acquired. If the male is being presented for a breeding soundness examination before first breeding, there may be no pertinent history. There are usually no apparent clinical signs. There may be no abnormal physical examination findings, or only those consistent with testicular degeneration, fibrosis, or atrophy.

Diagnostic Plan

A definitive diagnosis is based on the evaluation of an ejaculate. It may be impossible to determine the cause. A low baseline testosterone level may indicate testicular dysfunction, but multiple samples may be required to rule out normal fluctuations. Gonadotropin levels are abnormally high if there is a lack of testicular feedback (testosterone) on the hypothalamic-pituitary axis. GnRH stimulation tests may be run to evaluate pituitary-testicular interactions. Testosterone levels should increase within 1 hour of administration of GnRH. A biopsy may be indicated if these noninvasive procedures are not informative. Castration is recommended in nonbreeding animals.

Testicular Masses

A testicular mass can be any circumscribed nodule within the testicle. Testicular tumors include any neoplastic change, benign or malignant. Testicular tumors may be associated with any cell type present within the testicular parenchyma.[9] Other masses that can be found within the testicle include sperm granulomas and abscesses.

Pathophysiology

The pathophysiology of testicular tumors is unknown. Sperm granulomas form after one or more of the efferent ducts becomes occluded. The occlusion may be congenital or acquired. Because of the number of efferent ducts, sperm granulomas usually do not cause any reduction in fertility. Testicular abscesses may form any time bacteria are sequestered within the testicular parenchyma, whether from a penetrating wound or by hematogenous spread.

Clinical Signs

Clinical signs depend on the type of mass present. Most testicular masses are incidental findings on the physical examination. Abscesses cause pain that is evident on palpation and may cause gait aberrations. Sperm granulomas are asymptomatic. Tumors cause a variety of different clinical signs, depending on the cell type involved (see Testicular Tumors).

Diagnostic Plan

Ultrasonographic examination of the affected testicle may indicate the presence of a mass or fluid pocket of an abscess. As with any tumor, chest and abdominal radiographs are indicated to determine the presence of metastatic disease. Testicular biopsy may be obtained for histopathologic diagnosis, but castration is usually the treatment of choice.

Feminization

This syndrome is the clinical manifestation of hormonally active testicular tumors. Feminization is most commonly associated with Sertoli cell tumors but has been reported with seminomas.

Pathophysiology

The clinical signs seen with feminization result from increased production of estrogen from the tumor cells, increased conversion of testosterone to estrogen by tumor cells, or a hormonal imbalance. There is a 70% association between abdominally located testicular tumors and feminization syndrome.[10]

Clinical Signs

Mammary development and attraction of male dogs are common complaints. There may also be a history of bilateral alopecia on the abdomen in an animal that is cryptorchid. Animals affected are usually mature. On physical examination, a nonpruritic, symmetrical alopecia is present. This alopecia usually begins in the perineum and spreads to the ventral abdomen, flanks, thorax, and neck. Associated hyperpigmentation may be present. Gynecomastia, galac-

torrhea, and a pendulous prepuce may also be present in affected males. The animal is usually a cryptorchid. If both testicles are located in the scrotum, a palpable testicular mass or enlarged, firm testicle is noted. There may also be an enlarged prostate and a small scrotal, or opposite, testicle.

Diagnostic Plan

Hormonal analysis may prove helpful in identifying hormonally active tumors. Estrogens have been measured, but results are conflicting. Some studies show an increase in circulating levels of estrogens, but others do not. Radiographs are indicated in cryptorchid animals showing signs of feminization syndrome to determine the presence of an abdominal mass. Surgical exploratory of the abdomen may also be indicated.

Problem Identification (Females)

Frequent or Prolonged Estrus

Abnormal frequency of estrus in the bitch is defined as an interestrus period of less than 4 months (measured from the beginning of one cycle to the beginning of the next). Cycle frequency may be difficult to assess in the queen because of the lack of a diestrus and a discrete cycle pattern. Both bitches and queens may exhibit continuous estrus.

Pathophysiology

The abnormal frequency or duration of estrus may result from ovarian disorders such as follicular cysts, disruption of the pituitary-gonadal axis, or neoplasia. Follicular cysts are follicles that continue to be hormonally active without undergoing ovulation. The cause of follicular cysts is unknown but may be related to inadequate stores of LH, release of LH, or follicular response to LH from the pituitary. Follicular cysts in the queen have been induced by the exogenous administration of FSH. Neoplasias, particularly granulosa cell tumors, may be hormonally active and may produce sufficient quantities of estrogen to mimic the signs of estrus.

Clinical Signs

In the bitch, the presence of a hemorrhagic vulvar discharge with vulvar swelling that has persisted longer than 30 days may be noted. Alternatively, the bitch may demonstrate heat cycles at intervals that are shorter than every 4 months. These bitches usually attract males and exhibit standing behavior. Queens may show continuous signs of estrous behavior. On physical examination, the bitch may display standing behavior (flagging) on tactile stimulation of the perineal area. The vulva may be swollen in the bitch, and a hemorrhagic vulvar discharge may be noted. Queens show increased vocalization and assume the coital posture when the neck is grasped or the lumbosacral area is stroked. Increased mucus may be noted at the queen's vulva.

Diagnostic Plan

Vaginal cytology is evaluated to determine whether the animal is under estrogenic influence, which would be indicated by cornification of the squamous epithelial cells (see Fig. 22–1A). Cytology may also indicate the presence of any inflammatory process (see Fig. 20–4). Vaginoscopic examination may be used along with cytology to determine the origin of the vulvar discharge and the presence of any pathologic conditions ongoing in the vagina or uterus (see Chap. 22). Urinalysis helps to differentiate discharges of urinary tract origin. In cases of suspected ovarian cyst or neoplasia, ultrasonographic examination of the ovaries may confirm the diagnosis. Serum estrogen profiles may indicate abnormalities in hormonal production. Surgical exploration of the abdomen may be indicated in cases in which a diagnosis cannot be determined by other procedures.

Prolonged Anestrus

In the bitch, a prolonged interestral period is one of longer than 12 months in a postpubertal cycling animal. Pathologic anestrus in the queen is cessation of cycling that cannot be explained by season, pregnancy, or pseudopregnancy.

Pathophysiology

Prolonged anestrus may result from a disruption of the normal ovarian-pituitary interactions, unobserved heats, hypothyroidism, or a previous ovariohysterectomy. Normal ovarian-pituitary interactions involve the positive and negative feedback systems between the ovary and pituitary gland that allow the cyclic activity necessary for reproduction. Unobserved heats in the bitch are common in animals that show minimal external signs of estrus (e.g., vulvar swelling, bleeding), particularly in breeds with long hair. In households without intact male dogs, these bitches may cycle without the owner's knowing. Hypothyroidism can cause a complete cessation of ovarian activity. Occasionally, bitches stop cycling for no apparent reason. Apparently, in these cases, there has been some disruption in the ovarian-pituitary axis that normally stimulates cycling activity. There is no normal canine or feline equivalent of menopause.

Clinical Signs

In the bitch, the owners report no observable cyclic activity in the previous 12 months. In the animal with an incomplete history, it is difficult to rule out previous ovariohysterectomy. It is important to ascertain whether the animal has ever cycled in the past. The queen may or may not have exhibited any estrous behavior during the long daylight hours of March through September. Usually there are no abnormal physical examination findings. Signs associated with hypothyroidism may be seen if this condition is involved in the pathogenesis.

Diagnostic Plan

Hormone level analysis of T_4 is indicated to assess thyroid status. Progesterone levels may be determined to rule out the presence of ovarian luteal tissue, which would indicate an unobserved (silent) estrus. Serial monthly progesterone levels may be obtained over a period of 6 to 12 months to completely rule out the possibility of unobserved heats. Estrogen levels are not usually helpful. In the animal with an incomplete history, abdominal palpation may indicate the absence of a uterus (previous ovariohysterectomy). Simple observation of the animal for 6 to 12 months may be helpful in determining previous ovariohysterectomy. The ovaries may be examined ultrasonographically or through an exploratory laparoscopic incision. Ovarian biopsy is indicated if exploratory surgery is performed.

Diagnostic Procedures (Males)

Testicular Palpation

Testicular palpation is the manual examination of the scrotum and its contents to determine size, shape, symmetry, and consistency of both testes. Through palpation, gross abnormalities such as tumors or traumatic wounds may be identified, as may associated pain and swelling. Both the testes and the epididymides should be palpated. The testes should be smooth, firm, resilient, symmetrical in size and shape, and nonpainful. The epididymides should also be symmetrical and firm. The spermatic cord is evaluated for consistency and presence of pain. The scrotum and scrotal skin can be evaluated for dermatitis, abnormal thickening, or any other deviation from normal that may interfere with thermoregulation of the testes.

Ejaculation and Semen Collection

Semen from the dog is collected by use of the manual method. Different techniques have been described in the literature. They include the use of an artificial vagina or manual massage, or both. We use the manual method without an artificial vagina. The thumb and index finger are used gently but firmly, similar to a tourniquet, to encircle and apply pressure to the body of the penis, which is the region just caudal to the bulbus glandis. Gentle massage of the bulbus glandis while maintaining the constant but gentle tourniquet-like pressure on the penile body results in engorgement and ejaculation.

Pulsations, with intermittent pauses, may be felt in the urethra as the animal ejaculates the three fractions of the ejaculate. The first fraction is variable in volume and may have a slightly cloudy appearance. Most dogs give the first and second fractions at essentially the same time. There may be a slight discernible pause between the first and second fractions. The second fraction, which is the sperm-rich fraction, is cloudy and grayish-white. There is an obvious pause between the second and third fractions. The third fraction, the prostatic fluid, is collected if indicated for culture and cytologic analysis. Normal prostatic fluid should be clear. Any variance from the normal water-like appearance of prostatic fluid usually indicates prostatic disease and should be investigated.

When manually collecting from the male dog, distractions must be held to a minimum. Minimal personnel should be present. A quiet location with good footing for the dog is desirable. Success of collection increases if an estrous bitch is present. The semen can be collected into any container that is not contaminated with chemicals that may be spermicidal. Sterile disposable baby bottle liners make excellent collection containers. Plastic syringe cases, glass tubes, and polypropylene tubes can also be used. Rubber cones are helpful with glass or plastic tubes to direct the semen more easily into the tube.

Artificial semen collection from the male cat is not commonly done. General anesthesia is required if an electroejaculator is used. Male cats may be trained to serve an artificial vagina if time and facilities permit.

Semen Evaluation

Evaluation of a semen sample should include an analysis of volume, concentration, motility, and sperm morphology. Guidelines have been established by the Society for Theriogenology in Hastings, Nebraska. Motility and morphology are subjective analyses of sperm quality. Motility is assessed as a percentage of linearly progressive motile sperm cells. Motility should be assessed immediately after collection. A drop of semen is placed on a warm (37°C) microscope slide and evaluated at 100× magnification. A warm coverslip may be added to assess motility at 400× magnification. A drop of semen is stained with either eosin-nigrosin stain (a vital stain) or a modified Wright

stain (Diff-Quik). With eosin-nigrosin, a drop of semen is added to a drop of stain, which is then mixed and spread over a microscope slide like a blood smear. With Diff-Quik, the drop of semen is spread over a microscope slide and allowed to dry in air. The slide is then stained, with the modification that each stain is allowed 5 minutes of contact time with the specimen on the slide. Sperm morphology is assessed under an oil immersion objective (1000×). After a total of 100 individual sperm cells have been classified as normal or abnormal, the percentage of normal sperm is noted (Fig. 21–2). Common sperm abnormalities include detached heads (see Fig. 21–2B), head defects (see Fig. 21–2C), proximal and distal droplets (see Fig. 21–2D and E), abnormal midpieces (see Fig. 21–2D), and tightly coiled tails (see Fig. 21–2D and E).

Semen concentration may be determined with the use of a hemocytometer or a correctly calibrated automatic cell counter. Approximately 200 million normal spermatozoa per ejaculate are required for the dog to be considered fertile. This number is calculated by multiplying the volume of semen by the concentration and then by the percentage of normal cells. Volume is highly variable and depends on the size of the dog, the health of the prostate gland, and the degree of sexual excitement. Total numbers of sperm may be lower for the toy breeds without adversely affecting fertility. If the male is subfertile, normal fertility may be obtained if 200 million normal spermatozoa are inseminated into the bitch over a period of time.

Male cats normally produce low volumes of highly concentrated semen, which is technically difficult to evaluate. Motility and morphology are evaluated on a diluted sample, as described for the dog.

Ultrasonography

Ultrasonography may be used to visualize the internal structure of the testis. A 5- or 7.5-mHz linear or sector probe is used. Sound waves are transmitted through the organ and are reflected at different intensities or echogenicities, which are visualized as shades of gray. Denser areas reflect more waves and appear whiter or more hyperechoic. The testis is characterized by a coarse, medium echo pattern and should appear uniform throughout the stroma. The mediastinum testis is seen as a linear hyperechoicity in the central long axis of the testicle.[11] This procedure may be used to detect testicular tumors, masses, abscesses, or any condition that might change the density of the testes.

Serology

B. canis is an important reproductive pathogen that causes epididymitis and orchitis in the male dog.

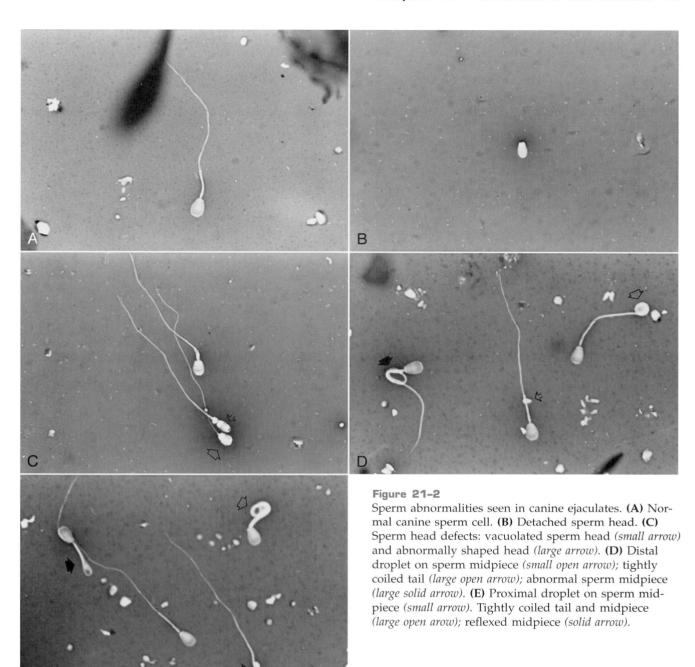

Figure 21–2
Sperm abnormalities seen in canine ejaculates. **(A)** Normal canine sperm cell. **(B)** Detached sperm head. **(C)** Sperm head defects: vacuolated sperm head *(small arrow)* and abnormally shaped head *(large arrow)*. **(D)** Distal droplet on sperm midpiece *(small open arrow)*; tightly coiled tail *(large open arrow)*; abnormal sperm midpiece *(large solid arrow)*. **(E)** Proximal droplet on sperm midpiece *(small arrow)*. Tightly coiled tail and midpiece *(large open arow)*; reflexed midpiece *(solid arrow)*.

Routine serology should be performed on all animals used for breeding. The rapid slide agglutination test is a good screening test. It is highly sensitive but not very specific, so false-positive results are possible. False-negative results are rare. A positive slide test should be verified by a tube agglutination test. Titers of 1:50 or less are usually considered to be not significant. The agar gel immunodiffusion test may be warranted if high titers are obtained, particularly in an asymptomatic animal. By testing for cytoplasmic antigens as well as cell surface antigens, the agar gel immunodiffusion test can distinguish between true- and false-positive test results. A positive blood or semen culture for *B. canis* gives a definitive diagnosis.

Biopsy

Gonadal biopsy is required to substantiate diagnoses of certain ovarian and testicular abnormalities. A testicular biopsy should be done only after a diagnosis of infertility has been made and all noninvasive procedures to determine a cause have been exhausted. Biopsy of the testicle may cause inflammation and the formation of spermatoceles, sperm granulomas, or testicular atrophy. Three techniques are described—fine-needle aspiration, punch, and incisional biopsy—all of which are preferably done with the patient under general anesthesia. The incisional technique is preferred because of less artifactual damage to the testicular sample. An incision is made into the tunica albuginea. The tissue that bulges through the incision is shaved off with a double-edged razor blade. This incision does not require closure. Bouin fixative is mandatory for tissue fixing because of the significant artifacts obtained if testicular biopsies are fixed with formalin.

Hormonal Analysis

Serum (or plasma) is submitted for determination of hormone concentrations (e.g., T_4, testosterone). T_4 levels within the established normal values rule out hypothyroidism. T_4 should be measured after stimulation with thyroid-stimulating hormone if baseline T_4 levels are low. Testosterone levels are quite variable in the male, and serial tests are necessary to determine whether the level is within normal limits (i.e., whether there is normal testicular function). GnRH stimulation tests also evaluate testicular function. Testosterone levels are determined from serum before and 1 hour after administration of GnRH at 3 µg/kg intramuscularly. Normal animals with functional testicles demonstrate a significant rise in testosterone in the second sample. Estrogen levels in males may be determined, but interpretation of their clinical significance is difficult.

Diagnostic Procedures (Females)

Hormonal Analysis

Serum (or plasma) is submitted for determination of hormone concentrations. Hormones to be analyzed include progesterone, T_4, and estrogen. Abnormal levels may correlate with clinical signs exhibited by the animal and may indicate imbalances of ovarian or hypothalamopituitary origin. Progesterone levels higher than 1 ng/mL in the female indicate the presence of functional luteal tissue and imply that the female has been through estrus and has ovulated within the last 60 days (in the dog) or 45 days (in the cat).

Ultrasonography

Using a 5- to 7.5-mHz linear probe, changes and abnormalities of the ovaries may be visualized by reflection of sound waves. The ovaries are located just caudal to the kidneys. In the normal animal, the ovary is difficult to visualize. Diagnosis of cystic or neoplastic conditions of the ovary is possible with this technique.

Exploratory Surgery and Biopsy

Complete visualization of the reproductive tract can be accomplished through a laparotomy incision. The ovarian bursa in the bitch should be incised to view the ovary or obtain a biopsy sample. Care must be taken to avoid damaging the uterine tubes (oviducts), which can be palpated through the bursal fat as cord-like structures similar to a vas deferens. A pie-shaped wedge is cut from the body of the ovary. This incision into the ovary does not require closure. Digital pressure is applied for hemostasis. Nonreactive suture material is used to close the bursa. Preplacement of sutures before the bursa is opened may prove helpful. Ovaries do not respond adversely to biopsy, as testicles may. Ovarian biopsies can be fixed with formalin.

Common Diseases of the Gonads

Testicular Tumors

Sertoli cell tumors, seminomas, and interstitial cell tumors are the most common testicular tumors, and they occur with similar frequency. Reportedly, 10% of all male dogs develop testicular tumors, and testicular tumors are the second most common type of tumor in the dog. The incidence of testicular neoplasia increases if the testicle is extrascrotal. Dogs with undescended testes are approximately 13 times more likely to develop testicular tumors, specifically Sertoli cell tumors and seminomas, than are normal animals.[12, 13] Testicular tumors are rare in male cats.[14]

Only intact male dogs are affected. Mean age of occurrence is approximately 7 to 10 years. Boxers, weimaraners, German shepherds, and Shetland sheepdogs are breeds most predisposed.[15, 16]

Pathophysiology

The exact mechanism of testicular tumors is unknown. Each tumor type is derived from its respective cell or component structure. Most are benign, slow-growing masses with no associated clinical signs. Sertoli cell tumors are usually large, firm, nodular, and fibrous. They are pale yellow or gray, with foci of necrosis, hemorrhage, and cystic degeneration. Seminomas are soft and dull white or gray.[17] Diameters range from 1 to 10 cm, but 75% are less than 2 cm wide.[18] Interstitial cell tumors are brownish-orange and soft. They may have foci of necrosis and may be hemorrhagic. Hormonally active tumors cause excess production of estrogens and androgens. Excess estrogen has a well-documented bone marrow toxicity in the dog. Aplastic anemia and thrombocytopenia result from the bone marrow suppression. Excess androgen production may stimulate the formation of perianal adenomas. If metastasis does occur, lymphatic and hematogenous routes are possible.

Clinical Signs

Signs associated with testicular tumors vary depending on tumor type and hormonal activity. Signs are related to tumor size and location and to secretion of estrogens or androgens. Sertoli cell tumors can cause feminization, enlargement of the involved testicle, atrophy of the noninvolved testicle, bilateral alopecia with hyperpigmentation, prostatic enlargement, and bone marrow dysfunction.[19, 20] If bone marrow involvement occurs, anemia and weakness may be seen, as well as bleeding problems associated with a decrease in platelets. Seminomas also may cause testicular enlargement, feminization, and prostatic enlargement. Interstitial cell tumors are of very little clinical significance. All can be associated with perianal adenomas.

Diagnostic Plan

Palpation of a testicular mass during physical examination with or without clinical signs suggests possible neoplastic changes. Ultrasonography of the affected testicle may prove helpful to identify the tumor as a discrete soft tissue mass and rule out the presence of an abscess. Definitive diagnosis is based on histopathologic analysis of a biopsy sample or the excised testicle. Abdominal and thoracic radiographs in cryptorchid animals aid in detection of abdominal masses, possible testicular tumors, and any metastases. A complete blood count identifies any anemia or decrease in platelet numbers.

Treatment

Surgical excision of the involved testicle is the treatment of choice. Care should be taken to remove a generous portion of the spermatic cord with the affected testicle. If cryptorchidism is present, both testes should be removed. Supportive therapy such as antibiotics, intravenous fluids, and blood transfusions may be necessary in cases complicated by bone marrow dysfunction. Chemotherapy with cyclophosphamide and vincristine or irradiation therapy may be attempted after surgery in metastatic cases. Seminomas are reportedly sensitive to irradiation therapy.[21]

Prognosis

With removal of the affected testis, the prognosis in uncomplicated cases is good. Clinical signs of male feminization should resolve within 4 to 6 weeks. The prognosis for cases complicated by bone marrow involvement is grave.

Infectious Orchitis and Epididymitis

Infectious orchitis and epididymitis are infection or inflammation of the testis and epididymis caused by ascending infection from normal urethral flora, bacterial prostatitis, or systemic disease. The incidence varies with the cause. Affected animals are usually intact male dogs. This condition is rare in the cat.

Pathophysiology

B. canis infection has the most reproductive significance. *B. canis* has a predilection for the epididymis. Other pathogens implicated in canine epididymitis and orchitis include *Blastomyces, Escherichia coli, Staphylococcus, Streptococcus,* and *Mycoplasma.* Inflammation inhibits spermatogenesis and damages seminiferous tubules. Epididymitis may result in occlusion of the ducts, preventing passage of sperm. Damage to the testicle or epididymis may be permanent, depending on the severity and duration of the insult.

Clinical Signs

Acute orchitis or epididymitis results in a swollen, painful, warm testicle and, in the dog, suggests *B. canis* infection. The animal is sometimes reluctant to walk. Pyrexia, anorexia, and depression may be present, as may peripheral lymphadenopathy. Animals with chronic disease may show only a small, soft testicle.

Diagnostic Plan

The diagnosis is based on history and physical examination. The cause may be determined by culture or by cytologic evaluation of semen or fine-needle aspiration of the affected organ. A complete blood count determines the degree of systemic involvement. A rapid slide agglutination test for *B. canis* is indicated in all cases of canine epididymitis or orchitis and rules in or rules out that specific infection. Ultrasonography may be useful in ruling out neoplasia. A prostatic examination may suggest the extension of a concurrent problem.

Treatment

Antibiotic therapy is indicated if bacteria are involved. Usually trimethoprim-sulfamethoxazole (30 mg/kg, every day or in divided doses twice a day) is used until results of culture and sensitivity are available. Cold compresses may be used to decrease intratesticular temperature. Anti-inflammatory agents such as aspirin and corticosteroids may be used to reduce inflammation. There is no successful treatment for *B. canis* infection. Although castration with long-term antibiotic therapy has been described, euthanasia is recommended as a control mechanism for this disease because of its highly infectious nature and the zoonotic implications. Unilateral infection from causes other than *B. canis* may be treated successfully by unilateral castration.

Prognosis

Prognosis in any case of orchitis or epididymitis is guarded. Fertility cannot accurately be determined until the disease process has resolved. Infertility may result from irreversible bilateral damage to germinal epithelium or to the ducts of the epididymes. Fertility may be maintained, even if the damage is irreversible, if the condition is unilateral.

Cryptorchidism

Cryptorchidism is the absence of one or both testicles in the scrotum owing to incomplete testicular descent through the inguinal rings. The cryptorchid testicle may be abdominal or inguinal in location. Incidence varies with breed and ranges from 1% to 15%. Most cases are unilateral, with involvement of the right testicle. Affected animals are usually intact young male dogs and cats. Breeds that appear to be at high risk include the boxer, Yorkshire terrier, poodle, Pomeranian, Siberian husky, miniature schnauzer, Shetland sheepdog, and Chihuahua.[1]

Pathophysiology

Cryptorchidism is thought to be caused by a dysfunction in the mechanism of testicular descent. In the process of testicular descent, cryptorchidism is brought on by failure of the gubernaculum to regress and pull the testis into the scrotum. The testicle may stop its descent anywhere from a location caudal to the kidney, where the gonads originate; to the inguinal ring within the abdomen; inside the inguinal ring itself; immediately outside the inguinal ring; in the subcutaneous tissue anterior to the scrotum; or in the neck of the scrotum. The condition may be associated with pseudohermaphroditism. In some animals, cryptorchidism is thought to be an inherited trait caused by a single recessive autosomal gene. The mode of inheritance for most cases is unknown, and recent evidence questions the hereditary component of this condition.

Clinical Signs

There are usually no clinical signs. Palpation of only one testicle or neither testicle in the scrotum is pathognomonic for cryptorchidism. If a scrotal testicle is present, spermatogenesis should be normal in that testicle, and the animal is fertile. Retained abdominal testes are at an increased risk for torsion and tumor formation. This may result in secondary clinical signs such as abdominal distention, abdominal pain, vomiting, or feminization.

Diagnostic Plan

There are no specific clinical signs other than the absence of two normally placed testicles within the scrotum. The condition is usually identified in the young animal at a physical examination. Because the canine testicle descends at or near the time of birth, the diagnosis can be made at any time the testicles are large enough to be detected by palpation, usually at 10 to 12 weeks of age. A definitive diagnosis may be delayed until the animal is 4 to 6 months of age to allow for complete descent, especially in the case of inguinally located testicles.

Treatment

The cryptorchid testicle does not produce spermatozoa because the testicle is maintained at body temperature. Testosterone production from this testicle is unaffected. Testosterone production and sperm production by the testicle within the scrotum remain normal. These animals are therefore fertile, but because of the possible genetic nature of this condition, surgical removal of both testicles is recommended. Serial injections of human chorionic gonadotropin (22 IU/kg intramuscularly, four times over a 2-week period before the age of 16 weeks) have been suggested to aid testicular descent. However, ethical concerns have been raised, and there is no proof that such injections work. We have had no success with such treatment. Orchiopexy has also been described as a treatment option[22] but would be considered unethical by American Veterinary Medical Association definitions.

Prognosis

The prognosis for correction (or reversal) of the condition is grave, with or without treatment. Because of the increase in incidence of neoplastic conditions in the retained testicle, it should be removed at a young age. Prognosis for fertility is essentially unaffected unless the condition is bilateral, in which case the animal is sterile.

Follicular Cysts

Cystic ovarian disease results from endocrine imbalances between the pituitary and the ovary. Cysts are thin-walled, fluid-filled structures that vary in size. They occur bilaterally or unilaterally. Incidence increases with increasing age. Ovarian cysts are fairly common, but most are nonfunctional and are incidental findings. Approximately 3% of all reported ovarian cystic structures are functional hormonally.[17] Affected animals are intact females aged 2 to 15 years.

Pathophysiology

Cysts may result from follicles that fail to ovulate during the normal reproductive cycle or from remnants of embryonic tissue. In other species, ovarian follicular cysts are believed to be a result of inadequate release or production of LH, the primary hormone of ovulation. The actual mechanism in the bitch and queen remains unknown.

Clinical Signs

Continuous or persistent signs of estrus are usually seen with functional cysts. Swollen, turgid vulva, bloody vaginal discharge, and attraction of male dogs are common associated signs in the bitch. Affected queens may also exhibit behavioral signs of persistent estrus if cysts are hormonally active.[23]

Diagnostic Plan

History, physical examination findings, vaginal cytology, and ultrasound findings are used to make a diagnosis. Vaginal cytology demonstrates the estrogenic influence on the vaginal epithelium by revealing increased numbers of cornified epithelial cells. Ultrasonography may detect the fluid-filled structures present on the ovary. In some instances, definitive diagnosis is made only after surgical exploration of the reproductive tract.

Treatment

Multiple intramuscular injections of human chorionic gonadotropin at 22 IU/kg or GnRH at 3 μg/kg once daily for 3 days cause luteinization of cysts. The animal then is under the influence of progesterone and should be monitored for pyometra during the following 2 months. Manual rupture of cystic structures during an exploratory surgery is also a described treatment. A biopsy should be obtained simultaneously.

Prognosis

The prognosis is considered fair to good for future reproductive function after successful treatment.

Ovarian Tumors

Ovarian tumors are neoplastic changes within the ovary that may arise from epithelial, germ cell, or sex-cord stromal origin. The most common tumor in the bitch is the granulosa cell tumor. Other tumors commonly seen include papillary adenoma and papillary adenocarcinoma. Ovarian tumors account for 0.5% to 1.2% of all neoplasms in the bitch. Primary ovarian neoplasia is uncommon in dogs and cats.[14, 24] Affected animals are intact females. The average age at occurrence is approximately 8 years.

Pathophysiology

The exact mechanism is unknown. Epithelial-type tumors include papillary adenoma and adenocarcinoma, cystadenoma, cystadenocarcinoma, and undifferentiated carcinoma. Sex-cord stromal tumors include granulosa cell tumors, which are lobulated, firm masses containing cysts that usually occur unilaterally. Granulosa cell tumors are usually benign but may infrequently metastasize by lymphatic vessels or by direct extension in the peritoneal cavity. Feline granulosa cell tumors are more aggressive and metastasize by lymphatic and hematogenous routes in 50% of cases. Dysgerminomas account for 15% of feline ovarian tumors, and they metastasize in approximately 20% of cases to the omentum and through the abdominal wall.[25]

Clinical Signs

Clinical signs vary with the type of tumor involved. Tumors in early stages of progression and small tumors may have no clinical signs. A large, palpable abdominal mass or abdominal distention may be seen with adenocarcinomas or granulosa cell tumors. Ascites and signs of hormone imbalance (persistent estrus) are common with adenocarcinomas (papillary), cystadenocarcinomas, and granulosa cell tumors. All may cause clinical signs of vomiting and gastrointestinal upset (anorexia, diarrhea) if they are large.

Diagnostic Plan

Diagnosis of small tumors may not be possible, or they may be diagnosed at ovariohysterectomy as incidental findings. Abdominal masses may be diagnosed by clinical signs, physical examination findings, and abdominal radiography or ultrasonography Fig.

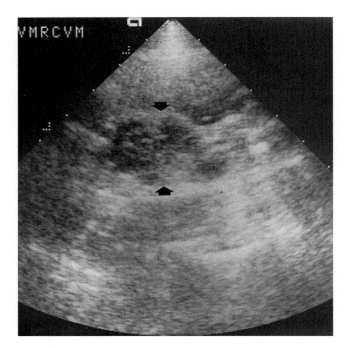

Figure 21-3
Canine granulosa cell tumor of the ovary depicted by ultrasonography. Tumor *(arrows)* shows characteristic cystic areas throughout.

21–3). In bitches that are exhibiting signs of prolonged estrus, hormonal analysis of estrogen or progesterone may reveal hormone-producing tumors. Definitive diagnosis is determined by histopathologic evaluation of the excised mass after exploratory surgery.

Treatment

Surgical excision of the affected ovary is the treatment of choice. Usually, complete ovariohysterectomy is performed. Unilateral removal of the affected ovary and ipsilateral uterine horn enables the bitch to be bred at a future time. Reduced litter size is expected because of reduction of uterine space. Unilateral removal of the affected ovary and ipsilateral uterine horn should not be considered if metastatic disease is present. Care should be taken not to rupture the tumor, because spread often occurs by implantation. Metastatic disease may be treated with cyclophosphamide at 50 mg/m^2 orally or intravenously, every 48 hours, three days a week. The animal should be monitored with repeated complete blood counts and urinalyses to prevent serious bone marrow depression and hemorrhagic cystitis. Drugs such as vincristine and doxorubicin or irradiation therapy may prove valuable.

Prognosis

For benign ovarian tumors, the prognosis is excellent. For malignant tumors, the prognosis is good if a complete oophorectomy is performed and there is no evidence of metastasis. In all other cases, the prognosis is grave.

Uncommon Diseases of the Gonads

Testicles may undergo torsion within the scrotal sac spontaneously. Testicular torsion is uncommon in the dog and rare in the cat. Torsions of 180° or less do not compromise the blood supply to the testicle and usually resolve spontaneously. Diagnosis of these mild testicular torsions in the dog occurs incidentally at physical examination with the finding of the tail of the epididymis anterior to the testicle instead of caudal. Torsions of 360° or more result in acute compromise of the testicle. Torsions are usually unilateral. The entire testicle and scrotum on the affected side are hard and very painful. Discoloration of the scrotal skin is observed, and the dog is reluctant to walk. If the condition is allowed to progress, systemic signs of shock may develop. Complete castration is the treatment of choice in the nonbreeding animal. Unilateral castration is the treatment of choice for the breeding animal.

References

1. Johnston SD. Anatomy and physiology of the normal female reproductive system. In: Proceedings 108: Reproduction in Small Companion Animals. JD Stewart Memorial Refresher Course for Veterinarians. Sydney, Australia: University of Sydney, August 1988.
2. Gilbert RO, Bosu WT. Clinical reproductive endocrinology of the dog and cat. In: Drazner FA, ed. Small Animal Endocrinology. New York, Churchill Livingstone, 1987: 341–371.
3. Amann RP. Reproductive physiology and endocrinology of the dog. In: Morrow DA, ed. Current Therapy in Theriogenology, 2nd ed. Philadelphia, WB Saunders, 1986:532–538.
4. Concannon PW, Lein DH. Hormonal and clinical correlates of ovarian cycles, ovulation, pseudopregnancy, and pregnancy in dogs. In: Kirk RW, ed. Current Veterinary Therapy X. Philadelphia, WB Saunders, 1989:1269–1282.
5. Wildt DE, Chan SYW, Seager SWJ, Chakraborty PK. Ovarian activity circulating hormones and sexual behavior in the cat: I. Relationships during coitus induced luteal phase and the estrous period without mating. Biol Reprod 1981;25:15–28.
6. Olson PN, Nett TM. Reproductive endocrinology and physiology of the bitch. In: Morrow DA, ed. Current Therapy in Theriogenology, 2nd ed. Philadelphia, WB Saunders, 1986:453–457.
7. Banks DR. Physiology and endocrinology of the feline estrus cycle. In: Morrow DA, ed. Current Therapy in

Theriogenology, 2nd ed. Philadelphia, WB Saunders, 1986:795.

8. Johnson CA. Disorders of the canine testicles and epididymis. In: Morrow DA, ed. Current Therapy in Theriogenology, 2nd ed. Philadelphia, WB Saunders, 1986:55l.

9. Cotchin E. Some tumors in dogs and cats of comparative veterinary and human interest. Vet Rec 1959;71:1040.

10. Morgan RV. Blood dyscrasias associated with testicular tumors in the dog. J Am Anim Hosp Assoc 1982;18:970–997.

11. Pugh CR, Konde LJ, Park RD. Testicular ultrasound in the normal dog. Vet Radiol 1990;31:195–199.

12. Hayes AN, Pendergrass TW. Canine testicular tumors: Pathologic features of 410 dogs. Int J Cancer 1976;l8:482.

13. Lipowitz AJ, Schwartz A, Wilson GP, Ebert JW. Testicular neoplasms and concomitant clinical changes in the dog. J Am Vet Med Assoc 1973; 163:1364.

14. Cotchin E. Neoplasia in the cat. Vet Rec 1957;69:425.

15. Howard EB, Nielson SW. Neoplasms of the boxer dog. Am J Vet Res 1965;26:1121–1131.

16. Theilen GH, Madewell BR. Tumors of the urogenital tract. In: Veterinary Cancer Medicine. Philadelphia, Lea & Febiger, 1979:357–381.

17. Herron MA. Tumors of the canine genital system. J Am Anim Hosp Assoc 1983;19:981–994.

18. Dow C. Testicular tumors in dogs. J Comp Pathol 1962;72:247–265.

19. Brodey RS, Martin JE. Sertoli cell neoplasms in the dog: The clinicopathologic and endocrinological findings in 37 dogs. J Am Vet Med Assoc 1958;133:244–257.

20. Sherding RG, Wilson GP, Kociba GJ. Bone marrow hypoplasia in eight dogs with Sertoli cell tumor. J Am Vet Med Assoc 1981;133:497–501.

21. Broadhurst J. Neoplasms of the reproductive system. In: Kirk RW, ed. Current Veterinary Therapy V. Philadelphia, WB Saunders, 1974:978.

22. Kawakami E, Tsutsui T, Yamada Y, et al. Spermatogenic function in cryptorchid dogs after orchiopexy. Jpn J Vet Sci 1988;50:227–235.

23. Herron MA. Infertility from noninfectious causes. In: Morrow DA, ed. Current Therapy in Theriogenology, 2nd ed. Philadelphia, WB Saunders, 1986:829.

24. Cotchin E. Further observations on neoplasms in dogs with particular reference to site of origin and malignancy. Br Vet J 1954;110:218–230.

25. Stein BS. Tumors of the feline genital tract. J Am Anim Hosp Assoc 1981;17:1022–1025.

Chapter 22

Diseases of the External Genitalia

Beverly J. Purswell

Anatomy

Female

The external genitalia of the bitch and queen includes the vulva, the vestibule, and the vagina. The vulvar lips are joined dorsally by the dorsal commissure and ventrally by the ventral commissure. The clitoral fossa and clitoris lie immediately cranial to the ventral commissure, within the vulvar opening. The vulva forms the distal opening of the vestibule. The vestibule is the common external opening of the urinary and reproductive tracts. The vestibule ends immediately anterior to the urethral papilla. In the bitch, this junction between the vestibule and vagina can be palpated digitally as a narrowing of the lumen, the vaginovestibular junction. The vagina extends from the vestibule to the cervix. The vagina originates embryologically from the paramesonephric ducts, whereas the vestibule and vulva originate from the urogenital sinus.[1, 2] Where these two embryologic structures join at the vaginovestibular junction, hymens may occur if the linkage is incomplete. There is a distinct downward slope to the vestibule from the vaginovestibular junction to the ventral commissure of the vulva. In the queen, the vagina has a very narrow lumen, only 1 mm in diameter, and is approximately 4 cm in length. The bitch has a relatively long vagina; the cervix is abdominal in location, situated underneath the fourth lumbar vertebra.

The vestibule is surrounded by the constrictor vestibuli and the constrictor vulvae muscles. The constrictor vestibuli muscle is responsible for the genital tie, which occurs during canine copulation. The constrictor vestibuli muscle, together with the weaker constrictor vulvae muscle, tightens behind the bulbus glandis after intromission and physically locks the male and female dogs together during copulation. The constrictor vulvae muscle, in response to tactile stimuli to the vulva during estrus, elevates the vulva to allow intromission to occur more easily. This elevation of the vulva is part of the standing reflex seen in the bitch during estrus.[3]

Male

The penis of the dog starts in the distal pelvic canal as paired roots that are attached to the ischial tuberosity of the pelvis. The paired roots of the penis join and become the body of the penis. The root and body are made up of the corpora cavernosa penis and are covered by the ischiocavernosus and bulbocavernosus muscles, respectively. The retractor penis muscle is a thin strip of smooth muscle that covers the corpus cavernosum urethrae and attaches to the fornix of the prepuce. The corpus cavernosum urethrae is located along the ventral portion of the penis and contains the penile urethra.[3] The glans penis consists of two parts, the bulbus glandis and the pars longa glandis. The roots and body of the penis are firmly attached to the body wall and are covered with skin along their ventral borders. Most of the glans penis is covered by a mucous membrane epithelium and is contained entirely within the prepuce in the nonerect state. The prepuce is attached to the ventral abdominal wall except at the distal, open end.[3] The dog has an os penis, which has its base in the body of the penis and ends with a fibrous tip in the pars longa glandis.

The male cat has a cone-shaped penis that contains a short os penis. The glans penis is totally contained within the prepuce in the nonerect state. The base of the glans penis is covered by multiple rows of mucosal barbs, which are more prominent in intact male cats. The penis of the tomcat is quite short in comparison with that of a dog of similar size, corresponding to the queen's vestibular and vaginal anatomy.

Physiology

Female

The vestibule and vagina are lined with nonglandular stratified squamous epithelium, which is highly responsive to estrogen and progesterone. In response to estrogen, the vaginal epithelium develops from several cell layers to 20 to 40 cell layers in thickness.[4] The outermost cells of this thickened lining of the vagina become cornified. Vaginal cytology during estrus indicates a high percentage (>90%) of cornified epithelial cells, demonstrating the estrogen influence. Under the influence of progesterone, the vaginal epithelium becomes quite thin.

Under the influence of estrogen, the vulva of the bitch becomes overtly swollen. This is a direct result of the estrogen-caused increase in blood supply as well as edema. These overt signs of estrogen influence on the vulva are indicative of similar changes throughout the entire reproductive tract. In addition, vaginal mucous glands become more active, adding to the moistness of the vagina. In queens, this may be seen in the form of a mucous discharge from the vulva. The bloody vulvar discharge seen in the bitch is caused by diapedesis of red blood cells into the uterus. The combined changes seen in the vulva, vestibule, and vagina (increased thickness in the vaginal epithelium, increased moisture) are designed to facilitate copulation with minimal damage to the female.

Male

At puberty, the male undergoes testosterone-related events. The testicles become functional by producing testosterone and spermatozoa. Secondary sexual characteristics become apparent because of the influence of testosterone, including libido, or interest in breeding. Male cats begin to look masculine, particularly noticeable as a thickening of the head and jowls, and begin sexual behaviors such as spraying. Male dogs develop behaviors such as marking territory and roaming; physically, the prostate gland enlarges. The changes in the external genitalia are subtle and may not be remarkable other than the development of the penile barbs in the male cat.

Copulation in the dog is a unique and complex process. Because of the os penis, the dog obtains intromission before erection. Erection occurs within the bitch, at which time her constrictor vulvae and constrictor vestibuli muscles contract around and behind the glans penis. The two animals become physically locked together during ejaculation. The presperm and sperm-rich fractions are ejaculated early in the ejaculation process. The third fraction, from the prostate gland, is ejaculated during the remainder of the copulatory tie. The end result is an efficient means of placing semen in the anterior vagina and flushing it into the uterus. As the dog gains intromission, the prepuce is reflected proximal on the glans penis until it is gathered around the body of the penis. In this process, the venous return from the penis is inhibited in a tourniquet-like manner, which promotes and maintains the erection. The body of the penis has great lateral flexibility. After the copulatory tie has been achieved, the dog dismounts from the bitch, throws a rear leg over her back, and stands facing away from her, bending the penis laterally by 180°. Erection, in general, is a parasympathetic function, and ejaculation is a sympathetic function.

The tomcat obtains intromission by grasping the neck of the queen in his mouth and positioning himself over her back. The size of the penis is well suited for semen deposition in the vestibule of the queen, the vagina being too narrow to allow penetration by the penis. The barbs on the penis are thought to cause local vulvar and vestibular stimulation, thus initiating the postcoital response from the queen (i.e., yowling, licking at the vulva, aggression toward the male cat). The postcoital response of the queen indicates that there has been a reflex release of luteinizing hormone from the queen's pituitary gland, resulting in the induction of ovulation.

Problem Identification

Vulvar Discharge

Discharge from the vulva refers to any fluid other than urine that is expelled from the vulvar lips. Purulent discharges indicate inflammatory processes occurring somewhere within the animal's reproductive tract. Hemorrhagic discharges indicate bleeding from some source, which may or may not be abnormal. Mucous discharges, originating from mucous glands, may also be normal or abnormal, depending on the source of the discharge and the situation. A foul-smelling discharge usually indicates a bacterial component to the problem (e.g., a gas-forming organism).

Pathophysiology

An attempt should be made to locate the origin of the vulvar discharge and thereby to rule out uterine or urinary tract sources. Purulent discharges are related to an inflammatory process in some portion of the reproductive tract. This inflammation may or may not be related to bacterial infections. Vaginal inflammation may be caused by trauma (breeding lacerations), abnormal vaginal environment (diabetes mellitus), viral infections (canine herpesvirus), bacterial infections, or neoplasia. Vaginal hemorrhagic discharges may come from vaginal trauma (breeding or dystocia), neoplasia, or estrus. Mucous discharges may be vaginal in origin; mucous glands are present in the vagina and are most commonly associated with estrus, particularly in the queen.

Clinical Signs

The animal may or may not have a previous history of ovariohysterectomy. All or part of the uterus may still be present in the animal. Estrus, breeding, or parturition may have occurred. Discharge from the vulva is unrelated to urination. The discharge may be of any consistency or color but is usually purulent or hemorrhagic and unrelated to signs of estrus. Mild discharges may be evident only by a crusty accumulation on hairs surrounding the vulva.

Diagnostic Plan

Vaginal cytology is indicated whenever a vulvar discharge is present. Vaginal cornification indicates the influence of estrogen. Vaginal cytology helps identify the location and degree of inflammation. An increased number of polymorphonuclear neutrophils (neutrophil/epithelial cell ratio ≥1:1) indicates an inflammatory process. Cytology samples taken from the vestibule and from the vagina help localize the disease process; inflammatory conditions may be distal or anterior in the reproductive tract. Inflammatory processes may involve the vulvar skin or the urinary tract. Vestibular inflammation is more pronounced than vaginal inflammation in these cases. Pure vaginal cytology samples may be obtained through a speculum. Vaginoscopy is necessary to identify the location and source of the discharge and any lesions present.

Vaginoscopy identifies the presence of lacerations, tumors, or hemorrhoidal vessels as well as evidence of inflammation such as lymphoid follicles, hyperemia of the mucosa, or pooling of discharges, urine, or blood. Vaginal cultures are indicated in cases of vaginal inflammation.

Masses

Masses originating from the vulva, vestibule, vagina, or penis may or may not protrude through the vulvar lips or preputial opening, respectively. These masses may deform the perineal or preputial area or simply be evident because of vulvar or preputial discharges.

Pathophysiology

The pathophysiology of most neoplastic conditions is unknown. Transmissible venereal tumors (TVTs) are passed by mucous membrane contact and are thought to be cells derived from a species other than the dog. Other common tumor types involving the external genitalia include leiomyomas and leiomyosarcomas in the female and papillomas and squamous cell carcinomas in the male. Vaginal fold prolapses occurring during estrus in the bitch are considered to be an exaggerated response to estrogen. The enlarged, penis-like clitoris associated with hermaphroditic conditions is caused by the testosterone production from the gonads, most commonly the testicles or ovatestes. Acquired clitoral enlargement may be caused by exogenous testosterone administration, as seen in the racing greyhound bitch: testosterone is routinely administered for estrus control. Any testosterone compound or anabolic steroid (e.g., Cheque Drops) has the potential to induce clitoral enlargement. Abscesses are usually caused by trauma, foreign bodies, or puncture wounds.

Clinical Signs

The enlarged clitoris of the pseudohermaphrodite is usually an incidental finding in the puppy or kitten. It may be visible as a protrusion from the vulvar lips but can be unfolded from the clitoral fossa to expose its full size. Extreme cases of clitoral enlargement may present as penile-like structures hanging from the vulva. Acquired clitoral enlargement has a gradual onset with varying degrees of enlargement. Vaginal fold prolapse is seen in young bitches during estrus. This condition tends to reoccur with each estrus cycle. Neoplasms may be seen on the vulva, protruding through the vulvar lips, or as a bulging in the perineal area. These conditions have a gradual onset. Vaginal tumors that are located internally may present with a vulvar discharge of a purulent or hemorrhagic nature. Penile or preputial tumors present as masses in the preputial area and usually exhibit a purulent (or hemorrhagic) preputial discharge.

Diagnostic Plan

The physical examination of the pseudohermaphrodite is diagnostic for that condition. Vaginal cytology, vaginoscopy, and biopsy of the mass all can help identify the location, size, and degree of involvement of the surrounding tissues. Vaginal cytology also helps identify the stage of estrous cycle and the degree of inflammation. The penis should be examined thoroughly by complete reflection of the prepuce.

Inability to Breed

The inability of the bitch to physically accommodate the dog's penis during copulation often accounts for the inability to breed. Queens are unlikely to experience this problem because of the extremely small size of the feline vagina, which is essentially uninvolved with copulation. Less commonly, the dog may be unable to completely extrude the penis from the prepuce because of physical restrictions of the penis or prepuce. Both species may experience psychological problems that may interfere with copulation and are unrelated to physically being unable to breed. The body of the queen may be too long for the male cat to accomplish intromission while maintaining the neck grasp essential to feline copulation.

Pathophysiology

Strictures of the vulva, vestibule, and vagina occur during embryologic development of the female. The paramesonephric duct must join the urogenital sinus to complete the reproductive tract. Incomplete linkage of the ducts with the sinus or of the paramesonephric ducts themselves may cause residual bands of tissue or strictures to remain. These strictures or bands of tissue physically impair the ability of the bitch to copulate. Other potential physical constraints of the vaginal lumen include vulvar, vestibular, or vaginal tumors and vaginal fold prolapse. Narrowing of the bony pelvic canal may result from genetic causes (brachycephalic breeds) or from previous pelvic fracture. Psychological problems with copulation are usually associated with dominance problems or the lack of proper socialization of the female as a puppy or kitten. Bitches that are more dominant than the male dog will not allow breeding. Queens may be too timid. Lack of socialization of the puppy with other dogs, preferably littermates, during the fifth through the seventh week of life may result in abnormal sexual behavior. In the male, inability to completely extend the penis from the prepuce may cause an inability to breed. Penile or preputial tumors may prevent intromission. Phimosis or partial phimosis prevents complete reflection of the prepuce anterior to the bulbus glandis, thus preventing complete intromission and the copulatory tie.

Clinical Signs

The history usually involves the inability of the bitch to tie with the male dog. This may be evident by a pain response associated with intromission or aggression toward the dog in general. No specific clinical signs are seen. The physical examination findings are strictures or bands of tissue found when a vaginal digital examination is performed. These strictures are typically at the dorsal commissure of the vulva or at the vaginovestibular junction. Pelvic abnormalities may be identified by a rectal digital examination and may include a genetically small pelvic canal (brachycephalic breeds) or previous pelvic fractures. In the male with penile or preputial tumors or partial or complete phimosis, attempts to breed may be painful and may eventually result in a lack of libido. Tumors may result in hemorrhagic preputial discharges. Pain may also be induced by musculoskeletal problems in the male, resulting in an inability to complete the copulatory tie or a lack of libido. If a short-bodied male cat attempts to breed a long-bodied queen, the male cat may be unable to reach the vulva with his penis while maintaining the necessary neck grasp. No copulatory cry is issued by the queen, and pregnancy does not ensue. The queen continues to cycle because of the lack of ovulation.

Diagnostic Plan

No further assessment is necessary if the problem is found by digital examination. If no problems are found, dominance issues or other physical problems (hip or back pain) may be explored. With dominance problems, the bitch may be bred by artificial insemination. If the queen is found to be too long for the male cat, another male cat may be chosen for breeding.

Phimosis and Paraphimosis

Phimosis is the inability to extrude the penis from the prepuce. Paraphimosis is the inability to retract the penis into the prepuce.[5]

Pathophysiology

Phimosis is normal in the young dog before puberty. As puberty is reached, the normal adhesions between the penis and prepuce break down and allow the penis to move freely within the prepuce. Postpubertal phimosis is caused by anatomic abnormalities, usually of a congenital nature, and is uncommon.

Partial phimosis is seen more commonly. Partial phimosis causes the dog to experience pain during copulation because of an inadequate preputial opening. Complete phimosis may cause partial or complete occlusion of urinary outflow with associated signs of dribbling urine or early death, respectively.

Paraphimosis is a problem in male dogs that is typically seen after copulation. During intromission, the prepuce is retracted anterior to the bulbus glandis before complete erection is achieved. The erect penis cannot be pulled through the preputial opening. After copulation, detumescence of the penis allows the penis to retract into the prepuce. On occasion, usually because of hair entanglement around the penis or penile trauma, detumescence is delayed, allowing the penis to experience drying, edema, and extreme congestion. These conditions prevent the penis from being retracted into the prepuce. Progressive changes occur that lead to necrosis of the penile tissue if left untreated. Occasionally, paraphimosis is seen in the neutered male, unrelated to copulation, usually associated with masturbation or excitement-induced erections. Paraphimosis is considered an emergency because of the potential for urinary obstruction. Conditions similar to paraphimosis but unrelated to the erection process may cause chronic exposure of the glans penis. In these cases, the glans penis is prolapsed in part or totally out of the prepuce. Causes for chronic penile prolapse include retractor penis muscle paralysis, abnormally large preputial opening, or congenital shortening of the prepuce.

Clinical Signs

Phimosis is most commonly diagnosed after attempted copulation results in pain and refusal to breed by the dog. Phimosis can be severe enough to interfere with urination, leading to urine-pooling within the prepuce. Urine leaking from the preputial opening may indicate a problem. Digital examination of the preputial opening is diagnostic for severe problems. Inability to extrude the flaccid penis from the prepuce or inability to extrude the penis without pain indicates phimosis.

With paraphimosis the animal presents with an engorged penis extending from the preputial opening. Depending on the extent of penile vascular occlusion and the duration of the problem, penile congestion to penile necrosis is evident. Penile extension from the prepuce without an erection indicates other, nonemergency problems such as congenital abnormalities of the penis and prepuce.

Diagnostic Plan

Phimosis is diagnosed by attempts to expose the glans penis and manually extrude the glans from the prepuce. Pain is induced at the point of overstretching of the preputial opening. It is obvious at this point that phimosis is present. In paraphimosis, the diagnosis is made by observing the protruding penis. After reduction of paraphimosis, assessment of urethral integrity is indicated. A urinary catheter may be placed to facilitate urination.

Preputial Discharge

Preputial discharge includes any fluid, other than urine, that is expelled from the preputial opening. Normal smegma is commonly seen as a small amount of yellowish-white, thick, mucoid discharge at the preputial opening. Purulent discharges indicate inflammation occurring somewhere anterior to the preputial opening. Hemorrhagic discharges may originate from the prepuce, penis, urethra, prostate gland, bladder, or testicles.

Pathophysiology

Any inflammatory process may produce a purulent discharge. Balanoposthitis, penile lacerations, and bacterial prostatitis or abscess are the most common sources of purulent preputial discharges. Hemorrhagic discharges may arise from preputial or penile abrasions or lacerations, urethral prolapse, neoplasia, urinary tract disease, or prostatic disease.

Clinical Signs

The dog may or may not have been neutered. Discharge from the prepuce is noted and is unrelated to urination. Increased frequency of licking may have been observed.

Diagnostic Plan

Cytologic examination may be performed on the discharge itself to determine its cellular nature. An attempt should be made to determine the source of the discharge. A thorough examination of the penis, with complete reflection of the prepuce, is necessary to rule out inflammatory, traumatic, and neoplastic lesions on the penis itself. The internal prepuce is visible only with endoscopic equipment. If the discharge is determined to originate from the urethra, the prostate gland and urinary tract should be considered possible sources for the discharge. The prostate gland should be palpated by digital rectal examination coupled with abdominal palpation. The prostate gland is trapped between the finger in the rectum and the hand on the abdomen so that an approximate size and shape can be determined. If the prostate gland is enlarged, irregularly shaped, or painful, prostate disease is probable. The prostatic fraction (third fraction) of the ejaculate

should be examined cytologically for evidence of inflammation, bacteria, or neoplasia. Urinalysis should be performed. Bacterial cultures should be made of both the prostatic fluid and the urine for comparison purposes. Bacterial prostatitis is commonly associated with bacterial cystitis.

Diagnostic Procedures

Vaginal Cytology

Vaginal cytology is the process of taking a superficial exfoliate sample of the vagina and evaluating the cell types present. Vaginal cytology is indicated whenever reproductive disease is suspected. Vaginal cytology is easy to perform. Because the vulva and vestibule are sensitive areas, gentle handling and adequate restraint of the animal are required. A cotton-tipped swab is introduced through the lips of the vulva at the dorsal commissure. The swab may be moistened with a few drops of sterile saline before it is inserted. This process is facilitated by spreading the lips of the vulva before insertion of the swab. After the cotton tip is within the vulvar lips, the swab is directed dorsally toward the tail. When the swab is at the dorsal-most aspect of the vestibule, the swab is then directed anteriorly into the vagina. The swab is rotated within the vagina one time in one direction to obtain an adequate exfoliated sample without leaving behind fibers from the swab. By this technique of spreading the lips of the vulva, introducing the swab at the dorsal commissure, and initially directing the swab dorsally, the keratinized skin, the clitoral fossa, and the sensitive urethral opening are avoided. The swab is withdrawn and immediately rolled firmly onto a slide. Some clinicians prefer to flush saline into and from the vagina with a pipette to obtain a cytology sample.[6]

The cytology sample is air-dried and stained using a rapid Wright-Giemsa stain (Diff-Quik).[7] In proestrus and estrus, estrogen influence is easily identified by the cornification pattern of the squamous epithelial cells. Cornified and superficial epithelial cells are large, angular cells with relatively small nuclei (Fig 22-1A). While the animal is under the influence of estrogen and the vaginal epithelium is thickened, cornified and superficial epithelial cells predominate in the cytology sample (>80%–90%). At any other time of the estrous cycle, parabasal and intermediate cells predominate. These two cell types are round cells with relatively large nuclei (Fig. 22-1B). The ratio of cytoplasm to nuclear material becomes larger as the cell type matures and becomes cornified. The high percentage of superficial and cornified cells drops dramatically as diestrus begins.

Because of the variability seen among individu-

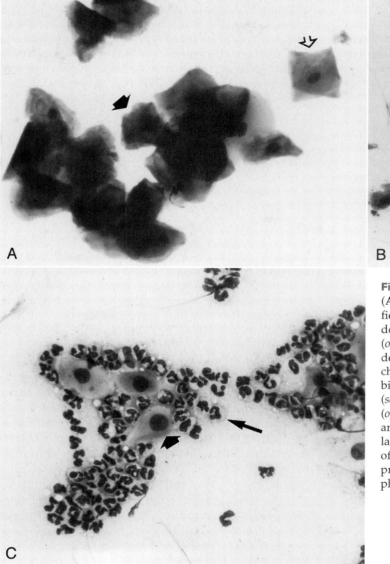

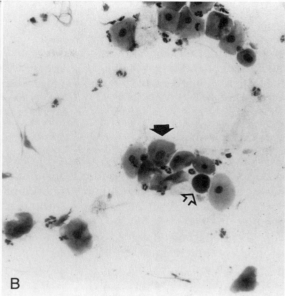

Figure 22–1

(**A**) Vaginal cytology of a bitch in estrus. Cornified squamous epithelial cells (*solid arrow*) predominate. A large superficial cell is also present (*open arrow*). Notice that the background is clear of debris and that no neutrophils are present; this is characteristic of estrus.(**B**) Vaginal cytology of a bitch in anestrus. Intermediate cells predominate (*solid arrow*). A parabasal cell is also present (*open arrow*). Notice the debris in the background and the presence of neutrophils, indicating the lack of estrogenic influence. (**C**) Vaginal cytology of a bitch in early diestrus. Intermediate cells predominate (*thick arrow*), and numerous neutrophils are present (*thin arrow*)

als, vaginal cytology as a breeding management tool is not reliable in every bitch. Inflammation is easily identified with the presence of numerous neutrophils (see Fig. 20-4). The only time numerous neutrophils are present normally on vaginal cytology samples is in the early diestrus period (Fig. 22-1C). Red blood cells are normally present in varying numbers during proestrus and estrus. In most bitches, the amount of red blood cells diminishes over time as the bitch progresses through proestrus into estrus. The amount of blood seen during proestrus and estrus may vary dramatically among normal individuals. The red blood cells seen during proestrus and estrus enter the uterus by diapedesis and are discharged through the cervix and vagina. Blood from vaginal sources may indicate the presence of vaginal pathologic changes such as lacerations or neoplasia.

Digital Examination

Digital examination of the vestibule and distal vagina is invaluable for detecting abnormalities in this area. A gloved finger lubricated with a water-soluble lubricant is inserted gently into the vestibule. This area is sensitive, and some bitches may react violently to this examination. In most bitches, the finger can be inserted to its full length, which enables the examination of the entire vestibule, the urethral opening, and the vaginovestibular junction. Many abnormalities often found in this area, such as strictures, may be missed by other methods of examination but are easily discerned by digital examination. Masses may be found and the extent and origin of growth delineated. Bitches 9 kg or less and queens are too small to allow this type of examination.

Vaginoscopy

Vaginoscopy is indicated whenever the vagina needs to be visualized in its entirety. Visualization of the vagina is helpful in identifying abnormalities, in locating the source of a discharge, and in routine breeding management.[8] Vaginoscopy is performed with an endoscope, proctoscope, or any flexible fiberoptic equipment with sufficient length (15 cm) to inspect the entire vagina. The procedure can be performed on the standing awake bitch, with sedation if necessary, or under anesthesia. Rigid instruments, such as a proctoscope, give better visualization of the vagina than the flexible fiberoptic endoscopes because of the difficulty of maintaining air insufflation to counteract the collapsing nature of the vaginal folds. When flexible endoscopes are used, air insufflation is accomplished by holding the vulva securely around the endoscope to prevent air from escaping. In order to observe the anterior vagina and paracervical area, the outside diameter of the endoscope must be 5 mm or less.[9] This small diameter may be necessary in smaller bitches to traverse the vaginovestibular junction. In prepubertal or ovariectomized bitches, body size does not always correlate with vestibular and vaginal diameter. Equipment with lengths of 5 cm or less, such as otoscopes, are inadequate to visualize the vagina. The technique for passing the scope is the same as that described for obtaining vaginal cytologic samples. The instrument is introduced at the dorsal commissure of the vulva, directed dorsally through the vestibule, and passed horizontally into the vagina, avoiding the clitoral fossa and the urethral opening. Vaginoscopy is not possible in the queen because of the small diameter (1 mm) of the feline vagina.[10]

Vaginoscopy is useful in evaluating the health of the vagina. The lining of the vagina can be evaluated for the presence of lesions indicative of inflammation (lymphoid follicular hyperplasia), discharges and their sources, masses, and anatomic abnormalities. Because the vaginal epithelium tends to become hyperemic when in contact with air, evaluation of vaginal hyperemia should be made early in the examination. Distinctive changes occur to the vaginal epithelium during proestrus and estrus that make vaginoscopy useful for routine breeding management. During proestrus, the vaginal mucosal folds become large, round, and edematous, and they fill the lumen of the vagina. At the onset of estrus, these folds take on a wrinkled appearance. During the most fertile period of estrus, the vaginal folds become lower and more crenated, and the borders of the folds become quite sharp and angular.[8, 9] At this time, the vaginal lumen appears open and wide. With the onset of diestrus, the vaginal folds become low and flat with red and white patches throughout. This change in vaginal appearance usually correlates with the change in vaginal cytology indicative of diestrus as well as the onset of rejection behavior toward the dog.

Vaginal Bacterial Cultures

Vaginal cultures are indicated if a bacterial problem is suspected within the reproductive tract. It also has become common for breeders to request vaginal cultures before breeding to screen for disease. Normal vaginal flora has been described in several reports in the literature.[11, 12] The aerobic bacterial flora of the bitch's vagina consists of common opportunistic pathogens whose presence does not influence fertility or necessarily lead to reproductive tract disease. Careful interpretation of culture results is essential when culturing an area that has been shown to have a normal flora. Obtaining vaginal cultures requires the use of a guarded swab culture instrument. After proper cleansing and drying of the vulva, the culture instrument is introduced into the vulva and passed into the anterior vagina. The inside swab is advanced until it contacts the vaginal lumen and then rotated. The swab is retracted within the guard before removal from the vagina. To further minimize contamination of the sample, the guarded swab may be introduced through a sterile speculum to reduce contact with the heavily contaminated vulva and vestibule. Minimal lubrication should be used. The swab should be processed immediately or placed in transport media and refrigerated until processing. Bacterial sensitivity determinations should be made on significant bacterial isolations.[13]

Bacterial isolations from the vagina should be interpreted carefully. *Brucella canis,* if isolated, is always significant and a definitive diagnosis. Most other bacteria may be normal flora. In the absence of reproductive tract disease, these organisms may not be pathogens. The known opportunistic pathogens, *Escherichia coli* and *Mycoplasma,* are routinely found in normal animals. Isolation of bacteria should be correlated with the presence of a purulent discharge, increased numbers of white blood cells on vaginal cytology, or heavy growth of a single organism. It is not unusual to find heavy growth of organisms during proestrus and estrus because of the hemorrhagic discharge normally seen at this time. Vaginal cytology reveals no inflammatory response in conjunction with

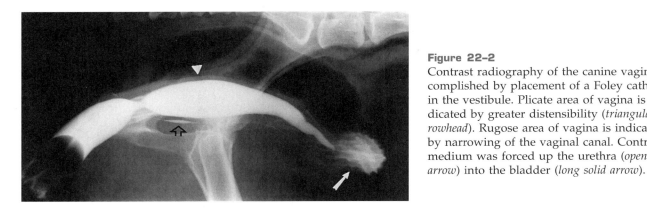

Figure 22-2
Contrast radiography of the canine vagina accomplished by placement of a Foley catheter in the vestibule. Plicate area of vagina is indicated by greater distensibility (*triangular arrowhead*). Rugose area of vagina is indicated by narrowing of the vaginal canal. Contrast medium was forced up the urethra (*open arrow*) into the bladder (*long solid arrow*).

the positive culture results or with large numbers of bacteria that may be seen on the cytologic sample in the normal animal. Research has shown that placing the normal animal on prophylactic antibiotics may predispose the vagina to colonization by organisms that are known opportunistic pathogens.[14]

Vaginal Contrast Radiography

Contrast radiography of the vaginal area is indicated if anatomic abnormalities are suspected and need further elaboration after other diagnostic techniques have been used.[15, 16] Contrast medium is introduced into the vagina through a Foley catheter whose balloon has been filled anterior to the vaginovestibular junction (Fig. 22-2). The volume necessary to fill the vaginal vault varies according to body weight and presence of an intact reproductive tract. In general, the vaginal volume in milliliters equals 1.14 times the body weight in kilograms. Animals previously ovariohysterectomized require less volume than similarly sized intact animals.[15] Radiographs may then reveal masses, diverticula, septal defects (double vagina), or other anatomic abnormalities. If the uterus is present, the contrast medium may diffuse up into the uterine body and horns and potentially into the abdominal cavity.

Common Diseases of the External Genitalia

Vaginitis

Vaginitis is inflammation affecting the epithelial lining of the vagina. Vaginitis can occur in a variety of situations and does not necessarily indicate an infectious process.

Pathophysiology

A variety of problems can cause vaginitis. Puppy vaginitis is poorly understood and is thought to

be caused by immaturity of the vagina. Trauma to the vagina may cause vaginitis as a result of breeding injuries, foreign bodies, or dystocias. Anatomic abnormalities may contribute to the development of vaginitis by allowing the pooling of discharge or urine in the vagina. Accumulation of urine in the vagina may present as urinary incontinence with urine dribbling from the vulva when the bitch changes position. Bacterial or chemical vaginitis is usually secondary to a predisposing anatomic abnormality such as vaginovestibular strictures, diverticula, ectopic ureters, or double vaginas.[16] Foreign bodies and tumors cause vaginitis when present in the vagina. Systemic disease (e.g., diabetes mellitus) may disrupt the normal local immunity and predispose the animal to vaginitis. Canine herpesvirus causes a nonirritating vesicular vaginitis in infected animals.[17] Canine herpesvirus is normally spread by mucous membrane contact with a virus-shedding animal. A common location of infection for canine herpesvirus is the upper respiratory tract; this causes a mild rhinitis that results in a serous nasal discharge. Both the rhinitis and the vaginitis are mild and are usually clinically inapparent. Canine herpesvirus may be spread venereally but more commonly is spread by casual dog-to-dog contact. Virus reactivation in bitches without clinical signs has been documented with the administration of prednisolone, indicating that latent canine herpesvirus infections do occur.[18]

Clinical Signs

Vaginitis is typically irritating to the animal and results in excessive licking of the perineal area. Vulvar discharges may be seen. Typically, male dogs are attracted to bitches with vaginitis. Some types of vaginitis cause no clinical signs, such as the vaginitis caused by canine herpesvirus.[17]

Diagnostic Plan

Inflammation is readily identified with vaginal cytology. Vaginoscopy may be useful in determining the extent and intensity of inflammation as well as any predisposing lesion such as a vaginal mass or laceration. Inflammation on vaginoscopy is noted by the presence of hyperemia, exudate, and mucosal lesions such as vesicles, ulcers, and lymphoid follicle hyperplasia. An attempt should be made to differentiate the clinical signs of vaginitis from those of urinary tract or skin disease. Urinary tract problems can cause vestibular irritation and attraction of male dogs. Skin disease may cause irritation in the perineal area, resulting in increased licking of the area. Comparison of vestibule cytology specimens with those obtained through a speculum for vaginal cytology may help to localize the area of inflammation. Digital examination of the vestibule and distal vagina identifies strictures or other anatomic abnormalities, particularly at the vaginovestibular junction, that may predispose the animal to vaginitis.

Treatment

The treatment of vaginitis depends on the inciting cause. Puppy vaginitis does not require any treatment. Antibiotic therapy for puppy vaginitis is contraindicated because of the possible disruption of normal flora and colonization of the vagina by potential pathogens. It is advisable to leave the animal intact until the vaginitis spontaneously resolves. This spontaneous resolution of puppy vaginitis may not occur until the bitch undergoes puberty and her first estrus. Anatomic abnormalities may be surgically corrected if possible. Foreign bodies and tumors may be removed if possible. Vaginal trauma usually resolves without treatment. Antibiotic therapy may speed the animal's recovery from vaginal lacerations and prevent deeper lacerations from becoming more serious, dissecting pelvic infections. Predisposing systemic disease, such as diabetes mellitus, should be treated appropriately. If a significant bacterial component to vaginitis is determined, vaginal cultures should be obtained, and the animal should be placed on an appropriate antibiotic. Lavage of the vagina may initially be beneficial to remove accumulated discharges. Lavage solutions should be mild and nonirritating (e.g., physiologic saline solution). Viral vaginitis is a self-limiting condition that requires no treatment. It is advisable to isolate bitches with active canine herpesvirus lesions from pregnant bitches and neonatal puppies.[19]

Prognosis

Prognosis for animals with vaginitis is variable. Puppy vaginitis has an excellent prognosis if allowed to regress spontaneously with the onset of puberty. Vaginal trauma caused by foreign bodies usually resolves without incident after the foreign body is removed. Vaginal trauma resolution depends on the extent of damage to the vagina. Most vaginal lacerations heal without incident with appropriate therapy. Vaginal scarring and adhesions must be evaluated later, after healing is complete. Prognosis for animals with vaginal tumors depends on the cell type involved and the degree of tissue invasion and metastasis. Treatment of vaginitis without having identified the cause can be quite frustrating.

Balanoposthitis

Balanoposthitis is inflammation of the penis and prepuce. Inflammation of these mucous membranes can occur in a variety of situations and does not necessarily indicate an infectious process.

Pathophysiology

A variety of problems can cause balanoposthitis. Most cases observed are mild and clinically insignificant.[20] Severe cases result most commonly from penile trauma, lacerations, foreign bodies, or neoplasia. Neoplasias seen most commonly are TVT, papillomas, and squamous cell carcinomas.[21] Abscess formation may result with trauma, lacerations, or foreign bodies and can lead to signs of systemic illness.

Clinical Signs

The most common sign is pus dripping from the preputial opening. In more severe cases, painful swelling of the prepuce and penis may be observed, usually with copious purulent preputial discharge. Examination of the mucus membranes reveals mucus membrane inflammation, follicular lymphoid hyperplasia, and possibly tissue necrosis. Inciting causes such as penile laceration or trauma, neoplasia, or foreign bodies may be found.

Diagnostic Plan

Cytology of the discharge identifies the presence of inflammation by large numbers of neutrophils. Complete extrusion of the penis from the prepuce allows examination of the entire glans penis up to the reflection of the prepuce. The inciting cause of the inflammation may be evident on visual examination of the penis. If the cause remains unclear, cytology or biopsy of any questionable lesions may be necessary.

Treatment

Treatment is not indicated in most cases of mild balanoposthitis. Penile lacerations usually heal spontaneously. Systemic antibiotics are indicated if signs of systemic illness have been observed. Any foreign bodies found should be removed. Neoplasia is most commonly treated by excision or chemotherapy. Abscesses should be opened and allowed to drain. Cleansing of the preputial cavity can be accomplished by lavage with sterile saline solution. If deemed necessary, antibiotic ointments may be infused into the preputial cavity until signs are alleviated. If possible, simple cleansing of the area is preferable to application of topical antibiotics because of disruption of the normal flora within the preputial cavity.

Prognosis

Prognosis is good if the inciting cause is identified and corrected. Prognosis for animals with neoplasia varies with the type of tumor and the degree of tissue invasion and metastasis. Treatment of balanoposthitis without identification of the cause can be frustrating because clinical signs commonly return after treatment.

Vaginal and Vestibular Anatomic Abnormalities

A variety of congenital abnormalities of the vagina and vestibule are found in the bitch. The incidence is unknown, but these abnormalities are not uncommon. Anatomic abnormalities may be incidental findings, or they may be the inciting cause of other problems such as vaginitis, chronic urinary tract infections, perineal irritation, or mating difficulties.

Pathophysiology

Most anatomic abnormalities of the external genitalia are caused by abnormal embryologic development in the fetus. Strictures and hymens at the vaginovestibular junction are caused by incomplete joining of the paramesonephric system with the urogenital sinus. With problems arising from paramesonephric duct organogenesis, the vulva and vestibule are usually normal. The incomplete fusion of the paramesonephric ducts results in a vertical septum within the vagina, a double vagina. The cause of some anatomic abnormalities, such as segmental hypoplasia or aplasia and vaginal diverticula, is unknown. The cause of vulvar strictures that do not relax sufficiently to allow copulation is unknown but may be related to an inadequate response to estrogen. Infantile vulvas are not necessarily an abnormality but a variation of normal. Clitoral abnormalities associated with pseudohermaphrodism are caused by the testosterone released from the testicles or ovotestes with this condition. Masculinization of the clitoris causes the structure to enlarge and take on penis-like characteristics.

Clinical Signs

The most common presenting complaint is the inability of the bitch to copulate with the male dog.

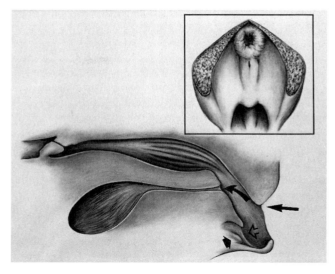

Figure 22–3

Drawing of canine vestibule and vagina. Vestibule is bordered caudally by the vulvar lips and anteriorly by the vaginovestibular junction. The dorsal commissure is indicated by the long solid arrow; the clitoral sinus by the open arrow; the clitoris by the short, solid arrow; and the urethral opening by the curved arrow. Insert demonstrates a 360° stricture at the vaginovestibular junction.

Usually, there are no clinical signs before the attempted breeding. Vaginitis, urinary incontinence, or other signs of irritation in the perineal area may indicate problems. Pseudohermaphrodites present with a soft tissue swelling protruding from the vulvar lips. Infantile inverted vulvas may cause irritation in the perineal area due to vaginitis, vulvar fold dermatitis, or urinary tract disease.

Diagnostic Plan

An enlarged clitoris in a young animal is essentially pathognomonic for pseudohermaphrodism. An acquired enlarged clitoris may be induced by administration of androgenic hormones such as Cheque Drops or testosterone. Infantile vulvas are found on physical examination. These vulvas are small and typically are inverted into the perineal area. Digital examination reveals the most common of the anatomic abnormalities, strictures. These common abnormalities occur most often at the dorsal commissure of the vulva or the vaginovestibular junction. Digital examination may reveal some abnormalities missed by other, more sophisticated techniques. Hymens are typically found at the vaginovestibular junction. Hymens may manifest as 360° annular strictures or vertical bands of tissue[22] (Fig. 22-3). Vaginoscopy may reveal abnormalities farther cranially than can be assessed by digital examination. Contrast radiography may help delineate the presence and extent of vaginal abnormalities such as vaginal septums or double vaginas.[16]

Treatment

Persistent hymens do not require treatment unless clinical signs are seen or the animal is to be used for breeding. The vertical bands are most easily treated by surgical removal. The annular ring strictures are very difficult to correct surgically. A variety of techniques have been described for removal or dilatation of these strictures, but in most cases the strictures return as healing takes place. If these rings prevent breeding, the bitch can be inseminated artificially. In many cases, at the time of parturition, these rings loosen sufficiently to allow a normal vaginal delivery of puppies. These animals should be examined 1 week before whelping for the assessment of this problem, and a cesarean section should be planned if sufficient relaxation has not occurred. Vaginal septal defects do not require treatment unless clinical signs are noted or the animal is to be used for breeding. Correction of these conditions may or may not be possible, depending on the extent of involvement. Surgical access to the vagina is technically difficult. Removal of the vagina has been described as a treatment for vaginal defects that are causing clinical signs. Surgical removal of the clitoris is indicated in hermaphrodites if excoriation of prolapsed tissue is a problem. Infantile vulvas are corrected by allowing the animal to undergo estrus. Neutering of these bitches should be postponed until after the first estrus. Eversion of the vulva occurs in most cases, under the influence of estrogen.

Prognosis

Prognosis varies depending on the condition and the existence of clinical signs. Some of the vaginitis and urine pooling problems associated with anatomic abnormalities are very resistant to correction. Surgical correction may be incomplete because of the inaccessibility of the area involved. Other problems are easily corrected without future sequelae.

Vaginal Fold Prolapse (Vaginal Hyperplasia)

Under the influence of estrogen, some bitches experience a proliferation of tissue to the extent of prolapse through the vulvar lips (Fig. 22-4). In some individuals, the mass does not regress at the end of estrus. This characteristic of nonregression may be related to the presence of a pregnancy. Predisposed breeds include the boxer, mastiff, Chesapeake Bay retriever, and many of the brachycephalic, mastiff-based breeds.

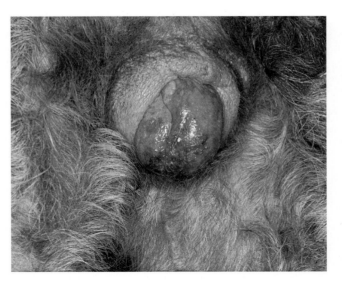

Figure 22-4
Vaginal fold prolapse during estrus in a Chesapeake Bay retriever. Edematous vaginal fold has prolapsed through the vulvar lips. Notice excoriation on the prolapsed tissue.

Pathophysiology

The influence of estrogen on the tissues of the reproductive tract is profound. Vaginal fold prolapse is an exaggerated response to estrogen. Traditionally, this condition has been called vaginal hyperplasia. Histologically, this tissue is not hyperplastic but rather edematous. The entire vagina usually does not prolapse, moving the cervix caudally, as occurs in other species. Typically, a fold of tissue from the ventral floor of the vagina grows and prolapses through the vulvar lips. The predisposition of certain breeds for this problem indicates a possible genetic component.[23]

Clinical Signs

Vaginal fold prolapse is seen almost exclusively when the bitch is in proestrus or estrus. The most obvious clinical sign is tissue prolapsing from the vulva. Problems with localized excoriation result from trauma to the prolapsed tissue. In less obvious cases, this tissue is evident only through a digital examination. An inability to breed may also be part of the presenting problem because of the lack of space to accommodate the dog's penis. There are usually no clinical signs other than the presence of estrus. The bitch usually exhibits the characteristic signs of estrus, including vulvar swelling, bleeding, and standing behavior.

Diagnostic Plan

Diagnosis is made based on examination of the tissue prolapsing through the vulvar lips during estrus. Vaginal cytology demonstrates the influence of estrogen by the high percentage of superficial and cornified epithelial cells present. An increase in inflammatory cells may be seen on vaginal cytology because of the localized trauma. If doubt still remains, a biopsy, incisional or excisional, may be performed.

Treatment

The condition usually disappears after the bitch proceeds from estrus to diestrus, but it recurs with each subsequent estrus because of the estrogen influence at those times. Treatment varies depending on the extent of tissue prolapse and whether the animal is to be used for breeding. An ovariohysterectomy permanently corrects the problem. If the swelling does not regress after the estrogen source is removed, surgical removal of the mass is performed, usually through an episiotomy incision. If the animal is to be used for breeding, the mass may be removed. This may permanently correct the problem, although some surgeons report recurrence. The animal may be artificially inseminated around the mass and rarely will have a problem at whelping. Supportive treatment, topical antibiotic creams, or bandaging of the mass may be considered to avoid or minimize the excoriation and drying that the prolapsed tissue undergoes. Reduction and stay sutures in the vulva are not advisable because of the potential damage to the vulva and the possibility of self-mutilation.

Prognosis

Prognosis is excellent with ovariohysterectomy. This treatment should be considered immediately or after any desired litters have been born to a bitch considered breeding stock. Because of the genetic potential, ovariohysterectomy should be recommended.

Vaginal and Penile Lacerations

Vaginal and penile lacerations may occur after any form of trauma. Most commonly, vaginal lacerations are a result of breeding or parturition injuries. Penile lacerations may result from breeding injuries, foreign bodies, or any injury to the ventral body wall.

Pathophysiology

Vaginal lacerations may occur during copulation with a dog that is too large for the bitch or in the case of animals that have been forcibly separated during the tie. Lacerations may also occur during parturition, particularly during an assisted birth. These lacerations may be of varying depth and consequence. Any time excessive bleeding transpires after copulation or delivery, vaginal lacerations must be considered. Foreign bodies or forced penetration of the bitch may also cause vaginal lacerations. In the male, penile lacerations are most commonly caused by foreign bodies that have entered the preputial opening or by trauma to the ventral abdominal wall. Forced separation during the copulatory tie may cause damage to the glans penis.

Clinical Signs

Excessive vaginal bleeding is the most common sign of vaginal lacerations. This bleeding may take place apparently spontaneously or in conjunction with a specific event such as copulation or whelping. Animals with penile lacerations present with bleeding from the preputial opening. Bleeding is not usually significant enough to cause signs of blood loss. In the male, differentiation must be made between internal and external sources of bleeding. With older lacerations, a purulent, malodorous discharge may be evident as healing occurs. The discharge may be profuse. Dissecting infection that progresses through the tissue planes of the pelvis and lower limbs is possible. A complete blood count may indicate a regenerative anemia, a hypoproteinemia, or a leukocytosis with a left shift in those patients that experience extreme blood loss or infection.

Diagnostic Plan

A digital examination of the vestibule and distal vagina may reveal the source of bleeding and the location of the vaginal laceration. Vaginoscopy may be necessary to ascertain the exact location and the extent of the laceration. Foreign bodies may be discovered at this time. The most common location for vaginal lacerations is the vaginovestibular junction. In the male, the penis should be examined by extruding the penis completely out of the prepuce to allow visualization of the entire glans penis.

Treatment

Because of the inaccessibility of the vaginal area, surgical correction is often difficult. Packing of the area to create pressure and reduce hemorrhage is indicated. Systemic antibiotics are indicated to reduce healing time and the possibility of infection's dissecting between the tissue planes. Topical therapy with a water-based antibiotic cream may be considered, depending on the location of the laceration.

Prognosis

Healing of lacerations of the vagina or penis is usually fast. After hemorrhage has been controlled, the prognosis is good. Scar tissue that would interfere with reproductive function may occur and should be assessed after healing is complete.

Vaginal and Vulvar Neoplasias

Vaginal and vulvar neoplasias represent 2.5% to 3% of all canine tumors.[24] Seventy percent to 80% of these tumors are benign, and they are typically found in older animals (average age, 11 years).

Pathophysiology

Leiomyomas are the most common benign tumors, and leiomyosarcomas are the most common malignant tumors. TVTs are more common in younger animals, especially in animals allowed to roam.

Clinical Signs

The clinical signs most often reported are perineal enlargement, masses protruding from the vulva, vulvar discharge, tenesmus, and dysuria.

Diagnostic Plan

Masses protruding from the vulva must be differentiated from vaginal fold prolapse by evaluation of the stage of estrous cycle and its relation to the onset of signs, the location of the mass, and the failure of the mass to regress after estrus. Other causes of vulvar discharge must be ruled out. Digital examination of the vestibule and distal vagina may reveal the presence of masses in the distal tract. Endoscopy is necessary to examine the entire vagina. As with any neoplastic process, evaluation for metastasis is advisable with abdominal and thoracic radiographs and aspiration cytology of regional lymph nodes.

Treatment

Surgical removal of the tumor is the treatment of choice. TVTs respond readily to chemotherapy (see next section). Ovariohysterectomy is recommended at the time of tumor removal because of the possibility of hormonal influence on the recurrence rate.

Prognosis

Prognosis is good provided that metastasis has not occurred prior to removal of the malignant tumors.

Penile and Preputial Neoplasias

The penis is rarely involved in tumorigenesis, but papillomas, squamous cell carcinomas, and TVTs are reported.[21] The TVT is the most common penile neoplasm of dogs, particularly in free-roaming animals. These tumors are found worldwide, most commonly in temperate climates, particularly areas with large populations of free-roaming dogs. The scrotum and prepuce are part of the integument and therefore may be affected by any neoplasm associated with the skin.

Pathophysiology

TVT is the most common tumor of the canine penis and prepuce. TVT is spread by cellular implants, primarily through venereal contact, but may involve the mucous membranes of the face. Other reported tumors include a long list of benign and malignant tumors.

Clinical Signs

A preputial discharge is frequently associated with penile or preputial tumors and may be purulent or hemorrhagic.[2] Swellings in the area of the prepuce are noted. Masses of variable size, color, and consistency are noted when the penis and prepuce are examined. TVTs may be found anywhere on the external genitalia and are usually cauliflower-like and friable.[25]

Diagnostic Plan

Biopsy of any tumor is necessary for diagnosis. Excisional biopsy may be indicated in many cases. Diagnosis of TVT may be based on cytologic or histologic examination of the tumor because of its distinctive cell type. The TVT cells are round to oval with abundant pale, granular cytoplasm that characteristically contains numerous vacuoles. The nuclei have clumped chromatin, visible nucleoli, and frequent mitotic figures.[26] Before surgery, the animal should be evaluated for metastatic disease by thoracic radiographs, abdominal radiographs, and regional lymph node evaluation.

Treatment

Surgical excision is the most effective treatment for penile and preputial neoplasms, excluding TVT. With large, invasive penile tumors, treatment may require penile amputation.[25] TVTs are best treated by chemotherapy. Weekly vincristine chemotherapy (0.5 mg/m[2] body surface area) is the most effective treatment, with a 90% cure rate reported.[27] Treatment should continue 2 weeks beyond clinical resolution of the tumor, which usually takes 4 to 6 weeks. A complete blood count and platelet count should be taken weekly to assess toxicity.

Prognosis

Prognosis with chemotherapy is very good. Complete remission in all dogs treated with vincristine is reported, with only a 10% recurrence rate at 12 months.[27] Without treatment, no spontaneous remission is expected, and tumor progression is likely.

Urethral Prolapse

Urethral prolapse is the prolapse of the urethral mucosa from the tip of the penis. The condition may have a hereditary component in the bulldog.

Pathophysiology

Urethral prolapse is seen in intact male dogs, particularly in the bulldog. Sexual excitement, multiple erections, and self-inflicted damage from licking are considered the inciting causes. Urinary tract disease leading to stranguria may also result in urethral prolapse.

Clinical Signs

The most common sign is blood dripping from the preputial opening. Blood may be seen during breeding, either in the ejaculate or on the penis itself. Physical examination of the glans penis reveals a mass of edematous, hyperemic tissue bulging from the tip of the penis.

Diagnostic Plan

The diagnosis is made on physical examination of the penis (Fig. 22-5). If surgery is performed, the tissue removed should be submitted for histologic examination to confirm the diagnosis.

Treatment

Manual replacement with or without a purse-string suture may correct the condition. In severe or recurring cases, surgical excision is considered the treatment of choice. Concurrent castration helps reduce the incidence of recurrence.

Prognosis

Prognosis is good after surgical correction and castration. Recurrence is common after more conservative treatment.

Uncommon Diseases of the External Genitalia

Hypospadia

Hypospadia is a congenital defect seen uncommonly in the dog. Hypospadia is defined as a defect in closure of the urethra that results in an abnormal opening in the urethra. The abnormal opening may be found anywhere from the glans penis to the perineal

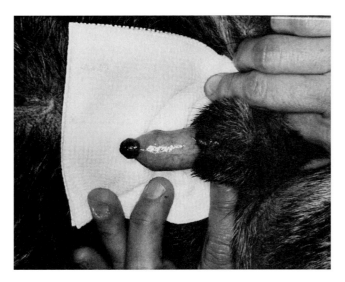

Figure 22-5
Urethral prolapse in a male English bulldog. The prepuce is pulled back to expose the distal portion of the glans penis.

area. Descriptions of hypospadia include the location of the opening. Openings in the distal glans penis are called glandular hypospadia. Openings in the mid-shaft of the penis are called penile hypospadia. Three other classifications are scrotal, perineal, and anal hypospadia.[28] Urinary incontinence and preputial abnormalities also may accompany hypospadia. Surgical correction of the abnormal urethral openings is indicated. Often, hypospadia is accompanied by other congenital abnormalities, particularly those of the urinary tract. Evaluation of the urinary tract is therefore indicated in cases of hypospadia. This evaluation may include urinalysis and contrast radiography of the bladder and kidneys.[29]

Priapism

Priapism is the presence of a persistent penile erection. In the dog, this condition is most commonly associated with a spinal cord lesion. Symptomatic treatment of the penis, cleansing, and lubrication are indicated until the spinal cord lesion is resolved. Thrombosis of the penis is a possibility, and penile amputation may be required in chronic cases.

References

1. Meyers-Wallen VN, Patterson DF. Disorders of sexual development in dogs and cats. In: Kirk RW, ed. Current Veterinary Therapy X. Philadelphia, WB Saunders, 1989: 1261–1269.

2. McEntee K. Reproductive Pathology of Domestic Mammals. San Diego, Academic Press, 1990:1–7.

3. Miller ME, Christensen GC, Evans HE. Anatomy of the Dog. Philadelphia, WB Saunders, 1964:751–778.

4. Banks WJ. Applied Veterinary Histology. Baltimore, Williams & Wilkins, 1986:513–517, 558–559.

5. Roberts SJ. Veterinary Obstetrics and Genital Diseases (Theriogenology). Woodstock, Vermont, SJ Roberts, 1986: 793–805.

6. Johnson CA. Vaginal disorders. In: Ettinger SJ, ed. Textbook of Veterinary Internal Medicine. Philadelphia, WB Saunders, 1989:1806–1813.

7. Holst PA. Vaginal cytology in the bitch. In: Morrow DA, ed. Current Therapy in Theriogenology. Phildelphia, WB Saunders, 1986:457–462.

8. Concannon PW, Lein DH. Hormonal and clinical correlates of ovarian cycles, ovulation, pseudopregnancy, and pregnancy in dogs. In: Kirk RW, ed. Current Veterinary Therapy X. Philadelphia, WB Saunders, 1989:1269–1282.

9. Lindsay FEF. Endoscopy of the reproductive tract in the bitch. In: Kirk RW, ed. Current Veterinary Therapy VIII. Philadelphia, WB Saunders, 1983:912–921.

10. Watson PF, Glover TE. Vaginal anatomy of the domestic cat (*Felis catus*) in relation to copulation and artificial insemination. J Reprod Fert Suppl 1993;47:355–359.

11. Olson PN, Mather ED: The use and misuse of vaginal cultures in diagnosing reproductive diseases in the bitch. In: Morrow DA, ed. Current Therapy in Theriogenology. Philadelphia, WB Saunders, 1986:469–475.

12. Bjurstrom L, Linde-Forsberg C. Long-term study of aerobic bacteria of the genital tract in breeding bitches. Am J Vet Res 1992;54:891–896.

13. Lein DH. Canine mycoplasma, ureaplasma, and bacterial infertility. In: Kirk RW, ed. Current Veterinary Therapy IX. Philadelphia, WB Saunders, 1986:1240–1242.

14. Strom B, Linde-Forsberg C. Effects of ampicillin and trimethoprim-sulfamethoxazole on the vaginal bacterial flora of bitches. Am J Vet Res 1993; 54:891–896.

15. Holt PE, Gibbs C, Latham J. An evaluation of positive contrast vagino-urethrography as a diagnostic aid in the bitch. J Small Anim Pract 1984; 25:531–549.

16. Root MV, Johnston SD, Johnston GR. Vaginal septa in dogs: 15 cases (1983–1992). J Am Vet Med Assoc 1995; 206:56–58.

17. Greene CE, Kakuk TJ: Canine herpesvirus infection. In: Greene CE, ed. Clinical Microbiology and Infectious Diseases of the Dog and Cat. Philadelphia, WB Saunders, 1984:419–429.

18. Okuda Y, Ishida K, Hashimoti A, et al. Virus reactivation in bitches with a medical history of herpesvirus infection. Am J Vet Res 1993; 54:551–554.

19. Evermann JF. Comparative clinical and diagnostic aspects of herpesvirus infections of companion animals with primary emphasis on the dog. Proceedings Annual Meeting Society for Theriogenology, 1989:335–343.

20. Feldman EC, Nelson RW. Disorders of the canine male reproductive tract. In: Canine and Feline Endocrinology and Reproduction. Philadelphia, WB Saunders, 1987: 481–524.

21. Herron MA. Tumors of the canine genital system. J Am Anim Hosp Assoc 1983; 19:981–994.

22. Wykes PM. Diseases of the vagina and vulva in the bitch. In: Morrow DA, ed. Current Therapy in Theriogenology. Philadelphia, WB Saunders, 1986:476–481.

23. Johnston SD. Vaginal prolapse. In: Kirk RW, ed. Current Veterinary Therapy X. Philadelphia, WB Saunders, 1989: 1302–1305.

24. Withrow SJ, Susaneck SJ. Tumors of the canine female reproductive tract. In: Morrow DA, ed. Current Therapy in Theriogenology. Philadelphia, WB Saunders, 1986: 521–528.

25. O'Keefe DA. Tumors of the genital system and mammary glands. In: Ettinger SJ, Feldman EC, eds. Textbook of Veterinary Internal Medicine. Philadelphia, WB Saunders, 1995:1699-1704.

26. MacEwen EG. Canine transmissible tumors. In: Withrow SJ, MacEwen EG, eds. Clinical Veterinary Oncology. Philadelphia, JB Lippincott, 1989:421–425.

27. Amber EI, Henderson RA, Adeyanju JB, et al. Single-drug chemotherapy of canine transmissible venereal tumor with cyclophosphamide, methotrexate, or vincristine. J Vet Intern Med 1990;4:144.

28. Ader PL, Hobson HP. Hypospadias: A review of the veterinary literature and a report of three cases in the dog. J Am Anim Hosp Assoc 1978;14:721.

29. Johnston SD. Disorders of the external genitalia of the male. In: Ettinger SJ, ed. Textbook of Veterinary Internal Medicine. Philadelphia, WB Saunders, 1989:1881–1889.

Chapter 23

Diseases of Pregnancy and Puerperium

Beverly J. Purswell

Anatomy and Physiology

The bitch and the queen have similar placental structure, which can be described as zonary endotheliochorial type. The placenta forms a zonary band or girdle, 2 to 7.5 cm in width, around the circumference of the uterine lumen in the middle of the oval sac containing the fetus, fetal membranes, and fetal fluids.[1] The placenta is a labyrinthine type, demonstrating complicated winding interdigitations rather than regularly spaced villi. Outside the central zonary band, the fetal placenta (chorion) is a bare, inactive structure that does not play a part in placental functions. Placental hematomas form along the margins of the zonary placenta and are thought to provide iron to the developing fetus as the blood is broken down. The maternal endothelium is directly apposed to the chorion of the fetal placenta. This allows the passage of small amounts of antibodies from the maternal circulation into the fetal circulation, although the major portion of passive transfer of immunity comes from the early mammary secretion of colostrum.[1]

Both the bitch and the queen have luteal-dependent pregnancies. Removal of the ovaries at any time during pregnancy results in the immediate loss of that pregnancy.[2, 3] Bitches spontaneously ovulate with each estrus and maintain the corpus luteum for the duration of a pregnancy ($\geq$60 days), whether or not they are pregnant. The queen ovulates only when mated or similarly stimulated. The duration of a pseudopregnancy in the queen is 40 to 45 days.[4] Parturition follows a rapid fall of progesterone levels at term or whenever progesterone drops below 2 ng/mL for longer than 24 hours. Owing to the thermogenic properties of progesterone, a decrease in body temperature can be detected in the bitch when this rapid decline of progesterone occurs.[5] Although the presence of ovarian-luteal progesterone is critical in the maintenance of both canine and feline pregnancies, there is evidence that prolactin plays a luteotropic role. Prolactin inhibitors, which are dopamine agonists, have been shown to lyse the corpus luteum and thus lower progesterone to baseline levels.[2, 6]

Progesterone is essential for maintenance of pregnancy because it stimulates growth of endometrial glands, creates a suitable uterine environment for the developing embryos and fetuses, and inhibits uterine motility. Progesterone also stimulates mammary development by cellular proliferation of the mammary ducts and alveoli.[1] Mammary development is seen during pseudopregnancies because of the similar progesterone profiles, but usually not to the extent seen during pregnancies.

Ovulation is stimulated by the release of luteinizing hormone (LH) from the pituitary gland. In the queen, the LH peak is induced by the copulatory reflex. Multiple copulations are usually necessary to ensure adequate release of LH and thereby stimulate complete ovulation in the queen. In one study, 100% of queens ovulated when bred four times, but only 50% ovulated after being bred once.[7] Bitches ovulate spontaneously. After a variable period of proestrus, when the animal is under the influence of estrogen only, LH is released and the ovulation process is initiated. In both the queen and the bitch, ovulation begins approximately 24 to 48 hours after the LH peak. The progesterone levels begin to rise concurrently with the LH peak. In the bitch, standing behavior of estrus is initiated by the joint influence of estrogen and progesterone. Ovulation occurs over a 24- to 72-hour time span. The bitch is unique in that she ovulates primary oocytes. It takes an additional 24 to 48 hours for the primary oocytes to undergo two meiotic divisions to become secondary oocytes. The secondary oocyte is the stage of oocyte development that is capable of being fertilized. The bitch experiences peak fertility approximately 3 to 6 days after the LH peak (see Fig. 21–1).

Timing of semen deposition in the queen is not usually a problem because of the interaction between copulation and ovulation. Induced ovulation ensures that semen is present when the oocytes are ovulated. The delay between copulation and fertilization can be extremely variable in dogs, and therefore the timing of copulation in dogs is much more susceptible to error. Proestrus may last from 2 to 21 days, and estrus from 2 to 21 days. Standing estrus should occur approximately at the LH peak, when progesterone levels begin to rise, but it may occur several days before or after the LH peak. The most accurate method for timing a canine breeding is to identify the LH peak directly or indirectly by measuring progesterone. For peak fertility, semen should be deposited between 3 and 6 days after the LH peak.

Gestation length in the bitch can be determined by two methods. Breeding dates are not a reliable way to predict gestation length. Normal pregnancies have been reported to occur anywhere from 57 to 72 days after the first of multiple matings and 57 to 70 days after single matings.[8] The first and most accurate method of determining gestation length is detection of the preovulatory LH peak. With the use of commercially available enzyme-linked immunosorbent assay (ELISA) kits, the LH peak can be detected indirectly by measurement of progesterone. The first rise in progesterone correlates with the occurrence of the preovulatory LH peak and, less accurately, with the onset of standing behavior. Whelping has reliably been shown to occur 65 days after the LH peak.[8] The second method to predict gestation length is the use of vaginal cytology. Whelping occurs 56 or 57 days after the onset of vaginal cytologic diestrus[9] (see Fig. 22-1C). In the queen, gestation length, defined as the interval between mating and parturition, is 64 to 69 days.[10] The variation is not as great in cats because of the induced ovulation.

Parturition is initiated by a fall of progesterone. Whelping (or queening) begins after the progesterone falls below 1 ng/mL or stays below 2 ng/mL for longer than 48 hours.[5] The first stage of labor averages 6 to 12 hours.[11] During this stage, the bitch appears restless and begins to nest. Panting, shivering, vomiting, and anorexia are common indicators of the first stage of labor. Queens usually seek solitude and exhibit nesting behavior. The second stage of labor is characterized by active abdominal contractions as each fetus is pushed out of the uterus and through the vaginal canal. The third stage of labor is the passing of the placenta. The second and third stages of labor are interspersed. Once active straining has started, a fetus should be delivered within 30 to 60 minutes. Rest periods of up to 4 hours with no abdominal contractions are considered normal. The duration of labor is quite variable, ranging normally from 2 to 36 hours. Queens usually complete parturition in 2 to 6 hours. In both species, breech presentations are considered normal.

Lochia (postpartum vulvar discharge) is expelled from the uterus in decreasing amounts over a period of several weeks. Release of endogenous oxytocin in response to suckling aids uterine involution by causing uterine contractions. Exogenous oxytocin is not indicated with the presence of suckling neonates. Most uterine lochia is expelled within the first 2 weeks. Normal lochia progresses from red to brown in color and from watery to mucoid in consistency; it has no odor.

Problem Identification

Infertility

Infertility is the failure of a bitch or queen to undergo normal pregnancy and parturition after breeding (i.e., failure to deliver live offspring). Infertility implies a temporary lack of fertility, whereas sterility implies a permanent condition (Table 23–1). The incidence of infertility is unknown, but normal fertility is considered to be in the range of 80%. In other words, 20% of the bitches and queens bred do not give birth to live offspring.

Pathophysiology

Lack of conception may occur because of incorrect or ill-timed semen deposition, absolute or relative lack of quality semen, inability of the semen to traverse the reproductive tract to the oviduct, or failure of ovulation. Ovulation failure may be caused by inadequate amounts of LH released from the pituitary gland or by some inherent dysfunction of the ovary itself. A relative lack of LH may be caused by an inadequate release of LH or inadequate pituitary stores of LH. There is no diestrus (luteal or progesterone phase) if ovulation failure occurs. Queens may not release adequate levels of LH to initiate ovulation after copulation because of inadequate stimulation.

Either species may begin follicular development and experience cystic degeneration of those follicles. Conception failure may result from the lack or relative lack of normal sperm reaching the oocytes at the proper time for fertilization or from the lack of normal oocytes. Early embryonic death or pregnancy reabsorption may cause infertility if all the embryos or fetuses are affected. Early embryonic death may result from chromosomal abnormalities inherent within the embryo, an aberration in normal development of the embryo, or a maternal environment that is incompatible with embryo viability. A hostile maternal environment may contribute to embryonic death either in the oviduct or in the uterus as a result of infection, hormone abnormalities or imbalances, cystic endometrial hyperplasia, or degenerative changes to the reproductive tract caused by any of those problems. Pregnancy reabsorption looks clinically like infertility and is differentiated from infertility by ultrasonography early in pregnancy. Pregnancy reabsorption results from fetal death during the first half of pregnancy. Fetal death can occur because of fetal abnormalities, genetic or acquired, or because of a hostile maternal environment (e.g., local intrauterine infection, cystic endometrial hyperplasia) or systemic disease in the female (e.g., endocrine, nutritional, neoplastic, or infectious disease).

Clinical Signs

The history includes a breeding of the female that does not result in a normal pregnancy carried to term with normal, viable offspring produced. Depending on the causative problem, there may be no other history than a breeding with no pregnancy resulting. Cycle abnormalities may be evident. The delivery of premature, diseased, stillborn, or weak neonates may also be part of the history. The only clinical sign with infertility may be the lack of parturition. In the case of abortion, a vulvar discharge is seen, with fetal tissues expelled (either fresh or autolyzed). There may be no fetal tissue observed because of the tendency for the females to ingest these as expelled. In the case of systemic female disease, the clinical signs vary with the condition involved.

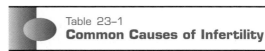

Table 23-1
Common Causes of Infertility

MALE	FEMALE	
	Normal Cycles	**Abnormal Cycles**
Testicular degeneration	Breeding management	Anestrus
High percentage of abnormal sperm	Uterine disease (cystic endometrial hyperplasia)	Prolonged estrus
Oligospermia	*Brucella canis* infection	Follicular cyst
Azoospermia	Feline leukemia virus infection	Granulosa cell tumor
Prostatitis (canine)	Feline infectious peritonitis	Hypothyroidism
Inability to breed		
Physical		
Behavioral		

Diagnostic Plan

In the female that is cycling normally, the two most common causes of infertility are male infertility and inadequate breeding management. The history should rule out cycle abnormalities of the female, which usually are related to ovarian-pituitary dysfunction (see Chap. 21). Physical examination should identify any systemic disease process that may be present. Abortion or delivery of dead fetuses should be evaluated aggressively (see Pregnancy Wastage and Dystocia).

Considerable variability is observed in the canine estrous cycle between and within individuals[8, 12]; therefore, timing of semen deposition is problematic. Breeding management must be addressed and maximized. The traditional breeding management recommendation in the dog is to breed on the first day of standing estrus and every other day until the bitch no longer stands. This should be done if possible or amenable to the client's situation. Ovulation timing kits are now available to aid in the timing of breedings. These are ELISA kits for progesterone. The first rise in progesterone correlates with the LH peak; ovulation should occur approximately 48 hours later. Another 48 to 72 hours is required for the primary oocyte to go through the two divisions required to become a fertilizable secondary oocyte. Serum samples should be tested every 2 to 3 days from the onset of proestrus to document this first rise in progesterone (2 µg/mL). The tentative plan would be to breed the bitch either 3 and 5 or 4 and 6 days after the first rise in progesterone. Progesterone testing and additional breedings should continue until the progesterone has risen above the upper limit of the ELISA kit (5–7.5 ng/mL). These higher levels of progesterone document that ovulation has taken place and therefore confirm that semen has been deposited in the bitch at the correct time. Peak fertility has been reported to occur when insemination takes place 0 to 5 days after the LH peak or within 2 to 3 days of ovulation.[13]

Breeding management in the queen differs from that in the bitch because of the characteristic of induced ovulation. When the male cat and queen are brought together in a breeding situation, an attempt should be made to observe the breeding to verify that it does take place. Multiple matings during the first 3 days of estrus are necessary to ensure that adequate LH is released from the pituitary. It has been shown that 100% of queens ovulated when bred four times consecutively (21–81 minutes).[7] Allowing unlimited matings over many days is not recommended because of compromise in the sperm output of the male and downregulation of the queen's pituitary LH release. Ovulation should take place approximately 48 hours after the induced LH peak. Serum progesterone levels can be determined in the queen 1 to 2 weeks after breeding to verify that ovulation has taken place. If it is suspected or confirmed that the queen is not ovulating at breeding, human chorionic gonadotropin (250 IU intramuscularly) or gonadotropin-releasing hormone (25 µg intramuscularly) given at breeding will help ensure that ovulation will take place.

Ultrasonography at 3 to 4 weeks determines the pregnancy status at that time and helps differentiate lack of conception from reabsorption or abortion of the pregnancy. Ultrasonography also is useful in detecting uterine diseases, which may be seen as a thickened uterus or uterine fluid (see Fig. 20–2).

The fertility of the dog and male cat should be evaluated and a fertile male chosen. Sperm quality (number, motility, morphology) influences whether adequate numbers of viable normal sperm cells reach the oocyte. A history of recent fertile matings is good circumstantial evidence of the male's fertility. A breeding soundness examination of the stud dog should be performed if fertility history is not available (see Chap.

21). Semen evaluation of the male cat is not often performed because of the difficulty in obtaining a semen sample. Trial breedings with the male dog or cat may help determine the animal's fertility status.

If breeding management and male fertility are determined to be adequate and pregnancy still does not result, the fertility of the bitch is then considered suspect. Estrous cycle regularity should be considered. In a bitch that is cycling normally (estrous cycle of 4–12 months, proestrus of 2–21 days, estrus of 2–21 days), an exploratory laparotomy to examine the bitch's reproductive tract should be considered as the next step in determining the cause of infertility. Surgery is best performed approximately 60 days after estrus, at the time when whelping should have occurred but did not. The uterus will still be under the influence of progesterone at that time, allowing an evaluation of the reproductive tract during diestrus. Biopsies of the ovary and uterus may reveal pathologic conditions undetectable by other means. A uterine culture should be obtained at surgery to determine the presence of potential pathogens. If severe or uncorrectable uterine or ovarian problems are detected at surgery, an ovariohysterectomy can be performed at this time. Treatment with prostaglandin $F_{2\alpha}$ (PGF) after surgery (0.05–0.1 mg/kg Lutalyse subcutaneously daily for 5 days) tends to improve fertility during the subsequent estrus in the bitch if mucometra or no obvious pathology is found.

An alternative approach to bitch infertility is surgical insemination (see Therapeutic Procedures). A cursory exploratory, visual examination of the uterus and ovaries without biopsy can be done at the same time as surgical insemination to rule out gross abnormalities of the reproductive tract. Pregnancies can be obtained by this method even after all other approaches have failed. Theories to explain the high success rate of surgical insemination include a possible hostile vaginal environment for semen or faulty sperm transport through the cervix.

Pregnancy Wastage

Pregnancy wastage is the death and elimination of any fertilized conceptus, whether by embryonic death, pregnancy reabsorption, or abortion (Table 23–2). Embryonic death involves death of the conceptus before closure of the thoracic cavity of the embryo, at which time the conceptus becomes a fetus. The incidence of embryonic death is not possible to determine with any accuracy because of the inability to detect pregnancies at this early stage of development.

Pregnancy reabsorption is the death and internal absorption of all fetal tissues with no vulvar discharge. Pregnancy reabsorption occurs if the pregnancy is lost before 30 days of gestation. Incidence of pregnancy reabsorption is difficult to determine but can accurately be documented with ultrasonography.

Abortion is the outward elimination of premature nonviable fetuses. Abortion occurs infrequently, though the incidence is unknown. The vulvar discharge seen with abortion may be difficult to differentiate from open-cervix pyometra. Pregnancy wastage can be seen in a bitch or queen of any age during the luteal phase that follows estrus.

Pathophysiology

Uterine infection, fetal infection, or placentitis may cause the death of fetuses and abortion. The most important cause of canine abortion is *Brucella canis* infection, which causes abortion during the last trimester. Toxoplasmosis can cause abortion in either species. Both *B. canis* and *Toxoplasma gondii* cause abortion by placentitis. Canine herpesvirus and canine distemper virus have been documented to cause abortion sporadically. Viral diseases may cause transplacental infection and death of the fetuses, which are not adequately immunocompetent. In the queen, both feline leukemia virus and feline infectious peritonitis are reported to cause pregnancy wastage, in the form of either abortion or pregnancy reabsorption.

Any systemic or debilitating disease process in the bitch or queen can adversely affect the outcome of a pregnancy. Any species of bacteria can cause abortion if not eliminated from the uterus before diestrus or if they gain access to the uterus through hematogenous routes or ascension through the cervix. Uterine bacteria cause an endometritis and metritis that can spread progressively throughout the uterus, undermining placental attachments. The most commonly reported

Table 23–2
Common Causes of Pregnancy Wastage

Uterine disease
  Cystic endometrial hyperplasia
  Pyometra
Infectious disease
  Brucella canis
  Feline leukemia virus
  Feline infectious peritonitis
  Toxoplasma
Endocrine disease
  Hypothyroidism
  Exogenous estrogen therapy
  Premature lysis of corpora lutea
Trauma

bacteria causing uterine infections are *Escherichia coli* and *Streptococcus* species. Trauma, particularly abdominal trauma, can cause abortion depending on the extent of damage to the dam, the uterus, placental attachments, and the fetuses.

Debilitating bacterial, viral, endocrine, or neoplastic conditions of the bitch can cause pregnancy wastage by a variety of mechanisms, not least of which is a negative energy balance. Adequate levels of thyroxine are critical for basal metabolism at all levels. Hypothyroidism is suspected to be a cause of pregnancy wastage, particularly in the bitch. Hypothyroidism is known to cause infertility in the bitch by adversely affecting the maternal environment (similarly to spontaneous abortion in the human female from this cause). Fetal reabsorption has been documented after estrogen therapy during estrus for misalliance.[14]

Adequate progesterone (>2 ng/mL) must be present to maintain the feline or canine pregnancy. If progesterone drops below 2 ng/mL, whether spontaneously or owing to induction by pharmaceuticals, the pregnancy is disrupted. Progesterone is necessary for the proper uterine environment for the maintenance of pregnancy, including endometrial gland development, quiescence of the myometrium, and closure of the cervix. Because both the queen and the bitch have luteal-dependent pregnancies, hypoluteoidism is a potential cause for pregnancy wastage.

Clinical Signs

The animal is intact and has had an estrus 4 to 7 weeks previously. A pregnancy, intended or not, has been observed or suspected. Systemic signs of disease may be evident with uterine infections (see Chap. 20). Clinical signs are seen only with abortion. Vulvar discharge, with or without fetal tissues, is a consistent sign with abortion. Abdominal contractions and expulsion of fetuses may also be seen. It is possible for part of a litter to be aborted and the remaining fetuses to be born normally at term. It is common for the bitch or queen to eat any tissue expelled from the uterus during an abortion. There are usually no abnormal physical examination findings other than a vulvar discharge and a palpable uterus.

Diagnostic Plan

Pregnancy diagnosis confirmed by ultrasonography early in gestation with no resultant parturition definitively diagnoses pregnancy reabsorption. With abortion, a physical examination should be performed to evaluate the systemic health of the animal. A complete blood count determines the presence of a systemic inflammatory response, particularly in toxemic patients. Serum chemistries aid in the diagnosis of endocrine abnormalities and the evaluation of liver and kidney function. Abdominal palpation may reveal the presence of additional fetuses, although it is difficult to differentiate them from an involuting uterus. Vaginoscopy may reveal an open cervix and the presence of other aborted fetuses. Digital examination detects the presence of a fetus only in the pelvic canal. Ultrasonography determines the presence of additional fetuses in the abdomen and their viability. Radiography is helpful only if the fetuses have undergone more than 40 days' gestation and therefore have sufficient skeletal calcification to been seen on a radiograph.

Vaginal cytology determines the presence of a uterine inflammatory response, indicating an infectious cause. Vaginal cultures obtained with the use of guarded culture instruments are helpful in determining which bacteria may be involved, primarily or secondarily. An aborting bitch should be isolated and handled carefully until *B. canis* has been ruled out. Serology for *B. canis* should be performed immediately. Serology for *T. gondii* may be considered and performed if deemed necessary. A second paired sample can be evaluated in 2 to 4 weeks to detect rising titers. Necropsy, including histopathology and appropriate bacterial culturing, should be performed on any fetus or fetal membranes available. Virus isolation for canine herpesvirus may be run at the time of necropsy.

Baseline thyroxine levels should be measured or thyroid-stimulating hormone response testing done to evaluate thyroid function. If all infectious causes of abortion or reabsorption have been ruled out, serial progesterone levels in subsequent pregnancies may be performed to document compatibility of progesterone levels with pregnancy. Progesterone must be above 2 ng/mL for a pregnancy to be maintained.

Dystocia

Dystocia is defined as a difficult birth (Table 23–3). Bitches experience dystocia at a higher rate than queens.

Pathophysiology

Many factors play a role in any dystocia. Uterine inertia is the inability of the uterus to contract sufficiently to push the fetuses through the birth canal. Primary uterine inertia is the failure of parturition to commence after the fall in progesterone that occurs at the end of pregnancy (see Primary Uterine Inertia). Aside from physiologic reasons, bitches have the ability to forestall parturition because of nervousness, undue distractions, or an aversion to pain. Incomplete uterine inertia is the cessation of uterine contractions during parturition. Fatigue plays a role, particularly in large litters. Secondary uterine inertia is the failure to push a fetus through the vagina and pelvic canal

Table 23-3
Causes of Dystocia

Fetopelvic Disproportion
Maternal
    Small pelvis (genetic, brachycephalic breeds)
    Pelvic canal compromise
        Obesity
        Pelvic fractures
    Vaginal or vestibular strictures
Fetal
    Oversized fetus
        Singleton litter, small litter size
        Genetic (brachycephalic breeds)
    Abnormal presentation

Uterine Inertia
Primary
    Hypocalcemia
    Hypoglycemia
    Genetic (familial tendency)
Incomplete
    Uterine fatigue, large litters
Secondary
    Fetal oversize
    Abnormal presentation
    Maternal blockage
        Soft tissue strictures
        Small pelvis

because of relative fetal oversize, abnormal presentation, or maternal blockage (i.e., soft tissue strictures or congenital or acquired pelvic narrowing).

Fetal-maternal disproportion is a primary cause of dystocia. Fetal oversize may result from a fetus that is too large or a pelvis that is too small (due to genetics, pelvic injury, pelvic fat in the obese dam). In some patients, particularly in brachycephalic breeds of dogs and cats, the pelvic canal may be proportionally too small to allow passage of the fetus. An oversized fetus may be unable to pass through the pelvic canal; this is more often seen in singleton litters. Fetal oversize in the case of a single fetus is caused by a lack of competition from other fetuses in a normally litter-bearing species. Occasionally, fetal presentation may cause a problem in fetal passage, such as hyperflexion of the neck or transverse presentation. Vaginal strictures may obstruct the passage of fetuses through the vagina or pelvis.

Clinical Signs

Incidence of dystocia is very high in brachycephalic breeds of dogs and cats, with English bulldogs

requiring cesarean section in almost all cases. Other brachycephalic breeds of dogs also have a high incidence of dystocia because of the tendency for large heads and shoulders with a proportionally small pelvis. Brachycephalic breeds of cats, Persians and Persian-based breeds, also exhibit a high incidence of dystocia. Pelvic fractures may cause a narrowing of the pelvic canal and predispose the bitch or queen to dystocia. Small toy breeds may exhibit a higher-than-normal incidence of dystocia because of their nervous temperaments, intolerance to pain, and tendency toward singleton litters. Giant-breed dogs tend to experience a higher-than-normal incidence of uterine inertia, taking many more hours to complete delivery than is compatible with fetal survival, particularly for the last pups delivered. Bitches that have very large litters, more than 10 or 12 pups, may experience fatigue requiring intervention. Patients that have had dystocias previously are at greater risk than those who have not. Most often, a patient with dystocia is presented after labor has begun with prolonged straining (>1 hour) or after a prolonged rest period (>4 hours) in which no pups or kittens have been delivered.

Diagnostic Plan

Radiographs should be taken to confirm the presence of fetuses within the abdomen. Abdominal palpation is an inaccurate method of confirming abdominal fetuses, because the uterus during labor is thickened and may feel like an additional fetus when none are there. A digital vaginal examination detects the presence of a fetus in the pelvic canal and, perhaps, the presence of a fetus in the vagina. A determination of fetal size compared to the maternal pelvis may be made at this time. If time permits, serum calcium and glucose may be measured.

Vulvar Discharge

Vulvar discharge is considered to be any discharge from the vulva excluding urine (see Chap. 22). Usually, no vulvar discharge is seen with embryonic death or pregnancy reabsorption. Vulvar discharges may be seen during a normal pregnancy. Clear mucoid discharges are considered normal. If the discharge is cloudy or has a foul odor, vaginal cytology should be performed to identify any inflammatory component to the discharge. Purulent discharges may be associated with bacterial abortions, pyometras, or diseases of the distal reproductive tract such as vaginitis. Hemorrhagic discharges during pregnancy may indicate an impending abortion. Vaginoscopy should be performed in purulent or hemorrhagic vulvar discharge to determine the extent and source of the discharge. Ultrasonography is helpful to determine the health of the uterus and the viability of the fetuses. If a pyometra exists in a pregnant bitch or queen, decisions must be made regarding treatment versus preservation of the pregnancy. Treatment for pyometra eliminates the pregnancy as well. Hemorrhagic discharges often are insignificant. If the pregnancy appears normal on ultrasonography, rest and exercise restriction may be the only treatment necessary (see Chap. 22 for a complete description of vulvar discharge).

Hypocalcemia

Hypocalcemia is defined as a serum calcium concentration lower than the normal range of 8 to 11 mg/dL. Clinical signs usually develop after calcium levels reach 7 mg/dL. Animals most often affected are bitches in late gestation or within the first 3 weeks of lactation (see Hypocalcemia and Eclampsia).

Diagnostic Procedures

Routine Laboratory Evaluation

A complete blood count helps detect systemic signs associated with uterine infections present during a pregnancy or a postpartum metritis. The most common finding with metritis and pyometra is leukocytosis with a regenerative left shift.[11] Biochemical profiles help detect metabolic abnormalities such as azotemia and dehydration and assess the health of other organ systems. Urinalysis, combined with the biochemical profile, evaluates renal function and screens for the presence of a concurrent urinary tract infection.

Abdominal Palpation

Abdominal palpation should allow for assessment of the size, consistency, and tone of the uterus. The technique is described in Chapter 20. Care must be taken when palpating a greatly enlarged uterus to avoid damage and rupture of the friable, thin-walled organ.

Brucella canis Serology

Serum should be tested for the presence of *B. canis* antibodies. The slide (or card) test is available to run in-hospital. These tests are very sensitive but not very specific. Therefore, false-positive results may occur. False-negative results are obtained only if the disease process is too early in its progression for antibody formation to have occurred or after long-term antibiotic therapy. Positive serology should be followed with a tube agglutination test, which is usually offered at diagnostic laboratories. A titer of less than 1:50 is considered nonsignificant. If the titer is greater than 1:50, an agar gel immunodiffusion test

should be run to differentiate the true-positive from the false-positive result. In the case of clinical signs, the animal should be isolated until results are confirmed.

Ultrasonography and Radiography

Ultrasonography can detect a pregnancy as early as 21 days after the LH peak. Multiple round, hypoechoic structures are seen, representing the amnionic vesicle and its fluid. The embryos can be seen as hyperechoic masses within the amnionic vesicle (see Fig. 20–1A). Heartbeats of fetuses are usually detectable in the fourth week of gestation. (Ultrasonography has the ability to assess fetal viability by visualizing fetal heartbeats, and with the more sophisticated machinery, fetal heart rates may be determined.) Fetal heart rates of 200 beats per minute or more are considered normal. Slower heart rates indicate fetal stress. Ultrasonography is not very accurate in assessing fetal numbers.

Radiography has the ability to detect uterine enlargement but is unable to differentiate that from pregnancy until after day 45, when the fetal skeletons are sufficiently calcified to be visible and accurate fetal counts may be performed (Fig. 23–1).

Serum Progesterone Assays

Progesterone levels can be easily measured from serum with ELISA kits available commercially or through laboratories that offer radioimmunoassay. If serum progesterone is ≥2 ng/mL, adequate progesterone levels are present to support a pregnancy, and luteal tissue is present on the ovaries. In the bitch, serum samples are taken within 60 days after estrus, and a progesterone level higher than 1 ng/mL confirms that ovulation has taken place. In the queen, pseudopregnancies do not last as long as pregnancies, and progesterone must be sampled 2 to 3 weeks after estrus (breeding) to confirm ovulation. Serum should be separated promptly after the blood has clotted. If the progesterone assay cannot be run immediately, the serum sample should be frozen.

Vaginal Cytology

Vaginal cytology is indicated whenever reproductive disease is suspected. Estrogen influence on the vaginal epithelium and inflammation or infection are easily detected with vaginal cytology (see Chap. 22).

Vaginoscopy

Vaginoscopy is indicated whenever vulvar discharges are present to determine the origin of these discharges. Vaginoscopy may help determine the

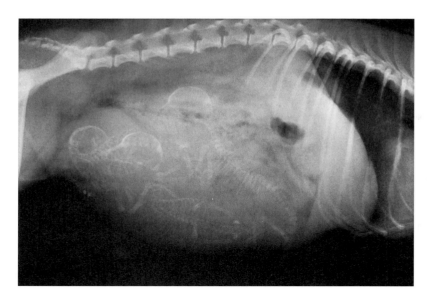

Figure 23-1
Prewhelping radiograph of a bitch at 64 days' gestation. Notice the three fully calcified fetal skeletons located between the diaphragm and the pelvic inlet.

degree of dilation of the cervix or detect the presence of fetuses during a dystocia. Vaginoscopy is used by some for breeding management because of the characteristic changes seen in the vaginal lining during estrus (see Chap. 22).

Vaginal Cultures

Bacterial cultures are indicated when purulent vulvar discharges are noted. *B. canis* requires special culture media and conditions; therefore, the laboratory should be advised if *B. canis* is suspected. Vaginal cultures should be obtained with a guarded culture instrument or carefully through a speculum. The distal part of the reproductive tract normally has high numbers of bacteria and should be avoided. For interpretation, see Chapter 22.

Therapeutic Procedures

Mismating and Pregnancy Termination

Unintentional pregnancies occur in the bitch and queen. Mismating, or misalliance, refers to the unwanted breeding of a female during estrus. Occasionally, it is desirable to end a pregnancy in a female whether or not the mating was intentional. The incidence of unintentional matings and pregnancies is difficult to determine, but considering the overpopulation problem of pets, the incidence can be considered high. If the bitch or queen is showing signs of estrus, the chance of a breeding's taking place is much higher. The incidence of pregnancies resulting from accidental matings has been reported as 38%.[15] Escape of the female while in estrus is frequently in the history. Witnessing of the breeding is proof that the female has

been exposed to semen but not proof of a pregnancy. Abdominal enlargement and a palpable, enlarged uterus are evident in most animals that are pregnant by 4 to 6 weeks after estrus. If the owner has not witnessed the breeding, the presence of sperm on vaginal cytologic examination is proof that the female has been mated (Fig. 23–2). Ultrasonography performed at 3 to 4 weeks after estrus determines whether a pregnancy is present.

Estrogen has traditionally been the treatment of choice for mismating. Estrogen causes aberrations in oviductal transport and changes in the uterine environment. Estrogen has fallen from favor because of the potential for permanent bone marrow suppression and development of pyometra in the dog.[16] Cats appear much more resistant to the harmful effects of estrogen therapy. Diethylstilbestrol has been shown to be ineffective in preventing pregnancies in the bitch, although it may reduce litter size owing to partial reabsorption of the litter.[17] Estradiol cypionate (ECP) has been demonstrated to be effective in preventing canine pregnancies at 44 µg/kg, but a 25% incidence of pyometra was observed in bitches given ECP during diestrus. ECP has a duration of action of 21 to 28 days[18] and should not be repeated more than once every 30 days. Estrogen therapy for mismating should be used only with great caution, complete client education, and the signing of a release form by the client. It is not recommended in breeding bitches because of the potential uterine changes that may follow estrogen administration. In nonbreeding bitches, an ovariohysterectomy should be considered during or immediately after estrus. In queens, an effective dose of ECP for mismating has been reported as 0.25 mg per animal.[19]

Because both canine and feline pregnancies

depend on ovarian progesterone, removal of this source of progesterone results in reabsorption or abortion of the litter. In bitches, it has been shown that prostaglandin $F_{2\alpha}$ (PGF) can be used to lyse the canine corpora lutea early in diestrus.[20] The onset of diestrus is documented with vaginal cytology, and PGF (Lutalyse) is administered between day 5 and day 10 of diestrus at a dosage of 0.25 mg/kg subcutaneously, twice a day for 4 days. Serum progesterone drops dramatically within several days of therapy. Serum progesterone levels should be measured within 1 week after the end of treatment to document baseline levels indicating complete luteolysis. If progesterone is higher than 2 ng/mL at this time, the treatment should be repeated.

PGF can be used later in diestrus in the bitch or queen. In the bitch, dosages of 0.1 to 0.25 mg/kg administered subcutaneously every 8 hours starting 30 to 35 days after breeding have been shown to be effective in aborting canine pregnancies. The pregnancy should be eliminated when the progesterone levels have been below 2 ng/mL for 36 to 48 hours. Abortion occurs within 9 days after initiation of therapy. Complete abortion should be documented by ultrasonography. Abdominal palpation alone is unreliable in determining completion of the abortion. If ultrasonography is not available, serum progesterone levels should be measured to document complete luteolysis. Serum progesterone levels should be measured 3 to 5 days after the abortion has been initiated to rule out the occurrence of possible luteal rebound.[21] In the queen, midgestation abortions can be accomplished by two subcutaneous injections of PGF, 0.5 to 1 mg/kg, administered 24 hours apart after day 40 of gestation.[22] Abortion occurs within 24 hours after the second injection. Another study reported 100% success in aborting fetuses in queens with intramuscular administration of 2 mg PGF daily for 5 days from day 33 of gestation.[23]

Side effects of prostaglandin therapy are dose related and are a result of its effects on smooth muscle. In the bitch, panting, salivation, vomiting, and defecation are typical side effects. The median lethal dose (LD_{50}) of PGF in the dog is 5 mg/kg. Because of the extreme physiologic effects of PGF, care must be taken in calculating the dosage for a dog. Only Lutalyse should be used, and dosages should never exceed 0.25 mg/kg. Side effects in queens are not as extreme and consist of panting, restlessness, and vocalization.

Alternative protocols for elective abortion involve the use of prolactin inhibitors. Prolactin is luteotropic in the bitch and queen during the last half of gestation.[6, 23] By use of prolactin inhibitors (dopamine agonists), luteolysis can be achieved and any existing pregnancy aborted. There is inadequate information to recommend use of prolactin inhibitors at this

time in the queen. In the bitch, these protocols are best started between day 30 and day 35 of gestation. Bromocriptine is administered orally, 0.01 mg/kg three times per day (t.i.d.) for 5 to 6 days or to effect. Bromocriptine is available in 2.5-mg tablets, which is a very stable form of this compound. After dilution in water, bromocriptine is not very stable and must be kept in brown glass at refrigerator temperatures for the duration of therapy. PGF is administered daily starting on day 3 of therapy at 0.1 mg/kg subcutaneously t.i.d. and continued for 2 days after the day of abortion. Abortion usually occurs on day 5 or 6 (range 3–8). With the use of a prolactin inhibitor, mammary development after the drop in progesterone is avoided. PGF has been added to this protocol for the smooth muscle contraction effect, which aids in uterine involution. A side effect of both bromocriptine and PGF is vomiting. If vomiting becomes a clinically significant problem, an antiemetic may be used sparingly.

Surgical Insemination

Surgical insemination has proven to be a legitimate treatment for infertility in the bitch. Timing must be accurate because of the radical nature of the insemination process. Insemination should take place approximately 4 to 5 days after the LH peak. The LH peak can be identified indirectly through the use of progesterone assays or directly by LH assays. If the former is used, it is important to run additional assays after the first rise of progesterone is detected to document that ovulation has proceeded as expected. If

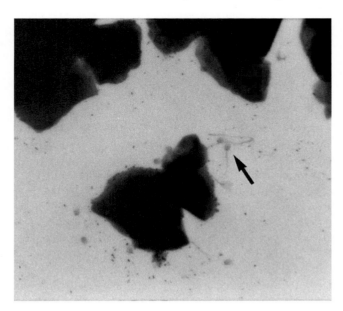

Figure 23–2

Vaginal cytology preparation from a bitch in estrus after breeding. Notice the cornified epithelial cells, indicative of estrus, and the presence of sperm (arrow).

LH assays are used, it is advisable to also run concurrent progesterone assays for the same reason. Surgical insemination should take place 48 hours after ovulation (4 days after LH peak) if fresh or fresh-cooled semen is used, and 72 hours after ovulation (5 days after LH peak) if frozen semen is used. Surgical insemination is considered mandatory for good conception rates when frozen semen is used.

Surgical insemination is a simple technique. The abdominal incision allows access to the uterine body. The uterine body is elevated out of the abdominal cavity. The semen can be injected directly into the uterine body through a 20- or 22-gauge needle or through a similar-sized intravenous catheter with a stylet. If a catheter is used, a hole is first blunt-punched into the uterine lumen with the distal end of the suture needle. The catheter is then inserted through the prepunched hole into the uterine lumen, and the stylet is removed. The semen is collected and placed into a syringe. The syringe is then attached to the catheter or needle, which has been placed into the uterine lumen. The semen is injected slowly into the uterine lumen. The uterus is seen (or felt) to fill and expand as the semen enters the uterine lumen. If semen is injected through a needle, the semen should flow easily into the uterus. If any resistance is felt, the location of the needle should be evaluated and the needle redirected until the semen flows easily into the uterine lumen.

As in any artificial insemination, the semen should be handled correctly and protected against any temperature, chemical, or mechanical damage. Frozen semen should be thawed according to the directions provided by the semen processor. Fresh or cooled shipped semen should be handled at room temperature and placed directly into the uterus without any attempt to heat the semen sample. Contact with spermicidal agents (e.g., water, detergents, detergent residues) should be avoided. Mechanical damage to the sperm cells can be avoided by slow aspiration and expression of the semen into and out of the syringe. Centrifugation of the semen sample should be avoided. The average volume inseminated is 4 to 5 mL.

Hand-rearing of Puppies and Kittens

Hand-rearing of neonates may be necessary in the event of death of the dam. Other situations that may dictate hand-rearing are severe mastitis, systemic illness of the bitch, or rejection of the neonates by the dam. It is desirable to leave the neonates with the dam, if possible, for assistance in heat regulation, urination and defecation, and species interaction and socialization. Complete nursing care of neonates is most intense during the first 3 weeks of life and requires 24-hour-per-day commitment from the caregiver.

The first consideration in hand-rearing neonates is the ingestion of colostrum during the first 12 hours after birth. In one study, the level of serum immunoglobulins (IgG) from puppies who were allowed to suckle and obtain colostrum measured in the range of 1700 mg/dL on day 2 after parturition, whereas the level in colostrum-deprived puppies that received subcutaneous serum was approximately 214 mg/dL.[24] It has been shown that partial protection can be obtained in puppies with the use of pooled canine serum injected subcutaneously at a dose of 22 mL/kg of body weight.[24] If this is injected slowly, the puppies tolerate the procedure well. However, it is preferable to allow the neonates to obtain colostrum by suckling, because serum immunoglobulin levels obtained by injection of canine serum are significantly lower than those obtained by colostrum ingestion. Because of gut closure, suckling should occur during the first 12 hours after birth, preferably during the first 4 hours. Subcutaneous serum produces significantly higher serum levels of immunoglobulin than oral administration of serum.

For the first 3 weeks of life, normal neonatal activity includes eating, sleeping, dreaming, urinating, and defecating. If neonates are being hand-reared, these vital functions should be monitored and assisted as necessary. Neonates are usually quiet; crying indicates problems, usually hunger or cold. The three most common causes of neonatal mortality are hypothermia, hypoglycemia, and hypovolemia. It is advisable to perform necropsies on all neonates that die in an attempt to ascertain the cause of death. If problems with septicemia are suspected, antibiotics may be administered orally (chloramphenicol, 50 mg/kg t.i.d.).

Hypothermia is, by far, the biggest killer of neonates. Puppies and kittens are poikilothermic for the first 2 weeks of life. They cannot regulate their body temperature with panting or shivering. Environmental ambient temperatures are not as life-threatening as are drafts. Care must be taken to protect the neonates from drafts. Heating pads and heat lamps are useful if used carefully. It is possible to overheat the neonates, and they must be able to move away from the heat source if they so desire. Once neonates become hypothermic, they cease to nurse. Hypoglycemia and hypovolemia result after oral intake of nutrients and fluids stops.

Daily weighing of neonates is the easiest way to assess adequate intake of nutrients. Both puppies and kittens should gain weight, approximately 5% to 10% of their birth weight, on a daily basis. If this does not occur, they have actually lost weight. Relative or actual weight loss precedes most serious and life-threatening neonatal conditions. Oral supplementation of commercial bitch or queen milk should be administered at 3- to 4-hour intervals at the recommended dose by stomach tube or by bottle. Most neonates are able to consume 45 to 50 mL/kg per feeding. Feeding of electrolyte solutions in between may be helpful in combating or preventing dehydration.

If it is not possible to leave the neonates with the dam, neonatal elimination must be assisted by stimulating urination and defecation by stroking over the perineal area using a warm, moist cloth. It is best to stimulate elimination after each feeding. Soft food can be offered as early as 3 weeks of age. After the neonates are eating on their own, supplementation can be discontinued.

Common Diseases of Pregnancy and Puerperium

Brucella canis Infection

B. canis is an intracellular organism that is highly contagious among dogs. The organism is passed venereally and is discharged in profuse numbers during abortion. Any mucous membrane contact with the organism, particularly oral contact, can establish infection in other dogs. Typically, the infection is inapparent in the bitch until she becomes pregnant and aborts. In the male dog, orchitis and epididymitis are common. The organism is spread rapidly throughout a kennel if a bitch aborts a pregnancy and other dogs come in contact with the abortion fluids. Human cases have been reported, primarily in people handling the aborting bitch or handling the organism in a laboratory setting.

Pathophysiology

B. canis is an intracellular organism that has a predilection for the placenta in the bitch and for the testis and epididymis in the male dog. This organism is highly contagious to other canids and renders both sexes essentially infertile. Abortion is caused by placentitis. Orchitis and epididymitis are seen in the acute phase of the disease process in the male, and testicular atrophy is seen in the chronic phase. Because of the intracellular location of the organism, treatment with antibiotics is difficult. Chronic *B. canis* disease often results in discospondylitis and periodic bacteremia.

Clinical Signs

In the bitch, no clinical signs are seen until a pregnancy is initiated. Abortion is typically seen during the last trimester. Less commonly, an abortion may occur late with apparently stillborn or weak puppies delivered. In the male dog, consistent clinical signs are orchitis and epididymitis initially with testicular degeneration and atrophy during the chronic stage of the disease process.

Diagnostic Plan

B. canis should be considered in any case of abortion in the bitch or orchitis or epididymitis in the dog. Culture of the organism provides the definitive diagnosis. Culture should be attempted from blood or from the abortion fluids. Special media are necessary, and the laboratory should be advised whenever this organism is suspected. Serologic tests for antibodies to *B. canis* provide the most common method of diagnosis. Slide tests for *B. canis* are available commercially and are accurate and reliable for screening. Tube agglutination tests are available through many diagnostic laboratories. Titers of 1:50 or less are considered insignificant. Both the slide and the tube tests are sensitive but not very specific. False-positive results are common. Agar gel immunodiffusion tests differentiate between false positives and true positives by testing for antibodies not only to cell surface antigens but to cytoplasmic antigens as well.

Treatment

The treatment of choice with *B. canis* is euthanasia of all infected animals. The only proven method of eradication from a kennel is testing and elimination of infected animals. Strict isolation and sanitation procedures have failed to protect uninfected animals in kennels where *B. canis*–positive animals are present.[25] The second treatment option is ovariohysterectomy of bitches and neutering of male dogs, followed by long-term antibiotic therapy (e.g., tetracycline 10 mg/kg per day for 30 days and streptomycin 4 mg/kg intramuscularly on days 1 through 7 and days 24 through 30).[26] Spread of *B. canis* is primarily related to the reproductive process. If the choice is made to retain the animal as a pet by neutering and treating with antibiotics, the animal should be tested yearly to detect any bacterial recrudescence. If recrudescence is detected, antibiotic therapy should be repeated.

Prognosis

Canine brucellosis is generally considered to be incurable,[27] and no antibiotic regimen has been shown to be 100% effective. A dog infected with *B. canis* should be eliminated from any breeding program, either by euthanasia or by neutering and long-term antibiotic therapy. If the infected animal is not killed, it is advisable to keep the dog away from children, immunocompromised individuals, and women of childbearing age to avoid infection of humans.

Canine Herpesvirus

Canine herpesvirus is reported to cause pregnancy reabsorption, abortion, and neonatal deaths in the dog. Canine herpesvirus is ubiquitous in the environment and in the general dog population.

Pathophysiology

Neonatal puppies are exposed to canine herpesvirus as they come through the birth canal, from other dogs in the environment including their own littermates, from oronasal secretions of the dam, or from fomites. Canine herpesvirus is a temperature-sensitive virus that grows best at 35° C to 36° C. Because adult dog body temperatures are above this ideal temperature, the virus grows best on mucous membranes. For the first 2 weeks of life, neonatal puppies are poikilothermic and unable to regulate their body temperature. In addition, they are unable to mount an adequate fever (inflammatory reponse).[28] Passive immunity obtained from the dam serves to protect the neonate. With seropositive dams, the puppies may become infected but remain asymptomatic. Severe clinical signs of canine herpesvirus occur only if the dam was exposed to the virus for the first time during the last 3 weeks of pregnancy or if the puppies were exposed during the first 2 to 3 weeks of life. If exposure occurs during this critical 5- to 6-week window, lethal neonatal infection ensues. Subsequent litters are unaffected because of seroconversion and adequate protection from the bitch.[28] Typically for herpesvirus, seroconversion with canine herpesvirus results in very low titers.

Clinical Signs

In dogs that are 2 to 3 weeks of age or older, typical infections with canine herpesvirus cause mild rhinitis or vaginitis. The physical symptoms seen with canine herpesvirus in the adult dog are mild, transitory, and usually missed by the client. Clinical signs in puppies typically occur between 7 and 14 days after birth and include depression, loss of interest in suckling, persistent crying, and abdominal discomfort, often accompanied by soft yellow-green feces. Petechial hemorrhages are widespread on mucous membranes. Rhinitis may be present with serous, mucopurulent to hemorrhagic nasal discharges. Puppies quickly lose consciousness, show seizure activity, and die within 24 to 48 hours after the onset of clinical signs. With intensive nursing, puppies may survive the acute infection but are typically affected with persistent neurologic signs such as ataxia, blindness, and cerebellar vestibular deficits.

Diagnostic Plan

Diagnosis of canine herpesvirus usually is made by identification of characteristic histopathologic lesions in the puppies or by virus isolation. Serology for titers to canine herpesvirus is possible but is usually unavailable.

Treatment

Treatment of affected neonatal puppies involves elevation of body temperature and intensive supportive therapy. Because of the persistent neurologic deficits in those puppies surviving systemic canine herpesvirus infections, treatment is unrewarding.

Prognosis

The prognosis of systemic neonatal infection is grave. However, bitches losing a litter to canine herpesvirus can subsequently give birth to normal litters.

Primary Uterine Inertia

Primary uterine inertia is the failure of parturition to commence after the fall in progesterone. It is poorly understood. After progesterone has fallen below 2 ng/mL, uterine motility should return. Rising estrogen levels, increased numbers of oxytocin receptors, and prostaglandin release should contribute to the increase in uterine motility and contractility.

Pathophysiology

Primary uterine inertia is thought to be caused, in part, by aberrations in calcium or glucose metabolism. There appears to be a hereditary component because uterine inertia occurs frequently in certain family lines or breeds. Aside from physiologic causes, bitches have the ability to forestall parturition because of nervousness, undue distractions, or an aversion to pain.

Clinical Signs

There may be no clinical signs. Abdominal enlargement and mammary development should accompany the pregnancy but may be seen in pseudopregnancies as well. Vulvar discharges may occur. Early, these discharges may be the normal allantoic fluid seen during parturition. If fetal death has occurred, the discharge may be black and tarry. Purulent discharges may be seen in cases of primary uterine inertia that have been ongoing longer than 24 to 48 hours as a result of ascending bacterial contamination of the uterus.

Diagnostic Plan

Primary uterine inertia is seen most commonly in patients presented because whelping should have occurred but has not (see Dystocia). Because pseudopregnancies may appear identical to pregnancies, radiography or ultrasonography is indicated. Abdominal radiographs confirm the presence, location, and number of fetuses. Ultrasonography determines fetal viability. The presence of a thick, tarry, black vulvar discharge is usually indicative of fetal death. Puppies that have not been delivered at the correct time (65 days after the LH peak) die quickly in utero.

Intervention in a pregnancy should never be done if gestation length is unknown. Determination of canine gestation length from breeding dates alone is highly inaccurate in many cases. Canine gestation lengths are predictably 65 days from the LH peak. A less accurate way to predict gestation is from the vaginal cytology. Bitches whelp 56 or 57 days after the change in vaginal cytology from estrus to diestrus. Feline gestation has been reported to vary from 58 to 70 days, with an average of 63 days from breeding, ovulation following breeding by 24 hours.

Owners that have been taking the bitch's temperature may become concerned when whelping has not taken place within 12 to 24 hours after a drop in temperature. Progesterone levels may be measured to determine whether the progesterone levels have truly decreased.

Treatment

If primary uterine inertia is suspected with prolonged gestation as a result, pregnancy should be confirmed by radiography. If fetuses are present, progesterone levels should be assessed as quickly as possible. Fetal viability can be assessed with ultrasonography. The presence of fetal heartbeats indicates fetal viability. Fetal stress is indicated if fetal heart rates are less than 200 beats per minute. If progesterone levels are baseline (<2 ng/mL) and fetal stress is present, cesarean section should be performed immediately. If progesterone is less than 2 ng/mL but no fetal stress is detected, calcium and glucose measurements may be made and deficits corrected. Bitches should be placed in a quiet area and monitored closely. If whelping does not occur within 24 hours after the progesterone has fallen below 2 ng/mL, a cesarean section is indicated. If progesterone levels are higher than 2 ng/mL, the bitch is not ready to whelp and no treatment is indicated.

Prognosis

Prognosis for the dam is usually good if intervention is prompt. Prognosis is variable for the offspring. Predelivery fetal stress makes the prognosis for neonatal survival poor. Patients that have had previous problems with uterine inertia have a greater chance for future problems.

Hypocalcemia and Eclampsia

Aberrations of calcium metabolism can cause hypocalcemia before or after parturition. In dogs, the incidence is highest in small breeds; the condition is seen only rarely in cats. Hypocalcemia is most commonly seen during the first 3 weeks of lactation but may occur before parturition or later in lactation.

Pathophysiology

The cause of the actual hypocalcemia is not well understood. The clinical signs result from the hypocalcemia, which causes aberrations in cell membrane potential that allow spontaneous discharge of nerve fibers. The heavy requirements for calcium associated with lactation may compromise the dam's ability to maintain adequate plasma levels because of relative parathyroid gland dysfunction. Gestational supplementation with calcium may predispose to hypocalcemia.

Clinical Signs

Behavioral changes may be seen first, including restlessness, panting, or whining. Progression to trembling, stiff or painful gait, increased salivation, ataxia, inability to stand, and profound hyperthermia (106° F–108° F) is seen. Muscle fasciculations, tonic-clonic muscle spasms, and seizure-like activity occur later in the disease progression. Death may result from respiratory arrest or hyperthermia.

Diagnostic Plan

Diagnosis is made initially from clinical signs in late gestation or in the lactating female. Confirmation of the diagnosis is made when serum calcium levels are determined to be less than 7 mg/dL.

Treatment

Calcium is administered intravenously as 10% calcium gluconate, to effect; the usual amount administered is 5 to 20 mL. This immediately corrects the serum deficit for calcium. Calcium is administered slowly, and the heart rate is monitored for bradycardia or arrhythmias. Clinical signs should immediately regress.[29] The same amount of calcium gluconate mixed with equal parts of saline may be administered subcutaneously to prevent immediate relapse. Calcium carbonate can be administered only intravenously or by mouth. After the body temperature and other clinical signs have returned to normal, the animal may be sent home on oral calcium supplementation (calcium carbonate 100 mg/kg of body weight, divided t.i.d.). The puppies should be removed from the dam for 12 to 24 hours. The animal should be monitored closely for any recurrence of clinical signs. The puppies should be weaned as soon as possible if they are older than 3 weeks of age. If the clinical signs recur, serious consideration should be given to hand-rearing the puppies until they can be placed on solid food. Milk production may be reduced by limiting puppy nursing and supplementing with hand-feeding.[11]

Prognosis

With immediate therapy, most animals should survive a hypocalcemic episode. Bitches can die from the acute effects of hypocalcemia or during treatment with intravenous calcium as a result of cardiac effects. There may be recurrence in the same lactation, at which time removal of the puppies is indicated. There is a tendency for recurrence with subsequent pregnancies as well as a hereditary component to the problem.

Postpartum Metritis

Postpartum metritis is an acute bacterial disease occurring in the immediate postpartum period. Postpartum metritis is a common occurrence after gestational intrauterine infections, retained placentas or fetuses, dystocias, or abortions. Unclean environmental conditions may also lead to ascending infections after parturition.

Pathophysiology

Postpartum metritis is caused by ascending bacterial contamination coupled with delayed uterine involution. Bacteria colonize the uterine lumen and are not expelled with the uterine lochia after parturition. Endometritis and metritis develop (see Chap. 20).

Clinical Signs

Purulent vulvar discharges, depression, fever, anorexia, and neglect of offspring are commonly seen.

Diagnostic Plan

Vaginal cytology demonstrates a purulent inflammatory discharge with neutrophils predominating. A firm, enlarged uterus can be felt on abdominal palpation. A complete blood count demonstrates leukocytosis, usually with a left shift.

Treatment

The treatment is described in Chapter 20.

Prognosis

Prognosis for the life of the dam is usually guarded to good, depending on the cause, extent of uterine damage, and response to therapy. With prompt therapy, most females respond and do well. Future fertility may be impaired, depending on the underlying cause of the metritis.

Subinvolution of Placental Sites

Subinvolution of placental sites (SIPS) is the failure of the zonary placental sites to involute in a normal fashion. There is no information on the incidence, but the condition occurs sporadically throughout the canine breeding population.

Pathophysiology

The underlying cause of SIPS is not understood. Histologically, the affected areas are erosions with trophoblastic (giant) cells embedded at the sites of placental attachment. Blood leaks from the erosions and produces the vulvar discharge.

Clinical Signs

A hemorrhagic, vulvar discharge that persists longer than 4 to 6 weeks after parturition in an otherwise normal animal is pathognomonic for SIPS.

Diagnostic Plan

Vaginal cytology reveals only red cells along with noncornified epithelial cells; there are no signs of inflammation. Abdominal palpation may reveal thickened areas throughout the uterus, but often these areas are not palpable. Ultrasonographic evidence of SIPS may be identified by thickened areas of the uterus that are evident because of uterine luminal fluid. The animal otherwise shows no signs of illness. Rarely, there may be enough blood loss to cause anemia.

Treatment

One option for therapy is to do nothing. SIPS is considered a self-limited problem. Monitoring of the animal is indicated for the duration of the vulvar discharge. Administration of prostaglandins may hasten resolution of the problem as a result of their effects on smooth muscle. Lutalyse, administered at 0.1 mg/kg subcutaneously once a day for 5 days, usually eliminates the discharge. If bleeding persists, this regimen may be repeated.

Prognosis

Prognosis after SIPS is excellent for the bitch as well as for its future fertility. Blood loss is rarely significant; if it is, evaluation for coagulopathies should be considered.

References

1. Roberts SJ. Veterinary Obstetrics and Genital Diseases: Theriogenology. North Pomfret, Vermont, David and Charles, 1986:45–47.
2. Verstegen JP, Onclin K, Silva LDM, et al. Regulation of progesterone during pregnancy in the cat: Studies on the roles of corpora lutea, placenta and prolactin secretion. J Reprod Fertil Suppl 1993;47:165–173.
3. Sokolowski JH. The effects of ovariectomy on pregnancy maintenance in the bitch. Lab Anim Sci 1971;21:696–699.
4. Verhage HG, Beamer NB, Brenner RM. Plasma levels of estradiol and progesterone in the cat during polyestrus, pregnancy and pseudopregnancy. Biol Reprod 1976;14: 579–585.
5. Concannon PW, Powers ME, Holder W, et al. Pregnancy and parturition in the bitch. Biol Reprod 1977;16:517–526.
6. Onclin K, Silva LDM, Donnay I, et al. Luteotrophic action of prolactin in dogs and the effect of a dopamine agonist, cabergoline. J Reprod Fertil Suppl 1993;47:403–409.
7. Concannon P, Hodgson B, Lein D. Reflex LH release in estrous cats following single and multiple copulations. Biol Reprod 1980;23:111–117.
8. Concannon PW. Clinical and endocrine correlates of canine ovarian cycles and pregnancy. In: Kirk RW, ed. Current Veterinary Therapy IX. Philadelphia, WB Saunders, 1986:1214–1224.
9. Holst PA, Phemister, RD. Onset of diestrus in the beagle bitch: Definition and significance. Am J Vet Res 1974;35: 401–406.
10. Lein DH, Concannon PW. Infertility and fertility treatments and management in the queen and tomcat. In: Kirk RW, ed. Current Veterinary Therapy VIII. Philadelphia, WB Saunders, 1983:936–942.
11. Feldman EC, Nelson RW. Canine and Feline Endocrinology and Reproduction. Philadelphia, WB Saunders, 1987:399–547.
12. Bouchard G, Youngquist RS, Vaillancourt D, et al. Seasonality and variability of the interestrous interval in the bitch. Theriogenology 1991;36:41–49.
13. Concannon PW, McCann JP, Temple M. Biology and endocrinology of ovulation, pregnancy and parturition in the dog. J Reprod Fertil Suppl 1989;39:3–25.
14. Bowen RA, Olson PN, Behrendt MD, et al. Efficacy and toxicity of estrogens commonly used to terminate canine pregnancy. J Am Vet Med Assoc 1985;186:783–788.
15. Feldman EC, Davidson AP, Nelson RW, et al. Prostaglandin induction of abortion in pregnant bitches after misalliance. J Am Vet Med Assoc 1993;202:1855–1858.
16. Crafts RC. The effects of estrogens on the bone marrow of adult female dogs. Blood 1948;3:276–285.
17. Bowen RA, Olson PN, Behrendt MD, et al. Efficacy and toxicity of estrogens commonly used to terminate canine pregnancy. J Am Vet Med Assoc 1985;186:783–788.
18. American Hospital Formulary Service. Am Soc Hosp Pharm 1983;2:68:16.
19. Schmidt PM. Feline breeding management. Vet Clin North Am Small Anim Pract 1986;16:435–451.
20. Romagnoli SE, Camillo F, Cela M, et al. Clinical use of prostaglandin F_{2a} to induce early abortion in bitches: Serum progesterone, treatment outcome and interval to subsequent estrus. J Reprod Fertil Suppl 1993;47:425–431.
21. Henderson RT. Prostaglandin therapeutics in the bitch and queen. Aust Vet J 1984;61:317–319.
22. Nachreiner RF, Marple DN. Termination of pregnancy in cats with prostaglandin F_{2a}. Prostaglandins 1974;7: 303–307.
23. Verstegen JP, Onclin K, Silva LDM, et al. Abortion induction in the cat using prostaglandin F_{2a} and a new anti-prolactinic agent, cabergoline. J Reprod Fertil Suppl 1993;47:411–417.
24. Poffenbarger EM, Olson PN, Chandler ML, et al. Use of adult dog serum as a substitute for colostrum in the neonatal dog. Am J Vet Res 1991;52:1221–1224.
25. Pickerill PA, Carmichael LE. Canine brucellosis: Control programs in commercial kennels and effect on reproduction. J Am Vet Med Assoc 1972;160:1607–1615.
26. Nicoletti P, Chase A. The use of antibiotics to control canine brucellosis. Compen Contin Educ Pract Vet 1987;9:1063–1066.
27. Johnson CA, Walker RD. Clinical signs and diagnosis of *Brucella canis* infection. Compen Contin Educ Pract Vet 1992;14:763–773.
28. Green CE, Kakuk TJ. Canine herpesvirus infection. In: Greene CE, ed. Clinical Microbiology and Infectious Diseases of the Dog and Cat. Philadelphia, WB Saunders, 1984:419–429.
29. Smith FO. Postpartum diseases in reproduction and periparturient care. Vet Clin North Am Small Anim Pract 1986;16:521–524.

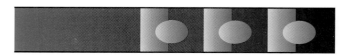

Neurologic
Diseases

Chapter 24

Diseases of the Cerebrum

Linda G. Shell

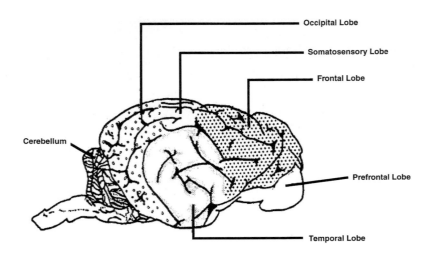

Figure 24–1
Diagrammatic lateral view of the dog brain demonstrating the relative positions of the four lobes of the cerebrum. (Modified with permission from McGrath JT. Neurologic Examination of the Dog. Philadelphia, Lea & Febiger, 1960.)

Anatomy

The cerebrum is the largest part of the brain. It consists of two equal hemispheres separated along the dorsal midline but united ventrally by a mass of white matter called the corpus callosum. Structurally, the cerebrum consists of a peripheral layer of gray matter or neurons called the cerebral cortex, white matter beneath the cortex, centrally located basal nuclei, and the phylogenetically older olfactory portions. The surface of the cerebrum is wrinkled by gyri (elevations) and sulci (depressions).[1, 2] Inside each cerebral hemisphere is a cavity, the lateral ventricle, which is filled with cerebrospinal fluid (CSF). The two lateral ventricles connect with the third ventricle, located in the midbrain, which connects with the fourth ventricle, located beneath the cerebellum in the pontine-medullary area.

Three membranes cover the surface of the brain and spinal cord and protect the nervous tissue. The outermost layer, the dura mater, adheres to the periosteum of the cranial vault. The next layer, the arachnoid membrane, has web-like projections connecting it to the innermost layer, the pia mater. CSF flows in the space between the arachnoid membrane and the pia mater. A large collection of CSF in the subarachnoid space is located between the caudal cerebellum and the medulla, the cerebellomedullary cistern,[2] and is the preferred site of CSF collection for patients with disorders of the cerebrum or brain stem.

The surface of each hemisphere is divided into four lobes with distinct functions yet indistinct anatomic boundaries; these are the frontal, somatosensory, temporal, and occipital lobes (Fig. 24–1). The frontal lobe has two sections: the prefrontal area, which contributes to behavior, and the motor area, which contributes to voluntary movements. The somatosensory lobe processes sensory information from peripheral receptors that detect pain, touch, and proprioception.[3, 4] Audition and behavioral activity are functions of the temporal lobe, and vision is the major function of the occipital lobe.

Physiology

Neurons are unable to use ketones or fatty acids to any extent and therefore require glucose for energy. Because neurons cannot store more than a minute amount of glucose, the brain must rely on readily available sources of glucose for energy production and oxygen for its metabolism.[5, 6] Thiamine (vitamin B_1) is also needed as a coenzyme for some of the biochemical reactions. Hypoxia, hypoglycemia, and thiamine deficiency can alter neural energetics and result in cerebral signs.

The blood-brain barrier is an anatomic and physiologic barrier between the systemic circulation and the brain. It exists between the plasma and extracellular fluid at the capillary level and consists of a thick basement membrane between central nervous system (CNS) capillaries and astroglial foot processes.[2] As long as this barrier functions normally, it is impermeable to proteins as well as many therapeutic agents (Table 24–1).[7] The blood-CSF barrier is similar to the blood-brain barrier except that it exists at the choroid plexus level, and fenestrations or pores make it semipermeable.[2] These barriers prevent antigens and antibodies in the circulation from reaching the CNS. Consequently, analysis of normal CSF reveals little albumin, almost no globulins, and only a few cells (lymphocytes).

CSF is continually produced by the choroid plexuses of the ventricles and circulates throughout the ventricular system, the central canal, and the subarachnoid space. CSF absorption occurs at the arachnoid villi in the venous sinuses or major cerebral veins.

The blood vessels of the brain are sensitive to blood carbon dioxide (CO_2) concentration, dilating with increased CO_2 levels and constricting with decreased levels. Increased CO_2 levels can result in cerebral edema, and decreased levels can result in ischemia. In acid-base imbalances, CO_2 easily passes the blood-CSF barrier, but bicarbonate exchange is slow because of the relative impermeability of this barrier to bicarbonate.[2] A rapid correction of metabolic acidosis may drive CO_2, but not bicarbonate, across the barrier; this can cause paradoxical CNS acidosis.

Problem Identification

Each lobe of the cerebrum has a distinct function that can be related to clinical signs. The most common clinical problems associated with cerebral disturbances are motor and sensory deficits, behavioral changes, seizures, and central blindness.

Motor and Sensory Deficits

Motor deficits are characterized by weakness or decreased strength of voluntary movements of the limbs and sometimes of the muscles of facial expression. Sensory deficits are characterized by impaired

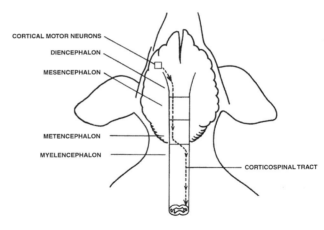

Figure 24-2
Diagrammatic representation of the origin and path of the corticospinal tract, one of the motor tracts. A lesion located in the left cerebrum or diencephalon should cause motor deficits on the right side of the body because the tracts cross over in the middle to the caudal brain stem region.

proprioception and reduced behavioral responses to noxious stimuli. Normally, for example, pinching of the upper lip of a dog or cat with a hemostat results in a whine, cry, or head turn as well as retraction of the lip. Proprioception deficits are sometimes difficult to differentiate from weakness of movement.

Pathophysiology

The motor area contains cell bodies (upper motor neurons) that give rise to the corticospinal system. This system, which is phylogenetically a newer acquisition of the nervous system, has its greatest physiologic expression in humans and higher primates. Although paralysis is a result of corticospinal lesions in humans, dogs and cats show only mild weakness. This is probably because the rubrospinal tract, located in the brain stem, is a more important motor tract in animals than is the corticospinal tract.[8]

In both animals and humans with unilateral motor cortex lesions, motor and sensory deficits are always found opposite the side of the lesion. Contralateral motor deficits are explained by the fact that corticospinal axons, descending from the cerebral cortex, cross in the lower brain stem and descend in the spinal cord on the side opposite their origin (Fig. 24-2).[9] Contralateral sensory deficits occur because afferent (sensory) neurons ascend the spinal cord through tracts that cross over in the brain stem before reaching the somatosensory lobe of the cerebrum (Fig. 24-3).[4]

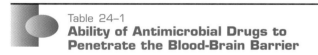

Table 24-1
Ability of Antimicrobial Drugs to Penetrate the Blood-Brain Barrier

GOOD	FAIR IF BLOOD-BRAIN BARRIER IS DAMAGED	POOR
Chloramphenicol	Tetracyclines*	Aminoglycosides
Trimethoprim	Flucytosine	Clindamycin
Sulfonamides	Ampicillin*	Amphotericin B
Metronidazole	Ticarcillin*	Erythromycin
Fluconazole	Penicillin G*	Ketoconazole
Rifampin	Nafcillin*	Amoxicillin-clavulanate
	Carbenicillin*	
	Methicillin*	First-generation
	Ureidopenicillins	cephalosporins
	Cefuroxine	Cefaclor
	Cefotaxime	Cefadroxil
	Ceftazidime	Cephalexin
	Ceftizoxime	Cephradine
	Ceftriaxone	Cefazolin
	Moxalactam	Cephapirin
	Vancomycin	Cephradine
	Pefloxacine	
	Ciprofloxacin	

*Intravenous preparation recommended for central nervous system infections.
Data from the Symposium on Antimicrobial Agents, Mayo Clin Proc 1991;66:942–1280.

Figure 24-3
Diagrammatic representation of the origin and path of the proprioceptive system, which carries sensory information from the limbs to the somatosensory cortex of the cerebrum (SS).
A lesion located in the left somatosensory cortex of the cerebrum should cause decreased proprioception or sensation on the right side of the body because the information crosses at the caudal brain stem level. However, a lesion to the left of the spinal cord should cause reduced proprioception on the left side because the tracts have not yet crossed.

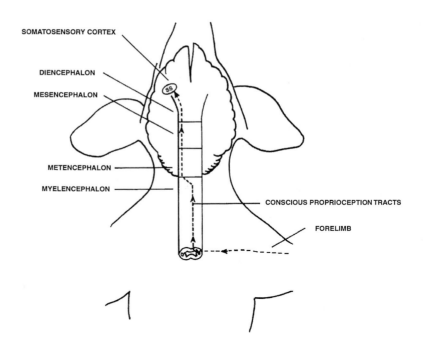

Clinical Signs

The owner's description of motor and sensory deficits may include weakness; inability or reluctance to jump, walk, or run; decreased activity level; or walking on the dorsal surface of the paws or dragging the paws. Decreased facial movements are frequently described as a change in facial expression, drooped ears, or drooling because of weakness of the upper lip muscles.

Motor and sensory deficits can be detected by observing the gait and the extent of limb or facial movements. Decreased ability to hop or hemiwalk on the limbs and decreased movements of the upper lip, eyelid, or ear may be found on neurologic examination. Asymmetrical motor deficits can often be confirmed by comparing movements on one side to those on the other. Sensory deficits, which are more difficult to detect than motor deficits, also are easier to detect if the lesion is asymmetrical. One of the best ways to judge reduced sensation to one side[4, 9] of the face is to gently insert a hemostat tip into the opening of each nostril. The normal response is a sudden jerking of the animal's head away from the instrument.

Because of the crossover of motor and sensory pathways in the brain, a focal lesion involving the left motor and somatosensory cortices would be expected to produce motor and sensory deficits on the right side.[4] Diffuse or bilateral deficits imply that both cerebral hemispheres are involved.

Diagnostic Plan

The history and the physical and neurologic examinations help to determine whether the weakness is neurologic, musculoskeletal, or metabolic in origin. Intermittent weakness should be pursued as a metabolic or musculoskeletal disorder first, because these are easier to investigate than nervous system disorders. Generalized weakness is more likely to be a neurologic or metabolic problem. Shifting leg weakness or lameness is probably a musculoskeletal problem. Weakness in conjunction with signs of systemic illness (e.g., fever, lymphadenopathy, dyspnea) is suggestive of inflammation, neoplasia, or a metabolic or toxic disorder.

The finding of motor and sensory deficits in conjunction with other cerebral signs, such as seizures or behavioral changes, implies a lesion of the brain. A complete history should establish the onset and course of the motor or sensory deficits. An acute onset with minimal to no progression of signs is suggestive of trauma or ischemia. Progressive signs, of either acute or insidious onset, are suggestive of neoplastic, inflammatory, metabolic, or toxic disorders.

A minimum database is the next part of the diagnostic plan, because some metabolic, inflammatory, or toxic disorders that cause cerebral disturbances are occasionally apparent on routine laboratory tests. For example, hypoglycemia, hepatic failure, or electrolyte disturbances such as hypocalcemia and hypokalemia can cause generalized weakness or other cerebral signs. Chest radiographs are recommended if the animal is middle-aged to older (because of the possibility of metastatic neoplasia) or if fungal diseases are in the differential diagnosis. Further work-up often includes skull radiographs to evaluate the possibility of trauma or bony neoplasia. CSF analysis may confirm the presence of inflammatory, neoplastic, or degenerative processes. Electroencephalography (EEG) could be beneficial in the diagnosis of hydrocephalus, encephalitis, or neoplasia. Computed tomography (CT) or magnetic resonance imaging (MRI) may also yield valuable information in cases of brain tumors, hydrocephalus, or vascular accidents.

Behavioral Changes

Decreased alertness, compulsive pacing or circling, loss of housebreaking or owner recognition, aggression, inability to learn, irritability, and hyperexcitability are examples of behavioral changes that are caused by cerebral dysfunction.

Pathophysiology

Prefrontal and temporal lobe lesions are often associated with behavioral changes. Destruction of the prefrontal area results in a wide variety of psychomotor disturbances, ranging from aggression and hyperactivity to dullness and inactivity. Parts of the temporal lobe, such as the pyriform area, are included in the limbic system, which governs emotions and innate survival behavior. Aggression has been observed with lesions located in the pyriform area. Cerebral and rostral thalamic lesions can cause leaning, circling, or head turning toward the side of the lesion (the adversive syndrome).[9, 10] The exact mechanism for these signs is not known.

Clinical Signs

The owners may report examples of behavioral changes such those that have been described.

Diagnostic Plan

A careful and thorough history can often establish the basis of the behavioral change. It is important to differentiate behavioral changes such as aggression or irritability related to neurologic dysfunction from non-neurologic behavioral disorders such as dominance aggression. As a general rule, a neurologic disorder is considered if behavioral changes occur in a previously well-adjusted adult pet in a stable household. If changes in residence, diet, household members, or schedules have occurred, the possibility of a non-neurologic behavioral disorder is given greater consideration. Some non-neurologic be-

havioral disorders are occasionally accompanied by focal alopecia or self-mutilation, but such changes may be observed with some cerebral disturbances as well. A neurologic cause for the behavioral change is supported by finding changes in gait, mentation, or cranial nerve (CN) function. Physical examination findings other than neurologic signs are usually normal unless an underlying systemic disorder is causing pain or discomfort and subsequent behavioral changes.

A minimum database should be obtained to rule out any obvious inflammatory or metabolic causes of behavioral disturbances such as abscesses causing pain, hepatic or renal disease causing mental depression, or hypoglycemia causing behavioral changes. In the middle-aged to older patient, chest radiographs should be considered to look for neoplastic lesions that may have metastasized to the brain to cause behavioral changes. Primary brain tumors rarely metastasize.[11, 12] The EEG can be useful in the diagnosis of hydrocephalus, encephalitis, and brain neoplasia but is not routinely available to many practitioners. CSF analysis is frequently helpful in diagnosing active brain processes such as encephalitis or neoplasia. Finally, skull radiographs or CT or MRI scans should be considered for disorders such as head trauma, brain neoplasia, brain infection, or hydrocephalus.

Central Blindness

Central blindness is lack of vision because of an abnormality in the optic radiations or visual (occipital) cortex; pupillary light responses are normal.

Pathophysiology

Visual deficits can be derived from several anatomic sites (Table 24–2). The optic nerve (CN II) contains sensory fibers for both vision and pupillary light reflexes (PLRs). Cell bodies, located in the ganglion layers of the retinas, converge to form the optic nerves, which in turn converge to form the optic chiasm located at the base of the diencephalon. The majority of the fibers decussate at the chiasm in both the dog and cat to form the optic tract. At this level, fibers take one of two pathways. Fibers of the visual pathway enter the lateral geniculate nucleus, the optic radiations, and the occipital or visual cortex, whereas those for the PLRs enter the pretectal and Edinger-Westphal nuclei in the midbrain. Blindness with abnormal PLRs suggests a lesion of the optic nerve, optic chiasm, or optic tract, whereas blindness with normal reflexes suggests a lesion of the optic radiations or occipital cortex.

Table 24–2
Lesions Causing Visual Deficits

LESION LOCATION	NEUROLOGIC EXAMINATION FINDINGS
Unilateral retina or optic nerve	Ipsilateral visual deficit or blindness with no direct or consensual pupil response to light from the ipsilateral eye
Bilateral retina, optic nerves, or optic chiasm	Bilateral visual deficit or blindness with no direct or consensual pupil response to light in either eye
Unilateral optic tract	Contralateral visual deficit with variable pupil responses depending on the part of the tract involved
Unilateral lateral geniculate nucleus, optic radiations, or occipital lobe cortex	Contralateral visual deficit with normal pupillary light responses
Bilateral lateral geniculate nucleus, optic radiations, and occipital lobe cortex	Bilateral visual deficit or blindness with normal pupillary light responses

Modified from Chrisman CL. Problems in Small Animal Neurology, 2nd ed. Philadelphia, Lea & Febiger, 1991:211.

Clinical Signs

The signs reported by owners may include a reluctance to jump or to go up and down stairs, a change in behavior such as aggression or lethargy, a change in gait (some dogs and cats pick their thoracic limbs up too high from the floor), or stumbling or walking into walls or obstacles. Some diseases that are insidious in onset may actually appear sudden in onset to the owner after the environment is changed, because animals tend to compensate well in a constant environment.

Clinical signs of a visual deficit are usually apparent on examination. The animal may walk into walls or obstacles when placed in a new environment. The menace response is absent or reduced.

Diagnostic Plan

After a visual deficit has been established by the history and examinations, its peripheral (optic nerve) or central (cerebrum) origin must be determined. Typically, peripheral lesions that cause visual deficits also produce slow or incomplete PLRs (see Chap. 26), whereas central lesions in the optic radiations and visual cortex are associated with normal PLRs. After a central location has been established, the diagnostic plan is the same as for motor and sensory deficits and behavioral changes.

Seizures

Seizures, fits, and convulsions are synonyms for transitory dysrhythmias of brain cells that begin suddenly and cease spontaneously.[13]

Pathophysiology

Transitory dysrhythmias of brain cells originate from either structural or functional damage to the cerebrum, particularly the frontal and temporal lobes.[14] The clinical appearance of a seizure varies with the location and severity of the dysrhythmia.

Seizures are classified into three categories: generalized, partial, or partial with secondary generalization. Generalized seizures are the most frequently recognized type of seizure in dogs and cats. During a generalized seizure, neurons on both sides of the cerebral cortex are discharging simultaneously to produce symmetrical involvement of the body. Although the initial seizure focus may involve only a small number of unstable neurons that spontaneously discharge, the surrounding normal neurons are induced to discharge, causing the seizure to spread or generalize. Specifically, the seizure generalizes when the electrical activity spreads to the diencephalon, which in turn discharges to both cerebral hemispheres to result in symmetrical involvement of the body.[15]

During a partial seizure, only one portion of the cerebral cortex is spontaneously discharging; therefore, the clinical appearance of the seizure varies with the function of the involved area. If motor areas of the cerebrum are affected, focal involuntary movements are observed during the seizure. For example, if the seizure focus is in the left motor cortex, involuntary movement or muscle jerking is observed on the right side of the body. Such seizure activity has also been referred to as a focal seizure. Partial seizures can become generalized.[13]

A seizure focus may occur in regions of the brain that affect behavior or autonomic nervous system activities as opposed to motor activity. Intermittent, bizarre behavioral activity with or without motor seizures in dogs and cats is commonly called psychomotor seizure activity[16]; other terms are temporal or pyriform lobe epilepsy, rhinencephalic seizure, limbic lobe epilepsy,[17] and autonomic epilepsy.[18] These types of seizures are usually classified as partial seizures with complex symptomatology in humans. Complex partial seizures is the recommended term to describe such intermittent bizarre activity in animals.[19]

Clinical Signs

Many seizures start while the pet is sleeping; the reason is unknown. The classic clinical description of a generalized tonic-clonic seizure is as follows: the pet usually falls over, loses consciousness, and manifests involuntary extension of the limbs (tonic phase) followed by paddling (clonic phase).[16] Chewing motions, pupillary dilation, and salivation may occur; they represent visceral motor activity. Defecation and urination may also occur during or after the seizure. This seizure description is frequently referred to as "grand mal" by owners.[15, 16]

Milder, generalized motor seizures are less dramatic, and the pet frequently remains conscious. It may act anxious, stumble or crawl, or fall over with little to no jerking of the limbs, head, or trunk. Owners refer to these signs as a "petit mal" seizure, although it is not related to such seizures in humans. Petit mal or absence seizures in humans consist of an extremely brief (seconds) loss of consciousness, generalized loss of muscle tone, a blank stare, and perhaps upward rotation of the eyes.[15, 20] Such seizures either are uncommon in dogs and cats or are uncommonly recognized because of their brief duration and mild signs. Myoclonic seizures are an uncommon form of generalized seizures characterized by massive, uncontrollable jerking of muscles.

Behavioral changes associated with psychomotor seizures vary and include fear, hysterical running, aggression, vocalization, cowering or hiding, licking or lip smacking, chewing motions, jaw snapping (fly biting), vomiting, diarrhea, excessive salivation, and flank biting. None of these is usually associated with a loss of consciousness, but there is an obvious lack of awareness in many cases. Such episodes may last minutes or hours and may be followed by a generalized motor seizure. There is no age or breed predilection.[18] Although such odd behaviors are likely to be produced by psychomotor seizure activity, abnormal stereotypic behavior should also be considered.

Some pets have an aura or preictal stage minutes or seconds before a seizure occurs. Some may appear restless, seek attention, attempt to hide, whine, salivate, or tremble. After the seizure (postictal stage), similar temporary changes may be observed, as may other changes such as disorientation, blindness, aggression, sleepiness, or dementia. The postictal stage lasts minutes to hours, or occasionally days, and is often unnoticed or confused with the seizure itself.

Diagnostic Plan

Getting an accurate description of the seizure or observing it firsthand is crucial to differentiate seizure from syncope. Syncope does not usually cause involuntary motor activity to the degree that is observed with generalized seizures. Syncope also does not usually cause autonomic signs such as urination or defecation, but some seizures do not manifest these signs either. However, if hypoxia occurs and lasts long enough, brain damage can result in unconsciousness as well as generalized involuntary limb movements that clinically appear to be seizure activity. The finding of cardiac arrhythmias or lung disorders can be of great help in establishing syncope as the clinical sign.

An accurate description or firsthand observation is also crucial to separate generalized seizures from partial seizures with secondary generalization. Subtle signs at the very beginning of generalized seizure activity (such as a turn of the head to one side, the lifting of one leg, or unilateral facial twitching) are important clues for classifying the seizure as partial with secondary generalization. It is likely that some generalized seizures are actually partial seizures with secondary generalization. Classification of the seizure is sometimes helpful in formulating a differential diagnosis. For example, generalized seizures are most often associated with primary epilepsy and toxic or metabolic disorders, whereas partial seizures are commonly associated with focal or multifocal structural damage to the cerebrum, as can occur with neoplasia, trauma, ischemia, or encephalitis.

Based on the history and the physical and neurologic examinations, the seizure is classified as having an extracranial or intracranial origin. Extracranial causes are easier to investigate and include such disorders as hypoglycemia, hepatic and uremic encephalopathy, lead intoxication, and organophosphate toxicity. The diagnostic work-up for extracranial disorders includes a hemogram (for evidence of lead intoxication), chemistry profile (to look for metabolic disturbance), and urinalysis. However, in the patient with clinically or historically obvious toxicity such as organophosphate exposure, a diagnostic work-up may not be warranted; response to appropriate treatment may be most reasonable.

Which diagnostic tests are chosen depends on the history and examinations as they pertain to the age of the animal, the presence or absence of other neurologic or physical signs, and the frequency of the seizures. For example, in a young animal with a history of one seizure and normal physical and neurologic examinations, a hemogram, chemistry profile, and urinalysis are indicated to help evaluate the possibility of inflammatory, toxic, or metabolic causes. If there is any chance of exposure to lead objects or any gastrointestinal signs, then a blood lead level should be obtained. If seizures persist, additional diagnostic tests are indicated; these may include liver function tests to help exclude a congenital portosystemic shunt or acquired liver disease. If seizures develop in a middle-aged to older patient or if any other systemic signs (e.g., fever, lymphadenopathy, weight loss, cough) are present, chest radiographs should be done to evaluate the possibility of primary or metastatic neoplasia. If such tests do not confirm an extracranial cause for the seizures, intracranial causes should be investigated. Skull radiographs occasionally reveal signs of trauma or bony neoplasia and are often done before more invasive or expensive tests such as CSF analysis, CT or MRI, or EEG. EEG can be of diagnostic benefit if the seizures were caused by hydrocephalus, encephalitis, or even neoplasia. CT or MRI may yield important information regarding the diagnosis of brain tumors, hydrocephalus, or sometimes, vascular accidents.

Diagnostic Procedures

Routine Laboratory Evaluation

A hemogram may show evidence of inflammation, suggesting an infectious cause. Occasionally, nucleated red blood cells or basophilic stippling are found, suggesting lead intoxication. A chemistry profile may show changes in renal or hepatic parameters or electrolytes. Elevation of globulins without evidence of dehydration is suggestive of inflammatory or neoplastic processes. A urinalysis may support a diagnosis of renal or hepatic disease.

Neurologic Examination

The neurologic examination[21, 22] consists of evaluation of (1) mental status, (2) cranial nerves, (3) gait and posture, (4) postural reactions, (5) spinal reflexes, (6) muscle mass and tone, (7) tactile and deep pain perception, and (8) miscellaneous features. Although some clinicians strongly advocate following the same sequence on all examinations, the sequence chosen is immaterial, except that tests to evaluate nociception should always be performed last. A complete examination should be done unless the animal is traumatized, in which case postural reactions and spinal manipulations are avoided. The examination is sometimes limited by the large size of the animal or an aggressive disposition. Cats often do not tolerate having the complete examination performed all at one time; performing sections of the examination at short intervals seems to work best. A sample neurologic examination form is presented in Table 24–3; the discussion here follows the outline presented on the form.

Part 1: Mental Status and Cerebral Signs

Evaluation of mental status includes observation of the state of consciousness and behavioral abnormalities. The state of consciousness is the level of the patient's awareness and how responsive the animal is to its environment and to impressions received through its special senses (e.g., taste, smell, sight). This state can be altered by disease in the cerebral cortex or in the ascending reticular activating system of the brain stem.[10] The normal animal should be alert and responsive to environmental stimuli. Depression is considered a state in which the animal is not as alert as usual or responds slowly.[10] Dementia is a state beyond depression in which the patient has a dull, emotionless, expressionless attitude.[14] The animal may not respond in appropriate ways, may walk into walls, or may be unable to get out of a corner. Stupor or semicoma is a state of partial or relative loss of response to the environment in which the animal appears to be asleep most of the time and is generally unresponsive except to vigorous and repeated stimuli that may necessarily be painful.[10] Coma is complete or almost complete loss of consciousness from which the animal cannot be aroused even by noxious stimuli.[23]

Behavioral changes of neurologic origin are usually caused by cerebral lesions and produce signs referred to as cerebral or head signs. Signs include compulsive walking or circling, head pressing, abnormal aggressiveness, changes in behavior toward the owner, disorientation, and confusion. Seizures are also the result of cerebral abnormalities and should be described as thoroughly as possible (see Seizures).

Part 2: Cranial Nerves

A quick but thorough CN examination[24] should be performed on every patient except those that are aggressive, for which an abbreviated examination suffices. Because the olfactory cranial nerve (CN I) is difficult to evaluate and because dysfunction is uncommon, it is not routinely evaluated. Disorders of the trochlear (CN IV) and trapezius (CN XI) nerves are also uncommon and difficult to appreciate.

Vision is the responsibility of the optic nerve (CN II) and can be evaluated by observing the animal ambulate in a new environment. If the animal tends to walk into walls or obstacles, there may be an abnormality of the eye or the visual pathway. Vision is further evaluated by testing of the menace response. This is performed by moving a hand briskly toward each eye as if to hit the animal's eye with the hand; the eye that is not being evaluated is covered by the examiner's other hand. The entire visual system must be intact to produce a positive response, an eye blink. Care must be taken not to create air currents with the

Table 24–3

PRACTICAL NEUROLOGIC EXAM
Linda G. Shell, D.V.M.

OWNER _____
ANIMAL _____
DATE _____

I.   MENTAL STATUS: Alert ____ Depressed ____ Demented ____ Stuporous ____ Comatose ____
     BEHAVIORAL CHANGE: Head pressing ____ Aggression ____ Circling ____ Pacing ____
     Other _____
     SEIZURE HISTORY:

II.   CRANIAL NERVES: Normal ____ Abnormal (describe below) ____

	Left	Right		Left	Right
Vision II			Facial movements VII		
Menace response II, VII			Vestibular strabismus VIII		
Pupil size II, PS, S			Oculocephalic III, IV, VI, VIII		
PLR II, PS, S			Head tilt VIII		
Lat strabismus III			Nystagmus VIII (describe direction and type)		
Med strabismus VI			Hearing VIII		
Masticatory mus motor V			Swallow IX, X, XI		
Facial sensation sensory V			Tongue movement/mass XII		

III. GAIT: Normal ____ Abnormal ambulatory ____ Nonambulatory ____

     Ambulatory: Ataxic ____ Mildly paretic ____ Severely paretic ____ Dysmetric ____ Vestibular ____
       Location: Forelimbs L ____ R ____ Hindlimbs L ____ R ____
     Nonambulatory: Voluntary movements present: Forelimbs L _____   R _____
                                        Hindlimbs L _____   R _____
                Voluntary movements absent: Forelimbs L _____   R _____
                                          Hindlimbs L _____   R _____

IV. POSTURAL REACTIONS: Normal ____ Abnormal (describe below) ____

                    Forelimbs
      Wheelbarrow   Ext postural thrust
      Hopping   Hopping
      Hemistand/hemiwalk   Hemistand/hemiwalk
      Proprioception   Proprioception

V.   SPINAL REFLEXES: Normal ____   Abnormal (describe below) ____

	Left	Right		Left	Right
Patellar			Triceps		
Sciatic			Ext carpi radialis		
Cr tibial			Biceps		
Gastrocnemius			Flexor		
Flexor			Crossed extensor		
Crossed extensor					

                    Perineal reflex

VI. MUSCLES: Normal ____ Atrophy ____ Hypertrophy ____ Painful ____
     Location of abnormality _____

VII. PAIN PERCEPTION: Behavioral response (crying, biting) to:
                            Superficial pain (hemostat on skin): Present ____ Absent ____
                            Deep pain (hemostat on lateral and medial toes): Present ____ Absent ____

VIII. MISC: Cutaneous trunci _____ Bladder control _____
         Bladder tone _____ Tail bone _____ Hyperpathia _____

LESION LOCATION, RULE-OUTS, PLANS:

rapid movement of the hand and to avoid touching the vibrissae, because either event could stimulate the sensory portion of CN V and result in an eye blink even if the animal is avisual. If the menace response is doubtful, the animal is observed in an obstacle course, or cotton balls are thrown in front of its eyes to determine whether it follows their movement. A complete ocular examination should be done to detect corneal opacities, cataracts, or retinal changes that can affect vision. Fundic examination also allows the optic nerve to be visualized for abnormalities such as edema and increased or decreased size.

Pupil size and response to light (PLR) is mediated by CN II and by the parasympathetic and sympathetic nerves to the eye. Both pupils should be of appropriate size for the environmental lighting. In bright light, the pupils should be small, and in dark areas, they should be enlarged or dilated. Anisocoria is the term used to describe unequal size of the pupils. It cases of anisocoria, it must be determined which pupil is normal and which is abnormal (see Chap. 19). Both pupils should constrict symmetrically when a direct and bright light is shone into one eye. If the PLR is questionable, it is sometimes helpful to darken the room and then shine a strong light into the pupil. Disorders of the iris (e.g., iris atrophy) can result in a dilated pupil that has a slow, incomplete, or absent PLR.

Strabismus, or deviation of the eyeball, occurs if one of the nerves that innervates the extraocular muscles is injured. These nerves are CNs III, IV, and VI. To evaluate them, the eyes are observed for symmetrical positioning and presence of strabismus. With a CN III deficit, the affected eyeball is usually deviated laterally and ventrally, and a CN VI deficit causes a medial deviation. Strabismus caused by a CN IV deficit is impossible to appreciate in animals with round pupils, but in cats it may be detected because the dorsal aspect of the vertical pupil is positioned laterally. Unilateral vestibular dysfunction results in a positional strabismus that is often best observed when the examiner elevates the animal's head; the affected eyeball tends to drop (eye drop) to a more ventral position than normal, but it is movable and is not paralyzed in this position.

The oculocephalic reflex is mediated by CNs III, IV, VI, and VIII. The examiner moves the animal's head from side to side to elicit brisk eyeball movements in the same direction as the head movement. Such eye movements are actually normal vestibular nystagmus with a fast phase (toward the direction of movement) and a slow phase. These eye motions should cease after head movement ceases. If nystagmus continues after head movement stops, positional nystagmus is present, reflecting dysfunction of the vestibular system (see Chap. 26).

The masticatory muscles (temporalis and masseter), which are innervated by the motor components of the trigeminal nerve (CN V), should be palpated for signs of swelling, pain, or atrophy. Jaw tone is also controlled by the trigeminal nerve. Jaw tone is evaluated by noting the resistance when an attempt is made to open the animal's mouth. A dropped jaw that will not stay closed implies bilateral dysfunction of the trigeminal nerve.

Facial sensation is mediated by sensory branches of CN V. The ophthalmic branch is evaluated by touching the medial canthus of the eye; this should result in closure of the eyelid. The maxillary branch is evaluated by pinching the upper lip, which causes lip retraction if sensation is intact and if CN VII is also functional (CN VII is responsible for movement of the lip). The mandibular branch is evaluated by touching the lower ear to elicit ear movement. In order to determine whether sensation is perceived at the thalamic or cerebral level, a behavioral response must be elicited with the stimuli. One of the best ways to evaluate cerebral perception of sensation is to gently insert a hemostat tip into the naris opening; the animal should withdraw its head or whine to indicate perception of the sensation.

Ear, eyelid, and lip movements are mediated by the facial nerve (CN VII). Signs of weakness or paralysis include drooping of the lip and ear, increased size of the palpebral fissure or opening, and poor palpebral reflex. The menace response may be weak or absent because the animal cannot close its eyelid. The ear may not move in response to touch, and the lip may not retract when it is pinched.

Head tilt and nystagmus are indications of vestibular dysfunction. The direction of the head tilt should be noted; it is usually toward the affected side. Resting nystagmus should be described in terms of the direction of the fast phase and the type (i.e., horizontal, vertical, or rotary). The direction of the fast phase of the nystagmus is opposite the side of the lesion. The oculocephalic response (described previously) is then evaluated in an attempt to elicit positional nystagmus. Other indications of vestibular dysfunction include ataxia and falling, leaning, or circling to one side.

Hearing is evaluated by calling the animal's name and observing its head turn or its ears move. The cochlear portion of the vestibulocochlear nerve is responsible for audition. Unilateral deficits are not usually detectable clinically.

The swallow or gag reflex is tested by opening the animal's mouth and inserting a gloved finger at the back of the throat or by pinching the throat or nose to elicit a swallow reflex. If there is the potential for rabies infection based on the history or examination, the fingers should not be inserted into the affected animal's mouth. If the animal is aggressive, it should be observed swallowing water or food instead. CNs IX and X contribute to this reflex.[24]

Tongue movement and muscle mass are evaluated by opening the animal's mouth and observing the tongue for movement and atrophy. A tongue with unilateral atrophy appears wrinkled on the affected side.

Part 3: Gait and Posture

Evaluation of gait and posture entails evaluation of four functional neuroanatomic systems: the motor system, the cerebellum, general proprioception, and the special proprioception-vestibular system. The somatic motor system innervates skeletal muscle and functions to initiate voluntary movement and to maintain postural antigravity support. Dysfunction results in weakness or paralysis of limb movement.

The cerebellum is concerned with integration of somatic motor activity and regulation of muscle tone and mechanisms that influence and maintain equilibrium. Because each movement requires the coordinated action (synergy) of a group of muscles, generalized cerebellar disease is characterized by inability to regulate rate, range, and force of movement activity. Normal strength is present, but integration is absent and movements may not be terminated at a proper time or distance (dysmetria). Head tremors, truncal sway, and nystagmus also may be present.

Conscious general proprioception is mediated through the dorsal columns (fasciculus gracilis and fasciculus cuneatus), which carry myotactic information from sensory receptors in the periphery to the contralateral sensory cortex.[4] Deficits anywhere in this system are characterized by malpositioning of the limbs such that the animal stands or walks with the dorsal paw surface touching the floor.

Subconscious or special proprioception is projected to the cerebellum from peripheral receptors by way of the spinocerebellar tracts. This information is influential in integration of the motor system. Deficits result in abnormal gait, which is especially noticeable during the nonsupport phase of progression. Dysmetria and circumduction of the outside pelvic limb on turning are commonly seen.

Vestibular proprioception is mediated by the vestibular system. Most cases affecting vestibular proprioception are unilateral, and asymmetrical signs are observed. Characteristically, the animal has a head tilt and leans, drifts, rolls, or collapses to the involved side. Nystagmus is frequently present. These signs are observed with lesions located both peripherally (vestibulocochlear nerve) and centrally (vestibular nuclei in brain stem or flocculonodular lobe of the cerebellum). Peripheral lesions do not cause limb weakness, although the animal may be so disoriented that

weakness is difficult to ascertain. Central lesions may cause weakness or decreased strength if the motor tracts located in the brain stem (e.g., rubrospinal, corticospinal tracts) are affected; likewise, other CN deficits may be detected because other CN nuclei are located near the vestibular nuclei in the brain stem. Animals that have bilateral vestibular involvement have a tendency to crouch, are reluctant to move, and usually have wide, sweeping head motions. Nystagmus is usually absent, and the oculocephalic reflex is weak or absent because both sides are affected.

For evaluation of gait, the animal should be placed on a surface with firm footing. The animal may be allowed to roam (if it is an enclosed area) or may be led on a leash. The normal gait of the species should be kept in mind as the gait is viewed, as should the many possible breed- and use-dependent variations of normal. Some normal dogs, such as poodles, tend to display hypermetria of the forelimbs as they walk; a few dogs pace (move the limbs on each side of the body forward simultaneously); some have an excessive roll or sway to the rear end. Yet, these same signs can be observed in other dogs with neurologic dysfunction.

The gait should be classified as ambulatory, ambulatory but abnormal, or nonambulatory. If the gait is abnormal, it is further described as ataxic, mildly paretic, severely paretic, dysmetric, or vestibular, and the affected limb or limbs are noted. If the animal is unable to support weight and ambulate, the presence or absence of voluntary motor activity should be recorded. A nonambulatory animal that lacks voluntary movements has a more guarded prognosis than one with voluntary movement. A good way to evaluate voluntary movement is to call the animal's name or offer it food from a distance and watch the limbs for movements as the animal responds.

Part 4: Postural Reactions

After observation of the gait for strength and coordination, postural reactions (e.g., hopping, wheelbarrowing, hemistanding, hemiwalking) are evaluated to help quantify gait deficits, to determine subtle deficits in strength, and to detect asymmetrical deficits. For example, an animal with a left cerebral lesion may have a normal-appearing gait, but postural reactions may show a subtle right-sided deficit. If the animal is nonambulatory, it will probably be unable to perform postural reactions.

Wheelbarrowing is performed by lifting the pelvic limbs to force complete weight bearing on the thoracic limbs. As the animal is gently urged to walk forward, head lifting should be followed by forward placement of one limb and then the other. Animals with cervical disease may have difficulty lifting the head, may be reluctant to move forward, or may actually walk on the dorsal paw surface. To accentuate subtle deficits, the head is elevated by the examiner and the dog is forced to walk forward; this procedure affects visual orientation and causes subtle weaknesses and asymmetries to become more obvious.

Extensor postural thrust reaction is performed by holding the animal in the air by the axillae and lowering the rear end to the ground so that the pelvic limb paws touch the floor and support weight. The normal animal takes one to three steps in a backward direction. If the animal is too big to lift in the air, the front end of the animal can be lifted by the axillae while the pelvic limbs are kept on the floor. The animal is then urged or gently pushed in a backward direction. This test is similar to wheelbarrowing in the thoracic limbs in that it can detect asymmetry in pelvic limb strength.

Hemistanding and hemiwalking also aid assessment of limb strength. These are performed by flexing the pelvic and thoracic limbs on the side of the examiner and forcing the animal to move either sideways away from the examiner or forward on the limbs of the other side. The normal animal's response is to keep the limbs extended when hemistanding and then to move them easily and symmetrically when forced to move in the hemiwalk position. The strength of each limb should be noted.

Hopping reactions are tested by lifting and holding the animal in a horizontal position. The animal is then forced to bear weight on one limb while the other three are in the air. The animal is forced to move on the one limb in a sideways (lateral) or forward direction. The normal response is for the limb to extend when it is completely weight bearing and to then smoothly and rather briskly to move or hop when forced.

Proprioceptive positioning is the animal's ability to detect limb position (sensory) and to correct that limb position (motor response). The animal should be standing bearing equal weight on all four limbs. The examiner places one hand under the pelvis (for pelvic limb testing) or thorax (for thoracic limb testing) to give the animal some sense of support when the test is performed. The animal's paw is placed so that its dorsal surface is in contact with the floor (knuckle position). The normal response is for the animal to immediately return the paw to the correct position.

Part 5: Spinal Reflexes

Spinal reflexes are involuntary responses to peripheral stimuli and are of value in determining the segmental integrity of the spinal cord and the peripheral nerves involved in the simple reflex arc. The components of the simple reflex arc are (1) a peripheral sensory receptor area, (2) the sensory portion of the peripheral nerve and dorsal spinal root, (3) a spinal cord segment, (4) the motor portion of the peripheral nerve, and (5) a muscle. If any of these components is nonfunctional, a depressed or negative response is seen when attempts to elicit a reflex are made. The reflex response is recorded as absent (0), hyporeflexic or decreased (+1), normal (+2), hyperreflexic or increased (+3), or clonic (+4). Lower motor neuron disease is characterized by hyporeflexia or areflexia, and upper motor neuron disease by hyperreflexia.

Reflexes are tested with the animal in lateral recumbence. Animals that are nervous may have a false hyperreflexia, and those that are tense and unrelaxed may have a false hyporeflexia. Nervousness or tenseness of the animal should be recorded so that an accurate interpretation of the results can be considered. As a general guideline, pelvic limb reflexes are easier to elicit than those of the thoracic limbs. Keeping the limb in slight flexion may result in more accurate reflex responses.

Pelvic Limb Reflexes

The patellar reflex is one of the most reliable tendon reflexes. With the animal in lateral recumbence and relaxed, the patellar tendon is tapped with a percussion hammer or instrument. The normal response is a brisk extension of the stifle joint. This reflex is mediated by the femoral nerve through lumbar spinal cord segments 4, 5, and 6.

The sciatic reflex is tested to evaluate the sciatic nerve, which originates from lumbar spinal cord segments VI and VII and sacral segments I and II. If the area between the trochanter major and ischial tuberosity is percussed, there should be reflex flexion of the stifle and hock joints.

The cranial tibial reflex is mediated by the peroneal branch of the sciatic nerve. To elicit this reflex, the muscle belly of the cranial tibial muscle, situated on the anterolateral aspect of the proximal tibial area, is percussed. The normal response is a flexion of the hock joint.

The gastrocnemius reflex is mediated by the tibial branch of the sciatic nerve and is elicited by percussion of the muscle belly of the gastrocnemius muscle located in the caudal angle of the stifle joint or by percussion of the tendon of insertion just proximal to the hock joint. The normal response is flexion of the stifle joint.

The flexor reflex is stimulated by gently pinching the toes to get the limb to flex. In the pelvic limbs, the flexor reflex is primarily mediated by the sciatic nerve.

The crossed extensor reflex is tested after the flexor reflex has been elicited. With the uppermost limb in the flexed position, the bottom limb is pinched gently (so as not to cause pain). The normal response is for the pinched limb to flex while the uppermost limb remains flexed. A positive crossed extensor reflex is present if the uppermost limb suddenly extends as the bottom limb is pinched. This is an abnormal response in the animal that is in lateral recumbence; it implies an upper motor neuron spinal cord lesion above the origin of the flexor reflex. If the stimulus is too intense, the animal tries to get away from the stimulus by extending the uppermost limb to right itself; this response should not be interpreted as a positive crossed extensor reflex.

The perineal reflex is elicited by gently pinching the anal sphincter and observing it contract; the tail also may move. This reflex is mediated by branches of the pudendal nerve, which originates at sacral spinal cord segments 2 and 3. If the sphincter is relaxed and areflexic, bladder denervation is usually present.

Thoracic Limb Reflexes

The triceps reflex is elicited by tapping the tendon of insertion of the triceps muscle, located at the olecranon, or by placing a finger on the tendon or muscle belly and tapping it with the percussion hammer. It is sometimes difficult to elicit this reflex, even in normal animals. The normal response is a slight extension of the elbow. This reflex is mediated by the radial nerve, which originates from cervical segments 7 and 8 and thoracic segments 1 and 2.

The extensor carpi radialis reflex is elicited by tapping the belly of the muscle on the craniolateral surface of the forearm, just distal to the elbow. The normal response is an extension of the carpus. This reflex is also mediated by the radial nerve.

The biceps reflex is mediated through the musculocutaneous nerve, which has origins at cervical spinal cord segments 6, 7, and 8. A slight flexion of the elbow is the normal response when the biceps tendon of insertion is tapped at the medial aspect of the elbow.

The flexor reflex in the thoracic limb is mediated by a number of nerves that arise from the sixth cervical to the second thoracic spinal cord segments. Minimal stimulation of pain receptors can be accomplished by compression of the foot pads or gentle pinching of the toes. The normal response is a reflex flexion or withdrawal of the limb. If the stimulus is too intense, behavioral responses, such as head turning or whining, may also occur.

Part 6: Muscle Mass and Tone

The animal should carefully be observed, preferably while it is standing symmetrically, for muscle atrophy or hypertrophy. The muscles should be palpated for tone or the presence of muscle pain. Atrophy and decreased muscle tone are associated with lower motor neuron disease, whereas minimal atrophy and normal to increased muscle tone are associated with upper motor neuron disease.

Part 7: Tactile and Deep Pain Perception

Evaluation of the sensory systems is often largely subjective because levels of pain perception vary from animal to animal, from species to species, and occasionally from day to day in the same animal. Pain perception may be interpreted somewhat differently among examiners. Nonetheless, hypalgesia and analgesia are important and usually accurate findings, and they are usually consistent from one examiner to another.

In order for deep pain and light touch (tactile) sensations to be perceived, sensory impulses must be carried from peripheral receptors or end organs to the thalamus and the somatosensory lobe of the cerebrum for conscious recognition. Superficial pain perception is evaluated by pinching the skin with hemostats in various places. Responses vary with the animal and its pain threshold, but most animals have a behavioral response (cry, whine, turn). If superficial pain sensation is present, deep pain perception may not need to be evaluated; however, it is imperative to evaluate deep pain perception in all paralyzed animals, because the prognosis becomes less favorable if deep pain perception is lacking. Perception of deep pain is tested by pinching the toes with a hemostat, gently at first and then harder if no behavioral response is elicited. Behavioral responses include the animal's trying to bite, crying out, or trying to get away from the painful stimulus. Involuntary (flexor) spinal reflexes should not be misinterpreted as an indication that the animal perceived deep pain.

Part 8: Miscellaneous Tests

The cutaneous trunci reflex test is performed by pinching the skin over the dorsum, starting at the rear and going forward. The normal response is a reflex movement or contracture of the subcutaneous musculature (crawling appearance). The sensory limb of this reflex is mediated by segmental sensory nerves near the area examined; the motor component is mediated by the lateral thoracic nerve, which originates at the eighth cervical and first thoracic spinal cord segments. In some cases of spinal cord disease, such as transverse myelopathies associated with trauma or disc herniations, this reflex disappears caudal to the lesion; superficial pain perception may also disappear.

Bladder control and tone are determined by observation of the animal during urination and by palpation of the bladder, respectively. A more complete description of micturition is found in Chapter 27.

Tail tone is evaluated by moving the tail upward

and noting the resistance and movement. Flaccid or paralyzed tails do not wag voluntarily, may be dropped instead of upright (depending on the breed), and seem to lack tone.

Hyperpathia refers to pain that can be elicited from a localized area by palpation.[25] The spine is evaluated by palpation of the dorsal spinous processes or the dorsolateral aspects of the paraspinal muscles. Because pain thresholds vary, light-intensity palpations should be used at first, with progression toward more forceful palpations.

Radiography

The radiographic anatomy of the skull is complex because of the superimposition of many bones and the marked differences in the shape and size among breeds. Because interpretation depends on positioning, skull radiographs are taken with the animal under general anesthesia. Lateral symmetry and precise superimposition should be achieved in positioning the animal. Lateral and dorsoventral or ventrodorsal views are routinely taken to evaluate intracranial disorders such as hydrocephalus, trauma, or neoplasia. Oblique views may add to localization and diagnosis of skull fractures and neoplasia.

Skull radiographs may be beneficial in diagnosing hydrocephalus, trauma, or neoplasia. Intraparenchymal brain tumors are not apparent unless mineralization or calcification occurs. Extraparenchymal tumors such as meningiomas may produce hyperostosis of the skull in cats. Bony tumors such as osteosarcomas or chondrosarcomas produce obvious signs of bony destruction or proliferation, or both. A dome-shaped skull with open suture lines and fontanelles is often observed on skull radiographs of hydrocephalic animals. Real-time B-mode ultrasonography has been used to diagnose congenital hydrocephalus if the fontanelle is open.[26]

CT of the brain provides an accurate method of localizing lesions and detecting soft tissue density changes.[27] The procedure is safe and noninvasive but has disadvantages of high cost and lack of availability. Animals must be anesthetized in order to position the head accurately within the unit. Ventrodorsal and occasionally lateral views are taken. Data are analyzed by a computer to produce cross-sectional images at various levels (slices) of the brain. An intravenous injection of an organic iodide contrast agent (e.g., meglumine iothalamate) frequently enhances neoplastic and other pathologic processes.

Like CT, MRI produces cross-sectional images, but although CT measures the radiographic attenuation of tissues, MRI, using a combination of magnetism and radio waves, measures nuclear magnetic resonance signals emitted from protons in the body. During scanning, the patient lies in the center of a powerful magnetic field; protons align themselves with or against the magnetic field. Radio waves at a specific frequency are then pulsed into the patient to cause a temporary disturbance to the alignment. Protons realign themselves over time and emit tiny radiofrequency signals that are detected and converted by a computer into an image using a mathematic process.[28] The complex anatomy of the nervous system is better defined with MRI than with any other current radiographic technique. The gray and white matter, CSF, and surrounding structures can easily be distinguished. Disadvantages include unavailability and high cost.

Spinal Fluid Analysis

Collection of CSF is performed for two major reasons: to examine the fluid and to perform subarachnoid myelographic procedures. The cerebellomedullary site is the preferred site of collection when evaluating brain and cervical spinal cord lesions. While the animal is under general anesthesia, the skin is aseptically prepared over the dorsal cervical area from the external occipital protuberance of the skull to the dorsal spine of the third cervical vertebra. After the patient is placed in lateral recumbence, its head is flexed by an assistant so that the nose is parallel to the table surface. Care must be taken to avoid restriction of the airway, and tracheal intubation is always performed. With the index finger of the left hand, the examiner palpates the occipital protuberance at the same time that the thumb and middle finger palpate the cranial borders of the wings of the atlas.

The right hand holds a 3.8-cm, 22-gauge spinal needle that is inserted directly on the midline about one half to two thirds of way between the protuberance and the wings of the atlas (Fig. 24–4). The needle should be held firmly and perpendicular to the spine. As each layer of skin, musculature, and ligament is approached, resistance is encountered before penetration. When learning the procedure, the examiner should withdraw the stylet from the needle to check for spinal fluid at each layer until enough experience is attained to know when the cistern has been penetrated. Movement of the needle at this stage could lacerate the cord and should be avoided. The fluid is allowed to drip into a sterile glass container (red-topped tube) until approximately 1.5 to 2.0 mL has been collected. Smaller amounts are usually obtained from small dogs and cats. Most laboratories require at least 1.0 mL for analysis; additional amounts are needed for cultures or titer determinations. If the fluid at first appears to be bloody, a few drops are allowed to collect in one tube and are saved for bacterial culture; then a different tube is used to collect the clearer CSF for analysis and titer

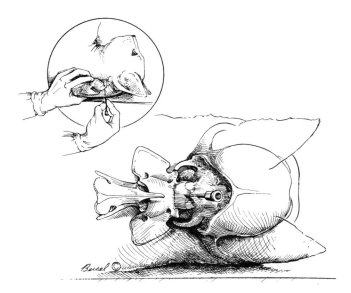

Figure 24–4
Landmarks for spinal fluid collection at the cerebello-medullary site. (From Greene CE, Oliver JE. Neurologic examination. In: Ettinger SJ, ed. Textbook of Internal Medicine: Diseases of the Dog and Cat, 2nd ed. Philadelphia, WB Saunders, 1983:419–460.)

evaluations. If the blood-tinged fluid does not become clear, the samples should be saved for analysis anyway, because the results must be interpreted in view of blood contamination. Another attempt at collection should be tried in a few days. If the dorsal venous sinuses that overlay the cistern are penetrated without entry to the cistern, the result is frank, undiluted blood in the hub of the needle. In this case, the head should be repositioned and the spinal tap attempted again with a new needle. A longer (6.3-cm) spinal needle is usually required for giant breeds of dogs.

Spinal fluid analysis must be performed within 0.5 hour of collection because the cells are unstable outside the body and begin to lyse. CSF is therefore analyzed on-site or at an adjacent human hospital laboratory. In-house analysis[29] is recommended only if CSF is analyzed frequently enough for the laboratory personnel to feel comfortable with the technique. In-house quantitation of CSF protein may not be possible because most instruments are not sensitive enough to accurately measure the low concentration of protein in CSF. A portion of the CSF sample should always be set aside for bacterial culture.

CSF analysis should include a physical description of the fluid (clear, opaque, xanthochromic, pink, or bloody), a white blood cell count, a red blood cell count, protein value, and cytologic description of the cell types. In most laboratories, normal CSF taken from the cerebellomedullary cistern usually has a red blood cell count of zero (unless iatrogenic blood contamina-

tion has occurred during the procedure), a white blood cell count of less than 5/µL, and a protein value of less than 25 mg/mL. Mononuclear cells predominate on cytologic evaluation.

Serologic Testing

Serum and CSF titers can be performed for canine distemper, toxoplasmosis, and some of the rickettsial diseases. Some laboratories offer titer determinations for other viruses as well. Positive serum titers do not necessarily differentiate exposure from disease, and CSF fluid titers can be difficult to interpret if the blood-brain barrier is broken (which happens with many infectious diseases) or if there is peripheral blood contamination of the CSF.[30] In both cases, leakage of circulating antibodies into the CSF can occur without the presence of actual CNS disease. Comparison of CSF with serum titers may be helpful in interpretation of CSF titers. Submission of serum and CSF samples for antibody titer analysis should be preceded by contact with the laboratory so that proper submission and accurate interpretation of the results can occur. A fluorescent antibody test to detect canine distemper virus antigens is available in some laboratories.

Electroencephalography

The EEG amplifies, filters, and graphically records the alterations over time of electrical potentials from the cerebral cortex.[31] Because of the cost of the unit and the expertise necessary to interpret the findings, availability is usually restricted to teaching hospitals and specialty practices. Although there are seldom specific changes for a particular disease, an EEG is indicated for many patients with signs of cerebral or head abnormalities. The EEG may be able to aid or confirm the localization of a lesion or to provide support for a diagnosis of hydrocephalus, encephalitis, asymmetrical lesion, acquired epilepsy, or brain death.

Common Diseases of the Cerebrum

Many neurologic, metabolic, systemic, and toxic disorders affect the cerebrum. Table 24–4 lists these disorders[32–85] and refers the reader to sources listed at the end of this chapter and to other chapters for disorders not discussed here.

Primary Epilepsy

Primary epilepsy is defined as recurrent seizure activity without an underlying structural cause. It has also been called idiopathic, genetic, true, or inherited epilepsy.[86] Primary epilepsy is the most

Table 24–4
The Differential Diagnosis of Cerebral Diseases in Dogs and Cats

CAUSE	USUAL AGE OF ONSET	BREED OR SPECIES PREDISPOSITION	REFERENCES	OTHER READINGS
Inherited or Congenital Disorders				
Congenital hydrocephalus	<1 y	Chihuahua, Boston terrier, Maltese, Yorkshire terrier, chow chow, Pomeranian, toy poodle, cats	26, 32, 33	This chapter
Portosystemic shunt	<1 y	Yorkshire terrier, miniature schnauzer, Lhasa apso, shih tzu, retrievers, Irish setter, Irish wolfhound		Chapter 34
Lissencephaly	<1 y	Lhasa apso, wirehaired fox terrier, Irish setter, cats	34	This chapter
Primary epilepsy	1–5 y	German shepherd, Saint Bernard, Irish setter, golden retriever, keeshond, Labrador retriever, Siberian husky, cocker spaniel, beagle, standard and miniature poodles, wirehaired fox terrier, border collie, others	15, 16, 20, 35–40	This chapter
Lysosomal storage diseases	<1 y	Beagle, basset hound, poodle, English setter, Chihuahua, spaniels, German short-haired pointer, others		Chapter 25
Metabolic Disorders				
Juvenile hypoglycemia (diet-related)	<1 y	Toy breeds		Chapter 48
Hypoglycemia (insulinoma)	>5 y	None		Chapter 48
Hyperlipoproteinemia	2–7 y	Miniature schnauzer		Chapter 50
Uremia	Any age	None		Chapter 16
Hypocalcemia	Any age	None		Chapter 49
Hypoxia	Any age	None		This chapter
Polycythemia	Any age	None		Chapter 41
Hepatic failure	Any age	None		Chapter 34
Neoplasms				
Primary brain tumors			11, 12, 41, 42	
Meningiomas	>5 y	Dolichocephalic dog breeds, cats		This chapter
Glial cell tumors	>5 y	Brachiocephalic dog breeds		
Metastatic brain tumors	>5 y	None		
Nutritional Problems				
Thiamine deficiency	Any age	Primarily cats	43–45	This chapter
Inflammatory Disorders (Dogs)				
Canine distemper virus	Any age but usually <1 y	None	30, 46, 47	This chapter and Chapter 38
Granulomatous meningoencephalitis	1–8 y	Any breed, but especially poodle and terrier	48–51	
Pug dog encephalitis	1–7 y	Pug	52	
Rickettsial meningoencephalitis	Any age	None	53	

Table 24–4
The Differential Diagnosis of Cerebral Diseases in Dogs and Cats *Continued*

CAUSE	USUAL AGE OF ONSET	BREED OR SPECIES PREDISPOSITION	REFERENCES	OTHER READINGS
Inflammatory Disorders (Cats)				
Feline infectious peritonitis	Usually <2 y	None	113, 114	Chapter 38 and this chapter
Feline immunodeficiency virus	Any age	None	54, 110	
Polioencephalomyelitis	Any age	None	55	
Spongioform encephalopathy	Any age	None	56–57	
Inflammatory Disorders				
Rabies	Any age	None	58	This chapter
Fungal encephalitis	>1 y	Primarily large-breed dogs; cats	59, 60	Chapter 39
Protozoal encephalitis	Any age	None		Chapter 40
Bacterial encephalitis	Any age	None	62, 63	Chapter 36
Pseudorabies	Any age	None	64, 65	
Idiopathic Conditions				
Feline hyperesthesia syndrome	Any age	None	111, 112	This chapter
Rage syndrome	3 mo to 3 y	Springer spaniel, golden retriever	66	This chapter
Toxicity				
Lead, organophosphates, ethylene glycol, many others	Any age, but usually <1 y	None	67–78	This chapter
Trauma				
Severe head trauma	Any age, but usually <1 y	None		Chapter 25
Vascular Disorders				
Feline ischemic encephalopathy	Any age	Cats	79–80	This chapter
Canine cerebrovascular disorders	Any age	None	81–84	This chapter
Parasitic Conditions				
Aberrant migration of *Cuterebra* or *Dirofilaria*	Any age	None	85	

Modified from Shell LG. The differential diagnosis of seizures. Vet Med 1993;88:629–640.

common cause of recurrent seizures in dogs; the incidence is 1% to 2%.[87] Although it has been reported to be a common cause of recurrent seizures in cats in the United Kingdom,[40] it appears to be uncommon in cats in the United States (Shell, unpublished observation). Any breed of dog, including mixed breeds, can be affected. Those most commonly affected are listed in Table 24–5. Age of onset of seizure activity is usually between 1 and 5 years, although seizures have been reported in much younger pups

if both parents have epilepsy.[35] Males have a slightly higher incidence rate than females.[37]

Pathophysiology

Primary epilepsy has been demonstrated to have a genetic component in beagles, German shepherds, keeshonds, and Belgian sheepdogs and probably has a genetic component in the other breeds listed in Table 24–5. The presumed abnormality is at the

Table 24–5
Breeds of Dogs With a High Incidence of Primary Epilepsy

Alaskan malamutes
American cocker spaniels
Beagles*
Collies
Dachshunds*
German shepherds (Alsatians)*
Golden retrievers
Irish setters
Keeshonds*
Labrador retrievers
Mastiffs
Miniature schnauzers
Poodles (standard and miniature)
Saint Bernards
Siberian huskies
Springer spaniels (English and Welsh)
Belgian Tervurens (Belgian sheepdogs)*
Wirehaired fox terriers

*A genetic or inherited basis is proven; in the other breeds, it is highly suspected.
From Shell LG. The differential diagnosis of seizures. Vet Med 1993;88:629–640.

physiologic or biochemical level; therefore, results of all diagnostic tests, including brain histopathology, are usually normal.[20]

Clinical Signs

Smaller breeds of dogs tend to have mild, generalized seizures and may not lose consciousness. In the larger breeds, seizures are usually severe and generalized and may develop into clusters of seizures occurring within a short time period. Most of the seizures begin during sleep, and lateralizing or asymmetrical signs are not usually evident. In between the periods of seizure activity (i.e., in the interictal period), the pet appears normal in all respects. The interictal period varies, but in the larger breeds there is a tendency for this period to become shorter with time.

Some of these patients experience status epilepticus. From a clinical perspective, status epilepticus is one continuous seizure lasting 30 minutes or longer, or a series of multiple seizures within a short period of time without intervening periods of consciousness.[88] The distinction between status epilepticus and clusters of seizures is not always clear if the intervals between seizures are short and the postictal changes alter consciousness. Both status epilepticus and clusters of seizures are emergency situations and should be treated because of the possible severe sequelae (Table 24–6),[89] including death.[38]

Diagnostic Plan

The diagnosis is based on the signalment (including age of onset), history (e.g., generalized seizures, no history of toxin or trauma exposure, no history of illness as a puppy that could have been canine distemper virus infection), normal interictal findings on physical and neurologic examination, and the elimination of other potential causes of seizures by routine laboratory testing. If primary epilepsy is suspected based on the above results, specialized tests (CSF analysis, CT scans, or EEG) may not be necessary. However, if the owner wants the diagnosis to be as accurate as possible, then specialized tests may be indicated. Results of such tests are likely to be normal or to show no consistent abnormalities.[20, 36]

Treatment

Anticonvulsant medication is the most acceptable treatment. It is recommended for any dog or cat that has had more than one seizure within 4 months, clusters of seizures without an identifiable cause, or increasing severity or frequency of seizures. Because smaller breeds tend to have less severe and less frequent seizures, they may not require treatment unless the severity or frequency increases. Larger breeds of dogs, particularly those breeds in which primary epilepsy has been proven or suggested, should be started on anticonvulsants after the second or third established seizure because of the severe nature of the seizure activity, the tendency for clusters to develop, and the increased risk of seizures that cannot be controlled well with anticonvulsants (refractory epilepsy). The pet owner must be committed to administering the medication as directed. Pertinent

Table 24–6
Possible Complications of Status Epilepticus

Acid-base imbalances
Brain herniation
Cardiac arrhythmias
Compromised respiratory function
Hyperglycemia
Hyperthermia
Hypoglycemia
Myoglobinuria
Neurogenic pulmonary edema
Permanent brain damage
Renal failure
Rhabdomyolysis

From Dyer KD, Shell LG. Managing patients with status epilepticus. Vet Med 1993;88:654–659.

Table 24–7
Client Education for Treating Pets With Epilepsy

1. Epilepsy cannot be cured, but it can usually be controlled with anticonvulsants. Control means that the frequency or severity of the seizures will be reduced with the anticonvulsant.
2. Medication may be required for the life of the pet.
3. No single drug or drug combinations will work in all pets. Every case is different. The dose may have to be adjusted from time to time. Successful management of some cases in dogs may require use of more than one anticonvulsant.
4. If the medication is to be effective, the usage directions must be followed.
5. Oral medication may take several days for therapeutic effect to occur. Do not be alarmed if the pet has a single, short seizure within the first few days of administering the anticonvulsant.
6. Common side effects of many anticonvulsants include sedation, uncoordination, excessive sleep, increased thirst, increased urination, and increased appetite. Many of these side effects disappear within a few weeks. If other side effects appear or if the above side effects do not disappear, they should be discussed with your veterinarian.
7. Never abruptly discontinue any anticonvulsant drug. A worsening of seizure activity (status epilepticus) could occur because many of the anticonvulsant drugs cause dependence or addiction.
8. A diary should be kept of all seizure activity, noting the date, the description and number of seizures, the drugs given and their doses, and any change in the pet's environment. This record or chart should be reviewed with the veterinarian every 6 to 12 months, or more often if seizure activity appears to increase.

client education must be given and is outlined in Table 24–7.

The goals of anticonvulsant therapy are to reduce the frequency, duration, and severity of seizures while producing minimal side effects. These goals are most often best achieved using primary anticonvulsants (Table 24–8). Secondary anticonvulsants are sometimes added to achieve better control in refractory cases.[39, 90]

In dogs and cats, the initial drug of choice is still phenobarbital, because it appears to be effective, economical, and safe and can be administered twice daily. Negative side effects include sedation, polydipsia, polyuria, and polyphagia, but some or all of these effects should disappear after 1 or 2 weeks of therapy. Occasionally, a dog appears hyperactive during the initial phase of treatment, but this effect can usually be overcome by increasing the dose. Phenobarbital can cause nonspecific, and presumably nonpathologic, increases in serum alkaline phosphatase and alanine aminotransferase concentrations.[91] Recent evidence has linked phenobarbital administration with idiosyncratic hepatotoxicity,[92] but the incidence does not appear to be frequent enough to prevent most clinicians from prescribing it to control seizures.

Primidone, an analog of phenobarbital that does not fall under US Drug Enforcement Agency controls, can also be used in dogs as a primary anticonvulsant. It is metabolized into two other compounds, both of which also have anticonvulsant activity: phenylethylmalonic acid and phenobarbital. Because phenobarbital is thought to account for at least 85% of the anticonvulsant effect, there may be little benefit gained

by using primidone instead of phenobarbital. Although it has not been used frequently in the cat, it can be used safely[93] (Table 24–9).

In cats, oral diazepam appears to be an effective anticonvulsant. Unpublished studies suggest that the halflife in cats is 15 to 20 hours. A standard dose of 2 to 5 mg per cat, or 0.25 to 0.5 mg/kg two or three times per day, is usually recommended. Unlike humans and dogs, cats do not appear to develop a tolerance to the anticonvulsant effects of diazepam.[94]

Client education is crucial to the success of therapy (see Table 24–7). The effectiveness of the chosen anticonvulsant requires that the owner be committed to giving the drug as instructed. A diary or record of all seizure activity should be maintained by the owner and reviewed by the veterinarian every 6 to 12 months, or more often if the seizures occur more than once every 2 months.

Unsatisfactory seizure control may include the persistence of clusters of seizures, severe or prolonged seizures that require intervention by the veterinarian to stop them, or seizures occurring more often than once a month. Possible reasons for apparent anticonvulsant failure are given in Table 24–10. The most reasonable approach is to determine whether appropriate serum levels of the drug have been reached. If the therapeutic concentration is in the low to middle range (see Table 24–8) and if most reasons for apparent anticonvulsant failure have been eliminated, an attempt can be made to gain better control of the seizures by increasing the dose of the anticonvulsant. Alternatively, a secondary anticonvulsant drug can be added to the protocol (see Table 24–8).

To date, the most satisfactory secondary anti-

Table 24-8
Anticonvulsant Drugs for Dogs

DRUG	ELIMINATION HALFLIFE	RECOMMENDED ORAL DOSAGE	THERAPEUTIC SERUM CONCENTRATION
Primary			
Phenobarbital	32–42 h	2 mg/kg b.i.d. (up to 10 mg/kg)	15–45 µg/mL
Primidone	5–10 h	5–10 mg/kg b.i.d. (up to 25 mg/kg)	15–45 µg/mL
Secondary			
Phenytoin	3–7 h	35 mg/kg t.i.d.	10–25 µg/mL
Clonazepam	Varies with dose (up to 5 or 6 h)	0.5 mg/kg t.i.d.	0.015–0.07 µg/mL*
Chlorazepate	5 h	2 mg/kg b.i.d.	500–1900 ng/mL*
Valproic acid	1.5–2 h	10–60 mg/kg t.i.d.	50–100 µg/mL*
Carbamazepine	1–2 h	40 mg/kg t.i.d.	4–12 µg/mL*
Potassium bromide	28 d	20–40 mg/kg/day	1–5 mg/mL*
Mephenytoin	27 h	10 mg/kg t.i.d.	25–40 µg/mL†

*Human values; canine values are unknown.
†Measurement of nirvanol, the active metabolite of mephenytoin.
b.i.d., twice per day; t.i.d., three times per day.
Modified from Dyer KR, Shell LG. Anticonvulsant therapy: A practical guide to medical management of epilepsy in pets. Vet Med 1993; 88:647–653.

convulsant has been bromide.[87, 95] About one half of dogs that have inadequate seizure control while receiving phenobarbital benefit from the addition of bromide. The recommended oral dose of potassium bromide is 20 to 40 mg/kg, once daily or divided twice daily. Serum concentrations increase for at least 4 months after maintenance therapy is started. To achieve more rapid therapeutic serum concentrations, a loading dose of 400 to 500 mg/kg can be divided into four doses and given orally over the course of 1 to 2 days. This loading dose should produce an immediate

Table 24-9
Anticonvulsant Drugs for Cats

DRUG	ELIMINATION HALFLIFE	RECOMMENDED ORAL DOSAGE
Primary		
Phenobarbital	34–43 h	1–2 mg/kg b.i.d. (up to 10 mg/kg)
Diazepam	15–20 h	0.25–0.5 mg/kg b.i.d. or t.i.d.
Secondary		
Primidone*	Not as rapidly metabolized as in dogs	12 mg/kg t.i.d. or 20 mg/kg b.i.d.
Phenytoin*	24–108 h	1.5 mg/kg per day

*Not recommended except in refractory cases.
b.i.d., twice per day; t.i.d., three times per day.
From Dyer KR, Shell LG. Anticonvulsant therapy: A practical guide to medical management of epilepsy in pets. Vet Med 1993; 88:647–653.

serum concentration of 1 to 1.5 mg/mL, but excessive sedation and ataxia may occur in some dogs,[96] especially those with concurrent phenobarbital concentrations higher than 20 µg/mL.[94] Some of the sedation and ataxia can be avoided if the dose of phenobarbital is reduced by 25% to 50% the day before the bromide loading. Such patients should be monitored closely, because rapid reductions in phenobarbital dosage can precipitate seizures. Potassium bromide is not currently commercially available and must be obtained from chemical supply houses as an American Chemical Society chemical grade reagent. Some pharmacies are willing to compound the chemical and dispense it for veterinarians. Because it is not a drug and not approved for use in animals, an investigational drug license from the Food and Drug Administration is necessary to legally dispense this reagent. Pet owners should be warned that it is toxic to humans.

The treatment of status epilepticus or clusters of seizures relies on stopping the seizure and correcting any systemic consequences (see Table 24–6). The approach to termination of a seizure is outlined in Figure 24–5. Diazepam, a short-acting benzodiazepine, is the first choice for those patients that have a history of recurrent seizures not caused by a metabolic cause. Glucose or calcium gluconate is used in selected cases (see Fig. 24–5).[88]

Prognosis

Although anticonvulsants may improve the quality of life in many patients, about 30% of canine

Table 24–10
Real or Apparent Antiepilepsy Drug Failure

REASONS	COMMENTS
Improper dose or frequency of administration	This is the most common cause of failure.
Drug interactions	Some drugs cause a decrease in the serum concentrations of the antiepilepsy drug. Always consult a drug interaction list.
Wrong diagnosis or progressive disease process	Diseases that produce seizures that are not usually controlled with antiepilepsy drugs include brain tumors, active encephalitis, portosystemic shunts, insulinomas or other causes of hypoglycemia.
Refractory epilepsy	The best example is primary epilepsy of large breed dogs.
Development of tolerance	Increasing the dose of the antiepilepsy drug can usually control the seizures again.
Use of drugs known to stimulate seizures	Avoid amphetamines and phenothiazine tranquilizers such as acepromazine, which can lower the seizure threshold.
Development of other diseases	Gastrointestinal or systemic diseases may alter the absorption of the antiepilepsy drug.
Estrus, stress, or excitement	Because seizures may increase in frequency or severity during estrus, ovariohysterectomy is suggested. Stress or excitement can also increase seizure episodes in some pets. Increasing the dose a few days before the anticipated excitement may alleviate the problem.

epileptics do not respond appropriately to anticonvulsant therapy and either die or are euthanized. This is particularly true for larger breeds of dogs, in which seizures may become refractory to anticonvulsant medication after several months to a few years.[38] Clusters of seizures and status epilepticus frequently develop in such cases.

Congenital Hydrocephalus

Hydrocephalus is the excessive accumulation of CSF within the ventricles or subarachnoid space of the brain. Congenital hydrocephalus accounts for about 3% of all congenital anomalies in hospital prevalence studies in dogs.[97] It is probably the most common anomaly of the nervous system. Affected dogs and cats are usually presented before 6 months of age. Breeds of dogs at increased risk are listed in Table 24–11.[16]

Pathophysiology

The primary defect is usually not known, although pathologic studies have found stenosis, atresia, or multiple branching of the mesencephalic aqueduct in some cases. Perinatal inflammation as well as genetic factors may contribute to the abnormal aqueduct and ventricular enlargement. A statistically significant correlation between small body size and hydrocephalus has been demonstrated in dogs.[16]

The extra CSF results in pressure-induced atrophy of the overlying white matter, which contributes to the clinical signs. If CSF volume increases rapidly, some of the excessive fluid enters surrounding brain tissue to cause edema; in such cases, clinical signs may become severe within a short period of time.

Clinical Signs

Behavioral changes are the most frequent complaint. In severe cases, learned responses such as house-breaking are difficult or impossible to achieve. Seizures are also common, with most beginning during the first year of life. Other nervous system signs include aggressive or irrational reactions, quadriparesis, and visual impairment. The menace response is often absent because of atrophy of the optic radiations or visual cortex; in such cases, the PLRs are normal. Head pain may be evident in some animals when the head is palpated.[16]

A dome-shaped skull and a palpable fontanelle are commonly present. One study found a significant relation between the presence of a palpable fontanelle and the presence of ventriculomegaly.[97] Sometimes the prominent or enlarged frontal areas encroach on the orbits, causing a mechanical ventrolateral deviation of the eyes (Fig. 24–6). However, not all animals with these physical abnormalities have clinical signs of hydrocephalus.[98] In addition, some patients with hydrocephalus may not have a prominent dome-shaped skull or a palpable fontanelle.

Diagnostic Plan

The diagnosis is suspected based on the signalment and results of physical and neurologic examinations. Skull radiographs often confirm a large, dome-

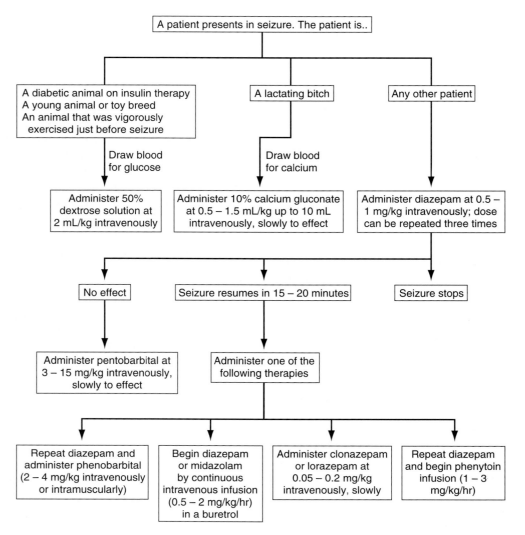

Figure 24–5

The approach to the termination of a seizure. (Modified from Dyer KR, Shell LG. Managing patients with status epilepticus. Vet Med 1993;88:656.)

shaped skull with a ground-glass appearance, open suture lines and fontanelles, and rostral displacement and thinning of the osseus tentorium cerebelli. Ultrasonography through a persistent fontanelle and CT scans are the most accurate and least invasive diagnostic tests for confirmation of an antemortem diagnosis of hydrocephalus. Both tests confirm the dilated ventricles.

Treatment

For patients with an acute onset of severe signs such as depression or stupor, immediate treatment with intravenous (IV) mannitol (0.25–1.0 g/kg, administered slowly), followed by corticosteroids, is necessary to reduce the cerebral edema. Mannitol acts as an osmotic diuretic, and the dose can be repeated twice, if necessary, at 6-hour intervals. Methylprednisolone

Table 24–11
Breeds of Dogs at an Increased Risk for Hydrocephalus

Maltese
Yorkshire terrier
English bulldog
Chihuahua
Lhasa apso
Pomeranian
Toy poodle
Cairn terrier
Boston terrier
Pug
Pekingese

Modified from Selby LA, Hayes HM, Becker SV. Epizootiologic features of canine hydrocephalus. Am J Vet Res 1979;40:411–413.

sodium succinate (30 mg/kg IV) is recommended in severe cases with an acute onset of signs. Methylprednisolone has been shown to be more effective than other drugs in cases of CNS trauma.[99] After clinical signs stabilize, dexamethasone (0.1 mg/kg daily) or prednisolone (0.25–1.0 mg/kg by mouth or intravenously, twice a day) can be used to decrease CSF production. Anticonvulsants are used if recurrent seizures develop. Phenobarbital (2.2 mg/kg twice daily by mouth) is the preferred anticonvulsant (see Primary Epilepsy).

Pets with chronic or more slowly progressive clinical signs can be treated medically, with the use of oral dexamethasone or prednisolone at the above dosages. Because corticosteroids reduce CSF production, improvement is usually noticed within several days. After 1 to 2 weeks, the dose should be reduced by 25% to 50%, and the clinical signs should be monitored closely. If the signs are stable and the pet is functional, this reduced dose can be tried every other day (prednisolone) or every third day (dexamethasone). The goal is to use the least amount of corticosteroid possible to control the signs and to use it as infrequently as the clinical signs allow. Because some animals require corticosteroids indefinitely, the long-term side effects must be discussed with the owners. Some patients stabilize and no longer need corticosteroids or need them only occasionally.

Surgical shunting of CSF to the peritoneal cavity can be attempted if stabilization cannot be achieved with medical treatment. The surgical procedure is described elsewhere.[32,33] Disadvantages include limited availability of surgical expertise, expense, and postoperative complications such as sepsis, occlusion of the drainage tube by fibrous tissue or clots, and the need to replace the tube as the animal matures.

Prognosis

Patients with the most severe signs at an early age have the most guarded prognosis. If such patients do not respond sufficiently to medical treatment, the prognosis is poor for an acceptable life. Those that have minor behavioral disturbances or periodic seizures often make acceptable pets but may require periodic treatments. It is likely that a significant number of animals with minimal hydrocephalus have no clinical signs.

Neoplasia

Brain tumors are masses of neoplastic cells. They arise either from the cells of the brain (primary neoplasias) or from surrounding structures such as meninges and skull or from hematogenous metastasis (secondary neoplasias). Brain tumors are a common cause of neurologic dysfunction in the middle-aged to

older patient and have been reported in 2.8% of necropsied dogs.[40] The incidence of intracranial neoplasia in dogs is approximately 14.5 per 100,000 at risk.[12] Middle-aged to older dogs (median age, 9 years[12]) and cats are most often affected, although brain neoplasms are occasionally found in younger patients as well. Brachycephalic breeds of dogs older than 5 years of age have the highest incidence of brain tumors among domestic animals; gliomas are the most numerous in such breeds, but pituitary adenomas are also frequently reported. Meningiomas tend to occur more frequently in dolichocephalic breeds of dogs (i.e., German shepherds and collies) and in older cats.

Pathophysiology

Although neurons are the most common cells in the brain, they have no significant ability to reproduce. Therefore, they have little potential for developing neoplastic changes. On the other hand, glial cells, the supporting cells of the brain, give rise to a variety of neoplasms. The most common gliomas are astrocytomas and oligodendrogliomas, and these actually invade adjacent normal tissue. Neoplasms may also develop from the meninges. Meningiomas do not usually invade brain parenchyma, but they do significantly compress the brain and thereby produce clinical signs. Recent studies suggest that meningiomas are the most common brain neoplasm.[12]

Many cancers can spread to the brain through blood-borne metastasis. Because the brain receives 20% of the cardiac output, it is not surprising to find metastases to the brain. In adult humans, metastatic tumors account for nearly 30% of all brain tumors[104]; the percentage in animals is not known.

Intracranial neoplasms take up space that

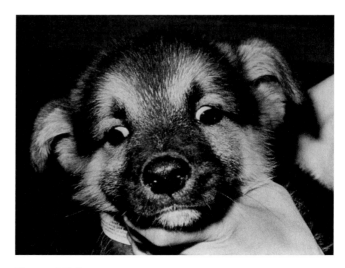

Figure 24–6
Ventrolateral deviation of eyes in a dog with congenital hydrocephalus.

should be occupied by brain tissue. Neurologic signs result not only from the primary effects of the mass (i.e., compression or invasion of brain tissue) but also from secondary side effects such as edema and increased intracranial pressure. Any increase in the volume of brain, be it from the mass directly or from the edema created by the mass, increases intracranial pressure because the brain is housed within a confined, nondistensible space.

Clinical Signs

Clinical signs depend on the size, location, and extent of the mass and its secondary side effects such as edema, elevated intracranial pressure, and displacement of brain tissue. Classically, the onset of signs has been described as gradually progressive, but one report has indicated that about one half of patients have an acute onset.[42] Cerebral masses can become relatively large (>1 cm in diameter) before clinical signs become apparent.[100] Many animals may have vague signs such as lethargy, decreased appetite, or subtle behavioral changes up to 1 year before showing obvious neurologic signs. Seizures, blindness,[101] dementia, and circling are common. If the neoplasm is located to one side of the cerebrum, one usually finds motor or sensory deficits of the limbs on the side opposite the mass. Signs of systemic illness (i.e., fever, weight loss, and coughing) may be found in cases of extracranial neoplasia with secondary cerebral involvement.

Diagnostic Plan

Any acute or slowly progressive behavioral change, seizure, visual deficit, or unilateral motor or sensory deficit in an older patient should arouse suspicions of a brain mass, but until localizing signs develop, the diagnosis of a brain tumor can be difficult. Metabolic disorders should be eliminated by evaluation of the hemogram, chemistry profile, and urinalysis. Chest radiographs should be taken to evaluate the possibility of metastatic neoplasia. The most useful diagnostic tests to confirm the presence of an intracranial tumor, to specify its exact location within the brain, and even sometimes to determine its nature are CT[27] and MRI scans. Both techniques are expensive and not always available to general practitioners. Certain diffuse neoplastic conditions, such as small tumor metastasis or lymphosarcoma,[102] may not be apparent on CT scans. CSF may be helpful[103] but provides limited information and could be rather risky in the patient with increased intracranial pressure. Brain neoplasias usually cause an increase in CSF pressure and protein content and occasionally an increase in the cell count, but similar CSF changes are found with encephalitis. EEG is occasionally helpful in localizing the side of the lesion if focal abnormalities are present, but the results are often nonspecific.

Treatment

The goals of treatment are to remove the mass, if possible, and to control secondary effects of edema and increased intracranial pressure. Surgical removal is not feasible unless a mass can be identified by CT or MRI scans and found to be in a location that is surgically accessible. Meningiomas are most amenable to surgery because they usually are well circumscribed, do not invade brain parenchyma, and are often located in an accessible area near the surface of a cerebral hemisphere.

Most often the secondary effects of brain tumors are treated with corticosteroids to reduce peritumoral edema. The growth of some tumors may also be reduced with corticosteroids. Signs that are acute and rapidly progressive should be managed with IV methylprednisolone sodium succinate (30 mg/kg) or dexamethasone (0.25–1 mg/kg). Mannitol may also be of benefit (1 g/kg IV bolus). Less acute and progressive signs can be managed with oral prednisolone (1–2 mg/kg daily). Anticonvulsant therapy may be needed to control seizures (see Primary Epilepsy treatment). Radiation,[12, 105] hyperthermia, and chemotherapy treatments are limited by availability, expense, experience, and tumor type.

Prognosis

The overall prognosis remains poor for most patients with brain tumors unless complete surgical excision can be performed. The use of irradiation combined with surgery or hyperthermia increased the lifespan of dogs to 4.9 months, compared with a 0.2-month survival time for those without therapy or those given only symptomatic therapy.[12]

Canine Distemper

Canine distemper is a severe, highly contagious infection caused by a species of *Morbillivirus* that can affect many organs. Although not as common as it was before the development of vaccines, canine distemper virus (CDV) infection remains a common cause of neurologic dysfunction. Canine distemper can occur in any age, breed, and sex of dog, regardless of vaccination status. However, unvaccinated, stray, or kennel pups are the most susceptible.

Pathophysiology

About one half of susceptible dogs exposed to CDV develop serum virus-neutralizing antibody titers and show no clinical signs. The other half do not produce sufficient antibody titers and therefore develop clinical signs and usually die during the acute stage of infection.[47] Of the 50% of dogs that develop a titer, neurologic signs occur in about 7%, suggesting that the virus infects epithelial tissue (brain, skin) before the animal is able to mount a sufficient protective response. The ability of CDV to remain in selected epithelial tissue in the presence of circulating antibody may account for nervous system signs in those dogs that seemed to have recovered from systemic disease. CNS infection may be initiated by migrating virus-infected lymphocytes. Both white and gray matter of the CNS can be affected.

Clinical Signs

Clinical signs are highly variable according to the virulence of the strain, the age and immunocompetence of the host, and the body systems affected.[30] The initial signs of viremia usually consist of lethargy, fever, and a decreased appetite; however, these signs may be subtle and may go unnoticed by the owner. A second fever spike may occur 7 to 10 days after the first. It is then that signs of systemic illness usually are noted. Clinical signs may involve the respiratory, ocular, gastrointestinal, integumentary, and nervous systems. The non-neurologic signs are discussed in Chapter 38.

A wide variety of neurologic signs can occur, including seizures, behavioral changes, ataxia and head tilt, nystagmus, tremors of the head and body, progressive weakness in one or more limbs, and rhythmic jerking or twitching of a muscle (myoclonus). Inflammation of the meninges may cause hyperesthesia, cervical rigidity, and pain. Occasionally, blindness occurs from inflammation or demyelination of the optic nerve. Any region of the CNS can be affected. Diffuse or multifocal nervous system involvement is typical, but signs referable to one site often predominate. Nervous system signs can occur simultaneously with the systemic signs or can occur any time after apparent recovery from systemic illness. Some dogs develop neurologic signs only.

Acute encephalitis is characterized by seizures, which can be partial or generalized. Classically, partial seizures are present and are described as "chewing gum" seizures, during which excessive chewing motions and salivation occur; consciousness may or may not be maintained. Other signs of a cerebral disorder include behavioral changes, circling, pacing, and changes in consciousness.

Cerebellar involvement is characterized by head tremors, generalized tremors, ataxia, or vestibular signs. Cranial nerve deficits are not commonly observed with CDV infections except for involvement of the vestibular system or the optic nerve.

Paraparesis or quadriparesis is almost always progressive, and paralysis is likely. Spinal reflexes are exaggerated because there is demyelination of white matter. Myoclonus, the rhythmic and repetitive nonvoluntary movements of a muscle or a group of muscles, is clearly associated with CDV. These movements may be sporadic in the early stages but become more repetitive and rhythmic over time. Limbs and facial muscles are most commonly affected. The pathogenic mechanism is not fully understood, but a "pacemaker" in the neurons of the brain or spinal cord may be involved.[9]

Diagnostic Plan

The antemortem diagnosis of CDV infection can be difficult to confirm. The key to the diagnosis relies on the clinician's ability to piece together the signalment, history, and physical and neurologic examination findings. Certainly, an unvaccinated dog with neurologic signs and coming from a kennel or pound would be suspected to have canine distemper. Chapter 38 discusses the laboratory results observed in systemic cases. Optic neuritis can be diagnosed if mild swelling of the optic disk is observed on fundic examination. Fundic examination may also show active or chronic retinitis (see Chap. 19).

Although anti-CDV antibody can be found in the serum of dogs with distemper, serology may not be beneficial because a single positive IgG titer does not distinguish current infection from previous infection or previous immunization. If the serum IgM titer is elevated or if a rising IgM titer can be established over a 2- to 3-week period, recent infection or vaccination is confirmed. Dogs that have had no prior exposure to CDV and that are severely immunosuppressed in the early stages of the disease may not have any detectable antibody.

In dogs with neurologic signs, routine CSF analysis can be helpful if CSF protein and cell counts (mostly lymphocytes) are elevated. However, during the acute demyelinating stage, inflammatory reactions may be absent. Some laboratories can determine albumin and immunoglobulin content in CSF and serum. The presence of intrathecally produced anti-CDV–specific antibody in spinal fluid supports the diagnosis, but the finding must be cautiously interpreted in view of results of routine CSF analysis. A positive CDV-specific antibody titer is difficult to interpret if the CSF was contaminated with peripheral blood.

Viral isolation is difficult and expensive, but it is the most definitive means to diagnose CDV infection. It can best be done at postmortem examination, because numerous tissues can be collected.

Treatment

There is no effective antiviral treatment; therefore, treatment of systemic canine distemper relies on supportive care (see Chap. 38). Anticonvulsants are used to control seizures but may not always be effective (see Primary Epilepsy). Corticosteroids are avoided if the dog is showing signs of systemic illness. Occasionally, prednisolone (1–2 mg/kg once daily for 3 days and then one half of this dose for another week) is administered if only neurologic signs are present; however, the efficacy is questionable. Although many drugs, such as procainamide, clonazepam, and diazepam, have been tried for treatment of myoclonus, none has proved to be successful.

Prognosis

Dogs with progressive neurologic signs have a poor prognosis, but those with only intermittent seizures, myoclonus, or visual impairment have a better prognosis. Mortality rate is variable and is highest in pups with severe systemic illness and patients with progressive neurologic disease. Dogs that recover from systemic illness can develop neurologic signs weeks to months later.

Granulomatous Meningoencephalitis

Granulomatous meningoencephalitis (GME) is a nonsuppurative, inflammatory disease of the canine CNS of unknown cause. The inflammation can be diffuse and microscopic, multifocal, or focal. It may appear grossly as a mass. Incidence figures have not been reported, but GME appears to be fairly common and is worldwide in distribution. Any age and any breed of dog can be affected. Most authors agree that the incidence is greatest among small purebred dogs and that the lowest incidence is among the very young and the very old.[48] In one study, poodles had a higher prevalence.[50] Some report that females may be affected more often,[106] but others report the opposite.[48]

Pathophysiology

Although many believe that GME is an infectious disease, experimental studies to transmit an infectious agent in dogs using GME-diseased brain tissue have failed.[106] No etiologic agent has been identified. Because similar histologic changes can be produced experimentally by stimulating an immune reaction against brain tissue, an immune-mediated pathogenesis has been proposed. What triggers this proliferation of reticulohistiocytic cells, primarily around blood vessels in the brain, is not known.[49]

Clinical Signs

The onset can be acute or slowly progressive over several weeks. Neurologic signs vary with the location of the changes within the brain or spinal cord. Behavioral changes and seizures have been observed with cerebral GME, and head tilt, nystagmus, and tremors of the head or limbs have been observed with GME of the posterior fossa. Other cranial nerve deficits and limb weakness have been observed with GME of the brain stem. Blindness, caused by GME optic neuritis, can also occur. Neck pain and quadriparesis can be expected if GME develops in the cervical region. Chronic and progressive signs are more likely to be associated with focal GME in which large masses may develop. Duration of clinical signs is variable; some dogs present with an acute onset of coma or status epilepticus from which they do not recover; others have signs that progress over weeks to months.

Diagnostic Plan

There are no typical hematologic or biochemical profile changes in dogs with GME. CSF analysis often reveals an increase in mononuclear cells and protein, with counts ranging from 100 to 1000 white blood cells/µL.[51] Occasionally, a large anaplastic mononuclear cell with lacy cytoplasm is found on cytologic examination. EEG analysis may show evidence of abnormalities, but they are not specific for GME. If lesions are focal or multifocal, they may be observed on CT or MRI scans but are impossible to differentiate from neoplasia without histology. Unfortunately, GME is difficult to differentiate from other types of encephalitis and may be hard to differentiate from neoplasia if a large focal lesion is present. The diagnosis can be confirmed definitively only by histopathology. Lesions are typically associated with the vasculature and consist of mononuclear perivascular cuffing. Eccentrically placed nodular foci of macrophages within these cuffs are characteristic of GME. Mononuclear perivascular cuffs may be found diffusely throughout the brain, or they may be localized to a particular area. If the cuffs become large or merge with adjacent cuffs, they can grossly appear as a mass.

Treatment

Corticosteroids (prednisolone 1–2 mg/kg daily) may temporarily improve signs in some patients, particularly those with a slower onset of clinical signs. If clinical signs improve, they tend to recur if the corticosteroids are discontinued. Anticonvulsants are used if recurrent seizures exist (see Primary Epilepsy).

Prognosis

The long-term prognosis is poor. Dogs that present in status epilepticus or coma usually never regain consciousness. Despite corticosteroid treatment, all confirmed cases have continued to progress to death.

Rabies

Rabies is a fatal viral infection of the nervous system transmitted by saliva of infected animals. The highest incidence of rabies in dogs and cats in the United States occurs in geographic locations in which wildlife rabies is epizootic.[58] Dogs and cats of any age, breed, or sex are susceptible if they have not had adequate vaccinations against the virus.

Pathophysiology

Rabies virus is a rhabdovirus that can infect any warm-blooded animal. The virus is transmitted through the saliva into a bite wound, where it replicates in the muscle cells. After a variable period (days to weeks), the virus spreads to the neuromuscular junction, enters the peripheral nerves, and spreads centripetally to the spinal cord and brain. It can then spread centrifugally from the cord or brain to peripheral nerves and other tissues such as salivary glands. In naturally occurring cases, the incubation period has ranged from 3 weeks to 6 months in dogs, 2 to 6 weeks in cats, and 3 weeks to 1 year in people.[58] The incubation period depends on the site of the bite wound, the amount of virus introduced, and the species that is bitten. The virus is shed in saliva shortly before clinical signs appear. Shedding continues until the animal dies.

Clinical Signs

The clinical course and signs are variable. Typically three phases may be observed. First, in the prodromal phase, the animal may show subtle behavioral changes or may chew at the bite site. This phase may go unnoticed. In the second phase, the animal may exhibit irritability, aggression, or barking. Pica, unexplained roaming, seizures, disorientation, or ataxia may develop. Animals are frequently described as excitable, photophobic, and hyperesthetic.[58] They may bark or snap at imaginary objects. This phase has been called the furious phase, and it lasts from 1 to 7 days. In the third and final phase, there is progressive lower motor neuron weakness and paralysis of the limbs as well as some of the cranial nerves. This "dumb" or paralytic phase may last 2 to 4 days. Spinal reflexes are reduced or absent, and muscles are flaccid and without tone. Inspiratory stridor and a change in the bark caused by laryngeal paralysis may develop. Drooling and dysphagia occur because of pharyngeal paralysis. The animal may make a choking sound that causes the owner to believe something is caught in the animal's throat.[58] The mouth may not close because of masticatory paralysis (dropped jaw). The animal is usually severely depressed and may become stuporous or comatose before death. Death usually occurs within 3 to 7 days from the onset of clinical signs.

Diagnostic Plan

Any animal with an acute onset of rapidly progressive neurologic signs that is not vaccinated for rabies must be considered a rabies suspect. Even in vaccinated animals, rabies should be on the differential diagnosis list if neurologic signs progress rapidly to death and another reasonable diagnosis has not been confirmed. No hematologic or serum biochemical changes are characteristic for rabies infection. Biochemical changes in CSF have been minimal in experimentally infected dogs.[58]

If rabies is suspected, precautions must be taken to prevent exposure of other pets and humans. Examinations are kept to a minimum and are performed by gloved individuals. If the animal is unvaccinated and human exposure has occurred, the animal should be humanely euthanized and the head submitted in a leak-proof, well-labeled container to the appropriate laboratory. Specimens may be refrigerated but not frozen, because thawing causes damage to the brain tissue. The direct fluorescent antibody test is used by most laboratories for confirmation of rabies virus in tissues. Routine histopathology of the brain may show neuronal inclusions called Negri bodies, but these are not observed in every case. Pathologic changes depend on the severity and duration of infection at the time of examination. Neuronal degeneration, lymphocytic and plasmacytic perivascular cuffing, and focal mononuclear cell infiltrates may be found.

Pursuit of an antemortem diagnosis of rabies is not recommended in suspected cases. The direct fluorescent antibody test has been used to detect rabies antigen in skin biopsies, but false-negative results can occur.

Treatment

There is no treatment for rabies. Supportive care is not recommended, because the virus can be excreted in the saliva for a variable and unknown amount of time.

Prognosis

The prognosis is poor for an animal with rabies. Some experimentally infected dogs have developed an atypical, abortive form of infection and showed clinical improvement for days to months.[107]

For rabies prevention and vaccination, the guidelines in the Compendium of Animal Rabies Control, published by the National Association of State Public Health Veterinarians, should be followed. The number of personnel handling or treating the patient with suspected rabies should be minimized, and a log of attending personnel should be maintained. Protective clothing (i.e., lab coat, mask, and gloves) should be worn. Local public health officials should be notified about suspected rabies cases.

Pseudorabies

Pseudorabies is a viral infection that predominantly affects pigs. It is uncommon in the general population but is observed sporadically in areas where the disease is enzootic in swine, the main reservoir of the virus.[64, 65] Dogs and cats of any age can become infected if they ingest contaminated raw pork.

Pathophysiology

The pseudorabies virus is a member of the α-herpesviruses. Although many mammals are susceptible to pseudorabies virus infection, the disease is predominantly observed in swine. Naturally acquired infections in dogs or cats almost always occur after ingestion of contaminated raw pork. Experimental studies in orally infected cats indicate that the virus replicates in the tonsils and enters nearby nerve endings such as the sensory branches of CN IX and CN X. Travelling in a retrograde fashion through the axoplasm of the nerve fibers, the virus enters the brain stem. Pathologic lesions are located predominantly in the brain stem at cranial nerve nuclei.

Clinical Signs

The initial signs are usually depression or anxiety (restlessness). In one study, 60.7% of 40 patients had increased salivation as the predominant sign[64]; in another study of 25 dogs, all had ptyalism.[65] Fever, ataxia, seizures, dyspnea, vomiting, and diarrhea are other clinical signs. Intense pruritus (hence the name "mad itch") and self-mutilation are characteristic signs but are not seen with every case. An animal may violently scratch or rub its faces and ears and then have a convulsion. Anisocoria and a hoarse voice have been noted in cats.[63] Duration of clinical signs is usually short, ranging from 6 to 96 hours.[65] Some animals die suddenly without observed clinical signs.[64] Death is preceded by severe depression, dyspnea, and coma in many cases.

Diagnostic Plan

The diagnosis relies on the acute progressive signs and a history of potential or confirmed exposure to raw pork. Certainly, rabies must be on the differential diagnosis list, especially if exposure to pork cannot be confirmed. Pseudorabies usually progresses more rapidly to death.

Laboratory test results are normal or reflect metabolic changes brought on by the disease (e.g., dehydration, azotemia, hypokalemia). CSF analysis may demonstrate increased protein and mononuclear cells, characteristic of a viral infection. Brain histopathology consists of perivascular cuffing and proliferation of astrocytes and microglial cells in the brain stem. Neuronal degeneration within cranial nerve nuclei and weakly eosinophilic viral inclusion bodies in the nuclei of astrocytes and neurons are also observed. The diagnosis of pseudorabies is confirmed by immunofluorescent testing of brain tissue or by viral isolation.

Treatment

There is no effective treatment, and the disease is almost always fatal. Prevention is the most important means of controlling infection in dogs and cats.

Prognosis

Pseudorabies is considered a fatal disease. Cats may be somewhat more resistant than dogs, but recovery is not common in either species.

Central Nervous System Toxins

There are many chemicals that cause CNS signs, either directly or indirectly.[69–78] Cases of toxicity are common, especially in emergency practices. Of 7326 calls to the Illinois Animal Poison Information Center in 1989, seizures alone were reported to occur in 8.2% of cases of intoxication involving dogs and cats.[69] Any age and breed may be affected. Younger animals may be more likely to ingest toxic materials because of their chewing habits. Cats are more susceptible than dogs to many toxins.

Pathophysiology

Each toxin has its own effect on the nervous system. For example, carbamates and organophosphates block acetylcholinesterase activity, leading to continuous neurostimulation. Ivermectin interferes with the inhibitory neurotransmitter γ-aminobutyric acid (GABA).[67] Toxicology textbooks should be consulted for further discussion on the pathophysiology of each toxin.

Table 24–12
Clinical Signs Associated With Exposure to Toxins

Seizures or Hyperactivity
Lead
Organophosphates
Chlorinated hydrocarbon
Carbamates
1080 (Sodium fluoroacetate)
Strychnine
Amphetamines
Pyrethrins
Rotenone
Organochlorines (lindane, chlordane)
Caffeine or chocolate
Bromethalin
Diethyltoluamide (DEET)

Depression, Stupor, or Coma
Ethylene glycol
α-Naphthylthiourea (ANTU)
Marijuana
Narcotics
Barbiturates
Tranquilizers
Ivermectin
Amitraz

Tremors (see Chap. 25)

Ataxia or Weakness
Lead
Organophosphates
Tranquilizers
Marijuana
Ethylene glycol
Bromethalin

Clinical Signs

Most common toxins that affect the nervous system produce one or more of the following signs: seizures, hyperactivity, ataxia or weakness, muscle tremors, depression, or stupor (Table 24–12).[67–78] Because more than 210 different toxins are reported to induce seizures,[69] it is important to determine exactly what the animal was exposed to. Some of the more common nervous system toxins and a summary of their clinical signs are as follows.

Pyrethrin and Pyrethroids. Signs include tremors, salivation, depression, excitability, ataxia, vomiting, seizures, and dyspnea. In cats, most cases are observed within hours of application of the insecticide. Sublethally exposed animals usually recover within 72 hours.

Organophosphates and Carbamates. These insecticides produce three categories of effects: muscarinic (salivation, lacrimation, vomiting, diarrhea, bronchial secretion), nicotinic (tremors, respiratory paralysis), and central nervous system (seizures, hyperactivity, miosis). Organophosphate compounds include chlorpyrifos, dichlorvos, fenthion, diazinon, chlorfenvinphos, malathion, phosmet, ronnel, and cythioate. Carbamate compounds include carbaryl, bendiocarb, propoxur, aldicarb, methomyl, and carbofuran.

Strychnine. This rodenticide produces clinical signs of seizures, opisthotonos, and extensor rigidity, usually within 2 hours after ingestion. Death occurs from apnea and hypoxia.

Organochlorines. Signs include sudden or progressive onsets of depression, hyperactivity, seizures, ataxia, salivation, hyperthermia, and coma. Liver damage may occur with lindane toxicity. Chlordane is another organochlorine.

Ivermectin. Toxicity is most profound in collies. Clinical signs consist of depression that progresses to coma, ataxia, salivation, mydriasis, and tremors.[78] Death results from bradycardia and respiratory failure.

Amitraz. This miticide can cause depression, hypothermia, ataxia, and seizures.

Caffeine and Methylxanthines. Toxicosis results in vomiting, hyperactivity, tremors, tachycardia, seizures, and arrhythmias. Caffeine toxicosis is most commonly the result of ingestion of caffeine-based stimulants (e.g., NōDōz) and chocolate. Methylxanthines include theophylline, aminophylline, and theobromine.

Lead. Common clinical signs of lead toxicity include a mixture of gastrointestinal signs (vomiting, diarrhea, constipation) and neurologic signs (depression, hyperactivity, seizures, vocalization, ataxia). Sources of lead include old paint, putties, artist paints, some tiles and linoleums, used motor oils, leaded gasoline, lead objects (e.g., fish sinkers, bullets, foil, drapery weights), and improperly glazed pottery.

Metaldehyde. Ingestion of molluscicides containing metaldehyde can produce tachycardia, salivation, tremors, vomiting, seizures, depression, and diarrhea within 3 hours. Death from respiratory failure can occur within 4 to 24 hours, and delayed deaths may occur from liver failure.[70]

Ethylene Glycol. Ingestion of antifreeze containing ethylene glycol can produce ataxia, tremors, depression, seizures, and coma before the onset of acute kidney failure (see Chap. 16).

Diagnostic Plan

Historical information is crucial in establishing the diagnosis of a specific toxicity. Most owners respond in a negative way if asked whether the pet has been exposed to toxins; many do not realize that insecticides and flea control products can be toxic. Intoxications are too frequently the result of the mindset, "If a little is good, a lot is better." Because owners are often unaware of all the potential toxins in the pet's environment, rather specific and direct questions must be asked:

1. What does the pet chew on? Does the pet chew on painted objects, linoleum, or caulking compounds, which could have lead in them?
2. What type of dishes does the pet drink and eat from?
3. What type of flea control is used, and how often?
4. Is the house, garden, or lawn treated with pesticides, and how often?
5. Have any other neighborhood animals been ill?
6. Has the antifreeze been changed in the car, and where?
7. Does the pet stay in the garage?
8. Could the pet have licked or ingested any automobile fluids (e.g., oil, antifreeze, transmission fluid)?
9. Could the pet have swallowed any human drugs accidentally?
10. Has anyone threatened the pet with harm?
11. Has anyone administered any pills or liquids to the pet? Or what medications is the pet receiving?
12. Does the pet get into garbage?

If organophosphate toxicity is suspected, evaluation of serum cholinesterase activity can help to establish a diagnosis. Likewise, elevated blood lead levels can confirm lead intoxication. The specific diagnosis of other toxins relies on the clinical signs and accurate historical information provided by the owner. For example, strychnine poisoning causes tetany and seizure-like activity, which are induced by noise, light, or handling.

Treatment

Treatment varies with the specific toxin. Supportive care usually consists of monitoring and maintaining a normal body temperature, providing respiratory support by ensuring a patent airway and adequate ventilation, stopping seizures or severe muscle tremors, providing cardiovascular support by treating bradycardia or arrhythmias, and maintaining blood pressure through fluid therapy.[67] Generally speaking, IV fluids may be helpful in eliminating some of the toxins (strychnine, caffeine, metaldehyde), but excessive use of fluids can contribute to cerebral edema. Injectable diazepam may be administered to stop seizures or tremors (see Primary Epilepsy). However, with some toxins (e.g., strychnine), general anesthesia is preferred because of the short-acting anticonvulsant effects of diazepam. If dermal exposure is suspected, a bath may prevent further dermal absorption of the toxin. The induction of emesis is valuable in limiting systemic absorption within the first 4 hours of ingestion. Apomorphine (0.04 mg/kg intravenously or intraocularly) is recommended. Gastric lavage is useful if it is initiated within 2 hours of toxin ingestion. A slurry of activated charcoal (1 g/kg), made by adding 1 g charcoal to 10 mL of water, acts to minimize gastric absorption.[67] For some of the more common toxins, the treatments are outlined as follows.

Pyrethrin and Pyrethroids. Treatment is directed at supportive care and prevention of further absorption from the skin and gastrointestinal tract.

Organophosphates and Carbamates. Treatment consists of supportive care, a mild detergent bath if the animal was dermally exposed, and atropine (0.1–0.2 mg/kg intravenously, as needed). Pralidoxime chloride (Protopam Chloride or 2-PAM, 20 mg/kg intramuscularly, two or three times per day until signs are resolved or benefit is no longer observed) is recommended in organophosphate toxicity, especially in dermally exposed animals.

Strychnine. Activated charcoal administration and forced diuresis are generally recommended. Pentobarbital or general anesthesia is used to control seizure activity. Urinary acidification (ammonium chloride, 100 mg/kg twice a day by mouth) may enhance renal excretion but is contraindicated if exertional acidosis or myoglobinuria is present.

Organochlorines. Bathing the animal with a mild detergent, administering activated charcoal, and giving supportive care are recommended.

Ivermectin. Supportive care and glycopyrrolate (0.01 mg/kg as needed) to treat bradycardia are recommended. Physostigmine (1 mg twice a day by slow IV administration) is recommended for patients with severe depression or coma. With supportive care, many survive.

Amitraz. Treatment is entirely supportive care.

Caffeine and Methylxanthines. Fluid therapy is recommended to enhance diuresis. Anticonvulsants may be needed to control seizures, and antiarrhythmics are recommended if necessary. Discontinuing of medications that contain methylxanthines, or decreasing the dose, is recommended.

Lead. Treatment is directed at chelation and removal of lead from body stores using EDTA (Calcium Disodium Versenate) at 100 mg/kg per day divided into four daily doses for 2 to 5 days and administered either intravenously or subcutaneously (10 mg EDTA in 1 mL of 5% dextrose). Chelation therapy may increase the severity and frequency of neurologic signs in the first several days of treatment. Oxygen, corticosteroids, and mannitol are recommended as possible means of decreasing cerebral edema associated with toxicity (see Chap. 25).

Metaldehyde. Treatment consists of anticonvulsants, activated charcoal, and fluid therapy to control acidosis.

Ethylene Glycol. See Chapter 16.

Prognosis

The prognosis varies with the toxin and the amount to which the animal was exposed. If the toxic agent can be identified, a more exact prognosis can be offered. It may take days to weeks for the animal to fully recover.

Feline Ischemic Encephalopathy

Feline ischemic encephalopathy (FIE) is a naturally occurring neurologic syndrome of acute, usually unilateral, necrosis of brain tissue.[108] The true incidence is unknown, but the syndrome appears to be common. In a retrospective study of seizures in cats by me and others, FIE was histopathologically diagnosed in 9.4% of cats presenting with seizures (Shell, unpublished observations). Any age, sex, and breed of mature cat can be affected.

Pathophysiology

The underlying cause for the ischemic necrosis is unknown.[80] Frequently, the major infarction lesion has been in the distribution of the middle cerebral artery on one side of the brain. Vascular abnormalities, such as venous thrombosis and vasculitis, have not been found consistently, nor have lesions been found consistently elsewhere. There has been no evidence of cardiomyopathy to date.[9]

Unilateral cerebral lesions often cause circling toward the affected side. Many such lesions are located in the frontal lobe or rostral thalamus, and the head turning and circling to the affected side is referred to as the adversive syndrome.[9] Involvement of the limbic system may contribute to behavioral changes.

Clinical Signs

All signs are peracute in onset. Generalized or partial seizures are commonly observed. Some cats have behavioral changes such as aggression, depression, dementia, or stupor. Many are ambulatory but ataxic and may circle toward the side of the lesion (adversive syndrome).[9] Blindness may be apparent. Cases can be found at any time during the year, but one author noted a tendency for more cases to occur during the summer months.[9]

The neurologic examination may show signs consistent with a unilateral cerebral lesion: circling to the side of the lesion, decreased facial movements (decreased eyelid closure or lip retraction), decreased facial sensation, or decreased menace response or impaired vision on the side opposite the lesion. Changes in the cat's behavior may be evident during the examination. Occasionally, bilateral blindness with dilated and unresponsive pupils occurs because of ischemic necrosis of the optic chiasm[9] if the cranial brain stem is affected.

Diagnostic Plan

The acute onset and asymmetry of clinical signs suggest FIE in adult cats. Differential diagnoses include trauma, neoplasia, and CNS infections. Routine laboratory data (hemogram, chemistry profile, urinalysis) should be evaluated for signs of systemic disease. Tests for the feline leukemia virus and feline immunodeficiency virus (FIV) should be performed before other expensive and sometimes invasive tests are pursued to evaluate the brain. If the cat is middle-aged to older, chest radiographs should be considered to evaluate the possibility of metastatic neoplasia that may have spread to the brain. Although an EEG may confirm brain dysfunction or even help to confirm a specific location, the results cannot differentiate vascular disease from neoplasia, trauma, or infection. CSF analysis may be normal or may show xanthochromia, erythrophagocytosis, an increase in protein, or, occasionally, an increase in cells. If severe necrosis of brain tissue occurs, increased numbers of white blood cells, mostly macrophages, are likely. CT or MRI scans may be the best antemortem means of diagnosing vascular disorders, but there have not been any published studies in cats to determine the value of such scans.

Treatment

Corticosteroids (prednisolone, 2 mg/kg subcutaneously, once daily for 1–2 days, or methylprednisolone sodium succinate, 30 mg/kg intravenously once, followed by 15 mg/kg at 3 and at 6 hours later) and hyperventilation (oxygen therapy) may help to reduce edema associated with the ischemia. Intravenous diazepam (see Primary Epilepsy) is usually needed to stop seizure activity. Because acquired epilepsy is a potential sequela, oral phenobarbital or diazepam (see Table 24–9) is recommended until it can be determined that the cat has not had seizures for at least 6 months after the onset of clinical signs.

Prognosis

The prognosis is guarded during the first several days until it can be determined that the clinical signs are not progressive and are not life-threatening. About one half of the cats that I have observed remained functional pets after the diagnosis was made. Permanent behavioral changes, especially aggressive behavior and recurrent seizures, are the two most common sequelae.

Canine Cerebrovascular Disorders

Cerebrovascular diseases encompass a variety of disorders that cause a pathologic change in cerebral blood vessels resulting in a decreased blood supply to the brain. These pathologic changes can be characterized as thrombosis, embolism, infarction, and hemorrhage. The true incidence is unknown. In one article, cerebrovascular disease was diagnosed in 17 dogs in a 1.5-year period.[82] Any breed and age of dog can be affected, but most cerebrovascular disease occurs in older dogs (mean age, 11.5 years).[82] See the previous section for a discussion of feline ischemic encephalopathy as a separate entity.

Pathophysiology

Thrombosis is a change in blood vessel diameter caused by formation of a mass (thrombus) derived from blood components. An embolus is also a mass that reduces vessel diameter, but it is formed elsewhere and travels to lodge in the affected vessel. Thrombosis or embolization results in obstruction of blood flow to a localized part of the brain; obstruction produces focal brain necrosis or infarction. Thromboembolic cerebrovascular occlusion can be caused by bacteria, neoplasia, parasites, or atherosclerosis associated with hypothyroidism.[81] Causes of primary cerebrovascular disease include vascular malformations, primary brain tumors, and trauma. Spontaneous hemorrhage of the CNS is rare; most hemorrhages are caused by trauma, blood dyscrasias, and neoplasia. Hemorrhage has been reported in association with vascular malformations.[82–84]

Clinical Signs

The onset is usually acute, with clinical signs that vary with the location and severity of the cerebrovascular lesion.[82] Most cases involve the cerebrum and produce ataxia, seizures, behavioral changes, stupor or coma, circling, and weakness. Nystagmus and head tilt are common findings if the brain stem is affected. Signs of systemic illness may precede the onset of neurologic deficits if cerebrovascular disease is secondary to sepsis, coagulopathy, metastatic tumor, diabetes mellitus, or hyperadrenocorticism.[82]

Diagnostic Plan

The diagnosis of cerebrovascular disease is usually difficult to make. Because it often occurs secondary to systemic disease, a thorough physical examination and evaluation of routine laboratory data are indicated. Chest radiographs and electrocardiographic monitoring may uncover abnormalities such as pathologic lung lesions and arrhythmias, respectively. In breeds known to have a high incidence of hypothyroidism, atherosclerosis of brain blood vessels has been associated with cerebral artery thrombosis.[81, 82] CT or MRI scans may be beneficial to help localize the lesion or suggest possible causes.

Treatment

Treatment should be directed at the underlying cause if one can be found. Hyperventilation with oxygen (see Chap. 25) may reduce elevated intracranial pressure and maintain the oxygen supply to the brain to prevent further hypoxia. Reduction of edema and intracranial pressure can be achieved with mannitol solution (1 g/kg IV bolus) or methylprednisolone sodium succinate (30 mg/kg intravenously, followed by 15 mg/kg at 3 and at 6 hours later).

Prognosis

The prognosis varies with the location of damage, the magnitude of vessel occlusion, and the rapidity of the occlusion[82] as well as the underlying cause. Because most patients have primary brain disease or underlying systemic illness, the prognosis is guarded.

Uncommon Diseases of the Cerebrum

Lissencephaly

Lissencephaly is a congenital absence of the convolutions (gyri and sulci) of the cerebral cortex. It has been reported in Lhasa apsos, Irish setters, wire-haired fox terriers, and cats. Progressive behavioral changes and seizures are common signs. There is no treatment. The diagnosis is made at necropsy, but with the advent of MRI scans, antemortem diagnosis may be possible.[34]

Storage Diseases

Storage disorders include a wide variety of inherited absences of enzymes necessary for normal cell metabolism. Many of these disorders affect the cerebrum and cause seizures and behavioral changes. Antemortem diagnosis is often difficult. There is no treatment, and clinical signs are progressive. Chapter 25 includes more discussion on these disorders.[109]

Rage Syndrome

Rage syndrome is characterized by sudden, unprovoked attacks of aggression; it occurs in male springer spaniels[66] and golden retrievers aged 3 months to 3 years (Shell, unpublished observation). The underlying cause is unknown, although it may be an extremely severe form of dominance aggression. A behaviorist should be consulted if the owner wishes to pursue treatment. Because of the unpredictable aggressive attacks by these animals and their lack of response to hormonal, behavioral, and anticonvulsant therapy, euthanasia must be a consideration.[66]

Thiamine Deficiency

A deficiency in vitamin B_1 (thiamine) can cause behavioral changes, stupor, seizures, pupil dilation, nystagmus and other vestibular signs, neck ventroflexion, and weakness of gait.[43–45] Thiamine deficiency has been associated with feeding dogs a diet of cooked meat and feeding cats an all-fish diet that contains thiaminase, an enzyme that destroys thiamine. It may also be associated with prolonged anorexia, extensive diuresis, or destruction of thiamine during the processing of commercial pet foods. Treatment with thiamine (50 mg intramuscularly, two or three times per day) before the onset of severe weakness or stupor usually results in partial or complete recovery within several days.

Pug Dog Encephalitis

Pug dog encephalitis is a granulomatous to necrotizing inflammatory disease of the white and gray matter of the cerebrum and sometimes of the meninges in dogs of the pug breed.[52] The cause is unknown. Signs consist of generalized or partial seizures, circling, staring into space, constant pacing, walking into objects, decreased awareness, or intermittent screaming. CSF analysis is abnormal in most cases. The prognosis for survival beyond several weeks to months is poor; seizures often become refractory to anticonvulsants, and behavioral changes are usually progressive. A recent report described similar clinical and histopathologic findings in Maltese.[110]

Mycotic, Protozoal, Bacterial, and Rickettsial Meningoencephalitis

Cryptococcus neoformans, Blastomyces dermatitidis, Histoplasma capsulatum, and *Cladosporium* spp. organisms probably enter the nervous system hematogenously or by extension from the upper respiratory tract through the cribriform plate. Seizures, behavioral changes, stupor, cranial nerve deficits, incoordination, nuchal rigidity, quadriparesis, or paraparesis can result. Some animals have systemic signs (pneumonia, lymphadenopathy, draining skin lesions). Diagnosis is usually made by finding the organism on aspiration cytology or histopathology. CSF cytology and culture are the definitive means to diagnose CNS infections. See Chapter 39 for a more complete discussion.

Prototheca, an achlorophyllous alga, affects immunocompromised hosts, producing bloody diarrhea and extensive retinal lesions. Nervous system signs include weakness, circling, blindness, and mental depression.[60]

Seizures, ataxia, limb weakness, and extensor rigidity of the pelvic limbs have been reported with *Toxoplasma* and *Neospora,* whereas disorientation, seizures, weight loss, behavioral changes, and circling have been reported in pups with encephalitozoonosis.[61] Affected animals may be immunosuppressed and may have signs of other diseases.

Bacterial infections causing meningitis, abscess, or subdural empyema occur through hematogenous spread from a systemic focus or by localized extension of infection. CSF should be cultured for aerobic as well as anaerobic bacteria.[62] Antibiotics that penetrate the blood-brain barrier should be used (see Table 24–1) until culture and sensitivity results return. The prognosis is guarded until the response to treatment can be ascertained.

Rickettsial meningoencephalitis in dogs is characterized by a rather acute onset of neurologic signs that rapidly progress to death unless treated. Lethargy, seizures, peripheral or central vestibular signs, ataxia, spinal hyperesthesia, and weakness can be observed[53] (see Chap. 37).

Feline Spongiform Encephalopathy

Feline spongiform encephalopathy is a type of transmissible spongiform encephalopathy[56–57] caused by an unconventional agent known as a prion, which has a long incubation period. Clinical signs in cats in the United Kingdom developed gradually over several weeks and often consisted of behavioral changes such as unprovoked aggression or increased timidity, ataxia, hypermetria, vestibular signs, marked hyperesthesia to touch and sound, and dementia. There is no treatment.

The diagnosis is based on histopathologic findings of vacuolation of the gray matter.

Feline Polioencephalomyelitis

Feline polioencephalomyelitis is a chronic, slowly progressive neurologic disease that is observed in both immature and mature cats. Neurologic signs vary and include seizures, weakness, head tremors, and aggressive behavior. Histologic findings suggest a viral cause, but viral isolation attempts have been unsuccessful.[55]

Feline Immunodeficiency Virus Encephalopathy

Neurologic abnormalities associated with FIV infection include seizures, dementia, social withdrawal, loss of toilet training, aggression, and twitching of the face and tongue. FIV antibodies have been reported in the CSF. Zidovudine (20 mg/kg twice daily, by mouth) may be an effective drug for managing such cats, but clinical trials have not been evaluated[54, 111] (see Chap. 38).

Feline Hyperesthesia Syndrome

Cats affected with feline hyperesthesia syndrome exhibit excessive twitching or crawling of the skin along the lumbar region; this may occur spontaneously or be induced by touching. In severe cases, seizures or seizure-like activity may occur when the lumbar region is vigorously rubbed. The cause is unknown, but contributing factors may include fleas, dermatitis, behavioral disorders, vertebral trauma, or food hypersensitivity. Treatments have included all-natural diets, anticonvulsants, and corticosteroids (prednisolone, 2 mg/kg once daily).[112, 113]

Hypoxia

Cerebral hypoxia or anoxia can occur with many disorders, but it is most commonly associated with cardiac and respiratory arrest. Results of oxygen deprivation to the brain depend on the duration and severity of the deprivation. Although different areas of the brain have different metabolic rates and oxygen needs, irreversible neuronal injury occurs within 15 minutes of anoxia. Neurons of the cerebral cortex, hippocampus, thalamus, and cerebellum tend to be more susceptible to the effects of hypoxia. Animals that survive arrests may show cerebral signs such as behavioral changes, blindness, and seizures or cerebellar signs such as head and body tremors.

Feline Infectious Peritonitis

The neurologic form of feline infectious peritonitis (FIP), including meningitis and encephalomyelitis, has been a clinical entity since FIP was originally recognized in the 1950s. Clinical signs referable to the CNS were observed in 29% of cases reviewed.[114] Neurologic involvement is about three times more prevalent in the noneffusive (dry) form as opposed to the effusive (wet) form. Common CNS signs include paraparesis, nystagmus, and seizures, but any neurologic sign may be seen. Most affected cats have other clinical signs suggesting systemic involvement. CSF examination often reveals increased protein and cells (both mononuclear and polymorphonuclear). On histopathologic examination, there is a pyogranulomatous leptomeningitis and encephalomyelitis.[115] Neurologic signs are progressive, and there is no good treatment (see Chap. 38).

Canine Herpesvirus Encephalitis

In newborn puppies, the canine herpesvirus can cause extensive inflammation in the brain. If a pup survives the encephalitis, residual signs such as seizures or cerebellar ataxia may be observed[116] (see Chap. 23).

References

1. Jenkins TW. Development and gross anatomy of the brain. In: Functional Mammalian Neuroanatomy. Philadelphia, Lea & Febiger, 1978:13–46.
2. de Lahunta A. Cerebrospinal fluid and hydrocephalus. In: de Lahunta A, Habel RE, eds. Veterinary Neuroanatomy and Clinical Neurology, 2nd ed. Philadelphia, WB Saunders, 1983:30–52.
3. Chrisman CL. Head tilt, circling, nystagmus and other vestibular deficits. In: Chrisman CL. Problems in Small Animal Neurology, 2nd ed. Philadelphia, Lea & Febiger, 1991:269–294.
4. de Lahunta A. General proprioception system GP. In: de Lahunta A, Habel RE, eds. Veterinary Neuroanatomy and Clinical Neurology, 2nd ed. Philadelphia, WB Saunders, 1983:156–165.
5. Chrisman CL. Signs related to other autonomic and somatic cranial nerve dysfunction. In: Chrisman CL. Problems in Small Animal Neurology, 2nd ed. Philadelphia, Lea & Febiger, 1991:235–293.
6. Cunningham JG. The neuron. In: Cunningham JG, ed. Textbook of Veterinary Physiology. Philadelphia, WB Saunders, 1992:38–45.
7. Dow SW, Papich MG. An update on antimicrobials: New uses, modifications and developments. Vet Med 1991;86:707–715.
8. Jenkins TW. Telencephalon. In: Jenkins TW. Functional Mammalian Neuroanatomy. Philadelphia, Lea & Febiger, 1978:269–301.
9. de Lahunta A. Upper Motor Neuron System. In: de Lahunta A, Habel RE, eds. Veterinary Neuroanatomy and Clinical Neurology, 2nd ed. Philadelphia, WB Saunders, 1983:130–155.

10. de Lahunta A. Diencephalon. In: de Lahunta A, Habel RE, eds. Veterinary Neuroanatomy and Clinical Neurology, 2nd ed. Philadelphia, WB Saunders, 1983: 344–355.
11. Schulman FY, Ribas JL, Carpenter JL, et al. Intracranial meningioma with pulmonary metastasis in three dogs. Vet Pathol 1992;29:196–202.
12. Heidner GL, Kornegay JN, Page RL, et al. Analysis of survival in a retrospective study of 86 dogs with brain tumors. J Vet Intern Med 1991;5:219–226.
13. Shell LG. Understanding the fundamentals of seizures. Vet Med 1993;88:622–628.
14. Chrisman CL. The functional neuroanatomy of the cerebrum and rostral brain stem. Prog Vet Neurol 1990;1:117–122.
15. de Lahunta A. Seizures-convulsions. In: de Lahunta A, Habel RE, eds. Veterinary Neuroanatomy and Clinical Neurology, 2nd ed. Philadelphia, WB Saunders, 1983: 326–343.
16. Oliver JE, Lorenz MD. Seizures and narcolepsy. In: Oliver JE, Lorenz MD, eds. Handbook of Veterinary Neurology. Philadelphia, WB Saunders, 1993: 296–313.
17. Breitschwerdt EB, Breazile FE, Broadhurst JJ. Clinical and electroencephalographic findings associated with ten cases of suspected limbic epilepsy in the dog. J Am Anim Hosp Assoc 1979;15:37–50.
18. Sorjonen DC. Psychomotor seizures in dogs. In: Kirk RW, Bonagura JD, eds. Current Veterinary Therapy XI. Philadelphia, WB Saunders, 1992:992–995.
19. Colter SB. Complex partial seizures: Behavioral epilepsy. Probl Vet Med 1989;1:619–627.
20. Chrisman CL. Seizures. In: Chrisman CL. Problems in Small Animal Neurology, 2nd ed. Philadelphia, Lea & Febiger, 1991:177–205.
21. de Lahunta A. Small animal neurologic examination and index of diseases of the nervous system. In: de Lahunta A, Habel RE, eds. Veterinary Neuroanatomy and Clinical Neurology, 2nd ed. Philadelphia, WB Saunders, 1983:365–387.
22. Braund KG. Neurological examination. In: Braund KG. Clinical Syndromes in Veterinary Neurology, St Louis, Mosby, 1994:1–36.
23. Colter SB. Stupor and coma. Prog in Vet Neuro 1990;1:137–145.
24. Shell LG. The cranial nerves of the brain stem. Prog in Vet Neuro 1990;1:233–245.
25. Withrow SJ. Localization and diagnosis of spinal cord lesions in small animals: Part 1. Compen Contin Educ Pract Vet 1980;2:464–474.
26. Hudson JA, Simpson ST, Buxton DF, et al. Ultrasonographic diagnosis of canine hydrocephalus. Vet Radiol 1990;31:50–58.
27. Turrel JM, Fike JR, LeCouteur RA, et al. Computed tomographic characteristics of primary brain tumors in 50 dogs. J Am Vet Med Assoc 1986;188:851–856.
28. Dennis R. Magnetic resonance imaging and its application to veterinary medicine. Vet Int 1993;2:3–10.
29. Mayhew IG, Beal CR. Techniques of analysis of cerebrospinal fluid. Vet Clin North Am Small Anim Pract 1980;10:155–176.

30. Shell LG. Canine distemper. Compen Contin Educ Pract Vet 1990;12:173–179.
31. Redding RW. Electroencephalography. Prog in Vet Neuro 1990;1:181–188.
32. Gage ED, Hoerlein BF. Surgical treatment of canine hydrocephalus by ventriculoatrial shunting. J Am Vet Med Assoc 1968;153:1418–1431.
33. Gage ED. Surgical treatment of canine hydrocephalus. J Am Vet Med Assoc 1970;157:1729–1740.
34. Greene CE, Vandevelde M, Braund K. Lissencephaly in two Lhasa apso dogs. J Am Vet Med Assoc 1976;169: 405–410.
35. Gerard VA, Conarck CN. Identifying the cause of an early onset of seizures in puppies with epileptic parents. Vet Med 1991;86:1060–1061.
36. Oliver JE. Seizure disorders in companion animals. Compend Contin Educ Pract Vet 1980;2:77–86.
37. Farnbach GC. Seizures in the dog: Part 1. Basics, classification, and predilection. Compen Contin Educ Pract Vet 1984;6:569–576.
38. Raw ME, Gaskell CJ. A review of one hundred cases of presumed canine epilepsy. J Small Anim Pract 1985;26: 645–652.
39. LeCouteur RA, Child G. Clinical management of epilepsy of dogs and cats. Probl Vet Med 1989;1:578–595.
40. Schwartz-Porsche D, Kaiser E. Feline epilepsy. Probl Vet Med 1989;1:628–649.
41. Zaki FA. Spontaneous central nervous system tumors in the dog. Vet Clin North Am Small Anim Pract 1977;7: 153–163.
42. Moreau PM, Vandvelde M, Fanuel-Barre D, et al. Old and new diagnostic and therapeutic methods for intracranial tumors. Proc Annu Meet Am Coll Vet Intern Med 1986;4:5–43.
43. Everett GM. Observations on the behavior and neurophysiology of acute thiamine deficient cats. Am J Physiol 1944;141:439–448.
44. Jubb KV, Saunders LZ, Coates HV. Thiamine deficiency encephalopathy in cats. J Comp Pathol 1956;66: 217–227.
45. Read DH, Jolly RD, Alley MR. Polioencephalomalacia of dogs with thiamine deficiency. Vet Pathol 1977;14: 103–112.
46. Thomas WB, Sorjonen DC, Steiss JE. A retrospective study of 38 cases of canine distemper encephalomyelitis. J Am Anim Hosp Assoc 1993;29:129–133.
47. Appel MJG. Pathogenesis of canine distemper. Am J Vet Res 1969;30:1167–1182.
48. Thomas JB, Eger C. Granulomatous meningoencephalitis in 21 dogs. J Small Anim Pract 1989;30:287–293.
49. Vandevelde M, Fatzer R, Fankhauser R. Immunohistologic studies in primary reticulosis of the canine brain. Vet Pathol 1981;18:577–588.
50. Braund KG. Granulomatous meningoencephalomyelitis. J Am Vet Med Assoc 1985;186:138–141.
51. Baily CS, Higgins RS. Characteristics of cerebrospinal fluid associated with granulomatous meningoencephalomyelitis: A retrospective study. J Am Vet Med Assoc 1986;188:418–421.
52. Cordy DR, Holliday TA. A necrotizing meningoencephalitis of pug dogs. Vet Pathol 1989;26:191–194.

53. Comer KM. Rocky Mountain spotted fever. Vet Clin North Am Small Anim Pract 1991;21:27–44.

54. Dow SW, Poss ML, Hoover EA. Feline immunodeficiency virus: A neurotrophic lentivirus. J Acquir Immune Defic Syndr 1990;3;658–668.

55. Vandevelde M, Braund KG. Polioencephalomyelitis in cats. Vet Pathol 1979;16:420–427.

56. Wyatt JM, Pearson GR, Gruffydd-Jones TJ. Feline spongiform encephalopathy. Fel Pract 1993;21:7–9.

57. Wyatt JM, Pearson, GR, Smerdon T, et al. Naturally occurring scrapie-like spongiform encephalopathy in five domestic cats. Vet Rec 1991;129:233–236.

58. Greene CE, Dreesen DW. Rabies. In: Greene CE, ed. Infectious Diseases of the Dog and Cat. Philadelphia, WB Saunders, 1990:365–383.

59. Fiske RA, Choyce PD, Whitford HW, et al. Phaeohyphomycotic encephalitis in two dogs. J Am Anim Hosp Assoc 1986;22:327–330.

60. Tyler DE. Protothecosis. In: Greene CE, ed. Infectious Diseases in the Dog and Cat. Philadelphia, WB Saunders, 1990:742–748.

61. Szabo JR, Pang V, Shadduck JA. Encephalitozoonosis. In: Greene CE, ed. Infectious Diseases of the Dog and Cat. Philadelphia, WB Saunders, 1990:786–791.

62. Dow SW, LeCouteur RA, Henik RA, et al. Central nervous system infection associated with anaerobic bacteria in two dogs and two cats. J Vet Intern Med 1988;2:171–176.

63. Vandevelde M. Pseudorabies. In: Greene CE, ed. Infectious Diseases of the Dog and Cat. Philadelphia, WB Saunders, 1990:384–388.

64. Hawkins BA, Olson GR. Clinical signs of pseudorabies in the dog and cat: A review of 40 cases. Iowa State Univ Vet 1986;47:116–119.

65. Monroe WE. Clinical signs associated with pseudorabies in dogs. J Am Vet Med Assoc 1989;195:599–602.

66. de Lahunta A. Nonolfactory rhinencephalon: Limbic system. In: de Lahunta A, Habel RE, eds. Veterinary Neuroanatomy and Clinical Neurology. Philadelphia, WB Saunders, 1983:318–325.

67. Greek JS, Moriello KA. Treatment of common parasiticidal toxicities in small animals. Fel Pract 1991;19:11–18.

68. Glauberg A, Blumenthal HP. Chocolate poisoning in the dog. J Am Anim Hosp Assoc 1983;19:246–248.

69. Dorman DC. Toxins that induce seizures in small animals. Proc Am Coll Vet Intern Med Forum 1990;8:361–364.

70. Firth AM. Treatment of snail bait toxicity in dogs: Literature review. Vet Emerg Crit Care 1992;2:25–30.

71. Clemmons RM. How do I treat? Acute and subacute organophosphate intoxication in the dog and cat. Prog in Vet Neuro 1990;1:102–103.

72. Dorman DC, Parker AJ, Buck WB. Bromethalin toxicosis in the dog: Part I. Clinical effects. J Am Anim Hosp Assoc 1990;26:589–594.

73. Dorman DC, Parker AJ, Buck WB. Bromethalin toxicosis in the dog: Part II. Selected treatments for the toxic syndrome. J Am Anim Hosp Assoc 1990;26:595–598.

74. Clemmons RM, Meyer DJ, Sundlof SF, et al. Correction of organophosphate-induced neuromuscular blockade by diphenhydramine. Am J Vet Res 1984;45:2167–2169.

75. Fikes JD, Dorman DC. Diagnosis and therapy of neurotoxicological syndromes in dogs and cats: Neurotoxic metals. Prog in Vet Neuro 1994;5:5–12.

76. Dorman DC. Diagnosis and therapy of neurotoxicological syndromes in dogs and cats: General concepts. Prog in Vet Neuro 1993;4:95–103.

77. Dorman DC, Fikes JD. Diagnosis and therapy of neurotoxicological syndromes in dogs and cats: Selected syndromes induced by pesticides. Prog in Vet Neuro 1993;4:111–120.

78. Paul AJ, Tranquilli WJ, Seward RL, et al. Clinical observations in collies given ivermectin orally. Am J Vet Res 1987;48:684–685.

79. de Lahunta A. Feline ischemic encephalopathy: A cerebral infarction syndrome. In: Kirk RW, ed. Current Veterinary Therapy VI. Philadelphia, WB Saunders, 1977:905–907.

80. Bernstein NM, Fiske RA. Feline ischemic encephalopathy in a cat. J Am Anim Hosp Assoc 1986;22:205–206.

81. Patterson JS, Rusley MS, Zachary JF. Neurologic manifestations of cerebrovascular atherosclerosis associated with primary hypothyroidism in a dog. J Am Vet Med Assoc 1985;186:499–503.

82. Joseph RJ, Greenlee PG, Carillo JM, et al. Canine cerebrovascular disease: Clinical and pathological findings in 17 cases. J Am Anim Hosp Assoc 1988;24:569–576.

83. Gorelick PB. Cerebrovascular disease-pathophysiology and diagnosis. Nurs Clin North Am 1986;21:275–287.

84. Hause WR, Helphrey ML, Green RW, et al. Cerebral arteriovenous malformation in a dog. J Am Anim Hosp Assoc 1982;18:601–607.

85. Cook JR, Levesque DC, Nuehring LP. Intracranial cuterebral myiasis causing acute lateralizing meningoencephalitis in two cats. J Am Anim Hosp Assoc 1985;21:279–284.

86. Shell LG. The differential diagnosis of seizures. Vet Med 1993;88:629–640.

87. Podell M, Fenner WR. Bromide therapy in refractory canine idiopathic epilepsy. J Vet Intern Med 1993;7:318–327.

88. Dyer KR, Shell LG. Managing patients with status epilepticus. Vet Med 1993;88:654–659.

89. Indieri RJ. Status epilepticus. Probl Vet Med 1989;1:606–618.

90. Frey HH. Anticonvulsant drugs used in the treatment of epilepsy. Probl Vet Med 1989;1:558–577.

91. Bunch SE, Baldwin BH, Hornbuckle WE, et al. Compromised hepatic function in dogs treated with anticonvulsant drugs. J Am Vet Med Assoc 1984;184:444–448.

92. Dayrell-Hart B, Steinberg SA, Van Winkle TJ, et al. Hepatotoxicity of phenobarbital in dogs: 18 cases (1985–1989). J Am Vet Med Assoc 1991; 199:1060–1066.

93. Sawchuk SA, Parker AJ, Neff-Davis C, et al. Primidone in the cat. J Am Anim Hosp Assoc 1985; 21:647–650.

94. Dyer KR, Shell LG. Anticonvulsant therapy: A practical guide to medical management of epilepsy in pets. Vet Med 1993;88:647–653.

95. Pearce LK. Potassium bromide as an adjunct to phenobarbital for the management of uncontrolled seizures in dogs. Prog in Vet Neuro 1990;1:95–101.

96. Yohn SE, Morrison WB, Sharp PE. Bromide toxicosis (bromism) in a dog treated with potassium bromide for refractory seizures. J Am Vet Med Assoc 1992;201: 468–470.

97. Spaulding KA, Sharp NJH. Ultrasonographic imaging of the lateral cerebral ventricles in the dog. Vet Radiol 1990;31:59–64.

98. Parent JM. Clinical management of canine seizures. Vet Clin North Am Small Anim Pract 1988;18:605–622.

99. Bracken MB, Shepard MJ, Collins WF, et al. Randomized controlled trial of methylprednisolone or naxolone in the treatment of acute spinal cord injury: Results of the second national acute spinal cord injury study. N Engl J Med 1990;322:1405–1411.

100. Laws ER, Thapar K. Brain tumors. CA Cancer J Clin 1993;43:263–271.

101. Oliver JE, Lorenz MD. Systemic or multifocal signs. In: Oliver JE, Lorenz MD, eds. Handbook of Veterinary Neurology, 2nd ed. Philadelphia, WB Saunders, 1993: 322–373.

102. Davidson MG, Naisse MP, Breitschwerdt EB, et al. Acute blindness associated with intracranial tumors in dogs and cats: Eight cases (1984–1989). J Am Vet Med Assoc 1991;199:755–758.

103. Couto CG, Cullen J, Pedroia V, et al. Central nervous system lymphosarcoma in the dog. J Am Vet Med Assoc 1984;184:809–813.

104. Bailey CS, Higgins RJ. Characteristics of cisternal cerebrospinal fluid associated with primary brain tumors in the dog: A retrospective study. J Am Vet Med Assoc 1986;188:414–417.

105. Turrel JM, Fike JR, LeCouteur RA, et al. Radiotherapy of brain tumors in dogs. J Am Vet Med Assoc 1984;1:82–86.

106. Vandevelde M. Neurologic diseases of suspected infectious origin. In: Greene CE, ed. Infectious Diseases of the Dog and Cat. Philadelphia, WB Saunders, 1990:862–870.

107. Fekadu M, Baer GM. Recovery from clinical rabies of 2 dogs inoculated with a rabies virus strain from Ethiopia. J Am Vet Med Assoc 1980;41:1632–1634.

108. Zaki FA, Nafe LA. Ischemic encephalopathy and focal granulomatous meningoencephalitis in the cat. J Small Anim Pract 1980;21:429–438.

109. Blakemore WF. Neurolipidoses: Examples of lysosomal storage diseases. Vet Clin North Am 1980;10:81–90.

110. Stalis IH, Chadwick B, Dayrell-Hart B, et al. Necrotizing meningoencephalitis of Maltese dogs. Vet Pathol 1995; 32:230–235.

111. Dow SW, Dreitz MJ, Hoover EA. Exploring the link between feline immunodeficiency virus infection and neurologic disease in cats. Vet Med 1992;87:1181–1184.

112. Parker AJ, O'Brien DP, Sawchuck SA. The nervous system. In: Pratt PW, ed. Feline Medicine. Santa Barbara, American Veterinary Publications, 1983:451–473.

113. Scott DW. The skin. In: Holzworth J, ed. Diseases of the Cat. Philadelphia, WB Saunders, 1987:654–655.

114. Kornegay JN. Feline infectious peritonitis: The central nervous system form. J Am Anim Hosp Assoc 1978;14: 580–584.

115. Slausen DO, Finn JP. Meningoencephalitis and panophthalmitis in feline infectious peritonitis. J Am Vet Med Assoc 1972;160:729–734.

116. Percy DH, Carmichael LE, Albert DM, et al. Lesions in puppies surviving infection with canine herpes virus. Vet Pathol 1971;8:37–53 .)

Chapter 25

Diseases of the Brain Stem and Cerebellum

Linda G. Shell

Anatomy

There are five basic regions of the brain: (1) the telencephalon, which consists of the cerebral cortex (see Chap. 24) and basal nuclei; (2) the diencephalon, which is composed of the hypothalamus and thalamus; (3) the mesencephalon or midbrain; (4) the metencephalon, which consists of the pons and cerebellum; and (5) the myelencephalon, or medulla oblongata. Together the diencephalon, midbrain, pons, and medulla oblongata constitute the brain stem (Fig. 25–1).[1] Within the brain stem are the third and fourth ventricles, nuclei (cell bodies), and tracts (axons) that descend or ascend to connect the brain stem to other parts of the brain and spinal cord. Nuclei that give rise to the cranial nerves (see Chap. 26) also originate here.

Various other ill-defined neuronal pools or nuclei also originate in the brain stem. Extending from the caudal diencephalon to the medulla is a diffuse collection of neurons and intermingled ascending and descending fibers called the reticular formation.[2] The ascending aspect (ascending reticular activating system, or ARAS) is located primarily in the midbrain and is involved in maintaining alertness. Other neuronal pools responsible for reflex control of cardiovascular and alimentary functions are found within the reticular formation of the pons and medulla.[2] The respiratory center, which controls respiration, is located near the fourth ventricle, and the cardiac center, which regulates heart rate and rhythm, is in the medulla.[3] The chemoreceptor trigger zone, sensitive to the presence of some drugs and toxins in the blood, is located near the third ventricle in the brain stem; if stimulated, it sends signals to the vomit center to induce vomiting.[4]

Nuclei of several significant motor tracts are also located in the brain stem. Axons of the red nucleus, located in the midbrain, cross over and descend the brain stem as the rubrospinal tract. This tract controls muscle tone in the flexor muscles and is considered an important voluntary motor tract in animals.[5] Another group of nuclei, the vestibular nuclei, give rise to motor tracts called the vestibulospinal tracts, which control muscle tone in the extensor muscles. Reticulospinal tracts also originate in the brain stem and aid in controlling extensor muscle tone. Although the corticospinal tract does not originate in the brain stem, it courses through it to reach the spinal cord to facilitate the flexor muscles.

Tracts that originate in the spinal cord and course to the cerebrum or cerebellum must travel through the brain stem. For example, information about position sense from the left side of the body enters the medulla on the left side, synapses at the nucleus gracilis and nucleus cuneatus, crosses to the right side to travel through the brain stem, and finally reaches the somatosensory cortex on the right side. Other sensory tracts that course from the spinal cord through the brain stem include the spinocerebellar tracts and the spinothalamic tracts.

The cerebellum is located dorsal to the fourth ventricle and is attached to the brain stem near the pons and medulla by three cerebellar peduncles. These peduncles constitute the afferent and efferent fibers that take information respectively to and from the cerebellum. Grossly, the cerebellum is composed of two lateral hemispheres that meet in a center portion called the vermis.[6, 7] The cerebellum contains a central medulla that consists primarily of white matter (axons) and an outer cortex of gray matter (cell bodies or neurons). Within the medulla are three pairs of nuclei (lateral, interpositus, and fastigial nuclei). Branches of white matter enter the overlying folds (folia) of the cerebellar cortex, and because of their resemblance to tree branches, they are called arbor vitae. The cerebellar cortex consists of three layers: the outer or molecular layer; the middle layer of Purkinje cells; and the inner or granule cell layer.

Although there are many functional subdivisions of the cerebellum, the three main regions are the rostral, caudal, and flocculonodular lobes. The rostral lobe has a descending inhibitory influence on motor neurons. The caudal lobe regulates skilled muscle movements. The flocculonodular lobe receives information from the vestibulocochlear cranial nerve and therefore functions to orient and balance the animal.[6–10]

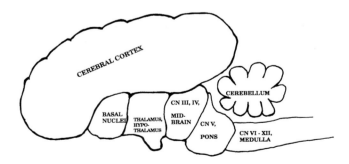

Figure 25–1
A schematic drawing of a sagittal cross section of the brain demonstrating the cerebellum, areas of the brain stem, and the origin of the cranial nerves. (Modified from Shell LG. The cranial nerves of the brain stem. Prog Vet Neurol 1990;1:234.)

Physiology

The hypothalamus, located in the diencephalon, has a variety of functions, including regulation of bladder

Table 25–1
The Clinical Signs Associated With Damage to Various Areas of the Cerebellum

CLINICAL SIGNS	CEREBELLAR AREA
Opisthotonos, forelimb hyperextension, hindlimb hip flexion, and hindlimb extension if the lesion reaches ventral aspect	Rostral lobe
Hypotonia, hypermetria, intention tremor	Caudal lobe
Dysequilibrium; drunken, broad-based, staggering gait; loss of balance; nystagmus	Flocculonodular lobe
Paradoxical vestibular signs (head tilt opposite to side of lesion, nystagmus toward lesion)	Cerebellar peduncles: mostly caudal, dorsal to the medulla
Dilated pupil, partial third eyelid protrusion, enlarged palpebral fissure	Cerebellar nuclei: fastigial, interposital

From de Lahunta A. Cerebellum. In: de Lahunta A. ed. Veterinary Neuroanatomy and Clinical Neurology, 2nd ed. Philadelphia, WB Saunders, 1983:255–278.

contraction, production and release of antidiuretic hormone, temperature regulation, hunger and thirst, expression of rage and aggression, sleep and sexual functions, and regulation of the adenohypophysis.[11] The thalamus, also located in the diencephalon, is involved in regulation of motor activity and maintenance of the alert conscious state. Rostral thalamic lesions may produce compulsive circling or turning toward the lesion (the adversive syndrome); the reason is not fully understood.

The cerebellum coordinates muscle activity and regulates muscle tone. In order to perform these functions, it must receive afferent information regarding where the limbs, trunk, and head are located in space. Therefore, tracts that carry proprioceptive information (e.g., spinocerebellar tracts) project to the cerebellum. The cerebellum must also receive information regarding the voluntary movements that are being induced by the upper motor neurons. Therefore, information from the cerebral cortex, basal nuclei, and voluntary motor tracts (e.g., rubrocerebellar tracts) also project to the cerebellum. All of this is integrated, and efferent cerebellar axons leave the cerebellum to carry information to the vestibular nuclei, the reticular formation, and the red nucleus. Very few efferent cerebellar axons project directly to the spinal cord to influence lower motor neurons[6]; instead, the cerebellum influences lower motor neurons indirectly through its effects on the upper motor neurons. The end result is that the cerebellum imposes fine control of all skeletal muscle activity.[6, 9–10]

Consciousness is maintained by the ARAS, located in the midbrain area, the thalamus, and the cerebral cortex.[12] The ARAS receives collaterals from every somatosensory and special sensory system in the body. Any disease that affects the midbrain, thalamus, or cerebrum can cause changes in consciousness such as depressed mentation, stupor, or coma. Lesions of the

medulla oblongata also cause stupor or coma if the respiratory and cardiovascular centers are affected severely enough to produce hypoxia.[13]

Problem Identification

Disorders of the brain stem frequently result in multiple signs because of the close proximity of the cranial nerve nuclei and the motor and sensory tracts (the long tracts). With brain stem disorders, one or more of the following signs is likely to be present: cranial nerve deficits (see Chap. 26), sleep disorders, changes in consciousness, or long tract signs. Long tract signs include changes in conscious proprioception or strength of limb movement (see Chap. 27) and imply damage to the ascending sensory tracts or descending motor tracts, respectively.

A lesion in the cerebellum does not cause the loss of any single function but does cause impaired motor responses. Usually, the cerebellum is affected by disease processes diffusely, and the patient presents with postural and gait changes characterized by ataxia and dysmetria, opisthotonos, tremors, or vestibular signs (e.g., loss of balance, head tilt, nystagmus). For most clinical purposes, signs of unilateral cerebellar damage are expected to be ipsilateral to the damaged side. Table 25–1 lists the clinical signs and the area of the cerebellum affected. Vestibular signs are discussed in more detail in Chapter 26.

Stupor and Coma

Coma is a severely altered state of consciousness in which the animal is unconscious and does not respond to any noxious stimuli except for reflex activity. Stupor is a reduction in consciousness such that the animal appears unconscious but can be aroused by a strong stimulus, such as pain.[12, 13]

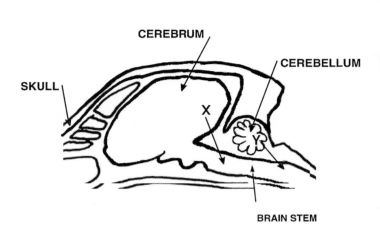

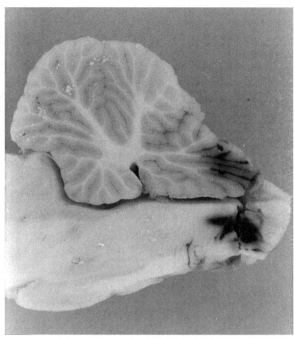

Figure 25-2

(A) A schematic drawing showing the two primary types of brain herniations. The area labeled X shows a caudal transtentorial herniation whereby part of the temporal lobe of the cerebrum moves ventrally to cause midbrain compression. The Y label shows herniation of the caudal cerebellum through the foramen magnum, causing compression of the medulla. **(B)** A sagittal cross section of a brain in which the cerebellum moved through the foramen magnum, causing medullary compression and death.

Pathophysiology

Coma and stupor are pathologic abnormalities caused by an interruption in the structural, metabolic, or physiologic integrity of the cerebrum or brain stem. Consciousness is maintained by the ARAS, the thalamus, and the cerebral cortex.[12] The ARAS receives collaterals from every somatosensory and special sensory system in the body. Any disease that affects the midbrain, thalamus, or cerebrum has the potential to produce a change in consciousness such as depressed mentation, stupor, or coma. Lesions of the medulla oblongata can also cause stupor or coma if respiratory and cardiovascular centers are affected severely enough to produce hypoxia.

Changes in consciousness are frequently caused by brain masses, cerebral edema, or increased intracranial pressure. Because the brain is immobilized within a nondistensible space (the skull), any increase in the volume of the brain raises the intracranial pressure and can potentially compress the brain stem, leading to coma. Masses (e.g., neoplasia, abscess, granuloma, blood clots) increase the volume of tissue within the skull by their physical presence and by the formation of edema.

Cerebral edema also increases intracranial pressure, which reduces cerebral perfusion, resulting in cellular hypoxia and even cell death; these effects in turn lead to more edema and greater increases in intracranial pressure. Eventually, a portion of the brain may herniate (Fig. 25–2), resulting in compression of vital brain stem structures. Subsequent life-threatening signs of coma or stupor, tetraplegia, and respiratory or cardiac difficulties often develop.[13]

Cerebral edema can be produced by vascular leakage (vasogenic edema) or by cellular hypoxia (cytotoxic edema). Vasogenic edema occurs if the tight junctions formed by the vascular endothelial cells are disrupted, resulting in increased permeability; water, sodium, and protein subsequently leak into the extracellular space. Cytotoxic edema occurs in hypoxic, hyperosmolar, and hyposmolar situations that cause failure of the adenosine triphosphate–dependent sodium pump. A rapid influx of sodium into the cells is followed by an influx of water to maintain osmotic equilibrium. Potassium leaves the cell, and the overall result is an increase in intracellular water and sodium and in extracellular potassium.

Clinical Signs

The stuporous or comatose patient is usually presented in lateral recumbence in a sleep-like state. The owner may report that the animal is not moving and cannot be awakened. Depending on the cause, the onset may be acute or gradual. It is difficult to separate the comatose patient from the stuporous one based on appearance only. The major difference is that stuporous patients can be aroused with external stimuli (e.g., loud sounds, noxious stimuli such as pinching the toe with a hemostat) but may lapse into the sleep-like state after the stimuli are withdrawn. Comatose patients do not respond to any external stimuli.[12]

A thorough neurologic examination should be performed on every stuporous or comatose patient to determine the location and severity of the lesion. Certain aspects of the neurologic examination should be repeated frequently, perhaps even hourly in some situations, in order to detect rapidly progressive changes and to begin treatment. These neurologic examinations should concentrate on the level of consciousness, pupil size and response to light, eye movements, and voluntary motor responses.

Level of Consciousness

As a general rule, a comatose condition has a less favorable prognosis than a stuporous one. Trends in the level of consciousness often yield more valuable prognostic information than does the information obtained on one examination.

Pupil Size

If the pupils are equal in size and respond normally to light and darkness, the integrity of the retinas, optic nerves, optic chiasm, and rostral brain stem can be assumed. Pupils that are unresponsive to light imply a grave to hopeless prognosis. As a general rule, lesions of the brain stem produce unilateral or bilateral pupil constriction or dilation, whereas lesions of the cerebrum produce normal or constricted pupils that respond to both light and darkness.

Eye Movements

If the animal's head is moved rapidly from side to side as it is held fixed in a forward position, several beats of horizontal nystagmus are elicited and disappear after the motion stops. This oculocephalic response requires the integrity of the vestibular nerves, the brain stem, and the cranial nerves that move the eyes (cranial nerves III, IV, and VI; Fig. 25–3). If the oculocephalic response is absent in a comatose patient, severe brain stem injury is likely and the prognosis for return of brain function is poor. The caloric test (see Diagnostic Procedures) can often confirm severe brain stem injury.

Skeletal Motor Responses

Comatose or stuporous patients do not have voluntary motor movements, are often tetraplegic, and may have extensor rigidity of the limbs (decerebrate rigidity) because of injury to the descending motor tracts in the brain stem. If opisthotonos or limb extensor rigidity develops, a lesion of the red nucleus or rubrospinal tract is likely. The prognosis is extremely grave in these patients because these structures are important for voluntary motor activity in animals and they are located near the ARAS and other important structures. Involuntary movements such as paddling may be associated with seizure activity.

Diagnostic Plan

The first consideration when approaching the stuporous or comatose patient is to determine whether the abnormality is the result of an extracranial or an intracranial disorder. Because there are numerous causes of stupor and coma (Table 25–2), historical data and physical and neurologic examination findings are critical for ranking the possible causes.

Head trauma is one of the most common causes of coma, and a quick but thorough history should ascertain this possibility if the owner does not volunteer the information. Signs of excoriations, scleral hem-

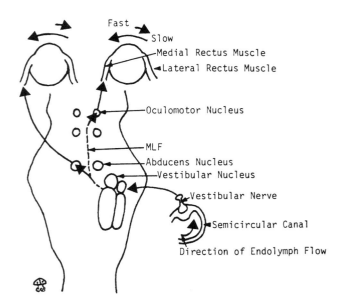

Figure 25–3

The neuroanatomic pathways involved in creating nystagmus and the oculocephalic response. MLF, medical longitudinal fasciculus. (From Chrisman CL. Vestibular disease. Vet Clin North Am Small Anim Pract 1980;10:106.)

orrhage, bruising, or shock should also be sought; all of these suggest a traumatic event. The owner should be questioned about any pre-existing medical problems. For example, an insulin overdose can result in hypoglycemia-induced coma in patients with diabetes mellitus.

Questions about potential toxin or drug exposure can be explored by asking whether the pet is known to chew or ingest plants, toys, metals, or other objects. Potential toxins include ethylene glycol, barbiturates, sleeping pills, insulin, and other drugs. Pre-existing neurologic problems such as hydrocephalus, encephalitis, or brain tumors may also be associated with coma.

Respiratory and cardiac rates and rhythms should be carefully evaluated for cardiopulmonary disease, which could secondarily cause neurologic signs by producing hypoxia. Alternatively, abnormal cardiac or respiratory rates or rhythms could be caused by damaged cardiac or respiratory centers in the medulla. The spine should be palpated carefully for deviations, crepitations, or fractures, and the abdomen for organomegaly, ascites, or masses that could indicate a systemic illness.

If a cause for the stupor or coma is not evident after a thorough history and physical and neurologic examinations, a hemogram, blood chemistry profile, and urinalysis should be evaluated to confirm or rule out metabolic causes. Signs of inflammation or toxicity may be evident on the hemogram; blood chemistry and urinalysis results help to evaluate the possibility of metabolic and endocrine disorders.

Lack of evidence of toxic or metabolic disorder or organ dysfunction may lead next to investigation of possible intracranial disease. If metastatic neoplasia or systemic infection is a possibility, chest or abdominal radiographs, or both, should be obtained. Likewise, skull radiographs may aid the diagnosis of cranial trauma if the history is unrewarding. In cases of coma or stupor of unknown cause, analysis of the cerebrospinal fluid (CSF) may be of benefit in the diagnosis of neoplasia (elevation of protein) or encephalitis (increased numbers of cells and protein), but there is a risk of brain herniation if the intracranial pressure is elevated, and this possibility should be considered. Magnetic resonance imaging (MRI) and computed tomography (CT) scans have proved useful in the diagnosis of neoplasia, hydrocephalus, vascular injury, and encephalitis, and they carry a reduced risk of brain herniation compared with spinal taps.

Sleep Disorders

Sleep disorders are characterized by abnormal patterns of sleep, often manifested as irresistible epi-

Table 25–2
Potential Causes of Stupor and Coma

Congenital or Familial Disorders
Hydrocephalus
Lysosomal storage disorders
Lissencephaly

Metabolic Disorders
Hepatic encephalopathy
Hypoadrenocorticism
Diabetes mellitus
Hypoglycemia
Hypothyroidism
Uremia
Hypoxia
Acid-base imbalance
Osmolality imbalance
Heatstroke
Hyperlipidemia

Nutritional Disorders
Thiamine deficiency (end stage)

Neoplasia
Primary lesions
Metastatic lesions

Inflammation
Canine distemper
Rabies
Rocky Mountain spotted fever
Ehrlichia spp.
Feline infectious peritonitis
Fungal, protozoal, and bacterial infections
Granulomatous meningoencephalitis

Toxins/Drugs
Ethylene glycol
Lead
Barbiturates
Mushroom poisoning
Alcohol
Cannabinoids
Hallucinogens
Ivermectin
Bromethalin

Trauma
Cranial trauma

Vascular
Coagulopathies
Hypertension
Cardiomyopathy
Bacterial emboli
Feline ischemic encephalopathy
Ischemia

Other
Status epilepticus

Adapted from Shell LG. Altered states of consciousness: Coma and stupor. In: Ettinger S, Feldman E, eds. Textbook of Veterinary Internal Medicine, 4th ed. Philadelphia, WB Saunders, 1995:151.

sodes of sleep or sudden attacks of loss of postural tone (cataplexy). They are uncommon (or uncommonly diagnosed) in animals.

Pathophysiology

Sleep is a state of cortical inactivity that is derived from a complex interplay between the cerebral cortex and the central reticular formation in the brain stem. Lesion and ablation studies in animals have shown that the pons is the area of the brain stem from which the sleep cycle is controlled. Normal sleep patterns occur as a result of decreased alerting influences of the reticular formation on the cerebral cortex.[14]

Normal mammalian sleep is usually divided into two stages. The first stage is slow-wave sleep or non–rapid eye movement phase, characterized by progressive decreases in muscle tone and heart and respiratory rates. The animal is quiescent, breathes regularly, and maintains muscle tone. The second stage is the rapid eye movement or fast-wave sleep, during which vivid dreaming occurs in humans. Rapid movements of the eyes, ears, vibrissae, and even limbs can occur in animals, but, paradoxically, muscle tone is depressed in this phase. Eyes may show nystagmiform movements behind the closed lids. The duration of these stages varies with the species,[14] but they are repeated several times during the sleep period.

Clinical Signs

The owner may report that the animal has excessive sleep activity, falls asleep when eating or excited, or collapses. The affected animal usually does not demonstrate the abnormal sleep pattern on examination and may not show it while hospitalized. If the reported behavior cannot be observed, the owners may be asked to make a videotape of the clinical signs.

Diagnostic Plan

First, excessive or inappropriate sleep must be differentiated from lethargy or depression caused by systemic illness or drug treatment. If the history indicates systemic disease, that possibility is pursued first, with the gathering of a minimum database. If the episodes are associated with signs such as urination, defecation, salivation, or paddling motions of the limbs, the possibility of seizure activity should be pursued (see Chap. 24). If the history is more suggestive of collapse, narcolepsy must be differentiated from syncope or metabolic-associated weakness. A hemogram, blood chemistry profile, and urinalysis are often helpful in diagnosing metabolic-associated weaknesses such as anemia, hypokalemia, hypoglycemia, hypocalcemia, and hypoadrenocorticism. If the history is suggestive of cardiovascular or respiratory disease (e.g., coughing, labored respirations, cyanosis), careful thoracic auscultation and palpation of femoral pulses may establish the need for electrocardiographic evaluation and chest radiography. A history of collapse when being fed or when excited is most consistent with narcolepsy; the food-elicited cataplexy test (see Narcolepsy) helps to confirm this diagnosis.

Dysmetria

Improper judgment of distance during movement or inability to control the range of movement during muscular actions is commonly called dysmetria.

Pathophysiology

Spatially organized, skilled movements and necessary adjustments of muscle tone and posture are regulated by the cerebellum. Disorders affecting the caudal lobe of the cerebellum result in dysmetria.

Clinical Signs

Owners frequently describe affected animals as having difficulty with walking, being unable to walk a straight line, having a drunken or wobbly gait, or picking the limbs up too high when walking. Usually, all limbs are affected, but occasionally the pelvic limbs are more affected than the thoracic limbs, or vice versa. Cat owners may report that the affected cat falls when it attempts to jump to or from objects. On examination, limb movements are uncoordinated. Animals that cannot judge distance or control their range of movements typically overstep (hypermetria) or understep (hypometria) when walking. In order to maintain balance, the affected animal must assume a broad-based stance.[10] Although cerebellar disease does not cause loss of strength, the patient may be so incapacitated by its condition that it falls to one side, forward, or backward. If severely affected, the patient may be unable to stand. Physical examination findings (other than neurologic findings) are usually normal in such animals. Observation of gait and postural reactions often reveals a raised threshold to response and, once the movement is initiated, an exaggerated response. With unilateral lesions, the signs of dysmetria or ataxia are usually ipsilateral to the lesion.[6]

Diagnostic Plan

If only one limb is showing signs of dysmetria, it should be examined carefully for signs related to

Table 25–3
Differential Diagnoses for Cerebellar Signs

DISORDER	NOTEWORTHY CHARACTERISTICS	PROGRESSIVE SIGNS	FURTHER READINGS
Immature Animals			
Viral-induced hypoplasia	Panleukopenia virus (cat), herpesvirus (dog)	No	This chapter; references 15, 16
Lysosomal storage disease	GM$_1$ gangliosidosis; breed predilection	Yes	This chapter; Table 25–9
Abiotrophy	Breed predilection	Yes	This chapter; Table 25–7
Congenital cerebellar malformations	Hypoplasia, vermian hypoplasia	No	This chapter; references 17, 18
Spongiform degeneration	Labrador retrievers aged 4–6 mo; extensor rigidity and opisthotonus	Yes	Reference 19
Neuroaxonal dystrophy	Collies and cats younger than 6 mo of age	Yes	References 20, 21
Dysmyelinogenesis	Chow chows, Dalmatians, springer spaniels, Samoyeds, weimaraners, Bernese mountain dogs, lurcher dogs	Variable and breed-dependent	This chapter; references 22–25
Mature Animals			
Neoplasia	Any age of animal	Yes	This chapter; references 10, 26
Granulomatous meningoencephalitis	Adult dogs	Yes	Chapter 24; reference 27
Feline ischemic encephalopathy	Acute onset	No	Chapter 24
Neuroaxonal dystrophy	Rottweilers aged 1–3 yr; slow onset	Yes	This chapter; references 7, 28
Any Age			
Canine distemper virus	Other neurologic signs likely	Yes	Chapter 24
Feline infectious peritonitis	Other systemic or neurologic signs likely	Yes	Chapter 38; reference 29
Other infections: protozoal, fungal, bacterial, rickettsial	Other systemic or neurologic signs likely	Yes	Chapters 36, 37, 39
Trauma	History or physical examination signs	No	This chapter
Toxins	Acute onset; other neurologic signs likely	Yes, unless treated	Table 25–4; references 30–44

musculoskeletal problems. If the thoracic or pelvic limbs are dysmetric, either hypermetric or hypometric, the cervical region should be evaluated carefully. Diseases in the cervical spinal cord, such as cervical vertebral malformation, atlantoaxial subluxation, and intervertebral disc herniation, can occasionally affect the spinocerebellar tract and result in dysmetria. In such cases, the animal usually also has pelvic limb weakness or neck pain caused by spinal cord compression. If only the pelvic limbs are dysmetric, a spinal cord lesion below the cervical area should be considered, again because of involvement of the spinocerebellar tract coursing from the pelvic limb area.

If the dysmetria is present in all limbs, a distinction must be made between cervical cord disease and cerebellar disease. In most cases, the animal with dysmetria caused by a cerebellar problem has other signs of cerebellar dysfunction, such as head tremors, opisthotonos, or vestibular signs. Table 25–3 lists disorders known to affect the cerebellum.[15–44] If dysmetria is localized to the cerebellum, CSF analysis could be of benefit in the diagnosis of neoplasia (protein elevation) or encephalitis (increased cell count and protein). MRI or CT scans may help to diagnose masses such as neoplasia or focal granulomatous meningoencephalitis (see Chap. 24).

Tremors

Tremors are involuntary trembles or quivers of the limbs or head. Those that become more obvious as the animal moves are called intention tremors.

Pathophysiology

Head tremors result from a lack of orientation of the head in space. Tremors caused by cerebellar dysfunction are often present at rest but may become more obvious as the animal attempts to perform a specific task.[7] Intention tremors are often associated with disorders of the caudal lobe of the cerebellum.[6]

Clinical Signs

Excessive head motions, shaking of the head, or bobbing may be described by the owner. Tremors of the body are sometimes described as shivering as if from cold, shaking, or twitching of the muscles.

A fine head tremor is characteristic of cerebellar cortical disease and is usually augmented by initiation of voluntary movements.[6] Head tremors are often accentuated when the patient approaches a food or water dish. Most often the head bobs up and down, and the patient may miss the food by over- or under-reaching or may plunge too deeply into the food, resulting in a faceful of food. In cats, head tremors often become more obvious as the cat stares at a moving object such as a piece of string being moved back and forth. If the cat pounces, its movements are erratic and uncoordinated.

Tremors can be constant with cerebellar disorders, or they can be so mild as to be unnoticed by the owner until the animal attempts to move. Such tremors usually disappear while the animal is sleeping.[45–47]

Diagnostic Plan

Tremors of cerebellar origin must be differentiated from those of noncerebellar origin. Noncerebellar causes of tremors are varied and include muscle disorders (see Table 28–2), hypoglycemia, hepatic encephalopathy, hyperthyroidism, hypoadrenocorticism, hypocalcemia, various toxins (Table 25–4), and congenital dysmyelinogenesis. A complete blood count, chemistry profile, and urinalysis are necessary to evaluate the possibilities of electrolyte disturbance or metabolic disease.

Depending on other possible differential diagnoses based on the history, physical examination, and results of routine laboratory determinations, other tests (e.g., creatine kinase, blood cholinesterase activity, muscle biopsy) may be pursued. An elevation of creatine kinase suggests a muscle disorder, which requires confirmation by muscle biopsy. If hypermetria, hypometria, nystagmus, or head tilt is also present, then a cerebellar origin is more likely. Tests that help evaluate the cerebellum include CSF analysis, skull radiographs, and CT or MRI scans. CSF analysis may show evidence of inflammation (elevated cell count and perhaps protein). Results of skull radio-

graphs and MRI or CT scans may support a diagnosis of trauma (fractures), neoplasia, or granulomatous meningoencephalitis (see Chap. 24).

Opisthotonos

Opisthotonos is a form of spasm in which the head is thrown upward (dorsiflexed); frequently, in animals, the limbs are held in extension.

Pathophysiology

The rostral portion of the vermis or the rostral lobe of the cerebellum is inhibitory to the stretch reflex mechanism of antigravity muscles.[6] If this inhibition is lost, the extensor muscle group, being stronger than the flexor muscle group, predominates, leading to increased extensor muscle tone and opisthotonos. Cerebellar ablation may also cause opisthotonos and tonic extension of all four limbs.[48]

Clinical Signs

Opisthotonos related to cerebellar dysfunction is not one of the more common signs of cerebellar disease observed in animals. It is most often observed after trauma to the brain and does not tend to occur in chronic progressive disorders. Owners may describe

Table 25–4
Toxins and Drugs That Can Cause Tremors

TOXINS	DRUGS
Organophosphates[30,40]*	Fentanyl/droperidol
Carbamates[30,40]†	Epinephrine
Hexachlorophene[36]	Isoproterenol
Chlorinated hydrocarbons	5-Fluorouracil[37]
Bromethalin[38,40]	Ivermectin[35]
Metaldehyde[40]	Tricyclic antidepressants[33]
Fluoroacetate[40]	Lithium[34]
Mycotoxins (penitrem A)	Piperazine[35]
Strychnine[40]	Sodium valproate
Organic mercuricals[34]	
Lead[34]	
Pyrethroids[40]‡	
Pyrethrins[40]	
Organochlorines[40]§	
Piperonyl butoxide	
Toluene/dichlorophen[39]	
Diethyl-*m*-toluamide (DEET)[31]	
D-Limonene[32]	
Thallium[34]	

*Chlorpyrifos, dichlorvos
†Aldicarb, methomyl, carbofuran
‡Permethrin, fenvalerate
§Lindane, endrin, dichlorodiphenyltrichloroethane (DDT)

Table 25–5
Location of Lesions Causing Opisthotonus

SITE	CLINICAL SIGNS
Rostral cerebellum (decerebellate rigidity)	Normal consciousness, nystagmus, head tremors
Midbrain (decerebrate rigidity)	Stupor or coma, no voluntary limb movements, pupils fixed and poorly responsive to light
T2–L4 (Schiff-Sherrington syndrome)	Normal consciousness, paraplegia, thoracic limb extensor rigidity

the animal as lying on its side with the head arched upward and the limbs stiff. Limb movements may or may not be present. If only the rostral part of the cerebellum is involved, the animal should remain alert and aware of its surroundings.

Diagnostic Plan

Opisthotonos that results from cerebellar disorders must be differentiated from that which occurs with midbrain injury (decerebrate rigidity) and spinal cord injury (Schiff-Sherrington syndrome). This differentiation is based on the clinical signs listed in Table 25–5. After opisthotonos has been determined to have a cerebellar origin, a minimal database (hemogram, chemistry profile, and urinalysis) is obtained to rule out possible metabolic disorders that could lead to brain hypoxia or swelling. Skull radiographs are diagnostic for trauma if fractures are visualized. Results of CSF analysis may support inflammatory diseases (e.g., canine distemper, granulomatous meningoencephalitis), whereas CT and MRI scans may aid the diagnosis of cerebellar neoplasia.

Paradoxical Central Vestibular Signs

Animals with central vestibular dysfunction that have a head tilt and vestibular ataxia away from instead of toward the side of the lesion are said to have paradoxical vestibular signs.[49, 50] Although the exact pathophysiology is not well understood, lesions causing paradoxical vestibular signs often involve the cerebellar medulla and caudal cerebellar peduncle. Such lesions are usually destructive mass lesions (i.e., neoplasia or granulomatous meningoencephalitis).

A lesion of the right caudal brain stem that affects the vestibular nuclei typically produces a right head tilt and a right-sided limb weakness. In cases of

paradoxical vestibular dysfunction, the head tilt and weakness or ataxia are on the opposite side. The position of the tilt is therefore unreliable as a localization clue. The rest of the clinical signs are similar to central vestibular signs, discussed in Chapter 26, and the diagnostic plan outlined in that chapter (under Head Tilt and Nystagmus) should be followed.

Diagnostic Procedures

Routine Laboratory Evaluation

Although routine laboratory tests do not usually contribute to a specific diagnosis of brain stem or cerebellar disease, they are helpful in establishing possible metabolic or inflammatory disorders that could contribute to the diagnosis, and they are recommended to ensure that other organs are functioning normally. In cases of systemic illness, such as feline infectious peritonitis or rickettsial disorders, inflammatory changes on the hemogram, elevated globulins, or changes in liver or kidney parameters may be seen. However, the most important information is derived from the signalment, onset and progression of signs, and neurologic examination.

Caloric Test

The caloric test can confirm severe brain stem injury in the comatose patient. Nystagmus should occur after 3 to 4 minutes of infusion of warm or cold water into the ear canals, if the pathway for the oculocephalic response is intact. Absence of nystagmus indicates severe damage to a large and significant portion of the brain stem and a poor to hopeless prognosis.

Electroencephalography

In specialty and referral practices an electroencephalogram (EEG) is often helpful in establishing the possibility of edema, encephalitis, or hydrocephalus as a cause for stupor or coma. Brain death can also be diagnosed by finding absent EEG activity. Cerebellar diseases do not typically produce changes in the EEG. See Chapter 24 for a more complete description of EEGs.

Spinal Fluid Analysis

Collection of CSF from the cerebellomedullary cistern is described in Chapter 24. In cases of known head trauma, CSF analysis is of no benefit to the diagnosis and could potentially harm the patient. In cases of coma or stupor of unknown cause, CSF analysis could be of benefit in the diagnosis of neoplasia (elevation of protein) or encephalitis (increased numbers of cells and protein), but the risk of brain herniation if intracranial pressure is elevated should be considered.

Radiography

Skull radiographs are not rewarding in the investigation of many disorders of the brain stem and cerebellum. Although the possibility of trauma can be investigated, skull fractures of the brain stem area can be difficult to visualize. MRI and CT scans have been useful in diagnosing cerebellar neoplasia, hypoplasia, inflammation, and brain stem masses.

Brain Stem Auditory Evoked Response

Although the brain stem auditory evoked response (BAER) test is most commonly used to evaluate deafness (see Chap. 26), it can also be used to evaluate brain stem integrity because the pathway for hearing courses through the brain stem before reaching the auditory cortex. Because this pathway is diffuse with multiple areas of crossover, the brain stem must be severely injured before BAER waveforms are abolished.

Common Diseases of the Brain Stem and Cerebellum

Head Trauma

Trauma to the head can result from road traffic accidents, falls, kicks or blows, fight injuries, or penetrating missile wounds.[12, 13, 51–53] Nonpenetrating brain trauma is commonly observed in veterinary medicine. Animals of any age and breed can be affected, but especially those that are allowed to roam.

Pathophysiology

Nonpenetrating brain trauma can be divided into contact injuries, produced by an object striking the skull, and acceleration injuries, produced by movement of the brain within the rigid calvaria. Contact injuries may cause contusions, skull fractures, or lacerations in the dura and brain parenchyma. Skull fractures may occur at the site of impact, or the compressive forces may be transmitted to weaker portions of the skull, creating fractures distant from the site of impact. Acceleration injuries, induced by rotational forces and pressure waves inside the skull, can cause contusions and hemorrhage.[13]

Acute consequences of head injury include brain edema and hemorrhage. The pathophysiology of brain edema has been discussed (see Stupor and Coma). Contusions may lead to subdural hemorrhage, which tends to be diffusely distributed over the cerebral cortex in animals. Hemorrhage into the brain tissue from damaged vessels is commonly observed. Both edema and hemorrhage can increase the size of the brain and predispose to herniation of the brain.

Clinical Signs

Clinical signs vary with the location and extent of the injury. Some animals are completely normal after a few seconds or minutes of unconsciousness; others have severe signs. Diffuse cerebral injury may cause delirium, seizures, stupor or coma, or pacing or circling; brain stem injury may cause stupor or coma, hemiparesis or quadriparesis, circling to the affected side, cranial nerve deficits, and changes in respiratory or cardiac rates or rhythms. Pulmonary contusions, pneumothorax, or shock can contribute to the progressive neurologic dysfunction. Animals that are conscious but have signs of tetraparesis or paraparesis should carefully be evaluated for concomitant spinal cord injury. Fractures, lacerations, and hemorrhage are direct, immediate effects of trauma that are usually noted on close observation and palpation. The location of injury and the expected clinical signs are given in Table 25–6.

Diagnostic Plan

The diagnosis is usually obvious from the history or from physical examination findings of lacerations, bruising, abrasions, hemorrhage, or fractures. Because of the possibility of systemic effects (e.g., shock, blood loss, cardiac or respiratory damage),

Table 25–6
Summary of the Possible Neurologic Signs Associated With Injury to the Medulla, Midbrain, and Cerebrum

LOCATION OF LESION	CLINICAL SIGNS*
Medulla	Stupor, coma, irregular respiration, tetraplegia
Midbrain	Stupor, coma, hyperventilation, decerebrate rigidity, tetraplegia, loss of oculocephalic response, ventrolateral strabismus, pupil constriction or dilation
Cerebrum	Stupor, coma, hyperpnea alternating with apnea, normal or constricted pupils, seizures

*Not all signs are present in every case.
From Shell LG, Dyer KR. Injuries to the brain. In: Bojrab MJ, Smeak DD, Bloomberg MS, eds. Disease Mechanisms in Small Animal Surgery, 2nd ed. Philadelphia, Lea & Febiger, 1993:1137.

routine laboratory work (hemogram, blood chemistry profile, urinalysis) is justified. Skull radiographs can support the diagnosis if fractures or bullet fragments are identified. Radiographs of the chest, abdomen, and spine may also be indicated in selected cases to more completely define the extent of injury.

Treatment

Treatment of the head trauma patient must be started at the time of presentation. The first step is to identify and correct any life-threatening non-neural problems such as hemorrhage, shock, obstructed airway, or thoracic trauma.[51, 52] A patent airway should be established and proper breathing and cardiac function ensured. An intravenous catheter should be placed and blood samples collected before any treatments are initiated. Valuable preliminary information such as packed cell volume, total solids, blood urea nitrogen (Azostix), blood glucose (Dextrostix or Chemstrip bG), and urine specific gravity can be obtained while the other laboratory tests are being processed.

If the animal is in shock, intravenous fluids are administered at a shock dose (see Chap. 31), but excessive amounts can contribute to cerebral edema.[13] If fluids are needed solely to correct dehydration, it is wiser to undercorrect rather than to overcorrect in the patient with head trauma.

There are three main treatments for cerebral trauma: corticosteroids, osmotic diuretics, and hyperventilation. Methylprednisolone sodium succinate is administered at an initial dose of 30 mg/kg, followed by repeated doses of 15 mg/kg at 3 and 6 hours later.[51-54] Because of corticosteroid-associated gastrointestinal ulceration and bleeding, injectable cimetidine (5–10 mg/kg by intravenous [IV] administration or by mouth, three times per day or four times per day), or sucralfate (250–1000 mg three times per day by mouth) should be considered. Other corticosteroids can be used, but studies in humans suggest that high doses of methylprednisolone are more effective in central nervous system trauma than are other drugs or other types of corticosteroids.[54, 55]

Osmotic agents, such as mannitol, reduce intracranial pressure by decreasing brain water content, but the therapeutic effect is short-lived. They should never be administered to a patient that is hypovolemic. The use of mannitol in head trauma cases is controversial because, if active brain hemorrhage is present, the reduction in the size of the brain and the resulting reduced intracranial pressure may allow more hemorrhage to occur. A 20% solution of mannitol is usually administered intravenously at 0.5 to 1.0 g/kg and repeated every 4 to 6 hours. In cases in which neurologic signs are focal, suggesting a discrete area of hemorrhage, some clinicians prefer to use IV furo-

semide at 2 to 4 mg/kg instead of mannitol to reduce cerebral water content.[6]

Hyperventilation (controlled ventilation) is probably the best emergency treatment for increased intracranial pressure. By increasing the partial pressure of oxygen (PO_2) and reducing the partial pressure of carbon dioxide (PCO_2) in the blood, cerebral blood flow and intracranial pressure are reduced. Disadvantages include the necessity for intubation and a short-lived effect. Putting the animal in an oxygen cage may be advantageous. If blood gas analysis is available, the arterial PCO_2 should be maintained between 35 and 40 mm Hg and the PO_2 higher than 60 mm Hg.[51]

Seizures can usually be controlled with injectable diazepam (0.5–1.0 mg/kg IV) on an as-needed basis. Anticonvulsants may complicate the neurologic assessment but are often necessary to prevent further brain damage secondary to seizures.[12] If more than three to four seizures occur daily, injectable phenobarbital (1–2 mg/kg three times per day, IV or intramuscularly) should be administered. After the pet is able to swallow, oral phenobarbital (2.2 mg/kg twice per day by mouth) is given until the pet has gone at least 6 months without a seizure (see Chap. 24 for more complete discussion of seizure management).

A craniotomy is indicated to remove depressed fractures that are compressing the brain or to control hemorrhage from lacerated meningeal vessels. Unless careful palpation or skull radiographs can confirm a depressed skull fracture, craniotomies are not routinely done in cases of head trauma. Readers are referred to a surgical text for a description of the procedure.[56]

Nursing care goals include prevention of hypostatic lung congestion by turning the patient every 3 to 4 hours, maintenance of fluid and electrolyte balances and proper nutrition, prevention of decubital ulcer formation by keeping the animal on soft cage padding or a waterbed, and prevention of urinary bladder overdistension by manual expression or catheterization three or four times daily. The eyes may need to be lubricated to prevent drying of the corneas and subsequent ulcerations. The head should be placed in a slightly elevated position to help prevent excessive blood flow to the brain.[51]

Prognosis

The prognosis for the animal with coma or stupor is generally guarded until serial neurologic examinations indicate improvement. If daily improvement is noted, partial or perhaps even complete recovery can be expected. The owner must be cautioned that the pet may have residual effects such as permanent motor or behavioral deficits or seizures. If improvement is not noted in 2 to 3 days despite appropriate treatment, the prognosis for return of function is extremely poor. Signs of deterioration include development of cardiac arrhythmias or bradycardia, impaired respiratory function, loss of the oculocephalic response, and lack of pupil responses to light.

Panleukopenia Virus-Associated Cerebellar Hypoplasia

Cerebellar hypoplasia is characterized by a failure of cerebellar cells to differentiate, resulting in a small and dysfunctional cerebellum. It is caused by in utero or perinatal inflammation of the developing brain by the panleukopenia virus. Although it is observed commonly in feral kittens, the incidence has not been reported. One or more kittens in a litter are commonly presented at 3 to 12 weeks of age.

Pathophysiology

The central nervous system, optic nerve, and retina are susceptible to damage by the panleukopenia virus during prenatal or early neonatal development.[15] The predilection for the cerebellum is explained by the fact that it develops during late gestation and the early neonatal period in cats,[6] and parvovirus has a cytopathic effect on rapidly dividing cells.[46] In utero or perinatal infection with the feline panleukopenia virus can destroy cells of the developing cerebellum. Although destruction is usually directed at the cells that are supposed to become granule neurons in the cerebellar cortex, pre-formed, growing Purkinje neurons are often also destroyed by the inflammation. In some cases, the destruction is so severe that the folia appear small and rudimentary. Grossly, the cerebellum is usually smaller than normal. Other central nervous system lesions (hydrocephalus or hydranencephaly) are occasionally present but are usually associated with earlier prenatal infections. The virus is found in the central nervous system for at least 22 days after neonatal infection.[16]

Clinical Signs

Clinical signs are usually evident to the owner when the kitten first begins to walk, but they may be interpreted as clumsiness. Signs do not progress, but some owners report progression when in fact the incoordination has just become more obvious to them and can no longer be attributed to clumsiness. Signs are more obvious if there are normal littermates or if the owner is experienced. Not all kittens in a litter may be affected.

Some affected kittens cannot walk without falling over; others can walk but demonstrate ataxia and dysmetria (particularly hypermetria) that is generally symmetrical and nonprogressive. The degree of incoordination varies. Most kittens have fine head and body tremors that become more obvious when they play with a string or attempt to eat or drink. Truncal swaying and loss of balance (the kitten falls from side to side) occur, but nystagmus is an unusual finding.[6] Some of the affected kittens tend to be aggressive and may hiss, bite, or resist manipulations. Queens infected during pregnancy do not manifest clinical signs of panleukopenia virus infection; however, some queens may abort dead or mummified fetuses.

Physical examination findings other than neurologic findings are usually normal. Occasionally, fundic examination reveals areas of retinal degeneration that appear as discrete gray foci with darkened margins. Retinal folding or streaking may also be observed.[16] Kittens with cerebellar damage do not typically have the systemic signs of gastrointestinal disease or leukopenia that are characteristic of the disease in postnatal infections. Postnatal infections with this virus rarely cause inflammation of the central nervous system.

Diagnostic Plan

The diagnosis is based on finding the cerebellar signs that have been described in a young kitten. Major differential diagnoses include lysosomal storage diseases and cerebellar abiotrophy, both of which show progression of clinical signs within a few weeks to months. The keys to diagnosing viral-associated cerebellar hypoplasia are the symmetrical cerebellar signs noted before 8 weeks of age and the nonprogressive nature of such signs.

Treatment

There is no treatment for the nervous system signs of this disease. The most effective method of prevention is to properly vaccinate the queen against the panleukopenia virus before breeding occurs.

Prognosis

The kitten with panleukopenia-induced cerebellar hypoplasia does not have progressive signs of dysfunction, but signs persist for the duration of its life. Compensation for the cerebellar deficits is usually minimal. If the kitten can walk, can get in and out of the litterbox, and is kept strictly indoors, it can function as a pet in some households. The owner must be aware of the cat's limitations, in particular its inability to adequately defend itself, and be willing to put up with the incoordination.

Idiopathic Generalized Tremor Syndrome

Idiopathic tremor is a clinical syndrome of unknown cause that is characterized by an acute onset of generalized tremors, which usually disappear within several weeks.[45, 47, 57] The true incidence is unknown. Any age, sex, and breed of dog can become affected. However, most cases occur in young adults of small breeds, particularly those breeds with white-haired coats; hence the term "little white shaker dog." Some of the more commonly affected breeds are Maltese, poodles, West Highland white terriers, beagles, and dachshunds.[57]

Pathophysiology

The observation that the tremors appear to worsen with voluntary motion implicates the cerebellum as a source. However, it is unlikely that the cerebellum is the sole source, because tremors of this nature have not been observed in numerous well-described clinical and experimental lesions of the cerebellum.[47, 48] Tremors can be generated from lesions in numerous other parts of the nervous system.

Histopathology in some cases has shown a diffuse, nonsuppurative encephalomyelitis, but serologic and viral isolation studies have not revealed a cause.[47, 57] Because of the high incidence in white-haired breeds, the presence of lymphocytes around blood vessels of the nervous system, and the clinical response to corticosteroids, an autoimmune reaction directed at tyrosine-producing cells has been proposed.[47, 57] Tyrosine is important in the production of the neurotransmitters dopamine and norepinephrine, as well as the production of melanin.

Clinical Signs

The onset of whole-body tremors is acute. Severity varies from mild to so severe that ambulation is difficult. The gait may be ataxic, but strength of movement is normal, as are the postural reactions. Tremors usually worsen with voluntary movement or excitement but tend to disappear with sleep. Affected dogs remain alert, but in some the menace response may be absent and nystagmus or dysconjugate, irregular, jerky eye movements may be present. Other inconsistent neurologic findings include paraparesis or quadriparesis, myoclonus, and seizures.[57] Body temperature may increase because of the tremors.

Diagnostic Plan

The tentative diagnosis is based on the signalment, acute onset, and clinical signs. Other possible causes of generalized tremors (see Tremors) must be considered. A thorough history may elucidate the possibility of exposure to toxins (see Table 25–4) or to drugs that can cause tremors. A blood chemistry profile helps to eliminate metabolic causes of tremors such as hypocalcemia and hypoglycemia. In the idiopathic generalized tremor syndrome, CSF analysis often shows an increase in protein and mild to moderate lymphocytic pleocytosis. CT of the brain has shown ventricular enlargement in some cases.[57]

Treatment

Corticosteroids seem to be the most effective treatment. Most dogs respond to immunosuppressive levels of prednisolone (2–4 mg/kg twice per day by mouth) within a few days. The dosage is reduced by one fourth after 2 to 4 weeks and reduced again by a fourth of the original dose every 2 weeks. Tremors have been reported to recur in a few dogs after prednisolone therapy was stopped. Some dogs may have to be maintained on low-dose alternate-day therapy, usually for 2 to 4 months.[47, 57]

Prognosis

The prognosis is generally favorable because of the response to corticosteroids. It is rare for the disease to progress to other signs of brain disease.[47]

Uncommon Diseases of the Brain Stem and Cerebellum

Neoplasia

In a recent review of 86 dogs with brain tumors, 19.7% were found to have a tumor located in the cerebellum.[26] Because primary and metastatic neoplasms of the cerebellum are often located at the cerebellomedullary or cerebellopontine angle, adjacent brain stem involvement may produce signs other than those produced by the cerebellar lesion: upper motor neuron weakness, proprioception deficits, ipsilateral cranial nerve deficits (especially of the trigeminal, facial, vestibulocochlear, glossopharyngeal, and vagus nerves), and mental depression owing to involvement of the reticular activating system. Astrocytomas and meningiomas are the most common tumors of the cerebellum. Although choroid plexus papillomas or carcinomas can involve any part of the ventricular system, they are commonly found in the fourth ventricle. Medulloblastomas have a tendency to selectively involve the cerebellum in young dogs, perhaps because they arise from the external germinal cell layer

Table 25–7
Breeds Reported to Have Cerebellar Abiotrophy

BREED	AGE OF ONSET	REFERENCES
Irish setter*	At ambulation	6, 8
Samoyed	At ambulation	6, 8
Beagle	At ambulation	66
Miniature poodle	At ambulation	58
Australian kelpie	4–12 wk	59
Bullmastiff*	6–9 wk	62
Airedale terrier	12 wk	60
Rough-coated and Border collies	4–12 wk	21, 61
Kerry blue terrier*	9–16 wk	63
Cairn terrier	2–6 mo	67, 68
Cocker spaniel	6–10 mo	69
Gordon setter*	6–30 mo	64
Brittany spaniel	7–13 yr	65

*Autosomal recessive mode of inheritance.

in utero.[10] Metastatic carcinomas may also affect the cerebellum.

Cerebellar Abiotrophy

In abiotrophies, a premature degeneration of cerebellar cells results in progressive signs of hypermetria, truncal ataxia, and tremors in dogs younger than 1 year of age. Progression of signs differentiates abiotrophy from hypoplasia but not from storage diseases. Breed predilections are noted in Table 25–7.[58–69] Most of the abiotrophies appear to be inherited by a non–sex-linked autosomal recessive manner. There is no treatment.

Neuroaxonal Dystrophy

Neuroaxonal dystrophy is a degenerative disease reported in young rottweilers,[7, 28] collie sheepdogs,[21] and cats.[20] Because all diagnostic test results are normal, a tentative diagnosis is based on the signalment and the slowly progressive cerebellar signs. There is no treatment. Histologically, swollen axons (axonal spheroids) are found in the gray matter, and there is a loss of Purkinje neurons. An autosomal recessive inheritance is suspected.

Toxins

Many toxins and drugs can cause tremors (see Table 25–4) as a result of cerebellar involvement or involvement of other parts of the nervous system. A history of exposure is crucial to the diagnosis. After exposure is confirmed, toxicology or pharmacology

textbooks or articles should be consulted regarding the treatment for each of these substances.[41, 42, 44]

Congenital Malformations

Congenital cerebellar hypoplasia, unrelated to virus-induced hypoplasia, has been reported in chow chows,[18] Irish setters, and wirehaired fox terriers.[8] No genetic basis has been determined, and the cause is unknown. Clinical signs of cerebellar disease are present as soon as the affected animal begins to ambulate.

Complete or partial absence of the cerebellar vermis also occurs in dogs.[17] Clinical signs are noted at about 2 weeks of age and consist of ataxia, dysmetria, and intention tremors. Congenital hydrocephalus is present in some of the patients.

Dysmyelinogenesis and Hypomyelinogenesis

Although this disorder is an abnormality of the myelin sheath within the central nervous system and not a primary cerebellar disorder, the predominant sign is a tremor that usually worsens with excitement and abates with rest. Tremors and hypermetria are usually noticed before 6 weeks of age in affected breeds (chow chows,[22] Dalmatians, springer spaniels, Samoyeds,[23] weimaraners, Bernese mountain dogs,[24] and lurcher dogs[25]). Hypomyelination in the springer spaniel is a sex-linked (males only) recessive trait. Clinical signs in the chow chow tend to plateau after 6 to 8 months of age and disappear altogether by 1 year of age, but this is not usually the case in the other breeds. All routine diagnostic test results are normal.

Table 25–8
Breeds of Dogs With Narcolepsy

Toy poodle
Miniature poodle
Doberman pinscher
Labrador retriever
Dachshund
Beagle
Wirehaired griffon
Saint Bernard
Cocker spaniel
Irish setter
Rottweiler
Cockapoo
Welsh corgi
Mixed breeds

From Shell LG. Sleep disorders. In: Ettinger S, Feldman E, eds. Textbook of Veterinary Internal Medicine, 4th ed. Philadelphia. WB Saunders, 1995:157.

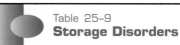

Table 25-9
Storage Disorders

ACCUMULATED SUBSTANCE	DISORDER	PREDOMINANT SIGNS	BREED OR SPECIES	REFERENCES
Lipid				
Gangliosides	GM$_1$ gangliosidosis	Dysmetria, head tremors	Beagle, cat, Siamese,* Korat, Portuguese waterdog*	71, 72
	GM$_2$ gangliosidosis	Seizures, dementia, blindness	German shorthaired pointer,* Japanese spaniel, cat	73, 74
Glucocerebroside	Glucocerebrosidosis (Gaucher's disease)	Ataxia, tremors	Silky terrier,* Abyssinian cat	75
Sphingomyelin	Sphingomyelinosis (Niemann-Pick disease)	Dysmetria, head tremors	Siamese cat, poodle, cat	76, 77
Galactocerebroside	Globoid cell leukodystrophy (Krabbe's disease)	Paresis, quadriparesis, tremors	Cairn and West Highland white terrier,* cat, beagle, poodle, blue-tick hound, Pomeranian, basset hound	78–81
Sulfatides	Metachromatic leukodystrophy	Seizures, weakness, opisthotonus	Cat	82
Carbohydrate				
Glycoprotein	Glycoproteinosis (Lafora's disease)	Seizures, dementia	Beagle, basset hound, poodle, mongrel	83
Mannoside	Mannosidosis	Head tremor, incoordination, aggression, opisthotonus	Persian cat	84–86
Glycogen	Glycogenosis (Pompe's disease)	Muscle weakness, seizures	Lapland dog, cat, German shepherd	87, 88
Mucopolysaccharide	Mucopolysaccharidosis	Lameness, facial dysmorphia	Siamese cat, domestic shorthair cat	89–91
Unknown	Ceroid lipofuscinosis (Batten's disease)	Seizures, dementia, blindness, tremors	English setter,* dachshund, Chihuahua, Siamese cat, cocker spaniel, Border collie, Saluki, Australian cattle dog, Tibetan terrier	92–98
	Fucosidosis	Behavioral change, seizures	Springer spaniel	99–101

*Autosomal recessive mode of inheritance.

Narcolepsy

Narcolepsy is characterized by hypersomnia or cataplexy, the sudden attack of flaccid paralysis often being precipitated by excitement.[70] Age of onset varies from 4 weeks to several years of age, and the various breeds reported to have narcolepsy are listed in Table 25–8. Petting the patient or making loud noises can often terminate the collapse, but the diagnosis is usually based on the results of a food-elicited cataplexy test. Ten 1-cm pieces of food are placed in a row 30.5 cm apart for small breeds or 50 cm apart for larger breeds. Normal dogs take less than 45 seconds to eat all pieces, whereas dogs with cataplexy take longer than 2.5 minutes and have more than two attacks.[70] The test is best performed in the dog's home environment, because the stress of being in a veterinary hospital may prevent an attack. Although the exact cause of narcolepsy is not known, inheritance plays a role in some breeds. Tricyclic antidepressants, such as imipramine (0.5–1.0 mg/kg three times per day by mouth) and protriptyline (5–10 mg/dog once or twice per day) may improve cataplectic signs.

Lysosomal Storage Diseases

Storage disorders[71–101] are inherited metabolic disorders resulting from a deficiency of a specific degradative lysosomal enzyme (Table 25–9). The biochemical substance that is normally degraded by the deficient enzyme accumulates in the cytoplasm of nervous system cells, disrupts their function, and results in subsequent clinical signs. Neurologic signs develop weeks to months after birth and become progressively more severe. Cerebellar signs are common, but other signs include seizures, dementia, upper or lower motor neuron weakness, aggression, blindness, and cranial nerve deficits. Some lysosomal enzyme activities can be measured antemortem from visceral biopsies, leukocytes, or skin fibroblast cultures. However, specialized laboratories are necessary to perform enzyme assays, and the cost can be expensive. Histopathology of affected organs may show changes characteristic of a storage disorder, but the exact disorder can be defined only with the use of enzymatic assays. There is no effective treatment, and the prognosis is poor because all storage disorders are progressive.

References

1. Shell LG. The cranial nerves of the brain stem. Prog Vet Neurol 1990;1:233–245.
2. Selcer RR. Functional neuroanatomy of the caudal brain stem and cerebellum. Prog Vet Neurol 1990;1:266–231.
3. Guyton AC. Regulation of respiration. In: Textbook of Medical Physiology, 6th ed. Philadelphia, WB Saunders, 1981:516–528.
4. Cunningham JG. Textbook of Veterinary Physiology. Philadelphia, WB Saunders, 1992:268.
5. Jenkins TW. Spinal cord. In: Jenkins TW, ed. Functional Mammalian Neuroanatomy, 2nd ed. Philadelphia, Lea & Febiger, 1978:166–198.
6. de Lahunta A. Cerebellum. In: de Lahunta A, ed. Veterinary Neuroanatomy and Clinical Neurology, 2nd ed. Philadelphia, WB Saunders, 1983:255–278.
7. Chrisman CL. Ataxia of the head and limbs. In: Chrisman CL, ed. Problems in Small Animal Neurology, 2nd ed. Philadelphia, Lea & Febiger, 1991:319–334.
8. de Lahunta A. Comparative cerebellar disease in domestic animals. Compend Contin Educ Pract Vet 1980; 2:8–17.
9. Selcer RR. Functional neuroanatomy of the caudal brain stem and cerebellum. Prog Vet Neurol 1990;1:226–231.
10. Kornegay JN. Ataxia of the head and limbs: Cerebellar diseases in dogs and cats. Prog Vet Neurol 1990;1: 255–274.
11. Chrisman CL. The functional neuroanatomy of the cerebrum and rostral brain stem. Prog Vet Neurol 1990;1:117–122.
12. Colter SB. Stupor and coma. Prog Vet Neurol 1990;1: 137–145.
13. Shell LG, Dyer KR. Injuries to the brain. In: Bojrab MJ, ed. Mechanisms of Surgical Disease of Small Animals, 2nd ed. Philadelphia, WB Saunders, 1993:1136–1139.
14. Hendrick JC, Morrison AR. Normal and abnormal sleep in mammals. J Am Vet Med Assoc 1981; 178:121–126.
15. Kilham L, Margolis G, Colby ED. Congenital infections of cats and ferrets by feline panleukopenia virus manifested by cerebellar hypoplasia. Lab Invest 1967; 17:465–480.
16. Greene CE, Scott FW. Feline panleukopenia. In: Greene CE, ed. Infectious Diseases of the Dog and Cat. Philadelphia, WB Saunders, 1990:291–299.
17. Kornegay JN. Cerebellar vermian hypoplasia in dogs. Vet Pathol 1986;23:374–379.
18. Knecht CD, Lamar CH, Schaible R, Pflum K. Cerebellar hypoplasia in chow chows. J Am Anim Hosp Assoc 1979;15:51–53.
19. O'Brien DP, Zachary JF. Clinical features of spongy degeneration of the central nervous system in two Labrador retriever littermates. J Am Vet Med Assoc 1985;186:1207–1210.
20. Woodard JC, Collins GH, Hessler JR. Feline hereditary neuroaxonal dystrophy. Am J Pathol 1974;74:551–560.
21. Clark RG, Hartley WJ, Burgess GS. Suspected neuroaxonal dystrophy in collie sheep dogs. N Z Vet J 1982;30:102–103.
22. Vandevelde M, Braund KG, Walker TL, Kornegay JN. Dysmyelination of the central nervous system in the chow chow dog. Acta Neuropathol (Berl) 1978;42: 211–215.
23. Cummings JF, Summers BA, de Lahunta A. Tremors in Samoyed pups with oligodendrocyte deficiencies and hypomyelination. Acta Neuropathol (Berl) 1986;71: 267–277.
24. Palmer AC, Blakemore WF, Wallace ME. Recognition of "trembler," a hypomyelinating condition in the Bernese mountain dog. Vet Rec 1986;120:609–612.
25. Mayhew IG, Blakemore WF, Palmer AC, Clarke CJ. Tremor syndrome and hypomyelination in lurcher pups. J Small Anim Pract 1984;25:551–559.
26. Heidner GL, Kornegay JN, Page RL, et al. Analysis of survival in a retrospective study of 86 dogs with brain tumors. J Vet Intern Med 1991;5:219–226.
27. Gearhart MA, de Lahunta A, Summers BA. Cerebellar mass in a dog due to granulomatous meningoencephalitis. J Am Anim Hosp Assoc 1986;22:683–686.
28. Chrisman CL, Cork LC, Gamble DA. Neuroaxonal dystrophy of rottweiler dogs. J Am Vet Med Assoc 1984;184:464–467.

29. Kline KL, Joseph RJ, Averill DR. Feline infectious peritonitis with neurologic involvement: Clinical and pathological findings in 24 cats. J Am Anim Hosp Assoc 1994;30:111–118.

30. Fikes JD. Organophosphorus and carbamate insecticides. Vet Clin North Am Small Anim Pract 1990;20: 353–367.

31. Dorman DC. Diethyltoluamide (DEET) insect repellent toxicosis. Vet Clin North Am Small Anim Pract 1990; 20:387–391.

32. Hooser SB. D-Limonene, linalool, and crude citrus oil extracts. Vet Clin North Am Small Anim Pract 1990;20: 383–385.

33. Johnson LR. Tricyclic antidepressant toxicosis. Vet Clin North Am Small Anim Pract 1990;20:393–403.

34. Fikes JD, Dorman DC. Diagnosis and therapy of neurotoxicological syndromes in dogs and cats: Neurotoxic metals, part 3. Prog Vet Neurol 1994;5:5–12.

35. Lovell RA. Ivermectin and piperazine toxicoses in dogs and cats. Vet Clin North Am Small Anim Pract 1990;20: 453–468.

36. Ward BC, Jones BD, Rubin GJ. Hexachlorophene toxicity in dogs. J Am Anim Hosp Assoc 1973;9;167–169.

37. Harvey HJ, MacEwen EG, Hayes AA. Neurotoxicosis associated with the use of 5-fluorouracil in five dogs and one cat. J Am Vet Med Assoc 1977;171:277–278.

38. Dorman DC, Parker AJ, Buck WB. Bromethalin toxicosis in the dog: Part 1. Clinical effects. J Am Anim Hosp Assoc 1990;26:589–594.

39. Lovell RA, Trammel HL, Beasley VR, Buck WB. A review of 83 reports of suspected toluene/dichlorophen toxicoses in cats and dogs. J Am Anim Hosp Assoc 1990;26:652–658.

40. Dorman DC, Fikes JD. Diagnosis and therapy of neurotoxicological syndrome in dogs and cats: Selected syndromes induced by pesticides, part 2. Prog Vet Neurol 1994;4:111–120.

41. Dorman DC. Diagnosis and therapy of neurotoxicological syndrome in dogs and cats: General concepts, part 1. Prog Vet Neurol 1993;4:95–103.

42. Greek JS, Moriello KA. Treatment of common parasiticidal toxicities in small animals. Fel Pract 1991;19: 11–18.

43. Mount ME. Toxicology. In: Ettinger SJ ed. Textbook of Veterinary Internal Medicine. Philadelphia, WB Saunders, 1989;456–483.

44. Beasley VR, Dorman CD. Management of toxicoses. Vet Clin North Am Small Anim Pract 1990;20:307–337.

45. Cuddon PA. Tremor syndromes. Prog Vet Neurol 1990;1:285–299.

46. Kornegay JN. Ataxia, dysmetria, tremor. Probl Vet Med 1991;3:410–416.

47. de Lahunta A. Upper motor neuron system. In: de LaHunta A, ed. Veterinary Neuroanatomy and Clinical Neurology, 2nd ed. Philadelphia, WB Saunders, 1983: 130–155.

48. Holliday TA. Clinical signs of acute and chronic experimental lesions of the cerebellum. Vet Sci Commun 1979;3:259–278.

49. Adamo PF, Clinkscales JA. Cerebellar meningioma with paradoxical vestibular signs. Prog Vet Neurol 1992;2: 137–142.

50. Shunck KL. Diseases of the vestibular system. Prog Vet Neurol 1990;1:247–254.

51. Kirby R. How do I treat? Dogs and cats with severe head injuries in the first 24 hours. Prog Vet Neurol 1994;5: 72–74.

52. Griffiths IR. Central nervous system trauma. In: Oliver JE, Hoerlein BF, Mayhew IG, eds. Veterinary Neurology. Philadelphia, WB Saunders, 1987:303–330.

53. Dewey CW, Budsburg SC, Oliver JE. Principles of head trauma management in dogs and cats: Part I. Compen Contin Educ Pract Vet 1992;14:199–207.

54. Bracken MB, Shepard MJ, Collins WF. A randomized controlled trial of methylprednisolone or naloxone in the treatment of acute spinal cord injury: Results of the second national acute spinal cord injury study. N Engl J Med 1990;322:1405–1411.

55. Anderson DK, Hall ED. Pathophysiology of spinal cord trauma. Ann Emerg Med 1993;22:987–992.

56. Indrieri RJ, Simpson ST. Intracranial surgery. In: Slatter DH, ed. Textbook of Small Animal Surgery, vol 1. Philadelphia, WB Saunders, 1985:1415–1429.

57. Bagley RS, Kornegay JN, Wheeler SJ, et al. Generalized tremors in Maltese: Clinical findings in seven cases. J Am Anim Hosp Assoc 1993;29:141–145.

58. Cummings JF, de Lahunta A. A study of cerebellar and cerebral cortical degeneration in the miniature poodle pups with emphasis on the ultrastructure of Purkinje cell changes. Acta Neuropathol (Berl) 1988;75:261–271.

59. Thomas JB, Robertson D. Hereditary cerebellar abiotrophy in Australian kelpie dogs. Aust Vet J 1989;66: 301–302.

60. Cordy DR, Snelbaker HA. Cerebellar hypoplasia and degeneration in a family of Airedale dogs. J Neuropathol Exp Neurol 1952;11:324–328.

61. Hartley WJ, Barker JSF, Wanner RA, Farrow BRH. Inherited cerebellar degeneration in the rough coated collie. Aust Vet Pract 1978;8:79–85.

62. Carmichael S, Griffiths IR, Harvey MJA. Familial cerebellar ataxia with hydrocephalus in bull mastiffs. Vet Rec 1983;112:354–358.

63. de Lahunta A, Averill DR. Hereditary cerebellar cortical and extrapyramidal nuclear abiotrophy in Kerry blue terriers. J Am Vet Med Assoc 1976;168:1119–1124.

64. Steinberg HS, Troncoso JC, Cork LC, Price DL. Clinical features of inherited cerebellar degeneration in Gordon setters. J Am Vet Med Assoc 1981;179:886–890.

65. LeCouteur RA, Kornegay JN, Higgins RJ. Late onset progressive cerebellar degeneration of Brittany spaniel dogs. Proc Annu Meet Am Coll Vet Intern Med 1988;6:657–658.

66. Yasuba M, Okimoto K, Iida M, Itakura C. Cerebellar cortical degeneration in beagle dogs. Vet Pathol 1988; 25:315–317.

67. Palmer AC, Blakemore WF. Progressive neuronopathy in the cairn terrier. Vet Rec 1988;123:39.

68. Palmer AC, Blakemore WF. A progressive neuronopathy in the young cairn terrier. J Small Anim Pract 1989;30:101.

69. Jaggy A, Vandevelde M. Multisystem neuronal degeneration in cocker spaniels. J Vet Intern Med 1988;2:117–120.

70. Katherman AE. A comparative review of canine and human narcolepsy. Compen Contin Educ Pract Vet 1980;11:818–822.

71. Shell LG, Potthoff A, Carithers R, et al. Neuronal-visceral GM1 gangliosidosis in Portuguese water dogs. J Vet Intern Med 1989;3:1–7.

72. Baker HJ, Mole JA, Lindsey JR, et al. Animal models of human ganglioside storage disease. Fed Proc 1976;35:1193–1201.

73. Cork LC, Munnell JF, Lorenz MD. The pathology of feline GM2 gangliosidosis. Am J Pathol 1978;90:723–734.

74. Cork LC, Munnell JF, Lorenz MD, et al. GM2 ganglioside lysosomal storage disease in cats with e-hexosaminidase deficiency. Science 1977;196:1014–1017.

75. Hartley WJ, Blakemore WF. Neurovisceral glucocerebroside storage (Gaucher's disease) in a dog. Vet Pathol 1973;10:191–201.

76. Bundza A, Lowden JA, Charlton KM. Niemann-Pick disease in a poodle dog. Vet Pathol 1979;16:530–538.

77. Cuddon PA, Higgins RJ, Duncan ID. Polyneuropathy in feline Niemann-Pick disease. Brain 1989;112:1429–1443.

78. Selcer ES, Selcer RR. Globoid cell leukodystrophy in two West Highland white terriers and one Pomeranian. Compen Contin Educ Pract Vet 1984;6:621–624.

79. Fletcher TF, Kurtz HJ, Low DG. Globoid cell leukodystrophy (Krabbe type) in the dog. J Am Vet Med Assoc 1966;149:165–172.

80. Luttgen PJ, Braund KG, Storts RW. Globoid cell leukodystrophy in a basset hound. J Small Anim Pract 1983;24:153–160.

81. Zaki F, Kay WJ. Globoid cell leukodystrophy in a miniature poodle. J Am Vet Med Assoc 1973;163:248–250.

82. Hegreberg GA, Thuline HC, Francis BH. Morphologic changes in feline leukodystrophy. Fed Proc 1971;30:341.

83. Cusick PK, Cameron AM, Parker AL. Canine neuronal glycoproteinosis: Lafora's disease in the dog. J Am Anim Hosp Assoc 1976;12:518–521.

84. Cummings JF, Wood PA, de Lahunta A, et al. The clinical and pathologic heterogenicity of feline alpha mannosidosis. J Vet Intern Med 1988;2:163–170.

85. Maenhout T, Kint JA, Dacremont G, et al. Mannosidosis in a litter of Persian cats. Vet Rec 1988;122:351–354.

86. Vandevelde M, Fankhauser R, Bichsel P, et al. Hereditary neurovisceral mannosidosis with associated mannosidase deficiency in a family of Persian cats. Acta Neuropathol (Berl) 1982;58:64–68.

87. Walvoort HC, Van Nes JJ, Stokhof AA. Canine glycogen storage disease type II: A clinical study of four affected Lapland dogs. J Am Anim Hosp Assoc 1984;20:279–286.

88. Sandstrom B, Westman J, Ockerman PA. Glycogenosis of the central nervous system in the cat. Acta Neuropathol (Berl) 1969;14:194–200.

89. Haskins ME, Jezyk PF, Desnick RJ, et al. Animal models of mucopolysaccharidosis. In: Desnick RJ, Patterson DF, Scarpelli DG, eds. Animal Models of Inherited Metabolic Diseases. New York, Alan R Liss, 1982;177–201.

90. Haskins ME, Aguirre GD, Jezyk PF. The pathology of the feline model of mucopolysaccharidosis I. Am J Pathol 1983;112:27–36.

91. Shull RM, Munger RJ, Spellacy E, et al. Animal model of human disease: Canine alpha-L-iduronidase deficiency, a model of mucopolysaccharidosis I. Am J Pathol 1982;109:244–248.

92. Barker CG. Fucosidosis in English springer spaniels: Results of a trial screening program. J Small Anim Pract 1988;29:623–630.

93. Taylor RM, Farrow BRH. Ceroid-lipofuscinosis in border collie dogs. Acta Neuropathol (Berl) 1988;75:627–631.

94. Vandevelde M, Fatzer R. Neuronal ceroid-lipofuscinosis in older dachshunds. Vet Pathol 1980;17:686–692.

95. Koppang N. Canine ceroid-lipofuscinosis in English setters. J Small Anim Pract 1970;10:639–644.

96. Appleby EC, Longestaffe JA, Bell FR. Ceroid lipofuscinosis in two Saluki dogs. J Comp Pathol 1982;92:375–380.

97. Green P, Little P. Neuronal ceroid-lipofuscin storage in Siamese cats. Can J Comp Med 1974;38:207–212.

98. Sisk DB, Levesque DC, Wood PA. Clinical and pathologic features of ceroid lipofuscinosis in two Australian cattle dogs. J Am Vet Med Assoc 1990;197:361–364.

99. Herrtage ME. Canine fucosidosis. Vet Annu 1988;28:223–227.

100. Taylor R, Farrow B, Healy P. Canine fucosidosis: Clinical findings. J Small Anim Pract 1987;28:291–300.

101. Kelly WR, Clague AE, Barns RJ. Canine-L-fucosidosis: A storage disease of springer spaniels. Acta Neuropathol (Berl) 1983;60:9–13.

Chapter 26

Diseases of the Cranial Nerves

Linda G. Shell

Anatomy and Physiology

There are twelve pairs of cranial nerves. Each cranial nerve enters or exits the central nervous system through a foramen in the skull; in some cases, several cranial nerves use the same foramen. Many cranial nerve nuclei are located near or adjacent to each other in the brain stem. For example, nuclei of cranial nerves III and IV are found in the midbrain, and those of cranial nerves VII through XII are located in the medulla. Some cranial nerves have more than one nucleus (e.g., cranial nerves V and VIII) and may encompass a larger portion of the brain stem. For these anatomic reasons, multiple cranial nerves can be injured at one site in the brain stem.[1-3]

Cranial nerves III, IV, VI, XI, and XII have a strictly motor function, with axons carrying information from the brain to muscles of the face, head, and neck. Cell bodies or nuclei for these motor axons are located in the gray matter of the brain stem. Cranial nerves I, II, and VIII are sensory and contain axons that relay information from sensory receptors of the head to the brain for processing. Cell bodies for these sensory axons are located in ganglia outside the central nervous system. The remaining cranial nerves (V, VII, IX, X) are mixed, containing both sensory and motor axons.

Clinical deficits related to cranial nerves are predominantly lower motor neuron signs such as decreased muscle tone, decreased reflexes, and weakness. Upper motor neuron signs, such as increased muscle tone, increased reflexes, and upper motor neuron weakness, are difficult to detect.[4] Table 26-1 lists the function of each cranial nerve as well as its course, method of testing, and common disease processes.[5, 6]

Problem Identification

Although most cranial nerves have more than one function, dysfunction often results in a specific, easily identifiable clinical sign (see Table 26-1). Common cranial nerve deficits include blindness with abnormal pupillary light reflexes (PLRs), anisocoria, strabismus, facial paralysis, masticatory muscle atrophy, dropped jaw, deafness, head tilt and nystagmus, laryngeal paralysis, dysphagia, and megaesophagus. Dysphagia and megaesophagus are discussed in Chapters 29 and 30, respectively.

Blindness With Abnormal Pupillary Light Reflexes

Visual deficits with pupils that do not respond appropriately to light imply a lesion of the optic nerve or its pathway to the midbrain region.

Pathophysiology

Because the optic nerve (cranial nerve II) contains sensory fibers for both vision and PLRs, the visual and pupillary light reflex pathways overlap to the level of the midbrain (Fig 26-1). Therefore, a lesion located at the optic nerve, optic chiasm, or optic tract to the level of the pretectal nucleus results in visual deficits as well as reduced or absent PLRs.[7-11]

Clinical Signs

Bilateral blindness of the pet is usually apparent to the owner, particularly if the pet is put into a new environment and bumps into objects. Because pets often compensate well in a familiar environment by learning where objects or obstacles are located, partial or gradual visual loss is more difficult for owners to appreciate. Clues may include a reluctance of the pet to travel up and down stairs or a reluctance to jump. Owners may report that the pet is always at their feet, refuses to move in the darkness, sniffs at the ground when walking, or is unable to locate moving objects.[8] Unilateral blindness may not be apparent to some owners; more observant owners may report that the pet bumps into objects on the blind side.

On examination, the blind pet bumps into people or objects in its path. The gait may be hesitant and cautious. Some dogs lift their forelimbs excessively high (goose-stepping or hypermetria). Others are hesitant to move around in a new environment. When the menace response is performed, the blind pet does not blink or close the eye because it does not see the threatening hand. However, the facial nerve (cranial nerve VII) must be functioning in order for the eye to close.[8] If cranial nerve VII is nonfunctional, vision can be evaluated by throwing cotton balls in front of the pet and observing whether it follows their movement.

With unilateral blindness caused by an optic nerve abnormality, the PLR on the affected side (the direct PLR) is poor to absent; the opposite unaffected pupil does not respond to this same light either, because the light impulse cannot travel in the affected optic nerve. If light is shined into the unaffected visual pupil, it constricts normally, and the pupil on the blind (affected) side also constricts (positive consensual response). In cases of bilateral blindness, the PLRs in both eyes are poor to absent. Blindness with normal PLRs implies a lesion in the brain beyond the level of the optic tract (see Chap. 24).

Diagnostic Plan

After blindness or visual deficits have been established and PLRs have confirmed that a peripheral origin is likely (see Chap. 24 for blindness of central origin), the next step is to determine whether the

Table 26-1
The Anatomic Course, Function, Method of Testing, and Clinical Signs of Dysfunction of Cranial Nerves

CRANIAL NERVE	ANATOMIC COURSE	FUNCTION	TEST	CLINICAL SIGNS OF DYSFUNCTION	DISORDERS
CN I Olfactory	Nasal mucosa to cribriform plate to olfactory bulbs and tract to pyriform cortex	Smell	Not routinely tested	Anosia; hyponosia	Nasal tumor or infection; canine distemper virus
CN II Optic	Retina to optic nerve to optic chiasm to optic tract to lateral geniculate nucleus to optic radiation to visual (occipital) cortex	Vision and pupillary light reflexes	Menace reflex; pupillary light reflex; avoids obstacles	Blindness with dilated pupils	Optic neuritis; neoplasia; trauma; granulomatous meningoencephalitis; fungal infection
CN III Oculomotor	Midbrain to cavernous sinus to orbital fissure to pupil and extraocular muscles	Motor to extraocular muscles; parasympathetic to pupil	Eye movement; pupillary light reflex	Dilated pupils that do not respond to light; ventrolateral strabismus; ptosis	Orbital trauma or neoplasia; brain herniations; feline leukemia virus-associated spastic syndrome; dysautonomia
CN IV Trochlear	Midbrain to cavernous sinus to orbital fissure and to extraocular muscle	Motor to dorsal oblique muscle	Not routinely tested	Dorsomedial strabismus in species with vertical pupil	Rarely observed
CN V Trigeminal	Motor: pons to trigeminal canal of petrosal bone to oval foramen to mandibular branch to masticatory muscles
Sensory: facial structures to trigeminal ganglion in trigeminal canal to pons	Motor to muscles of mastication; sensory to face	Jaw tone; muscle bulk; sensation to face	Masticatory muscle atrophy; decreased or absent facial sensation; dropped jaw if bilateral	Trigeminal neuritis; trauma; brain stem neoplasia or infection; peripheral nerve neoplasia
CN VI Abducent	Pons through cavernous sinus to orbital fissure to extraocular muscles	Motor to lateral rectus and retractor bulbi	Eye movement	Medial strabismus	Trauma; neoplasia; infection
CN VII Facial	Motor: medulla to internal acoustic meatus to facial canal and stylomastoid foramen to muscles of face	Motor to muscles of facial expression; parasympathetic to lacrimal glands; sensory (taste) to rostral tongue	Menace reflex or eye blink; retract lip; move ear; palpebral reflex; Schirmer tear test	Inability to close eyelid, move ear, or retract lip; dry eye	Idiopathic facial paralysis; middle ear infection; hypothyroidism; trauma; neoplasia; infection

Table continued on following page

Table 26-1
The Anatomic Course, Function, Method of Testing, and Clinical Signs of Dysfunction of Cranial Nerves *Continued*

CRANIAL NERVE	ANATOMIC COURSE	FUNCTION	TEST	CLINICAL SIGNS OF DYSFUNCTION	DISORDERS
CN VIII Vestibulo-cochlear	Inner ear through petrosal bone and internal acoustic meatus to medulla	Balance; hearing	Body posture; eye movement; hearing; head position	Head tilt; nystagmus; ataxia; eye drop (positional strabismus); deafness	Inner ear infection; idiopathic vestibular disease; neoplasia; hypothyroidism; ototoxicity
CN IX Glossopharyngeal	Medulla (ambiguus nucleus) through jugular foramen to pharynx	Sensory and motor to pharynx	Gag reflex; swallow	Dysphagia	Neoplasia; brain stem infection or trauma
CN X Vagus	Medulla (ambiguus nucleus) through jugular foramen to larynx, pharynx, viscera	Sensory and motor to pharynx, larynx, and viscera	Gag reflex; oculocardiac reflex	Dysphagia; laryngeal paralysis; megaesophagus	Neoplasia; brain stem infection or trauma
CN XI Accessory	Medulla (ambiguus nucleus) to cervical gray matter to cranial roots to jugular foramen	Motor to trapezius muscle	Normal muscle tone	Atrophy of trapezius muscle	Rarely observed
CN XII Hypoglossal	Medulla to hypoglossal canal to tongue	Motor to tongue muscles	Tongue movement	Atrophy of tongue; inability to retract tongue if bilateral	Trauma; brain stem infection; neoplasia

PUPILLARY LIGHT REFLEX PATHWAY

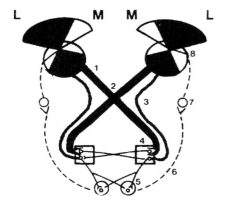

1. Optic nerve
2. Optic chiasm
3. Optic tract
4. Pretectal nucleus *
5. Edinger-Westphal nucleus *
6. Parasympathetic fibers in CN 3 *
7. Ciliary ganglion
8. Sphincter pupillae m.

L	= lateral visual field
M	= medial visual field
▬	= fibers that decussate at optic chiasm
▬	= fibers that do not decussate at optic chiasm
▪▪▪▪	= parasympathetic pathway to eye
*	= midbrain

CENTRAL VISUAL PATHWAY

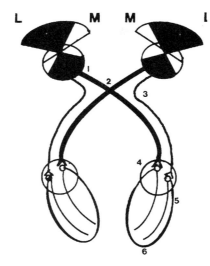

1. Optic nerve
2. Optic chiasm
3. Optic tract
4. Lateral geniculate *
5. Optic radiation
6. Occipital (visual) cortex

Figure 26-1
Pupillary light reflex pathways and central visual pathways overlap to the level of the midbrain. Lesions located at the optic nerve, optic chiasm, and optic tract cause pupillary light reflex changes in addition to visual deficits.

blindness is caused by disease of the eye or of the optic nerve and its pathway. A complete ocular examination should be done, including a fundic examination. Ocular lesions that can produce blindness with a change in the PLR include severe uveitis, sudden acquired retinal degeneration syndrome (SARDS), retinal atrophy, and retinal detachment. Many older dogs have concurrent iris atrophy, which decreases PLRs, and cataracts, which can impair vision. If anterior uveitis, retinitis, or other inflammatory ocular changes are noted, or if systemic signs are present, the possibility of inflammatory or neoplastic disorder should be pursued by obtaining a hemogram, chemistry profile, urinalysis, and possibly chest or abdominal radiographs (see Chap. 19). The optic nerve should be visualized on fundic examination for signs of atrophy, swelling, or discoloration, all of which suggest that optic nerve damage is causing the blindness. Although an electroretinogram (ERG) is a more objective means of assessing retinal disease and differentiating it from optic nerve disease, its use is usually limited to veterinary ophthalmologists.

If the eye itself is normal but the PLRs are abnormal, the location of the blindness is restricted to the optic nerves, optic chiasm, or optic tracts.[7] If neurologic signs are present (e.g., behavioral changes, seizures, concurrent cranial nerve signs), it can be assumed that the blindness is originating in the brain. The differential diagnosis includes neoplastic or inflammatory masses located at the optic chiasm and diffuse or multifocal neurologic diseases. Skull radiographs, spinal fluid analysis, electroencephalography, or computed tomography (CT) or magnetic resonance imaging (MRI) scans of the brain may be needed to identify a brain disease specifically (see Chap. 24).

Anisocoria

Gross inequality of pupil size is called anisocoria.[8]

Pathophysiology

The iris of the eye contains two sets of smooth muscle fibers. One set is arranged in a circular pattern around the pupil and causes the pupil to constrict or get smaller. These constrictor fibers are innervated by parasympathetic fibers that course with cranial nerve III, the oculomotor nerve. The second set of muscle fibers is arranged radially around the pupil; when they contract, the pupil dilates. These dilator muscles are innervated by sympathetic nerves. Stimulation of the sympathetic nerves excites the radial fibers of the iris and causes pupillary dilation or mydriasis.[9, 10]

The function of PLRs is to allow the eye to adapt rapidly to changing light conditions. When light hits the retina, the resulting impulses pass through the optic nerve and optic tract to the pretectal nuclei in the midbrain. Then impulses pass to the Edinger-Westphal nucleus and to the parasympathic nerves to constrict the sphincter of the iris (see Fig. 26–1).[9] Likewise, if the pet is in a darkened environment or if it is frightened, the sympathetic nervous system is activated to allow for dilation of the pupils. The sympathetic nervous system originates in the hypothalamus (Fig. 26–2). Axons from sympathetic cell bodies ascend and synapse in the gray matter of the spinal cord at thoracolumbar segments T1 to L3. Sympathetic preganglionic neurons at T1 and T2 give rise to axons that course cranially with the vago-sympathetic trunk to synapse at the cranial cervical ganglion in the neck. From here, postganglionic axons course to the eye to innervate the dilator muscles. Trauma, neoplasia, or inflammation at any point along this pathway can lead to lack of sympathetic tone and to anisocoria.

Pupil size varies with the intensity of the surrounding illumination, but both pupils should respond the same if they are normal. In lighting of average intensity, the pupils should neither be widely dilated nor very constricted.

Clinical Signs

Anisocoria can be very subtle or very marked. It is uncommon for owners to have a pet examined because of unequal pupil size unless there are marked differences between the two pupils. Because anisocoria can be caused by either a sympathetic or a parasym-

pathetic abnormality of the pupil, it must be determined which pupil is abnormal (see next section).

Diagnostic Plan

The diagnostic approach to anisocoria includes complete neurologic and ophthalmologic examinations. Ocular disorders can produce anisocoria. For example, anterior uveitis frequently causes a miotic pupil, whereas iris atrophy in older patients produces an enlarged pupil that responds weakly or slowly to light.[8]

After ocular disease is eliminated as a cause of the anisocoria, it must be determined whether parasympathetic or sympathetic innervation is affected. If sympathetic innervation is impaired, the affected pupil is miotic and responds more quickly and completely to light than does the normal pupil. Because sympathetic nerves also supply other parts of the eye, ptosis or drooping of the upper eyelid and enophthalmos may also be present, signs that constitute Horner's syndrome.[8] If parasympathetic innervation is impaired, the affected pupil is large and poorly responsive to light, either directly or indirectly. The unaffected pupil may be small because of the excessive amount of light entering the affected side.[8]

If a sympathetic lesion is suspected and other neurologic deficits do not exist, the location of the lesion is probably retrobulbar to the eye or in the vagosympathetic trunk or the middle ear cavity. An otoscopic examination may establish other signs of middle ear disease. Because the vagosympathetic trunk courses through the thorax and neck, radiographs of these areas and of the bullae may be indicated. In those patients with concurrent neurologic deficits, the location of the lesion can be anywhere from the brain stem, to the cervical to thoracic (T1–T3) spinal cord, to the T1 and T3 ventral nerve roots (Table 26–2; see Fig. 26–2).[11, 12] Of these sites,

Figure 26–2
The course of the sympathetic pathway from the brain to the eye. (Modified from Shell LG, Sponenberg P, Dallman M. Chondrosarcoma in a cat presenting with forelimb monoparesis. Compen Contin Educ Pract Vet 1987;9: 391–398.)

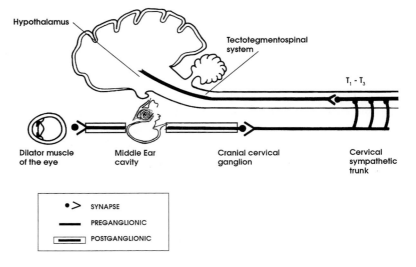

Table 26-2

Location, Causes, Pharmacologic Test Results, and Neurologic Deficits Associated With Lesions That Cause Horner's Syndrome

LOCATION	LESIONS	PREGANGLIONIC OR POSTGANGLIONIC	HYDROXY-AMPHETAMINE RESPONSE	PHENYLEPHRINE RESPONSE	ASSOCIATED NEUROLOGIC DEFICITS
Brain stem	Trauma, neoplasia, infectious agents	Preganglionic	Normal dilation	No dilation	Altered state of consciousness, cranial nerve deficits, motor deficits, respiratory difficulty, seizures
Cervical spinal cord	Trauma, focal ischemia, neoplasia	Preganglionic	Normal dilation	No dilation	Tetraparesis or tetraplegia, hemiparesis or hemiplegia
T1–T3 spinal segments	Trauma, neoplasia, fibrocartilaginous emboli	Preganglionic	Normal dilation	No dilation	Upper motor neuron weakness in pelvic limbs; weakness of thoracic limbs with mild lower motor neuron signs
T1–T3 ventral nerve roots	Avulsion of roots of brachial plexus; neural sheath tumor	Preganglionic	Normal dilation	No dilation	Weakness or paralysis of thoracic limb on same side as Horner's syndrome
Cranial thoracic sympathetic trunk	Lymphosarcoma; neural sheath tumor; cranial lung lobe disease	Preganglionic	Normal dilation	No dilation	None
Cervical sympathetic trunk	Bite wounds; neoplasia; surgical injury	Preganglionic	Normal dilation	No dilation	None if unilateral; bilateral vagal nerve lesions interfere with laryngeal and esophageal function
Middle ear	Otitis media; trauma; neoplasia	Postganglionic	Little to no dilation	Mydriasis is greater than in normal eye	Facial nerve palsy; peripheral vestibular signs if concurrent otitis interna present
Retrobulbar	Trauma; abscess; neoplasia	Postganglionic	Little to no dilation	Mydriasis is greater than in normal eye	None likely unless trauma is underlying cause, in which case a variety of neurologic signs are observed
Cavernous sinus	Neoplasia; trauma; abscess	Postganglionic	Little to no dilation	Mydriasis is greater than in normal eye	If oculomotor nerve is affected the pupil may be midposition

Modified from Neer TM. Horner's syndrome: Anatomy, diagnosis, and causes. Compen Contin Educ Pract Vet 1984:6:740–747.

lesions of the T1 to T3 spinal cord segments or ventral nerve roots are most common and often produce concurrent monoparesis of the thoracic limb. Cervical cord and brain stem lesions produce hemiparesis or quadriparesis. Brain stem lesions are likely also to cause other cranial nerve signs or mental depression or coma.[12] Spinal fluid analysis, radiographs of the skull or cervical spine, myelography, and electroencephalography are indicated if other neurologic signs are present.

In patients with a dilated pupil (parasympathetic) with no ophthalmologic explanation, with or without other neurologic signs, further evaluation of the parasympathetic pathway in the brain may be necessary, using such tests as electroencephalography, spinal fluid evaluation, skull radiographs, or CT or MRI scans. Cats should be checked for feline leukemia virus infection (see Spastic Pupil Syndrome).[8]

Strabismus

Strabismus is the deviation of one eye from its proper direction so that the visual axes of the two eyes cannot be directed simultaneously at the same objective point.

Pathophysiology

True strabismus is produced by disease of the extraocular cranial nerves: trochlear, oculomotor, abducent. These nerves control dorsal, ventral, medial, and lateral movements of the eye by innervating extraocular muscles that pull the eyeball in these directions (see Table 26–1). A positional strabismus, such as occurs with vestibular lesions, is not a true strabismus because the eyeball is not paralyzed or fixed in a deviated direction.

Clinical Signs

The owner may notice deviation of the eyes and describe the pet as being "cross-eyed." On examination, the deviation is usually obvious: ventrolateral deviation with oculomotor (cranial nerve III) injury and medial deviation with abducent (cranial nerve VI) injury. There is no observable deviation of the eyeball with trochlear nerve (cranial nerve IV) injury in species with round pupils; in cats, the dorsal portion of the vertical pupil is pulled laterally.[3] If the animal's head is moved from side to side (as in the oculocephalic response), the amount of eye movement, or lack thereof, in the various planes can be observed.

Positional strabismus is noted when the head is elevated. In normal dogs and cats, the eyes move so that they maintain a horizontal plane when the head is elevated. In animals with vestibular disease, the eye on

the affected side tends to move ventrally or ventrolaterally so that more sclera is visible in the upper portion of the orbit.[8] Because positional strabismus occurs with vestibular disease, other vestibular signs are likely to be present.

Diagnostic Plan

There are no other tests that can help to define the problem better than the neurologic examination, which should localize the abnormality and determine whether other signs are present. There are no known cranial nerve syndromes that cause strabismus; disease processes such as trauma, neoplasia, and inflammation are broad categories on which to base the differential diagnoses.[11] If other neurologic signs exist and the lesion is localized to the brain, then electroencephalography, spinal fluid analysis, and perhaps CT or MRI scans should be considered.

Facial Paresis or Paralysis

Facial paresis is weakness of the muscles of facial expression.

Pathophysiology

The facial nerve, cranial nerve VII, is predominantly a motor nerve, innervating the muscles of facial expression—the muscles of the eyelids, lips, ears, nose, and cheeks and the caudal portion of the digastric muscle.[3] In addition, it carries parasympathetic secretory fibers to the salivary and lacrimal glands and to the mucous membranes of the oral and nasal cavities. It also conveys sensation to the concave surfaces of the pinnae and the rostral part of the tongue.[6]

The nucleus of the facial nerve is located in the rostral medulla. Axons exit the brain stem, course with cranial nerve VIII through the internal acoustic meatus of the petrous bone, travel near the middle ear, exit the skull at the stylomastoid foramen, and finally course around the ramus of the mandible.[11] The facial nerve divides into several branches. The buccal branches innervate muscles of the cheek and lips; the auriculopalpebral branch divides into the auricular and palpebral nerves to innervate the ear and eyelid muscles, respectively.[13]

Clinical Signs

Unilateral facial paresis may go unnoticed by owners, but complete paralysis often results in obvious clinical signs. A lip droop on the affected side may be noted, as well as accumulation and dripping of saliva or food. The affected ear may droop, particularly in pets that normally have erect ears. The eyelid may not close, and the nictitans (third eyelid) may move across the eye when the menace response is evaluated. Passive protrusion of the third eyelid during globe retraction helps to distribute the tear film and protect the cornea from ulcerative keratitis.[8]

On neurologic examination, the menace response may be weak or absent, not because of a lack of vision but because of inability to blink or close the eyelid. Some pets retract the eye as a protective mechanism in response to the threat of the menace test. The eyelids on both sides should be palpated or touched simultaneously in order to detect strength of closure and to detect subtle weakness. Close inspection of the philtrum may reveal slight deviation from its normally vertical position, away from the side of the nerve deficit. During inspiration, the nostril on the affected side may not open or flare as much as that on the unaffected side.[3]

A Schirmer tear test should be done to determine whether the preganglionic parasympathetic fibers for lacrimal secretion have been injured as they course with the facial nerve. Tear production is not affected if the facial nerve is injured distal to the facial canal, because parasympathetic fibers leave the nerve during its course near the middle ear.[8]

Diagnostic Plan

After facial weakness has been established, it becomes important to distinguish between a lesion of the brain stem, where the origin of the facial nerve is located, and a lesion of the peripheral nerve itself. Lesions of the peripheral nerve have a more favorable prognosis for life than do those of the medulla.[1, 11] If all branches of the facial nerve are affected, weakness of the ear, lip, and eyelid muscles can be observed, and the lesion is probably located in the brain stem nucleus or in the nerve before it branches.[3]

It is also important to determine whether other cranial nerves are affected. Because of the close association of the facial and vestibulocochlear nerves, they often are affected simultaneously by the same lesion in the medulla or near the petrous bone.[3] With medullary lesions, other brain stem structures are likely to be affected to produce other cranial nerve deficits (e.g., vestibular signs, dysphagia), bradycardia, proprioception deficits, limb weakness, stupor, or severe depression.

If facial weakness or paralysis is thought to be peripheral in origin, possible causes include idiopathic facial paralysis,[14] trauma,[15] otitis media,[16] hypothyroidism,[17] and neoplasia. Thorough otoscopic examination, radiography of the bullae, and evaluation of thyroid function are in order. If a central or brain stem location is more likely than a peripheral one, spinal fluid analysis, skull radiography, and CT or MRI scans are in order (see Chaps. 24 and 25).

Masticatory Muscle Atrophy and Dropped Jaw

Decreased mass of the masseter and temporal muscles and lack of jaw tone (such that the mouth cannot be closed) are two clinical signs associated with dysfunction of the motor aspect of the trigeminal nerve (cranial nerve V).

Pathophysiology

The trigeminal nerve contains both sensory and motor fibers. It has three branches: maxillary, ophthalmic, and mandibular. The maxillary branch provides sensation to the ventral eyelids, face, and nasal area. The ophthalmic branch innervates the dorsal eyelids and corneas. The mandibular branch provides sensation to the lower jaw and also motor innervation to the muscles of mastication, which include the masseter, temporal, pterygoids, rostral digastric, and mylohyoid muscles.[1, 6]

Clinical Signs

The onset of a dropped jaw is usually acute, and it is a clinical sign that owners easily observe. There may a history of difficulty with food prehension or with keeping food in the mouth.[3] On examination, the jaw tone is slack and the jaw falls open immediately after it is manually closed. A dropped jaw implies a bilateral dysfunction of the mandibular branches; a unilateral lesion does not appear to interfere with jaw function.[18] Because a dropped jaw can be associated with rabies, gloves should be worn when first examining a patient with a dropped jaw.

Unilateral masticatory muscle atrophy is usually visually and palpably noticeable. With bilateral atrophy, lack of muscle mass results in a prominent occipital protuberance that owners sometimes mistake for a bony mass. Bilateral atrophy occasionally can be difficult to appreciate because the size of masticatory muscles is influenced by both breed and age. Larger breeds of dogs tend to have larger masticatory muscle mass than do smaller breeds. Muscle mass often decreases as part of aging. Palpation is often the best way of identifying atrophy, especially in dogs with long-haired coats.

Diagnostic Plan

After identification of a dropped jaw, it should be determined whether it is caused by a bilateral trigeminal nerve lesion or by temporomandibular joint (TMJ) luxation. With TMJ luxation, a thorough history may establish possible trauma, and careful palpation should elicit pain or excessive movement. Radiographs of the TMJ may confirm luxations or fractures. If joint disease is eliminated, the next step is to establish the origin of the nerve dysfunction (i.e., brain stem or peripheral nerve). If the origin is within the brain stem, other neurologic signs may be found, such as mental depression, upper motor neuron weakness, and other cranial nerve signs (e.g., facial weakness, vestibular signs, dysphagia). The presence of such signs is an indication for spinal fluid analysis, skull radiographs, and CT or MRI scans.

Localized peripheral nerve injury often does not produce other neurologic signs and is difficult to confirm with routine diagnostic tests. Inflammation, trauma, and neoplasia are possible diagnoses. Diffuse peripheral nerve disease can produce other cranial nerve deficits as well as diffuse muscle wasting, depressed spinal reflexes, and perhaps generalized weakness. If such signs are present in conjunction with a dropped jaw, polyradiculoneuritis, botulism, or other acquired polyneuropathies (see Chap. 28) should be considered. The presence of these signs is an indication for muscle or nerve biopsies and electrodiagnostic studies. Localized muscle disease is a common cause of masticatory muscle atrophy (see Chap. 28) and can be differentiated from peripheral nerve disease by muscle histopathology.

Deafness

The inability to hear or perceive sound is deafness.

Pathophysiology

The vestibulocochlear nerve, cranial nerve VIII, is composed of two fiber systems that are blended into a single nerve trunk.[16, 19, 20] These are the cochlear nerve, responsible for hearing, and the vestibular nerve, responsible for balance and orientation in space. These sensory nerves originate in separate peripheral receptors and have distinct and diffuse central connections. Although they are united along their course through the skull, they differ so greatly in their anatomic and functional relations that they should be considered separately.

The pathway for hearing begins with sound waves transmitted to the tympanum and across a chain of three ear ossicles to the vestibular window.[19, 20] Here the movement of perilymph stimulates movement of endolymph in the cochlear duct. Within the cochlear duct, hair cells or receptors are stimulated and trigger the generation of an action potential along cochlear nerve axons. These axons course to the internal acoustic meatus, where they join with the vestibular division of cranial nerve VIII. This nerve enters the medulla, where cochlear axons terminate on cochlear nuclei. From here, axons for audition follow one of two pathways that extend from the medulla to the midbrain, to the thalamus, and, finally, to the auditory cortex (temporal lobe of the cerebrum). These pathways cross numerous times, making it unlikely for a central or brain stem lesion to cause deafness without creating more serious and obvious deficits. Most deaf animals therefore have peripheral deafness, not central.

There are two kinds of peripheral deafness: conduction deafness and nerve deafness.[20, 21] Disorders that obliterate the external ear canal, destroy the tympanum, or damage the ear ossicles cause conduction deafness.[22] With conduction deafness, sound waves are unable to reach the receptor. With nerve deafness, the sound waves reach the receptor but cannot be conducted because of receptor or axonal impairment. Congenital deafness is an example of nerve deafness.[20, 21, 23] In older animals, hearing loss has been associated with a reduction in the number of spiral ganglion neurons.[24]

Clinical Signs

Partial or unilateral loss of hearing is usually unnoticed by pet owners and can be difficult to establish on clinical examination.[19] Bilaterally diminished hearing or complete hearing loss is noticed by most owners. The deaf pet sleeps through loud sounds that disturb others, and it does not hear the approach of people or other animals. If hearing loss occurs in a pet previously trained with voice commands, the owner may comment that the pet is no longer responsive to such commands. In older patients, deafness is frequently noted acutely when in fact the hearing loss or deficit progressed gradually and has been present for some time.

Diagnostic Plan

When taking the history for the problem of deafness, it must be ascertained whether the pet has had any previous ear infections, injuries, or surgery. Information on the use of topical or systemic drugs is important because ototoxicity can occur with various drugs (Table 26-3).[25] If the pet is younger than 6 months of age, the owner should be asked about the hearing ability of littermates or parents because of the possibility of congenital deafness.[26]

The two most important aspects of the physical examination are confirmation of the hearing loss and evaluation of the ear canals. Hearing loss can be crudely evaluated by producing loud sounds behind the pet and watching for such responses as a turn of the head or lifting of the ears. Care should be taken to avoid creating vibrations that the animal can feel.

A thorough otoscopic evaluation is necessary to evaluate the possibility of otitis externa[27] and to exclude conduction abnormalities. If an obvious reason for the hearing loss cannot be found, radiographs of the

Table 26–3
Ototoxic Drugs and Sites of Predominant Functional Impairment

DRUG	SITE OF IMPAIRMENT
Aminoglycosides	
Streptomycin	Vestibular
Netilmicin	Vestibular
Neomycin	Auditory
Dibekacin	Auditory
Kanamycin	Auditory
Amikacin	Auditory
Gentamicin	Vestibular; some auditory
Sisomicin	Vestibular and auditory
Tobramycin	Vestibular and auditory
Erythromycin	Vestibular and auditory
Hydromycin	Auditory
Polymyxin B	Auditory
Loop diuretics	Potentiates vestibular and auditory effects of aminoglycoside
Furosemide	
Ethacrynic acid	
Cisplatin	Unknown
Trialkyl tin compounds	Auditory
Chlorhexidine (local application)	Inner ear cell

Modified from Pickrell JA, Oehme FW, Cash WC. Ototoxicity in dogs and cats. Semin Vet Med Surg (Small Anim) 1993;8:42–49. See also references 50 and 66.

bullae should be considered as means to evaluate middle ear disease. Fluid or soft tissue densities in the middle ear can dampen sound waves and produce hearing deficits. If radiographic results are normal and the owner wants to pursue the deafness, a referral to a clinic that can perform brain stem auditory evoked responses (BAER) may be in order (see Diagnostic Procedures).

Head Tilt and Nystagmus

Head tilt (ear pointed to the ground), leaning, circling, rolling, and spontaneous jerking of the eyeballs (nystagmus) are signs of vestibular system imbalance.[28] Nystagmus is an involuntary, repetitive, to-and-fro movement of the eyes that can occur in any plane.[8]

Pathophysiology

The vestibular system alters the position of the eyes, trunk, and limbs in response to changes in head position.[28] It is divided into two aspects: peripheral and central. The peripheral vestibular system includes the inner ear receptors and the vestibulocochlear nerve (cranial nerve VIII). The central system includes the brain stem vestibular nuclei and a part of the cerebellum called the flocculonodular lobe.

The inner ear is located within the petrous temporal bone of the skull. It is a bony labyrinth containing a membranous labyrinth filled with endolymph. Perilymph, a fluid similar to cerebrospinal fluid, separates the two labyrinths. Receptors within the membranous labyrinth sense changes in endolymph flow and transmit these changes to the vestibular nuclei through cranial nerve VIII. Stimulation of receptors occurs with directional changes, angular acceleration, and deceleration. After velocity of movement becomes constant, receptors are no longer stimulated.[8, 28, 29]

Head movement causes stimulation of receptors and triggers impulses that travel through cranial nerve VIII to the vestibular nuclei in the brain stem.[28, 29] During head movements in normal animals, the eyes deviate slowly away from the direction the head is turning and then quickly jerk back to that direction. A normal vestibular nystagmus occurs with both slow and fast phases, which cease whenever head motions stop.

Clinical Signs

With vestibular disease, the primary complaint is often a head tilt, circling, loss of balance, or falling to one side. Head tilt, falling, and circling are usually toward the affected side; the exception is the paradoxical vestibular syndrome (described in Chap. 25). Spontaneous nystagmus is often present, and the fast phase is away from the side of the lesion. Nystagmus may occur in a horizontal, vertical, or rotary direction; vertical nystagmus is most often associated with central vestibular lesions. The head and body should be placed in various positions to determine whether the nystagmus changes direction; if so, a central vestibular lesion is more likely than a peripheral one. If spontaneous nystagmus is absent, changes in head and body position may elicit a "positional nystagmus," which is more often associated with a central vestibular lesion than a peripheral one. When the head and nose are elevated, the eye on the affected side usually drops (eye drop) more ventrally than the normal eye.[8, 28, 29] This observation is referred to as positional strabismus, and it can be seen with either central or peripheral vestibular lesions.

The gait of an animal with vestibular disease is ataxic and drunken-like. With acute onset of vestibular malfunction, the animal may not even be able to stand and prefers to lie down or roll to the affected side. Ambulatory patients are often hesitant to move and may stumble, fall, or appear clumsy.

Postural reactions in animals with vestibular signs can be difficult to assess; such tests should be performed slowly. With peripheral vestibular disease, strength and proprioception should be normal. Central vestibular disease causes proprioceptive deficits and hemiparesis, quadriparesis, or quadriplegia. With acute onset of vestibular disease, postural reactions are initially difficult to obtain and interpret because the animal is so disoriented. In such cases, daily serial examinations should be done until improvement or progression is noted.

Bilateral vestibular lesions are much less common than unilateral ones, and they are usually peripheral. With bilateral lesions, nystagmus and head tilt are usually absent.[28] Ataxia is prominent, with the animal falling to one side. Although the gait appears similar to that seen with cerebellar disorders, hypermetria, intention tremors, and head bobs are absent on closer evaluation. The tail is often held in an erect position. Wide, sweeping head movements from side to side and a poor to absent oculocephalic reflex (normal vestibular nystagmus) are two reliable signs of bilateral vestibular disease.

Diagnostic Plan

The onset (gradual versus acute), progression or regression, and duration of clinical signs should be established. Traumatic, vascular, and idiopathic vestibular diseases are usually more acute in onset and nonprogressive; neoplastic and inflammatory processes may have a more gradual onset and tend to produce progressive signs.

The history should also establish the possibility of ear infection, trauma, exposure to ototoxic drugs (see Table 26–3), and other systemic or neurologic signs. Physical examination should include palpation of the face, ear, and pharyngeal area for signs of discomfort or masses.[29] An otoscopic examination should evaluate the external ear canals for signs of otitis externa and the tympanic membrane for signs of middle ear disease. Middle ear disease can produce a ruptured, discolored, or bulging tympanic membrane, and infection can spread from the middle to the inner ear to produce otitis interna and vestibular signs.[16] Neurologic examination should establish the presence of vestibular dysfunction and whether it is peripheral or central (see Clinical Signs).

After peripheral vestibular signs have been identified, an otoscopic examination helps rule out otitis interna as a possible cause. Radiographs of the bullae are also indicated to assess the middle ear cavities and the possibility of otitis media that has spread to the inner ears. Although routine laboratory data are often unrewarding for assessment of neurologic disease, certain inflammatory and endocrine disorders can affect the vestibular system. A low or low-normal platelet count should raise suspicion of rickettsial infections (see Chap. 37), which can produce both central and peripheral vestibular signs. An increased cholesterol level may raise the possibility of hypothyroidism, which also can produce central or peripheral vestibular signs.[17] An older dog with an acute onset of peripheral vestibular signs without a history of trauma or signs of otitis externa or otitis media most likely has idiopathic vestibular disease.

If central vestibular signs are identified, a minimum database (hemogram, chemistry profile, urinalysis) is obtained and may suggest inflammatory or metabolic changes that could affect the brain. Chest radiographs can be assessed for signs of systemic mycosis or neoplasia that may have spread to the brain. Skull radiographs are not often helpful except in cases of trauma or skull tumors. In order to identify or confirm central vestibular lesions, CT or MRI scans and a spinal fluid analysis are required.

Laryngeal Paralysis

Laryngeal paralysis is a partial or complete loss of laryngeal muscle function associated with neurologic, muscular, or neuromuscular diseases.

Pathophysiology

Branches of the vagus nerve innervate the laryngeal muscles, which open the glottis on inspiration to allow air to pass to the trachea. Cell bodies for the vagus nerve are located in the nucleus ambiguus in the medulla. The nerve exits the skull through the jugular foramen and the occipitotympanic fissure. The cranial laryngeal nerve leaves the vagus nerve to innervate the cricothyroid muscle; the recurrent laryngeal nerve innervates the remainder of the laryngeal muscles.[3, 11] Multiple disease processes such as toxins, trauma, infection, neoplasia, polyneuropathies, and endocrine disorders may affect the neurologic pathway at a variety of locations by various mechanisms.

Clinical Signs

Classic signs are hoarse, raspy respiratory sounds, particularly during inspiration; decreased exercise tolerance; and cyanosis. Physical examination findings can be normal when the animal is at rest. As the activity level increases, dyspnea, inspiratory stridor, hyperthermia, and even collapse develop. If laryngeal paralysis is associated with diffuse neuromuscular disease, other neurologic signs (e.g., generalized muscle atrophy, reduced spinal reflexes) may be present.

Diagnostic Plan

The history should establish signs of systemic illness and potential exposure to toxins (e.g., lead, organophosphates). If the animal is younger than 1 year of age, the status of littermates should be ascertained because of the possibility of inherited laryngeal paralysis. Neck and laryngeal muscles should carefully be palpated for signs of masses or other objects that could obstruct the air passages or be a source or site of disease causing nerve damage and laryngeal paralysis.[3, 11, 30, 31]

Laryngeal paralysis is confirmed by performance of a laryngoscopic examination on a lightly anesthetized patient. Normal animals under a light plane of anesthesia have abduction of vocal folds on inspiration. In affected animals, these folds do not move or move poorly, either unilaterally or bilaterally. Once diagnosed, laryngeal paralysis should be categorized as either an inherited (congenital) or an acquired form. If the animal is younger than 1 year of age, if littermates are affected, and if toxins are eliminated as possible causes, an inherited form is likely. Because the paralysis is probably acquired in adult animals, generalized polyneuropathies should be considered (see Chap. 28). Possible causes include lead intoxication, myasthenia gravis, acute polyradiculoneuritis, and hypothyroidism.[17, 32, 33] Isolated cases of laryngeal paralysis have also been reported with foreign body penetration of the wall of the esophagus, iatrogenic nerve trauma as a postoperative complication of thyroidectomy and other neck surgeries, brain stem trauma or hemorrhage, rabies, and various other infections or inflammation of the medulla.[11] The great majority of acquired cases are idiopathic.

Diagnostic Procedures

Routine Laboratory Evaluation

Although routine laboratory test results are generally nonspecific for cranial nerve disorders, they should be evaluated before the affected patient is anesthetized because they identify factors that could affect the patient's response to anesthesia. Occasionally, metabolic, endocrine, toxic, or neoplastic disease processes can be supported by laboratory results.

Radiography

Although skull radiographs (see Chap. 24) are not generally rewarding for diagnosis of cranial nerve disorders, they can be helpful in some cases of trauma, bony neoplasia, or middle ear disease. Bullae radiographs are best taken with the animal under general anesthesia so that correct positioning for oblique lateral, open-mouth, and ventrodorsal views can be obtained.[16] Oblique lateral and open-mouth views are useful for evaluation of the air-filled tympanic cavity. Fluid, granulation tissue, or neoplasia in this cavity causes a soft tissue density. Walls of the tympanic bullae should be evaluated for thickening or sclerosis and bony proliferation or destruction.

Brain Stem Auditory Evoked Response

The BAERs are a group of five to seven waveforms recorded within 10 milliseconds after a click stimulus is applied to the ear. The impulse generated by the click travels from the ear through the brain stem to the auditory cortex.[19] These waves are recorded from subcutaneous electrodes placed on the head. Because of the considerable distance between the source and the recording site, the evoked potential is small compared with the surrounding electrical activity. Therefore, a signal averager must be used to average waveforms elicited by the click stimulus within a preset period after each click.

BAER testing has been used to evaluate hearing deficits caused by both conduction and neurologic abnormalities. It has also been used to evaluate brain stem function, because the hearing pathway traverses much of the brain stem (see Chap. 25).[34] The test requires special equipment, which is usually available only at referral centers.

Spinal Fluid Analysis

For cranial nerve diseases originating at the brain stem level, spinal fluid analysis may yield information to confirm brain stem disease and to give clues to its cause. Collection of spinal fluid from the cerebellomedullary cistern is described in Chapter 24.

Common Diseases of the Cranial Nerves

Optic Neuritis

Optic neuritis refers to inflammation of the optic nerve that produces impaired vision or loss of vision.[8, 35] The incidence is unknown. Any age, breed, or sex of dog can be affected; one author reported that most affected dogs were older than 3 years of age.[36] Cats are less commonly affected.

Pathophysiology

Underlying causes for most cases of optic neuritis are not usually determined, although inflammatory processes are probably most common.[8] Possible causes include canine distemper, the ocular form of granulomatous meningoencephalitis, systemic mycosis, toxoplasmosis, neoplasia, trauma, and acute toxication (lead or chlorinated hydrocarbon toxicity).[36]

Clinical Signs

Signs consist of a sudden onset of unilateral or bilateral blindness with dilated pupils that respond poorly to light or not at all. Blindness is often unassociated with other neurologic signs or obvious disease in other systems. [35]

Diagnosis

Ophthalmoscopy is necessary to differentiate optic neuritis from other retinal diseases that can cause blindness with impaired PLRs. With intrabulbar optic neuritis, the optic disk appears hazy, edematous, or elevated into the vitreous humor. Peripapillary vessels appear elevated, and portions may seem to disappear into the myelin as they exit the disk.[8] Retinal vessels may be engorged, and focal hemorrhage may be observed. In long-standing or chronic cases, the optic nerve atrophies. If optic nerve changes are not observed and there are no signs of retinal disease, the neuritis may be retrobulbar, meaning that changes are present behind the optic disk and cannot be seen on fundic examination. SARDS can present similarly and is differentiated from retrobulbar optic neuritis on ERG. With optic neuritis, the ERG waveforms are normal; with SARDS, the waveforms are absent.[37]

Because there are numerous inflammatory causes of optic neuritis, routine laboratory data (hemogram, chemistry profile, and urinalysis) should be evaluated. The results of neurologic examination is usually normal.

Treatment

Treatment should be directed at the underlying cause. If a cause cannot be determined at the initial examination, corticosteroids are often used to decrease inflammation. Oral prednisolone[8] is given at a dose of 2 mg/kg divided twice daily for 1 week, followed by half this dose for another 2 weeks, and then every other day for another 2 weeks.

Prognosis

The prognosis for return of vision is guarded because of the many potential causes and the unpredictable course. Some animals may have a return of some vision within days to weeks,[36] and others may remain permanently blind. Some may develop other clinical signs.

Horner's Syndrome

Horner's syndrome is an abnormality of the sympathetic innervation to the eye that results in one or more of the following clinical signs: miosis, prolapse of the third eyelid, ptosis, and relative enoph-

thalmos.[8, 12] The incidence in the general population is not known, but the syndrome appears to be common from literature reports.[38, 39] Any age, sex, and breed of cat or dog can be affected. One study showed that Horner's syndrome was associated with increasing age in dogs.[39]

Pathophysiology

Ocular sympathetic innervation maintains the normal smooth muscle tone of the eyelids, third membrane, periorbita, and iris constrictor muscles. Such tone maintains the palpebral fissure width and the normal anterior position of the globe within the orbit. The sympathetic pathway is a long, three-neuron pathway (see Fig. 26–2). The first or central neuron originates in the hypothalamus and descends the brain stem to synapse in gray matter at the level of T1 to T3. From there, second-order (preganglionic) neurons join the T1 to T3 ventral nerve roots and pass cranially in the neck as part of the vagosympathetic trunk. Near the tympanic bulla, sympathetic axons separate from the vagus and synapse on the cranial cervical ganglion. Axons from the third-order (postganglionic) neurons pass near the middle ear cavity and join the ophthalmic branch of cranial nerve V to enter the periorbita.[8, 11, 12] Although Horner's syndrome can be created with injury anywhere along this pathway, the most common sites are in the sections of the preganglionic and postganglionic neurons.

Clinical Signs

Classic signs of Horner's syndrome in dogs and cats are miosis, ptosis, enophthalmos, narrowed palpebral fissure, and prolapse of the third eyelid. Of these signs, miosis and prolapse of the third eyelid are most commonly recognized.[38, 40] Uncommon signs include iris color changes in cats and a change in the coat color of Siamese cats secondary to peripheral vasodilatation of the skin.[39, 40] Horner's syndrome most often occurs unilaterally, but it can occur bilaterally.

Diagnostic Plan

Diagnosis is made based on the findings of physical and neurologic examinations. With the use of indirect-acting and direct-acting sympathomimetic drugs, the lesion can be localized respectively to the preganglionic pathway (from the hypothalamus to T1 and T2 and then to the cranial cervical ganglion) or the postganglionic pathway (from the cranial cervical ganglion to the middle ear and then to the eye). If 1 to 2 drops of 1% hydroxyamphetamine causes the affected pupil to dilate within 1 hour, the lesion is located in the preganglionic pathway. In such cases, the nerve endings of the postganglionic neuron are not impaired and can liberate their stores of endogenous norepinephrine. If the lesion is postganglionic, norepinephrine stores are reduced or absent, and the affected eye does not dilate with hydroxyamphetamine. A sufficient number of drops must be administered equally to both eyes; mydriasis of the control eye must result to ensure a valid test. A direct-acting sympathomimetic agent such as 10% phenylephrine should be used 1 to 2 days after a positive hydroxyamphetamine test (i.e., one showing little to no dilation of the pupil) to confirm the presence of a postganglionic lesion. One to two drops of a 10% phenylephrine solution should produce dilation of the affected pupil within 10 minutes with postganglionic lesions; the normal pupil should not dilate.[11] Pharmacologic tests should be conducted on both eyes, using the normal eye as a control. The testing environment should be quiet; the patient should be calm to reduce the influence of any endogenously released neurohumoral substances.[8] At least 24 hours should elapse between tests, because the drugs could interfere with each other.

Table 26–2 lists disorders that can cause Horner's syndrome in dogs and cats. After the lesion has been localized to a degree, the history, palpation, radiographs, myelography, fine-needle aspirates, and spinal fluid analysis may be necessary to obtain a specific diagnosis of the actual cause.

Treatment

Clinical signs of Horner's syndrome do not need to be treated. Treatment should be directed at any underlying cause that is found.

Prognosis

Induced by a variety of causes, Horner's syndrome is rarely associated with serious or life-threatening disorders. If it is associated with trauma, the signs often disappear or subside, in many cases over weeks to months. Recovery appears to take longer or is incomplete in cases of idiopathic Horner's syndrome.[38] In those cases associated with masses, the prognosis depends on the biology of the mass and whether it can be treated or removed.

Trigeminal Neuritis

Trigeminal neuritis is a syndrome of unknown cause that produces an acute onset of inability to close the mouth.[41–43] The true incidence is unknown. Affected dogs have been mature and of various breeds. Cats also can be affected.[3]

Pathophysiology

The cause is unknown. Histopathology of the trigeminal nerve has shown bilateral nonsuppurative neuritis of all portions of the nerve and its ganglion. Demyelination is more prominent than axonal degeneration. The brain stem has not been affected. It is presumed that Horner's syndrome occurs from involvement of the postganglionic sympathetic axons coursing in the ophthalmic branch of the trigeminal nerve.[3]

Clinical Signs

The obvious abnormality is that the mouth hangs open and the animal is unable to close it even when it attempts to eat or drink. A few patients also have unilateral or bilateral ptosis, miosis, and enophthalmos (Horner's syndrome).[3] Sensation to the head is normal, and there is no atrophy of the muscles of mastication when clinical signs are first noticed. Affected animals are usually alert and have no other neurologic or physical examination deficits.

Diagnostic Plan

Clinical signs and history are the best diagnostic clues. Trauma, which can cause a fracture or luxation of the TMJ, should be eliminated by historical information and lack of physical evidence of TMJ pain or excessive movement. Other neurologic signs do not develop; this helps to eliminate rabies and other inflammatory diseases as possible causes. Needle electromyelography evaluation of temporal and masseter muscles may show denervation potentials, and muscle histopathology reflects neurogenic atrophy.[36]

Treatment

There is no specific treatment. Because affected dogs have difficulty with prehension of food, alimentation assistance is required. Available options include feeding an all-gruel diet and installing a nasogastric, pharyngostomy, or gastrostomy tube.

Prognosis

Prognosis is usually good to excellent because recovery is expected to occur in 2 to 3 weeks.[36] In a few cases, masticatory muscle atrophy has been observed in the recovery stage, but the muscles returned to normal mass after recovery was complete. Horner's syndrome is a permanent change in some dogs. Recurrence in the same dog has not been reported.

Idiopathic Facial Paralysis

Sudden onset of weakness or paralysis of the muscles of facial expression for which an underlying cause cannot be found has been named idiopathic facial paralysis. Although the incidence has not been evaluated, in one retrospective study of facial neuropathies, idiopathic facial nerve palsy was diagnosed in 74.7% of dogs and 25% of cats so affected.[44] Mature dogs and cats (>5 years of age) are most commonly affected,[36] and there appears to be an association with increased age. Breed predispositions include cocker spaniels,[14] Pembroke Welsh corgis, boxers, English setters, and domestic longhair cats.[44]

Pathophysiology

The cause of idiopathic facial paralysis is not known; clinical signs have been compared to those in humans with a facial neuritis called Bell's palsy. Although dogs with facial neuropathy are more likely to have otitis media or otitis interna than dogs in the reference population, a true association with idiopathic facial palsy has not been proved.[44] An association between idiopathic facial neuropathy and hypothyroidism has not been supported[44]; however, sporadic cases of dogs with hypothyroidism and facial palsy have been reported.[17]

Histopathologic findings have included degeneration of myelinated nerve fibers without associated inflammation. Ultrastructural findings have included Schwann cell proliferation and stages of remyelination.[45]

Clinical Signs

Onset is acute, and signs can be bilateral or unilateral. With unilateral involvement, a readily apparent asymmetry of the face is characterized by ear droop, lip droop, and inability to close the eye. The palpebral fissure may be widened because of decreased tone to the orbicular muscle of the eye. Food and saliva may accumulate on the inside of the affected lip. The affected nostril may not flare when the animal inhales; this is best recognized in patients with unilateral involvement because the unaffected side acts as a control. There is no evidence of Horner's syndrome in animals with idiopathic facial paralysis,[36] but some do have reduced tear production and possibly ulcerative keratitis.

Diagnostic Plan

Diagnosis is based on the history, clinical signs, and diagnostic tests to eliminate other common causes of facial neuropathy (see Facial Paresis or Paralysis). A thorough otoscopic examination should assess the possibility of otitis externa or otitis media. Radiographs of the tympanic bullae should be considered to evaluate for otitis media. Thyroid function tests (see Chap. 47) can be helpful in breeds predisposed to hypothyroidism. Needle electromyography can be used to confirm localization and rule out the possibility of other cranial nerve involvement or a generalized neu-

ropathy. If these test results return within normal limits, then the facial neuropathy is "idiopathic" in origin. A Schirmer tear test should be performed to determine whether parasympathetic fibers that innervate the lacrimal gland are involved, because these fibers course with the facial nerve.

Treatment

There is no specific treatment. Some clinicians administer systemic antibiotics for 2 weeks or longer, on the premise that the facial paralysis may be caused by early, undetectable otitis media. In humans with Bell's palsy, corticosteroids have been used, but they are not recommended to treat the syndrome in dogs. If tear production is affected, artificial tears should be used to prevent ulcerative keratitis.

Prognosis

The prognosis for life is good because this syndrome is not life-threatening. However, it is unlikely that the function of the facial nerve will return. Owners may report resolution of the signs, but close examination often reveals contracture of the affected lip or ear; denervated muscle is replaced by fibrous connective tissue, which contracts to pull the affected lip and ear muscles up. In some unilateral cases, the other side develops paralysis weeks to months later.

Otitis Media and Otitis Interna

The terms otitis media and otitis interna refer to inflammation of the middle and the inner ear structures, respectively.[46] The incidence of otitis media secondary to otitis externa is relatively high, with percentages varying from 16% in early cases of otitis externa to 50% in chronic cases.[47] The incidence of otitis interna is not known, but in one review of peripheral vestibular signs in dogs, 49% were determined to be caused by otitis interna.[48] Cats or dogs of any age, sex, or breed can develop otitis media or otitis interna. However, breeds that are predisposed to otitis externa because of conformation (e.g., long ears) are more commonly affected (see Chap. 4).

Pathophysiology

Inflammation of the middle ear cavity can be induced through one of three routes: across the tympanic membrane, through the auditory tube, or by hematogenous spread. It is assumed that otitis interna most commonly results from extension of middle ear infections.[16]

Most cases of otitis media and interna are caused by bacteria such as *Staphylococcus*, *Streptococcus*, *Pseudomonas*, *Proteus*, and *Clostridium* species. *Escherichia coli*, *Malassezia pachydermatis*, and *Candida* spp.

have also been reported to cause otitis media. Ear mites (*Otodectes cynotis*) occasionally cause rupture of the tympanic membrane and enter the middle ear. Trauma, polyps, neoplasms, and foreign bodies (e.g., grass or plant awns) may also enter the middle ear and cause signs of otitis media.[16]

Clinical Signs

Signs of otitis media include discharge from the external ear canal, pawing or rubbing of the affected ear, head shaking, decreased hearing, and, perhaps, pain when the head or ear is touched.[16] Sometimes, the pain can cause the pet to keep its head turned or tilted to one side. Decreased appetite, fever, and lethargy may also accompany otitis media. A facial neuropathy or Horner's syndrome may be present on the same side as the otitis media because the facial nerve and the sympathetic nerve supply to the eye course near the middle ear.

Signs of otitis interna are a head tilt to the affected side, spontaneous horizontal or rotary nystagmus, and ataxia. With an acute onset, the animal may be so severely disoriented that it is unable to walk or it circles, falls, or rolls toward the affected side. If the head is lifted, the eye on the affected side may deviate in a ventral or ventrolateral direction (positional strabismus). Vomiting can occur but is uncommon. Hearing loss is not usually detected. After several days, clinical signs become less pronounced and nystagmus may disappear. The head tilt may improve, but minor residual head tilts are common even with successful treatment.

The physical examination should include palpation of the base of the ears and the TMJs for signs of swelling, pain, or lumps. The pharyngeal area should be examined for signs of inflammation or masses that may have spread to the middle ear through the auditory tube. A thorough otoscopic examination is necessary to evaluate the external ear canals and tympanic membrane; sedation or general anesthesia is necessary in most cases. If the ear canals contain debris, warm normal saline solution can be used to lavage the ear canals to improve visibility of the tympanic membrane. Swabs for cytologic evaluation and culture and sensitivity should always be taken before the cleaning.

Diagnostic Plan

A diagnosis of otitis media is made based on clinical signs, observation of an abnormal tympanic membrane, or radiographic changes of the affected tympanic bullae. The normal pars tensa tympanic membrane is a glistening, transparent or pearl-gray translucent membrane through which the base of the malleus, one of the middle ear ossicles, can be observed. If the tympanic membrane is absent, torn, cloudy, or different in color from normal, middle ear disease should be suspected.

Oblique lateral and open-mouth radiographic views may show a soft tissue density in the normally air-filled tympanic cavity. The wall of the tympanic bulla may appear thickened or sclerotic, especially in cases of chronic otitis media. Bony proliferation, extending to the TMJ or petrous temporal bone, can sometimes be found in chronic cases. Radiographic changes may not be present for several weeks in acute cases, and some chronic cases may show only sclerosis of the bulla. CT scans may increase sensitivity for identification of middle ear disease radiographically.

In some cases (up to 25%), there are no otoscopic or radiographic signs of middle ear disease. If otitis media is suspected based on historical information, a 4- to 6-week course of antibiotics can be tried. If clinical signs progress and middle ear disease is still suspected, surgical exploration of the middle ear may be indicated.[49]

Treatment

If there is obvious fluid in the middle ear cavity (based on otoscopic observation or radiography) or if the tympanic membrane is intact but abnormal in appearance, a myringotomy is performed to obtain samples for cytology and culture and remove fluid from the middle ear cavity. After the tympanic membrane in the anesthetized patient is visualized with an otoscope and clean cone, a blunt probe is directed through the otoscope cone to perforate the tympanic membrane just caudal to the malleus. After the probe is removed, a 20-gauge spinal needle of adequate length with an attached syringe (plus extension tubing if necessary) is passed through the perforation, and fluid or material from the middle ear cavity is aspirated. If fluid cannot be retrieved, flushing with 0.5 to 1.0 mL of sterile saline solution may allow aspiration of material for cytologic analysis and culture.

Antibiotics should be administered for 4 to 6 weeks, and selection is based on culture results. If culture results are unavailable, a cephalosporin or trimethoprim-sulfonamide combination drug can be administered. Trimethoprim-sulfonamide should be avoided if there is decreased tear production, and owners should be warned of the potential for keratitis sicca with sulfa drugs. Topical therapy may be required if there is a significant otitis externa. However, many topical preparations contain aminoglycosides or antiseptics that could cause ototoxicity should they enter the middle and inner ear cavities (see Table 26–3). The ability of aminoglycosides to cause ototoxicity is controversial.[50] If clinical signs are not improving or if they become more severe during the course of treatment, surgical intervention is necessary to remove the infected material and to establish drainage. Surgical techniques are described elsewhere.[22, 49, 51–53]

Prognosis

The prognosis for medical management of otitis media is guarded because many patients require surgical intervention. With surgical intervention, signs often resolve, but any underlying causes of infection, such as otitis externa (see Chap. 4), must be addressed. Signs of otitis interna probably improve because of compensatory balance mechanisms. However, facial paralysis is often permanent regardless of medical or surgical intervention.

Idiopathic Vestibular Syndrome

Idiopathic vestibular syndrome is characterized by an acute onset of vestibular signs for which no underlying cause can be found. This syndrome is common in both dogs and cats. In one study of 75 affected cats, 80% were diagnosed in the months of July or August.[54] Older dogs of all breeds and any adult cat can be affected.

Pathophysiology

The cause is unknown. Microscopic lesions have not been documented in the inner ear receptors, in the vestibular nerve and ganglion, or within the brain stem of affected animals.[36]

Clinical Signs

An acute onset of head tilt, falling, rolling, or circling to the affected side is common.[55] Horizontal or rotary nystagmus is usually present, and the fast phase is directed away from the affected side. Spontaneous nystagmus may disappear or become less noticeable after a few days. In the acute stage, the animal may be so disoriented that a neurologic examination is difficult to perform. Other signs may include decreased appetite, positional strabismus on the affected side, and, less commonly, emesis.

Neurologic examination should confirm that the lesion is localized to the peripheral vestibular area (see Head Tilt and Nystagmus). No other cranial nerve deficits, hemiparesis, or proprioceptive deficits should be found on the neurologic examination.

Diagnostic Plan

The diagnosis is based on the acute onset of peripheral vestibular signs in a patient that does not have historical or physical examination findings consistent with trauma, systemic illness, or ear disease. The diagnosis is supported by clinical improvement of

signs within several days and by almost complete resolution of signs within several weeks. Because rickettsial infections can present as peripheral or central vestibular signs, a platelet count should be considered in any dog that presents with acute vestibular signs. However, signs are rapidly progressive with rickettsial diseases unless they are treated with tetracycline, doxycycline, or chloramphenicol (see Chap. 37).

Treatment

Although a variety of treatments have been tried, including antibiotics, anti-inflammatory drugs, and anti–motion sickness drugs, there is no evidence that any have changed the course of the disease.

Prognosis

The prognosis is good because most affected animals improve in 24 to 48 hours of presentation and make an almost complete recovery within several weeks. A residual head tilt and positional strabismus can sometimes be found on neurologic examination.

Idiopathic (Acquired) and Inherited Laryngeal Paralysis

Weakness or paralysis of the vocal folds is the result of hereditary (congenital) or acquired disorders of the recurrent laryngeal nerve.[56–62] Idiopathic laryngeal paralysis refers to a specific syndrome for which underlying causes cannot be found. The incidence is unknown. The acquired idiopathic form may develop in dogs and cats of any age; the hereditary form is usually found in 4- to 6-month-old dogs, especially Bouvier des Flandres, Siberian huskies, bull terriers, and Dalmatians. Castrated male dogs may be more frequently affected with the acquired form.[56] Castrated male cats also seem to be more commonly affected.[36]

Pathophysiology

The hereditary form in Bouvier des Flandres is transmitted as an autosomal dominant trait.[61] Preliminary observations in young Dalmatians suggest an autosomal recessive trait.[62] The cause for many cases of acquired laryngeal paralysis is not known. In both dogs and cats, some idiopathic cases may be part of a more generalized polyneuropathy.[60, 63] Histologic examination of the recurrent laryngeal nerve shows Wallerian degeneration.[60]

Clinical Signs

The most obvious clinical sign is inspiratory stridor or distress, as discussed previously in the section on laryngeal paralysis. Cyanosis, dyspnea, voice changes, and audible inspiratory sounds (stridor) become more apparent with exercise. Excessive head shaking and abnormal purring sounds have been observed in cats.[36, 62]

Diagnostic Plan

The clinical presentation of inspiratory dyspnea should alert the clinician to the possibility of upper airway obstruction such as laryngeal paralysis. Diagnosis is confirmed by observing lack of abduction of laryngeal muscles during inspiration under light anesthesia. The diagnosis of idiopathic laryngeal paralysis is made after ruling out other possible causes (see Laryngeal Paralysis).

Treatment

In animals with obvious and severe respiratory distress, a temporary tracheostomy tube or immediate surgery is often required. Surgical fixation of a vocal fold is the quickest and often the only means of alleviating the clinical signs, regardless of the underlying cause. Various techniques have been described, and most have had satisfactory results.[58, 63, 64] Although these procedures result in a permanently opened glottis, aspiration of food or water seems to be an uncommon sequela. A voice change or loss of voice is expected.

In those animals with minimal clinical signs, stress should be minimized and activity decreased until the diagnosis is made and testing for underlying diseases can be started. Even if an underlying cause can be found in adult animals, it may be best to surgically correct the paralysis and then direct treatment at the underlying cause to prevent degeneration of other nerves.

Prognosis

In many of the congenital forms, clinical signs are progressive because of presumed continued degeneration of nerve fibers.[57] For the acquired idiopathic form, the prognosis is usually good with surgical intervention. In both forms, the owner should be warned about underlying progressive neuropathies that could cause worsening of the laryngeal paralysis or other clinical signs.

Uncommon Diseases of the Cranial Nerves

Optic Nerve Hypoplasia

Lack of or incomplete development of the optic nerve, optic chiasm, and optic tracts results in blindness at birth.[8, 65] The optic disks are smaller than normal, and the pupils are widely dilated and nonresponsive to light if both optic nerves are affected. If only one is affected, the menace response is absent on the affected side, but the pupil is likely to be of normal size and responsive only if light is shined into the unaffected side.

Ototoxicity

Numerous drugs (see Table 26–3) have the potential to affect either the vestibular or the cochlear aspect of cranial nerve VIII. Effects may not be reversible.[25, 66] Metronidazole, a nitromidazole antibiotic used to treat anaerobic bacterial infections, giardiasis, hepatoencephalopathy, and inflammatory bowel disease, can cause vestibular signs in cats and dogs. However, the defect is at the brain stem vestibular nuclei level and not at the nerve or receptor level.[67, 68]

Congenital Peripheral Vestibular Syndrome

Unilateral or bilateral vestibular signs have been noted in German shepherds, beagles, collies, Akitas, Doberman pinschers,[39, 69, 70] smooth-haired fox terriers, and Siamese, Burmese, and Tonkinese cats.[28, 36] Signs may be present when the pet begins to ambulate, or they may develop at 3 to 14 weeks of age. Deafness may also be present. Affected animals usually do not improve but may make acceptable pets.[28]

Dysautonomic Polyganglionopathy (Key-Gaskell Syndrome)

Dysautonomic polyganglionopathy is a disease of unknown cause that affects cats and occasionally dogs, mostly in the United Kingdom.[71–74] Signs include vomiting or retching, lack of appetite, protrusion of the third eyelid, dilated pupils that respond poorly to light, decreased tear production, urinary and fecal incontinence, ataxia or paresis, megaesophagus, and bradycardia. Prognosis is guarded to poor; specific treatment is not available, and the need for nursing and supportive care can be prolonged.

Spastic Pupil Syndrome

The feline leukemia virus has been associated with dilated pupils that respond poorly to light.[8, 75] Miosis has also been noted in some cases. Signs can be intermittent. Histopathologic examination of the ciliary ganglion, or parasympathetic tract has shown lymphocytic infiltration.

Cranial Nerve Neoplasia

Peripheral nerve sheath tumors can occur along any peripheral nerve. Lymphosarcoma, squamous cell carcinoma, ceruminous adenocarcinoma, fibrosarcoma, and osteosarcoma can affect cranial nerves.[30, 31] Meningiomas of the calvarial floor can also compress cranial nerves before they exit the brain stem. Diagnosis of cranial nerve neoplasia can be difficult unless the mass can be palpated. The prognosis is guarded to poor.

Granulomatous Meningoencephalitis

Granulomatous meningoencephalitis is an inflammatory condition of the central nervous system of unknown cause.[76, 77] Occasionally, cranial nerves, particularly the optic nerves, are affected (see Chap. 24).

References

1. Shell L. Cranial nerve disorders in dogs and cats. Compen Contin Educ Pract Vet 1982;4:458–467.
2. Shell L. The cranial nerves of the brain stem. Prog Vet Neurol 1990;1:233–245.
3. de Lahunta A. Cranial nerve-lower motor neuron: General somatic efferent system, special visceral efferent system. In: de Lahunta A, ed. Veterinary Neuroanatomy and Clinical Neurology, 2nd ed. Philadelphia, WB Saunders, 1983:95–129.
4. Redding RW, Braund KG. Neurologic examination. In: Hoerlein BF, ed. Canine Neurology. Philadelphia, WB Saunders, 1978:53–70.
5. Oliver JE, Lorenz MD. Localization of lesions in the nervous system. In: Oliver JE, Lorenz MD. Handbook of Veterinary Neurology, 2nd ed. Philadelphia, WB Saunders, 1993:46–72.
6. Oliver JE, Lorenz MD. Disorders of the face, tongue, esophagus, larynx, and hearing. In: Oliver JE, Lorenz MD. Handbook of Veterinary Neurology, 2nd ed. Philadelphia, WB Saunders, 1993:229–244.
7. Chrisman CL. Visual dysfunction. In: Chrisman CL. Problems in Small Animal Neurology, 2nd ed. Philadelphia, Lea & Febiger, 1991:206–217.
8. Scagliotti RH. Neuro-ophthalmology. In: Gelatt KN, ed. Veterinary Ophthalmology, 2nd ed. Philadelphia, Lea & Febiger, 1991:706–743.
9. Guyton AC. The eye: 111. Central neurophysiology of vision. In: Guyton AC. Textbook of Medical Physiology, 7th ed. Philadelphia, WB Saunders, 1986:724–733.
10. Cunningham JG. The visual system. In: Cunningham JG, ed. Textbook of Veterinary Physiology. Philadelphia, WB Saunders, 1992:102–111.
11. Chrisman CL. Signs related to other autonomic and somatic cranial nerve dysfunction. In: Chrisman CL, ed. Problems in Small Animal Neurology, 2nd ed. Philadelphia, Lea & Febiger, 1991:235–266.
12. de Lahunta A. Lower motor neuron-general visceral efferent system. In: de Lahunta A, ed. Veterinary Neuroanatomy and Clinical Neurology, 2nd ed. Philadelphia, WB Saunders, 1983:115–129.
13. Evans HE, Kitchell RL. In: Evans HE, ed. Miller's Anatomy of the Dog, 3rd ed. Philadelphia, WB Saunders, 1993:953–987.
14. Braund KG, Luttgen PJ, Sorjonen DC, et al. Idiopathic facial paralysis in the dog. Vet Rec 1979;105:297–299.
15. Renegar WR. Auriculopalpebral nerve paralysis following prolonged anesthesia in a dog. J Am Vet Med Assoc 1979;174:1007–1009.
16. Shell LG. Otitis media and interna. Vet Clin North Am Small Anim Pract 1988;18:885–899.
17. Jaggy A, Oliver JE, Ferguson DC, et al. Neurological manifestations of hypothyroidism: A retrospective study of 29 dogs. J Vet Intern Med 1994;8:328–336.
18. Braund KG. Neurologic examination. In: Braund KG, ed. Clinical Syndromes in Veterinary Neurology, 2nd ed. St. Louis, Mosby, 1994:1–36.
19. Chrisman CL. Deafness and alterations in hearing. In: Chrisman CL, ed. Problems in Small Animal Neurology, 2nd ed. Philadelphia, Lea & Febiger, 1991:297–304.
20. de Lahunta A. Auditory system: Special somatic afferent system. In: de Lahunta A, ed. Veterinary Neuroanatomy and Clinical Neurology, 2nd ed. Philadelphia, WB Saunders, 1983:304–310.
21. Strain GM. Congenital deafness in dogs and cats. Compen Contin Educ Pract Vet 1991;13:245–254.
22. Beckman Sl, Henry WB, Cechner P. Total ear canal ablation combining bulla osteotomy and curettage in dogs with chronic otitis externa and media. J Am Vet Med Assoc 1990;196:84.
23. Bergsman DR, Brown KS. White fur, blue eyes and deafness in the domestic cat. J Hered 1971;62:166–174.
24. Knowles K, Blauch B, Leipold H, et al. Reduction of spiral ganglion neurons in the aging canine with hearing loss. J Vet Med 1989;36:188–199.
25. Pickrell JA, Oehme FW, Cash WC. Ototoxicity in dogs and cats. Semin Vet Med Surg (Small Anim) 1993; 8:42–49.
26. Hayes HM, Wilson GP, Fenner WR, et al. Canine congenital deafness: Epidemiologic study of 272 cases. J Am Anim Hosp Assoc 1981;17:473–476.
27. Rosychuk RAW, Luttgen P. Diseases of the ear. In: Ettinger SJ, Feldman EC, eds. Textbook of Veterinary Internal Medicine, 4th ed. Philadelphia, WB Saunders, 1994:533–550.
28. Chrisman CL. Head tilt, circling, nystagmus, and other vestibular deficits. In: Chrisman CL, ed. Problems in Small Animal Neurology, 2nd ed. Philadelphia, Lea & Febiger, 1991:269–294.
29. Chrisman CL. Vestibular disease. Vet Clin North Am Small Anim Pract 1980;10:103–129.
30. Saik JE, Toll SL, Diters RW, et al. Canine and feline laryngeal neoplasia: A 10 year study. J Am Anim Hosp Assoc 1986;22:359–365.
31. Schaer M, Zaki FA, Harvey HJ, et al. Laryngeal hemiplegia due to neoplasia of the vagus nerve in a cat. J Am Vet Med Assoc 1979;174:513–515.
32. Bichsel P, Jacobs G, Oliver JE. Neurologic manifestations

associated with hypothyroidism in four dogs. J Am Vet Med Assoc 1988;192:1745–1747.

33. Indrieri RJ, Whalen WR, Cardinet GH, et al. Neuromuscular abnormalities associated with hypothyroidism and lymphocytic thyroiditis in three dogs. J Am Vet Med Assoc 1987;190:544–548.

34. Fischer A, Obermaier G. Brain stem auditory-evoked potentials and neuropathologic correlates in 26 dogs with brain tumors. J Vet Intern Med 1994;8:363–369.

35. Nafe LA, Carter JD. Canine optic neuritis. Compen Contin Educ Pract Vet 1981;3:978–984.

36. Braund KG. Neurological diseases. In: Braund KG, ed. Clinical Syndromes in Veterinary Neurology, 2nd ed. St. Louis, Mosby, 1994:81–332.

37. Van der Woerdt A, Nasisse MP, Davidson MG. Sudden acquired retinal degeneration in the dog: Clinical and laboratory findings in 36 cases. Prog Vet Compar Ophthal 1991;1:11–18.

38. Morgan RV, Zanotti SW. Horner's syndrome in dogs and cats: 49 cases (1980–1986). J Am Vet Med Assoc 1989;194:1096–1099.

39. Kern TJ, Aromando MC, Erb HN. Horner's syndrome in dogs and cats: 100 cases (1975–1985). J Am Vet Med Assoc 1989;195:369–373.

40. Neer TM. Horner's syndrome: Anatomy, diagnosis, and causes. Compen Contin Educ Pract Vet 1984;6:740–747.

41. Hoelzle RJ. Idiopathic trigeminal neuropathy in a dog. Vet Med Small Anim Clin 1983;78:345.

42. Powell AK. Idiopathic trigeminal neuritis in a dog. Can Vet J 1991;32:265.

43. Robbins GM. Dropped jaw-mandibular neurapraxia in the dog. J Small Anim Pract 1976;17:753.

44. Kern TJ, Erb HN. Facial neuropathy in dogs and cats: 95 cases (1975–1985). J Am Vet Med Assoc 1987;192:1604–1609.

45. Wright JA. Ultrastructural findings in idiopathic facial paralysis in the dog. J Comp Pathol 1988;98:111–115.

46. Little CJL. Otitis media in the dog: A review. Vet Annu 1989;29:183–188.

47. Spruell JSA. Otitis media in the dog. In: Kirk RW, ed. Current Veterinary Therapy V. Philadelphia, WB Saunders, 1976:675–683.

48. Schunk KL, Averill DR. Peripheral vestibular syndrome in the dog: A review of 83 cases. J Am Vet Med Assoc 1983;182:1354–1357.

49. Remedios AM, Fowler JD, Pharr JW. A comparison of radiographic versus surgical diagnoses of otitis media. J Am Anim Hosp Assoc 1991;27:183–188.

50. Strain GM, Merchant SR, Neer TM, et al. Ototoxicity assessment of a gentamicin sulfate otic preparation in dogs. Am J Vet Res 1995;56:532–538.

51. Sharp NJH. Chronic otitis externa and otitis media treated by total ear canal ablation and ventral bulla osteotomy in thirteen dogs. Vet Surg 1990;19:162–166.

52. Mason LK, Harvey CE, Orsher RJ. Total ear canal ablation combined with lateral bulla osteotomy for end stage otitis in dogs: Results in thirty dogs. Vet Surg 1988;17:263–268.

53. Smeak DD, DeHoff WD. Total ear canal ablation. In:

Bojrab MJ, ed. Current Techniques in Small Animal Surgery. Philadelphia, Lea & Febiger, 1990:140.

54. Burke EE, Moise NS, de Lahunta A, et al. Review of idiopathic feline vestibular syndrome in 75 cats. J Am Vet Med Assoc 1985;187:941–943.

55. de Lahunta A. Vestibular system: Special proprioception. In: de Lahunta A, ed. Veterinary Neuroanatomy and Clinical Neurology, 2nd ed. Philadelphia, WB Saunders, 1983:238–254.

56. Gabor CE, Amis TC, LeCouteur RA. Laryngeal paralysis in dogs: A review of 23 cases. J Am Vet Med Assoc 1985;186:377–380.

57. Venker-van Haagen AJ, Hartman W, Goedegebuure SA. Spontaneous laryngeal paralysis in young Bouviers. J Am Anim Hosp Assoc 1978;14:714–720.

58. Love S, Waterman AE, Lane JG. The assessment of corrective surgery for canine laryngeal paralysis: A review of thirty-five cases. J Sm Anim Pract 1987;28:597–604.

59. Hardie EM, Kolata RJ, Stone EA, et al. Laryngeal paralysis in three cats. J Am Vet Med Assoc 1981;179:879–882.

60. Braund KG, Steinberg HS, Shores A, et al. Laryngeal paralysis in immature and mature dogs as one sign of a more diffuse polyneuropathy. J Am Vet Med Assoc 1989;194:1735–1740.

61. Venker-van Haagen AJ, Bouw J, Hartman W. Hereditary transmission of laryngeal paralysis in Bouviers. J Am Anim Hosp Assoc 1981;17:75–76.

62. Braund KG et al: Laryngeal paralysis in Dalmations. Am Coll Vet Intern Med Forum 1992;10:800.

63. White RAS, Littlewood JD, Herrtage ME, et al. Outcome of surgery for laryngeal paralysis in four cases. Vet Rec 1986;118:103–104.

64. Nelson AW, Wykes PM. Upper Respiratory System. In: Slatter DH, ed. Textbook of Small Animal Surgery. Philadelphia, WB Saunders, 1985;972–990.

65. Kern TJ, Riis RC. Optic nerve hypoplasia in three miniature poodles. J Am Vet Med Assoc 1981;178:49–54.

66. Mansfield PD. Ototoxicity in dogs and cats. Compen Contin Educ Pract Vet 1990;12:331–337.

67. Saxon B, Magne ML. Reversible central nervous system toxicosis associated with metronidazole therapy in three cats. Prog Vet Neurol 1993;4:25–27.

68. Dow SW, LeCouteur RA, Poss ML, et al. Central nervous system toxicity associated with metronidazole treatment of dogs: Five cases (1984–1987). J Am Vet Med Assoc 1989;195:365–368.

69. Forbes S, Cook JR. Congenital peripheral vestibular disease attributed to lymphocytic labyrinthitis in two related litters of Doberman pinscher pups. J Am Vet Med Assoc 1991;198:447–449.

70. Wilkes MK, Palmer AC. Congenital deafness and vestibular deficit in the Doberman. J Small Anim Pract 1992;33:218–224.

71. Key TJA, Gaskell CJ. Puzzling syndrome in cats associated with pupillary dilation. Vet Rec 1982;110:160.

72. Nash AS, Griffiths IR, Sharp NJH. The Key-Gaskell syndrome: An autonomic polyganglionopathy. Vet Rec 1982;111:307–308.

73. Sharp NJH, Nash AS, Griffiths IR. Feline dysautonomia (the Key-Gaskell syndrome): A clinical and pathological study of forty cases. J Sm Anim Pract 1984;25: 599–615.

74. Sharp NJH. Feline dysautonomia. Semin Vet Med Surg (Small Anim) 1990;5:67–71.

75. Brightman AH, Macy DW, Gosselin Y. Pupillary abnormalities associated with the feline leukemia complex. Fel Pract 1977;7:23–27.

76. Thomas JB, Eger C. Granulomatous meningoencephalo-myelitis in 21 dogs. J Sm Anim Pract 1989;30:287–293.

77. Sorjonen DC. Clinical and histopathological features of granulomatous meningoencephalomyelitis in dogs. J Am Anim Hosp Assoc 1990;26:141–147.

Chapter 27

Diseases of the Spinal Cord

Linda G. Shell
Karen Dyer

Anatomy

The spinal cord is that portion of the central nervous system contained within the vertebrae. It consists of a central region of gray matter surrounded by white matter tracts. Gray matter contains neuronal cell bodies and supporting glia; white matter is formed by densely packed axons that relay information to the brain (ascending or somatosensory axons) or transmit information from the brain to spinal neurons (descending or motor axons).[1]

At birth, the spinal cord extends from the foramen magnum into the sacrum. During postnatal development, bony portions of the spinal column continue to elongate, resulting in an apparent shortening of the spinal cord relative to surrounding vertebrae. This discrepancy is more marked in larger breeds of dogs than in either toy breeds or cats.[2] The result is that each spinal cord segment is not contained within the corresponding vertebra (i.e., the fifth cervical vertebra contains the sixth cervical spinal cord segment). In general, the spinal cord ends at the fifth or sixth lumbar vertebra in dogs and at the first or second sacral vertebra in cats.[1]

Functionally, the spinal cord contains elements of both the central and peripheral nervous systems. Sensory axons, relaying information about sensations and position, travel toward the spinal cord in peripheral nerves. These primary afferent axons enter the spinal cord and terminate on ascending somatosensory axons in the white matter or on neurons within spinal cord gray matter. There are three broad classes of neurons within the spinal cord gray matter: projection neurons, efferent neurons, and interneurons.[3] Projection neurons send axons into white matter to form additional ascending somatosensory tracts. Efferent neurons, sometimes referred to as lower motor neurons (LMNs), send axons to the periphery through the ventral nerve roots to innervate both muscles and glandular structures (autonomic neurons). Interneurons, interposed between other neurons, regulate information transmitted between cells.

Although each segment of spinal cord contains primary afferent axons and neurons, clinically only those portions that supply the limbs are easily evaluated. In general, these portions are located in spinal cord segments C6 through T2 (vertebrae C5–T1) for thoracic limbs and in spinal cord segments L4 through S2 (vertebrae L3–L5) for pelvic limbs. These regions of spinal cord are larger than other regions and are therefore referred to as cervical and lumbar intumescences (Fig. 27–1).

The dorsal and ventral nerve roots unite to form a spinal nerve near the intervertebral foramen before exiting the spinal canal. With the exception of C1, which exits through a foramen within the body of C1,

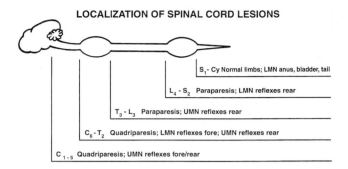

LOCALIZATION OF SPINAL CORD LESIONS

S$_1$- Cy Normal limbs; LMN anus, bladder, tail

L$_4$- S$_2$ Paraparesis; LMN reflexes rear

T$_3$- L$_3$ Paraparesis; UMN reflexes rear

C$_6$- T$_2$ Quadriparesis; LMN reflexes fore; UMN reflexes rear

C$_{1-5}$ Quadriparesis; UMN reflexes fore/rear

Figure 27–1
Schematic drawing showing how to localize spinal cord lesions based on limb movement and spinal reflexes. LMN, lower motor neuron; UMN, upper motor neuron. (From Shell LG. The basics of pelvic limb weakness. Vet Med 1996;91:222.)

the cervical spinal nerves exit rostral to the corresponding vertebrae (i.e., spinal nerve C6 exits the intervertebral foramen formed by the caudal border of C5 and the rostral border of C6). Because both dogs and cats have eight cervical spinal cord segments but only seven cervical vertebrae, the relation between spinal nerves and vertebrae changes at the cervicothoracic junction. The eighth cervical spinal nerve exits caudal to the seventh cervical vertebra, and all remaining nerve roots exit caudal to their corresponding vertebrae (e.g., the T1 spinal nerve exits through the foramen formed by the caudal border of T1 and the rostral border of T2).[4] Because the lumbosacral spinal cord terminates rostral to the corresponding vertebra, the dorsal and ventral nerve roots are much longer in this region. Because of visual similarities to a horse's tail, this intravertebral expanse of lumbosacral and caudal nerve roots was named the cauda equina.

Although each spinal nerve arises from a single spinal cord segment, each peripheral nerve is made up of branches from multiple spinal nerves (see Table 28–3). It is impossible to differentiate injury of the nerve cell body in the spinal cord from nerve root injury. Injury to either site causes loss of function, hypotonia, and rapid atrophy of muscles innervated by that nerve. Reflexes mediated by that nerve are also immediately diminished or abolished by these injuries.

Physiology

In order to provide fine control of movement, LMNs are under the control of neurons within the cerebrum and brain stem. These upper motor neurons (UMNs) send axons through the descending pathways in the spinal cord white matter to each spinal cord segment, where they modulate activities of LMNs. Injury to UMNs or their axons causes weak or absent voluntary movement and exaggerated spinal reflexes. Injury to LMNs also causes weak or absent voluntary movements, but spinal reflexes are diminished or absent. Muscle atrophy may occur with either LMN or UMN injury, but atrophy is faster in onset and more severe with LMN injury.[1, 4-6]

Problem Identification

Localization of Lesions

Differences in clinical signs produced by LMN or UMN injury have provided the basis for five recognized patterns of spinal cord injury: upper cervical, lower cervical, thoracolumbar, lower lumbar, and sacral-caudal (see Fig. 27–1). Lesions at the C1 through C5 cord segments produce quadriparesis and quadriplegia with UMN reflexes to all limbs. With lesions at the C6 through T2 cord segments, quadriparesis is present, but thoracic limb reflexes are either normal or depressed and pelvic limb reflexes are increased or normal. With lesions distal to the T2 cord segment, thoracic limbs are not impaired. Lesions of cord segments T3 through L3 produce weakness in the pelvic limbs with exaggerated (UMN) or normal pelvic limb reflexes. Lesions at cord segments L4 through S2 produce pelvic limb weakness with normal to depressed (LMN) pelvic limb reflexes. Lesions at or distal to the S1 cord segment produce urinary or fecal incontinence, or both, and weakness of tail movement. Clinical signs related to these areas include ataxia, quadriparesis and quadriplegia, paraparesis and paraplegia, incontinence, and dropped tail.

Ataxia

Ataxia is a sign of specific sensory dysfunction that produces wobbliness or incoordination of the limbs. For clinical purposes, there are three types of ataxia: sensory, vestibular, and cerebellar. Vestibular and cerebellar ataxia also produce changes in head movements (see Chaps. 26 and 25, respectively); sensory ataxia originates in the spinal cord and produces only limb incoordination.[7]

Pathophysiology

The nervous system is arranged so that the brain receives information about limb position (proprioception, or position sense) from muscle, joint, skin, and other receptors. This information travels to the brain through proprioceptive pathways (fasciculus gracilis and cuneatus and spinocerebellar tracts) located in the dorsal and dorsolateral portions of the spinal cord. These tracts are located more superficially in the white matter and contain larger-diameter axons; such features render them more susceptible to external compression. Therefore, proprioceptive deficits are usually one of the first clinical signs observed with compressive spinal cord injury.[5]

Clinical Signs

Ataxia can have an acute or gradual onset. It is more often noticeable in the pelvic limbs and when the animal is turning. Owners frequently describe the gait as "drunken-like" or comment that the animal does not seem to know "where its feet are." Limbs may cross one over the other (scissor cuts), and the pet may stand with its feet too close together or too far apart. When the pet walks on surfaces that conduct sound well, the observer may hear scraping of the dorsal aspects of the toenails. Physical examination findings may include worn toenails on the affected limbs.

Diagnostic Plan

Because ataxia may be caused by damage to the cerebellum, vestibular system, or sensory pathways in the spinal cord, the neurologic examination should establish the presence or absence of other cerebellar or vestibular signs. If ataxia is associated with a head tilt or nystagmus, vestibular diseases should be considered (see Chap. 26). If ataxia is associated with intention tremors of the head or hypermetria, cerebellar ataxia should be pursued (see Chap. 25). If only ataxia of the limbs is observed, spinal cord dysfunction is likely. If all four limbs are ataxic, the lesion either is in the cervical area or is multifocal to diffuse. If ataxia is confined to the pelvic limbs, the lesion is usually caudal to the T2 spinal cord segment. However, compressive cervical lesions often appear as pelvic limb ataxia before thoracic limb signs are observed. This observation occurs because tracts to the pelvic limbs are located more superficially than are those to the thoracic limbs. Externally compressive lesions compress the more superficial tracts first, causing clinical signs to be more obvious in the pelvic limbs.

Once the spinal cord lesion is localized, spinal radiographs of that area should be evaluated. Disc herniations, discospondylitis, vertebral fractures, bony neoplasia, or malformations may be evident. For unknown reasons, systemic illness and endocrine, cardiovascular, and metabolic disorders can cause ataxia, especially of the pelvic limbs. Therefore, a minimum database (hemogram, chemistry profile, and urinalysis) should be evaluated if spinal radiographs do not reveal a likely cause of the ataxia. If a diagnosis is not made and yet the clinical signs are progressing, analysis of the cerebrospinal fluid (CSF) and myelography may be necessary to identify inflammatory and compressive spinal cord diseases, respectively.

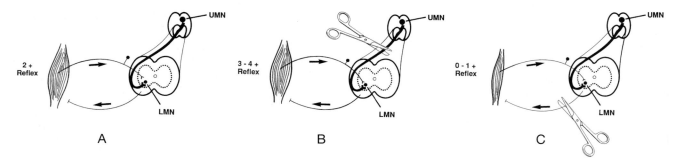

Figure 27–2
(A) A schematic drawing outlining the origin of the upper motor neuron (UMN) and lower motor neuron (LMN) systems. **(B)** If the UMN system *(larger bold lines)* is damaged, the spinal reflexes are no longer controlled and therefore become exaggerated or increased. **(C)** If the LMN system is damaged, the spinal reflexes can no longer function and become absent or depressed. (From Shell LG. The basics of pelvic limb weakness. Vet Med 1996;91:222.)

Paraparesis and Paraplegia

Paraparesis is weakness of voluntary movement in the pelvic limbs; paraplegia, or paralysis, is lack of voluntary movement.

Pathophysiology

In general, limb weakness can be caused by lesions in the UMN or the LMN system. Cell bodies or nuclei for the UMN system are located within the brain and are responsible for initiating voluntary movement (Fig 27–2). Axons from these cell bodies form tracts (e.g., rubrospinal, corticospinal, vestibulospinal) that descend from the brain to synapse on interneurons in the spinal cord. Interneuronal axons then synapse on the large (alpha) motor neurons in the ventral gray matter of the spinal cord. Such large motor neurons are the cell bodies of origin for the LMN system, which is responsible for spinal reflexes. Collections of large motor neurons in the cervical and lumbar intumescences provide innervation of limb muscles. Axons from these large motor neurons form ventral nerve roots, spinal nerves, and, ultimately, the peripheral nerves that innervate the limb muscles.[4–6] They also provide neural control of all limb movement, including spinal reflexes.

UMNs and their axons have an inhibitory influence on the large motor neurons of the LMN system. This inhibitory effect maintains normal muscle tone and normal spinal reflexes (see Fig. 27–2). If UMNs or their axons are injured, spinal reflexes are no longer inhibited or controlled,[4] and reflexes become exaggerated or hyperreflexic. If the large motor neurons or their processes (peripheral nerves) are injured, spinal reflexes cannot be elicited and are either reduced (hyporeflexic) or absent (areflexic).

Clinical Signs

Pelvic limb weakness can have an acute or gradual onset. Owners may describe their pets as being unable to move, walk, or get up. Many focal compressive spinal cord diseases begin with ataxia that progresses to reduced strength and finally to lack of any voluntary pelvic limb movements. Clinical signs often reflect severity of disease, with paralysis being more severe than weakness. Unless the disease process is systemic, most pets with paresis or paralysis are alert. Inflammatory processes such as meningitis and discospondylitis, which are described later in this chapter, and myelomalacia may cause an elevation of body temperature. If the disease process causes pain, many animals resent handling and manipulation during the examination. Atrophy of limb muscles from disuse (UMN disease) is mild, but it is severe with LMN disease.

Diagnostic Plan

Neurologic examination should confirm that the disease is restricted to the pelvic limbs and caudal to T2 (see Fig. 27–1). If pelvic limb reflexes are hyperreflexic or normal, the lesion is probably between T3 and L4. If pelvic limb reflexes are decreased or hyporeflexic, the lesion is probably distal to the L4 spinal cord segment. If pelvic limbs are paralyzed, the bladder is probably also paralyzed, and the pet cannot initiate voluntary urination. Because LMNs are vital to skeletal muscles, damage to them at the L4 spinal cord level and distally results in rapid and severe pelvic limb muscle atrophy, frequently called neurogenic atrophy. Disuse atrophy is often seen with lesions proximal to L4 spinal cord segments; however, the onset is not as rapid nor as severe as that of neurogenic atrophy.[5]

The history of onset can help determine cause; acute onsets are associated with trauma, disc herniations, and vascular accidents, whereas slower onsets are associated with inflammation, neoplasia, and cord degeneration. After localization of the lesion to the appropriate spinal cord area (see Localization of Lesions), radiographs of that area should be evaluated for obvious vertebral abnormalities such as discospondylitis, bony neoplasia, malformations, fractures, or luxations. Intervertebral disc disease and some herniations can also be sometimes diagnosed on survey spinal radiographs. Routine laboratory data (complete blood count, plasma chemistries, urinalysis) should be evaluated to assess other organ functions and the presence of other diseases that could cause weakness (e.g., hypocalcemia, lymphosarcoma).

If an obvious answer is not found on these tests and the animal is paralyzed or showing progressive weakness, myelography, CSF analysis, and perhaps surgery should be used to determine the location and type of lesion. Myelography is useful for detection of compressive spinal cord diseases such as disc herniation and neoplasia. CSF analysis is helpful in diagnosing inflammatory diseases such as meningomyelitis; an increased cell count and perhaps increased protein are seen. Surgical exploration with biopsy (if possible) is necessary in some cases of compressive cord lesions to get a diagnosis.

Quadriparesis and Quadriplegia

Quadriparesis (tetraparesis) is weakness of voluntary movements in all limbs; quadriparalysis or quadriplegia (tetraplegia) is absence of voluntary movement in all limbs.

Pathophysiology

The pathophysiology is the same as that of paresis and paraplegia.

Clinical Signs

If the animal is ambulatory, the owner may describe the gait as weak or wobbly. If the pet is nonambulatory, it is often described as being down and unable to get up and move around.

Because injury to spinal cord segments C1 through C5 damages UMN axons that regulate movement in all four limbs, clinical signs associated with injury in this region include paresis or paralysis of all four limbs and exaggerated (or normal) reflexes. Respiratory compromise may be produced by damage to the cell bodies that give rise to the phrenic nerve at segments C5 through C7. Respiratory paralysis can also result from severe cervical lesions that destroy the UMNs, which coordinate intercostal muscle movement.

Injury to spinal cord segments C6 through T2 damages LMNs to the thoracic limbs and UMNs to the pelvic limbs, resulting in weakness or paralysis of all limbs, thoracic limb muscle atrophy, diminished or absent thoracic limb reflexes, and hyperreflexia (or normal) pelvic limb reflexes. Clinical signs of Horner's syndrome (miosis, ptosis, and enophthalmos) may also be found with cervicothoracic injury, because cell bodies of the first-order neuron for sympathetic innervation to the head are located in the spinal cord gray matter at segments T1 and T2. Axons of these sympathetic neurons exit the spinal canal with the ventral roots before forming the vagosympathetic trunk. Also located at the area of C8 through T1 is the origin of the lateral thoracic nerve, which is responsible for the cutaneous trunci reflex. This reflex may also be absent with an upper thoracic lesion.

Diagnostic Plan

When presented with a quadriparetic or quadriplegic animal, the clinician must first establish whether the quadriparesis is caused by generalized LMN disease (see Chap. 28), cervical spinal cord disease, or brain stem disease. Historical information and neurologic examination should yield information to clarify this point. If cranial nerve signs, mental depression or stupor, and exaggerated (or normal) spinal reflexes are found, the quadriparesis is probably of brain stem origin (see Chap. 25). If the cranial nerves are normal and the spinal reflexes absent or reduced, an LMN quadriparesis is likely (see Chap. 28). If there are no cranial nerve signs or stupor, spinal reflexes are normal or exaggerated, and muscle tone is normal, UMN quadriparesis or quadriplegia (lesion at segments C1 through C5) is established.

The history should establish the onset. Acute onsets are more likely after traumatic or vascular injury, whereas more gradual onsets are associated with congenital or inherited diseases and with degenerative or inflammatory processes. Neoplasia and intervertebral disc herniations can have either acute or slowly progressive onsets. Routine laboratory data (complete blood count, plasma chemistries, and urinalysis) can be assessed for signs of systemic illnesses that could affect the spinal cord or vertebrae, including neoplasia, fungal or bacterial infections, and toxins. If the lesion has been localized to segments C1 through C5 based on the neurologic examination, survey cervical radiographs should be evaluated for signs of trauma, bony neoplasia, discospondylitis, or congenital malformations. If these diagnostic tests do not yield a reason for the UMN weakness, then CSF analysis and myelography are warranted, especially if the pet is paralyzed or if the weakness is progressing. CSF analysis usually demonstrates an increased white cell count and protein in cases of inflammatory disease such as myelitis. Myelography is useful for detecting compression of the cord from disc material, neoplasia, or trauma.

Fecal and Urinary Incontinence

Incontinence is the loss of voluntary control of urination and defecation.[8–13]

Pathophysiology

Fecal continence is maintained by the external anal sphincter, which is innervated by the pudendal nerve. This nerve arises from spinal cord segments S1 through S3. Damage to either the nerve or its cell bodies results in poor anal tone and inability to constrict the external anal sphincter. This is easily diagnosed by visual inspection or by rectal palpation. Injury to spinal cord segments rostral to S1 can result in loss of voluntary control of defecation, but reflex elimination can usually proceed.[8]

Urinary continence is more complex because there are three nerves that control the bladder and urethral sphincters (Fig. 27–3).[9–10] The hypogastric nerve is part of the sympathetic nervous system, and its first-order neuron arises from the L1 and L2 spinal cord segments. It provides innervation to β-receptors of the detrusor muscle located in the bladder wall for relaxation during filling, and to α-receptors located in the internal urethral sphincter for increased tone during filling. The pelvic nerve is part of the parasympathetic nervous system, and it originates at spinal cord segments S1 through S3. It innervates cholinergic receptors in the detrusor muscle. The pudendal nerve is part of the general somatic nervous system, and its cell bodies are located in spinal cord segments S1 through S3. It innervates nicotinic receptors in the external urethral sphincter. All of these nerves are under control of UMNs in the brain.

As the bladder fills with urine, stretch receptors in the bladder wall are stimulated and impulses are carried by sensory fibers of the pelvic nerve to the spinal cord. From the spinal cord, sensory impulses travel to UMNs in the brain stem, cerebral cortex (for conscious control), and cerebellum. These UMNs send messages to the lower spinal cord to inhibit the sympathetic and somatic nervous systems and to stimulate the parasympathetic nervous system. The pelvic nerve (parasympathetic) stimulates cholinergic receptors in the detrusor muscle to cause the bladder to contract and expel urine. Several local spinal reflexes facilitate voiding. As stretch receptors in the bladder wall are activated, sensory impulses stimulate the parasympathetic nervous system by reflex and simul-

taneously inhibit the somatic and sympathetic nervous systems. This reflex is the micturition or detrusor reflex, which is important in neonatal animals and in those with spinal cord dysfunction. However, in order to effectively empty the bladder, all portions of the nervous system must be working in concert.

Injury to spinal cord segments S1 through S3 damages the pudendal nerve and results in little to no contraction of the external urethral sphincter. Sphincter contraction is critical for maintaining urethral tone during the storage phase of urination. Urine leakage occurs if the pudendal nerve is injured. The pelvic nerve may also be affected, resulting in reduced or absent active bladder contraction. Urine accumulates in the bladder and is leaked out because of little to no urethral resistance.

Although hypogastric nerve injury should cause some impairment in urethral pressure because of denervation of the internal urethral sphincter, it is difficult to detect clinically. Instead, spinal cord injury rostral to S1 causes an "UMN bladder." The external urethral sphincter maintains urethral tone, allowing the bladder to fill with urine. When stretch receptors reach a critical level, the micturition reflex is stimulated and allows some urine to escape. Over time, this reflex becomes stronger, allowing a large volume of urine to escape. But without UMN control, the reflex is incomplete, and large amounts of urine are still retained within the bladder. Because spinal injury often prevents conscious perception of bladder distention or urethral pressure, the animal does not know it is urinating during reflex micturition. These animals seem to be spurting urine at inappropriate times. Bladders in these animals are difficult to compress. However, if overdistention occurs, damage to the detrusor muscle can cause a flaccid or LMN bladder (see later discussion).

Lesions in the brain do not abolish micturition but may affect voluntary control. Affected animals often urinate whenever threshold is reached, and they may not be aware that they are urinating. Mixed or partial lesions may result in a condition referred to as reflex dyssynergia, which is a failure in coordination between the detrusor muscle and the urethral sphincters. The bladder contracts, but the urethral sphincters fail to relax; the animal attempts to urinate but is unable to empty its bladder. It may strain and spurt a few drops of urine but is unable to maintain a normal stream. Many of these patients do not have other neurologic deficits.[10–11, 13]

If the bladder accumulates urine and overdistends, damage often occurs to the tight junctions of the detrusor muscle. Such damage causes poor or absent bladder contraction (bladder atony) and can be permanent. Bladder or detrusor atony can occur with either UMN or LMN injury as well as medical

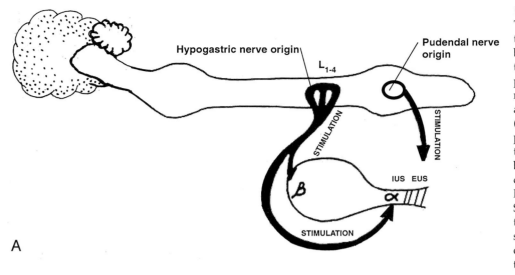

STORAGE PHASE OF MICTURITION

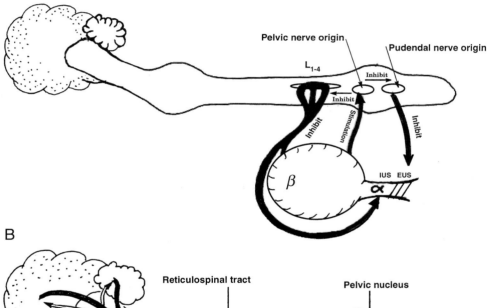

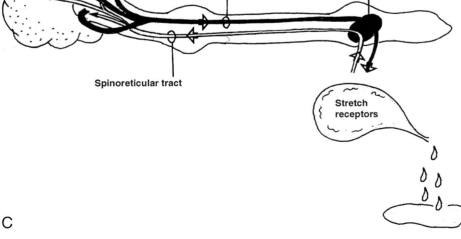

Figure 27-3
These diagrams outline the three nerves that control bladder continence and micturition. **(A)** The storage phase of micturition is dominated by the sympathetic and somatic nervous system (i.e., the hypogastric and pudendal nerves, respectively). β-receptors in the bladder wall are stimulated, causing the bladder to relax and expand with urine. Stimulation of the α-receptors in the internal urethral sphincter (IUS) and neck of the bladder cause contraction, thereby preventing urine leak from the bladder. The external urethral sphincter (EUS) is also stimulated to contract by the pudendal nerve. **(B)** As the bladder fills to capacity, the emptying stage begins. Stretch receptors in the bladder wall detect that the bladder is full and send impulses through the pelvic nerve to inhibit the hypogastric and pudendal nerves. This inhibition allows the bladder to contract in response to parasympathetic stimulation from the pelvic nerve and allows the EUS and IUS to relax. This is the reflex urination that often occurs in patients with damaged spinal cords. This reflex is overridden by the brain in most patients until an appropriate time and place can be found to voluntarily void. **(C)** Information about the bladder's fullness is sent from the pelvic nerve to the brain stem, cerebellum, and cerebrum through the spinoreticular tract. If the time and place are appropriate for urination to occur, information is relayed from the brain to the S1–S3 spinal cord area through the reticulospinal tract. The pelvic nerve (parasympathetic) initiates contraction of the detrusor muscle and continues to inhibit the hypogastric and pudendal nerves until voiding is complete.

Table 27–1
Pharmaceutical Treatment of Urinary Incontinence

DRUG	ACTION	DOSAGE
Bethanechol	Parasympathomimetic; increases detrusor contraction	5–15 mg t.i.d. PO (dog) 1.25–5.0 mg t.i.d. PO (cat)
Phenoxybenzamine	α-Blocker; relaxes internal sphincter	5–15 mg t.i.d. PO (dog) 2.5–7.5 mg t.i.d. PO (cat)
Diazepam	Skeletal muscle relaxant; relaxes external sphincter	2–10 mg t.i.d. PO (dog) 2–5 mg t.i.d. PO (cat)
Dantroline	Skeletal muscle relaxant; relaxes external sphincter	1–5 mg/kg b.i.d. PO (dog) 0.5 mg/kg b.i.d. PO (cat)
Phenylpropanolamine	α-Agonist; enhances internal sphincter tone	12.5–50 mg t.i.d. PO (dog) 12.5 mg t.i.d. PO (cat)
Diethylstilbestrol	Estrogen; enhances internal sphincter tone	0.1–1 mg daily PO for 3 days; then 0.1–1 mg once weekly (dog, female only)
Testosterone cypionate	Testosterone; enhances internal sphincter tone	2.2 mg/kg intramuscular every 30 days (dog, male only)
Propantheline bromide	Anticholinergic; decreases detrusor contraction	5–30 mg t.i.d. PO (dog) 5–7.5 mg t.i.d. PO (cat)

b.i.d., twice per day; t.i.d., three times per day; PO, by mouth.

conditions such as urethral obstructions. Table 27–1 lists the drugs that can be used to treat bladder and urethral sphincter dysfunctions.[12]

Clinical Signs

Inappropriate elimination habits are clinical signs that owners notice, especially in animals that have been housebroken. Dogs with congenital anomalies (ectopic ureters) usually are incontinent from birth. Because owners often confuse polyuria, dysuria, and stranguria with incontinence, history and physical examination are crucial for separating medical from neurologic and behavioral causes of incontinence. Owners may describe the pet as "embarrassed" because it looks at the mess and appears guilty or sheepish. The owners should be asked to describe what they have observed without labeling the event as incontinence until polyuria, dysuria, and stranguria have been eliminated. Pets with incontinence usually dribble urine in their sleep as well as when awake. They do not appear to have any conscious control of elimination and therefore do not usually posture to urinate or defecate while dribbling urine.

Diagnostic Plan

When presented with an animal that is urinating or defecating in an abnormal manner, the clinician must distinguish between medical, neurologic, and behavioral causes. The history and physical examinations should help with such diagnoses as diabetes mellitus (incontinence is not present but polyuria is), feline urologic syndrome (the pet urinates in strange places or shows frequent posturing or straining to

urinate), and bladder calculus (uroliths are felt on palpation). The bladder should be palpated to evaluate tone and estimate the size, and an attempt should be made to manually express urine. If the bladder tone is poor and urethral tone is easily overcome with manual compression of the bladder, an LMN lesion should be suspected. If the bladder tone is normal and urethral tone cannot be overcome with bladder compression, a UMN lesion, reflex dyssynergia, or urethral obstruction should be suspected.

If possible, the pet should be watched as it urinates. If it postures to urinate, the animal is not likely to be incontinent. If it strains to urinate, urethral obstructions (from masses, stones, scar tissue, or neoplasia) or reflex dyssynergia should be suspected. If it dribbles urine or feces while it walks, incontinence is likely. The finding of a weak perineal reflex or poor anal tone would further support a diagnosis of incontinence.

After the animal has been observed urinating, the bladder is palpated again and the size of the bladder is noted. This procedure gives a suggestion as to whether bladder emptying is complete. With UMN lesions, reflex dyssynergia, and partial urethral obstructions, the animal may not be able to empty its bladder.

In cases in which the history and physical examination (see Clinical Signs) do not clearly separate incontinence from other urinary tract disorders, a urinalysis (by cystocentesis), chemistry profile, and neurologic examination should be done. Urinalysis helps to establish medical disorders such as diabetes mellitus, urinary tract infection, liver disease, and some kidney diseases. A low urine specific gravity suggests polydipsia and polyuria (see Chap. 16). The chemistry profile may help evaluate for potential causes of excessive urination such as renal disease, liver disease, endocrine disorders, and metabolic disorders. If the neurologic examination reveals deficits in the pelvic limbs or pain over the lumbosacral area, spinal radiographs and CSF analysis should be pursued.

If the findings on history and physical examination clearly suggest incontinence, the clinician must try to separate neurogenic from non-neurogenic (estrogen- or testosterone-responsive) disorders using those findings and the results of a neurologic examination. Contrast urethrocystography may be required to rule out anatomic defects such as uroliths, neoplasia, or developmental anomalies. Excretory urography is required to confirm or exclude ectopic ureters.

Paralyzed or Dropped Tail

Inability to voluntarily move the tail results in a paralyzed or dropped tail.

Pathophysiology

The tail is innervated by the caudal spinal cord segments (located in vertebra L6), their nerve roots, and the nerves derived from them. UMN control over the LMNs in the caudal spinal cord segments exists and is responsible for the voluntary tail wag that usually occurs when a dog is offered food or spoken to in a pleasant tone.[13]

Clinical Signs

With UMN lesions (above vertebra L6), the tail is often paralyzed, with normal to increased tone. With LMN lesions of the tail, the tail is paralyzed but has little to no tone (flaccid). In breeds with a curled tail, there may be a loss of the curl, and the tail hangs limply. If the LMN lesion is located at L6, the pelvic limbs may also show LMN weakness (reduced spinal reflexes and muscle tone) and muscle atrophy. In addition, fecal or urinary incontinence, or both, may be present. If the LMN lesion is located at the sacral vertebrae, the sacral and caudal nerve roots are affected, producing fecal or urinary incontinence and a flaccid tail, respectively. If only the caudal nerve roots are affected, a flaccid and weak tail results.

Diagnostic Plan

With UMN tail paralysis, a lesion above vertebra L6 should be sought. If the onset is acute, trauma, type I disc herniation, neoplasia, and fibrocartilaginous embolism are possibilities. More gradual onsets are associated with type II disc herniation, inflammatory diseases (e.g., distemper myelitis, discospondylitis), or

degenerative cord disease. The results of the neurologic examination are used to localize the lesion, and then spinal radiographs may be used to rule in or out some of the disorders mentioned. If evidence of disc herniation, trauma, neoplasia, or discospondylitis is not present on survey radiographs, CSF analysis is recommended to evaluate for myelitis, and myelography to evaluate for compressive lesions such as disc herniation or neoplasia.

The procedure just described also applies to LMN lesions of the tail. In addition, lumbosacral stenosis should be considered in the middle-aged to older patient, and sacrococcygeal agenesis in the younger patient. Both of these conditions are discussed later in this chapter. Survey spinal radiographs of the lower lumbar, sacral, and tail vertebrae may show evidence of trauma, disc herniation, degenerative lumbosacral stenosis, sacrococcygeal agenesis, discospondylitis, or neoplasia. If a diagnosis is not reached, CSF analysis may indicate inflammation, and myelography or epidurography may reveal compressive lesions such as disc herniation, neoplasia, or lumbosacral stenosis. Magnetic resonance imaging (MRI) or computed tomography (CT) scans can also be helpful in such cases.[14]

Diagnostic Procedures

Routine Laboratory Evaluation

The major benefit of routine hematologic tests (hemogram, biochemical profile, and urinalysis) in animals with spinal cord disease is to rule out concurrent diseases that would influence case management. Occasionally, animals with infectious diseases have inflammatory changes on the hemogram. However, significant inflammation may occur in the nervous system without affecting any hematologic parameter. In cases of possible urinary incontinence, contrast urethrocystography may be needed to rule out anatomic defects such as uroliths, neoplasia, or developmental anomalies. Excretory urography is required to determine the presence or absence of ectopic ureters.

Spinal Fluid Analysis

CSF may be removed from either the cerebellomedullary cistern (see Chap. 24) or the lumbar cistern. Heavy sedation or general anesthesia is required to remove fluid from the lumbar cistern. The patient is placed in lateral recumbence with the hips and pelvic limbs flexed as far forward as possible. The dorsal spinous process of L7 is palpated between the wings of the ilium. By counting forward from L7, the more prominent dorsal spinous process of L6 is identified, and a 3.8- or 6.3-cm, 22-gauge spinal needle is inserted at its cranial aspect. If bone is reached, the needle is withdrawn slightly and redirected. Penetration of the dura matter and cauda equina is sometimes accompanied by tail or pelvic limb movement. If CSF is not observed after the stylet is removed, the needle should be slowly withdrawn while the hub is watched for fluid. It is usually possible to remove 1 mL of spinal fluid from the lumbar cistern in small patients. However, removal of CSF from this location is associated with an increased incidence of contamination with peripheral blood, which can make interpretation of the analysis difficult. Normal values for lumbar spinal fluid in most laboratories include a cell count of less than 8 cells/μL and a protein content of less than 45 mg/dL.[15, 16]

Interpretation of CSF changes is similar regardless of where the suspected injury is along the neuraxis. However, considerable overlap exists in cellular and biochemical responses of the nervous system to a broad range of insults. Protein is increased with any inflammatory condition of the nervous system, including inflammation associated with trauma or necrosis. Also, disorders that increase the permeability of the blood-brain barrier, such as vasculitis, infection, or trauma, can cause serum protein to "leak" into the CSF. Similarly, white blood cells migrate into the nervous system in response to inflammation regardless of the cause. In general, a mononuclear pleocytosis suggests viral infection or granulomatous meningoencephalitis (see Chap. 24), a neutrophilic pleocytosis suggests bacterial infection or immune-mediated meningitis, a mixed-cell or granulocytic pleocytosis suggests mycotic or protozoal disease, and an eosinophilic pleocytosis suggests a fungal or parasitic infection.[16, 17]

Radiography

Survey spinal films offer visualization of vertebrae, but because the spinal cord is a soft tissue completely surrounded by bone, it cannot be directly visualized on conventional radiographs. However, many congenital vertebral anomalies, fractures, osteolytic tumors, infections of the bone, or herniations of the intervertebral disc can be diagnosed reliably on survey radiographs.

In order to obtain diagnostic radiographs, attention to both patient positioning and proper radiographic technique is necessary. This is particularly important if intervertebral disc rupture is suspected. Precise positioning is facilitated by inhalation anesthesia. Unless vertebral instability is suspected, both lateral and ventrodorsal views should be included in all studies. Oblique views are accomplished by rotating the sternum approximately 45 degrees left and right from vertical in ventrodorsal posture. Such views isolate the intervertebral foramen and articular processes

and may aid the diagnosis of intraforaminal and lateral disc extrusions causing nerve root compression.[18] Most radiologists prefer a high-contrast technique for spinal films, accomplished with higher milliamperage and moderate kilovolt peak techniques.[19] High-detail film and screen combinations also enhance film detail. Regardless of the technique chosen, a technique chart is essential for consistent results.

Myelography is accomplished by injecting iodinated contrast material into the subarachnoid space and taking dorsoventral or ventrodorsal and lateral radiographic views. Newer, second-generation, nonionic, tri-iodinated media such as iopamidol (Isovue) and iohexol (Omnipaque) appear to produce fewer complications than earlier contrast agents.[20–23] Contrast material may be injected into either the cerebellomedullary or the lumbar cistern. The choice of injection site varies among clinicians, but most prefer to inject as close to the suspected lesion as possible. Doses range from 0.2 to 0.5 mL/kg.[18] Higher doses are recommended when the suspected lesion is a greater distance from the injection site. Anything that causes compression or displacement of nervous tissue influences the size and shape of the subarachnoid space. The pattern of displacement helps to determine the location of the lesion (extradural, intradural, extramedullary, or intramedullary).[18]

Epidurography involves injection of contrast material into the lumbosacral epidural space.[24, 25] Because the subarachnoid space rapidly narrows caudal to the termination of the spinal cord within the fifth or sixth lumbar vertebra in dogs, myelography has limited diagnostic value from L6 caudally. Epidurography may enhance visualization of mass lesions within the caudal lumbar and sacral spinal canal. However, it does not produce as consistent a result as myelography, and the presence of normal epidural fat and nerve roots can complicate interpretation.[18] The dosage is 0.1 to 0.2 mL/kg and the injection site is between the first caudal and third sacral vertebrae or the first and second caudal vertebrae. Lateral radiographs are made immediately with the pelvis in flexed, neutral, and hyperextended positions.[24, 25]

CT and MRI are the techniques most commonly used to visualize intracranial structures (see Chap. 24). They also hold promise in identifying intraspinal lesions and in gaining a better appreciation of the structures contributing to stenosis of the spinal canal, particularly in the regions caudal to the termination of the spinal cord.[14]

Electrophysiology

Conventional neuroimaging techniques provide useful information regarding the anatomic relations of neural tissues and surrounding bone. However, they provide little information regarding the functional integrity of the nervous tissue itself. Because nervous tissue is an electrically excitable tissue, it is possible to stimulate sensory nerves and record the electrical potential as it is conducted along spinal cord sensory pathways to the brain.[26] Incomplete spinal lesions may delay conduction and result in attenuated potentials; complete transection of the spinal cord abolishes these potentials.[27]

Common Diseases of the Spinal Cord

Intervertebral Disc Disease

Two types of disc herniation have been described.[28–31] Type I disc herniation involves tearing of the annulus fibrosis, which results in an acute extrusion or "explosion" of the nucleus pulposus into the spinal canal. Type II disc herniation occurs when the annulus fibrosis does not tear but bulges, together with the degenerated nucleus, into the floor of the spinal canal.[28–31] Both types are common. The incidence of clinical disc disease in the overall canine population is about 2%, but it is higher in chondrodystrophic breeds. In the dachshund population, the incidence is about 25%.[29] Chondrodystrophic breeds of dogs have a much higher incidence of type I disc disease, and clinical signs usually occur between 2 and 7 years of age. Dogs with type II disc disease tend to be older, nonchondrodystrophic breeds of dogs.

Pathophysiology

With the exception of the junction of C1 and C2, each adjacent pair of vertebral bodies is separated by an intervertebral disc. Each disc is composed of an outer sheath of fibrocartilaginous material, the annulus fibrosis, and a gelatinous center, the nucleus pulposus. Each annulus fibrosis is connected to the epiphyses of adjacent vertebral bodies by a rim of hyaline cartilage. These structures collectively form an amphiarthrodial joint between each vertebral body.[30] The nucleus pulposus is a readily compressible material at birth, but metaplastic changes occur with age and result in progressive loss of shock-absorbing properties.

Metaplastic changes may be either fibroid or chondroid in origin. Fibroid metaplasia occurs in most breeds of dogs and results in a gradual shift in glycosaminoglycan concentrations and loss of collagen so that, by 7 to 8 years of age, the entire nucleus has been replaced by fibrocartilage. Chondroid metaplasia occurs primarily in chondrodystrophoid breeds of dogs such as the dachshund, beagle, and Pekingese. In these breeds, the aging pattern begins at about 4 months of age, and degenerative changes are advanced by 12 months. Dystrophic calcification frequently ensues and results in replacement of the nucleus pulposus with nondistensible calcified material.[31–33] Aging changes occur in the annulus as well, increasing its friability. When the noncompressible nucleus is subjected to loading pressures, the dorsal annulus may stretch or tear, resulting in either extrusion or protrusion of the degenerative disc material. Because the annulus is thinner dorsally than either laterally or ventrally, the disc material typically moves dorsally into the spinal canal.

Type II disc protrusion produces a gradual deformation and compression of the spinal cord. After a critical degree of compression occurs, local hypoxia develops, and demyelination, axonal degeneration, and malacia ensue.[30] These changes result in gradual loss of proprioception and motor function.

Spinal injury with type I disc disease varies with the rate and volume of extruded disc material as well as the duration of spinal cord compression. If a large amount of disc material is rapidly extruded into the spinal canal, pathophysiologic changes typical of spinal trauma occur (see Spinal Cord Trauma). In addition, the extruded disc material initiates an inflammatory reaction that results in fibrous adhesions and contributes to meningeal irritation and hyperpathia.[30]

Clinical Signs

Clinical signs vary with both the type of herniation and the location of the degenerated disc. Onset of clinical signs may be acute (within minutes), subacute (within hours), or chronic (within days to weeks). Type I disc herniation tends to have a rapid onset and can result in severe spinal cord trauma, especially if the herniation occurs in the thoracolumbar area. Type II disc herniation is typically more chronic in onset, with a gradual worsening of spinal cord function over weeks to months.

Disc herniations occur most commonly in the cervical and thoracolumbar areas. Disc herniation in the cervical region is associated with minimal neurologic deficits because the extraspinal area is greater and can accommodate more foreign material before actual spinal cord compression occurs. Intense cervical pain is a common sign and is caused by meningeal and nerve root irritation.[34] Most affected animals have a history of being reluctant to move their necks. They may guard neck motions and keep their noses held close to the ground. When the wheelbarrow postural reaction is performed, many dogs hit their noses on the floor because of a weak or painful neck. Neck manipulation or palpation also results in pain. If one thoracic limb knuckles, appears lame, or is held in part flexion, the animal is demonstrating a "root signature" sign; in such cases, it is believed that nerve roots are entrapped or injured by the herniated disc material. If severe compression occurs, limb weakness develops as motor tracts become affected. Quadriplegia results in some cases. Pelvic limb spinal reflexes are hyperreflexic or occasionally normal. Thoracic limb reflexes are normal to hyperreflexic if the herniation occurs proximal to C5; distal to C5, the reflexes are normal to hyporeflexic (see Localization of Lesions). Atrophy of forelimb musculature may be noted with caudal cervical herniations.

Neurologic signs of thoracolumbar disc herniations are frequently more drastic than those observed with cervical herniations because of less space in the spinal canal to accommodate the herniated disc material. The earliest sign is pain or an arched back; this is followed by pelvic limb ataxia, paraparesis, and paraplegia. Type I herniations can cause an acute onset of paraplegia without any preceding neurologic signs. Hyperpathia near the site of the extrusion can usually be found on palpation of the dorsal spinous processes. The cutaneous trunci reflex may also be absent one or two segments caudal to the site of herniation. Acute thoracolumbar disc herniations are often associated with spinal trauma of such severity that complete loss of pain perception may occur in the pelvic limbs. Table 27–2 ranks the severity of clinical signs.

Some dogs may show a Schiff-Sherrington posture, which is characterized by paraplegia with extension of the thoracic limbs and opisthotonos. In some severe cases of acute disc extrusions, focal myelomalacia or spinal cord necrosis results in lack of cortical perception of deep pain (lack of a behavioral response such as whining, barking, or making attempts to bite) when pelvic limb toes are pinched vigorously with hemostats. These patients have a much poorer prognosis for regaining walking ability than do those that perceive painful stimuli.[6, 34, 35] If surgical intervention is being considered in these patients, it should

be done as soon as possible, preferably within minutes to hours after the loss of pain perception. Some surgeons do not advise surgery if there is loss of deep pain perception.

Patients that rapidly develop paraplegia and loss of deep pain perception are the ones most likely to develop ascending or descending myelomalacia, in which the initial focal hemorrhage and necrosis spread cranially or caudally (or both). If malacia descends, LMNs of the pelvic limbs become affected, causing pelvic limb reflexes to become areflexic. The anus may dilate, and the perineal reflex may be weak or absent. If malacia ascends, the level of the cutaneous trunci reflex and superficial pain perception over the dorsum progresses cranially. Fever, mental depression, inability to remain in sternal recumbence, and respiratory difficulty may develop.[36] The prognosis is grave in such cases.

Diagnostic Plan

A presumptive diagnosis is based on signalment, history, and clinical examination and is confirmed with radiography. Survey radiographs of type I disc extrusion often reveal narrowing, wedging, or collapse of the intervertebral disc space, collapse of the articular facets, and increased density or mineralized material within the intervertebral foramen (Fig. 27–4).[37] In cases of normal or nondiagnostic survey radiographs, myelography is necessary to confirm the diagnosis and locate the lesion. The most common myelographic finding is that of narrowing and dorsal deviation of the ventral contrast column at the site of the extrusion or protrusion. In cases with acute onset, spinal cord swelling can cause blockage of contrast media and prevent it from flowing past the obstruction.

If possible, CSF should be evaluated before myelography to rule out other diseases. Because of the net caudal flow of CSF, samples obtained at the lumbar cistern are more frequently abnormal than samples obtained from the cerebellomedullary cistern. With both acute and chronic disc herniations, normal or increased protein concentration and a normal or slightly increased number of white blood cells can be found. However, acute and clinically severe lesions tend to have more pronounced pleocytosis (8–20 leukocytes/μL, usually mononuclear cells) and higher protein concentration. Increased numbers of neutrophils may also be found, and their presence suggests acute inflammation.[38] Such CSF analysis results should not exclude myelography if the clinical signs and neurologic examination suggest disc herniation.

Treatment

With type I disc extrusion, appropriate therapy varies with severity and duration of clinical signs.

Table 27–2

A Grading Scale for Clinical Signs of Weakness *

SCORE	CLINICAL SIGNS
0	Normal
1	Hyperpathia only
2	Ataxia but effective voluntary movement of affected limbs
3	Ineffective voluntary movement of affected limbs
4	No voluntary movement of affected limbs, but can sense noxious stimuli applied to affected limbs
5	No voluntary movement of affected limbs and no conscious perception of noxious stimuli applied to affected limbs

*Score 5 is the most severe, and signs may not be reversible.

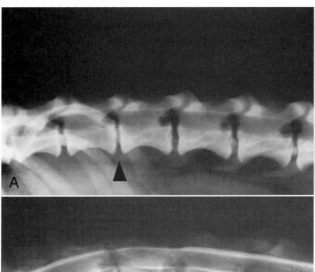
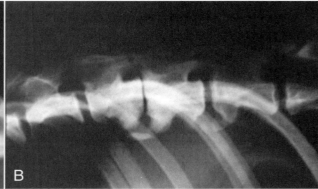

Figure 27–4

(A) A lateral radiograph showing an intervertebral disc herniation at L1–L2. The intervertebral disc space is narrow *(arrowhead)*. Note the calcified discs at T13–L1, L3–L4, and L4–L5 signifying degenerative disc disease but not herniation necessarily. (From Shell LG. Differential diagnoses for acute-onset paraparesis. Vet Med 1996;91: 234.) **(B)** A lateral radiograph of a chronic disc herniation at T12–T13. The disc space is very narrow, and there is significant spondylosis deformans at T12–T13 and T13–L1. **(C)** A lateral myelographic view shows mild attenuation of the dorsal dye column indicating slight cord compression.

Table 27–2 outlines the grading scale that is used by some surgeons and neurologists. Dogs that experience only hyperpathia or mild ataxia (score 1 or 2) usually respond to conservative management with strict cage rest for 2 to 4 weeks. Anti-inflammatory drugs such as prednisolone (1.0 mg/kg daily) relieve pain associated with extruded intervertebral discs but should be used with caution, because discomfort also effectively limits exercise. Surgical intervention should be considered for those dogs whose hyperpathia or ataxia persists for 2 to 4 weeks and for those whose clinical signs recur after an initial remission.

There is general agreement that if serious motor deficits (nonambulatory paraparesis or paraplegia) are present, prompt surgical decompression with removal of the herniated disc material results in the best clinical outcome. With cervical disc extrusions, a ventral slot procedure provides the best access to disc material in the spinal canal and usually results in adequate decompression of injured nervous tissue.[39, 40] With thoracolumbar disc extrusions, either hemilaminectomy or a modified dorsal laminectomy may be used.[34, 41, 42] Fenestration of the remaining intervertebral discs may reduce the incidence of future herniations,[43–45] but many authors consider recurrences too infrequent to warrant the additional surgical time and tissue trauma required for prophylactic fenestration.[39] Because trauma is an important aspect of type I disc extrusion, all patients with an acute onset of paresis or

paralysis should receive methylprednisolone sodium succinate therapy (see Spinal Cord Trauma).

With type II disc protrusion, corticosteroids and cage rest may result in temporary improvement for those dogs with pain, ataxia, or mild weakness. However, because many patients do seem to have progressive signs, surgical decompression, preferably with removal of the protruding mass, is the only definitive treatment.

With any paralyzed patient, conscientious nursing care is required. Passive flexion and extension of paralyzed limbs minimizes muscle fibrosis and joint stiffening, and soft, clean bedding and frequent turning help to prevent decubital ulcer formation. Attention should be given to urinary retention; antibiotics should be administered for urinary tract infections, as necessary.

Prognosis

Favorable outcomes are observed in most dogs with acute compressive injuries if deep pain sensation is retained. After deep pain perception is lost, the prognosis quickly declines. Recovery rates of 56% are reported for those patients that have lost deep pain but are surgically decompressed within 12 hours of developing clinical signs. This success rate drops to less than 5% if surgery is delayed for 48 hours or more.[34]

With type II disc protrusion, some authors

report worsening of clinical signs after release of chronic spinal cord compression[46]; the mechanism responsible for this change is not known. Others report improvement, but it usually takes weeks or months, presumably because of the time required for axonal remyelination to occur.

Degenerative Myelopathy

Degenerative myelopathy (chronic degenerative radiculomyelopathy) is a chronic, progressive, degenerative condition affecting spinal cord white matter tracts and, occasionally, the nerve roots.[47–51] The true incidence of this condition has never been documented, but it is a common diagnosis. It was originally reported in German shepherds,[48] and numerous large breeds of dogs appear susceptible.[48–50, 52] Most affected dogs are between 5 and 14 years of age.

Pathophysiology

Degenerative myelopathy is an idiopathic disease. A genetic predisposition has been suggested but not substantiated. Histologically, the disease is characterized by both demyelination and axonal loss, primarily in the dorsolateral and ventromedial funiculi of the thoracic spinal cord[51]; both ascending and descending tracts are affected. Lesions are similar to those seen with vitamin B_{12} deficiency in humans, but vitamin B supplementation in dogs does not ameliorate clinical signs. An immunodeficiency that is characterized by depressed proliferative response to thymus-dependent mitogens has been identified.[53] It is theorized that degenerative myelopathy may be an immune-mediated disease with the apparent immunodeficiency resulting from an ineffective host attempt to control the immune reaction.

Clinical Signs

Affected dogs present with progressive pelvic limb ataxia and mild weakness that is often confused with hip dysplasia. Proprioception deficits and weakness may be manifested (e.g., dragging or knuckling of the dorsal paw surface, standing or walking with pelvic limbs crossed, decreased extension of pelvic limbs). Occasionally, signs may be slightly worse on one side, resulting in asymmetrical postural reaction deficits. These dogs do not appear to be in pain, nor can hyperpathia be elicited on palpation of the spine. Pelvic limb reflexes are typically exaggerated, and there may be positive crossed extensor reflexes and positive Babinski signs. Occasionally, pelvic limb reflexes appear to be reduced because of

degenerative changes in dorsal nerve roots and peripheral nerves.[50]

Diagnostic Plan

Degenerative myelopathy is suspected in any older, large-breed dog with chronic, progressive paraparesis. The diagnosis can be confirmed only by histopathology. Other causes of progressive paraparesis, such as discospondylitis, type II disc protrusion, and spinal neoplasia, should be excluded with radiographs, CSF analysis, and myelography. An elevation in protein content of CSF collected from the lumbar subarachnoid space is the only typical finding in degenerative myelopathy. Results of radiographic studies, including myelography, show no changes associated with spinal cord degeneration. However, concurrent radiographic signs of hip dysplasia, degenerative lumbosacral stenosis, and mild type II disc protrusions can be found. If such changes are observed, the owner must be advised that degenerative myelopathy could be present concurrently with these changes and that these changes may not be responsible for the clinical signs. Because many dogs with hip dysplasia, disc herniation, and lumbosacral stenosis respond to anti-inflammatory doses of corticosteroids, failure to respond in such cases should raise the index of suspicion that the animal is suffering from degenerative myelopathy.

Treatment

No current therapy resolves the histologic changes associated with degenerative myelopathy. Clemmons[49] suggested in 1989 that an antiprotease agent, ε-aminocaproic acid (Amicar), may slow the progression of the disease; the recommended dosage is 500 mg by mouth, three times per day (t.i.d.). Side effects appear limited to gastrointestinal disturbances in a relative small percentage of dogs, but the costs may exceed $100 per month per patient. Because the course of the disease is variable, it is difficult to verify the efficacy of this treatment. Oral high-potency vitamin B complex twice daily has been suggested to support neuroregeneration.[47] Vitamin E (2000 IU/day) may provide nonsteroidal anti-inflammatory actions.[47] Most clinicians also recommend moderate amounts of daily exercise, consisting of short walks, swimming, or playing. There are no other treatment options for this incapacitating disease.

Prognosis

Clinical signs are slowly progressive over months. The rate of progression is variable, but most animals are unable to ambulate or are paralyzed within 6 to 12 months after the diagnosis is made.

Atlantoaxial Subluxation

Atlantoaxial subluxation is an instability of the atlantoaxial articulation caused by either a congenital malformation (hypoplasia of the dens) or traumatic injury to C1 or C2. Displacement of the axis dorsally into the vertebral canal results in subsequent spinal cord compression.[54–60] The actual incidence in dogs is unknown; the condition is rare in cats. Congenital malformations of the odontoid process (dens) occur most commonly in miniature and toy breeds of dogs; larger breeds are uncommonly affected. Dogs with congenital malformations are usually less than 1 year of age when initially presented. Fractures of C1 and C2 and subsequent atlantoaxial subluxation can occur in any age and in any breed of dog or cat.

Pathophysiology

Congenitally, there is no intervertebral disc between the first two cervical vertebrae. Instead, the vertebrae are joined by a series of ligaments, most of which attach the dens to either the occipital bone or C1. The dens arises from two separate ossification centers.[60, 61] In some dogs, one or both of these ossification centers fail to form. Alternatively, a vascular abnormality may prevent fusion of the dens to the remainder of the second cervical vertebra. Malformation or absence of the dens results in instability between the atlas and axis. Subsequent vertebral subluxation results in compression and trauma to the cervical spinal cord. Other congenital anomalies, such as abnormal angulation of the dens and absence of the transverse ligament of the atlas, have been reported.[55, 56, 59] Trauma may also cause atlantoaxial subluxation after fractures of C1 or C2, particularly the dens.

Clinical Signs

Clinical signs vary with the degree of luxation; they may develop slowly over weeks to months or be very sudden. Signs range from intermittent pain to quadriplegia to complete transection of the cervical spinal cord and death. Many affected ambulatory dogs have a spastic, hypermetric gait. When they are picked up, dorsiflexion of the head and neck may occur, and the thoracic limbs may extend. Pain may be evident on neck palpation, although if atlantoaxial subluxation is suspected, neck manipulations should be performed to avoid compression of the spinal cord. Pelvic and thoracic limb reflexes are exaggerated in most cases.

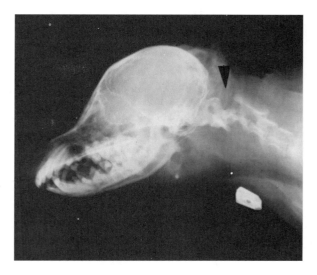

Figure 27–5
A lateral radiograph showing an atlantoaxial luxation (*arrowhead*) resulting from absence of the dens.

Diagnostic Plan

The diagnosis is usually made with radiography. Extreme caution should be exercised when anesthetizing and positioning these patients for radiographs; further spinal cord trauma must be prevented. A greater than normal distance between the vertebral arches of C1 and C2 is usually apparent on lateral views in cases of atlantoaxial subluxation or luxation (Fig. 27–5). In cases of congenital luxation, abnormal formation of the dens may be observed on survey radiographs in the ventrodorsal or oblique lateral view. In cases of traumatic luxation, dens fractures may be observed. Open-mouth views demonstrate the dens well, but compression of the spinal cord can occur during the positioning.

Treatment

For dogs with minimal neurologic deficits, prolonged (8–12 weeks), conservative management, consisting of rest and a neck brace, can be attempted. However, owners must be forewarned that the instability could result in severe spinal cord compression and even death at any time. Animals with acute onset of clinical signs should be treated for spinal trauma (see Spinal Cord Trauma). For those with motor deficits, internal stabilization by means of surgery is usually required to prevent further cord injury. Although surgical stabilization may be accomplished through either a dorsal or a ventral approach,[54, 57, 58, 62] stabilization through a ventral approach may be safer than dorsal stabilization. A neck brace may be beneficial during the initial phases of recovery, especially when severe spinal trauma has occurred.[60]

Prognosis

Without surgical stabilization, the prognosis is guarded for most cases because instability predisposes the pet to further spinal cord trauma. Surgical success of stabilization is variable.

Cervical Vertebral Stenosis (Wobbler Syndrome)

Wobbler syndrome describes a disorder with a variety of cervical bony and soft tissue lesions that result in spinal cord compression. It has also been called cervical malformation-malarticulation, cervical vertebral instability, caudal cervical spondylomyelopathy, and cervical spondylolisthesis.[63–78] The syndrome is common, although the actual incidence is unknown. Seventy percent to 90% of diagnosed cases are in Doberman pinschers and Great Danes. Dobermans are usually between 3 and 9 years of age when diagnosed,[67] but Great Danes are usually affected before 2 years of age. Males are affected three to four times more frequently than females.[67, 70–72] Other large breeds of dogs can also be affected.[65, 68]

Pathophysiology

As many as 11 different subtypes of compressive lesions have been associated with this syndrome.[77] Overall, most fit into one of four categories:

1. Vertebral malformation results in bony narrowing of the cervical vertebral canal.
2. Type II disc disease is often associated with buckling of the dorsal longitudinal ligament secondary to collapse of the disc space.[72, 77]
3. Increased range of motion (vertebral tipping) is interpreted as vertebral instability resulting in subluxation of adjacent vertebral segments.[64, 67]
4. Hypertrophy of the ligamentum flavum (yellow ligament) results in dorsal soft-tissue compression.

Most of the literature before 1970 emphasized vertebral malformations and attributed them to genetic predispositions,[63, 67, 68, 70] either alone or in conjunction with nutritional imbalances and rapid bone growth.[64, 66, 69, 78] Early identification of young dogs with vertebral malformations may have eliminated this trait from the breeding population, resulting in a decline in the incidence of overt vertebral malformations. More recent literature has concentrated on type II disc disease and ligamentous changes because these changes are now found more commonly than vertebral

malformations. Reasons for the compressive lesions are controversial. Many authors have emphasized instability, perhaps caused by subtle vertebral malformations. But instability has been difficult to prove because a substantial range of motion is present in normal animals.[79] Furthermore, it is difficult to determine whether malformation is the cause or the result of degenerative disc disease. Some believe that spinal cord compression often develops secondary to degenerative disc disease.[72]

Clinical Signs

Although the abnormality is located in the cervical area, clinical signs are most commonly observed in the pelvic limbs first. Most patients present with a history of insidious, chronic, progressive pelvic limb ataxia. Toenails of the pelvic limbs may be worn excessively because the pet does not lift the paw high enough from the floor's surface. Occasionally, the skin of the dorsal paw surface is abraded as well. Pelvic limbs may cross over (scissor-like) and circumduct, especially when the animal is turning. The stance may be widely based. Thoracic limb weakness is noted in more advanced cases, and atrophy of the triceps or scapular muscle groups can be found. Cervical hyperpathia is often found when the head and neck are extended, especially if intervertebral disc herniation is present. Occasionally, patients present with an acute onset of cervical pain, paraparesis, quadriparesis, or even quadriplegia; in such cases, intervertebral disc herniation is likely.

Diagnostic Plan

Rounding of the cranioventral aspect of the vertebral body, spondylosis deformans, and osteoarthritis of articular processes may be observed on survey spinal radiographs (Fig. 27–6).[74] The craniodorsal lip of a vertebral body may appear to be displaced dorsally. Variable degrees of collapsed disc spaces may be seen. In animals with primarily soft tissue changes, such as ligamentous hypertrophy, survey radiographs may be normal.[71–73, 75] Myelography is necessary to accurately localize the area of compression and to fully appreciate the contribution of soft tissue structures to the spinal stenosis. Malformation may occur anywhere in the vertebral canal, and at least 70% of animals have more than one area of compression.[70] The most commonly affected sites are the discs at C5 to C6 and C6 to C7; C4 to C5 and C3 to C4 are less commonly affected. In Basset hounds, C3 is the most commonly affected site.[76] CT and MRI have been used to further evaluate the diameter of the remaining spinal cord and to more thoroughly appreciate soft tissue changes.[73]

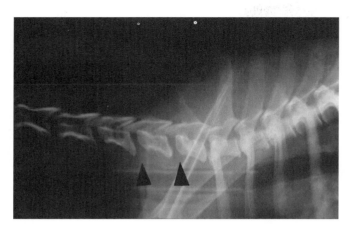

Figure 27-6
A lateral radiograph showing dorsal displacement of the craniodorsal lip of C6 and C7 cervical vertebrae *(arrowheads)* in a Doberman pinscher with quadriparesis. The dorsal displacements are suggestive of cervical vertebral stenosis, but the only way to determine spinal cord compression is with myelography.

Treatment

Because of the variety of lesions, no single therapeutic regimen can be recommended in all cases. Instead, treatment must be tailored to address the changes demonstrated in each case.[80–85] Conservative therapy consisting of restricted activity and anti-inflammatory agents such as prednisolone (1–2 mg/kg by mouth once daily) have successfully been used in some patients[80] and are recommended for those with minimal clinical signs. However, the owner should be advised that the lesions are frequently progressive and can result in gradual deterioration of neurologic function over time.

Surgical intervention is indicated if significant compression or instability can be demonstrated radiographically. Dogs with type II disc protrusion have been successfully treated with ventral decompression.[81, 82] If the compression appears radiographically to be alleviated by linear traction on the head and neck, fusion of the distracted vertebrae in extension may be of benefit.[83, 84] Fusion may be accomplished by a bone wedge held in place with a spinal plate or by using polymethyl methacrylate to bridge cancellous bone screws or Steinmann pins.[83, 84] Cases that have predominantly dorsal compression or bony stenosis of the spinal canal require dorsal decompression. Continuous dorsal laminectomy from C4 to T1 has been reported to result in excellent neurologic recovery in cases with multiple areas of compression.[85]

Prognosis

Prognosis varies with the duration and severity of spinal cord compression, the type of compression, and the ability to relieve it surgically. Dogs with relatively recent onset of type II disc protrusion respond well to ventral decompressive techniques with or without stabilization. Reported success rates for this type of lesion vary from 66% to 80%.[82, 84] Incomplete removal of disc material is the most common cause of therapeutic failure in these cases. Decompressive techniques are less successful if there are multiple levels of compression or if both dorsal and ventral compression are present. As with any chronic compressive myelopathy, the probability of successful return to function decreases with duration of the compression.

Lumbosacral Stenosis

Lumbosacral stenosis includes any type of acquired or congenital narrowing of the lumbosacral spinal canal or intervertebral foramina.[86–91] Based on the types of changes present, this syndrome has acquired many names, including lumbosacral instability, malformation-malarticulation, spondylopathy, or spondylolisthesis and cauda equina syndrome. Although incidence rates have not been reported, acquired degenerative lumbosacral stenosis is a frequently encountered syndrome. Congenital lumbosacral stenosis is a relatively rare condition. Acquired degenerative lumbosacral stenosis is seen primarily in large breeds of mature dogs, with a median age of 6 to 8 years and a range of 2 to 14 years at diagnosis. Males may be affected more commonly than females, and German shepherds may be predisposed to develop this syndrome.[90] Congenital lumbosacral stenosis occurs primarily in small to medium-sized dogs,[86] with clinical signs appearing in middle-aged and older dogs.[89]

Pathophysiology

Like cervical vertebral stenosis, lumbosacral stenosis can be produced by one or more pathologic changes. These include congenital vertebral malformations, type II disc protrusion, hypertrophy or hyperplasia of the interarcuate ligament, proliferation of the articular facets, and subluxation or instability of the lumbosacral junction. Acquired lumbosacral stenosis probably results from chronic mechanical stress. Biomechanically, the areas considered most susceptible to stress are the cervicothoracic, thoracolumbar, and lumbosacral junctions. Stresses exerted on the discs at these levels produce degenerative disc disease, narrowing of the interspace, instability, spondylosis, degenerative arthritis of the facets, and, ultimately, complete fusion of adjacent vertebrae.[88] These degenerative changes can reduce the canal diameter and cause compression of spinal nerve roots. If the canal is developmentally small, less stenosis is required before clinical signs appear.

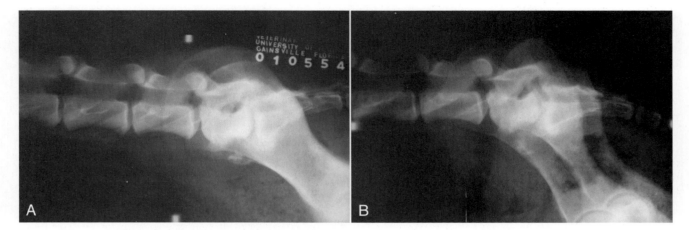

Figure 27-7
(A) A lateral radiograph of the lumbosacral vertebrae showing spondylosis deformans at the lumbosacral junction. **(B)** With hyperflexing of the pelvic limbs, the sacrum appears displaced relative to the lumbar vertebrae, suggesting instability. (From Shell LG. Differential diagnoses for progressive-onset paraparesis. Vet Med 1996;91:248.)

Although the reason for congenital lumbosacral stenosis is not clearly understood, it is considered similar to a congenital disease in humans.[86] Obvious vertebral malformation appears to be rare in most cases.[89]

Clinical Signs

Clinical signs with both forms are usually gradual in onset and progressive. Mildly affected patients may present with pain and lameness, and the disease is often difficult to differentiate from hip dysplasia or other musculoskeletal disturbances. As stenosis of the lumbosacral spinal canal progresses, compression of the seventh lumbar and caudal spinal nerve roots occurs, producing LMN signs to the tail, perineum, and sciatic nerves. Muscle atrophy in caudal thigh and distal limb muscles, paraparesis, tail weakness, and urinary and anal sphincter disturbances are common. Clinical signs may be asymmetrical, with one limb more severely affected than the other. Nerve root compression also typically causes sensory disturbances that vary from overt pain to paresthesias (unpleasant sensations that cause the pet to bite or chew on itself). Extension of the lumbosacral spine by caudal extension of the pelvic limbs or by dorsiflexion of the tail over the back reduces lumbosacral canal diameter and usually elicits a painful response from affected patients.

Diagnostic Plan

Survey radiographs may show spondylosis at the lumbosacral junction and a ventrally displaced sacrum relative to the lumbar vertebrae (Fig. 27–7). However, both of these changes should be interpreted with caution, because they can be seen in normal dogs to a degree.[91] In the congenital form, affected vertebrae characteristically have shortened pedicles (the lateral bony walls of the canal) and thickened and sclerotic laminae and articular processes.

Myelography is not always helpful because the subarachnoid space does not often extend to the lumbosacral junction; however, it does rule out lesions rostral to the sixth lumbar vertebra. Epidurography can identify a space-occupying mass over the lumbosacral disc space, but studies may be difficult to interpret without experience.[24, 25] Injection of contrast material into the coccygeal vertebral sinuses (intraosseous venography) is technically difficult and was the least reliable diagnostic procedure in several reviews.[24] Injection of contrast material into the disc space (discography) has helped to highlight elevation of the dorsal annulus fibrosis in cases with disc protrusion.[25] CT, MRI,[14] and electromyography may enhance the ability to diagnose this condition.

Treatment

Strict confinement and restricted leash walks, either alone or combined with corticosteroids (prednisolone, 1–2 mg/kg once daily), frequently alleviate the pain associated with this condition. However, clinical signs often return.[89, 90] Decompressive laminectomy of the L7 and S1 vertebrae has been effective at relieving compression in most cases.[86, 88, 89] If compression of the spinal nerves by spondylitic bone is suspected, a dorsal laminectomy can be combined with facetectomy or foraminotomy.[46, 88] In cases with instability that is demonstrated radiographically (on flexed and extended views) or visualized during surgery, fusion of the lumbosacral joint may be necessary.[92]

Prognosis

Prognosis varies with the severity of signs. Dogs with lameness or pain may respond to rest, but owners must be cautioned that clinical signs can progress. Dogs with hyperpathia and mild neurologic deficits have a good prognosis after surgery. The prognosis for functional return becomes less optimistic for those dogs with bladder atony and fecal incontinence.

Spinal Cord and Vertebral Neoplasia

Neoplasia affecting the spinal cord is divided into three types: intramedullary (within the spinal cord itself), extramedullary but intradural (outside the cord but within the dura mater), and extradural (outside the dura mater but within the spinal canal) (Table 27–3).[93] In humans, the overall incidence of primary brain tumors is approximately 10,000 per year, compared with 4000 for spinal cord tumors.[94] Although similar statistics are not available for veterinary medicine, the ratio of incidence appears to be similar. Any age, breed, and sex of dog and cat can be affected. The mean age of animals with spinal tumors is 5 to 6 years, although in one study 30% of patients were 3 years of age or younger.[95, 96] Spinal lymphosarcoma tends to affect young cats (<4 years of age).[97, 98] Most affected dogs are large breeds, with only 23.6% being small breeds.[95, 99]

Pathophysiology

Clinical signs of spinal tumors are the result of two mechanisms: physical destruction and derangement or compression of the nervous system. Intramed-ullary tumors cause dysfunction by direct physical destruction and by compression of adjacent normal nervous tissue. Tumors of the vertebrae, meninges, epaxial musculature, and vasculature cause clinical signs by compression of neural tissue; occasionally, they also invade nervous tissue. Because metastatic neoplasias can be either intramedullary or extramedullary in location, they can cause neurologic dysfunction by either mechanism.

Clinical Signs

Although most veterinary publications describe spinal tumors as producing slowly progressive spinal cord dysfunction, a critical review of the available literature suggests a marked variation in rate of progression, with many patients exhibiting an acute onset of signs.[93] Clinical signs vary with the tumor type,[95–106] the location, and the extent of spinal cord or nerve root involvement (see Localization of Lesions). In cases of spinal tumors, ataxia and weakness progress to paralysis either rapidly or somewhat slowly. Rate of progression is faster with intramedullary tumors than with other types.[95] In cases of peripheral nerve or nerve root tumors, lameness of the affected limb often occurs and progresses to severe limb weakness or complete monoplegia. Weakness of other limbs occurs if nerve root tumors invade or compress the spinal cord.[106]

Diagnostic Plan

Although results of the hemogram, blood chemistry profile, and urinalysis do not often contribute to the diagnosis of spinal tumors, such tests are useful for assessing the overall health of the animal before general anesthesia is used for radiographic studies and CSF analysis. CSF changes with spinal tumors mirror

Table 27–3
Types and Locations of Tumors That Affect the Spinal Cord and Surrounding Tissues

CELL OF ORIGIN	TUMOR	LOCATION
Tumors derived from primary neurologic cells	Astrocytoma	Intramedullary
	Ependymoma	Intramedullary
Tumors derived from supporting tissues	Meningioma	Intradural extramedullary
	Nerve sheath tumor	Intradural extramedullary
Tumors derived from vertebrae	Osteochondroma	Extradural
	Osteosarcoma	Extradural
	Chondrosarcoma	Extradural
	Fibrosarcoma	Extradural
Tumors of uncertain origin or metastatic	Medulloepithelioma	Intradural extramedullary
	Lymphosarcoma	Variable
	Hemangiosarcoma	Variable
	Prostatic tumor	Vertebral

those reported with brain tumors. Increased protein and minimal pleocytosis are characteristic of tumors outside the subarachnoid space. However, inflammatory changes (increased cell count and protein) are not uncommon with intramedullary tumors.[107] In cases of lymphosarcoma, neoplastic lymphocytes may be found on CSF analysis.[97]

Unlike brain tumors, tumors affecting the spinal cord may readily be diagnosed with conventional radiographic techniques. Primary bone tumors, such as multiple myeloma and osteosarcoma, often are apparent radiographically as lytic areas in either vertebral bodies or laminae (Fig. 27–8). Bone destruction occasionally results in pathologic fractures and an acute onset of spinal cord signs. Nerve root tumors may also cause an enlarged intervertebral foramen as a result of pressure necrosis of bone.[93] Soft tissue tumors require myelographic confirmation. Extradural tumors, located outside the dura, cause deviation and thinning of the myelographic dye column away from the mass. Because intradural extramedullary tumors are located outside the cord but within the dura, the dye column often flows around both sides of the tumor, creating a "golf tee" appearance. Intramedullary tumors, derived from spinal cord cells, classically create a bulging appearance to the spinal cord with attenuation (thinning) of surrounding dye columns. Problems arise if either the extradural or the intradural-extramedullary tumor is displaced to one side, in which case their patterns can be difficult to differentiate.[18]

Treatment

Although there are few large surveys evaluating the treatment of spinal tumors in small animals, it is generally agreed that the best treatment is surgical excision for those cases that are surgically accessible. Successful removal of some intradural-extramedullary tumors and extramedullary tumors is possible.[102, 103, 106] Adjunctive radiation therapy may extend survival after surgical removal of meningiomas.[105] Peripheral nerve and nerve root tumor removal often requires the removal of the affected nerve or nerve root, which can result in limb dysfunction. Complete amputation of the limb may be necessary if more than one nerve or nerve root is involved. Intramedullary and vertebral tumors are difficult to impossible to remove surgically. Although surgical removal of intramedullary tumors is not uncommon in human medicine, veterinary medicine is not as advanced.

Corticosteroids reduce edema around the tumor and may temporarily ameliorate clinical signs. They may also produce temporary regression of lymphoid masses. Prednisolone (1–2 mg/kg once daily) is rec-

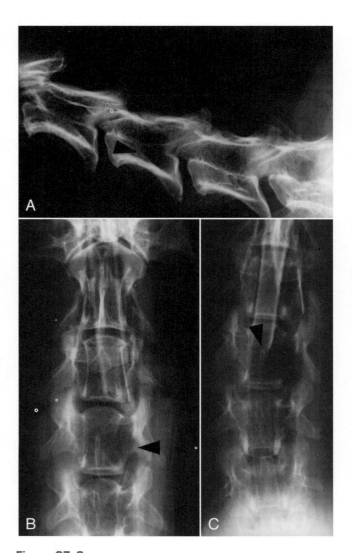

Figure 27–8
(A) Lateral and (B) ventrodorsal radiographs of the cervical spine in an aged briard with neck pain and quadriparesis worse on the left side. Notice the decreased density of the body of C4 (*arrow*) in (A) and (B). (C) The ventrodorsal myelographic film shows significant cord compression by a mass presumed to be neoplastic (*arrowhead*).

ommended. Chemotherapeutic agents are less effective against spinal cord tumors, probably because of their inability to penetrate the blood-brain barrier and the fact that many of these tumors are advanced when they are diagnosed. Nonetheless, the lifespan of dogs with vertebral multiple myeloma can be extended with chemotherapy (see Chap. 43). Cats with extradural lymphosarcoma may also improve with chemotherapy.[97]

Prognosis

Prognosis varies with the type of tumor, but in general a poor to guarded prognosis must be given. In one series, approximately 50% of dogs with spinal meningiomas were alive 6 months after surgical removal.[102] The survival interval may be extended to longer than 1 year with radiation therapy.[105]

Steroid-Responsive Meningitis

Inflammation of the meninges that is unassociated with an infectious cause and is responsive to corticosteroids has been called steroid-responsive meningitis.[108–111] Although the incidence has not been documented, numerous case reports have appeared in the literature since 1978.[108–116] It is difficult to prove whether these reports reflect an increased incidence or only increased awareness of this syndrome, but clinical impression suggests an increased frequency. Breed-specific syndromes occur in beagles,[112, 113] pointers,[114] boxers,[111] and Bernese mountain dogs.[109, 115] Large breeds of dogs as well as mixed breed dogs that weigh more than 18 kg are most commonly affected.[108–111] Most dogs are younger than 2 years of age. No sex predisposition is apparent.

Pathophysiology

Absence of an identifiable organism, unresponsiveness to antibiotics, and rapid response to corticosteroids all support an immune-mediated pathogenesis. Although antinuclear antibodies, lupus erythematous cells, and IgM rheumatoid factors may be found in some cases, widespread evidence of a systemic immune-mediated disease process has not been reported in the majority of affected dogs. All dogs in one series had been vaccinated with a multivalent modified live virus vaccine within 9 months of the onset of clinical signs.[108] Although an association is suggested, it is difficult to prove because most young dogs that receive routine veterinary care have been vaccinated within that time frame. A genetic predisposition has been suggested for beagles.[113]

Limited histopathologic data are available. Usually, no gross or microscopic lesions are found outside of the central nervous system. Inflammation of the meningeal arteries appears to be the common finding.[111] In chronic cases, meningeal fibrosis may occur and may lead to obstruction of spinal fluid flow and secondary hydrocephalus.[111]

Clinical Signs

Two clinical forms of the disease have been described.[111] One form is dominated by cervical pain, stiffness, and lethargy; the other has the added features of distinct neurologic signs such as atrophy of head or neck musculature, proprioception deficits, and impaired vision. The second form probably represents a chronic, protracted course of the disease.[111] Decreased appetite and intermittent fever can also be present. A spontaneously waxing and waning course early in the disease is observed in some dogs. Bernese mountain dogs and pointers tend to present with more neurologic deficits (e.g., weakness, blindness), probably because of a more intense inflammatory reaction that causes myelitis.[115]

Diagnostic Plan

Clinical pathologic abnormalities are confined to the hemogram and CSF analysis. A leukocytosis and occasionally a nonregenerative anemia have been reported. Elevated α_2-globulins have also been reported.[115] Occasionally, patients have a concurrent nonerosive polyarthritis. CSF analysis typically shows a marked leukocytosis (100 to >10,000 cells/mm^3), with nondegenerate neutrophils predominating. CSF culture results are negative, as are titers to various organisms. Most cases are antinuclear antibody–negative despite the suspected immune-mediated pathogenesis.

Treatment

Prednisolone (2–4 mg/kg per day) results in rapid resolution of clinical signs in many cases. Daily treatment can usually be tapered to 1 to 2 mg/kg per day after 2 to 4 weeks. Then alternate-day therapy is continued for 4 to 8 months. Monthly decreases of one eighth to one fourth of the prednisolone dose are recommended as long as clinical signs are stable or do not reappear. Neurologic deficits usually improve or resolve over several weeks. Clinical signs may recur if corticosteroids are withdrawn too rapidly. Readministration of prednisolone and more gradual tapering should be attempted in such cases. Ideally, periodic evaluation of CSF should be done to help decide when corticosteroids should be discontinued.[111] Occasionally, a patient requires corticosteroids for longer periods or has relapses that require treatment. Owners should be advised about the long-term side effects of corticosteroids.

Prognosis

There are insufficient numbers of reported cases in pointers and Bernese mountain dogs to accurately predict the outcome in these breeds. A high incidence of relapse has been reported in beagles after corticosteroid withdrawal, but complete resolution of clinical signs has been reported in some beagles and other dog breeds.

Spinal Cord Trauma

Spinal trauma occurs with any rapid deformation of the spinal cord such as from external trauma (e.g., automobile accidents, falls, fights with other animals), intervertebral disc extrusion, or luxation caused by congenital vertebral instability.[117–122] Spinal trauma is common. All ages and breeds of cats and dogs are affected.

Pathophysiology

The severity of the traumatic event is directly proportional to the speed and degree of deformation and the duration for which the spinal cord is displaced.[120] The immediate effect of mechanical forces acting on the spinal cord is commonly referred to as primary injury. Primary injury may vary in severity from mild contusion to complete severance of the spinal cord. Extensive evidence shows that primary injury initiates a series of pathophysiologic events that result in additional neurologic injury; this is referred to as secondary or delayed injury.[117–120]

Through experimental models of spinal trauma, a sequence of both histologic and biologic events that occur at specific intervals has been identified.[118–119] Petechial hemorrhage develops immediately after trauma, primarily in the gray matter. Within 30 minutes, attenuation of myelin in the surrounding white matter and enlargement of the periaxonal space develop. By 2 hours, these changes have progressed to gray matter necrosis and edema of the white matter. Chromatolysis and vacuolation of nerve cells and supporting glia are evident by 4 hours. Over the course of days, these changes evolve into necrotic cavitating lesions.

Histologic changes are accompanied by progressive reductions in spinal cord blood flow, which may be the underlying mechanism of secondary traumatic neural injury. The exact mechanisms responsible for this progressive vascular collapse are not known, but several chemical mediators have been identified that function alone or in concert to enhance vascular spasm and thrombosis of microvessels. Experimental evidence supports the role of endogenous opioids and excitatory amino acids released after injury, as well as eicosanoids and leukotrienes, compounds generated from the byproducts of cellular membrane damage.[123–125] All of these changes stimulate the generation of unstable free radicals, which in turn cause further membrane damage and perpetuation of the cycle.

Clinical Signs

Clinical signs vary with location and severity of the trauma. Ataxia, weakness, and paralysis of one or more limbs are common. Spinal reflexes vary with the location of injury (see Fig. 27–1 and Localization of Lesions). With severe injury to the thoracolumbar spinal cord, the Schiff-Sherrington syndrome may

occur. It is characterized by flaccid paralysis of the rear limbs and involuntary extension of the thoracic limbs and neck. Forelimb rigidity results from loss of inhibitory interneurons in the spinal cord that normally limit forelimb extensor tonus. Postural reactions are intact in the front limbs despite their apparent rigidity. The presence of Schiff-Sherrington syndrome indicates severe but not irreversible injury to the spinal cord. The prognosis becomes very guarded to poor if deep pain perception is lost.

Diagnostic Plan

Spinal cord trauma should be suspected in any animal with an acute onset of paraparesis, quadriparesis, or paralysis. Spinal cord injury or vertebral fracture or luxation should be considered in all animals with external evidence of trauma. These animals should be immobilized on a stretcher or another rigid surface while the full extent of their injuries is evaluated. Neurologic examination should be restricted to assessment of consciousness, cranial nerves, and spinal reflexes until a fracture can be ruled out radiographically. In most cases, survey radiographs are sufficient to rule out fractures and displacement of the vertebral segments. Concussive injuries, including traumatic disc herniations, can occur without obvious radiographic vertebral trauma. Myelography is necessary to fully evaluate the extent of these injuries in the patient with paraparesis or quadriparesis and to determine whether decompressive surgery is warranted.

Treatment

Because spinal trauma is a biphasic phenomenon, treatment should be directed at correcting the primary event and preventing any further mechanical trauma, as well as mitigating the effects of secondary spinal trauma. A number of clinical trials have been conducted to evaluate specific antagonists for each of the punitive chemical mediators of secondary neural trauma. The only compound that has been found consistently useful is methylprednisolone sodium succinate.[122, 126–128] Methylprednisolone, a potent antioxidant, inhibits free radical–induced membrane injury as well as the formation of eicosanoids and leukotrienes. It may also directly support cellular energy metabolism, and it inhibits vasospasm.

Methylprednisolone sodium succinate should be administered at 30 mg/kg intravenously as soon as possible after the injury. Higher and lower doses are not as efficacious.[129] Current recommendations are to administer IV doses of 15 mg/kg at 2 and 6 hours after the initial dose, followed by a constant infusion of 2.4 mg/kg per hour for the next 42 hours.[128] High doses of methylprednisolone have been associated with increased wound contamination in human patients.[126]

This finding, together with other undesirable characteristics of corticosteroids, has prompted the development of nonglucocorticoid 21-aminosteroid compounds that have antioxidant properties similar to those of methylprednisolone. One of these, U74006F (tirilazad mesylate), has shown promise in experimental studies and is currently undergoing clinical trials.[123, 129]

Conscientious nursing care is required. Passive flexion and extension of paralyzed limbs minimizes muscle fibrosis and joint stiffening, and soft, clean bedding and frequent turning help to prevent decubital ulcer formation. Attention should be given to urinary retention; antibiotics should be administered for urinary tract infections as necessary.

Prognosis

Prognosis varies with the severity of the injury and the ability to prevent further injury if significant vertebral instability is present. In general, the same guidelines described for acute type I disc disease apply to spinal trauma (see Intervertebral Disc Disease). The absence of deep pain perception for longer than 24 hours warrants a poor prognosis. However, dogs that retain sensation and are not at risk for further injury from unstable vertebral fragments are likely to improve if given appropriate nursing care and time.

Fibrocartilaginous Embolism

Fibrocartilaginous embolism is an ischemic necrosis of the spinal cord caused by lodging of fibrocartilaginous emboli in arteries and veins.[130–134] In a review of 1,074,329 entries into the veterinary medical database at Purdue University, 730 (0.06%) of patients were diagnosed as having fibrocartilaginous emboli.[132] Although this would suggest that emboli are relatively rare, the disorder appears to be common if only those patients that present with cord disease are considered.

Although it has been reported in horses,[135] pigs,[136] and cats,[137] the syndrome appears most commonly in dogs. Larger breeds such as Labrador retrievers, German shepherds, golden retrievers, Great Danes, and Doberman pinschers appear to be at greater risk, but the syndrome is also seen in miniature schnauzers and shelties and other small breeds.[133] Chondrodystrophic breeds of dogs are notably spared. Males and females appear to be equally affected, usually in middle age (3–7 years).[130, 133]

Pathophysiology

Although the embolic material is histochemically identical to fibrocartilage in the nucleus pulposus, the mechanism by which this material gains access to the vascular supply of the spinal cord remains a mystery. Theories include disc protrusion directly into a radicular, ventral spinal, or lumbar artery[131]; disc protrusion into a venous structure with retrograde flow through the vascular anastomotic network into spinal arteries[134]; or disc protrusion into an anomalous vessel that was the result of chronic inflammation or a remnant of embryonal arteries.[132] A final possible mechanism suggests that disc material penetrates vertebral end plates and enters cancellous bone, where it then gains access to the spinal vascular supply. The material may be found in spinal arteries, veins, or both.

Clinical Signs

Fibrocartilaginous emboli can affect any area of the spinal cord. Clinical manifestations vary with location and severity of the lesion (see Localization of Lesions and Fig. 27–1). The infarcted area may primarily involve gray or white matter and is often significantly asymmetrical. Clinical signs rarely worsen after the initial 24 hours, so the syndrome is best classified as acute in onset and nonprogressive. Many owners describe an acute painful episode when the animal first shows clinical signs, but hyperpathia is notably absent after the first 24 hours. Spinal reflexes are hyperreflexic if white matter is involved and hyporeflexic if gray matter is involved.

Diagnostic Plan

Fibrocartilaginous embolism is diagnosed on the basis of an acute onset of weakness in the absence of other processes that could cause acute, nonprogressive spinal cord dysfunction (i.e., intervertebral disc disease, trauma, neoplasia, or acute myelitis). Survey radiograph results are normal. Myelography may show intramedullary cord swelling if it is performed within hours of injury. CSF analysis may be normal or may demonstrate albuminocytologic dissociation (i.e., an increase in protein without an increase in cell count) or xanthochromia, or both. Occasionally, a mild elevation in CSF white blood cells may be found within the first 24 hours of the infarct.[130]

Treatment

Treatment is similar to that recommended for spinal trauma. Because both edema and hemorrhage are significant components of the syndrome, the treatment recommended for spinal trauma is presumed to be beneficial. Conscientious nursing care is required, with passive flexion and extension of paralyzed limbs to minimize muscle fibrosis and joint stiffening and soft, clean bedding and frequent turning to help prevent decubital ulcer formation. Attention should be given to urinary retention; antibiotics should be administered for urinary tract infections as necessary.

Prognosis

Prognosis varies with location and severity of the infarct. Gray matter lesions that affect the cervical or lumbar intumescences usually result in permanent dysfunction of the affected limb or limbs. There appear to be significantly more compensatory mechanisms for white matter lesions. Therefore, the prognosis is much better for animals with upper motor signs and intact pain perception.[130]

Discospondylitis

Discospondylitis is an inflammatory process involving intervertebral discs and adjacent vertebral bodies.[138–143] The incidence of discospondylitis in dogs has not been documented, but, based on clinical experience, it is relatively common. Discospondylitis occurs most commonly in young to middle-aged, large breeds of dogs. Males are affected twice as often as females.[139]

Pathophysiology

The most common route of infection is thought to be hematogenous. Bacteremia may occur secondary to dental disease, urinary tract infections, endocarditis, or other infections. Foreign body migration is another route of infection, reported most frequently in areas where migrating plant awns are common. In one report, immunosuppression probably contributed to establishment of discospondylitis in a kennel of Airedale terriers.[140, 144]

Coagulase-positive *Staphylococcus* is the most commonly identified organism, but *Streptococcus, Brucella, Pasteurella, Proteus, Corynebacterium, Actinomyces, Nocardia, Bacteroides,* and *Mycobacterium* species have also been isolated.[141, 142] Fungal organisms have included *Aspergillus, Paecilomyces,* and *Coccidioides.*

Clinical Signs

Clinical signs are variable and depend on the site of infection. In the early stages, dogs may show only vague evidence of pain, such as reluctance to jump, lameness, or a stiff gait. Mental depression, inappetence, and fever may be present. Hyperesthesia or hyperpathia may also be noted in one or more areas on spinal palpation. The development of ataxia and weakness is usually attributable to either spinal cord compression or extension of the infection into the spinal canal. Compression may be secondary to ruptured disc, pathologic vertebral fracture, or connective tissue proliferation in response to chronic inflamma-

tion. Subluxations of the affected vertebrae may also cause spinal cord compression. Common sites of infection include the caudal cervical, midthoracic, thoracolumbar, and lumbosacral regions.[139] Spinal reflexes reflect the site or sites of involvement (see Fig. 27–1 and Localization of Lesions). Systemic evidence of inflammation (e.g., fever, leukocytosis) is variable.

Diagnostic Plan

Discospondylitis is diagnosed on survey radiographs by finding characteristic lysis of adjacent vertebral end plates (Fig. 27–9). Variable degrees of spondylosis and sclerosis are often present, especially in more chronic cases. Multiple sites may be infected simultaneously, especially in the thoracic region. Unfortunately, radiographic changes may not appear for several weeks after the onset of clinical signs. Lesions may be diagnosed earlier, before they are visible by conventional radiology, with the use of radionuclide imaging techniques.[145] Many dogs have evidence of a urinary tract infection on urinalysis. Blood cultures are positive in about 75% of dogs with bacterial discospondylitis, and urine cultures are positive in about 25% of cases.[139] Although fluoroscopic-guided fine-needle aspiration of the infected disc space has been recommended if other cultures are negative,[138] the diagnostic yield from these aspirates has not been reported. *Brucella canis* is responsible for discospondylitis in approximately 10% of patients[141, 142]; a slide agglutination serum test for that organism is recommended for all patients diagnosed with discospondylitis because of potential human health considerations.

Treatment

Antibiotics are the mainstay of therapy for discospondylitis caused by bacterial infections.[139, 141, 142] The choice of antibiotic should be based on culture and sensitivity results if possible. If the causative organism cannot be identified, a broad-spectrum, bactericidal antibiotic effective against coagulase-positive staphylococci should be administered. Cephalosporins (e.g., cephalexin 22 mg/kg by mouth t.i.d.) and β-lactamase penicillins (dicloxacillin, 20–50 mg/kg by mouth t.i.d.; cloxacillin, 10–15 mg/kg by mouth four times per day [q.i.d.]; oxacillin, 15–25 mg/kg by mouth t.i.d. or q.i.d.; Clavamox, 11–22 mg/kg twice per day [b.i.d.]) has been used with good success. Treatment duration is 6 weeks or longer.

For dogs with evidence of spinal cord compression (weakness or paralysis) and those that do not respond to antibiotic therapy, surgical exploration should be considered. Curettage and culture of the infected disc material may be needed to identify resistant organisms. Spinal cord compression can be

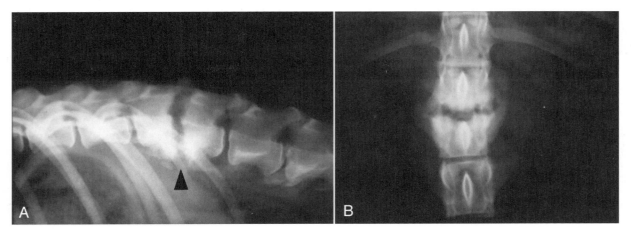

Figure 27-9
(A) Lateral and **(B)** ventrodorsal radiographs demonstrating lysis of vertebral end plates and mild sclerosis caused by discospondylitis. Notice the proliferation of bone ventrally in **A** *(arrowhead)* and laterally in **B**. (Courtesy of Martha L. Moon, DVM, MS, Blacksburg, Virginia.) (From Shell LG. Differential diagnoses for progressive-onset paraparesis. Vet Med 1996;91:245.)

relieved with a dorsal laminectomy or hemilaminectomy, but stabilization of affected vertebrae may be necessary after surgical decompression. If fungal organisms are found or suspected, antifungal therapy (e.g., fluconazole) may be effective (see Chap. 39).

Prognosis

Dogs without neurologic deficits usually respond to antibiotics quickly. If marked improvement in hyperpathia is not observed within 1 week of starting therapy, fungal infection or a resistant strain of bacteria should be considered. The prognosis for dogs with neurologic dysfunction is more guarded. However, most do respond favorably, and treatment should be considered in all cases. The prognosis for fungal-induced discospondylitis is less favorable, and the expense and duration of treatment are greater than for bacterial discospondylitis.

Uncommon Diseases of the Spinal Cord

Infectious Meningitis and Meningomyelitis

The terms meningitis and myelitis refer to inflammation of the meninges and spinal cord, respectively.[146–148] Meningomyelitis is the most appropriate term when the two occur together. Reported infectious causes of meningomyelitis are outlined in Table 27–4.[146–167] Most of these organisms cause systemic or multifocal neurologic disease and are discussed in more detail in other chapters. Occasion-

ally, these agents localize to the meninges and spinal cord, causing pain and weakness, respectively. Viral, protozoal, and parasitic diseases tend to affect the spinal cord, whereas rickettsial and fungal diseases most commonly affect the meninges. Bacterial diseases most commonly affect meninges but can spread to spinal cord parenchyma.[148] Diagnosis is based on CSF analysis and culture as well as serum and CSF titers.

Block Vertebrae

Block vertebrae result from improper segmentation of somites and often appear radiographically as fusion of adjacent vertebrae. Clinical signs are not usually present because this malformation is usually very stable. Block vertebrae can be confused with fusions resulting from trauma, instability, or discospondylitis.[60]

Hemivertebrae

Hemivertebrae are shortened, wedge-shaped vertebrae that result from incomplete development of vertebral bodies, because of either displacement of left and right somatic halves or incomplete formation of the adjacent half.[60, 168] Hemivertebrae are common incidental findings on spinal radiographs of brachycephalic breeds of dogs; clinical signs are not usually present. If clinical signs are present, myelography is recommended to demonstrate that the hemivertebra is responsible for the clinical signs through cord compression. Hemivertebrae occur in German shorthaired pointers as an autosomal recessive disorder.[169]

Table 27–4
Infectious Agents That Can Cause Meningomyelitis

AGENT	AFFECTED SPECIES	INCIDENCE OF MENINGO-MYELITIS*	EXPECTED SPINAL FLUID RESULTS	TREATMENT
Bacterial[146,148,152,160]				
Staphylococci, *Pasteurella* anaerobes	Canine, feline	Rare	Extreme polymorpho-nuclear pleocytosis; increase protein (100 + mg/dL)	Antibiotics that cross blood-brain barrier (see Chap. 24)
Viral				
Rabies[154,162]	Canine, feline	Rare	Mild to severe mono-nuclear pleocytosis with lymphocytes predominating ex-cept in FIP cases where neutrophils predominate; in-creased protein	Supportive care
Canine distemper[158,164]	Canine, ferret	Common		
Parainfluenza	Canine	Rare		
Feline infectious perito-nitis (FIP)	Feline	Common		
Feline leukemia virus[159]	Feline	Rare		
Protozoan				
Toxoplasma gondii[147,149,157]	Canine, feline	Rare	Mixed mononuclear and polymorpho-nuclear pleocytosis; increased protein	Clindamycin or trimethoprim-sulfonamide
Neospora caninum[153]	Canine	Rare		
Fungal				
Blastomycosis[150,161]	Canine, feline	Rare	Mixed mononuclear and polymorphonu-clear pleocytosis; in-creased protein; may find organisms	Fluconazole (see Chap. 39)
Cryptomycosis[165]	Canine, feline	Rare		
Aspergillosis	Canine	Rare		
Histoplasmosis[166]	Canine	Rare		
Rickettsial				
Ehrlichia canis[155,167]	Canine	Rare	Mild mononuclear pleocytosis and pro-tein elevation	Tetracycline or chloramphenicol (see Chap. 37)
Rocky Mountain spotted fever[151,155,156,163,167]	Canine	Rare		

*The incidence of meningomyelitis does not reflect the incidence of the disease, only the frequency with which this diagnosis is made in an animal presented for meningitis.

Butterfly or Cleft Vertebrae

These appear radiographically on dorsoventral films as butterfly-shaped vertebrae and are usually incidental findings. Abnormal persistence of the noto-chord is thought to contribute to this malformation.[60]

Spina Bifida

Spina bifida refers to a condition whereby the vertebral arches fail to fuse, resulting in a bony defect in the dorsal portions of the vertebrae.[60] Spina bifida may occur alone or in conjunction with spinal cord and meningeal defects. A portion of the meninges or spinal cord may protrude through the bony defect. Occasion-ally such defects are open to the environment, increas-ing the risk of meningitis or myelitis. The relatively high incidence of spina bifida in bulldogs and Manx cats is probably related to genetic selection for kinked or absent tails in these breeds. Teratogens and nutri-tional deficiencies may be responsible for the sporadic incidence of spina bifida in other breeds.[60]

Clinical signs vary with both location and severity of the anomaly. Spina bifida occulta usually produces no neurologic deficits, but spina bifida aperta may appear as an open, draining wound over the dorsum. Less severe lesions may result in palpable depressions of the vertebral canal, often with whorls of misdirected hair growth. Although survey radio-graphs usually demonstrate vertebral arch defects, myelography is often necessary to outline any associ-ated neural or meningeal abnormality. Surgical correc-tion of the existing defect may be possible in selected cases, but because other neural deficits may not be radiographically apparent, the prognosis is guarded.

Spinal Dysplasia

Spinal dysplasia refers to a congenital defect whereby abnormal migration of cells in the developing lumbosacral spinal cord results in disorganization of the normal cytoarchitecture.[170, 171] Such spinal cord malformations are not visible with conventional radiographic procedures. Typical clinical signs include a symmetrical hopping gait, hindlimb abduction, and slow postural reactions in the pelvic limbs. Withdrawal reflex typically produces flexion of both pelvic limbs. In weimaraners, the defect is inherited as a codominant gene with variable expressivity.[172] No treatment is available for such intrinsic spinal cord malformations, but clinical signs rarely progress beyond a few months of life.

Occipitoatlantoaxial Malformations

Occipitoatlantoaxial malformation refers to a collective group of uncommon malformations involving the occipital bones, atlas, and axis.[60] Frequently, the atlas is fused to the occipital bones, and the axis is misshapen, often with a hypoplastic dens. Such malformations are usually apparent on survey radiographs.

Granulomatous Meningoencephalitis

This inflammatory disorder of unknown cause affects the brain more commonly than the spinal cord (see Chap. 24). Signs of spinal cord involvement vary from quadriparesis to paraparesis or paralysis.[173] The only means of obtaining a definitive diagnosis is to review spinal cord histopathology. Prednisolone (1–2 mg/kg by mouth once daily) may temporarily ameliorate the clinical signs, but the prognosis for a long life span is poor.

Multiple Cartilaginous Exostoses

This disorder is a proliferation of cartilage and bone that can occur in both young and adult dogs and cats.[60] Bony masses may be palpated or observed radiographically on long bones, ribs, digits, and the spine. A familial basis is suspected in dogs, but in cats electron microscopy has identified viral particles in affected bone.[174]

Spontaneous Cord Hemorrhage

Intraspinal hemorrhages may be observed with arteriovenous vascular malformations,[175] trauma, and intrinsic and extrinsic clotting defects.[36] Diagnosis is usually made at the time of surgery or on histopathologic review.

Lysosomal Storage Diseases

Many storage diseases affect the spinal cord as well as the brain (see Chap. 25), and limb ataxia and weakness are observed. Signs of brain disturbances are usually noted or more prominent than those related to spinal cord disease. The exception is globoid cell leukodystrophy, in which the predominant clinical sign is progressive pelvic limb weakness.[176]

Afghan Myelopathy

This disorder in young Afghan hounds presents as pelvic limb ataxia and weakness that progresses to quadriparesis within weeks. Diagnosis is based on the signalment, history of clinical signs, normal radiographic (including myelography) findings, and histologic findings consisting of necrosis of white matter in the cervical to thoracic regions.[177] There is no treatment, and the prognosis is poor.

Leukoencephalomyelopathy of Rottweilers

This disorder is probably inherited as an autosomal recessive trait.[178] Clinical signs include progressive ataxia and weakness of limbs, hypermetria, and increased to normal spinal reflexes. All diagnostic test results, including myelography, are within normal limits. Diagnosis is based on histopathology of the nervous system. There is no treatment, and progression over 6 to 12 months is typical.[179]

Tetanus

Tetanus is caused by the localization of *Clostridium tetani* spores in an anaerobic environment, such as a wound, and the subsequent production of exotoxins.[180] Tetanospasm exotoxin binds the release of an inhibitory neurotransmitter (glycine) from interneurons, resulting in hyperexcitability. Within 5 to 10 days of infection, gait stiffness, increased extensor rigidity, and spasms of muscles are observed. Affected animals are hypersensitive to external stimuli. Death results from respiratory failure. Diagnosis is based on the characteristic signs. Treatment consists of penicillin G (20,000 to 100,000 U/kg q.i.d., IV or intramuscularly [IM]) to kill any remaining vegetative organisms; tetanus antitoxin (100–1000 IU/kg IV) to neutralize any toxin that remains unbound; debridement and excision of all infected or necrotic-appearing tissue; and chlorpromazine (0.5–2.0 mg/kg IM, IV, or by mouth, b.i.d. or t.i.d.) or pentobarbital (3–15 mg/kg IV as needed) to control reflex spasms and seizure activity.

Sacrocaudal Agenesis

Manx and other tailless cats and Old English Sheepdogs, bulldogs, Boston terriers, and other short-tailed or tailless dogs are sometimes affected with a congenital malformation or agenesis of the sacral and caudal vertebrae and spinal cord. If neurologic deficits are present, they are present at birth in the pelvic limbs and anus. Deficits may include excessive flexion of hips and hocks, hopping type of gait, proprioception deficits, large and easily compressed bladder, dilated and atonic anal sphincter, and fecal or urinary incontinence. There is no treatment.[13]

References

1. Chrisman CL. Introduction to the nervous system. In: Chrisman CL. Problems in Small Animal Neurology. Philadelphia, Lea & Febiger, 1991:3–24.

2. Morgan JP, Atilola M, Bailey CS. Vertebral canal and spinal canal mensuration: A comparative study of its effect on lumbosacral myelography in the dachshund and German shepherd dog. J Am Vet Med Assoc 1987;191:951–957.

3. Walton, J. Structure and function of the nervous system. In: Introduction to Clinical Neuroscience. London, Bailliere Tindall, 1987:1–52.

4. de Lahunta A. Lower motor neuron-general somatic efferent system. In: Veterinary Neuroanatomy and Clinical Neurology. Philadelphia, WB Saunders, 1983: 53–93.

5. Oliver JC, Lorenz MD. Handbook of Veterinary Neurologic Diagnosis. Philadelphia, WB Saunders, 1993:46–55.

6. Withrow SJ. Localization and diagnosis of spinal cord lesions in small animals: Part 1. Compen Contin Educ Pract Vet 1980;2:464–474.

7. Oliver JC, Lorenz MD. Handbook of Veterinary Neurologic Diagnosis. Philadelphia, WB Saunders, 1993:208.

8. Guilford WG. Fecal incontinence in dogs and cats. Compen Contin Educ Pract Vet 1990;12:313–326.

9. Michell AR. Ins and outs of bladder function. J Small Anim Pract 1984;25:237–247.

10. Moreau PM. Neurogenic disorders of micturition in the dog and cat. Compen Contin Educ Pract Vet 1982;4: 12–22.

11. O'Brien D. Neurogenic disorders of micturition: Common neurologic problems. Vet Clin North Am Small Anim Pract 1988;18:529.

12. Rosin AM, Ross L. Diagnosis and pharmacological management of disorders of urinary continence in the dog. Compen Contin Educ Pract Vet 1981;3:601–608.

13. Chrisman CL. Problems in Small Animal Neurology. Philadelphia, Lea & Febiger, 1991:457–458.

14. Jones JC, Cartee RE, Bartels JE. Computed tomographic anatomy of the canine lumbosacral spine. Vet Radiol Ultrasound 1995;36:91–99.

15. Bailey CS, Higgins RJ. Comparison of total white blood cell count and total protein content of lumbar and cisternal cerebrospinal fluid in healthy dogs. Am J Vet Res 1985;46:1162–1165.

16. Thompson CE, Kornegay JN, Stevens JB. Analysis of cerebrospinal fluid from the cerebellomedullary and lumbar cisterns of dogs with focal neurologic disease: 145 cases (1985–1987). J Am Vet Med Assoc 1990;196: 1841–1844.

17. Vandevelde M, Spano JS. Cerebrospinal fluid cytology in canine neurologic disease. Am J Vet Res 1977;38:1827–1832.

18. Barber DL, Oliver JE, Mayhew IG. Neuroradiology. In: Oliver JE, Hoerlein BF, Mayhew IG, eds. Veterinary Neurology. Philadelphia, WB Saunders, 1987:65–110.

19. Sande RD. Radiography, myelography, computed tomography, and magnetic resonance imaging of the spine. Vet Clin North Am Small Anim Pract 1992;22: 811–832.

20. Widemer WR. Iohexol and iopamidol: New contrast media for veterinary myelography. J Am Vet Med Assoc 1989;194:1714–1716.

21. Spencer CP, Chrisman CL, Mayhew IG, Kaude JV. Neurotoxic effects of the nonionic contrast agent iopamidol on the leptomeninges of the dog. Am J Vet Res 1982;43:1958–1962

22. Lewis DD, Hosgood G. Complications associated with the use of iohexol for myelography of the cervical vertebral column in dogs: 66 cases (1988–1990). J Am Vet Med Assoc 1992;200:1381–1384.

23. Puglisi TA, Green RW, Hall CL, Read WK, et al. Comparison of metrizamide and iohexol for cisternal myelographic examination of dogs. Am J Vet Res 1986;47:1863–1869.

24. Hathcock JT, Prechman RD, Dillon AR, et al. Comparison of three radiographic contrast procedures in the evaluation of the canine lumbosacral spinal canal. Vet Radiol 1988;29:4–15.

25. Sisson AF, LeCouteur RA, Ingram JT, et al. Diagnosis of cauda equina abnormalities by using electromyography, discography, and epidurography in dogs. J Vet Intern Med 1992;6:253–263.

26. Holiday TA. Electrodiagnostic evaluation: Somatosensory evoked potentials and electromyography. Vet Clin North Am Small Anim Pract 1992;22:833–858.

27. Shores A, Redding RW, Knecht CD. Spinal-evoked potentials in dogs with acute compressive thoracolumbar spinal cord disease. Am J Vet Res 1987;48:1525–1530.

28. Hoerlein BF. Intervertebral disk disease. In: Oliver JE, Hoerlein BF, Mayhew IG, eds. Veterinary Neurology. Philadelphia, WB Saunders, 1987:321–341.

29. Simpson ST. Intervertebral disc disease. Vet Clin North Am Small Anim Pract 1992;22:889–897.

30. Toombs JP, Bauer MS. Intervertebral disc disease. In: Slatter D, ed. Textbook of Small Animal Surgery, 2nd ed. Philadelphia, WB Saunders, 1985:1070–1087.

31. Braund KG. Intervertebral disc disease. In: Bojrab MJ, Smeak DD, Bloomberg MS, eds. Disease Mechanisms in Small Animal Surgery, 2nd ed. Philadelphia, Lea & Febiger, 1993:960–970.

32. Ghosh P, Taylor TKF, Braund KG, Larsen LH. A comparative chemical and histochemical study of chon-

drodystrophoid and nonchondrodystrophoid canine intervertebral disc. Vet Pathol 1976;13:414–427.

33. Braund KG, Ghosh P, Taylor TKF, Larsen LH. Morphological studies of the canine intervertebral disc: The assignment of the beagle to the achondroplastic classification. Res Vet Sci 1975;19:167–172.

34. Gambardella PC. Dorsal decompressive laminectomy for treatment of thoracolumbar disc disease in dogs: A retrospective study of 98 cases. Vet Surg 1980;9:24–26.

35. Morgan PW, Parent J, Holmberg DL. Cervical pain secondary to intervertebral disc disease in dogs: Radiographic findings and surgical implications. Prog Vet Neurol 1993;4:76–80.

36. Chrisman CL. Problems in Small Animal Neurology. Philadelphia, Lea & Febiger, 1991:396–431.

37. Burk RL. Problems in the radiographic interpretation of intervertebral disc disease in the dog. Probl Vet Med 1989;1:381–401.

38. Thompson CE, Kornegay JN, Stevens JB. Canine intervertebral disc disease: Changes in the cerebrospinal fluid. J Small Anim Pract 1989;30:685–688.

39. Seim HB, Prata RG. Ventral decompression for the treatment of cervical disc disease in the dog: A review of 54 cases. J Am Anim Hosp Assoc 1982;18:233–240.

40. Fry TR, Johnson AL, Hungerford L, Toombs J. Surgical treatment of cervical disc herniations in ambulatory dogs: Ventral decompression vs. fenestration 111 cases (1980–1988). Prog Vet Neurol 1991;2:165–173.

41. Black AP. Lateral spinal decompression in the dog: A review of 39 cases. J Small Anim Pract 1988;29:581–588.

42. Schulman A, Lippincott CL. Dorsolateral hemilaminectomy in the treatment of thoracolumbar intervertebral disc disease in dogs. Compen Contin Educ Pract Vet 1987;9:305–310.

43. Butterworth SJ, Denny HR. Follow-up study of 100 cases with thoracolumbar disc protrusions treated by lateral fenestration. J Small Anim Pract 1991;32:443–447.

44. Davies JV, Sharp NJH. A comparison of conservative treatment and fenestration for thoracolumbar intervertebral disc disease in the dog. J Small Anim Pract 1983;24:721–729.

45. Levine SH, Caywood DD. Recurrence of neurological deficits in dogs treated for thoracolumbar disk disease. J Am Anim Hosp Assoc 1984;20:889–894.

46. LeCouteur RA, Child G. Diseases of the spinal cord. In: Ettinger SJ, ed. Textbook of Veterinary Internal Medicine. Phliadelphia, WB Saunders, 1989:624–701.

47. Clemmons RM. Degenerative myelopathy. Vet Clin North Am Small Anim Pract 1992;22:965–971.

48. Averill DR. Degenerative myelopathy in the aging German shepherd dog: Clinical and pathologic findings. J Am Vet Med Assoc 1973;162:1045–1051.

49. Clemmons RM. Degenerative myelopathy. In: Kirk RW, Bonagura JD, eds. Current Veterinary Therapy X. Philadelphia, WB Saunders, 1989:830–833.

50. Griffiths IR, Duncan ID. Chronic degenerative radiculomyelopathy in the dog. J Small Anim Pract 1975;16: 461–471.

51. Braund KG, Vandevelde M. German shepherd dog myelopathy: A morphologic and morphometric study. Am J Vet Res 1978;39:1309–1315.

52. Bichsel P, Vandevelde M. Degenerative myelopathy in a family of Siberian husky dogs. J Am Vet Med Assoc 1983;183:998–1000.

53. Waxman FJ, Clemmons RM, Johnson G, Everman JF, et al. Progressive myelopathy in older German shepherd dogs: I. Depressed response to thymus-dependent mitogens. J Immunol 1980;124:1209–1215.

54. Denny HR, Gibbs C, Waterman A. Atlanto-axial subluxation in the dog: A review of thirty cases and an evaluation of treatment by lag screw fixation. J Small Anim Hosp Assoc 1988;29:37–47.

55. Parker AJ, Park RD, Cusick PK. Abnormal odontoid process angulation in a dog. Vet Rec 1973;93:559.

56. Watson AG, de Lahunta A. Atlantoaxial subluxation and absence of transverse ligament of the atlas in a dog. J Am Vet Med Assoc 1989;15:235–237.

57. LeCouteur RA, McKeown D, Johnson J, Eger CE. Stabilization of atlantoaxial subluxation in the dog using the nuchal ligament. J Am Vet Med Assoc 1980;177:1011–1018.

58. Sorjonen DC, Shires PD. Atlanto-axial instability: A ventral surgical technique for decompression, fixation, and fusion. Vet Surg 1981;10:22–29.

59. Swaim SF, Greene CE. Odontoidectomy in a dog. J Am Anim Hosp Assoc 1975;11:663–667.

60. Bailey CS, Morgan JP. Congenital spinal malformations. Vet Clin North Am Small Anim Pract 1992;22:985–1015.

61. Watson AG, Stewart JS. Postnatal ossification centers of the atlas and axis in miniature schnauzers. Am J Vet Res 1990;51:264–268.

62. Chambers JN, Betts CW, Oliver JE. The use of nonmetallic suture material for stabilization of atlanto-axial subluxation. J Am Anim Hosp Assoc 1977;13:602–604.

63. Selcer RR, Oliver JE. Cervical spondylopathy: Wobbler syndrome in dogs. J Am Anim Hosp Assoc 1975;11: 175–179.

64. Trotter EJ, de Lahunta A, Geary JC, Brasmer TH. Caudal cervical vertebral malformation-malarticulation in Great Danes and Doberman pinschers. J Am Vet Med Assoc 1976;168:917–930.

65. Wright F, Rest JR, Palmer AC. Ataxia of the Great Dane caused by stenosis of the cervical vertebral canal: Comparison of similar conditions in the basset hound, Doberman pinscher, ridgeback, and the thoroughbred horse. Vet Rec 1973;92:1–6.

66. Hedhammer A, Wu FM, Krook L, Schryver HF, et al. Overnutrition and skeletal disease: An experimental study in growing Great Dane dogs. Cornell Vet 1974; 64(Suppl 5):58–71.

67. Chambers JN, Betts CW. Caudal cervical spondylopathy in the dog: A review of 20 clinical cases and the literature. J Am Anim Hosp Assoc 1977;13:571–576.

68. Jaggy A, Gaillard C, Lang J, Vandevelde M. Hereditary cervical spondylopathy (Wobbler syndrome) in the borzoi dog. J Am Anim Hosp Assoc 1988;24:453–460.

69. Mason TA. Cervical vertebral instability (Wobbler syndrome) in the dog. Vet Rec 1979;104:142–145

70. Raffe MR, Knecht CD. Cervical vertebral malformation: A review of 36 cases. J Am Anim Hosp Assoc 1980;16: 881–883.

71. Read RA, Robbins GM, Carlisle CH. Caudal cervical

spondylomyelopathy: Wobbler syndrome in the dog. A review of thirty cases. J Small Anim Prac 1983;24: 605–621.

72. Seim HB, Withrow SJ. Pathophysiology and diagnosis of caudal cervical spondylo-myelopathy with emphasis on the Doberman pinscher. J Am Anim Hosp Assoc 1982;18:241–251.

73. Sharp NJH, Wheeler SJ, Cofone M. Radiological evaluation of "wobbler" syndrome: Caudal cervical spondylomyelopathy. J Small Anim Pract 1992;33:491–499.

74. VanGundy T. Canine wobbler syndrome: Part I. Pathophysiology and diagnosis. Compen Contin Educ Pract Vet 1989;11:144–158.

75. Geary JC. Canine spinal lesions not involving discs. J Am Vet Med Assoc 1969;155:2038–2044.

76. Palmer AC, Wallace ME. Deformation of cervical vertebrae in basset hounds. Vet Rec 1967;80:430–433.

77. VanGundy TE. Disc-associated wobbler syndrome in the Doberman pinscher. Vet Clin North Am Small Anim Pract 1988;18:667–696.

78. Olsson SE, Stavenborn M, Hoppe F. Dynamic compression of the cervical spinal cord: A myelographic and pathologic investigation in Great Dane dogs. Acta Vet Scand 1982;23:65–78.

79. Wright JA. A study of the radiographic anatomy of the cervical spine of the dog. J Small Anim Pract 1977;18: 341–357.

80. Hurov LI. Treatment of cervical vertebral instability in the dog. J Am Vet Med Assoc 1979;175:278–285.

81. Chambers JN, Oliver JE, Kornegay JN, Malnati GA. Ventral decompression for caudal cervical disk herniation in large- and giant-breed dogs. J Am Vet Med Assoc 1982;180:410–414.

82. Chambers JN, Oliver JE, Bjorling DE. Update on ventral decompression for caudal cervical disk herniation in Doberman pinschers. J Am Anim Hosp Assoc 1986;22: 775–778.

83. Bruecker KA, Seim HB, Blass CE. Caudal cervical spondylomyelopathy: Decompression by linear traction and stabilization with Steinmann pins and polymethyl methacrylate. J Am Anim Hosp Assoc 1989;25:677–683.

84. Ellison GW, Seim HB, Clemmons RM. Distracted cervical spinal fusion for management of caudal cervical spondylomyelopathy in large-breed dogs. J Am Vet Med Assoc 1988;193:447–453.

85. Lyman R. Continuous dorsal laminectomy for treatment of Doberman pinschers with caudal cervical vertebral instability and malformations. Proc Annu Meet Coll Vet Intern Med 1987;5:303–308.

86. Tarvin G, Prata RG. Lumbosacral stenosis in dogs. J Am Vet Med Assoc 1980;177:154–159.

87. Watt PR. Degenerative lumbosacral stenosis in 18 dogs. J Small Anim Pract 1991;32:125–134.

88. Tarvin GB, Prata RG. Cauda equina compression syndrome. In: Bojrab MJ, ed. Current Techniques in Small Animal Surgery, 2nd ed. Philadelphia, Lea & Febiger, 1983:594–598.

89. Schulman AJ, Lippincott CL. Canine cauda equina syndrome. Compen Contin Educ Pract Vet 1988;10: 835–844.

90. Oliver JE Jr, Selcer RR, Simpson S. Cauda equina compression from lumbosacral malarticulation and malformation in the dog. J Am Vet Med Assoc 1978;173: 207–214.

91. Morgan JP, Bailey CS. Cauda equina syndrome in the dog: Radiographic evaluation. J Small Anim Pract 1990;31:69–77.

92. Slocum B, Devine T. L7-S1 fixation-fusion for treatment of cauda equina compression in the dog. J Am Vet Med Assoc 1986;188:31–35.

93. Luttgen PJ. Neoplasms of the spine. Vet Clin North Am Small Anim Pract 1992;22:973–984.

94. Kornblith PL, Walker MD, Cassady JR. Neoplasms of the central nervous system. In: DeVita VT Jr, Hellman S, Rosenberg SA, eds. Cancer Principles and Practice of Oncology. Philadelphia, JB Lippincott, 1985;1437–1510.

95. Luttgen PJ, Braund KG, Brawner WR, Vandevelde M. A retrospective study of twenty-nine spinal tumours in the dog and cat. J Small Anim Pract 1980;21:213–226.

96. Braund KG. Neurological diseases. In: Braund KG, ed. Clinical Syndromes in Veterinary Neurology. St. Louis, Mosby, 1994:81–332.

97. Lane SB, Kornegay JN, Duncan JR. Feline spinal lymphosarcoma: A retrospective evaluation of 23 cats. J Vet Intern Med 1994;8:99–104.

98. Spodnick GJ, Berg J, Moore FM, et al. Spinal lymphosarcoma in cats: 21 cases (1976–1989). J Am Vet Med Assoc 1992;200:373–376.

99. Morgan JP, Ackerman N, Bailey CS, Pool RR. Vertebral tumors in the dog: A clinical, radiologic, and pathologic study of 61 primary and secondary tumors. Vet Radiol 1980;21:197–212.

100. Gilmore DR. Neoplasia of the cervical spinal cord and vertebrae in the dog. J Am Anim Hosp Assoc 1983;19: 1009–1014.

101. Gilmore DR. Intraspinal tumors in the dog. Compen Contin Educ Pract Vet 1983;5:55–66.

102. Fingeroth JM, Prata RG, Patnaik AK. Spinal meningiomas in dogs: 13 cases (1972–1987). J Am Vet Med Assoc 1987;191:720–726.

103. Bailey CS. Long-term survival after surgical excision of a schwannoma of the sixth cervical spinal nerve in a dog. J Am Vet Med Assoc 1990;196:754–756.

104. Fenner WR. Metastatic neoplasms of the central nervous system. Semin Vet Med Surg (Small Anim) 1990;5:253–261.

105. Bell FW, Feeney DA, O'Brien TJ, et al. External beam radiation therapy for recurrent intraspinal meningioma in a dog. J Am Anim Hosp Assoc 1992;28:318–322.

106. Brehm DM, Vite CH, Steinberg HS, et al. A retrospective evaluation of 51 cases of peripheral nerve sheath tumors in the dog. J Am Anim Hosp Assoc 1995;31:349–359.

107. Bailey CS, Higgins RJ. Characteristics of cisternal cerebrospinal fluid associated with primary brain tumors in the dog: A retrospective study. J Am Vet Med Assoc 1986;188:414–417.

108. Meric SM, Perman V, Hardy RM. Corticosteroid-responsive meningitis in ten dogs. J Am Anim Hosp Assoc 1985;21:677–684.

109. Meric SM. Breed-specific meningitis in dogs. In: Kirk RW, Bonagura JD, eds. Kirk's Current Veterinary Therapy XI. Philadelphia, WB Saunders, 1992:1007–1009.

110. Russo EA, Lees GE, Hall CL. Corticosteroid-responsive aseptic suppurative meningitis in three dogs. Southwestern Vet 1983;35:197–201.

111. Tipold A, Jaggy A. Steroid responsive meningitis-arteritis in dogs: Long term study of 32 cases. J Small Anim Pract 1994;35:311–316.

112. Harcourt RA. Polyarteritis in a colony of beagles. Vet Rec 1978;102:519–522.

113. Scott-Moncrief JCR, Snyder PW, Glickman LT, et al. Systemic necrotizing vasculitis in nine young beagles. J Am Vet Med Assoc 1992;201:1553–1558.

114. Braund KG. Encephalitis and meningitis. Vet Clin North Am Small Anim Pract 1980;10:31–63.

115. Meric SM, Child G, Higgins RJ. Necrotizing vasculitis of the spinal pachyleptomeningeal arteries in three Bernese mountain dog littermates. J Am Anim Hosp Assoc 1986;22:459–465.

116. Hoff EJ, Vandevelde M. Necrotizing vasculitis of the central nervous system of two dogs. Vet Pathol 1981; 18:219–223.

117. Braund KG. Acute spinal cord trauma. In: Bojrab MJ, ed. Disease Mechanisms in Small Animal Surgery, 2nd ed. Philadelphia, Lea and Febiger, 1993:1140–1151.

118. Tator CH, Fehlings MG. Review of the secondary injury theory of acute spinal cord trauma with emphasis on vascular mechanisms. J Neurosurg 1991;75:15–26.

119. Anderson DK, Hall ED. Pathophysiology of spinal cord trauma. Ann Emerg Med 1993;22:987–992.

120. Hall ED, Wolf DL. A pharmacological analysis of the pathophysiological mechanisms of posttraumatic spinal cord ischemia. J Neurosurg 1986;64:951–961.

121. Colter S, Rucker NC. Acute injury to the central nervous system. Vet Clin North Am Small Anim Pract 1988;18: 545–563.

122. Rucker NC, Lumb WV, Scott RJ. Combined pharmacologic and surgical treatments for acute spinal cord trauma. Am J Vet Res 1981;42:1138–1142.

123. Hall ED. Lipid antioxidants in acute central nervous system injury. Ann Emerg Med 1993;22:1022–1027.

124. Gentile NT, McIntosh TK. Antagonists of excitatory amino acids and endogenous opioid peptides in the treatment of experimental central nervous system injury. Ann Emerg Med 1993;22:1028–1034.

125. Geisler FH, Dorsey FC, Coleman WP. Past and current clinical studies with GM-1 ganglioside in acute spinal cord injury. Ann Emerg Med 1993;22:1041–1047.

126. Bracken MB, Collins WF, Freemen DF, et al. Efficacy of methylprednisolone in acute spinal cord injury. J Am Med Assoc 1984;251:45–52.

127. Bracken MB, Shepard MJ, Collins WF, et al. A randomized, controlled trial of methylprednisolone or naloxone in the treatment of acute spinal cord injury: Results of the second national acute spinal cord injury study. N Engl J Med 1990;322:1405–1411.

128. Hall ED, Braughler JM. Effects of intravenous methylprednisolone on spinal cord lipid peroxidation and Na$^+$ + K$^+$ ATPase activity: Dose-response analysis during 1st hour after contusion injury in the cat. J Neurosurg 1982;57:247–253.

129. Brown SA, Hall ED. Role of oxygen-derived free radicals in the pathogenesis of shock and trauma, with focus on central nervous system injuries. J Am Vet Med Assoc 1992;200:1849–1858.

130. de Lahunta A, Alexander JW. Ischemic myelopathy secondary to presumed fibrocartilaginous embolism in nine dogs. J Am Anim Hosp Assoc 1976;12:37–48.

131. Griffiths IR. Spinal cord infarction due to emboli arising from the intervertebral discs in the dog. J Comp Path 1973;83:225–232.

132. Hayes MA, Creighton SR, Boyson BG, Holfeld N. Acute necrotizing myelopathy from nucleus pulposus embolism in dogs with intervertebral disc degeneration. J Am Vet Med Assoc 1978;173:289–295.

133. Neer TM. Fibrocartilaginous emboli. Vet Clin North Am Small Anim Pract 1992;22:1017–1026.

134. Zaki FA, Prata RG. Necrotizing myelopathy secondary to embolization of herniated intervertebral disk material in the dog. J Am Vet Med Assoc 1976;169:222–228.

135. Taylor HW, Vandevelde M, Fih EC. Ischemic myelopathy caused by fibrocartilaginous emboli in a horse. Vet Pathol 1977;14:479–481.

136. Pass DA. Posterior paralysis in a sow due to cartilaginous emboli in the spinal cord. Aust Vet J 1978;54: 100–101.

137. Zaki FA, Prata RG. Necrotizing myelopathy in a cat. J Am Vet Med Assoc 1976;169:228–229.

138. Kornegay JN. Diskospondylitis revisited. Proc Am Coll Vet Intern Med Forum 1991;9:291–293.

139. Kornegay JN. Diskospondylitis. In: Kirk RE, ed. Current Veterinary Therapy IX. Philadelphia, WB Saunders, 1986:810–814.

140. Turnwald GH, Shires PK, Turk MAM, et al. Diskospondylitis in a kennel of dogs: Clinicopathologic findings. J Am Vet Med Assoc 1986;188:178–183.

141. Kornegay JN, Barber DL. Diskospondylitis in dogs. J Am Vet Med Assoc 1980;177:337–341.

142. Hurov L, Troy G, Turnwald G. Diskospondylitis in the dog: 27 cases. J Am Vet Med Assoc 1978;173:275–281.

143. Kerwin SC, Lewis DD, Hribernik TN, et al. Discospondylitis associated with Brucella canis infection in dogs: 14 cases (1980–1991). J Am Vet Med Assoc 1992;201:1253–1257.

144. Barta O, Turnwald GH, Shaffer LM, Po SS. Blastogenesis-suppressing serum factors, decreased immunoglobulin A, and increased β-1-globulins in Airedale terriers with diskospondylitis. Am J Vet Res 1985;46: 1319–1322.

145. Bruschwein DA, Brown ML, McLeod RA. Gallium scintigraphy in the evaluation of disk-space infections: Concise communication. J Nucl Med 1980;21:925–927.

146. Fenner WR. Bacterial infections of the central nervous system. In: Greene CE, ed. Infectious Diseases of the Dog and Cat. Philadelphia, WB Saunders, 1990:184–196.

147. Braund KG. Encephalitis and meningitis. Vet Clin North Am Small Anim Pract 1980;10:31–56.

148. Luttgen PJ. Inflammatory disease of the central nervous system. Vet Clin North Am Small Anim Pract 1988;18: 623–640.

149. Averill DR, de Lahunta A. Toxoplasmosis of the canine nervous system: Clinicopathologic findings in 4 cases. J Am Vet Med Assoc 1971;159:1134–1147.

150. Breider MA, Walker TL, Legendre AM, et al. Five cases

of feline blastomycosis. J Am Vet Med Assoc 1988;193: 570–572.

151. Comer KM. Rocky mountain spotted fever. Vet Clin North Am Small Anim Pract 1991;21:27–44.

152. Dow SW, LeCouteur RA, Henik RA, et al. Central nervous system infection associated with anaerobic bacteria in two dogs and two cats. J Vet Intern Med 1988;2:171–176.

153. Dubey JP, Carpenter JL, Speer CA, et al. Newly recognized fatal protozoan disease of dogs. J Am Vet Med Assoc 1988;192:1269–1285.

154. Esh JB, Cunningham JG, Wiktor TJ. Vaccine-induced rabies in four cats. J Am Vet Med Assoc 1982;180:1336–1339.

155. Greene CE, Burgdorfer W, Cavagnolo R, Philip RN, et al. Rocky mountain spotted fever in dogs and its differentiation from canine ehrlichiosis. J Am Vet Med Assoc 1985;186:465–472.

156. Greene CE. Update on neurologic and serologic findings of RMSF in dogs. Proc Am Coll Vet Intern Med Forum 1987;5:691–692.

157. Hass JA, Shell L, Saunders G. Neurological manifestations of toxoplasmosis: A literature review and case summary. J Am Anim Hosp Assoc 1989;25:253–260.

158. Higgins RJ, Child G, Vandevelde M. Chronic relapsing demyelinating encephalomyelitis associated with persistent spontaneous canine distemper infection. Acta Neuropathol (Berl) 1988;77:441–444.

159. Kornegay JN. Feline infectious peritonitis: The central nervous system form. J Am Anim Hosp Assoc 1978;14: 580–584.

160. Kornegay JN, Lorenz MD, Zenoble RD. Bacterial meningoencephalitis in two dogs. J Am Vet Med Assoc 1978;173:1334–1336.

161. Legendre AM. Blastomycosis. In: Greene CE, ed. Infectious Diseases of the Dog and Cat. Philadelphia, WB Saunders, 1990:669–678.

162. Pederson NC, Emmons RW, Selcer R, et al. Rabies vaccine virus infection in three dogs. J Am Vet Med Assoc 1978;172:1092–1096.

163. Rutgers C, Kowalski J, Cole CR, et al. Severe Rocky Mountain spotted fever in five dogs. J Am Anim Hosp Assoc 1895;21:361–369.

164. Summers BA, Greisen HA, Appel MJG. Canine distemper encephalomyelitis: Variation with virus strain. J Comp Pathol 1984;94:65–75.

165. Wilkinson GT. Feline cryptococcosis: A review and seven case reports. J Small Anim Pract 1979;20:749–768.

166. Wolf AM. Histoplasmosis. In: Greene CE, ed. Infectious Diseases of the Dog and Cat. Philadelphia, WB Saunders, 1990:679–686 .

167. Woody BJ, Hoskins JD. Ehrlichial diseases of dogs. Vet Clin North Am Small Anim Pract 1991;21:75–98.

168. Done SH, Drew RA, Robins GM, Lane JG. Hemivertebrae in the dog: Clinical and pathological observations. Vet Rec 1975;96:313–317.

169. Kramer JW, Schiffer WP, Sande RD, et al. Characterization of heritable thoracic hemivertebra of the German shorthaired pointer. J Am Vet Med Assoc 1982;15: 814–815.

170. Engle HN, Draper DD. Comparative prenatal development of the spinal cord in normal and dysraphic dogs: Embryonic stage. Am J Vet Res 1982;43:1729–1734.

171. Engle HN, Draper DD. Comparative prenatal development of the spinal cord in normal and dysraphic dogs: Fetal stage. Am J Vet Res 1982;43:1735–1743.

172. van den Broek AHM, Else RW, Abercromby R, France M. Spinal dysraphism in the weimaraner. J Small Anim Prac 1991;32:258–260.

173. Thomas JB, Eger C. Granulomatous meningoencephalomyelitis in 21 dogs. J Small Anim Pract 1989;30: 287–293.

174. Pool RR, Carrig CB. Multiple cartilaginous exostoses in a cat. Vet Pathol 1972;9:350–359.

175. Cordy DR. Vascular malformations (cavernous angiomas) of the spinal cord in a dog. Vet Pathol 1979;16: 275–282.

176. Blakemore WF. Neurolipidoses: Examples of lysosomal storage diseases. Vet Clin North Am Small Anim Pract 1980;10:81–90.

177. Cummings JF, de Lahunta A. Hereditary myelopathy of Afghan hounds, a myelinolytic disease. Acta Neuropathol (Berl) 1978;42:173–181.

178. Slocombe RF, Mitten R, Mason TA. Leukoencephalomyelopathy in Australian rottweiler dogs. Aust Vet J 1989;66:147–150.

179. Gamble DA, Chrisman CL. A leukoencephalomyelopathy of rottweiler dogs. Vet Pathol 1984;21:174–180.

180. Greene CE. Tetanus. In: Greene CE, ed. Infectious Diseases of the Dog and Cat. Philadelphia, WB Saunders, 1990:521–529.

Chapter 28

Diseases of Peripheral Nerve, Neuromuscular Junction, and Muscles

Linda G. Shell

Anatomy

The peripheral nervous system is composed of 12 pairs of cranial nerves that arise from the brain stem and 36 pairs of spinal nerves that arise from the spinal cord. Most nerves contain both ascending (afferent) and descending (efferent) fibers. Bundles of nerve fibers within a peripheral nerve are called fascicles. In most nerves, the fascicles contain a mixture of myelinated and unmyelinated axons. Myelin allows for faster impulse transmission.

Although the structural unit of the nervous system is the neuron, the functional unit is the reflex arc. The somatic reflex arc is the mechanism by which the animal reacts to external stimuli. A simple reflex arc begins at the receptor ending of the afferent axon. The receptor ending continues into the axon of the afferent neuron, whose cell body is in the sensory ganglion. After leaving the sensory ganglion, the afferent axon continues through the dorsal root into the spinal cord (or brain stem for cranial nerves), where it ends in terminal filaments that form synaptic connections with the efferent neurons or lower motor neurons (LMNs) located in the ventral gray matter of the cord. The LMNs receive information from the periphery and also from upper motor neurons (UMNs) through the descending long tracts (e.g., rubrospinal, vestibulospinal) in the brain.

Axons from the LMNs pass out of the spinal cord through the ventral nerve root and join with others to form motor or efferent axons of the peripheral nerves (Fig. 28–1).[1, 2] Terminal filaments of these motor axons end at the neuromuscular junction, where they enter muscle and branch so that one nerve fiber may innervate many myofibers. Transmission of electrical signals from nerve to muscle occurs at this junction (Fig. 28–2).[3]

The motor unit includes the cell body in the gray matter of the spinal cord (for peripheral nerves) or the brain stem (for cranial nerves), its axons, the neuromuscular junction, and the myofibers innervated by those axons. The cell body and its axon are collectively called the motoneuron.[4]

Physiology

Afferent or sensory axons carry information, such as proprioception, pain, touch, and temperature, from the periphery to the spinal cord and brain. This information is "processed," and efferent or motor axons carry responses from the brain and spinal cord to other parts of the brain and spinal cord and finally to the muscles that perform movement. Electrical signals continuously ascend and descend along peripheral nerves and are dependent on the resting membrane potential of the cell and its ability to develop an action potential.

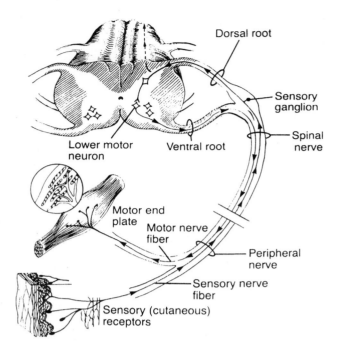

Figure 28–1

Schematic diagram of sensory and motor impulse pathways in peripheral and spinal nerves. (From Shell LG, Dyer KR. Peripheral nerve disorders. In Birchard SJ, Sherding RG. Saunders Manual of Small Animal Practice. Philadelphia, WB Saunders, 1993:1165.)

The resting membrane potential is caused by the relative permeability of the cell membrane to potassium (K^+) ions and its relative impermeability to sodium (Na^+) ions; an electrical potential exists whereby the inside of the cell is negative with respect

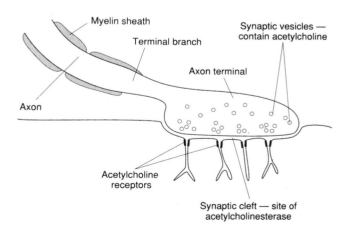

Figure 28–2

Transmission of an impulse from nerve to muscle occurs at the neuromuscular junction. (From Wheeler SJ. Disorders of the neuromuscular junction. Prog Vet Neurol 1991; 2:129–135.)

Table 28–1
Differential Diagnosis for Clinical Signs Associated with Common Motor Unit Abnormalities

PROBLEM	DIFFERENTIAL DIAGNOSIS
Acute monoparesis or monoplegia	Trauma to nerve root or peripheral nerve Fibrocartilaginous embolism Lateral intervertebral disc herniation
Chronic monoparesis or monoplegia	Tumor of nerve root or peripheral nerve Lateral intervertebral disc herniation Severe arthritic disease (pseudoparesis)
Acute lower motor neuron quadriplegia	Acute polyradiculoneuritis (coonhound paralysis) Tick paralysis Botulism Protozoal myositis or neuritis Myasthenia gravis crisis

Chronic progressive lower motor neuron quadriparesis	Immature animal
	    Congenital or inherited nerve disorder
	    Congenital or inherited muscle disorder
	Mature animal
	    Acquired neuropathies
	        Toxins
	        Metabolic or endocrine disorder
	        Inflammatory or infectious origin
	        Neoplasia
	    Acquired myopathies
	        Metabolic or endocrine disorder
	        Inflammatory or infectious origin
	        Immune-mediated disorder

Exercise-induced or episodic weakness	Myasthenia gravis Hypoglycemia Anemia Cardiovascular disease Respiratory disease Narcolepsy Polymyopathies Electrolyte disturbances

to the outside. Conduction begins with the loss of the resting membrane potential.

At the neuromuscular junction (see Fig. 28–2), conduction results in the release of acetylcholine (ACH) from the terminal axon. ACH diffuses across the synapse and attaches to a muscle receptor, causing an influx of Na^+ ions and depolarization of the muscle membrane. An action potential spreads over the muscle fiber to cause muscle contraction.[3] ACH is then released from the muscle receptor into the synaptic cleft and degraded by acetylcholinesterase into acetyl and choline, which are recycled into ACH.

Problem Identification

The four most common problems associated with the motor unit are acute LMN quadriparesis, chronic LMN

quadriparesis, monoparesis, and episodic or exercise-induced weakness (Table 28–1). Less common problems include muscle wasting, muscle hypertrophy, muscle pain, and cranial nerve deficits (see Chap. 26).

Lower Motor Neuron Quadriparesis

LMN quadriparesis is weakness of all limbs that originates from disease of the LMNs located in the gray matter of the spinal cord, their axons within nerve roots or peripheral nerves, the neuromuscular junction, or muscle.

Pathophysiology

Voluntary movement originates with nuclei of UMNs in the brain stem and cerebrum. Axons from these nuclei group together to form tracts (e.g.,

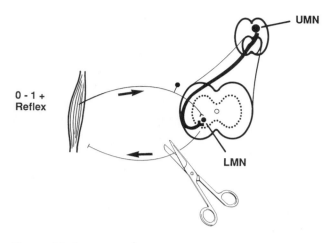

0 - 1 +
Reflex

UMN

LMN

Figure 28-3

Schematic diagram demonstrating how reflexes become reduced or absent with disorders affecting the lower motor neuron. (From Shell LG. The basics of pelvic limb weakness. Vet Med 1996;91:222.)

rubrospinal tract, vestibulospinal tract, corticospinal tract) that traverse the brain stem and spinal cord to control the spontaneous reflexive actions of the LMNs located in the ventral gray matter of the spinal cord. If UMNs or tracts are not functioning properly, voluntary movements are impaired and spinal reflexes become exaggerated because the calming influence of the UMNs on the LMNs is lacking. Muscle tone may also be increased for the same reason. These signs are referred to as upper motor neuron signs.

Although the UMNs initiate voluntary movement, they can effect movement only through the LMNs and their axons. Weakness of movement and decreased strength are also observed if LMNs or their axons or receptors (i.e., muscle) are injured. With LMN injury, the spinal reflexes become diminished to absent, and muscle tone is reduced because the effector side of the reflex arc is not functioning properly (Fig. 28-3). These signs are referred to as lower motor neuron signs.[5, 6]

Clinical Signs

Patients with LMN weakness in all four limbs may present acutely "down," unable to rise and walk. Such patients can be differentiated from those with UMN dysfunction by evaluation of muscle tone and spinal reflexes. If muscle tone and spinal reflexes are decreased or absent, causes of acute LMN quadriparesis must be pursued (see Table 28-1).

In ambulatory animals, the gait may be described as clumsy or drunken-like. Decreased muscle tone and wasting or atrophy may also be noted and may be described as lack of strength and weight loss, respectively. Polyuria, polydipsia, hair loss, weight loss, coughing, vomiting, or diarrhea may be noted if systemic illnesses such as neoplasia, endocrine disorders, or inflammatory diseases are contributing to the quadriparesis. Likewise, fever, lymphadenopathy, or abdominal masses may be found on physical examination if systemic illness is present. Except for the patient with severe muscle atrophy, it is difficult to differentiate LMN weakness from UMN weakness until spinal reflexes and muscle tone are evaluated.

Diagnostic Plan

If an animal is presented for weakness, the clinician must first differentiate neurologic disease from systemic disease causing weakness. The physical and neurologic examinations should help with the differentiation. The neurologic examination should also distinguish between LMN and UMN weakness. LMN weakness is established by finding reduced muscle tone and spinal reflexes. The rapidity of onset must then be established, because the causes of acute LMN quadriparesis are different from those of chronic and progressive LMN quadriparesis. The owner should be questioned about the possibility of the patient's having been exposed to carrion or other foodstuffs that could contain toxins produced by *Clostridium botulinum*. If the patient is a hunting dog, exposure to a raccoon 1 to 2 weeks before the onset of signs should be ascertained because of the possibility of acute polyradiculoneuritis (coonhound paralysis). If the patient has had a history of intermittent weakness that resolves with rest, myasthenia gravis becomes a possible cause. The patient must be examined carefully for the presence of ticks, which can cause tick paralysis. If the owner reports a gradual or progressive weakening of the patient's limbs, causes of chronic, progressive LMN weakness should be pursued (see Table 28-1). Because many toxins can cause chronic polyneuropathies, the environment should be examined carefully for toxins.

Causes of LMN quadriparesis are also different in immature and mature animals. Congenital or inherited muscle and nerve disorders manifest most commonly in the immature animal, whereas metabolic and endocrine disorders occur most often in the mature animal. For those cases involving a mature animal with a progressive and chronic course, routine laboratory information is indicated to help investigate the possibility of systemic or generalized illness. If hypothyroidism is suggested by the signalment (mature dog, especially in a middle- to large-sized breed), history (e.g., lethargy, seeks heat), or physical examination findings (e.g., symmetrical hair loss or thin hair coat, obesity), a resting thyroid hormone level should be evaluated. If it is lower than normal, the possibility of hypothyroidism should be investigated, along with performance of other tests (see Chap. 47), or a trial therapy of replacement hormone should be administered.

If there is suspicion of organophosphate exposure, a blood cholinesterase level can be evaluated, but the results can be normal in cases of chronic exposure. Thoracic radiographs can help to assess the potential for neoplastic or inflammatory processes causing a secondary neuropathy or myopathy. Muscle and nerve biopsies may help establish the diagnosis of a neuropathy or a myopathy, but results are often nonspecific when it comes to identifying the cause. Occasionally, protozoal cysts, associated with *Neospora caninum* or *Toxoplasma gondii*, can be found in such samples (see Chap. 40). Electrophysiologic testing may help confirm muscle or nerve disease, but it is not readily accessible to many practitioners unless a specialty practice or teaching hospital is nearby.

If the onset is progressive in the immature animal, congenital or inherited and inflammatory polyneuropathies or polymyopathies should be considered. A minimum database may help to identify inflammation, but results will probably be normal in cases of congenital or inherited diseases. If the creatine kinase level is greatly increased, a muscle disorder may be more likely than nerve disease. However, muscle and nerve biopsies are ultimately needed to better define the abnormality.

If the onset is acute in the mature or immature animal, a minimum database should be pursued to ensure that the weakness is not caused by a metabolic abnormality such as hypocalcemia, hypoglycemia, or hypokalemia. If there is no evidence of systemic or metabolic disease and if the pet is nonambulatory with minimal to no voluntary movements, tick paralysis, acute polyradiculoneuritis, botulism, acute myasthenia gravis crisis,[7] and protozoal neuritis or myositis[8] should be considered. Historical information or physical examination findings may help to narrow this list. If it is springtime or summer, treatment for tick paralysis may be justified (i.e., insecticide dips or sprays). If muscle or nerve biopsies or electrophysiologic testing is not feasible, treatment for protozoal myositis or neuritis can be started with clindamycin (see Polymyositis).

Monoparesis

Monoparesis is weakness of one limb.

Pathophysiology

Although monoparesis can be caused by a selective UMN lesion in the spinal cord, it is most commonly a result of a lesion located at one of the following sites: at the LMNs of the spinal cord at C5 to T2 (thoracic limbs) or L3 to S2 (pelvic limbs), at the nerve roots that exit at these sites, at the peripheral nerves that supply the limbs, or, least likely, at the muscle level.

Clinical Signs

Owners may observe that the pet drags the paw or does not use the affected limb. They may also describe the pet as favoring the affected limb or being lame. On examination, the limb may be weight bearing but weak, in which case the animal may appear lame. If the limb is able to bear weight, the pet either carries the limb or lets it dangle loosely to scrape the floor, depending on which nerves are injured. If the injury is more than 1 week old, appreciable muscle atrophy may be found. Atrophy of affected muscles is likely to become more extensive the longer the condition exists.

If the radial nerve in the thoracic limb or the femoral nerve in the pelvic limb is injured, the patient is not able to bear full weight on the injured limb. However, the animal should be able to withdraw or flex the limb, provided that the musculocutaneous nerve in the thoracic limb or the sciatic nerve in the pelvic limb is intact. Therefore, the animal may be able to lift the affected limb from the floor enough to prevent abrasions to the dorsal paw surface. If the injury or disease is located at the cervical intumescence or at the C5 through T2 nerve roots, a concurrent ipsilateral Horner's syndrome (miosis, ptosis, enophthalmos) or lack of the ipsilateral cutaneous trunci reflex may be also found on neurologic examination.

Diagnostic Plan

As a general rule, the limb that has no voluntary movement and no flexor (withdrawal) reflex has an abnormality at the LMN (spinal cord gray matter), at the nerve root, or at the peripheral nerve level. A thorough history and neurologic examination often give insight into the possible causes. An acute onset of monoparesis suggests trauma or ischemia, whereas progressive limb weakness is more suggestive of neoplasia or disc herniation (see Table 28–1). Muscles should be palpated for tone and resistance to flexion and compared with muscles on the normal, unaffected limb. The entire limb should be palpated carefully for masses. Neoplasia occasionally develops along the nerves or in the soft tissues of the axillary area, and masses can sometimes be palpated.

The limb that continues to bear weight but appears weak is more difficult to assess, because a musculoskeletal problem could present in a similar manner. Monoparesis in this instance must be differentiated from lameness. Spinal reflexes should be critically assessed in such patients, keeping in mind that it is sometimes difficult to elicit reflexes in the thoracic limbs; comparison of the affected limb's reflexes with reflexes on the normal side becomes crucial for accurate interpretation of the results. Those patients with a musculoskeletal disease should not have reflexes that vary from one side to the other, particularly the flexor (withdrawal) reflex. Thorough palpation of the limb, including extension and flexion of all joints, is also indicated; joint pain, swelling, or increased warmth suggests arthritis as a cause of the limb weakness. If pain is found, radiographs of the limb should be taken. Even if changes are not noted on the musculoskeletal examination, radiographs of the entire limb may help to establish musculoskeletal disorders such as degenerative or inflammatory joint disease, bony neoplasia, or osteomyelitis. Radiographs of the spine, limb, or chest may show evidence of trauma to the bones or soft tissues. Radiographs can also delineate soft tissue or bony masses. However, radiographs are normal in cases of spinal cord ischemia (i.e., fibrocartilaginous embolus) and in many cases of nerve root tumors. Myelography and analysis of cerebrospinal fluid (CSF) are required for such patients.

Exercise-Induced Weakness

Exercise-induced weakness is weakness that occurs as the animal is walking or running; strength usually returns to normal after a period of rest.

Pathophysiology

Although mechanisms vary for specific disorders, the ultimate result is the generation of an end-plate potential of insufficient amplitude to trigger a propagated muscle action potential. Factors that interfere with presynaptic Ca^{++} channel function or ACH release, binding, or degradation can result in inadequate synaptic transmission and clinical weakness.[9]

Clinical Signs

The affected pet may be described as having weakness or an inability to move during exercise. Stiffness of gait, progressively shorter steps, and a reluctance to move may be followed by episodes of collapse.[10] With certain disorders, such as myasthenia gravis and polymyositis, gagging motions or regurgitation associated with esophageal dysfunction may be described, although owners frequently describe regurgitation as vomiting.

Diagnostic Plan

There are several categories or disease mechanisms for exercise-induced weakness, and each should be given consideration as the history, physical, and neurologic examination results are evaluated (see Table 28–1). Historical questions and a thorough physical examination should help to establish a cardiogenic or respiratory basis for the weakness. A history of coughing or dyspnea or auscultation of a heart murmur, arrhythmia, or abnormal lung sounds is important enough to warrant further evaluation of the chest with radiographs. An electrocardiogram and appropriate heartworm tests should also be considered. Intermittent cardiac arrhythmias, such as heart blocks, can be difficult to diagnose without continuous 24-hour electrocardiogram monitoring.

Metabolic-induced weaknesses usually can be excluded by evaluation of a chemistry profile taken preferably when the animal is in the weakened or collapsed state. Because intermittent hypoglycemia can be difficult to diagnose, a 24-hour fasting blood sample with patient observation should be evaluated for hypoglycemia (see Chap. 48). Some metabolic or endocrine disorders, such as hypothyroidism and hypoadrenocorticism, require special hormonal studies for confirmation of the diagnosis (see Chaps. 46 and 47). Occasionally, anemia can cause or contribute to weakness; therefore, a hemogram should be evaluated, especially if there are other indications of anemia such as pale mucous membranes.

If weakness occurs with excitement or is associated with eating, narcolepsy should be considered (see Chap. 25). If weakness occurs with exercise, myasthenia gravis can tentatively be diagnosed if an intravenous (IV) injection of 1 to 10 mg edrophonium chloride (Tensilon) temporarily alleviates the weakness. Anticholinesterase antibodies can also be measured in serum (see Myasthenia Gravis).[11]

The possibility that the weakness is caused by a myopathy can be investigated by palpation of muscles for signs of pain, hypertrophy, or atrophy. Creatine kinase level is sometimes elevated in cases of polymyositis or some inherited myopathies, but a muscle biopsy is required for confirmation. There are no blood tests to confirm neuropathies; needle electromyography (EMG), nerve conduction studies, and biopsies of nerves and muscles are required.

Muscle Wasting

Muscle wasting or atrophy is a decrease in the size of muscle. There are three types: neurogenic atrophy, myogenic atrophy, and disuse atrophy.

Pathophysiology

Under normal circumstances, each muscle receives a rhythmic volley of motor impulses from the LMNs of the gray matter. These stimuli are responsible for the trophic state of the muscle. As long as the motor unit is intact, the nutrition to and tone of the muscle are maintained. If these stimuli no longer reach the muscle, owing to disease or injury to the LMNs or their axons, the muscles lack tone and strength. There is an alteration in the electrical excitability and chemical irritability. All affected muscle fibers decrease in weight and size. Associated with the loss of muscle mass, there may be an increase in connective tissue leading to fibrosis, and the atrophied muscles may be infiltrated with fat. This type of atrophy is called neurogenic atrophy. The more abrupt or extensive the interruption of the nerve supply, the more rapid the wasting.[12]

Myogenic atrophy occurs as a result of disease within the muscle. Disuse atrophy occurs if the muscles have not been used because of weakness or paralysis or because of prolonged immobilization, such as occurs with the application of a cast to repair a fracture. In contrast to myogenic atrophy, no degeneration of muscle fibers or nerves and no changes in the electrical responses of the muscles occur in disuse atrophy.

Clinical Signs

Owners may describe the pet as being thin or losing weight when in fact the muscle mass has decreased. Weakness or exercise intolerance may be noted. On examination, reduced muscle mass and tone are observed; these signs may be localized or diffuse. Spinal reflexes may be normal or reduced, depending on the cause.

Diagnostic Plan

Diffuse neurogenic muscle atrophy must be differentiated from the cachexia associated with many systemic illnesses. Ribs tend to be more prominent in cachectic or systemically ill animals, but this can be a subjective finding. A thorough physical examination as well as evaluation of routine laboratory data are often necessary to distinguish between the two conditions.

If localized appendicular atrophy is present, the neurologic examination may allow localization of the problem to the cervical or lumbosacral intumescences of the spinal cord, the peripheral nerves of the affected limb, or the muscles. If EMG is available, a more accurate localization (specific muscles or nerves) may be possible. Spinal radiographs, CSF analysis, muscle and nerve biopsies, or contrast studies of the spinal cord may then be pursued after the lesion is localized by neurologic examination.

Generalized appendicular muscle atrophy that is not of metabolic origin is more compatible with a diffuse myopathy or neuropathy than with a spinal cord abnormality. Creatine kinase levels, EMG, nerve conduction studies, and muscle or nerve biopsies are indicated.

Muscle Hypertrophy

Muscle hypertrophy is an increase in the bulk or volume of muscle tissues.

Pathophysiology

Hypertrophy can be the result of excessive use of muscles, or it can occur on a pathologic basis, as in some muscle disorders called myotonias.[12, 13] In myotonia, the muscles are enlarged because of sustained muscle contraction after stimulation.

Clinical Signs

Owners do not often present their pet because of a perceived increase in muscle mass. Rather, hypertrophy is a sign found by the astute clinician on physical examination. Owners may present the pet because of a stiff or hopping gait, a sawhorse type of posture, or hyperextension of the limbs.[13] It can be difficult to appreciate muscle hypertrophy in dogs with long or curly coats and in breeds for which large muscles are characteristic.

Diagnostic Plan

If hypertrophy cannot be appreciated on palpation, an area can be clipped and the firm, rigid, and well-defined muscles visualized, especially in the proximal limb and neck areas. If such muscles are gently percussed with a pleximeter, a dimple or depression is created in the percussed area. EMG can be helpful, especially because hypertrophy is most often associated with myotonia or pseudomyotonia. If the patient is immature, a congenital myotonic myopathy is the most likely cause. Mature patients should be evaluated for electrolyte disturbances (hypokalemia, hyperkalemia) and hyperadrenocorticism, which can lead to acquired myotonia.[14, 15]

Muscle Pain

Because animals cannot verbalize sensations, muscle pain is difficult to define. It can be subjectively described as signs of discomfort at rest or especially when the muscles are palpated or touched.

Pathophysiology

It is assumed that muscle disorders associated with inflammation cause pain by stimulation of nociceptors in and around muscle fibers.

Clinical Signs

Although pain is a common complaint made by pet owners, they often have difficulty describing the location of the pain or discomfort in their pets.

Behavioral responses that indicate pain or discomfort include vocalization, biting or snarling at the examiner, and movements away from noxious stimuli. A reluctance to walk upstairs, jump into vehicles or on furniture, or walk across thresholds is another possible sign of discomfort. Some pets may seem to have a stiff or very careful stepping gait ("walks on eggs"), similar to that of an animal with joint disease. Others keep their heads held low and may be reluctant to lift them.

Diagnostic Plan

A thorough physical examination and careful palpation of the joints, muscles, bones, and spine are required to localize the pain. Muscle pain can be evaluated by gently palpating each group of muscles and determining whether the animal's response is normal. Extreme or intense palpation may cause even mild-mannered normal animals some discomfort. Because animals have different levels of pain tolerance, caution should be used in interpreting the palpation results. However, if pain can be consistently produced by palpation of a specific area or structure, then a pathologic abnormality of that area is likely. After pain is localized to the muscles, other signs of muscle disease, such as atrophy and reduced tone or reflex changes, should be investigated. Muscle diseases associated with muscle pain are primarily inflammatory or neoplastic. Muscle enzyme evaluations, muscle biopsy, and perhaps EMG should be considered. Because some inflammatory muscle conditions such as protozoal myositis and immune-mediated polymyositis have a systemic effect, routine laboratory tests (hemogram, chemistry profile, and urinalysis) should be evaluated. If systemic signs (e.g., fever, decreased appetite, inflammatory leukogram findings) are present, titers for protozoal diseases (*Toxoplasma* and *Neospora*) and an antinuclear antibody test should be considered.

Diagnostic Procedures

Routine Laboratory Evaluation

A hemogram, blood chemistry profile, and urinalysis are recommended in all cases of LMN weakness because of the potential for metabolic, endocrine, or neoplastic disorders to cause changes in muscles and nerves.

Specialized Laboratory Tests

Muscle enzyme evaluations (creatine kinase, aldolase, lactate dehydrogenase, and aspartate aminotransferase) can usually be done at commercial laboratories and may help differentiate muscle disorders from peripheral neuropathies. Muscle enzymes are located within myofibrils, and their concentrations in the serum of normal dogs are usually low unless the muscle membrane has been damaged. Creatine kinase is the most specific of the muscle enzymes, but an increase in creatine kinase does not necessarily indicate muscle disease because mild, transient elevations have been observed in nonmuscle disorders.[16, 17] Intramuscular injections, trauma, and prolonged recumbence can also increase serum concentrations of creatine kinase.

Cholinesterase determinations are also offered by most commercial laboratories and are used to confirm the diagnosis of acute organophosphate toxicity. Cholinesterase is an enzyme located at the muscle membrane that inactivates ACH. Organophosphates and carbamates inhibit cholinesterase and therefore prolong the attachment of ACH at the muscle membrane. A reduction of more than 50% in cholinesterase activity in plasma is necessary to confirm the diagnosis of organophosphate or carbamate toxicity.[18]

Spinal Fluid Analysis

Analysis of CSF is occasionally beneficial in disorders of the nerve roots such as acute polyradiculoneuritis or protozoal infections. Descriptions of the procedures and analysis are presented in Chapters 24 and 27.

Electrodiagnostics

Needle Electromyography

EMG, the recording of electrical activity in skeletal muscle,[19] is used to determine the presence and distribution of peripheral nerve and muscle disorders. Normal muscle is electrically silent. Five to seven days after denervation has occurred, spontaneous denervation potentials can be found on insertion of an electrode in the muscle innervated by the damaged nerve.[20] Similar changes are observed in muscle diseases, making it difficult sometimes to separate muscle from nerve disorders on EMG examination.[21] Because of the cost of the instrument and the training needed to interpret the findings, this test is usually offered only at veterinary teaching hospitals or certain specialty practices.

Nerve Stimulation Studies

Nerve stimulation studies[19, 22] are used to determine the location and nature of a peripheral nerve abnormality. Such studies are recorded under general anesthesia. The conduction velocity of motor nerves is tested by stimulating a nerve at two separate sites and recording the time it takes an evoked muscle potential to appear in a muscle supplied by the stimulated nerve. Reduction of the conduction velocity or a change in amplitude, duration, or waveform of the evoked action potential suggests pathologic conditions. In conjunction with the EMG, nerve stimulation studies may be able to provide information to help distinguish between axonal and myelination disorders.[19]

Muscle and Nerve Biopsies

Muscle biopsy samples can easily be taken, provided that the biopsy does not injure peripheral nerves, blood vessels, or tendons.[23, 24] Muscle histopathology can help to distinguish different muscle disorders and can also differentiate nerve from muscle disorders if histochemical staining* is used.[25] Routine histology (hematoxylin and eosin stain) may reveal inflammatory or neoplastic changes or etiologic agents such as protozoal organisms.

Sensory and motor nerve biopsies involve removing a fascicle of the nerve several centimeters in length, leaving the rest of the nerve trunk intact. Because they are easily accessible and would not result in severe clinical signs if inadvertently damaged by the biopsy procedure, the common peroneal and the ulnar nerves are usually the ones selected for biopsy. Because special handling and processing are required, these biopsies are best performed at a specialty practice or a teaching hospital. Before taking muscle or nerve biopsies, it is important to communicate with the pathology laboratory or pathologist to determine the methods of fixation or storage of the samples.

Common Diseases of Peripheral Nerve, Neuromuscular Junction, and Muscles

Most motor unit disorders fall into one of three areas: peripheral nerve, neuromuscular junction, or muscle (Table 28–2). Disorders of peripheral nerves or muscle usually cause muscle wasting and a slow onset of LMN weakness, whereas disorders of the neuromuscular junction usually cause episodic weakness or acute quadriparesis.

Acute Polyradiculoneuritis

Acute polyradiculoneuritis, or coonhound paralysis,[26] is a condition of acute-onset LMN ascending paralysis characterized by inflammatory demyelination of nerve roots and peripheral nerves and degeneration of axons. Although this is the most commonly recognized peripheral neuropathy in North America, its true incidence is unknown. Any age, sex, and breed of dog can be affected, but hunting dogs are most

*Available from Neuromuscular Diagnostic Laboratory, Scott-Ritchey Research Center, Auburn University, Auburn, Alabama, or Comparative Neuromuscular Laboratory, School of Veterinary Medicine, University of California at San Diego, La Jolla, California.

commonly affected. A similar rare condition may exist in cats.

Pathophysiology

Acute polyradiculoneuritis bears a close resemblance to Guillain-Barré syndrome in humans, for which there appear to be triggering factors such as viral or bacterial infections, vaccinations, surgery, or fever-reduction therapy. In dogs, the precise relation between raccoon saliva and cell-mediated and humoral responses that contribute to the demyelination is not defined.[27] Genetic susceptibility probably plays a role, because only one dog in a group of dogs bitten by the same raccoon may develop the disease. Pathologic changes are usually prominent in ventral roots and spinal nerves, with fewer changes in peripheral nerves. Leukocytic infiltration, demyelination, and degeneration of axons and myelin are found.[28]

Clinical Signs

The initial sign may be a stiff, stilted gait that rapidly (in 24–48 hours) progresses to weakness in the pelvic limbs and then in the thoracic limbs. Although some dogs may show only a mild weakness, most dogs are nonambulatory and quadriparetic rather than quadriplegic.[26] As the cervical muscles become weakened, the dog has difficulty raising its head. Occasionally, intercostal muscles become involved and breathing becomes labored. Spinal reflexes are generally decreased to absent except for perineal and cutaneous trunci reflexes, which are usually normal. Pain sensation remains intact, and most dogs seem to be hyperesthetic in response to painful stimuli. For example, during testing of the flexor reflex, most affected dogs whine or cry with even a gentle pinch of the toes. Muscle tone is reduced, and within a few days muscle atrophy becomes apparent. Cranial nerves are occasionally involved, causing facial weakness or a hoarse bark.

Diagnostic Plan

A raccoon bite 7 to 10 days before the onset of clinical signs has been a common historical finding in many but not all cases. In animals with a history of raccoon exposure, the clinical diagnosis is based on the history, the acute onset of LMN paralysis, and the absence of other diseases as determined by history, physical examination, and routine laboratory work. In patients that do not have a history of exposure to raccoons, the diagnosis can be more difficult because other disorders can have a similar appearance, including tick paralysis, botulism, protozoal myositis or neuritis[8, 29] and myasthenia gravis crisis.[7] EMG can help to differentiate acute polyradiculoneuritis from

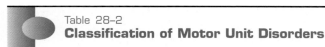

Table 28–2
Classification of Motor Unit Disorders

CATEGORY	MUSCLE DISORDERS	NEUROMUSCULAR JUNCTION DISORDERS	PERIPHERAL NERVE DISORDERS
Metabolic or endocrine	Hyperadrenocorticism Hypothyroidism Malignant hyperthermia Hypokalemic polymyopathy		Diabetes mellitus Hypothyroidism Hyperinsulinism Paraneoplastic neuropathy
Inflammatory or infectious	*Toxoplasma gondii* *Neospora caninum* *Clostridium* *Leptospira* *Dirofilaris immitis* *Hepatozoon canis*		*Toxoplasma gondii* infection *Neospora caninum* infection
Immune-mediated	Masticatory myositis Polymyositis Acquired myasthenia gravis	Acquired myasthenia gravis	
Inherited	Dermatomyositis Muscular dystrophy Myotonic myopathy Hereditary myopathy	Congenital myasthenia gravis	See Table 28–4
Neoplastic	Rhadomyosarcoma		Nerve sheath tumors Lymphosarcoma
Toxic		Organophosphates Carbamates Tick paralysis Botulism	Organophosphates Heavy metals Vincristine
Traumatic	Traumatic myopathy		Nerve root or brachial plexus avulsion Peripheral nerve injury
Idiopathic	Myositis ossificans		Dysautonomia

botulism and tick paralysis because of the presence of denervation potentials in coonhound paralysis. However, this test may not be readily available. Motor nerve conduction velocity is often normal in coonhound paralysis, but it can be slowed if there is significant demyelination of the more distal parts of the peripheral nerves. CSF analysis from the lumbar cistern shows an increase in total protein without pleocytosis. If none of these tests is available, the tentative diagnosis of coonhound paralysis can be made based on the history, the clinical signs, and the fact that coonhound paralysis occurs more frequently than does botulism, protozoal myositis or neuritis, or myasthenia gravis.[27, 28]

Treatment

Supportive care is critical and includes frequent turning and the use of soft bedding to help prevent decubital ulcer formation; daily flexion and extension of limb joints to maintain flexibility; and assistance with eating, urination (bladder compression or catheterization), and defecation (enemas). Corticosteroids are used by some clinicians in the early course of the disorder if there are no contraindications such as decubital ulcers, urinary tract infections, or aspiration pneumonia. Appropriate antibiotics are used to treat any such secondary infections.

Prognosis

Because most dogs recover spontaneously, the prognosis is generally good if supportive care can be given over weeks to several months. Occasionally, the bladder is paralyzed for several weeks or the dog retains urine until it is taken outside. Either of these situations can make a urinary tract infection a likely sequela. Respiratory muscle weakness occasionally results in death unless ventilation is assisted, but this is an uncommon sequela. Recovery does not prevent the dog from having another episode; in fact, some dogs have experienced up to seven bouts.[26]

Tick Paralysis

Tick paralysis is an LMN ascending paralysis caused by a neurotoxin produced by ticks of the genera *Dermacentor* (in United States) and *Ixodes* (in Australia). Although the disorder appears to be common, especially in the spring and summer months when ticks are most evident, the true incidence is not known. Any age, sex, and breed of dog can be affected. Cases have been described in cats in Australia[30] but not in the United States.

Pathophysiology

Adult ticks, especially female ones, produce a salivary neurotoxin that circulates in the host animal and interferes with ACH liberation at the neuromuscular junction, creating a neuromuscular blockade. Various species of ticks are incriminated in different parts of the world, with subsequent variation in the severity of the disease produced. For *Ixodes* spp., the paralysis is caused by a temperature-dependent inhibition of the evoked release of ACH at the neuromuscular junction.[9, 31]

Clinical Signs

In the United States, the clinical signs cannot reliably be differentiated from those of acute polyradiculoneuritis (see previous section). Dogs with tick paralysis are not as hyperesthetic in response to touch or other noxious stimuli as those with acute polyradiculoneuritis. In Australia, affected animals may have sensory and autonomic involvement in addition to the motor deficits.[3] Hypothermia, dilated pupils with poor to no response to light, regurgitation or vomiting, and increasing dyspnea are other prominent signs.[30] Clinical signs tend to be more severe with *Ixodes* spp. tick paralysis.

Diagnostic Plan

History, clinical signs, evidence of ticks on the animal, and a return of function after ticks are removed help to establish the diagnosis. If ticks are not observed but tick paralysis is suspected, the dog should be treated with an appropriate insecticide. If electrophysiologic testing is available, EMG and motor nerve conduction velocity studies can aid the diagnosis and may differentiate tick paralysis from polyradiculoneuritis.

Treatment

Removal of ticks manually or by the application of an insecticide usually results in recovery within hours to 1 day in the United States. In Australia, removal of ticks is not sufficient because the disease can progress up to 48 hours even after tick removal. A hyperimmune serum must be administered intravenously to neutralize circulating tick toxin. The efficacy varies from batch to batch, but a general dosage recommendation is 0.5 to 1.0 mL/kg.[30]

Prognosis

Prognosis is excellent in the United States after the ticks are removed. The prognosis for tick paralysis in Australia is guarded even after treatment with hyperimmune serum.

Myasthenia Gravis

Myasthenia gravis is a neuromuscular disorder characterized by an acquired or congenital decrease in the number of ACH receptors. The incidence is unknown, but acquired myasthenia gravis appears to be one of the most common disorders of the neuromuscular junction in dogs.[9] Both acquired and congenital forms are rare in cats. Although various breeds of dogs have been affected with the acquired form, the German shepherd is overrepresented.[3] For the acquired form, there are peaks of incidence at 2 to 3 and at 9 to 10 years of age, with females more frequently affected in the older group.[3] The congenital form has been recognized in Jack Russell terriers, springer spaniels, and smooth-haired fox terriers at 6 to 9 weeks of age.[32] Acquired and congenital forms have been also observed in cats.[33–35]

Pathophysiology

Acquired myasthenia gravis is caused by an immune-mediated interference of neuromuscular transmission. Antibodies made against the postsynaptic ACH receptor attach to and cause immune-mediated destruction of the receptor. The initiating event that leads to antibody formation is unknown. A high proportion of humans with myasthenia gravis have thymic abnormalities, but thymic disease has been observed in only a small number of animals with myasthenia gravis.[9]

The congenital form is caused by a deficiency or abnormality of the postsynaptic ACH receptor rather than an immune-mediated destruction. Therefore, circulating anti-ACH receptor antibodies are not observed and cannot be demonstrated in muscle. The congenital form is probably inherited as an autosomal recessive trait.[9, 32, 36]

Clinical Signs

Exercise-induced weakness to the point of collapse, increased fatigue, and regurgitation from reduced esophageal motility are among the most common signs. Muscle tremors, a short choppy gait,[9] and hindlimb weakness are often observed before collapse. Weakness often improves after rest. The neurologic examination is unremarkable during periods of normality after rest. Occasionally, animals present with regurgitation or secondary aspiration pneumonia without a history of collapse or weakness.[11]

Diagnostic Plan

A tentative diagnosis can be based on the signalment, history, and observation of exercise-induced weakness. Other possible causes of exertional weakness (see Table 28–1) should be considered and excluded by a thorough physical examination (cardiac arrhythmias or murmurs, abnormal lung sounds), fasting blood chemistry profile (electrolyte abnormalities, hypoglycemia, hypocalcemia), and hemogram (anemia). A normal creatine kinase level decreases the possibility of polymyositis.

After these other possibilities have been eliminated, pharmacologic testing may support the diagnosis of acquired myasthenia gravis. After the dog or cat is in the collapsed state, an immediate IV injection of 1 to 10 mg of the short-acting anticholinesterase edrophonium chloride (Tensilon)[9] should reverse the collapse. Within 30 seconds of the injection, the animal arises and walks or runs without weakness for approximately 5 to 10 minutes. However, the test is not completely reliable[7] and should not be used as the sole method of diagnosing myasthenia gravis. An assay for circulating ACH receptor antibody* can confirm the diagnosis of acquired myasthenia gravis in many cases. However, approximately 15% of myasthenic dogs do not have an elevated ACH receptor antibody concentration, and immunologic tests on muscle samples are necessary to identify immune complexes at the neuromuscular junction.[4, 37]

Teaching hospitals or neurology specialty practices may be able to perform repetitive nerve stimulation studies as another means of diagnosing myasthenia gravis.[22] Most myasthenia gravis cases show a decremental response to repetitive nerve stimulation because of rapid and progressive failure of neuromuscular junction transmission. Normal animals do not show such a response. Animals diagnosed with the acquired form should have chest radiographs performed to evaluate for the presence of a thymic mass, because a few cases have been associated with a thymoma.[9] Such radiographs should also yield information about the possibility of aspiration pneumonia, a common sequela to the megaesophagus that is associated with many myasthenic cases.

Treatment

Longer-acting anticholinesterase drugs, such as pyridostigmine or neostigmine, are used to treat both forms of the disease. If the animal can tolerate oral medication, 0.5 to 3.0 mg/kg pyridostigmine bromide syrup, diluted in water, is administered by mouth in divided doses two times (b.i.d.) or three times (t.i.d.) per day,[9, 34] beginning at the lower dose and gradually increasing it to the point at which clinical signs are not improved any further. If oral medication is not possible because of dysphagia or regurgitation, injectable neostigmine at a dosage of 0.04 mg/kg can be can be administered intramuscularly four times per day until oral medications can be tolerated. The treatment of aspiration pneumonia is discussed in Chapter 54.

Because the acquired form has an immune-mediated basis, immunosuppressive doses of prednisolone (1.0–1.5 mg/kg b.i.d. by mouth)[9] are used if muscle strength does not improve significantly after anticholinesterase treatment. After a clinical response is observed, the dose is reduced by one eighth to one fourth every 2 weeks to get to the lowest dose every other day that controls the clinical signs. The long-term side effects of corticosteroids should be discussed with the owner. Prednisolone must be avoided if aspiration pneumonia is present. If megaesophagus is present, the animal should be fed and allowed to drink water in an upright position that is maintained for 15 to 20 minutes after eating to help avoid aspiration pneumonia.

Prognosis

If aspiration pneumonia is present, the prognosis is guarded because this complication can result in death. With appropriate treatment, the prognosis is fair to good in cases of acquired myasthenia gravis. Megaesophagus may resolve, but resolution may take longer than the weakness.[9] In some acquired cases, there is spontaneous remission within variable periods of time. The prognosis in congenital cases is guarded because the condition is permanent.

Traumatic Neuropathies

Traumatic neuropathies are those nerve disorders produced by injuries such as tearing, stretching, or compression of nerves. Although statistics are not available, trauma is a common cause of neuropathy. Any age, sex, or breed of dog or cat can be injured.

---

* Available from Comparative Neuromuscular Laboratory, School of Veterinary Medicine, University of California at San Diego, La Jolla, California.

Pathophysiology

Nerve trauma is most commonly associated with automobile accidents, but other sources of injury include intramuscular injections, fractures and their repair, bite wounds, and lacerations. In cases of automobile or falling accidents, nerve roots at the spinal cord level are more likely to be pulled or avulsed than are nerves at the brachial plexus.[38, 39]

There are three degrees of nerve injury: axonotmesis, neurotmesis, and neurapraxia. Axonotmesis is severance of nerve fibers (axons) within the nerve bundle, and neurotmesis is severance of axons as well as their connective tissue sheath. Neurotmesis is the more severe injury, because axonal regeneration is hampered by the lack of the scaffold of connective tissue to guide the direction of axonal growth. Neurapraxia is a physiologic rather than a physical disruption of nerve fibers. Sensory and motor deficits usually exist with axonotmesis and neurotmesis, but only motor deficits are present with neurapraxia. Motor function usually returns to normal within days to weeks with neurapraxia; with axonotmesis and neurotmesis, it takes weeks to months. It can be difficult to separate these three degrees of injury without serial neurologic examinations and electrodiagnostic studies.

Clinical Signs

With most peripheral nerve injuries, the history reflects a sudden onset of disuse or paralysis of the affected limb; spinal reflexes are reduced (Fig. 28–4).[40] Table 28–3 lists signs associated with specific nerve injuries. If an injury occurs at the nerve root level in the cervical area, other signs may be found on neurologic examination. For example, damage to the T1 nerve root may cause an ipsilateral Horner's syndrome, and damage to C8 and T1 nerve roots results in lack of cutaneus trunci reflex on the affected side. Occasionally, the ipsilateral pelvic limb may also show conscious proprioceptive deficits or subtle weakness because of injury to white matter near the entrance or exit of nerve roots. Damage to nerve roots C5 through C7 can cause ipsilateral paralysis of the diaphragm, which may be noted on fluoroscopic examination.

Diagnostic Plan

A history or clinical signs of trauma, monoparesis, and reduced spinal reflexes are suggestive of nerve root or peripheral nerve trauma. Muscles on the affected limb lack tone, and a significant amount of atrophy develops in 1 to 2 weeks after trauma. Denervation potentials can be found on EMG examination 5 days after injury, and changes in motor nerve conduction velocity can be found within 3 days of

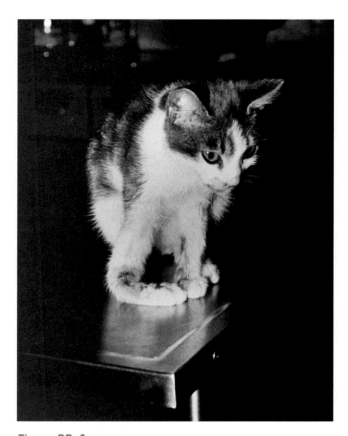

Figure 28–4
A cat with nerve root avulsion at the C8 to T2 nerve root level. The limb cannot support weight because of radial nerve damage.

injury. Radiographs of the affected area may indicate evidence of bone damage or muscle swelling associated with the trauma.

Treatment

There is no specific treatment other than physical therapy to prevent tendon and muscle contracture. Gentle muscle massage and flexion and extension of all joints several times a day are recommended. To prevent abrasions, particularly if the animal drags the foot when walking, the foot should be protected with a thick sock, boot, or bandage. If the pet begins to lick or chew at the limb, an Elizabethan collar may help to prevent more damage. It is important to warn the client that self-mutilation can be severe if the animal cannot feel pain sensations. If abrasions become infected, systemic antibiotics and soaking of the area in astringents or antibacterial solutions may be of benefit.

Prognosis

The prognosis is depends on severity of damage. The patient with radial nerve paralysis and lack of deep pain perception to the digits has a guarded

Table 28–3
Signs of Individual Nerve Injury

NERVE	ORIGIN	CLINICAL SIGNS	REFLEXES AFFECTED
Radial	C6–T1	Injury proximal to branches that supply triceps muscle; unable to support weight; limb collapses; may carry the limb if musculocutaneous nerve is functional; triceps muscle atrophy Injury distal to branches that supply triceps muscle: can support some weight but stands on dorsum of paw	Reduced to absent triceps and extensor carpi radialis reflexes
Musculocutaneous	C6–C8	No gait changes; slight straightening of angle to elbow joint	Reduced withdrawal and biceps reflexes
Median and ulnar	C8–T2	Slight carpal extension ("dropped carpus")	Reduced carpal flexion on withdrawal reflex
Femoral	L4–L6	Unable to support weight; limb collapses or may be carried; short stride; lack of pain perception on medial surface of thigh, stifle, leg, and paw; atrophy of quadriceps muscle	Reduced to absent patellar reflex
Sciatic	L6–S2	Supports weight on limb but stands on dorsum of paw; unable to flex or extend hock; atrophy of biceps femoris, semimembranous, semitendinous, cranial tibial, and gastrocnemius muscles; lack of pain perception on caudal and lateral sides of leg	Reduced to absent withdrawal reflex
Peroneal	L6–S2	Straightening of hock; stands on dorsum of paw and hock	Reduced to absent flexion on withdrawal reflex
Tibial	L6–S2	Increased flexion of hock ("dropped" hock)	—
Obturator	L5–L6	Abduction of limb on slippery surface	—

prognosis; the patient with some pain perception has a more favorable prognosis. The patient with a more proximally located injury has a more guarded prognosis than one with a distal injury because of the time and distance it takes the nerve to regenerate and reach the muscles. Regrowth of injured nerves (axonotmesis or neurotmesis) is slow (about 2.5 cm/month).[20] If self-mutilation occurs or if acceptable improvement does not occur, amputation should be considered.

Acquired Polyneuropathies

Acquired polyneuropathies are disorders of peripheral nerves that result from toxic, metabolic, endocrine, neoplastic, or idiopathic disorders (see Table 28–2). Some idiopathic acquired polyneuropathies have been given descriptive names because they have characteristic signs. The incidence is probably higher than what is recognized because some cases may be subclinical or the neurologic signs may be attributed to the disease rather than to a neuropathy created by the disease. Any age, sex, or breed of dog or cat can be affected.

Pathophysiology

The exact pathophysiology for nerve fiber degeneration or demyelination for most endocrine disorders is not fully understood. For paraneoplastic neuropathies, there is probably an immune reaction to antigens shared by the tumor on a peripheral nerve. Toxins can affect nerves in many ways. For other disorders, there have not been any reasonable explanations for the nerve damage.

Clinical Signs

Progressive weakness of limbs with reduction in spinal reflexes and muscle mass are hallmark signs for most acquired polyneuropathies. Pelvic limbs are usually more noticeably affected. Cranial nerve deficits may develop in some cases. Some disorders have a characteristic history or clinical sign that allows the disorder to be more easily recognized. For example, the classic sign of diabetic neuropathy in cats is that of a plantigrade stance (dropped hock).[41] Chronic relapsing polyradiculoneuritis is characterized by an insidious onset of LMN weakness with periods of remission and subsequent relapses.[42, 43] Distal polyneuropathy in Doberman pinschers ("dancing Doberman disease")[44] is a slowly progressive distal axonopathy that begins with persistent pelvic limb flexion or bicycling motions noted when the dog is standing.[45]

Diagnostic Plan

Historical information and signs of systemic illness should yield clues for beginning the investigation of possible causes of the LMN weakness. Animals with diabetic neuropathy should have a history of polyuria, polydipsia, and weight loss in addition to the LMN weakness. Those with hypothyroid neuropathy may have historical or physical examination changes suggestive of hypothyroidism; breed predilection should also be considered. Routine laboratory evaluation (hemogram, blood chemistry profile, and urinalysis) should aid the primary diagnosis of an endocrine disorder, but electrodiagnostic tests (EMG and nerve conduction studies) and muscle and nerve biopsies are required to confirm the polyneuropathy.

If routine laboratory data are normal, the possibility of neoplasia should be considered in the older patient. Thoracic radiographs, careful abdominal palpation, abdominal radiographs, or abdominal ultrasound may reveal a mass. Toxic disorders are more difficult to diagnose unless the owner knows that the animal was exposed to a specific toxin; careful inquiry into potential toxin exposure is necessary. Toxins or drugs that could cause a neuropathy include organophosphorus compounds[18]; heavy metals such as mercury, arsenic, lead, or thallium[46]; and vincristine.[47]

In cases in which an underlying cause cannot be found, the diagnosis of idiopathic polyneuropathy is made. In such cases, an underlying cause may become more obvious at a later date, and it is therefore important to pursue follow-up examinations and testing.

Treatment

Treatment is directed at removal or correction of the underlying abnormality if one can be identified. If an underlying cause for the neuropathy cannot be identified, prednisolone (2 mg/kg once daily by mouth) can be used cautiously with gradual dose reduction, after clinical response is noted, by one eighth to one fourth every 2 weeks until the lowest alternate-day dose that provides control is reached.

Prognosis

The prognosis is good to guarded if the underlying condition (e.g., diabetes mellitus) can be identified and treated. The prognosis for cases without any identifiable cause is guarded because many of them are progressive.

Peripheral Nerve Neoplasia

Peripheral nerve sheath neoplasias are malignant transformations of Schwann cells (schwannoma, neurinoma, or neurilemmoma) or endoneural and epineural fibroblasts (neurofibroma or neurofibrosarcoma). Other tumors that can affect peripheral nerves include lymphosarcoma, chondrosarcoma,[39] and osteosarcoma. In one study, peripheral nerve tumors represented 26.6% of canine nervous system tumors.[48] Although any breed or either sex of mature dog or cat can be affected, middle-aged to older animals are most commonly affected.[49–51]

Pathophysiology

Reasons for malignant transformation of Schwann cells or fibroblasts are not known. Lymphosarcoma, chondrosarcoma, and osteosarcoma can affect peripheral nerves either by diffusely infiltrating them or by entrapping them.

Clinical Signs

Signs vary with the location of the tumor. Many involve the spinal nerve roots that make up the brachial plexus, the cervical or thoracolumbar nerve roots, or, less commonly, the roots of cranial nerves. Vague lameness progressing to monoparesis is the most common clinical sign if the nerve roots or peripheral nerves of limbs are involved.[49] Muscle atrophy occurs and is usually significant. If the brachial plexus is involved, neoplastic cells can invade the adjacent spinal nerve roots and proliferate within the spinal canal, causing subsequent spinal cord compression and weakness of the ipsilateral pelvic limb followed by quadriparesis or quadriparalysis. Tumors of individual nerves produce clinical signs associated with dysfunction of the particular nerve (see Table 28–3).

Diagnostic Plan

In early stages, peripheral nerve tumors are difficult to diagnose. For patients presenting with lameness, other causes of lameness must be investigated first. If orthopedic examination, joint aspiration, and radiography of the affected limb do not yield a diagnosis, then a nerve root tumor in the early growth stage should be considered. EMG may show denervation potentials and may be able to localize the abnormality to a specific nerve or even a specific location on a nerve. Exploratory surgery of the brachial plexus area is in order if the condition has been documented to be progressing, if orthopedic diseases have been eliminated, and if there are EMG changes. If the neurologic examination shows lack of ipsilateral cutaneous trunci reflex or weakness or proprioceptive deficits in the rear limbs or the opposite thoracic limb, cervical radiographs, CSF analysis, and myelography are indicated. CSF analysis can potentially show neoplastic cells, especially in cases of lymphosarcoma. The newer techniques of computed tomography and magnetic resonance imaging may yield more specific and diagnostic information, possibly allowing the diagnosis of these tumors before they invade the spinal canal. Definitive diagnosis requires cytologic analysis of fine-needle aspirates or biopsy of masses palpated or delineated by imaging techniques.

Treatment

The recommended treatment is surgical excision of the tumor, which may not be possible without amputation of the affected limb or excision of nerve roots or nerves. Exploration of the brachial plexus area may reveal that the mass cannot be removed without damage to nerves, which may then render the limb nonfunctional. Excision of nerve roots that are not associated with either the cervical or lumbosacral intumescence should not result in limb weakness. Chemotherapy can be attempted for tumors such as lymphosarcomas, but chemotherapy and radiation treatment have not been effective for nerve sheath tumors.[51]

Prognosis

Although peripheral nerve and nerve root tumors can sometimes be resected, the prognosis is guarded until the extent of the mass is known. Even if the mass can be surgically removed, the nerves surrounding it may be damaged, causing further neurologic deficits. A poorer prognosis is given for patients that have signs of spinal cord compression; surgery is not likely to improve their condition for any long period of time.

Masticatory Myositis

Masticatory myositis, a focal inflammation of the muscles of mastication, has been called eosinophilic and atrophic myositis, idiopathic inflammatory muscle disease, and polymyositis.[52, 53] Masticatory myositis is distinct from polymyositis in that only the masticatory muscles are involved. The true incidence is unknown, but in my experience the disease is fairly common. Dogs of any age and breed can be affected, although large breeds of dogs predominate. Samoyeds, Doberman pinschers, and German shepherds appear

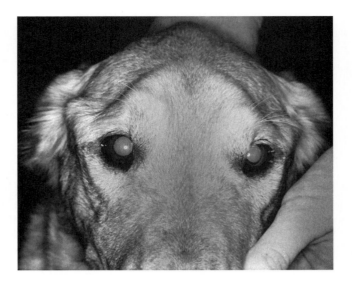

Figure 28–5
A dog with severe atrophy of the temporalis and masseter muscles from masticatory myositis. (Courtesy of Karen Dyer, DVM, Blacksburg, Virginia.)

to be more commonly affected than other breeds. The condition has not been reported in cats.

Pathophysiology

Documented histochemical and biochemical differences between canine masticatory and limb muscles provide a basis for a selective immune-mediated response. Autoantibodies against cytoplasmic and sarcolemmal proteins of masticatory muscle fibers have been demonstrated.[4] In addition, an immune-mediated pathogenesis has been suspected because of the response to immunosuppressive doses of corticosteroids.

Clinical Signs

In the initial stage, masseter and temporal muscles may be visibly swollen and painful on palpation. The dog is often reluctant to open its mouth, and the owner may have the pet examined because of its reluctance to eat, decreased appetite, or even weight loss. Some dogs are febrile and have enlarged tonsils or mandibular lymph nodes.[16] A few patients have presented with exophthalmos because of pressure on retrobulbar tissue by the swollen muscles.[52] Repeated bouts of inflammation result in atrophy of the muscles and replacement of myofibers with connective tissue (Fig. 28–5). In this later stage, trismus occurs, not because of pain but because of muscle fibrosis. Again, the owner's complaint may be related to inability of the dog to eat or lack of appetite. A few animals have been presented because of a lump on top of the head; this was actually the occipital protuberance, which had become more noticeable after the surrounding temporal muscles atrophied.

Diagnostic Plan

A tentative diagnosis can be based on findings of trismus and painful or swollen masticatory muscles in the initial stage, or trismus and atrophy of these muscles in the chronic stage. Creatine kinase may be elevated in the initial stage, but this is an unreliable finding. EMG may show mild changes in both stages but tends to be abnormally silent in the fibrotic stage because so few normal muscle fibers remain. The disease is confirmed by histopathologic evaluation of muscle and immunocytochemical staining (available from Comparative Neuromuscular Laboratory, School of Veterinary Medicine, University of California at San Diego, La Jolla, California) for the detection of immune complexes.[52, 53]

Treatment

Prednisolone (1.0–1.5 mg/kg, by mouth b.i.d.) should be used for 3 to 4 weeks, followed by tapering of the dose by one fourth every 2 weeks until one half of the original dose is reached. One half of the original dose is then administered every other day for 2 weeks, at which time the dosage can be tapered by one eighth to one fourth every 2 weeks. Should clinical signs recur while the dose is being tapered, the dose is increased to the level that last appeared to control the signs. Some dogs require prednisolone treatment indefinitely; others can be weaned from it after several months of treatment. A common mistake is to treat for too short a time or to wean too fast. After atrophy and fibrosis develop, prednisolone is often not as effective.

Prognosis

The prognosis is fair to good in the initial, acute stage, because clinical signs can usually be significantly improved with prednisolone. The prognosis becomes more guarded after atrophy and fibrosis develop. Because some dogs may have relapses that require reinstitution of prednisolone, the prognosis for complete recovery is guarded.

Polymyositis

Polymyositis is a generalized inflammatory disease of skeletal muscles with many possible causes, including parasites, bacteria, neoplasia, and autoimmune disorders. It is a condition that occurs occasionally and may actually be more common than is recognized. Any age and breed of dog can be affected, but mature adults of large breeds seem to be more commonly diagnosed with polymyositis than others.[54]

Pathophysiology

There are numerous causes of polymyositis. Parasitic agents presently recognized as causing myositis include *Trypanosoma cruzi, T. gondii, Neospora caninum, and Hepatozoon canis.*[55] *T. cruzi* infections are more common in the Gulf Coast states and tend to affect the myocardium of puppies. Cases of hepatozoonosis have been limited to the southern United States and have been characterized by fever, muscle pain and atrophy, and a leukocytosis. *N. caninum* is a newly recognized protozoan that can cause meningoencephalitis, neuritis, and myositis in dogs. In retrospect, some cases reported to be toxoplasmosis may have actually been neosporosis. Although other parasites, such as *Trichinella spiralis, Ancylostoma caninum, Sarcocystis* spp.,[56] and *Hammondia* spp., have been found in muscles, they are probably more of an incidental finding than an indication of disease.[57] *Dirofilaria immitis* adults can occlude vessels, especially those in the pelvic limbs, and produce myofiber degeneration or necrosis as well as wallerian-type degeneration of peripheral nerves.[58, 59]

Bacterial agents include streptococci, staphylococci, *Pasteurella, Leptospira icterohaemorrhagiae,* and *Clostridium* spp.[58] Such organisms may cause a local myositis after direct implantation into wounds.

In many cases of polymyositis, an immune-mediated pathogenesis is suspected based on histopathologic findings and response to immunosuppressive therapy. What triggers the immune response is usually not known. Polymyositis has been reported in conjunction with systemic lupus erythematosus and neoplasia in dogs.[60, 61]

Clinical Signs

Clinical signs can be variable but usually include weakness that may be exacerbated by exercise. Owners may report that the affected animal is reluctant to move or appears to have pain when moving. Muscle stiffness or wasting, lameness, and a stilted gait can be observed. In severe cases, the animal may be recumbent and unable to support weight. Depression, fever, and lymphadenopathy may also be observed, especially with infectious, immune, or neoplastic causes. Regurgitation may occur if esophageal muscles are involved. Involvement of laryngeal muscles can cause a voice change or inspiratory dyspnea. Spinal reflexes are usually normal but can be reduced in those animals with severe disease.[54] The pet may show evidence of atrophy or pain on muscle palpation.

In pups younger than 4 months of age, a characteristic, irreversible pelvic limb extensor rigidity may develop with *N. caninum* or *T. gondii* infection.[62–64] Joints cannot be flexed or extended normally, even when the dog is anesthetized.

Diagnostic Plan

An elevated white blood cell count has been reported in some dogs, but this is not a consistent finding.[54] Although an elevation in the serum levels of muscle enzymes should increase the index of suspicion of polymyositis, elevations do not necessarily correlate with the severity of the disease,[65] and some patients do not demonstrate such elevations. EMG changes are usually present but cannot be distinguished from those found with neuropathies.[54] Definitive diagnosis of polymyositis is based on muscle biopsy results.[54] Serum titers for *Toxoplasma* or *Neospora* spp. can be helpful (see Chap. 40).

Histologic changes consist of a perivascular cellular infiltrate that may extend into the perimysium. Cell type varies with the disease process, but lymphocytes, macrophages, and plasma cells are commonly observed with many polymyositides, especially those that are immune-mediated. Eosinophils may be found with parasitic processes, and parasitic agents may occasionally be observed. Myofiber necrosis and regenerating fibers can also be observed.

Treatment

If infectious or parasitic causes are identified, appropriate antibiotic or antiparasitic drugs should be administered. If protozoal myositis is diagnosed or suspected, clindamycin (10–40 mg/kg per day, in divided doses three to four times per day) should be administered for at least 2 weeks. Trimethoprim-sulfadiazine (15 mg/kg b.i.d.) and pyrimethamine (1 mg/kg daily) can also be used for 2 weeks.

Treatment of idiopathic or immune-mediated polymyositis consists of prednisolone (1–2 mg/kg b.i.d. by mouth) for several weeks, followed by a gradual reduction in dosage over several months. It is wise to taper the dose slowly, because relapses are common. Some dogs, such as those with systemic lupus erythematosus, must be maintained on alternate-day corticosteroid therapy indefinitely. Other immunosuppressive drugs, such as azathioprine (2.2 mg/kg by mouth daily to remission then every other day) or cyclophosphamide (1 mg/kg by mouth daily for 4 days per week), can be added if there is no response to corticosteroids.

Prognosis

The prognosis is guarded for most patients until the underlying cause can be found and appropriately treated. If extensor limb rigidity develops because of protozoal infection, the prognosis for regaining normal function of the affected limbs is poor.

Uncommon Diseases of Peripheral Nerve, Neuromuscular Junction, and Muscles

Botulism

Botulism is a disease of acute LMN weakness caused by ingestion of spoiled food or carrion containing a preformed exotoxin (type C) produced by the bacteria *Clostridium botulinum*.[66] The ingested preformed exotoxin blocks or interferes with the release of ACH from the neuromuscular junction, producing neuromuscular blockade. Clinically, botulism is difficult to differentiate from acute polyradiculoneuritis or tick paralysis, but botulism may have more obvious cranial nerve involvement (i.e., dysphagia, dysphonia, mydriasis, and facial weakness). Treatment is essentially supportive, although administration of laxatives and enemas may help to remove unabsorbed toxin from the gastrointestinal tract.[9] Duration of clinical signs is usually 1 to 2 weeks, but occasionally recovery takes longer.[67]

Congenital and Inherited Myopathies

Clinical signs of congenital and inherited myopathies are usually noted during the first few months of life and consist of weakness or stiffness, decreased exercise tolerance, and muscle atrophy or hypertrophy (Table 28–4).[68–77] Although the creatine kinase level may be elevated, the diagnosis relies on results of EMG and muscle histopathology examinations. Prognosis is guarded because there are no specific treatments, although mildly affected animals can make acceptable pets (see Table 28–4).

Congenital and Inherited Neuropathies

Congenital or inherited polyneuropathies include disorders that affect peripheral nerves or lower motor neurons in the gray matter of the spinal cord.[78–86] The overall incidence is low, and such disorders are usually breed-specific and evident by 1 year of age (see Table 28–4). Because there are no known treatments for these disorders, the prognosis is poor and signs are often progressive.

Table 28–4
Classification of Congenital and Inherited Muscle and Nerve Disorders in Dogs and Cats

DISEASE AND REFERENCE	SIGNALMENT	BRIEF DESCRIPTION
Nemaline myopathy[68]	Young cats	Hypermetric gain; depressed patellar reflexes
Myotonic myopathy[69,70]	Immature chow chows, Staffordshire terriers, Great Danes	Stiffness; rigidity; hypertrophy of proximal limb and neck muscles; worse in cold weather; suspected to be inherited
Muscular dystrophy[70–72,76,77]	Golden retrievers, Irish terriers, Samoyeds, rottweilers, Bouvier des Flandres, cats; males	Stunted growth; weakness; hypertrophy of proximal limb muscles; dysphagia; elevated creatine kinase; similar to Duchenne muscular dystrophy in humans
Dermatomyositis[74,75]	2- to 12-month-old collies, Shetland sheep dogs	Dermatitis of face, tail tip, ears, and distal extremities; inflammatory myopathy of distal limb muscles and masticatory muscles; inherited in collies
Hereditary myopathy (type II myofiber deficiency)[73]	2- to 6-month-old Laborador retrievers	Progressive exercise and cold intolerance; muscle atrophy; bunny-hoping gait; signs improve with rest and often stabilize before 1 year of age; autosomal recessive inheritance
Globoid cell leukodystrophy[78]	Young West Highland white and cairn terriers, Pomeranians, beagles, poodles, blue-tick hounds, basset hounds, cats	Inherited storage disease; paraparesis that progresses to quadriparesis
Hypomyelinating polyneuropathy[79]	Young golden retrievers	Pelvic limb ataxia and atrophy; may stabilize
Boxer neuropathy[80,81]	Young boxers	Slowly progressive pelvic limb ataxia
Spinal muscular atrophy[82,83]	Brittany spaniels, rottweilers, Swedish Laplands, English pointers	Lower motor neuron weakness and muscle atrophy
Hypertrophic polyneuropathy[84]	7- to 12-month-old Tibetan mastiffs	Hyporeflexia; quadriparesis; inherited metabolic defect of Schwann cells
Giant axonal neuropathy[85,86]	14- to 16-month-old German shepherds	Paraparesis; decreased patellar reflexes; megaesophagus; muscle atrophy distal to stifles; diminished bark; autosomal recessive inheritance likely

Sensory Neuropathies

Sensory neuropathies can be acquired or inherited (familial). Inherited sensory neuropathies have been reported in 3- to 4-month-old pointers, who bit and licked at their paws, resulting in mutilation.[87] Signs in 3-month-old long-haired dachshunds have included progressive pelvic limb ataxia, urinary incontinence, and decreased pain perception over the entire body.[88] There are no treatments for such disorders. Signs associated with acquired sensory neuropathies have included progressive ataxia, decreased patellar reflexes, variable degrees of reduced facial sensation, dysphagia, and prehension difficulty.[89–91]

Dysautonomia (Key-Gaskell syndrome) is a type of sensory neuropathy reported in cats and dogs in the United Kingdom in the 1980s.[92] The frequency of occurrence of the disease appears to have reduced markedly in recent years. Clinical signs included mydriasis, regurgitation, constipation, dry mucous membranes, bradycardia, and prolapse of the nictitating membrane. Recovery was possible with months of supportive care. Histopathologically, there was a loss of neurons in all autonomic ganglia, some cranial nerve ganglia, and some ventral horn cells in the spinal cord.[92]

Acquired Myopathies

Acquired metabolic myopathies[93] include exertional myopathy, malignant hyperthermia, and electrolyte imbalances. Malignant hyperthermia can be

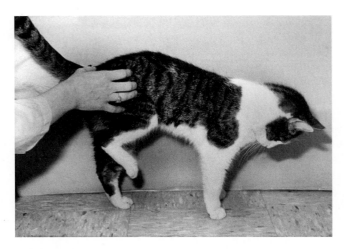

Figure 28-6
A cat with ventroflexion of the neck because of hypokalemia. This cat had chronic renal failure.

related to either exercise or anesthesia (halothane anesthesia in particular). Breeds affected include greyhounds,[94] English springer spaniels, Labrador retrievers, Saint Bernards, Border collies, pointers,[93] and Chesapeake Bay retrievers. Temperature elevation, tachycardia, tachypnea, rigidity of limbs, trismus, and possibly respiratory and cardiac arrest are common features.[93]

Electrolyte abnormalities, such as alterations in the concentrations of K^+ or Ca^{++}, can cause muscle weakness.[95] A hypokalemic polymyopathy related to renal disease, diuresis, or certain diets with insufficient potassium has been documented in cats,[96] in whom a characteristic ventroflexion of the neck is observed clinically (Fig. 28-6). Supplementation with potassium reverses the clinical signs.

Subclinical as well as clinical myopathies can be found in dogs with endocrine disorders. Endocrinopathies that have been reported to affect muscles include hyperadrenocorticism,[15, 97] hyperthyroidism, hypothyroidism, hypoadrenocorticism, hypopituitarism, primary aldosteronism, primary hyperparathyroidism, and hypoparathyroidism.[93]

Ischemic Neuropathy Resulting From Thromboembolism

Embolus formation associated with cardiomyopathy in cats can occlude one or more branches of the aorta to cause paraparesis, paraplegia, loss of femoral pulses, cold limbs, and pale or cyanotic foot pads and nails. Acute ischemia of nerve and muscle is caused by the release of serotonin and not by an actual loss of blood supply. Prognosis depends on the degree of ischemia, the stage of cardiac disease, and whether gangrene develops (see Chap. 12).[58]

Myositis Ossificans

Non-neoplastic bone formation in muscle and other soft tissue structures exists in localized and generalized forms. Trauma is often associated with the development of the localized form, whereas the cause of the generalized form is unknown. Signs include stiffness, weakness, and swollen, painful muscles with firm, palpable lumps. Radiographs may reveal linear bone densities in affected muscles. No specific treatment exists.[62]

Traumatic Myopathy

Muscles can be physically lacerated or their blood supply damaged, causing ischemia. Swelling of muscles within their heavy aponeurotic sheaths can result in increased intramuscular pressure, decreased venous outflow, and ischemia (compartment syndrome).[62]

Muscle Neoplasia

Primary tumors of striated muscle are rare. Rhabomyosarcomas are malignant striated muscle tumors that appear as hard, spheric masses. Malignant melanoma, angiosarcoma, and lymphoreticular system tumors can metastasize to muscle.[62]

References

1. de Lahunta A. Lower motor neuron-general somatic efferent system. In: Veterinary Neuroanatomy and Clinical Neurology, 2nd ed. Philadelphia, WB Saunders, 1983:53–54.
2. Duncan ID. Peripheral nerve disease in the dog and cat. Vet Clin North Am Small Anim Pract 1980;10:177.
3. Wheeler SJ. Disorders of the neuromuscular junction. Prog Vet Neurol 1991;2:129–135.
4. Shelton GD. Differential diagnosis of muscle diseases in companion animals. Prog Vet Neurol 1991;2:27–33.
5. Withrow SJ. Localization and diagnosis of spinal cord lesions in small animals: Part 1. Compen Contin Educ Pract Vet 1980;2:464–474.
6. Oliver JC, Lorenz MD. Handbook of Veterinary Neurologic Diagnosis. Philadelphia, WB Saunders, 1993:46–55.
7. Chrisman CL. Clinical manifestations of multifocal peripheral nerve and muscle disorders in dogs. Compen Contin Educ Pract Vet 1985;7:355–360.
8. Braund KG. Toxoplasma polymyositis/polyneuropathy: A new clinical variant in two mature dogs. J Am Anim Hosp Assoc 1988;24:93–97.
9. Shelton GD. Disorders of neuromuscular transmission. Semin Vet Med Surg (Small Anim) 1989;4:126–132.
10. Berry WL. Episodic weakness in dogs. Compen Contin Educ Pract Vet 1990;12:141–154.
11. Shelton GD, Willard MD, Cardinet GH III, Lindstrom J. Acquired myasthenia gravis: Selective involvement of

esophageal, pharyngeal, and facial muscles. J Vet Intern Med 1990;4:281–284.

12. Dejong RN. Muscle volume and contour. In: Dejong RN, ed. The Neurologic Examination, 4th ed. Hagerstown, Maryland, Harper & Row, 1975:386–392.
13. Kortz G. Canine myotonia. Semin Vet Med Surg (Small Anim) 1989;4:141–145.
14. Griffiths IR, Duncan ID. Myotonia in the dog: A report of four cases. Vet Rec 1973;93:184–188.
15. Duncan ID, Griffiths IR, Nash AS. Myotonia in canine Cushing's disease. Vet Rec 1977;100:30–31.
16. Scott-Moncrieff, Hawkins EC, Cook JR. Canine muscle disorders. Compen Contin Educ Pract Vet, 1990;12:31–39.
17. DiBartola SP, Tasker SB. Elevated serum creatine phosphokinase: A study of 53 cases and a review of its diagnostic usefulness in clinical veterinary medicine. J Am Anim Hosp Assoc 1977;13:744–753.
18. Fikes JD. Organophosphorus and carbamate insecticides. Vet Clin North Am Small Anim Pract 1990;20: 353–367.
19. Niederhauser UB, Holliday TA. Electrodiagnostic studies in diseases of muscles and neuromuscular junction. Semin Vet Med Surg (Small Anim) 1989;4:116–125.
20. Chrisman CL. Peripheral nerve disorders. In: Ettinger SJ, ed. Textbook of Veterinary Internal Medicine, 3rd ed, vol 1. Philadelphia, WB Saunders, 1989:708–732.
21. Griffiths IR. Introduction to the diagnosis and management of neuromuscular disorders in small animals. Prog Vet Neurol 1991;2:21–25.
22. Sims MH, McLean RA. Use of repetitive nerve stimulation to assess neuromuscular function in dogs. Prog Vet Neurol 1990;1:311–319.
23. Braund KG, Walker TL, Vandevelde M. Fascicular nerve biopsy in the dog. Am J Vet Res 1979;40:1025–1030.
24. Braund KG. Diagnostic techniques. In: Braund KG, ed. Clinical Syndromes in Veterinary Neurology. St. Louis, Mosby, 1994:376–421.
25. Braund KG. Nerve and muscle biopsy techniques. Prog Vet Neurol 1991;2:35–56.
26. Duncan ID. Peripheral neuropathy in the dog and cat. Prog Vet Neurol 1991;2:111–128.
27. Cuddon PA. Electrophysiological and immunological evaluation in coonhound paralysis. Proc Am Coll Vet Intern Med Forum 1990;8:1009–1012.
28. Cummings JF. Ganglioradicular diseases in the dog. Proc Am Coll Vet Intern Med Forum 1990;8:1017–1024.
29. Cummings JP, de Lahunta A, Suter MM, et al. Canine protozoan polyradiculoneuritis. Acta Neuropathol (Berl) 1988;76:46–54.
30. Malik R, Farrow BRH. Tick paralysis in North America and Australia. Vet Clin North Am Small Anim Pract 1991;21:157–171.
31. Cooper BJ, Spence I. Temperature-dependent inhibition of evoked acetylcholine release in tick paralysis. Nature 1979;263:693–695.
32. Miller LM, Lennon VA, Lambert EH, et al. Congenital myasthenia gravis in 13 smooth fox terriers. J Am Vet Med Assoc 1983;182:694–697.
33. Indrieri RJ, Creighton SR, Lambert EH, Lennon VA. Myasthenia gravis in two cats. J Am Vet Med Assoc 1983;182:57–60.

34. Joseph KJ, Carillo JM, Lennon VA. Myasthenia gravis in the cat. J Vet Intern Med 1988;2:75–79.
35. Mason KV. A case of myasthenia gravis in a cat. J Small Anim Pract 1979;17:467–472.
36. Johnson RP, Watson ADJ, Smith J, et al. Myasthenia in springer spaniel littermates. J Small Anim Pract 1979;16: 641–647.
37. Pflugfelder CM, Cardinet GH, Lutz H, et al. Acquired myasthenia gravis: Immunocytochemical localization of immune complexes at neuromuscular junctions. Muscle Nerve 1981;4:289–295.
38. Griffiths IR. Avulsion of the brachial plexus: 1. Neuropathology of the spinal cord and peripheral nerves. J Small Anim Pract 1974;15:165–176.
39. Wheeler S, Jones C, Wright J. The diagnosis of brachial plexus disorders in dogs: A review of twenty-two cases. J Small Anim Pract 1986;27:147–157.
40. Griffiths IR, Duncan ID, Lawson DD. Avulsion of the brachial plexus: 2. Clinical aspects. J Small Anim Pract 1984;15:177–182.
41. Kramek BA, Moise NS, Cooper B, et al. Neuropathy associated with diabetes mellitus in the cat. J Am Vet Med Assoc 1984;184:42–45.
42. Cummings JF, de Lahunta A. Chronic relapsing polyradiculoneuritis in a dog: A clinical, light and electron microscope study. Acta Neuropathol (Berl) 1974;28: 191–204.
43. Flecknell PA, Lucke VM. Chronic relapsing polyradiculoneuritis in a cat. Acta Neuropathol (Berl) 1978;41: 81–84.
44. Chrisman CL. Distal polyneuropathy of Doberman pinschers. Proc Am Coll Vet Intern Med Forum 1985; 3:164.
45. Chrisman CL. Dancing Doberman disease. Prog Vet Neurol 1990;1:83–90.
46. Zook BC, Gilmore CE. Thallium poisoning in dogs. J Am Vet Med Assoc 1967;151:206–217.
47. Hamilton TA. Vincristine-induced peripheral neuropathy in a dog. J Am Vet Med Assoc 1991;198:635–638.
48. Hayes HM, Priester WA, Pendergrass TW. Occurrence of nervous-tissue tumors in cattle, horses, cats and dogs. Int J Cancer 1975;15:39–47.
49. Bradley RL, Withrow SJ, Synder SP. Nerve sheath tumors in the dog. J Am Anim Hosp Assoc 1982;18:915–921.
50. Carmichael S, Griffiths IR. Brachial plexus tumors in seven dogs. Vet Rec 1981;108:435–437.
51. Brehm DM, Vite CH, Steinberg HS, et al. A retrospective evaluation of 51 cases of peripheral nerve sheath tumors in the dog. J Am Anim Hosp Assoc 1995;15:349–359.
52. Brogdon JD, Brightman AH, McLaughlin SA. Diagnosing and treating masticatory myositis. Vet Med 1991;86:1164–1170.
53. Shelton GD, Cardinet G, Bandman E. Canine masticatory muscle disorders: A study of 29 cases. Muscle Nerve 1987;10:753–766.
54. Smith MO. Idiopathic myositides in the dog. Semin Vet Med Surg (Small Anim) 1989;4:156–160.
55. Craig TM, Jones LP, Nordgren RM. Diagnosis of *Hepatozoon canis* by muscle biopsy. J Am Anim Hosp Assoc 1984;20:301–303.

56. Hill JE, Chapman WL, Prestwood AK. Intramuscular *Sarcocystis* sp in two cats and a dog. J Parasitol 1988;74: 724–727.

57. Craig TM. Parasitic myositis of dogs and cats. Semin Vet Med Surg (Small Anim) 1989;4:161–167.

58. Luttgen PJ. Miscellaneous myopathies. Semin Vet Med Surg (Small Anim) 1989;4:168–176.

59. Stuart BP, Hoss HE, Root CR, et al. Ischemic myopathy associated with systemic dirofilariasis. J Am Anim Hosp Assoc 1978;14:36–39.

60. Griffiths IR, Duncan ID, McQueen A, et al. Neuromuscular disease in the dog: Some aspects of its investigation and diagnosis. J Small Anim Pract 1973;14:533–554.

61. Krum SH, Cardinet GH, Anderson BC, Holliday TA. Polymyositis and polyarthritis associated with systemic lupus erythematosus in a dog. J Am Vet Med Assoc 1977;170:61–64.

62. Cuddon P, Lin D-S, Bowman DD, et al. *Neospora caninum* infection in English springer spaniel littermates. J Vet Intern Med 1992;6:325–332.

63. Hass, JA, Shell LG, Saunders G. Neurologic manifestations of toxoplasmosis: A literature review and case summary. J Am Anim Hosp Assoc 1989;25:253–260.

64. Hay WH, Shell LG, Lindsay DS, et al. Diagnosis and treatment of *Neospora caninum* infection in a dog. J Am Vet Med Assoc 1990;197:87–89.

65. Kornegay JN, Gorgacz EJ, Dawe DL, Bowen JM, et al. Polymyositis in dogs. J Am Vet Med Assoc 1980;176: 431–438.

66. Cornelissen JM, Haagsma J, van Nes JJ. Type C botulism in five dogs. J Am Anim Hosp Assoc 1985;21:401–404.

67. Barsanti JA, Walser M, Hatheway CL, et al. Type C botulism in American fox hounds. J Am Vet Med Assoc 1978;172:809–813.

68. Cooper BJ. Nemaline myopathy in cats. Muscle Nerve 1986;9:618–625.

69. Jones BR. Hereditary myotonia in the chow chow. Vet Annu 1984;24:286–291.

70. Braund KG. Neurological diseases. In: Braund KG, ed. Clinical Syndromes in Veterinary Neurology. St. Louis, Mosby, 1994:81–332.

71. Sharp NJH, Kornegay JN, Lane SB. The muscular dystrophies. Semin Vet Med Surg (Small Anim) 1989;4: 133–140.

72. Wentink GH, van der Linde-Sipman JS, Meijer AEF, et al. Myopathy with a possible recessive x-linked inheritance in a litter of Irish terriers. Vet Pathol 1972;9:328–349.

73. Kramer JW, Hegreberg GA, Bryan GM, et al. A muscle disorder of Labrador retrievers characterized by deficiency of type II muscle fibers. J Am Vet Med Assoc 1976;169:817–820.

74. Hargis AM, Haupt KH, Hegreberg GA, et al. Familial canine dermatomyositis: Initial characterization of the cutaneous and muscular lesions. Am J Pathol 1984;116: 234–244.

75. Kunkle GA, Chrisman CL, Gross TL, et al. Dermatomyositis in collie dogs. Compen Contin Educ Pract Vet 1985;7:185–192.

76. Peeters MC, Haagen AJ V-V, Goedegebuure SA. Dysphagia in Bouviers associated with muscular dystrophy: Evaluation of 24 cases. Vet Q 1991;13:65–73.

77. Vos JH, van der Linde-Sipman JS, Goedegebuure SA. Dystrophy-like myopathy in the cat. J Comp Pathol 1986;96:335–341.

78. Kurtz HJ, Fletcher TF. The peripheral neuropathy of canine globoid-cell leukodystrophy (Krabbe-Type). Acta Neuropathol (Berl) 1970;16:226–232.

79. Matz ME, Shell L, Braund KG. Peripheral hypomyelinization in two golden retriever littermates. J Am Vet Med Assoc 1990;197:228–230.

80. Griffiths IR, Duncan ID, Barker J. A progressive axonopathy of boxer dogs affecting the central and peripheral nervous system. J Sm Anim Pract 1980;21:29–43.

81. Cummings JF, Cooper BJ, de Lahunta A, et al. Canine inherited hypertrophic neuropathy. Acta Neuropathol (Berl) 1981;53:137–143.

82. Lorenz MD, Cork LC, Griffin JW, et al. Hereditary canine spinal muscular atrophy in Brittany spaniels. J Am Vet Med Assoc 1979;175:833–839.

83. Shell LG, Jortner BS, Leib MS. Spinal muscular atrophy in two rottweiler littermates. J Am Vet Med Assoc 1987;190:878–880.

84. Cooper BJ, de Lahunta A, Cummings JF, et al. Canine inherited hypertrophic neuropathy: Clinical and electrodiagnostic studies. Am J Vet Res 1984;45:1172–1177.

85. Duncan ID, Griffiths IR. Canine giant axonal neuropathy. Vet Rec 1977;101:438–441.

86. Duncan ID, Griffiths IT, Carmichael S, et al. Inherited canine giant axonal neuropathy. Muscle Nerve 1981;4: 223–227.

87. Cummings JF, de Lahunta A, Winn SS. Acral mutilation and nociceptive loss in English pointer dogs. Acta Neuropathol (Berl) 1981;53:119–127.

88. Duncan ID, Griffiths IR, Munz M. The pathology of a sensory neuropathy affecting long haired dachshund dogs. Acta Neuropathol (Berl) 1982;58:141–151.

89. Steiss JE. Sensory neuropathy in a dog. J Am Vet Med Assoc 1987;190:205–208.

90. Cummings JF, de Lahunta A, Mitchell WJ. Ganglioradiculitis in the dog. Acta Neuropathol (Berl) 1983;60:29–39.

91. Wouda W, Vandevelde M, Oettli P, et al. Sensory neuronopathy in dogs: A study of four cases. J Comp Pathol 1983;93:437–450.

92. Sharp NJH, Nash AS, Griffiths IR. Feline dysautonomia (the Key-Gaskell syndrome): A clinical and pathological study of forty cases. J Small Anim Pract 1984;25:599–615.

93. LeCouteur RA, Dow SW, Sisson AF. Metabolic and endocrine myopathies of dogs and cats. Semin Vet Med Surg (Small Anim) 1989;4:146–155.

94. Gannon JR. Exertional rhabdomyolysis (myoglobinuria) in the racing greyhound. In: Kirk RW, ed. Current Veterinary Therapy VII. Philadelphia, WB Saunders, 1980:783–787.

95. Jezyk PF. Hyperkalemic periodic paralysis in a dog. J Am Anim Hosp Assoc 1982;18:977–980.

96. Dow SW, LeCouteur RA, Fettman MJ, et al. Potassium depletion in cats: Hypokalemic polymyopathy. J Am Vet Med Assoc 1987;191:1569–1575.

97. Braund KG, Dillon AR, Mikeal RL, August JR. Subclinical myopathy associated with hyperadrenocorticism in the dog. Vet Pathol 1980;17:134–148.

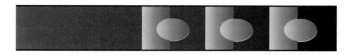

Gastrointestinal, Pancreatic, and Hepatobiliary Diseases

Chapter 29

Diseases of the Oral Cavity, Pharynx, and Salivary Glands

Michael S. Leib

Anatomy

The external opening of the oral cavity is surrounded by the lips, which are lined by stratified squamous epithelium.[1] The muscles of the cheeks aid in the transport of food to the pharynx and are innervated by the facial nerve. The tongue (also covered by stratified squamous epithelium) lies on the floor of the oral cavity, and its root is formed by muscles that arise from the hyoid apparatus.[1] It is innervated by the hypoglossal nerves and is important in bolus formation and transport to the pharynx and in taste sensation. The hard and soft palates form the dorsal roof of the oral cavity and separate it from the nasal cavity.[1]

The confines of the oropharynx are indistinct.[1] The palatine arches reflect from the mandible and can be considered the most caudal aspect of the oral cavity. The tonsils are paired lymph nodes within crypts along the lateral wall of the oropharynx.

The major paired salivary glands are the parotid, mandibular, sublingual, and zygomatic.[1-3] The parotid is located below the horizontal ear canal, and its duct enters the cheek at the level of the upper fourth premolar.[2, 3] Ventral to the parotid lies the mandibular gland, caudal to the angle of the jaw.[3] It shares a capsule with the caudal, monostomatic portion of the sublingual gland.[2, 3] Its duct courses along the sublingual gland and opens on the lateral aspect of the sublingual frenulum.[1-3] The sublingual gland courses from the rostral aspect of the mandibular gland to the root of the tongue.[1] Its duct opens just cranial to the mandibular gland or joins the mandibular gland's duct.[2, 3] The zygomatic gland lies on the floor of the orbit, ventrocaudal to the eye. Its duct opens lateral to the last upper molar.[1-3]

The gingivae, or gums, form a collar around the neck of each tooth.[4] The attached gingiva is firmly fixed to the alveolar bone, in which the teeth are seated. The gingiva courses buccally and labially to join the mucosa of the oral cavity. The gingiva surrounding the tooth that is not attached forms the gingival sulcus, which normally is not more than 2 to 3 mm deep.[4] The periodontal ligament is a thin layer of connective tissue that surrounds the tooth root and helps support its attachment into bone.

Physiology

Deglutition

The most important function of the oral cavity and oropharynx is in the initial stages of deglutition, the transport of food and water from the mouth to the stomach. Prehension (grasping the food) and mastication (chewing) precede swallowing. The teeth, tongue, and mandible are responsible for prehension. Cranial nerves I, II, V, and XII and the cerebral cortex are important in these processes.[5] After the food is grasped, the teeth cut and grind the material to decrease the size of ingesta, which increases the surface area for digestion. Chewing is a reflex that is under voluntary control. The food bolus stimulates sensory receptors within the oral cavity that initiate transmission to the brain stem through cranial nerve V, leading to inhibition of the muscles of mastication, the temporalis, masseter, pterygoid, and digastricus muscles. The lower jaw drops, which stimulates stretch receptors in the muscles of mastication, initiating a rebound contraction.

Swallowing can be divided into three phases: oropharyngeal, esophageal (see Chap. 30), and gastroesophageal.[5, 6] The oropharyngeal phase is also divided into three stages: oral, pharyngeal, and pharyngoesophageal.[5, 7, 8] The oral stage is voluntary; a food bolus is moved to the base of the tongue by the cheek muscles and tongue, under the control of cranial nerves V, VII, and XII. The bolus is propelled into the pharynx by the plunger-like activity of the base of the tongue.[5, 7]

The pharyngeal phase is involuntary. The food bolus stimulates sensory receptors that initiate impulses through cranial nerves V, IX, and X.[5] A reflex through the swallowing center in the medulla ensues, causing progressive contraction of the pharyngeal muscles through cranial nerves V, VII, IX, X, and XII and propulsion of the bolus through the pharynx.[5, 7, 9] The respiratory center is inhibited to prevent aspiration. The soft palate is elevated to seal off the nasopharynx, and the trachea is covered by the glottis and the tipping of the epiglottis.

The final stage is the pharyngoesophageal phase, which is also involuntary. The normally closed upper esophageal or cricopharyngeal sphincter (composed of the cricopharyngeus and thyropharyngeus muscles) relaxes to accept the food bolus moving through the pharynx.[7] This phase is controlled through the swallowing center and mediated by cranial nerves IX and X.[5] After the bolus enters the esophagus, the sphincter closes to prevent aerophagia during respiration and to aid retention of the bolus within the esophagus.[8] The bolus initiates a primary peristaltic wave within the esophagus (see Chap. 30).

Salivary Glands

The salivary glands function to produce saliva, which helps to soften and lubricate the food.[1] Saliva also helps to moisten the oral cavity, which is helpful for heat loss.

Problem Identification

Gingivitis and Stomatitis

Inflammation of structures within the oral cavity is a very common problem encountered in small animal practice. Gingivitis is defined as inflammation of the gingival surfaces of the oral cavity. Stomatitis is a broader term and denotes inflammation of any of the mucosal surfaces within the oral cavity. Inflammation of the tongue or lips is termed glossitis or cheilitis, respectively.

Pathophysiology

The causes of gingivitis and stomatitis in dogs and cats are numerous (Table 29-1).[10-14] The most common cause is periodontal disease resulting from accumulation of plaque and tartar. Periodontal disease is a progressive disorder that can lead to tooth and gum destruction. Initially, it is a reversible process. The initiating substance, plaque (consisting of food, saliva, bacteria, and cellular debris), accumulates within the gingival sulcus and results in inflammation.[15] The bacteria associated with the plaque change to a predominantly gram-negative anaerobic flora.[16] Release of bacterial toxins adds to the inflammatory process. Inflammation results in loosening of the periodontal ligament attachments and deepening of the gingival sulcus (allowing accumulation of more plaque and tartar). The inflammatory process proceeds along the tooth root, causing recession of the gum, exposure of the root, and loosening of its attachments in alveolar bone.[15]

Regardless of the cause of gingivitis or stomatitis, the large and varied microbial population of the oral cavity contributes to the inflammatory process. Partial clinical improvement after antibiotic therapy is a result of reduction in the secondary bacterial component of inflammation. Other mechanisms of disease are related to the specific cause of the gingivitis or stomatitis. Immunosuppression caused by infectious agents such as feline leukemia virus (FeLV) or feline immunodeficiency virus (FIV), neutropenia of any cause, immunosuppressive drug therapy, or diabetes mellitus can initiate gingivitis or stomatitis or worsen existing mild periodontal disease. Caustic agents, thermal burns, and plant awns can directly damage the mucosa.[13] The pathophysiology associated with other viral agents is unknown but may involve direct infection of epithelial cells.[17] The gingivitis and stomatitis associated with uremia may be caused by metabolism of urea by oral bacteria to ammonia, which is irritating to the mucosa.[14] Vasculitis also accompanies uremia. Necrotizing ulcerative stomatitis occurs when normal oral bacteria cause infection of tissues after the

Table 29-1
Differential Diagnosis for Gingivitis and Stomatitis

Periodontal disease
Idiopathic plasmacytic lymphocytic gingivitis-stomatitis-pharyngitis
Immunosuppression
    Feline leukemia virus or feline immunodeficiency virus
    Neutropenia
    Corticosteroids
    Cancer chemotherapy
Caustics
    Lye
    Acids
    Phenols
Foreign material
    Plant awns
    Fiberglass
    Porcupine quills
    Bones
    Sticks
Thermal burns
Virus
    Calicivirus
    Rhinotracheitis
    Canine distemper
Uremia
Diabetes mellitus
House plants
    Dieffenbachia
Autoimmune skin disease
Necrotizing ulcerative stomatitis
    Nocardia
    Fusobacterium
    Borrelia
Candida albicans
Thallium

oral cavity has been damaged.[14] Yeast infections with the opportunistic pathogen *Candida albicans* are associated with immunosuppression.[14] Autoimmune disorders may produce direct mucosal damage and ulceration.[14]

Clinical Signs

Common clinical signs of gingivitis and stomatitis, regardless of the cause, are anorexia, halitosis, bleeding within the oral cavity, dysphagia, ptyalism, pain associated with opening or examinination of the mouth, and submandibular lymphadenopathy.[18, 19] The mucosal surfaces are often erythematous, friable, ulcerated, necrotic, proliferative, or covered by pseu-

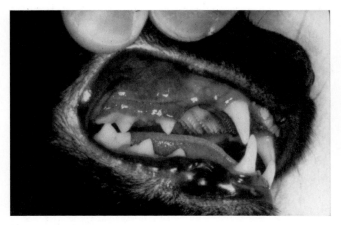

Figure 29-1
Marginal gingivitis along the maxillary teeth in a 4-year-old domestic shorthair cat with plasmacytic lymphocytic stomatitis. The gingiva is swollen and red. A proliferative lesion on the buccal mucosa and submandibular lymphadenopathy were also present.

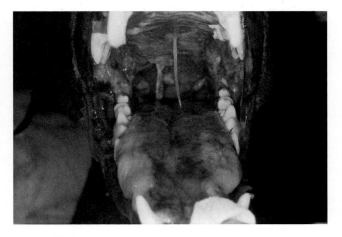

Figure 29-3
Ulcerative glossitis and pharyngitis in a 6-year-old Doberman pinscher that ingested caustic drain cleaner. Some tissue along the lateral rostral surface of the tongue is not as severely affected.

domembranes (Figs. 29-1 and 29-2). Changes may be limited to one region or may involve multiple areas such as the gingiva, the tongue, beneath the tongue, the hard palate, the glossopalatine arches, and the pharynx.[18]

Other clinical signs relate to the primary underlying condition. The history may include exposure to chemicals, hot liquids, or foreign materials. Polyuria with polydipsia is associated with uremia or diabetes mellitus. Cats with FeLV or FIV often have a variety of signs such as diarrhea, rhinitis, weight loss, fever, lymphadenopathy, conjunctivitis, abscesses, other chronic infections, lethargy, dermatitis, vomiting, or neoplasia. Other erosive, crusting, or bullous skin lesions may be present in patients with autoimmune disease.

Diagnostic Plan

Because of the many causes of gingivitis and stomatitis, a thorough diagnostic plan must be followed to arrive efficiently at an accurate diagnosis. The history and physical examination should identify administration of immunosuppressive drugs, exposure to caustic agents or foreign materials, or evidence of systemic disorders associated with gingivitis and stomatitis. In cases of caustic ingestion, lesions are often present along the dorsal surface of the tongue and the hard palate (Fig. 29-3). Plant awn ingestion often causes lesions along the edge of the tongue and the rostral lips and gingiva (Fig. 29-4).[13, 14] Plant material can sometimes be seen protruding from the lesions. A complete blood count, biochemical profile, urinalysis, and enzyme-linked immunosorbent assay (ELISA) tests for FeLV and FIV can identify most underlying systemic diseases. If a diagnosis is not reached, mucosal biopsy may be indicated. In most cases, general anesthesia is necessary to obtain biopsy samples and perform a complete oral examination. If autoimmune disorders are suspected, mucosal samples should be collected for immunofluorescence.

Dysphagia

Dysphagia is defined as difficulty in swallowing. It is encountered in small animal practice, but not as commonly as regurgitation, vomiting, or diarrhea. Difficulty in the esophageal phase of swallowing is better termed regurgitation (see Chap. 30). For the

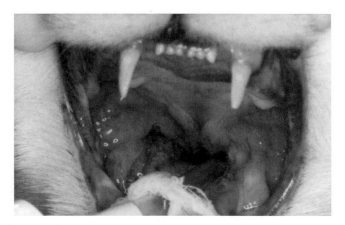

Figure 29-2
Severe ulcerative oropharyngitis in a 5-year-old domestic shorthair cat with plasmacytic stomatitis. The molars and premolars had previously been extracted, reducing the severity of lesions along the gum line.

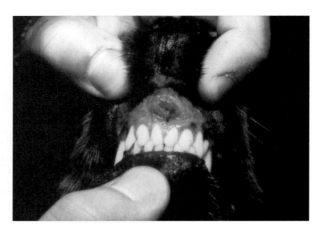

Figure 29–4
Plant burr gingivitis in a 1-year-old English cocker spaniel. The rostral gingiva is granular, hyperemic, friable, and proliferative. Lesions were also present on the tongue and along the rostral mandibular gingiva.

purposes of this section, dysphagia pertains to difficulties in the oropharyngeal phase of swallowing.

Pathophysiology

Dysphagia can be associated with structural or functional abnormalities within the mouth or pharynx (Table 29–2).[5, 7] Structural problems physically interfere with the process of swallowing. Neuromuscular problems cause dysphagia by altering the neurologic reflex that controls swallowing, resulting in paresis or paralysis, failure to relax (achalasia), or asynchrony between different regions.

Defects within the oral phase of swallowing decrease bolus formation and transmission to the pharynx.[7] Tongue movement is often abnormal. In pharyngeal phase dysphagia, there is ineffective transmission of the bolus through the pharynx. Pharyngoesophageal dysphagia is associated with failure of the bolus to pass into the esophagus because of obstruction or asynchrony of pharyngeal contraction with the opening of the cricopharyngeal sphincter.[6] Mixed-phase dysphagia is common.

Pneumonia is common with pharyngeal and pharyngoesophageal dysphagia because pharyngeal retention of food leads to aspiration into the trachea.[7]

Clinical Signs

The clinical signs associated with dysphagia include excessive salivation, difficulty in lapping water or prehension of food, gagging, food's falling from the mouth, decreased tongue movement, weight loss, repeated and exaggerated swallowing movements, nasal regurgitation of food, and respiratory signs associated with aspiration pneumonia (e.g., cough,

pyrexia, tachypnea, mucopurulent nasal discharge, crackles on thoracic auscultation).[5–7]

Diagnostic Plan

The most important initial step to be taken in cases of suspected dysphagia is to distinguish between dysphagia, regurgitation, and vomiting (see Chaps. 30 and 31). In cases of dysphagia, food may fall from the mouth immediately after ingestion and before swallowing. Repeated swallowing attempts are often made before a bolus successfully passes into the esophagus. Regurgitation or vomiting returns food after swallowing has successfully occurred, and it can be delayed for hours. If the history does not clarify this distinction, observation of the animal while it eats often correctly identifies the problem.

After it has been determined that the animal is having dysphagia, a thorough oral and pharyngeal examination should be performed. Sedation or general anesthesia may be necessary to evaluate these areas thoroughly if the animal is uncooperative. Diagnosis and removal of foreign bodies and biopsy of masses can be accomplished. If lesions are not detected, a complete neurologic examination and dynamic radiographic studies should be performed. If neurologic deficits are detected, further evaluation is indicated (see Chap. 26). If the neurologic examination is normal, most patients need to be referred to a specialty center for a barium swallow observed under fluoroscopy to identify deficits in tongue movement and bolus formation, pharyngeal transport, or passage into the esophagus.[6, 7]

Table 29–2
Differential Diagnosis of Dysphagia

Structural problems
  Trauma
    Fractured mandible or maxilla
    Luxated temporomandibular joint
    Soft tissue laceration or swelling
  Foreign body
  Gingivitis or stomatitis
  Neoplasia
  Indolent ulcer
  Salivary mucocele
  Feline nasopharyngeal polyp
Neurologic problems
  Cranial nerve deficit (V, VII, IX, X, XI, or XII)
  Medullary swallowing center
  Neuromuscular junction (myasthenia gravis)
  Striated muscle (masticatory myositis)

Diagnostic Procedures

Routine Laboratory Evaluation

A complete blood count, biochemical profile, and urinalysis are never diagnostic of specific oropharyngeal disorders, but they do allow detection of underlying or concurrent illnesses, help assess the animal's risk for general anesthesia, and provide supportive information for a diagnosis. In cases of gingivitis or stomatitis, renal failure, diabetes mellitus, or neutropenia may be detected as underlying causes. A neutrophilia, with or without a left shift, may occur in cats with plasmacytic stomatitis, in dogs or cats with ulcerative gingivitis or stomatitis from any cause, in animals with an oronasal fistula, or in any dysphagic animal with aspiration pneumonia. Hyperglobulinemia may be present in cats with plasmacytic stomatitis.[18] Animals with oropharyngeal neoplasia may have a nonregenerative anemia.

Oropharyngeal Examination

A complete and thorough examination should be performed whenever signs of oropharyngeal disease exist. In most cases, a cursory examination of the oral cavity and pharynx can be accomplished in the awake animal. Palpation of the pharynx should initiate a gag reflex. However, a thorough evaluation, especially of the pharynx or the area under the tongue, or examination in an animal that is fractious or in pain, requires sedation or general anesthesia.

The gingival surfaces and teeth should be examined for masses, gingivitis, and periodontal disease. The oral mucosa should be smooth, pink or slightly pigmented, and glistening.[1] The hard palate should be carefully examined for masses or fistulae into the nasal cavity. The entire surface of the tongue should be evaluated for signs of glossitis, masses, or fluctuant swellings beneath the tongue (ranulas) (Fig. 29–5). The area under the tongue should be examined for a linear foreign body that may have penetrated into the tissue and become surrounded by an inflammatory mass.[20, 21] Normally, the tonsils are contained within their crypts and are pink to tan. Foreign bodies may be seen in the pharynx, along the hard palate, or over the rostral mandible. The submandibular lymph nodes and the pharyngeal area should be palpated carefully.

Biopsy

Many oropharyngeal lesions require histologic assessment of tissue to establish a definitive diagnosis. Usually, heavy sedation or general anesthesia must be used to obtain diagnostic tissue specimens. A cuffed endotracheal tube should be placed before biopsy to protect the airway from hemorrhage.

Gingival masses and fluctuant swelling should

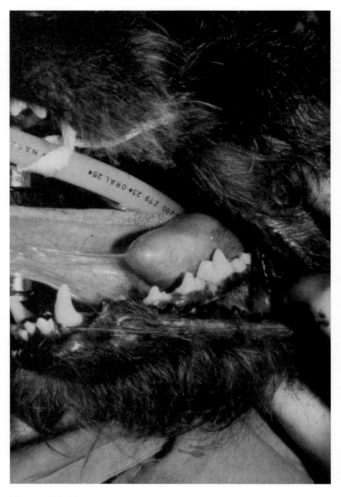

Figure 29–5
Ranula along the ventral surface of the tongue in a dog. (Courtesy of Robert Martin, DVM, Blacksburg, Virginia.)

be evaluated by fine-needle aspiration cytology before biopsy. Fine-needle aspiration of gingival masses may be diagnostic of malignant melanomas. Fluctuant swellings such as mucoceles and abscesses can be diagnosed easily.

Biopsy samples can be obtained from large masses with Tru-Cut needles (see Chap. 34 for a detailed description of technique) or with incisional or excisional techniques. Gingival samples can be obtained by excision. Abnormalities of the buccal mucosa or palatine arches are best sampled with skin biopsy punches.

Radiography

Survey radiographs of the pharynx are indicated for patients with pharyngeal swellings or oropharyngeal dysphagia, especially if complicated by inspiratory stridor or dyspnea. Bony or metallic foreign bodies, a gas pocket within the tissues (abscess), or loss of visualization of detail of soft tissue (cellulitis) may be seen.[22, 23]

In cases of suspected neoplasia, thoracic radiographs should be made to evaluate the presence of metastatic lesions. A ventrodorsal or dorsoventral view and right and left lateral recumbent views should be taken. Thoracic radiographs should also be made of patients with dysphagia, coughing, fever, or mucopurulent nasal discharge to evaluate for aspiration pneumonia. Aspiration pneumonia appears as peribronchial and alveolar densities, most commonly in the ventral aspects of the cranial and middle lung lobes (see Fig. 30–6). However, any lung lobe may be involved, and large areas of lung can become consolidated.

If gingival masses are present, the mandible or maxilla should be radiographed to evaluate bony involvement, which appears as bone destruction (Fig. 29–6). General anesthesia is required to allow careful positioning of the patient.[24] Open-mouth oblique projections (rotated 30°–45° from lateral position) of the mandible allow visualization of each hemimandible. A ventrodorsal intraoral projection is best for the rostral mandible. Open-mouth oblique views of the maxilla demonstrate lesions in the area of the premolars or molars. Ventrodorsal open-mouth or dorsoventral intraoral projections show lesions of the central maxilla.

Contrast studies to evaluate swallowing are best performed with fluoroscopy and usually require referral.[5–7] Administration of liquid barium and barium mixed with food localizes the defect responsible for dysphagia. Static radiographs after administration of enough barium to initiate a swallow may demonstrate nasal regurgitation, tracheal aspiration,

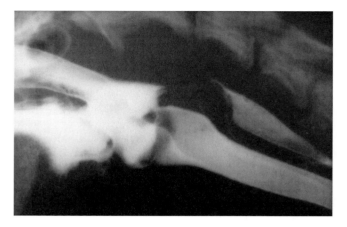

Figure 29–7
Lateral pharyngeal radiograph of a 6-month-old mixed breed dog with cricopharyngeal dysphagia, after administration of liquid barium sulfate. Reflux of barium into the nasal pharynx and tracheal aspiration are present. Barium remains in the pharynx because it is unable to pass through a closed cricopharyngeal sphincter into the esophagus.

and retention of barium within the oral cavity or pharynx in animals with dysphagia (Fig. 29–7).[5, 6]

Common Diseases of the Oral Cavity, Pharynx, and Salivary Glands

Plasmacytic Lymphocytic Gingivitis-Stomatitis-Pharyngitis

An idiopathic gingivitis-stomatitis-pharyngitis complex commonly occurs in middle-aged cats of all breeds, although purebred cats may be affected more commonly.[10, 17–19]

Pathophysiology

The cause of this condition is unknown, although calicivirus has been isolated from affected cats.[11, 17] The mucosa responds to an unknown insult with an inflammatory reaction. Inflammation is perpetuated by continued exposure to the inciting cause, secondary bacterial infection, periodontal disease (if present), and the mediators of inflammation released from the plasma cells and lymphocytes.

Clinical Signs

The clinical signs in cats with plasmacytic lymphocytic gingivitis-stomatitis-pharyngitis are similar to those described for gingivitis (see Problem Identification). Weight loss is common. Proliferative, cobblestone-like lesions often occur along the glossopalatine arches and the gingivae, and they can occur

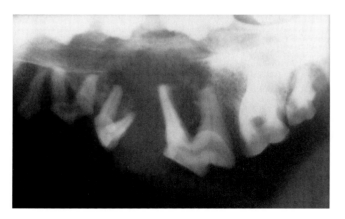

Figure 29–6
Radiograph of the maxilla of a dog with a malignant tumor, showing a soft tissue mass, severe destruction of bone, and displacement of teeth. (Courtesy of Don Barber, DVM, MS, Blacksburg, Virginia.)

anywhere within the oral cavity (see Fig. 29–2).[18, 19] Mild or moderate dental tartar is present in approximately 25% of cases.[18]

Diagnostic Plan

The diagnosis requires excluding the many causes of gingivitis and stomatitis (see Table 29–1) and obtaining biopsy samples that are infiltrated with large numbers of plasma cells or plasma cells and lymphocytes within the mucosa and submucosa.[18, 19] Hyperglobulinemia is often present.[18, 19] Leukocytosis is present in approximately 40% of cases. Most cats are negative for FeLV or FIV on ELISA.[17–19]

Treatment

No treatment is universally effective, so the response to therapy should be monitored carefully, and other treatments should be initiated if improvement does not occur. The teeth should be cleaned and polished and diseased teeth extracted. Home hygiene should be initiated.[16] Dry foods should be fed to reduce calculus formation.[10, 25] Antibiotic therapy for 3 to 6 weeks (amoxicillin, 10–20 mg/kg twice per day [b.i.d.]; clindamycin, 22 mg/kg once per day [s.i.d.]; metronidazole, 10–25 mg/kg s.i.d.; or tetracycline, 15–20 mg/kg three times per day [t.i.d.]) helps to reduce the secondary bacterial component.[10, 18] Concurrent immunosuppressive therapy with prednisone (1–2 mg/kg b.i.d.) or repositol prednisone acetate (2 mg/kg every 1–4 weeks subcutaneously) improves the clinical signs.[18] After the lesions resolve, the prednisone dosage should be reduced slowly every 2 weeks to the lowest alternate-day dose that controls clinical signs. Patients that do not respond may benefit from gold salt (aurothioglucose, 1 mg/kg intramuscularly every 7 days), from megestrol acetate (1 mg/kg every 1–4 days or 2.5 mg per cat s.i.d. for 10 days, then every 48 hours for 10 days, then twice per week, and finally reduced to the lowest frequency necessary to control signs), or occasionally from removal of all teeth.[10, 18, 19] Caution is needed with megestrol because of frequent serious side effects such as development of diabetes mellitus, mammary hyperplasia, and adrenal suppression. During the initial phases of gold salt therapy, a complete blood count and platelet count should be performed weekly to monitor for bone marrow suppression.

Prognosis

The prognosis for complete resolution of clinical signs is guarded.[19] Improvement often occurs with the treatments described, but mild clinical signs often persist, and relapses are common after withdrawal of therapy.[18] Because of oral pain, cats are difficult for owners to medicate.

Oral Neoplasia

The oral cavity is the fourth most common site for neoplasia in dogs.[24, 26] Oral tumors occur less commonly in cats. In dogs, the most common tumors are squamous cell carcinomas, malignant melanomas, fibrosarcomas, and epulides.[27] The most common tumors of cats are squamous cell carcinomas, fibrosarcomas, and fibromatous epulides.[28–31] Some studies have shown that males dogs are affected more often than females, but others have shown equal frequencies.[24, 26, 29, 32–35] Commonly affected dog breeds include German shorthaired pointers, weimaraners, golden retrievers, and boxers.[24, 26] Fibrosarcomas are more common in large-breed dogs.[26, 36] Most tumors develop in middle-aged or older animals.[26, 28, 29, 33–35]

Pathophysiology

Malignant melanomas arise from melanocytes within the gingiva and are locally invasive to bone and highly metastatic to regional lymph nodes, tonsils, and the lungs.[26, 27, 34, 35, 37] Squamous cell carcinomas arise from the gingiva and are locally invasive to bone, but they are relatively slow to metastasize to distant locations.[26, 27, 34, 35, 37, 38] The more rostrally located squamous cell carcinomas are not as metastatic as the caudally located tumors.[36] Fibrosarcomas arise from submucosal stroma and are highly invasive locally, with distant metastatic potential between melanomas and squamous cell carcinomas.[26, 27, 34, 35, 37]

Based on histologic evaluation, there are three types of epulides: fibromatous, ossifying, and acanthomatous.[27] All arise from the periodontal ligament. The fibromatous type consists mostly of periodontal ligament stoma, the ossifying type has large amounts of osteoid matrix, and the acanthomatous type consists of epithelial cells.[27] The acanthomatous type frequently invades bone.

Clinical Signs

Clinical signs associated with oral tumors include anorexia, dysphagia, excessive salivation, halitosis, dyspnea, loose teeth, and blood-tinged saliva.[26, 29] Submandibular lymphadenopathy may be present.[29] In some asymptomatic cases, a mass may be noticed by owners or found on physical examination. Coughing or tachypnea may occur if pulmonary metastasis is present.

Most tumors are large (2–6 cm) at the time of diagnosis. Malignant melanomas often are dome-shaped, ulcerated, or necrotic, and they vary in color from pink to white, gray, or black (Fig. 29–8). Squamous cell carcinomas are red, friable, and eroded, and they appear inflamed (Fig. 29–9).[24] In cats, they often originate in the sublingual area.[28] Fibrosarcomas often

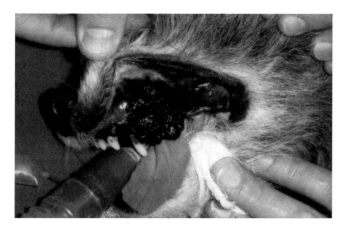

Figure 29-8
Gingival malignant melanoma in the area of the maxillary premolars in a mixed breed dog. The mass and adjacent gingiva are black. (Courtesy of Steve Susaneck, DVM, MS, Houston, Texas.)

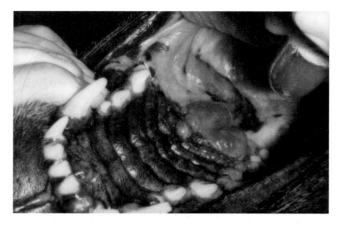

Figure 29-10
Fibrosarcoma in the area of the maxillary molars extending medially across the midline at the junction of the hard and soft palates in an 8-year-old mixed breed dog. (Courtesy of Steve Susaneck, DVM, MS, Houston, Texas.)

arise along the maxillary gingiva between the canine tooth and the fourth premolar or the hard palate and are firm, ulcerated, and necrotic (Fig. 29–10).[27] Epulides are benign tumors that are firm and often pedunculated and commonly occur along the incisors (Fig. 29–11).[39]

Diagnostic Plan

The clinical appearance of many tumors may be identical to that of some inflammatory conditions; definitive diagnosis requires aspiration cytology or biopsy of the mass and histopathologic evaluation.[27] Complete staging of the tumor is important to establish a prognosis and plan the most effective therapy.[27, 34] A laboratory minimum database should be collected to

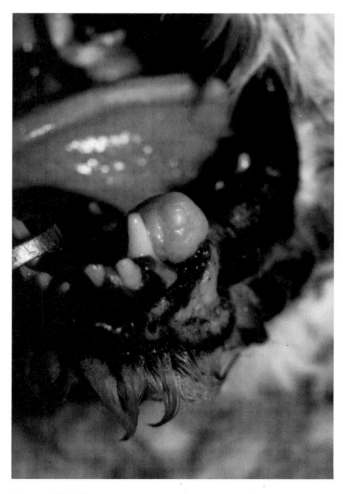

Figure 29-11
Mandibular epulis caudal to the canine tooth in a dog. (Courtesy of Steve Susaneck, DVM, MS, Houston, Texas.)

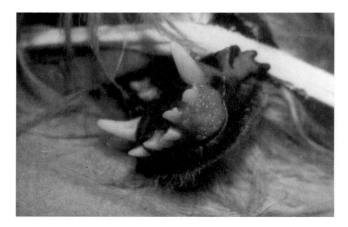

Figure 29-9
Squamous cell carcinoma in the area of the mandibular incisors in a dog. The mass is red and granular. (Courtesy of Robert Martin, DVM, Blacksburg, Virginia.)

evaluate any concurrent problems and to assess the animal's risk for general anesthesia. A nonregenerative anemia may be present as a result of chronic inflammatory disease. Regional lymph nodes should be aspirated. Thoracic radiographs should be evaluated for metastases. Radiographs of the mandible or maxilla should be made to assess local bony invasion (bone destruction) by the tumor (see Fig. 29–6).[40] Fine-needle aspiration of the mass can be diagnostic in cases of malignant melanoma. Most other tumor types require incisional, excisional, or needle biopsy for diagnosis. Non-neoplastic masses can be diagnosed by aspiration or biopsy, or both; these include indolent ulcers in cats, plasmacytic gingivitis and stomatitis in cats, gingival hyperplasia, eosinophilic granulomas in huskies, mucoceles, and abscesses.

Treatment

Early surgical excision remains the most effective treatment for oral tumors. However, other modes of therapy have been evaluated and can be effective in some cases. Radiation has been shown to be effective against acanthomatous epulides, although malignant transformation at the radiation site can occur.[24, 41] Hyperthermia combined with radiation is effective for squamous cell carcinomas and some fibrosarcomas.[24, 42, 43] Radiation therapy and mandibulectomy in cats with squamous cell carcinoma was more effective than surgery alone.[44] Cryosurgery is effective for some epulides.[24]

Adequate resection of neoplastic tissue usually requires at least a 1-cm margin, necessitating partial mandibulectomy and maxillectomy in most cases. These procedures have been well described in the literature and have resulted in prolonged survival times, compared with more conservative surgeries.[30–33, 35, 37, 45–48] Despite the radical nature of this type of surgery, acceptable cosmetic results are usually obtained, and the animal is usually free of pain and discomfort.[36, 37] The animal can often eat and drink within 2 to 3 days of surgery.[30, 36, 37] Complications include partial dehiscence, tumor recurrence, oronasal fistula, drooling, mandibular malocclusion, and prehension dysfunction.[29, 30, 32, 33, 35, 37]

Adequate treatment of epulides requires removal of the tumor and affected teeth with the alveoli and periodontal ligaments.[39] Because of frequent bony invasion with acanthomatous epulides, partial bony resection is necessary.[49]

Prognosis

Epulides respond very favorably to wide surgical resection with long survival periods.[35, 39] However, recurrence is common if only local excision is used.

The prognosis for malignant tumors is poor, with median survival times of 8 to 26 months reported.[32, 33, 35] Malignant melanomas carry a poor prognosis because of early distant metastasis and frequent recurrence.[24, 26, 27] Median survival time in some studies is only 7 to 10 months, and 1-year survival rates vary between 0 and 21%.[34, 35, 45] Small melanomas, tumors located on the rostral mandible or caudal maxilla, and those with a low mitotic index are associated with longer remissions and longer survival times.[48]

The prognosis for squamous cell carcinoma in dogs is more favorable than for other malignancies because it is slow to metastasize.[24] However, unless it is located in the rostral mandible, local recurrence is common. Mean survival time in some studies is 16 to 26 months, and 1-year survival rates vary between 44% and 91%.[34, 35, 46] Among dogs receiving radiation therapy, the tumor-free interval was longest with maxillary tumors, and survival time was longest in dogs younger than 6 years of age, those with rostrally located tumors, and those without local recurrence.[38] Squamous cell carcinoma warrants a poorer prognosis in cats than in dogs, with median survival times of 5 months or less.[29–31] Radiation therapy after surgery has prolonged the median survival time to 14 months in cats.[44]

Fibrosarcomas carry a guarded prognosis, because most are advanced at the time of diagnosis. Recurrence is common, and distant metastasis occurs. Mean survival time in some studies was 7 to 10 months, although 1-year survival rates varied between 22% and 50%.[24, 30, 34, 35, 45]

With any malignant tumor, demonstration of lymph node involvement or distant metastasis to the lungs is a poor prognostic indicator.[26] The presence of tumor cells at the margins of resected tissue is also associated with reduced survival.[32, 33] Prognosis is worse for all tumors located caudal to the first mandibular or third maxillary premolar.[32, 33]

Foreign Body

Foreign bodies within the oral cavity and pharynx are commonly encountered in small animal practice. Wooden stick injuries are most commonly seen in young, large-breed dogs.[23] Linear foreign bodies wrapped under the tongue are most common in cats (Fig. 29–12).[20, 21]

Pathophysiology

Bones, fishhooks, and wooden sticks are the most common foreign bodies encountered in the oral cavity and pharynx.[22, 23] Foreign bodies cause clinical signs by interfering with swallowing or respiration, irritating the mucosa, or lacerating the mucosa and

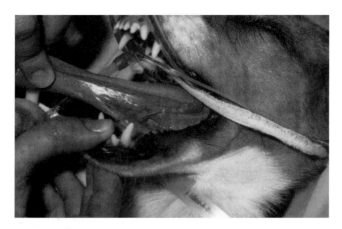

Figure 29–12
Linear foreign body wrapped under the tongue of a dog. (Courtesy of Don Waldron, DVM, Blacksburg, Virginia.)

causing cellulitis or abscess formation.[22] Plant awns can penetrate the mucosa and cause gingivitis and stomatitis. Fishhooks can imbed into the mucosa and cause pain, dysphagia, and oral hemorrhage. Bones can become lodged between the upper teeth along the hard palate and cause dysphagia. Occasionally, a hollow bone can become trapped caudal to the canine teeth on the mandible, causing discomfort and dysphagia. Thin poultry bones can become wedged in the pharynx and cause dysphagia or dyspnea.[22] Poultry bones, needles, pins, or wooden sticks can penetrate the pharynx and produce cellulitis or an abscess.[23] Linear foreign bodies that wrap under the tongue can result in plication of small intestines (Fig. 32–7), perforation, and peritonitis (see Chap. 32).[20, 21]

Clinical Signs

The clinical signs associated with foreign body ingestion vary greatly depending on the size and shape of the foreign body and its location. Many foreign bodies pass through the oral cavity and pharynx without causing any clinical signs. Salivation, pain, pawing or rubbing the face, reluctance to eat or drink, gingivitis or stomatitis, coughing, gagging, dysphagia, and dyspnea are common signs.[22, 50] Penetrating injuries can cause fever, localized cellulitis, abscess formation, or draining cervical wounds that do not heal.[23] Linear foreign bodies (see Chap. 32) can be wrapped under the tongue or passed into the stomach and small intestines and may be associated with vomiting, depression, fever, and plicated bowel loops.[20, 21]

Diagnostic Plan

In most cases, careful oral and pharyngeal examination is all that is necessary to make a diagno-

sis.[50] The foreign body is often visible on physical examination. Bones can be wedged between the teeth or across the hard palate, caudal to the maxillary canine teeth, or caught in the pharynx.[22, 50] Fishhooks are usually embedded in the mucosa of the tongue, cheeks, or lips.[50] Fishing line may be attached and may protrude from the mouth. Needles are often stuck within the tongue.[50] Gingivitis associated with a granular mucosa along the rostral gingiva, lips, and tongue may be present in cases of plant awn ingestion (see Fig. 29–4). Wooden sticks may be visible within the pharynx.[23]

The area under the tongue should be inspected carefully, because a linear foreign body can penetrate into the soft tissue. Sedation or anesthesia may be necessary to facilitate complete examination. If dyspnea is present, curved hemostats should be available to quickly remove a foreign body in the pharynx should airway obstruction become worse during induction of anesthesia. Survey radiographs of the pharynx can identify bones or metal objects, cellulitis (loss of detail of soft tissue structures), or abscess (gas pocket within the tissues).[23]

Treatment

Removal of the foreign body is usually curative.[22] Mucosal lacerations may have to be sutured.[23] Broad-spectrum antibiotics for 5 to 7 days may be indicated if there is severe mucosal damage.[22] Soft tissue exploration should be performed in cases of stick penetrations into the pharynx.[23] Plant awn gingivitis or stomatitis can be treated by scraping and debridement of the mucosa. To remove embedded fishhooks, the tip of the hook (containing the barb) should be passed through the mucosa and cut off, and the remainder of the hook removed. Bones wedged across the hard palate can be removed by passing a Gigli-saw wire under the bone and cutting it in half or using a bolt cutter to cut the bone. The same techniques can be used to remove a hollow bone wedged over the rostral mandible. A curved hemostat is usually sufficient to remove foreign bodies embedded in the pharynx.

Prognosis

The prognosis for recovery is excellent after removal of the foreign body and treatment of lacerations.

Pharyngitis and Tonsillitis

Inflammation of the pharynx and tonsils is commonly seen in dogs but is less common in cats. Primary tonsillitis occurs in young dogs.[1, 50] In most cases, pharyngitis and tonsillitis occur together and are secondary to other diseases.

Pathophysiology

After the pharyngeal mucosa is damaged, the oral bacterial flora promotes secondary inflammation. The tonsils respond to infective agents by initiating an immune response, which results in hyperemia and hyperplasia. Localized inflammation within the tonsillar crypt and tonsils can cause pain, especially in association with swallowing.

Many of the causes of gingivitis and stomatitis (see Table 29–1) can also produce a concurrent pharyngitis. Trauma may be caused by wooden sticks that damage the pharynx while dogs are retrieving.[23] Foreign bodies, especially bones or needles, can lodge within the pharynx or create damage as they pass into the esophagus. Small foreign bodies can be caught within the tonsillar crypt, causing unilateral tonsillitis. Diseases that cause vomiting or regurgitation can result in inflammation of the pharyngeal mucosa because of the irritant nature of the ingesta. Many viral diseases (e.g., parvoviruses, infectious canine hepatitis, canine distemper, canine herpesvirus, feline calicivirus, feline herpesvirus, pseudorabies) cause pharyngitis and tonsillitis as they replicate within regional lymphoid material. Respiratory disorders result in pharyngitis or tonsillitis as discharges with infective and inflammatory components are coughed up from the bronchial tree or swallowed from the nose and nasopharynx. The cause of idiopathic tonsillitis is unknown.[50]

Clinical Signs

Affected animals present with pyrexia, inappetence, dysphagia, gagging, retching, excessive salivation, and stomatitis.[50] The pharynx may be hyperemic, may be eroded or ulcerated, and may contain hyperplastic mucosa. A foreign body or signs of pharyngeal trauma may be observed. Submandibular lymph nodes may be enlarged. In cases of tonsillitis, both tonsils are usually nodular, red, enlarged, and protruding from their crypts.[1, 50] Small hemorrhages may be present. Occasionally, purulent material can be seen within the tonsillar crypts or on the surface of the tonsil.

Other clinical signs relate to the primary underlying problem (e.g., vomiting, regurgitation, coughing, nasal discharge). Pharyngitis and tonsillitis occur secondary to many viral diseases; the clinical signs of these infections are varied and usually are more prominent than the secondary pharyngitis and tonsillitis.

Diagnostic Plan

Thorough examination of the pharynx confirms the diagnosis. In some cases, the animal must be sedated or anesthetized to perform a complete evaluation. In most cases, diagnostic evaluation of concurrent problems (vomiting, regurgitation, cough, nasal discharge, or systemic signs associated with viral diseases) allows identification of the cause of the secondary pharyngitis or tonsillitis. In cases of stomatitis and pharyngitis, mucosal biopsy may be necessary. In young dogs with no other signs of disease, the diagnosis of idiopathic tonsillitis may be made after the condition resolves without therapy or after a short course of antibiotic therapy.[50]

A biopsy should be performed in cases of persistent tonsillar enlargement without an underlying cause, because neoplasia could be present (Fig. 29–13).[51–53]

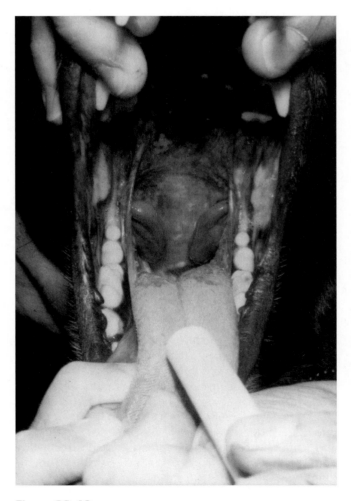

Figure 29–13
Bilateral tonsillar enlargement in an 11-year-old English pointer with multicentric lymphosarcoma. (Courtesy of Steve Susaneck, DVM, MS, Houston, Texas.)

Treatment

Most cases of pharyngitis and tonsillitis require treatment of the underlying cause. Foreign bodies should be removed. Large or deep lacerations should be sutured. Broad-spectrum antibiotics should be administered for 7 days to reduce the secondary bacterial component of the inflammation. Persistent tonsillitis in young dogs with extreme hyperplasia may require tonsillectomy.[1, 50]

Prognosis

The prognosis for most patients with pharyngitis or tonsillitis is related to the underlying cause. Tonsillitis in young dogs often resolves on its own or responds to antibiotic therapy. Clinical signs in cases requiring surgery often resolve after treatment.[50]

Salivary Mucocele

Salivary mucoceles are accumulations of saliva outside of the salivary glands and ducts.[54–56] They often occur in the submandibular region, ventral to the tongue, or in the pharynx. They are more common in dogs than in cats. Most cases occur in young animals, 2 to 4 years of age.[3, 56–58] German shepherds and miniature poodles may be predisposed.[3, 54, 57]

Pathophysiology

Saliva accumulates outside of salivary glands and flows along the path of least resistance.[58, 59] Usually, it leaks from the sublingual gland or its duct.[3, 55, 56, 59] The cause is unknown, although trauma is suspected.[54, 57] The saliva causes inflammation and stimulates the formation of a connective tissue lining of the mucocele.[54, 55, 57–59]

Clinical Signs

The clinical signs depend on the size of the mucocele and its location. Mucoceles are soft, fluctuant, nonpainful swellings. Mucoceles in the submandibular region (or upper cervical region) usually do not produce any clinical signs.[56, 58, 59] Sublingual mucoceles (also called ranulas) may interfere with the tongue and cause dysphagia or pain if they are bitten (see Fig. 29–5).[56, 59] Pharyngeal mucoceles can cause dysphagia, inspiratory stridor, cough, or dyspnea.[3, 54, 55] Submandibular and sublingual mucoceles often occur together.[56]

Diagnostic Plan

The diagnosis is based on the characteristic location and appearance.[54] Fine-needle aspiration produces a viscid fluid with the appearance of saliva.[54–59] The fluid may be tinged with blood. Cytology helps to exclude the presence of an abscess.

Treatment

The best treatment is to remove the affected salivary gland and drain the mucocele.[54, 56, 59] Although the sublingual gland is most commonly affected, it cannot be resected without removal of the submandibular gland.[3, 57] If surgery cannot be performed because of the client's wishes or anesthetic risk to the animal, the swelling can be lanced and drained periodically.[59]

Prognosis

The prognosis is excellent after removal of the salivary glands.[54, 56, 57] If the mucocele is simply drained, it will return and have to be drained repeatedly.[56]

Gingival Hyperplasia

Gingival hyperplasia occurs as nodular swellings of the attached gingiva. It can occur in any breed but is common in boxers, collies, Great Danes, Doberman pinschers, and Dalmatians.

Pathophysiology

The cause of the hyperplasia is unknown, but it is not related to primary gingivitis and periodontal disease. There may be a hereditary component in some breeds.

Clinical Signs

Often, clinical signs do not occur.[1] The nonpainful swellings may involve some or most of the gingival surfaces. The swellings are similar in color to the surrounding epithelium. Periodontitis can develop.

Diagnostic Plan

If the changes diffusely affect the gingiva, the diagnosis is based on clinical examination. Localized hyperplasia must be differentiated from neoplasias, especially epulides, by biopsy.

Treatment

In most cases, no treatment is needed. If secondary gingivitis and periodontal disease develop, gingivectomy is indicated.[1]

Prognosis

The hyperplasia continues to be present and will recur after gingivectomy.

Oronasal Fistula

Abnormal communications between the oral and nasal cavities are termed oronasal fistulae.[15] They occur most commonly in animals with severe periodontal disease. However, they can be seen in any animal that suffers severe trauma. In puppies and kittens, they occur as congenital abnormalities (cleft palates). Commonly affected breeds include miniature schnauzers, cocker spaniels, beagles, and brachycephalic breeds.[60, 61]

Pathophysiology

Oronasal fistulae occur most commonly in animals with severe periodontal disease and apical root abscesses; lysis occurs through the thin layer of bone that separates the tooth from the nasal cavity or maxillary sinus. They may also develop after tooth removal, other types of oral surgery, or severe trauma, or they may be associated with neoplasia.[15, 62]

Congenital cleft palates consist of cleft lip or cleft hard or soft palate.[63] Often both types of clefts are present, even though the palates develop at different times.[63] The defects occur because of failure of the embryonic nasal or palatal processes to unite; they are inherited traits.

Clinical Signs

Sneezing (especially after eating or drinking) and mucopurulent nasal discharge often occur. Gingivitis with plaque and tartar accumulation or apical root abscesses are found in patients with periodontal disease. In some patients, an ulcerated mass may be present.

Puppies and kittens with cleft palates have difficulty in nursing and do not gain weight. Coughing, gagging, milk exuding from the nostrils, and aspiration pneumonia are common. A cleft lip is often present along with a defect in the hard or soft palate.

Diagnostic Plan

The diagnosis is based on identification of the palatal defect during physical examination (Fig. 29–14). Sedation or general anesthesia may be necessary to facilitate complete examination and probing to determine their full extent. A leukocytosis may be present because of rhinitis.

Treatment

Definitive treatment often requires surgical correction with mucoperiosteal flaps.[15] Puppies and kittens with congenital cleft palates need nutritional management with nasoesophageal, oroesophageal, or gastrostomy tubes to allow sufficient growth before

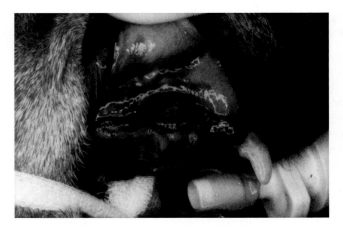

Figure 29–14
Oronasal fistula caused by severe periodontal disease in a 15-year-old dachshund.

surgery. Broad-spectrum antibiotics should be administered.

Prognosis

The prognosis is variable and depends on the size and location of the defect.

Uncommon Diseases of the Oral Cavity, Pharynx, and Salivary Glands

Eosinophilic Granuloma of Dogs

Eosinophilic granulomas of dogs occur most commonly in young, male Siberian huskies on the tongue or in the palatine arch region.[64, 65] Diagnosis requires biopsy. Initial treatment with prednisone, 0.5 to 2.2 mg/kg per day, usually results in resolution of the mass after 2 to 3 weeks. The prednisone dose should be reduced slowly and withdrawn.

Cricopharyngeal Dysphagia

Cricopharyngeal dysphagia (also called achalasia) occurs in young dogs soon after weaning and is caused by asynchronous contraction of the pharynx and relaxation of the cricopharyngeal sphincter.[6, 8, 66] Clinical signs include dysphagia, failure to thrive, and aspiration pneumonia. Diagnosis requires a barium swallow observed with fluoroscopy (see Fig. 29–7). Treatment involves cricopharyngeal myotomy.

Oral Plasmacytoma

Extramedullary plasmacytomas can occur on the gingiva or tongue in middle-aged or older dogs.[67] Most tumors are single, smooth, raised, pink nodules. Surgical resection can be curative, but recurrence is likely with some gingival tumors, and mandibulectomy or maxillectomy may be necessary.

Tonsillar Tumors

Squamous cell carcinoma, lymphosarcoma, or benign polyps can occur on the tonsils. They may be discovered as incidental findings or in association with dysphagia, inappetence, coughing, or gagging. Polyps arise from one tonsil, and removal improves clinical signs.[68] Squamous cell carcinomas usually involve one tonsil, grow rapidly, infiltrate regional tissue, and readily metastasize to lymph nodes and the lungs.[52, 53] Surgery followed by chemotherapy and radiation therapy improves survival, usually to longer than 6 months. Lymphosarcoma usually involves both tonsils (see Fig. 29–13) and is part of the multicentric form of the disease (see Chap. 43).[51]

Tongue Tumors

Tumors of the tongue may be discovered as incidental findings or in association with salivation, halitosis, dysphagia, inappetence, hemorrhage, or stertorous respiration. Squamous cell carcinomas, plasmacytomas, granular cell myoblastomas, malignant melanomas, and mast cell tumors can be found.[69] Surgical removal of granular cell myoblastomas and plasma cell tumors results in long-term survival, and removal of melanomas can result in survival times longer than 1 year.[69, 70]

Oral Papillomatosis

Oral papillomas in young dogs are caused by a papillomavirus.[71] They can occur anywhere within the oral cavity. Often 50 to 100 masses are present. They can cause hemorrhage and pain if the dog bites the masses. They spontaneously regress after 4 to 8 weeks of growth. If necessary, surgery, cryosurgery, or electrosurgery is an effective treatment.

Sialadenitis

Inflammation of the salivary glands, with or without necrosis and infarction, can be associated with trauma, infection, or mucoceles.[2, 72] The mandibular glands are most commonly affected. Swelling, pain, and fever may occur. Retrobulbar abscesses with exophthalmos, strabismus, and reluctance to open the mouth may be associated with zygomatic sialadenitis.[2] Treatment for abscesses should include ventral drainage caudolateral to the last maxillary molar and broad-spectrum antibiotic therapy.[3] Treatment for other cases of sialadenitis is empiric and includes broad-spectrum antibiotics, anti-inflammatory drugs, and surgical debridement of necrotic tissue.

Salivary Tumors

Many types of salivary tumors have been reported in old dogs and cats, but adenocarcinoma is most common.[72, 73] The parotid gland is commonly affected.[73] Most animals present with an asymptomatic mass.[73] Most tumors are locally invasive, making surgical resection difficult; if surgery can be accomplished, recurrence is common. Radiation therapy after the surgery may be beneficial.[74]

References

1. Harvey CE. Oral, dental, pharyngeal, and salivary disorders. In: Ettinger SJ, ed. Textbook of Veterinary Internal Medicine, 3rd ed. Philadelphia, WB Saunders, 1989:1203–1254.
2. Knecht CD. Diseases of the salivary glands in the dog. Compen Contin Educ Pract Vet 1980;1:932–938.
3. Smith MM. Surgery of the canine salivary system. Compen Contin Educ Pract Vet 1985;7:457–480.
4. Wiggs RB. Canine oral anatomy and physiology. Compen Contin Educ Pract Vet 1989;11:1475–1482.
5. Shelton GD. Swallowing disorders in the dog. Compen Contin Educ Pract Vet 1982;4:607–616.
6. Watrous BJ, Suter PF. Oropharyngeal dysphagias in the dog: A cinefluorographic analysis of experimentally induced and spontaneously occurring swallowing disorders. II: Cricopharyngeal stage and mixed oropharyngeal dysphagias. Vet Radiol 1983;24:11–24.
7. Suter PF, Watrous BJ. Oropharyngeal dysphagias in the dog: A cinefluorographic analysis of experimentally induced and spontaneously occurring swallowing disorders. I: Oral stage and pharyngeal stage dysphagias. Vet Radiol 1980;21:24–39.
8. Goring RL, Kagan KG. Cricopharyngeal achalasia in the dog: Radiographic evaluation and surgical management. Compen Contin Educ Pract Vet 1982;4:438–447.
9. Venker-van Haagen A, Hartman W, Wolvekamp W. Contributions of the glossopharyngeal nerve and the pharyngeal branch of the vagus nerve to the swallowing process of dogs. Am J Vet Res 1986;47:1300–1307.
10. Harvey CE. Oral inflammatory diseases in cats. J Am Anim Hosp Assoc 1991;27:585–591.
11. Knowles JO, Gaskell RM, Gaskell CJ, et al. Prevalence of feline calicivirus, feline leukaemia virus and antibodies to FIV in cats with chronic stomatitis. Vet Rec 1989;124:336–338.
12. Waters L, Hopper CD, Gruffydd-Jones TJ, et al. Chronic gingivitis in a colony of cats infected with feline immunodeficiency virus and feline calicivirus. Vet Rec 1993;132:340–342.
13. McKeever PJ, Klausner JS. Plant awn, candidal, nocardial, and necrotizing ulcerative stomatitis in the dog. J Am Anim Hosp Assoc 1986;22:17–24.
14. Anderson JG. Approach to diagnosis of canine oral lesions. Compen Contin Educ Pract Vet 1991;13:1215–1219,1222–1226.
15. Bojrab MJ, Tholen MA, Constantinescu MG. Oronasal

fistulae in dogs and cats. Compen Contin Educ Pract Vet 1986;8:815–819.

16. Aller S. Dental home care and preventive strategies. Semin Vet Med Surg (Small Anim) 1993;8:204–212.

17. Thompson RR, Wilcox GE, Clark WT, et al. Association of calicivirus infection with chronic gingivitis and pharyngitis in cats. J Small Anim Pract 1984;25:207–210.

18. White SD, Rosychuk RAW, Janik TA, et al. Plasma cell stomatitis-pharyngitis in cats: 40 cases (1973–1991). J Am Vet Med Assoc 1992;200:1377–1380.

19. Johnessee JS, Hurvitz AI. Feline plasma cell gingivitis-pharyngitis. J Am Anim Hosp Assoc 1983;19:179–181.

20. Felts JF, Fox PR, Burk RL. Thread and sewing needles as gastrointestinal foreign bodies in the cat: A review of 64 cases. J Am Vet Med Assoc 1984;184:56–59.

21. Basher AWP, Fowler JD. Conservative versus surgical management of gastrointestinal linear foreign bodies in the cat. Vet Surg 1987;16:135–138.

22. Rendano VT, Zimmer JF, Wallach MS, et al. Impaction of the pharynx, larynx, and esophagus by avian bones in the dog and cat. Vet Radiol 1988;29:213–216.

23. White RAS, Lane JG. Pharyngeal stick penetration injuries in the dog. J Small Anim Pract 1988;29:13–35.

24. Oakes MG, Lewis DD, Hedlund CS, et al. Canine oral neoplasia. Compen Contin Educ Pract Vet 1993; 15:15–30.

25. Golden AL, Stoller N, Harvey CE. A survey of oral and dental diseases in dogs anesthetized at a veterinary hospital. J Am Anim Hosp Assoc 1982;18:891–899.

26. Hoyt RF, Withrow SJ. Oral malignancy in the dog. J Am Anim Hosp Assoc 1982;20:83–92.

27. Richardson RC, Jones MA, Elliott GS. Oral neoplasms in the dog: A diagnostic and therapeutic dilemma. Compen Contin Educ Pract Vet 1983;5:441–448.

28. Stebbins KE, Morse CC, Goldschmidt MH. Feline oral neoplasia: A ten-year survey. Vet Pathol 1989; 26: 121–128.

29. Bradley RL, MacEwen EG, Loar AS. Mandibular resection for removal of oral tumors in 30 dogs and 6 cats. J Am Vet Med Assoc 1984;184:460–463.

30. Emms SG, Harvey CE. Preliminary results of maxillectomy in the dog and cat. J Small Anim Pract 1986;27:291–306.

31. Penwick RC, Numamaker DM. Rostral mandibulectomy: A treatment for oral neoplasia in the dog and cat. J Am Anim Hosp Assoc 1987;23:19–25.

32. Schwarz PD, Withrow SJ, Curtis CR, et al. Mandibular resection as a treatment for oral cancer in 81 dogs. J Am Anim Hosp Assoc 1991;27:601–610.

33. Schwarz PD, Withrow SJ, Curtis CR, et al. Partial maxillary resection as a treatment for oral cancer in 61 dogs. J Am Anim Hosp Assoc 1991;27:617–624.

34. White RAS, Jefferies AR, Freedman LS. Clinical staging for oropharyngeal malignancies in the dog. J Small Anim Pract 1985:26:581–594.

35. Kosovsky JK, Matthiesen DT, Manfra Marretta S, et al. Results of partial mandibulectomy for the treatment of oral tumors in 142 dogs. Vet Surg 1991;20:397–401.

36. Donner GS. The role of surgery in the treatment of common tumors of the nose and mouth. Vet Med 1992;87:993–998.

37. Salisbury SK, Richardson DC, Lantz GC. Partial maxillectomy and premaxillectomy in the treatment of oral neoplasia in the dog and cat. Vet Surg 1986;15:16–26.

38. Evans SM, Shofer F. Canine oral nontonsillar squamous cell carcinoma: Prognostic factors for recurrence and survival following orthovoltage therapy. Vet Radiol 1988;29:133–137.

39. Bjorling DE, Chambers JN, Mahaffey EA. Surgical treatment of epulides in dogs: 25 cases (1974–1984). J Am Vet Med Assoc 1987;190:1315–1318.

40. Frew DG, Dobson JM. Radiological assessment of 50 cases of incisive or maxillary neoplasia in the dog. J Small Anim Pract 1992;33:11–18.

41. Thrall DE. Orthovoltage radiotherapy of acanthomatous epulides in 39 dogs. J Am Vet Med Assoc 1984;184: 826–829.

42. Thompson JM, Gorman NT, Bleehen NM, et al. Hyperthermia and radiation in the management of canine tumours. J Small Anim Pract 1987;28:457–477.

43. Brewer WG, Turrel JM. Radiotherapy and hyperthermia in the treatment of fibrosarcomas in the dog. J Am Vet Med Assoc 1982;181:146–150.

44. Hutson CA, Willauer CC, Walder EJ, et al. Treatment of mandibular squamous cell carcinoma in cats by use of mandibulectomy and radiotherapy: Seven cases (1987–1989). J Am Vet Med Assoc 1992;201:777–781.

45. White RAS. Mandibulectomy and maxillectomy in the dog: Long term survival in 100 cases. J Small Anim Pract 1991;32:69–74.

46. White RAS, Gorman NT, Watkins SB, et al. The surgical management of bone-involved oral tumours in the dog. J Small Anim Pract 1985;26:693–708.

47. Withrow SJ, Holmberg DL. Mandibulectomy in the treatment of oral cancer. J Am Anim Hosp Assoc 1983;19:273–286.

48. Hahn KA, DeNicola DB, Richardson RC, et al. Canine oral malignant melanoma: Prognostic utility of an alternative staging system. J Small Anim Pract 1994;35: 251–256.

49. White RAS, Gorman NT. Wide local excision of acanthomatous epulides in the dog. Vet Surg 1989;18:12–14.

50. Hallstrom M. Surgery of the canine mouth and pharynx. J Small Anim Pract 1970;11:105–111.

51. Couto CG. Canine lymphomas: Something old, something new. Compen Contin Educ Pract Vet 1985;7: 291–302.

52. MacMillan R, Withrow SJ, Gillette EL. Surgery and regional irradiation for treatment of canine tonsillar squamous cell carcinoma: Retrospective review of eight cases. J Am Anim Hosp Assoc 1982;18:311–314.

53. Brooks MB, Matus RE, Leifer CE, et al. Chemotherapy versus chemotherapy plus radiotherapy in the treatment of tonsillar squamous cell carcinoma in the dog. J Vet Intern Med 1988;2:206–212.

54. Weber WJ, Hobson HP, Wilson SR. Pharyngeal mucoceles in dogs. Vet Surg 1986;15:5–8.

55. Harvey HJ. Pharyngeal mucoceles in dogs. J Am Vet Med Assoc 1981;178:1282–1283.

56. Glen JB. Canine salivary mucocoeles: Results of sialographic examination and surgical treatment of fifty cases. J Small Anim Pract 1972;13:515–526.

57. Harvey CE. Canine salivary mucocele. J Am Anim Hosp Assoc 1969;5:155–165.
58. Spreull JSA, Head KW. Cervical salivary cysts in the dog. J Small Anim Pract 1967;8:17–35.
59. Harvey CE. Salivary gland disorders. In: Bojrab MJ, ed. Disease Mechanisms in Small Animal Surgery. Philadelphia, Lea & Febiger, 1993:197–199.
60. Howard DR, Davis DG, Merkley DF, et al. Mucoperiosteal flap technique for cleft palate repair in dogs. J Am Vet Med Assoc 1974;165:352–354.
61. Edmonds L, Stewart RW, Selby L. Cleft lip and palate in Boston terrier pups. VMSAC 1972;67:1219–1222.
62. Salisbury SK, Richardson DC. Partial maxillectomy for oronasal fistula repair in the dog. J Am Anim Hosp Assoc 1986;22:185–192.
63. Sinibaldi KR. Cleft palate. Vet Clin North Am Small Anim Pract 1979;9:245–257.
64. Madewell BR, Stannard AA, Pulley LT, et al. Oral eosinophilic granuloma in Siberian husky dogs. J Am Vet Med Assoc 1980;177:701–703.
65. Potter KA, Tucker RD, Carpenter JL. Oral eosinophilic granuloma of Siberian huskies. J Am Anim Hosp Assoc 1980;16:595–600.
66. Weaver AD. Cricopharyngeal achalasia in cocker spaniels. J Small Anim Pract 1983;24:209–214.
67. Clark GN, Berg J, Engler SJ, et al. Extramedullary plasmacytomas in dogs: Results of surgical excision in 131 cases. J Am Anim Hosp Assoc 1992;28:105–111.
68. Lucke VM, Pearson GR, Gregory SP, et al. Tonsillar polyps in the dog. J Small Anim Pract 1988;29:373–379.
69. Beck ER, Withrow SJ, McChesney AE, et al. Canine tongue tumors: A retrospective review of 57 cases. J Am Anim Hosp Assoc 1986;22:525–532.
70. Rakich PM, Latimer KS, Weiss R, et al. Mucocutaneous plasmacytomas in dogs: 75 cases (1980–1987). J Am Vet Med Assoc 1989;194:803–810.
71. Calvert CA. Canine viral papillomatosis. In: Greene CE, ed. Infectious Diseases of the Dog and Cat. Philadelphia, WB Saunders, 1990:288–290.
72. Spangler WL, Culbertson MR. Salivary gland disease in dogs and cats: 245 cases (1985–1988). J Am Vet Med Assoc 1991;198:465–469.
73. Carberry CA, Flanders JA, Harvey HJ, et al. Salivary gland tumors in dogs and cats: A literature and case review. J Am Anim Hosp Assoc 1988;24:561–567.
74. Evans SM, Thrall DE. Postoperative orthovoltage radiation therapy of parotid salivary gland adenocarcinoma in three dogs. J Am Vet Med Assoc 1983;182:993–994.

Chapter 30

Diseases of the Esophagus

Michael S. Leib

Anatomy

The esophagus is a muscular tube that connects the pharynx to the stomach. It consists of three regions; the cervical esophagus extends from the pharynx to the thoracic inlet; the thoracic portion continues to the hiatus of the diaphragm; and a short abdominal segment connects with the cardia of the stomach. The cranial cervical esophagus lies dorsal to the trachea but courses to the left as it approaches the thoracic inlet. In the cranial mediastinum, the esophagus lies to the left of the trachea. The esophagus lies dorsal to the tracheal bifurcation and to the right of the aorta as it leaves the thorax. The esophageal hiatus of the diaphragm is on the midline, ventral to the aortic hiatus.

Histologically, the canine esophagus comprises four layers: an inner mucosa, consisting of an epithelial lining of stratified squamous epithelium, lamina propria, and muscularis mucosa; a submucosa, which contains mucous glands, blood vessels, nerves, and connective tissue; a thick, muscular layer composed of two oblique intertwining layers of striated muscle; and an outer layer of loose connective tissue.[1-3] The esophagus is bounded by two sphincters, the cricopharyngeal sphincter and the gastroesophageal sphincter (GES). The cricopharyngeal sphincter is composed of the cricopharyngeal and thryropharyngeal muscles and functions to prevent aerophagia and esophageal-pharyngeal reflux. The GES consists of an inner layer of smooth muscle that functions in concert with an outer, longitudinal layer of striated muscle to prevent gastroesophageal (GE) reflux.

The innervation to the orad portion of the esophagus is supplied by the glossopharyngeal nerve and pharyngeal branches of the vagus nerve. Innervation to the remainder of the esophagus is supplied by branches of the vagus nerve.[3]

The anatomy of the feline esophagus differs from that of the dog.[1] The muscular layer of the middle and most of the aboral portions of the feline esophagus consists of a mixture of smooth and striated muscle, whereas the terminal section (approximately 35%) is entirely smooth muscle, with an inner circular layer and an outer longitudinal layer. A myenteric nervous plexus, important in control of motility, exists between the smooth muscle layers.

Physiology

The function of the esophagus is to transport ingesta from the mouth to the stomach in an orderly fashion.[2, 3] As the pharyngeal muscles contract and propel a food bolus aborally, the cricopharyngeal sphincter relaxes to accept the bolus. After passage of the bolus into the esophagus, the cricopharyngeal sphincter contracts, preventing esophageal-pharyngeal reflux.

Distention of the orad esophagus initiates a progressive wave of muscular contraction, termed primary peristalsis.[1] As the bolus is propelled aborally, the wave of peristalsis is maintained by stimulation associated with esophageal distention. As the bolus approaches the distal esophagus, the GES relaxes to allow passage of the ingesta into the stomach. The GES then contracts, preventing GE reflux. If the wave of primary peristalsis fails to propel the bolus into the stomach, esophageal distention stimulates a wave of secondary peristalsis that begins orad to the bolus and moves the bolus toward the stomach.

Normal esophageal motility in dogs requires reflex control by the central nervous system. Sensory receptors in the esophagus are stimulated by distention and relay information to the swallowing center in the brain stem by means of the vagus nerves and the nucleus solitarius. Inhibitory impulses are sent to the respiratory center, preventing inspiration during swallowing. The swallowing center connects to the nucleus ambiguus, which contains the cell bodies of the lower motor neurons that travel in the vagus nerves and innervate the esophageal striated muscle.

Control of the GES is complex. Release of an inhibitory neurotransmitter results in relaxation of the sphincter. Sphincter function is controlled by a combination of neurologic input, circulating hormones, and intrinsic smooth muscle myogenic factors.

Because of differences in anatomy, the feline esophagus functions differently from that of the dog. Control of the striated muscle is similar to that in dogs. Control of the smooth muscle relies on local intramural reflexes mediated through the myenteric plexus, but it is influenced by cholinergic neurons contained in the vagus nerve.

Problem Identification

Regurgitation

Regurgitation of food or water is the most common problem associated with esophageal disorders in dogs and cats.[1] Regurgitation is defined as the passive backward movement of food or water from the esophagus to the pharynx, where a gag reflex is triggered and results in expulsion of the matter from the mouth.

Pathophysiology

Regurgitation is not associated with a neurologic reflex or reverse esophageal peristalsis. Food or fluid that is retained in the esophagus because of obstruction or because of ineffective, decreased, or absent motility is propelled along the path of least resistance by increased intrathoracic pressure associated with excitement, changes in body position, respiration, muscular activity, or extreme esophageal dilation.

Regurgitation must be differentiated from oropharyngeal dysphagia, vomiting, or, in some instances, expectoration. Often, owners have not observed the act but describe finding "vomitus." Even if they observe the event, owners often describe all of these processes as vomiting. A careful history is necessary to distinguish between them. Accurate problem identification is important because the differential diagnosis, diagnostic plan, and therapeutic plan are different for each of these problems. Oropharyngeal dysphagia results in food, or sometimes water, falling from the mouth soon after chewing. Repeated swallowing attempts often occur (see Chap. 29). Expectoration is always preceded by coughing (see Chaps. 9 and 54). Vomiting is associated with nausea and is manifested by frequent swallowing and licking of the lips, retching, and abdominal contractions (see vomiting in Chap. 31). If the owner is unable to provide an accurate description, it is necessary to observe the animal eating.

Both regurgitation and vomiting can occur soon after swallowing or can be delayed 24 hours or more after a meal. The longer food is retained within the esophagus, the more "digested" it appears. If the owner does not observe the event, a urine dipstick placed into the material may help differentiate regurgitation from vomiting. A low pH indicates gastric contents and vomiting. The presence of bilirubin indicates small intestinal contents and confirms vomiting.[4]

Clinical Signs

A careful review of the signalment and history can help establish the differential diagnoses (Table 30–1), allowing a final diagnosis to be obtained efficiently. Regurgitation that begins soon after weaning is common in cases of megaesophagus and vascular ring anomalies. These two disorders may also affect multiple littermates. Puppies that begin regurgitating acutely may have ingested a foreign body that has become lodged in the esophagus. Regurgitation that begins 5 to 14 days after an esophageal foreign body has been removed after general anesthesia has been used, or after a severe vomiting episode has occurred may be caused by stricture formation. An animal that can retain water but regurgitates food may have a partial esophageal obstruction caused by stricture, foreign body, extraluminal esophageal compression, or, rarely, neoplasia.

The history may include observation of or the possibility of ingestion of a foreign body, ingestion of hot food or fluids, or exposure to caustic substances,

Table 30–1
Causes of Regurgitation

Foreign body
Megaesophagus
Vascular ring anomaly
Esophagitis
Stricture
Extraluminal esophageal obstruction
Esophageal neoplasia
Hiatal hernia
Secondary megaesophagus
Spirocerca lupi
Gastroesophageal intussusception
Segmental motility disorder
Diverticulum
Bronchial esophageal fistula
Esophageal deviation

such as drain cleaners, that can cause esophagitis. If adult dogs also demonstrate generalized muscle weakness, megaesophagus secondary to myasthenia gravis may be present.

Coughing, nasal discharge, tachypnea, or dyspnea can occur secondary to aspiration pneumonia associated with regurgitation. A history of respiratory signs before the onset of regurgitation may indicate an extraluminal esophageal obstruction. In cases of mediastinal or multicentric lymphosarcoma, enlarged mediastinal or hilar lymph nodes can partially obstruct the esophagus.

Odynophagia, or pain associated with swallowing, may occur with foreign bodies, esophagitis, or strictures. Animals with megaesophagus or vascular ring anomalies maintain excellent appetites unless moderate or severe aspiration pneumonia is present. A poor appetite is often associated with foreign bodies, esophagitis, extraluminal esophageal compression, or moderate or severe aspiration pneumonia, which may occur with any cause of regurgitation.

Physical examination demonstrates failure to thrive in puppies and kittens and weight loss in adults. Pain detected on palpation of the cervical region suggests the presence of esophagitis or a foreign body. Ingestion of caustic or hot substances usually results in oral erosion in addition to esophagitis. Auscultation of the thorax may detect crackles, most commonly in the cranioventral lung fields, associated with aspiration pneumonia. Compression of the thorax with the mouth closed and nares occluded may produce a bulging of the cervical region; this is caused by a dilated, air-filled esophagus and is associated with megaesophagus, vascular ring anomaly, or a long-standing stricture or extraluminal esophageal obstruction. Postprandial esophageal distention may be detected near the tho-

Table 30–2
Causes of Secondary Megaesophagus

Myasthenia gravis
Dysautonomia
Systemic lupus erythematosus
Polymyositis
Polyneuritis
Familial canine dermatomyositis
Giant axonal neuropathy
Hypoadrenalcorticism
Polyradiculoneuritis
Familial reflex myoclonus
Ganglioradiculitis
Glycogen storage disease, type II
Medullary disease—canine distemper, trauma, neo-
    plasia
Anticholinesterase intoxication
Bronchoesophageal fistula
Spinal muscle atrophy
Thallium poisoning
Botulism
Lead poisoning

racic inlet in these disorders. Extraluminal esophageal obstruction caused by lymphosarcoma may be associated with a noncompressible thorax or muffled heart and lung sounds (pleural effusion) in cats or generalized lymphadenopathy in dogs. Generalized muscle weakness or other neurologic deficits suggest that myasthenia gravis or other neuromuscular disorders may have resulted in secondary megaesophagus. Other abnormalities found on physical examination may help identify a systemic disease that uncommonly causes a secondary megaesophagus (Table 30–2).

Diagnostic Plan

After confirmation that an animal is regurgitating, the most important diagnostic step is to make survey thoracic radiographs. If a diagnosis cannot be made, a barium contrast esophagram should be performed. If an intramural mass or irregular mucosal surface is demonstrated on the esophagram, histologic examination of biopsies obtained by endoscopy is necessary for diagnosis. If radiographic studies are normal, endoscopic examination should always be performed, because esophagitis and some strictures can be difficult to confirm radiographically.

Cough

Regurgitation is often associated with an acute, chronic, or intermittent cough. In most cases, a history of regurgitation preceding the development of cough is present and suggests that the cough is secondary to aspiration pneumonia. Evaluation of the primary problem of regurgitation should lead to a definitive diagnosis. Thoracic radiographs and a complete blood count can help assess the severity of the aspiration pneumonia. Occasionally, in a coughing animal, a history of regurgitation cannot be obtained because regurgitation is infrequent or not observed by the owner. Diagnostic evaluation of the cough with survey thoracic radiographs often demonstrates aspiration pneumonia and evidence of esophageal disease. Any time thoracic radiographs indicate that aspiration pneumonia may be present, a careful review of the history and thoracic radiographs for evidence of esophageal disease should be performed. A barium contrast esophagram may be necessary to eliminate the presence of esophageal disorders causing regurgitation and aspiration pneumonia. See Chapters 9 and 54 for a complete diagnostic approach to the problem of cough.

Diagnostic Procedures

Routine Laboratory Evaluation

A complete blood count, biochemical profile, and urinalysis contribute little to the diagnosis of esophageal diseases. Aspiration pneumonia can cause a mature neutrophilia, a neutrophilia with a left shift, or, in severe cases, an inappropriate left shift. A foreign body that has perforated the esophageal wall and caused mediastinitis can produce similar changes. Cats with thymic lymphosarcoma, which causes extraluminal esophageal obstruction, may test positive for feline leukemia virus (FeLV). Other laboratory abnormalities may be associated with systemic disorders that rarely result in secondary megaesophagus (see Table 30–2).

Radiography

The normal esophagus is not usually visualized on survey thoracic radiographs unless air is present within the lumen.[5] Survey thoracic radiographs are helpful in the diagnosis of esophageal disease if a radiodense foreign body is present or if the esophagus is dilated with air, fluid, or food. Generalized esophageal dilation occurs with megaesophagus; regional dilation may be caused by stricture, foreign body, extraluminal esophageal obstruction, or a vascular ring anomaly. In some cases, a dilated esophagus may not be visualized but can be suspected if a widened mediastinum or a displaced trachea (ventrally and to the right) can be seen. A thymic mass or mediastinal, hilar, or sternal lymphadenopathy causing extraluminal esophageal obstruction may also be noted. Cats with mediastinal lymphosarcoma may have pleural effusion. Aspiration pneumonia is a common complication of esophageal disease and appears as peribronchial and alveolar densities, most commonly in the ventral aspects of the cranial and middle lung lobes. However, any lung lobe can be involved, and large areas of lung can become consolidated.

If survey radiographs appear normal, a barium contrast esophagram is necessary for diagnosis. Esophageal size, lumen, mucosal characteristics, and motility can be better assessed by contrast studies. Barium sulfate paste (1–2 mL/kg) allows good definition of the mucosa and can be administered slowly into the mouth with a syringe.[6] The animal should be rolled over several times to help coat the esophagus with barium. Lateral and ventrodorsal oblique (sternum rotated to left) radiographs should be made. Radiolucent foreign bodies, intraluminal masses, or roughened and irregular mucosa caused by esophagitis may be identified.

If a dilated esophagus is suspected on survey radiographs, the esophagus should be distended to determine whether dilation is generalized or regional. Approximately 20 mL of barium sulfate suspension should be mixed with one third of a can of food and enough fed to distend the esophagus. Lateral and ventrodorsal oblique radiographs should be made. If the esophagus is not fully distended, additional boluses should be administered. Megaesophagus or esophageal obstruction secondary to foreign body, stricture, vascular ring anomaly, or extraluminal obstruction can be visualized.

If esophageal perforation is suspected, barium is probably contraindicated, because free barium can cause a severe mediastinitis. Oral aqueous iodine contrast agents are safer.

After administration of barium to a normal animal, only the smooth and parallel longitudinal folds of the esophagus remain coated with a small amount of barium (Fig. 30–1). Most of the contrast medium should be present in the stomach within seconds after administration. In cats, the caudal one third of the esophagus has a herringbone appearance associated with transverse folds because of the presence of smooth muscle[5, 6] (Fig. 30–2). The diameter of the empty esophagus should not exceed the diameter of the aorta.[6] The esophagus normally tapers as it passes through the diaphragm, and this area should not be misinterpreted as a stricture, extraluminal obstruction, or foreign body.

Esophagoscopy

Instrumentation

A flexible endoscope with a working length of 1 m, an outside diameter less than 10 mm, and a biopsy channel of 2.8 mm is appropriate for examination of the esophagus in most dogs and cats.[7, 8] Four-way, distal-tip deflection and automatic water-air insufflation are important characteristics of a useful endoscope. A separate suction pump is necessary.

Although not optimal, rigid proctosigmoidoscopes can be used to examine the proximal esophagus. These inexpensive instruments are available in a variety of diameters. Longer, rigid esophagoscopes are also available.[9, 10] A rigid biopsy forceps allows procurement of large tissue samples. Care must be taken to grasp only mucosa and submucosa, to avoid penetrating the esophageal wall. With rigid endoscopes, the ability to visualize the entire circumference of the esophagus is hampered by lack of mobility. In addition, the clarity of mucosal visualization and forceps dexterity are reduced with rigid equipment. Rigid endoscopes can be beneficial in removing foreign bodies lodged in the esophagus.

Patient Preparation and Restraint

Examination of the esophagus requires withholding of food for at least 12 hours.[11] If esophageal dilation or obstruction is present, endoscopy should be delayed until the esophagus is empty, which may

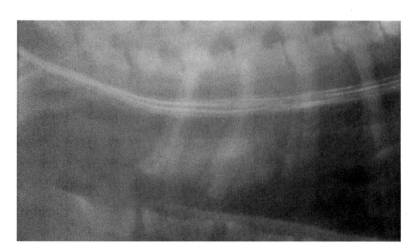

Figure 30–1
Lateral barium esophagram in a normal cat. Only longitudinal stripes of barium are retained within the esophagus.

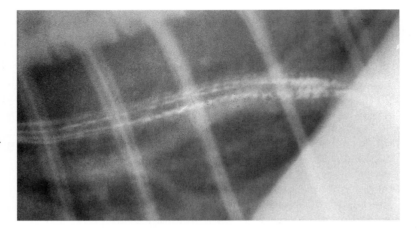

Figure 30-2
The caudal esophagus of a lateral barium esophagram in a normal cat. The transverse folds retain barium in a herringbone pattern.

require a fast of 24 hours or longer. Animals should be allowed free access to water. Examination of the esophagus requires general anesthesia to prevent biting of the endoscope.[12, 13]

Procedure

The animal should be positioned in left lateral recumbence.[14] A mouth speculum must be placed on the left upper and lower canine teeth to protect the endoscope. The tongue should be grasped and the head and neck extended by an assistant. A flexible endoscope is passed over the base of the tongue, through the pharynx dorsal to the endotracheal tube, and into the proximal esophagus. During passage of a flexible endoscope, the tip should be deflected slightly downward to follow the normal anatomic bend between the mouth and pharynx. Lubrication is usually not necessary.

The esophageal mucosa is usually collapsed and appears in longitudinal folds.[11, 12, 15] It should be distended by insufflation of air. The endoscope tip should be centralized within the lumen by adjustment of the control knobs. Only minor tip adjustments are necessary, because the esophagus is a relatively straight tube. By advancing the endoscope only when the lumen is clearly visible, the endoscopist can dramatically reduce the risk of esophageal perforation.

Normal esophageal mucosa is pale pink, smooth, and very tough. Normally, the esophagus should be empty and not contain fluid or food. The trachea indents the distended esophagus, and the tracheal rings should be clearly visible. At the tracheal bifurcation, it is common to see pulsation of the heart or aorta. The GE junction is normally closed and often assumes a stellate mucosal pattern. A small amount of red gastric mucosa can be seen within the distal esophageal lumen.

Because the esophagus is lined by tough, stratified squamous epithelium, it is often difficult to obtain mucosal samples in a normal animal with flexible biopsy forceps. However, obtaining tissue samples from an intraluminal mass or roughened mucosa is relatively easy. To obtain a biopsy, the endoscope tip should be placed 1 to 2 cm from the area to be sampled. The biopsy forceps is advanced through the biopsy channel until it is visible through the endoscope. The forceps should be opened by an assistant, and the endoscopist should advance the forceps until mucosal contact is made. The forceps should then be advanced gently until a slight bowing of the forceps can be seen. The assistant closes the forceps and the endoscopist snaps off the tissue sample by withdrawing the forceps into the biopsy channel. Usually, a small amount of hemorrhage is produced at the biopsy site.

During passage of a rigid endoscope, the animal's head and neck should be fully extended, and the endoscope should be lubricated. The obturator should be in place to facilitate passage into the proximal esophagus. The obturator should then be removed, the viewing lens closed, and air manually insufflated with the bulb to distend the esophagus. The endoscope should be advanced slowly, as long as the lumen is clearly visible. To obtain a biopsy, the endoscope should be placed within 1 cm of the lesion, the viewing lens opened, and the forceps placed into the endoscope. The esophageal mucosa should be grasped gently and the forceps moved back and forth within the endoscope. If the grasped tissue moves easily, it is safe to completely close the forceps and cut off the sample. If the grasped tissue remains fixed to the esophageal wall, the forceps should be opened, because a full-thickness tissue sample may be grasped.

In addition to the obvious length and diameter differences between dogs and cats, there are several striking differences encountered when performing esophagoscopy in cats.[15] First, transverse folds are normally evident in the distal one third of the feline esophagus. Second, it is common to visualize submucosal blood vessels throughout the feline esophagus.

Common Diseases of the Esophagus

Foreign Body Ingestion

Most foreign material ingested by dogs and cats passes uneventfully through the gastrointestinal tract, causes mild vomiting or diarrhea or both, or is dissolved by gastric acid. However, lodging of foreign bodies in the esophagus should be considered an emergency. The longer entrapped foreign bodies are present, the greater the chances of severe esophageal wall damage and perforation.[16] Sharp-pointed objects can penetrate the esophageal wall, leading to mediastinitis or, occasionally, to bronchoesophageal fistula.[17] The most commonly encountered esophageal foreign bodies are bones, rawhide chew toys, fishhooks, and hair balls.

Because of their indiscriminate eating habits and incomplete mastication, dogs ingest more foreign bodies than cats do.[17, 18] Hair balls can obstruct the esophagus in cats. Foreign bodies can be seen in animals of any age but are most common in young pets and dogs routinely given bones or rawhide chew toys.[9] Foreign body entrapment may be more common in small dogs.[17]

Pathophysiology

The esophagus is very distensible, and most ingested foreign objects are passed into the stomach.

Foreign bodies commonly lodge where the esophagus is restricted from distending: at the thoracic inlet, the base of the heart, or the diaphragmatic hiatus. The entrapped foreign body stimulates secondary peristalsis, which can augment pressure necrosis of the esophageal wall.[19, 20] Even though the esophagus is lined by tough stratified squamous epithelium, erosion, ulceration, and perforation can develop if the foreign body is not removed promptly.

Clinical Signs

The most common clinical signs associated with esophageal foreign bodies are regurgitation, excessive salivation, anorexia, odynophagia, and respiratory signs caused by aspiration pneumonia. Foreign body ingestion may be observed or suspected by the owner. Clinical signs develop acutely. With obstructive lesions, regurgitation of water occurs, and dehydration can develop quickly. Perforation of the esophageal wall may result in pyrexia and depression. Mediastinitis and extension into the pleural cavity lead to production of pleural effusion and progressive respiratory difficulty.

Diagnostic Plan

Most esophageal foreign bodies are radiodense and clearly visible on survey radiographs (Fig. 30–3). Other common radiographic findings include a soft

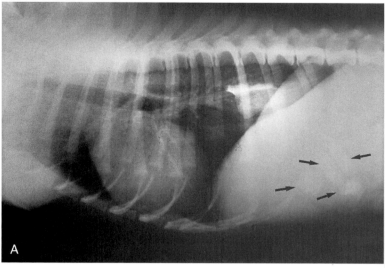
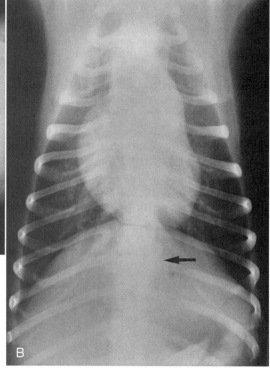

Figure 30–3
(A) Lateral survey thoracic radiograph from a 7-month-old male West Highland white terrier showing a bone density cranial to the diaphragmatic hiatus. Several other bone fragments are visible in the stomach *(arrows)*. **(B)** Ventrodorsal survey thoracic radiograph from the same dog as in **A.** The bone is difficult to see *(arrow)* because it is superimposed over the vertebral bodies.

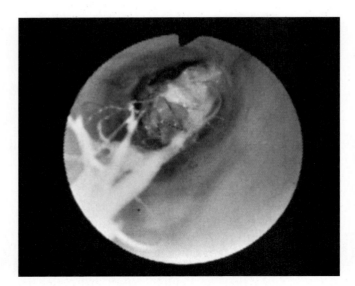

Figure 30–4
Endoscopic appearance of a bone lodged within the esophagus.

tissue density surrounding the foreign body (fluid in the esophagus, thickened wall, or localized mediastinitis) and an air-filled, dilated esophagus cranial to the foreign body.[10] Thin poultry bones can easily be missed because they silhouette with ribs and vertebrae.

Although difficult to diagnose in cases with large entrapped bones, mediastinitis is highly suspicious of esophageal perforation. Radiographic findings associated with mediastinitis include increased mediastinal opacity and widening, extensive fluid density surrounding the foreign body, loss of detail around the mass, and obliteration of the shadow of the caudal vena cava.[17]

Thoracic radiographs taken after endoscopy may demonstrate pneumomediastinum if perforation has occurred. If perforation is suspected on survey radiographs but cannot be confirmed, an iodine contrast study should be performed. Aqueous organic iodide contrast medium at 0.5 to 1.0 mL/kg can be administered.[6] Contrast studies should be performed after foreign body removal, because while the foreign body is still in place it may obstruct the perforation site, blocking leakage of contrast material.[17]

Treatment

Most esophageal foreign bodies can be removed successfully with the use of an endoscope (Fig. 30–4).[10] Surgery of the esophagus should be avoided, if possible, because of difficult exposure in the thorax, postoperative morbidity, and frequent complications. If foreign bodies cannot be extracted endoscopically from the esophagus, they can often be pushed carefully into the stomach. In the stomach, gastric acid acts to

dissolve many foreign bodies; they can also be removed with gastrotomy or removed endoscopically (because more room is available for endoscopic manipulation).[10, 18, 19]

Most foreign bodies can be removed with the use of flexible endoscopic techniques. Large foreign bodies may be so tightly lodged in the esophagus that flexible endoscopic forceps cannot grasp the object tightly enough for removal. These objects can often be retrieved by a rigid uterine or rectal biopsy forceps passed alongside the flexible endoscope.[16] During removal, large foreign bodies may lodge at the pharynx, but they can be removed by grasping with curved Carmalt forceps. Foreign bodies can also be removed with the use of a rigid endoscope and rigid forceps.[9, 10, 18]

During retrieval of an esophageal foreign body, air should be insufflated as the endoscope is withdrawn, to help dilate the esophagus and prevent damage to the esophageal mucosa as the foreign body is pulled out.

Fishhooks can be very difficult to remove. If the tip of the hook is protruding into the lumen, it can be grasped and the entire hook pulled through the mucosa and removed. If the tip of the hook is not visible but appears to be embedded in only the mucosa or submucosa, the hook can gently be torn through the mucosa, creating a superficial laceration that usually heals without complication. If the hook appears to have passed through the esophageal wall, it should be surgically removed.

Hair balls, which are most common in cats, often fall apart when grasped with forceps. Multiple attempts may be necessary to retrieve them. Sometimes, it is easier to push the hair ball into the stomach, where there is more room for endoscopic manipulation and where it can be grasped with a basket or snare forceps and removed.

Perforation with mediastinitis is a severe complication of esophageal foreign bodies. Small perforations can be managed medically (as described for mild esophagitis), but large perforations require surgical repair.[9]

Mild esophagitis and erosion heal quickly and without complications. Food should be withheld for 24 hours, after which frequent feedings of small quantities of gruel are given for 2 or 3 days. The gruel can gradually be thickened, the meal volume increased, and the feeding frequency decreased if regurgitation does not occur. Moderate or severe esophagitis and ulceration require medical management (see Esophagitis).

Prognosis

The overall prognosis is good but is dependent on the type of foreign body, the duration it is present, the degree and severity of esophageal damage, and the development of perforation. The longer a foreign body is present, the harder it is to remove and the greater the chance for perforation. Large perforations warrant a poor prognosis, despite aggressive surgical care.[17] Most patients with esophagitis that receive appropriate medical care heal without complications.[10, 19] In some cases, strictures can develop after foreign body retrieval. Patients with severe esophagitis or ulceration should be re-evaluated by endoscopy after 7 to 10 days to assess stricture formation, which, if present, can be dilated with balloon catheters.

Megaesophagus

Megaesophagus is the most common cause of chronic regurgitation in dogs. It is a syndrome in which the esophagus becomes dilated because of neuromuscular dysfunction, which produces decreased motility.[2] Megaesophagus is most often idiopathic. Although traditionally it was thought to occur most often in puppies, several reports have found that as many as 50% of patients are adults at the time of diagnosis.[21–24] Development of megaesophagus secondary to a systemic or neuromuscular disorder occurs more commonly in adults.[25] Myasthenia gravis is the most common cause of secondary megaesophagus in adult dogs.[26]

Megaesophagus may affect one puppy, multiple littermates, or, on rare occasions, the entire litter.[24, 27] Megaesophagus occurs in most breeds of dogs, but an increased prevalence has been noted among German shepherds, Great Danes, miniature schnauzers, wirehaired fox terriers, Labrador retrievers, and Irish setters.[21, 24] The disorder has been shown to be hereditary in wirehaired fox terriers and miniature schnauzers and most likely can be inherited in many other breeds.[22, 28] Megaesophagus is uncommon in cats and is most frequently described with the neurologic condition dysautonomia.[29, 30]

To avoid confusion, a dilated esophagus caused by obstruction from a foreign body, stricture, extraluminal compression, intraluminal mass, or vascular ring anomaly should not be termed megaesophagus.

Pathophysiology

Animals with megaesophagus have decreased or absent esophageal peristalsis, which results in retention of ingesta within the esophagus, esophageal distention, and regurgitation. After swallowing, the GES remains closed, because it has not received the proper stimulus for relaxation, which is normally stimulated by an aborally moving peristaltic wave. The GES is not hypertensive; rather, it is thought to function asynchronously, not in coordination with the presence of a bolus in the distal esophagus.[31, 32] The mechanisms responsible for sporadic relaxation of the GES in cases of megaesophagus are unknown.

The pathophysiology of idiopathic megaesophagus has not been studied in large numbers of dogs.[27, 33, 34] However, it appears that the lower motor neuron portion of the esophageal peristaltic reflex is intact. The neurologic defect in idiopathic megaesophagus resides in the ascending sensory arm of the peristaltic reflex or within interconnections in the brain stem.

Secondary megaesophagus can occur with dysfunction in any portion of the peristaltic reflex; mucosal receptors (esophagitis), neuromuscular junction (myasthenia gravis), striated muscle (polymyositis), peripheral nerve (polyneuropathy), or central nervous system (inflammatory, toxic, or neoplastic disorders).[24, 25]

Clinical Signs

Regurgitation of food or water is the most common clinical sign. Regurgitation may occur immediately after eating or may be delayed up to 24 hours. The frequency of regurgitation waxes and wanes without a detectable cause and varies greatly among affected dogs. Puppies often start regurgitating after solid food is instituted but occasionally may regurgitate milk through the nostrils while nursing. Affected puppies fail to grow normally and develop poor hair coats. Adult dogs with megaesophagus usually exhibit rapid weight loss. Other signs of an underlying primary disorder may also be apparent (see Table 30–2). In some cases of myasthenia gravis, signs of generalized episodic weakness are apparent, but in others only esophageal weakness occurs.[26] In adult cats with dysautonomia regurgitation, constipation, bradycardia, decreased lacrimal and nasal secretion, and dilated pupils occur. Although this perplexing disorder appeared in the United Kingdom in the early 1980s, it was never commonly recognized in the United States.[29, 30] Presently, dysautonomia is rarely seen in the United Kingdom.

Approximately 60% of dogs with megaesophagus have aspiration pneumonia at the time of diagnosis.[21, 23, 24] Aspiration pneumonia is often the cause of death or euthanasia. On occasion, respiratory signs occur without historical evidence of regurgitation.[23] Uncommonly, dogs are asymptomatic and megaesophagus is discovered incidentally.[23]

Diagnostic Plan

Survey radiographs often show an esophagus uniformly dilated with gas, fluid, or ingesta (Fig. 30–5) but on occasion may identify only a partially dilated esophagus.[24, 25] The trachea may be depressed cranial to the heart on the lateral view.[5, 6, 24, 25] A prominent

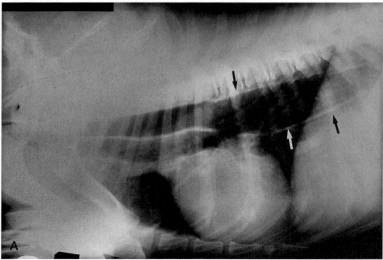
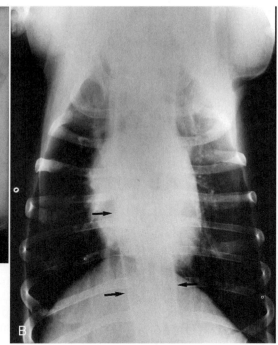
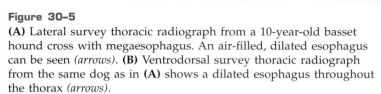

Figure 30-5
(A) Lateral survey thoracic radiograph from a 10-year-old basset hound cross with megaesophagus. An air-filled, dilated esophagus can be seen *(arrows)*. **(B)** Ventrodorsal survey thoracic radiograph from the same dog as in **(A)** shows a dilated esophagus throughout the thorax *(arrows)*.

tracheal stripe may be present, caused by the air-filled, dilated esophagus silhouetting with the tracheal wall.[24] Peribronchial and alveolar infiltration and pulmonary consolidation suggest aspiration pneumonia (Fig. 30–6). Retention of barium mixed with food within a dilated, hypomotile esophagus without evidence of obstruction is diagnostic of megaesophagus. Most often, the entire thoracic esophagus is uniformly dilated (see Fig. 30–6). If examined, the cervical esophagus is usually also dilated, but not to the same magnitude as the thoracic esophagus. On occasion, cranial to the heart, the esophagus gravitates ventrally and forms a large sacculation.[24] This radiographic pattern can be differentiated from a vascular ring anomaly because a dilated esophagus is also present caudal to the heart.

Radiographic signs do not correlate well with clinical signs, and dogs with identical fluoroscopic motility patterns can have vastly different clinical signs.[24, 25] In addition, waxing and waning clinical signs in an individual dog are not associated with changing radiographic findings.

After megaesophagus is diagnosed in an adult dog, a thorough investigation for an underlying primary disorder should be undertaken (see Table 30–1).[24, 25] A careful neurologic examination should be performed because many neuromuscular disorders can cause a secondary megaesophagus. Any identifiable neurologic abnormalities should be evaluated by appropriate ancillary tests. Even if the neurologic examination is normal, an antibody titer for acetylcho-

line receptors should be determined, because myasthenia gravis can be localized to the striated muscle of the esophagus without causing other signs of weakness.[26]

A thorough laboratory evaluation should be performed to identify any of the diseases that can cause a secondary megaesophagus (see Table 30–2).[24, 25]

Treatment

Dietary management is the most universally accepted therapy for megaesophagus.[21, 24, 25] Elevated feedings of a liquid diet are tolerated by many dogs. Dogs can easily be trained to eat from an elevated platform. Large dogs can be trained to sit after eating. Small dogs should be held upright for 15 minutes after eating. Elevated feeding allows gravity to assist delivery of food into the stomach. The GES still functions asynchronously, so some ingesta may be retained within the esophagus.

Small volumes (to reduce esophageal distention) of a high-protein, calorie-dense canned food, mixed approximately 1:1 with water into a gruel consistency, should be fed frequently. The feeding frequency can be decreased, the volume increased, and the consistency of the gruel gradually thickened if regurgitation does not occur. Other types of food should be tried if regurgitation persists, because some dogs tolerate dry or semimoist foods better. Small (1–2 cm in diameter) "meatballs" of canned food work well in some patients.

Aspiration pneumonia often becomes a serious complication. Antibiotic therapy should be based on culture and sensitivity testing on samples obtained by transtracheal aspiration. However, if a transtracheal aspirate is not performed, chloramphenicol, ampicillin, trimethoprim-sulfonamides, or cephalosporins may be effective. Consistent absorption of orally administered medication is difficult to achieve because of regurgitation. Parenteral administration of antibiotics should be used initially in the hospital. Because regurgitation can lead to further aspiration, it may be necessary to withhold food and water until aspiration pneumonia improves. Fluid therapy can be administered parenterally to maintain hydration. Because many dogs with megaesophagus are already in a state of negative nitrogen balance, food should not be withheld for more than a few days. Placement of a percutaneous endoscopic gastrostomy (PEG) tube allows delivery of food and medication directly into the stomach, reducing the risk of further aspiration pneumonia[35] (see Chap. 34). The major drawback of placing a PEG tube is the necessity of general anesthesia in a dog with respiratory compromise.

If an underlying cause for megaesophagus can be identified, treatment of the primary disorder may result in improvement in clinical signs. See Chapter 28 for a discussion of the treatment of myasthenia gravis.

Most authorities agree that surgical managment to weaken the GES has resulted in greater morbidity and mortality in dogs with megaesophagus than has dietary management alone.[21] Surgical therapy has probably not been fairly evaluated in the veterinary literature. In many instances, surgery was performed only on severely ill dogs with little chance for survival, whereas mildly affected dogs were treated medically. Surgical weakening of the GES aids gravity in delivering food into the stomach but does not improve peristalsis. Further investigation of surgical management of megaesophagus in dogs should be undertaken.

Because megaesophagus is thought to be hereditary in some breeds, dogs with idiopathic megaesophagus and their sires and dams should not be bred.

Prognosis

The prognosis for dogs with megaesophagus is poor.[21, 23–25] Most patients continue to regurgitate, lose weight, and aspirate food material. Owners often become unwilling to continue dietary management or to tolerate clinical signs. Commonly, animals that recover from aspiration penumonia clinically improve for a limited time, but they often undergo recurrent

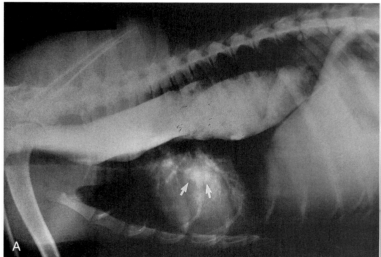
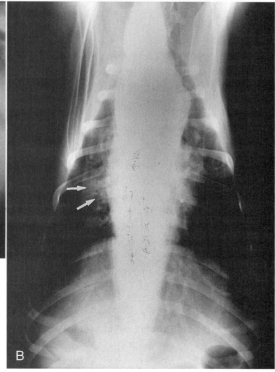

Figure 30–6
(A) Lateral barium esophagram from a 9-year-old Dalmatian with megaesophagus. The entire thoracic esophagus is distended with barium. No motility was observed with fluoroscopy. Patchy interstitial and alveolar infiltrate can be seen over the heart, consistent with aspiration pneumonia *(arrows).* **(B)** Ventrodorsal barium esophagram from the same dog as in **A.** The entire thoracic esophagus is distended with barium. Patchy interstitial and alveolar infiltrate can be seen lateral to the heart, consistent with aspiration pneumonia *(arrows).*

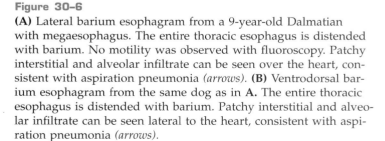

episodes of aspiration and frequent regurgitation. With dietary therapy, some may improve and become acceptable pets.[23, 24] In rare cases, clinical signs can completely resolve.[36] Most affected miniature schnauzers in one research colony ceased regurgitating by 4 to 6 months of age.[28]

Animals that have a primary underlying condition have a better prognosis if the primary problem can be successfully treated and if aspiration pneumonia is not severe.[24–26]

Vascular Ring Anomaly

Vascular rings are congenital embryologic malformations of the great vessels that encircle the esophagus and cause obstruction and regurgitation.[37, 38] Many types of anomalies occur, but persistent right aortic arch (PRAA) is most common. Although vascular ring anomalies occur in cats, they are more frequently encountered in dogs. German shepherds, Irish setters, and Boston terriers are predisposed. PRAA has been shown to be hereditary in German shepherds. Most cases occur in dogs with expected adult body weights greater than 15 kg.[39] Diagnosis is usually made by 6 months of age, but on occasion adults may develop acute clinical signs.[39]

Pathophysiology

Six pairs of aortic arches connect the paired dorsal and ventral aortas in the embryo. As the heart and great vessels develop, involution of most of the arches frees the esophagus from entrapment.[38] Normally, the left fourth aortic arch becomes the aorta, and the right fourth arch becomes the right subclavian artery. If the right fourth arch is retained as the aorta, the esophagus is encircled by the ligamentum arteriosum on the left, the aorta on the right, and the pulmonary trunk and heart base ventrally. In a few cases, a patent ductus arteriosus is present, but minimal blood flow usually occurs through it.[37] Extraluminal esophageal obstruction results in retention of esophageal contents, regurgitation, and gradual esophageal enlargement. Progressive enlargement stretches esophageal muscle, resulting in diminished peristalsis. Reduced esophageal motility may be permanent after the obstruction is removed.

Clinical Signs

Regurgitation usually is observed soon after weaning to solid food. Initially, regurgitation occurs immediately after eating, but as the esophagus dilates, food may be retained for many hours after a meal. Affected animals are thin and smaller than their littermates. Aspiration pneumonia may be chronically present, be intermittent, or cause severe acute signs.

Appetite is excellent if moderate or severe pneumonia is not present.

Diagnostic Plan

An air-, fluid- or food-filled cranial esophagus may be visible on survey thoracic radiographs (Fig. 30–7).[5, 6] An increased alveolar pattern, suggesting aspiration pneumonia, is often visible (see Fig. 30–6). Distention of the esophagus with barium localizes the dilation cranial to the heart. On the ventrodorsal radiograph, an asymmetrical tapering of the esophagus with indentation on the right side from the PRAA may be seen (Fig. 30–8). The esophagus caudal to the vascular ring should be normal, and contrast material passing the obstruction should be propelled quickly into the stomach. The trachea may be deviated ventrally and to the left.[38] A symmetrical esophageal obstruction suggests the possibility of an uncommon anomaly, and angiographic studies are required to define the defect and plan therapy.[37, 38]

Treatment

Definitive management requires surgical correction of the obstruction. In cases of PRAA, ligation and transection of the ligamentum arteriosum and dissection of the fibrous bands in the esophageal wall serve to relieve the obstruction. In severely affected animals, nutritional support and treatment for aspiration pneumonia (see Megaesophagus) should be initiated before surgery is performed. Elevated feeding of gruel should be continued postoperatively. If regurgitation does not occur, the gruel can slowly be thickened and the animal gradually switched to normal feedings.

Prognosis

Although surgery can resolve the obstruction, the prognosis for patients with vascular ring anomalies remains guarded. Esophageal dilation with loss of motility often persists after surgery. Continued regurgitation and bouts of aspiration pneumonia are common. In a large study of PRAA in dogs, 80% survived surgery; of the survivors, 24% died or were euthanized because of continued problems, 67% continued to have clinical signs but were considered acceptable pets by their owners, and only 9% were clinically normal.[39] If a diagnosis can be made before moderate or severe esophageal dilation occurs, normal esophageal motility may remain, and the prognosis is brighter.

Esophagitis

Inflammation, erosion, and ulceration of the esophagus are recognized more frequently today in

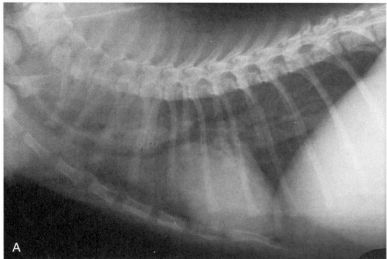

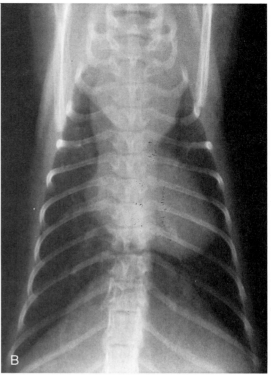

Figure 30-7
(A) Lateral survey thoracic radiograph from a 4-month-old Siamese kitten with a persistent right aortic arch. The trachea is displaced ventrally, and the esophagus cranial to the heart is dilated with air and fluid. **(B)** Ventrodorsal survey thoracic radiograph from the same kitten as in **A.** The cranial mediastinum is widened, and the cardiac apex is displaced to the left because of the fluid-distended esophagus.

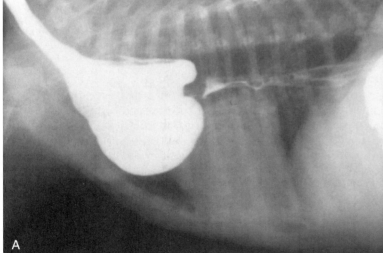

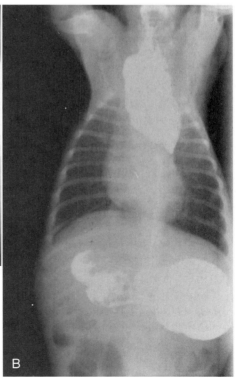

Figure 30-8
(A) Lateral barium esophagram from a 3-month-old mixed breed puppy with a persistent right aortic arch. The esophagus cranial to the heart is greatly distended. **(B)** Ventrodorsal barium esophagram from the same puppy as in **A.** The esophagus is greatly dilated cranial to the heart. The esophagus is indented on the right side, which is typical for persistent right aortic arches.

dogs and cats because of the widespread use of endoscopy. Usually, moderate or severe esophagitis must be present for clinical signs to be apparent. In most cases of esophagitis, a predisposing factor can be identified.

Pathophysiology

Caustic substances directly damage the esophageal mucosa and deeper structures.[40] In animals that vomit or have GE reflux, gastric acid, pepsin, bile acids, and pancreatic enzymes contribute to esophageal injury.[41, 42] Mucosal or muscular damage results in decreased peristalsis, esophageal distention, and regurgitation. Severe esophagitis interferes with GES function, resulting in GE reflux and worsening esophagitis and creating a vicious circle of esophageal damage.

GE reflux occurs in normal animals and does not usually result in esophageal damage. The normal esophagus rapidly clears acid by secondary peristalsis, and remaining acid is neutralized by swallowed saliva.[43] The development of esophagitis depends on the frequency of reflux and the length of contact time. Anesthetic agents can relax the GES, reduce peristalsis, and decrease salivation.[44–49] During anesthesia, refluxed gastric contents remain in the esophagus and can cause damage. Lowering the animal's head by tilting the surgical table increases the incidence of anesthesia-related GE reflux. Food in the stomach at the time of anesthesia can also predispose to GE reflux. Inflammation that occurs in the deeper layers of the esophagus can heal by fibroplasia, resulting in stricture formation.

Some medications that are retained in the esophagus cause esophagitis (e.g., tetracycline, doxycycline, potassium chloride, propranolol, quinidine).[50] Predisposing factors include large tablets, administration with little water, abnormal esophageal transport, and administration when the animal is not fully awake.[51]

Esophagitis can also be associated with feeding tubes that are placed through a pharyngostomy incision or the nares and enter the stomach. Reflux of gastric contents along the tube and direct irritation caused by the tube have been incriminated.[52] To reduce this possibility, feeding tubes should be made of soft material and should be advanced only to the distal one third of the esophagus.

Clinical Signs

Regurgitation is often accompanied by excess salivation, odynophagia, and anorexia. Recent ingestion of caustic chemicals (e.g., household drain cleaners that contain lye or strong acids) or hot food or fluids

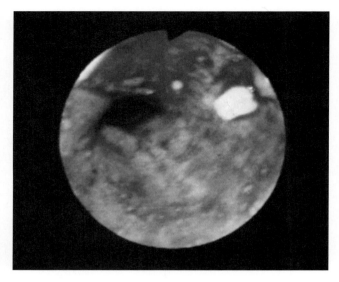

Figure 30–9
Endoscopic appearance of esophagitis in a 7-year-old field spaniel. The mucosa is ulcerated, hemorrhagic, and friable. The cause was acid reflux due to vomiting caused by pyloric hypertrophy.

may have occurred. In cases of caustic or thermal ingestion, the tongue, lips, and pharynx are often involved and are hyperemic, eroded, or ulcerated. A recent anesthetic episode that resulted in reduced GES pressure and esophageal motility may have promoted GE reflux and esophagitis. A history of eating bones or swallowing other foreign objects may be present. Esophagitis may also develop after a severe vomiting episode, insertion of a feeding tube, or administration of medications.

Diagnostic Plan

The diagnosis of esophagitis is often suspected based on the history of identifying a potential underlying cause. Survey thoracic radiographs are often normal. Disruption, irregularity, and smudging of the normally smooth mucosal folds can be seen with barium contrast studies.[6] Endoscopic examination is the preferred way to diagnose esophagitis. The affected mucosa is hyperemic, eroded, or ulcerated (Fig. 30–9). If lesions are located in the distal esophagus and predisposing factors cannot be identified in the history, idiopathic GE reflux or hiatal hernia should be suspected. These patients may benefit from referral, because fluoroscopic examination with application of abdominal pressure may be necessary for diagnosis.

Treatment

The first step in effectively treating esophagitis is to identify and remove any predisposing conditions.

For mild or moderate cases, the esophagus should be rested for 1 to 5 days, because feeding can irritate the healing mucosa. Hydration can be maintained by parenteral fluid administration. Small, frequent feedings of a liquid gruel or of canned food can then be initiated. If regurgitation does not occur, the feeding frequency can be decreased, the meal volume increased, and the consistency thickened until normal feeding is gradually reinstituted over a period of 3 to 7 days.

Severe esophagitis may require a longer period of rest. A PEG tube (see Chap. 34) may be needed to supply nutrition. After the esophagus has healed, oral feeding can be started as described previously. Cimetidine (10 mg/kg three times per day) or ranitidine (2 mg/kg two or three times per day) should be given to reduce gastric acid production and prevent further esophageal damage from reflux. Metoclopramide (0.2–0.4 mg/kg three times per day) can be administered to help increase GES tone and reduce reflux. If severe mucosal damage is present, broad-spectrum antibiotics should be given for 1 to 2 weeks. These drugs should be continued for 1 week after normal feeding has been resumed. Until oral feeding begins, they must be given parenterally or in the PEG tube.

Prognosis

The prognosis is dependent on the severity of esophageal lesions. Extensive lesions caused by caustic or thermal ingestion and lesions severe enough to cause perforation carry a poor prognosis. Stricture, which can be a sequela to deep lesions, requires aggressive therapy. Mild or moderate cases of esophagitis often heal without further complication.

Stricture

Narrowing of the esophageal lumen secondary to fibrous contraction of the esophageal wall can be caused by injury to the submucosa or muscularis. Strictures most commonly occur after esophagitis.

Pathophysiology

Damage to the deeper layers of the esophagus heals by fibroplasia and contraction, narrowing the esophageal lumen. The most common predisposing factor for stricture formation is the use of anesthetic agents that relax the GES, reduce peristalsis, and decrease salivation (see Esophagitis).[44, 46–49, 53] Strictures are relatively uncommon after foreign body entrapment.[10, 19] Regurgitation of solid food often begins after the esophageal lumen narrows to 1 cm or less. Regurgitation of liquids occurs if the lumen becomes less than 4 mm in diameter.

Clinical Signs

Regurgitation usually develops 5 to 14 days after the onset of esophagitis. Odynophagia, anorexia, and weight loss often occur. Historical and clinical findings associated with the underlying cause of esophagitis may be apparent.

Diagnostic Plan

The diagnosis of stricture is based on barium contrast radiography and endoscopic examination. The presence of a stricture should be considered if regurgitation develops or becomes more frequent 5 to 14 days after any of the predisposing factors of esophagitis occurs. If a stricture has been present for many weeks, survey radiographs may show an esophagus dilated with air, fluid, or food cranial to the stricture.[6] Barium contrast studies may identify a localized narrowing of the lumen (Fig. 30–10). Barium suspension may pass through a relatively large stricture, yielding a falsely negative study. Barium mixed with food is often necessary to demonstrate luminal compromise. It may be possible to determine the length of the stricture or to identify the presence of multiple strictures if the barium passes caudally to the obstruction.

Endoscopically, the esophageal lumen is usually narrowed by smooth, glistening, tough, whitish fi-

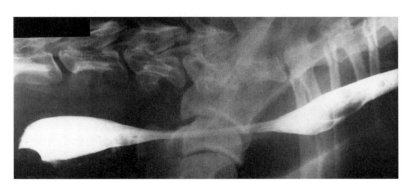

Figure 30–10
Lateral barium esophagram from a 3-year-old chow chow with esophageal strictures. The esophagus is narrowed at the thoracic inlet. Endoscopy showed the esophageal diameter to be approximately 3 mm and the stricture to be 5 cm in length. A second stricture was present 6 cm caudal and caused retention of barium distal to the proximal stricture.

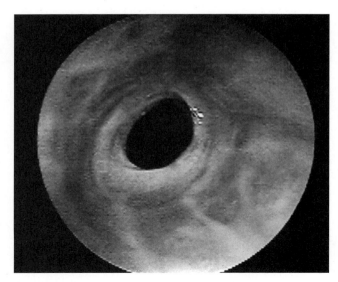

Figure 30-11
Endoscopic appearance of an esophageal stricture in a 7-year-old cocker spaniel. The lumen is symmetrically narrowed to 9 mm by a tough band of white fibrous tissue. Streaks of fibrosis can be seen cranial to the stricture. The cause of the stricture was acid reflux during general anesthesia for a dental procedure.

brous tissue (Fig. 30-11). If granularity is present, samples should be collected for histopathology, because malignant strictures do occur. It is often not possible to measure the length of the stricture or determine whether multiple strictures exist, because the esophagus is usually narrower than the outer diameter of the endoscope. If the stricture is thought to be secondary to vomiting, complete evaluation of the stomach and duodenum should be performed.

Treatment

Dilation of strictures with instruments of increasing diameter passed down the esophagus through the stricture (bougienage) and surgical resection and anastomosis have been used in dogs and cats. However, balloon catheters appear to offer a better success rate with fewer complications. Dilation with balloon catheters under fluoroscopic control is successful but requires referral for fluoroscopy.[44, 53] Dilation with balloon catheters placed through an endoscope is currently the most practical treatment available. Sequentially larger balloons can be placed within the lumen of the stricture and inflated for 60 to 90 seconds. If severe esophageal trauma does not develop, it is often possible to dilate the esophagus with an 18-mm balloon. Multiple dilations are often necessary. The optimal dilation interval has not been determined in dogs or cats; however, anywhere from 5 to 28 days between dilations has been rec-

ommended. After the stricture has been dilated, the remainder of the esophagus should be examined thoroughly to measure the length of the stricture and to evaluate for the presence of multiple strictures.

Postdilation care is similar to that described for treatment of esophagitis. Many clinicians add an anti-inflammatory dose of prednisone (1.0 mg/kg daily) for several weeks to reduce the likelihood of fibroplasia and restricture.[40]

Prognosis

Clinical improvement occurs soon after balloon catheter dilation. The owner must understand that multiple endoscopic procedures are often necessary. In some cases, a liquid or soft diet must be fed for the animal's entire life because some degree of narrowing of the esophageal lumen remains.[44, 53] These animals are very susceptible to foreign body entrapment, so owners must prevent dietary indiscretion.

Extraluminal Obstruction

Obstruction of the esophagus resulting from impingement by periesophageal structures produces regurgitation and, if long-standing, esophageal dilation and decreased motility. Common causes of obstruction include vascular ring anomalies, cranial mediastinal masses, and hilar lymphadenopathy, although lesions anywhere along the esophagus can result in obstruction.[54–56]

Pathophysiology

Extraluminal masses compress the esophagus and result in obstruction. Because the normal esophagus is distensible, development of clinical signs requires a large degree of luminal compromise. With slowly enlarging masses, esophageal dilation with progressive loss of motility can develop. In some cases, an inflammatory or neoplastic mass can invade the esophageal wall.

Clinical Signs

The predominant clinical signs often reflect the underlying disorder. However, in some cases, regurgitation may be the most obvious sign. Concurrent compression of the trachea results in cough and may progress to dyspnea. Cats with mediastinal lymphosarcoma often have a noncompressible thorax. Concurrent pleural effusion results in muffled heart and lung sounds. Generalized lymphadenopathy or hepatosplenomegaly, or both, may be detected in dogs with multicentric lymphosarcoma. Hilar lymphadenopathy may be associated with systemic mycoses, and coughing with respiratory disease. A palpable cervical mass may be detected in dogs with thyroid adenocarcinoma.[57]

Diagnostic Plan

The cause of the obstruction usually can be palpated in the cervical region or is obvious on thoracic radiographs. A cranial mediastinal mass, sternal or hilar lymphadenopathy, or pleural effusion may be observed on thoracic radiographs. Barium contrast studies clearly demonstrate the location of the obstruction (Fig. 30–12).

Cats with lymphosarcoma may test positive for FeLV. In addition, nonregenerative anemia, hypercalcemia, or circulating lymphoblasts may be detected on routine laboratory evaluation in dogs or cats with lymphosarcoma. Fine-needle aspiration of a cervical or cranial mediastinal mass or analysis of pleural fluid usually provides a diagnosis. Rarely, a biopsy obtained under ultrasonographic guidance or with exploratory surgery is necessary to identify the cause of the obstruction.

Treatment

The treatment should be directed toward the primary disorder. If an endoscope can be passed through the obstruction, a PEG tube can be placed to provide nutrition (see Chap. 34). The treatment of lymphosarcoma can be found in Chapter 43.

Prognosis

The prognosis depends on the primary disorder. Esophageal dilation with loss of motility is a poor prognostic sign, because function may not return after the obstruction is removed.

Uncommon Diseases of the Esophagus

Neoplasia

Squamous cell carcinoma is the most common primary esophageal tumor. Sarcoma may develop in association with *Spirocerca lupi* granulomas. Local extension of thyroid adenocarcinoma may occur.[58] Diagnosis requires biopsy.

Hiatal Hernia

A sliding hiatal hernia occurs when the GE junction intermittently moves into the thoracic cavity. Clinical signs include regurgitation, vomiting, and dyspnea. Chinese shar-peis may be predisposed.[59] Hiatal hernias may not produce clinical signs unless GE reflux is present. Diagnosis can be made if a soft tissue density is seen in the dorsal caudal thorax on thoracic radiographs. Because of the intermittent nature of the hernia, fluoroscopy, after application of external pressure to the abdomen, may be necessary for diagnosis. If medical management for esophagitis does not improve clinical signs, surgery to stabilize the GE junction is indicated.[59–61]

Secondary Megaesophagus

Table 30–2 lists some of the uncommon primary disorders associated with megaesophagus. These disorders should be suspected based on abnormal findings on physical examination, neurologic examination, or routine laboratory evaluation.

Segmental Motility Disorder

Reduced or absent peristalsis, limited to one area and without dilation of the esophagus, may result

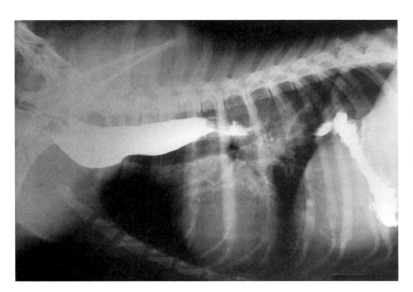

Figure 30–12
Lateral barium esophagram of a 4-year-old Samoyed with extraluminal esophageal compression. There is increased perihilar density in the area lacking barium. Some barium has entered the stomach. The mass occupied the area of the heart base and was composed of inflammatory tissue and reactive lymph nodes.

in regurgitation. Fluoroscopy is necessary for diagnosis. Esophagitis can result in decreased motility, but the cause in most cases is unknown.

Spirocerca lupi

S. lupi are large, reddish worms (3–8 cm in length) that form granulomatous masses in the esophagus and sometimes in the aorta. Small, thick-shelled, larvated eggs with parallel sides may be found in the feces or in regurgitated material. Sarcomas can develop at the granuloma sites. The infection is most common in the Gulf Coast states. One or two doses of disophenol, 7.7 mg/kg, taken 7 days apart, kills the adult worms.[62]

Gastroesophageal Intussusception

Invagination of the stomach into the esophagus occurs predominantly in puppies, most of which have megaesophagus or other esophageal disorders. Clinical signs include vomiting, regurgitation, dyspnea, hematemesis, and abdominal pain. Affected dogs rapidly deteriorate and die. Diagnosis is based on radiographic evidence of esophageal obstruction, increased soft tissue density in the dorsal caudal thorax, and lack of an abdominal gastric gas bubble. Prompt diagnosis and surgical correction are necessary for survival.[63]

Diverticulum

Diverticula are pouches in the esophageal wall. They can be congenital, but they most commonly form secondary to esophageal trauma or obstruction of peristalsis by foreign bodies, strictures, or extraluminal obstructions.[64] Small diverticula do not cause clinical signs; large ones require surgical resection.

Bronchial Fistula

A fistulous connection between the esophagus and a bronchus occurs most commonly because of foreign body entrapment in the esophagus. Coughing may occur shortly after drinking of liquids. Diagnosis requires barium contrast radiography. Surgical correction is necessary for resolution of clinical signs.[65]

Esophageal Deviation

Esophageal redundancy with a prominent ventral deviation in the cranial mediastinum may be a normal finding in young dogs, especially Chinese shar-peis.[66] On occasion, this deviation is associated with regurgitation. In several English bulldogs, esophageal deviation was associated with vascular compression. Surgical redirection of the subclavian artery resulted in remission of clinical signs.[67]

References

1. Zawie DA. Medical diseases of the esophagus. Compen Contin Educ Pract Vet 1987; 9:1145–1154.
2. Leib MS. Megaesophagus. In: Bojrab MJ, ed. Disease Mechanisms in Small Animal Surgery. Philadelphia, Lea & Febiger, 1993:205–209.
3. Leib MS. Megaesophagus in the dog: I. Anatomy, physiology, and pathophysiology. Compen Contin Educ Pract Vet 1983; 5:825–833.
4. Willard M. Clinical manifestations of gastrointestinal disorders. In: Nelson RW, Couto CG, eds. Essentials of Small Animal Internal medicine. St Louis, Mosby–Year Book, 1992:257–279.
5. Stickle RL, Love NE. Radiographic diagnosis of esophageal diseases in dogs and cats. Semin Vet Med Surg (Small Anim) 1989; 4:179–187.
6. Moon M, Myer W. Gastrointestinal contrast radiology in small animals. Semin Vet Med Surg (Small Anim) 1986;1:121–143.
7. Jones BD, Gross ME. Introduction to endoscopy. Vet Clin North Am Small Anim Pract 1990; 20:1199–1208.
8. Jones BD. Choosing an endoscope. Vet Med Rep 1990; 2:175–178.
9. Ryan WW, Greene RW. The conservative management of esophageal foreign bodies and their complications: A review of 66 cases in dogs and cats. J Am Anim Hosp Assoc 1975; 11:243–249.
10. Houlton EF, Herrtage ME, Taylor PM, et al. Thoracic oesophageal foreign bodies in the dog: A review of ninety cases. J Sm Anim Pract 1985; 26:521–536.
11. Guilford W, Jones BD. Gastrointestinal endoscopy of the dog and cat. Vet Med Rep 1990; 2:140–150.
12. Guilford WG. Upper gastrointestinal endoscopy. Vet Clin North Am Small Anim Pract 1990; 20:1209–1227.
13. Happe RP. Gastrointestinal endoscopy in the dog. Vet Q 1985; 7: 231–234.
14. Leib MS. Endoscopic examination of the dog and cat. In: Jensen SL, Gregersen H, Moody FG, et al, eds. Essentials of Experimental Surgery: Gastroenterology. Amsterdam, Harwood Academic Publishers, 1996:10/1–10/17.
15. Tams TR. Esophagoscopy. In: Tams TR, ed. Small Animal Endoscopy. St Louis, CV Mosby, 1990:47–88.
16. Jones BD. Management of esophageal foreign bodies. In: Kirk RW, Bonagura JD, ed. Current Veterinary Therapy IX. Philadelphia, WB Saunders, 1992:577–580.
17. Parker NR, Walter PA, Gay J. Diagnosis and surgical management of esophageal perforation. J Am Anim Hosp Assoc 1989; 25:587–594.
18. Pearson H. Symposium on conditions of the canine oesophagus: I. Foreign bodies in the oesophagus. J Sm Anim Pract 1966; 7:107–116.
19. Spielman BL, Shaker EH, Garvey MS. Esophageal foreign body in dogs: A retrospective study of 23 cases. J Am Anim Hosp Assoc 1992;28:570–574.
20. Zimmer JF. Canine esophageal foreign bodies: Endo-

scopic, surgical, and medical management. J Am Anim Hosp Assoc 1984; 20:669–677.

21. Harvey CE, O'Brien JA, Durie VR, et al. Megaesophagus in the dog: A clinical survey of 79 cases. J Am Vet Med Assoc 1974; 165:443–446.

22. Osborne CA, Clifford DH, Jessen C. Hereditary esophageal achalasia in dogs. J Am Vet Med Assoc 1967; 151:572–581.

23. Boudrieau RJ, Rogers WA. Megaesophagus in the dog: A review of 50 cases. J Am Anim Hosp Assoc 1985; 21:33–40.

24. Leib MS, Hall RL. Megaesophagus in the dog: II. Clinical aspects. Compen Contin Educ Pract Vet 1984; 6:11–17.

25. Guilford WG. Megaesophagus in the dog and cat. Semin Vet Med Surg (Small Anim) 1990; 5:37–45.

26. Shelton GD, Willard MD, Cardinet GH III, et al. Acquired myasthenia gravis. J Vet Intem Med 1990; 4:281–284.

27. Knowles KE, O'Brien DP, Amann JF. Congenital idiopathic megaesophagus in a litter of Chinese shar-peis: Clinical, electrodiagnostic, and pathological findings. J Am Anim Hosp Assoc 1990; 26:313–318.

28. Cox VS, Wallace LJ, Anderson VE, et al. Hereditary esophageal dysfunction in the miniature schnauzer dog. Am J Vet Res 1980; 41:326–330.

29. Rochlitz I. Feline dysautonomia (the Key-Gaskell or dilated pupil syndrome): A preliminary review. J Sm Anim Pract 1984; 25:587–598.

30. Sharp NJH, Nash AS, Griffiths IR. Feline dysautonomia (the Key-Gaskell syndrome): A clinical and pathological study of forty cases. J Sm Anim Pract 1984; 25:599–615.

31. Diamant N, Szczepanski M, Mui H. Manometric characteristics of idiopathic megaesophagus in the dog: An unsuitable animal model for achalasia in man. Gastroenterology 1973; 65:216–223.

32. Hoffer RE, MacCoy DM, Quick CB, et al. Management of acquired achalasia in dogs. J Am Vet Med Assoc 1979; 175:814–817.

33. Strombeck DR, Troya L. Evaluation of lower motor neuron function in two dogs with megaesophagus. J Am Vet Med Assoc 1976; 169:411–414.

34. Rogers WA, Fenner WR, Sherding RG. Electromyographic and esophagomanometric findings in clinically normal dogs and in dogs with idiopathic megaesophagus. J Am Vet Med Assoc 1979; 174:181–183.

35. Bright RM. Percutaneous endoscopic gastrostomy. Vet Clin North Am Small Anim Pract 1993; 23:531–545.

36. Hendricks JC, Maggio-Price L, Dougherty JF. Transient esophageal dysfunction mimicking megaesophagus in three dogs. J Am Vet Med Assoc 1984; 185:90–92.

37. Ellison GW. Vascular ring anomalies in the dog and cat. Compen Contin Educ Pract Vet 1980; 2:693–706.

38. VanGundy T. Vascular ring anomalies. Compen Contin Educ Pract Vet 1989; 11:35–45.

39. Shires PK, Liu W. Persistent right aortic arch in dogs: A long term follow-up after surgical correction. J Am Anim Hosp Assoc 1981; 17:773–776.

40. Knox WG, Scott JR, Zintel HA, et al. Bouginage and steroids used singly or in combination in experimental corrosive esophagitis. Ann Surg 1967; 166:930–941.

41. Eastwood GL, Castell DO, Higgs RH. Experimental esophagitis in cats impairs lower esophageal sphincter pressure. Gastroenterology 1975; 69:146–153.

42. Henderson RD, Mugashe F, Jeejeebhoy KN, et al. The role of bile and acid in the production of esophagitis and the motor defect of esophagitis. Ann Thorac Surg 1972; 14:465–473.

43. Johnson SE, Zelner A, Sherding RG. Esophageal acid clearance test in healthy dogs. Can J Vet Res 1989; 53:244–247.

44. Burk RL, Zawie DA, Garvey MS. Balloon catheter dilation of intramural esophageal strictures in the dog and cat: A description of the procedure and a report of six cases. Semin Vet Med Surg (Small Anim) 1987; 2:241–247.

45. Pearson H, Darke PGG, Gibbs C, et al. Reflux oesophagitis and stricture formation after anaesthesia: A review of seven cases in dogs and cats. J Sm Anim Pract 1978; 19:507–519.

46. Strombeck DR, Harrold D. Effects of atropine, acepromazine, meperidine, and xylazine on gastroesophageal sphincter pressure in the dog. Am J Vet Res 1985; 46:963–965.

47. Strombeck DR, Harrold D. Effect of gastrin, histamine, serotonin, and adrenergic amines on gastroesophageal sphincter pressure in the dog. Am J Vet Res 1985; 46:1684–1690.

48. Hall J, Magne M, Twedt D. Effect of acepromazine, diazepam, fentanyl-droperidol, and oxymorphone on gastroesophageal sphincter pressure in healthy dogs. Am J Vet Res 1987; 48:556–558.

49. Johnson SE, Zelner A, Sherding RG. Effect of lenperone hydrochloride on gastroesophageal sphincter pressure in healthy dogs. Can J Vet Res 1989; 53:248–250.

50. Carlborg B, Densert O. Esophageal lesions caused by orally administered drugs: An experimental study in the cat. Eur Surg Res 1980; 12:270–282.

51. Delpre G, Kadish U, Stahl B. Induction of esophageal injuries by doxycycline and other pills: A frequent but preventable occurrence. Dig Dis Sci 1989; 34:797–800.

52. Lantz GC, Cantwell HD, VanVleet JF, et al. Pharyngostomy tube induced esophagitis in the dog: An experimental study. J Am Anim Hosp Assoc 1983; 19:207–212.

53. Sooy TE, Adams WM, Pitts RP, et al. Balloon catheter dilatation of alimentary tract strictures in the dog and cat. Vet Radiol 1987; 28:131–137.

54. Gruffydd-Jones TJ, Gaskell CJ. Clinical and radiological features of anterior mediastinal lymphosarcoma in the cat: A review of 30 cases. Vet Rec 1979; 104:304–307.

55. Bellah JR, Stiff ME, Russell RG. Thymoma in the dog: Two case reports and review of 20 additional cases. J Am Vet Med Assoc 1983; 183:306–311.

56. Crow SE. Lymphosarcoma (malignant lymphoma) in the dog: Diagnosis and treatment. Compen Contin Educ Pract Vet 1982; 4:283–292.

57. Harari J, Patterson JS, Rosenthal RC. Clinical and pathologic features of thyroid tumors in 26 dogs. J Am Vet Med Assoc 1986; 188:1160–1164.

58. Ridgway RL, Suter PF. Clinical and radiographic signs in primary and metastatic esophageal neoplasms of the dog. J Am Vet Med Assoc 1979; 174:700–704.

59. Callan MB, Washabau RJ, Saunders HM, et al. Congenital

esophageal hiatal hernia in the Chinese shar-pei dog. J Vet Intern Med 1993; 7:210–215.

60. Bright RM, Sackman JE, DeNovo C, et al. Hiatal hernia in the dog and cat: A retrospective study of 16 cases. J Small Anim Pract 1990; 31:244–250.

61. Ellison GW, Lewis DD, Phillips L, et al. Esophageal hiatal hernia in small animals: Literature review and a modified surgical technique. J Am Anim Hosp Assoc 1987; 23:391–399.

62. Fox SM, Burns J, Hawkins J. Spirocercosis in dogs. Compen Contin Educ Pract Vet 1988; 10:807–822.

63. Leib MS, Blass CE. Gastroesophageal intussusception in the dog: A review of the literature and a case report. J Am Anim Hosp Assoc 1984; 20:783–790.

64. Pearson H, Gibbs C, Kelly DF. Oesophageal diverticulum formation in the dog. J Sm Anim Pract 1978; 19:341–355.

65. Park RD. Bronchoesophageal fistula in the dog: Literature survey, case presentations, and radiographic manifestations. Comp Cont Educ Pract Vet 1984; 6:669–677.

66. Stickle R, Sparschu G, Love N, et al. Radiographic evaluation of esophageal function in Chinese shar-pei pups. J Am Vet Med Assoc 1992; 201:81–84.

67. Woods CB, Rawlings C, Barber D, et al. Esophageal deviation in four English bulldogs. J Am Vet Med Assoc 1978; 172:934–939.

Diseases of the Stomach

Michael S. Leib

Anatomy

The C-shaped stomach lies in a transverse plane across the abdomen, more to the left of the median plane. It is bound laterally by the ribs. It is in contact with the liver cranially and with the left limb of the pancreas caudally. The stomach consists of five anatomic regions.[1] The cardia connects with the short intra-abdominal esophagus. The fundus is the outpouching dorsal and to the left of the cardia. The body is the largest section; it is bound by the greater and lesser curvatures. The greater omentum attaches along the greater curvature. The concave lesser curvature forms the angularis incisura, an important endoscopic landmark (Fig. 31–1). The distal one third of the stomach consists of the antrum and its connection to the duodenum, the pyloric sphincter.

The position of the stomach is relatively fixed by the diaphragmatic hiatus of the esophagus, the gastrohepatic ligament, and the common bile duct. In an empty dog stomach, the antrum lies to the right of midline,[2, 3] but in cats, the pyloric region lies on the midline and the lesser curvature forms a more acute angle, giving a V configuration.[2, 3] The body of the stomach is capable of tremendous enlargement and expansion to the left and caudoventrally.[2]

Microscopically, the stomach consists of four layers: an inner mucosa, a submucosa, a muscular layer, and an outer serosa.[1] The mucosa and submucosa form rugal folds in the nondistended stomach. The mucosa is lined with columnar epithelial cells (surface mucous cells), which invaginate to form many gastric pits that connect to one or more gastric glands. The surface mucous cells secrete a thick mucus. The mucosal surface is replaced every 3 to 7 days.

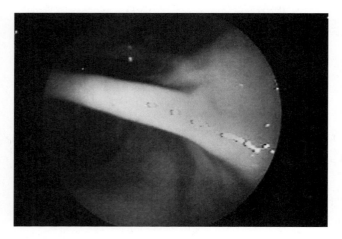

Figure 31–1
Endoscopic view of the angularis incisura, the reflection of the lesser curvature. The antrum is below the "shelf," and the gastric body and cardia are above. The angularis is an important endoscopic landmark. The white areas along the "shelf" are photographic reflections.

The epithelial cells lining the glands vary in the different regions of the stomach.[4] In the cardia, the cells lining the glands secrete an alkaline mucus. In the fundus and body, four types of epithelial cells line the glands: the chief cells, which produce pepsinogen; the parietal cells, which secrete acid; the mucous neck cells, which secrete mucus, divide and mature into other cell types, and migrate up or down the gland to replace epithelial cells; and the argentaffin cells, which produce serotonin and histamine. The glands in the antrum contain mucous neck cells and gastrin-containing cells (G cells).

The submucosa contains elastic areolar tissue and the small branches of blood vessels and nerves. The muscular layer consists of smooth muscle in an inner circular layer, an outer longitudinal layer, and some oblique fibers in the gastric body. A circular muscular sphincter exists at the pylorus. The serosa that covers the stomach is thin and elastic.

A vast enteric nervous system lies within the stomach wall. The myenteric plexus innervates the muscular layers and regulates motor function, and the submucosal plexus regulates secretion and absorption.[5, 6] Many excitatory and inhibitory transmitters have been identified. Parasympathetic and sympathetic neurons interconnect with the enteric nervous system. The vagus nerve supplies parasympathetic innervation, and the celiac plexus provides sympathetic connections. Arterial blood supply to the stomach is carried by the celiac artery. Venous drainage enters the portal vein.

Physiology

The functions of the stomach are to serve as a reservoir for food, to control the delivery of ingesta into the small intestine at a rate appropriate for digestion and absorption, and to begin the digestive process by secreting acid and a proteolytic enzyme precursor, pepsinogen.[6]

Motility

The proximal stomach, consisting of the cardia, fundus, and body, serves to store ingesta by a process called receptive relaxation, wherein dilation occurs without an increase in intraluminal pressure.[7] The proximal stomach is also important in the regulation of gastric emptying of liquids, which is dependent on the pressure gradient between the stomach and duodenum.[6, 8] The distal stomach, composed of the antrum and pylorus, is responsible for grinding and mixing ingesta and reducing particle size.[8] The pylorus allows only small particles (<2 mm) to enter the duodenum and prevents reflux of duodenal contents into the stomach. Between meals, during the interdigestive period, vigorous gastric contractions help to move larger, nondigestible particles through an open pylorus into the duodenum; this is known as the migrating motor complex or intestinal "housekeeper."[6, 8]

Electrical potentials, termed slow waves or pacesetter potentials, are generated in the smooth muscle along the greater curvature and control the frequency, velocity, and direction of muscular contractions (peristalsis).[6, 7] Peristaltic waves often occur 3 to 5 times per minute in the dog.[7] As the wave of contraction moves toward the antrum, a small amount of ingesta is propelled through the pylorus, and the majority is retropulsed, which results in mixing and grinding.[7, 8] It often takes 8 to 10 hours for a meal to empty from the stomach.

The control of gastric emptying is complex and involves neural and hormonal input. Liquids empty faster than solids. Receptors in the duodenum monitor contents, and increases in osmolarity, viscosity, acidity, fatty acids, tryptophan, and energy density slow the rate of gastric emptying.[6, 8]

Secretion

The stomach is a very efficient secretor of acid. The gastric mucosal barrier protects the mucosa from digestion (see Gastritis). Acid secretion contributes to protein digestion by helping to convert pepsinogen to pepsin. Acid also reduces the number of ingested bacteria that reach the intestine. Hydrogen ions are produced in the parietal cells by carbonic anhydrase. At the apical cell membrane, a proton pump exchanges intraluminal potassium for the hydrogen. Gastric acid secretion can be inhibited by blocking this proton pump with omeprazole (see Gastric Ulceration). Within the lumen, the pH of gastric secretion can be less than 1.

The parietal cell has receptors for gastrin, histamine (type 2 receptor), and acetylcholine.[4, 5] Maximum stimulation occurs when all three receptors are occupied. Acetylcholine is released from parasympathetic neurons, histamine is released from mast cells in the gastric mucosa and submucosa and from argentaffin cells in the gastric mucosa, and gastrin is released into the circulation by the G cells.[5] Gastric acid secretion can be inhibited by administration of H_2-receptor antagonists (see Gastric Ulceration). As the pH of the gastric lumen falls, negative feedback (release of somatostatin) inhibits release of gastrin by G cells, decreasing gastric acid secretion.[5, 9]

The chief cells synthesize pepsinogens, which are secreted into the stomach, where, in an acid environment, they are converted to pepsin. Pepsin initiates protein digestion. The mechanisms that stimulate and inhibit acid secretion probably also affect pepsinogen secretion.

Surface mucous cells secrete bicarbonate, which helps to buffer the region immediately adjacent to the mucosa. Bicarbonate secretion increases as acid secretion increases. Prostaglandins and cholinergic stimulation increase bicarbonate secretion.

The control of gastric secretion is complex.[4] The cephalic phase of secretion is initiated by the anticipation of eating and the sight and smell of food.[5] It is mediated by the parasympathetic system, which releases acetylcholine, which in turn also causes release of gastrin. As food enters the stomach, the gastric or main phase of secretion begins. Gastric distention and intraluminal proteins cause the release of gastrin.[5, 9] As the pH of the stomach and duodenum decreases, gastric secretion is inhibited by hormonal and neural mechanisms.

Problem Identification

Acute Vomiting

Vomiting is defined as the forceful ejection of gastric and duodenal contents through the mouth. Although a clear distinction cannot always be made between acute and chronic vomiting, a practical definition of acute vomiting includes cases in which clinical signs have persisted for 1–7 days. Vomiting must be differentiated from regurgitation and oropharyngeal dysphagia, based on a description by a witness, because each problem has a different differential diagnosis and requires a different diagnostic plan (see Chaps. 29 and 30). Acutely vomiting animals should be classified as having a self-limited problem or a potentially life-threatening problem, based on the severity of their clinical signs (discussed later in this section). These two groups have different differential diagnoses and diagnostic plans and require different levels of therapy.[10]

Pathophysiology

Vomiting is a centrally mediated reflex controlled by the vomiting center in the medulla.[10, 11] Input can reach the vomiting center by four pathways.[12–15] First, efferent impulses from receptors in the pharynx, stomach, duodenum, jejunum, liver, gallbladder, and other abdominal organs can travel to the vomiting center by vagal and sympathetic pathways. These receptors are stimulated by distention, irritation, hyperosmolarity, and certain chemicals. Second, circulating substances can stimulate the vomiting center through the chemoreceptor trigger zone (CRTZ). The CRTZ is located on the floor of the fourth ventricle and is not protected by the blood-brain barrier. Free nerve endings are in direct contact with cerebral spinal fluid.[16] Stimulation of the CRTZ results in dopamine release and subsequent activation of the vomiting center. Substances such as digoxin, apomorphine, cancer chemotherapeutics (doxorubicin, cisplatin, and mitoxantrone[17-19]), and uremic toxins can stimulate the CRTZ. Third, input from the semicircular canals is responsible for vomiting associated with motion sickness and, rarely, otitis media. Finally, the vomiting center may be stimulated by input from the cerebral cortex or limbic system. This route appears to be of minor importance in small animals.

Regardless of the stimulus, the vomiting center initiates the complex act of vomiting.[13, 15] Nausea, the initial event, is an imprecisely defined, unpleasant sensation believed to be caused by mild activation of the same pathways that mediate vomiting. Nausea results in salivation, depression, anxiety, and frequent swallowing efforts. Retching precedes the expulsion of gastric and duodenal contents and is associated with deep inspiration, elevation of the soft palate, closure of the glottis, inhibition of esophageal and proximal gastric motility, and relaxation of the gastroesophageal sphincter. Expulsion occurs as the duodenum, antrum and pylorus, abdominal musculature, and diaphragm vigorously contract, forcing gastric and duodenal contents into the pharynx and triggering a gag reflex, which expels ingesta from the mouth. The respiratory center is inhibited, preventing aspiration.

Occasional vomiting results in few pathophysiologic consequences to the animal but may be unpleasant and inconvenient for owners. Profuse and protracted vomiting can lead to dehydration, loss of electrolytes (chloride, sodium, and potassium), and acid-base derangement.[11] Mildly vomiting dogs and cats usually maintain normal acid-base status, but severe vomiting can lead to metabolic acidosis from loss of duodenal bicarbonate and contraction of the extracellular fluid space.[13, 15, 20] Animals vomiting because of an obstructed pylorus can develop metabolic alkalosis, because vomitus is limited to gastric contents, and these animals do not lose duodenal bicarbonate.[15, 20, 21] Vomiting can result in aspiration pneumonia.

Clinical Signs

Acute self-limited vomiting is often characterized by a history of infrequent vomiting of food, mucus, bile, or foreign material and by ingestion of table scraps or other forms of dietary indiscretion. Questioning of the owner may uncover a history of administration of drugs (aspirin, ibuprofen, erythromycin) or exposure to chemicals (herbicides, fertilizers, cleaning agents) or plants that may be the cause of the acute vomiting. The presence of acute vomiting and diarrhea may indicate dietary indiscretion or gastrointestinal parasites, such as roundworms, hookworms, or whipworms.

Physical examination is often normal. However, mild depression and signs of mild or moderate dehydration may be evident; these are characterized by slight changes such as dry mucous membranes, a loss of skin turgor, prolonged capillary refill time, or enophthalmos. Abdominal palpation is often normal, although evidence of mild abdominal pain may be found.

Animals thought to have a life-threatening cause of acute vomiting have a history of profuse or persistent vomiting that may be increasing in frequency. The vomitus may be bloody (hematemesis) or have the appearance of coffee grounds (partially digested blood). Vaccination status may be incomplete, supporting the possibility of an infectious cause of acute vomiting, especially in the puppy or kitten. Owners may report evidence of moderate to severe abdominal pain, depression, or diarrhea in the animal. Melena may occur in hookworm-infested puppies, and mucoid diarrhea may be seen with whipworm infection.

Physical examination in animals with potentially life-threatening causes of acute vomiting may reveal moderate to severe depression and dehydration (dry mucous membranes, loss of skin turgor, prolonged capillary refill time, enophthalmos, and cold extremities). A linear foreign body may be found wrapped around the base of the tongue, especially in cats.[22] Abdominal palpation often demonstrates moderate to severe pain and may identify abnormalities such as a distended and enlarged stomach, thickened small intestinal walls, distended loops of bowel, bunched intestines, intestinal foreign body, or abdominal mass. Metabolic diseases that can cause vomiting may be associated with pyrexia, lymphadenopathy, icterus, or respiratory crackles.

Diagnostic Plan

The most important initial distinction to be made is to accurately determine whether the dog or cat is vomiting, is regurgitating, or has oropharyngeal dysphagia.[11, 15, 22] These problems have distinct differential diagnoses and diagnostic plans. Most owners describe regurgitation or oropharyngeal dysphagia as vomiting. A thorough description of the actual event usually enables differentiation among these problems. Oropharyngeal dysphagia usually results in food's falling from the mouth soon after mastication (see Chap. 29). Regurgitation, the ejection of esophageal contents, is a passive process, often associated with changes in body position or excitement (see Chap. 30). Vomiting is accompanied by retching and forceful abdominal contractions.[11] Yellow discoloration of vom-

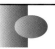

Table 31–1
Differential Diagnosis of Acute Vomiting

Self-limited
Acute gastritis
  Dietary indiscretion
  Drugs
  Chemicals
  Foreign material
Parasites
  Roundworms
  Hookworms
  Whipworms
Motion sickness
Canine coronavirus

Life-threatening
Hookworms
Acute gastritis
Gastric dilatation–volvulus
Gastric-duodenal foreign body
Gastric-duodenal ulcer
Intussusception
Canine distemper
Feline panleukopenia
Canine parvovirus
Leptospirosis
Salmon poisoning
Hemorrhagic gastroenteritis
Acute pancreatitis
Acute renal failure
Acute hepatic failure
Hypoadrenocorticism
Ketoacidotic diabetes mellitus
Peritonitis
Pyometra
Septicemia

itus suggests the presence of bile and confirms that vomiting has occurred.

Once the animal's problem has been defined as acute vomiting, the next important step is to determine whether the animal has a self-limited or a possibly life-threatening problem.[10] This assessment is crucial and must be based on a thorough history, careful physical examination, clinical experience and judgment, and a sound understanding of the differential diagnosis of acute vomiting (Table 31–1).[11, 15] Animals should be considered to have a potential life-threatening problem if some of the following are present: moderate or severe abdominal pain, lethargy, dehydration or pyrexia, enlarged and distended stomach, frequent and severe diarrhea, hematemesis, frequent vomiting or increasing frequency of vomiting, signs of systemic disease, or an incomplete vaccination history in a puppy or kitten. If a clear distinction cannot be reached, it is better to err on

the cautious side and consider a potentially life-threatening problem.

Animals with a self-limited problem require minimal diagnostic testing and symptomatic treatment; they often cease vomiting within 12 to 24 hours after initial presentation.[11] A minimum database for animals with self-limited vomiting should include determination of packed cell volume and total solids, zinc sulfate fecal flotation, and digital rectal examination. The packed cell volume and total solids help to assess hydration and also provide a baseline reference if clinical signs persist or progress. The digital rectal examination allows immediate collection of feces for flotation and verifies the presence or absence of diarrhea. If diarrhea is present, it can intensify dehydration, and more aggressive fluid therapy may be required. Reclassification to life-threatening status may be indicated if an animal initially assessed as having self-limited, acute vomiting continues to vomit despite appropriate symptomatic therapy.

Life-threatening cases of acute vomiting require an in-depth diagnostic evaluation, vigorous symptomatic management, and often specific therapy directed at the underlying cause.[11] The initial minimum database for life-threatening acute vomiting includes a complete blood count (CBC), biochemical profile with amylase and lipase, urinalysis, zinc sulfate fecal flotation, and survey abdominal radiographs. Complete laboratory evaluation helps to eliminate metabolic causes of acute vomiting (see Table 31–1) and allows assessment of fluid, electrolytes, and acid-base status. Fecal examination identifies parasites such as roundworms, hookworms, and whipworms. Survey abdominal radiographs help rule out radiopaque foreign bodies, small intestinal obstructions from foreign bodies or intussusceptions, linear foreign bodies, peritonitis, an enlarged uterus, or a case of gastric dilatation-volvulus (GDV) that has not yet progressed to abdominal distention but involves gastric distention.[23] After the initial evaluation, additional diagnostic studies may be indicated, such as upper gastrointestinal (GI) endoscopy, upper GI barium contrast series, abdominal ultrasonography, adrenocorticotropic hormone response testing, or surgical exploration of the abdomen.

Chronic Vomiting

If vomiting continues for more than 5 to 7 days or if episodes occur periodically, it should be classified as chronic. Occasional vomiting (2 or 3 times per week) in an otherwise healthy pet may require only dietary adjustment and simple management changes. However, vomiting associated with weight loss, inappetence, and lethargy should be considered serious and thoroughly evaluated. Also, frequent vomiting (2 or 3 times per day for 2 or 3 days per week) in an animal

Table 31–2
Causes of Chronic Vomiting

Systemic
Chronic renal failure
Chronic hepatobiliary diseases
Systemic mastocytosis
Diabetes mellitus
Feline hyperthyroidism
Feline heartworm disease
Lead poisoning

Gastrointestinal
Parasites

    Roundworms
    Hookworms
    Whipworms

Chronic gastritis
Gastric or duodenal foreign body
Gastric or duodenal ulcer
Chronic hypertrophic pyloric gastropathy
Gastric or duodenal neoplasia
Inflammatory bowel disease
Partial intestinal obstruction

without systemic signs warrants a thorough diagnostic work-up. Because there are so many causes of chronic vomiting (Table 31–2), a logical and organized diagnostic plan is necessary to allow a correct diagnosis to be reached efficiently.[24] Information in the history, physical examination, and routine laboratory evaluation can be used to guide the diagnostic plan.

Pathophysiology

The vomiting reflex is discussed in the section on acute vomiting. Occasional vomiting does not result in serious consequences for the animal. However, frequent vomiting can cause severe dehydration, electrolyte aberration, acid-base disturbance, and weight loss from decreased nutrient assimilation.

Clinical Signs

The frequency of vomiting can be variable and is dependent on the underlying cause. An increasing frequency of vomiting is often associated with progressive disease.

The time interval between eating and vomiting may be helpful in establishing the differential diagnosis. Vomiting of "undigested" food 8 or more hours after eating suggests delayed gastric emptying.[15, 22] Vomiting occurring immediately after eating may indicate gastritis or duodenitis. An inconsistent relation between vomiting and eating may be associated with a systemic disorder.[15]

The history should be carefully reviewed be-

cause many drugs, such as nonsteroidal anti-inflammatory drugs (NSAIDs), can cause vomiting. Hair ingestion can cause vomiting and should be suspected if the owner reports vomiting of hair balls, material containing hair, or excessive grooming by a dog or cat. Ingestion of a foreign body may have been observed or suspected. Dietary indiscretion is very common in dogs but less common in cats. The occasional feeding of table scraps or other forms of dietary indiscretion could be the underlying cause of recurrent vomiting. A careful environmental history may uncover a source for dietary indiscretion. A description of the nature of the vomiting act may be helpful, because projectile vomiting has been associated with pyloric diseases.[15, 25]

Chronic vomiting may be associated with weight loss, an unthrifty appearance, and a dull, dry hair coat. Clinical signs such as loss of skin turgor, dry mucous membranes, delayed capillary refill time, cold extremities, or enophthalmos indicate moderate or severe dehydration. Dehydration occurs most often with frequent, severe episodes of vomiting. Diarrhea, if present, contributes to dehydration. Many animals with chronic intermittent vomiting can retain water or food between episodes. Evidence of weight loss and dehydration may not be present in these dogs or cats.

The importance of thorough abdominal palpation cannot be overemphasized. Abnormalities detected help to narrow the diagnostic plan and properly rank the differential diagnoses. The normal stomach cannot be palpated abdominally.[15] However, gastric enlargement secondary to chronic outflow obstruction can be severe enough to allow detection by abdominal palpation. Thickened bowel wall (inflammatory bowel disease or diffuse lymphosarcoma), a dilated loop of bowel (partial intestinal obstruction), a foreign body, a neoplastic mass, bunched (plicated) intestines, abdominal pain, or enlarged mesenteric lymph nodes may be detected.[23, 26–28] However, many animals with chronic vomiting have a normal physical examination.

Diagnostic Plan

The most important initial distinction to be made is to accurately confirm that the dog or cat is vomiting.[11, 22] The distinction between regurgitation and oropharyngeal dysphagia is discussed in the section on acute vomiting.

Multiple fecal examinations for parasites should be performed, especially if diarrhea is present. If the physical examination is normal, the fecal examination is negative, and other predisposing causes of vomiting cannot be identified in the history, treatment for hair ingestion (especially in cats) and for dietary indiscretion (if suspected or possible) may resolve clinical signs before further diagnostic evaluation is performed.

Lubrication therapy with petroleum-based products and grooming to remove hair should be instituted or intensified. Elimination of the source of dietary indiscretion and, in some cases, institution of an easily digested diet may resolve the vomiting.

If vomiting continues despite this protocol, systemic causes of vomiting (see Table 31–2) should be evaluated. Suspicion of a systemic disorder should be increased if a thorough history and careful physical examination reveal signs of any systemic disease that can cause vomiting. Most systemic diseases can be identified by a CBC, biochemical profile, and urinalysis. In older cats, serum thyroxine should be evaluated.[22, 29] In endemic areas, an occult test for heartworms should be performed on cats.[22, 30] After evaluation of the routine laboratory data, additional diagnostic procedures may be necessary to confirm a diagnosis.

Other diagnostic tests are indicated to evaluate gastrointestinal causes of vomiting (see Table 31–2) if an underlying systemic disease has not been identified, if symptomatic therapy (including an easily digested diet trial) has not resulted in improvement, or if abnormalities are detected during abdominal palpation. The most direct and sensitive diagnostic approach involves gastroduodenoscopy with mucosal biopsy.[22, 31] Endoscopic examination is minimally invasive, can be performed rapidly, and only rarely fails to identify a gastrointestinal cause for vomiting. It allows identification and removal of foreign bodies; detection and directed biopsy of intramural masses and irregular, eroded, or ulcerated mucosa; and discovery of retained ingesta (delayed gastric emptying).

Some clinicians routinely make survey abdominal radiographs or perform abdominal ultrasound examinations before an endoscopic examination is performed. The diagnostic utility of these tests in comparison with endoscopy has not been demonstrated. My choice is to make abdominal radiographs and perform ultrasound if endoscopic examination does not lead to a diagnosis.

If a diagnosis is not reached after endoscopic examination and biopsy, or if endoscopic equipment is not available, the diagnostic plan should include survey abdominal radiographs and abdominal ultrasound, an upper GI barium contrast study, and, possibly, exploratory laparotomy. Survey radiographs may reveal a dilated, fluid-filled stomach (delayed gastric emptying); radiopaque foreign body; dilated, gas-filled loop of small bowel (obstruction by foreign body, intraluminal mass, or intussusception); bunched intestines suggesting a linear foreign body; hepatomegaly; or a soft tissue mass.[3] Ultrasound may identify an abdominal mass, thickened gastric or intestinal wall, gastric or intestinal tumor, mesenteric lymphadenopathy, or hepatomegaly.[32, 33]

Although not as valuable a diagnostic tool as endoscopy in the chronically vomiting animal, a barium contrast upper GI series offers several potential advantages over endoscopy: it is noninvasive; it does not require general anesthesia; it allows evaluation of gastric size and position within the abdomen; it allows assessment of wall thickness; it demonstrates gastric motility and emptying; and it allows evaluation of the entire small bowel.[3] Abnormalities that may be detected include plicated bowel (linear foreign body), barium-coated radiolucent foreign body, delayed gastric emptying (gastric outflow obstruction or motility disorder), intraluminal filling defect (neoplasia or hyperplasia), ulcer, irregular smudged mucosal surface with flocculation of barium (gastritis or duodenitis), obstruction (foreign body, intraluminal mass, or intussusception), or a thickened stomach or duodenal wall (neoplasia, inflammation, hyperplasia).

Exploratory laparotomy is often necessary in chronically vomiting animals if endoscopy is not available.[22] A diagnostic approach using exploratory surgery is more invasive and time-consuming than endoscopy. Surgery should be performed after survey and contrast radiography and abdominal ultrasonography. During surgery, biopsies can be taken, foreign bodies removed, and neoplastic or hyperplastic masses resected. Even if gastric and duodenal abnormalities are not detected with inspection and palpation, multiple biopsy samples should always be collected from these areas. After thorough exploration of the entire abdomen, the liver and hepatic and mesenteric lymph nodes should be examined and biopsied.

Hematemesis

Hematemesis is defined as vomiting of blood. The vomitus may be reddish or contain flecks of blood, blood clots, or "coffee grounds" (blood mixed with gastric acid). In most cases, the presence of blood results from erosive or ulcerative disease of the stomach or proximal small intestine (Fig. 31–2).[22] Melena (digested blood) is often present in the feces. The diagnostic approach is similar to that used with any case of acute or chronic vomiting. In acute vomiting, the presence of blood is a factor that suggests a potentially life-threatening cause of vomiting. Endoscopy is performed in many of these animals with life-threatening disease to provide a definitive diagnosis and to evaluate the depth of an ulcer, if present, so that immediate exploratory surgery may be undertaken if necessary. If severe blood loss has occurred, transfusion of red blood cells is necessary before institution of anesthesia.

Blood can also be present in the vomitus in patients with a bleeding disorder (see Chap. 44). Other evidence of bleeding may be detected on the physical

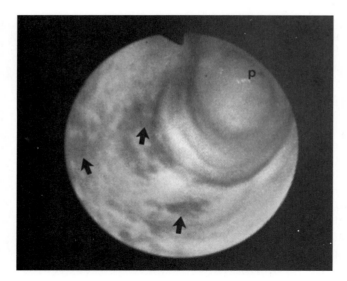

Figure 31–2
Endoscopic appearance of erosions and superficial ulcers *(arrows)* in the antrum of a 4-year-old Irish wolfhound that was vomiting blood. The pylorus (p) can be seen at 2 o'clock.

examination. Mucous membranes should be carefully evaluated for petechial hemorrhages. Prolonged bleeding from venipuncture sites, acutely developing subcutaneous masses, painful and swollen joints, or thoracic or abdominal effusion suggests the presence of a generalized bleeding disorder. Thrombocytopenia can be evaluated with a platelet count. If other evidence of bleeding is detected, coagulation can be evaluated with prothrombin and partial thromboplastin times.

It is also possible for blood to originate outside the stomach or small intestine. Blood coughed up from the lower respiratory tract can be swallowed and then vomited. In these cases, a history of coughing is usually present. Blood from the posterior nasal cavity, nasopharynx, oropharynx, or esophagus can also be swallowed and vomited. In these cases, sneezing or nasal discharge, dysphagia, or regurgitation should be evident.

Delayed Gastric Emptying

Delayed gastric emptying is associated with acute or chronic vomiting of "undigested" food more than 8 hours after eating, postprandial abdominal distention, and abdominal pain. If it is chronic, severe weight loss may be present. In some cases, classic clinical signs are not present, and delayed gastric emptying is discovered during evaluation of a vomiting patient. Delayed gastric emptying may be suspected if liquid barium sulfate remains in the stomach for more than 4 hours in dogs or 30 minutes in cats, or if ingesta is found during endoscopy after an overnight fast (Fig. 31–3).[3]

Two general causes for delayed gastric emptying exist: mechanical obstruction and abnormal gastric motility (Table 31–3). A diagnosis can usually be reached by following the diagnostic plan for acute or chronic vomiting. If causes of mechanical obstruction are not identified with endoscopy or barium contrast studies, a motility disorder can be diagnosed by exclusion.

Acute Abdominal Distention

Acute abdominal distention is most often caused by gastric distention in cases of GDV. Usually, large-breed dogs are affected, and they may have had a previous episode. The abdomen is usually very hard and tympanic (from gas distention), and it is difficult to palpate intra-abdominal structures, although splenomegaly may be detected. Respiratory distress and shock are usually present. The diagnosis is confirmed after passage of an orogastric tube that relieves the gastric and abdominal distention.

Sometimes, a poorly observed animal with chronic abdominal distention (see Chap. 34) is presented with the complaint of acute abdominal distention. These cases can be distinguished from GDV by the presence of abdominal fluid or a large abdominal mass. The abdomen is not tympanic, and respiratory distress and shock are uncommon. Rarely, a severe case of acute small intestinal obstruction may cause a tympanic abdominal distention. Respiratory distress does not occur in these cases, and a history

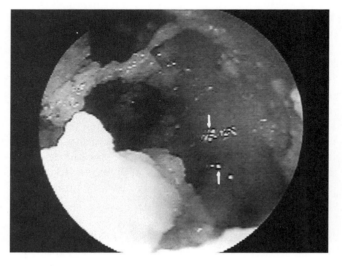

Figure 31–3
Endoscopic appearance of food in the gastric body 18 hours after eating in a 6-year-old Old English sheepdog. The delayed gastric emptying was thought to be caused by chronic gastritis. The white areas *(arrows)* are photographic reflections.

Table 31–3
Delayed Gastric Emptying

Mechanical Obstruction
Gastric or duodenal foreign body
Gastric or duodenal neoplasia
Chronic hypertrophic pyloric gastropathy
Extraluminal compression

Abnormal Motility
Idiopathic
Sympathetic stimulation
Hypokalemia
Anticholinergics
Narcotics
Gastritis or ulcer
Neoplasia
Peritonitis
Atony after gastric surgery

of vomiting, diarrhea, anorexia, lethargy, and depression is often present. If a thorough history cannot be obtained from the owner, a lateral abdominal radiograph clearly distinguishes between GDV and intestinal obstruction.

A ruptured intra-abdominal tumor with severe hemorrhage can cause acute nontympanic abdominal distention, shock, and tachypnea. Most commonly, this occurs with hemangiosarcoma of the spleen.[34] A higher prevalence occurs in German shepherds, a breed that is also predisposed to GDV. Fluid should be ballotted during abdominal palpation.

Diagnostic Procedures

Routine Laboratory Evaluation

A CBC, biochemical profile, and urinalysis are important components in the evaluation of dogs and cats with life-threatening acute vomiting or chronic vomiting. Laboratory evaluation can help assess the severity of dehydration, blood loss, electrolyte changes, and acid-base aberrations; identify a systemic disease that is the cause of vomiting (Table 31–4)[21]; and provide information to help rank the differential diagnoses for gastric diseases that cause vomiting (Table 31–5).

Elevated total protein, hematocrit, blood urea nitrogen (BUN), creatinine, and phosphorus, along with a concentrated urine specific gravity, indicate dehydration. Because of the wide range of normal values for these tests, results may be normal in a dog or cat with mild or moderate dehydration. Interpretation can also be difficult if concurrent anemia or hypoproteinemia exists. However, sequential evaluation may provide valuable information regarding

hydration status. With severe vomiting and fluid loss, hypochloremia and metabolic acidosis can occur. Although potassium is lost in the vomitus, serum levels are often normal or only slightly low. Uncommonly, hyponatremia may occur.

Gastroscopy

Instrumentation, Patient Preparation, and Restraint

The intrumentation, patient preparation, and restraint required for gastroscopy are similar to those used for esophagoscopy (see Chap. 30) except for the following differences. First, rigid endoscopy has little usefulness in the vomiting patient. Second, if delayed gastric emptying is suspected (e.g., vomiting of "undigested" food more than 8 hours after eating), a longer fasting period is necessary (see Fig. 31–3). Third, narcotics should not be used as premedications, because they affect pyloric tone and hinder the ability to enter the duodenum.[35] Finally, biopsies are easier to obtain in the stomach than in the esophagus. In most instances, the endoscope tip can be placed perpendicular to the area to be sampled, allowing a head-on view and secure purchase of the forceps.

Procedure

The endoscope is passed through the esophagus (see Chap. 30) to the gasatroesophageal sphincter, which is usually closed. A slight directional change is needed to advance the endoscope into the stomach. The endoscope tip is centralized into the gastroesophageal sphincter and insufflated with air, and the insertion tube is gently advanced, moving the tip into the stomach.

The following describes examination of the canine stomach.[36] Differences encountered in cats are discussed at the end of this section. After the endoscope has entered the stomach, it is important to view the rugal folds along the greater curvature before gastric distention.[37] Normal rugal folds should be equally wide and tall (Fig. 31–4). After evaluation of rugal folds, a small amount of air is insufflated, and the endoscope is advanced along the greater curvature. As the endoscope approaches the antrum, the reflection of the lesser curvature, the angularis incisura, becomes visible (see Fig. 31–1). This structure serves as a gastric landmark. Deflection of the endoscope tip downward (inside control knob away from endoscopist's face) allows the antrum, which lacks rugal folds, to be seen (Fig. 31–5). Deflection of the tip upward (inside control knob toward endoscopist's face) creates a retroflexed position and a view of the gastric body (Fig. 31–6).

The endoscope should be advanced into the antrum with minimal air insufflation. The appearance

Table 31–4

Laboratory Abnormalities Associated With Systemic Diseases That Cause Vomiting

ABNORMALITY	SYSTEMIC DISEASE
Neutropenia	Canine and feline parvovirus
Eosinophilia	Feline heartworms
Nucleated red blood cells and basophilic stippling	Lead poisoning
Neutrophilia with a left shift	Acute pancreatitis
	Peritonitis
	Pyometra
	Septicemia
Normal neutrophil, lymphocyte, and eosinophil count in a stressed animal (lack of stress leukogram)	Hypoadrenocorticism
Elevated alkaline phosphatase and elevated alanine aminotransferase	Hyperthyroidism
	Infectious canine hepatitis
	Leptospirosis
	Acute and chronic liver disease
Elevated amylase and lipase	Acute pancreatitis
Hyponatremia and hyperkalemia	Hypoadrenocorticism
Elevated blood urea nitrogen, creatinine, and phosphorus	Acute and chronic renal failure
	Leptospirosis
	Moderate dehydration from any cause
Hyperglycemia and glucosuria	Diabetes mellitus

of the pylorus is variable and can change during an examination. The pyloric canal may be open, closed, or surrounded by a mucosal rosette. The pylorus may be located centrally within the antrum, located off-center along the lateral antral wall, tipped away from the gastric lumen, or hidden behind a flap of mucosa. The duodenum should be entered and inspected and diagnostic samples collected before the remainder of the stomach is observed (see Chap. 32).

The endoscope is withdrawn into the gastric antrum, and a careful, systematic evaluation is begun. With mild distention, the entire antrum can usually be seen. The walls are smooth and lack rugal folds. Further withdrawal of the endoscope, coupled with

mild upward deflection of the tip, creates a direct frontal view of the angularis incisura. The endoscope tip can now be retroflexed 180° by full upward deflection. The stomach should be moderately distended with air to allow visualization of the mucosa between the rugal folds. A deep, retroflexed view of the

Table 31–5

Laboratory Abnormalities Associated With Gastric Diseases That Cause Vomiting

ABNORMALITY	GASTRIC DISEASE
Elevated hematocrit	Hemorrhagic gastroenteritis
Regenerative anemia	Ulcer and erosive gastritis
Nonregenerative anemia	Neoplasia
	Chronic hemorrhage caused by erosion and ulceration
Eosinophilia	Gastritis (inflammatory bowel disease)
Metabolic alkalosis and paradoxical aciduria	Pyloric obstruction

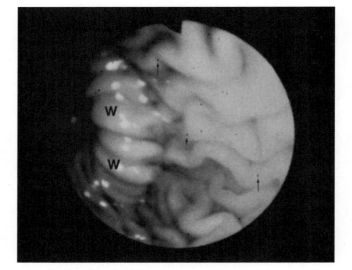

Figure 31–4

Endoscopic appearance of rugal folds in the gastric body of a normal dog. They are smooth and glistening and are wide as tall. A wave of contraction can be seen (W). The black dots (*arrows*) are broken endoscopic fibers. The larger white areas along the wave of contraction are photographic reflections.

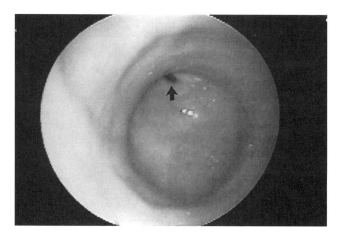

Figure 31-5
Endoscopic appearance of the antrum of a normal dog. The pylorus can be seen at 12 o'clock *(arrow)*. The white areas are photographic reflections.

gastric body, cardia, and lesser curvature can be obtained by advancing the insertion tube slightly. This view is extremely important, because the lesser curvature is not seen in other endoscopic positions. The insertion tube can be withdrawn slowly, in the retroflexed position, allowing closer inspection of the cardia. Torque should be applied to the insertion tube in both clockwise and counterclockwise directions in order to examine the mucosal surface behind the endoscope. Submucosal blood vessels should be seen in the cardia as the overlying mucosa is stretched during gastric distention.

It is very easy to overdistend the stomach, especially in small dogs. Excessive gastric distention

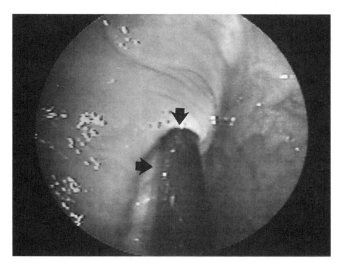

Figure 31-6
Endoscopic retroflexed appearance of the gastroesophageal junction. The endoscope *(arrows)* can be seen entering the stomach at the center of the photograph.

can interfere with effective ventilation or trigger vagal reflexes, leading to bradycardia.[38-40] The endoscopist should constantly evaluate the degree of gastric distention and immediately remove air with suction if the stomach becomes too distended.

By deflection of the endoscope tip downward, the retroflexed position is removed, and the endoscope can be withdrawn slowly, allowing examination of the greater curvature. Normal gastric mucosa is pale red, smooth, and glistening. It is tougher than small intestinal mucosa and, if normal, does not bleed on contact with the endoscope.

Biopsy and cytologic samples should be collected from any abnormal areas, and biopsy samples from the pylorus, angularis, cardia, and midway along the greater curvature. (The technique is described in Chap. 30.) After all samples have been collected and the entire gastric mucosal surface has been examined, all air is removed with suction and the endoscope is withdrawn into the esophagus.

The biggest difference between endoscopy in dogs and in cats is the small size of the feline stomach and duodenum.[40, 41] There is much less room available for maneuvering the endoscope in cats, especially in the antrum, pylorus, and duodenum. Because of the relatively small size, the feline stomach is easily overdistended, creating respiratory distress and activating vagal reflexes that may cause bradycardia. The endoscopist should constantly monitor the degree of gastric distention when performing endoscopy in cats.

The antral portion of the feline stomach is attached to the gastric body at a more acute angle than in dogs, making it difficult to directly maneuver the endoscope into the antrum (Fig. 31-7). Often, as the endoscope tip moves along the greater curvature, it retroflexes into the gastric body. Because of the small size, it is often difficult to obtain a direct frontal view of the angularis incisura. The antrum is often hidden behind a foldlike angularis. To enter the antrum, it is often necessary to advance the endoscope along the greater curvature with moderate pressure and a slight tip deflection downward. In this position, the advancing endoscope may deflect off the greater curvature into the antrum, or, in some instances, it may retroflex into the body. If the latter occurs, the endoscope should be withdrawn and the maneuver repeated. The pylorus is often slightly open. The direct, head-on, frontal view of the angularis incisura, which is commonly seen in dogs, can usually be accomplished in cats as the endoscope is withdrawn from the antrum.

Radiography

Lateral and ventrodorsal survey radiographs of the abdomen should be made in cases of acute, life-threatening vomiting and in some cases of chronic

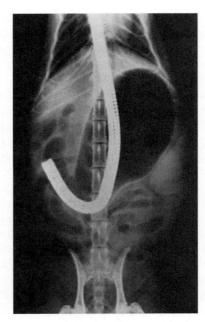

Figure 31–7
Ventrodorsal radiograph showing the endoscope tip at the antral-body junction in a cat. The acute angle of attachment of the antrum can be clearly seen. (From Leib MS. Gastrointestinal endoscopy. In: August JR. Consultations in Feline Internal Medicine 2. Philadelphia, WB Saunders, 1994.)

vomiting. The animal should be fasted for 12 hours and receive a warm-water enema before radiography is performed.[42] Abdominal radiographs are often normal but may demonstrate radiopaque foreign bodies, an air- or fluid-distended stomach (delayed gastric emptying or GDV), small intestinal lesions (see Chap. 32), signs of generalized or localized peritonitis (ground-glass appearance and loss of serosal surface visualization; see Chap. 33), hepatomegaly, enlarged uterus, or other abdominal mass.[42]

After survey radiographs have been made, a barium contrast study can be performed. Ten to 12 mL/kg of 30% micronized barium sulfate suspension is administered with an orogastric tube.[3, 42] Ventrodorsal, dorsoventral, and right and left lateral views are immediately taken. Additional lateral and ventrodorsal views are taken at 15, 30, and 60 minutes, and hourly thereafter until the stomach is empty and barium has reached the large intestine. In a normal dog, barium should begin to reach the duodenum within 30 minutes. The stomach should be empty in 4 hours, and barium should reach the large intestine within 4 hours. Transit is usually much faster in cats than in dogs. In many cats, gastric emptying begins immediately, the stomach is empty in 30 minutes, and barium reaches the colon within 1 hour.[3] In cats, peristaltic activity is usually brisk in the

duodenum, producing a "string of pearls" appearance.[3, 42]

On the ventrodorsal view in normal dogs, the stomach is perpendicular to the spine, with the cardia and fundus to the left and the antrum to the right. The cat's stomach is more oblique, with the antrum on the left of midline.[3] Rugal folds appear as uniform and parallel radiolucent lines separated by contrast-containing spaces. Gastritis may cause a smudged and irregular appearance of the rugal folds. Ulcers may have adhered contrast or a mucosal defect filled with contrast. Gastric tumors appear as filling defects associated with a thickened wall.[3] A radiolucent foreign body may initially appear as a filling defect in the barium but may remain coated as the barium leaves the stomach.[42] Changes in the small intestine are discussed in Chapter 32.

Because the upper GI series can be an insensitive test to detect gastric mucosal diseases, a normal study does not eliminate the presence of gastritis, gastric erosions or ulcers, and even small or infiltrative gastric tumors.[22, 31, 42, 43] In addition, because control of gastric emptying is different for liquids and solids, failure to demonstrate delayed gastric emptying with liquid barium does not rule out a gastric motility defect or partial obstruction.

Ultrasonography

Technologic advancements and improved expertise have resulted in the capability of sonographic evaluation of the gastrointestinal tract. Ultrasonic evaluation of the abdomen can provide valuable information in the vomiting patient. Organomegaly (liver, pancreas, spleen, uterus) can be detected and evaluated, and ultrasound-guided biopsy of the liver, spleen, or other intra-abdominal mass can be performed. Normal wall thicknesses, motility patterns, and sonographic layers of the stomach, small intestine, and colon have been identified.[44] Sonographic patterns consistent with gastric neoplasia, gastritis with ulceration, and pyloric stenosis have been described.[32, 33] Intestinal findings are described in the next chapter.

Common Diseases of the Stomach

Gastritis

Inflammation of the gastric mucosa is one of the most common causes of both acute and chronic vomiting (see Fig. 31–2).[45] Gastritis is not a specific disease but rather a syndrome with many causes. A single exposure to a potential causative agent can result in self-limited or life-threatening acute vomiting, whereas chronic ingestion can result in chronic gastritis or ulceration. Inflammation may be limited to the stomach or involve the small or large intestine (gastroenteritis or gastroenterocolitis, respectively). Gastritis occurs in dogs and cats of all ages. The signalment and history may reflect the underlying cause—for example, foreign bodies in young animals or dietary indiscretion (table scraps) in the pampered house pet.

Pathophysiology

Gastric mucosa is normally well protected from the harsh environment of gastric acid, pepsin, refluxed bile, and pancreatic enzymes.[46, 47] Gastric epithelial cells are connected by tight junctions that help to provide a mucosal barrier that prevents autodigestion. The apical surface is hydrophobic, with low permeability to water and ions. The epithelial cells secrete mucus and bicarbonate to protect the mucosa. Mucus lubricates the epithelium and helps maintain an unstirred water layer in close proximity to the epithelium. The thick mucus layer impedes movement of acid and pepsin to the mucosa. Bicarbonate is secreted into this layer and maintains a pH gradient that provides a diffusion barrier, protecting the mucosa from the low pH of the gastric lumen. Abundant mucosal blood flow helps to maintain mucosal health. Mucus and bicarbonate secretion are dependent on blood flow. In addition, any acid that back-diffuses across the mucosa is removed by local blood flow. Cellular turnover and repair of mucosal damage are rapid. Locally active prostaglandins of the E type are necessary for normal mucus and bicarbonate secretion, mucosal blood flow, and cellular repair.[46]

Most cases of gastritis are associated with decreased mucosal cytoprotection. Any agent that damages the mucosal barrier increases its permeability to luminal acid. In addition, decreases in mucus and bicarbonate secretion, mucosal blood flow, or local prostaglandin synthesis also increase permeability and back-diffusion of acid. Acid causes further mucosal, subepithelial, and vascular damage and stimulates mucosal mast cells to degranulate.[48] Release of histamine stimulates further gastric acid secretion. Damaged mucosal blood flow further decreases mucosal cytoprotection. A self-perpetuating cycle occurs, wherein increased permeability to acid leads to further epithelial damage and increased permeability.

Occasionally, hypersecretion of acid may overwhelm mucosal protection and result in gastritis. This occurs most commonly in cases of mastocytosis.[49-51]

Dietary Indiscretion

Ingestion of many substances can cause gastritis by irritation of and damage to the gastric mucosa. Foreign bodies and swallowed hair (Fig. 31–8) can abrasively erode the mucosa. Toxins and putrefactive factors in ingested garbage can chemically disrupt the mucosal barrier. A similar mechanism occurs with many other chemicals, toxins, and plants.

Nonsteroidal Anti-inflammatory Drugs

NSAIDs are common causes of gastritis and ulceration.[52-55] These drugs inhibit prostaglandin synthesis, severely decreasing mucosal cytoprotection.[46] Aspirin also causes direct mucosal damage.[56, 57]

Corticosteroids

Corticosteroids decrease mucosal cell growth and repair, decrease mucus production and viscosity, and increase acid secretion.[46, 58] Although corticosteroids can cause gastritis by themselves,[59] they may be more important in the pathogenesis of gastritis because they enhance the effects of other drugs or factors.[52]

Decreased Mucosal Blood Flow

Because of the importance of mucosal blood flow in gastric cytoprotection, anything that severely reduces it can result in gastritis or ulcers.[46] Common causes include hypovolemia and hypotension associated with severe dehydration, trauma, anesthesia, surgery, or sepsis. Thrombosis of blood vessels can have the same effect; it occurs in cases complicated with disseminated intravascular coagulation (DIC).

Renal Failure

Renal failure can cause gastritis by direct damage by uremic toxins to gastric mucosal cells and blood vessels[60] or by decreased renal metabolism of gastrin, which leads to increased gastric acid secretion.[46]

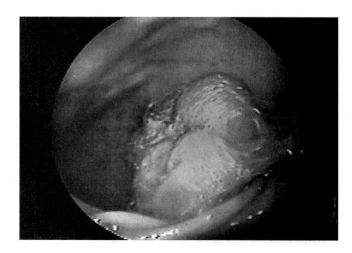

Figure 31–8
Endoscopic appearance of a large hair ball in the antrum of an adult dog. Hair can irritate the gastric mucosa, resulting in gastritis and vomiting.

Liver Disease

Chronic liver diseases can also cause gastritis as a result of a negative nitrogen balance that alters cytoprotection, reduced gastric mucosal blood flow associated with portal hypertension, and elevated gastrin and gastric acid secretion.[57, 61]

Duodenogastric Reflux

Chronic reflux of duodenal contents (bile, pancreatic enzymes, and short-chain fatty acids) into the stomach can cause gastritis in dogs. Factors that contribute to reflux include delayed gastric emptying from any cause, hyposecretion of acid, and disturbed duodenal motility.[62]

Helicobacter *Infection*

A bacterium, *Helicobacter pylori,* has been shown to be a major cause of gastritis and peptic ulcers in humans.[63] Preliminary evidence in laboratory dogs showed that *Helicobacter felis* can cause a lymphofollicular gastritis.[64] The importance of this pathogen in clinical cases of gastritis in dogs and cats is unknown, but it may prove to be an important cause in dogs and cats.

Clinical Signs

Acute, intermittent, or chronic vomiting is the most common clinical sign of gastritis. Small or large bowel diarrhea, anorexia, depression, lethargy, hematemesis, abdominal pain, and pyrexia can also be present. Weight loss can occur in chronic cases. Vomiting within 30 minutes of eating is common.

Dehydration is common in cases of gastritis, and its severity is related to the frequency of vomiting, the animal's ability to retain food and water between vomiting episodes, and the presence of diarrhea. An animal must be at least 5% dehydrated before dehydration can be clinically detected by mild changes in skin turgor, mucous membrane moisture, eye position, capillary refill time, or extremity temperature. More pronounced alterations in these parameters indicate moderate dehydration (7%–9%), and extreme alterations denote severe dehydration (10%–12%). Mild dehydration may be present in acute self-limited cases of gastritis. Animals with life-threatening acute gastritis may be moderately or severely dehydrated. Chronic gastritis does not often lead to dehydration unless an acute bout of severe vomiting occurs.

Other clinical signs are dependent on the underlying cause of the gastritis (Table 31–6). The history may reveal dietary indiscretion or exposure to foreign bodies (more common in dogs than in cats), drugs, plants, chemicals, or other toxins. Canine distemper should be suspected in unvaccinated puppies if vomiting occurs along with conjunctivitis,

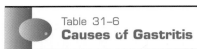

Table 31–6
Causes of Gastritis

Dietary indiscretion
Drugs—aspirin, ibuprofen, phenylbutazone, flunixin, corticosteroids
Foreign body
Plants
Chemicals
Lead poisoning
Decreased gastric blood flow—stress, hypotension, shock, sepsis, disseminated intravascular coagulation
Canine distemper
Inflammatory bowel disease
Mastocytosis
Liver diseases
Renal failure

cough, pyrexia, and mucopurulent nasal discharge.[65] If inflammatory bowel disease is present, thickened intestinal walls may be palpated.[26, 27] Signs of other systemic disorders, such as renal and liver diseases, may accompany the vomiting. A cutaneous nodule, enlarged lymph nodes, or splenomegaly may be associated with systemic mast cell disease.[49, 50]

Diagnostic Plan

In acute self-limited gastritis, a causative factor may be evident in the history. If present, removal of the underlying cause and symptomatic therapy should result in rapid clinical recovery. In cases in which an obvious cause is not apparent from the history or physical examination, symptomatic care often results in clinical recovery. A presumptive diagnosis of acute gastritis is made based on response to therapy. Further diagnostic evaluation is not necessary unless repeated episodes occur.

In cases of acute life-threatening gastritis, history and clinical signs may suggest an underlying cause (see Table 31–6). The minimum database (CBC, biochemical profile, urinalysis, fecal examination, and survey abdominal radiographs) should provide a diagnosis in most cases (e.g., acute renal failure, acute liver disease, radiopaque foreign body). Additional diagnostic tests are sometimes indicated. As an example, a history of potential foreign body ingestion in a cat with normal laboratory evaluation and survey radiographs warrants endoscopic examination or an upper GI barium contrast series. The diagnosis of acute gastritis is based on identification of an underlying cause, or, if one is not found, on the response to therapy.

Results of routine laboratory evaluation are often normal in cases of chronic gastritis, unless an underlying systemic disorder such as renal failure or liver disease is present. Patients with inflammatory bowel disease may have peripheral eosinophilia. Survey abdominal radiographs are usually normal, unless a radiopaque foreign body is seen. The diagnosis of chronic gastritis requires mucosal biopsy. Endoscopic examination may identify a foreign body or reveal mucosal hyperemia or hemorrhage, increased friability (bleeding on contact with the endoscope), or mucosal erosions or ulcerations (see Fig. 31–2). Histologic findings include epithelial necrosis, erosion, edema, hemorrhage, infiltration of inflammatory cells into the lamina propria, mucosal atrophy, and fibrosis.[45]

If an underlying cause of chronic gastritis cannot be identified, a diagnosis of idiopathic gastritis is made. Various histologically classified types of gastritis have been recognized: atrophic, superficial, diffuse, follicular, and hypertrophic.[45, 66] However, the clinical significance of this classification scheme remains unknown. Chronic idiopathic cases of gastritis may be part of the inflammatory bowel disease complex (see Chap. 32). Repeated exposure to causative factors may generate an immune-mediated process in these cases.[48]

Treatment

Primary Therapy

In all cases of gastritis, treatment should be directed at the underlying cause, if one is identified. Acute self-limited cases of gastritis require only symptomatic care and correction of the underlying cause. Food and water should be withheld (food in the stomach stimulates gastric secretion and motility) until the animal stops vomiting for 12 to 24 hours (nothing per os, or NPO).[15, 67] If mild dehydration is present, a balanced isotonic, polyionic fluid can be administered subcutaneously. The animal's deficit from dehydration can be calculated by multiplying the estimated percentage of dehydration (from physical examination) by the body weight (in kilograms). Dehydration should be corrected within 24 hours. Maintenance fluids (44–66 mL/kg per day) should be added to the deficit.[20] After the animal has not vomited for 12 to 24 hours, gradual oral alimentation can be started. Initially, ice cubes or small amounts of water are frequently offered. If vomiting does not occur, small amounts of a highly digestible diet can be frequently offered. On day 1, one third of maintenance caloric requirements can be divided into 3 to 6 feedings. If vomiting does not occur, two thirds can be given on day 2, and full maintenance on day 3. This diet should be soft and low in fiber (so as not to irritate the gastric mucosa), highly digestible, high in carbohydrates, low in fat (fat delays gastric emptying), and low in protein (proteins can stimulate gastric acid secretion).[67] Boiled rice, rice with chicken,

low-fat cottage cheese, Prescription Diet i/d, or CNM EN is effective. The size of the meals should slowly be increased and the frequency of feeding decreased if vomiting does not recur. If the dog or cat does not vomit for 3 days, the normal diet can slowly be added over several days. If at any time vomiting returns, the animal should be re-evaluated and further diagnostics performed, a longer NPO period instituted, or antiemetic medication administered (see later discussion of antiemetics).

Animals with acute life-threatening gastritis require more vigorous therapy. If an underlying condition exists, it should be specifically treated. The animal should be kept NPO until vomiting ceases for 24 hours. Moderate or severe dehydration is usually present, and intravenous fluid therapy is indicated. The volume of fluid to be infused is made up of three components: the deficit caused by dehydration, maintenance requirements, and the volume of fluids lost in the vomitus. A balanced polyionic fluid, such as Ringer's or lactated Ringer's solution, should be infused over as long a time period as practical. In many practices, 24 hours of fluid requirements must be administered during a 12-hour workday, but this is not as physiologic as continuous 24-hour infusion. Automatic infusion pumps provide accurate and uniform infusion rates and reduce the human effort needed to provide fluid therapy. Dehydration should be corrected within 24 hours.

Even if serum potassium remains normal, a total body deficit probably exists because of loss in the vomitus and urine and lack of food intake.[67] Before laboratory results are received, 20 mEq potassium chloride should be added to each liter of fluid, provided urine output is judged to be adequate.[15] Additional potassium should be added to the fluids based on serum potassium levels (Table 31–7).[20] Potassium must always be administered slowly, diluted into the 12- or 24-hour fluid volume, to avoid cardiotoxicity.

The animal should be monitored carefully during fluid therapy. The physical examination find-

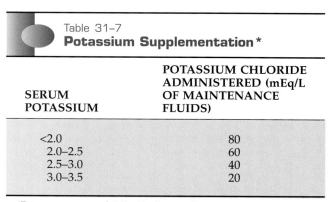

Table 31–7
Potassium Supplementation*

SERUM POTASSIUM	POTASSIUM CHLORIDE ADMINISTERED (mEq/L OF MAINTENANCE FLUIDS)
<2.0	80
2.0–2.5	60
2.5–3.0	40
3.0–3.5	20

*Rate not to exceed 0.5 mEq/kg per hour.

ings that indicated dehydration should gradually improve as the patient is rehydrated during the first 24 hours of therapy. The hematocrit and total protein should fall. Body weight should be measured frequently, because changes accurately reflect hydration. After hydration has been re-established, body weight should remain relatively stable throughout the treatment period. A falling weight suggests dehydration, and an increasing weight may indicate overhydration. Serum electrolytes should be monitored daily for several days in animals with profuse vomiting or severe electrolyte abnormalities on initial laboratory evaluation. After no vomiting has occurred for 24 hours, the animal can gradually be reintroduced to water and food, as described previously. If vomiting continues and causes a large fluid loss, or if it is frequent enough to interfere with the animal's ability to rest, antiemetic therapy is indicated.

Therapy for chronic gastritis is directed at the underlying cause. If dehydration is present, it should be managed as described previously. Idiopathic chronic gastritis should be treated according to the guidelines for treating inflammatory bowel disease (see Chap. 32). Briefly, feeding of a hypoallergenic diet or immunosuppression with prednisone is often indicated. If erosions are seen endoscopically, treatment with an H_2-receptor blocker is beneficial (see Gastric Ulceration). The diet should be soft, low in fiber, highly digestible, high in carbohydrates, and low in fat. Treatment should continue for at least 4 to 6 weeks. All forms of dietary indiscretion must be avoided during the recovery period. At the time of this writing it is premature to suggest treatment of suspected *Helicobacter* infection. However, in humans a combination of amoxicillin, metronidazole, and bismuth with an H_2-receptor antagonist for 2 weeks is usually effective.

Antiemetics

Antiemetics should be used cautiously, because continued vomiting is an important sign that the underlying condition may be progressing or that an incorrect diagnosis has been made. Masking of this important parameter may give the clinician a false sense of security that the animal is improving, when actually heightened surveillance and therapy are indicated. I am most comfortable prescribing antiemetics after a definitive diagnosis has been reached or for only a brief period in animals with self-limited gastritis.

Phenothiazines. Phenothiazines are potent, centrally acting drugs that block both the vomiting center and the CRTZ.[11, 14, 68] They are dopamine antagonists with antihistaminic and weak anticholinergic properties. They cannot be administered until the animal has been rehydrated, because they are α-adrenergic recep-

tor blockers and can cause hypotension.[12] Even at low doses, they produce tranquilization, which has the benefit of promoting rest and reducing stress but the disadvantage of interfering with monitoring of the animal's attitude. They should not be used in animals with epilepsy because they may lower the seizure threshold. They can be given intramuscularly or subcutaneously, and several are available in suppository form. Recommended dosages of commonly used drugs include chlorpromazine (Thorazine), 0.2 to 0.5 mg/kg three times (t.i.d.) or four times (q.i.d.) per day, and prochlorperazine (Compazine), 0.5 mg/kg t.i.d. or q.i.d.[11, 67, 68]

Metoclopramide. Metoclopramide (Reglan) is a highly effective antiemetic with both central and peripheral effects.[67–69] Metoclopramide is a dopamine antagonist that very effectively blocks the CRTZ and raises the threshold of the vomiting center. Peripherally, it augments acetylcholine release from postganglionic nerves, increases the tone and amplitude of gastric contractions, and increases gastroesophageal sphincter pressure.[69] These actions oppose some of the physical events necessary for the vomiting reflex to occur.[14] Short-term side effects are uncommon and include depression, nervousness, and restlessness. Metoclopramide is contraindicated in gastric or intestinal obstructions. Dosages of 0.2 to 0.4 mg/kg t.i.d. subcutaneously are often effective. Because it has a short halflife, it may need to be administered by constant infusion at 1.0 to 2.0 mg/kg per day intravenously.

Anticholinergics. Anticholinergics are often used as antiemetics, but I prefer using phenothiazines or metoclopramide. Peripherally, anticholinergics may decrease afferent stimulation of the vomiting center by relieving smooth muscle spasm or by inhibiting gastric secretion.[14, 68] However, these drugs are potent inhibitors of GI motility. Gastric and duodenal ileus can cause vomiting.[67] Recovery from gastritis often requires re-establishment of normal gastric and duodenal motility. Other side effects include xerostomia, mydriasis, tachycardia, and urinary retention.[68]

Anticholinergics are often combined with other drugs that can contribute to their effectiveness. Isopropamide is combined with the phenothiazine prochlorperazine (Darbazine, 0.14–0.22 mg/kg twice per day [b.i.d.] intramuscularly or subcutaneously). Aminopentamide (Centrine, 0.01–0.03 mg/kg b.i.d. or t.i.d., intramuscularly or subcutaneously) crosses the blood-brain barrier and may have some central antiemetic effects in the vomiting center.[68]

Antihistamines. Antihistamines are primarily used to prevent motion sickness. These drugs possess both antihistaminic and anticholinergic effects and block vomiting at the vestibular apparatus.[68] They cause sedation and xerostomia. Dimenhydrinate (Dramamine, 25–50 mg total dose in dogs, 12.5 mg total dose in cats) or diphenhydramine (Benadryl 2–4 mg/kg) can be given 30 to 60 minutes before automobile travel.[68]

Prognosis

The prognosis for most cases of acute gastritis is good. Life-threatening cases require prompt diagnosis and aggressive fluid therapy. The prognosis for chronic gastritis depends on the underlying cause. Idiopathic chronic gastritis has a favorable prognosis, but long-term, possibly lifelong therapy may be necessary.

Gastric Ulceration

An ulcer is defined as a mucosal defect through the muscularis mucosae. Ulcers occur more commonly in dogs than in cats. The incidence of gastric or duodenal ulcer disease (GDUD) seems to be increasing, most likely because of increased availability and use of NSAIDs in animals with chronic arthritis.[52–54] Any of the causes of gastritis can lead to GDUD (see Table 31–6). The most common predisposing causes in dogs are NSAIDs and liver diseases.[55, 70]

Pathophysiology

Most GDUD in dogs and cats is related to decreased mucosal cytoprotection, which is discussed in the section on gastritis. If continued mucosal damage exceeds the reparative process, erosions can progress to ulcers. It is unknown why only single or several ulcers form, instead of widespread mucosal changes.[57] Ulcers caused by NSAIDs are commonly found in the stomach, whereas those associated with liver diseases commonly occur in the duodenum.[54, 55, 70]

Dogs with neurologic disease (usually intervertebral disc herniation) treated with corticosteroids and surgery have a high incidence of GDUD, and death occurs in approximately 2% of cases.[58] Some of these dogs also develop colonic ulcers.[71, 72] The pathophysiology is related to the detrimental effects on mucosal cytoprotection by corticosteroids; the stress of disease and surgery, which causes release of endogenous corticosteroids and epinephrine; and autonomic imbalance, which causes decreased gastric blood flow and increased gastric acid secretion.

Two serious complications of GDUD are possible: GI hemorrhage and perforation.[57] As the ulcerative process progresses, erosion into blood vessels can occur, resulting in hemorrhage into the GI tract. Moderate amounts of hemorrhage result in a regenerative anemia, hematemesis, melena, progressive weakness, and pallor of the mucous membranes. With continued loss of iron from the body, the anemia becomes nonregenerative, and weakness and lethargy become pronounced. Severe hemorrhage can be associated with collapse, shock, and death. Perforation leads to peritonitis, sepsis, and death. In some cases, clinical signs of GDUD are not present until perforation occurs.[70]

Clinical Signs

Acute or chronic vomiting with or without hematemesis is the most common sign associated with GDUD.[54, 55, 57] A history of NSAID administration may be present. Other signs are related to the underlying cause and may mask the clinical signs associated with the ulcer (e.g., renal failure, liver diseases, mast cell tumor, neurologic disease treated with corticosteroids, and surgery).[57] Moderate or severe abdominal pain is common, but some animals may not demonstrate any discomfort.[55] Melena often accompanies hematemesis. If severe GI hemorrhage has occurred, weakness and pale mucous membranes or circulatory shock may be present. Perforation of the stomach or duodenum may result in sudden onset of severe weakness, severe abdominal pain, fever, shock, abdominal distention, and death.[55, 70]

Diagnostic Plan

The diagnosis of GDUD requires either direct visualization of the ulcer with endoscopy or indirect identification with a barium contrast study. Ulcers can vary in size from several millimeters to 4 cm in diameter.[70] Barium may adhere to the mucosal defect or penetrate into the crater.[3] Neoplastic ulcers may be associated with a thickened gastric wall. However, a barium contrast upper GI series is relatively insensitive, and small ulcers or larger defects filled with blood or debris may not be identified.[55, 57]

Endoscopic examination is the best way to diagnose GDUD (Fig. 31–9).[54, 57] Round or oval ulcers, often with raised borders, can be seen along the greater curvature, angularis incisura, antrum, or duodenum. Evidence of gastritis or duodenitis may also be present in nonulcerated mucosa (i.e., increased mucosal granularity and friability). If a blood clot is present in the ulcer crater, it should not be disturbed. Multiple biopsy samples should be collected from the edge of the ulcer to eliminate the presence of neoplasia. Deeper tissues should be collected by repeatedly placing the forceps in the same location, because superficial inflammation often accompanies neoplasia. Nonulcerated mucosa should also be sampled to identify diffuse gastritis or duodenitis. If perforation is suspected or severe bleeding is encountered, the animal should undergo exploratory laparotomy with resection of the lesion. Perfo-

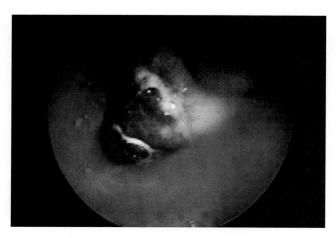

Figure 31-9
Endoscopic appearance of a large and deep ulcer in the antrum of a 9-month-old dachshund that ate three tablets of the owner's prescription nonsteroidal anti-inflammatory drug (flurbiprofen). The white adherent material at the top and bottom of the ulcer is sucralfate that was instilled through the endoscope.

ration may be difficult to detect endoscopically, because small lesions often seal over with omentum and fibrin. Perforation should be suspected if abdominal distention remains after the stomach has been deflated. A survey abdominal radiograph may demonstrate free gas in the abdomen if perforation has occurred.

Blood loss may result in a regenerative anemia.[54] Chronic loss of blood may lead to an iron deficiency anemia that is nonregenerative, microcytic, and hypochromic.[55] Hypoproteinemia accompanies severe blood loss. A leukocytosis with a left shift may accompany perforation and peritonitis. Other laboratory abnormalities are associated with the underlying cause of the GDUD (see Table 31-6).

Treatment

Successful management of GDUD requires identification and correction of the underlying cause, supportive therapy (see discussion of life-threatening acute gastritis), and specific antiulcer therapy. In most cases, either an H_2-receptor antagonist or sucralfate is adequate. If moderate or severe anemia is present, transfusion with whole blood or packed red blood cells is indicated. Antiulcer therapy should be continued for 4 to 6 weeks. Severe hemorrhage or perforation requires resection and anastomosis.

Histamine₂-Receptor Blockade

Back-diffusion of acid across a damaged mucosa leads to further damage and retards healing processes. Reduction of gastric acid secretion promotes healing of GDUD. Drugs such as cimetidine (Tagamet),

ranitidine (Zantac), famotidine (Pepcid), and nizatidine (Axid) block the H_2-receptor on the gastric parietal cell and dramatically decrease acid production.[46, 57, 73] Cimetidine (5–10 mg/kg t.i.d. or q.i.d.) and ranitidine (2 mg/kg b.i.d. or t.i.d.) have been used most commonly in veterinary medicine. Both can be given orally or parenterally, and neither has been commonly associated with adverse effects. Cimetidine can inhibit hepatic cytochrome P-450 enzymes, potentially interfering with the metabolism of other drugs.

Antacids

Antacids are safe and effective compounds that neutralize acid, inactivate pepsin, bind bile acids, and stimulate release of prostaglandins.[46, 57, 73, 74] Most products contain aluminum, magnesium, or calcium. Because they must be administered every 2 to 4 hours and are unpalatable, they are impractical for treatment of GDUD in dogs and cats.

Sucralfate

Sucralfate (Carafate) is a sulfated disaccharide that forms an adherent gel and binds to an ulcer crater, protecting it from acid and pepsin.[57, 73, 74] It also stimulates the synthesis of prostaglandin, increases mucosal cytoprotection, and binds epithelial growth factor at the ulcer, where it stimulates cellular proliferation.[46] It has been shown to be as effective as H_2-receptor blockers in healing ulcers in humans. Because sucralfate can bind other drugs, medications should be given 1 to 2 hours before sucralfate is administered.[74] The recommended dose is 1 g/25 kg t.i.d. or q.i.d. Because absorption is minimal, toxicity is uncommon. Long-term use may lead to constipation because of its aluminum content.[73] There is no evidence to support an added benefit for combination therapy with sucralfate and an H_2-receptor antagonist compared with use of either drug alone.[74]

Misoprostol

Misoprostol (Cytotec) is a synthetic prostaglandin that prevents or heals ulcers associated with administration of NSAIDs by directly increasing mucosal cytoprotection.[73–76] The suggested dose is 3 µg/kg t.i.d. The most common side effect is diarrhea, although the drug can also cause abortion. Its major indication is in preventing GI mucosal injury in dogs with arthritis that require long-term NSAID therapy. It can also be used to treat cases of GDUD caused by NSAIDs.

Proton Pump Inhibitors

Omeprazole (Prilosec) inhibits action of the proton pump at the apical portion of the parietal cell, which exchanges hydrogen ions for luminal potassium, and thereby prevents secretion of acid.[46, 73, 74, 77, 78]

As a weak base, it accumulates in the acid compartment of the parietal cell, necessitating only once-daily (s.i.d.) administration. The recommended dose is 0.7 mg/kg s.i.d. The enteric-coated granules (20 mg) are packaged in gelatin capsules to resist degradation by gastric acid. If less than one capsule is to be administered, the granules should be repackaged in gelatin capsules.[46, 77] Omeprazole also inhibits hepatic P-450 enzymes.[74] Prolonged use may induce mucosal hyperplasia and tumor formation in laboratory species. Omeprazole is indicated if GDUD is unresponsive to therapy with H_2-blockers or sucralfate and in gastric acid hypersecretory conditions such as systemic mast cell disease.

Prognosis

The prognosis for GDUD is variable and depends on the underlying cause, size and depth of ulcer, and presence of complications such as severe hemorrhage or perforation and peritonitis. Most NSAID-induced ulcers heal within 4 to 6 weeks after withdrawal of the drug and appropriate antiulcer therapy.[54] Ulcers associated with chronic diseases benefit from antiulcer therapy, but the overall prognosis depends on that of the primary disorder.

Gastric Foreign Bodies

Foreign body ingestion is very common in dogs and less so in cats. Many foreign objects reaching the stomach are removed by the vomiting reflex, are dissolved by gastric acid, or pass through the remainder of the GI tract without serious consequences. Approximately 50% of objects retained in the stomach cause vomiting. The remainder of foreign bodies are detected in asymptomatic animals, as incidental findings or because the owner has observed or suspects ingestion. Foreign body ingestion is most common in puppies. Hair balls form in cats of all ages.

Pathophysiology

Many objects (especially bone and cartilage) can be partially digested by gastric acid, facilitating passage into the small intestine. Small, smooth-surfaced objects often do not cause any pathophysiologic effects. However, rough-surfaced foreign bodies in the stomach cause clinical signs (gastritis) by physical abrasion of the mucosa. Dogs and cats ingest a wide variety of foreign bodies: sewing needles, fishhooks, bones, rocks, Popsicle sticks, balls, marbles, articles of clothing, coins, toys, batteries, and a variety of plastic or metal household items.[79] Ingested hair can irritate the mucosa. The pathogenesis of hair ball (trichobezoar) formation is perplexing. Hair should empty from the stomach during the interdigestive motility complex.[6]

Gastric retention of hair, with subsequent formation of hair balls, may reflect abnormal gastric motility.[80]

Lead or zinc objects (including pennies minted after 1983) can produce systemic toxicity (lead poisoning or hemolytic anemia, respectively); gastric acid enhances availability and absorption of these metals. Batteries are corrosive after interaction with gastric acid and can cause severe mucosal changes and even perforation. Large, sharp objects can cause perforation and peritonitis.

An object can mechanically obstruct the pylorus as gastric motility attempts to move it into the duodenum. Occasionally, a foreign body that obstructs the pylorus and causes severe clinical signs may become dislodged during vomiting and remain in the stomach, producing few clinical signs. Cyclic signs may develop as the foreign body reobstructs the pylorus.

Clinical Signs

Gastric foreign bodies often cause acute or chronic vomiting. Hematemesis is sometimes present. Owners may observe or suspect foreign body ingestion. Obstruction of the pylorus occurs uncommonly and is associated with life-threatening acute vomiting. Chronic partial pyloric obstruction can cause delayed gastric emptying with postprandial gastric and abdominal distention and discomfort, vomiting of food 8 or more hours after eating, and weight loss. Many gastric foreign bodies remain in the stomach for long periods (months) without causing clinical signs.

Physical examination is often normal. Mild abdominal pain may be detected. Pyrexia may be present if gastric perforation and peritonitis are present. Depending on the severity of vomiting, dehydration may be evident on physical examination, and routine laboratory tests may reveal electrolyte abnormalities.

Diagnostic Plan

Owners may observe or suspect foreign body ingestion, making diagnosis relatively easy. Other cases are discovered by following the diagnostic plans for acute or chronic vomiting. Survey abdominal radiographs demonstrate radiopaque foreign bodies (Fig. 31–10) and may show signs of outflow obstruction—that is, an air-, fluid-, or food-dilated stomach. Some foreign bodies may be visible by their soft tissue appearance and abnormal gas patterns.[42] If a suspected foreign body cannot be visualized, a barium contrast study is necessary. The foreign body may cause a filling defect in the barium, or contrast may adhere to it after most of the barium has left the stomach.[42]

The best method to diagnose (and treat) a gastric foreign body is with endoscopic examination

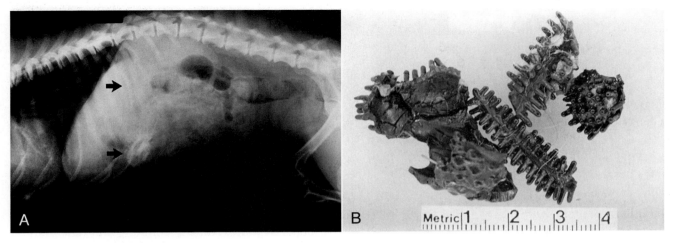

Figure 31–10

(A) Lateral abdominal radiograph of a 12-year-old dachshund that shows radiodense material within the stomach *(arrows)*. The dog was being evaluated for intervertebral disc disease. The gastric foreign body was an incidental finding. **(B)** Pieces of a plastic toy removed endoscopically from the dog in A.

(Fig. 31–11). False-negative procedures are very uncommon, because thorough endoscopic examination of the entire stomach should identify the foreign body. If the foreign body cannot be located, the cardiac region should be carefully evaluated with the endoscope in a retroflexed position. In most cases, endoscopic retrieval is possible.

Treatment

Certain foreign bodies recently ingested are best treated by inducing vomiting with syrup of ipecac (2–6 mL total dose, by mouth). Vomiting should not be induced if large, long, irregularly shaped, or sharp-pointed objects have been swallowed, because these objects may penetrate the gastric or esophageal walls during vomiting. If a foreign body remains in the stomach despite vomiting (spontaneous or induced) or if, by entering the small intestine, it could cause obstruction or perforation, it should be removed. Endoscopic removal is the treatment of choice because it avoids the morbidity and risks associated with surgery. Before general anesthesia is induced, dehydration and electrolyte abnormalities should be corrected and radiographs taken to confirm the location of the foreign body.

Various types of endoscopic retrieval forceps are available. I have had best results with rat-tooth, snare, and basket forceps. After the foreign body has been grasped by the forceps, the foreign body and forceps should be withdrawn against the endoscope, air insufflated to dilate the gastroesophageal sphincter, and the endoscope slowly withdrawn. The foreign body may dislodge at the gastrointestinal sphincter. Repositioning of the forceps to obtain a firmer pur-

chase or use of a different type of forceps should allow successful delivery. Resistance is also met in the pharynx. Additional treatment is not usually indicated, but medical management is warranted if the foreign object has induced severe gastritis (see Gastritis). If endoscopic equipment is not available, the foreign body can be removed with gastrotomy.

Often, acute foreign body ingestion occurs into

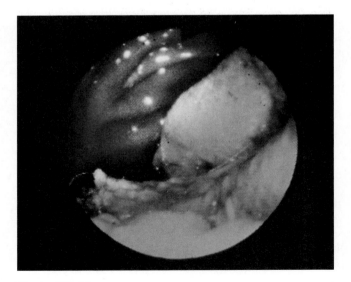

Figure 31–11

Endoscopic appearance of a large white athletic sock in the gastric body of a 6-month-old puppy. The sock was grasped with a rat-tooth forceps and removed during endoscopy. The dog was released from the hospital the same afternoon and enjoyed its normal evening meal. The large white areas at the top of the photograph are light reflections.

a stomach full of food. General anesthesia of an animal with a food-distended stomach carries an increased risk of aspiration pneumonia. A full stomach also may obscure visualization of the foreign body. Allowing time for the food to empty from the stomach may facilitate identification and retrieval of the foreign body and reduce the risk of aspiration, but it may also result in perforation or small intestinal obstruction, depending on the nature of the foreign body. The endoscopist must make a decision based on the type of foreign body, clinical signs, and other predisposing factors.

Hair balls are often recurring problems, and vigorous preventative therapy with petroleum-based lubricants and frequent grooming is necessary to avoid repeated bouts.

Prognosis

The prognosis for most cases of gastric foreign bodies is excellent. Many dissolve or pass uneventfully through the GI tract. If foreign bodies need retrieval, endoscopy is safe and effective. Cases with gastric perforation carry a guarded prognosis, and outcome is related to the severity and duration of peritonitis. The prognosis is also guarded for lead and zinc ingestion if systemic signs of toxicity are present at the time of diagnosis.

Gastric Dilatation-Volvulus

GDV is an acute life-threatening syndrome with a high mortality rate that occurs primarily in adult, large, deep-chested breeds of dogs.[81–85] The clinical signs can intensify very rapidly and, if the condition is untreated, progress to death. GDV should not be confused with dietary indiscretion and engorgement, which occur most commonly in puppies and cause acute vomiting.

Pathophysiology

The pathophysiology of GDV has been extensively studied in experimental models of disease. The cause is probably multifactorial; proposed mechanisms include body conformation, chronic gastric distention (single daily feeding and consumption of large volumes of water), postprandial exercise, hereditary predisposition, aerophagia, abnormal gastric emptying and eructation, hypergastrinemia, stress, processed dry foods, and intragastric bacterial fermentation.[86–94]

Regardless of the cause, the stomach becomes distended with atmospheric air, secondary to aerophagia.[90] Rapid swallowing of food increases aerophagia, as do nervousness, pain, excitement, and exercise.[95] As the stomach dilates, it rotates 90° to 360°, usually clockwise when viewed from caudal to the stomach.[82, 96–98] There is speculation that the stomach may first rotate and then dilate, but this is an impossible question to answer in spontaneous cases.[99] It is postulated that before volvulus develops, a failure of the eructation and vomiting mechanisms occurs. It is theorized that after volvulus develops, swallowed air can pass the twisted gastroesophageal junction but cannot escape the stomach. The spleen follows the stomach, and, as it becomes congested, it can act as a weight and pull the stomach further.

As intraluminal gastric pressure increases, venous return is compromised, producing vascular stasis and hypoxia. Gastric mucosal edema, hemorrhage, and necrosis occur.[95] Severe distention damages intramural neurons, and muscle contractile properties are lost.[100] Volvulus occludes the arterial blood supply.[101] The dilated stomach occludes the portal vein, leading to splenic congestion and, in some cases, to thrombus formation.[95] Splenic volvulus occludes its arterial blood supply, resulting in hypoxia and necrosis.

The greatly distended stomach impinges on the thoracic cavity, preventing expansion and causing decreased tidal volume and decreased lung compliance.[95] Inadequate alveolar ventilation leads to generalized hypoxia.

Gastric distention compresses the vena cava, decreasing venous return to the heart, and subsequently decreasing cardiac output.[102–105] Compression of the portal vein leads to intestinal stasis and the potential development of endotoxemia.[95, 106]

A wide variety of acid-base disturbances have been documented.[103, 107] Some dogs develop metabolic acidosis (because of decreased tissue perfusion and anaerobic metabolism with lactic acid production) or metabolic alkalosis (from outpouring of hydrochloric acid into the stomach), whereas others maintain a normal arterial pH as a result of a combination of both processes.[108, 109]

Cardiac arrhythmias develop in approximately 50% of dogs with GDV.[83, 110, 111] The most common arrhythmia is ventricular tachycardia, which usually develops within 36 hours of admission to the hospital. Approximately 20% of cardiac arrhythmias are present on admission, 20% develop during surgery, and the remaining arrhythmias develop in the immediate postoperative period. The cause is multifactorial and includes myocardial ischemia, autonomic imbalance, alterations in electrolytes, acid-base derangement, gastric necrosis, and endotoxemia.[83, 110–114]

Other pathophysiologic changes may lead to DIC or release of cardiostimulatory and depressant substances (e.g., myocardial depressant factor).[95, 115, 116] There is a relation between gastric necrosis and DIC.[116] Recent experimental investigation has suggested that reperfusion injury is important in the pathophysiology of GDV.[117, 118]

Clinical Signs

Dogs with GDV acutely develop severe gastric and abdominal distention.[81, 82] Initially, the dogs are restless and uncomfortable and manifest abdominal pain. Acute vomiting quickly progresses to nonproductive retching and excessive salivation. As the stomach continues to distend, tachypnea progresses to dyspnea. Shock develops and is manifested by weakness, depression, tachycardia, weak peripheral pulses, pale mucous membranes, delayed capillary refill, and cold extremities. Severe splenomegaly develops, but the spleen often cannot be palpated because of the extreme tympanic abdominal distention.

Diagnostic Plan

In most cases, a diagnosis of GDV can easily be made based on signalment, history, physical examination, and clinical response to gastric decompression.[96] No other condition causes such acute and severe abdominal distention (see Acute Abdominal Distention).

Abdominal distention may not be obvious if a patient is examined early in the course of the disease, because the mildly distended stomach remains within the rib cage. For this reason, an abdominal radiograph should be made in large and giant breeds of dogs that have vague signs of acute pain and restlessness. In early cases of GDV, radiographs show a gas-distended stomach. The right lateral view is best to demonstrate gastric volvulus; a soft tissue fold (antral wall folding back) appears to compartmentalize the stomach, and the air-filled pylorus is located dorsal and cranial to the fundus.[81, 119]

As soon as practical, a lead II ECG should be taken, because ventricular arrhythmias may be present.[83]

Treatment

Prompt recognition of GDV and vigorous emergency management are the cornerstones of successful therapy.[97, 120] Intravenous volume expansion and gastric decompression need to be accomplished simultaneously.[121]

Before decompressive efforts, several large-bore intravenous catheters are placed and a large volume (90 mL/kg during the first hour) of isotonic fluids (e.g., lactated Ringer's solution) is infused.[81, 98, 120, 122, 123] Because shock is a dynamic condition, the animal should be monitored closely. The fluid administration rate should be decreased if clinical improvement occurs. Recent experimental evidence suggests that a small volume (5 mL/kg) of 7% sodium chloride in 6% dextran 70 is effective in treating the initial stages of shock in GDV.[124] Although controversial, corticosteroids (dexamethasone, 4 mg/kg, or prednisone sodium succinate, 20 mg/kg, intravenously) are usually administered because of their beneficial effects in endotoxemia and their potential effects in stabilizing lysosomal membranes and increasing cardiac output.[81] Bactericidal antibiotics (ampicillin, 5–10 mg/kg q.i.d.) should also be administered intravenously.

There are many ways to accomplish gastric decompression, and individual preference is based on experience. I prefer to pass a stiff foal orogastric tube into the stomach. The tube should be premeasured from the incisor teeth to the 13th rib to ensure that an excessive length of tube is not inserted.[96, 122] Resistance is met at the gastroesophageal junction. The tube should be advanced with firm pressure and a twisting motion. As the tube enters the stomach, a large amount of gas, and sometimes fluid, passes through the tube from the stomach. As the stomach decompresses, respiratory effort should decrease and cardiovascular status improve. The stomach should be lavaged with warm water to remove any particulate matter.[82, 122]

Elevation of the animal's forequarters may facilitate tube passage by reducing the weight of the abdominal viscera on the gastroesophageal junction.[121, 125] If the tube still cannot be successfully passed, percutaneous needle decompression should be attempted.[81, 82, 96, 120] The left and right paracostal regions should be "pinged," using a stethoscope to determine where the spleen is located. The side lacking the spleen is surgically prepared, and a 14-gauge, 15-cm catheter is passed through the body wall into the stomach. Often, an orogastric tube can be placed after some decompression has occurred.

If the animal becomes severely stressed during decompressive efforts, or if decompression cannot be achieved, mild sedation may be administered. Some clinicians prefer sedation before orogastric intubation.[82, 121] Oxymorphone, 0.05 to 0.1 mg/kg intravenously, often reduces stress and allows intubation.[120] Narcotics can cause respiratory distress, so they should be used with caution and narcotic antagonists should be available. One vial (0.4 mg) of naloxone is diluted with 9 mL saline and injected at a rate of 1 mL/min to effect. Finally, if decompression cannot be achieved, a temporary gastrostomy should be performed in the right paracostal region.[98, 126]

If ventricular tachycardia persists after gastric decompression and fluid therapy, it should be treated (see discussion of postoperative therapy).

The time necessary to stabilize a patient is variable.[120] If prolonged temporary decompression (up to 48 hours) is indicated, a pharyngostomy tube can be placed to maintain gastric decompression.[98, 127–129] Benefits of prolonged temporary decompression include the following: it allows a longer period for stabilization; surgery can be done at a convenient time; the dog can safely be transported to a referral center; and a full preoperative diagnostic evaluation can be performed.[121, 122] Disadvantages include failure to immediately inspect the stomach to detect necrosis or leakage of gastric contents, and postponement of surgery to a time at which cardiac arrhythmias may have developed.[121, 125] Blood flow is reduced, and reversible mucosal changes (edema and hemorrhage) can occur in a twisted but non-distended stomach.[101] The period of temporary decompression should be shortened if splenomegaly does not resolve or if evidence of hemorrhage is seen in gastric lavage fluid.

After the dog has stabilized, exploratory surgery is indicated to inspect and reposition the stomach and spleen, resect devitalized tissue, and perform a gastropexy to prevent recurrence.[96, 120, 121, 125] In most cases, splenectomy is not indicated.[81] If gastric wall devitalization is present or suspected, resection should be performed.[112]

Many surgical procedures have been developed to permanently attach the stomach to the body wall and prevent recurrence of GDV. These procedures include tube gastrostomy, circumcostal gastropexy, incisional gastropexy, belt loop gastropexy, and muscular flap gastropexy.[130–142] Although previously recommended, pyloric surgery has not been shown to alter the long-term complications of GDV and is not currently recommended unless pyloric obstruction can be demonstrated.[142, 143]

Postoperative care includes treatment for acute gastritis, monitoring for infection, routine wound care, and treatment of cardiac arrhythmias.[120] If vomiting is severe, an H$_2$-receptor antagonist (cimetidine, 5–10 mg/kg t.i.d. or q.i.d. intramuscularly, subcutaneously, or intravenously) may be administered.[122] Hypokalemia often develops and can promote cardiac arrhythmias and gastrointestinal atony.[109, 120, 122] Maintenance fluid therapy should include potassium supplementation (see Table 31–7).[144] Because gastric distention and hypoxia interfere with gastric motility, metoclopramide may benefit the dog with unresponsive vomiting.[145, 146]

Cardiac arrhythmias, especially ventricular tachycardia, are common in the postoperative period. These arrhythmias are often difficult to manage and may require intravenous lidocaine boluses, continuous lidocaine infusion, and a longer-acting agent, such as procainamide (see Chap. 10).[81, 96, 111, 120–122, 125, 144]

All dogs with a typical GDV episode should undergo exploratory surgery with gastropexy to prevent recurrence of GDV.[120, 121, 125] A common mistake is to radiograph the abdomen after the dog has been decompressed, find the stomach in normal position, diagnose simple gastric distention, and suggest that surgery is not necessary. These dogs are at risk for recurrence of GDV.[82, 85] Most patients do have volvulus on admission, and spontaneous repositioning of the stomach can occur after decompression.[147, 148]

Long-term management in postoperative patients and dogs susceptible to development of GDV should include frequent feeding to minimize gastric distention, reduction of postprandial exercise, and avoidance of short-term consumption of large volumes of water.[96]

Prognosis

The prognosis for GDV is guarded. Dogs that can be successfully stabilized have a greater chance of survival. Gastric leakage, infarction, necrosis, and peritonitis carry a poor prognosis.[81, 112, 130] Dogs surviving surgery have a brighter prognosis. Most postoperative deaths occur within the first 4 days after surgery.[149] Dogs surviving the postoperative period that have received an appropriate gastropexy have an excellent prognosis with little risk of recurrence of GDV.[130]

Chronic Hypertrophic Pyloric Gastropathy

Chronic hypertrophic pyloric gastropathy (CHPG) is associated with mucosal or muscularis hypertrophy that causes gastric outflow obstruction, delayed gastric emptying, chronic vomiting, and weight loss. It was originally described during the 1980s and is being recognized with increasing frequency. It occurs primarily in middle-aged, small breeds of dogs but has been seen in young large breeds. More males than females seem to be affected.[150–152]

Pathophysiology

The cause of the hypertrophy is unknown, although hypergastrinemia has been speculated.[153] Three histologic forms have been recognized: hypertrophy of the smooth muscle, hypertrophy of the smooth muscle and the mucosa, and, most commonly, hypertrophy of the mucosa, with or without inflammation.[151, 152] The hypertrophy results in a narrowing of the pyloric canal, gastric outflow obstruction, and chronic vomiting.

Clinical Signs

The most common clinical sign of CHPG is chronic vomiting.[150–152] The frequency of vomiting progresses as the obstruction worsens. A classic presentation of delayed gastric emptying may occur (e.g., vomiting of food many hours after eating, postprandial

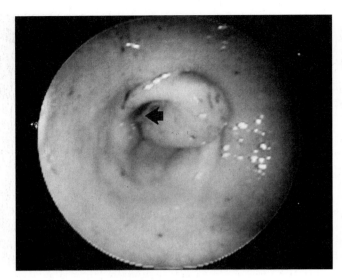

Figure 31–12
Endoscopic appearance of chronic hypertrophic pyloric gastropathy in an 11-year-old Lhasa apso. A large mucosal fold can be seen surrounding the entire pyloric orifice *(arrow)*. The black specs are adherent flecks of blood. The larger white areas are light reflections.

abdominal distention and discomfort, weight loss). Projectile vomiting can occasionally occur.[151] An enlarged stomach may be detected on abdominal palpation. Routine laboratory evaluation is often normal, although hypokalemia, hypochloremia, and metabolic alkalosis have been reported.[150, 151]

Diagnostic Plan

Survey radiographs may demonstrate a fluid- or food-distended stomach. Delayed gastric emptying, pyloric filling defects, or a narrow and blunted pyloric canal may be detected with a barium contrast series.[150–152, 154] Recently, ultrasonography has been used to help confirm diagnosis by identifying a thick hypoechoic layer of pyloric muscle and a thickened gastric wall.[33]

The diagnosis can be made on endoscopic examination of the stomach. The pyloric orifice is surrounded by a single, or several, enlarged mucosal folds (Fig. 31–12).[151, 155, 156] The duodenum usually can be entered and should be evaluated thoroughly to eliminate the presence of a mass that is distorting the pyloric area. Mucosal samples of the pylorus help eliminate the possibility of neoplasia.

The diagnosis can be confirmed during exploratory surgery, with the finding of a firm, thickened pylorus with thickened mucosal folds.[154, 157]

Treatment

Successful treatment requires surgical resection of the obstructive lesions. Mucosal resection,

pyloroplasty, and gastroduodenostomy have been used.[151, 152, 156, 157] In long-standing cases, extreme gastric distention can result in abnormal gastric motility, and vomiting may persist after surgery. Metoclopramide (0.2–0.4 mg/kg t.i.d. by mouth, subcutaneously, or intramuscularly) can be helpful in re-establishing gastric motility in these cases.

Prognosis

The prognosis for animals with CHPG is excellent.[150, 154, 155, 157] Most dogs respond to surgery rapidly and cease vomiting. The prognosis is more guarded in dogs with persistently abnormal motility. In these cases, intermittent vomiting can continue despite metoclopramide therapy.

Neoplasia

Gastric tumors are not as common as intestinal tumors.[158–160] The most common tumors that involve the stomach of dogs are adenomatous polyp, adenocarcinoma, and lymphosarcoma; adenocarcinoma occurs most commonly.[161] In cats, lymphosarcoma is most common, and the other tumor types are rare.[158] Most tumors occur in middle-aged or older dogs and cats.[162] Malignant tumors in dogs occur more commonly in males than in females.[43, 161, 163, 164]

Pathophysiology

Malignant tumors cause clinical signs by interfering with gastric motility, inducing inflammation, causing ulceration and hemorrhage, obstructing the pylorus, or metastasizing to other organs. The most common sites for metastasis of adenocarcinoma are the liver, lungs, regional lymph nodes, omentum, and mesentery.[163–169] Adenocarcinomas are sessile or polyploid masses that often ulcerate, occur as annular lesions, or diffusely invade the gastric wall.[166, 168, 170] They occur most commonly in the pyloric region or along the greater or lesser curvature.[43, 165, 170, 171] Ulceration is most often caused by interference in blood supply because of invasion of neoplastic cells within blood vessels or compression of blood vessels by adjacent neoplastic masses.[170]

Lymphosarcoma may occur as single or multiple intramural masses or as diffuse involvement of the mucosa. Dogs and cats with diffuse lymphosarcoma may develop diarrhea or small intestinal obstruction as a result of nodular or diffuse mucosal involvement of the small or large intestine.[167, 172] Dogs with gastric lymphosarcoma often have involvement of the liver.[173]

Adenomatous polyps often appear as single or multiple mucosal masses, usually 0.5 to 1 cm in diameter. They occur most commonly in the antral region.

Clinical Signs

The most common clinical signs associated with gastric neoplasia are chronic vomiting, anorexia, and weight loss.[43, 164–166, 170, 171] Hematemesis and melena can occur if ulceration is present. Abdominal pain sometimes occurs.[166] Vomiting may become profuse if the neoplastic mass becomes large enough to obstruct the pylorus. Occasionally, a cranial abdominal mass can be palpated. Other clinical signs (e.g., ascites, icterus, dyspnea) may reflect sites of metastasis.[171]

Adenomatous polyps are often discovered as incidental findings during endoscopy or necropsy.[162, 165] Polyps can produce clinical signs if they obstruct the pylorus.[166, 174] Lymphosarcoma often affects multiple areas of the GI tract, and small or large bowel diarrhea may accompany vomiting. Mesenteric lymphadenopathy, thickened bowel walls, or neoplastic intestinal masses can be palpated in many patients with lymphosarcoma.

Diagnostic Plan

Routine laboratory evaluation may demonstrate anemia, leukocytosis, and hypoproteinemia. The anemia may be regenerative, resulting from blood loss, or nonregenerative, resulting from chronic inflammatory disease. Most cats with gastric lymphosarcoma test negative for feline leukemia virus at the time of diagnosis.[172]

Survey abdominal radiographs are often normal, but a thickened gastric wall or cranial abdominial mass may be visualized. Barium contrast studies may show an ulcer, roughened irregular mucosal surfaces, intramural mass, luminal filling defect, thickened gastric wall, derangement of rugal folds, and delayed gastric emptying.[43, 166, 167, 170, 171, 173] In many cases, radiographic findings do not support the presence of neoplasia or may only be consistent with it.[43, 166, 171]

Thoracic radiographs should be taken in a patient in which gastric neoplasia is suspected, because 30% of dogs with gastric adenocarcinoma have visible pulmonary metastases at the time of diagnosis.[167]

The definitive diagnosis of gastric neoplasia requires examination of biopsy samples, obtained by endoscopy or exploratory surgery. Endoscopically, a single, large, oblong ulceration is commonly seen in adenocarcinoma cases.[43] Thickened rugal folds that do not disappear during insufflation of air may be visualized extending up to the raised rim of the ulcer crater (Fig. 31–13). In other cases, the rugal fold pattern is completely absent. In cases with diffuse involvement, the mucosa appears abnormal, with increased friability, granularity, and erosions.[171] Multiple nodular masses are often found throughout the stomach in cats with lymphosarcoma (Fig. 31–14). In cases of diffuse lymphosarcoma, the mucosa appears thickened and granular, and biopsy samples that are larger than

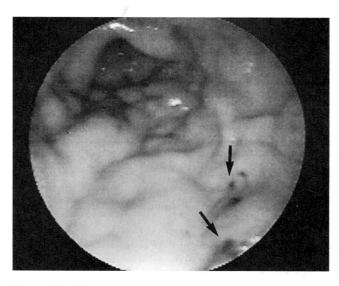

Figure 31–13
Endoscopic appearance of thickened rugal folds in the gastric body of an 11-year-old chow chow with adenocarcinoma. The folds persisted despite maximal insufflation of air into the stomach. The dark spots (arrows) are bleeding erosions. The larger white areas are light reflections.

usual can be readily obtained. Diagnosis in some cases may be reached by percutaneous fine-needle aspiration of an intestinal mass, enlarged mesenteric lymph node, or infiltrated liver in cases of diffuse lymphosarcoma.

Treatment

Adenomatous polyps that obstruct the pylorus can be removed by submucosal resection.[174] The most

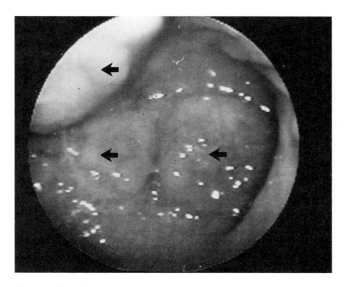

Figure 31–14
Endoscopic appearance of three masses (arrows) at the junction of the gastric body and antrum in a 10-year-old domestic shorthair cat with lymphosarcoma. The white areas are light reflections.

effective treatment for adenocarcinoma is surgical resection.[175] Because many adenocarcinomas in dogs occur in the pyloric region, gastroduodenostomy may be necessary. During surgery, thorough exploration of the abdomen should always be performed to search for metastases. Biopsy samples should be collected from regional lymph nodes and the liver. Solitary lymphosarcoma is best treated with surgical resection followed by multiagent chemotherapy. Diffuse lymphosarcoma should be treated with multiagent chemotherapy (see Chap. 43).[167, 172] In other instances, surgery in lymphosarcoma patients should be reserved for those with pyloric obstruction, intestinal obstruction, and moderate or severe hemorrhage caused by gastric ulceration.

Prognosis

The prognosis for patients with adenomatous polyps that obstruct the pylorus is excellent after surgical resection. The prognosis for adenocarcinoma is guarded to poor. Small lesions that are detected early, have not metastasized, and can be surgically excised warrant a better prognosis.[171, 175] However, most cases of adenocarcinoma are advanced at the time of diagnosis.[43, 163, 170, 171] In most cases, surgical resection is not possible; in others, it may relieve clinical signs for only a short period. Solitary lymphosarcoma carries a better prognosis if treated with surgery and multiagent chemotherapy, compared with either treatment alone or with other types of GI lymphosarcoma. Diffuse lymphosarcoma warrants a poor prognosis.[167]

Uncommon Diseases of the Stomach

Bilious Vomiting Syndrome

Bilious vomiting syndrome is a poorly defined condition of dogs that may be more common than the literature suggests. Vomiting of bile or bile-stained mucus often occurs in the early morning or many hours after eating. It has been postulated to be caused by abnormal pyloric function. Diagnosis is based on the history and response to treatment. Feeding of a small meal or administration of metoclopramide (0.2–0.4 mg/kg) before bedtime often prevents vomiting.

Abnormal Gastric Motility

Abnormalities in gastric myoelectric activity and motility can cause chronic vomiting and delayed gastric emptying.[176] The diagnosis is made in a patient with delayed gastric emptying by exclusion of the mechanical obstructive causes (see Fig. 31–3). There are many possible underlying causes of abnormal gastric motility (see Table 31–3). Idiopathic causes are probably more common than was previously thought.

Treatment should be directed at a primary cause, if one is found. Idiopathic cases can be treated with metoclopramide, 0.2 to 0.4 mg/kg by mouth t.i.d.

Leiomyoma

Benign tumors of gastric smooth muscle, leiomyomas, occur in older and very old dogs.[162] The tumors, which can be as large as 5 cm, often originate in the area of the gastroesophageal junction. They do not usually cause clinical signs but rarely can cause vomiting or result in megaesophagus. In patients with clinical signs, diagnosis can be made by following the diagnostic plans for vomiting or regurgitation. Surgical resection should be curative.

Parasites

Several parasites can uncommonly infect the stomachs of dogs and cats and may cause clinical signs. *Ollulanus tricuspis* is a small nematode (adults 1 mm long) found in cat stomachs.[177] Although it may not cause clinical signs in all cats, occasionally it has been associated with gastritis, fibrosis, and lymphoid aggregates.[178] The parasite is transmitted by larvae passed in the vomitus. Diagnosis is based on histologic examination of gastric mucosa or microscopic examination of vomitus. No successful treatment has been described.

Physaloptera spp. are stout nematodes (1–5 cm long) that infect the stomach and duodenum of both dogs and cats. Adults attach to the mucosa and cause localized gastritis. The parasites can be incidental findings during endoscopy or can cause chronic vomiting. The intermediate hosts are beetles, crickets, and cockroaches. The spiruroid eggs are not often observed in the feces when examined by routine flotation techniques. Treatment with fenbendazole, 50 mg/kg s.i.d. for 3 days, or pyrantel pamoate, 5 mg/kg once, is effective.

Aonchotheca (Capillaria) putorii are thin nematodes (2.5–7.5 mm long) that have been identified in the stomachs and small intestines of cats.[179] Their pathogenicity has not been firmly established. It is clinically important to distinguish their eggs in the feces from those of the capillarids that occur in the respiratory and urinary tracts.

Eosinophilic Granulomatous Gastritis

Eosinophilic granulomatous gastritis is an uncommon condition seen in dogs. Lesions with eosinophils, fibrosis, and granulation tissue occur throughout the wall of the stomach.[180] Areas of the stomach become very thick and appear similar to neoplasia. The small and large intestines can also be involved. The cause is unknown, and successful treatment has not been reported. If it is diagnosed early, surgical removal of small lesions could theoretically be curative.

Hypertrophic Gastropathy

A syndrome in dogs and cats characterized by epithelial cell hyperplasia and mucosal inflammation results in marked enlargement of rugal folds and chronic vomiting.[181] Anemia and hypoalbuminemia are common. The syndrome has been described in basenji dogs and may be part of their immunoproliferative bowel disease.[182] The relation of this hypertrophic gastropathy syndrome to CHPG is unknown. Diagnosis is based on radiographic, endoscopic, and histologic findings. If the lesion is small when it is diagnosed, surgical resection may be curative.

Pyloric Muscular Hypertrophy

Hypertrophy of the pyloric musculature leads to delayed gastric emptying and vomiting. Congenital and acquired forms have been described.[183] In adult dogs, concurrent mucosal involvement occurs in CHPG. However, isolated muscular hypertrophy does occur in some cases.[152] Diagnosis requires demonstration of delayed gastric emptying in a barium contrast series, followed by exploratory surgery and biopsy. Pyloroplasty is curative in most cases. The relation of this syndrome to CHPG is unknown.

Gastrinoma

Production of the hormone gastrin by a pancreatic tumor causes gastric hypersecretion of acid, leading to gastric and duodenal ulceration, chronic vomiting, and diarrhea.[184–186] This rare syndrome has been diagnosed in both dogs and cats. Diagnosis is suspected in patients with recurrent GI ulcers that do not respond to conventional therapy. Ultrasonographic examination may identify masses in the pancreas. Elevated gastrin levels in serum should be found. Treatment requires resection of the pancreatic tumor. Because of frequent metastasis, prognosis is poor.

Phycomycosis

Infection with the ubiquitous fungus *Pythium* results in pyogranulomatous inflammation in the stomach, small intestine, or colon of young, male, large-breed dogs.[187–189] The most common clinical signs are vomiting, diarrhea, and weight loss; in some cases, an abdominal mass can be palpated. Diagnosis is based on finding the organisms in biopsy samples. Most cases are very advanced at the time of diagnosis, so surgical therapy is often not possible. Medical therapy has not been successful.

Chronic Gastric Volvulus

Partial gastric volvulus, without massive dilation, can cause chronic vomiting, weight loss, postprandial abdominal distention, and discomfort.[190, 191] The volvulus may be intermittent. Diagnosis is based on barium contrast radiographs. Gastropexy is curative. The relation to typical GDV is unclear, but dogs with chronic volvulus are at risk to develop GDV.

References

1. Strombeck DR, Guilford WG. Small Animal Gastroenterology. Davis, California, Stonegate Publishing, 1990: 167–186.
2. Kleine LJ. Radiology of the stomach in the dog and cat. Compen Contin Educ Pract Vet 1979;1:936–945.
3. Moon M, Myer W. Gastrointestinal contrast radiology in small animals. Semin Vet Med Surg 1986;1:121–143.
4. Herdt T. Secretions of the gastrointestinal tract. In: Cunningham JG, ed. Textbook of veterinary physiology. Philadelphia, WB Saunders, 1992:275–285.
5. Schubert ML, Shamburek RD. Control of acid secretion. Gastroenterol Clin North Am 1990;19:1–25.
6. Hall JA, Burrows CF, Twedt DC. Gastric motility in dogs: Part I. Normal gastric function. Compen Contin Educ Pract Vet 1988;10:1281–1291.
7. Kelly KA. Gastric emptying of liquids and solids: Roles of proximal and distal stomach. Am J Physiol 1980;239: G71–G76.
8. Minami H, McCallum RW. The physiology and pathophysiology of gastric emptying in humans. Gastroenterology 1984;86:1592–1610.
9. Schubert ML, Makhlouf GM. Neural, hormonal, and paracrine regulation of gastrin and acid secretion. Yale J Biol Med 1992;65:553–560.
10. Leib MS. Acute vomiting: A diagnostic approach and symptomatic management. In: Kirk RW, Bonagura JD, eds. Kirk's Current Veterinary Therapy XI. Philadelphia, WB Saunders, 1992:583–587.
11. Thayer GW. Vomiting: A clinical approach. Compen Contin Educ Pract Vet 1981;3:49–52.
12. Davis LE. Pharmacologic control of vomiting. J Am Vet Med Assoc 1980;176:241–242.
13. Kirby R, Jones BD. Gastrointestinal emergencies: Acute vomiting. Semin Vet Med Surg (Small Anim) 1988;3: 256–264.
14. Forrester SD, Boothe DM, Willard MD. Clinical pharmacology of antiemetic and antiulcer drugs. Semin Vet Med Surg (Small Anim) 1989;4:194–201.
15. Twedt DC. Differential diagnosis and therapy of vomiting. Vet Clin North Am Small Anim Pract 1983;13: 503–520.
16. Willard MD. Some newer approaches to the treatment of vomiting. J Am Vet Med Assoc 1984;184:590–592.
17. Ogilvie GK, Obradovich JE, Elmslie RE, et al. Toxicosis associated with administration of mitoxantrone to dogs with malignant tumors. J Am Vet Med Assoc 1991;198: 1613–1617.

18. Ogilvie GK, Moore AS, Curtis CR. Evaluation of cisplatin-induced emesis in dogs with malignant neoplasia: 115 cases (1984–1987). J Am Vet Med Assoc 1989;195:1399–1403.
19. Ogilvie GK, Richardson RC, Curtis CR, et al. Acute and short-term toxicoses associated with the administration of doxorubicin to dogs with malignant tumors. J Am Vet Med Assoc 1989;195:1584–1587.
20. Twedt DC, Grauer GF. Fluid therapy for gastrointestinal, pancreatic, and hepatic disorders. Vet Clin North Am Small Anim Pract 1982;12:463–485.
21. Moore FM. The laboratory and pathologic assessment of vomiting animals. Vet Med (Prague) 1992;87:796–805.
22. Tams TR. A diagnostic approach to vomiting in dogs and cats. Vet Med (Prague) 1992;87:785–793.
23. Felts JF, Fox PR, Burk RL. Thread and sewing needles as gastrointestinal foreign bodies in the cat: A review of 64 cases. J Am Vet Med Assoc 1984;184:56–59.
24. Leib MS. Chronic vomiting: A diagnostic approach. In: August JR, ed. Consultations in Feline Internal Medicine. Philadelphia, WB Saunders, 1991:403–407.
25. Pearson H, Gaskell CJ, Gibbs C, et al. Pyloric and oesophageal dysfunction in the cat. J Small Anim Pract 1974;15:487–501.
26. Tams TR. Chronic feline inflammatory bowel disorders: Part II. Feline eosinophilic enteritis and lymphosarcoma. Compen Contin Educ Pract Vet 1986;8:464–471.
27. Tams TR. Chronic feline inflammatory bowel disorders: Part I. Idiopathic inflammatory bowel disease. Compen Contin Educ Pract Vet 1986;8:371–378.
28. Leib MS. Stagnant loop syndrome in the dog and cat. Semin Vet Med Surg (Small Anim) 1987;2:257–265.
29. Peterson ME, Kintzer PP, Cavanagh PG, et al. Feline hyperthyroidism: Pretreatment clinical and laboratory evaluation of 131 cases. J Am Vet Med Assoc 1983;183:103–110.
30. Dillon R. Feline dirofilariasis. Vet Clin North Am Small Anim Pract 1984;14:1185–1199.
31. Bonneau NH, Reed JH, Pennock PW, et al. Comparison of gastrophotography and contrast radiography for diagnosis of aspirin-induced gastritis in the dog. J Am Vet Med Assoc 161:1972;190–198.
32. Penninck D, Nyland T, LY K, et al. Ultrasonographic evaluation of gastrointestinal diseases in small animals. Vet Radiol 1990;31:134–141.
33. Biller DS, Partington BP, Miyabayashi T, et al. Ultrasonographic appearance of chronic hypertrophic pyloric gastropathy in the dog. Vet Radiol Ultrasound 1994;35:30–33.
34. Brown NO, Patnaik AK, MacEwen EG. Canine hemangiosarcoma: Retrospective analysis of 104 cases. J Am Vet Med Assoc 1985;186:56–58.
35. Donaldson LL, Leib MS, Boyd C, et al. The effect of preanesthetic medication on ease of endoscopic intubation to the duodenum of dogs anesthetized with halothane and oxygen. Am J Vet Res 1993;54:1489–1495.
36. Leib MS. Endoscopic examination of the dog and cat. In: Jensen SL, Gregersen H, Moody FG, et al., eds. Essentials of Experimental Surgery: Gastroenterology. Amsterdam, Harwood Academic Publishers, 1996:10/1–10/17.
37. Sullivan M, Miller A. Endoscopy (fibreoptic) of the oesophagus and stomach in the dog with persistent regurgitation or vomiting. J Small Anim Pract 1985;26:369–379.
38. Guilford WG. Upper gastrointestinal endoscopy. Vet Clin North Am Small Anim Pract 1990;20:1209–1227.
39. Guilford W, Jones BD. Gastrointestinal endoscopy of the dog and cat. Vet Med Rep 1990;2:140–150.
40. Tams TR. Gastroscopy. In: Tams TR ed. Small Animal Endoscopy. St Louis, CV Mosby, 1990:89–166.
41. Leib MS. Gastrointestinal endoscopy. In: August JR ed. Consultations in Feline Internal Medicine. Philadelphia, WB Saunders, 1994:119–126.
42. Kantrowitz B, Biller D. Using radiography to evaluate vomiting in dogs and cats. Vet Med (Prague) 1992;87:806–813.
43. Sullivan M, Lee R, Fisher EW, et al. A study of 31 cases of gastric carcinoma in dogs. Vet Rec 1987;120:79–83.
44. Penninck DG, Nyland TG, Fisher PE, et al. Ultrasonography of the normal canine gastrointestinal tract. Vet Radiol 1989;30:272–276.
45. van der Gaag I. The histological appearance of peroral gastric biopsies in clinically healthy and vomiting dogs. Can J Vet Res 1988;52:67–74.
46. DeNovo RC. Medical management of gastritis, ulcers, and erosions. Waltham/OSU Symposium. Columbus, Ohio, 1993:17;108–116.
47. Shorrock CJ, Rees WDW. Overview of gastroduodenal mucosal protection. Am J Med 1988;84:25–34.
48. Twedt DC, Magne ML. Chronic gastritis. In: Kirk RW ed. Current Veterinary Therapy IX. Philadelphia, WB Saunders, 1986:852–856.
49. O'Keefe DA, Couto CG, Burke-Schwartz C, et al. Systemic mastocytosis in 16 dogs. J Vet Intern Med 1987;1:75–80.
50. Howard EB, Sawa TR, Nielsen SW, et al. Mastocytoma and gastroduodenal ulceration: Gastric and duodenal ulcers in dogs with mastocytoma. Vet Pathol 1969;6:146–158.
51. Fox LE, Rosenthal RC, Twedt DC, et al. Plasma histamine and gastrin concentrations in 17 dogs with mast cell tumors. J Vet Intern Med 1990;4:242–246.
52. Dow SW, Rosuchuk RAW, McChesney AE, et al. Effects of flunixin and flunixin plus prednisone on the gastrointestinal tract of dogs. Am J Vet Res 1990;51:1131–1138.
53. Vonderhaar MA, Salisbury SK. Gastroduodenal ulceration associated with flunixin meglumine administration in three dogs. J Am Vet Med Assoc 1993;203:92–95.
54. Wallace MS, Zawie DA, Garvey MS. Gastric ulceration in the dog secondary to the use of nonsteroidal antiinflammatory drugs. J Am Anim Hosp Assoc 1990;26:467–472.
55. Stanton ME, Bright RM. Gastroduodenal ulceration in dogs: Retrospective study of 43 cases and literature review. J Vet Intern Med 1989;3:238–244.
56. Lipowitz AJ, Boulay JP, Klausner JS. Serum salicylate concentrations and endoscopic evaluation of the gastric mucosa in dogs after oral administration of aspirin-containing products. Am J Vet Res 1986;47:1586–1589.

57. Moreland KJ. Ulcer disease of the upper gastrointestinal tract in small animals: Pathophysiology, diagnosis, and management. Compen Contin Educ Pract Vet 1988;10:1265–1280.

58. Moore RW, Withrow SJ. Gastrointestinal hemorrhage and pancreatitis associated with intervertebral disk disease in the dog. J Am Vet Med Assoc 1982;180:1443–1447.

59. Sorjonen DC, Dillon AR, Powers RD, et al. Effects of dexamethasone and surgical hypotension on the stomach of dogs: Clinical, endoscopic, and pathologic evaluation. Am J Vet Res 1983;144:1233–1237.

60. Cheville NF. Uremic gastropathy in the dog. Vet Pathol 1979;16:292–309.

61. Twedt DC. Cirrhosis: A consequence of chronic liver disease. Vet Clin North Am Small Anim Pract 1985;15:151–176.

62. Happe RP, van den Brom WE, van der Gaag I. Duodenogastric reflux in the dog: A clinicopathological study. Res Vet Sci 1982;33:280–286.

63. Tytgat GNJ, Noach L, Rauws EAJ. *Helicobacter pylori.* Scand J Gastroenterol 1991;26:1–8.

64. Lee A, Krakowka S, Fox JG, et al. Role of *Helicobacter felis* in chronic canine gastritis. Vet Pathol 1992;29:487–494.

65. Shell LG. Canine distemper. Compen Contin Educ Pract Vet 1990;12:173–179.

66. Van der Gaag I, Happe RP. Follow-up studies by peroral gastric biopsies and necropsy in vomiting dogs. Can J Vet Res 1989;53:468–472.

67. Richter KP. Treating acute vomiting in dogs and cats. Vet Med (Prague) 1992;87:814–818.

68. Johnson SE. Clinical pharmacology of antiemetics and antidiarrheals. In: Eighth Annual Kal Kan Symposium on the Treatment of Small Anim Diseases, Columbus, Ohio, 1984.

69. Burrows CF. Metoclopramide. J Am Vet Med Assoc 1983;183:1341–1343.

70. Murray M, Robinson PB, McKeating FJ, et al. Peptic ulceration in the dog: A clinico-pathological study. Vet Rec 1972;91:441–447.

71. Toombs JP, Caywood DD, Lipowitz AJ, et al. Colonic perforation following neurosurgical procedures and corticosteroid therapy in four dogs. J Am Vet Med Assoc 1980;177:68–72.

72. Toombs JP, Collins LG, Graves GM, et al. Colonic perforation in corticosteroid-treated dogs. J Am Vet Med Assoc 1986;188:145–150.

73. Richter KP. Therapy for vomiting patients with gastrointestinal ulcers. Vet Med (Prague) 1992;87:819–824.

74. Papich MG. Antiulcer therapy. Vet Clin North Am Small Anim Pract 1993;23:497–512.

75. Johnston SA, Leib MS, Forrester SD, et al. The effect of misoprostol on aspirin induced gastroduodenal lesions in dogs. J Vet Intern Med 1995;9:32–38.

76. Murtaugh RJ, Matz ME, Labato MA, et al. Use of synthetic prostaglandin E1 (misoprostol) administration for prevention of aspirin induced gastroduodenal ulceration in arthritic dogs. J Am Vet Med Assoc 1993;202:251–256.

77. Jenkins CC, DeNovo RC. Omeprazole: A potent antiulcer drug. Compen Contin Educ Pract Vet 1991;13:1578–1582.

78. Jenkins CC, DeNovo RC, Patton CS, et al. Comparison of effects of cimetidine and omeprazole on mechanically created gastric ulceration and on aspirin-induced gastritis in dogs. Am J Vet Res 1991;52:658–661.

79. Antonin J, Guitart P, Rodón J. Fibroendoscopy of the gastro-intestinal tract: Oesophagogastric foreign bodies. Vet Int 1991;2:29–39.

80. Twedt DC. Disorders of gastric retention. In: Eighth Annual Kal Kan Symposium on the Treatment of Small Animal Diseases, Columbus, Ohio, 1984.

81. Matthiesen DT. The gastric dilatation-volvulus complex: Medical and surgical considerations. J Am Vet Med Assoc 1983;19:925–932.

82. Dann JR. Medical and surgical treatment of canine acute gastric dilatation. J Am Anim Hosp Assoc 1976;12:17–22.

83. Muir WW. Gastric dilatation-volvulus in the dog, with emphasis on cardiac arrhythmias. J Am Vet Med Assoc 1982;180:739–742.

84. Pass MA, Johnston DE. Treatment of gastric dilation and torsion in the dog. Gastric decompression by gastrostomy under local analgesia. J Small Anim Pract 1973;14:131–142.

85. Betts CW, Wingfield WE, Greene RW. A retrospective study of gastric dilatation-torsion in the dog. J Small Anim Pract 1974;15:727–734.

86. Burrows CF, Ignaszewski LA. Canine gastric dilatation-volvulus. J Small Anim Pract 1990;31:495–501.

87. Leib MS, Wingfield WE, Twedt DC, et al. Plasma gastrin immunoreactivity in dogs with acute gastric dilatation-volvulus. J Am Vet Med Assoc 1984;185:205–208.

88. Rogolsky B, Van Kruiningen HJ. Short-chain fatty acids and bacterial fermentation in the normal canine stomach and in acute gastric dilatation. J Am Anim Hosp Assoc 1978;14:504–515.

89. Warner NS, Van Kruiningen HJ. The incidence of *Clostridia* in the canine stomach and their relationship to acute gastric dilatation. J Am Anim Hosp Assoc 1978;14:618–623.

90. Caywood D, Teague HD, Jackson DA, et al. Gastric gas analysis in the canine gastric dilatation-volvulus syndrome. J Am Anim Hosp Assoc 1977;13:459–462.

91. Van Kruiningen HJ, Gregoire K, Meuten DJ. Acute gastric dilatation: A review of comparative aspects, by species, and a study in dogs and monkeys. J Am Anim Hosp Assoc 1974;10:294–324.

92. Funkquist B, Garmer L. Pathogenetic and therapeutic aspects of torsion of the canine stomach. J Small Anim Pract 1967;8:523–532.

93. Hall JA, Willer RL, Seim HB, et al. Gastric emptying of nondigestible radiopaque markers after circumcostal gastropexy in clinically normal dogs and dogs with gastric dilatation-volvulus. Am J Vet Res 1993;53:1961–1965.

94. Hall JA, Solie TN, Seim HB, et al. Gastric myoelectric and motor activity in dogs with gastric dilatation-volvulus. Am J Physiol 1993;265:G646–653.

95. Wingfield WE, Betts CW, Rawlings CA. Pathophysiology associated with gastric dilatation-volvulus in the dog. J Am Anim Hosp Assoc 1976;12:136–141.

96. Morgan RV. Acute gastric dilatation-volvulus syndrome. Compen Contin Educ Pract Vet 1982;4:677–682.

97. DeHoff WD, Greene RW. Gastric dilatation and the gastric torsion complex. Vet Clin North Am Small Anim Pract 1972;2:141–153.

98. Todoroff RJ. Gastric dilatation-volvulus. Compen Contin Educ Pract Vet 1979;1:142–148.

99. Hall JA. Canine gastric dilatation-volvulus update. Semin Vet Med Surg (Small Anim) 1989;4:188–193.

100. Stampley AR, Burrows CF, Ellison GW, et al. Gastric myoelectric activity after experimental gastric dilatation-volvulus and tube gastrostomy in dogs. Vet Surg 1992;21:10–14.

101. Lantz GC, Bottoms GD, Carlton WW, et al. The effect of 360 degree gastric volvulus on the blood supply of the nondistended normal dog stomach. Vet Surg 1984;13:189–196.

102. Wingfield WE, Cornelius LM, Ackerman N, et al. Experimental acute gastric dilatation and torsion in the dog: 2. Venous angiographic alterations seen in gastric dilation. J Small Anim Pract 1974;15:55–60.

103. Merkley DF, Howard DR, Eyster GE, et al. Experimentally induced acute gastric dilatation in the dog: Cardiopulmonary effects. J Am Anim Hosp Assoc 1976;12:143–148.

104. Orton EC, Muir WW. Hemodynamics during experimental gastric dilatation-volvulus in dogs. Am J Vet Res 1983;44:1512–1515.

105. Wingfield WE, Cornelius LM, DeYoung DW. Pathophysiology of the gastric dilatation-torsion complex in the dog. J Small Anim Pract 1974;15:735–739.

106. Davidson JR, Lantz GC, Salisbury SK, et al. Effects of flunixin meglumine on dogs with experimental gastric dilatation-volvulus. Vet Surg 1992;21:113–120.

107. Wingfield WE, Cornelius LM, DeYoung DW. Experimental acute gastric dilatation and torsion in the dog: 1. Changes in biochemical and acid-base parameters. J Small Anim Pract 1974;15:41–53.

108. Wingfield WE, Twedt DC, Moore RW, et al. Acid-base and electrolyte values in dogs with acute gastric dilatation-volvulus. J Am Vet Med Assoc 1982;180:1070–1072.

109. Muir WW. Acid-base and electrolyte disturbances in dogs with gastric dilatation-volvulus. J Am Vet Med Assoc 1982;180:229–231.

110. Muir WW, Lipowitz AJ. Cardiac dysrhythmias associated with gastric dilatation-volvulus in the dog. J Am Vet Med Assoc 1978;172:683–689.

111. Muir WW, Bonagura JD. Treatment of cardiac arrhythmias in dogs with gastric distention-volvulus. J Am Vet Med Assoc 1984;184:1366–1371.

112. Matthiesen DT. Partial gastrectomy as treatment of gastric volvulus: Results in 30 dogs. Vet Surg 1985;14:185–193.

113. Muir WW, Weisbrode SE. Myocardial ischemia in dogs with gastric dilatation-volvulus. J Am Vet Med Assoc 1982;181:363–366.

114. Horne WA, Gilmore DR, Dietze AE, et al. Effects of gastric distention-volvulus on coronary blood flow and myocardial oxygen consumption in the dog. Am J Vet Res 1985;46:98–104.

115. Orton EC, Muir WW. Isovolumetric indices and humoral cardioactive substance bioassay during clinical and experimentally induced gastric dilatation-volvulus in dogs. Am J Vet Res 1983;44:1516–1520.

116. Millis DL, Hauptman JG, Fulton RB. Abnormal hemostatic profiles and gastric necrosis in canine gastric dilatation-volvulus. Vet Surg 1993;22:93–97.

117. Lantz GC, Badylak SF, Hiles MC, et al. Treatment of reperfusion injury in dogs with experimentally induced gastric dilatation-volvulus. Am J Vet Res 1992;53:1594–1598.

118. Badylak SF, Lantz GC, Jeffries M. Prevention of reperfusion injury in surgically induced gastric dilatation-volvulus in dogs. Am J Vet Res 1990;51:294–299.

119. Hathcock JT. Radiographic view of choice for the diagnosis of gastric volvulus: The right lateral recumbent view. J Am Anim Hosp Assoc 1984;20:967–969.

120. Whitney WO. Complications associated with the medical and surgical management of gastric dilatation-volvulus in the dog. Probl Vet Med 1989;1:268–280.

121. Leib MS, Martin RA. Therapy of gastric dilatation-volvulus in dogs. Compen Contin Educ Pract Vet 1987;9:1155–1165.

122. Wingfield WE. Acute gastric dilatation-volvulus. Vet Clin North Am Small Anim Pract 1981;11:147–155.

123. Rawlings CA, Wingfield WE, Betts CW. Shock therapy and anesthetic management in gastric dilatation-volvulus. J Am Anim Hosp Assoc 1976;12:158–161.

124. Allen DA, Schertel ER, Muir WW, et al. Hypertonic saline/dextran resuscitation of dogs with experimentally induced gastric dilatation-volvulus shock. Am J Vet Res 1991;52:92–96.

125. Davidson JR. Acute gastric dilatation-volvulus in dogs: Surgical treatments. Vet Med 1992;87:118–126.

126. Walshaw R, Johnston DE. Treatment of gastric dilatation-volvulus by gastric decompression and patient stabilization before major surgery. J Am Anim Hosp Assoc 1976;12:162–167.

127. Leib MS, Blass CE. Acute gastric dilatation in the dog: Various clinical presentations. Compen Contin Educ Pract Vet 1984;6:707–716.

128. Crowe DT, Downs MO. Pharyngostomy complications in dogs and cats and recommended technical modifications: Experimental and clinical investigation. J Am Anim Hosp Assoc 1986;22:493–503.

129. Lantz GC. Pharyngostomy tube installation for the administration of nutritional and fluid requirements. Compen Contin Educ Pract Vet 1981;3:135–142.

130. Leib MS, Konde LJ, Wingfield WE, et al. Circumcostal gastropexy for preventing recurrence of gastric dilatation-volvulus in the dog: An evaluation of 30 cases. J Am Vet Med Assoc 1985;187:245–248.

131. Parks JL, Greene RW. Tube gastrostomy for the treatment of gastric volvulus. J Am Anim Hosp Assoc 1976;12:168–172.

132. Fox SM. Results from 31 surgical cases circumcostal gastropexy vs. tube gastrostomy. Calif Vet 1985;39:8–11.

133. Fallah AM, Lumb WV, Nelson AW, et al. Circumcostal gastropexy in the dog: A preliminary study. Vet Surg 1982;11:9–12.

134. Fox SM, McCoy CP, Cooper RC, et al. Circumcostal

gastropexy versus tube gastrostomy: Histological comparison of gastropexy adhesions. J Am Anim Hosp Assoc 1988;24:273–279.

135. Fox SM, Ellison GW, Miller GJ, et al. Observations on the mechanical failure of three gastropexy techniques. J Am Anim Hosp Assoc 1985;21:729–734.

136. Schulman AJ, Lusk R, Lippincott CL, et al. Muscular flap gastropexy: A new surgical technique to prevent recurrences of gastric dilatation-volvulus syndrome. J Am Anim Hosp Assoc 1986;22:339–346.

137. Whitney WO, Scaveli TD, Matthiesen DT, et al. Belt-loop gastropexy: Technique and surgical results in 20 dogs. J Am Anim Hosp Assoc 1989;25:75–83.

138. Woolfson JM, Kostolich M. Circumcostal gastropexy: Clinical use of the technique in 34 dogs with gastric dilatation-volvulus. J Am Anim Hosp Assoc 1986;22:825–830.

139. Johnson RG, Barrus J, Greene RW. Gastric dilatation-volvulus: Recurrence rate following tube gastrostomy. J Am Anim Hosp Assoc 1984;20:33–37.

140. MacCoy DM, Sykes GP, Hoffer RE, et al. A gastropexy technique for permanent fixation of the pyloric antrum. J Am Anim Hosp Assoc 1982;18:763–768.

141. Flanders JA, Harvey HJ. Results of tube gastrostomy as treatment for gastric volvulus in the dog. J Am Vet Med Assoc 1984;185:74–77.

142. Ellison GW. Gastric dilatation volvulus: Surgical prevention. Vet Clin North Am Small Anim Pract 1993;23:513–530.

143. Greenfield CL, Walshaw R, Thomas MW. Significance of the Heineke-Mikulicz pyloroplasty in the treatment of gastric dilatation-volvulus: A prospective clinical study. Vet Surg 1989;18:22–26.

144. Leib MS, Blass CE. Gastric dilatation-volvulus in dogs: An update. Compen Contin Educ Pract Vet 1984;6:961–969.

145. Graves GM, Becht JL, Rawlings CA. Metoclopramide reversal of decreased gastrointestinal myoelectric and contractile activity in a model of canine postoperative ileus. Vet Surg 1989;18:27–33.

146. Stampley AR, Burrows CF, Ellison GW. The use of retrievable electrodes for recording gastric myoelectric activity after spontaneous gastric dilatation volvulus in dogs. Cornell Vet 1992;82:423–434.

147. Funkquist B. Gastric torsion in the dog: I. Radiological picture during nonsurgical treatment related to the pathological anatomy and to the further clinical course. J Small Anim Pract 1979;20:73–91.

148. Funkquist B. Gastric torsion in the dog: Non-surgical reposition. J Small Anim Pract 1969;10:507–511.

149. Wingfield WE, Betts CW, Greene RW. Operative techniques and recurrence rate associated with gastric volvulus in the dog. J Small Anim Pract 1975;16:427–432.

150. Bellenger CR, Maddison JE, MacPherson GC, et al. Chronic hypertrophic pyloric gastropathy in 14 dogs. Aust Vet J 1990;67:317–320.

151. Matthiesen DT, Walter MC. Surgical treatment of chronic hypertrophic pyloric gastropathy in 45 dogs. J Am Anim Hosp Assoc 1986;22:241–247.

152. Sikes RI, Birchard S, Patnaik A, et al. Chronic hypertrophic pyloric gastropathy: A review of 16 cases. J Am Anim Hosp Assoc 1986;22:99–104.

153. DeNovo RC. Antral pyloric hypertrophy syndrome. In: Kirk RW ed. Current Veterinary Therapy X. Philadelphia, WB Saunders, 1989:918–921.

154. Walter MC, Matthiesen DT. Acquired antral pyloric hypertrophy in the dog. Vet Clin North Am Small Anim Pract 1993;23:547–554.

155. Leib MS, Saunders GK, Moon ML, et al. Endoscopic diagnosis of chronic hypertrophic pyloric gastropathy in dogs. J Vet Intern Med 1993;7:335–341.

156. Happe RP, Van Der Gaag I, Wolvekamp WTC. Pyloric stenosis caused by hypertrophic gastritis in three dogs. J Small Anim Pract 1981;22:7–17.

157. Walter MC, Goldschmidt MH, Stone EA, et al. Chronic hypertrophic pyloric gastropathy as a cause of pyloric obstruction in the dog. J Am Vet Med Assoc 1985;186:157–161.

158. Brodey RS. Alimentary tract neoplasms in the cat: A clinicopathologic survey of 46 cases. Am J Vet Res 1966;27:74–80.

159. Turk MAM, Gallina AM, Russell TS. Nonhematopoietic gastrointestinal neoplasia in cats: A retrospective study of 44 cases. Vet Pathol 1981;18:614–620.

160. Cribb AE. Feline gastrointestinal adenocarcinoma: A review and retrospective study. Can Vet J 1988;29:709–712.

161. Patnaik AK, Hurvitz AI, Johnson GF. Canine gastrointestinal neoplasms. Vet Pathol 1977;14:547–555.

162. Culbertson R, Branam JE, Rosenblatt LS. Esophageal/gastric leiomyoma in the laboratory Beagle. J Am Vet Med Assoc 1983;183:1168–1171.

163. Scanziani E, Giusti AM, Gualtieri M, et al. Gastric carcinoma in the Belgian shepherd dog. J Small Anim Pract 1991;32:465–469.

164. Lingeman C, Garner F, Taylor D. Spontaneous gastric adenocarcinomas of dogs: A review. J Nat Cancer Inst 1971;47:137–153.

165. Hayden DW, Nielsen SW. Canine alimentary neoplasia. Zbl Med A 1973;20:1–22.

166. Murray M, Robinson PB, McKeating FJ, et al. Primary gastric neoplasia in the dog: A clinico-pathological study. Vet Rec 1972;91:474–479.

167. Couto CG. Gastrointestinal neoplasia in dogs and cats. In: Kirk RW, Bonagura JD, ed. Kirk's Current Veterinary Therapy XI. Philadelphia, WB Saunders, 1992:595–601.

168. Patnaik AK, Hurvitz AI, Johnson GF. Canine gastric adenocarcinoma. Vet Pathol 1978;15:600–607.

169. Roth L, King JM. Mesenteric and omental sclerosis associated with metastases from gastrointestinal neoplasia in the dog. J Small Anim Pract 1990;31:28–31.

170. Sautter JH, Hanlon GF. Gastric neoplasms in the dog: A report of 20 cases. J Am Vet Med Assoc 1975;166:691–696.

171. Fonda D, Gualtieri M, Scanziani E. Gastric carcinoma in the dog: A clinicopathological study of 11 cases. J Small Anim Pract 1989;30:353–360.

172. Davenport DJ. Gastrointestinal lymphosarcoma. In: August JR, ed. Consultations in Feline Internal Medicine. Philadelphia, WB Saunders, 1991:419–423.

173. Couto CG, Rutgers HC, Sherding RG, et al. Gastrointes-

tinal lymphoma in 20 dogs: A retrospective study. J Vet Intern Med 1989;3:73–78.

174. Happe RP, Van Der Gaag I, Wolvekamp WTC, et al. Multiple polyps of the gastric mucosa in two dogs. J Small Anim Pract 1977;18:179–189.

175. Douglas SW, Hall LW, Walker RG. The surgical relief of gastric lesions in the dog: Report of seven cases. Vet Rec 1970;86:743–746.

176. Hall JA, Twedt DC, Burrows CF. Gastric motility in dogs: Part II. Disorders of gastric motility. Compen Contin Educ Pract Vet 1990;12:1373–1391.

177. Hargis AM, Prieur DJ, Wescott RB. A gastric nematode (*Ollulanis tricuspis*) in cats in the Pacific Northwest. J Am Vet Med Assoc 1981;178:475–478.

178. Hargis AM, Prieur DJ, Blanchard JL. Prevalence, lesions, and differential diagnosis of *Ollulanus tricuspis* infection in cats. Vet Pathol 1983;20:71–79.

179. Greve JH, Kung FY. *Capillaria putorii* in domestic cats in Iowa. J Am Vet Med Assoc 1983;182:511–513.

180. Hayden DW, Fleischman RW. Scirrhous eosinophilic gastritis in dogs with gastric arteritis. Vet Pathol 1977;14:441–448.

181. Clark WA. Canine gastric hyperplasia. Vet Annu 1985; 25:245–247.

182. Van Kruiningen HJ. Giant hypertrophic gastritis of Basenji dogs. Vet Pathol 1977;14:19–28.

183. Pearson H. Pyloric stenosis in the dog. Vet Rec 1979; 105:393–394.

184. Happe RP, van der Gaag I, Lamers CBHW, et al. Zollinger-Ellison syndrome in three dogs. Vet Pathol 1980;17:177–186.

185. Drazner FH. Canine gastrinoma: A condition analogous to the Zollinger-Ellison syndrome in man. Calif Vet 1981;11:6–11.

186. Shaw DH. Gastrinoma (Zollinger-Ellison syndrome) in the dog and cat. Can Vet J 1988;29:448–452.

187. Troy GC. Canine phycomycosis: A review of twenty-four cases. Calif Vet 1985;39:12–17.

188. Miller RI. Gastrointestinal phycomycosis in 63 dogs. J Am Vet Med Assoc 1985;186:473–478.

189. Ader PL. Phycomycosis in fifteen dogs and two cats. J Am Vet Med Assoc 1979;174:1216–1222.

190. Frendin J, Funkquist B, Stavenborn M. Gastric displacement in dogs without clinical signs of acute dilatation. J Small Anim Pract 1988;29:775–779.

191. Leib MS, Blass CE. Acute gastric dilatation volvulus in the dog: Various clinical presentations. Compen Contin Educ Pract Vet 1984;6:707–716.

Chapter 32

Diseases of
the Intestines

Michael S. Leib
Michael E. Matz

Anatomy

The small intestine begins at the pylorus and terminates at the ileocolic junction.[1] It varies in length from 1 to 1.5 m in cats and from 2 to 5 m in dogs. The first portion of the small intestine, the duodenum, is approximately 25 cm long and is fixed in position by the pylorus and the duodenocolic ligament. From the pylorus, the proximal duodenum turns caudally at the cranial duodenal flexure and descends along the right side of the abdomen toward the pelvic inlet, where a U-shaped turn, the caudal duodenal flexure, occurs. The ascending duodenum courses left and caudal to the root of the mesentery to join the longest section of the small intestine, the jejunum. The right limb of the pancreas lies in close contact to the descending portion of the duodenum. The ascending duodenum is near the descending colon. Both the pancreatic and the bile ducts empty into the descending duodenum.

The jejunum is the midportion of the small intestine and is very mobile, allowing the abdomen to change shape and capacity.[1] It is suspended by the mesentery, hanging from the root of the mesentery beneath the first lumbar vertebra. The mesentery supports the coils of jejunum and carries blood vessels and nerves. Anatomically, the duodenojejunal and the jejunoileal junctions are indistinct. The ileum is the terminal 15 cm of the small intestine and joins the large intestine at the ileocolic junction, in the right cranial portion of the abdomen.

The large bowel ranges in length from 28 to 90 cm in dogs and from 20 to 45 cm in cats.[2] It begins at the ileocolic junction and terminates at the anus. Anatomically, the large bowel is divided into the cecum, colon, and rectum. The cecum is a sigmoid diverticulum of the proximal colon and joins the colon through the cecocolic orifice. This junction is near the ileocolic orifice. The cecum is variable in length in dogs (8–30 cm) and short in cats (2–4 cm).

The colon is divided into ascending, transverse, and descending portions and their connecting flexures. The ascending colon is a short segment that begins at the ileocolic sphincter and courses craniad to the right (hepatic) colic flexure. The cecum and ascending colon lie to the right of the median plane and are in close association with the descending duodenum, the right limb of the pancreas, and the stomach. From the right colic flexure, the transverse colon runs across the abdomen, cranial to the root of the mesentery, to the left (splenic) colic flexure, where it becomes continuous with the descending colon. The transverse colon is near the left limb of the pancreas, the stomach, and the loops of jejunum. The descending colon, the longest segment, passes caudally, following the left lateral abdominal wall into the pelvic inlet, where the rectum begins. It is usually covered by the greater omentum and lies adjacent to the ascending portion of the duodenum. The uterus or prostate and bladder lie ventral to its terminal portion. The rectum continues through the pelvic cavity to the anus.

Histologically, the intestines are composed of four layers: mucosa, submucosa, muscularis, and serosa.[1] In the small intestine, the mucosal wall is folded, which increases the surface area three times.[3] Finger-like projections, the villi, protrude into the lumen and increase the surface area an additional 10 times. The villi are covered with a single layer of columnar enterocytes, as well as scattered mucus-secreting goblet cells and endocrine cells. The enterocytes are connected with tight junctions and provide a mucosal barrier that protects the submucosa from the macromolecular contents of the bowel lumen. Water and some electrolytes can pass through the tight junctions. The surface of each enterocyte is covered with thousands of folds, microvilli, that increase the surface area another 20 times. The remainder of the mucosa consists of the lamina propria, which contains a population of inflammatory cells, and the muscularis mucosae. The submucosa supports the mucosa and contains blood vessels, lymphatics, and nervous plexi. The muscular layer consists of a thin longitudinal layer and a thicker circular layer of smooth muscle. The serosa covers the intestines with the visceral peritoneum.

The colonic mucosa is devoid of villi, and the microvilli of the colonic epithelial cells are less abundant than their counterparts in the small bowel.[2] Despite the absence of villi, there are numerous crypts that extend from the absorptive surface through the entire thickness of the mucosa. These crypts, called crypts of Lieberkühn, contain epithelial, mucous, and endocrine cells.

In the small intestine at the base of the villi are crypts that contain undifferentiated cells, which rapidly divide.[3] Crypt cells are responsible for the majority of intestinal secretion. Crypt cells migrate toward the tip of the villus, lose the ability to divide and secrete, and develop a brush border with digestive enzymes and carrier proteins necessary for digestion and absorption of nutrients. After 3 to 5 days, the cells are sloughed into the lumen, where they are digested and their components absorbed. Migration of epithelial cells is similar in the large intestine, where the lower halves of the crypts consist mainly of undifferentiated cells that migrate along the crypts as they proliferate and mature, ultimately giving rise to epithelial, mucous, and endocrine cells. Cell turnover in the colon is slower than in the small intestine, requiring 4 to 7 days.

Both intrinsic and extrinsic nervous systems regulate intestinal function.[2] Intrinsic innervation occurs through the intramural network of neurons contained in the myenteric plexus, which lies between the longitudinal and circular muscle layers, and the submucosal plexus. Intrinsic control allows the intestines to autonomously regulate functions based on intraluminal conditions, such as the degree of distention and type and amount of contents. Extrinsic neural control occurs through the autonomic nervous system. Parasympathetic innervation to the majority of the intestines is through the vagus nerve; the distal large intestine is supplied by the pelvic nerves. Sympathetic innervation arises from the paravertebral ganglia and follows splanchnic nerves to the intestines.

Physiology

The major functions of the intestines in the dog and cat are digestion and absorption of nutrients, extraction of water and electrolytes from the lumen, storage of feces, and defecation.

Digestion and Absorption

Proteins, fats, and carbohydrates must be converted into molecules that can cross the brush border of the small intestine and be absorbed into the enterocytes.[3] Many carbohydrates are split by pancreatic enzymes into polysaccharides, which are hydrolyzed by brush border enzymes into monosaccharides and transported by carriers into the enterocytes.[3] Protein digestion begins in the stomach with the action of acid and pepsins and is continued within the small intestine by the action of pancreatic enzymes. Oligopeptides are hydrolyzed at the brush border of the enterocyte into dipeptides and amino acids, which cross the mucosal barrier on specific carriers. Fat digestion begins with gastric lipase and continues with pancreatic enzymes within the small intestine. Monoglycerides and free fatty acids form water-soluble micelles with bile acids, allowing fats to be transported to the mucosa, where they cross the cell membrane by diffusion. Medium- and short-chain fatty acids can directly enter the portal blood, whereas long-chain fatty acids enter the lymphatics.

In addition to pancreatic, biliary, and gastric secretions, the small intestine secretes fluids into the lumen to help mix ingesta with digestive enzymes. The intestines absorb approximately 98% of the fluid contained within the lumen. Most nutrient and water absorption occurs in the proximal small intestine by facilitated diffusion. Approximately 90% of the water entering the large intestine is absorbed.[4] The large intestine has a maximum absorptive capacity for water. If fluid flow from the small intestine exceeds this absorptive capacity, if there is increased colonic fluid secretion, or if colonic absorption is decreased, diarrhea occurs. The capacity of the large bowel to absorb water principally determines whether diarrhea is present with diseases of either the small or large intestine.

Motility

The functions of intestinal motility are to mix ingesta with digestive secretions, bring luminal contents in contact with the absorptive surface, move ingesta toward the large intestine at a rate appropriate for digestion and absorption, promote storage of feces, and facilitate defecation. When ingesta are present in the small intestine, two types of muscular contractions, called peristalsis, occur.[5] Segmentation is a localized contraction of circular smooth muscle (approximately 1 cm) that functions to mix ingesta and slow their passage along the small intestine, allowing optimal digestion and absorption. Progressive peristalsis results from contraction of the longitudinal smooth muscle; it moves ingesta 1 to 4 cm toward the large intestine with each contraction.

During fasting, another type of motility, called the migrating motor complex, occurs. It consists of powerful contractions that move from the stomach to the colon in approximately 5 minutes and recur every 120 minutes. This type of motility functions as an intestinal housekeeper to remove indigestible solids and the debris of digestion and to sweep bacteria toward the large intestine.[6] The migrating motor complex does not occur in cats, but a somewhat similar process, the migrating spike complex, occurs.[6]

Most muscular contractions arising in the proximal colon are retrograde peristaltic contractions that are initiated in the transverse colon and propagate toward the cecum.[2] Termed antiperistalsis, this motility pattern slows the transit of colonic contents and enhances mucosal absorption of fluid and electrolytes. Throughout the colon, rhythmic segmentation similar to that in the small intestine moves contents short distances in both antegrade and retrograde directions, preventing rapid transit. This activity aids absorption of water and electrolytes.

Motility in the distal colon is characterized by spontaneous, giant migrating contractions or mass movements. These powerful smooth muscle contractions originate in the proximal colon and migrate in an aboral direction over a segment or over the entire length of the colon, moving colonic contents toward the rectum in preparation for defecation.[7]

Intestinal contractile activity is influenced by smooth muscle properties, intrinsic neurons, extrinsic nerves, and peptides. Control of peristalsis and rhythmic segmentation is determined by slow-wave activity, which is an inherent myoelectric property of smooth muscle. Oscillation of resting membrane potential is initiated in a series of pacemakers throughout the intestines. The frequency of slow-wave activity determines the rate of contraction.[6] Additional stimuli (facilitory impulses from the intramural plexuses, extrinsic innervation, or local or systemic peptides) can cause the membrane potential to exceed the excitation threshold and produce spike activity, which is usually accompanied by muscular contraction.[6] The number of spike potentials generated during the depolarization phase determines the strength of contraction. Slow-wave frequency is slower in the proximal colon than in the distal colon, which helps to impede transit and contributes to the extraction of water and electrolytes. The proximal colon is dominated by a single pacemaker in the transverse colon, from which slow waves are spread most often orad and are associated with antiperistalsis, once again facilitating storage of feces and extraction of water.[8] Giant migrating contractions result from prolonged bursts of electrical activity that span several slow-wave cycles and appear to be independent of slow-wave activity.

The intrinsic nervous system is essential for normal intestinal motility and can function independently from the extrinsic nervous system.[2] Reflexes mediated through efferent cholinergic neurons stimulate segmental contractions and peristalsis. Stimulus for contraction occurs through mechanoreceptors in the muscular layers in response to distention or through chemoreceptors located within the mucosa in response to changes in luminal conditions.

The major function of the extrinsic nervous system is in the distal colon, where it participates in the defecation reflex.[2] The defecation reflex is initiated in response to luminal distention in the distal colon and rectum. Increased tension in the rectal wall stimulates extrarectal receptors, which transmit impulses along afferent parasympathetic pathways within the pelvic nerve to the sacral spinal cord. Efferent nerve fibers contained within the pudendal, hypogastric, and pelvic nerves complete the reflex arc. Stimulation of these fibers initiates a motor response that causes contraction of colonic and rectal smooth muscle and relaxation of the internal and external anal sphincters, allowing evacuation of the rectum and distal colon. Defecation is usually preceded by giant migrating contractions of the distal colon.[7] The defecation reflex can be inhibited by voluntary contraction of the external anal sphincter. Receptive relaxation of the distal colon and rectum accommodates fecal storage until the next defecation reflex is initiated.

Immune Function

Natural defense mechanisms of the intestines include mechanical and immunologic facets, which act in concert to protect the host.[2, 9] These mechanisms are particularly important because of the extensive bacterial flora contained within the intestines. Important mechanical factors include motility, mucus, and normal bacterial flora. The intestinal immune system consists of three main compartments that contain lymphocytes: gut-associated lymphoid tissue (GALT), the intestinal epithelium, and the mucosal lamina propria.[10]

GALT consists of mucosal lymphoid follicles and mesenteric lymph nodes. The function of the lymphoid follicles is to capture (trap) and process antigens to initiate an appropriate immune response. GALT contains B and T lymphocytes (mainly helper T cells) and antigen-processing cells, including macrophages and dendritic cells. Germinal centers of the lymphoid follicles contain B cells that produce immunoglobulin A (IgA). Specialized epithelial cells, termed membranous or M cells, overlie the lymphoid follicles. These cells trap antigens and channel them toward antigen-processing cells.[11]

Intraepithelial lymphocytes are principally suppressor T cells.[11, 12] Mast cell progenitors are also found in this compartment.

The mucosal lamina propria contains B and T cells. IgA-producing B cells predominate the B cell subtype, and the majority of the T cells are of the helper subset. Plasma cells, mast cells, macrophages, and eosinophils are also present in the lamina propria. Besides mediating immediate hypersensitivity, mast cells also may play a role in delayed hypersensitivity, inflammation, cytotoxicity, and immunoregulation.[13]

Plasma cells within the mucosa produce primary IgA, which is bound to a secretory component on the epithelial cell membrane and released into the gut lumen. By binding to antigens, the secretory IgA prevents their attachment to and uptake by the intestinal mucosa.[9, 11] IgA in combination with mechanical factors serves to exclude antigenic material from the mucosa.

Antigens that penetrate the mucosal epithelium initiate an immune response. After antigen processing, the immune system undergoes regulated expansion to produce clones responsible for cell-mediated immunity, humoral immunity, immune memory, and immunoregulation. The immune response results in sensitivity (elimination) or tolerance to the antigen.

Cell-mediated immunity involves cellular cytotoxicity and synthesis of biologically active compounds called cytokines. Lymphocytes in the epithelial and mucosal compartments possess cytotoxic potential. Macrophages also may become cytotoxic.

Lymphokines are produced by T lymphocytes and macrophages after stimulation by antigens or other inflammatory cells. Lymphokines, including interleukins, leukotrienes, and interferons, promote cellular functions such as macrophage activation, T-cell proliferation and maturation, IgA production, and cytotoxic activity.[11]

After antigen penetration of the mucosal barrier, non-IgA immunoglobulins also become involved in the humoral immune response. IgM, IgG, and IgE may participate in host defense by the processes of opsonization, complement fixation, and promotion of an inflammatory response, all properties that IgA lacks. IgE is also important in the mediation of immediate hypersensitivity. After antigen binds to IgE molecules fixed to mast cells, degranulation of the mast cells occurs, releasing inflammatory mediators (e.g., histamine, serotonin, leukotrienes). The release of inflammatory mediators may be important in the expulsion of parasites.[14]

Oral immunologic tolerance is a prominent feature of the gastrointestinal (GI) immune system. Tolerance results from suppression of cell-mediated and IgG, IgM, and IgE humoral immune responses to ingested luminal antigens and microbial flora. This response is thought to be caused by suppressor T cells generated by the GALT. Most antigens processed by M cells induce tolerance, whereas antigens that penetrate the mucosal barrier can induce potentially harmful local or systemic reactions. Oral tolerance is necessary to prevent mucosal and systemic injury as a result of a continuous inflammatory response to benign, persistent intraluminal antigens. A breakdown of this tolerance response may be involved in the pathogenesis of inflammatory bowel disease.

Microflora

The intestines are inhabited by hundreds of species of bacteria, with anaerobes outnumbering aerobes by 1000 to 1.[15] Microflora serve as a barrier between pathogenic organisms and the host and help condition the immunologic response to respond to antigens efficiently and appropriately. Fermentation in the colon also provides some energy to the colonocytes. The orad small bowel contains relatively few bacteria, but their numbers increase in the distal small intestine.[16, 17] The orad small bowel contains mostly *Clostridium*, *Streptococcus*, *Lactobacillus*, and *Staphylococcus* spp., whereas the aboral portion contains mostly coliforms and enterococci.

The large bowel contains the highest concentration of bacteria in the GI tract, with 1 g of feces containing up to 10^{11} organisms.[2] Almost 50% of the dry weight of feces consists of bacteria. Anaerobic (spore-forming and nonspore-forming) bacteria predominate and account for up to 90% of the microflora. *Bifidobacterium* and *Bacteroides* spp. are found in the highest numbers, with lesser numbers of clostridia and lactobacilli. Enterobacteria and streptococci are the predominant aerobic bacteria found in the large bowel.

The physiologic mechanisms that maintain normal colonic microflora and prevent disease associated with bacterial overgrowth or colonization by pathologic organisms include the presence of normal intestinal motility, maintenance of the mucosal barrier, and local immune factors. Environmental factors that influence intestinal microflora include interrelations of resident microflora, diet, and orally administered or enterohepatically circulated antibacterial agents.

Normal resident microflora resist colonization by other organisms by producing metabolic inhibitory products and competing for mucosal attachment sites and nutrients. The use of antibiotics with anaerobic spectrums or broad spectrums may upset this sensitive balance and result in overpopulation of pathogens.

Carbohydrates, proteins, and lipids are metabolized by colonic bacteria. Carbohydrates are transformed into short-chain fatty acids (acetate, propionate, butyrate) and gases (hydrogen, methane, and carbon dioxide). Luminal bicarbonate neutralizes most of the acids, resulting in the production of carbon dioxide and water. Absorbed fatty acids are either metabolized by colonic epithelium (butyrate) or transported to other tissues and used as an energy source (acetate, propionate, butyrate).

Problem Identification

Acute Diarrhea

Diarrhea can be defined as increased fluidity of the feces, often accompanied by an increased frequency and volume. Dogs and cats frequently develop diarrhea of abrupt onset, lasting for less than 7 days. Most cases are mild and self-limited, requiring minimal diagnostic testing and therapy, but are unpleasant for the animal and inconvenient for the owner. The most common causes of acute diarrhea are dietary indiscretion and GI parasites. However, life-threatening cases occur, and these animals need intensive diagnostic testing and therapy.

Pathophysiology

There are four major mechanisms that can cause diarrhea: osmotic forces, increased secretory activity, increased permeability, and abnormal motility.[4, 18, 19] Osmotic forces and changes in permeability are the most important mechanisms in small animals.[4] However, in most diseases, multiple mechanisms contribute to the diarrhea.

The number of osmotically active particles in feces determines water content.[4] Osmotic diarrhea occurs when increased numbers of osmotically active particles are retained in the intestinal lumen.[20] This occurs with pancreatic exocrine insufficiency (see Chap. 33) and with many malabsorptive disorders in which nutrients are not digested and absorbed nor-

mally, remain within the GI lumen, and osmotically attract water.[4] This can lead to bacterial overgrowth and fermentation of carbohydrates, which can further increase the number of osmotically active particles. Osmotic diarrhea can also occur with overeating and ingestion of spoiled foods containing poorly absorbed nutrients.[4]

Stimulation of crypt enterocytes can result in secretion of large volumes of fluid that exceed the absorptive ability of the intestine. This occurs most commonly with infectious diseases such as colibacillosis and salmonellosis, but byproducts of bacterial overgrowth can also stimulate intestinal secretion.[4, 20] Increased permeability of the intestine causes loss of fluids, electrolytes, proteins, and blood into the intestinal lumen. It commonly accompanies erosive, ulcerative, and inflammatory processes such as inflammatory bowel disease and hookworm infection.[4, 20] Abnormal motility is often a secondary problem in disorders causing diarrhea. Decreased segmental contractions result in transport of ingesta at a rate too fast for digestion and absorption. Byproducts of bacterial overgrowth can cause abnormal motility.

Mild diarrhea causes few metabolic consequences. However, moderate or severe diarrhea can lead to profound dehydration and electrolyte and acid-base disturbance.[19] A tremendous loss of fluid can occur if the intestine does not function normally because of the large amount of daily physiologic secretion from the salivary glands, stomach, and small and large intestines.[18] Hypokalemia, hypochloremia, and hyponatremia can develop.[21] Metabolic acidosis develops secondary to loss of intestinal bicarbonate and dehydration, which leads to hypovolemia and to production of lactic acid because of anaerobic metabolism by tissues. When death accompanies severe diarrhea, often it is not due to the primary cause of diarrhea but is secondary to dehydration and to electrolyte and acid-base disturbance resulting from the diarrhea.

Clinical Signs

The history may reveal dietary indiscretion, including potential exposure to foreign materials, chemicals, or toxins; administration of drugs, especially antibiotics; an incomplete vaccination or deworming status; or recent exposure to other animals with diarrhea. The diarrhea may have characteristics of small intestinal disease or signs of mixed small and large bowel disease. On occasion, signs of only large bowel disease are present. Signs of small bowel diarrhea include melena, normal or moderately increased frequency of defecation, and production of a large volume of feces per defecation.[22–24] Signs of large bowel diarrhea include hematochezia, tenesmus, ex-

Table 32-1
Clinical Signs Associated With Systemic Diseases That Cause Acute Diarrhea

SIGN	DISEASE
Pyrexia	Parvoviruses
	Acute pancreatitis
	Infectious canine hepatitis
	Canine distemper
	Leptospirosis
	Acute liver failure
Icterus	Leptospirosis
	Acute pancreatitis
	Acute liver failure
Lymphadenopathy	Infectious canine hepatitis
	Salmon poisoning
Oliguria or anuria	Acute renal failure
	Leptospirosis
Ocular and nasal discharge	Canine distemper
Cough	Canine distemper
	Infectious canine hepatitis

cess fecal mucus, moderate to greatly increased frequency of defecation, and reduced volume of feces per defecation.[22–25]

In many cases of acute diarrhea, vomiting and abdominal pain occur. Other clinical signs can be related to the cause of diarrhea, including pyrexia, icterus, lymphadenopathy, oliguria or anuria, hepatomegaly, ocular and nasal discharge, and coughing (Table 32–1).[26–30] Physical examination may detect an abdominal mass, dilated loop of bowel, foreign body, or intussusception.[15, 31, 32] Dry mucous membranes, a loss of skin turgor, prolonged capillary refill time, or enophthalmos indicates dehydration.[33, 34]

Diagnostic Plan

Because there are so many causes of acute diarrhea, a thorough diagnostic plan must be followed to reach a diagnosis efficiently. Often, a cause can be identified after evaluation of the history, physical examination, and screening laboratory tests. The most important initial step is to determine if the animal with acute diarrhea has a self-limited or a potentially life-threatening problem. This distinction is crucial and should be based on a thorough history, careful physical examination, clinical experience and judgment, and sound knowledge of the differential diagnosis of acute diarrhea (Table 32–2). Animals should be considered to have a potentially life-threatening problem if some of the following are present: moderate to severe dehydration, abdominal pain or depression; melena or hematochezia; palpation of an abdominal mass or dilated loop of bowel; frequent vomiting; or signs of systemic diseases such as pyrexia, lymphadenopathy, ocular and nasal discharge, cough, oliguria or anuria, or icterus. If the distinction is not clear, it is better to be cautious and treat the animal initially as if it has a life-threatening problem.

A minimum database for self-limited diarrhea includes several fecal examinations, fecal cytology, and measurement of total protein and hematocrit, which help to assess hydration and provide a baseline reference if clinical signs persist or progress. If dietary indiscretion is present, removal of the incriminating factors or feeding a highly digestible diet for 3 to 5 days, or both, often resolves the diarrhea.[35, 36] If parasites are detected (e.g., hookworms, roundworms, coccidia, *Giardia* spp., whipworms), diarrhea should improve in 2 to 3 days after appropriate treatment has been administered.[37–41] Fecal cytology may identify many safety pin–shaped bacterial spores (Fig. 32–1), suggesting the presence of *Clostridium perfringens* enterotoxicosis.[42] If these are present, a fecal sample should be submitted for enterotoxin identification. If a cause is not detected, a diagnosis of acute idiopathic self-limited diarrhea may be made. Symptomatic therapy (see Dietary Indiscretion) often relieves clinical signs in 1 to 3 days. If diarrhea persists or other clinical signs develop or intensify, a life-threatening problem that requires more thorough evaluation and intensive therapy may exist.

Patients with potentially life-threatening disorders require multiple fecal examinations, rectal cytology, complete blood count, biochemical profile, urinalysis, and abdominal radiographs (Table 32–3). Fecal examination may identify parasites, which could be the cause of the diarrhea or simply contribute to its severity. If rectal cytologic examination shows increased numbers of neutrophils, sea gull–shaped bacteria *(Campylobacter)*, or safety pin–shaped spores *(Clostridium perfringens)*, a fecal sample should be submitted for bacterial culture or enterotoxin analysis.[42, 43] The laboratory evaluation should help to eliminate the presence of systemic disorders that can cause diarrhea (e.g., acute hepatitis, acute pancreatitis, acute renal failure) and to assess the severity of electrolyte disorders, guiding rational fluid therapy.[27, 28, 44] Survey abdominal radiographs may demonstrate an abdominal mass, dilated loop of bowel, ileocolic intussusception, or foreign body obstruction, any of which requires surgical therapy (Fig. 32–2).[15, 31, 32] In some cases, additional diagnostic tests may be indicated to definitively diagnose a specific disorder, such as a fecal enzyme-linked immunosorbent assay (ELISA) for parvovirus or a liver biopsy for acute hepatic failure, or to pursue diagnosis if a cause of the diarrhea is not evident (e.g., barium upper GI series, abdominal ultrasound, fecal culture).[45–48]

Chronic Diarrhea

Chronic diarrhea can be defined as the presence of loose stools for at least 2 to 4 weeks. It is a common problem in dogs and cats of all ages and breeds, although the incidence in German shepherds and basenjis appears to be higher than in other breeds.[17, 49, 50] Because animals with chronic diarrhea can be uncomfortable, clients are often inconvenienced, and veterinarians become frustrated, it is necessary that a definitive diagnosis be reached and appropriate therapy instituted.

Pathophysiology

The pathophysiology of diarrhea is described in the section on acute diarrhea. Because the condition is chronic, dehydration and electrolyte abnormalities occur less frequently than in acute diarrhea, unless there is a sudden intensification of clinical signs. The pathophysiologic aspects of individual causes of chronic diarrhea are covered in the sections on specific diseases.

Clinical Signs

During the history, specific attention should be given to the animal's diet (including supplements, changes, snacks, and treats), environment (free-roaming), and previous deworming.[22, 36] Assessment of previous treatments and the response to therapy can help rank the differential diagnoses.

Diarrhea in chronic cases may be continuous, but often it is intermittent or cyclic. It may be associated with or intensified by stressful conditions. Intermittent vomiting often occurs. Characteristics associated with diarrhea caused by small intestinal disease include normal or moderately increased frequency of defecation, large volume of feces per defecation, melena, and weight loss. Diarrhea associated with diseases of the large intestine is characterized by a moderate to greatly increased frequency of defecation, reduced volume of feces per defecation, tenesmus, excess fecal mucus, and hematochezia (Table 32–4).[22–25]

Other clinical signs can relate to underlying systemic diseases, including polyuria and polydipsia (chronic renal failure, liver diseases, feline hyperthyroidism), severe vomiting (chronic pancreatitis, liver diseases, feline hyperthyroidism), polyphagia or hyperactivity (feline hyperthyroidism), or stomatitis (feline immunodeficiency virus [FIV] or feline leukemia virus [FeLV]).[27, 51–54]

Physical examination may be normal. Weight

Table 32–2
Differential Diagnosis of Acute Diarrhea

Self-Limited Disorders
Dietary indiscretion
  Diet change
  Garbage
  Table scraps
  Foreign material
  Chemicals and toxins
Parasites
  Hookworms
  Roundworms
  Giardia
  Coccidia
  Whipworms
Coronavirus
Drugs
  Nonsteroidal anti-inflammatory drugs
  Digoxin
  Antibiotics
  Corticosteroids
  Magnesium antacids
  Cancer chemotherapeutics
Idiopathic

Life-Threatening Disorders
Severe dietary indiscretion
Severe parasitism
  Hookworms
  Whipworms
  Giardia
Intestinal obstruction
  Foreign body
  Intussusception
Parvoviruses
Hemorrhagic gastroenteritis
Systemic diseases
  Acute pancreatitis
  Acute liver failure
    Infectious canine hepatitis
  Acute renal failure
    Leptospirosis
  Canine distemper
  Salmon poisoning
Bacteria
  Salmonella
  Campylobacter
  Clostridium perfringens

loss or evidence of emaciation can be detected. Animals often appear unthrifty and have a dull, lusterless hair coat. Abdominal palpation may detect a mass, thickened bowel walls, a dilated segment of intestine, or evidence of ascites.[15] Rectal examination

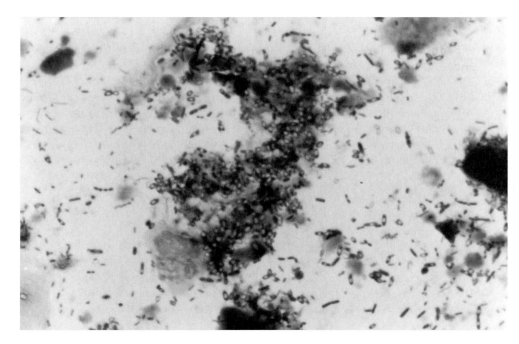

Figure 32–1
Rectal cytology specimen showing a large number of clostridial spores. The spores are similar in appearance to safety pins, with a clear center and dark ends. Magnification, ×500.

may reveal rough, corrugated mucosae, a colonic mass, enlarged sublumbar lymph nodes, or rectal pain.[25]

Diagnostic Plan

Because there are so many causes of chronic diarrhea, a thorough and logical diagnostic plan should be followed to efficiently arrive at an accurate diagnosis so effective therapy can be prescribed.[25] The most important initial step is to localize the origin of diarrhea to the small or large intestine, based on descriptions of the feces and of the act of defecation obtained from the history (see Table 32–4).[22–25] Localization should not be based solely on observations made during hospitalization, because fecal characteristics often vary owing to stress or dietary and environmental changes. Localization is important because the differential diagnosis and diagnostic plans are different for small intestinal and large intestinal causes of diarrhea (Table 32–5). In some cases, signs of both small and large intestine diarrhea exist because the animal has a disease that affects both the small and large intestines.

In many cases, the history and physical examination do not suggest a specific cause for diarrhea. The animal's signalment and anthelmintic treatment history are important in ranking the differential diagnoses. GI parasites are a common cause of chronic diarrhea in patients that have not been recently tested or treated for parasites or do not receive monthly heartworm prophylaxis.[37–40] In addition, specific disorders may have an age or breed association, such as pancreatic exocrine insufficiency and bacterial over-

growth in young German shepherds, immunoproliferative small intestinal disease in basenjis, and partial small intestinal obstructions caused by intussusceptions and foreign bodies in young dogs.[17, 31, 32, 49, 50]

If systemic diseases (e.g., renal failure, hepatic diseases, hyperthyroidism, FeLV or FIV, chronic pancreatitis) are suspected because of polyuria and polydipsia, severe vomiting, icterus, ascites, stomatitis, polyphagia, or hyperactivity, laboratory evaluation should be performed immediately.[27, 51–54]

If an abdominal mass or dilated loop of bowel is palpated in a patient with small bowel diarrhea, the diagnostic plan should include survey abdominal radiographs, an upper GI contrast study, abdominal ultrasonography, a laboratory database, thoracic radiographs to detect metastasis (in older animals), and exploratory surgery.[15] If a rectal mass is detected in a patient with large bowel diarrhea, the diagnostic plan should include thoracic radiographs and abdominal ultrasonography to detect metastasis, a laboratory database, and colonoscopy. However, in the absence of these historical and physical examination findings, a slower, less aggressive plan may be followed.

The two most common causes of chronic small bowel diarrhea are dietary indiscretion and GI parasites. If dietary indiscretion is present, it should be corrected. If the diet cannot be implicated, multiple fecal examinations for parasites should be performed. If a parasite is identified, appropriate therapy should be instituted and diarrhea should rapidly resolve. Although three fecal examinations by zinc sulfate flotation can identify most cases of *Giardia* infection, it may be prudent to treat for *Giardia* infection with

Table 32–3
Laboratory Abnormalities for Causes of Life-Threatening Diarrhea

LABORATORY VALUE	DISEASE
Decreased total protein	Hookworms Whipworms Canine parvovirus Hemorrhagic gastroenter- itis (late) Salmonellosis
Anemia	Canine parvovirus Hemorrhagic gastroenter- itis (late)
Elevated hematocrit	Hemorrhagic gastroenter- itis Moderate to severe dehy- dration from any cause
Neutrophilia	Acute pancreatitis Liver diseases Infectious canine hepatitis (late) Salmonellosis (late) Leptospirosis (late) *Campylobacter* infection Salmon poisoning
Neutropenia	Canine parvovirus Feline parvovirus Leptospirosis Infectious canine hepatitis Salmonellosis Salmon poisoning
Lymphopenia	Canine parvovirus Feline parvovirus Canine distemper Infectious canine hepatitis Salmonellosis
Eosinophilia	Gastrointestinal parasites
Hypoglycemia	Canine parvovirus Salmonellosis
Increased alanine trans- aminase and alkaline phosphatase	Acute pancreatitis Acute liver failure Infectious canine hepatitis Leptospirosis
Hyperbilirubinemia	Acute pancreatitis Acute liver failure Leptospirosis
Increased blood urea ni- trogen, creatinine, and phosphorus	Acute renal failure Leptospirosis Moderate to severe dehy- dration from any cause
Hypocalcemia	Acute pancreatitis
Increased amylase and lipase	Acute pancreatitis Acute renal failure
Increased prothrombin and partial thrombo- plastin times	Infectious canine hepatitis Acute liver failure
Proteinuria	Acute renal failure Infectious canine hepatitis Leptospirosis

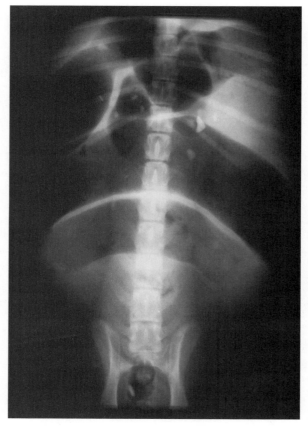

Figure 32–2
Ventrodorsal abdominal radiograph showing massive dilation of small intestine in a 1-year-old Akita. The cause of
the obstruction was an intussusception, foreign body, and
mesenteric torsion through a mesenteric rent.

metronidazole in some cases despite negative fecal
examinations.[37] Rectal cytology should be performed
and may show increased numbers of neutrophils,
safety pin–shaped spores, or sea gull–shaped bacteria;
if so, fecal samples should be submitted for *C.
perfringens* enterotoxin or bacterial culture.[25, 42, 43] If
diarrhea continues or a diagnosis has not been reached,
a 4-week trial with a highly digestible diet should be
instituted, even if dietary indiscretion cannot be
identified.[35, 36] During this trial period, the animal
should not receive any other foods or snacks. If severe
weight loss or profuse diarrhea is present, a 4-week
diet trial is not appropriate because, if it fails to resolve
the diarrhea, the animal's condition may further
deteriorate. In our experience, many cases of chronic
diarrhea resolve after these simple steps are followed,
avoiding unnecessary expense for the client and
inappropriate diagnostic testing for the patient.

If diarrhea continues, pancreatic exocrine function should be evaluated in young dogs by submitting
a serum sample for trypsin-like immunoreactivity (see
Chap. 33).[55, 56] In all other animals, a laboratory

Table 32–4
Localization of Chronic Diarrhea

SIGN	SMALL BOWEL	LARGE BOWEL
Weight loss	Common	Uncommon
Frequency of defecation	Normal or mildly increased	Moderate to largely increased
Volume per defecation	Normal or increased	Normal or decreased
Tenesmus	Negative	Positive
Blood	Melena	Hematochezia
Mucus	Negative	Positive

database should be assessed to evaluate for systemic disorders and to help assess the animal's risk for general anesthesia, which may be necessary for additional diagnostic testing. This database should include a complete blood count, biochemical profile, urinalysis, and, in cats, a serum thyroxine and FeLV and FIV ELISAs.

If a diagnosis is not apparent, the animal probably has a malabsorption disorder and requires intestinal biopsy for diagnosis. Survey abdominal

Table 32–5
Differential Diagnosis of Chronic Diarrhea

Chronic Small Bowel Diarrhea
Giardia, hookworms, roundworms
Highly digestible diet–responsive diarrhea
Pancreatic exocrine insufficiency
Inflammatory bowel disease
Stagnant loop syndrome
Feline hyperthyroidism
Lymphosarcoma (diffuse)
Lymphangiectasia
Feline leukemia virus
Feline immunodeficiency virus
Neoplasia
Histoplasmosis
Bacterial overgrowth
Intussusception

Chronic Large Bowel Diarrhea
Whipworms
Highly digestible diet–responsive diarrhea
Plasmacytic lymphocytic colitis
Irritable bowel syndrome
Neoplasia
Clostridium perfringens enterotoxicosis
Fiber-responsive diarrhea
Ulcerative colitis
Eosinophilic colitis
Histoplasmosis
Intussusception

radiographs or abdominal ultrasonography can discover abnormalities not detected during abdominal palpation. D-Xylose and fat absorption tests can add information on small bowel function, but the tests lack sensitivity.[57, 58] Bacterial overgrowth can be indirectly evaluated with serum folate and vitamin B_{12} determinations.[17, 56] However, many of these tests can be omitted and a diagnosis obtained after histologic assessment of mucosal biopsy. Biopsy samples can be collected during endoscopic examination or exploratory laparotomy. Limitations of endoscopic biopsy are that samples can be collected only from the proximal small intestine and that biopsy samples are small and contain only mucosa. Surgery offers the potential to collect large, full-thickness biopsies from the duodenum, jejunum, ileum, and mesenteric lymph nodes and allows exploration of the entire abdomen. Morbidity is higher with surgery than with endoscopy. In addition, hypoproteinemic animals are at increased risk of dehiscence after surgery; these patients should receive endoscopic biopsies. If a diagnosis is not reached, some of the tests that were omitted (described above) can be performed and a fecal sample submitted for bacterial culture.

Because the two most common causes of chronic large bowel diarrhea are dietary indiscretion and *Trichuris vulpis* infection, the same considerations apply for the initial approach to large bowel diarrhea as for small bowel diarrhea in regard to dietary indiscretion, trial with a highly digestible diet, fecal examination, and rectal cytology. In dogs, treatment for whipworms should be administered even if fecal examinations are negative, because *T. vulpis* can shed eggs intermittently.[38] Many cases of chronic large bowel diarrhea resolve after these simple procedures are followed.

If large bowel diarrhea persists, further diagnostic testing is indicated. A complete blood count, biochemical profile, and urinalysis should be evaluated to eliminate the presence of systemic diseases that can be associated with chronic large bowel diarrhea and to identify concurrent illnesses that can increase the risk of anesthesia.[25] If a cause for the diarrhea cannot be identified, colonoscopy and mucosal biopsy should be performed.[59, 60] If endoscopic examination fails to identify a cause for the diarrhea, a fecal sample should be submitted for bacterial culture.[25]

Partial Intestinal Obstruction

Partial obstruction of the small intestinal lumen, or stagnant loop syndrome (SLS), can be identified in dogs and cats based on progressive clinical signs, abdominal palpation, and survey and contrast radiography. It differs from complete intestinal obstruction because the disorder develops slowly, only a portion of the small intestinal lumen is compromised, strangulation of bowel usually does not occur (although partial venous strangulation can occur with intussusceptions), and it is not a surgical emergency.

Pathophysiology

The most common causes of SLS in dogs and cats are foreign bodies, neoplasia, and intussusceptions.[15] Partial small intestinal obstruction leads to altered intestinal motility, stagnation of intestinal contents, and overgrowth of normal bacterial flora.[61, 62] Bacterial overgrowth can cause both functional and morphologic damage to the mucosa, leading to malabsorption.[17, 61, 63] Bacterial overgrowth causes deconjugation of bile acids. Deconjugated bile acids either precipitate within the intestinal lumen or are absorbed and do not function properly in fat digestion; as a result, fat malassimilation develops.[64] Deconjugated bile acids can also cause bowel damage, alter absorption, and stimulate secretion.[61, 62, 64] Bacteria hydroxylate the increased intraluminal concentration of free fatty acids (caused by malabsorption), which become toxic to the intestines and can alter intestinal motility, increase secretion, increase permeability, and decrease absorption.[62, 64] Bacterial fermentation of carbohydrates contributes to osmotic diarrhea.[61] Protein malassimilation can also develop because of utilization of enteric protein.[61]

Protein-losing gastroenteropathy (PLE) and GI hemorrhage may be associated with some causes of SLS. Hypoalbuminemia leads to decreased serum osmotic pressure and edema, or body cavity effusion can develop (see Hypoproteinemia).

Clinical Signs

The clinical signs associated with SLS vary depending on the cause, the location along the small intestine, and the degree and duration of obstruction. Chronic small bowel diarrhea, weight loss, and poor general condition are common. Vomiting occurs with involvement of the proximal small intestine. A history of foreign body ingestion may be present.[15]

An abdominal mass, dilated loop of bowel, or foreign body may be palpated. Mild to moderate dehydration may be detected. If hypoalbuminemia develops, ballottement of the abdomen may reveal ascitic fluid; in addition, crackles caused by pulmonary edema or muffled heart and lung sounds from pleural effusion may be detected, and pitting edema may be seen along the extremities or ventrum.

Diagnostic Plan

The problem of SLS may be identified in two ways in an animal with chronic small bowel diarrhea: (1) abdominal palpation reveals a dilated loop of bowel, or (2) abdominal radiographs detect a dilated loop that could not be palpated.[15] If a dilated loop of bowel can be palpated, survey abdominal radiographs, thoracic radiographs to detect metastasis (in older animals), a laboratory database, and exploratory surgery are indicated. Abdominal ultrasonography and a barium contrast examination may be helpful in reaching a diagnosis but are not necessary in many cases. If the dilated loop cannot be palpated, the diagnostic plan for patients with chronic small bowel diarrhea should be pursued. Because these animals have severe weight loss, a 4-week dietary trial with a highly digestible diet is not indicated. Multiple fecal examinations, fecal cytology, laboratory database, and abdominal radiographs should be performed. Once the dilated loop is identified, the diagnostic work-up previously described should be followed.

Survey abdominal radiographs may show a dilated section of bowel, lack of intra-abdominal contrast because of loss of fat or ascites formation, or a radiopaque foreign body (Fig. 32–3).[15] If the dilated segment of intestine cannot be identified to be small bowel, air can be placed in the colon and an abdominal radiograph taken. An upper GI barium contrast examination may demonstrate delayed small bowel transit, a radiolucent foreign body, an intussusception, or eccentric or annular narrowing of bowel lumen.[47] Because of bacterial overgrowth, D-xylose absorption may be decreased and serum folate may be increased while serum vitamin B_{12} is decreased.[17]

Complete Intestinal Obstruction

Complete obstruction of the small intestine occurs when there is total occlusion of the lumen. Obstructions can be simple, with the blood supply to the intestinal wall not affected, or can be strangulated, with the blood supply compromised.[65–67] Complete obstructions are surgical emergencies. Dogs can die within 3 days of a proximal simple obstruction and within 12 hours of a strangulating obstruction.

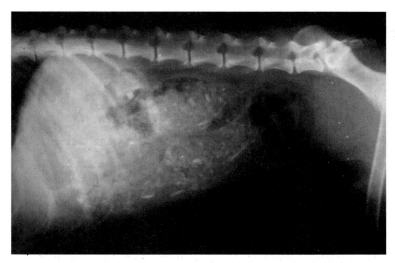

Figure 32-3
Lateral survey abdominal radiograph from a middle aged Siberian husky with a partial small bowel obstruction, chronic diarrhea, and weight loss. A very dilated loop of bowel is filled with fecal-type material. The cause of the partial small bowel obstruction was an adenocarcinoma of the proximal colon. (From Leib MS. Stagnant loop syndrome in the dog and cat. Sem Vet Med Surg 1987;2:257–265.)

Pathophysiology

The most common cause of simple intestinal obstruction is foreign body ingestion.[65] Distention of the bowel orad to the obstruction results from accumulation of fluid and gas.[65, 66] Intestinal secretion is stimulated, absorption of fluid is reduced, and GI secretions (salivary, gastric, pancreatic, biliary, and intestinal) accumulate within the lumen. Most of the gas is caused by aerophagia, but some diffuses from blood or is produced by intestinal bacteria. Increased intraluminal pressure leads to capillary and lymphatic stasis, bowel wall edema, abdominal effusion, and bowel wall ischemia.[65, 66] Devitalization can lead to peritonitis.[66] The small bowel responds to distention by increasing neuromuscular activity, which causes cramping and pain.[65] Damage to the normal mucosal barrier allows absorption of bacteria and toxins into the systemic circulation. Fluid loss from vomiting and sequestration of fluid within the bowel lead to severe dehydration, which can progress to hypovolemic shock.[66] Hypochloremia, hyponatremia, hypokalemia, and metabolic acidosis frequently develop.[65]

Strangulated obstructions occur less frequently and are most commonly seen with intussusceptions, intestinal volvulus, and incarcerated bowel in diaphragmatic, inguinal, or abdominal hernias or mesenteric rents.[65, 68–70] The pathophysiologic changes relate to the degree of vascular compromise: partial venous, complete venous, or complete arterial occlusion.[65] Strangulation of intestinal blood supply results in severe damage to the bowel wall and, eventually, necrosis. Severe blood loss into the lumen can occur.[66] Massive bacterial overgrowth occurs within the strangulated portion of bowel. Endotoxin released from *Escherichia coli* and exotoxin from *C. perfringens* cause severe hypotension.[65, 66] Abdominal fluid accumulates with high concentrations of bacteria and toxins.[66] Reperfusion injury and generation of oxygen-derived free radicals can contribute to the pathophysiology after relief of the obstruction.[65]

Clinical Signs

Vomiting, abdominal pain, anorexia, and depression are the most common clinical signs with proximal (high) simple obstruction.[66, 67] Severe dehydration (delayed capillary refill time, enophthalmos, decreased skin turgor, tachycardia, pale mucous membranes, and cold extremities) can rapidly progress to hypovolemic shock (tachycardia and weak peripheral pulses).[33, 34, 65] Animals may have a history of potential foreign body ingestion. Abdominal palpation may detect a dilated segment of intestine or an intestinal mass. Clinical signs develop more slowly in animals with a distal (low) simple obstruction.[66, 67] Anorexia and lethargy may be the only initial signs.[65]

Clinical signs develop more rapidly in animals with strangulated obstructions. However, partial venous obstruction, as occurs in most intussusceptions, can mimic simple obstruction. With complete venous or arterial obstruction, abdominal pain, vomiting (sometimes hematemesis), abdominal bloating, hematochezia, recumbence, collapse, and death can occur within 12 hours.[68–70]

Diagnostic Plan

Most patients with complete intestinal obstruction present with acute life-threatening vomiting and abdominal pain (see Chap. 31). The diagnosis of obstruction can be confirmed with radiography. Survey radiographs may demonstrate dilation of the small intestine proximal to the obstruction, with gas and fluid (see Fig. 32–2).[47] A radiopaque foreign body may be present. If the degree of bowel distention is only moderate and a definitive diagnosis cannot be reached, an upper GI contrast study can be performed. Movement of contrast ends abruptly at the obstruction.[47, 71] After administration of fluid therapy to correct fluid, electrolyte, and acid-base derangement, exploratory surgery should be performed to relieve the obstruction.[65, 66]

If vomiting is not severe, the predominant clinical sign may be abdominal pain (see Chap. 33). The intestinal obstruction can be identified by palpation of the abdomen and radiographic studies. The diagnostic plan should be carried out as rapidly as possible in animals that are rapidly deteriorating, because these patients could have a strangulating obstruction.

Hypoproteinemia

Low serum protein can be caused by hypoalbuminemia, hypoglobulinemia, or both. Low serum protein and anemia occur with hemorrhage. The most common causes of hypoproteinemia without anemia are PLE, protein-losing nephropathy, and liver disease. Protein loss into the GI tract as a result of PLE differs from the other two mechanisms because it leads to a panhypoproteinemia, loss of both albumin and globulins.[72] PLE is not a specific disease but rather a syndrome that accompanies many GI disorders that primarily cause small bowel diarrhea but may on occasion cause vomiting, large bowel diarrhea, or no GI signs.

Pathophysiology

The GI tract is a site for plasma protein catabolism.[73] Proteins leak through large fenestrations in capillaries into the mucosa and the intestinal lumen.[74] Protein digestion and absorption of peptides and amino acids occur, and the components are used to synthesize new proteins in the liver. If mucosal permeability is increased because of disease, protein loss can exceed the intestine's ability to reassimilate the protein, resulting in fecal loss. If mucosal disease is severe, producing malabsorption, fecal protein loss is even greater. If loss exceeds the liver's ability to increase synthesis, hypoalbuminemia develops. Lymphangiectasia, with dilation and possibly rupture of lacteals, can accompany disorders causing increased intestinal permeability or can occur without other lesions. Lymphangiectasia causes loss of proteins, cholesterol, and lymphocytes into the bowel lumen.[75]

Normal levels of albumin are necessary to maintain serum osmotic pressure. If albumin declines to 1.5 g/dL or less, edema, ascites, and pleural effusion can develop.

Clinical Signs

The clinical signs associated with hypoproteinemia relate to the underlying cause and the severity of the hypoalbuminemia. In cases of PLE, acute or chronic small bowel diarrhea and weight loss are most common, although vomiting and large bowel diarrhea can occasionally occur.[72, 76] Abdominal palpation may detect an intestinal mass, dilated loop of bowel, or thickened bowel wall. Hypocalcemia, hypocholesterolemia, and lymphopenia may be present. In some cases, GI signs are very mild or do not occur.[74] In protein-losing nephropathy (see Chap. 16), polyuria and polydipsia, weight loss, lethargy, or decreased appetite may be evident; however, in many cases only the manifestations of the hypoalbuminemia occur. Decreased synthesis of albumin as a result of liver disease (see Chap. 34) is always accompanied by other signs, such as decreased appetite, lethargy, weight loss, vomiting, diarrhea, polyuria and polydipsia, encephalopathy, ascites, icterus, microhepatia or hepatomegaly, and hemorrhage. If hemorrhage is the cause of hypoalbuminemia, pale mucous membranes, a cardiac murmur, a source of bleeding, melena, hematochezia, or hematuria may be detected.

Regardless of the cause, hypoalbuminemia can lead to dyspnea and muffled heart and lung sounds (pleural effusion); cough, dyspnea, and crackles (pulmonary edema); abdominal distention (ascites); or subcutaneous edema (Fig. 32–4).[74, 76] Because a portion of serum calcium is bound to albumin, hypocalcemia is often present.[72] In most cases, ionized calcium remains normal and clinical signs of hypocalcemia do not occur. The adjusted calcium level in dogs is often normal after one of several correction formulas is applied: measured calcium − serum albumin + 3.5.[77] This formula is not appropriate for cats.[78]

Diagnostic Plan

If hypoproteinemia and anemia are present, hemorrhage should be suspected. Occult sources, such as the GI and urinary tracts, should be investigated by looking for melena and hematuria. Obvious external sources of hemorrhage can easily be identified. If panhypoproteinemia (without anemia) occurs along with diarrhea, the diagnostic plan for acute or chronic small bowel diarrhea should be followed.[74] Because of the severity of the problem (hypoproteinemia), a diagnosis must be reached rapidly, and there is no time for a dietary trial. Occasionally, large bowel diarrhea or vomiting is present without small bowel diarrhea, and the diagnostic plans for these problems should be followed. If there are no GI signs and hypoalbuminemia and normal serum globulins are present, primary attention should be directed to liver or kidney diseases (see Chaps. 16 and 34).[74, 76] If proteinuria is found, a urine protein/creatinine ratio should be obtained. Abnormally high values should be followed by renal biopsy. If signs or biochemical evidence of hepatic

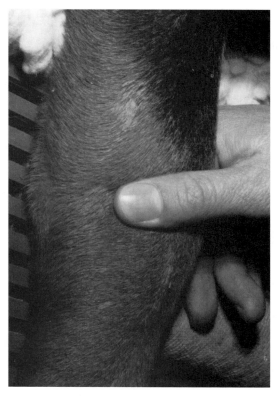

Figure 32-4
Pitting edema in the distal limb in a dog with hypoalbuminemia caused by protein-losing gastroenteropathy.

disease occurs, serum bile acids or ammonia concentrations should be assessed. Abnormal hepatic function should be followed by biopsy. If liver function appears adequate and proteinuria is not present, the plan for chronic small bowel diarrhea should be followed, because some patients with PLE have mild diarrhea or normal-appearing feces.

Melena

Melena is the presence of digested blood in the stool; it causes a dark, tarry, and sticky appearance. It is usually caused by bleeding into the stomach or small intestine. Vomiting (hematemesis), diarrhea, or both often accompany melena. Abdominal pain may be present. If blood loss is acute and severe, signs of hypovolemic shock may be present. If hemorrhage occurs slowly, weakness, depression, and anorexia are often present. Initially, a regenerative anemia is present, but with continued loss of iron into the GI tract a microcytic, hypochromic, nonregenerative anemia develops.[79]

A diagnosis in most cases of melena can be reached by pursuing either acute or chronic vomiting or acute or chronic diarrhea. Animals with mild or no vomiting or diarrhea should be evaluated for a coagulopathy by measurement of the platelet count and prothrombin and partial thromboplastin times. If a coagulopathy is not present, following the diagnostic plans for vomiting or diarrhea usually facilitates a diagnosis. If a diagnosis still cannot be made, the blood may be originating from an oral, nasopharyngeal, or pulmonary lesion. In these cases, other clinical signs such as dysphagia, sneezing, nasal discharge, gagging, or coughing are usually present.

Hematochezia

Hematochezia is the presence of bright red blood in the feces. It is often associated with large bowel diarrhea and tenesmus.[23, 25] Diagnosis can be reached by following the plan for acute or chronic large bowel diarrhea.

Sometimes hematochezia occurs along with formed feces. Excess fecal mucus and tenesmus often occur. These animals often have disease of the rectum (polyps, malignant tumors, or proctitis), and diagnosis can be made by proctoscopic examination and biopsy.[25] Some lesions of anal sacculitis or perianal fistula may bleed onto normal feces as they are passed. Careful physical examination reveals the diagnosis. Rarely, a coagulopathy or strangulated intestinal obstruction may be present.[69, 70, 80]

Tenesmus

Tenesmus, or straining to defecate, often accompanies large bowel diarrhea.[23, 25] Inflammation from rectal disease stimulates the defecation reflex even when the colon is practically empty. Diagnosis can be made by pursuing the diagnostic plan for acute or chronic large bowel diarrhea. Tenesmus, hematochezia, and excess fecal mucus can occur along with formed feces. These animals often have disease of the rectum (polyps, malignant tumors, proctitis, or foreign body), and diagnosis can be made by proctoscopic examination and biopsy.[25] Tenesmus can also be caused by anal sacculitis, perianal fistula, perineal hernia, or perirectal abscess or neoplasia. Diagnosis can be made after careful physical examination.

Tenesmus can also be associated with disorders causing constipation.[81, 82] In these cases, the cause of tenesmus can be determined by following the diagnostic plan for constipation.

Owners may confuse tenesmus with dysuria. Abdominal palpation may reveal a distended bladder. Rectal examination eliminates the presence of diarrhea or constipation. Further diagnosis requires survey abdominal radiographs, a contrast urethrogram, and passage of a urinary catheter (see Chap. 17).

Ascites, Pleural Effusion, and Subcutaneous Edema

Ascites and pleural effusion, the accumulation of fluid within the abdomen and pleural space, and subcutaneous edema (see Fig. 32–4 and Chap. 43) occur in animals with diseases of the intestines caused by PLE and resultant hypoalbuminemia. Fluid analysis reveals a pure transudate. The serum albumin level is usually less than 1.5 g/dL. In most cases, signs of small bowel diarrhea are present. Pleural effusion may be severe enough to cause dyspnea (see Chap. 53).

Constipation

Constipation can be defined as absent or infrequent defecation.[83, 84] Feces are usually hard and dry. Defecation is often associated with tenesmus (straining) or dyschezia (difficulty). It occurs commonly in small animals. Most cases are acute, have easily identifiable causes, and can be managed simply. Chronic cases are more difficult to manage and can result in stretching of the colon and irreversible loss of motility (megacolon). Obstipation is defined as intractable constipation, in which defecation cannot occur.[83, 84]

Pathophysiology

Constipation can be caused by any disorder that delays the passage of feces through the colon (Table 32–6).[81, 83–86] Regardless of the cause, the longer feces remain within the large intestine, the harder and drier they become, making defecation more difficult.[82–84] Chronic distention from any cause can result in stretching of the colon and reduction or irreversible loss of motility (megacolon).[82, 83]

Retention of feces may result from intraluminal or extraluminal obstruction, suppression of the defecation reflex because of pain or lack of appropriate environmental conditions, neurologic disease, administration of motility-altering drugs, or, rarely, metabolic conditions (the most common being dehydration).

Clinical Signs

Absent or infrequent defecation associated with tenesmus, dyschezia, and the production of hard, dry feces is characteristic of constipation. Small volumes of watery feces, sometimes with mucus and blood, may be passed during episodes of tenesmus.[82–84] This results from inflammation associated with the impacted fecal mass. Moderately or severely affected animals are depressed, lethargic, anorexic, in pain, and dehydrated, and they may vomit or be pyrexic.[82, 83] The abdomen may appear distended. Abdominal palpation usually reveals a large, hard, tubular mass.[84, 86] Rectal examination often elicits pain and identifies hard feces or foreign material. Rectal examination may also

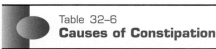

Table 32–6
Causes of Constipation

Dietary and Environmental
Bones
Hair
Foreign material: rocks, cloth, cat litter
Inadequate water intake
Dirty litterbox
Inadequate defecation opportunity or location
Prolonged inactivity
Changes in daily routine

Painful Defecation
Anorectal disease

    Anal sacculitis or abscess
    Perianal fistula
    Proctitis
    Perianal dermatitis
    Perianal soft tissue injury
Orthopedic

    Pelvic injury or fracture
    Spinal column injury or fracture
    Pelvic limb injury or fracture

Mechanical Obstruction
Extraluminal

    Prostatomegaly
    Sublumbar lymphadenopathy
    Healed malaligned pelvic fracture
    Perianal neoplasia
    Perineal hernia
    Atresia ani
Intraluminal
    Neoplasia
    Stricture
    Foreign body

Neurologic
Spinal cord disease
Idiopathic megacolon
Dysautonomia

Drugs
Anticholinergics
Antihistamines
Barium sulfate
Diuretics
Opiates
Aluminum hydroxide
Iron

Metabolic
Dehydration
Hypokalemia
Hypothyroidism

detect pelvic fractures, perineal hernia, prostatomegaly, sublumbar lymphadenopathy, or other intrapelvic mass.[81, 85] Perianal disorders may be obvious but can be missed in an animal that is uncooperative and in pain. Routine laboratory evaluation may reveal an increased hematocrit and total protein (dehydration), leukocytosis, or electrolyte abnormalities (hypokalemia, hyponatremia, and hypochloremia).[86]

Diagnostic Plan

Animals with mild signs presenting with their first episode do not require in-depth evaluation. Usually, an obvious cause can be identified (e.g., dietary indiscretion, hair balls, perianal disorders, neurologic disorders, pelvic fractures). Further diagnostic evaluation and treatment depend on the abnormality identified. If a precipitating cause cannot be found, symptomatic therapy often alleviates clinical signs (see Megacolon).

Constipation in animals with moderate or severe clinical signs or recurrent episodes deserves more complete evaluation. These patients often need vigorous treatment with intravenous (IV) fluids and breakdown of the fecal impaction (see Megacolon) while diagnostic tests are being performed. A complete blood count, biochemical profile, and urinalysis should be performed to evaluate electrolyte aberration and the severity of dehydration.[83] Abdominal radiographs should be made to assess the degree of colonic distention, determine the presence of foreign material, identify a localized area of obstruction, or identify malaligned pelvic fractures (Fig. 32–5).[81, 86] A complete neurologic examination should be performed to identify any subtle spinal cord deficits.[81] Colonoscopy may be indicated to evaluate an area of localized obstruction seen on radiographs.[81, 82] A diagnosis of idiopathic megacolon requires demonstration of persistence or return of the severe colonic distention after evacuation of feces and appropriate symptomatic care.

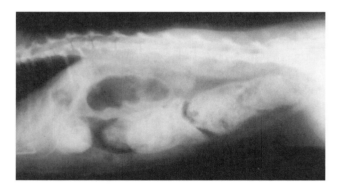

Figure 32–5
Lateral survey abdominal radiograph of a cat with idiopathic megacolon. A very distended, feces-filled colon is evident. (From Leib MS, Matz ME. Diseases of the large intestine. In: Ettinger SJ, Feldman EC, eds. Textbook of Veterinary Internal Medicine. Philadelphia, WB Saunders, 1995:1232–1260.)

Abdominal Pain

Abdominal pain (see Chap. 33) commonly occurs with many intestinal diseases. However, it is not a specific sign and can be caused by diseases of any of the abdominal viscera, the parietal peritoneum, or abdominal wall.[87] In addition, pain from extra-abdominal locations, such as intervertebral disc disease, can also mimic abdominal pain. Intestinal diseases should be considered possible causes of abdominal pain if vomiting, diarrhea, or constipation is a prominent clinical sign.

Mild abdominal pain may be associated with acute enteritis caused by dietary indiscretion. Intestinal disorders associated with moderate to severe abdominal pain include intestinal obstruction (foreign body, intussusception, neoplasia), parvoviral infection, peritonitis (penetrating intestinal foreign body, ruptured intestinal neoplasia, perforating duodenal ulcer, linear foreign body), hemorrhagic gastroenteritis, whipworm infection, irritable bowel syndrome, and megacolon.[32, 38, 45, 65, 88–93]

Diagnostic Procedures

Routine Laboratory Evaluation

A complete blood count, biochemical profile, and urinalysis rarely identify a specific intestinal disorder but can help to rank the differential diagnoses, provide information on the severity of the disorder, guide fluid therapy, and help assess the overall health of the patient. Anemia may be caused by GI blood loss from erosive or ulcerative conditions, or it may be associated with chronic inflammatory disease. Hemorrhage initially causes a regenerative anemia, which can become nonregenerative (microcytic and hypochromic) because of iron loss. The anemia associated with chronic inflammatory disease is nonregenerative. An elevated hematocrit can occur because of dehydration or in cases of hemorrhagic gastroenteritis. Hypoproteinemia can occur as a result of GI hemorrhage or PLE (see Hypoproteinemia). Neutrophilia can accompany inflammatory bowel disease, GI neoplasia, duodenal ulceration, and bacterial infection. Neutropenia is commonly seen with canine or feline parvovirus and may occur with *Salmonella* infection. Lymphopenia may be found in patients with parvovirus, lymphangiectasia, or *Salmonella* infection. Eosinophilia occurs with GI parasites or eosinophilic enterocolitis and in some cases of plasmacytic lymphocytic enterocolitis (PLEC).

Elevations in serum liver enzymes (alanine aminotransferase and alkaline phosphatase) occur with inflammatory bowel disease and GI lymphosarcoma (with liver involvement). Hypercalcemia can be found in cases of anal sac adenocarcinoma. Hypocalcemia can occur with hypoalbuminemia. In most cases, a normal adjusted value for calcium is present (see Hypoproteinemia). However, lymphangiectasia can cause true hypocalcemia.

Fecal Examination

Fecal examination is simple, quick, inexpensive, and one of the most important diagnostic procedures to perform when evaluating disorders of the intestines. Examination of a fresh fecal saline smear may yield a diagnosis in some cases. Several drops of saline can be applied to a fresh thin fecal smear, a coverslip added, and the slide examined microscopically. Motile trophozoites of *Giardia* can be identified from a saline smear.[94] In addition, large numbers of highly motile corkscrew-shaped bacteria may indicate an infection with *Campylobacter* spp. A fecal culture should be submitted to confirm this diagnosis.

Zinc sulfate fecal flotation is the most accurate and practical fecal flotation test available to identify *Giardia* cysts.[37, 94-96] In addition, eggs of common parasites can also be found. Approximately 2 g of feces are mixed with 15 mL of a 33% solution of zinc sulfate and strained. The tube is filled with additional zinc sulfate and centrifuged for 3 to 5 minutes at 1500 rpm. If a free-swinging head centrifuge is available, additional zinc sulfate is added to create a meniscus, and the tube is covered with a coverslip. The coverslip can be transferred to a microscope slide for examination after centrifugation. If a fixed-head centrifuge is used, the surface layer of fluid can be transferred to a microscope slide with the bottom of a small glass blood or serum tube, pipette, or bacteriologic loop.[37] The microscope slide is then examined.

Examination of a rectal cytology specimen may yield a diagnosis. A gloved finger can be scraped across the rectal mucosa and gently rolled along a microscope slide. The slide is air dried, stained with Wright stain, and examined microscopically. A normal rectal cytology specimen should contain colonic epithelial cells and a mixed population of bacteria. An increased number of neutrophils suggests the presence of inflammatory or infectious disease and warrants culturing of feces. Eosinophils may be found in cases of eosinophilic enterocolitis. On occasion, clumps of neoplastic cells or *Histoplasma* organisms within macrophages are found (Fig. 32–6). Numerous safety pin–shaped spores support a diagnosis of *Clostridium perfringens* enterotoxicosis (see Fig. 32–1).[42] A large population of sea gull–shaped bacteria may be indicative of a *Campylobacter* infection.

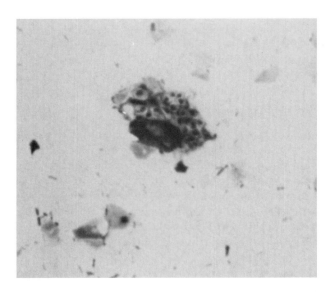

Figure 32-6
Rectal cytology specimen from a dog showing *Histoplasma* organisms within the cytoplasm of a macrophage. (From Leib MS, Matz ME. Diseases of the large intestine. In: Ettinger SJ, Feldman EC, eds. Textbook of Veterinary Internal Medicine. Philadelphia, WB Saunders, 1995:1232–1260.)

Radiography

Survey Radiography

Although survey abdominal radiographs may be normal in many intestinal disorders, abnormalities can be detected. Poor intra-abdominal detail may be present because of lack of intra-abdominal fat or presence of ascites.[15, 97] Dilation of bowel with gas or fluid occurs orad to a partial or complete small intestinal obstruction (see Fig. 32–2). Linear foreign bodies result in plication of intestines (Fig. 32–7).[47, 88] In addition, a radiopaque foreign body, neoplastic or granulomatous masses, or sublumbar lymphadenopathy can be identified.[98] Gas within the bowel lumen may allow identification of intramural masses, a thickened bowel wall, or intestinal compression.[99-101] A dilated, feces-filled colon is present in patients with constipation or megacolon (see Fig. 32–5).[102] Extraluminal compression of the colon caused by pelvic fractures may be seen.[85]

Contrast Radiography

Endoscopic examination of the duodenum and colon greatly reduces the need to perform contrast examination of the intestines. However, an upper GI series is indicated if a partial or complete intestinal obstruction is suspected but cannot be definitively diagnosed from survey radiographs. If an obstruction is present, contrast examination may demonstrate delayed small bowel transit, a radiolucent foreign body, intussusception, or eccentric or annular narrowing of the bowel lumen.[47, 71, 100] An upper GI series is also indicated if endoscopic examination of the small intestine has not resulted in a diagnosis in a vomiting patient. Enteritis may be associated with smudging of the contrast-mucosa interface, flocculation of barium, and rapid transport.[47] Intramural masses (not associated with partial or complete obstructions) appear as lucent filling defects in the barium.[47] Intestinal ulcers result in adherence and penetration of contrast medium into a mucosal defect.[47] Pseudoulcers occur in dogs and appear as regular outpouchings of barium in the descending duodenum, caused by filling of normal lymphoid follicles (Peyer's patches) (Fig. 32–8).[47, 97]

An upper GI series is often performed in conjunction with a gastrogram (see Chap. 31). Preparation of the animal includes withholding of food for 12 hours and removal of feces from the colon with enemas. Survey radiographs should always be made to determine correct radiographic technique and to ensure adequate preparation.[47] Ten to 12 mL/kg of 30% micronized barium sulfate should be administered through an orogastric tube.[47] In dogs, lateral and ventrodorsal radiographs should be made at 0, 15, 30, 60, 120, 180, and 240 minutes, or until barium has reached the colon. Transit in cats is much faster, and radiographs should be made at 0, 15, 30, and 60 minutes. Barium should reach the colon within 3 to 4 hours in dogs and often in 1 hour in cats.[47, 100] Peristaltic contractions of the duodenum are prominent in cats and should not be misdiagnosed as indicating a linear foreign body.[47] The normal diameter of the small bowel is 1 to 2 rib-widths in dogs and approximately 12 mm in cats.[47]

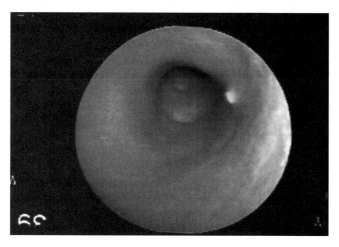

Figure 32–8
Endoscopic appearance of the normal duodenum in a dog. The mucosa is slightly granular. The white mass at the 10 o'clock position is the major duodenal papilla. Two smooth, depressed areas in the center of the photograph are Peyer's patches.

Complete barium enema is indicated in cases in which (1) luminal narrowing of the colon prohibits passage of an endoscope, (2) only a rigid endoscope is available and examination of the descending colon is normal, (3) abdominal palpation or survey radiographs identify a mural or extramural mass associated with the colon and the mucosa is found to be normal on endoscopic examination, or (4) an ileocolic intussusception is suspected. Abnormalities detected with barium enema include mural masses, extramural colonic compression, intussusceptions, strictures, and severe mucosal irregularities associated with inflammatory bowel disease.[47, 100]

For a complete barium enema examination, patients should be prepared in a similar manner as for flexible colonoscopy. Heavy sedation or general anesthesia is necessary. Narcotic premedication should be avoided because of its spasmogenic properties. Survey radiographs should always be made to determine correct radiographic technique and to ensure adequate preparation.[47] An inflatable cuffed catheter should be positioned with the balloon inflated in the distal rectum. Premixed, micronized barium sulfate, 11 to 33 mL/kg, should be infused slowly with the dog in left lateral recumbence.[47] After 65% of the barium has been given, the animal should be positioned in right lateral recumbence to fill the transverse and ascending colons and cecum. A radiograph can be taken to check the extent of colonic filling. The barium should distend the entire colon and cecum but should not enter the small intestine, because superimposition of the small intestine on the colon can make evaluation difficult.

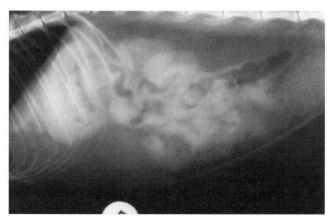

Figure 32–7
Lateral survey abdominal radiograph from a cat with a linear small intestinal foreign body. The small bowel is plicated and bunched within the abdomen.

Multiple exposures should be made, including left lateral, ventrodorsal, and left and right ventrodorsal oblique views. In some cases, removal of as much barium as possible and addition of an equivalent volume of room air creates a double contrast study that may enhance the detection of subtle mucosal lesions.[101] If colonic perforation is suspected, a 15% to 20% concentration of water-soluble, organic iodide contrast medium should be substituted for barium.[97]

A small amount of barium or room air can be instilled into the rectum and descending colon to help delineate changes seen on survey radiographs. This is much simpler to perform than a complete barium enema and can help evaluate the location of the colon, the relation of extraluminal masses to the colon, and the presence of intramural masses and strictures.

Ultrasonography

The diagnostic utility of ultrasonographic evaluation of the intestines has only recently been explored.[46, 103–106] The limiting factor is the presence of air within the intestines. Assessment of wall thickness and symmetry, identification of wall layers and intraluminal contents, frequency of peristalsis, and examination of regional lymph nodes or other abdominal organs are possible.[103] Bowel wall thickness of 5 mm or more (normal 2–3 mm) is highly indicative of disease.[103] Diffuse thickening of the bowel wall is usually associated with an inflammatory process, whereas neoplasia is most often characterized by localized and asymmetrical wall thickening.[46, 104] Intussusception is readily identified by a multilayered series of concentric rings.[46] Ultrasound-guided fine-needle aspirate and biopsies of lesions can be performed safely.[105, 106] Intestinal foreign bodies and obstructions can be identified.[46]

D-Xylose Absorption

D-Xylose absorption is the most commonly used quantitative test to characterize small intestinal carbohydrate absorption in dogs.[57, 58] It is not a valuable test in cats because absorption is too variable in normal cats.[107, 108] D-Xylose is a 5-carbon monosaccharide that is absorbed by the jejunum, not metabolized, and excreted by the kidney. It is a simple test to perform. After the dog is fasted for 12 to 18 hours, 500 mg/kg of a 5% solution of D-xylose is administered by orogastric intubation. Serum samples are obtained at 0, 30, 60, 90, 120, and 180 minutes. Serum D-xylose levels can be measured at most commercial laboratories. Normal dogs should have values greater than 45 mg/dL at 60 minutes.

D-Xylose absorption is not a sensitive test; animals with malabsorption can have normal D-xylose results.[49, 109–113] However, dogs with decreased D-xylose absorption often have moderate or severe malabsorption.[111, 114, 115] Delayed gastric emptying, ascites, bacterial overgrowth, and impaired intestinal circulation can lead to falsely low D-xylose levels.[17, 116] Animals with renal disease can have falsely high D-xylose values.

Plasma Turbidity

Lipid assimilation can easily be tested with the plasma turbidity test. After an overnight fast, a hematocrit tube is evaluated to ensure that the serum is clear. Two to 3 mL/kg of corn oil should be administered. Most animals readily drink the oil. Hematocrit tubes should be collected at 1, 2, 3, and 4 hours for lipemia. If lipemia is present, adequate digestion and absorption of fat has occurred. In dogs, if the test is negative, the corn oil should be preincubated with 2 to 3 teaspoons of pancreatic enzymes for 30 minutes and the test repeated. If the second test remains negative, malabsorption of lipid has occurred. If lipemia develops, pancreatic exocrine insufficiency may be present (see Chap. 33). Because this is a qualitative test, there may be only subtle differences between a negative and a positive result. Serum triglycerides can be measured before and after administration of oil. A large increase in triglyceride content indicates adequate assimilation of fat.

Vitamin B_{12} and Folate

Measurement of serum vitamin B_{12} (cobalamin) and folic acid concentration can be beneficial in the diagnosis of bacterial overgrowth of the small intestine. The increased numbers of bacteria bind and metabolize vitamin B_{12} and produce additional folic acid, which can be absorbed by the host, resulting in decreased serum B_{12} levels and increased folic acid levels in blood.[17, 56, 116, 117] However, small intestinal bacterial overgrowth can occur in the presence of normal serum concentration of cobalamin or folate, or both.[16] Normal values vary depending on the laboratory. When assayed by competitive binding, normal values in one laboratory are cobalamin, 300 to 800 ng/L, and folate, 7.5 to 17.5 μg/L.[56]

Cobalamin is a water-soluble vitamin that is plentiful in canine diets.[56] The absorption of cobalamin is complex and involves multiple steps. In the small intestine, free cobalamin is bound to intrinsic factor, and absorption of the complex occurs in the distal small intestine.[56] Folate is also a water-soluble vitamin abundant in canine diets. It is absorbed after binding to specific carriers in the proximal small intestine.[56]

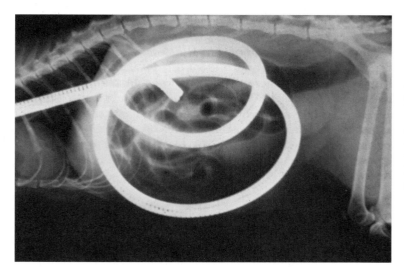

Figure 32-9
Lateral survey abdominal radiograph of a cat showing advancement of the endoscope into the orad jejunum. (From Leib MS. Gastrointestinal endoscopy. In: August JR, ed. Consultations in Feline Internal Medicine 2. Philadelphia, WB Saunders, 1994:119–126.)

Endoscopic Examination

Endoscopic examination of the small intestine and colon are extremely useful diagnostic procedures in dogs and cats with intestinal diseases.

Enteroscopy

Endoscopic examination of the small intestine is a minimally invasive method of obtaining tissue samples for histopathologic evaluation. It offers advantages over exploratory surgery in hypoproteinemic patients, in which delayed healing of surgical incisions and dehiscence can occur. An aspirate of duodenal contents can be collected for identification of *Giardia* trophozoites.[37, 118] Instrumentation, patient preparation, and restraint are similar to that described in Chapters 30 and 31.

As the endoscope advances past the pylorus, an acute directional change is encountered; this is the cranial duodenal flexure, which is the junction with the descending duodenum. The major duodenal papilla occurs in this area and is often better seen as the endoscope is withdrawn (see Fig. 32–8). In addition, the minor duodenal papilla can be seen several centimeters distal in some cases. To enter the descending duodenum, the tip of the endoscope should be deflected, torque applied to the insertion tube, air insufflated, and the endoscope gently advanced. The duodenal mucosa slides across the lens of the endoscope for 2 to 3 cm. The tip can then be centralized within the lumen of the duodenum by adjustment of the control knobs. As long as mucosa is seen sliding across the lens equidistant to the length of endoscope inserted, it is safe to perform this maneuver. However, if the insertion tube is advanced and the endoscope tip does not move a corresponding distance, the maneuver

should be discontinued, the endoscope withdrawn, and the lumen visualized before further advancement. If sufficient insertion tube length is still available after the descending duodenum has been entered, the endoscope can be advanced to the caudal duodenal flexure and into the ascending duodenum, as previously described. In small dogs and cats, it is possible to continue advancing the endoscope into the orad jejunum. The junction between the ascending duodenum and orad jejunum is indistinct.

The normal small intestinal mucosa is granular, pale pink, and more friable than that of the stomach or esophagus. In dogs, multiple Peyer's patches can often be seen as depressed areas (1–2 cm) along the descending duodenum (see Fig. 32–8). They should not be confused with duodenal ulcers, which are not covered by epithelium and are not as uniform in appearance as Peyer's patches. Examination of the mucosa and procurement of biopsy and cytologic samples (described in Chap. 30) are performed as the endoscope is withdrawn. A duodenal aspirate for *Giardia* can be obtained by flushing 10 mL of saline through polyethylene tubing placed in the biopsy channel and aspirating with a syringe. The fluid can be centrifuged and the sediment evaluated for motile trophozoites.[118, 119]

The biggest difference between dogs and cats is the small diameter of the feline duodenum, which provides less room for maneuvering the endoscope.[120] Cats differ from dogs in having only a single duodenal papilla that transports both bile and pancreatic secretions. Peyer's patches are not seen endoscopically in cats. The jejunum can be reached in most cats (Fig. 32–9). A smaller-diameter endoscope (<8 mm) may facilitate entering the duodenum, and subsequently the jejunum, if difficulty is encountered with larger endoscopes.[121]

Colonoscopy

Instrumentation, Patient Preparation, and Restraint

Because many colonic diseases diffusely affect the large intestine, examination with a rigid endoscope, which allows visualization of the descending colon, can retrieve diagnostic tissue samples in approximately 80% of cases. Examination of the transverse colon, ascending colon, and cecum requires a more expensive flexible endoscope (described in Chap. 30).

Rigid proctosigmoidoscopes are inexpensive, easy to use, and available in a variety of diameters.[59, 122] The 9-mm endoscopes are useful in small dogs and cats. Rigid biopsy forceps allow procurement of large tissue samples. Mucosal visualization and forceps maneuverability are attenuated with rigid equipment, compared to flexible endoscopes.

Preparation of the descending colon for rigid examination is relatively easy. Food should be withheld for 12 to 24 hours, and two or three warm-water enemas (20 mL/kg) should be administered. The enema tube should be well lubricated and premeasured from the anus to the 13th rib. Examination of the colon with a flexible endoscope requires more extensive preparation. Mucosal surfaces must be free of fecal material, and a clear ileal effluent should be present.[59] Food should be withheld for 24 to 36 hours. Use of a GI lavage solution greatly improves colonic evacuation.[123, 124] We administer two doses of 66 mL/kg GoLYTELY in dogs (33 mL/kg in cats) 2 hours apart during the afternoon before a morning endoscopy. GI lavage solutions must be administered by orogastric intubation in dogs and nasoesophageal intubation in cats. A warm-water enema, 20 mL/kg, should accompany each GoLYTELY dose, and a third enema should be given in the morning before endoscopy. Administration of metoclopramide, 0.2–0.4 mg/kg subcutaneously, 30 minutes before the first GoLYTELY dose reduces the frequency of vomiting.

Patients experience little discomfort when the descending colon is examined with rigid endoscopes because minimal stretching of mesenteric attachments occurs. Patients can be tranquilized (acepromazine, 0.05 mg/kg intramuscularly) or lightly sedated (oxymorphone, 0.05 mg/kg intravenously) along with physical restraint.

Flexible colonoscopy requires the use of heavy sedation or general anesthesia.[59, 122, 125] Passage of the endoscope into the transverse and ascending colon and into the cecum causes stretching of mesenteric attachments and pain. We have found that narcotic premedications increase colonic tone, allowing the cecum to be reached more efficiently.

Procedure

Rigid Colonoscopy. Rigid colonoscopy can be performed with the dog in sternal or right lateral recumbence.[59, 122, 125] Before insertion of the endoscope, a digital rectal examination should be performed to rule out the presence of an obstruction or diverticulum into which placement of the endoscope could lead to perforation. Rigid endoscopes have a smooth obturator that should be inserted into the endoscope to assist advancement through the anal sphincters into the rectum. The tip of the endoscope should be well lubricated. The obturator should be removed, the viewing lens tightly closed over the end of the endoscope, and the endoscope advanced slowly under direct visualization. Distention of the colon with air with the hand-operated insufflator assists advancement. The rigid endoscope should be advanced as far as possible into the descending colon. The mucosa is carefully evaluated as the endoscope is slowly withdrawn.

To obtain biopsies with a rigid endoscope, the tip of the endoscope should be placed approximately 1 cm from the area to be sampled. The viewing lens is removed, allowing the colon to collapse as air moves out through the open end of the endoscope. The area to be biopsied should be visible at the tip of the endoscope. A rectal or uterine biopsy forceps is advanced through the endoscope and opened, and the area to be biopsied is gently grasped. Care must be taken to grasp only mucosa and submucosa with these forceps, to prevent perforation of the colonic wall. Before the tissue is broken off, the biopsy forceps should be moved gently back and forth. If only mucosa and submucosa have been grasped, the tissue should be freely moveable. If the grasped tissue remains firmly attached to the colonic wall, the forceps may have gathered muscular tunics, and colonic perforation is possible. The forceps should be opened, and a new site, at least 1 to 2 cm distant, should be selected. Samples should be collected from all abnormal areas and from the orad, middle, and distal descending colons.

Flexible Colonoscopy. Flexible colonoscopy allows evaluation of the entire colon and cecum.[59, 122, 125] The anesthetized dog is positioned in left lateral recumbence. After a digital rectal examination has ruled out abnormalities, the endoscope tip is inserted into the rectum. An assistant digitally tightens the perianal tissue around the endoscope to improve the seal and allow insufflated air to distend the colon. The endoscope is advanced only when the lumen is clearly visible. Blind advancement of the endoscope can lead to colonic trauma and possibly to perforation. The distal colon in dogs contains a large amount of mucosal folding, which can make this area difficult to traverse.

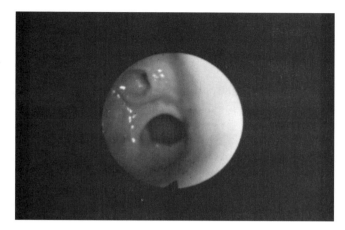

Figure 32–10
Endoscopic appearance of the normal ileocecocolic junction in a dog. The cecocolic sphincter is in the center of the photograph. The ileocolic sphincter is at the 10 o'clock position. Both sphincters are wide open. Normally, the cecocolic sphincter is open and the ileocolic sphincter is closed.

After advancement of the flexible endoscope through the descending colon, a fold (at the junction of the transverse colon) is encountered. The tip of the endoscope should be deflected up and advanced slowly through the splenic flexure into the transverse colon. Visualization of the lumen is lost for approximately 1 to 2 cm as the endoscope tip contacts the colonic wall. Visualization returns as the transverse colon is entered and distended with air. During this maneuver, colonic mucosa should be seen sliding across the lens. As long as the tip of the endoscope advances an amount equal to the length of insertion tube advanced, this slide-by technique can be performed safely. However, if the endoscope tip stops advancing, the endoscope should be withdrawn and the maneuver started again. The transverse colon is only 5 to 8 cm long in dogs. Another fold is reached at the orad portion of the transverse colon. The tip of the endoscope must be deflected caudally and slowly advanced past the hepatic flexure into the ascending colon, which is very short in the dog (3–6 cm). The same mucosal slide-by technique used at the entrance to the transverse colon should be performed. The ileocecocolic junction may now be visualized (Fig. 32–10). The cecocolic junction usually appears straight ahead and can be entered. It may be partially opened, or it may appear as a flat sphincter if closed. The endoscope should be advanced into the cecum, which is a spiral structure, 8 to 30 cm in length, until the blind end is reached. The ileocolic sphincter is visible as it enters the ascending colon near the cecocolic sphincter. It often protrudes into the lumen and appears as a thick sphincter. If signs of small bowel diarrhea are present,

the endoscope can be passed into the ileum, and mucosal samples obtained.

Complete evaluation of the colon is performed as the endoscope is slowly withdrawn. The tip of the endoscope should be maneuvered to ensure that the entire circumference of the colonic mucosa is observed. Normal colonic mucosa is pale pink, smooth, and glistening. Submucosal blood vessels should be clearly visible (Fig. 32–11). Scattered lymphoid follicles, 2 to 3 mm in diameter, with umbilicated centers, are commonly seen in the distal colon and cecum. The colonic mucosa normally is tough and resists trauma associated with the endoscope. Multiple biopsies from all abnormal areas and from each segment of the colon should be taken (cecum, ascending colon, transverse colon, and orad, middle, and aborad descending colon). Multiple biopsy samples should always be obtained (see Chap. 30), even if the mucosa appears normal, because histologic abnormalities can be present.[126, 127] Biopsy samples should be obtained as deeply as possible and ideally should include the muscularis mucosae.[128] Examination and biopsy should continue until the endoscope nears the rectum. In dogs weighing more than 10 kg, the flexible endoscope should be retroflexed 180° to allow better visualization of the terminal rectum. This site is often incompletely examined during initial placement of the endoscope.

The major difference encountered with colonoscopy in cats is the small diameter of the colon.[120] This restricts the maneuverability of the endoscope for biopsy procurement. However, biopsy sampling is not difficult so long as the tip of the endoscope is deflected toward the colonic wall and suction is applied to

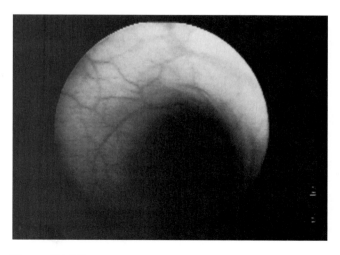

Figure 32–11
Endoscopic appearance of the normal descending colon in a dog. Submucosal blood vessels are clearly visible. The mucosa is smooth and glistening.

partially collapse the mucosa. The rectal folds are not as prominent in cats as they are in dogs. The transverse colon and the ascending colon are shorter in cats than in dogs: 2 to 4 cm and 1 to 2 cm, respectively. The cecum is approximately 1 cm in length. The retroflex view of the distal rectum cannot be obtained in cats.

Common Diseases That Involve Both the Small and Large Intestines

Dietary Indiscretion

Dietary indiscretion can be defined as the consumption of inappropriate foodstuffs.[2] This can encompass a wide variety of causes, including over-consumption of food, abrupt dietary change (even from one high-quality commercial food to another), feeding of table scraps or supplements, and ingestion of garbage. Dogs are more prone to dietary indiscretion than are cats because of their indiscriminate eating habits.

Pathophysiology

There are many possible mechanisms by which dietary indiscretion can lead to diarrhea. Abrupt dietary changes, even to a high-quality diet, do not allow time for brush border enzymes to adapt to a different nutrient profile. The feeding of homemade diets can cause diarrhea because of variations in ingredients or cooking time, by the use of raw egg whites, which contain a trypsin inhibitor, or by overcooking of meat, which can decrease its digestibility.[129]

Diarrhea in cases of garbage-can enterocolitis may be caused by bacterial, fungal, and other toxins, vasoactive amines, large quantities of decomposing and poorly digestible nutrients, indigestible abrasive foreign material, or poisonous plants. Excessive amounts of poorly digestible carbohydrates and fats may overwhelm the small intestine's ability to digest and absorb nutrients. These substances can pass into the large intestine, where colonic bacteria ferment carbohydrates, producing many small, osmotically active molecules that draw water into the lumen of the colon, resulting in diarrhea. Bacterial metabolism of fatty acids results in production of hydroxy fatty acids, which can stimulate colonic secretion, inhibit fluid absorption, and alter motility.[15, 130] Bacterial enterotoxins can also stimulate intestinal secretion. Nondigestible abrasive material can cause intestinal inflammation, alter mucosal surfaces, and result in increased permeability with loss of water, electrolytes, and proteins.

Clinical Signs

Dietary indiscretion is a common cause of vomiting and acute or chronic diarrhea.[25, 130] The diarrhea may have characteristics of either small or large intestinal dysfunction, or both (see Table 32–4).

Diagnostic Plan

Dietary indiscretion should be strongly suspected in any free-roaming dog presenting with diarrhea. In strictly supervised animals, a thorough history may identify the source of indiscretion. Clinical signs of acute diarrhea should promptly resolve after removal of the offending substance and appropriate symptomatic care. However, it may take up to 14 days to see a response in cases of chronic diarrhea. Fecal examination should be performed in all suspected cases to evaluate concurrent parasitism.

Treatment

Food should be withheld for 24 hours and subcutaneous or IV fluids administered if moderate or severe dehydration is present (see treatment of gastritis in Chap. 31). In some cases, it may be beneficial to administer opioids to prolong intestinal transit time, allowing increased fluid absorption and reducing the frequency of diarrhea. However, if toxins or pathogenic bacteria are suspected as being the cause of the diarrhea, opioids should not be used, because they may increase absorption of toxins or allow more time for bacterial proliferation.[131] Opioids act by increasing colonic segmentation, decreasing propulsive peristaltic contractions, increasing fluid absorption, decreasing secretion, and increasing anal tone.[132] Drugs such as loperamide (0.1–0.2 mg/kg, twice [b.i.d.] or four times [q.i.d.] per day) or diphenoxylate (0.05–0.1 mg/kg, b.i.d. to q.i.d.) are very effective in reducing the frequency of diarrhea. Both are available as elixirs, which are convenient for dosing small dogs and cats. Loperamide has been shown to be more potent, and it has a faster onset of action and a longer duration of effect than diphenoxylate. Loperamide does not cross the blood-brain barrier, so addiction is unlikely.[131, 132] At recommended doses, both drugs are safe and have few side effects. In cats, excitatory behavior can occur, but it is rare in our experience.

Normal fecal consistency can often be re-established within 3 to 5 days of feeding a highly digestible diet. Highly digestible diets are mostly assimilated in the small intestine, resulting in a reduced residue's reaching the colon.[133] The diet should be low in fat (<15% dry matter), contain a highly digestible carbohydrate (50% dry matter) such as rice, and contain protein of high biologic value.[35, 36, 133, 134]

Diets such as Prescription Diet i/d, CNM EN, and Waltham Low Fat are effective in dogs. Although higher in fat content than these three diets, a ration with high-quality nutrients and moderate fiber concentration, such as Eukanuba, may be as effective in some animals with large bowel diarrhea. Although highly digestible diets contain little fiber, the ideal amount of dietary fiber for animals with large bowel diarrhea remains unknown. Fiber can help normalize colonic myoelectrical activity and motility, which results in improved fecal consistency. In addition, water-adsorbing properties decrease free fecal water.[135]

Recurrent dietary indiscretion may lead to chronic or intermittent bouts of diarrhea. Confining a free-roaming dog or permanently removing the source of dietary indiscretion may be necessary to relieve clinical signs. In some instances, minor asymptomatic GI disorders can be aggravated by dietary indiscretion and result in diarrhea. Eliminating the source of dietary indiscretion or feeding an easily digested diet may correct clinical signs.

Although dietary indiscretion does not occur as commonly in cats as in dogs, it can be the cause of acute or chronic diarrhea. Modifying the behavior of outdoor cats is very difficult. However, feeding a diet with high-quality, easily digestible nutrients may alleviate clinical signs. Most cats do not find low-fat diets very palatable, so diets higher in fat content must be used in these cases. We have had success with Prescription Diet c/d, Iams Cat Food, and Tender Vittles. A lower-fat feline diet, CNM EN, has recently been marketed and appears to be effective in cats.

Prognosis

The prognosis for dietary indiscretion is excellent if the cause can be identified and removed. Free-roaming dogs and cats are prone to repeated episodes.

Inflammatory Bowel Disease: Plasmacytic Lymphocytic Enterocolitis

Inflammatory bowel disease (IBD) is a very common cause of chronic vomiting or diarrhea in dogs and cats.[2] A diagnosis of IBD requires finding excessive numbers of inflammatory cells in mucosal samples of the stomach, small intestine, or colon in animals that do not have evidence of other disorders. Mucosal inflammation similar to that seen in IBD can occur in a diverse group of disorders, such as bacterial, viral, and parasitic infections; bacterial overgrowth; metabolic diseases; food allergy; and neoplasia.[136] Because mucosal inflammation is nonspecific, there is danger that

IBD can become a convenient, abused, and inaccurate diagnosis in veterinary medicine.[137] Only after thorough diagnostic evaluation can an accurate diagnosis of IBD be made in dogs and cats.

The specific type of IBD diagnosed is based on the area of the GI tract affected and the predominant type of inflammatory cell found in the mucosa. The most common form of IBD in dogs and cats is plasmacytic lymphocytic infiltration in the small intestine (plasmacytic lymphocytic enteritis), but eosinophilic, suppurative, granulomatous, and mixed forms occur. Mucosal inflammation may be limited to the stomach, small intestine, or large intestine or may involve multiple regions. Clinical signs are dependent on the area affected.

The following discussion pertains to plasmacytic lymphocytic enterocolitis (PLEC), although many sections also apply to other forms of IBD. Eosinophilic colitis, histiocytic ulcerative colitis, and the immunoproliferative enteropathy of basenjis are discussed in subsequent sections.

IBD usually occurs in middle-aged dogs and cats, although animals of any age can be affected.[127, 136, 138–148] There does not appear to be a sex predilection, but purebred cats may be at a greater risk.[127, 141, 142]

Pathophysiology

The pathophysiology of IBD has been intensely studied in humans without emergence of a unified explanation. It is unknown whether IBD is caused by an inflammatory response to a foreign agent or by an abnormal immunologic response to a normal intraluminal antigen (such as food or bacteria).[149] Most likely, IBD is multifactorial, with infectious agents, immunologic mechanisms, genetic influences, and psychosocial factors participating.[150–152]

In humans, increased mucosal permeability appears to be a central component of IBD. A breakdown in the mucosal barrier results in increased access of antigens to the mucosa and the development of a self-perpetuating inflammatory process.[136, 153] Inflammation leads to recruitment of additional inflammatory cells with release of potent inflammatory mediators that cause further damage to the mucosal barrier; these include prostaglandins, leukotrienes, platelet activating factor, interleukins, reactive oxygen metabolites, and several GI peptides.[154–157] Mucosal damage permits entry of additional intraluminal antigens across the mucosal surface, which stimulates further inflammation and damage, and so on.

Increased permeability may result from a primary mucosal defect or from damage secondary to infectious, metabolic, allergic, or toxic insults.[150, 155]

Alternatively, faulty immunoregulation (decreased suppressor T-lymphocyte function) may occur in which normal intraluminal antigens induce an exaggerated immune response that is not dampened and controlled by normal suppressor mechanisms.[158]

Regardless of the cause of increased permeability, luminal antigens that normally are tolerated by the mucosal immune system (i.e., do not induce an inflammatory response) are capable of inciting a severe immune response. The therapeutic response to a hypoallergenic diet or broad-spectrum antibiotics that occurs in some dogs and cats may be caused by limitation or reduction of luminal antigens that are secondarily involved in the pathogenesis of IBD.[136, 138, 139, 143, 155]

Mucosal inflammation results in the clinical signs associated with IBD. Intestinal inflammation disrupts tight junctions between epithelial cells and reduces the absorption and promotes the loss of nutrients, electrolytes, and water.[159] Some inflammatory mediators stimulate intestinal secretion. Inflammation adversely affects motility by inhibiting segmental contractions and causing decreased fecal storage and frequent elimination of colonic contents.[160] Goblet cells respond to inflammation by increasing secretion of mucus. The inflamed rectum becomes sensitized to stretch, initiating the urge to defecate and tenesmus. Inflammation in the duodenum and stomach stimulates receptors that trigger the vomiting reflex. Severe vomiting or profuse diarrhea can lead to dehydration because of loss of fluid and electrolytes.

Clinical Signs

The most common clinical signs in dogs and cats with IBD are vomiting, diarrhea, and weight loss.[127, 136, 138–148, 161, 162] Affected animals may vomit food, water, mucus, or bile-stained fluid. Vomiting may not be temporally related to the ingestion of food or water. Diarrhea may have characteristics associated with the small intestine (increased fecal volume per defecation or weight loss), those associated with the large intestine (increased frequency, reduced fecal volume per defecation, tenesmus, hematochezia, and excess mucus), or both (see Table 32–4). Appetite is usually normal or depressed, although some animals may exhibit increased appetite.[144, 161] In the early stages of IBD, clinical signs often are mild and intermittent, and they may occur cyclically.[127, 148, 161] As the condition progresses, clinical signs often gradually increase in frequency and intensity and may become continuous.[136, 148] In some cases, the first stool of the day may be normal or near normal, and successive bowel movements become looser.[136] During severe episodes, mild pyrexia, depression, and anorexia may occur.[148, 161]

Physical examination may be unremarkable.[162]

Weight loss may be present, and it may be severe in some cases.[140, 141, 144] Thickened segments of bowel wall or bowel distended with gas or fluid may be detected during abdominal palpation.[139–142, 144] Mild-to-moderate dehydration may be detected if vomiting or diarrhea is severe. Digital rectal examination may produce pain or detect roughened mucosa.[136] Fresh blood may be visible on the glove after it is removed from the rectum.

Diagnostic Plan

The definitive diagnosis of IBD requires histopathologic assessment of GI mucosal samples and elimination of other diseases that result in mucosal inflammation.[161] Mucosal samples may be obtained during endoscopic examination or, if endoscopy is not available, by exploratory surgery. In order to identify other causes of mucosal inflammation, a thorough diagnostic evaluation, following the guidelines described for chronic vomiting (see Chap. 31) and chronic diarrhea, must be followed in all cases.

Routine Laboratory Evaluation

Routine laboratory evaluation may be normal in cases of IBD.[145, 162, 163] However, a wide variety of mild and nonspecific hematologic or biochemical abnormalities may occur.[127, 140–142, 144] No consistent or diagnostic pattern of laboratory abnormalities in animals with IBD has been identified.

Radiography

Survey abdominal radiographs do not usually contribute to the diagnosis of IBD but may be helpful in excluding other causes of vomiting, diarrhea, or weight loss.[141, 142, 161] They may demonstrate gas- or fluid-filled loops of bowel.[127, 136, 140, 144, 148] Upper and lower barium contrast studies may demonstrate mucosal irregularity and possibly ulceration or thickened intestinal walls, but these findings are not specific for IBD.[127, 144]

Endoscopy

Endoscopic abnormalities include hyperemia, mucosal hemorrhage, increased mucosal granularity, increased mucosal friability, loss of visualization of colonic submucosal blood vessels, and, in some cases, ulceration or inability to adequately distend the intestinal lumen (Fig. 32–12).[127, 141, 142, 145, 161, 163, 164] Multiple biopsy samples should always be obtained, even if the mucosa appears normal, because histologic abnormalities may be present.[126, 127] The clinical signs should indicate which portion of the GI tract to examine (for vomiting, stomach and duodenum; for small bowel diarrhea, duodenum and possibly ileum; for large bowel diarrhea, cecum and colon). Because

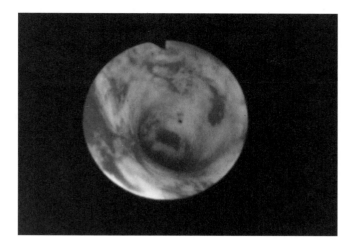

Figure 32-12
Endoscopic appearance of the descending colon in a 9-year-old domestic shorthair cat with plasmacytic lymphocytic colitis. Multiple bleeding erosions are visible. The mucosa was very friable, and bleeding occurred with only minimal endoscope trauma. (From Leib MS, Matz ME. Diseases of the large intestine. In: Ettinger SJ, Feldman EC, eds. Textbook of Veterinary Internal Medicine. Philadelphia, WB Saunders, 1995:1232–1260.)

histologic changes may be present in regions without producing classic clinical signs, some authors recommend examining and obtaining biopsy samples from both the upper and lower GI tracts in all cases of suspected IBD.[144]

Histopathology

The histologic criteria for establishing a diagnosis of IBD in dogs and cats remain controversial. Classification schemes that provide some objective criteria and that can be applied to the diagnosis of cases of IBD have recently been proposed.[127, 141, 142, 144, 165]

All diagnostic classification schemes have as a central criterion the presence of increased numbers of plasma cells and lymphocytes within the lamina propria. Lesser numbers of eosinophils and scattered neutrophils and macrophages often are found. Other histologic changes that occur in IBD include edematous separation of crypts, increased numbers of intraepithelial lymphocytes, blunting or fusion of villi, obliteration of crypts, cryptal abscessation, basophilia with flattening of surface epithelium, and erosion.[127, 128, 141, 142, 144, 165] The major difficulty in interpreting the histopathologic changes in cases of IBD lies at both ends of the spectrum: mild lesions must be differentiated from normal tissue, and severe lesions from lymphosarcoma.[128, 166, 167] Inflammatory infiltrates commonly are found near neoplastic cells in cases of lymphosarcoma.[168] A small, flexible endoscopic forceps biopsy may miss a neoplastic lesion.

Treatment

Optimal therapy for dogs and cats with IBD often requires a combination of dietary and pharmacologic management that should be modified specifically for each case. If initial therapeutic management does not improve clinical signs, other drugs and drug combinations should be instituted. Compared with administration of a single drug, combination therapy often allows decreased drug dosages to be used, which reduces adverse drug effects. The initial treatment of choice varies greatly among authors; some prefer dietary manipulations, and others use sulfasalazine, prednisone, or metronidazole.[127, 138, 139, 141–147]

Dietary Management

Because of the potential role of dietary antigens as either a primary or a secondary factor in the pathogenesis of IBD, hypoallergenic diets have been recommended as the initial treatment.[35, 36, 136, 138, 139, 143, 148, 159] Successful management of dogs and cats with plasmacytic lymphocytic colitis has been documented with a diet of rice and low-fat cottage cheese or a hypoallergenic diet with lamb or chicken as a protein source.[138, 139, 143]

A hypoallergenic diet must contain protein and carbohydrate sources novel to the patient. A thorough dietary history should be obtained to determine which ingredients the animal has not been previously exposed to. Many hypoallergenic diets are commercially available and use lamb, egg, rabbit, venison, fish, or chicken as a protein source.[35, 36, 159] A homemade diet can be formulated using these protein sources, or others such as cottage cheese or tofu, with rice or potatoes as a carbohydrate source.[136, 169] Homemade diets can be deficient in vitamins and minerals. They can be safely fed for trial periods but must be balanced for long-term use. Vitamin and mineral supplements must be carefully selected because many contain extracts and flavorings.

The hypoallergenic diet should be fed for 4 to 8 weeks and must be the only nutrient source that the dog or cat receives.[170–172] The food of other household pets, table scraps, treats, and flavored vitamin and heartworm preventatives must be avoided. Free-roaming animals must be strictly supervised to avoid the potential for dietary indiscretion. If the diarrhea resolves when the hypoallergenic diet is fed, the animal should be challenged with its original diet.[170, 172] Diarrhea should rapidly return if dietary hypersensitivity is a component of the IBD.

The owner can continue feeding the hypoallergenic diet or can pursue antigen identification by adding single ingredients to the hypoallergenic diet for 7 to 10 days. Although hypersensitivity can occur to any dietary constituent, common offending allergens include beef, cow's milk, eggs, fish, wheat, soybeans, oats, and corn.[36, 169, 171–174] After the ingredient that causes diarrhea is identified, a commercial or home-made ration that lacks the offending antigen can be used. There is some evidence that patients can subsequently develop hypersensitivity to other antigens. Some authors have advocated rotation of diets to prevent this from occurring.[175] In addition, use of a "sacrificial" hypoallergenic diet along with anti-inflammatory medications until the mucosal barrier is repaired, followed by a different hypoallergenic diet, has been suggested.[176] This recommendation is based on development of hypersensitivity to the newly administered diet while the mucosal barrier is healing. Poorly digestible novel proteins may induce hypersensitivity in patients with increased mucosal permeability, because protein digestion usually renders them nonallergenic. Cooked eggs and cottage cheese are assimilated more readily than many meats and may be more hypoallergenic to intestinal mucosa than meat-based diets.[4] Although elimination testing is the current diagnostic procedure of choice, preliminary experience with gastroscopic food sensitivity testing indicates that it may be a useful method to identify the offending food antigen in patients with IBD.[177, 178]

In addition to hypoallergenic diets, other types of diets may be beneficial in the management of IBD. In cats with plasmacytic lymphocytic colitis, a high-fiber diet (Prescription Diet r/d) or psyllium supplementation (Metamucil) has been documented to relieve or improve diarrhea.[142] Even if diarrhea does not completely resolve with a hypoallergenic or high-fiber diet, concurrent dietary and medical therapy may achieve control of clinical signs with lower dosages of medication, and potentially with fewer side effects, than medical management alone.[141, 142, 144, 179] If diarrhea continues despite feeding of a hypoallergenic or high-fiber diet, the animal may benefit from a highly digestible diet (see Dietary Indiscretion) along with medical management.

Corticosteroids

Corticosteroids are the drugs of choice for cats with colitis and for dogs and cats with enteritis that have failed to respond to dietary management.[146, 147, 161] They are used less frequently in dogs with colitis because most cases can be managed by diet, sulfasalazine, or the newer mesalamine products. In dogs showing adverse effects associated with sulfasalazine, addition of corticosteroids may allow reduction of the sulfasalazine dosage.

The efficacy of corticosteroids is thought to result from their anti-inflammatory, antiprostaglandin, antileukotriene, and immunosuppressive effects. They inhibit cell membrane phospholipase A, suppressing production of arachidonic acid and, subsequently,

synthesis of prostaglandins and leukotrienes.[180] Corticosteroids also increase sodium and water absorption and help regulate colonic electrolyte transport.[136]

An initial dose of 2.0 mg/kg prednisone or prednisolone per day often improves clinical signs within 7 to 10 days.[141, 144, 148, 161] After normal feces have been produced for approximately 2 to 4 weeks, the dosage should be decreased by 50%. As long as diarrhea does not return, the dosage can gradually be reduced (at intervals of 2–4 weeks) until the least amount given every other day that controls clinical signs is reached. Typical maintenance therapy is 0.5 to 1.0 mg/kg every 48 hours. Some animals require long-term treatment, but in others it is possible to discontinue prednisone within 3 to 4 months. If prednisone and sulfasalazine are used in a dog, it may be possible to reduce the dosage of sulfasalazine after the prednisone dosage declines to 1.0 mg/kg every 48 hours. Dietary management with a hypoallergenic, high-fiber, or highly digestible diet often has a corticosteroid-sparing effect.

In cats that cannot tolerate daily oral medication, injectable long-acting methylprednisolone acetate, 20 mg subcutaneously, can be administered every 2 to 4 weeks.[161] Injectable therapy, however, has not been as successful as daily medication in controlling clinical signs. Adverse effects of corticosteroids are uncommon in cats.[179] Side effects are common in dogs and often are dosage related. They include polyuria and polydipsia, polyphagia, iatrogenic hyperadrenocorticism, hypothalamic-pituitary suppression, GI bleeding, acute pancreatitis, steroid hepatopathy, and predisposition to bacterial or fungal infections.[136]

Sulfasalazine

The treatment of choice for dogs with colitis that do not respond to dietary management is sulfasalazine.[35, 136, 159, 163, 179] Sulfasalazine consists of mesalamine (previously called 5-aminosalicylic acid) linked by an azo bond to sulfapyridine.[131–185] This linkage prevents absorption by the small intestine and allows delivery of approximately 70% of the drug to the colon.[180] Bacteria in the distal small intestine and the colon break the azo bond, liberating both components. Sulfapyridine is absorbed, metabolized in the liver, and excreted by the kidney. It is not thought to have therapeutic effects in IBD and is responsible for some of the adverse reactions associated with sulfasalazine. Mesalamine acts topically in the colon to reduce mucosal inflammation. Although the mechanism of action was once believed to be related to antiprostaglandin activity, recent evidence supports its antileukotriene activity.[181, 182, 184]

The recommended dosage range for sulfasalazine in dogs is 20 to 50 mg/kg, to a maximum of 1 g three times per day (t.i.d.).[35, 159, 163] High dosages may be needed in chronic cases. For initial treatment of a dog, a dosage of 20 to 30 mg/kg t.i.d. usually is effective.[136] One of the most common therapeutic mistakes is discontinuation of therapy too soon after resolution of clinical signs, which can lead to diarrhea that may be refractory to the dosage that previously controlled clinical signs. After the dog has normal feces for 2 to 4 weeks, the dosing frequency should be reduced to twice per day. After an additional 2 to 4 weeks without diarrhea, maintenance dosages should be decreased by 50%, still given twice per day. If diarrhea returns, the dosage should be increased to the amount that previously controlled clinical signs. In some dogs, sulfasalazine can be discontinued; other patients require long-term therapy. Concurrent dietary management with a hypoallergenic or highly digestible diet may help control clinical signs with a lower dosage of sulfasalazine.

In dogs, vomiting and keratoconjunctivitis sicca are common side effects.[35, 136, 163, 179] Vomiting can usually be controlled by administration of medication with food or by use of an enteric-coated preparation. If decreased tear production is detected early, reduction of the dosage or discontinuation of the drug may restore tear production and prevent progression to keratoconjunctivitis sicca.[186] However, if decreased tear production is not detected early, it becomes irreversible. The mechanism of action for toxicity is unknown, but sulfapyridine may directly damage the lacrimal and nictitans tear glands, reducing production of the aqueous component of tears.[186] When initiating sulfasalazine treatment, especially with high dosages, tear production should be measured at 2-week intervals. If therapy is continued long term, tear production should be measured monthly. Treatment of keratoconjunctivitis sicca that is associated with sulfasalazine administration with cyclosporine has been shown, in a limited number of cases, to be less successful compared to other causes.[187]

Sulfasalazine should be used with caution in cats because of their sensitivity to salicylates. Prednisone is the drug of choice for cats with colitis that fail to respond to hypoallergenic, high-fiber, or highly digestible diets. Sulfasalazine has been used in cats at a dosage of 10 to 20 mg/kg once a day (s.i.d.) or b.i.d. Side effects include anorexia and anemia.[148, 188] The oral suspension (50 mg/mL) allows accurate measurement of doses for cats.

Newer Mesalamine Preparations

In order to reduce the toxicity associated with sulfasalazine, new drugs have been developed that deliver mesalamine to the colon without linkage to sulfapyridine. These drugs have been shown to be safe and effective for treatment of humans with IBD.[181, 182] Two have been approved for use in humans in the United States. Olsalazine (Dipentum) consists of two molecules of mesalamine linked with an azo bond.[189, 190] Asacol consists of mesalamine coated with an acrylic resin that dissolves at pH 7 or greater, usually in the terminal ileum and colon.[191, 192] Although there are no established guidelines for using these drugs in dogs with colitis, 10 to 20 mg/kg t.i.d. of Dipentum or 10 mg/kg t.i.d. of Asacol has been suggested.[136]

These newer agents are less toxic than sulfasalazine; approximately 80% to 90% of humans with sulfasalazine intolerance can be treated with these drugs without adverse effects.[181, 193] The most common adverse effect of olsalazine in humans is watery diarrhea, which may be minimized by taking the drug with food and gradually increasing the dosage.[190, 193]

Although these new drugs have not been used extensively in dogs, keratoconjunctivitis sicca has been associated with Asacol in a limited number of cases.[194, 195] The mechanism of toxicity is unknown. Dipentum or Asacol should not be the initial drug used in dogs with colitis but should to be reserved for patients that develop side effects associated with sulfasalazine.

Metronidazole

Metronidazole possesses several properties thought to be beneficial in dogs and cats with IBD. In addition to its antiprotozoal effects, it is a broad-spectrum antibiotic with impressive activity against anaerobic bacteria, it inhibits cell-mediated immunity, it alters neutrophil chemotaxis, and it may have other immunosuppressive effects.[136, 179, 188, 196] Although most veterinary authors suggest that it be used in conjunction with sulfasalazine or prednisone, it can be used as a single agent to manage dogs and cats with IBD.[188] Dosages of 10 to 20 mg/kg b.i.d. or t.i.d. have been recommended in dogs and cats.[161, 188] Adverse effects at this dosage are uncommon, but severe neurologic toxicity has been reported with higher dosages.[197] Peripheral neuropathy has been reported in humans receiving long-term therapy. Combination therapy with metronidazole may have a sulfasalazine- or prednisone-sparing effect, often resulting in fewer adverse drug reactions. We have found that the addition of metronidazole to maintenance therapy for 2 to 4 weeks may be beneficial in dogs or cats with IBD that experience an unexplained bout of vomiting or diarrhea.

Azathioprine

Other immunosuppressive drugs can be used in dogs and cats with IBD. Azathioprine (Imuran) is the most commonly used drug of this group. Azathioprine is a purine analog that competes with natural purines in the synthesis of DNA and RNA, resulting in nonfunctional nucleic acid strands and preventing proliferation of rapidly dividing cells. Azathioprine is metabolized to 6-mercaptopurine in the liver.[136, 182, 198, 199] Most veterinary authors recommend azathioprine for cases of refractory IBD that have not responded to the previously described treatments.[136, 159, 161, 179, 188] In our experience, azathioprine and other immunosuppressive agents are infrequently needed in cases of IBD. The initial dose in dogs is 2.0 mg/kg s.i.d., and in cats it is 0.3 mg/kg every 48 hours. It may take several months of therapy for this drug to be effective.[183, 198] The dosage can often be reduced to 2 mg/kg every 48 hours in dogs. Side effects seen in dogs and cats include myelosuppression, hepatic disease, and acute pancreatitis.[179, 199]

Tylosin

Tylosin is a macrolide antibiotic that has been recommended for the treatment of IBD in dogs and cats.[136, 200] Its mechanism of action is unknown. In our experience, it is not often beneficial in refractory cases of IBD. The recommended dose range is broad, although 10 to 20 mg/kg b.i.d. is commonly used.[42] It currently is available as a powder for use in poultry (Tyspolan Soluble) in a formulation that contains approximately 2.25 g per teaspoon.[42, 136] Clinical experience suggests that it is safe for long-term administration.[42] Tylosin can be used in cases that do not respond to dietary management, sulfasalazine, prednisone, or metronidazole, or if adverse effects of these medications are encountered.

Prognosis

The prognosis for most patients with PLEC is good. In some animals, medication can be discontinued, whereas others require long-term or lifelong treatment. Some patients develop recurrent clinical signs and must be retreated.

Inflammatory Bowel Disease: Eosinophilic Enterocolitis

Eosinophilic enterocolitis (EEC) is the second most common form of IBD that occurs in dogs and cats.[166] However, it occurs much less frequently than PLEC. The clinical features of both of these forms of IBD are similar (see Inflammatory Bowel Disease: Plasmacytic Lymphocytic Enterocolitis). This section emphasizes the differences between these two forms of IBD.

EEC is an idiopathic inflammatory disease that causes vomiting and diarrhea in dogs and cats. Histopathologic lesions are characterized by increased numbers of eosinophils in any layer of the GI tract.[201] Affected dogs tend to be younger than those with PLEC.

Pathophysiology

There has been an association between cases of eosinophilic gastroenteritis and migrating larvae of *Toxocara canis* in both naturally occurring and experimentally induced disease.[202, 203] Food allergy and *Ancylostoma caninum* have been incriminated as the cause of eosinophilic enterocolitis in some humans.[201, 204, 205] As in other forms of IBD, food antigens may not be the inciting cause of mucosal damage, but they may amplify the immune reaction as increased mucosal permeability allows access to gut-associated lymphoid tissue.

Clinical Signs

Cases of EEC are often indistinguishable from cases of PLEC. Mucosal ulceration is more common in dogs with this form of IBD, and hematemesis, melena, or hematochezia can occur.[201] Extreme thickening of the small bowel can sometimes be detected in affected cats.[146] Rarely, a granulomatous form in dogs may be associated with a large mass that can be palpated abdominally or, if it involves the distal colon, rectally.[201, 206–208] An uncommon condition, hypereosinophilic syndrome in cats, can be associated with EEC. In these cases, hepatosplenomegaly and mesenteric lymphadenopathy are also present.[209]

Diagnostic Plan

Definitive diagnosis of EEC requires biopsy of affected tissue and elimination of other causes of chronic vomiting (see Chap. 31) and diarrhea. In most cases of EEC, multiple areas of the GI tract are affected. Eosinophilic infiltration into the submucosa, or deeper layers, is common and characteristic of the disease.[128] This differs from PLEC, in which infiltration occurs in the mucosa.

Mucosal ulceration may be visible during endoscopy or exploratory surgery.[201] A mild to moderate peripheral eosinophilia is often found, but not always. Blood loss can lead to a regenerative anemia and hypoproteinemia. Microscopic evaluation of rectal cytologic scrapings often reveals increased numbers of eosinophils.

Treatment

Treatment requires a combination of dietary and medical management. Because this condition occurs primarily in young dogs, parasites should always be considered potential causative agents, because they have the ability to attract eosinophils into mucosa. Treatment for adult whipworms, roundworms, and hookworms or migrating *T. canis* larvae should be instituted before other means of therapy are explored. Fenbendazole (Panacur Granules, 25 mg/kg b.i.d. for

14 days) may be effective against migrating larvae of *T. canis*.[201] Although not approved for this indication, ivermectin (Ivomec), 200 μg/kg subcutaneously, kills larval stages of *T. canis*.[210] This dosage of ivermectin should not be used in collies or related breeds because of potential toxicity. Hypoallergenic diets rarely control clinical signs by themselves, but they may allow reduction of the dosage of concurrently used medication.[201] If diarrhea continues despite feeding of a hypoallergenic diet, a highly digestible diet should be used. Prednisone can be given to dogs at a dosage of 2 mg/kg per day, and to cats at 4 to 6 mg/kg per day.[146, 201] Prednisone dosages should be slowly tapered at 2- to 4-week intervals until the lowest dosage that controls clinical signs when given every other day is reached. Prednisone can be withdrawn from some dogs; in others, relapses occur. Cats often require aggressive and long-term therapy.[146] If adverse effects of glucocorticoids occur or diarrhea cannot be controlled, the antimetabolite azathioprine (Imuran) can be used. Initial dosage in dogs is 2 mg/kg s.i.d., and in cats it is 0.3 mg/kg every 48 hours (see Inflammatory Bowel Disease: Plasmacytic Lymphocytic Enterocolitis).

Prognosis

The prognosis for dogs with EEC is good because most patients rapidly respond to therapy.[201] The prognosis for cats is guarded.[146] Many cats continue to show clinical signs despite intensive therapy. The prognosis for the rare forms of EEC, hypereosinophilic syndrome and transmural granuloma, is grave.

Adenocarcinoma

Adenocarcinoma is a malignant tumor of epithelial origin that occurs most commonly in middle-aged to older dogs and older cats.[90, 101, 154, 211–220] Siamese cats appear to have a higher incidence of intestinal adenocarcinoma than other breeds.[211, 213, 216, 218, 221] Adenocarcinomas are the most common malignant intestinal tumor in dogs and the second most common in cats (lymphosarcoma is first).[101, 166, 214, 215, 217]

Pathophysiology

Adenocarcinomas are found with equal frequency in the colon and in the small bowel in dogs but are much more common in the small bowel of cats.[211, 213, 218, 219, 221] In the colon, most tumors are located within the rectum.[212, 214]

Grossly, the appearance of adenocarcinoma is variable: a single, pedunculated, polypoid mass; multiple nodular masses; or an annular or intramural mass

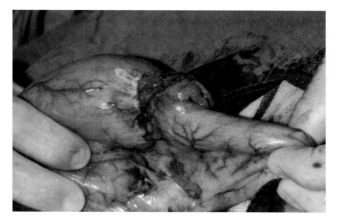

Figure 32–13
Annular transmural adenocarcinoma in the ascending colon in the dog shown in Figure 32–3. The mass caused a partial small intestinal obstruction, dilation of the small bowel, chronic diarrhea, and weight loss.

with stricture or obstruction may be seen (Fig. 32–13). Common metastatic sites for adenocarcinoma are regional lymph nodes, liver, lungs, and omentum.[213, 218, 220] Adenocarcinoma is a highly aggressive tumor, and metastasis often occurs before diagnosis.[213, 216] In cats, metastatic lesions have been found at necropsy in at least 75% of cases.[213, 218]

Clinical Signs

Clinical signs include anorexia, weight loss (which may be profound), vomiting, and occasional diarrhea.[211, 213, 216, 218, 221, 222] If present, diarrhea usually is associated with large bowel involvement. Dogs with rectal lesions may produce formed feces associated with hematochezia, tenesmus, or dyschezia, abnormally shaped stools, or rectal bleeding not associated with defecation.[212, 217, 219] Obstructive lesions of the colon may cause constipation.[221]

An abdominal mass can often be detected on physical examination.[211, 213, 216] Masses can be identified on digital rectal palpation in dogs with rectal neoplasia.[212]

Diagnostic Plan

The majority of cats are negative for FeLV.[211, 213] Nonregenerative anemia and neutrophilia are often present.[216] A microcytic, hypochromic anemia secondary to chronic GI blood loss can be present.

Survey abdominal radiographs may demonstrate an abdominal mass or, less commonly, a pattern consistent with small bowel obstruction (see Fig. 32–3).[211, 213, 216, 222] With some colonic tumors, the mass can be highlighted by air in the rectum, or sublumbar lymphadenopathy can be detected.[101] Abdominal ultrasonography may identify an abdominal mass or

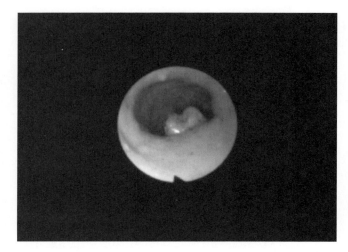

Figure 32-14
Sessile mass in the distal descending colon in a 10-year-old West Highland white terrier. Biopsy revealed adenocarcinoma.

lymphadenopathy. Barium contrast radiographs may identify an intramural mass or intestinal obstruction.[211, 216, 218, 222] Thoracic radiographs are usually negative for metastasis at initial diagnosis.[211, 213, 216]

In cases with small bowel involvement, endoscopic examination often fails to identify the lesion because many tumors are located distal to the duodenum and proximal jejunum, out of range for the endoscope.[211, 216] If an abdominal mass can be palpated, diagnosis can be reached by fine-needle aspiration cytology or by exploratory surgery and biopsy. If signs of large bowel disease are present, the most direct diagnostic approach involves colonoscopic examination, which not only identifies the presence and location of a lesion but also provides tissue for microscopic evaluation. A sessile mass, ulcerated mucosa, or an annular mass can be seen (Fig. 32-14).

Treatment

Treatment consists of surgical resection and anastomosis. Mesenteric lymph nodes should be biopsied, and the entire abdominal cavity should carefully be examined for metastatic lesions.

Prognosis

Overall, the prognosis for animals with intestinal adenocarcinoma is guarded. Local recurrence of disease is common. Mean survival times of as long as 6 to 12 months have been described in dogs.[101, 212] In dogs with colonic lesions, survival was longer in patients with single masses and much shorter in those with annular masses.[212] However, a group of 23 dogs with colonic adenocarcinoma that did not undergo surgery had a mean survival time of 15 months.[212] The

prognosis for intestinal adenocarcinoma in cats is more guarded, with mean survival times after surgery often less than 20 weeks.[211, 213, 216, 221] However, long-term survival can occur in individual cases in dogs and cats, even in those with metastasis at the time of initial surgery.[212, 216, 223]

Lymphosarcoma

Lymphosarcoma is a malignant neoplasm that arises from the submucosa, often within multiple locations in the GI tract. It is the second most common malignant GI tumor in dogs (adenocarcinoma is most common) but the most common in cats.[101, 166, 214, 215, 217] Primary GI lymphosarcoma represents between 15% and 40% of feline lymphomas and is considered to be the second most common form in cats.[168, 224] Intestinal lymphosarcoma occurs most commonly in middle-aged male dogs and older cats.[101, 225, 226]

Pathophysiology

Lymphosarcoma involves the GI tract in two ways. Primary GI lymphosarcoma is present when neoplastic tissue occurs primarily within the stomach, small intestine, or large intestine; it may also involve the liver, kidneys, or bone marrow. In the other form, the GI tract may be secondarily involved in multicentric lymphosarcoma.[225] GI lymphosarcoma can assume many forms: a solitary mass, multiple discontinuous masses, or diffuse mucosal infiltration, which results in a corrugated, thickened, irregular, and friable surface (Fig. 32-15).

Although in cats lymphosarcoma is caused by FeLV, most cats with GI lymphosarcoma have a negative FeLV ELISA at the time of diagnosis.[226]

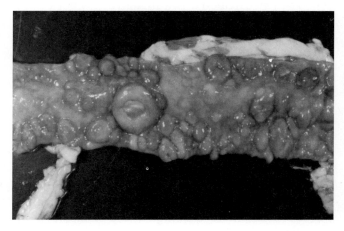

Figure 32-15
Necropsy appearance of the small intestine in a 4-year-old Labrador retriever with chronic vomiting. Nodules were as large as 3 cm in diameter. Diagnosis was multifocal lymphosarcoma.

Malignant transformation of cells is thought to be followed by neutralization of the virus, with tumor development occurring later.

Clinical Signs

The clinical signs are mainly those of malabsorption or colitis caused by diffuse mucosal infiltration of the small or large bowel or by obstructive masses within the stomach or intestine.[226] Diffuse small bowel infiltration can lead to obstructive lymphangiectasia and PLE. Hepatic, renal, or bone marrow involvement, GI blood loss, or, rarely, intestinal perforation can cause additional clinical signs.

Clinical signs of intestinal lymphosarcoma are often similar to those of IBD. Vomiting, diarrhea, decreased appetite, lethargy, and weight loss are most common.[168, 223, 225, 226] Diarrhea can have characteristics of small bowel or large bowel involvement, or both, although small bowel signs are most common (see Table 32–4).[214] Mesenteric lymphadenopathy commonly occurs. Hepatomegaly in dogs and cats and renomegaly in cats may be present.[224] Ascites caused by PLE and lymphangiectasia, secondary to diffuse small bowel infiltration, can occasionally occur. If small bowel obstruction is present, severe vomiting, profound depression, severe dehydration, and abdominal pain occur.

Abdominal palpation may reveal an abdominal mass, mesenteric lymphadenopathy, or thickened small bowel.[226] Digital rectal examination may identify a rectal mass, sublumbar lymphadenopathy, or thickened, corrugated, friable mucosa.

Diagnostic Plan

Diagnosis frequently requires histologic assessment of mucosal samples obtained during endoscopy or, if endoscopy is not available, during exploratory surgery. Exploratory surgery should be performed to obtain a biopsy if a palpable small intestinal mass is present, because these lesions are usually beyond the range of small intestinal endoscopy. Impression smears of biopsy samples, brush cytology of infiltrated mucosa or masses, or fine-needle aspiration of intestinal masses, enlarged mesenteric lymph nodes, or the liver may also be diagnostic.[168]

Routine laboratory evaluation may reveal a nonregenerative anemia associated with chronic disease or bone marrow involvement or a regenerative anemia and hypoproteinemia caused by loss of blood.[226] Liver enzymes (alanine aminotransferase and alkaline phosphatase) may be elevated if the tumor has invaded the liver. Hypoalbuminemia may be present in cases of diffuse small bowel infiltration and lymphangiectasia. Most cats test negative for FeLV by ELISA at the time of diagnosis.[168, 226]

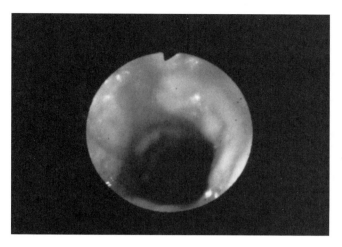

Figure 32–16

Endoscopic appearance of the duodenum in a 7-year-old golden retriever with chronic vomiting and weight loss. The mucosa is very thickened in places. Diagnosis was diffuse lymphosarcoma. The liver was also infiltrated with malignant lymphocytes.

Survey radiographs may detect an abdominal mass, mesenteric lymphadenopathy, or, in some cases, signs of small bowel obstruction (segments of bowel distended with fluid and gas).[222, 223] A thickened rectal wall may occasionally be visible.[101] Barium contrast radiographs may demonstrate an intramural mass, multiple masses, small bowel obstruction, a thickened intestinal wall, or a roughened, irregular, and possibly ulcerated mucosa.[222] Abdominal ultrasonography may demonstrate segmental thickening of the intestinal wall with loss of normal wall layering or mesenteric lymphadenopathy.[46, 104]

Endoscopic examination of the duodenum or colon may identify a mass lesion or a granular, thickened, friable mucosa (Fig. 32–16).[101, 215, 226] Diagnosis of lymphosarcoma by small flexible endoscopic biopsies can be difficult in some cases because of the submucosal origin of the tumor and the frequent association of inflammatory cells with neoplastic cells.[166, 225] Diagnosis is aided by obtaining deeper tissue by repeated sampling of the same location with flexible forceps or by use of a large, rigid forceps in the colon.

Treatment

Treatment involves surgical resection of any obstructing or solitary masses, ulcerated masses causing severe GI hemorrhage, or masses associated with intestinal perforation.[226] Surgery should be followed by chemotherapy. For GI lymphosarcoma with nonresectable lesions, multiple-agent chemotherapy is indicated.

We have had limited success with standard

protocols for multicentric lymphosarcoma using prednisone, cyclophosphamide, and vincristine (see Chap. 43). Some authors have suggested debulking masses before initiating chemotherapy to reduce the risk of intestinal perforation.[101] Concurrent use of sulfasalazine in dogs with colonic lymphosarcoma may help to resolve the clinical signs associated with colitis and proctitis.[101]

Prognosis

Prognosis is generally poor, but isolated cases may respond to treatment with prolonged remission.[225] In several small studies of cats and dogs, chemotherapy resulted in a mean survival time of 4.5 to 6.5 months, during which resolution of clinical signs occurred.[101] More favorable results may occur with multiagent chemotherapy in cases in which lymphosarcoma is confined to the colon or cases of solitary masses after surgical resection.[168]

Intussusception

Intestinal intussusceptions occur when one portion of the intestine invaginates into an adjacent section, causing a partial obstruction of the bowel (Fig. 32–17). Ileocolic and enteroenteric intussusceptions are the most common types in dogs and cats.[227–230] Intussusceptions occur more commonly in dogs than in cats; they occur more commonly in animals 1 year of age or younger, with no apparent breed or sex predilection.[31, 228–230]

Pathophysiology

Intussusceptions have been associated with intestinal parasitism, linear foreign bodies, infectious diseases, recent adoption of a puppy with diarrhea, prior abdominal or thoracic surgery, and neoplasia.[31, 227–230] Most cases, however, are idiopathic. The exact pathophysiologic events involved in the development of intussusceptions are unknown. Intussusceptions have been proposed to result from differences in motility or bowel diameter between adjacent segments (e.g., at the ileocolic junction) or from mechanical linkage of nonadjacent bowel segments (e.g., linear foreign bodies, adhesions). Intussusceptions usually occur in the direction of normal peristalsis, with the proximal segment (intussusceptum) invaginating into the distal segment (intussuscipiens). Because the mesentery and blood supply are included in the invaginating segment, vascular compromise can occur; this initially leads to intramural hemorrhage and edema and eventually to ischemia and necrosis of the bowel. Fibrin exuded from the serosal surfaces may lead to the development of adhesions between the segments; this occurs more commonly in cats.[31]

Clinical Signs

Clinical signs are referable to partial or complete intestinal obstruction and may be acute or chronic. Vomiting, anorexia, weight loss, and depression are observed in most cases in dogs and cats. Diarrhea, often containing blood and mucus, is commonly observed in dogs.[31, 227–231] Intussusceptions frequently can be palpated in the cranial abdomen, usually as a cylindric or sausage-shaped abdominal mass.[227, 229, 230]

Diagnostic Plan

Detection of an elongated, cylindric mass on abdominal palpation suggests the possibility of an intussusception.[228] Abdominal ultrasound may be the best means for confirming a diagnosis. Intussusceptions are usually characterized by a multilayered series of concentric rings representing the bowel wall layers.[46] Intussusceptions can also be identified by barium contrast studies (distention of bowel with a space-occupying mass), pneumocolonography, or endoscopy.[227] Specific diagnosis on survey radiographs is difficult, but typically, signs of partial bowel obstruction are observed.[31, 229–231] Fecal examination for parasites and a thorough abdominal exploration should be performed to identify potential underlying causes.

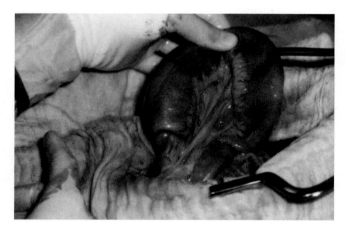

Figure 32–17
Surgical appearance of ileocolic intussusception in an 18-month-old weimaraner. (Courtesy of Don Waldron, DVM, Blacksburg, Virginia.)

Treatment

Treatment involves manual reduction and possibly intestinal resection and anastomosis or enteroplication.[227–231]

Prognosis

The prognosis depends on the predisposing cause, anatomic location, duration, degree of obstruction, and amount of intestinal damage. Recovery rates vary from 35% to 74%.[31, 227, 231] Recurrence is seen in approximately 10% to 20% of cases, often in the immediate postoperative period.[227, 229, 230]

Histoplasmosis

Histoplasmosis, caused by the dimorphic fungus *Histoplasma capsulatum*, typically results in subclinical infection of the respiratory tract after inhalation of the soil-borne organism (see Chap. 39). Involvement of the intestinal tract appears to result from dissemination of the organism from the respiratory tract. Intestinal histoplasmosis is the most common form of disseminated disease in dogs, whereas intestinal involvement is rare in cats.[232–238] It occurs most commonly in young dogs living in endemic regions.[237]

Pathophysiology

Infection may involve the small intestine, large intestine, or both. Infiltration of *H. capsulatum* into the bowel wall results in a severe granulomatous inflammatory response that disrupts the normal architecture and function. In the small intestine, lymphangiectasia can occur secondary to obstruction of lymphatics and can result in PLE.

Clinical Signs

The most common clinical manifestations of GI histoplasmosis are chronic diarrhea, anemia, intestinal blood loss, and weight loss.[232–238] Signs of large bowel diarrhea usually predominate. Malabsorption and PLE can develop with severe small bowel involvement.[237] Anorexia, lethargy, fever, and labored breathing may also be noted.[232, 237, 238]

Physical examination often reveals that the animal is emaciated. Focal or diffuse intestinal wall thickening, omental or mesenteric thickening, mesenteric lymphadenopathy, hepatosplenomegaly, or ascites may be present on abdominal palpation.[237, 238] With colonic involvement, a thickened and corrugated mucosa may be detected on digital rectal examination.[237]

Diagnostic Plan

Diagnosis requires finding the organism in cytologic or histopathologic samples. Routine laboratory evaluation is nonspecific but may show a nonregenerative anemia, neutrophilia, thrombocytopenia,

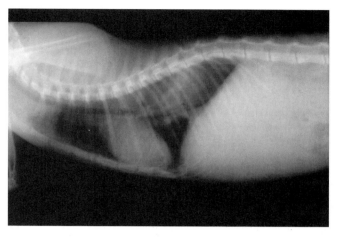

Figure 32–18
Lateral thoracic and cranial abdominal radiograph in a 7-month-old domestic shorthair cat with disseminated histoplasmosis. Massive hepatomegaly is present. Increased interstitial density is present in the dorsal lung fields.

and hypoalbuminemia. Survey abdominal radiographs may demonstrate mesenteric lymphadenopathy or hepatomegaly (Fig. 32–18). Barium contrast studies may show a thickened bowel wall with an irregular or ulcerated mucosa.[237]

Cytologic examination of intestinal mucosal scrapings (see Fig. 32–6), impression smears of biopsy specimens, or fine-needle aspirations of enlarged mesenteric lymph nodes or thickened bowel wall are often diagnostic.[232, 237, 238] The organisms are usually demonstrated within macrophages using routine hematologic stains. If evaluation of cytologic specimens is not diagnostic, tissue biopsy is required.

Endoscopically, intestinal lesions appear as areas of irregular mucosal thickening and proliferation that impart a corrugated appearance, with or without mucosal hemorrhage and ulceration.[237] Histopathologic identification of the organism may require the use of special stains.

Treatment

Treatment requires long-term administration of amphotericin B, ketoconazole, itraconazole, or a combination of amphotericin and an oral azole (see Chap. 39).[237]

Prognosis

The prognosis is guarded for all patients with disseminated histoplasmosis. Long-term remission can be achieved.

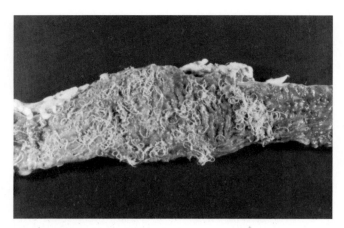

Figure 32-19
Necropsy specimen of the small intestine of a dog with massive hookworm infection. (Courtesy of Geoff Saunders, DVM, MS, Blacksburg, Virginia.)

Common Diseases That Involve Primarily the Small Intestine

Hookworms

Studies have shown that between 11% and 87% of dogs in the United States harbor hookworms.[239, 240] Four species infect dogs and cats. *Ancylostoma caninum* is the most common and pathogenic in dogs and is a common cause of hemorrhagic enteritis and anemia in puppies. *A. tubaeforme*, the most common hookworm in cats, causes less intestinal damage than *A. caninum*. Other hookworms that are less pathogenic than *A. caninum* and infect both dogs and cats include *A. braziliense* (southern United States) and *Uncinaria stenocephala* (northern United States and Canada).

Pathophysiology

Hookworm infection can be acquired by five routes: prenatal, lactogenic, ingestion of infective larvae, skin penetration by infective larvae, and ingestion of a paratenic host. Ingestion of larvae and skin penetration are probably most common. Some larvae may reach maturity within the small intestine; others migrate through the lungs before reaching the small intestine (Fig. 32–19). Some migrating larvae are diverted to skeletal muscle or other organs, where they serve as a source for future intestinal infections or lactogenic transmission in bitches.[241] Adult worms are between 3 and 21 mm in length and have a slightly hooked anterior end. They embed their mouth parts into the mucosa and suck blood and tissue fluids.[39, 242] Blood loss from an *A. caninum* infection can be heavy, but with other types of hookworms blood loss is insignificant. As the worms detach, they leave small, bleeding lesions. The severity of blood loss peaks 10 to 14 days after infection. Massive numbers of eggs are released 2 to 4 weeks after infection. Free-living larvae rapidly hatch, develop into infective stages in 3 to 22 days, and can survive for 3 to 4 months in warm, moist environments.[242] Older animals are more resistant to infection than younger animals.[242] Acquired resistance results in decreased worm burden and pathogenicity.[241]

Severe clinical signs do not commonly occur in kittens because transplacental and lactogenic transmissions probably do not occur.[242] However, infection with a large number of worms can cause death in cats.[242]

Hookworms can cause larva migrans in humans. *A. braziliense* is the most common cause of cutaneous larva migrans. *A. caninum* can cause visceral larva migrans.[243] Recently, *A. caninum* has been implicated as a cause of eosinophilic enteritis in humans.[205]

Clinical Signs

Hookworm infection may not cause clinical signs in adults, but in puppies it can cause diarrhea with melena, vomiting, anorexia, weakness, and failure to thrive. GI hemorrhage can be fatal. Severe clinical signs in cats are very uncommon.

Diagnostic Plan

The diagnosis of hookworms is easily made by finding, on fecal examination, pale and thin-shelled eggs, with free space between the shell wall and morula (Fig. 32–20).[39] Eggs range from 55 to 95 µm in length and from 34 to 55 µm in width.[39] In very young puppies, development of severe clinical signs can occur before passage of eggs, because the prepatent period is approximately 2 weeks. Regenerative anemia

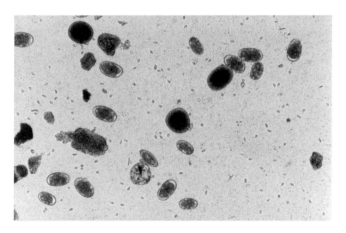

Figure 32-20
Fecal flotation showing many *Ancylostoma caninum* eggs, three large, dark *Toxocara canis* eggs, a single bipolar *Trichuris vulpis* egg at bottom center, and a single *Giardia* cyst next to the *Trichuris* egg. Magnification, ×100. (Courtesy of Anne Zajac, DVM, PhD, Blacksburg, Virginia.)

and eosinophilia are common. Chronic blood loss can result in iron deficiency anemia, which is microcytic, hypochromic, and nonregenerative.[79]

Treatment

Many anthelmintics are effective against hookworms. Pyrantel pamoate (Nemex, 4.5 mg/kg once by mouth) is safe and effective. Animals should be re-treated in 2 to 3 weeks, because larvae that have been arrested in the tissues migrate to the intestine. Severely anemic animals need transfusion of red blood cells. Because of potential zoonotic disease, hookworms should be aggressively treated. Puppies from hookworm-infested environments should be treated every 2 weeks, starting at 2 weeks of age until 8 to 10 weeks. Proper sanitation and removal of feces help reduce the number of infective larvae in the environment. Larvae do not survive freezing. Sodium borate, 0.5 kg/m^2, controls larval growth in the environment but kills grass.[242]

Broader-spectrum anthelmintics are indicated in dogs with concurrent whipworm infection. Fenbendazole (Panacur, 50 mg/kg s.i.d. for 3 days), dichlorvos (Task, 30 mg/kg once), febantel (Rintal, 10 mg/kg s.i.d. for 3 days and 15 mg/kg s.i.d. for 3 days in puppies less than 6 months of age), and mebendazole (Telmintic, 22 mg/kg s.i.d. for 3 days) are effective. Dichlorvos should not be used in debilitated dogs or dogs with heartworm.

Transmammary migration can be prevented in pregnant female dogs by administration of fenbendazole, 100 mg/kg daily, from day 40 of pregnancy to postpartum day 14.[244] Ivermectin, 0.5 to 1.0 mg/kg, also prevents transmammary migration when given 2 to 10 days before whelping, although it is not approved for this use. This dosage should not be used in collies and related breeds because of toxicity.[245] In addition, two doses of 0.5 mg/kg given 4 to 9 days before whelping, and repeated 10 days later, prevents infection in puppies.[242]

Heartworm preventatives such as diethylcarbamazine citrate/oxibendazole (Filarabits Plus), milbemycin oxide (Interceptor), and pyrantel (Heartgard Plus) also treat *A. caninum* and may be beneficial in chronically infected animals kept in contaminated environments that cannot be cleaned properly.[246, 247–250]

Prognosis

The prognosis for hookworm infection is related to the condition of the animal at the time of diagnosis. Puppies with heavy infections of *A. caninum* and severe anemia can die before treatment with anthelmintics and blood transfusion can be effective. If severely affected puppies survive the initial treatment stage, prognosis for recovery is good. The prognosis in older animals and in animals infected with other types of hookworms is good.

Roundworms

Most puppies and kittens have roundworm infections.[251] Studies have shown that up to 91% of dogs and 24% to 75% of cats are infected.[240, 251, 252] Infection is most common in animals younger than 1 year of age. Two species commonly infect dogs, *Toxocara canis* and *Toxascaris leonina*; *Toxocara cati* and *Toxascaris leonina* infect cats. *Toxocara canis* is an important cause of the zoonotic disease visceral larva migrans.

Pathophysiology

Roundworms can be acquired by four routes: transplacental migration, which occurs commonly with *T. canis*; milk-borne transmission, which occurs with both *T. canis* and *T. cati*; ingestion of infective eggs, which occurs with all three species; and ingestion of a paratenic or intermediate host, which also occurs with all three species. After ingestion of *T. canis* or *T. cati* eggs, larvae are released in the stomach and small intestine, enter the liver through the portal system, migrate within the liver, are carried with blood to the lungs, migrate within the lungs, are coughed up and swallowed, and return to the small intestine, where they mature and produce large numbers of eggs.[40, 253] In older puppies, larvae do not enter the trachea but are carried to somatic tissues, where they remain dormant.[251] In pregnant female dogs, these larvae are activated and migrate to the liver and lungs of the puppies.[251] After the puppies are born, the larvae complete their migration to the intestine, where they develop into adult worms and can begin shedding eggs when the puppies are 3 weeks of age.[253] After birth, larvae can migrate to the mammary glands, and transmission in the milk can occur. Migration of *Toxascaris leonina* is confined to the mucosa of the intestine, and this organism does not cause liver or lung damage.[251]

In cats, somatic migration does occur after ingestion of eggs but does not result in transplacental infection. During lactation, larvae migrate to the mammary gland. The major route of infection in kittens is through the milk. Adult cats acquire *Toxocara cati* through ingestion of paratenic hosts (rodents, birds, and insects).[251] Most larvae obtained in this manner develop directly into adults in the intestinal lumen.[40]

Adult worms can be as large as 20 cm in length and 3 mm in width. They do not attach to the mucosa but live on intestinal contents.[40] Inflammation is caused by migration of larvae within the intestinal wall and may involve a hypersensitivity reaction. Some cases of eosinophilic gastroenteritis may be associated with migrating *T. canis* larvae.[202, 203] Eggs are unembryonated when passed in the feces. Infected animals can shed millions of eggs each day.[251] In a suitable environment, eggs can remain infective for years.

Humans become infected by ingesting eggs from the environment. Most infections do not result in clinical signs.[254] Somatic migration causes mechanical damage and inflammation. Common sites involved are liver, lungs, heart, brain, and eyes.[252, 254] Visceral larva migrans is most common in young children who have ingested large numbers of larvae or are repeatedly infected. Ocular larva migrans often affects children older than 7 years of age; they probably have ingested only a few larvae that have by chance migrated to the eye.[252]

Clinical Signs

Many animals infected with roundworms remain asymptomatic. Clinical signs are most common in puppies and kittens and include vomiting, diarrhea, abdominal pain, pot-bellied appearance, and failure to thrive.[40, 251] The vomitus and feces may contain worms. Occasionally, intestinal obstruction can occur. A cough, fever, mucopurulent nasal discharge, and respiratory distress can accompany pneumonia in young puppies as a result of extensive migration of larvae. Heavy infection can lead to stillbirth or to pneumonia in newborn puppies.[40]

Diagnostic Plan

Roundworm infection should be suspected in all puppies and kittens. Diagnosis is confirmed on fecal examination by finding eggs that are 65 to 90 × 75 μm and have a thick, pitted shell with dark brown to black contents that fill it entirely (Fig. 32–21; see Fig. 32–20).[40] *Toxascaris leonina* eggs are distinct from those of the other two species; they are oval and have smooth, colorless shells, and their contents occupy only part of the shell.[40] Severe clinical signs can occur in prepatent infections, so diagnosis must be based on signalment, history, and physical examination in some cases. Eosinophilia may be present.

Treatment

Many common anthelmintics are effective against roundworms. In dogs, pyrantel pamoate (Nemex, 4.5 mg/kg, by mouth once) is safe and effective; although this drug is not approved for cats, 20 mg/kg appears to be safe and efficacious.[255–257] Heavily infected puppies should be treated at 2-week intervals from 2 weeks of age until 8 weeks.[40, 253] Kittens can be treated several times at 2- to 3-week intervals up to 3 to 4 months of age.[255] Sanitation and

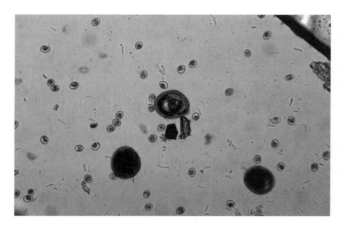

Figure 32–21

Fecal flotation showing several *Toxocara cati* eggs and numerous *Isospora* spp. cysts. Magnification, ×100. (Courtesy of Anne Zajac, DVM, PhD, Blacksburg, Virginia.)

removal of feces help to reduce environmental contamination.

Broader-spectrum anthelmintics are indicated in dogs with concurrent whipworm infection. Fenbendazole (Panacur, 50 mg/kg by mouth s.i.d. for 3 days), dichlorvos (Task, 30 mg/kg by mouth once), febantel (Rintal, 10 mg/kg by mouth s.i.d. for 3 days and 15 mg/kg s.i.d. in puppies less than 6 months of age), and mebendazole (Telmintic, 22 mg/kg by mouth s.i.d. for 3 days) are effective. Dichlorvos should not be used in debilitated dogs or those with heartworms.

Fenbendazole, 50 mg/kg, given to pregnant female dogs from day 40 of gestation until 14 days after birth, can prevent infection of puppies.[244] In addition, fenbendazole at 150 mg/kg for 3 days is effective in killing dormant second-stage larvae in the tissues.[258]

Heartworm preventatives diethylcarbamazine citrate/oxibendazole (Filarabits Plus), milbemycin oxide (Interceptor), pyrantel (Heartgard Plus), and diethylcarbamazine are effective in treating or preventing roundworms and may be beneficial in chronically infected animals kept in contaminated environments that cannot be cleaned properly and in dogs that ingest paratenic hosts.[246, 259] One percent bleach solutions strip the outer sticky layer of the eggs, allowing them to be washed away more easily.

Prognosis

The prognosis for most dogs and cats with roundworm infection is excellent. Mixed parasitic infections (especially with hookworms) or concurrent viral infection can dramatically worsen the prognosis. However, the outlook for eliminating the possibility of human infection is not as good, because environmental contamination often has occurred by the time puppies or kittens are first presented to the veterinarian.

Coccidia

Coccidia are obligate intracellular parasites that infect dogs and cats.[41] *Isospora* spp. are most common in both animals. *Toxoplasma gondii* (see Chap. 40) and *Besnoitia* spp. can be found in cats, and *Hammondia* spp., *Sarcocystis* spp., and *Cryptosporidium parvum* (see Uncommon Disorders) occur in both dogs and cats.

Pathophysiology

The life cycles of coccidia are complex.[41, 260, 261] Dogs and cats become infected with *Isospora* spp. by ingestion of oocysts from the environment or by ingestion of infected paratenic hosts (mice). Sporozoites are liberated in the small intestines, where they enter mucosal cells and develop further. After several asexual stages, microgametes (sperm) and macrogametes (eggs) are produced. Fertilization yields a zygote, and an oocyst wall is produced. The oocyst is then excreted in the feces. The prepatent period varies from 3 to 11 days.[261] Oocyst shedding can continue for up to 9 weeks in some animals.[261] Sporulation occurs in several days (two sporocysts, each with four sporozoites). The sporulated oocysts survive in the environment for long periods.

Clinical Signs

Many animals remain asymptomatic after infection by *Isospora* spp.[260] When clinical signs do occur, they are most often seen in young puppies and kittens, especially those that have been recently stressed, are immunocompromised, or are infected with other GI parasites.[41] The most common signs are acute diarrhea, sometimes with blood or mucus, and abdominal pain.[261–263] Sometimes, dehydration can become severe, especially if other GI parasites or viral disorders are present.

Sarcocystis spp., *Besnoitia* spp., and *Hammondia* spp. do not cause clinical signs in dogs and cats. *T. gondii* may cause a mild, self-limited, acute diarrhea. The role of *C. parvum* as a cause of diarrhea in dogs and cats is unknown but is currently being investigated.[261]

Diagnostic Plan

The diagnosis of coccidial infection requires identification of ovoid or subspherical oocysts in feces (see Fig. 32–21).[41] Unsporulated *Isospora* oocysts range in size from about 23 to 44 × 20 to 33 μm. Smaller unsporulated oocysts (10 × 10 μm) may indicate *T. gondii* or *Besnoitia* spp. in cats or *Hammondia* spp. in dogs or cats. *Sarcocystis* produces small, sporulated oocysts that can rupture, and free sporocysts may be found in the feces. Very small, sporulated oocysts of *C. parvum* (4 × 5 μm) appear as pinkish bodies that contain a dark dot in sugar solutions.[41]

The role of *Isospora* spp. in diarrhea in dogs and cats is unknown. Animals with clinical signs and a positive fecal examination should be carefully assessed for other GI parasites, viral infections, and environmental and dietary causes of diarrhea. If diarrhea does not resolve after appropriate treatment for coccidia, a more in-depth diagnostic work-up should be pursued.

Treatment

Treatment with sulfadimethoxine, 55 mg/kg for the first day, followed by 27.5 mg/kg daily for 10 to 20 days, should alleviate clinical signs. Combination of sulfadimethoxine (55 mg/kg) and ormetoprim (11 mg/kg) for 23 days has been shown to be an effective treatment.[264] Trimethoprim-sulfonamide combinations have also been recommended at 30 to 60 mg/kg per day (or 15–30 mg/kg in animals weighing less than 4 kg) for 6 days.[260, 261] Dehydrated animals require fluid therapy.[263] Prompt removal of feces and appropriate sanitation help prevent outbreaks in kennels and catteries.[41, 261]

Prognosis

The prognosis for puppies and kittens infected with coccidia is excellent. Failure to respond to treatment suggests the presence of immunosuppression or other GI diseases.

Giardia

Giardia is a flagellate protozoan parasite commonly associated with acute small bowel diarrhea, but in some cases, acute large bowel diarrhea, chronic small or large bowel diarrhea, or, rarely, acute or chronic vomiting may occur. Some infected animals do not develop any clinical signs. Studies throughout the world have found infection rates in dogs and cats ranging from 1% to 39%.[96, 265–270] Younger animals have a higher rate of infection.

Various strains possess different degrees of pathogenicity.[96] Clinical signs may be self-limited in some patients.[271] Severe disease most often occurs in puppies or kittens, animals with other GI parasites or diseases, or debilitated animals, but it can occur in otherwise healthy patients.

Pathophysiology

The life cycle of *Giardia* is direct.[95] Cysts (9–13 μm) may be ingested from contaminated water, but direct transmission between animals is also possible, especially where animals are in close contact, as in catteries or kennels.[96, 272] Cysts are oval and contain two or four nuclei.[273] Excystation occurs in the small intestine, and each cyst releases two trophozoites. Maturation and division of the motile trophozoite

(12–17 μm long and 7–10 μm wide) occur in the small bowel.[96, 273, 274] Trophozoites are shaped like teardrops, have four pairs of flagella and a pair of dark median bodies, and are binucleated.[273, 275] Trophozoites attach to the brush border, where they absorb nutrients.[273, 275] The prepatent period in dogs and cats varies from 5 to 16 days. Little is known about encystation, but it probably occurs in the ileum or colon. Although cysts are susceptible to desiccation, they are hardy and can survive for weeks to months in a cool, moist environment.

Little is known about the pathogenesis of *Giardia* infection in dogs and cats. Studies in laboratory animals and humans have demonstrated malabsorption of nutrients, decreased intestinal disaccharidases, increased enterocyte turnover, lymphocytic infiltration, and villous atrophy.[37, 96, 275, 276] The wide variation of pathogenicity may be related to the host's immune response or nutritional status, presence of other parasites or GI diseases, or strain variation.[37] Because younger animals are more commonly affected, it is possible that some degree of protective immunity develops.[96, 275]

Giardia should be considered potentially zoonotic, and adequate precautions should be taken when handling feces.[37, 275] Cysts are susceptible to drying and to many common disinfectants.[37, 277] Dog and cat feces should be disposed of promptly, and hands should be washed immediately after contact.[275] Children and immunocompromised adults should avoid contact with feces.

Clinical Signs

Most dogs and cats infected with *Giardia* remain asymptomatic.[37, 95] If clinical signs occur, acute small bowel diarrhea is most common. Diarrhea may be self-limited in some patients. Severe diarrhea may be accompanied by dehydration, lethargy, and anorexia. However, most affected patients remain bright, alert, and afebrile and maintain a normal appetite. Occasionally, acute vomiting may accompany diarrhea.

Chronic small intestinal diarrhea accompanied by weight loss can occasionally occur. Acute or chronic large bowel diarrhea with hematochezia, excessive fecal mucus, and tenesmus may develop on occasion. Excessive fecal mucus is often seen in infected cats.[272, 278]

Diagnostic Plan

Diagnosis of *Giardia* can often be made by appropriate fecal examination techniques. *Giardia* cysts are not routinely identified by commonly used fecal flotation solutions, because cysts become shriveled and cannot be identified. If giardiasis is suspected but cannot be confirmed, a therapeutic trial may be indicated. However, cessation of diarrhea after treatment does not confirm a definitive diagnosis of giardiasis.

Motile trophozoites may be found in a fresh saline fecal smear.[37] Trophozoites can be identified by their rapid motion and concave ventral surface. Trophozoites are not often found in semiformed or firm feces. One study in dogs showed that examination of fresh feces on three separate days identified approximately 40% of dogs infected with *Giardia*.[94] Examination of feces by zinc sulfate flotation (see Fecal Examination) is considered to be the most accurate practical diagnostic test available (Fig. 32–22).[37, 94–96] Duodenal aspiration of fluid with examination of the sediment for motile trophozoites was at one time considered the gold standard for diagnosis of *Giardia* in dogs.[279] However, this requires either endoscopy or exploratory laparotomy. Several studies in experimental dogs have demonstrated that one to three zinc sulfate fecal flotations are as sensitive as or more sensitive than duodenal aspiration in identifying *Giardia* cysts.[118]

Recently, several fecal ELISAs have been marketed for human use.[37] These tests identify *Giardia*-specific antigens. Preliminary use of one of these tests showed that a falsely negative ELISA can occur, emphasizing that a negative ELISA does not eliminate the possibility of *Giardia* infection.[37, 280, 281] It is possible that the ELISA may be a more sensitive test than zinc sulfate flotation, but further investigation is necessary to establish the value of ELISA in diagnosing giardiasis in dogs and cats.

Treatment

Our drug of choice in treating giardiasis is metronidazole, 50 mg/kg s.i.d. for 5 days. It has been suggested to split the dosage and administer it b.i.d. Metronidazole was effective in clearing 67% of infected dogs at 22 mg/kg b.i.d. for 5 days.[273, 282] Tablets should not be divided, because the medication is bitter and unpalatable.[37, 274, 275] Some authors have found that a lower dosage, 10 mg/kg b.i.d., is effective in cats.[274] Severe neurologic side effects, including seizures and coma, have been reported in dogs receiving higher dosages or prolonged treatment.[197] Mild neurologic signs can occur with lower dosages but are usually reversible if the drug is discontinued. Metronidazole is a potential mutagen and carcinogen, so treatment of pregnant animals should be avoided.[37, 275]

Furazolidone (Furoxone Suspension) is available as a suspension and is convenient to administer to cats and small dogs (4 mg/kg b.i.d. for 7 days). It has been shown to be effective in cats.[272, 274] Recently, albendazole (Valbazen Suspension), 25 mg/kg b.i.d. for 2 days, and fenbendazole, 50 mg/kg s.i.d. for 3 days, were shown to be safe and effective in dogs.[283, 284]

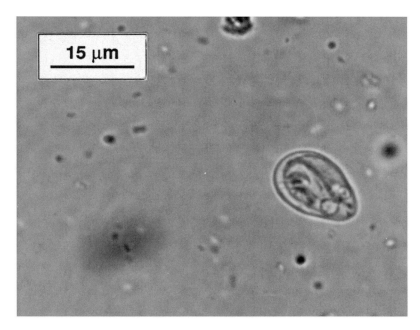

Figure 32–22
Giardia cyst in a zinc sulfate flotation. Two nuclei are visible. (From Zajac AM. Giardiasis. In: August JR. Consultations in Feline Internal Medicine 2. Philadelphia, WB Saunders, 1994:85.)

Persistent clinical signs after treatment may suggest treatment failure, lack of client compliance, reinfection, underlying GI disease, or incorrect diagnosis. If clinical signs continue, treatment for a prolonged period (i.e., metronidazole for 6–10 days), use of a different agent, or further diagnostic testing to identify a primary GI disorder is indicated.

Prognosis

Most patients with giardiasis promptly recover after therapy. If another GI disorder is present concurrently, the prognosis for clearing the *Giardia* organisms is related to the primary condition. Recurrent infection is possible if re-exposure to the source of infection cannot be prevented.

Tapeworms

Tapeworms commonly parasitize the small intestines of dogs and cats but do not cause serious clinical signs.[240] Owners may become alarmed after noticing motile proglottids in the feces. The common tapeworms include *Dipylidium caninum* (dogs and cats), *Taenia pisiformis* (dogs), and *Taenia taeniaeformis* (cats).

Two small tapeworms (1–10 mm in length) that can be found in dogs *(Echinococcus granulosus)* and in dogs or cats *(Echinococcus multilocularis)* are important because serious disease can develop in an intermediate host (humans).[285–287]

Pathophysiology

Dogs and cats become infected by ingestion of the intermediate hosts of the tapeworm: fleas *(Dipy-lidium),* rabbits *(T. pisiformis),* or rodents *(T. taeniaeformis).* Adult tapeworms can grow from 10 to 100 cm in length.[288, 289] They attach to the mucosa with a scolex, which has four oval suckers and many spines. They absorb nutrients from the GI lumen through the integument.[289] Gravid proglottids containing eggs *(Taenia)* or egg packets *(Dipylidium)* pass out with the feces. Eggs hatch after ingestion by an intermediate host. An infective larva develops in 1 to 3 weeks.

Dipylidium infection can be transmitted to humans by ingestion of infected fleas. This occurs most commonly in children.[288, 289]

E. granulosus occurs most commonly in the sheep-rearing areas of the Southwest. Besides dogs, foxes, wolves, coyotes, dingoes, and jackals can serve as definitive hosts.[285, 286, 290–292] *E. multilocularis* is enzootic in the north central United States and south central Canada and appears to be spreading southeast.[286] The common definitive hosts for *E. multilocularis* are wolves, foxes, and coyotes, but dogs and cats can also serve this function.[285] Besides humans, other intermediate hosts for these two parasites include sheep, moose, caribou, field voles, and deer mice.[286] In humans, the larval stages of both tapeworms can produce large hydatid cysts in the liver or, less commonly, in the lungs, kidney, spleen, bone, or central nervous system.[286]

Clinical Signs

The common tapeworms of dogs and cats do not usually cause clinical signs. Occasionally, anal pruritus may be produced by motile proglottids.

Diagnostic Plan

Diagnosis of common tapeworms is based on observation of the proglottids in the feces or on the perianal region. Proglottids of *Dipylidium* are similar in shape to cucumber seeds; those of *Taenia* are rectangular (Fig. 32–23). Proglottids can be examined microscopically to differentiate *Dipylidium* from *Taenia* spp. by demonstrating the two genital pores of *Dipylidium*.[289] In addition, the proglottid can be squashed on a microscope slide to free the characteristic egg packet of *Dipylidium*.[289]

Because of their small size, proglottids are not visible in the feces of animals infected with *Echinococcus* spp. Single taeniid eggs can be identified in feces but cannot be differentiated from nonpathogenic *Taenia* spp.[285, 286] In endemic areas, eggs found without evidence of *Taenia* proglottids should be considered potentially to be *Echinococcus* spp., and care should be taken when handling feces. Development of serodiagnostic tests is currently underway.[293–296]

Treatment

Treatment with praziquantel (Droncit, 5 mg/kg by mouth once) or epsiprantel (Cestex, 2.75 mg/kg by mouth once in cats; 5.5 mg/kg by mouth once in dogs) is effective in eliminating common tapeworms.[288, 289, 297, 298] Both mebendazole and fenbendazole are effective against *Taenia* spp. Long-term control depends on eliminating the intermediate hosts through vigorous flea control methods or abolishing hunting and scavenging behavior. Praziquantel is effective against *Echinococcus* spp.[285, 286, 299, 300]

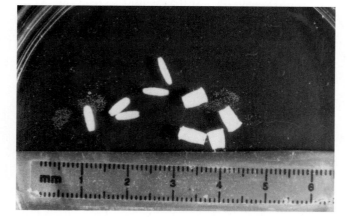

Figure 32–23

Tapeworm proglottids from *Dipylidium caninum* (cucumber seed–shaped) and *Taenia* (rectangular-shaped). (Courtesy of Anne Zajac, DVM, PhD, Blacksburg, Virginia.)

Prognosis

The prognosis for removal of the tapeworms after therapy is excellent.

Canine Parvovirus

In the late 1970s, canine parvovirus type 2 emerged as a common cause of acute life-threatening vomiting and diarrhea in dogs. Presently, disease occurs most commonly in unvaccinated puppies. Doberman pinschers and rottweilers are at increased risk to develop infection.[301]

Pathophysiology

Affected dogs shed large numbers of viral particles in their feces for 1 to 2 weeks. The virus is extremely hardy and may persist in the environment for 5 to 6 months.[45, 302, 303] Fomites are important in the transmission of disease. Most infections are subclinical or result in mild clinical signs that do not require treatment by the veterinarian. However, severe disease can occur in unprotected animals.[304] Other stresses, parasites, and viral diseases are important in the development of clinical signs.[304–306]

Dogs ingest infective virus particles. Relatively few particles are necessary for infection.[45] Virus replication occurs in the lymphoid tissues of the oropharynx. Viremia occurs by 3 to 5 days, and virus is spread to rapidly dividing tissues (i.e., intestinal crypt epithelium and bone marrow).[307–312] Infection of crypt epithelium leads to villous collapse, malabsorption, and PLE.[313–315] Vomiting and diarrhea occur 5 to 6 days after infection.[315] Fecal excretion of virus reaches a peak by day 6 and declines by day 12.[45, 303, 306, 307] Secondary bacterial infection is common because of an altered small intestinal mucosal barrier, leukopenia, and lymphoid depletion.[316, 317] Sepsis is suspected to be the cause of hypoglycemia.[21] With continued diarrhea, progressive anemia and hypoproteinemia develop. An immune response develops rapidly.[306–308, 318] Animals that can limit the magnitude and duration of viremia have milder disease.[45, 313]

In the past, infection of puppies near the time of birth led to a fatal myocardial form of the disease, with severe myocarditis and heart failure. The frequency of this syndrome has dramatically decreased, most likely because of higher antibody levels in the adult population.[45]

Clinical Signs

The initial clinical signs are vague and nonspecific; puppies are often lethargic and anorexic.[313, 319] Vomiting and profuse hemorrhagic diarrhea soon develop. Physical examination reveals pyrexia, moderate or severe depression, dehydration (delayed capillary refill time, enophthalmos, decreased skin turgor, tachycardia, pale mucous membranes, and cold extremities), generalized abdominal pain, gas-filled bowel loops, and thickened intestinal walls.[301, 314, 315, 320]

Occasionally, littermates may show signs of acute severe heart failure at 4 to 12 weeks of age.[321, 322] Affected puppies are weak and dyspneic and may have a pink frothy nasal discharge, or they may be found dead.[323] Sick puppies quickly die, and litter mortality may approach 100%. Surviving puppies often develop congestive heart failure. Currently, this form of the disease is very rare.[45]

Diagnostic Plan

Parvovirus should be suspected in any unvaccinated puppy with typical clinical signs. Fecal examination should be performed to assess parasites as a cause of the vomiting and diarrhea or as complicating factors in a case of parvovirus. Routine laboratory evaluation may reveal an elevated total protein and hematocrit and prerenal azotemia (dehydration), leukopenia, neutropenia, lymphopenia, hypoglycemia, hypokalemia, hypochloremia, hyponatremia, and metabolic acidosis or alkalosis.[313, 315, 324, 325] Anemia and hypoproteinemia can develop during hospitalization. Classic changes in the hemogram support the diagnosis but are not confirmatory. Fecal antigen testing by ELISA is definitive.[326] Modified live vaccines lead to fecal viral shedding and can cause a false-positive result 4 to 10 days after vaccination.

Abdominal radiographs may be made to eliminate the presence of small bowel obstruction. Signs consistent with parvovirus include gas and fluid distention of the bowel, flocculation of barium, delayed transit of barium, and marked irregularity to the small intestinal mucosa.[327]

Treatment

Vigorous fluid therapy is necessary to combat dehydration and extensive fluid loss as well as to provide maintenance requirements. The IV route is usually necessary.[319] Parenteral broad-spectrum antibiotics should also be administered (ampicillin, 22 mg/kg intravenously t.i.d. or q.i.d.). If life-threatening sepsis may be present, addition of gentamicin (2–4 mg/kg intravenously t.i.d.) or enrofloxacin (2.5–5.0 mg/kg intramuscularly b.i.d.) has been recommended by some clinicians. Severely depressed puppies should be suspected of being hypoglycemic. Serum glucose should be evaluated with a glucometer, and if it is low or if a glucometer is not available, the puppy should receive an IV bolus of 25% dextrose (0.5–1.0 g/kg). The amount of fluid required should be calculated, admin-

istered, and monitored as described in Chapter 31 for treatment of gastritis. Particular attention must be given to the amount of continued losses from vomiting and diarrhea. These losses represent a substantial portion of the daily fluid requirement and must be estimated and immediately replaced. Lactated Ringer's solution with 2.5% to 5% glucose and potassium supplementation is an appropriate fluid in most cases (see Table 31–7). During the first few days of therapy, fluids should be administered over as long a period as possible, preferably 24 hours a day. This is especially important in puppies that are hypoglycemic, because as little as 4 to 8 hours without glucose supplementation can lead to fatal hypoglycemia in these animals.

Oral food and water should be withheld until vomiting ceases for 24 hours; then gradual oral alimentation can be started (see treatment of gastritis in Chap. 31). Most patients need 3 to 5 days of fluid therapy, although occasionally up to 10 days are needed. GI parasites should be treated as soon as possible. Because of vomiting, oral medications for hookworms and roundworms are not appropriate. Although not approved for this purpose, ivermectin (Ivomec, 200 μg/kg once subcutaneously) is effective. This dosage should not be used in collies or related breeds because of toxicity.[245] Antiemetics may be indicated if the vomiting is severe (see Chap. 31). In cases in which diarrhea is especially profuse, motility modification with opioids may be necessary (see Dietary Indiscretion). Because loperamide and diphenoxylate are available only in oral formulations, vomiting must be controlled before they can be effective. In severe cases, blood transfusion may be necessary to treat the anemia and hypoproteinemia that develop. Antiendotoxin plasma was shown to reduce morbidity and shorten hospitalization in one study.[328] Disinfection with chlorine bleach (1:30) kills virus on appropriate surfaces after organic material has been removed.[320, 329]

Vaccination

Appropriate vaccination programs can dramatically reduce the incidence of parvoviral infections. Vaccination should start at 6 weeks of age and continue every 3 to 4 weeks until 18 weeks of age.[330] Vaccination cannot completely protect a puppy from disease, because there exists a 1- to 3-week window during which the puppy's maternal antibody prevents an immune response to vaccination but does not protect the puppy against virulent viral exposure.[45, 303, 331–333] Recent introduction of high-titer vaccines may break through maternal immunity and provide protection earlier, reducing a puppy's susceptibility to infection. Until the puppy reaches 18 weeks of age, it should be isolated from all sources of exposure, especially public parks and other areas frequented by dogs that may contain infected feces. Adults should be revaccinated yearly.

Three closely related subtypes of parvovirus have been identified, CPV-2, CPV-2a, and CPV-2b. Currently used vaccines protect against all three types.[45] Apparent vaccination failures are probably a result of maternal immunity interference.

Prognosis

With prompt diagnosis and vigorous fluid therapy, most puppies with parvovirus survive. Clients must be prepared for an extensive hospitalization and intensive care. Puppies presented moribund have a much poorer prognosis.

Feline Parvovirus

Infection with feline parvovirus results in a disease that has been called panleukopenia, feline infectious enteritis, or feline distemper.[334] Unlike canine parvovirus, the disease has been present for a long time. The clinical syndromes caused by the canine and feline viruses have many similarities. The development of clinical signs in unvaccinated kittens is common, although subclinical infections are most prevalent.[335]

Pathophysiology

Transmission occurs by ingestion or inhalation of the virus, which is excreted in the feces, saliva, urine, and nasal discharge of infected cats. Replication occurs in the lymphoid tissue of the oropharynx.[334] Viremia develops, and the virus replicates in rapidly dividing cells in lymphoid tissue, bone marrow, small and large intestinal crypts, and the central nervous system of the fetus.[336, 337] Infection of intestinal crypts leads to villous collapse and atrophy. Surviving cats rapidly develop an antibody response.[335] Pyrexia, vomiting, and diarrhea lead to dehydration and electrolyte changes. Secondary infection is common because of an altered mucosal barrier that allows the absorption of bacteria, neutropenia, and generalized lymphoid depletion. Disseminated intravascular coagulation (DIC) may be a terminal event.[335]

The virus is extremely stable in the environment and may remain alive for 1 year or longer.[335] Infected animals can shed virus in the feces and urine for up to 6 weeks. Fomites are important in transmission.

Clinical Signs

The most common clinical signs are anorexia, lethargy, depression, and vomiting.[334, 338] Diarrhea may develop as the disease progresses. Unlike with canine parvovirus, signs of large bowel involvement may also be present (i.e., mucus, hematochezia, and tenesmus). Usually, diarrhea and vomiting are not as profuse in cats as in dogs. Physical examination may reveal pyrexia, abdominal pain, thickened bowel walls, enlarged mesenteric lymph nodes, and signs of secondary infection. Oral ulceration develops in some cats as the disease progresses.[338]

Infection of a pregnant queen can cause severe reproductive abnormalities. Infection early in pregnancy can result in fetal resorption. Mummification and abortion can result from infection acquired in midgestation. Stillbirth, abortion, neonatal death, and cerebellar hypoplasia in kittens can follow infection in the third trimester or in the neonatal period. Kittens with cerebellar hypoplasia have severe static ataxia, incoordination, and tremors (see Chap. 25).[334, 335, 339] Usually only part of the litter is affected.[335]

Diagnostic Plan

Diagnosis is based on finding the classic clinical signs in an unvaccinated kitten. Routine laboratory evaluation often reveals leukopenia, characterized by neutropenia, and lymphopenia.[338] Dehydration may cause an elevated total protein and hematocrit and prerenal azotemia. Electrolyte changes are less common and milder than in dogs with parvovirus but are proportional to the severity of clinical signs. There are no commercially available definitive diagnostic tests. A fecal examination should be performed to exclude the presence of parasites, which can mimic some of the clinical signs or intensify the severity of a parvoviral infection. Thrombocytopenia and prolonged clotting times accompany DIC. A survey abdominal radiograph helps eliminate the presence of an intestinal obstruction from a foreign body or intussusception.

Treatment

Prompt diagnosis, fluid therapy, and administration of antibiotics to combat secondary infection are the cornerstones of effective therapy. Because vomiting and diarrhea may not be as profuse as in dogs with parvovirus, fluids may be able to be administered subcutaneously.[336] Kittens that are severely dehydrated and those with profuse losses require IV fluid administration. Guidelines for calculating dehydration, providing maintenance, and replacing losses are similar to those used for dogs with parvovirus (see treatment of gastritis in Chap. 31). In most cases, a balanced polyionic fluid such as lactated Ringer's solution is appropriate. Glucose (2.5%–5%) and potassium supplementation are also important (see Table 31–7).

Broad-spectrum parenteral antibiotics are important to prevent or treat secondary infections (ampicillin, 22 mg/kg intravenously t.i.d. or q.i.d.).[336] Food and water should be withheld until vomiting has ceased for 12 to 24 hours, and then gradual oral alimentation can be started (see treatment of gastritis in Chap. 31). Most animals require 2 to 5 days of therapy. The virus can be killed by dilute bleach (6% sodium hypochlorite).[335]

Vaccination

Both killed and modified live vaccines can protect kittens from infection. Vaccinations should be administered at 8 to 10 weeks of age and should be repeated at 12 to 14 weeks of age. Adults should receive a yearly booster. Most kittens have lost maternal immunity by 12 weeks of age. Although not as well documented, a situation similar to that in canine parvovirus probably exists in which maternal immunity blocks a response to vaccination but cannot protect the kitten against virulent viral challenge.[334, 336]

Prognosis

Survival is common for most kittens that receive timely veterinary attention. Kittens that are moribund on presentation or have signs of severe secondary infection or DIC have a poor prognosis. There is no effective treatment for cerebellar hypoplasia, although kittens can survive with good nursing care.

Canine Coronavirus

Subclinical infection with canine coronavirus is common in the dog population, but the incidence of clinical disease is unknown.[340–343] Puppies 6 to 12 weeks of age appear to be most susceptible to developing clinical signs.

Pathophysiology

Canine coronavirus is highly contagious.[344–346] Transmission occurs after oral ingestion of virus from feces. The incubation period is short, 1 to 4 days. Viral replication takes place in the mature epithelial cells of the small intestinal villi, leading to villous blunting, but because the crypt cells are spared, crypt hypertrophy rapidly leads to repair of the villi. A brief period of loss of absorptive and digestive surface area leads to maldigestion and diarrhea.[320] Local intestinal immunity is probably responsible for protection.[346] The development and severity of clinical signs may be affected by stress and by the presence of parasites, bacteria, or other viruses.[347, 348] Infected dogs can shed virus for several months.

Mixed infections with canine parvovirus and coronavirus are common and may result in increased morbidity and mortality.[349, 350] Coronavirus-induced crypt cell hyperplasia provides more cells for parvovirus to infect, which worsens the severity of infection.

Clinical Signs

The clinical signs associated with coronavirus infection are highly variable.[347] The most common sign is mild, self-limited diarrhea.[351] Feces have been described as yellow to orange, and fresh blood may occasionally be present.[344, 352, 353] Anorexia, lethargy, and vomiting can occur.[320, 345–347] Pyrexia is not consistently produced. Loose stools may persist for 3 to 4 weeks.[348, 353] Deaths in young puppies have been reported, but concurrent diseases may have been responsible for the intensification of clinical signs.[352] In contrast to parvoviral diarrhea, leukopenia is not present.[353]

Diagnostic Plan

The definitive diagnosis requires electron microscopic examination of feces.[343, 347] Because this test is not universally offered at diagnostic laboratories, it is often very difficult to confirm a diagnosis. In most dogs, clinical signs resolve without intensive treatment, and it is difficult to differentiate coronavirus from other causes of self-limited vomiting and diarrhea. Laboratory evaluation in cases involving mild dehydration reveal elevated total protein and hematocrit and prerenal azotemia. Fecal examinations should be performed to identify concurrent parasitic infections. Because concurrent infections with parvovirus occur, a fecal ELISA for parvovirus should be evaluated, especially if severe clinical signs or leukopenia is present.

Treatment

Cases of suspected coronavirus can effectively be treated by following the guidelines for treatment of dietary indiscretion. In many cases, it may not be possible to determine which of these two disease processes is responsible for clinical signs. Withholding of food and water until vomiting ceases for 12 to 24 hours, followed by gradual oral alimentation and use of a highly digestible diet, may be sufficient in many cases.[344, 352] Motility modification with opioids is not often necessary but may be beneficial for patients with severe diarrhea. If mild to moderate dehydration is present, subcutaneous fluids should be administered. If moderate to severe dehydration and profuse diarrhea are present, IV fluids should be administered in a manner similar to that used in treating canine parvovirus.

Vaccination

Several killed virus vaccines that markedly reduce viral replication in the small intestine are available.[354] We do not routinely administer coronavirus vaccines to puppies because the incidence and significance of clinical disease are presently unknown and because, in most cases, only mild clinical signs are attributed to coronavirus infection. We do vaccinate higher-risk puppies such as show, field trial, and kenneled puppies.

Prognosis

The prognosis for dogs infected with coronavirus is excellent. Most dogs recover with minimal treatment. Severely affected patients that die may have had concurrent parvovirus or other infectious disease.

Feline Coronavirus

An enteric coronavirus, similar to the virus that causes feline infectious peritonitis (FIP), is very common in the cat population.[355, 356] It appears to cause mild, self-limited diarrhea, vomiting, and low-grade fever in kittens younger than 12 weeks of age.[355, 357] The virus acts like other coronaviruses and attacks the villous epithelial cells.[356] The diagnosis is difficult to establish, but confirmation is rarely needed because of the mild clinical signs and transient nature of the infection. Treatment may not be necessary or may consist of subcutaneous fluids if dehydration has occurred. Cats develop a positive antibody titer, which is important when assessing FIP serologic tests (see Chap. 38).[356] Infection may sensitize the cat to future infection with the FIP virus and may accelerate the disease process.[355, 356]

Hemorrhagic Gastroenteritis

Hemorrhagic gastroenteritis is a syndrome of unknown origin that causes life-threatening acute vomiting and diarrhea. Schnauzers, dachshunds, Yorkshire terriers, and poodles may be at increased risk to develop the syndrome.[92, 358] Middle-aged dogs are affected most commonly.[92] Relapses are uncommon.[92, 358]

Pathophysiology

Hemoconcentration leads to increased blood viscosity, sludging of red blood cells, and hypoxia. The mechanism causing hemoconcentration is unknown, but intestinal hypersecretion has been proposed.[92] Anemia develops because of the loss of blood into the GI tract. Damage to the intestinal mucosal barrier makes the dog susceptible to sepsis and endotoxemia.[359] The generation of oxygen-derived free radicals may also participate in the pathogenesis. The syndrome has not been linked to dietary or bacterial causes.[92] An allergic reaction to bacterial endotoxin

and an abnormal immune response have been proposed as causes.[92, 358]

Clinical Signs

Acute profuse hemorrhagic diarrhea and vomiting occur.[358] The stool often assumes a "raspberry jam" consistency. Dogs initially are bright and alert and appear well hydrated.[92] Physical examination may reveal generalized abdominal pain.[358] Occasionally, ventricular premature contractions develop.[92] The syndrome rapidly progresses, and hypovolemic shock and anemia can develop.

Diagnostic Plan

Massive increases in the hematocrit occur (as high as 86%).[92, 358] Thrombocytopenia and prolonged clotting times occur in cases that progress to DIC.[358] The diagnosis is based on the clinical signs, characteristic appearance of the feces, and massively elevated hematocrit, often with a normal or only slightly elevated total protein.[92, 358]

Treatment

Successful treatment requires prompt recognition of the syndrome, vigorous fluid therapy, and administration of parenteral bactericidal antibiotics (ampicillin, 22 mg/kg intravenously t.i.d. or q.i.d.).[92] A balanced polyionic electrolyte solution (i.e., lactated Ringer's solution) should be administered intravenously as rapidly as possible until the hematocrit falls below 60%. The rate of fluid therapy can then be slowed to correct for maintenance, continued losses, and any remaining dehydration (see treatment of gastritis in Chap. 31). Administration and monitoring of therapy is similar to that used in treating parvovirus. Most patients require 2 to 3 days of intensive fluid therapy; those with severe blood loss require transfusion. If vomiting is profuse, antiemetic therapy is indicated (see Chap. 31). Phenothiazines should not be administered until the dog has become rehydrated. Metoclopramide should not be used until GI obstruction has been ruled out.

Prognosis

A guarded prognosis should be given on admission until the response to treatment can be assessed. Most dogs improve rapidly after initial fluid therapy and completely recover.[92, 358]

Foreign Body

Most foreign materials entering the small intestine pass without causing clinical signs or cause only

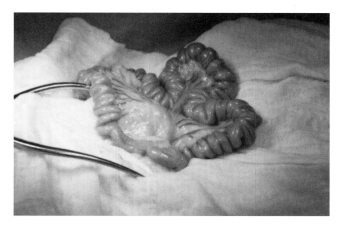

Figure 32–24
Surgical appearance of plicated small bowel in a 1-year-old domestic longhair cat with a linear foreign body. (Courtesy of Robert Martin, DVM, Blacksburg, Virginia.)

mild diarrhea and abdominal pain. However, foreign bodies that become lodged in the small intestine can produce a partial or complete obstruction (see sections under Problem Identification). Sharp objects can penetrate the intestinal wall and cause peritonitis. Linear objects (e.g., thread, string, dental floss) can cause intestinal plication and perforation. Younger animals are more prone to ingesting foreign materials, and cats swallow linear objects more commonly than do dogs.[32, 88, 360, 361]

Pathophysiology

A variety of foreign objects are ingested by animals and either lodge in or pass through the small intestine. Common objects include stones, fruit pits, rubber balls, other rubber objects, cloth, metal objects, coins, sponges, hair balls, corn cobs, bottle caps, chew toys, string, thread, dental floss, marbles, and bones.[32, 362] Many foreign bodies pass through the intestines and cause mild abrasion of mucosal surfaces, leading to self-limited enteritis or colitis, or both. The pathophysiology of partial and complete obstructions is covered in the Problem Identification section. Linear foreign bodies can become lodged at the base of the tongue or pylorus.[88, 360, 361] As peristalsis propels the linear object, the intestines become plicated (Fig. 32–24). Continued peristaltic activity can result in intestinal perforation and peritonitis.[88] Intussusceptions can be found concurrently in some dogs with linear foreign bodies.[361]

Clinical Signs

An owner may report suspicion or observation of ingestion of foreign material. The clinical signs

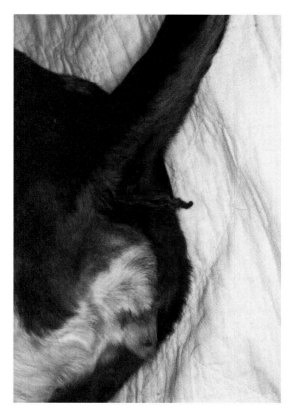

Figure 32–25
Linear foreign body protruding from the anus of a 9-year-old basset hound that ate carpet. A large amount of the fiber was caught at the pylorus. The entire small bowel was plicated.

associated with intestinal foreign bodies are variable and range from none to severe vomiting, diarrhea, and abdominal pain.[360, 361] Chronic diarrhea and weight loss can result from a partial obstruction.[15] The foreign object or a dilated loop of intestine may be palpated.[32] A linear foreign body can be wrapped around the base of the tongue (see Fig. 29–12) or protrude from the rectum (Fig. 32–25); bunched and plicated intestines can be palpated.[88, 360]

Animals with complete obstruction may be moderately to severely dehydrated (delayed capillary refill time, enophthalmos, decreased skin turgor, tachycardia, pale mucous membranes, and cold extremities).[362] Hypovolemic or endotoxic shock, or both, can also develop. Intestinal perforation may lead to pyrexia. Foreign bodies that have passed through the small and large intestines may become lodged at the rectum and cause tenesmus and hematochezia.

Diagnostic Plan

The diagnosis of intestinal foreign body requires radiographic confirmation. Radiopaque foreign objects are easy to visualize.[32] Linear foreign bodies cause pleating of bowel, eccentric tapered intestinal gas bubbles, gathering of intestines to the right of midline, and signs of peritonitis (see Fig. 32–7).[88, 363] Indirect evidence that radiolucent objects have caused an obstruction include dilation of the small bowel proximal to the obstruction with gas and fluid.[47, 71] The distinction between paralytic ileus and obstructive disease is not always clear-cut.[364] However, the degree of intestinal dilation is usually more severe with obstruction. An upper GI barium contrast series may be necessary to identify a radiolucent object. In cases of partial obstruction, the barium should outline the foreign body as it passes around it. If a complete obstruction is present, the barium abruptly stops.[47]

Routine laboratory evaluation often reflects the degree of dehydration. Elevations in the hematocrit and total protein and prerenal azotemia are common. Hypokalemia, hyponatremia, hypochloremia, and either metabolic acidosis or alkalosis can be seen.[362] Perforation and peritonitis may causes a leukocytosis with a left shift.

Treatment

Intervention is not required for all objects radiographically identified in the small intestine, because many spontaneously pass in the feces. The severity and progression of clinical and radiographic signs should be monitored closely. It may be necessary to make sequential radiographs before an appropriate decision can be made to remove the foreign object. Linear foreign bodies that have lodged under the tongue can be freed and allowed to pass (usually in 1–3 days), so long as the cat is monitored carefully for worsening of clinical signs.[360]

Foreign bodies that become lodged in the small intestine and cause obstruction, those that have perforated the bowel wall, and linear foreign bodies associated with prolonged vomiting, severe abdominal pain with pyrexia, or a degenerative left shift need to be removed by exploratory surgery and enterotomy or intestinal resection and anastomosis.[88, 360] Fluid therapy should be instituted before surgery to correct dehydration and electrolyte and acid-base abnormalities.[21] Endoscopic retrieval is usually unrewarding, because most foreign bodies lodge beyond the reach of the endoscope or are too tightly wedged to be removed. Objects lodged at the rectum can usually be removed manually. Sedation or anesthesia, rectal dilation, or colonoscopy may be necessary.

Prognosis

The prognosis for most patients with intestinal foreign bodies is good.[362] A guarded prognosis is warranted if perforation and peritonitis have devel-

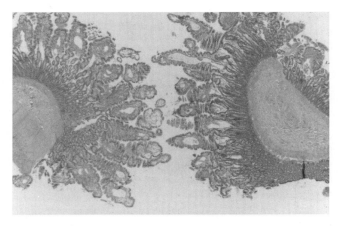

Figure 32–26

Microscopic appearance of lymphangiectasia of the small bowel of a Pomeranian with chronic intermittent vomiting and diarrhea and hypoalbuminemia. Dilation of the lacteals in the tips of many villi is present. Full-thickness small bowel biopsy samples were obtained during exploratory laparotomy.

oped or if complete obstruction has resulted in severe bowel damage or endotoxemia.[32, 88, 361]

Lymphangiectasia

Lymphangiectasia is dilation of the lymphatics of the small intestine (Fig. 32–26). Leakage of lymph or rupture of lymphatics leads to loss of protein-rich lymph into the small intestine and PLE. Lymphangiectasia can be idiopathic or secondary to lymphatic obstruction, most commonly caused by disease of the small bowel. It occurs in dogs.

Pathophysiology

The cause of idiopathic lymphangiectasia is unknown. A hereditary syndrome in the Lundehund has been proposed.[72] Obstructive lymphangiectasia results from diseases that obstruct lymphatic flow and produce dilation with leakage or rupture of lymphatic vessels. Lymph can escape into the GI lumen or into the bowel wall, where it can cause granulomatous inflammation.[110, 365] The most common causes of obstructive lymphangiectasia are inflammatory bowel disease, infiltrative lymphosarcoma, and histoplasmosis.

The loss of both albumin and globulins into the GI tract exceeds the intestines' ability for reabsorption and the liver's ability for synthesis; panhypoproteinemia develops. With decreased plasma osmotic pressure, edema, ascites, and pleural effusion can develop.

Clinical Signs

Most cases of lymphangiectasia are associated with chronic small bowel diarrhea, vomiting, weight loss, and PLE. With severe protein loss, edema, ascites, or pleural effusion can develop (see Fig. 32–4).[72, 110, 366]

Diagnostic Plan

The diagnostic plan for chronic small bowel diarrhea should be followed (see Chronic Diarrhea). The definitive diagnosis requires intestinal biopsy, although gross evidence can be seen endoscopically or during exploratory surgery as white dilated villi and engorged lymphatics (Fig. 32–27).[365] In small, endoscopically obtained mucosal biopsy samples, the thin-walled lymphatic vessels may collapse, and the characteristic ballooning dilation of lymphatic vessels may not be seen. However, the presence of an underlying cause of obstruction can be determined. The histologic features of lymphangiectasia are better preserved in full-thickness biopsy samples. However, exploratory surgery is not recommended because of the increased risks associated with hypoproteinemia.

Routine laboratory evaluation reveals hypoalbuminemia, hypoglobulinemia, hypocholesterolemia, hypocalcemia, and lymphopenia.[72, 74, 75, 110] Hypocalcemia can persist after correction for hypoalbuminemia because of malabsorption of vitamin D and calcium.[110, 366] Other laboratory changes associated with the primary cause of lymphatic obstruction may be evident.

Treatment

If an underlying cause of obstruction is present, it should be treated.[366] If lymphangiectasia is idiopathic, dietary management with a low-fat diet is indicated to reduce lymphatic flow and loss into the GI tract.[366] Both commercial low-fat diets and homemade recipes are available. Medium-chain triglyceride oil should be added to the diet to supply calories. Medium-chain triglycerides are absorbed directly into the enterocyte; they are transported to the liver by means of the portal system and do not require lymphatic absorption.[74, 75, 366] The dose should be increased gradually over 2 to 4 weeks, because diarrhea can be intensified and the drug can be unpalatable, until 1 to 2 mL/kg per day is reached. An anti-inflammatory dose of prednisone (1 mg/kg per day) can be added to reduce the inflammation within the intestinal wall resulting from leaking lymph.[76] If improvement occurs, the lowest dose that can be given every other day should be used.

Animals with edema, pleural effusion, or ascites benefit from plasma transfusion to temporarily raise serum albumin during the diagnostic period and to give the therapy a chance to become effective.

Prognosis

The prognosis for lymphangiectasia is guarded. The prognosis in cases caused by obstructive disorders is related to the underlying cause. Some patients with idiopathic disease respond well to dietary management, but most respond either partially or not at all. Sequential measurement of total protein is a convenient test to assess response to therapy.

Bacterial Overgrowth

Overgrowth of the normal bacterial flora of the small intestine can cause chronic diarrhea and weight loss. Bacterial overgrowth can occur secondary to partial intestinal obstruction (see Problem Identification), secondary to pancreatic exocrine insufficiency (see Chap. 33), or as an idiopathic condition. The idiopathic disorder has been recognized most commonly in young German shepherds but can occur in other breeds.[16, 367]

Pathophysiology

The effects of bacterial overgrowth are described in the Problem Identification section on partial intestinal obstruction. In dogs with idiopathic disease, overgrowth of many species of normal intestinal inhabitants occurs, with *E. coli*, enterococci, and *Clostridium*, *Staphylococcus*, *Corynebacterium*, *Proteus*, *Peptostreptococcus*, and *Actinomyces* spp. most commonly found.[16, 17, 63, 367–369] The numbers and types of bacteria isolated in individual dogs vary over time.[16] Minimal morphologic changes in the small intestine usually occur, but partial villous atrophy and infiltration of plasma cells and lymphocytes and reversible damage to the brush border membrane have been demonstrated.[16, 63, 368] The cause is unknown but has

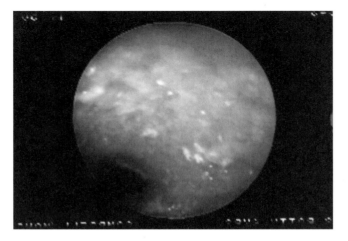

Figure 32–27
Endoscopic appearance of lymphangiectasia of the duodenum in a 6-year-old rottweiler with chronic diarrhea and hypoproteinemia. White dilated lacteals are visible.

been postulated to be related to reduced serum IgA levels in German shepherds. [16, 371, 372]

Clinical Signs

Idiopathic bacterial overgrowth results in chronic small bowel diarrhea and weight loss.[367] The diarrhea may initially be intermittent. However, some dogs with bacterial overgrowth may not develop clinical signs.[16]

Diagnostic Plan

Diagnosis of idiopathic bacterial overgrowth is difficult for the practitioner. Quantitative aerobic and anaerobic duodenal cultures and breath hydrogen analysis are not routinely available.[62, 134, 367, 368] Indirect assessment by measurement of serum vitamin B_{12} and folic acid is the most practical method currently available.[56] In patients with bacterial overgrowth, serum B_{12} should be reduced and folate increased.[17, 367] However, vitamin B_{12} may be normal and folate increased.[16] D-Xylose absorption may be reduced in approximately 50% of cases.[367] Finally, response to treatment provides indirect evidence of bacterial overgrowth.[16]

If bacterial overgrowth is suspected, predisposing conditions such as partial intestinal obstruction or pancreatic exocrine insufficiency should be evaluated with a barium contrast upper GI series and measurement of serum trypsin-like immunoreactivity, respectively.[15, 55, 56, 370]

Treatment

Treatment should be directed primarily against an underlying cause, if one is present. In idiopathic disease, a 3- to 4-week course of antibiotics is often effective. Tetracyclines (doxycycline, 3–5 mg/kg by mouth b.i.d.), amoxicillin (11–22 mg/kg by mouth b.i.d. or t.i.d.), and tylosin (7–15 mg/kg by mouth t.i.d.) have been recommended.[62]

Prognosis

Most dogs with idiopathic bacterial overgrowth respond favorably to antibiotic therapy. However, in the absence of a correctable cause, relapses are possible.

Duodenal Ulceration

Ulceration of the stomach or duodenum can cause acute or chronic vomiting, hematemesis, melena, and abdominal pain. Profuse GI hemorrhage can lead to anemia and profound weakness. Duodenal ulcers occur in dogs with liver diseases and mast cell

neoplasia.[373] The syndrome of gastric and duodenal ulcer disease is described in Chapter 31.

Feline Leukemia Virus-Associated Diarrhea

Enteritis associated with FeLV occurs in approximately 10% to 20% of infected cats.[54] Histologically, small intestinal lesions appear similar to those caused by feline panleukopenia virus, but lesions do not occur in the bone marrow and other lymphoid tissues. The mean age of affected cats is 2 years. Vomiting and hematemesis also occur.[374] Other FeLV-associated conditions are commonly found, including anemia, emaciation, rhinitis, and bronchitis (see Chap. 38).[375] Diagnosis is based on a positive FeLV ELISA and the absence of other common causes of diarrhea (e.g., parasites, dietary indiscretion, inflammatory bowel disease). Supportive therapy may be beneficial in the short term.

Feline Immunodeficiency Virus-Associated Diarrhea

Chronic or intermittent diarrhea is common in cats infected with FIV (12%–18%).[54, 376–378] Other clinical signs include lethargy, weight loss, pyrexia, lymphadenopathy, gingivitis or stomatitis, rhinitis, abscesses, and ocular discharge (see Chap. 38). Most cats with clinical signs are middle-aged. The pathogenesis of the diarrhea is unknown, but it may be related to immunosuppression. Histologically, diffuse enterocolitis, enterocyte necrosis, and villous atrophy and fusion occur.[379] Diagnosis is based on a positive FIV ELISA, the presence of other clinical signs, and the absence of other common causes of diarrhea (e.g., parasites, dietary indiscretion, inflammatory bowel disease, hyperthyroidism). Supportive therapy may be beneficial in the short term.

Common Diseases That Involve Primarily the Large Intestine

Whipworms

Trichuris vulpis infection is one of the most common causes of acute or chronic large bowel diarrhea in dogs.[2, 25] Puppies and dogs that live in contaminated environments are commonly affected. Cats only rarely have whipworms.

Pathophysiology

The parasite's life cycle is direct. Adult worms shed eggs intermittently, which can result in false-negative fecal examinations. The eggs have thick, yellow-brown shells, are barrel-shaped, have polar plugs, and are approximately 80 × 35 μm (see Fig. 32–20). They can persist for years in the environment. Prolonged sunlight kills whipworm eggs. A horticultural flame gun can kill eggs on concrete surfaces.[38, 380] Areas that cannot be easily cleaned, such as lawns and dirt kennels, can become contaminated, providing a source for reinfection. The eggs embryonate in as few as 10 days in optimal environmental conditions. After a dog ingests the infective eggs, the larvae hatch in the small intestine and burrow into the mucosa for 2 to 10 days, emerge, and attach to the mucosa in the cecum and ascending colon, where they complete maturation.[380] Females begin producing eggs 70 to 107 days after the infection has been acquired. Estimates of daily egg production range from 1000 to 4000. Adult worms may live up to 18 months.

Pathogenicity is related to tunneling of the thin anterior portion of the adult worm into the epithelium of the cecum or ascending colon, which produces localized inflammation, mucosal hyperplasia, and, in some cases, focal granulomatous reactions.[38, 380, 381] Adult worms measure 45 to 75 mm in length. The worms feed on tissue fluid, blood, and cellular debris. The parasites may be found throughout the large intestine in dogs harboring large numbers of worms.

Many infected dogs do not show any clinical signs. The factors contributing to the development of clinical signs include the number of worms present, location of worms, degree of inflammation produced, level of anemia or hypoproteinemia, nutritional status of the host, and presence of other GI parasites.[380]

Although controversial and unproven, infections of humans with *T. vulpis* may occur.[38, 380] Clients should be warned of the possible public health significance, and appropriate sanitary measures should be taken when disposing of fecal material.

Clinical Signs

Feces typically contain frank blood and excess mucus. Abdominal pain, inappetence, and weight loss can also occur.[380] Diarrhea may be intermittent in some cases.

Diagnostic Plan

Whipworm eggs can be identified with the use of routine fecal flotation procedures. However, if multiple fecal examinations fail to identify eggs, treatment for whipworms should be instituted before additional diagnostic tests are performed. A presumptive diagnosis of whipworm infection can be made if clinical signs improve within 2 or 3 days of institution of appropriate anthelmintic therapy. Adult worms may be seen in the cecum and ascending colon during

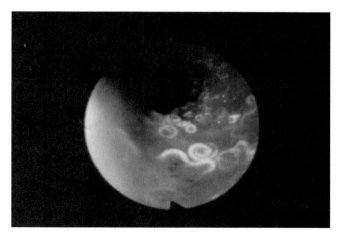

Figure 32-28
Endoscopic appearance of adult *Trichuris vulpis* in the ascending colon of a dog.

colonoscopic examination in a dog with an occult infection if the animal was not treated before colonoscopy was performed (Fig. 32–28).[382] Eosinophilia may be present; in severe cases, anemia and hypoproteinemia may develop.

Treatment

There are numerous therapeutic agents that are effective against whipworms in dogs.[38, 381] Commonly used treatments include fenbendazole (Panacur, 50 mg/kg by mouth s.i.d. for 3 days), butamisole (Styquin, 2.2 mg/kg subcutaneously), febantel with praziquantel (Vercom, 10 mg/kg by mouth s.i.d. for 3 days in adult dogs, or 15 mg/kg by mouth s.i.d. for 3 days in puppies younger than 6 months of age), and febantel without praziquantel (Rintal, 10 mg/kg by mouth s.i.d. for 3 days, or 15 mg/kg by mouth s.i.d. for 3 days in puppies).

Fenbendazole is a safe and efficacious drug with broad-spectrum activity against common GI nematodes and some tapeworms. Febantel is converted to fenbendazole. When combined with praziquantel, it offers broad-spectrum activity against common GI nematodes and tapeworms. Butamisole has the advantage of being given subcutaneously, ensuring that the entire dose is administered. However, it has a relatively low therapeutic index and should not be used in heartworm-positive or debilitated dogs.

Treatment should be repeated in 3 weeks and again in 3 months. The effects of most anthelmintics on the larval stages of whipworms remain unknown.[380] After anthelmintic administration has removed adult worms, larvae develop into adult parasites and reestablish infestation. Frequent disposal of feces helps reduce the risk of reinfection. In severe, recurrent cases, heartworm prophylaxis with milbemycin oxide (Interceptor, 0.5 mg/kg by mouth once a month) or diethylcarbamazine/oxibendazole (Filarabits Plus, 4.5 mg/kg [oxibendazole] by mouth s.i.d.) helps control whipworm infection.[248, 250, 383] Oxibendazole has been linked to idiosyncratic hepatic toxicity in dogs (see Chap. 34).[384]

Prognosis

Clinical signs rapidly resolve after appropriate therapy is instituted. Reinfestation is common in dogs that live in contaminated environments.

Irritable Bowel Syndrome

Irritable bowel syndrome (IBS) is a commonly diagnosed but poorly described functional disorder of dogs.[2] Synonyms include spastic colon, nervous colitis, and mucus colitis.[90] It has been estimated that 10% to 15% of dogs with chronic large bowel diarrhea have IBS.[385] Colonic dysfunction exists in the absence of structural, biochemical, or microbiologic abnormalities.[386]

In dogs, IBS is a diagnosis of exclusion. Before a diagnosis of IBS can be made, known causes of large bowel diarrhea must be eliminated as diagnostic possibilities. It is possible that dogs diagnosed with IBS may have (1) a true syndrome similar to IBS in humans, (2) another colonic disorder that has not been correctly diagnosed, (3) one of several newly described conditions, such as fiber-responsive large bowel diarrhea or *Clostridium perfringens* enterotoxicosis, that may be related to IBS, or (4) an idiopathic condition.

Pathophysiology

There have been no pathophysiologic studies concerning IBS in dogs. Studies in humans have investigated the roles of low-fiber diet, food allergy or intolerance, abnormal GI motility, altered pain perception, and psychologic factors.[386] Abnormal myoelectrical activity causes abnormal intestinal motility, which is the probable cause of clinical signs.[90, 386, 387]

Clinical Signs

In dogs, the most common clinical sign is intermittent large bowel diarrhea with excess fecal mucus, dyschezia, urgency to defecate, and increased frequency of defecation.[90] Hematochezia is uncommon. Intermittent bloating, nausea, vomiting, and abdominal pain may occur. Often, stresses can be identified and associated with cyclic clinical signs. Affected dogs are not necessarily hyperexcitable or unmanageable.[385]

Diagnostic Plan

IBS in dogs is an exclusion diagnosis. A thorough diagnostic plan must be followed without finding evidence of any other known disorder before a diagnosis of IBS can be made. Fecal examinations must be negative for parasites; laboratory evaluation should eliminate the possibility of a systemic disorder; an easily digested or high-fiber diet and deworming for whipworms should not relieve clinical signs; and finally, colonoscopic examination and mucosal biopsy must be normal. In some cases of IBS, spasm of the colonic wall may occur after contact with the endoscope. A response to a high-fiber diet does not eliminate the possibility of IBS, but it may support a diagnosis of fiber-responsive large bowel diarrhea or *C. perfringens* enterotoxicosis. The potential relation of these three syndromes is discussed in the following sections.

Treatment

Treatment for dogs with IBS must be individually planned for each patient. The intermittent nature of clinical signs often makes assessment of therapy difficult. Multiple treatments may be tried before control of clinical signs is obtained. If a stress factor can be identified, removal or modification may be beneficial. However, most stressors cannot be modified, and dietary or pharmacologic therapy is indicated. Diets high in fiber are often helpful in eliminating or reducing clinical signs in dogs. We have recommended commercially available high-fiber diets or supplementation of highly digestible diets with a source of soluble fiber. In many cases, feeding of high-fiber diets can reduce the dosage and frequency of administration of pharmacologic agents. An in-depth discussion of dietary fiber can be found in the section on fiber-responsive large bowel diarrhea.

Episodes of diarrhea can be controlled with the use of motility-modifying agents such as loperamide or diphenoxylate. These agents reduce diarrhea by increasing colonic segmentation. They can often be used for several days to a week and discontinued after the diarrhea resolves.[90] These drugs are discussed in detail in the section on dietary indiscretion. Pain can often be relieved by antispasmodic agents, and the effects of stressors can be reduced by sedatives. Librax contains the sedative chlordiazepoxide (5 mg) and clidinium bromide (2.5 mg), an anticholinergic agent. A suggested dosage is 0.1 to 0.25 mg/kg of clidinium, or 1 to 2 capsules by mouth b.i.d. or t.i.d.[90, 388] The drug can be given when the owner first notices abdominal pain or diarrhea in the animal or when stressful conditions are encountered and can usually be discontinued after a few days. Other anticholinergics, such as propantheline (Pro-Banthine, 0.25 mg/kg by mouth b.i.d. or t.i.d.), hyoscyamine (Levsin, 0.003–0.006 mg/kg by mouth b.i.d. or t.i.d.), or dicyclomine (Bentyl, 0.15 mg/kg by mouth b.i.d. or t.i.d.) have been suggested.[90] Anticholinergics can decrease or inhibit GI motility, which may worsen diarrhea. In humans, side effects include xerostomia, urinary retention, blurred vision, headache, psychosis, nervousness, and drowsiness. On occasion, nausea and vomiting preclude the use of oral medications. Parenteral antiemetics such as chlorpromazine (Thorazine, 0.2–0.5 mg/kg t.i.d. or q.i.d., intramuscularly or subcutaneously) can be given to relieve nausea and vomiting and allow administration of oral medications in 1 or 2 days.[90]

Prognosis

The prognosis for cure of IBS in dogs is guarded. Affected dogs may have intermittent clinical signs for years. Environmental, dietary, and pharmacologic therapy often results in control or reduction of clinical signs.

Fiber-Responsive Large Bowel Diarrhea

We have successfully managed a group of dogs with chronic idiopathic large bowel diarrhea with the use of a highly digestible diet supplemented with soluble fiber. Most dogs are middle-aged.[2, 389]

Pathophysiology

Some of the dogs with fiber-responsive large bowel diarrhea (FRLBD) could have IBS. However, the relation between IBS and FRLBD is unclear. Many of the dogs have hematochezia, a clinical sign considered uncommon in dogs with IBS.[90, 385] In addition, only rarely do dogs with IBS respond to dietary fiber supplementation alone.[90] Thus, it is possible that dogs with FRLBD may represent a separate syndrome or a subset of IBS patients that respond to dietary fiber supplementation. Some of the dogs with FRLBD may have had *C. perfringens* enterotoxicosis, a newly reported syndrome that is discussed in the next section.

Dietary fiber is a collective term for a wide variety of plant polysaccharides and lignins that are resistant to mammalian digestive enzymes.[135, 390] There are many types of dietary fiber, each with diverse chemical, physical, and physiologic properties. Water-soluble fibers include pectin, gums, mucilages, and some hemicelluloses.[135, 390] They are found in the parenchymatous portions of fruit and vegetables and in the seeds of leguminous plants. Water-insoluble fibers include cellulose, lignin, and some hemicelluloses. They are found in cereal grains and seed coats.

There are several potential mechanisms by which dietary fiber supplementation may result in clinical improvement in dogs with FRLBD. Soluble fiber absorbs a large quantity of water, improving fecal consistency. Colonic bacteria, which make up approximately 40% to 55% of the dry stool mass, ferment soluble fiber, which results in a vast increase in the numbers (but not types) of colonic bacteria and the quantity of bacterial byproducts.[391, 392] Insoluble fiber greatly adds to fecal volume. Thus, dietary fiber can increase fecal bulk, which increases colonic distention, the major stimulus for normal colonic motility. With increased colonic distention, an improved motility pattern in dogs with FRLBD may result in resolution of clinical signs. Dietary fiber has been shown to normalize colonic myoelectrical activity and colonic motility in humans. Bacterial fermentation of fiber leads to the production of short-chain fatty acids, of which butyrate serves as an energy source for colonocytes.[391–393]

Psyllium comes from the seeds or husks of the plant ispaghul and consists of approximately 90% soluble fiber. Although there are no other studies evaluating the use of soluble fibers in dogs with diarrhea, psyllium was found to be beneficial in treating a group of children with an idiopathic condition, chronic nonspecific diarrhea of childhood.[394] Because the beneficial effects persisted after the withdrawal of fiber supplementation, the authors postulated that an alteration of normal colonic flora may have occurred. This possibility could be important in understanding the pathogenesis of the next disorder to be discussed, *C. perfringens* enterotoxicosis.

Clinical Signs

The predominant clinical sign is chronic intermittent or continuous large bowel diarrhea, with hematochezia, excess fecal mucus, and tenesmus. Occasional vomiting and decreased appetite can occur. Only rarely did owners describe their dogs as nervous or high-strung.

Diagnostic Plan

The diagnosis is based on exclusion of known causes of large bowel diarrhea with a thorough diagnostic evaluation, including colonoscopy and mucosal biopsy.

Treatment

A highly digestible diet (Prescription Diet i/d) supplemented with psyllium hydrophilic mucilloid (Metamucil, 1–3 tablespoons) benefits most affected dogs. In our cases, the mean amount of Metamucil added to the diet was 2 tablespoons per day (range, 0.7–6.0).

Prognosis

The prognosis is excellent in dogs that respond to fiber supplementation. There have been no clinical findings identified that help predict whether an individual patient will respond to therapy. Some dogs can have the amount of fiber added to the diet reduced and finally withdrawn entirely, but others require long-term supplementation.

Clostridium perfringens Enterotoxicosis

A preliminary report has associated diarrhea and *C. perfringens* type A enterotoxin.[42] The disorder occurs most commonly in dogs but is seen occasionally in cats. Both naturally occurring and hospital-acquired cases have been detected.[395] The relation of this syndrome to IBS or FRLBD remains to be determined. It is possible that some dogs with either IBS or FRLBD may have *C. perfringens* enterotoxicosis.[2]

Pathophysiology

A vegetative form of *C. perfringens* is a normal inhabitant of the colon. The enterotoxin is a component of the spore coat and causes intestinal fluid accumulation, mucosal damage, and diarrhea.[396] The stimuli for sporulation and enterotoxin production are unknown. Enterotoxin has also been identified in some cases of hemorrhagic gastroenteritis syndrome, parvovirus, giardiasis, and IBD.[42, 397]

Clinical Signs

Acute or chronic large bowel diarrhea occurs commonly. Vomiting, weight loss, flatulence, and abdominal pain occur less frequently.

Diagnostic Plan

Diagnosis can be confirmed by identifying enterotoxin in a fecal sample with the use of a reverse latex agglutination test (PET-RPLA Kit). The test is available at many human diagnostic laboratories. In animals with intermittent signs, fecal samples should be collected when clinical signs are present, because enterotoxin may not be found during asymptomatic periods. Diagnosis should also be suspected if more than two spores per oil-immersion field are found in a rectal cytology specimen. The spores are larger than most bacteria and assume a safety-pin appearance (see Fig. 32–1). Endoscopic examination of affected animals may show hyperemic, hemorrhagic,

or ulcerated mucosa. Histopathologic findings include catarrhal or suppurative colitis.[42]

Treatment

Acute cases may resolve spontaneously. Chronic cases resolve with antibiotic therapy in 3 to 5 days. Metronidazole at 6 mg/kg b.i.d. to t.i.d. for 7 days is often effective.[42] Ampicillin (22 mg/kg by mouth t.i.d.) and amoxicillin (11–22 mg/kg by mouth b.i.d. or t.i.d.) are also effective treatments. Patients that show intermittent clinical signs require long-term therapy. Tylosin can be used in these cases at 10 to 20 mg/kg b.i.d. A more detailed description of tylosin administration can be found in the section on IBD. Some patients respond to a high-fiber diet. Proposed mechanisms of action for dietary fiber include acidification of the colon, which may inhibit sporulation, or an alteration of bacterial flora that inhibits *C. perfringens* proliferation.

Prognosis

The prognosis is excellent. Most affected animals respond to therapy within several days. At the present time, clinical findings have not been identified that predict which animals need long-term therapy.

Adenomas

Adenomas are the most common benign tumors found in the colons of dogs. Adenomas arise from the mucosal layer of the colon. Middle-aged to older dogs are most commonly affected. They are uncommon in cats.[101, 166, 214, 215, 217, 398, 399]

Pathophysiology

Adenomas frequently occur in the distal colon and rectum, often within 3 cm of the anus. In most cases only a single mass occurs, but occasionally multiple tumors are present.[215, 398, 399] Clinical signs are caused by interference with the fecal stream, hemorrhage from trauma associated with defecation, and inflammation. Malignant transformation to adenocarcinoma is possible and is thought to be more likely in larger tumors.[101, 219]

Clinical Signs

The most common clinical sign is hematochezia.[101, 215, 398] Feces may be well formed but on occasion are soft and contain excess mucus. Tenesmus is occasionally present and may result in protrusion of the mass through the anus. Digital rectal examination often identifies a mass and may result in discomfort and hemorrhage.

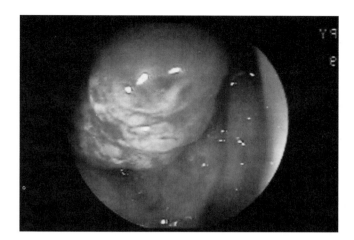

Figure 32–29
Endoscopic appearance of a 4-cm diameter adenomatous polyp in the rectum of a 9-year-old English setter.

Diagnostic Plan

Diagnosis requires histopathologic evaluation. The mass can be identified by visualization as it protrudes through the anus, by rectal palpation, or during endoscopy. Endoscopically, most adenomas appear as raised, sessile masses with smooth surfaces, although some have a granular and friable surface (Fig. 32–29). On occasion, a pedunculated mass with a stalk can be encountered. The average polyp is 2 cm in diameter.[101, 215, 398]

Treatment

Many adenomas can be extruded through the anus and removed with submucosal resection.[101, 399] In rare instances, adenomas can be found in the descending colon, and exploratory laparotomy is necessary for removal.

Prognosis

Prognosis for long-term survival is excellent, although recurrence has been reported.[101, 215, 398, 399]

Megacolon

Megacolon occurs more frequently in cats than dogs and is characterized by diffuse colonic dilation with ineffective motility. It often occurs in middle-aged cats. Megacolon may be idiopathic or associated with an underlying cause. Idiopathic megacolon may be congenital, but more commonly it is acquired later in life. No age, breed, or sex predilection is observed.[102]

Pathophysiology

Megacolon can occur secondary to mechanical or functional obstructions that prevent defecation for prolonged periods. Mechanical obstruction secondary to malunion of pelvic fractures occurs principally in cats.[85] Intramural and extramural masses, strictures, and, rarely, foreign bodies can also result in obstruction. Functional obstruction secondary to metabolic diseases (e.g., hypokalemia, hypothyroidism), trauma resulting in damage to colonic innervation, and neuromuscular disorders are infrequent causes of acquired megacolon. Megacolon may result from congenital anomalies such as anal or rectal atresia or sacral spinal deformity in Manx cats. Prolonged, severe colonic dilation from any cause disrupts coordinated motility patterns responsible for the storage and evacuation of feces. Smooth muscle degeneration results in a dilated, flaccid colon. Even when an underlying cause · of megacolon can be identified and treated, the functional changes in the dilated colon are often irreversible.

Clinical Signs

Constipation is the predominant clinical sign in animals with megacolon. Tenesmus and frequent attempts to defecate are commonly observed. Passage of liquid feces, which may contain mucus or blood, may occur secondary to colonic inflammation. If intractable constipation (obstipation) develops, dehydration, weakness, and vomiting may occur. Anorexia, weight loss, and a poor hair coat are frequently observed in long-standing cases.[82, 91, 102]

Abdominal palpation and digital rectal examination identify a markedly distended colon packed with hard feces. Occasionally, obstructive causes of megacolon may be identified (e.g., rectal mass, fractured pelvis, extraluminal mass causing compression of the colon).

Diagnostic Plan

Neurologic examination should be performed to evaluate lumbosacral function. Laboratory evaluation may identify underlying metabolic causes or secondary electrolyte changes. Survey abdominal radiographs confirm the presence of megacolon and may identify abdominal masses, pelvic fractures, or vertebral lesions (see Fig. 32–5). Contrast radiography, abdominal ultrasound, or endoscopy may be necessary to rule out obstructive diseases such as intramural masses or strictures.

Treatment

If an underlying cause is identified, it should be corrected. A diagnosis of idiopathic megacolon can be made if an underlying cause cannot be established. Initially, medical management of idiopathic megacolon should be attempted. If only mild to moderate constipation is present, bisacodyl (Dulcolax, 5 mg per cat or 5–20 mg per dog, by mouth s.i.d.) or docusate sodium suppositories (Colace) may be given.[82, 84] In most cases, the animal fails to respond, and enemas must be administered. If systemic signs are present, such as vomiting, weakness, and anorexia, fluid and electrolyte balance should be restored before the stool is evacuated. To remove impacted feces, warm water or saline enemas (20 mL/kg) should be infused slowly. The addition of 5 to 10 mL of an emollient laxative, such as docusate sodium (Colace) or docusate calcium (Surfak), or equal parts of sterile lubricant jelly to the enema solution may be helpful.[81, 82] Phosphate enemas should be avoided in cats and small dogs because they can induce fatal electrolyte disturbances.[400]

In severely obstipated animals, manual removal of the feces under general anesthesia is usually necessary. Broad-spectrum antibiotics should be administered, because the colonic mucosal barrier is probably damaged, increasing the potential for invasion of bacteria.[401] Feces can be massaged and broken apart by abdominal palpation after enema infusion. After the fecal mass is broken down, the contents can be manipulated into the rectum and removed digitally. Sponge forceps, passed rectally, help break down and remove impacted feces. Manipulations should be performed carefully to avoid further damage to the colonic wall or perforation.

After complete removal of the feces, long-term medical management consists of dietary modifications combined with laxatives, periodic administration of enemas, and use of the prokinetic agent cisapride.[81–84, 86] Commercially available high-fiber diets (Prescription Diet w/d and r/d) or the addition of fiber (psyllium, wheat bran, or canned pumpkin at 1 to 3 tablespoons per meal) to an easily assimilated diet is recommended. Laxatives that may be useful adjuncts to dietary management include lubricants, stimulants, emollients, and osmotic agents. Lubricants coat feces and decrease colonic water resorption. Petroleum jelly (1–3 inches per cat per 24 hours) is commonly used. Bisacodyl (5 mg/cat or 5–20 mg/dog by mouth s.i.d.) is an irritant that stimulates defecation and decreases intestinal water absorption. It should be used only intermittently, because long-term use can damage the myenteric plexus.[83, 84] Because of bisacodyl's stimulatory effect on colonic motility, it should be avoided if severe obstipation or obstructive lesions are present. Emollient laxatives, docusate sodium or docusate calcium (50 mg/cat or 50–200 mg/dog by mouth s.i.d.), are surfactants that soften stools by mixing aqueous and fatty substances, and they also stimulate colonic secretion. Lactulose

(Duphalac syrup, 0.5–1.0 mL/kg by mouth b.i.d. or t.i.d.) is a synthetic disaccharide that is metabolized by colonic bacteria to form organic acids, which are osmotically active, drawing water into the colonic lumen to soften feces and stimulate colonic motility. Lactulose also lowers colonic pH, which stimulates motility. We have found that lactulose may relieve constipation when other laxatives have failed.

Recently, the prokinetic agent cisapride has been licensed in the United States. Preliminary information indicates it is beneficial in the management of megacolon in cats. Cisapride acts by releasing acetylcholine from the enteric nervous system, which stimulates the colonic smooth muscle to contract.[402] Doses of 0.5 mg/kg by mouth b.i.d. or t.i.d. may be effective, if the stools are kept soft. Lactulose should be used concurrently and its dosage adjusted to produce two to three soft stools per day.

If medical management is ineffective or repeated episodes of constipation become frustrating, time-consuming, and expensive for clients, subtotal colectomy should be considered.[82, 84, 91, 102, 403] This technique has been used successfully in cats and in a limited number of dogs.[85, 91, 102, 401, 403] Complications have been minimal, and formed feces are usually noted within 6 weeks of surgery.[404]

Prognosis

The prognosis for secondary megacolon is related to the underlying disease and the degree of colonic distention that has occurred. The prognosis for idiopathic megacolon is guarded. However, improvements in therapy with cisapride and colectomy have greatly improved the quality of life for cats with idiopathic megacolon. It is not possible to judge the long-term response to cisapride at this time.

Perianal Tumors

Perianal tumors are slow-growing masses of the circumanal hepatoid glands located in the subcutaneous area of the outer cutaneous zone of the anus.[405] They are much more common in older, intact male dogs than in female dogs, and they are one of the most common tumors found in male dogs.[406–409] Adenomas are 4 to 30 times more common than adenocarcinomas.[408, 410] Cocker spaniels, English bulldogs, Samoyeds, and beagles are predisposed to develop perianal adenoma.[406, 408, 409] Arctic Circle breeds, German shepherds, and dogs of greater than 35 kg body weight are predisposed to develop adenocarcinoma.[410]

Pathophysiology

Perianal adenomas are often hormonally mediated, and many cases in intact males have been associated with testicular tumors.[406, 410] Androgenic stimulation causes proliferation of the circumanal hepatoid glands.[406, 410] The function of these glands is unknown.[406, 410] Adenomas may slowly progress to adenocarcinoma under the influence of androgens, but growth of carcinomas does not seem to be hormonally mediated.[406, 410]

Clinical Signs

Adenomas often cause few clinical signs. A single mass or multiple tumors may be present.[407] Masses can vary from 0.5 to 10 cm in diameter.[408] The firm masses can become large and ulcerate, bleed, or necrose.[407] An owner may notice the mass because of the dog's persistent licking of the perianal area.

Adenocarcinomas often metastasize and can result in tenesmus and constipation.[406, 410] However, they can also be discovered as incidental findings or because the dog licks its perianal region excessively. Rectal examination may reveal masses or enlarged lymph nodes in the ventral lumbar and sacral region.[406]

Often, in cases of perianal gland neoplasia, careful palpation of the testicles may detect large or irregular testicles caused by testicular neoplasia.[406, 409, 410]

Diagnostic Plan

A diagnosis of perianal adenoma should be strongly suspected in any older intact male dog with a characteristic perianal lesion. Fine-needle aspiration often provides diagnosis (Fig. 32–30). Diagnosis should be confirmed with surgical biopsy.

If a narrowed pelvic canal can be detected on rectal palpation, adenocarcinoma should be suspected. Thoracic radiographs should be evaluated for metastasis. Diagnosis is confirmed by fine-needle aspiration or surgical biopsy. Adenocarcinomas should be suspected if castration has not greatly reduced tumor size or if regrowth has occurred after surgical removal of a mass.[406, 410]

Treatment

Treatment of perianal adenomas requires castration in intact males, with or without excision or cryosurgery. In females or neutered males, surgical excision or cryosurgery is indicated.[406, 407] Treatment for adenocarcinoma requires surgical excision, although in many cases complete removal is not possible.[410] Castration does not help the tumor to regress but removes testicles that may be neoplastic.[410]

Prognosis

The prognosis for perianal adenoma is excellent. The prognosis for adenocarcinoma is guarded.[406, 407]

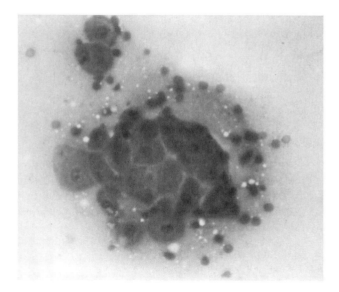

Figure 32–30
Cytologic appearance of a perineal adenoma. A cluster of hyperchromatic hepatoid epithelial cells with discrete nuclei and some pleomorphism is present in the center of the photograph.

Masses larger than 5 cm in diameter and those with identifiable metastases are associated with a poor prognosis.[410]

Anal Sac Impaction, Sacculitis, and Abscess

Disorders of the anal sac are very common in dogs of all ages but rare in cats.[405] Surveys have indicated that between 2% and 12.5% of dogs examined at veterinary clinics are affected.[411, 412] Anal sac disease is most common in dogs that weigh less than 15 kg.[412] Poodles and Chihuahuas may be overrepresented.[412]

Pathophysiology

The anal sacs lie underneath and between the muscle fibers of the external anal sphincter.[405, 413] Normal fluid can be clear and slightly yellow or brownish.[413, 414] A small amount of secretion is released with normal defecation. Diarrhea, constipation, recent estrus, and poor muscle tone associated with obesity can predispose an animal to anal sac problems.[405, 412, 414] Duct obstruction and bacterial infection are responsible for most anal sac diseases. Inflammation increases secretion, providing an excellent medium for bacterial growth.[405] Common bacteria isolated clinically include micrococci, *E. coli*, *Streptococcus fecalis*, *Clostridium welchii*, and *Proteus* spp.[414, 415] Impaction, sacculitis, and abscess probably represent variations of the same pathophysiologic process.[413]

Clinical Signs

Clinical signs often recur in affected dogs. Common signs include licking or biting of the anal region, tail chasing, scooting or rubbing the anal region on the floor, pain, and tenesmus.[412, 413, 415] Usually both glands are affected.[412] The anal sacs may be enlarged, painful on palpation, and obstructed, or they may contain a malodorous, purulent, discolored, or bloody fluid with yellow granules.[405] A draining, ruptured abscess may be present, or the gland may be fluctuant and ready to burst.[413] The skin overlying the abscessed gland may be discolored and warm. Localized cellulitis may be present. Depression, anorexia, and pyrexia often accompany abscess.

Diagnostic Plan

Visual examination and rectal examination should confirm the diagnosis. The distinction between impaction and anal sacculitis is not always clear. In patients with sacculitis, cytologic evaluation of fluid reveals increased numbers of neutrophils and bacteria. Animals with anal sacculitis are often in more pain than those with simple impaction. Anal sac tumors are not usually painful. Fine-needle aspiration helps to diagnose neoplasia if the distinction is not clear.

Treatment

Anal gland impaction is managed by frequent expression and removal of the viscous fluid. This is best accomplished by placing a finger in the rectum and applying internal pressure while another finger compresses the gland externally.[414] Clients can be trained to apply pressure to the affected glands externally. If the contents are too thick to be expressed, saline can be infused to soften contents. Chronic cases require anal sacculectomy.[415]

Anal sacculitis is treated by expression of the gland and cannulation of the duct for infusion with topical antiseptics, antibiotics, or antibiotic-corticosteroid preparations.[413] Systemic antibiotic therapy is not often needed, but metronidazole (7.5–10 mg/kg b.i.d. or t.i.d.) and amoxicillin clavulanic acid (12.5–25 mg/kg by mouth b.i.d.) are effective.[416] Chronic cases respond to anal sacculectomy.[415]

Abscesses should be treated by ventral drainage.[415] If the gland has already ruptured, the aperture should be enlarged to facilitate drainage. If the gland has not ruptured, it should be lanced. The abscess cavity should be flushed with antiseptic solution.[413] Systemic antibiotics should be administered if the animal is pyrexic, anorexic, or severely depressed.

Prognosis

The prognosis for anal sac diseases is variable; many cases become chronic and may require surgical therapy.[405, 413] Anal sacculectomy often cures the problem.[405]

Anal Sac Adenocarcinoma

Adenocarcinoma of the apocrine glands of the anal sac is a highly malignant tumor that occurs most commonly in older female dogs.[417–419] The incidence is low.

Pathophysiology

Anal sac adenocarcinoma metastasizes readily to both regional lymph nodes (external iliac) and distant sites (liver, spleen, and lungs).[405, 417–419] The hypercalcemia is thought to be associated with production of an osteolytic substance by the tumor.[419] Hypercalcemia and its associated renal disease is responsible for the polyuria and polydipsia (see Chap. 16).[419]

Clinical Signs

Common clinical signs include tenesmus, constipation or abnormally shaped stools, perianal swelling, and polyuria with polydipsia.[101, 418, 419] The tumor is often discovered incidentally.[101, 417, 418] Tumors can be palpated rectally and can vary in size from 0.2 to 10.0 cm.[417, 419] Tumors can affect either gland, and occasionally both are involved.[417–419]

Diagnostic Plan

Diagnosis requires histopathologic assessment of excised tissue. From 25% to 90% of patients are hypercalcemic and hypophosphatemic.[101, 417, 419] Abdominal radiographs often reveal a sublumbar mass (iliac lymphadenopathy). Thoracic radiographs can show evidence of metastasis.[417] The differential diagnosis should include perianal adenoma, perianal adenocarcinoma, and anal sacculitis.

Treatment

Surgical resection of the mass, with or without removal of metastatic tissue, has been suggested.[417, 418] Complications associated with surgery include fecal incontinence, local infection or sepsis, and urinary incontinence.[417] Hypercalcemia and hypophosphatemia often resolve after surgery (see Chap. 49 for discussion of treatment for hypercalcemia).[101, 419]

Prognosis

The prognosis for patients with this highly aggressive tumor is guarded.[418] Early treatment with complete excision offers the best prognosis. Incomplete surgical resection, recurrence of the primary tumor or metastatic lesions, and development of additional metastatic lesions are common. Mean survival time after surgery has been approximately 10 to 12 months.[101, 417] The presence of hypercalcemia and detectable metastasis at the time of diagnosis is associated with a poorer prognosis.[417]

Perianal Fistula

Perianal fistula, or anal furunculosis, is an ulcerative fistulating disease of the anus and perianal skin that occurs most commonly in middle-aged and sexually intact dogs.[420–425] However, it can occur in any dog older than 6 months of age.[413] German shepherds and Irish setters are commonly affected.[415, 421, 422, 424–426]

Pathophysiology

The cause of perianal fistula is unknown. A genetic predisposition is thought to exist.[427] One theory is that a broad tail base with low tail carriage potentiates the retention of a fecal film over the anus, leading to dermatitis and deeper inflammation.[415, 427] Another theory is based on an increased density of apocrine sweat glands in the cutaneous zone of the anus in German shepherds.[427, 428] Self-mutilation, caused by pain, irritation, and inflammation, aids development of bacterial infection and results in production of granulation tissue. Regardless of the cause, bacterial infection occurs after epidermal ulceration.[427] Many types of bacteria have been cultured from deep perianal tissue, with *E. coli, Staphylococcus aureus,* streptococci, and *Proteus mirabilis* found most commonly.[422]

Clinical Signs

The history may include pain, weight loss, anorexia, tenesmus, diarrhea, constipation, fecal incontinence, hemorrhage, licking of the anal region, and malodorous discharge.[415, 421, 424–427] The severity of clinical signs varies greatly, from a single fistula to 360° involvement of the perianal tissue (Fig. 32–31).[427] Complete physical examination may require sedation because the animal is in pain.[415] Rectal examination can reveal stenosis of the anal region.

Diagnostic Plan

The diagnosis can be made after careful physical examination and, in some cases, histologic assessment of biopsy specimens. The differential diagnosis should include anal sac abscess and rupture with cellulitis and ulcerated anal sac or perianal adenocarcinoma.[427] The locations commonly seen with anal sac abscess (the 4 o'clock and 8 o'clock positions) and the cytologic

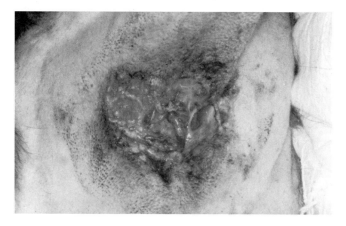

Figure 32–31
Close-up photograph of a 9-year-old German shepherd with severe perianal fistula involving 360° of the anus.

characteristics of adenocarcinomas usually make diagnosis simple.

Treatment

Successful treatment usually requires surgery. Preoperative therapy consists of systemic antibiotics, hydrotherapy, and topical antiseptic treatment of the perianal region. There is no consensus regarding the most effective surgery. Procedures that have been suggested include cauterization of fistulas, excision of affected tissue, cryosurgery, anal sacculectomy, radical excision of the anal ring, deroofing and fulguration, tail setting, and tail amputation.[420, 421, 423–427, 429]

Prognosis

In mild cases, many surgical procedures are effective.[421] Severe cases require radical treatment and are associated with a higher failure rate and more complications.[415, 427] Complications include fecal incontinence, tenesmus, anal stricture, failure to heal, and recurrence of disease.[420, 421, 423–427]

Rectal and Anal Prolapse

Prolapse of the rectum, anus, or both can accompany tenesmus from any cause.[405] Prolapse occurs most commonly in puppies and kittens with GI parasites.

Pathophysiology

In partial rectal prolapse, only mucosa everts through the anus. In anal prolapse, only anal mucosa everts. In complete prolapse, all the layers of the rectum evert.[405] Besides GI parasites, foreign bodies, enteritis, colitis or proctitis, rectal or pelvic masses, perineal hernias, congenital spinal deformity (in Manx cats), prostatitis, dystocia, and urolithiasis can be underlying causes.[405]

Clinical Signs

A tube-like protrusion of rectal tissue can be identified on physical examination.[430] Often, there is a history of acute or chronic diarrhea with tenesmus. Rectal examination may reveal the presence of colonic or pelvic masses.

Diagnostic Plan

The diagnosis of rectal or anal prolapse is made on physical examination. Differential diagnosis includes a prolapsed ileocolic intussusception.[405] In cases of rectal prolapse, a finger placed between the prolapsed mucosa and the mucocutaneous junction can be inserted only a short distance.[430] The underlying cause of the prolapse should carefully be investigated. Multiple fecal examination specimens should be evaluated for parasites. If parasites are not identified, the diagnostic approaches for acute or chronic diarrhea should be followed.

Treatment

Treatment of the primary cause is mandatory for successful resolution of the prolapse. Incomplete prolapses can often be manually replaced with the aid of lubricants and hypertonic glucose compresses, to help shrink the everted tissue. A purse-string suture helps prevent recurrence while the underlying cause is treated. If mucosal necrosis has occurred, mucosal resection is necessary.[405] Severely affected patients require rectoanal anastomosis.[405] Recurrent cases are best managed with colopexy.[430]

Prognosis

The prognosis for most patients with prolapse is good if the underlying cause can be identified and treated. Recurrence is common if the underlying cause cannot be found. The prognosis is worse if there is severe mucosal damage, if a large amount of rectum has prolapsed, or if the prolapse is long-standing.

Uncommon Intestinal Diseases

Immunoproliferative Enteropathy of Basenjis

Immunoproliferative enteropathy is a form of IBD that commonly occurs in basenjis.[49, 152, 431] Clinical signs include severe small bowel diarrhea, anorexia, and weight loss, which usually develop by 3 years of age. Skin lesions of the pinnae are common. A poorly responsive anemia, hypoalbuminemia, and hyperglobulinemia with increased serum IgA often occur. Treatment includes removal of stressors, dietary modification, systemic antibiotics, and immunosuppressive therapy, as used in other cases of IBD. Prognosis is poor, and most patients die or are euthanized within 3 years of developing signs.

Wheat-Sensitive Enteropathy

Gluten-sensitive enteropathy results in chronic small bowel diarrhea and weight loss or failure to thrive in Irish setter puppies, usually those younger than 6 months of age.[114, 432–434] Sensitivity to wheat gluten results in partial villous atrophy and lymphocytic enteritis. Feeding of a wheat-free diet resolves the clinical signs.

Rotavirus

Rotavirus has been implicated as a cause of mild diarrhea in newborn puppies. Puppies remain bright and alert and have normal appetites.[435, 436] The virus infects the epithelial cells on the villous tips. The clinical significance of this viral disorder is unknown.

Leiomyosarcoma

Leiomyosarcomas are slow-growing, malignant tumors that arise from the smooth muscle layers of the GI tract, most commonly in the jejunum or cecum. These tumors are very rare in cats. Clinical signs with jejunal tumors include vomiting, diarrhea, anorexia, and weight loss.[437] Signs associated with cecal perforation include fever and collapse.[89, 98, 437] Some patients with cecal rupture and peritonitis do not have any clinical signs before developing peritonitis.[89] In many cases of intestinal leiomyosarcoma, an abdominal mass can be palpated or visualized on survey radiographs. Cecal rupture is associated with a poor prognosis. Metastasis can occur to the omentum, liver, and lungs. Patients with intestinal leiomyosarcoma that survive surgery have a good long-term prognosis.[437]

Duodenal Adenoma

Adenomatous polyps occur in the duodenum of old cats and cause vomiting, often with hematemesis, and anemia.[438] Diagnosis is based on endoscopic examination of the duodenum (or barium contrast radiography) and histopathologic assessment of tissue. Treatment consists of mucosal resection. The prognosis is excellent, and recurrence is uncommon.

Intestinal Volvulus

Intestinal volvulus is an acute and often fatal cause of strangulated intestinal obstruction in dogs.[69, 70, 80] Clinical signs include an abrupt onset of vomiting, bloody diarrhea, depression, abdominal pain, abdominal distention, circulatory shock, and collapse. Intestinal rotation at the root of the mesentery causes bowel obstruction and occlusion of the cranial mesenteric artery. Treatment requires prompt recognition of the condition by the veterinarian and surgical correction. Most patients die in the perioperative period. A relatively large number of reported cases have involved German shepherds with pancreatic exocrine insufficiency.[68]

Salmon Poisoning

Salmon poisoning occurs in the Pacific northwest. It is caused by the rickettsia *Neorickettsia helminthoeca* and is spread by the fluke *Nanophyetus salmincola*.[439] The dog obtains the fluke by eating an infected salmon. The adult fluke attaches to the dog's intestinal mucosa. Clinical signs include anorexia, pyrexia, vomiting, diarrhea, peripheral and mesenteric lymphadenopathy, splenomegaly, and weight loss. Diagnosis is based on clinical signs, geographic location, finding large fluke eggs in the feces (90 × 45 μm), or identifying rickettsia on lymph node or splenic aspirates stained with Giemsa stain. Treatment requires vigorous fluid therapy and systemic antibiotics such as trimethoprim-sulfonamide, penicillins, tetracyclines, or chloramphenicol.

Tropical Sprue–like Syndrome

This rare condition of unknown cause has been described in dogs with chronic diarrhea and weight loss.[115] Marked villous atrophy and infiltration of inflammatory cells occur in the small intestine. No specific therapy is available, and the prognosis is poor.

Regional Enterocolitis

Regional enterocolitis is a rare, chronic, progressive, and usually fatal inflammatory bowel disease of unknown cause that occurs most commonly in young male dogs.[440–442] It is characterized by a transmural granulomatous inflammatory response, which can involve the distal ileum, cecum, proximal colon, distal colon and rectum, or stomach.

The diagnosis requires a biopsy specimen, which can be obtained by endoscopy or exploratory surgery. Radiographic signs of intestinal obstruction can be present. Treatment requires intestinal resection and anastomosis. Corticosteroids have been used in some cases with generally poor results.

Phycomycosis

Infection with the ubiquitous fungus *Pythium* spp. results in pyogranulomatous inflammation in the stomach, small intestine, or colon, most often in young, male dogs of large breeds.[443, 444] The most common clinical signs are vomiting, diarrhea, and weight loss. In some cases, an abdominal mass can be palpated. Diagnosis is based on finding the organisms in biopsy samples. Most cases are very advanced at the time of diagnosis, so surgical therapy often is not possible.

Histiocytic Ulcerative Colitis of Boxers

Histiocytic ulcerative colitis is an uncommon, chronic, idiopathic disease characterized by progressive colonic ulceration that is histologically associated with an inflammatory mucosal infiltrate of plasma cells, lymphocytes, and distended macrophages that are positive on periodic acid–Schiff (PAS) staining.[445, 446] The disease occurs most commonly in boxers younger than 2 years of age.

Weight loss and debilitation occur as a result of chronic intestinal loss of blood and protein. A corrugated, thickened mucosa, hemorrhage, or pain may be evident on digital rectal examination.

Treatment is similar to that described for IBD, with sulfasalazine the drug of choice. If histiocytic colitis is advanced at the time of diagnosis, treatment often does not improve clinical signs, and a poor prognosis is warranted. However, if management is instituted early in the course of the disease, the prognosis is more favorable, although the disease is usually progressive, and lifelong therapy is required.

Colonic Ulceration Associated With Neurologic Disease

Most affected dogs are middle-aged males. The onset of clinical signs occurs at a mean of 5 days after neurosurgery.[447–449] Depression, anorexia, vomiting, diarrhea, melena, and abdominal pain are the most common clinical signs, but they are not always observed. Even with surgical intervention, colonic perforation is usually fatal.

Preventative measures include using short-acting corticosteroids (prednisolone or methylprednisolone) and limiting their duration of administration, avoiding the concurrent use of other drugs with ulcerogenic properties, managing urine and fecal retention, avoiding enemas after surgery, and using antibiotics judiciously to reduce the incidence of bacterial overgrowth.[450]

Parasitic Diseases

Strongyloides

Strongyloides stercoralis infects the small intestines of dogs, and *Strongyloides tumefaciens* can occasionally be found in cats.[38] A complex life cycle exists, with both free-living and parasitic stages. The very small females, 2 to 5 mm long and 34 to 109 μm wide, parasitize animals. In dogs, the eggs hatch and the first-stage larva can be identified by direct saline smears of the feces or by Baermann flotation. In cats, the large ova, 120 × 65 μm, can be identified in fecal flotations. Infection occurs by skin penetration by the third-stage larva. Clinical signs (diarrhea, cough, and dermatitis) are most common in puppies in kennels and occur in hot, humid weather.[451] Fenbendazole, 50 mg/kg s.i.d. for 5 days, is probably effective therapy. Ivermectin, 200 to 800 μg/kg by mouth, may also be effective in eliminating adults from the small intestine.[452] Ivermectin is not approved for this indication and should not be used in collies or related breeds because of toxicity.[245] *S. stercoralis* can infect humans, and appropriate sanitary measures should be recommended.

Cryptosporidium

Cryptosporidiosis most commonly affects ruminants and produces a self-limited enteritis in most cases. Recently, *C. parvum* has been identified in dogs and cats.[41, 261, 453] The life cycle is similar to that of other coccidia, except that the thin-walled oocysts can rupture within the small intestine and autoinfection can occur. It is not clear whether these organisms are pathogenic in dogs and cats, but they have been associated with diarrhea.[454] Diagnosis is difficult because the oocysts are transparent and very small (5 μm). Cysts float in zinc sulfate or saturated sucrose solutions but dehydrate and become collapsed and unrecognizable. Flotation with Sheather's sugar solution is more reliable. There is no proven effective therapy. As in humans, immunocompromised hosts may be most susceptible. The organism should be considered zoonotic.

Trichomoniasis

Pentatrichomonas hominis is a protozoan that can inhabit the colon and cecum of normal dogs, cats, and humans.[455] *P. hominis* is most often considered an asymptomatic commensal, but it has been observed in association with diarrhea.[456, 457] Direct fecal-oral transmission occurs. There is no cyst stage. Microscopic examination of fresh fecal smears reveals tiny, motile, pyriform, flagellated trophozoites that are characterized by an undulating membrane. They can be confused with *Giardia* trophozoites. Metronidazole, 22

mg/kg by mouth b.i.d. for 5 days, has been shown to eliminate the organism if treatment is desired.[282]

Entamoeba

Entamoeba histolytica is a protozoal parasite of the large bowel that primarily infects humans and rarely infects dogs and cats.[455] Trophozoites colonize the large intestine, where the organisms may inhabit the lumen as commensals or invade the bowel wall as pathogens.[458] Animals may be asymptomatic or may demonstrate signs ranging from mild chronic large bowel diarrhea to fulminant bloody diarrhea.

Diagnosis requires demonstration of *E. histolytica* trophozoites or cysts in fresh feces or colonic tissue. Little is known about treatment of *E. histolytica* in dogs and cats. Metronidazole may be the drug of choice, based on its efficacy in the treatment of humans with amebiasis. Dosages similar to those used for giardiasis (25 mg/kg by mouth b.i.d. for 5–10 days) are recommended.

Balantidium

Balantidium coli is a large, ciliated protozoan parasite commonly found as a commensal in the large bowel of swine. Clinical signs associated with *B. coli* infections in the dog are uncommon. Trophozoites inhabit the large bowel, either as commensals or as invasive parasites.[455]

Most infections are probably asymptomatic, but in some cases, infection may result in ulcerative colitis or severe diarrhea. Diagnosis of *B. coli* is based on identification of trophozoites in fresh fecal smears, rectal scrapings, or colonic mucosal biopsies, or identification of cysts in zinc sulfate fecal flotations.

Optimum therapy for *B. coli* has not been determined. Tetracycline (22 mg/kg by mouth t.i.d. for 10 days) or metronidazole (25 mg/kg by mouth b.i.d. for 5 to 10 days) is recommended for treatment based on guidelines for humans.

Bacterial Diseases

Salmonellosis

Salmonella spp. are gram-negative bacilli that can cause acute enterocolitis. Other clinical signs include fever, vomiting, anorexia, malaise, abdominal pain, and dehydration.[459–463] Asymptomatic carriage commonly occurs.[464] *S. typhimurium* is the most common serotype isolated from dogs and cats with diarrhea.[459, 460, 464, 465]

Young dogs and cats, especially those with concurrent disease (e.g., viral enteritis), stress, and overcrowded or unsanitary kennel conditions, are most commonly affected.[460–462] The infection is acquired through fecal-oral spread with food-borne, water-borne, or fomite transmission. Among hospitalized animals, stress associated with severe disease, prolonged hospitalization or surgery, immunosuppression due to glucocorticoid therapy or anticancer chemotherapy, and antibiotic therapy that disrupts the normal microflora predisposes animals to salmonellosis.[459, 465]

Diagnosis is based on fecal culture. *Salmonella* infections limited to the intestinal mucosa should not be treated with antibiotics because treatment may prolong fecal shedding and encourage development of a carrier state. Antibiotic therapy is warranted in animals with hemorrhagic diarrhea, a history of immunosuppression, evidence of bacteremia, or positive culture from nonintestinal sources.

Antibiotics that are most effective against *Salmonella* are trimethoprim-sulfonamide (30 mg/kg b.i.d. by mouth or subcutaneously), ampicillin (22 mg/kg t.i.d. by mouth or intravenously), and enrofloxacin (5 mg/kg b.i.d. by mouth, intravenously, or subcutaneously). A 10-day course of therapy is recommended.

Salmonellosis is of public health significance. Infected animals should be isolated during hospitalization, and strict hygiene must be practiced for at least 6 weeks.

Campylobacteriosis

Campylobacter are small, curved, motile, gram-negative rods that may act as primary pathogens (with predisposing factors), act as opportunistic pathogens, or be associated with asymptomatic carriers. *Campylobacter* is most commonly isolated from young or kenneled animals.[466–473]

Fecal-oral inoculation is the principal route for infection. *Campylobacter* typically colonize the jejunum, ileum, and colon, with the majority of pathologic changes occurring in the colon.[462, 474]

Most dogs and cats infected with *Campylobacter* remain asymptomatic. Acute diarrhea, ranging from intermittent soft stools to continuous watery or mucoid stools containing blood, is the most common clinical sign.[43, 462, 471, 472, 475] Other clinical manifestations include vomiting, anorexia, fever, dehydration, and depression. Clinical signs are usually self-limited within 3 to 15 days if untreated. Chronic diarrhea can also occur.[461–463, 472, 474, 475]

Diagnosis is based on a positive fecal culture. Small, curved or sea gull–shaped bacteria, neutrophils, and red blood cells may be observed on rectal cytology specimens. Fresh saline fecal smears may reveal the corkscrew shape and darting motility characteristic of *Campylobacter*.

Erythromycin, 10 mg/kg by mouth t.i.d. for 5 to 12 days, is the drug of choice in dogs.[469, 473, 476]

Antibiotic therapy administered early in the course of disease reduces the severity of diarrhea and eliminates fecal shedding.

Infection with *Campylobacter* can be transmitted from both normal and diarrheic dogs and cats to humans.

Yersiniosis

Yersinia enterocolitica is a motile, gram-negative coccobacillus that is an infrequent cause of enterocolitis in young dogs.[477] Infection is thought to be contracted principally through ingestion of contaminated food and water, although direct fecal-oral transmission can occur.

Diagnosis requires culture of the organism from feces. Administration of trimethoprim-sulfonamide (Tribrissen, 30 mg/kg b.i.d. by mouth), tetracycline (22 mg/kg t.i.d. by mouth), and cephalosporins (cefadroxil, Cefa-Tabs, 22 mg/kg b.i.d. by mouth for 7–10 days) is usually effective for treatment.[478] Because humans are susceptible to infection with *Y. enterocolitica*, zoonotic potential exists.[463]

Colibacillosis

E. coli, a gram-negative coccobacillus, is a component of the normal GI flora.[479] Pathogenic *E. coli* subtypes are a well-recognized cause of acute diarrhea in many animal species and humans, but their role as primary enteric pathogens in dogs and cats remains unknown. Enterotoxigenic, enteropathogenic, and enterohemorrhagic *E. coli* have been isolated from dogs or cats with diarrhea.[480–482]

Diagnosis cannot be made by routine fecal culture. Documentation of pathogenic strains of *E. coli* requires serotyping and in vivo and in vitro testing, which are not commonly available to practitioners. Fluoroquinolones are the antibiotic of choice in humans infected with pathogenic *E. coli*. Zoonotic potential appears to be low because many pathogenic strains are host specific.

Pseudomembranous Colitis

Clostridium difficile is the primary cause of pseudomembranous colitis in humans. The prevalence of this condition in dogs and cats is not known.[483] Overgrowth of this organism in the colon most often occurs secondary to the use of antibiotics that suppress the normal colonic bacterial flora. Clindamycin, ampicillin, and cephalosporins are most often incriminated. The diagnosis of pseudomembranous colitis is based on endoscopic and histopathologic criteria and isolation of *C. difficile* or its toxin from the feces. Metronidazole and vancomycin are effective treatments in humans.

Tyzzer's Disease

Tyzzer's disease is caused by an obligate intracellular bacterium, *Bacillus piliformis*.[461] This rare condition is characterized by a fatal hemorrhagic necrotizing enterocolitis and hepatic necrosis, most commonly in puppies and kittens. Diagnosis requires histopathologic identification of the organism in the intestines or the liver. There is no known treatment.

Heterobilharziasis

Heterobilharzia americana is the primary causative organism of canine schistosomiasis.[484] The life cycle of this trematode is complex. In the United States, heterobilharziasis is confined to the Southern Atlantic and Gulf Coast states. Chronic disease in dogs is manifested by intermittent diarrhea containing fresh blood and mucus, tenesmus, and progressive weight loss. Anemia, eosinophilia, hypoalbuminemia, and hyperglobulinemia may be observed. Acute heavy infestation is characterized by profuse bloody mucoid diarrhea, dehydration, and anorexia. Diagnosis is confirmed by demonstration of ova on direct fecal examination or tissue biopsy. Fenbendazole, 50 mg/kg s.i.d. by mouth for 10 days alone, or in combination with praziquantel (40 mg/kg by mouth once), appears to be effective treatment.

Protothecosis

Protothecosis is an uncommon cause of colitis in dogs that is caused by an achlorophyllous (colorless), unicellular alga of the genus *Prototheca*.[485] Colonization of the bowel wall causes diffuse nodular mucosal thickening with ulceration and hemorrhage. The organism eventually disseminates by hematogenous and lymphatic routes to other tissues, such as the eyes, central nervous system, kidneys, and mesenteric lymph nodes. Diagnosis of protothecosis requires demonstration of the organism in rectal scrapings, colonic biopsies, or urine sediment or culture of vitreous humor or cerebral spinal fluid. Successful treatment of disseminated disease has not been reported.

References

1. Evans HE, Christensen GC. Miller's Anatomy of the Dog. Philadelphia, WB Saunders, 1979:479–492.
2. Leib MS, Matz ME. Diseases of the large intestine. In: Ettinger SJ, Feldman EC, eds. Textbook of Veterinary Internal Medicine. Philadelphia, WB Saunders, 1995: 1232–1260.
3. Burrows CF, Batt RM, Sherding RG. Diseases of the small intestine. In: Ettinger SJ, Feldman EC, eds. Textbook of Veterinary Internal Medicine. Philadelphia, WB Saunders, 1995:1169–1232.
4. Strombeck DR, Guilford WG. Small Animal Gastroenterology. Davis, California, Stonegate, 1990:277–295.
5. Herdt T. Movements of the gastrointestinal tract. In: Cunningham JG, ed. Textbook of Veterinary Physiology. Philadelphia, WB Saunders, 1992:259–274.
6. Roussel AJ. Intestinal motility. Compen Contin Educ Pract Vet 1994;16:1433–1442.
7. Karaus M, Sarna SK. Giant migrating contractions during defecation in the dog colon. Gastroenterology 1987;92:925–933.
8. Christensen J. Motility of the colon. In: Johnson LR, ed. Physiology of the Gastrointestinal Tract. New York, Raven Press, 1987:665–693.
9. Doe WF. The intestinal immune system. Gut 1989;30: 1679–1685.
10. Willard MD. Normal immune function of the gastrointestinal tract. Semin Vet Med Surg (Small Anim) 1992;7:107–111.
11. Keren DF. Gastrointestinal immune system and its disorders. In: Appleman HD, Kaufman N, eds. Gastrointestinal Pathology. Baltimore, Williams & Wilkins, 1990:247–285.
12. Carman PS, Ernst PB, Rosenthal KL, et al. Intraepithelial leukocytes contain a unique population of NK-like cytotoxic cells active in the defense of gut epithelium to enteric murine coronaviruses. J Immunol 1986;136: 1548–1553.
13. Befus D, Fijimaki H. Mast cell polymorphisms: Present concepts, future directions. Dig Dis Sci 1988;33(Suppl): 16S–22S.
14. Targan SR, Kagnoff MF, Brogan MD, et al. Immunologic mechanisms in intestinal disease. Ann Intern Med 1978;106:853–870.
15. Leib MS. Stagnant loop syndrome in the dog and cat. Semin Vet Med Surg (Small Anim) 1987;2:257–265.
16. Willard MD, Simpson RB, Fossum TW, et al. Characterization of naturally developing small intestinal bacterial overgrowth in 16 German shepherd dogs. J Am Vet Med Assoc 1994;204:1201–1206.
17. Batt RM, Needham JR, Carter MW. Bacterial overgrowth associated with a naturally occurring enteropathy in the German shepherd dog. Res Vet Sci 1983;35: 42–46.
18. Moon HW. Mechanisms in the pathogenesis of diarrhea: A review. J Am Vet Med Assoc 1978;172:443–448.
19. Whipp SC. Physiology of diarrhea. J Am Vet Med Assoc 1978;173:662–666.
20. Field M, Rao MC, Chang EB. Intestinal electrolyte transport and diarrheal disease. N Engl J Med 1989;321: 879–883.
21. Twedt DC, Grauer GF. Fluid therapy for gastrointestinal, pancreatic, and hepatic disorders. Vet Clin North Am Small Anim Pract 1982;12:463–485.
22. Burrows CF. Chronic diarrhea in the dog. Vet Clin North Am Small Anim Pract 1983;13:521–540.
23. Sherding RG. Canine large bowel diarrhea. Compen Contin Educ Pract Vet 1980;2:279–290.
24. Van Kruiningen HJ, Hayden DW. Interpreting problem diarrhea of dogs. Vet Clin North Am Small Anim Pract 1972;2:29–47.

25. Leib MS, Codner EC, Monroe WE. A diagnostic approach to chronic large bowel diarrhea in dogs. Vet Med (Prague) 1991;86:892–899.

26. Shell LG. Canine distemper. Compen Contin Educ Pract Vet 1990;12:173–179.

27. Meyer DJ, Center SA. Approach to the diagnosis of liver disorders in dogs and cats. Compen Contin Educ Pract Vet 1986;8:880–888.

28. Forrester SD, Brandt KS. The diagnostic approach to the patient with acute renal failure. Vet Med (Prague) 1994;89:212–218.

29. Sherding RG. Acute hepatic failure. Vet Clin North Am Small Anim Pract 1985;15:119–133.

30. Baldwin CJ, Atkins CE. Leptospirosis in dogs. Compen Contin Educ Pract Vet 1987;9:499–508.

31. Levitt L, Bauer MS. Intussusception in dogs and cats: A review of thirty-six cases. Can Vet J 1992;33: 660–664.

32. Clark WT. Foreign bodies in the small intestine of the dog. Vet Rec 1968;83:115–119.

33. Finco DR. Fluid therapy: Detecting deviations from normal. J Am Anim Hosp Assoc 1972;8:155–165.

34. Schall WD. General principles of fluid therapy. Vet Clin North Am Small Anim Pract 1982;12:453–462.

35. Leib MS, Monroe WE, Codner EC. Management of chronic large bowel diarrhea in dogs. Vet Med (Prague) 1991;86:922–929.

36. Leib MS. Dietary management of chronic large bowel diarrhea in dogs. Vet Econ 1992;34:26–32 (nutr suppl).

37. Zajac AM. Giardiasis. Compen Contin Educ Pract Vet 1992;14:604–611.

38. Hendrix CM, Blagburn BL, Lindsay DS. Whipworms and intestinal threadworms. Vet Clin North Am Small Anim Pract 1987;17:1355–1375.

39. Kalkofen U. Hookworms of dogs and cats. Vet Clin North Am Small Anim Pract 1987;17:1341–1354.

40. Parsons JC. Ascarid infections of cats and dogs. Vet Clin North Am Small Anim Pract 1987;17:1307–1339.

41. Lindsay DS, Blagburn BL. Coccidial parasites of cats and dogs. Compen Contin Educ Pract Vet 1991;13: 759–765.

42. Twedt DC. *Clostridium perfringens*–associated enterotoxicosis in dogs. In: Kirk RW, Bonagura JD, eds. Kirk's Current Veterinary Therapy XI. Philadelphia, WB Saunders, 1992:602–604.

43. Dillon AR, Boosinger TR, Blevins WT. *Campylobacter* enteritis in dogs and cats. Compen Contin Educ Pract Vet 1987;9:1175–1183.

44. Schaer M, Holloway S. Diagnosing acute pancreatitis in the cat. Vet Med (Prague) 1991;86:782–795.

45. Pollock RVH, Coyne MJ. Canine parvovirus. Vet Clin North Am Small Anim Pract 1993;23:555–568.

46. Penninck D, Nyland T, Ly K, et al. Ultrasonographic evaluation of gastrointestinal diseases in small animals. Vet Radiol 1990;31:134–141.

47. Moon M, Myer W. Gastrointestinal contrast radiology in small animals. Semin Vet Med Surg (Small Anim) 1986;1:121–143.

48. Jones BD, Hitt M, Hurst T. Hepatic biopsy. Vet Clin North Am Small Anim Pract 1985;15:39–65.

49. Breitschwerdt EB, Waltman C, Hagstad V, et al. Clinical and epidemiologic characterization of diarrheal syndrome in basenji dogs. J Am Vet Med Assoc 1982;180: 914–920.

50. Rimaila-Parnanen E, Westermarck E. Pancreatic degenerative atrophy and chronic pancreatitis in dogs. Acta Vet Scand 1982;23:400–406.

51. Hill FWG. Persistent diarrhoea. Br Vet J 1984;140: 150–158.

52. Peterson ME, Kintzer PP, Cavanagh PG, et al. Feline hyperthyroidism: Pretreatment clinical and laboratory evaluation of 131 cases. J Am Vet Med Assoc 1983;183: 103–110.

53. Friend SCE, Birch CJ, Lording PM, et al. Feline immunodeficiency virus: Prevalence, disease associations and isolation. Aust Vet J 1990;67:237–243.

54. O'Conner TP, Tonelli QJ, Scarlett JM. Report of the national FeLV/FIV awareness project. J Am Vet Med Assoc 1991;199:1348–1353.

55. Williams DA, Batt RM. Diagnosis of canine exocrine pancreatic insufficiency by the assay of serum trypsin-like immunoreactivity. J Small Anim Pract 1983;24: 583–588.

56. Williams DA. New tests of pancreatic and small intestine function. Compen Contin Educ Pract Vet 1987;9:1167–1174.

57. Nix BE, Leib MS, Zajac A, et al. The effect of dose and concentration on D-xylose absorption in healthy, immature dogs. Vet Clin Pathol 1993;22:10–16.

58. Hill FWG, Kidder DE, Frew J. A xylose absorption test for the dog. Vet Rec 1970;87:250–255.

59. Leib MS, Monroe WE, Codner EC. Performing rigid or flexible colonoscopy in dogs with chronic large bowel diarrhea. Vet Med (Prague) 1991;86:900–912.

60. Simpson KW. Gastrointestinal endoscopy in the dog. J Small Anim Pract 1993;34:180–188.

61. Banwell JG, Kistler LA, Giannella RA, et al. Small bowel bacterial overgrowth syndrome. Gastroenterology 1981; 80:834–845.

62. Willard MD. Chronic intestinal bacterial overgrowth. In: Kirk RW, ed. Current Veterinary Therapy X. Philadelphia, WB Saunders, 1989:933–938.

63. Batt RM, McLean L. Comparison of the biochemical changes in the jejunal mucosa of dogs with aerobic and anaerobic bacterial overgrowth. Gastroenterology 1987; 93:986–993.

64. King CE, Toskes PP. Small intestinal bacterial overgrowth. Gastroenterology 1979;76:1035–1055.

65. Ellison GW. Intestinal obstruction. In: Bojrab MJ, ed. Disease Mechanisms in Small Animal Surgery. Philadelphia, Lea & Febiger, 1993:252–257.

66. Lantz GC. The pathophysiology of acute mechanical small bowel obstruction. Compen Contin Educ Pract Vet 1981;3:910–916.

67. Lipowitz AJ. Intestinal obstruction in the dog. Calif Vet 1980;34:8–13.

68. Westermarck E, Rimaila-Parnanen E. Mesenteric torsion in dogs with exocrine pancreatic insufficiency: 21 cases (1978–1987). J Am Vet Med Assoc 1989;195:1404–1406.

69. Harvey HJ, Rendano VT. Small bowel volvulus in dogs: Clinical observations. Vet Surg 1984;13:91–94.

70. Shealy PM, Henderson RA. Canine intestinal volvulus: A report of nine new cases. Vet Surg 1992;21:15–19.

71. Gibbs C, Pearson H. The radiological diagnosis of

gastrointestinal obstruction in the dog. J Small Anim Pract 1973;14:61–82.

72. Flesja K, Yri T. Protein-losing enteropathy in the Lundehund. J Small Anim Pract 1977;18:11–23.

73. Glenert J, Jarnum S, Riemer S. The albumin transfer from blood to gastrointestinal tract in dogs. Acta Chir Scand 1962;124:63–74.

74. Tams TR. Canine protein-losing gastroenteropathy syndrome. Compen Contin Educ Pract Vet 1981;3:105–118.

75. Lorenz MD. Canine malabsorption syndromes. Compen Contin Educ Pract Vet 1980;2:885–893.

76. Fossum TW. Protein-losing enteropathy. Semin Vet Med Surg (Small Anim) 1989;4:219–225.

77. Meuten DJ, Chew DJ, Capen CC, et al. Relationship of serum total calcium to albumin and total protein in dogs. J Am Vet Med Assoc 1982;180:63–67.

78. Flanders JA, Scarlett JM, Blue JT, et al. Adjustment of total serum calcium concentration for binding to albumin and protein in cats: 291 cases (1986–1987). J Am Vet Med Assoc 1989;194:1609–1611.

79. Harvey J, French T, Meyer D. Chronic iron deficiency anemia in dogs. J Am Anim Hosp Assoc 1982;18:946–960.

80. Nemzek JA, Walshaw R, Hauptman JG. Mesenteric volvulus in the dog: A retrospective study. J Am Anim Hosp Assoc 1993;29:357–362.

81. Dimski DS. Constipation: Pathophysiology, diagnostic approach, and treatment. Semin Vet Med Surg (Small Anim) 1989;4:247–254.

82. DeNovo RC, Bright RM. Chronic feline constipation/obstipation. In: Kirk RW, Bonagura JD, eds. Kirk's Current Veterinary Therapy XI. Philadelphia, WB Saunders, 1992:619–626.

83. Sherding RG. Management of constipation and dyschezia. Compen Contin Educ Pract Vet 1991;13:677–685.

84. Burrows CF. Constipation, obstipation, and megacolon. In: August JR, ed. Consultations in Feline Internal Medicine. Philadelphia, WB Saunders, 1991:445–450.

85. Matthiesen DT, Scavelli TD, Whitney WO. Subtotal colectomy for the treatment of obstipation secondary to pelvic fracture malunion in cats. Vet Surg 1991;20:113–117.

86. Hoskins JD. Management of fecal impaction. Compen Contin Educ Pract Vet 1990;12:1579–1585.

87. Macintire DK. The acute abdomen: Differential diagnosis and management. Semin Vet Med Surg (Small Anim) 1988;3:302–310.

88. Felts JF, Fox PR, Burk RL. Thread and sewing needles as gastrointestinal foreign bodies in the cat: A review of 64 cases. J Am Vet Med Assoc 1984;184:56–59.

89. Gibbons GC, Murtaugh RJ. Cecal smooth muscle neoplasia in the dog: Report of 11 cases and literature review. J Am Anim Hosp Assoc 1989;25:191–197.

90. Tams TR. Irritable bowel syndrome. In: Kirk RW, Bonagura JD, eds. Kirk's Current Veterinary Therapy XI. Philadelphia, WB Saunders, 1992:604–608.

91. Rosin E. Megacolon in cats: The role of colectomy. Vet Clin North Am Small Anim Pract 1993;23:587–594.

92. Spielman BL, Garvey MS. Hemorrhagic gastroenteritis in 15 dogs. J Am Anim Hosp Assoc 1993;29:341–344.

93. Stanton ME, Bright RM. Gastroduodenal ulceration in dogs: Retrospective study of 43 cases and literature review. J Vet Intern Med 1989;3:238–244.

94. Zimmer JF, Burrington DB. Comparison of four techniques of fecal examination for detecting canine giardiasis. J Am Anim Hosp Assoc 1986;22:161–167.

95. Kirkpatrick CE, Farrell JP. Giardiasis. Compen Contin Educ Pract Vet 1982;4:367–378.

96. Kirkpatrick CE. Feline giardiasis: A review. J Small Anim Pract 1986;27:69–80.

97. Kleine LJ, Lamb CR. Comparative organ imaging: The gastrointestinal tract. Vet Radiol 1989;30:133–141.

98. Bruecker KA, Withrow SJ. Intestinal leiomyosarcomas in six dogs. J Am Anim Hosp Assoc 1988;24:281–284.

99. McPherron MA, Withrow SJ, Seim HB, et al. Colorectal leiomyomas in seven dogs. J Am Anim Hosp Assoc 1992;28:43–46.

100. Kleine LJ. Interpreting radiographic signs of abdominal disease in dogs and cats: 3. Vet Med (Prague) 1985;80:73–85.

101. White RAS, Gorman NT. The clinical diagnosis and management of rectal and pararectal tumours in the dog. J Small Anim Pract 1987;28:87–107.

102. Rosin E, Walshaw R, Mehlhaff C, et al. Subtotal colectomy for treatment of chronic constipation associated with idiopathic megacolon in cats: 38 cases (1979–1985). J Am Vet Med Assoc 1988;193:850–853.

103. Penninck DG, Nyland TG, Fisher PE, et al. Ultrasonography of the normal canine gastrointestinal tract. Vet Radiol 1989;30:272–276.

104. Penninck DG, Moore AS, Tidwell AS, et al. Ultrasonography of alimentary lymphosarcoma in the cat. Vet Radiol Ultrasound 1994;35:299–304.

105. Penninck DG, Crystal MA, Matz ME, et al. The technique of percutaneous ultrasound guided fine-needle aspiration biopsy and automated microcore biopsy in small animal gastrointestinal diseases. Vet Radiol Ultrasound 1993;34:433–436.

106. Crystal MA, Penninck DG, Matz ME, et al. Use of ultrasound-guided fine-needle aspiration biopsy and automated core biopsy for the diagnosis of gastrointestinal diseases in small animals. Vet Radiol Ultrasound 1993;34:438–444.

107. Sherding RG, Stradley RP, Rogers WA, et al. Bentiromide: Xylose test in healthy cats. Am J Vet Res 1982;43:2272–2273.

108. Hawkins E, Meric S, Washabau R, et al. Digestion of bentiromide and absorption of xylose in healthy cats and absorption of xylose in cats with infiltrative intestinal disease. Am J Vet Res 1986;47:567–569.

109. Hayden DW, Van Kruiningen HJ. Lymphocytic-plasmacytic enteritis in German shepherd dogs. J Am Anim Hosp Assoc 1982;18:89–96.

110. Finco DR, Duncan JR, Schall WD, et al. Chronic enteric disease and hypoproteinemia in 9 dogs. J Am Vet Med Assoc 1973;163:262–271.

111. Hill FWG. Malabsorption syndrome in the dog: A study of thirty-eight cases. J Small Anim Pract 1972;13:575–594.

112. Batt RM. Chronic small intestinal disease in the dog. In: Proc Annu Kal Kan Symp Treat Small Anim Dis 1984;8:93–103.

113. Hall EJ, Batt RM. Enhanced intestinal permeability to 51 Cr-labeled EDTA in dogs with small intestinal disease. J Am Vet Med Assoc 1990;196:91–95.

114. Batt RM, Carter MW, McLean L. Morphological and biochemical studies of a naturally occurring enteropathy in the Irish setter dog: A comparison with coeliac disease in man. Res Vet Sci 1984;37:339–346.

115. Batt RM, Bush BM, Peters TJ. Subcellular biochemical studies of a naturally occurring enteropathy in the dog resembling chronic tropical sprue in human beings. Am J Vet Res 1983;44:1492–1496.

116. Batt RM, Hall EJ, McLean L, et al. Small intestinal bacterial overgrowth and enhanced intestinal permeability in healthy beagles. Am J Vet Res 1992;53:1935–1940.

117. Batt RM, Morgan JO. Role of serum folate and vitamin B_{12} concentrations in the differentiation of small intestinal abnormalities in the dog. Res Vet Sci 1982;32:17–22.

118. Zajac AM, Leib MS, Burkholder WJ. *Giardia* infection in a group of experimental dogs. J Small Anim Pract 1992;33:257–260.

119. Roudebush P, Delivorias MH. Duodenal aspiration via flexible endoscope for diagnosis of giardiasis in a dog. J Am Vet Med Assoc 1985;187:162–163.

120. Leib MS. Gastrointestinal endoscopy. In: August JR, ed. Consultations in Feline Internal Medicine. Philadelphia, WB Saunders, 1994:119–126.

121. Tams TR. Gastrointestinal endoscopy: Instrumentation, handling technique, maintenance. In: Tams TR, ed. Small Animal Endoscopy. St Louis, CV Mosby, 1990: 31–46.

122. Guilford W, Jones BD. Gastrointestinal endoscopy of the dog and cat. Vet Med Rep 1990;2:140–150.

123. Burrows CF. Evaluation of a colonic lavage solution to prepare the colon of the dog for colonoscopy. J Am Vet Med Assoc 1989;195:1719–1721.

124. Richter KP, Cleveland MV. Comparison of an orally administered gastrointestinal lavage solution with traditional enema administration as preparation for colonoscopy in dogs. J Am Vet Med Assoc 1989;195: 1727–1731.

125. Jones BD. Endoscopy of the lower gastrointestinal tract. Vet Clin North Am Small Anim Pract 1990;20: 1229–1242.

126. Roth L, Leib MS, Davenport DJ, et al. Comparisons between endoscopic and histologic evaluation of the gastrointestinal tract in dogs and cats: 75 cases (1984–1987). J Am Vet Med Assoc 1990;196:635–638.

127. Jergens AE, Moore FM, Haynes JS, et al. Idiopathic inflammatory bowel disease in dogs and cats: 84 cases (1987–1990). J Am Vet Med Assoc 1992;201:1603–1608.

128. Wilcock B. Endoscopic biopsy interpretation in canine or feline enterocolitis. Semin Vet Med Surg (Small Anim) 1992;7:162–171.

129. Murdoch DB. Diarrhoea in the dog and cat: 1. Acute diarrhoea. Br Vet J 1986;142:307–316.

130. Simpson JW. Role of nutrition in aetiology and treatment of diarrhoea. J Small Anim Pract 1992;33:167–171.

131. Kruth SA. Infectious diarrhea in the dog and cat. In: Kirk RW, Bonagura JD, eds. Kirk's Current Veterinary Therapy XI. Philadelphia, WB Saunders, 1992:237–245.

132. Johnson SE. Loperamide: A novel antidiarrheal drug. Compen Contin Educ Pract Vet 1989;11:1373–1375.

133. Guilford WG. New ideas for the dietary management of gastrointestinal tract disease. J Small Anim Pract 1994; 35:620–624.

134. Washabau RJ, Strombeck DR, Buffington CA, et al. Evaluation of intestinal carbohydrate malabsorption in the dog by pulmonary hydrogen gas excretion. Am J Vet Res 1986;47:1402–1406.

135. Dimski DS. Dietary fiber in the management of gastrointestinal disease. In: Kirk RW, Bonagura JD, eds. Kirk's Current Veterinary Therapy XI. Philadelphia, WB Saunders, 1992:592–595.

136. Richter KP. Lymphocytic-plasmacytic enterocolitis in dogs. Semin Vet Med Surg (Small Anim) 1992;7:134–144.

137. Leib MS. Forward: Inflammatory bowel disease. Semin Vet Med Surg (Small Anim) 1992;7:105–106.

138. Nelson RW, Stookey LJ, Kazacos E. Nutritional management of idiopathic chronic colitis in the dog. J Vet Int Med 1988;2:133–137.

139. Nelson R, Dimperio M, Long G. Lymphocytic-plasmacytic colitis in the cat. J Am Vet Med Assoc 1984;184:1133–1135.

140. Jacobs G, Collins-Kelly L, Lappin M, et al. Lymphocytic-plasmacytic enteritis in 24 dogs. J Vet Intern Med 1990;4:45–53.

141. Dennis JS, Kruger JM, Mullaney TP. Lymphocytic/plasmacytic gastroenteritis in cats: 14 cases (1985–1990). J Am Vet Med Assoc 1992;200:1712–1718.

142. Dennis JS, Kruger JM, Mullaney TP. Lymphocytic/plasmacytic colitis in cats: 14 cases (1985–1990). J Am Vet Med Assoc 1993;202:313–318.

143. Simpson JW, Maskell IE, Markwell PJ. Use of a restricted antigen diet in the management of idiopathic canine colitis. J Small Anim Pract 1994;35:233–238.

144. Hart JR, Shaker E, Patnaik AK, et al. Lymphocytic-plasmacytic enterocolitis in cats: 60 cases (1988–1990). J Am Anim Hosp Assoc 1994;30:505–514.

145. Leib MS, Hiler LA, Roth L, et al. Plasmacytic lymphocytic colitis in the dog. Semin Vet Med Surg (Small Anim) 1989;4:241–246.

146. Tams TR. Chronic feline inflammatory bowel disorders: Part II. Feline eosinophilic enteritis and lymphosarcoma. Compen Contin Educ Pract Vet 1986;8:464–471.

147. Tams TR. Chronic feline inflammatory bowel disorders: Part I. Idiopathic inflammatory bowel disease. Compen Contin Educ Pract Vet 1986;8:371–378.

148. Wolf AM. Feline lymphocytic-plasmacytic enterocolitis. Semin Vet Med Surg (Small Anim) 1992;7:128–133.

149. Riis P. Extension of indications of immunosuppression in inflammatory bowel disease. J Autoimmun 1992; 5 (Supp A):289–291.

150. Barkin R, Lewis JH. Overview of inflammatory bowel disease in humans. Semin Vet Med Surg (Small Anim) 1992;7:117–127.

151. Van Kruiningen HJ. Granulomatous colitis of boxer dogs: Comparative aspects. Gastroenterology 1967;53: 114–122.

152. Breitschwerdt EB. Immunoproliferative enteropathy of basenjis. Semin Vet Med Surg (Small Anim) 1992;7: 153–161.

153. Magne ML. Pathophysiology of inflammatory bowel disease. Semin Vet Med Surg (Small Anim) 1992;7:112–116.

154. Eliakim R, Rachmilewitz D. Inflammatory mediators and the pathogenesis of inflammatory bowel disease. Ital J Gastroenterol 1992;24:361–368.

155. Jayanthi V, Probert CS, Sher KS, et al. Current concepts of the etiopathogenesis of inflammatory bowel disease. Am J Gastroenterol 1991;86:1566–1572.

156. Sartor RB. Pathogenetic and clinical relevance of cytokines in inflammatory bowel disease. Immunol Res 1991;10:465–471.

157. Schreiber S, Raedler A, Stenson WF, et al. The role of the mucosal immune system in inflammatory bowel disease. Gastroenterol Clin North Am 1992;21:451–502.

158. Nagura H. Mucosal defense mechanism in health and disease. Role of the mucosal immune system. Acta Pathol Jpn 1992;42:387–400.

159. Burrows CF. Canine colitis. Compen Contin Educ Pract Vet 1992;14:1347–1354.

160. Sethi AK, Sarna SK. Colonic motor activity in acute colitis in conscious dogs. Gastroenterology 1991;100:954–963.

161. Tams TR. Feline inflammatory bowel disease. Vet Clin North Am Small Anim Pract 1993;23:569–586.

162. Tams TR. Chronic canine lymphocytic plasmacytic enteritis. Compen Contin Educ Pract Vet 1987;9:1184–1194.

163. Leib MS, Hay WH, Roth L. Plasmacytic-lymphocytic colitis in dogs. In: Kirk RW, ed. Current Veterinary Therapy X. Philadelphia, WB Saunders, 1989:939–944.

164. Jergens AE, Moore FM, March P, et al. Idiopathic inflammatory bowel disease associated with gastroduodenal ulceration-erosion: A report of nine cases in the dog and cat. J Am Anim Hosp Assoc 1992;28:21–26.

165. Roth L, Walton AM, Leib MS, et al. A grading system for lymphocytic plasmacytic colitis in dogs. J Vet Diag Invest 1990;2:257–262.

166. van der Gaag I. The histological appearance of large intestinal biopsies in dogs with clinical signs of large bowel disease. Can J Vet Res 1988;52:75–82.

167. van der Gaag I, Happe RP. Follow-up studies by large intestinal biopsies and necropsy in dogs with clinical signs of large bowel disease. Can J Vet Res 1989;53:473–476.

168. Couto CG. Gastrointestinal neoplasia in dogs and cats. In: Kirk RW, Bonagura JD, eds. Kirk's Current Veterinary Therapy XI. Philadelphia, WB Saunders, 1992:595–601.

169. Merchant SR, Taboada J. Food allergy and immunologic diseases of the gastrointestinal tract. Semin Vet Med Surg (Small Anim) 1991;6:316–321.

170. Halliwell REW. Management of dietary hypersensitivity in the dog. J Small Anim Pract 1992;33:156–160.

171. Jeffers JG, Shanley KJ, Meyer EK. Diagnostic testing of dogs for food hypersensitivity. J Am Vet Med Assoc 1991;198:245–250.

172. Wills JM. Diagnosing and managing food sensitivity in cats. Vet Med (Prague) 1992;87:884–892.

173. White SD. Food hypersensitivity in 30 dogs. J Am Vet Med Assoc 1986;188:695–698.

174. White SD, Sequoia D. Food hypersensitivity in cats: 14 cases (1982–1987). J Am Vet Med Assoc 1989;194:692–695.

175. Guilford WG. Adverse reactions to food. In: Kirk RW, Bonagura JD, eds. Kirk's Current Veterinary Therapy XI. Philadelphia, WB Saunders, 1992:587–591.

176. Guilford WG. Dietary therapy for gastrointestinal tract diseases. In: Proc World Cong World Small Anim Vet Assoc, Durban, South Africa, 1994.

177. Guilford WG, Strombeck DL, Rogers QR, et al. Development of gastroscopic food sensitivity testing in dogs. J Vet Intern Med 1994;8:414–422.

178. Elwood CM, Rutgers HC, Batt RM. Gastroscopic food sensitivity testing in 17 dogs. J Small Anim Pract 1994;35:199–203.

179. Willard MD. Inflammatory bowel disease: Perspectives on therapy. J Am Anim Hosp Assoc 1992;28:27–32.

180. Kirsner JB. Inflammatory bowel disease. Part II: Clinical and therapeutic aspects. Dis Mon 1991;37:669–746.

181. Linn FV, Peppercorn MA. Drug therapy for inflammatory bowel disease: Part I. Am J Surg 1992;164:85–89.

182. Geier DL, Miner PJ. New therapeutic agents in the treatment of inflammatory bowel disease. Am J Med 1992;93:199–208.

183. Shanahan F, Targan S. Medical treatment of inflammatory bowel disease. Ann Rev Med 1992;43:125–133.

184. Gaginella TS, Walsh RE. Sulfasalazine: Multiplicity of action. Dig Dis Sci 1992;37:801–812.

185. Arvind AS, Farthing MJ. Review: New aminosalicylic acid derivatives for the treatment of inflammatory bowel disease. Aliment Pharmacol Ther 1988;2:281–289.

186. Sansom J, Barnett KC. Keratoconjunctivitis sicca in the dog: A review of two hundred cases. J Small Anim Pract 1985;26:121–131.

187. Morgan RV, Bachrach A. Keratoconjunctivitis sicca associated with sulfonamide therapy in dogs. J Am Vet Med Assoc 1982;180:432–434.

188. Jergens AE. Feline idiopathic inflammatory bowel disease. Compen Contin Educ Pract Vet 1992;14:509–520.

189. Meyers S, Sachar DB, Present DH, et al. Olsalazine sodium in the treatment of ulcerative colitis among patients intolerant of sulfasalazine: A prospective, randomized, placebo-controlled, double-blind, dose ranging clinical trial. Gastroenterology 1987;93:1255–1262.

190. Sandberg-Gertzen H, Jarnerot G, Kraaz W. Azodisal sodium in the treatment of ulcerative colitis: A study of tolerance and relapse-prevention properties. Gastroenterology 1986;90:1024–1030.

191. Riley SA, Mani V, Goodman MJ, et al. Comparison of delayed-release 5-aminosalicylic acid (mesalazine) and sulfasalazine as maintenance treatment for patients with ulcerative colitis. Gastroenterology 1988;94:1383–1389.

192. Sninsky CA, Cort DH, Shanahan F, et al. Oral mesalamine (Asacol) for mildly to moderately active ulcerative colitis. Ann Intern Med 1991;115:350–355.

193. Cole AT, Hawkey CJ. New treatments in inflammatory bowel disease. Br J Hosp Med 1992;47:581–590.

194. Houston DM, Keller CB. Keratoconjunctivitis sicca in

the dog following prolonged use of Salazopyrin and other 5-ASA containing drugs for treatment of canine colitis. Can Vet J 1989;30:437.

195. Barnett KC, Joseph EC. Keratoconjunctivitis sicca in the dog following 5-aminosalicylic acid administration. Human Toxicol 1987;6:377–383.

196. Sutherland L, Singleton J, Sessions J, et al. Double blind, placebo controlled trial of metronidazole in Crohn's disease. Gut 1991;32:1071–1075.

197. Dow SW, LeCouteur RA, Poss ML, et al. Central nervous system toxicosis associated with metronidazole treatment of dogs: Five cases (1984–1987). J Am Vet Med Assoc 1989;195:365–368.

198. Linn FV, Peppercorn MA. Drug therapy for inflammatory bowel disease: Part II. Am J Surg 1992;164:178–185.

199. Beale KM. Azathioprine for treatment of immune-mediated diseases of dogs and cats. J Am Vet Med Assoc 1988;192:1316–1318.

200. Van Kruiningen HJ. Clinical efficacy of tylosin in canine inflammatory bowel disease. J Am Anim Hosp Assoc 1976;12:498–501.

201. Johnson SE. Canine eosinophilic gastroenterocolitis. Semin Vet Med Surg (Small Anim) 1992;7:145–152.

202. Hayden DW, Van Kruiningen HJ. Eosinophilic gastroenteritis in German shepherd dogs and its relationship to visceral larva migrans. J Am Vet Med Assoc 1973;162:379–384.

203. Hayden DW, Van Kruiningen HJ. Experimentally induced canine toxocariasis: Laboratory examinations and pathologic changes, with emphasis on the gastrointestinal tract. Am J Vet Res 1975;36:1605–1614.

204. Wershil BK, Walker WA. The mucosal barrier, IgE-mediated gastrointestinal events, and eosinophilic gastroenteritis. Gastroenterol Clin North Am 1992;21:387–404.

205. Croese J, Loukas A, Opdebeeck J, et al. Occult enteric infection by *Ancylostoma caninum*: A previously unrecognized zoonosis. Gastroenterology 1994;106:3–12.

206. van der Gaag I, Happe RP, Wolvekamp WTC. Eosinophilic gastroenteritis complicated by partial ruptures and a perforation of the small intestine in a dog. J Small Anim Pract 1983;24:575–581.

207. van der Gaag I, van der Linde-Sipman JS. Eosinophilic granulomatous colitis with ulceration in a dog. J Comp Pathol 1987;97:179–185.

208. van der Gaag I, van der Linde-Sipman JS, van Sluys FJ, et al. Regional eosinophilic coloproctitis, typhlitis and ileitis in a dog. Vet Q 1990;12:1–6.

209. Neer TM. Hypereosinophilic syndrome in cats. Compen Contin Educ Pract Vet 1991;13:549–555.

210. Anderson D, Roberson E. Activity of ivermectin against canine intestinal helminths. Am J Vet Res 1982;43:1681–1683.

211. Birchard SJ, Couto CG, Johnson S. Nonlymphoid intestinal neoplasia in 32 dogs and 14 cats. J Am Anim Hosp Assoc 1986;22:533–537.

212. Church EM, Mehlhaff CJ, Patnaik AK. Colorectal adenocarcinoma in dogs: 78 cases (1973–1984). J Am Vet Med Assoc 1987;191:727–730.

213. Cribb AE. Feline gastrointestinal adenocarcinoma: A review and retrospective study. Can Vet J 1988;29:709–712.

214. Head KW, Else RW. Neoplasia and allied conditions of the canine and feline intestine. Vet Ann 1981;21:190–207.

215. Holt PE, Lucke VM. Rectal neoplasia in the dog: A clinicopathological review of 31 cases. Vet Rec 1985;116:400–405.

216. Kosovsky JE, Matthiesen DT, Patnaik AK. Small intestinal adenocarcinoma in cats: 32 cases (1978–1985). J Am Vet Med Assoc 1988;192:233–235.

217. Patnaik AK, Hurvitz AI, Johnson GF. Canine gastrointestinal neoplasms. Vet Pathol 1977;14:547–555.

218. Patnaik AK, Liu SK, Johnson GF. Feline intestinal adenocarcinoma. Vet Pathol 1976;13:1–10.

219. Patnaik AK, Hurvitz AI, Johnson GF. Canine intestinal adenocarcinoma and carcinoid. Vet Pathol 1980;17:149–163.

220. Schaffer E, Schiefer B. Incidence and types of canine rectal carcinomas. J Small Anim Pract 1968;9:491–496.

221. Turk MAM, Gallina AM, Russell TS. Nonhematopoietic gastrointestinal neoplasia in cats: A retrospective study of 44 cases. Vet Pathol 1981;18:614–620.

222. Feeney DA, Klausner JS, Johnston GR. Chronic bowel obstruction caused by primary intestinal neoplasia: A report of five cases. J Am Anim Hosp Assoc 1982;18:67–77.

223. Gibbs C, Pearson H. Localized tumours of the canine small intestine: A report of twenty cases. J Small Anim Pract 1986;27:507–519.

224. Loar AS. The management of feline lymphosarcoma. Vet Clin North Am Small Anim Pract 1984;14:1299–1330.

225. Couto CG, Rutgers HC, Sherding RG, et al. Gastrointestinal lymphoma in 20 dogs: A retrospective study. J Vet Intern Med 1989;3:73–78.

226. Davenport DJ. Gastrointestinal lymphosarcoma. In: August JR, ed. Consultations in Feline Internal Medicine. Philadelphia, WB Saunders, 1991:419–423.

227. Wilson GP, Burt JK. Intussusception in the dog and cat: A review of 45 cases. J Am Vet Med Assoc 1974;164:515–518.

228. Weaver AD. Canine intestinal intussusception. Vet Rec 1977;100:524–527.

229. Bellenger CR, Beck JA. Intussusception in 12 cats. J Small Anim Pract 1994;35:295–298.

230. Oakes MG, Lewis DD, Hosgood G, et al. Enteroplication for the prevention of intussusception recurrence in dogs: 31 cases (1978–1992). J Am Vet Med Assoc 1994;205:72–75.

231. Lewis DD, Ellison GW. Intussusception in dogs and cats. Compen Contin Educ Pract Vet 1987;9:523–534.

232. Clinkenbeard K, Cowell RL, Tyler RD. Disseminated histoplasmosis in dogs: 12 cases (1981–1986). J Am Vet Med Assoc 1988;193:1443–1447.

233. Clinkenbeard KD, Cowell RL, Tyler RD. Disseminated histoplasmosis in cats: 12 cases (1981–1986). J Am Vet Med Assoc 1987;190:1445–1448.

234. Clinkenbeard KD, Wolf AM, Cowell RL, et al. Feline disseminated histoplasmosis. Compen Contin Educ Pract Vet 1989;11:1223–1233.

235. Clinkenbeard KD, Tyler RD, Cowell RL. Thrombocytopenia associated with disseminated histoplasmosis

in dogs. Compen Contin Educ Pract Vet 1989;11:301–308.

236. Clinkenbeard KD, Wolf AM, Cowell RL, et al. Canine disseminated histoplasmosis. Compen Contin Educ Pract Vet 1989;11:1347–1360.

237. Sherding RG, Johnson SE. Intestinal histoplasmosis. In: Kirk RW, Bonagura JD, eds. Kirk's Current Veterinary Therapy XI. Philadelphia, WB Saunders, 1992:609–613.

238. Wolf AM. Histoplasmosis. In: Greene CE, ed. Infectious Diseases of the Dog and Cat. Philadelphia, WB Saunders, 1990:679–686.

239. Roberson E, Cornelius LM. Gastrointestinal parasitism. In: Kirk R, ed. Current Veterinary Therapy VII. Philadelphia, WB Saunders, 1980:935–948.

240. Hass DK, Collins JA, Flick SC. Canine parasitism. Canine Pract 1975;2:42–47.

241. Zajac AM. The role of gastrointestinal immunity in parasitic infections of small animals. Semin Vet Med Surg (Small Anim) 1989;2:274–281.

242. Bowman DD. Hookworm parasites of dogs and cats. Compen Contin Educ Pract Vet 1992;14:585–595.

243. Harvey JB, Roberts JM, Schantz PM. Survey of veterinarians' recommendations for treatment and control of intestinal parasites in dogs: Public health implications. J Am Vet Med Assoc 1991;199:702–707.

244. Burke TM, Roberson EL. Fenbendazole treatment of pregnant bitches to reduce prenatal and lactogenic infections of *Toxocara canis* and *Ancylostoma caninum* in pups. J Am Vet Med Assoc 1983;183:987–990.

245. Paul A, Tranquilli W, Seward R, et al. Clinical observations in collies given ivermectin orally. Am J Vet Res 1987;48:684–686.

246. Clark JN, Daurio CP, Plue RE, et al. Efficacy of ivermectin and pyrantel pamoate combined in a chewable formulation against heartworm, hookworm, and ascarid infections in dogs. Am J Vet Res 1992;53:517–520.

247. Wade CG, Mercer SH, Hepler DI, et al. Effect of milbemycin oxime against *Ancylostoma caninum* in dogs with naturally acquired infection. Am J Vet Res 1991;52:951–953.

248. Blagburn BL, Hendrix CM, Lindsay DS, et al. Efficacy of milbemycin oxime against naturally acquired or experimentally induced *Ancylostoma* spp and *Trichuris vulpis* infections in dogs. Am J Vet Res 1992;53:513–516.

249. Bowman D, Lin D-S, Johnson R, et al. Effects of milbemycin oxime on adult *Ancylostoma caninum* and *Uncinaria stenocephala* in dogs with experimentally induced infections. Am J Vet Res 1991;52:64–67.

250. Bowman D, Johnson R, Hepler D. Effects of milbemycin oxime on adult hookworms in dogs with naturally acquired infections. Am J Vet Res 1990;51:487–490.

251. Schantz PM, Glickman LT. Roundworms in dogs and cats: Veterinary and public health considerations. Compen Contin Educ Pract Vet 1981;3:773–784.

252. Kazacos KR. Visceral and ocular larva migrans. Semin Vet Med Surg (Small Anim) 1991;6:227–235.

253. Barriga OO. Rational control of canine toxocariasis by the veterinary practitioner. J Am Vet Med Assoc 1991;198:216–221.

254. Schantz PM, Stehr-Green JK. Toxocaral larva migrans. J Am Vet Med Assoc 1988;192:28–32.

255. Zajac A. Treatment of gastrointestinal parasitic infections. In: August JR, ed. Consultations in Feline Internal Medicine. Philadelphia, WB Saunders, 1991:425–433.

256. Reinemeyer CR. Feline gastrointestinal parasites. In: Kirk RW, Bonagura JD, eds. Kirk's Current Veterinary Therapy XI. Philadelphia, WB Saunders, 1992:626–630.

257. Reinemeyer C, DeNovo R. Evaluation of the efficacy and safety of two formulations of pyrantel pamoate in cats. Am J Vet Res 1990;51:932–934.

258. Lloyd S, Soulsby EJL. Prenatal and transmammary infections of *Toxocara canis* in dogs: Effect of benzimidazole-carbamate anthelmintics on various developmental stages of the parasite. J Small Anim Pract 1983;24:763–768.

259. Bowman DD, Parsons JC, Grieve RB, et al. Effects of milbemycin on adult *Toxocara canis* in dogs with experimentally induced infection. Am J Vet Res 1988;49:1986–1990.

260. Dubey JP, Greene C. Enteric coccidiosis. In: Greene CE, ed. Infectious diseases of the dog and cat. Philadelphia, WB Saunders, 1990:835–846.

261. Kirkpatrick CE, Dubey JP. Enteric coccidial infections. Vet Clin North Am Small Anim Pract 1987;17:1405–1420.

262. Oduye OO, Bobade PA. Studies on an outbreak of intestinal coccidiosis in the dog. J Small Anim Pract 1979;20:181–184.

263. Correa WM, Correa CNM, Langoni H, et al. Canine isosporosis. Can Pract 1983;10:44–46.

264. Dunbar MR, Foreyt WJ. Prevention of coccidiosis in domestic dogs and captive coyotes (*Canis latrans*) with sulfadimethoxine-ormetoprim combination. Am J Vet Res 1985;46:1899–1902.

265. Collins GH, Pope SE, Griffen DL, et al. Diagnosis and prevalence of *Giardia* spp in dogs and cats. Aust Vet J 1987;64:89–90.

266. Hahn NE, Glaser CA, Hird DW, et al. Prevalence of *Giardia* in the feces of pups. J Am Vet Med Assoc 1988;192:1428–1429.

267. Simpson JW, Burnie AG, Miles RS, et al. Prevalence of *Giardia* and *Cryptosporidium* infection in dogs in Edinburgh. Vet Rec 1988;123:445.

268. Swan JM, Thompson RCA. The prevalence of *Giardia* in dogs and cats in Perth, Western Australia. Aust Vet J 1986;63:110–112.

269. Winsland JKD, Nimmo S, Butcher PD, et al. Prevalence of *Giardia* in dogs and cats in the United Kingdom: Survey of an Essex veterinary clinic. Trans R Soc Trop Med Hyg 1989;83:791–792.

270. Sykes TJ. Patterns of infection with *Giardia* in dogs in London. Trans R Soc Trop Med Hyg 1989;83:239–240.

271. Belosevic M, Faubert GM, Guy R, et al. Observations on natural and experimental infections with *Giardia* isolated from cats. Can J Comp Res 1984;48:241–244.

272. Kirkpatrick CE, Laczak JP. Giardiasis in a cattery. J Am Vet Med Assoc 1985;187:161–162.

273. Barlough JE. Canine giardiasis: A review. J Small Anim Pract 1979;20:613–623.

274. Kirkpatrick C, Farrell J. Feline giardiasis: Observation on natural and induced infections. Am J Vet Res 1984;45:2182–2188.

275. Kirkpatrick CE. Giardiasis. Vet Clin North Am Small Anim Pract 1987;17:1377–1387.

276. Tanowitz HB, Weiss LM, Wittner M. Diagnosis and treatment of protozoan diarrheas. Am J Gastroenterol 1988;83:339–350.

277. Zimmer JF, Miller JJ, Lindmark DG. Evaluation of the efficacy of selected commercial disinfectants in inactivating *Giardia muris* cysts. J Am Anim Hosp Assoc 1988;24:379–385.

278. Brightman AH. A review of five clinical cases of giardiasis in cats. J Am Anim Hosp Assoc 1976;12:492–497.

279. Pitts RP, Twedt DC, Mallie KA. Comparison of duodenal aspiration with fecal flotation for diagnosis of giardiasis in dogs. J Am Vet Med Assoc 1983;182:1210–1211.

280. Leib MS, Zajac AM. Giardia infection in dogs and cats. In: Waltham/OSU Symposium for the Treatment of Small Animal Diseases. Columbus, Ohio, 1993;17:90–93.

281. Barr SC, Bowman DD, Erb HN. Evaluation of two test procedures for diagnosis of giardiasis in dogs. Am J Vet Res 1992;53:2028–2031.

282. Zimmer JF, Burrington DB. Comparison of four protocols for the treatment of canine giardiasis. J Am Anim Hosp Assoc 1986;22:168–172.

283. Barr SC, Bowman DD, Heller RL, et al. Efficacy of albendazole against giardiasis in dogs. Am J Vet Res 1993;54:926–928.

284. Barr SC, Bowman DD, Heller RL. Efficacy of fenbendazole against giardiasis in dogs. Am J Vet Res 1994;55:988–990.

285. Hildreth MB, Johnson MD, Kazacos KR. *Echinococcus multilocularis*: A zoonosis of increasing concern in the United States. Compen Contin Educ Pract Vet 1991;13:727–741.

286. Bryan RT, Schantz PM. Echinococcosis (hydatid disease). J Am Vet Med Assoc 1989;195:1214–1217.

287. Walters TMH. Echinococcosis/hydatidosis and the South Powys control scheme. J Small Anim Pract 1986;27:693–703.

288. Boreham RE, Boreham PFL. *Dipylidium caninum*: Life cycle, epizootiology, and control. Compen Contin Educ Pract Vet 1990;12:667–671, 674–676.

289. Georgi JR. Tapeworms. Vet Clin North Am Small Anim Pract 1987;17:1285–1305.

290. Baldock FC, Thompson RCA, Kumaratilake LM, et al. *Echinococcus granulosus* in farm dogs and dingoes in south eastern Queensland. Aust Vet J 1985;62:335–336.

291. Obendorf DL, Matheson MJ, Thompson RCA. *Echinococcus granulosus* infection of foxes in south-eastern New South Wales. Aust Vet J 1989;66:123–124.

292. Morrison P, Stanton R, Pilatti E. *Echinococcus granulosus* infection in wild dogs in south-eastern New South Wales. Aust Vet J 1988;65:97–98.

293. Gasser RB, Lightowlers MW, Rickard MD. *Echinococcus granulosus*: Antigenic proteins in oncospheres and on the surface of protoscoleces identified by serum antibodies from infected dogs. Res Vet Sci 1991;50:340–345.

294. Gasser RB, Lightowlers MW, Obendorf DL, et al. Evaluation of a serological test system for the diagnosis of natural *Echinococcus granulosus* infection in dogs using *E. granulosus* protoscolex and oncosphere antigens. Aust Vet J 1988;65:369–373.

295. Gasser RB, Lightowlers MW, Rickard MD, et al. Serological screening of farm dogs for *Echinococcus granulosus* infection in an endemic region. Aust Vet J 1990;67:145–147.

296. Jenkins DJ, Rickard MD. Specific antibody responses to *Taenia hydatigena*, *Taenia pisiformis* and *Echinococcus granulosus* infection in dogs. Aust Vet J 1985;62:72–78.

297. Manger BR, Brewer MD. Epsiprantel, a new tapeworm remedy: Preliminary efficacy studies in dogs and cats. Br Vet J 1989;145:384–388.

298. Corwin RM, Green SP, Keefe TJ. Dose titration and confirmation tests for determination of cesticidal efficacy of epsiprantel in dogs. Am J Vet Res 1989;50:1076–1077.

299. Anderson FL, Short JA, McCurdy HD. Efficacy of a combined paste formulation of praziquantel/febantel against immature *Echinococcus granulosus* and immature *Echinococcus multilocularis*. Am J Vet Res 1985;46:253–255.

300. Arru E, Garippa G, Manger BR. Efficacy of epsiprantel against *Echinococcus granulosus* infections in dogs. Res Vet Sci 1990;49:378–379.

301. Glickman LT, Domanski LM, Patronek GJ, et al. Breed-related risk factors for canine parvovirus enteritis. J Am Vet Med Assoc 1985;187:589–594.

302. Gordon JC, Angrick EJ. Canine parvovirus: Environmental effects on infectivity. Am J Vet Res 1986;47:1464–1467.

303. Pollock RVH, Carmichael LE. Newer knowledge about canine parvovirus. Gaines Vet Symp 1981;30:36–40.

304. Brunner CJ, Swango LJ. Canine parvovirus infection: Effects on the immune system and factors that predispose to severe disease. Compen Contin Educ Pract Vet 1985;7:979–989.

305. McAdaragh JP, Eustis SL, Nelson DT, et al. Experimental infection of conventional dogs with canine parvovirus. Am J Vet Res 1982;43:693–696.

306. Pollock RVH. Experimental canine parvovirus infection in dogs. Cornell Vet 1982;72:103–119.

307. Macartney L, McCandlish IAP, Thompson H, et al. Canine parvovirus enteritis: 2. Pathogenesis. Vet Rec 1984;115:453–460.

308. O'Sullivan G, Durham PJK, Smith JR, et al. Experimentally induced severe canine parvoviral enteritis. Aust Vet J 1984;61:1–4.

309. Carman PS, Povey RC. Pathogenesis of canine parvovirus-2 in dogs: Haematology, serology and virus recovery. Res Vet Sci 1985;38:134–140.

310. Meunier PC, Cooper BJ, Appel MJG, et al. Pathogenesis of canine parvovirus enteritis: Sequential virus distribution and passive immunization studies. Vet Pathol 1985;22:617–624.

311. Meunier PC, Cooper BJ, Appel MJG, et al. Pathogenesis of canine parvovirus enteritis: The importance of viremia. Vet Pathol 1985;22:60–71.

312. Boosinger TR, Rebar AH, DeNicola DB, et al. Bone marrow alterations associated with canine parvoviral enteritis. Vet Pathol 1982;19:558–561.

313. Mason MJ, Gillett NA, Muggenburg BA. Clinical, pathological, and epidemiological aspects of canine parvoviral enteritis in an unvaccinated closed beagle colony: 1978–1985. J Am Anim Hosp Assoc 1987;23: 183–192.

314. Stann SE, DiGiacomo RF, Giddens WE, et al. Clinical and pathologic features of parvoviral diarrhea in pound-source dogs. J Am Vet Med Assoc 1984;185: 651–655.

315. Macartney L, McCandlish IAP, Thompson H, et al. Canine parvovirus enteritis: 1. Clinical, haematological and pathological features of experimental infection. Vet Rec 1984;115:201–210.

316. Turk J, Miller M, Brown T, et al. Coliform septicemia and pulmonary disease associated with canine parvoviral enteritis: 88 cases (1987–1988). J Am Vet Med Assoc 1990;196:771–773.

317. Carmen PS, Povey RC. Pathogenesis of canine parvovirus-2 in dogs: Histopathology and antigen identification in tissues. Res Vet Sci 1985;38:141–150.

318. Nara PL, Winters K, Rice JB, et al. Systemic and local intestinal antibody response in dogs given both infective and inactivated canine parvovirus. Am J Vet Res 1983;44:1989–1995.

319. Woods CB, Pollock RVH, Carmichael LE. Canine parvoviral enteritis. J Am Anim Hosp Assoc 1980;16: 171–179.

320. Moreau PM. Canine viral enteritis. Compen Contin Educ Pract Vet 1980;11:540–547.

321. Robinson WF, Huxtable CR, Pass DA. Canine parvoviral myocarditis: A morphologic description of the natural disease. Vet Pathol 1980;17:282–293.

322. Hayes MA, Russell RG, Babiuk LA. Sudden death in young dogs with myocarditis caused by parvovirus. J Am Vet Med Assoc 1979;174:1197–1203.

323. Jezyk PF, Haskins ME, Jones CL. Myocarditis of probable viral origin in pups of weaning age. J Am Vet Med Assoc 1979;174:1204–1207.

324. Heald RD, Jones BD, Schmidt DA. Blood gas and electrolyte concentrations in canine parvoviral enteritis. J Am Anim Hosp Assoc 1986;22:745–748.

325. Jacobs RM, Weiser MG, Hall RL, et al. Clinicopathologic features of canine parvoviral enteritis. J Am Anim Hosp Assoc 1980;16:809–814.

326. Mildbrand MM, Teramoto YA, Collins JK, et al. Rapid detection of canine parvovirus in feces using monoclonal antibodies and enzyme-linked immunosorbent assay. Am J Vet Res 1984;45:2281–2284.

327. Farrows CS. Radiographic appearance of canine parvovirus enteritis. J Am Vet Med Assoc 1982;180:43–47.

328. Wessels BC, Gaffin SL. Anti-endotoxin immunotherapy for canine parvovirus endotoxaemia. J Small Anim Pract 1986;27:609–615.

329. McGavin D. Inactivation of canine parvovirus by disinfectants and heat. J Small Anim Pract 1987;28: 523–535.

330. O'Brien SE. Serologic response of pups to the low-passage, modified-live canine parvovirus-2 component in a combination vaccine. J Am Vet Med Assoc 1994; 204:1207–1209.

331. Pollock RVH, Carmichael LE. Maternally derived im-munity to canine parvovirus infection: Transfer, decline, and interference with vaccination. J Am Vet Med Assoc 1982;180:37–42.

332. Burtonboy S, Charlier P, Hertoghs J, et al. Performance of high titre attenuated canine parvovirus vaccine in pups with maternally derived antibody. Vet Rec 1991; 128:377–381.

333. Macartney L, Thompson H, McCandlish IAP, et al. Canine parvovirus: Interaction between passive immunity and virulent challenge. Vet Rec 1988;122: 573–576.

334. Pollock RVH. The parvoviruses: Part I. Feline panleukopenia virus and mink enteritis virus. Compen Contin Educ Pract Vet 1984;6:227–241.

335. Greene CE, Scott FW. Feline panleukopenia. In: Greene CE, ed. Infectious Diseases of the Dog and Cat. Philadelphia, WB Saunders, 1990:291–299.

336. Shindel NM, Van Kruiningen HJ, Scott FW. The colitis of feline panleukopenia. J Am Anim Hosp Assoc 1978;14: 738–747.

337. Langheinrich KA, Nielsen SW. Histopathology of feline panleukopenia: A report of 65 cases. J Am Vet Med Assoc 1971;158:863–871.

338. Carpenter JL. Feline panleukopenia: Clinical signs and differential diagnosis. J Am Vet Med Assoc 1971;158: 857–862.

339. Kilham L, Margolis G, Colby ED. Cerebellar ataxia and its congenital transmission in cats by feline panleukopenia virus. J Am Vet Med Assoc 1971;158:888–900.

340. Tennant BJ, Gaskell RM, Jones RC, et al. Studies on the epizootiology of canine coronavirus. Vet Rec 1993; 132:7–11.

341. Tennant BJ, Gaskell RM, Jones RC, et al. Prevalence of antibodies to four major canine viral diseases in dogs in a Liverpool hospital population. J Small Anim Pract 1991;32:175–179.

342. Helfer-Baker C, Evermann JF, McKeirnan AJ, et al. Serological studies on the incidence of canine enteritis viruses. Canine Pract 1980;7:37–42.

343. Marshall JA, Healey DS, Studdert MJ, et al. Viruses and virus-like particles in the faeces of dogs with and without diarrhoea. Aust Vet J 1984;61:33–38.

344. Halnan CRE. Vomiting and diarrhoea in dogs. Vet Rec 1972;91:571–572.

345. Appel MJG, Meunier P, Greisen H, et al. Enteric viral infections of dogs. Gaines Vet Symp 1979;29:3–8.

346. Appel M, Meunier P, Pollack R, et al. Canine viral enteritis. Canine Pract 1980;7:22–34.

347. Carmichael LE, Binn LN. New enteric viruses in the dog. Adv Vet Sci Comp Med 1981;25:4–11.

348. Vandenberghe J, Ducatelle R, Debouck P. Coronavirus infection in a litter of pups. Vet Q 1980;2:136–141.

349. Appel MJG. Does canine coronavirus augment the effects of subsequent parvovirus infection? Vet Med 1988;83:360–366.

350. Tingpalapong M, Whitmore R, Watts D, et al. Epizootic of viral enteritis in dogs in Thailand. Am J Vet Res 1982;43:1687–1690.

351. Tennant BJ, Gaskell RM, Kelly DF, et al. Canine coronavirus infection in the dog following oronasal inoculation. Res Vet Sci 1991;51:11–18.

352. Carmichael LE. Infectious canine enteritis caused by a corona-like virus. Canine Pract 1978;5:25–27.

353. Appel MJG, Cooper BJ, Greisen H, et al. Status report: Canine viral enteritis. J Am Vet Med Assoc 1978;173:1516–1518.

354. Edwards BG, Fulker RH, Acree WM, et al. Evaluating a canine coronavirus vaccine through antigen extinction and challenge studies. Vet Med 1985;85:28–33.

355. Grahn BH. The feline coronavirus infections: Feline infectious peritonitis and feline coronavirus enteritis. Vet Med 1991;86:376–393.

356. Pedersen NC, Boyle JF, Floyd K, et al. An enteric coronavirus infection of cats and its relationship to feline infectious peritonitis. Am J Vet Res 1981;42:368–377.

357. Pedersen N, Everman J, McKeirnan A, et al. Pathogenicity studies of feline coronavirus isolates 79–1146 and 79–1683. Am J Vet Res 1984;45:2580–2585.

358. Burrows CE. Canine hemorrhagic gastroenteritis. J Am Anim Hosp Assoc 1977;13:451–458.

359. Wessels BC, Gaffin SL, Wells MT. Circulating plasma endotoxin (lipopolysaccharide) concentrations in healthy and hemorrhagic enteric dogs: Antiendotoxin immunotherapy in hemorrhagic enteric endotoxemia. J Am Anim Hosp Assoc 1987;23:291–295.

360. Basher AWP, Fowler JD. Conservative versus surgical management of gastrointestinal linear foreign bodies in the cat. Vet Surg 1987;16:135–138.

361. Evans KL, Smeak DD, Biller DS. Gastrointestinal linear foreign bodies in 32 dogs: A retrospective evaluation and feline comparison. J Am Anim Hosp Assoc 1994;30:445–450.

362. Koikem T, Otomo K, Kudo T, et al. Clinical cases of intestinal obstruction with foreign bodies and intussusception in dogs. Jpn J Vet Res 1981;29:8–15.

363. Root CR, Lord PF. Linear radiolucent gastrointestinal foreign bodies in cats and dogs: Their radiographic appearance. Vet Radiol 1971;12:45–52.

364. Kantrowitz B, Biller D. Using radiography to evaluate vomiting in dogs and cats. Vet Med 1992;87:806–813.

365. Suter MM, Palmer DG, Schenk H. Primary intestinal lymphangiectasia in three dogs: A morphological and immunopathological investigation. Vet Pathol 1985;22:123–130.

366. Burns MG. Intestinal lymphangiectasia in the dog: A case report and review. J Am Anim Hosp Assoc 1982;18:97–105.

367. Batt RM. New approaches to malabsorption in dogs. Compen Contin Educ Pract Vet 1986;8:783–794.

368. Batt RM, Hall EJ. Chronic enteropathies in the dog. J Small Anim Pract 1989;30:3–12.

369. Delles EK, Willard MD, Simpson RB, et al. Comparison of species and numbers of bacteria in concurrently cultured samples of proximal small intestinal fluid and endoscopically obtained duodenal mucosa in dogs with intestinal bacterial overgrowth. Am J Vet Res 1994;55:957–964.

370. Williams DA, Batt RM, McLean L. Bacterial overgrowth in the duodenum of dogs with exocrine pancreatic insufficiency. J Am Vet Med Assoc 1987;191:201–206.

371. Batt RM, Barnes A, Rutgers HC, et al. Relative IgA deficiency and small intestinal bacterial overgrowth in German shepherd dogs. Res Vet Sci 1991;50:106–111.

372. Whitbread T, Batt RM, Garthwaite G. Relative deficiency of serum IgA in the German shepherd dog: A breed abnormality. Res Vet Sci 1984;37:350–352.

373. Stanton MLE. Gastric ulceration and neoplasia. In: Bojrab MJ, ed. Disease Mechanisms in Small Animal Surgery. Philadelphia, Lea & Febiger, 1993:232–234.

374. Reinacher M. Feline leukemia virus-associated enteritis: A condition with features of feline panleukopenia. Vet Pathol 1987;24:1–4.

375. Reinacher M. Infections with feline leukaemia virus detected upon post-mortem examination. J Small Anim Pract 1987;28:640–649.

376. Ishida T, Washizu T, Toriyabe K, et al. Feline immunodeficiency virus infection in cats of Japan. J Am Vet Med Assoc 1989;194:221–225.

377. Yamamoto JK, Hansen H, Ho EW, et al. Epidemiologic and clinical aspects of feline immunodeficiency virus infection in cats from the continental United States and Canada and possible mode of transmission. J Am Vet Med Assoc 1989;194:213–220.

378. Hopper CD, Sparkes AH, Gruffydd-Jones TJ, et al. Clinical and laboratory findings in cats infected with feline immunodeficiency virus. Vet Rec 1989;125:341–346.

379. Sparger EE, Yamamoto JK. Feline immunodeficiency virus infection. In: Kirk RW, ed. Current Veterinary Therapy X. Philadelphia, WB Saunders, 1989:530–534.

380. Campbell BG. Trichuris and other trichinelloid nematodes of dogs and cats in the United States. Compen Contin Educ Pract Vet 1991;13:769–780.

381. Dryden MW, Gaafar SM. Whipworm infection in small animals. Comp Anim Pract 1988;2:17–22.

382. Leib MS, Codner EC, Monroe WE. Common colonoscopic findings in dogs with chronic large bowel diarrhea. Vet Med 1991;86:913–921.

383. Zajac AM. Developments in the treatment of gastrointestinal parasites of small animals. Vet Clin North Am Small Anim Pract 1993;23:671–681.

384. Hardy RM, O'Brien T, Adams LG, et al. Periportal hepatitis associated with the use of a heartworm-hookworm preventative (diethylcarbamazine-oxibendazole) in 13 dogs. J Am Anim Hosp Assoc 1989;25:419–429.

385. Burrows CF. Medical diseases of the colon. In: Jones BD, Liska WD, eds. Canine and Feline Gastroenterology. Philadelphia, WB Saunders, 1986:221–256.

386. van Wijk HJ, Smout JPM. The puzzling pathogenesis of the irritable bowel syndrome. Scand J Gastroenterol 1988;23(Suppl 154):66–71.

387. Kellow JE, Phillips SF. Altered small bowel motility in irritable bowel syndrome is correlated with symptoms. Gastroenterology 1987;92:1885–1893.

388. Johnson SE. Clinical pharmacology of antiemetics and antidiarrheals. In: Proc Kal Kan Sym Treat Small Anim Dis, Columbus, Ohio, 1984;8:7–15.

389. Leib MS. Fiber-responsive large bowel diarrhea. In: Proc Annu Meet Am Coll Vet Intern Med 1990;9:817–819.

390. Dimski DS, Buffington CA. Dietary fiber in small animal therapeutics. J Am Vet Med Assoc 1991;199:1142–1146.

391. Cranston D, McWhinnie D, Collin J. Dietary fibre and gastrointestinal disease. Br J Surg 1988;75:508–512.

392. Eastwood MA. The physiological effect of dietary fiber: An update. Annu Rev Nutr 1992;12:19–35.

393. Bergman EN. Energy contributions of volatile fatty acids from the gastrointestinal tract in various species. Physiol Rev 1990;70:567–589.

394. Smalley JR, Klish WJ, Campbell MA, et al. Use of psyllium in the management of chronic nonspecific diarrhea of childhood. J Pediatr Gastroenterol Nutr 1982;1:361–363.

395. Kruth SA, Prescott JF, Welch MK, et al. Nosocomial diarrhea associated with enterotoxigenic *Clostridium perfringens* infection in dogs. J Am Vet Med Assoc 1989;195:331–334.

396. Niilo L. *Clostridium perfringens* in animal disease: A review of current knowledge. Can Vet J 1980;21:141–148.

397. Turk J, Fales W, Miller M, et al. Enteric *Clostridium perfringens* infection associated with parvoviral enteritis in dogs: 74 cases (1987–1990). J Am Vet Med Assoc 1992;200:991–994.

398. Seiler RJ. Colorectal polyps of the dog: A clinicopathologic study of 17 cases. J Am Vet Med Assoc 1979;174:72–75.

399. Palminteri A. The surgical management of polyps of the rectum and colon of the dog. J Am Vet Med Assoc 1966;148:771–777.

400. Atkins CE, Tyler R, Greenlee P. Clinical, biochemical, acid-base, and electrolyte abnormalities in cats after hypertonic sodium phosphate enema administration. Am J Vet Res 1985;46:980–988.

401. Bertoy RW. Megacolon. In: Bojrab MJ, ed. Disease Mechanisms in Small Animal Surgery. Philadelphia, Lea & Febiger, 1993:262–265.

402. McCallum RW. Cisapride: A new class of prokinetic agent. Am J Gastroenterol 1991;86:135–149.

403. Bertoy RW, MacCoy DM, Wheaton LG, et al. Total colectomy with ileorectal anastomosis in the cat. Vet Surg 1989;18:204–210.

404. Gregory CR, Guilford WG, Berry CR, et al. Enteric function in cats after subtotal colectomy for treatment of megacolon. Vet Surg 1990;19:216–220.

405. Niebauer GW. Rectoanal disease. In: Bojrab MJ, ed. Disease Mechanisms in Small Animal Surgery. Philadelphia, Lea & Febiger, 1993:271–284.

406. Wilson G, Hayes HM. Castration for treatment of perianal gland neoplasms in the dog. J Am Vet Med Assoc 1979;174:1301–1303.

407. Liska WD, Withrow SJ. Cryosurgical treatment of perianal gland adenomas in the dog. J Am Anim Hosp Assoc 1978;14:457–463.

408. Nielsen SW, Aftosmis J. Canine perianal gland tumors. J Am Vet Med Assoc 1964;144:127–135.

409. Hayes HM, Wilson GP. Hormone-responsive neoplasms of the canine perianal gland. Can Res 1977;37:2068–2071.

410. Vail DM, Withrow SJ, Schwarz PD, et al. Perianal adenocarcinoma in the canine male: A retrospective study of 41 cases. J Am Anim Hosp Assoc 1990;26:329–334.

411. Halnan CRE. The frequency of occurrence of anal sacculitis in the dog. J Small Anim Pract 1976;17:537–541.

412. Harvey CE. Incidence and distribution of anal sac disease in the dog. J Am Anim Hosp Assoc 1974;10:573–577.

413. van Duijkeren E. Disease conditions of canine anal sacs. J Small Anim Pract 1995;36:12–16.

414. Halnan CRE. The diagnosis of anal sacculitis in the dog. J Small Anim Pract 1976;17:527–535.

415. Washabau RJ, Brockman DJ. Recto-anal disease. In: Ettinger SJ, Feldman EC, eds. Textbook of Veterinary Internal Medicine. Philadelphia, WB Saunders, 1995:1398–1409.

416. Jones RL, Godinho KS, Palmer GH. Clinical observations on the use of oral amoxicillin/clavulanate in the treatment of gingivitis in dogs and cats and anal sacculitis in dogs. Br Vet J 1994;150:385–388.

417. Ross JT, Scavelli TD, Matthiesen DT, et al. Adenocarcinoma of the apocrine glands of the anal sac in dogs: A review of 32 cases. J Am Anim Hosp Assoc 1991;27:349–355.

418. Goldschmidt MH, Zoltowski C. Anal sac adenocarcinoma in the dog: 14 cases. J Small Anim Pract 1981;22:119–128.

419. Meuten DJ, Cooper BJ, Capen CC, et al. Hypercalcemia associated with an adenocarcinoma derived from the apocrine glands of the anal sac. Vet Pathol 1981;18:454–471.

420. Elkins AD, Hobson HP. Management of perianal fistulae: A retrospective study of 23 cases. Vet Surg 1982;11:110–114.

421. Goring RL, Bright RM, Stancil ML. Perianal fistulas in the dog: Retrospective evaluation of surgical treatment by deroofing and fulguration. Vet Surg 1986;15:392–398.

422. Killingsworth C, Walshaw R, Dunstan R, et al. Bacterial population and histologic changes in dogs with perianal fistula. Am J Vet Res 1988;49:1736–1741.

423. Vasseur PB. Results of surgical excision of perianal fistulas in dogs. J Am Vet Med Assoc 1984;185:60–62.

424. Van Ee RT, Palminteri A. Tail amputation for treatment of perianal fistulas in dogs. J Am Anim Hosp Assoc 1987;23:95–100.

425. Harvey CE. Perianal fistula in the dog. Vet Rec 1972;91:25–33.

426. Vasseur PB. Perianal fistulae in dogs: A retrospective analysis of surgical techniques. J Am Anim Hosp Assoc 1981;17:177–180.

427. van Ee RT. Perianal fistulas. In: Bojrab MJ, ed. Disease Mechanisms in Small Animal Surgery. Philadelphia, Lea & Febiger, 1993:285–286.

428. Budsberg S, Spurgeon T, Liggitt H. Anatomic predisposition to perianal fistulae formation in the German shepherd dog. Am J Vet Res 1985;46:1468–1472.

429. Ellison GW. Treatment of perianal fistulas in dogs. J Am Vet Med Assoc 1995;206:1680–1682.

430. Seim HB III. Diseases of the anus and rectum. In: Kirk RW, ed. Current Veterinary Therapy IX. Philadelphia, WB Saunders, 1986:916–921.

431. Breitschwerdt EB, Ochoa R, Barta M, et al. Clinical and laboratory characterization of basenjis with immuno-

proliferative small intestinal disease. Am J Vet Res 1984;45:267–273.

432. Hall EJ, Batt RM. Development of wheat-sensitive enteropathy in Irish setters: Morphologic changes. Am J Vet Res 1990;51:978–982.

433. Hall EJ, Batt RM. Development of wheat-sensitive enteropathy in Irish setters: Biochemical changes. Am J Vet Res 1990;51:983–989.

434. Batt RM, Carter MW, McLean L. Wheat-sensitive enteropathy in Irish setter dogs: Possible age-related brush border abnormalities. Res Vet Sci 1985;39:80–83.

435. Johnson CA, Fulton RW, Henk WG, et al. Inoculation of neonatal gnotobiotic dogs with a canine rotavirus. Am J Vet Res 1983;44:1682–1686.

436. Johnson CA, Snider TG, Fulton RW, et al. Gross and light microscopic lesions in neonatal gnotobiotic dogs inoculated with a canine rotavirus. Am J Vet Res 1983;44:1687–1693.

437. Kapatkin AS, Mullen HS, Matthiesen DT, et al. Leiomyosarcoma in dogs: 44 cases (1983–1988). J Am Vet Med Assoc 1992;201:1077–1079.

438. MacDonald JM, Mullen HS, Moroff SD. Adenomatous polyps of the duodenum in cats: 18 cases (1985–1990). J Am Vet Med Assoc 1993;202:647–651.

439. Gorham JR, Foreyt WJ. Salmon poisoning disease. In: Greene CE, ed. Infectious Diseases of the Dog and Cat. Philadelphia, WB Saunders, 1990:397–403.

440. Fletcher WD. Advanced granulomatous colitis in a Siberian husky: A case report. Vet Med Sm Anim Clin 1978;73:1409.

441. Van Kruiningen HJ. Canine colitis comparable to regional enteritis and mucosal colitis of man. Gastroenterology 1972;62:1128–1142.

442. Strande A, Sommers SC, Petrak M. Regional enterocolitis in cocker spaniel dogs. Arch Pathol 1954;57:357–362.

443. Troy GC. Canine phycomycosis: A review of twenty-four cases. Calif Vet 1985;39:12–17.

444. Ader PL. Phycomycosis in fifteen dogs and two cats. J Am Vet Med Assoc 1979;174:1216–1222.

445. Ewing GO, Gomez JA. Canine ulcerative colitis. J Am Anim Hosp Assoc 1973;9:395–406.

446. Hall EJ, Rutgers HC, Scholes SFE, et al. Histiocytic ulcerative colitis in boxer dogs in the UK. J Small Anim Pract 1994;35:509–515.

447. Moore RW, Withrow SJ. Gastrointestinal hemorrhage and pancreatitis associated with intervertebral disk disease in the dog. J Am Vet Med Assoc 1982;180:1443–1447.

448. Toombs JP, Caywood DD, Lipowitz AJ, et al. Colonic perforation following neurosurgical procedures and corticosteroid therapy in four dogs. J Am Vet Med Assoc 1980;177:68–72.

449. Toombs JP, Collins LG, Graves GM, et al. Colonic perforation in corticosteroid-treated dogs. J Am Vet Med Assoc 1986;188:145–150.

450. Toombs JP, Kelley LC, Tyler DE. Corticosteroid-associated colonic perforation in dogs. In: Bojrab MJ, ed. Disease Mechanisms in Small Animal Surgery. Philadelphia, Lea & Febiger, 1993:266–270.

451. Gibbons LM, Jacobs DE, Pilkington JG. Strongyloides in British greyhounds. Vet Rec 1988;122:114.

452. Mansfield LS, Schad GA. Ivermectin treatment of naturally acquired and experimentally induced *Strongyloides stercoralis* infections in dogs. J Am Vet Med Assoc 1992;201:726–730.

453. El-Ahraf A, Tacal JV, Sobih M, et al. Prevalence of cryptosporidiosis in dogs and human beings in San Bernardino County, California. J Am Vet Med Assoc 1991;198:631–634.

454. Moore JA, Blagburn BL, Lindsay DS. Cryptosporidiosis in animals including humans. Compen Contin Educ Pract Vet 1988;10:275–287.

455. Kirkpatrick CE. Enteric protozoal infections. In: Greene CE, ed. Infectious Diseases of the Dog and Cat. Philadelphia, WB Saunders, 1990:804–814.

456. Burrows RB, Hunt GR. Intestinal protozoan infections in cats. J Am Vet Med Assoc 1970;157:2065–2067.

457. Burrows RB, Lillis WG. Intestinal protozoan infections in dogs. J Am Vet Med Assoc 1967;150:880–883.

458. Swatzwelder JC. Immunity to amebic infections in dogs. Am J Trop Med Hyg 1952;1:567–575.

459. Calvert CA. *Salmonella* infections in hospitalized dogs: Epizootiology, diagnosis, and prognosis. J Am Anim Hosp Assoc 1985;21:499–503.

460. Greene CE. Salmonellosis. In: Greene CE, ed. Infectious Diseases of the Dog and Cat. Philadelphia, WB Saunders, 1990:542–549.

461. Sherding RG, Burrows CF. Diarrhea. In: Anderson NV, ed. Veterinary Gastroenterology. Philadelphia, Lea & Febiger, 1992:399–477.

462. Strombeck D, Guilford WG. Small Animal Gastroenterology. Davis, California, Stonegate Publishing. 1990:320–337.

463. Willard MD, Sugarman B, Walker RD. Gastrointestinal zoonoses. Vet Clin North Am Small Anim Pract 1987;17:145–194.

464. Ikeda J, Hirsh D, Jang S, et al. Characteristics of *Salmonella* isolated from animals at a veterinary medical teaching hospital. Am J Vet Res 1986;47:232–235.

465. Uhaa I, Hird D, Hirsh D, et al. Case-control study of risk factors associated with nosocomial *Salmonella krefeld* infection in dogs. Am J Vet Res 1988;49:1501–1505.

466. Newton CM, Newell DG, Wood M, et al. *Campylobacter* infection in a closed dog breeding colony. Vet Rec 1988;123:152–154.

467. Nair GB, Sarkar RK, Chowdhury S, et al. *Campylobacter* infection in domestic dogs. Vet Rec 1985;116:237–238.

468. Macartney L, Al-Mashat RR, Taylor DJ, et al. Experimental infection of dogs with *Campylobacter jejuni*. Vet Rec 1988;122:245–249.

469. Boosinger TR, Dillon AR. *Campylobacter jejuni* infections in dogs and the effect of erythromycin and tetracycline therapy on fecal shedding. J Am Anim Hosp Assoc 1992;28:33–38.

470. Fox JG, Claps M, Beaucage CM. Chronic diarrhea associated with *Campylobacter jejuni* infection in cats. J Am Vet Med Assoc 1986;189:455–456.

471. Fox JG, Krakowka S, Taylor NS. Acute-onset *Campylobacter*-associated gastroenteritis in adult beagles. J Am Vet Med Assoc 1985;187:1268–1271.

472. Olson P, Sandstedt K. *Campylobacter* in the dog:

A clinical and experimental study. Vet Rec 1987;121: 99–101.

473. Junttila J, Schildt R, Myllys V, et al. *Campylobacter* associated epidemic in cats. Comp Anim Pract 1987;1: 16–18.

474. Fox JG. Campylobacteriosis. In: Greene CE, ed. Infectious Diseases of the Dog and Cat. Philadelphia, WB Saunders, 1990:538–542.

475. Davenport DJ. *Campylobacter* enteritis. In: Kirk RW, ed. Current Veterinary Therapy X. Philadelphia, WB Saunders, 1989:944–947.

476. Monfort JD, Donahoe JP, Stills HF, et al. Efficacies of erythromycin and chloramphenicol in extinguishing fecal shedding of *Campylobacter jejuni* in dogs. J Am Vet Med Assoc 1990;196:1069–1072.

477. Fantasia M, Mingrone MG, Martini A, et al. Characterisation of *Yersinia* species isolated from a kennel and from cattle and pig farms. Vet Rec 1993;132:532–534.

478. Greene CE. Yersiniosis. In: Greene CE, ed. Infectious Diseases of the Dog and Cat. Philadelphia, WB Saunders, 1990:551.

479. Greene CE. Gastrointestinal and intra-abdominal infections. In: Greene CE, ed. Infectious Diseases of the Dog and Cat. Philadelphia, WB Saunders, 1990:125–145.

480. Olson P, Hedhammar A, Faris A, et al. Enterotoxigenic *Escherichia coli* (ETEC) and *Klebsiella* pneumoniae isolated from dogs with diarrhoea. Vet Microbiol 1985;10: 577–589.

481. Pospischil A, Mainil JG, Baljer G, et al. Attaching and effacing bacteria in the intestines of calves and cats with diarrhea. Vet Pathol 1987;24:330–334.

482. Abaas S, Franklin A, Kuhn I, et al. Cytotoxin activity on Vero cells among *Escherichia coli* strains associated with diarrhea in cats. Am J Vet Res 1989;50:1294–1296.

483. Berry AP, Levett PN. Chronic diarrhoea in dogs associated with *Clostridium difficile* infection. Vet Rec 1986; 118:102–103.

484. Slaughter J, Billups LH, Acor GK. Canine heterobilharziasis. Compen Contin Educ Pract Vet 1988;10:606–612.

485. Tyler DE. Prototheosis. In: Greene CE, ed. Infectious Diseases of the Dog and Cat. Philadelphia, WB Saunders, 1990:742–748.

Chapter 33

Diseases of the Exocrine Pancreas

Michael S. Leib

Anatomy

The pancreas of the dog and cat is a pinkish-gray, lobulated gland that consists of right and left lobes joined by a small central body. It is located in the right cranial portion of the abdomen.[1] The right lobe lies close to the stomach; the body and left lobe lie along the descending duodenum.[2] In dogs, two pancreatic ducts drain secretions into the duodenum. The pancreatic duct enters the duodenum at the major duodenal papilla, in close proximity to the bile duct. Most secretions pass through the accessory duct, which enters the duodenum at the minor duodenal papilla (several centimeters distal to the major papilla).[1] In some dogs, only the accessory duct is present. In most cats, only one duct carries secretions to the duodenum. The pancreatic duct joins the common bile duct before it enters the major duodenal papilla. A small percentage of cats retain both ducts.[2]

Microscopically, the pancreas is arranged in lobules that contain tubuloacinar glands. A single row of acinar cells forms a cluster around a ductule and forms a unit called an acinus. Acinar cells synthesize and store enzymes. Scattered among the acinar tissue are the islets of Langerhans, which secrete insulin and glucagon (see Chap. 48).

Physiology

The major function of the exocrine pancreas is to secrete a fluid rich in digestive enzymes and bicarbonate to aid digestion of proteins, fats, and carbohydrates within the small intestine.[3] Acinar cells synthesize and store, in vesicles called zymogen granules, at least 19 digestive enzymes.[4, 5] When the acinar cell is stimulated, the granules fuse with the cell membrane, and their contents enters the ductal system, eventually reaching the duodenum. The cells lining the ducts produce a watery secretion rich in bicarbonate.

Cholecystokinin (CCK) is the primary hormonal stimulus for acinar cells, and secretin is the primary hormonal stimulus for the ductal cells.[4] Acinar and ductal cells have receptors for both of these hormones and for acetylcholine. Maximal stimulation occurs when all three receptors are occupied. Pancreatic stimulation occurs in three stages. The cephalic stage is stimulated by the sight, smell, and anticipation of food and is mediated by the vagus nerve and acetylcholine release. The gastric stage is stimulated by gastric distention and is also mediated by vagal reflexes. These preliminary stages begin pancreatic stimulation in anticipation of an arriving meal. The most intense phase is the intestinal stage, which is initiated by the arrival of food in the duodenum.[4] Duodenal distention activates vagal reflexes that release acetylcholine within the pancreas. Peptides and fats within the duodenum stimulate the release of CCK, and gastric acid stimulates the release of secretin. Both of these hormones are synthesized and stored within endocrine cells in the duodenal mucosa. These hormones circulate through blood to the pancreas and stimulate the release of digestive enzymes and bicarbonate. As the nutrients are absorbed and the acid neutralized, the stimulus for secretion ends.

There are many safeguards to prevent damage from occurring within the pancreas from these digestive enzymes.[3] Many are synthesized as inactive proenzymes.[5] Under normal conditions, they are activated within the lumen of the duodenum. Enterokinase is contained within the duodenal brush border. It activates the proteolytic enzyme trypsin by converting the inactive proenzyme trypsinogen to trypsin.[5] Active trypsin then converts many of the other proenzymes into their active forms (chymotrypsin, elastase, carboxypeptidase A and B, colipase, and phospholipase). Some enzymes are not stored as proenzymes but require a cofactor that is present in the duodenum for full activity. Lipase requires colipase to function. Procolipase is secreted as a zymogen and is activated to colipase in the duodenum by trypsin.[5] Other enzymes that require cofactors include amylase (chloride and calcium), ribonuclease (phosphate or citrate), and deoxyribonuclease (divalent ions).[5] Another safeguard is the storage of enzymes, especially lysosomal enzymes, within granules that segregate them from the rest of the cell. Finally, a pancreatic secretory trypsin inhibitor is present to bind any trypsin that becomes prematurely activated.[5] If active trypsin reaches the circulation, several protease inhibitors are present to bind it. α_1-Protease inhibitor transiently binds proteases in the serum and transfers them to one of the two α-macroglobulins that irreversibly bind the protease.[3] The complex is removed by the monocyte-macrophage system.[3] It is the depletion of the macroglobulins that is associated with the intensification of systemic signs, and often death, in patients with severe pancreatitis.

Problem Identification

Acute Vomiting

The differential diagnosis for animals with acute vomiting is extensive (see Chap. 31). Acute pancreatitis can cause both self-limited and life-threatening vomiting. Signs that should increase the index of suspicion that the vomiting is caused by acute pancreatitis include signalment (middle-aged female dog), abdominal pain in the right anterior quadrant, pyrexia, leukocytosis with a left shift, and increased serum amylase and lipase (elevated at least three to five times normal). Abdominal ultrasound can be very helpful in establishing a diagnosis.

Chronic Diarrhea

The differential diagnosis for animals with chronic diarrhea is extensive (see Chap. 32). Pancreatic exocrine insufficiency results in severe diarrhea and weight loss and is associated with polyphagia. Pancreatic exocrine insufficiency should be considered a possible diagnosis in young dogs, especially German shepherds, with severe weight loss or failure to thrive and signs of small bowel diarrhea and that do not have gastrointestinal parasites. The characteristics of the stool include an increased frequency (three to eight times per day) and increased quantity of feces per defecation. Diagnosis is based on demonstration of reduced serum trypsin-like immunoreactivity (STLI).

Weight Loss Despite Polyphagia

Weight loss accompanies many diseases. However, weight loss associated with polyphagia is less common (see Chap. 47). A differential diagnosis includes hyperthyroidism, severe gastrointestinal parasites, exocrine pancreatic insufficiency, diabetes mellitus, and starvation. Exocrine pancreatic insufficiency should be suspected in young dogs, especially German shepherds, with severe weight loss and signs of small bowel diarrhea and that do not have gastrointestinal parasites. Diagnosis is based on demonstration of reduced STLI.

Abdominal Pain

Abdominal pain is not a specific sign and can be caused by disease of any of the abdominal viscera, of the parietal peritoneum, or of the abdominal wall.[6] In addition, referred pain from extra-abdominal disorders (e.g., intervertebral disc disease, myositis, discospondylitis) can also mimic abdominal pain.

Animals with acute and severe abdominal pain are said to have an acute abdomen. Many of these patients have disorders that require immediate surgical intervention. Performing unnecessary surgery in a critically ill patient can be detrimental, although delaying surgery in a patient that needs it can be disastrous.[7] The decision to perform surgery can be very difficult to make.

Pathophysiology

The specific causes of abdominal pain vary, although pain is generally associated with distention of a hollow viscus, stretching of an organ's capsule, ischemia, inflammation, or traction on the mesentery or omentum.[6] Visceral pain fibers are located within abdominal organs and connect to the sympathetic chain and the spinal cord. This overlapping and multisegmental arrangement leads to poorly localized and dull pain sensation.[6] Somatic pain fibers originate within the parietal peritoneum. Impulses are transmitted to the thoracolumbar spinal cord, producing a sharper and more localized pain sensation.[6]

Clinical Signs

Besides abdominal pain, other clinical signs relate to the cause of the acute abdomen. Common signs include vomiting, diarrhea, abdominal distention, pyrexia, anorexia, lethargy, dehydration, and shock.[6] A history or external signs of recent trauma may be evident. Urethral obstruction causes pollakiuria, stranguria, hematuria, anuria, or oliguria. Peritonitis caused by leakage of gastric or intestinal contents, bile, or urine, pancreatitis, or intra-abdominal hemorrhage results in abdominal distention and fluid accumulation within the abdomen that may be ballotted. Dilated loops of bowel can be palpated in cases of intestinal obstruction. A mass may be palpated in cases of splenic neoplasia, splenic torsion, uterine torsion or rupture, or intra-abdominal neoplasia. The kidneys may be enlarged in acute pyelonephritis. Rectal examination may detect a prostatic abscess. Obstipated animals have a feces-filled colon.

Different animals manifest abdominal pain very differently. Reluctance to move and reduced appetite are often the initial signs. The animal may grunt, whine, or cry. It may attempt to bite or scratch when picked up or examined, behavior that is atypical for the individual. Dogs may demonstrate a position of relief in which the forelimbs are outstretched, the sternum is on the floor, and the hind limbs are raised.[3, 8] The animal may tense the abdominal musculature, making palpation difficult or impossible.

Diagnostic Plan

The differential diagnosis for abdominal pain is extensive (Table 33–1).[6, 7, 9–11] Only with a thorough knowledge of the differential diagnosis, careful consideration of the signalment and history, a thorough physical examination, and evaluation of diagnostic procedures with rapid turnaround times can appropriate decisions be made about the necessity of immediate surgical intervention and initiation of other life-saving therapy. Gastrointestinal diseases should be considered as possible causes of abdominal pain if vomiting, diarrhea, or constipation is a prominent clinical sign.

Animals with mild pain can be observed for 12 to 24 hours and evaluated further if pain persists or worsens. The initial diagnostic plan in those with moderate or severe pain should include a complete blood count, biochemical profile, urinalysis, fecal

Table 33–1
Differential Diagnosis for Abdominal Pain

Gastrointestinal
Acute gastritis or enteritis
Gastric dilatation or volvulus
Gastric or duodenal ulcer
Pyloric foreign body
Intestinal obstruction
  Foreign body
  Intussusception
  Neoplasia
Parvovirus
Peritonitis
  Penetrating gastrointestinal foreign body
  Perforating gastric or duodenal ulcer
  Ruptured gastric or intestinal neoplasia
  Linear foreign body
  Pancreatitis
  Ruptured stomach caused by gastric dilatation or volvulus
  Gastrointestinal surgical site dehiscence
  Biliary tract rupture
Acute hepatitis
Hemorrhagic gastroenteritis
Whipworms
Irritable bowel syndrome
Obstipation or megacolon
Trauma to liver or bowel
Hernia with incarcerated bowel

Urinary
Acute pyelonephritis
Urethral obstruction
Trauma
Ruptured bladder or ureter

Genital
Pyometra
Ruptured uterus
Acute prostatitis
Prostatic abscess

Splenic
Trauma
Ruptured neoplasia
Torsion

examination, and survey abdominal radiographs. Abdominal ultrasound can be helpful.[12] If fluid is detected on abdominal palpation or ultrasound, or if signs of increased intra-abdominal density, loss of serosal surface visualization, or free intra-abdominal gas are seen on radiographs, abdominocentesis should be performed (see Chap. 34). Abdominal radiographs may also show signs of intestinal obstruction, gastric distention, an abdominal mass, organomegaly, a gastrointestinal foreign body, or urinary calculi. Ultrasound may identify abdominal fluid, stomach or intestinal wall thickening, lymphadenopathy, biliary obstruction, urinary calculi, intestinal obstruction, organomegaly, or an intra-abdominal mass.[12]

If laboratory results will be delayed, a packed cell volume, total solids, and reagent strips for blood urea nitrogen and glucose should be collected.[6] Other tests are indicated to evaluate specific problems that have been identified—for example, endoscopic examination of the stomach in cases of pyloric foreign body, contrast urethrogram in animals with urinary obstruction or suspected ruptured bladder, abdominal ultrasound in suspected pancreatitis, enzyme-linked immunosorbent assay (ELISA) for parvovirus in puppies with acute diarrhea, and complete neurologic examination in cases with potential intervertebral disc disease.

Diagnostic peritoneal lavage can be performed if radiographic or ultrasonographic signs of peritonitis or intra-abdominal fluid exist but abdominocentesis fails to retrieve a sample or in cases of penetrating abdominal wounds.[6, 7, 13, 14] It is a sensitive test to determine which animals require immediate surgical intervention.[7] Local anesthesia is used, and a long, 14-gauge intravenous catheter (to which additional very small holes are added) is placed within the abdomen, 1 to 2 cm caudal to the umbilicus. Warm saline (22 mL/kg) is infused into the abdomen. The animal is rocked back and forth, and the fluid is aspirated and evaluated cytologically. Degenerate neutrophils, bacteria, vegetable fibers, or more than 1000 leukocytes indicate that septic peritonitis is present, and immediate surgical exploration is indicated.[6, 7] Retrieval of bloody fluid indicates intra-abdominal hemorrhage. Fluid can also be evaluated for creatinine (urinary tract rupture), bilirubin (biliary tract rupture), or amylase (pancreatitis).[7]

In some cases, diagnosis can be reached only with an exploratory laparotomy. The decision to perform surgery for diagnosis (as well as definitive treatment for many of the diseases listed in Table 33–1) is based on test results and on the severity and progression of clinical signs.

Diagnostic Procedures

Routine Laboratory Evaluation

A complete blood count, biochemical profile, and urinalysis do not lead to a definitive diagnosis of pancreatic diseases but can supply information supportive of a diagnosis, screen for concurrent diseases, and help evaluate the risk if general anesthesia becomes necessary for diagnostic procedures. Animals with pancreatitis can have a leukocytosis with a left shift; elevated hematocrit and total protein; prerenal azotemia (dehydration); elevated alanine aminotransferase (ALT) and alkaline phosphatase (AP);

hyperbilirubinemia; hyperglycemia; hypercholesterolemia; hypocalcemia; and hypokalemia, hyponatremia, and hypochloremia (vomiting and diarrhea). Urine is often concentrated (dehydration), and bilirubinuria and glucosuria may be present. Anemia and hypoglycemia can occur in cats with pancreatitis. Hypoalbuminemia and hypoproteinemia can be seen in some dogs with pancreatic exocrine insufficiency caused by severe malnutrition.

Pancreatic Enzymes

Evaluation of serum amylase, lipase, and STLI can be very helpful in the diagnosis of pancreatic diseases. These enzymes leak from normal tissues and are present in the blood in low concentrations. Larger quantities leak from an inflamed pancreas or other organs. Increased serum levels of these enzymes should occur in cases of pancreatitis. Normal values vary, and a specific reference range should be available from the laboratory performing the assay.

Amylase is actually made up of a group of amylolytic isoenzymes that hydrolyze glycoside linkages in monosaccharides and disaccharides in the small intestine. Although contained in large quantities in the pancreas, these isoenzymes can also be found in many other body tissues, especially within the small intestine.[15] Because amylase is excreted by the kidneys, azotemia also causes hyperamylasemia.[16] Many vomiting animals without pancreatitis are dehydrated, and mild to moderate hyperamylasemia is often present, complicating diagnosis. Renal failure may result in values up to four times higher than normal ranges.[17] Hyperamylasemia is therefore not specific for pancreatitis, and normal serum amylase does not eliminate it.[3, 18] In fact, the sensitivity and specificity of hyperamylasemia in dogs with pancreatitis are less than 80%.[19] The magnitude of serum elevation is not proportional to the severity of pancreatitis. Hyperamylasemia is found inconsistently in cats with pancreatitis.[20, 21]

Lipase is a lipolytic enzyme. Although previously thought to be pancreas specific, it has been identified in the stomach.[22] Although hyperlipasemia may be a better determinant of pancreatitis than hyperamylasemia, it should always be evaluated in view of amylase levels and other clinical factors (see Pancreatitis). The magnitude of serum elevation is not proportional to the severity of pancreatitis. Administration of dexamethasone and prednisone can increase serum lipase without causing pancreatitis.[23, 24] Lipase can also increase threefold after exploratory laparotomy.[25] Because it is also excreted by the kidneys, azotemia from any cause can lead to increased serum levels of lipase. Serum lipase is increased up to fourfold in renal failure.[17] Hyperlipasemia is inconsistently found in cats with pancreatitis.[20, 21]

For the most accurate results in diagnosing pancreatitis, serum amylase concentration should always be determined in concert with serum lipase levels. A diagnosis of pancreatitis should not be made based on amylase or lipase values alone but on many other clinical factors as well (see Pancreatitis).

STLI is a measurement of trypsinogen that leaks from the pancreas. A small amount leaks into serum from the normal pancreas. It is a pancreas-specific marker.[26–28] It greatest utility is in the diagnosis of pancreatic exocrine insufficiency, in which low serum levels are consistently measured. Recently, an assay for cats has been developed.[29]

Because it is pancreas specific, STLI has been evaluated as a test for pancreatitis. In experimental studies, it was found to increase before serum amylase and lipase did.[30] However, its utility in clinical cases has not yet been established. Azotemia can also cause increases in the serum concentration.[26]

Radiography

Survey abdominal radiographs rarely provide help in diagnosing pancreatitis but may demonstrate a mass in patients with advanced pancreatic cancer (Fig. 33–1). Radiographs are normal in cases of pancreatic exocrine insufficiency but can help exclude the presence of other conditions that can cause chronic diarrhea (e.g., small bowel obstruction from foreign body, intussusception, neoplasia).

Radiographic signs of acute pancreatitis are nonspecific but may help to rule out the presence of a foreign body or intestinal obstruction, which can also cause vomiting. Radiographic findings of pancreatitis include signs of duodenal ileus (displaced to the right, fixed in position on multiple views, widened angle between the pylorus and duodenum), localized peritonitis (increased density in the anterior right quadrant and decreased serosal surface visualization), increased density caused by saponification of fat, and displacement of the stomach to the right or of the transverse colon caudally.[3, 5, 31–37]

Ultrasonography

Abdominal ultrasonography can be very helpful in establishing a diagnosis of pancreatitis or identifying pancreatic cancer. Ultrasound-guided biopsy can be used to definitively diagnose a mass as adenocarcinoma. Imaging of the pancreas is difficult and requires skill and experience. Changes that can be found in cases of pancreatitis include a pancreatic mass, a hypoechoic pancreas, abscesses and cysts, and increased echodensity associated with fibrosis (Fig. 33–2).[3, 32, 35, 38] Positive findings are very reliable, but a normal abdominal ultrasound study does not rule out pancreatitis. In the future, ultrasound may

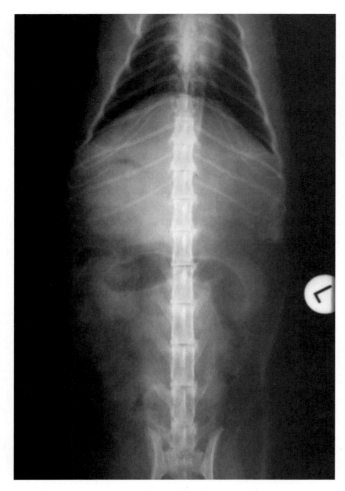

Figure 33-1
Ventrodorsal radiograph of a 6-year-old domestic shorthair cat showing a right cranial abdominal soft tissue mass, which was shown to be a 3 × 6 cm pancreatic adenocarcinoma. The mass caused biliary obstruction and icterus. The mass was palpable on physical examination.

prove to be very beneficial in helping to accurately diagnose pancreatitis in cats.

Common Diseases of the Exocrine Pancreas

Acute Pancreatitis in Dogs

Acute pancreatitis is a common cause of vomiting and abdominal pain in dogs. Although it can occur in dogs of any signalment, middle-aged obese females may be predisposed.[1, 3, 21, 32, 34, 36, 37, 39, 40] Acute pancreatitis is difficult to diagnose. Most patients respond favorably to treatment, but some severely affected dogs die despite intensive therapy.

Pathophysiology

The cause of acute pancreatitis in most cases remains unknown.[32] Risk factors include obesity, high-fat diets, hyperlipidemia, drugs (e.g., corticosteroids, chlorpromazine, furosemide, azathioprine, L-asparaginase, sulfonamides, tetracycline, thiazide diuretics), toxins (e.g., anticholinesterase insecticides), hypercalcemia, duct obstruction, duodenal reflux, pancreatic trauma, and pancreatic ischemia.[1, 3, 5, 32, 35, 41, 42]

Pathologically, two forms of acute pancreatitis are recognized.[32, 34] The mild, edematous form is often associated with a mild course of illness and rapid recovery. It is characterized by interstitial edema and a mild inflammatory exudate consisting of neutrophils or lymphocytes. Acinar tissues and ducts remain intact.[34] The hemorrhagic necrotic form is usually associated with severe and prolonged clinical signs (Fig. 33-3). Grossly, the pancreas contains hemorrhages, has soft necrotic areas, and may be attached to adjacent organs by fibrous adhesions.[3, 21, 35, 37, 43] Hemorrhages may be present within the omentum, and chalky areas of fat necrosis are present adjacent to the pancreas and throughout the abdomen.[34] A hemorrhagic peritoneal effusion may be present. Microscopically, edema, hyperemia, necrosis, and leukocyte infiltration are seen.[37] Many animals with this form of pancreatitis die despite vigorous therapy. The factors that control progression from one form to another are not known but may relate to the integrity of pancreatic circulation.

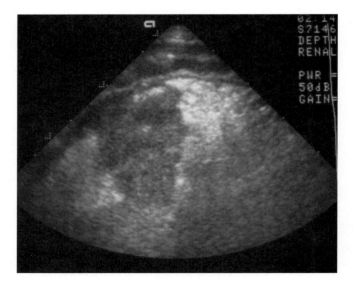

Figure 33-2
Ultrasonographic appearance of pancreatitis in a 6-year-old miniature schnauzer. The duodenum is on top of the photograph. The large hypoechoic area is the inflamed pancreas. The hyperechoic areas surrounding the pancreas are inflamed or necrotic fat. (Courtesy of Martha L. Moon, DVM, MS, Blacksburg, Virginia.)

The pathogenesis of acute pancreatitis is complex. If defense mechanisms intended to prevent pancreatic autodigestion fail, enzymes are activated within the pancreas, and a self-perpetuating autodigestive process ensues.[44] Potent digestive enzymes are released into the parenchyma of the pancreas, the blood vessels, and the adjacent abdominal cavity. This causes severe localized inflammation and hemodynamic alterations and can occasionally trigger disseminated intravascular coagulation (DIC), acute renal failure, or respiratory distress syndrome. Depletion of circulating and tissue antiproteases occurs and is followed by an intensification of the systemic signs.[45] Vascular collapse results from a combination of fluid loss from vomiting and diarrhea, release of vasoactive substances, release of cardiodepressant substances, fluid sequestration within the abdominal cavity, and blood loss from DIC.[1]

The cause of trypsin activation remains speculative, but activation appears to occur intracellularly and may involve a disturbance in cellular metabolism or increase in the permeability of lipoprotein membranes that results in fusion of zymogen granules with lysosomes.[35] Complement activation may alter membrane permeability.[5, 44] Trypsinogen is converted to trypsin, and, after saturating the pancreatic secretory trypsin inhibitors, it activates the other zymogens.[1, 5, 44] Elastase and phospholipase further pancreatic damage and increase the severity of the inflammation.[35] Consumption of serum antiproteases leads to intensification of the systemic signs by activation of the kinin, coagulation, fibrinolytic, and complement cascades, resulting in vascular collapse

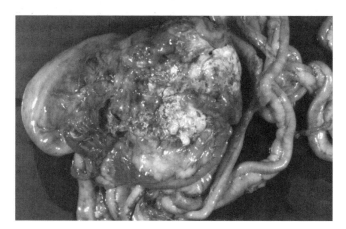

Figure 33–3
Necropsy appearance of severe pancreatitis in a 7-year-old miniature schnauzer. The pancreas, omentum, duodenum, and colon are adherent with extensive necrosis and fibrin deposition. The pancreas is obliterated. Disseminated intravascular coagulation was present. (Courtesy of Geoff Saunders, DVM, MS, Blacksburg, Virginia.)

and DIC.[1, 3, 5, 34, 35, 41, 45] Reperfusion injury is also believed to play a role in the pathophysiology.[44]

Abdominal pain is the result of the inflamed pancreas, chemical or septic peritonitis, or inflammation of the stomach, intestines, or liver.[1] Elevations in serum ALT and AP are caused by hepatic ischemia, exposure of the liver to toxic and inflammatory portal venous drainage of the pancreas, or posthepatic biliary obstruction of the common bile duct as it passes near the pancreas on its way to the duodenum.[35] Obstructions occur because of fibrous tissue within the inflamed pancreas.[46, 47] A transient and mild diabetes mellitus can develop as a result of pancreatic inflammation. Hyperglycemia is also fostered by hyperglucagonemia and release of stress hormones such as cortisol and catecholamines.[3, 5, 21, 35] The cause of hypocalcemia is unknown. Clinical signs attributed to hypocalcemia do not usually occur.[35] Potential causes include saponification of intra-abdominal fat, altered response to parathormone, delayed release or increased destruction of parathormone, increased calcitonin secretion, hyperglucagonemia, hypomagnesemia, and formation of free fatty acid–calcium complexes.[32]

Clinical Signs

The most common clinical sign associated with acute pancreatitis is vomiting.[1, 34, 36, 37, 48] The severity varies greatly; some patients develop only mild vomiting that is self-limited, similar to cases of dietary indiscretion, whereas others have vomiting that is life-threatening. Other clinical signs include depression, anorexia, abdominal pain, which may be localized to the right cranial quadrant, pyrexia, and diarrhea.[1, 3, 32, 34–37, 40, 43, 49] Dehydration may be undetectable or very severe. Signs include dry mucous membranes, loss of skin turgor, prolonged capillary refill time, and enophthalmos; if hypovolemic shock develops, tachycardia and weak peripheral pulses are also observed.[1]

Historically, clinical signs may be associated with recent ingestion of a high-fat meal or administration of a medication associated with acute pancreatitis, such as corticosteroids (see Pathophysiology).[3, 34] Some patients with acute pancreatitis develop icterus as a result of posthepatic biliary obstruction, often 5 to 8 days after initial presentation.[34, 46, 47]

Diagnostic Plan

It is difficult to definitively diagnose cases of acute pancreatitis, and misdiagnosis is common.[32] Because the therapy for many other causes of acute vomiting is similar to that used in cases of acute pancreatitis, misdiagnosis of acute pancreatitis as another disorder often does not have consequences.

However, an incorrect diagnosis of acute pancreatitis may lead to failure to perform additional diagnostic tests or institute specific therapy for another condition. If this occurs in a patient with gastric or duodenal ulcer disease, foreign body intestinal obstruction, or intussusception, there can be dramatic consequences.

Patients with acute pancreatitis often have inconsistent laboratory parameters. Diagnosis should be based not on any single test but on assessment of all tests, the history, and the physical examination. Common findings include leukocytosis with a left shift; elevated hematocrit and total protein; prerenal azotemia (caused by dehydration); elevated ALT, AP, amylase, and lipase; and hyperglycemia.[1, 3, 5, 21, 32, 34, 35, 40, 43, 49–51] Although elevated amylase and lipase are considered by many practitioners to be pathognomonic for acute pancreatitis, they are not. Both enzymes are present in other body tissues, and serum levels can be normal in cases of acute pancreatitis at the time of diagnosis if the inflamed pancreas is depleted of stored enzymes.[3, 5, 15, 21, 22, 50] STLI is also increased, and in experimental acute pancreatitis it rises before amylase and lipase levels do.[3, 30, 35] Electrolyte changes are associated with vomiting and diarrhea and include hypokalemia, hyponatremia, and hypochloremia.[21] Anemia, hypercholesterolemia, hyperlipidemia, and hypocalcemia occur less frequently.[5, 21, 35] Hyperbilirubinemia, bilirubinuria, and extreme elevations in serum ALT and AP occur in patients that develop biliary obstruction.[5] If DIC develops (see Chap. 44), thrombocytopenia, prolongation of prothrombin and partial thromboplastin times, and elaboration of fibrin degradation products occur.[50, 52]

Radiographic signs of acute pancreatitis are nonspecific and seldom confirm a diagnosis, but they may help to eliminate the presence of a foreign body or intestinal obstruction. Radiographic findings include signs of duodenal ileus (e.g., displaced to the right, fixed in position on multiple views, widened angle between the pylorus and duodenum), localized peritonitis (e.g., increased density in the anterior right quadrant, decreased serosal surface visualization), increased density because of saponification of fat, or displacement of the stomach to the right or of the transverse colon caudally.[3, 5, 31–37] Ultrasonographic evaluation can be very helpful in establishing a diagnosis and may identify a pancreatic mass, a hypoechoic pancreas, abscesses and cysts, or increased echodensity associated with fibrosis (see Fig. 33–2).[3, 32, 35, 38]

Although many other tests (phospholipase A, serum amylase isoenzymes, serum methemalbumin, serum antiproteases, trypsin complexed with antiproteases, serum pancreatic polypeptide, and clearance of amylase and creatinine) have been evaluated, none has proved to be practical, convenient, or consistent enough to aid the clinician.[3, 5, 15, 19, 32, 37, 44, 45, 52, 53] Recently, measurement of serum or urine trypsinogen activation peptide has demonstrated promise as a diagnostic aid.[3, 35]

The gold standard for diagnosis is histopathologic evaluation of tissue samples. Because samples cannot be retrieved noninvasively, biopsy is used only if the diagnosis remains unclear and other intraabdominal disorders that require surgical therapy may be present. Biopsy can also confirm a diagnosis if a patient tentatively diagnosed as having acute pancreatitis does not respond to therapy or has an expanding pancreatic mass, abscess, or cyst identified with ultrasonography.

Because the diagnosis is so difficult to make, a thorough evaluation of other causes of acute vomiting (see Chap. 31) should always be performed. In addition, I use a series of six major diagnostic criteria to help establish a diagnosis. The index of suspicion is higher for acute pancreatitis the more criteria are present. However, patients with most of these criteria may not have acute pancreatitis, and those with few or none of them can have it. The major criteria are acute vomiting, cranial abdominal pain, pyrexia, leukocytosis with a left shift, elevated serum amylase and lipase, and ultrasonographic findings of a hypoechoic pancreas. Clearly present ultrasonographic findings are very supportive of a diagnosis of acute pancreatitis, but negative findings do not eliminate it. Amylase and lipase values must be elevated at least three to five times above normal to be suggestive of acute pancreatitis, but this is not as strong a criterion as ultrasonographic findings.[17, 35, 50]

Treatment

The objectives of therapy are to prevent pancreatic secretion and manage hypovolemia, thus supporting pancreatic circulation.[1, 3, 5, 35, 40, 44] If drug-induced acute pancreatitis is suspected, the offending agent should immediately be discontinued.[3, 35] The dog should be maintained on nothing by mouth, and fluid therapy should be administered.

If vomiting is mild and dehydration minimal, the withholding of food and water for 12 to 24 hours, administration of fluids subcutaneously, and slow introduction of water and a highly digestible, low-fat diet may be all that is necessary (see Chap. 31 on treatment of acute, self-limited gastritis).[34] Patients with more severe signs require a longer period on nothing by mouth and must receive intravenous fluid therapy (see Chap. 31 on treatment of acute, life-threatening gastritis).[1, 3, 34] Lactated Ringer's solution is an appropriate fluid to use at a volume necessary to correct dehydration, to provide maintenance (44–66 mL/kg per day), and to replace losses from vomiting and diarrhea. Potassium supplementation, initially at 20 mEq/L KCl, is necessary to replace losses in diarrhea, vomitus, and urine and to supplement the lack of food intake.[3, 35] Potassium supplementation should be based on assessment of serum potassium levels (Table 31–7). Antibiotic therapy is usually administered and may help to prevent secondary infection of the inflamed pancreas.[1, 34, 35] Commonly used antibiotics include ampicillin (22 mg/kg, three [t.i.d.] or four [q.i.d.] times per day, either intravenously, intramuscularly, or subcutaneously) or enrofloxacin (2.5–5 mg/kg b.i.d. intramuscularly). Plasma transfusion has been recommended for severely affected patients to provide a fresh source of protease inhibitors and to supply albumin, which helps to maintain blood volume and support pancreatic circulation.[3, 34, 35, 44]

Treatment should continue until the parameters used to make the diagnosis of acute pancreatitis return toward normal and vomiting has stopped for 24 to 48 hours.[1, 5] A biochemical profile should be repeated every 1 or 2 days, depending on the severity of clinical signs. Most severely affected patients require 3 to 5 days of fluid therapy, although some require much longer treatment. These very severely affected patients may need referral and institution of total parenteral nutrition if vomiting continues for more than 7 days.

After vomiting stops, gradual oral alimentation can be initiated.[1, 3, 5, 35, 40] Ice cubes or small amounts of water are offered frequently. If vomiting does not occur, small amounts of a highly digestible, low-fat diet are offered frequently (see Chap. 31). A low-fat diet and control of obesity have been recommended to prevent relapse.[1, 3, 40]

If vomiting is severe, antiemetics can be used (see Chap. 31). Chlorpromazine (0.5 mg/kg every 4–6 hours intramuscularly or subcutaneously) or metoclopramide (0.2–0.4 mg/kg every 8 hours intramuscularly or subcutaneously) can be used. Because phenothiazines cause vasodilation, they cannot be started until the dog has been rehydrated. Metoclopramide is contraindicated if gastrointestinal obstruction is present, so this possibility must be eliminated before it is used.

If severe abdominal pain persists, analgesic therapy may be necessary.[3] Meperidine (5–10 mg/kg b.i.d. or t.i.d. intramuscularly or subcutaneously) has been recommended.[1, 34] Morphine should be avoided because it may induce pancreatic duct spasm and contribute to the pathogenesis of acute pancreatitis. The effects of buprenorphine on the pancreatic duct are unknown, but I have used it at 5 to 15 µg/kg intramuscularly or subcutaneously every 4 to 12 hours in several cases.

Surgical intervention remains controversial, and firm guidelines do not exist to appropriately guide surgical intervention.[3, 32, 34] Patients that are not responding to therapy and those that have an expanding mass (demonstrable by palpation, radiography, or ultrasonography) should undergo exploratory surgery with the intent of draining and lavaging the abdomen, removing necrotic tissue, and draining abscesses or cysts.[5, 34, 54, 55] Most patients with acute pancreatitis do not require surgery.[32] Those with posthepatic biliary obstruction rarely need surgical intervention, because the obstruction usually resolves spontaneously.

Prognosis

The prognosis for patients with acute pancreatitis is highly variable.[1, 3, 35] Mildly affected dogs with edematous acute pancreatitis respond to minimal therapy. Life-threatening cases of hemorrhagic necrotic acute pancreatitis warrant a guarded prognosis. Response to therapy in 3 to 5 days is a favorable prognostic sign. Dogs requiring intensive therapy for longer than 7 days carry a more guarded prognosis. Extrapancreatic manifestations such as DIC, acute renal failure, or respiratory distress syndrome are associated with a much poorer prognosis.[32] Because the cause is unclear, recurrent episodes can occur. Destruction of the pancreas can result in pancreatic exocrine insufficiency and diabetes mellitus.[1, 34]

Pancreatitis in Cats

Much less is known about pancreatitis in cats than in dogs. This section briefly summarizes the major differences between dogs and cats. Definitive diagnosis of pancreatitis is difficult and is not often made before necropsy.[20, 56] Commonly, it is a subclinical condition, recognized as chronic pancreatitis at necropsy.[2, 57] However, it can mimic the acute illness in dogs.[20, 40, 58] If clinical signs are present, pancreatitis often causes a mild chronic illness.[57] There does not appear to be an age or sex predilection, although Siamese cats may be over-represented.[2, 20, 59]

Pathophysiology

Blunt abdominal trauma, especially that seen with high-rise syndrome, can cause acute pancreatitis.[59, 60] Other associated conditions include fluke infection, feline infectious peritonitis, and toxoplasmosis.[2, 61]

One necropsy series classified cases into acute (33%), chronic active (25%), and chronic (41%) forms.[58] Pancreatitis may occur in conjunction with cholangitis, cholangiohepatitis, or hepatic lipidosis.[20, 56–59, 62, 63] The clinical signs of pancreatitis in these cases may be obscured by the more obvious signs of liver disease. Pancreatitis may contribute to the pathophysiology of the hepatic disease. In addition, renal failure is commonly found in conjunction with pancreatitis, but a cause-and-effect relation has not been proposed.[58] Once again, the obvious clinical signs of renal failure may obscure the more subtle signs of pancreatitis.

Clinical Signs

Clinical signs are highly variable and include anorexia, weight loss, dehydration, vomiting, icterus, abdominal pain, pyrexia, hypothermia, shock, and polyuria with polydipsia if concurrent diabetes mellitus exists.[2, 20, 59, 64, 65] In experimental acute pancreatitis, clinical signs are very mild.[61] Diabetes mellitus that resolves soon after diagnosis may be associated with acute pancreatitis.[59] Vomiting, diarrhea, and abdominal pain occur much less frequently in cats than in dogs with acute pancreatitis.[20, 59, 61, 65] Pleural, abdominal, or pericardial fluid may be present.[20, 56, 57]

Diagnostic Plan

The antemortem diagnosis of pancreatitis in cats is very difficult. Continued development of ultrasonographic skills may be the best hope for diagnosis in the future. In many cases, exploratory surgery remains the only practical antemortem tool.

Laboratory findings can be similar to those seen in dogs.[21] Anemia and hypokalemia may be more common.[20, 61] Although reported in only a few clinical cases, serum amylase and lipase can be normal.[20, 21, 64, 65] However, lipase is elevated in experimental pancreatitis.[61] Hypoglycemia occurs in cats with suppurative acute pancreatitis.[20] Icterus appears to be more common in cats.[20] Coagulation abnormalities are commonly encountered in cats with pancreatitis and hepatic lipidosis.[56] Pulmonary thrombi have also been found in this group of cats.[56]

Treatment

The recommended therapy for cats suspected of having pancreatitis is similar to that for dogs. Concurrent pancreatitis and hepatic lipidosis represent a challenge: the former requires fasting and resting of the pancreas, and the latter requires feeding.[56] In several of these cases, I have initiated feeding after 3 to 5 days of fasting or used total parenteral nutrition.

Prognosis

The prognosis is poor for cats with severe acute pancreatitis despite intensive therapy.[20] Until more cats with pancreatitis can be studied, establishment of an accurate prognosis is very difficult.

Exocrine Pancreatic Insufficiency

In exocrine pancreatic insufficiency (EPI), deficiency of pancreatic enzymes leads to maldigestion,

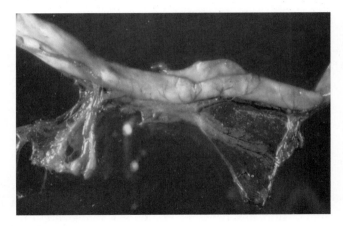

Figure 33–4
Necropsy specimen of a Norwegian elkhound puppy with exocrine pancreatic insufficiency. Almost no exocrine tissue is present, and mostly fibrous stroma and islets of Langerhans remain. (Courtesy of Geoff Saunders, DVM, MS, Blacksburg, Virginia.)

small bowel diarrhea, and weight loss. It occurs most commonly in young German shepherds (<5 years old) but can occur in any breed up to 5 years of age.[27, 66–73] It is rare in cats. Occasionally, it can develop as a sequela to acute pancreatitis in middle-aged or older dogs or cats.[66]

Pathophysiology

The clinical signs of EPI are caused by atrophy of the pancreatic acinar tissue (Fig. 33–4).[69] The cause of the atrophy is unknown. Endocrine tissue is spared, so diabetes mellitus does not occur.[66] A genetic predisposition occurs in German shepherds and in rough-coated collies.[66] Because of the great functional reserve of the pancreas, approximately 85% to 90% of function must be lost before clinical signs develop.[66, 74] In cases that arise secondary to acute pancreatitis, acinar tissue is destroyed by the inflammation and fibrosis associated with the acute or chronic smoldering disease.

Lack of pancreatic enzymes leads to malabsorption of carbohydrates and fats.[74, 75] Unabsorbed carbohydrates remain within the intestinal lumen, attracting water because of osmotic forces, and resulting in diarrhea as the colon's ability to absorb water is exceeded.[72, 74] The unabsorbed carbohydrates are fermented by intestinal bacteria, producing many more osmotically active particles, which contribute to diarrhea. Malabsorbed fats remain within the intestinal lumen and are converted to hydroxy fatty acids by intraluminal bacteria. Hydroxy fatty acids promote diarrhea by decreasing fluid absorption, increasing fluid secretion, and altering gastrointestinal motility.[76–78] Lack of pancreatic bicarbonate alters the intraluminal pH and adversely affects enzymatic processes.[74] The malabsorption of nutrients and diarrhea leads to severe weight loss or failure to thrive.

A secondary bacterial overgrowth (see Chap. 32) develops in many cases of EPI and contributes to the diarrhea and malnutrition.[79, 80] In addition to fermentation of nonabsorbed carbohydrates, other proposed causes of bacterial overgrowth include decreased intraluminal pH, decreased intestinal immunity or abnormal gastrointestinal motility caused by malnutrition, and lack of an antibacterial component in pancreatic juice.[66, 79, 80]

Decreased cobalamin absorption occurs in experimental disease and does not resolve after enzyme supplementation.[81] It is possible that a pancreatic intrinsic factor is necessary for the absorption of cobalamin in the distal small intestine.

The cause of mesenteric volvulus in German shepherds with EPI is unknown. Possibilities include abnormal intestinal motility, excessive gas within the intestinal lumen, and abnormal intraluminal contents.[82]

Clinical Signs

The most common clinical signs in dogs with EPI are severe weight loss (or failure to thrive), chronic diarrhea, and polyphagia.[48, 66, 72–74] Stools are typical of small bowel diarrhea and are voluminous, rancid, possibly greasy, and often gray or yellowish.[70, 72] Frequency of defecation is increased (three to eight times per day). Coprophagia is common. Vomiting and polydipsia can occur.[70] Affected dogs are normal before manifesting the signs of EPI.[70] Physical examination reveals a thin or emaciated dog with normal abdominal palpation.

In one report, approximately 10% of German shepherds with EPI treated for an average of 1.2 years developed fatal mesenteric volvulus.[82] Clinical signs included vomiting, abdominal pain, bloody mucoid diarrhea, bloating, recumbence, and death.

Diagnostic Plan

The diagnosis of EPI is reached by following the diagnostic plan for chronic diarrhea (see Chap. 32). It should be strongly suspected in young dogs (especially German shepherds) with severe weight loss, profound diarrhea, and ravenous appetites that do not have gastrointestinal parasites. Definitive diagnosis requires finding a low STLI (<2.5 µg/L).[26–28, 66] Although some practitioners use radiographic film digestion or Sudan staining of feces to make a diagnosis, these qualitative tests are inconsistent and inaccurate.[66] Assessment of plasma turbidity (see Chap. 32) after incubation with pancreatic enzymes provides supportive evidence for the diagnosis.[72] I strongly recommend that STLI be used as the gold standard for diagnosis. Some confirmed cases (low STLI) that do not respond to therapy should be evaluated for secondary bacterial overgrowth of the small intestine by measurement of serum vitamin B_{12} and folic acid.

Treatment

Supplementation of each meal with powdered extracts of beef or pork pancreas (Viokase-V) usually results in resolution of diarrhea and rapid weight gain. The initial dose of 2 teaspoons per 20 kg body weight in each meal can be reduced slowly after formed stools are produced.[66, 72] If improvement does not occur, the dose should be increased. Most dogs should be fed twice per day. Enzyme powder should be mixed into food shortly before feeding; preincubation does not improve digestibility.[75] Cobalamin therapy (250 µg intramuscularly or subcutaneously, once a week for 4 weeks and then once every 6–12 months) is necessary in some dogs.[66]

If rapid clinical improvement does not occur, a highly digestible, low-fat diet may improve fecal consistency.[68, 83, 84] If diarrhea continues, bacterial overgrowth should be suspected. Three weeks of treatment with tetracycline (20 mg/kg t.i.d. by mouth) should result in prompt resolution of diarrhea.

Prognosis

The prognosis for dogs with EPI is excellent. Most dogs respond dramatically to therapy, gain weight, and produce normal stools.[68] Owners should be warned about the potential for development of mesenteric volvulus and the poor prognosis associated with it. The prognosis is guarded for dogs that develop EPI after acute pancreatitis, because these dogs often develop diabetes mellitus, and regulation is very difficult with concurrent EPI.

Uncommon Diseases of the Exocrine Pancreas

Pancreatic Acinar Adenocarcinoma

Malignant tumors of the exocrine pancreas occur in older dogs and cats but are uncommon.[85] The condition is usually advanced by the time of diagnosis, and treatment is not often possible. Clinical signs include anorexia, weight loss, depression, vomiting, and icterus.[86] Occasionally, an abdominal mass can be palpated (see Fig. 33–1) or fluid can be detected within the abdomen.[57, 86] Multifocal steatitis has been described in some dogs and progressive, nonscarring alopecia (caused by unknown mechanisms) in some cats.[87, 88] Diagnosis is based on radiographic and ultrasonographic findings and on biopsy obtained under ultrasonographic guidance or during exploratory surgery. Some animals have elevated serum amylase and lipase. Biliary obstruction or liver metastasis may cause hyperbilirubinemia and elevated serum ALT and AP. Metastasis commonly occurs to the duodenum, omentum, mesentery, liver, regional lymph nodes, and lungs.[57, 86] The prognosis is grave.

Pancreatic Flukes

Infection with the pancreatic fluke *Eurytrema procyonis* usually does not cause any clinical signs in cats. The 1- to 2-mm flukes live within the small and medium-sized pancreatic ducts and cause duct obstruction.[86, 89] Atrophy and fibrosis of the pancreas can develop.[90] Although flukes result in reduced pancreatic secretion of enzymes and bicarbonate, clinical signs of EPI usually do not occur.[90] Operculated eggs can be found during fecal examination.

References

1. Mulvany MH, Feinberg CK, Tilson DL. Clinical characterization of acute necrotizing pancreatitis. Compen Contin Educ Pract Vet 1982;394:394–407.
2. Smith FWK. Feline pancreatitis: A review. Comp Anim Pract 1987;1:4–13.
3. Williams DA. Diagnosis and management of pancreatitis. J Small Anim Pract 1994;35:445–454.
4. Herdt T. Secretions of the gastrointestinal tract. In: Cunningham JG, ed. Textbook of Veterinary Physiology. Philadelphia, WB Saunders, 1992:275–285.
5. Hall JA, Macey DW. Acute canine pancreatitis. Compen Contin Educ Pract Vet 1988;10:403–417.
6. Macintire DK. The acute abdomen: Differential diagnosis and management. Semin Vet Med Surg (Small Anim) 1988;3:302–310.
7. Crowe DT. The first steps in handling the acute abdomen patient. Vet Med 1988;83:652–674.
8. Thrall DE, Bovee KC, Biery DN. Demonstration of a "position of relief" in dogs with lesions of the stomach or small bowel. J Am Anim Hosp Assoc 1978;14: 343–347.
9. King LG. Postoperative complications and prognostic indicators in dogs and cats with septic peritonitis: 23 cases (1989–1992). J Am Vet Med Assoc 1994;204:407–414.
10. Hosgood G, Salisbury SK. Generalized peritonitis in dogs: 50 cases (1975–1986). J Am Vet Med Assoc 1988;193:1448–1450.
11. Greenfield CL, Walshaw R. Open peritoneal drainage for treatment of contaminated peritoneal cavity and septic peritonitis in dogs and cats: 24 cases (1980–1986). J Am Vet Med Assoc 1987;191:100–105.
12. Penninck D, Nyland T, LY K, et al. Ultrasonographic evaluation of gastrointestinal diseases in small animals. Vet Radiol 1990;31:134–141.
13. Bjorling DE, Crowe DT, Kolata RJ, et al. Penetrating abdominal wounds in dogs and cats. J Am Anim Hosp Assoc 1982;18:742–748.
14. Crowe DT. Diagnostic abdominal paracentesis techniques: Clinical evaluation in 129 dogs and cats. J Am Anim Hosp Assoc 1984;20:223–230.
15. Murtaugh RJ, Jacobs RM. Serum amylase and isoamylases and their origins in healthy dogs and dogs with experimentally induced acute pancreatitis. Am J Vet Res 1985;46:742–747.
16. Wagner AE, Macy DW. Nephelometric determination of serum amylase and lipase in naturally occurring azotemia in the dog. Am J Vet Res 1982;43:697–699.
17. Polzin DJ, Osborne CA, Stevens JB, et al. Serum amylase and lipase activities in dogs with chronic primary renal failure. Am J Vet Res 1983;44:404–410.
18. Strombeck DR, Farver T, Kaneko JJ. Serum amylase and lipase activities in the diagnosis of pancreatitis. Am J Vet Res 1981;42:1966–1970.
19. Jacobs RM, Swenson CL, Davenport DJ, et al. Sensitivity and specificity of canine serum total amylase and isoamylase activity determinations. Can J Vet Res 1988; 52:473–475.
20. Hill RC, Van Winkle TJ. Acute necrotizing pancreatitis and acute suppurative pancreatitis in the cat: A retrospective study of 40 cases (1976–1989). J Vet Intern Med 1993;7:25–33.
21. Schaer M. A clinicopathologic survey of acute pancreatitis in 30 dogs and 5 cats. J Am Anim Hosp Assoc 1979;15:681–687.
22. Carrire F, Raphel V, Moreau H, et al. Dog gastric lipase: Stimulation of its secretion in vivo and cytolocalization in mucous pit cells. Gastroenterology 1992;102: 1535–1545.
23. Fittschen C, Bellamy JEC. Prednisone treatment alters the serum amylase and lipase activities in normal dogs without causing pancreatitis. Can J Comp Med 1984;48: 136–140.
24. Parent J. Effects of dexamethasone on pancreatic tissue and on serum amylase and lipase activities in dogs. J Am Vet Med Assoc 1982;180:743–746.
25. Bellah J, Bell G. Serum amylase and lipase activities after exploratory laparotomy in dogs. Am J Vet Res 1989;50: 1638–1641.
26. Williams DA. New tests of pancreatic and small intestine function. Compen Contin Educ Pract Vet 1987;9:1167–1174.
27. Williams DA, Batt RM. Sensitivity and specificity of radioimmunoassay of serum trypsin-like immunoreactivity for the diagnosis of canine exocrine pancreatic insufficiency. J Am Vet Med Assoc 1988;192:195–201.
28. Williams DA, Batt RM. Diagnosis of canine exocrine pancreatic insufficiency by the assay of serum trypsin-like immunoreactivity. J Small Anim Pract 1983;24: 583–588.
29. Steiner JM, Williams DA. Feline trypsin-like immunoreactivity as a diagnostic tool for diseases of the exocrine pancreas in the cat. Vet Prev 1995;2:7–9.
30. Simpson K, Batt R, McLean L, et al. Circulating concentrations of trypsin-like immunoreactivity and activities of lipase and amylase after pancreatic duct ligation in dogs. Am J Vet Res 1989;50:629–632.
31. Gibbs C, Denny HR, Minter HM, et al. Radiological features of inflammatory conditions of the canine pancreas. J Small Anim Pract 1972;13:531–544.

32. Murtaugh RJ. Acute pancreatitis: Diagnostic dilemmas. Semin Vet Med Surg 1987;2:282–295.

33. Kleine LJ. Acute pancreatitis: The radiographic findings in 182 dogs. Vet Radiol 1978;19:102–106.

34. Schaer M. Acute pancreatitis in dogs. Compen Contin Educ Pract Vet 1991;13:1769–1781.

35. Williams DA. Acute pancreatitis. In: Kirk RW, Bonagura JD, eds. Kirk's Current Veterinary Therapy XI. Philadelphia, WB Saunders, 1992:631–639.

36. Kleine LJ. Clinical and radiographic aspects of acute pancreatitis in the dog. Compen Contin Educ Pract Vet 1980;2:295–302.

37. Westermarck E, Rimaila-Parnanen E. Serum phospholipase A2 in canine acute pancreatitis. Acta Vet Scand 1983;24:477–487.

38. Murtaugh RJ, Herring DS, Jacobs RM, et al. Pancreatic ultrasonography in dogs with experimentally induced acute pancreatitis. Vet Radiol 1985;26:27–32.

39. Cook AK, Breitschwerdt EB, Levine JF, et al. Risk factors associated with acute pancreatitis in dogs: 101 cases (1985–1990). J Am Vet Med Assoc 1993;203:673–679.

40. Pidgeon G. Exocrine pancreatic disease in the dog and cat: Part 1. Acute pancreatitis. Comp Anim Pract 1987;1:67–71.

41. Simpson KW. Current concepts of the pathogenesis and pathophysiology of acute pancreatitis in the dog and cat. Compen Contin Educ Pract Vet 1993;2:247–254.

42. Moriello KA, Bowen D, Meyer DJ. Acute pancreatitis in two dogs given azathioprine and prednisone. J Am Vet Med Assoc 1987;191:695–696.

43. Strombeck DR, Wheeldon E, Harrold D. Model of chronic pancreatitis in the dog. Am J Vet Res 1984;45:131–136.

44. Stewart AF. Pancreatitis in dogs and cats: Cause, pathogenesis, diagnosis, and treatment. Compen Contin Educ Pract Vet 1994;16:1423–1430.

45. Murtaugh RJ, Jacobs RM. Serum antiprotease concentrations in dogs with spontaneous and experimentally induced acute pancreatitis. Am J Vet Res 1985;46:80–84.

46. Matthiesen DT, Rosin E. Common bile duct obstruction secondary to chronic fibrosing pancreatitis: Treatment by use of cholecystoduodenostomy in the dog. J Am Vet Med Assoc 1986;189:1443–1446.

47. Martin RA, MacCoy DM, Harvey HJ. Surgical management of extrahepatic biliary tract disease: A report of eleven cases. J Am Anim Hosp Assoc 1986;22:301–307.

48. Holroyd JB. Canine exocrine pancreatic disease. J Small Anim Pract 1968;9:269–281.

49. Attix E, Strombeck DR, Wheeldon EB, et al. Effects of an anticholinergic and a corticosteroid on acute pancreatitis in experimental dogs. Am J Vet Res 1981;42:1668–1674.

50. Whitney MS. The laboratory assessment of canine and feline pancreatitis. Vet Med 1993;88:1045–1052.

51. Jacobs RM, Murtaugh RJ, DeHoff WD. Review of the clinicopathological findings of acute pancreatitis in the dog: Use of an experimental model. J Am Anim Hosp Assoc 1985;21:795–800.

52. Feldman BF, Attix EA, Strombeck DR, et al. Biochemical and coagulation changes in a canine model of acute necrotizing pancreatitis. Am J Vet Res 1981;42:805–809.

53. Murtaugh R, Jacobs R, Sherding R, et al. Serum pancreatic polypeptide and amylase concentrations in dogs with experimentally induced acute pancreatitis. Am J Vet Res 1985;46:654–656.

54. Edwards DF, Bauer MS, Walker MA, et al. Pancreatic masses in seven dogs following acute pancreatitis. J Am Anim Hosp Assoc 1990;26:189–198.

55. Salisbury SK, Lantz GC, Nelson RW, et al. Pancreatic abscess in dogs: Six cases (1978–1986). J Am Vet Med Assoc 1988;193:1104–1108.

56. Akol KG, Washabau RJ, Saunders HM, et al. Acute pancreatitis in cats with hepatic lipidosis. J Vet Intern Med 1993;7:205–209.

57. Owens JM, Drazner FH, Gilbertson SR. Pancreatic disease in the cat. J Am Anim Hosp Assoc 1975;11:83–89.

58. Macy DW. Feline pancreatitis. In: Kirk RW, ed. Current Veterinary Therapy X. Philadelphia, WB Saunders, 1989:893–896.

59. Garvey MS, Zawie DA. Feline pancreatic disease. Vet Clin North Am Small Anim Pract 1984;14:1231–1246.

60. Suter PF, Olsson SE. Traumatic hemorrhagic pancreatitis in the cat: A report with emphasis on the radiological diagnosis. J Am Vet Rad Soc 1969;10:4–11.

61. Kitchell B, Strombeck D, Cullen J, et al. Clinical and pathologic changes in experimentally induced acute pancreatitis in cats. Am J Vet Res 1986;47:1170–1173.

62. Center SA, Rowland PH. The cholangitis/cholangiohepatitis complex in the cat. Proc Annu Meet Am Coll Vet Intern Med 1994;12:766–771.

63. Center SA, Crawford MA, Guida L, et al. A retrospective study of 77 cats with severe hepatic lipidosis: 1975–1990. J Vet Intern Med 1993;7:349–359.

64. Simpson KW, Shiroma JT, Biller DS, et al. Ante mortem diagnosis of pancreatitis in four cats. J Small Anim Pract 1994;35:93–99.

65. Duffel SJ. Some aspects of pancreatic disease in the cat. J Small Anim Pract 1975;16:365–374.

66. Williams DA. Exocrine pancreatic insufficiency. Waltham Int Focus 1992;2:9–14.

67. Westermarck E, Junttila JT, Wiberg ME. Role of low dietary fat in the treatment of dogs with exocrine pancreatic insufficiency. Am J Vet Res 1995;56:600–605.

68. Simpson JW, Maskell IE, Quigg J, et al. Long term management of canine exocrine pancreatic insufficiency. J Small Anim Pract 1994;35:133–138.

69. Rimaila-Parnanen E, Westermarck E. Pancreatic degenerative atrophy and chronic pancreatitis in dogs. Acta Vet Scand 1982;23:400–406.

70. Raiha M, Westermarck E. The signs of pancreatic degenerative atrophy in dogs and the role of external factors in the etiology of the disease. Acta Vet Scand 1989;30:447–452.

71. Hall EJ, Bond PM, McLean C, et al. A survey of the diagnosis and treatment of canine exocrine pancreatic insufficiency. J Small Anim Pract 1991;32:613–619.

72. Sherding RG. Canine exocrine pancreatic insufficiency. Compen Contin Educ Pract Vet 1979;1:816–821.

73. Hill FWG. Pancreatic disorders of dogs. Vet Ann 1978;18:198–203.

74. Moore RP. Pathophysiology of canine exocrine pancreatic insufficiency. Compen Contin Educ Pract Vet 1980;2:657–661.

75. Pidgeon G, Strombeck DR. Evaluation of treatment for

pancreatic exocrine insufficiency in dogs with ligated pancreatic ducts. Am J Vet Res 1982;43:461–464.

76. Leib MS. Stagnant loop syndrome in the dog and cat. Semin Vet Med Surg (Small Anim) 1987;2:257–265.

77. King CE, Toskes PP. Small intestinal bacterial overgrowth. Gastroenterology 1979;76:1035–1055.

78. Willard MD. Chronic intestinal bacterial overgrowth. In: Kirk RW, ed. Current Veterinary Therapy X. Philadelphia, WB Saunders, 1989:933–938.

79. Williams DA, Batt RM, McLean L. Bacterial overgrowth in the duodenum of dogs with exocrine pancreatic insufficiency. J Am Vet Med Assoc 1987;191:201–206.

80. Simpson K, Batt R, Jones D, et al. Effects of exocrine pancreatic insufficiency and replacement therapy on the bacterial flora of the duodenum in dogs. Am J Vet Res 1990;51:203–206.

81. Simpson K, Morton D, Batt R. Effect of exocrine pancreatic insufficiency on cobalamin absorption in dogs. Am J Vet Res 1989;50:1233–1236.

82. Westermarck E, Rimaila-Parnanen E. Mesenteric torsion in dogs with exocrine pancreatic insufficiency: 21 cases (1978–1987). J Am Vet Med Assoc 1989;195:1404–1406.

83. Pidgeon G. Effect of diet on exocrine pancreatic insufficiency in dogs. J Am Vet Med Assoc 1982;181:232–235.

84. Westermarck E, Wiberg M, Junttila J. Role of feeding in the treatment of dogs with pancreatic degenerative atrophy. Acta Vet Scand 1990;31:325–331.

85. Anderson NV, Low DG. Diseases of the canine pancreas: A comparative summary of 103 cases. Anim Hosp 1965;1:189–195.

86. Dill-Macky E. Pancreatic diseases of cats. Compen Contin Educ Pract Vet 1993;15:589–598.

87. Brooks DG, Campbell KL, Dennis JS, et al. Pancreatic paraneoplastic alopecia in three cats. J Am Anim Hosp Assoc 1994;30:557–563.

88. Brown PJ, Mason KV, Merrett DJ, et al. Multifocal necrotizing steatitis associated with pancreatic carcinoma in three dogs. J Small Anim Pract 1994;35:129–132.

89. Sheldon WG. Pancreatic flukes (*Eurytrema procyonis*) in domestic cats. J Am Vet Med Assoc 1966;148:251–253.

90. Fox JN, Mosley JG, Vogler GA, et al. Pancreatic function in domestic cats with pancreatic fluke infection. J Am Vet Med Assoc 1981;178:58–60.

Chapter 34

Hepatobiliary Diseases

Michael S. Leib

Anatomy

The liver is the largest gland in the body.[1, 2] It consists of six lobes, arranged into three regional divisions: right (right lateral lobe and caudate process of caudate lobe), central (quadrate and right medial lobes), and left (left lateral lobe, left medial lobe, and papillary process of caudate lobe).[3] The left division comprises approximately 50% of total hepatic mass. The porta hepatis is the area on the ventral surface of the liver where the portal vein, hepatic artery, common bile duct, and lymphatic vessels enter or leave the liver.[4]

The liver has a great storage capacity for blood. Hepatomegaly associated with right-sided heart failure is simply caused by increased blood storage.[4] The liver receives approximately 20% to 25% of cardiac output from a dual blood supply.[2, 3] The portal vein carries approximately 70% to 75% of the hepatic blood supply.[2] The portal vein receives venous drainage from the stomach, pancreas, spleen, and intestines.[1] At the hilus of the liver, the portal vein divides into two or three branches before branching further to supply each hepatic lobe.[3] The portal vein supplies about 50% of the liver's oxygen. The common hepatic artery is a branch of the celiac artery.[3] It divides into multiple hepatic arteries, with at least one going to each hepatic division. There are usually six to eight hepatic veins. Two large veins, one draining the left and one draining the central division, are consistent in location.[3] The other hepatic veins vary in number, size, location, position, and portion of the liver that they drain. The hepatic veins enter the caudal vena cava after exiting from the liver at the level of the diaphragm.[3]

The gallbladder is located on the visceral surface of the liver between the quadrate and right medial lobes.[5] Interlobular bile ducts unite to form hepatic bile ducts, which emerge from the lobes and enter the common bile duct. The cystic duct is the section of the bile duct between the gallbladder and the point at which the first hepatic duct enters.[5] The distal end of the common bile duct lies near the pancreas and enters the duodenum at the major duodenal papilla. A small muscular sphincter, the sphincter of Oddi, is present at the papilla and controls bile flow. It is this anatomic relation that is responsible for the biliary obstruction that occurs in some cases of pancreatitis.[5] In cats, the pancreatic duct joins the bile duct, and they enter the duodenum together as a common duct; in dogs, each duct enters separately. The cystic artery, from the left branch of the proper hepatic artery, supplies blood to the gallbladder.[3]

Nodular hyperplasia of the liver is a common finding in old dogs.[6] Nodules can range from 2 to 50 mm in diameter. Multiple nodules can be found in all liver lobes. The nodules are variable in color and can be yellow, pink, tan, or red. The nodules cause compression and atrophy in surrounding parenchyma. Nodular hyperplasia is an incidental finding that should be considered normal. It is a clinically significant finding because it must be differentiated by biopsy from neoplasia and the nodular regeneration that occurs in cirrhosis.[7, 8]

An understanding of the microscopic anatomy of the liver is necessary to appreciate hepatic function and to interpret histopathologic changes found on biopsy. The basic anatomic unit is the hexagonal lobule, composed of a central vein bounded by plates or cords of hepatocytes, which are surrounded on two sides by blood-filled sinusoids.[1, 9] Sinusoids form a greatly anastomosing vascular network among the hepatocytes.[2] Sinusoids are lined by fenestrated endothelial cells, allowing hepatocytes access to the filtrate of portal blood. The space of Disse separates the sinusoidal epithelium from the hepatocytes.[2] Microvilli project from the hepatocyte membrane into the space of Disse, greatly increasing the surface area for interaction with the fluid.[10] At the periphery of the lobule are portal tracts, each of which contains a bile duct, a branch of the portal vein, a branch of the hepatic artery, and lymphatics.[2, 9] The cell membranes between hepatocytes form small bile canaliculi, which converge into larger intrahepatic ductules. Bile flow within the lobule is opposite that of blood flow.[9] This anatomic arrangement explains why periportal inflammation can result in icterus.

Using the classic lobular arrangement, the area around the central vein is called centrolobular zone; the area at the circumference is called the peripheral lobular zone, or the periportal zone if it is near a portal triad; and the midzonal area lies between the two.[2] These zones are important in interpretation of histologic changes because various pathologic processes can affect different zones (see Hepatitis and Necrosis).

Physiology

The liver normally performs more than 1500 functions.[11] Because of this complexity, only some of the major, clinically significant hepatic functions are reviewed here. The liver has a great functional reserve. Often, only 10% to 20% of function is necessary to maintain homeostasis.[1] In addition, hepatocytes retain the ability to divide. Up to 70% of hepatic mass can be regenerated in 10 to 14 days in normal dogs.[1]

Protein, Carbohydrate, and Fat Metabolism

The liver plays the central role in the inter-related metabolism of proteins, fats, and carbohydrates. After a meal, the liver receives amino acids, monosaccharides, short-chain fatty acids, and B-complex vitamins from portal blood and long-chain fatty acids and fat-soluble vitamins from arterial circulation (through the lymphatics).[12] Hepatic metabolism of these substances is complex and is influenced by nutrient concentrations and many endocrine factors.

Along with insulin and glucagon, the liver helps prevent fluctuations of blood glucose.[4] Glucose is used within the hepatocyte for energy, stored as glycogen to be released when needed, or converted into fatty acids.[1, 13] The liver can also manufacture glucose from proteins or fats (gluconeogenesis). The liver is the primary organ for the metabolism of lactate, which is produced during anaerobic conditions.[1] Hypoglycemia can occur in animals with liver disease, but the liver often maintains blood glucose levels despite reduced function.[4] The liver is an important site for the degradation of insulin.[4] In steroid hepatopathy of dogs, accumulation of glycogen occurs within hepatocytes and causes hepatomegaly.

The liver can convert excess carbohydrates and proteins into fatty acids and extract fatty acids from blood.[10] Fatty acids may be oxidized for energy, re-esterified into triglycerides, converted to phospholipids, used for formation of cholesterol esters, or packaged with apoproteins for dispersal as very-low-density lipoproteins.[13, 14] The liver also synthesizes cholesterol and synthesizes and degrades lipoproteins. Excess accumulation of lipid within the hepatocytes occurs in hepatic lipidosis, a common disorder in cats.

The liver maintains a pool of free amino acids.[10] Abnormalities in the serum concentrations of amino acids occur with many hepatic diseases and participate in the pathophysiology of hepatic encephalopathy. Amino acids are used within the liver for protein synthesis.[13] Hepatic catabolism of excess amino acids provides carbon for gluconeogenesis, ketogenesis, or fatty acid synthesis.[10] The liver can also synthesize amino acids from intermediates of carbohydrate and lipid metabolism.[10]

Bile

Bile provides a route for bilirubin, cholesterol, and drug elimination and is important in fat assimilation from the intestine.[15] Bile is an iso-osmotic alkaline solution of bile salts, bile pigments (see

Bilirubin), phospholipids, and cholesterol.[10] Bile acids are the predominant component of bile (see Bile Acids).[15] Bile salts are actively secreted from the hepatocyte into the bile canaliculi; water and electrolytes follow passively.[10] Bile is modified with the addition of electrolytes as it is transported through the ductules. Bile is stored within the gallbladder and is concentrated by absorption of sodium. Bile flow can be stimulated by substances termed cholerectics. Absorption of bile acids from the intestine is a major stimulus for bile synthesis. During a meal, fats within the duodenum stimulate the release of cholecystokinin from intestinal epithelial cells, which stimulates contraction of the gallbladder, relaxation of the sphincter of Oddi, and delivery of bile into the duodenum.[10]

In the intestinal lumen, bile salts aid emulsification of lipid by their detergent action, reducing lipid droplets to a size that forms stable suspensions in water.[16] In emulsified droplets, lipids are acted on by lipase and colipase, resulting in free fatty acids and monoglycerides. These products join with phospholipids and bile acids to form water-soluble micelles, which allow fats to be transported to the mucosa, where they cross the cell membrane by diffusion. Medium- and short-chain fatty acids can enter portal blood directly; long-chain fatty acids are packaged into chylomicrons and enter the lymphatics.

Plasma Proteins

The liver is the site of synthesis of most plasma proteins, excluding γ-globulins.[1] Albumin is the major contributor to plasma osmotic pressure and serves as a carrier and transport protein. Albumin production represents about 25% of hepatic protein synthesis.[10] In liver disease, the ability to synthesize albumin is preserved; decreased synthesis is associated only with very severe hepatic dysfunction.[9, 17, 18] Hypoalbuminemia can contribute to ascites formation.

Many of the other proteins synthesized by the liver have diverse and important functions.[10] Examples include thyroid-binding globulin (transports thyroxine in serum), α-protease inhibitor and α-macroglobulins (protease inhibitors; see Chap. 33), ceruloplasm (carries copper), haptoglobin (binds hemoglobin), transferrin (transports iron), and components of the complement system C3 and C4 (mediates inflammation). Severe hepatic disease compromises these functions, resulting in additional pathophysiologic consequences of liver disease.

Coagulation

The liver synthesizes most of the clotting factors (see Chap. 44).[10] In addition, factors II, VII, IX, and X require vitamin K as a cofactor for activation. Fat-soluble vitamin K (from dietary sources or as a product of gastrointestinal [GI] bacterial metabolism) requires bile for absorption from the intestines. Fat malassimilation can occur with severe and prolonged cholestasis. The liver also synthesizes fibrinogen, coagulation inhibitors such as antithrombin III, and plasminogen (precursor of plasmin, which is responsible for degradation of fibrin clots) and removes active clotting factors from circulation.[10] For these reasons, a wide range of coagulation abnormalities often accompany severe liver disease.

Urea Cycle

The most important mechanism for the detoxification of ammonia is the urea cycle, which occurs only within the liver.[10] Ammonia is metabolized to urea, which is excreted in the urine.[19] Intermediates of the cycle include ornithine, citrulline, and arginine. Hepatic insufficiency can cause increased serum ammonia, which is one of the toxins of hepatic encephalopathy. In cats, arginine is an essential amino acid. Anorexia can result in arginine deficiency and hyperammonemia as the efficiency of the urea cycle is reduced. Rarely, a deficiency of urea cycle enzymes can occur, resulting in hyperammonemia and signs of hepatic encephalopathy.

Vitamins

The liver produces bile to aid absorption of the fat-soluble vitamins A, D, E, and K; stores most vitamins; and converts many of them to active compounds.[4, 10] Many water-soluble vitamins must be phosphorylated to become active cofactors in metabolic processes.[10] The effect of cholestasis on vitamin K has been discussed previously.

Reticuloendothelial Function

Motile Kupffer cells line the sinusoids and function to remove and degrade substances contained in portal blood.[10] They represent the largest accumulation of fixed macrophages in the body.[4] They are also important antigen-presenting cells in the immune response to foreign substances.[4] Because the liver receives all portal blood flow, the liver serves as a filter to remove bacteria, endotoxins, enterotoxins, exotoxins, nutrients, and chemicals.[11] In addition, Kupffer cells can remove and degrade GI hormones and chylomicrons. With hepatic dysfunction, increased concentrations of these substances reach systemic circulation and can cause inflammation, septicemia, or endotoxemia or contribute to hepatic encephalopathy. Hyperglobulinemia often develops in animals with liver disease because of increased systemic antigenic stimulation. The administration of broad-spectrum antibiotics is often indicated in animals with severe liver disease to treat or prevent bacterial infection.

Drug Metabolism

The liver plays a central role in drug metabolism. Phase I enzymes of the smooth endoplasmic reticulum (microsomal enzymes) are responsible for the initial stages of drug metabolism.[20, 21] Three major consequences of hepatic phase I metabolism of a drug are possible: inactivation, conversion from an inactive drug to an active metabolite, and conversion from an active drug to an active metabolite.[21] Phase II metabolism involves conjugation with glutathione, glucuronate, sulfate, and several amino acids to produce drugs that are more water soluble, making elimination from the body easier.[20, 21]

Some drugs that can cause liver disease are discussed in the section on hepatotoxic drugs. For treatment of an animal with liver disease, drugs that require the liver for metabolism should not be used, to avoid causing toxicity. Liver disease can affect drug metabolism by alterations in hepatic blood flow, availability of transport proteins, decreased hepatocellular function, and cholestasis.[21] Because of these variables, it is often difficult to predict how a patient's specific hepatic disease will affect drug metabolism. In general, sedatives and anesthetics should be avoided because they can contribute to the signs of encephalopathy.[22] In addition, many sedatives and anesthetics require hepatic metabolism, so a "relative overdose" is common. Some antibiotics require hepatic clearance and should be avoided; these include chloramphenicol, erythromycin, lincomycin, and sulfonamides.[21, 23, 24] Some tetracyclines are potentially hepatotoxic.[21]

Problem Identification

The initial clinical signs of hepatobiliary diseases are often subtle and vague.[25] The intensity of signs often waxes and wanes. Decreased appetite, lethargy, depression, and mild weight loss may be the only signs present. If no other clues can be detected during physical examination, a complete blood count (CBC), biochemical profile, and urinalysis can often suggest the presence of hepatobiliary disease.[25]

As the severity of hepatobiliary diseases progress, other clinical signs usually develop. Although these signs can often be associated with extrahepatic disorders, following the diagnostic plans for vomiting, polyuria and polydipsia, coagulation deficits, or diarrhea should reveal evidence of hepatobiliary disorders.

The classic findings of icterus, hepatomegaly, ascites, and encephalopathy often develop as the consequences of hepatobiliary disorders intensify.

These findings are not specific for hepatobiliary disorders, but, when associated with hepatobiliary disease, they indicate severe disease.

Icterus

Icterus, or jaundice, is defined as yellowish discoloration of the skin and mucous membranes.[26] It is caused by excessive amounts of bilirubin, which occurs when the rate of production exceeds the rate of elimination.[26] Bilirubin is a waste product of red blood cell metabolism without benefit to the body, but it has major diagnostic implications in disease. Serum bilirubin must be approximately 2.5 to 3.0 mg/dL or higher to produce icterus.[9]

Pathophysiology

Bilirubin levels in the blood can increase because of impaired excretion into bile or excessive production from hemolysis (see Chap. 41). The liver has a tremendous ability to metabolize excessive bilirubin, so prehepatic or hemolytic icterus results only when moderate or severe red blood cell destruction is present.[17] Impaired excretion is caused by cholestasis; by stagnation of bile, either within the liver parenchyma (intrahepatic) or in the extrahepatic biliary system; or, less commonly, by rupture of the biliary system, which is usually associated with trauma[27] (see Bilirubin).

Obstruction of bile flow within the liver or during its extrahepatic transport results in regurgitation of conjugated bilirubin into the sinusoids and into systemic circulation. Hepatocellular swelling, inflammation, necrosis, or fibrosis, especially in the periportal area, can obstruct bile flow.[26, 27] Hepatocyte dysfunction may interfere with the uptake, conjugation, or secretion process and cause icterus.[27, 28] Most hepatic disorders discussed in this chapter can cause intrahepatic icterus.

Several surveys of icteric cats have shown that the most common causes of icterus include lipidosis, cholangiohepatitis, feline infectious peritonitis, toxic hepatopathy, hepatic neoplasia, sepsis, and hemolytic anemia.[29, 30] Posthepatic disorders that obstruct bile flow occur more commonly in dogs than cats; examples include biliary carcinoma, pancreatitis, pancreatic adenocarcinoma, cholelithiasis, cholecystitis, and duodenal neoplasia.[5, 31–33] Trauma to the biliary system (gallbladder, common bile duct, cystic duct, or intrahepatic bile ducts) can result in leakage of bile into the abdomen, bile peritonitis, reabsorption of the bilirubin into plasma, and icterus.

Bile retained within the liver is toxic and leads to hepatocellular degeneration.[27] Prolonged extrahepatic cholestasis can lead to hepatic disease and complicate the distinction between hepatic and posthepatic icterus.

Clinical Signs

Owners may notice icterus, or it may be identified by the veterinarian during physical examination. It is easiest to detect icterus in the sclera, conjunctiva, gingiva, hard palate, vulva, or penis.[28] It is more difficult to detect discoloration of the skin, but it can be noticed on the inside surfaces of the ears or on the caudoventral abdomen. The history may reveal exposure to potentially hepatotoxic drugs or chemicals.[26] Abdominal trauma, often 5 to 10 days previously, may have occurred and resulted in leakage of bile.

Other clinical signs are dependent on the cause of icterus. Patients with prehepatic or hemolytic icterus are often weak, lethargic, and tachypneic and have dark, discolored urine, a systolic heart murmur not previously detected, or hepatosplenomegaly. Animals with hepatic or posthepatic disorders may have some of the following signs: anorexia, weight loss, pyrexia, vomiting, diarrhea, abdominal distention, encephalopathy, polyuria and polydipsia, or bruising or bleeding tendencies. Abdominal distention caused by hepatomegaly or ascites or cranial abdominal pain may be detected during physical examination.

Diagnostic Plan

The most important initial diagnostic step with the icteric patient is to evaluate the hematocrit to determine if prehepatic (hemolytic) icterus is present. Moderate or severe anemia with a normal total protein level suggests hemolysis (see Chap. 41). The presence of hemolysis is also supported by a finding of hemoglobinuria or autoagglutination, although neither must be present. Further evaluation of hemolysis should include a review of red blood cell (RBC) morphology for spherocytosis and hemoprotozoa, determination of the reticulocyte count, a Coombs test, and an enzyme-linked immunosorbent assay (ELISA) for feline leukemia virus (FeLV) in cats.

If the hematocrit is normal or mild anemia is present, the icterus is a result of either hepatic or posthepatic causes.[34] The distinction between hepatic and posthepatic disease is important, because hepatic disease can be diagnosed with a minimally invasive closed liver biopsy, whereas with posthepatic disorders more invasive exploratory surgery is often needed to diagnose and potentially relieve the obstruction. To obtain a liver biopsy by exploratory laparotomy when less invasive methods are available is not in the animal's best interests. The best method to differentiate hepatic from posthepatic disorders is ultrasonography. Posthepatic disorders are associated with a distended

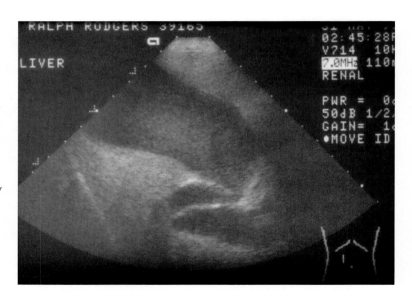

Figure 34-1
Longitudinal ultrasonographic appearance of biliary obstruction caused by a duodenal metastatic adenocarcinoma obstructing the common bile duct in a 10-year-old mixed breed dog. A large dilated gallbladder can be seen in the center of the photograph. A dilated and tortuous cystic duct is visible below the gallbladder. The primary tumor is pancreatic adenocarcinoma. (Courtesy of Martha L. Moon, DVM, MS, Blacksburg, Virginia.)

gallbladder, and enlarged and tortuous cystic, common bile, or intrahepatic bile ducts (Fig. 34–1).[35–37] A potentially neoplastic mass of the biliary system or pancreas, signs of pancreatitis (a pancreatic mass, a hypoechoic pancreas, abscesses and cysts, or increased echodensity associated with fibrosis),[38–41] an echogenic cholelith, or a thickened gallbladder wall may be found. With intrahepatic disorders, the liver may be enlarged and diffusely hyperechoic or hypoechoic or contain focal or multifocal abnormalities (Fig. 34–2).[42–47]

Without ultrasonographic assistance, the distinction between hepatic and posthepatic disorders is much more difficult. If the animal is relatively bright and alert, posthepatic disease is probably present. Elevated resting or posttolerance serum ammonia levels support hepatic disease. Very high serum alkaline phosphatase (AP) with only mildly elevated alanine aminotransferase (ALT) suggests posthepatic cholestasis. Finally, very high serum bilirubin levels (>10–15 mg/dL) are most often associated with posthepatic disorders.[48] None of these criteria are absolutely reliable, but they do provide some assistance in making the decision of closed liver biopsy versus exploratory surgery.

The complete diagnostic evaluation of a case of hepatic icterus should include a CBC, biochemical profile, urinalysis, FeLV and feline immunodeficiency virus (FIV) ELISAs in cats, abdominocentesis and fluid analysis (if ascites is suspected), coagulation profile, hepatic ultrasound, and liver biopsy using the least invasive method available. If examination of the ascitic fluid suggests bile peritonitis (see Ascites), diagnosis and treatment requires exploratory laparotomy. The pivotal step in evaluation of a suspected case of posthepatic disease is ultrasonography. A laboratory

minimum database should be collected to evaluate concurrent disease as well as the metabolic effects of the primary disorder. Additional diagnostic tests depend on sonographic findings but may include thoracic radiographs for metastasis, serum amylase and lipase, and exploratory laparotomy for definitive diagnosis and relief of the obstructing process.

Ascites

Ascites is defined as the accumulation of fluid within the abdominal cavity.[49] For diagnostic purposes, I prefer to limit the definition to fluids classified as transudates or modified transudates (Table 34–1). Ascites associated with liver disease is less common in cats than in dogs.[25] Exudates are produced by a different group of diseases and can easily be characterized by fluid evaluation.[50] Examples of exudates include bacterial peritonitis, chemical peritonitis (pancreatitis or bile or urine peritonitis), feline infectious peritonitis, chylous effusions, and some intra-abdominal neoplasms. Hemorrhage can also cause blood to accumulate within the abdominal cavity.[49]

Pathophysiology

The pathophysiology of ascites formation associated with liver disease is not completely understood. Portal hypertension associated with ascites in dogs and cats develops secondary to obstruction of portal blood flow or increased volume of portal blood flow.[51] Obstruction occurs either within the liver (hepatic) or in hepatic veins, the vena cava, or the right side of the heart (posthepatic).[51] Portal hypertension leads to vascular stasis and increased capillary filtration pressure.

One of the current theories describing ascites

formation is called the overflow theory.[52] The initial event is renal sodium retention.[53] Although the initiating cause is not known, it is postulated that hepatic disease results in decreased availability of a natriuretic hormone, which leads to sodium retention.[54] Natriuretic factors, atriopeptins, have been identified in the cardiac atria. Reduced atrial content or insensitivity to the actions of these compounds may be responsible for renal sodium retention associated with liver disease.[55] Sodium retention leads to expansion of extracellular volume and portal hypertension secondary to an increased volume of portal blood flow.[51] It is also possible that the initiating factor may be some other abnormal signal received by the kidney that results in sodium retention.

Another theory of ascites formation is called the classic theory.[52] It suggests that resistance to portal blood flow (due to compressed sinusoids) leads to splanchnic pooling, which results in decreased cardiac output, decreased renal blood flow, activation of the renin-angiotensin system, and increased aldosterone secretion resulting in sodium retention.[49, 51, 53] Although compatible endocrine changes have been observed in humans with cirrhosis and ascites, experimental production of liver disease and ascites in dogs has been shown to result from the initial retention of sodium and water.[53, 56-59] In some studies, plasma renin and aldosterone remained within normal limits before ascitic fluid accumulation.[57]

Animals with liver disease may develop obstruction of portal blood flow secondary to distortion and compression of hepatic sinusoids due to fibrosis, formation of regenerative nodules, inflammation, necrosis, or neoplastic masses.[51] In right-sided congestive heart failure, posthepatic obstruction results in intrahepatic portal hypertension. Regardless of the initiating event, sinusoidal hypertension leads to fluid accumulation within the space of Disse at a rate greater than the capacity of hepatic lymphatics to remove the fluid.[51, 53, 60] Lymph exudes across the hepatic capsule, resulting in ascites.[49, 53] Sinusoidal hypertension may progress to prehepatic portal hypertension and cause leakage of intestinal lymph into the abdomen. Prehepatic portal hypertension is relatively short-lived, because it is a potent stimulus for development of portosystemic shunts, which reduce portal pressure. Excess fluid accumulated within the abdomen is initially removed by abdominal lymphatics, especially along the diaphragm.[51] As fluid production exceeds lymphatic drainage capacity, fluid accumulates within the abdomen.

In cases of liver disease, congestive heart failure, or intra-abdominal neoplasia, hypoalbuminemia contributes to the forces favoring fluid accumulation because of decreased plasma osmotic pressure.[49, 51, 53] If serum albumin reaches 1.5 g/dL or less (often <1.0 g/dL), it can lead to ascites formation without other causes.[49]

Intra-abdominal neoplasia can cause ascites by obstructing venous and lymphatic return. In addition, the tumors may outgrow vascular and lymphatic channels and fluid may exude from their ulcerated surfaces.

Clinical Signs

A large amount of abdominal effusion can cause tachypnea or dyspnea by impinging on the diaphragm and can lead to anorexia and lethargy because of the physical discomfort caused by the fluid. Dogs and cats with ascites exhibit various findings on history and physical examination, depending on the underlying cause of the ascites. Animals with liver disease may have a history of vomiting, diarrhea, anorexia, leth-

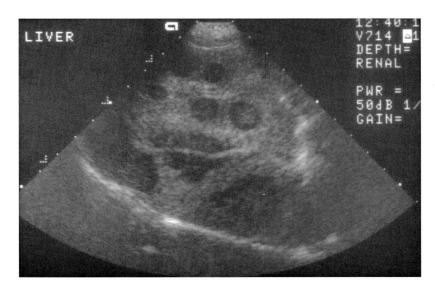

Figure 34-2
Longitudinal ultrasonographic appearance of metastatic carcinoma in a 7-year-old Labrador retriever. Multiple target lesions consisting of nodules with hyperechoic centers and hypoechoic peripheries are present. The primary tumor was not discovered. (Courtesy of Martha L. Moon, DVM, MS, Blacksburg, Virginia.)

Table 34–1
Common Causes of Ascites

Liver diseases
    Chronic hepatitis
    Chronic active hepatitis
    Cirrhosis
    Diffuse hepatic neoplasia
Congestive heart failure (right-sided)
    Congestive cardiomyopathy
    Heartworm disease
    Pericardial disease
    Tricuspid endocardiosis
Hypoalbuminemia
    Protein-losing enteropathy
    Glomerular diseases
    Liver failure
Intra-abdominal neoplasia

argy, weight loss, icterus, encephalopathy, or bleeding tendencies. The history may reveal exposure to potentially hepatotoxic drugs or chemicals.[26] Clinical signs seen in animals with right-sided heart failure and ascites may include weight loss, anorexia, exercise intolerance, cough, tachycardia, weak femoral pulses, pulse deficits, cyanosis, jugular pulses, venous distention, muffled heart and lung sounds, hepatomegaly, cardiac murmurs, or gallop rhythms.[49, 61] If hypoalbuminemia is the cause of ascites, the animal may have peripheral edema, muffled heart and lung sounds (pleural effusion), chronic vomiting or diarrhea, polyuria and polydipsia, weight loss, anorexia, or the signs associated with liver disease (listed previously).[49] Neoplastic ascites may be associated with a palpable abdominal mass or a history of vomiting, diarrhea, weight loss, anorexia, and lethargy.

Diagnostic Plan

Animals with ascites are usually presented to the veterinarian with a complaint of abdominal distention (Table 34–2) or for evaluation of one of the obvious associated clinical signs (e.g., vomiting, diarrhea, icterus, polyuria and polydipsia).[49] Detection of a fluid wave by ballottement (tapping the abdominal wall on one side and feeling waves of fluid movement on the other side[49]) during careful abdominal palpation identifies the presence of fluid within the abdominal cavity.

A sample of fluid should be collected (see Abdominocentesis) and analyzed for total protein, nucleated cell count, and cytologic differential, and a sample should be saved for bacterial culture.[50] Ascitic fluid is clear, has a total protein less than 3.5 g/dL

(often < 2.5 g/dL[61]), and has fewer than 5000 nucleated cells, with mononuclear cells predominating. A fluid with a very low total protein (<2.5 g/dL) and few nucleated cells (<1000) is found in cases of hypoproteinemia.[49] Exudative conditions can easily be distinguished by their high protein content (>3.5 g/dL) and their high nucleated cell count (>5000), often with a high percentage of degenerate neutrophils and, in some cases, bacteria. Chylous effusions are pink or creamy white and contain large quantities of triglycerides.[62] Hemorrhagic effusions are red and have a high RBC count.

Once the presence of ascites is confirmed by fluid analysis, the diagnostic plan is dependent on the clinical signs identified in the history and physical examination. If cardiovascular disease is suspected, an occult heartworm test, thoracic radiography, electrocardiography, and echocardiography should be performed. Depending on the results of these tests, pericardiocentesis may be indicated. If evidence of liver disease is present, a laboratory minimum database should be evaluated.[61] Liver function should be evaluated with either an ammonia tolerance test or determination of serum bile acids.[61] Hepatic ultrasonography can be very beneficial in describing the contour and texture of the liver.[61] After a coagulation profile has been evaluated, hepatic biopsy helps to identify the specific disease process.[61]

If severe hypoalbuminemia (<1.5 g/dL) is identified on the biochemical profile, glomerular disease, liver failure, or protein-losing gastroenteropathy is probably present.[60] Initial evaluation of renal function should include urinalysis and determination of serum urea nitrogen, creatinine, and electrolyte values. If proteinuria is detected, calculation of the ratio of urine protein to creatinine, renal ultrasonography, and renal biopsy may be indicated (see Chap. 16). The presence of diarrhea suggests the need for multiple fecal examinations to detect gastrointestinal parasites,

Table 34–2
Causes of Abdominal Enlargement

Ascites
Extreme obesity
Pregnancy
Canine Cushing's disease
Splenomegaly
Hepatomegaly
Gastric distention
Pyometra
Obstipation
Urinary obstruction
Small intestinal obstruction
Intra-abdominal neoplasia

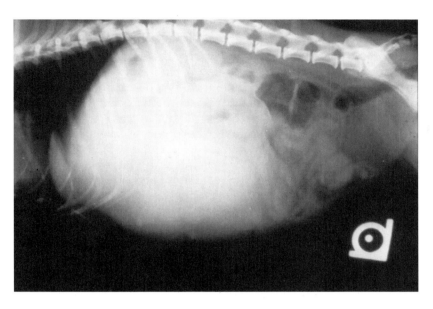

Figure 34-3
Lateral abdominal radiograph of a dog showing massive hepatomegaly caused by a hepatocellular carcinoma. Hepatomegaly was detected on physical examination.

D-xylose testing, determinations of serum vitamin B_{12} and folic acid concentrations, and mucosal biopsy by endoscopy or exploratory laparotomy (see Chap. 32). If signs of liver disease are present, or if renal or gastrointestinal disease cannot be found, evaluation of the liver should be performed as described previously.

Failure to identify the underlying cause of ascites should prompt the search for an occult intra-abdominal neoplasm. If careful abdominal palpation does not reveal an intra-abdominal mass, abdominal ultrasonography may identify one. Abdominal radiography in the presence of abdominal fluid is usually not rewarding, but removal of most of the fluid before radiography may increase the diagnostic yield.[49] Finally, exploratory laparotomy may be indicated to locate the underlying neoplasm.

Hepatomegaly

Hepatomegaly is defined as enlargement of the liver. It is a problem that is identified most commonly during physical examination. However, in some cases it is discovered during radiography, ultrasonography, or exploratory laparotomy (Fig. 34-3).

Pathophysiology

The most common causes of hepatomegaly are vascular congestion (right-sided congestive heart failure), infiltration of inflammatory or neoplastic cells, excessive storage of lipid (hepatic lipidosis) or glycogen (steroid hepatopathy), hepatocyte inflammation (canine infectious hepatitis), and Kupffer cell hyperplasia (systemic mycosis).[63–71] The enlargement can be diffuse or focal. Clinical signs are not caused by the excessive hepatic size but are related to the effects of the underlying disease on liver function or

other body systems (e.g., thin skin in hyperadreno-corticism).

Clinical Signs

In some cases, hepatomegaly can be present without any clinical signs. If clinical signs occur, they include the signs of liver diseases (anorexia, weight loss, pyrexia, vomiting, diarrhea, abdominal distention, encephalopathy, icterus, polyuria and polydipsia, bruising or bleeding tendencies) or the systemic effects of nonhepatic disorders that cause hepatomegaly. Clinical signs in animals with right-sided heart failure include weight loss, anorexia, exercise intolerance, cough, tachycardia, weak femoral pulses, pulse deficits, cyanosis, jugular pulses, venous distention, muffled heart and lung sounds, cardiac murmurs, and gallop rhythms.[49, 61, 66] Dogs with steroid hepatopathy (iatrogenic or secondary to hyperadreno-corticism) may have polyuria and polydipsia, alopecia, polyphagia, thin skin, pot-bellied appearance, and recurrent urinary tract and skin infections.[63, 71] Animals with hepatomegaly caused by systemic mycosis commonly have weight loss, anorexia, pyrexia, tachypnea, cough, and vomiting or diarrhea (see Chap. 39).[64, 65]

Diagnostic Plan

Normally, the liver lies within the costal arch and cannot be palpated. If the liver can be felt during physical examination, it should be considered to be enlarged, and hepatomegaly is present. If a cranial abdominal mass is detected but it is not possible to determine whether it is the liver, the spleen, or something else, abdominal radiographs or ultrasound can help make the distinction. There is less merging of the silhouettes of the liver and spleen on a left lateral abdominal radiograph than on a right lateral view.[72] Radiographically, generalized hepatomegaly is characterized by projection of the liver caudal to the costal arch, caudal displacement of the stomach, or enlargement and rounding of the caudal liver margin (see Fig. 34–3).[73] Localized hepatic enlargement is radiographically characterized by caudal displacement of the fundus (left side), caudal displacement of the ventral fundus and gastric body (central), and displacement of the right kidney, duodenum, pyloric antrum, and gastric body (right side).[73] Administration of a small volume of barium helps to outline the stomach (Fig. 34–4).

The significance of mild hepatic enlargement detected on abdominal radiographs but not found during careful abdominal palpation is questionable. Various radiographic and ultrasonographic methods have been studied to objectively quantitate liver size.[72, 74–77] Some studies have revealed measurements and ratios that can help assess the radiographic size of the liver.[75–77] However, unless veterinarians use these measurements frequently, unreliable information may be obtained. If a suspicion of mild hepatomegaly is detected radiographically or ultrasonographically (with normal-appearing parenchyma) but clinical signs of liver disease, congestive heart failure, hyperadrenalcorticism, or systemic mycosis are not present, no further diagnostic evaluation is indicated. The animal should be reassessed in 3 months, or sooner if clinical signs develop.

After hepatomegaly is identified, the diagnostic approach is determined by the presence of additional signs suggesting liver disease, right-sided congestive heart failure, hyperadrenalcorticism, or systemic mycosis. Abdominal radiographs can help determine whether focal or diffuse involvement is present. Ultrasonography is very useful to rank the differential diagnoses. A high index of suspicion can be obtained for lipidosis, metastatic neoplasia, lymphosarcoma, steroid hepatopathy, and primary neoplasia (Fig. 34–5).[42, 44–46, 78]

If clinical signs of liver disease are present, a diagnostic plan should include CBC, biochemical profile, urinalysis, FeLV and FIV ELISAs in cats, measurement of serum ammonia and ammonia tolerance or bile acids, abdominocentesis and fluid analysis (if ascites is suspected), hepatic ultrasound, coagulation profile, and liver biopsy using the least invasive method available.

If clinical signs of right-sided congestive heart failure are present, the diagnostic plan should include thoracic radiography, an occult heartworm test, electrocardiography, and echocardiography (see Chaps. 9 and 10). Depending on these results, pericardiocentesis (see Chap. 15) may be indicated.

The diagnostic plan for potential steroid hepatopathy should include a CBC, a biochemical profile, urinalysis, an abdominal ultrasound, and an adrenocorticotropic hormone response test (see Chap. 46). If systemic mycosis is suspected, a complete ocular examination (see Chap. 19), CBC, biochemical profile, urinalysis, and thoracic radiographs should be performed (see Chap. 39). In many instances, diagnosis is based on identification of the organism in either a cytologic sample of a percutaneous fine-needle aspirate of the lungs or a liver biopsy specimen. Before hepatic biopsy is performed, the results of hepatic ultrasound and a coagulation panel should be assessed.

Figure 34–4
Lateral abdominal radiograph of the dog in Figure 34–3 after administration of a small volume of barium sulfate. The stomach and pylorus are displaced dorsally.

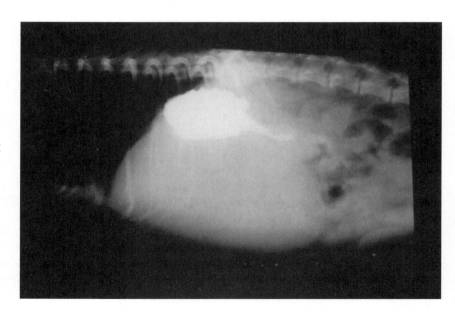

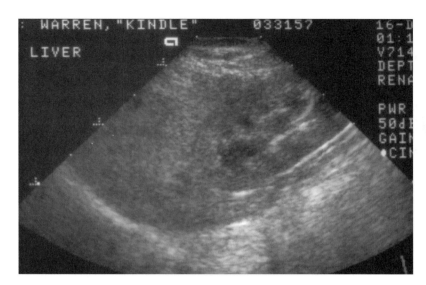

Figure 34-5
Longitudinal ultrasonographic appearance of steroid hepatopathy in an 11-year-old toy poodle. Patchy hyperechoic areas are present throughout the liver. The right kidney is on the left side of the photograph. The ultrasonographic pattern is consistent with many diffuse hepatic disorders. (Courtesy of Martha L. Moon, DVM, MS, Blacksburg, Virginia.)

Hepatic Encephalopathy

Hepatic encephalopathy is a syndrome associated with neurologic signs caused by the failure of the liver (because of severe disease or portosystemic shunting) to properly metabolize nutrients or toxins.[22, 79-81] These nutrients or toxins circulate in blood and enter the central nervous system (CNS), where they interfere with neural function and neurotransmission.

Pathophysiology

The pathophysiology of hepatic encephalopathy is complex and incompletely understood.[22, 80] The diseased liver is unable to remove toxins from portal blood and to properly perform metabolic functions.[22] In cases with portosystemic shunting, the liver does not receive all of the portal blood flow, so it cannot adequately perform its metabolic activities. Abnormal substances or substances in altered concentrations circulate in blood and affect the blood-brain barrier or enter the CNS and interfere with neurotransmission, alter membrane activity, or affect metabolism.[79, 82] Normal neurotransmission is decreased because of reduced concentrations of neurotransmitters or reduced receptor density.[79] Hepatic encephalopathy is a reversible metabolic condition (i.e., histologic changes are minimal) if hepatic function can be improved or portosystemic shunting attenuated.[79, 80, 83] Although many substances are believed to participate, only a few clinically relevant and illustrative toxins are described here.

Ammonia

Ammonia is produced by metabolism of protein by intestinal bacteria, the action of bacterial urease on urea, and hepatic metabolism of proteins and amino acids.[19, 22] Un-ionized ammonia from the intestines readily crosses cell membranes and enters portal circulation. In health, 90% is removed by the liver, which uses it for amino acid synthesis and metabolism to urea by the urea cycle.[9, 17, 19] With hepatic disease or portosystemic shunting, the liver is unable to remove the ammonia, and it accumulates in blood.[17] Ammonia concentration does not correlate with the degree of encephalopathy.[22, 80] The exact mechanisms causing encephalopathy are unknown, but ammonia is neurotoxic.[19, 22, 79, 84]

Other toxins involved in hepatic encephalopathy, mercaptans and short-chain fatty acids decrease the conversion of ammonia to urea. Alkalosis increases intestinal absorption of ammonia and increases the entry of ammonia into the CNS.[80] Azotemia increases ammonia production because of increased urea concentrations that can be metabolized by urease-containing bacteria.[22] Gastrointestinal hemorrhage also increases ammonia production because more protein is available for bacterial metabolism.[22] Stored blood products contain increased levels of ammonia.[22] Arginine is an essential amino acid in cats; anorexia results in decreased arginine availability for the urea cycle and decreased urea production, promoting hyperammonemia.[19] Therefore, anorexia associated with hepatic diseases in cats can worsen signs of hepatic encephalopathy.

Ammonia metabolism within the CNS depletes levels of α-ketoglutamate, which is necessary for normal CNS metabolism, and results in increased glutamine.[22, 80] This contributes to altered CNS amino acid concentrations and leads to abnormal neurotransmitter synthesis.[82]

Amino Acids

The liver plays a central role in the maintenance of plasma amino acid levels. Normally, a ratio of approximately 3:1 of branched chain to aromatic amino acids is found in blood. The ratio can approach 1:1 in animals with chronic liver disease as hepatic catabolism of aromatic amino acids is reduced.[12, 22, 84–87] Reduced hepatic metabolism of insulin and glucagon also participate. Because amino acids cross the blood-brain barrier in proportion to plasma levels, liver disease results in increased CNS concentration of aromatic amino acids.[22, 80] Increased concentrations of aromatic amino acids are used to synthesize inhibitory transmitters, which contribute to clinical signs of encephalopathy.[79]

γ-Aminobutyric Acid

γ-Aminobutyric acid (GABA) is one of the most potent inhibitory neurotransmitters.[22, 82, 84] Increased CNS metabolism of ammonia causes increased GABA production. In hepatic encephalopathy, increased GI bacterial production of GABA occurs. Normally, increased concentrations would be removed by the liver, but increased serum levels occur with liver disease and portosystemic shunts.[22, 84] In addition, increased passage through the blood-brain barrier occurs.[82] Increased concentrations of GABA contribute to some of the clinical signs of encephalopathy.

The GABA receptor is complexed with a receptor for benzodiazepines and barbiturates.[79, 80, 84] Treatment with diazepam or barbiturates can inhibit neurotransmission and worsen the signs of encephalopathy.[22]

Mercaptans

Mercaptans are formed from bacterial metabolism of sulfur-containing amino acids in the GI tract.[22, 79, 80] The liver normally removes these toxins from portal blood. With hepatic disease, increased levels of mercaptans circulate in blood and can induce coma.[22, 79] Increased levels of short-chain fatty acids and ammonia decrease hepatic metabolism of mercaptans.

Several "liver-sparing" drugs or dietary supplements contain methionine, which can be metabolized into mercaptans.[84] The classic response to criticism that these drugs were not beneficial in treating liver disease was that they caused no harm. However, an understanding of the pathophysiology of hepatic encephalopathy clearly demonstrates the risk associated with administration of large dosages of these potential toxins. These drugs should not be used in dogs or cats with hepatic disease.[24]

Short-Chain Fatty Acids

Short-chain fatty acids (5, 6, or 8 carbon atoms) are normally removed by the liver from portal blood and metabolized. Increased serum levels occur in liver disease. They have a barbiturate-like effect. Increased levels also interfere with the detoxification of ammonia and mercaptans.[22]

Clinical Signs

Clinical signs can be associated with acute hepatic failure, chronic hepatic disease, or portosystemic shunts.[22] The clinical signs of hepatic encephalopathy vary. They occur suddenly and are rapidly progressive in patients with acute hepatic failure.[22, 83] In chronic disease, signs are often episodic and may worsen after ingestion of a high-protein meal, development of GI bleeding or azotemia, or administration of sedatives or anesthetics.[22, 83] Animals may appear normal between episodes. Clinical signs include weakness, ataxia, stupor, head pressing, circling, pacing, blindness, ptyalism, behavioral changes, dementia, hysteria, aggression, seizures, and coma.[22, 24, 83]

In addition to the neurologic changes, clinical signs of the underlying hepatic disease can be present; they include anorexia, weight loss, pyrexia, vomiting, diarrhea, abdominal distention, icterus, polyuria and polydipsia, and bruising or bleeding tendencies.[22, 24, 83]

Diagnostic Plan

A complete neurologic examination should be performed to localize the lesions. Whenever signs of diffuse cerebral cortical disease are present, hepatic encephalopathy should be considered in the differential diagnosis. A high index of suspicion of hepatic disease can be reached after reviewing the results of a laboratory minimum database. Abnormalities suggesting liver disease include poikilocytosis, microcytic anemia, elevated AP and ALT, hyperbilirubinemia, hyperammonemia, hypoalbuminemia, low blood urea nitrogen (BUN), bilirubinuria, and ammonium biurate crystalluria.[24, 83] The minimum database helps to rule out other metabolic conditions that can cause similar signs, such as hypoglycemia, hyperglycemic coma, uremia, and polycythemia. If liver disease is suspected, further evaluation should include liver function tests (bile acids or ammonia tolerance), hepatic ultrasound, and liver biopsy (after assessing coagulation).[24, 83] If metabolic disorders are ruled out, further evaluation should include analysis of the cerebrospinal fluid.[83] There are many neurologic causes of encephalopathy including bacterial, viral, fungal, and protozoal encephalitis; neoplasia; thiamine deficiency; hydrocephalus; ischemic encephalopathy; and lead toxicity (see Chap. 24).

Vomiting

Vomiting (see Chap. 31) commonly occurs in animals with acute or chronic liver disease. Chronic gastritis or gastric or duodenal ulcer disease may be present in patients with liver disease.[88, 89] Abnormal metabolism of GI peptides or stimulation of the chemoreceptor trigger zone by circulating toxins associated with hepatic encephalopathy may be involved in the pathophysiology.[90]

In a vomiting dog or cat, liver disease should be suspected if some of the following clinical signs are also present: anorexia, weight loss, pyrexia, diarrhea, abdominal distention, encephalopathy, icterus, polyuria or polydipsia, or bruising or bleeding tendencies. Confirmation of liver disease can be found on a laboratory minimum database: elevated AP and ALT, hyperbilirubinemia, reduced BUN, hypoalbuminemia, anemia, and bilirubinuria. A further diagnostic plan includes determination of ammonia and ammonia tolerance or serum bile acids, hepatic ultrasound, coagulation profile, and hepatic biopsy by the least invasive method available.

Coagulopathy

Because the liver synthesizes most of the coagulation factors, animals with liver disease can hemorrhage as a result of factor deficiency.[91] Prolonged bile duct obstruction can lead to fat malabsorption and vitamin K deficiency. Vitamin K is necessary for activation of coagulation factors II, VII, IX, and X. Some liver diseases are also associated with platelet function defects. In most cases of liver disease, spontaneous hemorrhage does not occur, but the tendency to hemorrhage is increased.[67, 91–93] Prolonged bleeding from venipuncture sites, excessive hemorrhage after intravenous catheterization or biopsy procedures, bleeding into the GI tract from gastritis or ulcers (hematemesis and melena), and bruising associated with minor trauma can occur.

Disseminated intravascular coagulation (DIC) may accompany liver disease and promote hemorrhagic tendencies because of thrombocytopenia and additional coagulation factor deficiency. Hemorrhage can occur within most organs. Bleeding is often observed from skin and mucous membranes, and into the eye, joints, and body cavities. Epistaxis, hematemesis, melena, hematochezia, and hematoma formation commonly occur.[94] Causes of DIC in liver disease include release of thromboplastic substances from damaged hepatocytes, decreased clearance of endotoxins and activated coagulation factors, reduced anti-thrombin III, and stagnation of blood in mesenteric circulation.[4] Further evaluation of coagulation should include a platelet count, prothrombin time, partial thromboplastin time, mucosal bleeding time, and measurement of fibrinogen, fibrin degradation products, and antithrombin III (see Chap. 44).

Liver disease should be suspected if coagulation defects are associated with other clinical signs that suggest liver disease (i.e., anorexia, weight loss, pyrexia, vomiting, diarrhea, abdominal distention, encephalopathy, icterus, or polyuria and polydipsia). Confirmation of liver disease can be found on a laboratory minimum database: elevated AP and ALT, hyperbilirubinemia, hypoalbuminemia, reduced BUN, anemia, and bilirubinuria. A further diagnostic plan includes determination of ammonia and ammonia tolerance or serum bile acids, hepatic ultrasound, and hepatic biopsy by the least invasive method available.

Polyuria and Polydipsia

Increased water consumption with increased urine volume (see Chap. 16) occurs in animals with liver disease.[92, 95] The pathogenesis may involve decreased urea production from ammonia (decreased medullary hypertonicity), decreased metabolism of aldosterone (sodium and water retention), decreased metabolism of cortisol (polyuria), psychogenic polydipsia, alterations in portal vein osmoreceptors, or potassium depletion.[96, 97]

Liver disease should be suspected if some of the following clinical signs are also present: anorexia, weight loss, pyrexia, vomiting, diarrhea, icterus, abdominal distention, encephalopathy, icterus, or bruising or bleeding tendencies. Confirmation of liver disease can be found on a laboratory minimum database: elevated AP and ALT, hyperbilirubinemia, hypoalbuminemia, reduced BUN, anemia, and bilirubinuria. A further diagnostic plan includes determination of ammonia and ammonia tolerance or serum bile acids, hepatic ultrasound, coagulation profile, and hepatic biopsy by the least invasive method available.

Diagnostic Procedures

The accurate diagnosis of hepatobiliary disorders requires a thorough and logical diagnostic plan.[25] Suspicion of hepatobiliary disease may be based on clinical signs (anorexia, weight loss, pyrexia, vomiting, diarrhea, icterus, abdominal distention, encephalopathy, icterus, polyuria and polydipsia, or bruising or bleeding tendencies) or on evidence obtained on a routine CBC, biochemical profile, and urinalysis (elevated AP and ALT, hyperbilirubinemia, hypoalbuminemia, reduced BUN, anemia, and bilirubinuria).

Many times benefit is obtained from the use of hepatic function tests (i.e., ammonia and ammonia tolerance or serum bile acids). Ultrasonographic evaluation has developed into a vital diagnostic procedure. After a coagulation panel has been obtained, a liver biopsy by the least invasive method available is indicated in most patients.

One of the major difficulties encountered during evaluation of hepatobiliary diseases is the presence of secondary hepatic disease, wherein the liver is an innocent bystander.[11] The liver's central role in metabolism, dual blood supply (it receives approximately 25% of cardiac output through the portal blood flow and arterial supply), and active reticuloendothelial function promote the development of secondary liver disease with associated laboratory abnormalities.[25] Because 70% to 80% of hepatic function must be compromised before clinical signs occur, many primary disorders result in only biochemical evidence of hepatic dysfunction.[11] A thorough diagnostic plan helps to identify the underlying primary disease in these cases.

Routine Laboratory Evaluation

Complete Blood Count

A nonregenerative anemia may be present as a result of chronic inflammatory disease.[17] A regenerative anemia may occur secondary to blood loss. With chronic GI blood loss, this can develop into a nonregenerative, microcytic, hypochromic anemia as a result of iron deficiency. Hypoproteinemia may be present because of decreased production of albumin and many globulins or because of hemorrhage. Hyperproteinemia may be associated with dehydration or inflammation associated with decreased reticuloendothelial function. A leukocytosis characterized by a neutrophilia with or without a left shift is often present, associated with inflammation within the liver.[17] Abnormal RBC morphology may be present in some hepatic diseases (i.e., target or spur cells). Microcytosis may occur with congenital portosystemic shunts in dogs.[98–100]

Biochemical Profile

Hepatic Enzymes

Although there are many hepatic enzymes that can be measured in serum, in most cases only ALT and AP are very beneficial in the evaluation of hepatobiliary diseases. A third enzyme, γ-glutamyl transpeptidase (GGT), has received a great deal of attention in the literature, and is briefly discussed here.

Alanine Aminotransferase. ALT, formerly called serum glutamic-pyruvic transaminase (SGPT), is contained within the hepatocyte cytoplasm at levels 10,000 times greater than in serum.[34, 101] Although it is present in low levels in other tissues, increased serum concentrations are usually secondary to hepatic disease.[18, 101] Rarely, mild serum increases may be caused by muscle necrosis.[102] This enzyme leaks into serum because of increased permeability of hepatocellular membranes.[34] The concentration in serum is proportional to the number of hepatocytes affected.[9, 34] Serum levels often remain elevated 2 to 4 days after an acute insult.[101] There is also increased release of ALT during hepatocellular repair.[34] Persistently elevated levels indicate ongoing leakage.[34]

Although it is released from necrotic hepatocytes, elevated serum concentration of ALT indicates not irreversible necrosis but only hepatocellular leakage.[101] Corticosteroids can induce hepatic production of ALT and can produce pathologic changes (steroid hepatopathy) that cause leakage.[101] Measurement of ALT is considered highly specific but only moderately sensitive for detection of hepatobiliary diseases.[103] It is therefore possible to have hepatobiliary disease without increased serum ALT.[48]

Alkaline Phosphatase. AP is bound to cytoplasmic and microsomal membranes within the epithelial cells of the bile ducts, ductules, periportal bile canaliculi, and sinusoids.[17, 104, 105] Production is increased in the presence of cholestasis, perhaps because of the effects of retained bile acids.[17, 103, 104, 106–111] In general, extrahepatic cholestasis is associated with higher levels of AP than is intrahepatic disease.[48] Corticosteroids induce production of a unique isoenzyme from the liver in dogs.[17, 18, 34, 103, 104, 109, 112] Elevated serum AP can persist long after corticosteroid administration.[9] Corticosteroids and anticonvulsants can also induce production of the liver isoenzyme.[17, 18, 104, 112–115]

AP is contained in various other tissues. However, because of very short serum halflives, increased serum concentrations occur only as a result of cholestasis, corticosteroid induction, or bone lysis (levels are usually increased only twofold to fivefold with bony lysis).[17, 104, 112] Young, growing animals have slightly increased serum levels of AP because of osteoblast activity.[17, 34, 104, 112]

Cats differ from dogs in several respects: the halflife of AP in cats is only 6 hours, versus 3 days in dogs; the total liver content is 50% less in cats; and there is no corticosteroid isoenzyme.[9, 17, 34] Any elevation of serum AP in a cat should be considered significant and investigated further. Elevations in serum AP precede bilirubinuria and hyperbilirubinemia in dogs and cats with cholestatic disease.

In several studies, it has been shown that serum AP has poor specificity but high sensitivity (few false-negative results) in hepatobiliary diseases in dogs.[116] However, in cats it has high specificity (few false-positive results) but lower sensitivity.[117] Concurrent evaluation of GGT has been shown to increase the specificity in dogs and the sensitivity in cats.[116, 117] Although it is possible to measure the corticosteroid-induced isoenzyme, it has limited diagnostic significance.[118]

γ-Glutamyl Transpeptidase. GGT is a membrane-bound enzyme contained in high concentrations in the kidney, pancreas, and small intestine and in lower amounts in the liver.[34, 119, 120] Serum increases in dogs and cats are caused by cholestatic liver disease or, in dogs, by induction by corticosteroids and possibly anticonvulsants.[17, 18, 34, 107–110, 119] It is not contained in bone.

I have not found this enzyme to be particularly useful when evaluating dogs and cats with hepatobiliary disorders. It often parallels serum AP activity. However, other authors have found it useful because it may be more sensitive (fewer false-negative results) in the cat and more specific (fewer false-positive results) in the dog for detecting hepatobiliary disorders.[9, 17, 34, 116, 117, 121] Concurrent evaluation of both AP and GGT provides greater sensitivity in the detection of hepatobiliary disorders in cats and greater specificity in dogs.[116, 117]

Bilirubin

Bilirubin is a waste product of RBC metabolism that has major diagnostic implications in animals with hepatobiliary diseases (see Icterus). Most bilirubin is derived from the normal breakdown process of hemoglobin from senescent RBCs.[17, 26–28, 122, 123] Hemoglobin is phagocytosed by the reticuloendothelial system and converted into bilirubin.[26] It is bound to albumin and transported to the liver, where it is taken up by the hepatocyte, conjugated with glucuronic acid, and secreted into bile canaliculi by active transport, which is the rate-limiting step.[17, 26–28, 122, 124] Bile is stored within the gallbladder until feeding, when it enters the duodenum. Bacterial metabolism occurs in the small intestine and produces several urobilins.[27, 123] One of these, urobilinogen, is reabsorbed within the small intestine, but most of it is removed from the portal blood by the liver and excreted back into bile.[17, 27, 28, 122] Urobilinogen, which remains in circulation, is removed by the kidney. In dogs, the renal tubules can convert hemoglobin to bilirubin, conjugate it, and excrete it into the urine.[122, 124] Urobilinogen remaining within the bowel may be passed in the feces or metabolized to stercobilins, which impart color to the feces.[26, 28, 123] Cats differ from dogs in that their renal threshold is considerably higher, and bilirubinuria does not occur in normal cats.[26, 124, 125]

Elevated serum bilirubin is commonly found in hemolytic disease and in intrahepatic or extrahepatic cholestasis.[48, 111, 126] In general, higher levels are found in patients with extrahepatic cholestasis than in those with intrahepatic cholestasis.[48] However, it is possible to have normal serum bilirubin in a variety of hepatobiliary disorders.[48, 126] In cholestatic disorders, elevated serum AP occurs before any changes in bilirubin metabolism in both dogs and cats. As the cholestatic process progresses, bilirubinuria precedes hyperbilirubinemia in dogs, but hyperbilirubinemia precedes bilirubinuria in cats. Icteric plasma can usually be detected after bilirubin reaches 1.5 to 2.0 mg/dL.[28] Serum bilirubin level must be higher than 2.5 to 3.0 mg/dL to reveal clinical icterus. Although it is possible to measure conjugated levels (and thereby determine unconjugated levels) with the van den Bergh test, I have found little clinical significance for this test.

Albumin

Albumin is synthesized entirely within the liver.[9] It is the major contributor to osmotic pressure within the circulation and serves as a carrier and transport protein. Decreased synthesis is associated with very severe hepatic dysfunction.[9, 17, 18] Because the halflife is 7 to 10 days, severe hypoalbuminemia does not commonly accompany acute liver disease.[18] Decreased albumin contributes to the formation of ascites and can cause ascites if serum levels become lower than 1.0 to 1.5 g/dL.[18] Other causes of hypoalbuminemia include glomerular diseases and protein-losing enteropathy.

Globulins

The liver synthesizes most serum globulins, except for immunoglobulins.[17, 18] Thus, with severe liver disease, the serum concentration of many globulins is decreased. However, in severe hepatic diseases, the serum concentration of total globulins is often normal or increased.[17] Inflammation associated with hepatic disease or immune stimulation that occurs because the liver is not performing its reticuloendothelial function causes increased synthesis of immunoglobulins, increasing the total serum concentration of globulins.[18]

Coagulation Profile

Most animals with hepatobiliary disease have normal prothrombin and partial thromboplastin times.[93] However, because the liver synthesizes most coagulation factors, their serum levels are reduced.[91] The sensitivity of prothrombin and partial thromboplastin times can be increased by dilution of the plasma, which often results in prolongation.[93] If DIC develops (see Coagulopathy), prolongation of undiluted prothrombin and partial thrombo-plastin times is common, as are thrombocytopenia, hypofibrinogenemia, and elevated fibrin degradation products. Prolonged biliary obstruction can lead to vitamin K deficiency and prolongation of the pro-thrombin and partial thromboplastin times.[9, 17]

Urea Nitrogen

The BUN may be elevated in animals with hepatobiliary disease because of dehydration. With severe hepatic disease, the BUN may be reduced because of decreased conversion of ammonia to urea in the urea cycle.[9, 17, 34] Decreased renal medullary urea concentration may promote polyuria, which is associ-ated with some liver diseases.

Glucose

Because of the liver's central role in the metabo-lism of carbohydrates, hypoglycemia can be present in animals with severe liver disease or portosystemic shunts.[12, 18, 34] It may be caused by reduced glycogen storage or by decreased gluconeogenesis or glyco-genolysis.[12] Hypoglycemia may also be associated with hepatocellular adenomas as a paraneoplastic syndrome.[70]

Cholesterol

The liver is the major site of cholesterol synthe-sis and excretion.[17] Serum cholesterol can be normal, decreased, or increased in animals with hepatobiliary diseases. Increased levels can be associated with cholestasis as a result of decreased excretion and increased production.[17, 111] Decreased levels may be caused by decreased synthesis, malabsorption of fat from the small intestine, or increased synthesis of bile acids.[17]

Urinalysis

Bilirubinuria often occurs in dogs and cats with hepatobiliary disorders. Slight bilirubinuria in dogs, especially in concentrated urine, is normal. Biliru-binuria is always abnormal in cats, because they have a higher threshold for bilirubin excretion than dogs.[26, 124, 125]

The presence of urobilinogen in the urine indicates at least partial patency of the biliary system. However, the absence of urobilinogen is not indicative of complete biliary obstruction; it can occur because of altered GI flora, diarrhea, dilute urine, acid urine, or exposure of urine to light.[17]

Bilirubin crystals can often be seen in the urine of animals with hepatobiliary disorders. Ammonium biurate crystals can occur in animals with portosys-temic shunts.[127, 128]

Bile Acids

Measurement of total serum bile acids has been shown to be a very effective test (with high sensitivity and specificity) of hepatobiliary dysfunction in dogs and cats.[48, 103, 126, 129–132] Values in excess of established cutoff levels (which, in one laboratory, were fasting, >20 µmol/L in dogs and >15 µmol/L in cats, and post-prandial, >25 µmol/L in dogs and >20 µmol/L in cats) indicate the need for hepatic biopsy and suggest that morphologic changes will be histologically identi-fied.[34, 103, 129, 130] Serum should be collected after food has been withheld for 12 hours and 2 hours after feed-ing a small meal (Prescription Diet c/d in cats and p/d in dogs).[103] Serum bile acids that are increased above a laboratory's established normal (or cutoff) values indi-cate hepatic dysfunction, portosystemic shunting, or cholestasis.[103, 133] It is not necessary to measure serum bile acids in an animal with icterus caused by hepatic or posthepatic cholestasis; in these cases, assessment of serum bilirubin provides similar information.[34] Al-though determination of serum bile acids does not distinguish between the types of hepatobiliary dis-eases, certain trends have been identified.[15, 133] Ani-mals with portosystemic shunts and cirrhosis can have relatively low fasting values but have very elevated postprandial levels (>200 µmol/L). Those with bile duct obstruction have very high fasting and postpran-dial levels (250 µmol/L). Moderately high fasting lev-els (125 µmol/L) that increase only slightly after feed-ing are characteristic of intrahepatic cholestasis.

To understand the implications of abnormal bile acids, it is important to review physiology. Bile acids are synthesized in the liver from cholesterol.[15, 18] The most common ones are cholic acid and chenodeox-ycholic acid.[15, 103] They are conjugated with taurine and excreted into bile.[15] In the small intestine, they aid in the digestion and absorption of fat.[15] They assist lipid assimilation as they move down the small bowel toward the ileum, where 95% are absorbed by active transport.[15, 18, 103] They are bound to plasma proteins and transported to the liver in the portal blood. They are extracted by the liver (often the step that fails in liver disease), reconjugated, and re-secreted into bile.[17, 103] The bile acid pool may recirculate two or three times per meal. Serum levels remain stable in health. Bile acids not reabsorbed in the ileum are metabolized by colonic bacteria to secondary acids, deoxycholate and lithocholate.[15] These secondary acids become toxic in large amounts and can cause diarrhea.

Ammonia

Measurement of blood ammonia with fasting or after ammonium chloride challenge is a useful test of hepatic function.[103] Difficult sample handling has limited its usefulness in practice. With the growth of in-office dry chemistry analyzers, many of the problems previously experienced can be avoided. A fasting blood sample should always be analyzed before a tolerance test is performed because, if ammonia is elevated, hepatic dysfunction is present and a challenge test is not necessary. If the fasting sample is within laboratory-established normal values, a challenge test should be performed. Ammonium chloride, 100 mg/kg, mixed into a 5% solution, should be given by orogastric intubation. A blood sample should be collected 30 minutes later. Levels after challenge should return to within 130% of baseline values.[17] Hyperammonemia indicates hepatic dysfunction or portosystemic shunting. Blood samples should be placed on ice after collection and analyzed within 30 minutes.[9, 17] One additional reason practitioners have been hesitant to perform ammonia challenge testing is the possibility of potentiating hepatic encephalopathy with the administered ammonia. In my experience, this is an extremely rare event, and the risk is offset by the beneficial information gained about hepatic function.[134, 135] If vomiting is present or orogastric intubation is too difficult to perform, ammonium chloride can be given rectally, 30 minutes after an enema; 2 mL/kg of a 5% solution is infused, and blood samples measured at 20 and 40 minutes[135] (see Hepatic Encephalopathy).

Radiography

Standard preparation for abdominal radiography should include withholding of food for 12 hours (empty stomach) and administration of a warm-water enema (20 mL/kg) to cleanse the colon.[73] Survey abdominal radiographs may detect hepatomegaly (see Fig. 34–3), microhepatica, loss of intra-abdominal detail because of ascites or carcinomatosis, or, occasionally, radiopaque choleliths.[73, 136, 137] Generalized hepatomegaly is characterized by projection of the liver caudal to the costal arch, caudal displacement of the stomach, or enlargement and rounding of the caudal liver margin.[73] A small liver may be associated with a reduced distance between the diaphragm and the stomach, cranial displacement of the stomach, vertical or cranial angle to the stomach (instead of being parallel to the ribs), or cranial displacement of the pyloric antrum.[73] Localized hepatic enlargement is characterized by caudal displacement of the fundus (left side), caudal displacement of the ventral fundus and gastric body (central), and displacement of the right kidney, duodenum, pyloric antrum, and gastric body (right side).[73] Administration of a small volume of barium helps to outline the stomach (see Fig. 34–4).

Radiographs may also help identify a cranial abdominal mass detected on physical examination as being either liver or spleen.[72] Survey radiographs can also help eliminate disorders of other organs that can cause signs similar to liver disease (e.g., vomiting caused by gastric or intestinal foreign body).

Because of breed variation, positioning, and respiration, radiographic assessment of hepatic size is subjective and often imprecise.[73] Numerous radiographic studies have been conducted to investigate objective criteria of liver size.[72, 75–77] Some of these studies have proposed measurements and ratios that can help the clinician to objectively assess the radiographic size of the liver (see Hepatomegaly).

Ultrasonography

Abdominal ultrasonography has become an invaluable diagnostic tool for the assessment of hepatobiliary disorders in dogs and cats.[73, 138] Abnormalities in hepatic size, shape, and architecture, parenchymal echogenicity, or blood vessels (portosystemic shunt) and distention of the gallbladder, cystic duct, common bile duct, and hepatic ducts can be noninvasively detected.[7, 36, 37, 42, 43, 45–47, 78, 139] Ultrasonographic examination is probably the best way to differentiate between hepatic and posthepatic icterus (see Icterus).[37] Ultrasound-guided hepatic biopsy has become the procedure of choice to obtain a liver biopsy (see Hepatic Biopsy) because it is easy, safe, and rapid to perform and allows guided sampling of discrete lesions.[140–142]

The normal liver has a homogeneous echogenicity and smooth, sharp borders. Its echogenicity is less than the spleen's and slightly greater than or equal to the renal cortex's.[37] Hepatic and portal veins appear as branching, anechoic structures. Portal veins have bright periportal echoes and hepatic veins do not. The caudal vena cava is ventral and to the right of the aorta and dorsal and to the left of the portal vein.[37] The gallbladder is an anechoic, round to pear-shaped structure on the right of midline, with a wall 2 to 3 mm thick.[37, 143] Normal intrahepatic and extrahepatic bile ducts cannot be visualized.

Many diffuse hepatic diseases do not produce detectable sonographic changes until they become advanced, when either an increase or a decrease in echogenicity is present.[37] Hyperechogenicity is indicated by increased echogenicity compared with the renal cortex, spleen, or falciform fat and poor visualization of the deep portion and intrahepatic portal vein borders.[37, 42] Hepatic lipidosis, steroid hepatopathy, and cirrhosis are associated with hyperechogenicity (see Fig. 34–5; Fig. 34–6). Decreased heptatic echogenicity is associated with hypoechogenicity compared

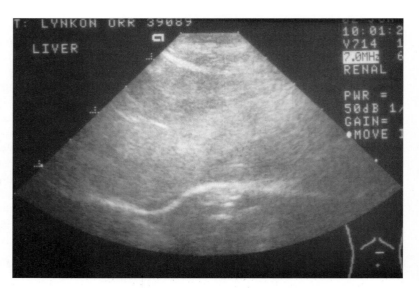

Figure 34-6
Transverse cross-sectional ultrasonographic appearance of hepatic lipidosis in an 8-year-old Siamese cat. The liver is diffusely hyperechoic compared with falciform fat. (Courtesy of Martha L. Moon, DVM, MS, Blacksburg, Virginia.)

with the renal cortex and increased prominence of portal vein walls.[37] Suppurative hepatitis, passive congestion, and lymphosarcoma are associated with hypoechogenicity.[37, 42]

Focal hepatic diseases (cysts, abscess, hyperplastic nodules, and neoplasia) are more easily recognized by differences in acoustic impedance between the normal liver and the abnormality.[37] Hyperplastic nodules appear as hypoechoic to isoechoic nodules and are indistinguishable from neoplasia.[37] Neoplasia can appear as a diffuse inhomogeneity with areas of mixed echogenicity or as focal or multifocal areas of variable echogenicity.[37] Findings associated with a portosystemic shunt include a small liver, a decrease in the number and size of portal and hepatic veins, and identification of a vessel connecting the portal and systemic circulations.[37] A more detailed description of specific abnormalities can be found in the sections on specific disorders.

Abdominocentesis

The presence of fluid within the abdomen should be detected with abdominal ballottement (taping the abdominal wall on one side and feeling waves of fluid movement on the other side).[49] In cases with minimal fluid accumulation, it may be detected with abdominal radiographs or ultrasound. Many acceptable techniques have been described to aseptically obtain a sample of fluid for complete analysis, and personal preference should dictate which technique is commonly used. With the animal standing, an area 2 to 4 cm caudal to the umbilicus and 1 to 2 cm to the right of the midline should be clipped and surgically scrubbed. I prefer to insert a 21-gauge butterfly needle into the abdomen. Alternatively, a 22-gauge needle can be placed into the abdomen and fluid collected into a

purple-topped tube via gravity. Fluid should be evaluated for a total nucleated cell count. The sample should be centrifuged, the supernate evaluated for total protein with a refractometer, and the sediment examined cytologically. In addition, a sample should be saved and submitted for bacteriologic culture if cytology reveals increased numbers of neutrophils or the presence of bacteria.

Ascitic fluid is clear, has a total protein level of less than 3.5 g/dL (often <2.5 g/dL[61]), and has less than 5000 nucleated cells, with mononuclear cells predominating. A fluid with a very low total protein level (<2.5 g/dL) and few nucleated cells (<1000) is found in cases of hypoproteinemia.[49] Exudative conditions can easily be distinguished by their high protein content (>3.5 g/dL) and their high nucleated cell count (>5000), often with a high percentage of degenerate neutrophils and, in some cases, bacteria. Chylous effusions are milky white and contain large quantities of triglycerides. Hemorrhagic effusions are red and have a high RBC count (see Ascites).

Hepatic Biopsy

The definitive diagnosis of many hepatic disorders requires histologic evaluation of hepatic tissue. Although biopsy is an invasive procedure with potentially serious complications, the risks of a properly performed biopsy are offset by the benefits associated with establishing a definitive diagnosis.[144] There are many methods available to obtain hepatic tissue samples. The most commonly used are ultrasound-guided percutaneous, blind percutaneous (transabdominal or transthoracic), keyhole, or exploratory laparotomy. Because animals with hepatic disease have many metabolic derangements and are very susceptible to stress, biopsy samples should be obtained by the least invasive method available. Frequently, patients thought to be stable decompensate after liver biopsy obtained by exploratory laparotomy.

A coagulation profile should be assessed before performing hepatic biopsy.[25] A mucosal bleeding time should be performed in Doberman pinschers and other breeds that are prone to von Willebrand's disease.[144] If coagulation times are prolonged, a transfusion of fresh plasma provides additional coagulation factors to aid hemostasis.[25] If prolonged cholestasis is present, vitamin K deficiency caused by fat malassimilation can be corrected by administration of vitamin K_1, 2 mg/kg subcutaneously in dogs or 5 mg subcutaneously per cat twice per day (b.i.d.) for 1 to 2 days before biopsy.[25]

Before the biopsy procedure, the animal should be fasted overnight. A small amount of a fatty meal can be given to stimulate gallbladder contraction; a smaller gallbladder is harder to puncture.[145] Sedation (acepromazine, 0.05 mg/kg, and oxymorphone, 0.05 mg/kg intravenously or 2–5 mg/kg meperidine intramuscularly in dogs; 1–4 mg/kg ketamine intravenously or intramuscularly in cats) or light anesthesia (intravenous thiamylal to effect) is usually necessary to provide restraint for percutaneous procedures. General anesthesia is necessary for keyhole and laparotomy techniques. The area of penetration should be clipped and surgically scrubbed and a stab incision made through the skin for percutaneous techniques.

Although there are various needles available for use in hepatic biopsy, I prefer the cutting Tru-Cut needle. The needle consists of an inner obturator with a distal tissue notch and an outer cannula with a distal cutting edge (Fig. 34–7).[144] With the obturator fully retracted and covered by the outer cannula, the needle is advanced until the tip lies in proximity to the area to be sampled. The inner obturator is advanced into the

liver, filling the tissue notch with hepatic tissue. The outer cannula is then advanced over the inner obturator, cutting off the tissue present within the notch. The entire needle is withdrawn, and the hepatic tissue is gently removed from the notch with a 25-gauge needle. Samples for histopathology are placed in a tissue cassette, which is immersed in formalin. Automated biopsy guns are available and simplify the procedure. Regardless of the method used, several samples should be collected and submitted for histopathology and bacterial culture. In selected cases, analysis of hepatic copper concentration should be performed.

Although it is not available in all practices, ultrasound-guided hepatic biopsy is my technique of choice for obtaining hepatic tissue samples.[140, 141] Ultrasound-guided biopsy procedures are quick to perform, allow focal abnormalities to be sampled, usually require only sedation and local anesthesia, are safe, and usually retrieve diagnostic samples.[140, 141, 144] It may not be possible to use this technique in an animal with a very small liver.

If ultrasound-guided biopsy is not available, other techniques should be used. If the liver can be palpated, subcostal transabdominal percutaneous biopsy is easy to perform.[146] Sedation is usually necessary. If the liver cannot be palpated, "blind" percutaneous techniques through the abdomen or caudal thorax can be used. Although veterinarians experienced with these techniques report that they are easy to perform, result in diagnostic specimens, and are associated with few side effects, I have had poor results and have never become proficient in their use.[146–148] "Blind" techniques can retrieve nondiagnostic samples if focal or multifocal disease is present.

To perform a transthoracic percutaneous biopsy,

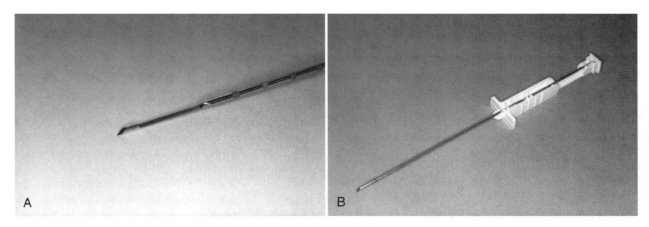

Figure 34–7
(A) Distal tissue notch of the inner obturator of a Tru-Cut biopsy needle. **(B)** The outer cannula has been advanced over the inner obturator, cutting off the tissue sample contained within the notch.

the animal is placed in left lateral recumbence with the forelimbs extended.[144, 146] The biopsy needle is passed through the sixth intercostal space, dorsal to the costochondral junction, into the pleural space. The tip of the needle is then directed caudally until it reaches the diaphragm.[145] The movement of the diaphragm can be felt against the needle tip. After full expiration, the needle is advanced through the diaphragm into the liver and the sample is quickly collected before the next respiratory cycle, to avoid diaphragmatic movement and laceration of the liver. The animal should be placed in right lateral recumbence for 5 minutes so the weight of the liver and intra-abdominal viscera will help compress the biopsy site.

For the transabdominal approach, the animal should be placed in oblique dorsal recumbence with the right side rotated 30° to 45° toward the table-top.[144, 147] The needle is introduced through a small stab incision between the tip of the xyphoid and the left costal arch and directed dorsad, craniad (20% from perpendicular), and to the left (20°–30°).[146–148] In cats, the needle is positioned more perpendicular to the skin.[148] The needle should also be placed more vertically in deep-chested dogs.[147] It may be possible to feel the needle pass through the subcutaneous and fatty tissue before reaching the liver. If not, the needle should initially be advanced 1 to 2 cm. If liver tissue is not retrieved, the needle can be placed deeper, up to 5 cm, and the direction slightly modified.[147] If firm resistance to advancement of the needle is encountered, it should be withdrawn and redirected, because the resistance may be caused by the diaphragm. The biopsy procedure should be initiated at the end of inspiration and the needle removed before the next respiratory cycle to avoid diaphragmatic movement and laceration of the liver.[147] After the procedure, the animal should be placed in sternal recumbence for 5 minutes so that the liver and abdominal viscera will compress the biopsy site.[147]

Minilaparotomy, or keyhole, techniques provide limited exposure of the liver, are quicker to perform, and require a much smaller incision than laparotomy. General anesthesia is usually needed. A small incision caudal to that used for the transabdominal percutaneous approach provides access for a finger to be inserted into the abdomen.[144, 146] The liver is palpated and stabilized for biopsy. A sterilized otoscope cone can be used as a minilaparoscope to view the liver to be biopsied. In this manner, some focal lesions can be sampled.

Exploratory laparotomy can be performed in all practices. It does require general anesthesia, is more time-consuming to perform, and is associated with greater morbidity and mortality than closed biopsy procedures.[144] Exploratory laparotomy should be used cautiously in patients with hypoalbuminemia, because wound healing may be delayed.[144] It offers advantages in that the surgeon can sample focal abnormalities, obtain larger tissue samples, assist coagulation at the biopsy site, and explore the entire abdomen and extrahepatic biliary system.[149] The latter advantage is useful if ultrasonography is not available and a distinction between hepatic and posthepatic icterus cannot be made. In addition, exploratory laparotomy allows assessment of a primary disease process when secondary hepatic disease may be present (e.g., inflammatory bowel disease, pancreatitis, primary intraabdominal neoplasia). If the area to be biopsied is near the edge of the liver lobe, it can be fractured with a suture ligature.[149] If the area to be sampled is not near the edge, a biopsy needle can be used to obtain tissue. Solitary lesions can be resected.

The complications associated with hepatic biopsy vary with the technique used and the skill and experience of the operator. Potential complications include hemorrhage from the biopsy site or laceration of blood vessels; puncture of the gallbladder, pancreas, bile duct, diaphragm, lung, or other adjacent organs; leakage of bile from rupture of intrahepatic ducts; pneumothorax; encephalopathy from anesthetic agents; and hemorrhage associated with surgical incisions.[141, 146] One major advantage of ultrasound-guided biopsy is that if it is performed by a skilled operator, it rarely causes any serious side effects.[140, 141]

Therapeutic Procedures

Treatment of Hepatic Encephalopathy

Hepatic encephalopathy can accompany many of the disorders discussed in this chapter, and treatment directed at the mechanisms responsible for encephalopathy is critically important for the animal's well-being and survival. The overall goals of therapy are to treat the primary hepatic disease, reduce the signs of encephalopathy, and provide supportive care to allow time for the liver to regenerate and recover its functions. Supportive care consists of providing adequate nutrition, fluid therapy to maintain hydration and electrolyte balance, and antibiotics to assist reduced reticuloendothelial function.

Precipitating factors in hepatic encephalopathy should be corrected to avoid intensification of clinical signs.[22, 24, 84] Many of these factors are discussed in the section on ammonia metabolism (see Hepatic Encephalopathy). Prerenal azotemia should be addressed by correcting dehydration and maintaining hydration. Gastrointestinal hemorrhage caused by gastritis or ulceration should be treated with a histamine$_2$-receptor antagonist such as cimetidine, 5 to 10 mg/kg three (t.i.d.) or four (q.i.d.) times per day subcutaneously or intramuscularly, or sucralfate, 1.0 g/25 kg t.i.d. or q.i.d. by mouth in dogs or 0.25 g t.i.d. or q.i.d. by mouth in cats. If a coagulopathy is caused by cholestasis and decreased absorption of vitamin K, therapy with vitamin K_1, 2 mg/kg in dogs (or 5 mg per cat) subcutaneously b.i.d., may help arrest bleeding.[25, 150] If transfusion is necessary, fresh blood products should be used, because stored blood has higher levels of ammonia. The use of sedatives and anesthetics should be avoided if possible, or used in very low dosages.[22]

Fluid therapy is vital to ensure adequate hepatic blood flow and delivery of oxygen and nutrients, to aid elimination of toxins, and to prevent complications such as DIC, shock, and renal failure.[150] Fluid therapy should correct dehydration, supply maintenance requirements, and replace losses from vomiting and diarrhea (see Chap. 31). A good initial fluid is half-strength saline (0.45%) and 2.5% dextrose.[22, 24, 151] Dextrose is necessary to help maintain blood glucose, because the diseased liver may have decreased glycogen stores and reduced capacity for gluconeogenesis.[12, 24, 151] If hepatic disease is accompanied by portal hypertension, total body sodium is increased, and full-strength saline or lactated Ringer's solution could cause or worsen ascites.[8, 151] Anorexia, losses from diarrhea and vomiting, and intracellular shifts associated with alkalosis promote hypokalemia.[8, 24, 83, 151] In addition, hypokalemia can promote alkalosis, which can increase the production of ammonia and its movement into the CNS. Potassium should initially be supplemented at 20 mEq/L in maintenance fluids and readjusted based on serum levels (see Table 31–7).[24, 151]

Hepatic disease is accompanied by decreased hepatic reticuloendothelial function, increasing the risk of septicemia from absorbed intestinal bacteria. Parenteral antibiotic therapy (i.e., ampicillin, 22 mg/ kg, t.i.d. or q.i.d.) is indicated to prevent septicemia.

If seizures occur frequently, if they are long-lasting, or if status epilepticus develops, they should be treated. Initially 25% to 50% glucose should be given in a bolus at 0.5 to 1.0 g/kg intravenously, to rule out hypoglycemia as a cause.[84] If seizures continue despite glucose administration, a very low dose of diazepam should be given intravenously to effect.[24, 84]

Reduction of the production and absorption of GI toxins is necessary if severe signs of encephalopathy are present. The animal should be fasted to remove sources of dietary protein.[22, 24, 84] The colon should be cleansed by administration of a dilute (10%) provodone iodine enema, 20 mL/kg.[22, 24, 84] This form of enema physically removes feces and bacteria, kills bacteria, and, because it is acidic, donates a proton to the ammonia molecule, ionizing it and trapping it in the colon. Intestinal bacteria can be killed by administration of a nonabsorbable antibiotic such as neomycin (10–20 mg/kg b.i.d. to q.i.d. by mouth). If the animal is too depressed to safely be administered oral medications (i.e., because of risk of aspiration), neomycin can be given in the enema solution. Other orally administered antibiotics, such as metronidazole (7.5–10 mg/kg t.i.d.) or ampicillin (22 mg/kg t.i.d. or q.i.d.) are effective against ammonia-producing anaerobes.[22, 84] Lactulose, a semisynthetic disaccharide that is not metabolized by mammalian digestive enzymes, can be given orally to cause osmotic diarrhea (0.5–1.0 mg/kg t.i.d.).[22, 24, 84] The dose should be adjusted to produce two to three soft stools per day. When lactulose reaches the colon, it is fermented by bacteria into many organic acids, which cause osmotic diarrhea. The production of acids also ionizes ammonia, trapping it in the colon. If the drug cannot be given orally, 10 to 20 mL/kg can be given by enema in a 30% solution.[22]

Dietary therapy can reduce the clinical signs of encephalopathy in animals with portosystemic shunts or severe hepatic disease. An appropriate diet is also necessary to provide the nutrients necessary for hepatic regeneration.[12] Diets should be highly digestible and palatable, contain protein of high biologic value with high concentrations of branched-chain amino acids, have readily available carbohydrates (e.g., rice) as the primary energy source, contain low levels of fat and sodium, and be supplemented with vitamins A, C, E, D, K, and B complex.[12, 23, 152, 153] Ideally, small meals should be fed b.i.d. or t.i.d. to maximize assimilation and reduce the amount of nutrients reaching the colon.[23, 154]

High digestibility results in fewer nutrients being presented to the colonic bacteria for metabolism.[12] Excess protein is metabolized and increases production of ammonia; protein deficiency can lead to catabolism of body proteins and increased ammonia production.[152] Milk proteins are higher in branched-chain amino acids than are meat proteins. Cholestatic disorders may be accompanied by reduced fat assimilation, which can cause diarrhea or increased absorption of short-chain fatty acids. However, most short-chain fatty acids are derived from the metabolism of carbohydrates, not from absorption of fats.[12] Vitamins are important, because hepatic metabolism and storage may be deficient.[12] Salt should be restricted to minimize sodium retention and the development of ascites. Although homemade diets can be fashioned to meet many of these requirements, long-term preparation is often difficult and impractical for owners. The recipes of some homemade diets have been reviewed.[12] Prescription Diet k/d or the Waltham low-protein diet is suitable for dogs and cats with hepatic disease.[153–155]

Palatability can be improved by warming the food.[156] Tube feeding (by a nasoesophageal or gastrostomy tube) is indicated if anorexia continues (see Hepatic Lipidosis and Percutaneous Endoscopic Gastrostomy Tube Placement).

Percutaneous Endoscopic Gastrostomy Tube Placement

Percutaneous endoscopic gastrostomy (PEG) tubes provide a convenient and nonstressful avenue for enteral nutritional support. Blended, nutritionally balanced pet foods can easily be administered through their large diameter.[157] They are well tolerated by the animal during long-term use.[158] They are indicated whenever prolonged anorexia is anticipated or if bypass of the oral cavity, pharynx, or esophagus is needed, so long as vomiting does not occur and gastric and intestinal function is normal. Gastrointestinal diseases that may benefit from their use include hepatic lipidosis, oronasal fistula, trauma or surgery, megaesophagus, esophageal foreign body, severe esophagitis, and esophageal stricture.[159] Most owners can manage tube feeding at home.[157] They can remain in place for months without complications.[157, 159]

Surgical and nonendoscopic techniques have been described, and several applicators have been developed.[160–162] Endoscopic placement does not require a surgical incision, is fast and easy, is done under direct visualization, is associated with few complications, and allows examination of the stomach and duodenum and collection of biopsy samples. A 20- to 24-Fr, mushroom-tipped urinary catheter (Pezzer-model drain) is prepared by removing the tip of the mushroom, which adds a large hole to the two preplaced holes and allows a thicker gruel to be fed, and adding a piece of the catheter 2 to 3 cm long as an internal stent (Fig. 34–8). Several veterinary kits are available commercially (e.g., Percutaneous Endoscopic Gastrostomy System, Pezzer catheter assembly). However, I prefer to make my own PEG kits, because they are less expensive and require little preparation time.

Minor variations in the following placement procedure exist.[158, 159, 163–165] Food is withheld for 12 hours, and the animal is placed under general anesthesia in right lateral recumbence. A longer period of fasting may be necessary in animals with esophageal dilation to prevent regurgitation during anesthesia and aspiration pneumonia. An area 15 × 15 cm centered caudal to the costal arch on the left side is clipped, surgically scrubbed, and draped. The stomach is distended with air to displace the liver, spleen, and colon from the gastrostomy site. An assistant depresses the skin and musculature caudal to the last rib, producing a depression visible with the endoscope inside the stomach. The area should not be too close to the pyloric antrum.

A 3-mm stab incision is made into the skin, and a 5-cm long, 14-gauge over-the-needle catheter (Sov-

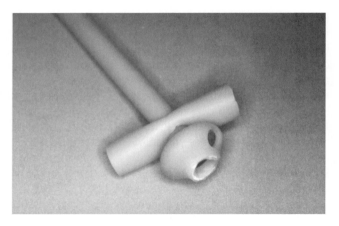

Figure 34–8
Distal end of a mushroom catheter. The tip has been cut off to increase the area for food delivery, and an internal stent has been placed on the tube.

ereign Indwelling Catheter) is inserted into the stomach. The needle is removed. The end of a 1.5-m long 0 suture is passed through the catheter, grasped by an endoscopic foreign body forceps, and withdrawn into the endoscope. The endoscope is slowly withdrawn (as the suture is fed through the catheter), and the suture is removed from the endoscopic forceps when the endoscope exits the mouth. The suture now passes through the left-sided skin incision and exits through the mouth. The catheter is removed from the flank and threaded onto the suture at the animal's mouth with the thin, tapered end placed on first. The suture is tied onto the feeding tube; this is facilitated by cutting the tip of the tube into a tapered V and passing the suture through it with an 18-gauge needle. The catheter–feeding tube assembly is then pulled together (Fig. 34–9). The feeding tube should be lubricated.

The suture is slowly withdrawn through the flank, pulling the feeding tube into the stomach and through the body wall and leaving the mushroom tip within the stomach. The endoscope is placed back into the stomach to observe the final placement of the mushroom tip. The tube should be placed gently against the mucosa; a placement that is too tight can cause necrosis, and one that is too loose can allow the stomach to move away from the body wall and interfere with adhesion formation (Fig. 34–10). The tube must be left in place for a minimum of 7 to 10 days. During this time, the stomach remains against the body wall, and localized inflammation results in a fistulous adhesion.

I place an external stent, similar to the internal stent, against the skin. The position of the tube as it exits the skin is carefully marked to ensure that it does not move into the abdomen, allowing the stomach to move away from the body wall. The junction of the tube and stent is glued, and the stent is glued or sutured to the skin. The feeding tube is lightly

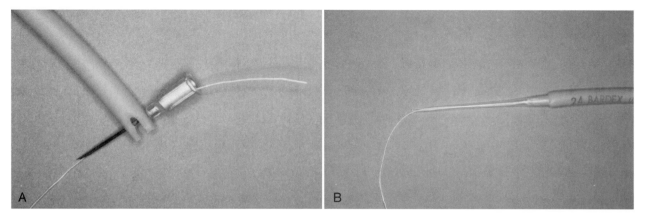

Figure 34-9
(A) The proximal end of the catheter has been tapered, and an 18-gauge needle is passed through to allow a suture to be tied to the tube. **(B)** The suture and proximal end of the tube are pulled into an intravenous catheter. The feeding tube assembly is ready to be pulled into the stomach.

bandaged to protect it from the animal's teeth. Feeding can begin the following day and is described in the treatment section of hepatic lipidosis. When no longer needed, the tube can be endoscopically removed.[166] In large dogs, endoscopic removal is not always necessary because the mushroom can be pulled through the skin by inserting a wooden cotton-tipped swab and elongating the mushroom (only if the tip was not cut off; see Fig. 34-10).[158] The internal stent falls into the stomach and should be passed in the feces within 4 days.[164] The wound quickly closes and needs to be kept clean for 2 to 4 days.[166]

Complications associated with the procedure are uncommon and usually minor.[157-159, 163] The most common complication I have seen is caused by excessive tension on the external flange, which results in necrosis of skin. Loosening of the stent and topical wound care are all that is needed. Mild pyrexia may occur for several days.[157, 163] Serious complications include excessive tension on the internal flange, which leads to gastric necrosis and peritonitis; inadvertent removal of the tube by the animal; pulling of the tube through the stomach into the abdominal cavity, which results in delivery of food into the abdominal cavity and peritonitis; leakage of food around the tube into the abdomen; obstruction of the pylorus if the tube is placed too far distally; pyloric or duodenal obstruction after tube removal from the internal stent; and splenic hemorrhage associated with insertion.

Common Hepatobiliary Diseases

Infectious canine hepatitis is described in Chapter 38. Other common hepatobiliary disorders are discussed here.

Hepatitis and Necrosis

Hepatitis and necrosis are pathology terms indicating inflammation of the liver and death of hepatocytes, respectively. There are numerous causes of hepatitis (Tables 34-3 and 34-4). Some are well-defined syndromes, such as infectious canine hepatitis and chronic active hepatitis of Doberman pinschers, and others are nonspecific, such as toxic or idiopathic hepatitis. Acute hepatitis occurs in dogs and cats of all ages and breeds and produces a variable syndrome that ranges from only biochemical abnormalities to

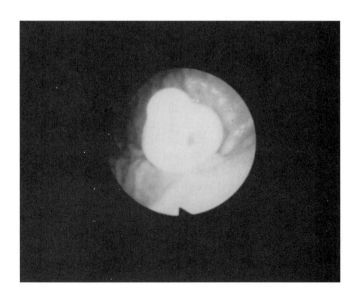

Figure 34-10
Endoscopic appearance of a mushroom tip pulled against the gastric mucosa. An internal stent is not present, and the distal tip has not been removed from the mushroom to facilitate stretching during percutaneous removal (personal preference of the endoscopist).

Table 34–3
Hepatotoxic Chemicals

Aflatoxins
Arsenic
Blue-green algae
Carbon tetrachloride
Chlordane
Chlorinated hydrocarbons
Chlorinated naphthalenes
Chlorinated biphenyls
Chloroform
Cinchophen
Coal tar pitch
Copper
Dieldrin
Dimethylnitrosamine
Gossypol
Iron
Mercury
Mushrooms
Pyrrolidine alkaloids
Phosphorus
Selenium
Tannic acid
Tetrachlorethane
Tetrachloroethylene
Trinitrotoluene

acute hepatic failure and death. Chronic hepatitis also occurs in small animals and is associated with persistent hepatic inflammation. Many of the common specific causes of hepatitis are described further in this chapter.

Pathophysiology

Because of the liver's central role in metabolism, its dual blood supply, and its reticuloendothelial function, it is susceptible to inflammation from a wide variety of causes. Acute hepatitis results from short-term exposure to an offending agent; chronic disease usually results from continuous or intermittent exposure. There are a large number of industrial chemicals, organic solvents, pesticides, and heavy metals to which dogs and cats can be exposed that can cause hepatitis (Table 34–3 is a partial list).[150] Drugs can cause hepatotoxicity and are described in the section on drug-induced hepatotoxicity.[167–172] Many drugs not discussed in that section have the potential to cause hepatotoxicity and should be included in the differential diagnosis if the clinical signs and laboratory abnormalities can be temporally related to drug therapy.[21]

Many metabolic disorders can produce a secondary hepatitis. In animals with acute pancreatitis, inflammatory products, vasoactive amines, and toxins are carried to the liver in the portal blood.[11, 39, 150]

Direct extension of enzymatic digestion from the pancreas to the liver can also occur. Inflammatory bowel disease is associated with increased permeability of the mucosal barrier.[173] Increased absorption of bacteria, endotoxins, and the products of digestion occurs, and these are delivered directly to the liver by portal blood flow.[11] Acute anemia, caused by blood loss or hemolysis, and hypovolemic shock can cause hypoxia and hepatocyte necrosis. They can also disrupt the intestinal mucosal barrier, allowing increased delivery of bacteria and endotoxins to the liver.[8, 11, 150] Hyperthyroidism in cats is often associated with mild hepatic degeneration and necrosis, as a result of unknown mechanisms.[29] Septicemia can lead to bacterial hepatitis through the arterial circulation. Right-sided heart failure and vena caval syndrome can produce acute hepatic congestion, hypoxia, and hepatitis.[8, 11, 150] Chronic passive congestion can be accompanied by hepatic fibrosis.[11] High body temperatures,

Table 34–4
Metabolic and Infectious Causes of Hepatitis

Acute anemia
Acute pancreatitis
Hypovolemic shock
Inflammatory bowel disease
Acute right heart failure
Septicemia and endotoxemia
Heatstroke
Vena caval syndrome
Viral

    Infectious canine hepatitis
    Canine herpes virus
    Feline infectious peritonitis

Bacterial

    Leptospirosis
    Bacillus piliformis
    Secondary to septicemia
    Ascending from duodenum
    Through portal blood because of increased intestinal mucosal permeability

Histoplasmosis
Toxoplasmosis
Granulomatous hepatitis

    Histoplasmosis
    Lymphangiectasia
    Lymphosarcoma
    Dirofilariasis
    Visceral larval migrans
    Lungworms
    Cryptococcosis
    Coccidioidomycosis
    Sporotrichosis
    Tuberculosis
    Heterobilharzia americana
    Prototheocosis

hypovolemia, hypoxia, and DIC associated with heatstroke can damage hepatocytes.[11, 174]

Cholestasis resulting from any extrahepatic biliary obstruction can cause a secondary hepatitis, because hydrophobic bile acids are toxic to hepatocytes.[8, 27] Common causes of extrahepatic biliary obstruction include biliary carcinoma, pancreatitis, pancreatic adenocarcinoma, cholelithiasis, cholecystitis, and duodenal neoplasia.[5, 31–33]

Infectious diseases can localize within the liver or infect the liver as part of a systemic process. Viral agents that can cause hepatitis include infectious canine hepatitis, canine herpes virus, and feline infectious peritonitis (see Chap. 38).[150, 175, 176] Fungal diseases, especially histoplasmosis, can cause hepatitis (see Chap. 39).[150, 177] Hepatitis can be a prominent feature of toxoplasmosis (see Chap. 40).[150] Bacterial hepatitis can result from septicemic processes or ascending infection from the small intestine through the biliary tree or portal blood. Bacterial hepatitis can also be caused by leptospirosis or *Bacillus piliformis*.[150] Granulomatous hepatitis is associated with a variety of infectious and noninfectious disorders (see Table 34–4).[178]

If mild or focal hepatitis is produced, clinical signs may not occur and only biochemical evidence of inflammation (i.e., elevated ALT) may be present. Moderate, diffuse inflammation and necrosis causes clinical signs; severe inflammation and necrosis can result in hepatic failure and death.

Gastric ulceration or gastritis can develop in animals with hepatitis. Although the mechanism is unknown, the following are thought to participate: a negative nitrogen balance altering cytoprotection, reduced gastric mucosal blood flow associated with portal hypertension, and elevated gastrin concentration and gastric acid secretion.[8, 179]

Clinical Signs

The clinical signs of acute hepatitis include anorexia, depression, icterus, hepatomegaly, vomiting, diarrhea, polyuria and polydipsia, dark urine, a bleeding diathesis (hematemesis, melena, hematochezia, hematuria, petechiation, or cutaneous hemorrhage), and signs of hepatic encephalopathy.[150] Clinical signs of chronic hepatic disease may be mild and episodic, but they often progress and become continuous. Ascites and weight loss may accompany the acute signs listed here.

Additional clinical signs may be associated with a primary disease that has caused a secondary hepatitis.[150] Pale mucous membranes and a recently detected heart murmur suggest anemia. Tachycardia, weak peripheral pulses, pale mucous membranes, delayed capillary refill, and cold extremities are associated with hypovolemic shock. Coughing or abnormal lung sounds suggest heartworm disease, systemic mycosis, feline infectious peritonitis, or toxoplasmosis. Anterior uveitis or chorioretinitis are often associated with feline infectious peritonitis, toxoplasmosis, and systemic mycosis. Hepatitis secondary to sepsis or endotoxemia can be associated with bacterial infection elsewhere in the body or with severe enteritis. Hyperthermia and exposure to high temperatures are associated with heatstroke. A history of severe vomiting or diarrhea or a thickened bowel loop on abdominal palpation support the presence of inflammatory bowel disease. Oliguria can occur with leptospirosis.

Diagnostic Plan

Because there are so many possible causes of hepatitis, the diagnosis in most cases requires a thorough history, complete physical examination, assessment of routine laboratory parameters and liver function tests, hepatic ultrasound, and microscopic sections of liver. The history may indicate administration of potentially hepatotoxic drugs (see Drug-Induced Hepatotoxicity) or exposure to hepatotoxic chemicals (see Table 34–3).[150] Review of the vaccination history helps assess the possibility of leptospirosis or infectious canine hepatitis.[150] The biochemical profile reveals elevated ALT, evidence of damage to hepatocyte membranes.[150] If intrahepatic cholestasis accompanies hepatitis and necrosis, elevated serum AP, hyperbilirubinemia, and bilirubinuria occur.[150] Hypoglycemia, hyperammonemia, and elevated bile acids are found if liver function is severely affected.[48, 126, 129, 130] Anemia (secondary to blood loss) and poikilocytosis can be found. Prolonged prothrombin and partial thromboplastin times can occur. Respiratory and metabolic acidosis can be present.[150] Chronic cases may exhibit hypoalbuminemia, hypocholesterolemia, and a low BUN.

Assessment of the history, physical examination, and routine laboratory parameters may suggest a metabolic or infectious cause for the hepatitis (see Table 34–4).[11, 150] Anemia may be detected on the CBC. Dogs with heartworms often have eosinophilia. Septicemia, pancreatitis, or leptospirosis may be accompanied by a neutrophilia with a left shift. Cats with feline infectious peritonitis (FIP) often have hyperglobulinemia. Elevated BUN and creatinine associated with a dilute urine specific gravity may occur in leptospirosis. Elevated amylase and lipase often occurs in dogs with pancreatitis. However, in many cases, despite a thorough diagnostic evaluation, a specific cause or well-defined syndrome cannot be identified (Fig. 34–11).[150]

In acute cases, hepatic biopsy may not be indicated if only laboratory abnormalities or mild clinical signs occur. These animals can be re-evaluated

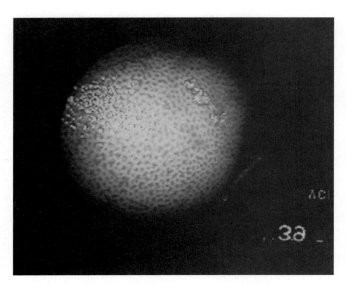

Figure 34-11
Laparoscopic appearance of the liver in a 7-year-old Siberian husky with nonspecific suppurative hepatitis. The liver is yellow, and a pronounced lobular or reticulated pattern is present.

in 2 to 4 weeks; if abnormalities improve or resolve, a clinical diagnosis of nonspecific hepatitis can be made and further evaluation is not necessary. At the other end of the spectrum are patients with severe hepatic failure that may be too metabolically unstable to withstand hepatic biopsy. If supportive care results in clinical improvement, biopsy may be performed. If the animal greatly improves, a clinical diagnosis of nonspecific acute hepatitis may be made based on response to therapy. These animals should be re-evaluated in 2 to 4 weeks and a biochemical profile obtained. Patients with chronic hepatitis with persistent clinical signs and laboratory abnormalities should undergo liver biopsy.

Hepatic biopsy may be diagnostic of histoplasmosis, toxoplasmosis, infectious canine hepatitis, herpesvirus infection, or leptospirosis.[2] Biopsy may indicate granulomatous hepatitis, which has been associated with many disorders (see Table 34-4).[178] Histologic patterns of several drug toxicities have been described and may suggest a diagnosis. Anatomic distribution of nonspecific histologic findings (hepatocyte swelling, hydropic degeneration, and necrosis) can suggest certain causes.[2] Centrolobular changes may occur with passive congestion, hypoxia, steroid administration, and toxicities. Peripheral lobular changes accompany biliary disease, chronic active hepatitis, and aflatoxicosis.[2] Locally extensive lesions may result from massive toxic injury or infarction.

Treatment

Treatment should be directed at the underlying cause, if identified. Potential hepatotoxic drugs should be discontinued.[150] Fluid therapy, administration of antibiotics, control of GI bleeding, and reduction in the absorption and production of GI toxins involved in hepatic encephalopathy are important components of successful treatment of hepatitis (see Treatment of Hepatic Encephalopathy).

Although less common than chronic hepatic failure, acute hepatic failure can accompany many types of hepatitis. In animals with acute hepatic failure, severe cerebral edema develops and is a major cause of death.[22] It is difficult to separate the clinical signs of encephalopathy from those caused by edema. Treatment of edema requires administration of a 20% solution of mannitol, 1 g/kg intravenously over 30 minutes, and furosemide, 1 to 2 mg/kg intravenously t.i.d.[22] Other beneficial treatments include plasma transfusion to increase serum osmotic pressure, systemic antibiotics to control sepsis, management of GI hemorrhage, supplemental glucose administration, and vigorous support of blood pressure to prevent development of renal failure.[22]

Prognosis

The prognosis for animals with hepatitis is variable and depends on the underlying cause and severity of inflammation and necrosis. The prognoses for recognized hepatitis syndromes are discussed elsewhere in this chapter.

Portosystemic Shunts

Portosystemic shunts are vascular connections between the portal system and the systemic circulation that partially divert portal blood around the liver.[128, 180] They occur most commonly in young purebred dogs and domestic shorthair and domestic longhair cats as congenital abnormalities.[181, 182] Yorkshire terriers, miniature schnauzers, Himalayans, and Persians may be predisposed.[127, 134, 181, 183, 184] About 30% of shunts are contained within the liver parenchyma (intrahepatic). Intrahepatic shunts occur more commonly in large-breed dogs, whereas extrahepatic shunts are more common in small-breed dogs.[183, 185] Intrahepatic shunts are found more frequently in dogs than cats.[128, 180, 181, 186, 187] Acquired multiple extrahepatic shunts develop as a consequence of severe liver disease and portal hypertension (see Ascites). They produce the same pathophysiologic changes as congenital shunts and are discussed further in the section on cirrhosis.

Pathophysiology

Most congenital shunts are single vessels.[127, 128, 180, 187] A persistent ductus venosus results in an intrahepatic shunt. The ductus venosus carries oxygenated fetal blood from the placenta to systemic circulation and bypasses the liver (Fig. 34–12). Normally, it closes within 2 to 3 days after birth as a result of decreased blood pressure and oxygen content.[134, 187–189] The most common types of extrahepatic shunts are splenic to vena cava, portocaval, and portoazygos.[127, 183, 187, 190, 191] It is not known whether these vessels are anomalies or fetal alternatives to the ductus venosus.[181]

Lack of blood flow to the liver results in hypoplasia because of underperfusion and insufficiency of trophic pancreatic hormones.[128, 134, 192] Histologic changes include compressed hepatic cords with dilated sinusoids, close proximity of portal triads, portal vein hypovascularity, proliferation of small vessels and lymphatics, and mild hepatocellular degeneration.[181, 182] The hepatic atrophy and diverted portal blood cause signs of liver failure and hepatic encephalopathy (see Hepatic Encephalopathy). Clinical signs can be most severe after a meal, because nutrients, toxins, bacteria, and drugs are not removed and metabolized by the liver and enter systemic circulation and the CNS.[134, 180, 193] Intrahepatic shunts have been associated with an earlier onset and greater severity of clin- ical signs, as a result of larger shunt volumes that by- pass hepatic circulation.[181] After shunt ligation, increased portal blood flow to the liver delivers trophic factors that stimulate regeneration of the liver.[188]

Hepatic insufficiency leads to accumulation of ammonia and uric acid (decreased conversion to allantoin). Increased urine concentrations of these substances causes precipitation of ammonium biurate crystals or formation of urate calculi.[181]

Clinical Signs

The clinical signs of congenital portosystemic shunt are usually evident before 12 months of age, but diagnosis may be delayed for many years if signs are subtle.[96, 128, 134, 180, 182, 185, 190, 194] Affected animals do not grow as well as littermates.[182, 194] Signs of hepatic encephalopathy are most common, and they often occur episodically, sometimes after ingestion of a high-protein meal.[134, 181, 182, 188, 190, 194, 195] Clinical signs often progressively become more severe. Common findings include weakness, ataxia, stupor, head pressing, circling, pacing, blindness, ptyalism, behavioral changes, dementia, hysteria, aggression, seizures, and coma.[96, 127, 128, 134, 181, 182, 186, 189] Clinical signs often resolve, and animals can appear normal between episodes.[128] Ptyalism (excessive salivation) is common in cats.[128, 134, 181, 182, 186, 195] Other, less common signs include vomiting, diarrhea, constipation, polyphagia, pica, polyuria and polydipsia, fever, pruritus, and anesthetic intolerance.[96, 128, 181, 182, 189, 190] In some cases, urolithiasis (ammonium urate) may be present, and signs of cystitis or urethral obstruction (hematuria, pollakiuria, or dysuria) occur.[127, 134, 181, 186] Physical examination may reveal renomegaly, cryptorchidism, or heart murmurs in cats.[96, 127, 181, 182]

Diagnostic Plan

The diagnosis of congenital portosystemic shunt should be suspected if classic clinical signs and laboratory changes are present in a puppy or kitten.[128, 181] The diagnosis is confirmed by ultrasonography, contrast radiographic techniques, or nuclear scintigraphy (which usually require referral to a specialty center) or during exploratory laparotomy. Common laboratory abnormalities include microcytic nonregenerative anemia, poikilocytosis, target red blood cells, mildly increased ALT and AP (perhaps of bone origin in young animals), hypocholesterolemia, hypoalbuminemia, reduced BUN, hypoglycemia, increased partial thromboplastin time, ammonium urate crystalluria, proteinuria, and hematuria.[96, 100, 127, 128, 134, 181, 182, 188, 195] Electrolyte changes can occur as a result of vomiting and diarrhea. Elevated serum ammonia and postchallenge serum ammonia and increased fasting and postprandial bile acids are present.[182, 195–198]

Survey abdominal radiographs may demonstrate a small liver, large kidneys, or both.[128, 134, 182, 186, 194, 195, 199] A small liver may be associated with a reduced distance between the diaphragm and the stomach, cranial displacement of the stomach, vertical or cranial angle to the stomach (instead of being parallel to the ribs), or cranial displacement of the pyloric antrum.[73] Visualization of intra-abdominal structures is often reduced because of lack of intra-abdominal fat.[186, 199] Ultrasonographic evaluation often reveals a small hypovascular liver and may identify the anomalous vessel.[47, 181, 199, 200] The

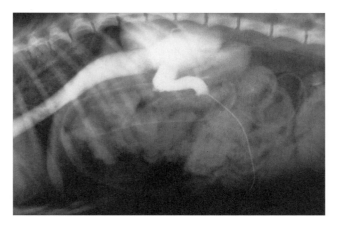

Figure 34–12
Contrast jejunal venogram in an 8-month-old mixed breed dog showing a single extrahepatic portocaval shunt. Contrast medium fills the portal vein and vena cava but does not enter the liver. (Courtesy of Don Barber, DVM, MS, Blacksburg, Virginia.)

renal pelves and bladder should carefully be evaluated for urate calculi.[181]

Although not performed at most veterinary clinics, contrast radiographic procedures such as mesenteric venography, trans-splenic venography, or venous or per rectal portal scintigraphy definitively provide the diagnosis.[128, 134, 181, 188, 199, 201–208.]

Treatment

Medical management (see Treatment of Hepatic Encephalopathy) may improve the clinical signs or temporarily resolve them, but long-term successful management usually requires surgical attenuation of the shunt.[134] The patient should be stabilized before surgery by treating for hepatic encephalopathy, if present.[128, 188, 192, 209] In most cases, diagnosis and treatment require referral to a specialty center.

During surgery, a catheter is placed within the portal system to measure pressure and to perform radiographic procedures.[128, 210] The shunt should be attenuated until the pressure increases by 7 to 10 cm H_2O or reaches 19 to 20 cm H_2O.[128, 180, 181, 210] Objective pressure measurements alone are not sufficiently sensitive to judge the degree of ligation and should be correlated with visual signs of portal hypertension. Signs of portal hypertension include splanchnic vascular distention and pulsation, visceral cyanosis, and bowel hypermotility.[128, 181, 184] The pancreas is most easily assessed for congestion caused by portal hypertension.[180] In most cases, the shunt can be attenuated by 60% to 80%.[181, 184] Complete ligation is accomplished less frequently in cats than in dogs.[128, 181, 186] During surgery, extrahepatic shunts can be visualized, and intrahepatic shunts can often be detected as soft dilations within the hepatic tissue.[181] Intrahepatic shunts should be dissected from hepatic parenchyma at their junction with the hepatic vein or vena cava on the diaphragmatic surface of the liver and attenuated at that site.[181] Postoperative portography should be performed to confirm shunt ligation, identify additional shunts, and assess hepatic portal circulation. If clinical signs do not vastly improve after surgery in cases in which partial ligation was performed, follow-up assessment of portal circulation and additional shunt ligation should be performed, unless multiple acquired shunts are identified.[181, 186, 210]

Complications of surgery, radiography, and anesthesia can be caused by impaired drug metabolism, hypotension, hypothermia, hypoglycemia, portal hypertension, hemorrhage from the catheter site, portal vein thrombosis, or acute pancreatitis.[127, 181, 184, 194] Portal hypertension can result in bowel edema, ascites, or acute cardiovascular collapse and death. Other clinical signs include abdominal pain, hemorrhagic diarrhea, systemic hypotension, hypovolemia, and

endotoxemia.[128, 188, 210] The shunt ligature should promptly be removed if these signs are present.[128, 209] Intraoperative complications are more common with ligation of intrahepatic shunts.[181]

Ascites may develop postoperatively as a result of portal hypertension but should resolve within 3 weeks.[180, 183, 184, 210] Postligation seizures can occur up to 5 days after surgery, possibly because of the rapid changes in metabolism.[209, 211] Older dogs may be more likely to develop seizures.[181, 212]

After surgery, a low-protein diet should be fed.[188] Treatment for hepatic encephalopathy should be continued if it was instituted before surgery.[128, 180] Animals with complete ligation of the shunt and some with partial ligation can gradually be switched to normal diets and other treatments can be stopped, often by 3 months after surgery. If clinical signs develop after institution of a normal diet, the low-protein diet should be reinstated.

Prognosis

Surgical mortality has been reported to vary from 14% to 21%.[181, 185] Animals that survive surgery and have had a complete shunt ligation have an excellent prognosis.[127, 181, 190, 210] A more guarded but still optimistic prognosis is offered for animals with a partial ligation.[127, 184, 194, 213] Overall, results in cats are not as good as in dogs.[128] Dogs with intrahepatic shunts may have a poorer prognosis.[213] Persistent or recurrent clinical signs after surgery (in cases in which partial ligation was performed) suggest that further attenuation of the shunt is necessary. Dogs older than 2 years of age at the time of surgery may have a poorer prognosis, although a recent report contradicted this finding.[181, 190, 213] Postligation seizures are a poor prognostic sign.[184, 212]

Hepatic Lipidosis

Hepatic lipidosis is the most common liver disease recognized in cats.[214] It is characterized by the massive accumulation of lipid within hepatocytes and clinical signs of liver disease. It occurs in cats of all ages but is most common in those between 2 and 8 years of age, often after a 1- to 2-week period of anorexia.[14, 67, 214–218] Obese cats may be predisposed.[14, 216, 217, 219] In some cats, a primary disorder or stress causing inappetence can be identified; in others, the condition is idiopathic. Fatty infiltration of hepatocytes is a nonspecific histologic finding and occurs commonly with reduced food intake, a variety of metabolic illnesses, obesity, toxicity, and other types of hepatic disorders.[11, 14, 220] A clinical diagnosis of hepatic lipidosis requires demonstration that at least 50% of hepatocytes are filled with lipid.[67]

Pathophysiology

Hepatic lipidosis develops most commonly in obese cats after a period of prolonged anorexia. Anorexia leads to lipolysis and increased delivery of fatty acids to the liver. Many cases of hepatic lipidosis are idiopathic, and a primary disorder cannot be identified. In some of these cases, a stressful event may initiate anorexia; in others, a stressor cannot be discovered. Many diseases have been associated with concurrent hepatic lipidosis in cats. Some common examples include other hepatic diseases, neoplasia, renal diseases, hyperthyroidism, inflammatory bowel disease, pancreatitis, and diabetes mellitus.[67, 221] Inappetence, caused by the primary disease, may initiate the lipidosis. The role that obesity plays is unclear, but it could relate to altered hormonal interactions. Obese cats may be insulin resistant (insulin inhibits lipolysis), possibly predisposing them to massive release of free fatty acids from adipose tissue during anorexia.[14, 67, 215]

It is thought that excessive triglyceride accumulation within the hepatocyte is only one manifestation of a broader metabolic derangement.[67, 215] In health, fatty acids are taken up by the liver, metabolized for energy, or converted to triglycerides, phospholipids, or cholesterol.[222] These three products can be bound to apoproteins to form very-low-density lipoproteins, which are excreted from the liver and enter circulation.[214, 222] The normal liver can extract fatty acids from the blood and form triglycerides at a rate that exceeds the capacity for dispersal.[14] Lipidosis occurs if fatty acids are presented to the hepatocytes faster than they can be oxidized or packaged into lipoproteins and excreted.[214, 223] Although carnitine is necessary for the transfer of fatty acids across mitochondrial membranes, it was shown not to be deficient in cats with lipidosis.[224] Ultrastructural studies of hepatocytes in cats with lipidosis suggest that the number of organelles necessary for oxidation and lipoprotein dispersal may be reduced.[14, 225] Triglyceride deposition is a reversible process in most cases.[67] In diabetes mellitus, disrupted lipid metabolism occurs, but most diabetic cats do not develop the clinical syndrome of hepatic lipidosis.[14, 67, 215]

Clinical Signs

Clinical signs include anorexia, weight loss, icterus, hepatomegaly, and, in some instances, hepatic encephalopathy, vomiting, or diarrhea.[14, 67, 214, 216, 223] If a primary disease is present, additional clinical signs occur (e.g., vomiting or diarrhea in inflammatory bowel disease, polyuria and polydipsia in renal diseases). Historically, many cats have previously been obese.[214–216, 223] The history may contain a stressful episode that initiated inappetence. Stressful events include moving to a new household, the addition of a new dog or cat, the arrival of a new baby, and absence of an owner.[214, 215, 223] Physical examination often reveals evidence of muscle wasting but preservation of the intra-abdominal fat pad.[214, 215, 226]

Diagnostic Plan

Cats with hepatic lipidosis have extremely elevated serum AP levels.[214, 216, 223] Other common laboratory findings include elevated ALT and hyperbilirubinemia, anemia, poikilocytes, microcytosis, a mature neutrophilia, abnormal coagulation profiles, and bilirubinuria.[14, 67, 214, 216, 217, 219, 223] Hypercholesterolemia, hypoglycemia, hyperglycemia, and hypoalbuminemia are found less commonly.[215, 223] Serum bile acids and ammonia levels are increased. Liver function tests should be performed only if hyperbilirubinemia is not present.[14]

Ultrasonographic examination of the liver can be very helpful in establishing a diagnosis. In cats with lipidosis, the liver is usually diffusely hyperechoic compared with falciform fat, has smooth borders, and may be enlarged (see Fig. 34–6).[42, 44] Other findings include isoechogenicity to omental fat and poor visualization of intrahepatic blood vessel margins.[44]

A fine-needle aspirate of the liver is often diagnostic of lipidosis: samples contain vacuolated, fat-filled hepatocytes.[214, 215] Few inflammatory cells should be present.[14] If hepatomegaly is present, a 23- to 25-gauge needle can be directed into the liver toward the diaphragm at a 45° angle, caudal to the last rib on the left side.[214] If the liver cannot be palpated, the aspiration can be done with ultrasound guidance or by following the procedure for transabdominal percutaneous biopsy described elsewhere in this chapter. Although more invasive than aspiration, hepatic biopsy also confirms the diagnosis.[214, 215]

Grossly, the liver is enlarged and yellow and has a reticulated pattern.[215] The tissue is greasy on cut section and very friable.[14, 67, 215, 222] Microscopically, at least 50% of hepatocytes are highly vacuolated (Fig. 34–13). Canalicular bile stasis is present.[223] A lipid stain, such as oil red O, confirms the presence of lipid within the vacuoles.[215]

After confirmation of a diagnosis of lipidosis, the cat should be evaluated carefully for any of the common primary disorders associated with hepatic lipidosis.[67]

Treatment

Fluid therapy should be administered to correct dehydration and electrolyte abnormalities. Supplementation of potassium is extremely important (see Chap. 31). If signs of hepatic encephalopathy are present, the cat should be treated as described previously in this chapter.

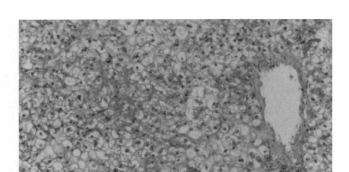

Figure 34–13

Microscopic appearance of hepatic lipidosis in a 7-year-old domestic shorthair cat. The hepatocytes are vacuolated and filled with lipid. A central vein is visible on the left side of the photograph.

Successful treatment of hepatic lipidosis involves supplying adequate calories and high levels of high-quality protein and managing concurrent diseases.[223] Most cats without concurrent disorders (idiopathic lipidosis) begin eating on their own within 3 to 8 weeks. Improvement in biochemical parameters should parallel clinical improvement.

I prefer to insert a PEG tube and to feed blenderized, balanced, calorie-dense cat foods, such as Prescription Diet a/d or p/d.[157, 159, 164] The cat should be carefully monitored for signs of encephalopathy, and if signs develop, a lower-protein diet should be substituted. On the first day of feeding, one third of the cat's maintenance caloric requirement (approximately 60 kcal/kg) should be fed, with meals given every 2 to 4 hours. Two thirds of the caloric requirements should be given on day 2, and full maintenance on day 3.[156, 227] If vomiting occurs, metoclopramide, 0.2 to 0.4 mg/kg subcutaneously t.i.d., can be used as an antiemetic. The volume of the meal is gradually increased until the entire daily volume can be administered in three or four feedings. The cat can be discharged and feeding continued at home. After 2 weeks of tube feedings, the owner should offer the cat canned food before feeding. The amount consumed should be subtracted from the amount fed by tube.[156] After the cat consumes at least 75% of maintenance calories for 5 consecutive days, the tube can be removed.

It is also possible to feed cats with hepatic lipidosis by nasoesophageal tube.[219, 222] Only liquid diets can be passed through nasoesophageal tubes.[153, 156, 227] Most cats tolerate gastrostomy tubes better than nasoesophageal tubes.[14, 227] Human enteral products, such as Pulmocare, must be supplemented with protein and taurine.[153, 222] Veterinary products, such as CliniCare and RenalCare, do not require supplementation.[153]

Prognosis

The prognosis for animals with idiopathic lipidosis is good, approximately 50% to 75% making a full recovery, if owners are able to tube feed for up to 8 weeks.[14, 215, 216, 219, 221] Relapses are uncommon. The prognosis for cases associated with other diseases depends partly on the prognosis of the primary disorder.[221]

Chronic Active Hepatitis

Chronic active hepatitis is a term adopted from the human literature that is commonly used to describe a diverse group of chronic canine hepatic disorders characterized by inflammation and fibrosis.[228] Strict clinical and pathologic criteria are not available in veterinary medicine, and many dogs diagnosed with chronic active hepatitis do not have a syndrome similar to that in humans. Some authors do not think a disease similar to the human disorder occurs in dogs.[229] Others have suggested that the term active be deleted from the literature and that chronic cases be classified as idiopathic, as drug-induced, as breed-related, or based on morphologic characteristics of the hepatic biopsy.[230]

Regardless of terminology and definitions, a classic example of what is considered chronic active hepatitis in veterinary medicine is the hepatopathy recognized in middle-aged female Doberman pinschers.[92, 95] Syndromes in several other breeds and affected individuals of many other breeds have been recognized. Middle-aged dogs are affected most commonly.[231] An increased incidence may occur in male American and English cocker spaniels, female Labrador retrievers, and West Highland white terriers of both sexes.[231] In one report, chronic active hepatitis represented approximately 20% of hepatic diseases diagnosed by biopsy and occurred in 1.2 out of 1000 dogs seen at a university teaching hospital.[232] A brief discussion of several other syndromes of chronic hepatitis follows this section to broaden the reader's concept of chronic hepatitis.

Pathophysiology

In humans, chronic active hepatitis is initiated by viruses or drugs or is an autoimmune disease.[233] A genetic predisposition probably occurs. The pathophysiology is as follows. An inciting event causes damage to hepatocytes.[233] An immune response is directed against the altered hepatocyte membrane, causing further damage or cell death. Hepatocyte-specific antigens (not previously exposed to the immune system) are released, and additional immunologic reactions occur, leading to complement-mediated cytotoxic reactions and further damage to hepatocytes. A self-perpetuating immunologic process develops.

In dogs, the inciting event is usually not discovered. The pathophysiology of the disease is unknown, and few immunologic studies have been performed. In a limited number of cases, spirochetes believed to be leptospiral organisms were identified in histologic sections of liver. A serologic study of the involved kennel revealed exposure to *Leptospira interrogans* serovar *grippotyphosa*.[234] Infectious canine hepatitis virus has been associated with chronic active hepatitis in a group of experimentally infected dogs with low levels of antibodies to the virus.[175] Recently, anti-hepatic membrane protein and cell nuclei antibodies were detected in dogs with chronic hepatitis.[235, 236] However, it was not possible to determine whether the autoantibodies were primary (causative) or secondary to chronic liver disease.

Excessive hepatic copper levels have been demonstrated in Doberman pinschers with chronic active hepatitis.[92] The predominantly held theory is that copper accumulation is secondary to cholestasis and is not a primary inciting event, as it is in Bedlington terriers (see Copper-Associated Hepatitis). However, cases have been documented that did not involve fibrosis or cholestasis but involved elevated hepatic copper content.[237]

Clinical Signs

Initially, intermittent and mild clinical signs may occur, but they often progress until continuous advanced signs of liver disease are present. Some patients may present with acute signs of liver failure, despite histopathologic findings that support the presence of chronic disease.[92] Common signs include weight loss, vomiting, anorexia, icterus, ascites, polyuria and polydipsia, bleeding tendencies, and hepatic encephalopathy.[92, 95, 228, 232, 238, 239] Some cases are asymptomatic and are identified after finding abnormalities on routine laboratory evaluation.

Diagnostic Plan

The diagnosis of chronic active hepatitis is based on signalment, clinical signs, laboratory evaluation, hepatic ultrasonography, and histopathologic evaluation of hepatic tissue (after evaluation of coagulation). Common laboratory abnormalities include elevated serum AP and ALT (mean values approximately 500–600 IU/L), hyperbilirubinemia, hypoalbuminemia, anemia, reduced BUN, and prolonged coagulation tests.[92, 228, 232, 238, 239] Serum bile acids and resting serum ammonia or ammonia tolerance test results are usually abnormal.[92] Abdominal radio-

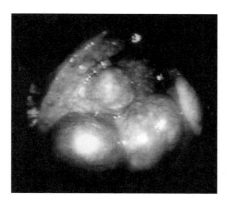

Figure 34–14
Laparoscopic appearance of the liver in a 5-year-old female Doberman pinscher with chronic active hepatitis. Several regenerative nodules are present. The liver is small, is yellow-tan, and has an irregular surface. The edges are rounded.

graphic findings include loss of intra-abdominal detail, microhepatica, and ascites.[92]

Grossly, affected livers are usually small, with irregular or nodular surfaces (Fig. 34–14).[95, 238] Acquired portosystemic shunts may be present.[238] Microscopically, piecemeal necrosis, bridging necrosis, inflammatory infiltrates of neutrophils and macrophages, and fibrosis are present.[92, 95, 232] Intrahepatic and intracanalicular bile stasis and bile duct hyperplasia are present.[95] Portal tracts are infiltrated with plasma cells and lymphocytes.[238] Accumulation of copper and iron can be seen in hepatocytes, and their concentration in hepatic tissue is moderately elevated.[92, 95, 228]

Treatment

Animals with severe signs of liver failure require vigorous intravenous fluid therapy to manage dehydration from anorexia, vomiting, and diarrhea (see Chap. 31). Broad-spectrum antibiotics, such as ampicillin (22 mg/kg intravenously t.i.d. or q.i.d.) should be administered to combat secondary infection from reduced hepatic reticuloendothelial function.[23] Treatment of hepatic encephalopathy may be necessary (see Therapeutic Procedures).

Long-term management of chronic active hepatitis requires prednisone, 1 to 2 mg/kg per day, for its anti-inflammatory, immunosuppressive, and antifibrotic activity.[23, 92, 228, 232, 239, 240] It may be possible in some cases to reduce the dosage to alternate-day therapy or eventually to discontinue drug therapy. Azathioprine has been recommended in combination with prednisone at 2 mg/kg once daily (s.i.d.). The drug should be slowly reduced to 0.5 mg/kg every 48 hours. Azathioprine prevents cell division in rapidly dividing cells and inhibits immunologic response.[241] Azathioprine can inhibit the bone marrow, and the

CBC and platelet count should be monitored frequently during therapy.[23] Monitoring the response to therapy is often difficult because prednisone causes increased liver enzymes. Decisions to reduce dosages should be based on improvement in clinical signs and liver function test results and, in some instances, repeat biopsy. Most patients require lifelong treatment. Dietary management should include the use of a low-protein diet composed of high-quality nutrients.[23, 239]

If elevated hepatic copper content can be identified, chelation with D-penicillamine, 10 to 15 mg/kg b.i.d., may be beneficial.[23, 92, 228] D-penicillamine promotes urinary excretion of copper and also prevents or reverses hepatic fibrosis and suppresses T-lymphocyte function.[23] Common side effects include vomiting and anorexia. Recently, ursodeoxycholic acid (Actigall), 10 to 15 mg/kg s.i.d., has been used with apparent benefit. In humans, it improves the biochemical markers of cholestasis and inflammation in cholestatic liver diseases.[242] As a hydrophilic bile acid, it alters the bile acid milieu, replacing hepatotoxic bile acids and reducing the adverse effects of retained bile on hepatocytes. It also promotes bile flow and may act as a hepatoprotectant by membrane stabilization or immunomodulatory effects.[242] Side effects are uncommon.

Some authors suggest using colchicine, 0.03 mg/kg s.i.d., to help decrease fibrosis.[23] It also possesses anti-inflammatory effects.[233] Side effects are uncommon and include vomiting, diarrhea, abdominal pain, and bone marrow depression.

If a large volume of ascitic fluid is present, causing respiratory distress or abdominal discomfort, abdominal paracentesis should be performed to provide relief. If a moderate level of ascitic fluid remains after treatment of the hepatic disease, diuretic therapy with furosemide, 1 mg/kg b.i.d., is indicated.[23] A low-sodium diet may be instituted in these cases. However, many restricted-sodium diets contain excessive protein or a lower quality of protein than in protein-restricted diets. If signs of hepatic encephalopathy develop after the diet change, the restricted-protein diet should be reinstituted. Serum electrolytes should be carefully monitored while furosemide is administered, because hypokalemia can lead to metabolic alkalosis, which can increase production and absorption of ammonia and worsen hepatic encephalopathy.[23]

There are no published controlled studies that have evaluated treatment of this disorder. I most commonly use prednisone, ursodeoxycholic acid, and a protein-restricted diet in cases of chronic active hepatitis. If moderate or severe copper accumulation is present, I add D-penicillamine. Additional treatment of hepatic encephalopathy is used if signs occur. I rarely use azathioprine and colchicine.

Prognosis

The overall prognosis for cases of chronic active hepatitis is guarded. Doberman pinschers do very poorly; other breeds can fair better.[92, 95, 232, 238, 240] In one study, hypoalbuminemia and bridging fibrosis on hepatic biopsy were associated with shorter survival times.[240] Early diagnosis of the disease, coupled with ursodeoxycholic acid treatment, has resulted in improved survival and reduced clinical signs in my experience.

Hepatitis in Skye Terriers

A hepatitis syndrome in Skye terriers has been described, with histologic lesions ranging from hepatocellular degeneration and necrosis, with cholestasis and mild inflammation, to chronic hepatitis and cirrhosis.[243] Clinical signs and laboratory findings are typical of hepatitis, although several dogs were asymptomatic at the time of liver biopsy. The disorder does not appear to be a familial copper storage disease (see Copper-Associated Hepatitis), because copper accumulation is an inconsistent finding and is not uniformly present early in the disease. Intrahepatic cholestasis is the early and characteristic lesion, suggesting that copper accumulation occurs secondary to cholestasis. The disorder appears to be inherited with a defect in metabolism that interferes with bile secretion, resulting in cholestasis and copper accumulation. Prognosis appears to be poor, but results of treatment have not been reported.

Lobular Dissecting Hepatitis

A syndrome of chronic hepatitis has been described in young dogs (median age, approximately 1 year) that is characterized histologically by diffuse infiltration of inflammatory cells and fibrotic dissection of the lobular parenchyma into individual and small groups of hepatocytes.[244, 245] Standard poodles may be predisposed.[245, 246] Portal hypertension is common, and almost all reported cases involve ascites. Other clinical and laboratory findings are typical of chronic hepatitis. On necropsy, the liver is small and acquired portosystemic shunts are present. Prognosis appears to be poor, but results of treatment have not been reported.

Canine Acidophil Cell Hepatitis

A transmissible hepatitis that can cause acute and chronic disease and progresses to cirrhosis has been histologically described in which hepatocytes have strongly acidophilic cytoplasm, condensed nuclei, and contracted cell outlines causing an angular or polygonal form.[247, 248] The acute phase can cause severe clinical signs and death or persist for months, and it is associated with intermittent pyrexia and elevations of ALT. Other clinical and laboratory findings are those typical of acute or chronic hepatitis. The etiologic agent has not been identified, but evidence suggests it may be a virus. The prognosis is poor, but results of treatment have not been reported.

Cholangitis and Cholangiohepatitis

Cholangitis and cholangiohepatitis (cholangitis complex) is a common hepatic disease of cats but is relatively uncommon in dogs. It is characterized histologically by inflammation within the portal triads and extension into surrounding hepatocytes. Suppurative, plasmacytic-lymphocytic, lymphocytic, and mixed forms have been identified.[68, 249, 250] Biliary cirrhosis is believed by some to be the end stage of the cholangitis complex.[68] It is not known whether these histologic types are separate diseases or are stages of a single disorder. Cholangitis complex occurs in cats of all ages.[249, 250]

Pathophysiology

Initially, inflammation is localized to the bile ducts (cholangitis). Few clinical signs, if any, are present at this stage. Extension to surrounding hepatocytes (cholangiohepatitis) is associated with the development of clinical signs.[68]

Many cats with suppurative cholangitis and cholangiohepatitis have underlying disorders that favor the development of a septic process (e.g., inflammatory bowel disease, pancreatitis, extrahepatic biliary duct obstruction, cholecystitis).[68, 249, 251] However, in many of these cats it may not be possible to culture bacteria.[249, 251]

Lymphocytic and lymphocytic-plasmacytic infiltration is a response to chronic nonseptic inflammation. Inflammatory bowel disease and pancreatitis may participate in the development of these forms of cholangitis because inflammatory products and toxins may enter the liver through the portal blood.[249] Recently, the presence of increased portal infiltrates of plasma cells and lymphocytes was found to be a very common lesion in older cats with a wide variety of chronic disorders.[252]

Clinical Signs

Clinical signs include icterus, pyrexia, vomiting, diarrhea, dehydration, weight loss, and hepatomegaly.[68, 249–251, 253] Less common signs are abdominal pain, ascites, signs of hepatic encephalopathy, and generalized lymphadenopathy.[68, 254] Some cats maintain good appetites.[249, 254]

Diagnostic Plan

Diagnosis requires evaluation of clinical signs, laboratory abnormalities, abdominal ultrasonography, bacterial culture of bile or hepatic tissue, and histologic examination of hepatic tissue (after assessment of a coagulogram). Common laboratory abnormalities include increased ALT and AP, hyperbilirubinemia, poikilocytosis, leukocytosis with a left shift and toxic neutrophils (suppurative form), and abnormal coagulation tests (lymphocytic form).[68, 249–251] Hyperglobulinemia occurs in some cases.[254] Serum bile acids are often abnormally elevated.[250] On occasion, ultrasonography may demonstrate choleliths.[249]

Grossly, the liver has fine nodularity and an accentuated lobular pattern giving a reticulated appearance (see Fig. 34–11).[254] The histologic form of cholangitis complex is characterized by the type of inflammatory cells present in biopsy specimens. Histopathologic findings include infiltration of neutrophils, of plasma cells and lymphocytes, of lymphocytes, or of mixtures of cell types around the portal triads and into the surrounding hepatic parenchyma.[68] Dilation of intrahepatic bile ducts, periportal edema, and accumulation of exudate within the biliary lumen occur.[249, 251] Periductal fibrosis, swelling and degeneration of bile duct cells, bile duct hyperplasia, bridging fibrosis between portal triads, cholecystitis, cholelithiasis, and interstitial pancreatic fibrosis also occur.[249, 251, 253, 254] Bacteria culture may be positive, especially in the suppurative form, for *Escherichia coli*, *Clostridium*, *Bacteroides*, *Actinomyces*, and α-streptococcal species.[249, 251]

After histopathologic review of a biopsy specimen confirms a diagnosis of cholangitis complex, further evaluation of the cat for inflammatory bowel disease or pancreatitis is indicated (see Chaps. 32 and 33).

Treatment

Treatment of the suppurative form should include fluid therapy to correct dehydration and electrolyte abnormalities and antibiotic therapy. Initial antibiotic selection (pending culture and sensitivity) should include gentamicin (3 mg/kg t.i.d. intravenously, intramuscularly, or subcutaneously) and ampicillin (22 mg/kg t.i.d. or q.i.d., intravenously, intramuscularly, or subcutaneously) or gentamicin and metronidazole (7.5–10 mg/kg b.i.d. or t.i.d. intravenously or by mouth).[249] An alternative choice is chloramphenicol, which is effective against intestinal bacteria and undergoes enterohepatic circulation. Anorexia is a common side effect, but a dose of 50 mg per cat b.i.d. rarely causes inappetence.[68] If gentamicin is used, adequate hydration and renal perfusion must be maintained. Once culture and sensitivity results are obtained, gentamicin should be discontinued, if possible, and other antibiotics used. Other antibiotics should be continued for at least 3 to 6 weeks, with some authors suggesting 3 to 6 months.[249] If choleliths are causing extrahepatic biliary obstruction, surgical removal and decompression of the biliary tree should be performed (usually at a referral center).

If biliary obstruction is not present, or after the cholelith is removed, ursodeoxycholic acid, 10–15 mg/kg s.i.d., should be started.[249] Ursodeoxycholic acid is a choleretic that promotes bile flow and may prevent recurrence of cholelithiasis. It also replaces hydrophobic bile acids, reducing hepatic damage associated with cholestasis, and functions as a hepatoprotectant.[242]

Cats with the lymphocytic, lymphocytic-plasmacytic, or mixed forms should be treated with prednisone at 2 to 4 mg/kg per day.[68, 249, 253, 254] Glucocorticoids initiate some choleresis and help to treat concurrent inflammatory bowel disease, if present.[249] In addition to prednisone, metronidazole may be beneficial, 7.5 to 10 mg/kg b.i.d. It helps to modify the immune response and is effective against many anaerobic bacteria.[249] Ursodeoxycholic acid (already described) is also beneficial.[249]

Prognosis

The prognosis for cats with the cholangitis complex is variable.[250, 253, 254] Cats with the suppurative form caused by cholelithiasis can return to normal after surgical management and medical therapy.[249] Many cats with other forms can do well for long periods of time with treatment.[253] Some cats can be weaned off therapy without relapsing.[254] Much more needs to be learned about this syndrome before a more accurate prognosis can be offered.

Steroid Hepatopathy

A reversible hepatopathy develops in some dogs treated with glucocorticoids and in those with spontaneous hyperadrenalcorticism.[71] Any age or breed is susceptible to the iatrogenic disorder. Spontaneous hyperadrenalcorticism occurs most commonly in older dogs, especially dachshunds and poodles.[63] Hepatic failure or clinical signs of hepatic disease do not commonly develop in cases of steroid hepatopathy. The importance of recognizing this disorder is threefold: (1) if signs of hepatic dysfunction develop, they are reversible after withdrawal of corticosteroids; (2) clinical signs and laboratory changes may indicate spontaneous hyperadrenalcorticism, requiring additional diagnostic testing and therapy; and (3) identification of steroid hepatopathy in a dog receiving corticosteroids rules out other, more serious hepatic disorders. There can be difficulty separating cortico-

steroid-induced elevations in liver enzymes and steroid hepatopathy from another hepatic disorder in a dog that has received corticosteroids. Cats do not develop steroid hepatopathy.

Pathophysiology

Corticosteroids increase hepatic glycogen storage and gluconeogenesis and decrease glucose uptake and use by peripheral tissues.[255] Susceptibility of an individual dog to develop steroid hepatopathy is variable and also depends on the type, dose, and duration of corticosteroid administered. Some dogs develop hepatopathy after a single injection of glucocorticoids, others only after long-term administration, and many never develop hepatic changes.[71] Glucocorticoids can be given by any route, including oral, subcutaneous, intramuscular, intravenous, or topically applied to the eyes, ears, or skin.[255, 256] The rate of resolution of the hepatopathy is also variable.

Clinical Signs

The clinical signs associated with glucocorticoid administration or excess predominate. Polyuria, polydipsia, and polyphagia occur commonly.[71, 257] Moderate to severe hepatomegaly is commonly present.[71] Mild signs of liver disease, such as inappetence, vomiting, lethargy, and weight loss, rarely occur. Other signs of spontaneous hyperadrenocorticism (see Chap. 46), such as bilaterally symmetrical nonpruritic alopecia, a pot-bellied appearance, thin skin, hyperpigmentation, and recurrent pyoderma and urinary tract infections, may be present.[63]

Diagnostic Plan

The diagnosis of iatrogenic steroid hepatopathy should be based on a history of glucocorticoid administration, clinical signs, laboratory abnormalities, and re-evaluation after discontinuation or reduction of glucocorticoid administration. Rarely, if clinical signs of hepatic dysfunction are present, further evaluation should include abdominal ultrasonography, liver function testing (bile acids or serum ammonia), and hepatic biopsy (after assessment of coagulation).

Dogs with steroid hepatopathy can have massively increased AP and normal or mildly or moderately increased ALT.[48, 71, 116, 257–259] Lymphopenia and eosinopenia can be present.[258, 260] Serum bile acids may be normal or mildly increased.[48, 130] Hepatic ultrasound reveals diffusely increased echogenicity (see Fig. 34–5).[42]

Grossly, the liver is enlarged, smooth, and friable.[257] Histologically, the liver is characterized by hydropic degeneration and centrilobular vacuolization.[259] Glycogen accumulates within the vacuoles.[257, 258] Focal necrosis may be present.[71]

The diagnosis of spontaneous hyperadrenocorticism requires evaluation of the pituitary-adrenal axis with an adrenocorticotropic hormone response test (see Chap. 46).

Treatment

Usually, treatment is not indicated. Rarely, if clinical signs of hepatic dysfunction are present, it may be necessary to withdraw or reduce corticosteroid therapy. If corticosteroids are needed to treat a primary disease, the dosage should be reduced to the lowest alternate-day amount necessary to control the primary condition. Addition of other immunosuppressive drugs, such as azathioprine or cyclophosphamide, may allow reduction or elimination of the corticosteroid dose. Hyperadrenalcorticism should be treated as described in Chapter 46.

Prognosis

The prognosis for steroid hepatopathy is excellent. Withdrawal of corticosteroids or treatment of hyperadrenocorticism resolves the clinical signs, laboratory abnormalities, and histologic findings. Because most dogs with steroid hepatopathy do not develop clinical signs, the clinician needs to recognize the presence of the disorder and accept it as a common side effect of glucocorticoid therapy.

Drug-Induced Hepatotoxicity

In humans, drug-induced liver disease is a common cause of icterus and acute hepatic failure.[21] The frequency in dogs and cats is unknown, but it is believed to be greater than reported because of the difficulty of establishing a definitive diagnosis and the absence of routine biochemical monitoring during drug therapy. Many drugs commonly used in small animal practice have the potential to cause acute or chronic hepatic disease in individual patients. Drugs that often cause hepatic toxicity are rarely used or are used with extreme caution, often at lower dosages.

Drug-induced hepatic disease should be considered in the differential diagnosis in any dog or cat with clinical signs or laboratory findings consistent with hepatic disease that received drug therapy before developing signs.[21] The most commonly used drugs associated with toxicity are anticonvulsants (phenobarbital, primidone, phenytoin), anthelmintics (oxibendazole and mebendazole), glucocorticoids (see Steroid Hepatopathy), antimicrobials (trimethoprim-sulfonamides, tetracycline, ketoconazole, and griseofulvin), anesthetics (halothane and methoxyflurane), acetaminophen, thiacetarsamide, and phenylbuta-

zone.[20, 21] A discussion of several clinically important examples of drug-induced hepatotoxicity follows the Prognosis section.

Pathophysiology

Hepatotoxins can be classified as either intrinsic or idiosyncratic.[21] Intrinsic hepatotoxins produce a predictable reaction: toxicity in a large number of treated individuals. The injury produced by intrinsic hepatotoxins is dose dependent and is reproducible in experimental animals. Idiosyncratic hepatotoxins produce injury in a very small percentage of animals treated. Induction of toxicity is unpredictable and cannot reliably be produced in experimental animals. There is little if any dose dependency. Intrinsic hepatotoxins are not routinely used in veterinary practice, or they are administered in doses that do not produce toxicity.

How and why idiosyncratic hepatotoxicity develops in an individual animal is unknown. Possible factors influencing toxicity include age, sex, genetic variation in drug metabolism, pre-existing hepatic disease, administration of other drugs, environmental factors, nutritional status, and concurrent diseases.[20] Hepatotoxins can be cytotoxic, induce cholestasis, or, rarely, result in neoplasia.[171] Hepatotoxins can directly damage the hepatocyte membrane or can enter the cell and disrupt metabolic pathways.[21] In cats, deficiency of glucuronic acid and reduced ability to conjugate drugs may participate in the pathogenesis of toxicity.[20]

Clinical Signs

Hepatic drug-induced toxicity may cause only elevated liver enzymes or may cause clinical signs of acute or chronic liver disease. Acute hepatic disease usually develops during drug treatment or shortly after completion of therapy. Signs associated with acute hepatic disease include anorexia, depression, icterus, hepatomegaly, vomiting, diarrhea, polyuria and polydipsia, dark urine, a bleeding diathesis, and signs of hepatic encephalopathy.[150] Clinical signs of chronic hepatic disease are usually associated with long-term drug administration. Initially, signs may be mild and episodic, but they often progress and become continuous. In addition to the signs listed for acute disease, ascites, weight loss, and peripheral edema may develop.

Diagnostic Plan

The diagnosis of drug-induced hepatotoxicity is easy to suspect but difficult to prove. Drug-induced hepatic injury does not produce pathognomonic clinical, laboratory, or histologic changes.[20] Ideally, diagnosis should be based on challenge with the potential agent.[20] This is dangerous and impractical and should not be performed routinely in veterinary practice. A tentative diagnosis can be made if clinical signs or laboratory abnormalities develop in association with administration of a known hepatotoxic drug and resolve after discontinuation of the medication. If the drug in question has not commonly caused hepatotoxicity in dogs and cats, arriving at a tentative diagnosis is more difficult. If only laboratory abnormalities or mild clinical signs occur, the animal can be reassessed 2 to 4 weeks after discontinuance of the drug. However, if moderate or severe clinical signs occur, a further diagnostic work-up is indicated (i.e., liver function tests, hepatic ultrasound, and liver biopsy, after assessment of coagulation).

Laboratory abnormalities associated with drug-induced hepatic toxicity include elevated ALT (hepatocyte injury), elevated AP and hyperbilirubinemia (intrahepatic cholestasis), hypoalbuminemia, reduced BUN, hyperammonemia, and elevated bile acids (liver failure).[167–172] Histologic findings are variable and nonspecific and have been defined for only a few drugs.[167–172] However, histologic patterns can aid diagnosis, especially the decision as to whether drug toxicity is present or clinical findings are caused by another hepatic disorder in an animal that is coincidentally receiving a potentially hepatotoxic drug.

Treatment

If only laboratory abnormalities or mild clinical signs are present, the only treatment required is discontinuation of the drug.[20] The drug should not be given to the animal for the remainder of its life. If moderate or severe clinical signs are present, supportive care as described in the section on hepatitis and necrosis should be instituted.

Prognosis

The prognosis for hepatic drug toxicity is variable and depends on the agent administered, the severity of hepatic disease, and the duration of the drug-induced hepatotoxicity. Animals with only laboratory abnormalities or mild clinical signs should completely recover after withdrawal of the drug. The prognosis is guarded in patients with more severe clinical signs. Progression to cirrhosis is a poor prognostic sign.

Anticonvulsants

It has been estimated that between 6% and 15% of dogs receiving anticonvulsants for at least 6 months develop hepatic disease (Fig. 34–15).[170, 261] Increased serum enzymes (ALT up to 150 IU/L and AP up to 300 IU/L) commonly occur in dogs receiving long-term anticonvulsants, usually because of enzyme induction,

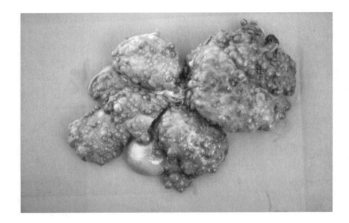

Figure 34–15
Necropsy specimen from a 9-year-old Lhasa apso that received primidone for 4 years to treat seizures. The liver is small, tan, and nodular. Histologically, the parenchyma is collapsed and contains dense bands of fibrous connective tissue. Nodular regeneration is present.

and they are not necessarily associated with serious hepatic disease.[113, 114, 262]

Hepatic abnormalities occur more often in dogs treated with high dosages of primidone, primidone and phenytoin, and phenobarbital for at least 6 months.[169, 170, 172, 262] Liver enzymes are commonly elevated, liver function tests (bile acids or sulfobromophthalein sodium [Bromsulfalein retention]) abnormal, and histologic changes common in the livers of dogs receiving primidone and phenytoin alone or in combination.[170, 262] However, clinical signs of hepatic failure (weakness, lethargy, anorexia, ataxia, weight loss, ascites, icterus, and coagulopathy), hypoalbuminemia, hyperbilirubinemia, hypocholesterolemia, and cirrhosis of the liver occur less commonly.[169–172, 262] In one review, 31% of dogs with cirrhosis had received long-term anticonvulsant medications.[170] In both clinical and experimental studies, laboratory abnormalities are reversible if the dosage is reduced or the drug discontinued.[113, 172, 262] Use of alternative anticonvulsants, such as potassium bromide, may allow reduction in drug dosage without intensification of seizures (see Chap. 24).

Hepatotoxicity associated with administration of phenobarbital can occur when serum levels are within the therapeutic range (<40–45 µg/mL).[172] It has been suggested that maximum serum levels not exceed 35 µg/mL.[172]

Histologic findings in dogs receiving primidone or phenytoin, or both, without signs of hepatic failure are hepatocellular hypertrophy, single cell necrosis, multifocal lipidosis, dilated bile canaliculi, and damaged sinusoidal epithelium.[262] A syndrome of intrahepatic cholestasis also occurs in dogs receiving phenytoin in combination with other anticonvulsants. In these dogs, hepatomegaly with diffuse hepatocellular swelling and cytoplasmic vacuolization occurs.[171] Primidone and phenobarbital are associated with small, firm, nodular livers, nodular regeneration, fibrosis, bile duct hyperplasia, cholestasis, and mild inflammation (see Fig. 34–15).[169, 172]

Oxibendazole

Periportal hepatitis has been identified in some dogs that received diethylcarbamazine-oxibendazole as a heartworm-hookworm preventative.[20, 167] Clinical signs included anorexia, depression, vomiting, weight loss, icterus, ascites, behavioral changes, and seizures; these signs developed from 4 days to 10 months after starting therapy. Laboratory findings included elevated liver enzymes, hyperbilirubinemia, hypoalbuminemia, borderline reduced BUN, and hyperammonemia. Hepatocellular swelling, vesicular nuclei, thickened and disorganized hepatic cords, infiltration of neutrophils in periportal areas, portal or bridging fibrosis, and bile duct proliferation were found histologically. Clinical improvement occurred within 21 days of stopping the medication, although biochemical resolution required up to 6 months in some dogs. Challenges in two dogs resulted in return of clinical signs, laboratory findings, and histopathologic changes.

Mebendazole

Acute hepatic necrosis has been reported in dogs receiving mebendazole for routine GI parasite control.[168] Acute hepatic failure occurred and was characterized by anorexia, depression, vomiting, icterus, hemorrhagic diarrhea, and death in some dogs. Clinical signs appeared as soon as the first day of treatment or as long as 2 weeks after administration of mebendazole. Laboratory abnormalities include elevated hepatic enzymes and hyperbilirubinemia. Severe generalized centrilobular necrosis was found histologically. Biochemical changes returned to normal in surviving dogs. Experimentally, administration of repeated and exaggerated mebendazole dosages did not induce clinical or laboratory findings of hepatic disease in normal dogs.[263] In addition, mebendazole had no effect on carbon tetrachloride hepatotoxicity and did not cause hepatic disease in dogs with glutathione depletion or in those pretreated with barbiturates or fed a high-protein diet. These studies suggest that the uncommon occurrence of mebendazole-induced hepatotoxicity must be caused by unrecognized factors.[263]

Cirrhosis

Cirrhosis is the end stage of many inflammatory diseases.[8] It accounted for 15% of hepatic biopsy samples evaluated at one institution.[8] It is characterized by widespread fibrosis and loss of normal hepatic architecture.[8] On the basis of histopathologic findings, it is usually not possible to determine the cause of the liver disease at this stage.

Pathophysiology

Fibrosis is part of the normal repair process of inflammation.[8] Severe acute inflammation or chronic inflammation leads to the deposition of so much fibrous tissue that it interferes with hepatic function. The process can become self-perpetuating. Regenerative nodules form as remaining hepatocytes undergo hyperplasia to restore hepatic functions.[8] Contracting fibrous tissue and regenerative nodules compress sinusoids and bile ducts, leading to hypoxia, further inflammation, and subsequent fibrosis and cholestasis.[8, 264] Prolonged cholestasis adds to hepatic damage.[8, 27] As the condition becomes advanced, there is an increase in hepatic collagen synthesis and reduction in hepatic collagenase activity.[8] Interference with hepatic blood flow leads to development of bridging vascular channels from the portal tracts to the central veins, bypassing the sinusoidal system.[8]

As portal hypertension (see Ascites) develops as a result of obstruction of sinusoidal flow, extrahepatic shunts between the portal vein and systemic venous circulation develop.[8, 78] These acquired shunts promote bypass of portal blood around the liver and result in pathophysiologic effects similar to those that occur with congenital shunts (see Portosystemic Shunts). Shunts are often multiple and commonly occur in the region of the left kidney.[8] However, unlike congenital shunts, acquired shunts do not benefit from attenuation, because this would cause fatal portal hypertension. Acquired portosystemic shunts represent the body's compensation to life-threatening portal hypertension caused by severe hepatic disease.

Clinical Signs

The clinical signs of cirrhosis indicate severe chronic hepatic disease and liver failure. Weight loss is usually profound.[8] Icterus, ascites, edema, and signs of hepatic encephalopathy are very pronounced.[8] Other signs of liver disease also occur: vomiting, diarrhea, polyuria and polydipsia, and coagulopathy.[8]

Diagnostic Plan

Diagnosis of cirrhosis requires evaluation of the clinical signs, routine laboratory evaluation, liver function tests, hepatic ultrasound, and histopathologic changes (after assessment of coagulation). Serum ALT may be mildly to moderately elevated.[8] It is often lower than expected with this severity of disease because of the lack of active inflammation. AP is often elevated, and hyperbilirubinemia, hypoalbuminemia, reduced BUN, and bilirubinuria are present.[8, 48] Liver function tests are abnormal.[48, 130] Radiographically, the liver appears small. An exception to this is in biliary cirrhosis of cats, which is associated with hepatomegaly.[8, 68] Ultrasound may reveal a highly irregular hepatic border, nodules, increased superficial echogenicity, and markedly diminished echogenicity deep within the liver.[42]

Definitive diagnosis requires hepatic biopsy.[48, 130] Grossly, the liver is small, misshapen, nodular, and covered with fibrous bands (see Fig. 34–15).[8] Histologically, loss of normal architecture, widespread fibrosis, regenerative nodules, and scattered areas of inflammation and necrosis are seen.

Treatment

Treatment for cirrhosis is very difficult and usually supportive. If an underlying hepatic disorder can be identified, it should be treated.[8] Potentially hepatotoxic medications should be withdrawn. Fluid therapy should be administered as described in the section on hepatitis. Signs of encephalopathy should be treated medically and nutritionally, as previously described. A broad-spectrum antibiotic, such as ampicillin, 22 mg/kg t.i.d. or q.i.d., should be administered intravenously, intramuscularly, subcutaneously, or by mouth, because of the reduced reticuloendothelial cell function of the liver.[8] Ascites may need to be managed by intermittent abdominocentesis, a low-salt diet, and diuretic therapy (see Chronic Active Hepatitis).

If gastritis and gastric ulceration develop (see Hepatitis and Necrosis), they should be treated with a histamine$_2$-receptor antagonist, such as cimetidine (5–10 mg/kg t.i.d. or q.i.d.) or sucralfate (1 g/25 kg b.i.d. or t.i.d. subcutaneously, intravenously, intramuscularly, or by mouth in dogs; 0.25 g b.i.d. or t.i.d. by mouth in cats).[8]

Although not commonly used in veterinary medicine, treatment to arrest fibrogenesis has been beneficial in humans with chronic hepatic diseases.[264] Colchicine (0.03 mg/kg s.i.d. by mouth) blocks the secretion of collagen into the fibrous matrix, is also anti-inflammatory, and may have a direct hepatoprotectant effect.[264] Toxic effects include vomiting, diarrhea, and abdominal pain. D-penicillamine (10–15 mg/kg b.i.d. by mouth) inhibits collagen cross-linking, chelates copper and promotes urinary excretion, and has immunomodulating effects.[264] The most common toxic effect is vomiting. Further investigation into the use of these and other promising agents is necessary to demonstrate benefit in animals with chronic inflammatory and fibrotic hepatic disorders.

Prognosis

The prognosis for patients with cirrhosis is very poor. Liver function is irreversibly destroyed, and the available treatments are only supportive.

Neoplasia

Primary and metastatic hepatobiliary neoplasia occurs in middle-aged to older dogs and cats.[69, 70, 136, 265–268] Metastatic tumors are more common than primary tumors.[269] Primary tumors account for approximately 1% of cancers in dogs.[70] Malignant primary tumors occur more often than benign tumors. Lymphosarcoma can occur in younger animals. Male dogs may be predisposed to develop hepatocellular carcinomas and females to develop biliary carcinomas.[70, 268]

Pathophysiology

Hepatocellular Adenoma

Hepatocellular adenoma, or hepatoma, is a benign tumor of hepatocytes that occurs in older dogs. It usually is a single, large, well-circumscribed mass that may become massive.[70] It often does not cause clinical signs but can cause abdominal distention, hypovolemic shock from rupture and intra-abdominal hemorrhage, and, occasionally, hypoglycemia resulting from a paraneoplastic syndrome.[70] The tumor is uncommon in cats and is usually discovered as an incidental finding at necropsy.[267]

Hepatocellular Carcinoma

Hepatocellular carcinoma is a malignant tumor of hepatocytes that occurs most commonly in older male dogs (Fig. 34–16). It occurs in three forms: (1) a single large mass originating from a single lobe (left lobes are most common), which is the most common type, (2) multiple nodules throughout the liver, or (3) a diffuse, nonencapsulated mass infiltrating a large area of the liver.[70, 265, 268] It is a highly metastatic tumor spreading to other hepatic lobes, regional lymph nodes, omentum, and the lungs.[70, 268]

Biliary (Cholangiocellular) Adenoma

Biliary adenoma is a benign tumor of biliary epithelium that occurs in older cats.[69, 267] It usually is found as an incidental finding at necropsy and does not cause clinical signs.[267]

Biliary (Cholangiocellular) Carcinoma

Biliary carcinoma is a malignant tumor originating from biliary epithelium in older dogs and cats (Fig. 34–17). It can arise from intrahepatic bile ducts, extrahepatic bile ducts, or the gallbladder, but the intrahepatic location is most common.[70, 270] Within the

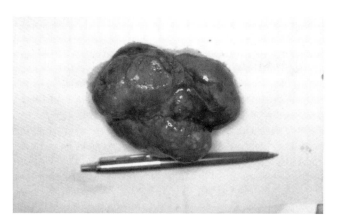

Figure 34–16
Resected solitary hepatocellular carcinoma from the left lateral liver lobe of an 11-year-old miniature schnauzer.

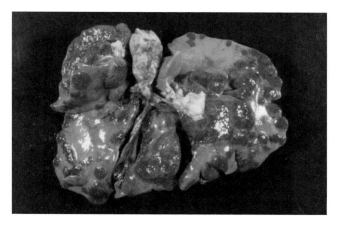

Figure 34–18
Necropsy specimen of the liver from an 18-month-old domestic shorthair cat with lymphosarcoma showing diffuse multifocal nodules of various sizes. The nodules are red.

liver, it can assume the same three forms as does hepatocellular carcinoma.[70, 268] It commonly causes cholestasis and icterus. It is also a highly metastatic tumor, spreading to regional lymph nodes, omentum, and the lungs.[70, 270]

Lymphosarcoma

If lymphosarcoma (Fig. 34–18) involves the liver, it often is present in the stomach and small or large intestines as well (see Chaps. 31 and 32). Occasionally, it may affect only the liver.

Metastatic Tumors

Tumors may spread to the liver through the portal system, arterial blood supply, or lymphatics, or

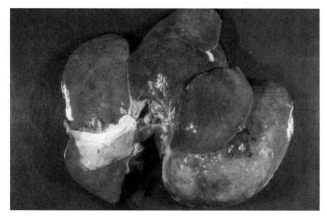

Figure 34–17
Necropsy specimen of a solitary biliary carcinoma from a 13-year-old Labrador retriever. The mass is in the left lateral lobe, measures approximately 10 × 15 cm, is mottled tan to dark green, and is cystic in some areas. Small foci (<4 mm) of metastasis are present throughout the other lobes.

by direct extension. Adenocarcinoma or undifferentiated carcinoma originating in the mammary glands, spleen, pancreas, stomach, and intestines is most common. Metastatic tumors often appear as multifocal nodules (Fig. 34–19; see Fig. 34–2).

Clinical Signs

The clinical signs associated with hepatobiliary neoplasia are variable and depend on the tumor type, its location, and the extent of disease. A mass, hepatomegaly, or ascites may be detected during physical examination in an asymptomatic animal or during the evaluation of another problem.[265] Mild signs of liver disease are most commonly seen: anorexia, weight loss, lethargy, or occasional vomiting or diarrhea.[70, 136, 265, 267–269, 271] Icterus is common with biliary carcinomas. Signs of hepatic failure can occur with diffuse infiltration of the liver and include ascites, hepatic encephalopathy, icterus, severe weight loss, vomiting, diarrhea, polyuria and polydipsia, and coagulopathy. Rupture of a large hepatic mass can lead to hemoperitoneum and hypovolemic shock. This can occur spontaneously or, often, after minor trauma or physical activity. Other signs relate to the site of metastasis of the hepatobiliary tumor. Tachypnea, cough, or dyspnea may occur secondary to pulmonary metastasis.

The clinical signs associated with metastatic neoplasia of the liver are often related to the primary tumor.[271] Mammary neoplasia is associated with palpable mammary masses. Splenic neoplasia often causes a palpable abdominal mass and may rupture and result in abdominal hemorrhage and hypovolemic shock. Pancreatic tumors cause profound weight loss, vomiting, and icterus. Tumors of the stomach and intestines can cause vomiting or diarrhea, or both.

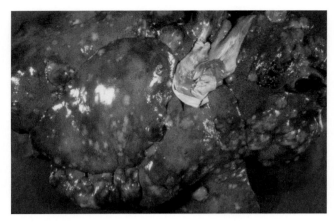

Figure 34-19

Necropsy specimen of the liver from a 7-year-old mixed breed dog with metastatic pancreatic adenocarcinoma. The liver has extensive coalescing tan nodules 5 mm to 3 cm in diameter involving approximately 80% of the liver.

Diagnostic Plan

Suspicion of hepatic neoplasia is based on the animal's age, the presence of clinical signs, or, in many cases, abnormalities found on the biochemical profile. Hepatic ultrasound is very helpful in establishing a tentative diagnosis. Thoracic radiographs (ventrodorsal, right lateral, and left lateral) should be evaluated for the presence of metastasis if neoplasia is suspected.[136] A definitive diagnosis requires hepatic biopsy (after evaluation of coagulation). This is especially important to differentiate neoplastic nodules from hyperplastic nodules, which frequently occur in the livers of older dogs.[6] If metastatic neoplasia is suspected after hepatic ultrasound, a thorough search for the primary tumor should be performed. All mammary glands in females should be palpated carefully. Careful abdominal palpation should be performed, and intra-abdominal structures, especially the spleen and pancreas, should be evaluated with abdominal ultrasound.

Common laboratory findings associated with hepatic neoplasia include anemia, neutrophilia, elevated ALT and AP, and hyperbilirubinemia and bilirubinuria in cholestatic diseases.[48, 70, 126, 265, 267–269, 272] Diffuse infiltration of the liver can be associated with hepatic failure and hypoalbuminemia, reduced BUN, and abnormal liver function tests.[48, 126, 130, 272] Measurements of serum α-fetoprotein (a protein produced by the fetus and by some malignant tumors) have demonstrated that high levels can be associated with the common primary hepatic malignant tumors in dogs.[272]

The most common radiographic changes associated with hepatic neoplasia are a right cranial abdominal mass, causing left gastric displacement and loss of intra-abdominal detail, resulting from ascites or carcinomatosis (see Fig. 34–3).[136, 265] Other radiographic findings associated with localized hepatic enlargement include caudal displacement of the fundus (left side) and caudal displacement of the ventral fundus and gastric body (central).[73] Administration of a small volume of barium helps to outline the stomach (see Fig. 34–4).

Ultrasound evaluation can identify neoplasia as focal, large mixed hyperechoic and hypoechoic masses or multifocal hypoechoic masses (Fig. 34–20).[138] Metastatic neoplasia may appear as focal areas of decreased echogenicity, areas with both increased and decreased echogenicity (target lesions with an echo-dense center surrounded by a sonolucent rim), or areas of diffuse involvement without focal masses (see Fig. 34–2).[37, 47] Lymphosarcoma has several patterns: a normal parenchyma or a slight reduction in echogenicity, anechoic or hypoechoic and poorly marginated lesions, or multiple round echodensities surrounded by sonolucency.[46]

Treatment

Surgical resection of hepatocellular adenomas and the massive forms of hepatocellular and biliary carcinoma can be accomplished.[70, 265] Lymphosarcoma can be treated with chemotherapy (see Chap. 43).

Prognosis

The prognosis for most animals with malignant (primary and metastatic) hepatobiliary tumors is

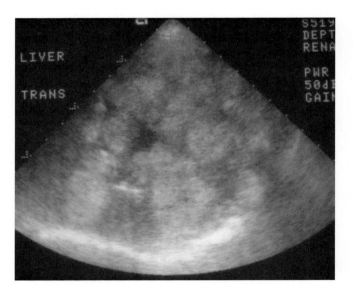

Figure 34-20

Transverse cross-sectional ultrasonographic appearance of hepatic carcinoma in a 13-year-old toy poodle. Multiple hyperechoic nodules are present. Histologically, evidence of both hepatocellular and cholangiocellular neoplasia is present. (Courtesy of Martha L. Moon, DVM, MS, Blacksburg, Virginia.)

poor.[70, 267] In dogs, some hepatocellular adenomas can be resected and long-term survival expected.[70] In cats, cholangiocellular adenomas rarely cause clinical signs, and the prognosis without treatment is good. Massive forms of hepatocellular and biliary carcinomas that can be resected surgically have a good long-term prognosis because some of these are slow to metastasize.[265]

Uncommon Hepatobiliary Diseases

Copper-Associated Hepatitis

Copper-associated hepatitis (copper storage disease) is a hereditary disorder of Bedlington terriers that results in the inability to excrete copper in bile, accumulation of copper by hepatocytes, and hepatitis.[273] A similar disease also occurs in West Highland white terriers.[274] Copper-associated hepatitis can cause acute hepatic failure in young adult dogs, often after a stressful event. More commonly, however, chronic progressive hepatitis occurs. Asymptomatic carriers pass the disease to their offspring as an autosomal recessive trait.[275] At one time, it was estimated that as many as 65% of Bedlington terriers carried the gene.

Clinical signs and laboratory findings are those typical of hepatitis. Diagnosis requires biopsy and determination of hepatic copper content. Histopathologic findings may include normal morphology, focal hepatitis, chronic active hepatitis, or cirrhosis. Hepatic copper concentrations are often greater than 2000 μg/g (normal, <350 μg/g). Carriers may have elevated hepatic copper levels at 5 to 7 months that return to normal by 14 to 15 months.[276] Fecal excretion of radioactive copper was shown to be a noninvasive method of diagnosis.[277]

Specific therapy requires removal of the excess copper from the liver. D-Penicillamine (10–15 mg/kg b.i.d. by mouth) or trientine (10–15 mg/kg b.i.d. by mouth) chelates copper and promote urinary excretion.[278] It often takes 12 months or longer to reduce hepatic copper. Zinc acetate (4–10 mg/kg b.i.d. by mouth) decreases intestinal copper absorption.[279] Vitamin C (500–1000 mg/day by mouth) promotes urinary excretion of copper. Ursodeoxycholic acid (see Chronic Active Hepatitis) has been recommended, but results of therapy are not yet published. The prognosis for clinically affected dogs is guarded, but early diagnosis and vigorous treatment can improve clinical signs.

Hepatic Abscesses

Hepatic abscesses occur in neonates in association with omphalophlebitis and in adults because of hematogenous spread of bacteria from septic foci or septicemia.[11, 280] Clinical signs relate to the underlying disorder. Signs associated with abscesses include anorexia, depression, vomiting, persistent fever, and hepatomegaly. Laboratory findings include leukocytosis with a left shift, hyperglobulinemia, elevated liver enzymes, hyperbilirubinemia, and hypoglycemia. Radiographs may reveal hepatomegaly or focal radiolucent areas within the liver (gas formation). Ultrasound may reveal a hypoechoic or anechoic structure containing mixed echoes.[281] Treatment consists of exploratory surgery to drain fluid or remove abnormal tissue, supportive care, antibiotic therapy based on culture and sensitivity, and treatment of the underlying process.

Idiopathic Hepatic Fibrosis

Idiopathic hepatic fibrosis has been described in a group of young dogs (many were German shepherds).[282] Common findings included ascites, anorexia, weight loss, hepatic encephalopathy, vomiting, diarrhea, microcytosis, increased liver enzymes, hyperbilirubinemia, hypoalbuminemia, abnormal liver function tests, and microhepatica on radiographs. Several dogs survived for long periods and were treated for encephalopathy and with prednisolone or colchicine.

Platynosomum concinnum

The biliary trematode of cats has a complex life cycle that requires three intermediate hosts.[283] The fluke measures approximately 5 to 6 mm × 2 mm. Adults live in the gallbladder and bile ducts. In the United States, it is most common in Florida and Hawaii.[284, 285] Cats with low fluke burdens remain asymptomatic; those with heavier infection develop vague clinical signs such as anorexia, depression, and weight loss. Vomiting, diarrhea, hepatomegaly, icterus, and ascites can develop in patients with biliary obstruction. Operculated eggs can be identified in direct fecal smears or by formalin-ether sedimentation. Laboratory findings include eosinophilia, elevated ALT, and, in patients with biliary obstruction, elevated AP, hyperbilirubinemia, and bilirubinuria. Ultrasound may demonstrate distention of the gallbladder and bile duct. Animals with chronic cases with heavy infection can develop cholangiohepatitis and fibrosis. Pancreatic atrophy can develop if flukes migrate into pancreatic ducts. Treatment with praziquantal (20 mg/kg by mouth) is effective and should be repeated at 12-week intervals.

Peliosis Hepatis

Peliosis hepatis is characterized by blood-filled cystic spaces in the hepatic parenchyma and is often accompanied by telangiectasis and dilation of sinusoids.[286] It has been described in a group of cats with abdominal hemorrhage, anemia, weakness, and hepatomegaly.

Amyloidosis

Deposition of amyloid within the liver is an uncommon cause of hepatomegaly. Familial renal amyloidosis has been described in Chinese shar-peis.[287] Many of these dogs also had deposition into the liver. Other findings included chronic renal failure, fever, swollen tibiotarsal joints, vomiting, anorexia, ascites, and edema. No treatment has been proven to be effective, but colchicine has been recommended. Clinical signs of hepatic disease and rupture of the liver causing intra-abdominal hemorrhage have been reported.[288, 289]

Tyzzer's Disease

Infection with *Bacillus piliformis* results in fatal multifocal, periportal hepatitis in dogs and cats.[290] The organism is a normal inhabitant of the GI tract of rodents. Most affected animals are immunosuppressed. Clinical signs of the peracute hepatitis include depression, anorexia, hypothermia, hepatomegaly, abdominal pain, icterus, and abdominal enlargement. Laboratory findings may include anemia, neutropenia, elevated ALT, and hyperbilirubinemia. The organisms can be identified in tissue samples but cannot be cultured on artificial media. No effective treatment is available.

Carcinoids

Hepatic carcinoids, malignant tumors of neuroectodermal origin, occur in old dogs.[291] Clinical signs include anorexia, ascites, weight loss, polyuria and polydipsia, icterus, and diarrhea. Laboratory abnormalities include anemia, leukocytosis, elevated liver enzymes, and hyperbilirubinemia. All liver lobes are usually affected and contain nodules. Metastasis to the mesentery, omentum, and lymph nodes is common. Prognosis is very poor.

Cystadenomas

Cystic hepatic masses can be benign or malignant. A slow-growing, benign tumor has been described in old cats.[292] Clinical signs occur when the masses get large and include abdominal enlargement, lethargy, vomiting, polydipsia, hepatomegaly, and ascites. Ultrasound reveals cystic hepatic masses. Exploratory surgery to resect the masses and establish a definitive diagnosis is indicated. Long-term prognosis is excellent.

Hepatic Microvascular Dysplasia

Hepatic microvascular dysplasia describes the histologic findings in the liver of animals with portosystemic shunts and some without a macroscopic shunt.[230, 293] Dogs and cats in the latter group have clinical signs similar to those with a congenital shunt, although signs are usually less severe and diagnosis often is reached at a later age. Serum bile acids are often elevated, but not as high as in those patients with congenital shunts. Contrast radiographic studies are usually normal. Treatment with a low-protein diet is often successful. Hepatic microvascular dysplasia may represent a congenital disorder wherein portal blood is shunted directly to the central vein, bypassing the sinusoids. The importance of diagnosing this syndrome is to rule out the presence of a macroscopic shunt that can be surgically attenuated.

Arteriovenous Fistula

Hepatic arteriovenous fistulae can occur as congenital defects (in puppies) or, rarely, secondary to trauma or neoplasia.[294] Clinical signs often develop suddenly. Ascites, pyrexia, cardiac murmur, vomiting, diarrhea, and signs of encephalopathy are common. A continuous murmur can often be auscultated over the liver through the abdominal wall. Laboratory abnormalities include anemia, leukocytosis, elevated AP and ALT, hypoalbuminemia, low BUN, and abnormal liver function tests. Acquired portosystemic shunts develop commonly. Diagnosis can be based on angiography, scintigraphy, or surgical exploration, whereby the fistula is usually visible as a tortuous vessel in the involved liver lobe. Treatment requires lobectomy and, in some cases, additional surgery to attenuate the acquired portosystemic shunts. Medical management of hepatic encephalopathy may be needed. The overall prognosis is guarded, but dogs that survive surgery often do well.

Veno-occlusive Disease

Multiple acquired portosystemic shunts have been described in a group of young cocker spaniels. Clinical signs and laboratory results were similar to those of dogs with congenital portosystemic shunts. Histologically, prominent muscular sphincters were present in small hepatic venules and appeared to be in spasm; perivenous fibrous tissue was also observed. Prognosis was poor.

Urea Cycle Enzyme Deficiency

A congenital deficiency of urea cycle enzymes can cause hyperammonemia and signs of hepatic encephalopathy.[19] Diagnosis requires enzyme assay of frozen tissue. Treatment for hepatic encephalopathy may improve clinical signs.

Glycogen Storage Diseases

A group of inherited disorders causing deficiencies of enzymes necessary for normal glycogen metabolism occurs in dogs and cats and can result in glycogen accumulation within tissues.[295, 296] In addition to the liver, the CNS, kidney, heart, and skeletal muscle can be affected. Clinical signs occur in young animals and reflect the organs involved. In some forms of the disease, hepatomegaly and hypoglycemia are common. Diagnosis requires enzymatic assay of affected tissue. There is no effective treatment available.

Hepatocutaneous Syndrome

Superficial necrolytic dermatitis (hepatocutaneous syndrome) has been described in dogs. Crusting lesions of the foot pads, mucocutaneous junctions, ears, elbows, and hocks occur in association with a severe hepatopathy.[297] The syndrome has been seen in dogs with glucagon-producing pancreatic tumors or diabetes mellitus, but neither of these conditions must be present. Livers are often small and nodular and have hepatocellular degeneration.

Chylous Ascites

The leakage of chyle into the abdomen is an uncommon cause of ascites.[62, 298] Fluid is pink to creamy white and contains a high concentration of triglycerides. It has been associated with intraabdominal neoplasia, lymphosarcoma, biliary cirrhosis, steatitis, rupture of a mesenteric lymph vessel, lymphatic obstruction, and surgical ligation of the thoracic duct.

Kinking of the Vena Cava

Kinking of the intrathoracic caudal vena cava is an uncommon cause of ascites.[299] Possible causes of kinking include trauma, pulmonary neoplasia, and cardiomegaly. Treatment includes surgical correction of the defect and management of the primary condition.

Biliary Tract Rupture

Perforation, avulsion, or rupture of the bile duct, hepatic ducts, gallbladder, or cystic duct occasionally occurs as a result of blunt or penetrating trauma of the abdomen or secondary to cholelithiasis or cholecystitis.[5, 300–302] Diagnosis is usually not reached until 10 to 14 days after the traumatic event. Other injuries causing serious clinical signs often occur.

Clinical signs of biliary tract rupture include lethargy, depression, anorexia, icterus, ascites, vomiting, and gray stools. Laboratory abnormalities include elevated AP and ALT, hyperbilirubinemia, and bilirubinuria. Abdominal fluid contains a higher level of bilirubin than serum contains. Bilirubin crystals can sometimes be seen. Surgical repair of the defect or cholecystoduodenostomy is necessary.

Cholelithiasis

Choleliths commonly develop within the biliary tree in dogs but only rarely cause clinical signs, usually associated with cholecystitis, biliary obstruction, or biliary tree rupture.[137, 303] In cats, they have been associated with the cholangiohepatitis syndrome. Calculi can be found within the gallbladder, cystic duct, and common bile duct. Multiple calculi are often present. Common clinical signs, if they occur, include vomiting, anorexia, weakness, and icterus. Laboratory abnormalities include neutrophilia, greatly increased AP and mildly increased ALT, severe hyperbilirubinemia, and bilirubinuria. About 50% of calculi are radiopaque. Bacterial culture of bile is usually positive. Calculi can often be identified with ultrasound. Calculi consist mainly of bilirubin pigments. Treatment requires antibiotic therapy based on culture and sensitivity, removal of calculi, cholecystectomy, or, in some instances, cholecystoduodenostomy or jejunostomy.

Cholecystitis

Cholecystitis is thought to develop as a result of bacterial infection, most often from reflux of intestinal bacteria.[5] E. coli is the most common organism isolated. Cholecystitis is often associated with cholelithiasis or inspissated bile.[304] It occurs most commonly in older dogs. Clinically, several forms have been recognized: necrotizing cholecystitis, acute cholecystitis with gallbladder rupture, and chronic cholecystitis.[304] Clinical signs include lethargy, pain, anorexia, vomiting, diarrhea, and pyrexia. If gallbladder rupture occurs, peritonitis, sepsis, and shock follow. Laboratory abnormalities include leukocytosis with a left shift, hypoproteinemia, hypoglycemia, elevated AP and ALT, hyperbilirubinemia, and elevated amylase and lipase.[304] Ultrasonography may demonstrate a thickened gallbladder wall, inspissated bile, or choleliths. Treatment for the necrotizing and acute forms with bladder rupture includes cholecystectomy and antibiotic therapy (ampicillin or first-generation cephalosporin until results of culture and sensitivity are available). A delay in surgery is associated with a poorer prognosis.[304] Histologic abnormalities are often found in the liver concurrently.[304] Treatment of chronic cholecystitis requires long-term antibiotic therapy.

Emphysematous cholecystitis occurs if gas develops within the wall or lumen of the gallbladder as a result of infection with *E. coli* or clostridia.[305] It frequently occurs in animals with diabetes mellitus.

Portal Vein Thrombosis

Thrombosis of the portal vein has been found in association with lymphangiectasia, glomerular amyloidosis, hepatitis, pancreatic necrosis, peritonitis, neoplasia, and corticosteroid administration and after surgical correction of portosystemic shunts.[306] Clinical signs associated with thrombosis include depression, ascites, icterus, and death.[307]

References

1. Raffe MR, Hardy R. Anesthetic management of the hepatic patient. Compen Contin Educ Pract Vet 1982;4: 841–851.
2. Roth L. Hepatic pathophysiology and biopsy interpretation. Semin Vet Med Surg (Small Anim) 1989;2: 296–301.
3. Blass CE, Seim HB. Surgical techniques for the liver and biliary tract. Vet Clin North Am Small Anim Pract 1985;15:257–275.
4. Center SA. Pathophysiology, laboratory diagnosis, and diseases of the liver. In: Ettinger SJ, Feldman EC, eds. Textbook of Veterinary Internal Medicine. Philadelphia, WB Saunders, 1995:1261–1312.
5. Neer TM. A review of disorders of the gallbladder and extrahepatic biliary tract in the dog and cat. J Vet Intern Med 1992;6:186–192.
6. Bergman JR. Nodular hyperplasia in the liver of the dog: An association with changes in the ito cell population. Vet Pathol 1985;22:427–438.
7. Stowater JL, Lamb CR, Schelling SH. Ultrasonographic features of canine hepatic nodular hyperplasia. Vet Radiol 1990;31:268–272.
8. Twedt DC. Cirrhosis: A consequence of chronic liver disease. Vet Clin North Am Small Anim Pract 1985;15: 151–176.
9. Meyer DJ. The liver: Part 1. Biochemical tests for the evaluation of the hepatobiliary system. Compen Contin Educ Pract Vet 1982;4:663–674.
10. Strombeck DR, Guilford WG. Small Animal Gastroenterology. Davis, California, Stonegate Publishing, 1990: 465–518.
11. Dillon R. The liver in systemic disease: An innocent bystander. Vet Clin North Am Small Anim Pract 1985;15:97–117.
12. Bauer JE. Nutrition and liver function: Nutrient metabolism in health and disease. Compen Contin Educ Pract Vet 1986;8:923–932.
13. Herdt T. Postabsorptive nutrient utilization. In: Cunningham JG, ed. Textbook of Veterinary Physiology. Philadelphia, WB Saunders, 1992:345–365.

14. Center SA. Hepatic lipidosis. In: August JR, ed. Consultations in Feline Internal Medicine 2. Philadelphia, WB Saunders, 1994:87–101.
15. Center SA. Serum bile acids in companion animal medicine. Vet Clin North Am Small Anim Pract 1993; 23:625–657.
16. Herdt T. Digestion and absorption: The non-fermentative process. In: Cunningham JG, ed. Textbook of Veterinary Physiology. Philadelphia, WB Saunders, 1992:286–315.
17. Hall RL. Laboratory evaluation of liver disease. Vet Clin North Am Small Anim Pract 1985;15:3–19.
18. Sutherland RJ. Biochemical evaluation of the hepatobiliary system in dogs and cats. Vet Clin North Am Small Anim Pract 1989;19:899–927.
19. Dimski DS. Ammonia metabolism and the urea cycle: Function and clinical implications. J Vet Intern Med 1994;8:73–78.
20. Bunch SE. Hepatotoxicity associated with pharmacologic agents in dogs and cats. Vet Clin North Am Small Anim Pract 1993;23:659–670.
21. Papich MG, Davis LE. Drugs and the liver. Vet Clin North Am Small Anim Pract 1985;15:77–95.
22. Hardy RM. Hepatic coma. Semin Vet Med Surg (Small Anim) 1988;3:311–320.
23. Magne ML, Chiapella AM. Medical management of canine chronic hepatitis. Compen Contin Educ Pract Vet 1986;8:915–921.
24. Tams TR. Hepatic encephalopathy. Vet Clin North Am Small Anim Pract 1985;15:177–195.
25. Meyer DJ, Center SA. Approach to the diagnosis of liver disorders in dogs and cats. Compen Contin Educ Pract Vet 1986;8:880–888.
26. Anderson JG, Washabau RJ. Icterus. Compen Contin Educ Pract Vet 1992;14:1045–1059.
27. Meyer DJ, Chiapella AM. Cholestasis. Vet Clin North Am Small Anim Pract 1985;15:215–227.
28. Rogers KS, Cornelius LM. Feline icterus. Compen Contin Educ Pract Vet 1985;7:391–402.
29. Twedt DC. Feline liver disease. Vet Int 1995;6:33–43.
30. Cornelius LM, DeNovo RC. Icterus in cats. In: Kirk RW, ed. Current Veterinary Therapy VIII. Philadelphia, WB Saunders, 1983:822–829.
31. Fahie MA, Martin RA. Extrahepatic biliary tract obstruction: A retrospective study of 45 cases (1983–1993). J Am Anim Hosp Assoc 1995;31:478–482.
32. Martin RA, MacCoy DM, Harvey HJ. Surgical management of extrahepatic biliary tract disease. A report of eleven cases. J Am Anim Hosp Assoc 1986;22: 301–307.
33. Boothe HW, Boothe DM, Komkov A, et al. Use of hepatobiliary scintigraphy in the diagnosis of extrahepatic biliary obstruction in dogs and cats: 25 cases (1982–1989). J Am Vet Med Assoc 1992;201:134–141.
34. Meyer DJ, Williams DA. Diagnosis of hepatic and exocrine pancreatic disorders. Semin Vet Med Surg (Small Anim) 1992;4:275–284.
35. Reed AL. Ultrasonographic findings of diseases of the gallbladder and biliary tract. Vet Med (Praha) 1995;90: 950–958.
36. Nyland TG, Gillett NA. Sonographic evaluation of

experimental bile duct ligation in the dog. Vet Radiol 1982;23:252–260.

37. Biller DS, Grooters AM. Ultrasound examination of the liver, pancreas, and gastrointestinal tract. In: Proc Waltham/OSU Symposium, Columbus, Ohio, 1993;17: 33–42.

38. Williams DA. Acute pancreatitis. In: Kirk RW, Bonagura JD, eds. Kirk's Current Veterinary Therapy XI. Philadelphia, WB Saunders, 1992:631–639.

39. Williams DA. Diagnosis and management of pancreatitis. J Small Anim Pract 1994;35:445–454.

40. Murtaugh RJ, Herring DS, Jacobs RM, et al. Pancreatic ultrasonography in dogs with experimentally induced acute pancreatitis. Vet Radiol 1985;26:27–32.

41. Murtaugh RJ. Acute pancreatitis: Diagnostic dilemmas. Semin Vet Med Surg (Small Anim) 1987;2:282–295.

42. Biller DS, Kantrowitz B, Miyabayashi T. Ultrasonography of diffuse liver disease. J Vet Intern Med 1992;6: 71–76.

43. Lamb CR. Abdominal ultrasonography in small animals: Examination of the liver, spleen and pancreas. J Small Anim Pract 1990;31:6–15.

44. Yeager AE, Mohammed H. Accuracy of ultrasonography in the detection of severe hepatic lipidosis in cats. Am J Vet Res 1992;53:597–599.

45. Voros K, Vrabely T, Papp L, et al. Correlation of ultrasonographic and pathomorphological findings in canine hepatic diseases. J Small Anim Pract 1991;32:627–634.

46. Nyland RG. Ultrasound patterns of canine hepatic lymphosarcoma. Vet Radiol 1984;25:167–172.

47. Nyland TG, Park RD. Hepatic ultrasonography in the dog. Vet Radiol 1983;24:74–84.

48. Center SA, Baldwin BH, Erb HN, et al. Bile acid concentrations in the diagnosis of hepatobiliary disease in the dog. J Am Vet Med Assoc 1985;187:935–940.

49. King LG, Gelens HCJ. Ascites. Compen Contin Educ Pract Vet 1992;14:1063–1075.

50. Meyer DJ, Franks PT. Effusion: Classification and cytologic examination. Compen Contin Educ Pract Vet 1987;9:123–128.

51. Johnson SE. Portal hypertension: Part I. Pathophysiology and clinical consequences. Compen Contin Educ Pract Vet 1987;9:741–750.

52. Epstein FH. Underfilling versus overflow in hepatic ascites. N Engl J Med 1982;307:1577–1578.

53. Grauer GF, Nichols CER. Ascites, renal abnormalities and electrolyte and acid-base disorders associated with liver disease. Vet Clin North Am Small Anim Pract 1985;15:197–214.

54. Naccarato R, Messa P, D'Angelo A, et al. Renal handling of sodium and water in early chronic liver disease. Gastroenterology 1981;81:205–210.

55. Jimenez W, Martinez-Pardo A, Arroyo JG, et al. Atrial natriuretic factor: Reduced cardiac content in cirrhotic rats with ascites. Am J Physiol 1986;250:F749–F752.

56. Levy M. Sodium retention and ascites formation in dogs with experimental portal cirrhosis. Am J Physiol 1977; 233:F572–F585.

57. Levy M. Sodium retention in dogs with cirrhosis and ascites: Efferent mechanisms. Am J Physiol 1977;233: F586–F592.

58. Unikowsky B, Wexler MJ, Levy M. Dogs with experimental cirrhosis of the liver without intrahepatic hypertension do not retain sodium or form ascites. J Clin Invest 1983;72:1594–1604.

59. Levy M, Allotey JBK. Temporal relationships between urinary salt retention and altered systemic hemodynamics in dogs with experimental cirrhosis. J Lab Clin Med 1978;92:560–576.

60. Greene CE. Ascites: Diagnostic and therapeutic considerations. Compen Contin Educ Pract Vet 1979;1: 712–718.

61. Johnson SE. Portal hypertension: Part II. Clinical assessment and treatment. Compen Contin Educ Pract Vet 1987;9:917–928.

62. Gores BR, Berg J, Carpenter JL, et al. Chylous ascites in cats: Nine cases (1978–1993). J Am Vet Med Assoc 1994;205:1161–1164.

63. Ling GV, Stabenfeldt GH, Comer KM, et al. Canine hyperadrenocorticism: Pretreatment clinical and laboratory evaluation of 117 cases. J Am Vet Med Assoc 1979;174:1211–1215.

64. Clinkenbeard KD, Wolf AM, Cowell RL, et al. Feline disseminated histoplasmosis. Compen Contin Educ Pract Vet 1989;11:1223–1233.

65. Clinkenbeard K, Cowell RL, Tyler RD. Disseminated histoplasmosis in dogs: 12 cases (1981–1986). J Am Vet Med Assoc 1988;193:1443–1447.

66. Hill BL. Canine idiopathic congestive cardiomyopathy. Compen Contin Educ Pract Vet 1981;3:615–621.

67. Center SA, Crawford MA, Guida L, et al. A retrospective study of 77 cats with severe hepatic lipidosis: 1975–1990. J Vet Intern Med 1993;7:349–359.

68. Zawie DA, Garvey MS. Feline hepatic disease. Vet Clin North Am Small Anim Pract 1984;14:1201–1230.

69. Post G, Patnaik AK. Nonhematopoietic hepatic neoplasms in cats: 21 cases (1983–1988). J Am Vet Med Assoc 1992;201:1080–1082.

70. Magne ML. Primary epithelial hepatic tumors in the dog. Compen Contin Educ Pract Vet 1984;6:506–515.

71. Rogers WA, Ruebner BH. A retrospective study of probable glucocorticoid-induced hepatopathy in dogs. J Am Vet Med Assoc 1977;170:603–606.

72. van Bree H, Sackx A. Evaluation of radiographic liver size in twenty-seven normal deep-chested dogs. J Small Anim Pract 1987;28:693–703.

73. Wrigley RH. Radiographic and ultrasonographic diagnosis of liver diseases in dogs and cats. Vet Clin North Am Small Anim Pract 1985;15:21–37.

74. Godshalk CP, Badertscher RR, Rippy MK, et al. Quantitative ultrasonic assessment of liver size in the dog. Vet Radiol 1988;29:162–167.

75. van Bree H, Jacobs V, Vandekererckhove P. Radiographic assessment of liver volume in dogs. Am J Vet Res 1989;50:1613–1616.

76. Cockett PA. Radiographic anatomy of the canine liver: Simple measurements determined from the lateral radiograph. J Small Anim Pract 1986;27:577–589.

77. Godshalk C, Kneller S, Badertscher R, et al. Quantitative noninvasive assessment of liver size in clinically normal dogs. Am J Vet Res 1990;51:1421–1426.

78. Nyland TG, Fisher PE. Evaluation of experimentally

induced canine hepatic cirrhosis using duplex Doppler ultrasound. Vet Radiol 1990;31:189–194.

79. Basile AS, Jones EA, Skolnick P. The pathogenesis and treatment of hepatic encephalopathy: Evidence for the involvement of benzodiazepine receptor ligands. Pharmacol Rev 1991;43:27–71.

80. Maddison JE. Hepatic encephalopathy. Current concepts of the pathogenesis. J Vet Intern Med 1992;6: 341–353.

81. Hardy RM. Pathophysiology of hepatic encephalopathy. Semin Vet Med Surg (Small Anim) 1990;5:100–106.

82. Fraser CL, Arieff AI. Hepatic encephalopathy. N Engl J Med 1985;313:865–873.

83. Tyler JW. Hepatoencephalopathy. Part I. Clinical signs and diagnosis. Compen Contin Educ Pract Vet 1990;12: 1069–1073.

84. Tyler JW. Hepatoencephalopathy. Part II. Pathophysiology and treatment. Compen Contin Educ Pract Vet 1990;12:1260–1270.

85. Strombeck DR, Harrold D, Rogers Q, et al. Plasma amino acid, glucagon, and insulin concentrations in dogs with nitrosamine-induced hepatic disease. Am J Vet Res 1983;44:2028–2036.

86. Rutgers C, Stradley R, Rogers W. Plasma amino acid analysis in dogs with experimentally induced hepatocellular and obstructive jaundice. Am J Vet Res 1987; 48:696–702.

87. Strombeck DR, Rogers Q. Plasma amino acid concentrations in dogs with hepatic disease. J Am Vet Med Assoc 1978;173:93–96.

88. Stanton ME, Bright RM. Gastroduodenal ulceration in dogs: Retrospective study of 43 cases and literature review. J Vet Intern Med 1989;3:238–244.

89. Murray M, Robinson PB, McKeating FJ, et al. Peptic ulceration in the dog: A clinico-pathological study. Vet Rec 1972;91:441–447.

90. Leib MS. Chronic vomiting: A diagnostic approach. In: August JR, ed. Consultations in Feline Internal Medicine. Philadelphia, WB Saunders, 1991:403–407.

91. Badylak SF, Dodds WJ, Van Vleet JF. Plasma coagulation factor abnormalities in dogs with naturally occurring hepatic disease. Am J Vet Res 1983;44:2336–2340.

92. Crawford MA, Schall WD, Jensen RK, et al. Chronic active hepatitis in 26 Doberman pinschers. J Am Vet Med Assoc 1985;12:1343–1350.

93. Badylak SF, Van Vleet JF. Alterations of prothrombin time and activated partial thromboplastin time in dogs with hepatic disease. Am J Vet Res 1981;42:2053–2056.

94. Drazner FH. Clinical implications of disseminated intravascular coagulation. Compen Contin Educ Pract Vet 1982;4:974–981.

95. Johnson GF, Zawie DA, Gilbertson SR, et al. Chronic active hepatitis in Doberman pinschers. J Am Vet Med Assoc 1982;180:1438–1442.

96. Center SA, Magne ML. Historical, physical examination, and clinicopathologic features of portosystemic vascular anomalies in the dog and cat. Semin Vet Med Surg (Small Anim) 1990;5:83–93.

97. Grauer GF, Pitts RP. Primary polydipsia in three dogs with portosystemic shunts. J Am Anim Hosp Assoc 1987;23:197–200.

98. Bunch SE, Jordan HL, Sellon RK, et al. Characterization of iron status in young dogs with portosystemic shunt. Am J Vet Res 1995;56:853–858.

99. Meyer DJ, Harvey JW. Hematologic changes associated with serum and hepatic iron alterations in dogs with congenital portosystemic vascular anomalies. J Vet Intern Med 1994;8:55–56.

100. Laflamme DP, Mahaffey EA, Allen SW, et al. Microcytosis and iron status in dogs with surgically induced portosystemic shunts. J Vet Intern Med 1994;8:212–216.

101. Hall RL. Laboratory evaluation of gastrointestinal diseases. In: August JR, ed. Consultations in Feline Internal Medicine. Philadelphia, WB Saunders, 1991: 471–477.

102. Valentine BA, Blue JT, Shelley SM, et al. Increased serum alanine aminotransferase activity associated with muscle necrosis in the dog. J Vet Intern Med 1990;4: 140–143.

103. Schlesinger DP, Rubin SI. Serum bile acids and the assessment of hepatic function in dogs and cats. Can Vet J 1993;34:215–220.

104. Milne EM. The diagnostic value of alkaline phosphatase in canine medicine: A review. J Small Anim Pract 1985;26:267–278.

105. Sanecki RK, Hoffmann WE, Gelberg HB, et al. Subcellular location of corticosteroid-induced alkaline phosphatase in canine hepatocytes. Vet Pathol 1987;24: 296–301.

106. McLain DL, Nagode LA, Wilson GP, et al. Alkaline phosphatase and its isoenzymes in normal cats and in cats with biliary obstruction. J Am Anim Hosp Assoc 1978;14:94–99.

107. Spano JS, August JR, Henderson RA, et al. Serum gamma-glutamyl transpeptidase activity in healthy cats and cats with induced hepatic disease. Am J Vet Res 1983;44:2049–2053.

108. Meyer DJ. Serum gamma-glutamyl transferase as a liver test in cats with toxic and obstructive hepatic disease. J Am Anim Hosp Assoc 1983;19:1023–1026.

109. DeNovo RC, Prasse KW. Comparison of serum biochemical hepatic functional alterations in dogs treated with corticosteroids and hepatic duct ligation. Am J Vet Res 1983;44:1703–1709.

110. Guelfi JF, Braun JP, Benard P, et al. Value of so-called cholestasis markers in the dog: An experimental study. Res Vet Sci 1982;33:309–312.

111. Center SA, Baldwin BH, King JM, et al. Hematologic and biochemical abnormalities associated with induced extrahepatic bile duct obstruction in the cat. Am J Vet Res 1983;44:1822–1829.

112. Hoffmann WE. Diagnostic value of canine serum alkaline phosphatase and alkaline phosphatase isoenzymes. J Am Anim Hosp Assoc 1977;13:237–241.

113. Meyer DJ, Noonan NE. Liver tests in dogs receiving anticonvulsant drugs (diphenylhydantoin and primidone). J Am Anim Hosp Assoc 1981;17:261–264.

114. Sturtevant F, Hoffmann WE, Dorner JL. The effect of three anticonvulsant drugs and ACTH on canine serum alkaline phosphatase. J Am Anim Hosp Assoc 1977;13: 754–757.

115. Solter PF, Hoffmann WE, Chambers MD, et al. Hepatic

total 3-alpha-hydroxy bile acids concentration and enzyme activities in prednisone-treated dogs. Am J Vet Res 1994;55:1086–1092.

116. Center SA, Slater MR, Manwarren T, et al. Diagnostic efficacy of serum alkaline phosphatase and gamma-glutamyltransferase in dogs with histologically confirmed hepatobiliary disease: 270 cases (1980–1990). J Am Vet Med Assoc 1992;201:1258–1264.

117. Center SA, Baldwin BH, Dillingham S, et al. Diagnostic value of serum gamma-glutamyl transferase and alkaline phosphatase activities in hepatobiliary disease in the cat. J Am Vet Med Assoc 1986;188:507–510.

118. Wilson SM, Feldman EC. Diagnostic value of the steroid-induced isoenzyme of alkaline phosphatase in the dog. J Am Anim Hosp Assoc 1992;28:245–250.

119. Braun JP, Benard P, Burgat V, et al. Gamma glutamyl transferase in domestic animals. Vet Res Commun 1983;6:77–90.

120. Milne EM, Doxey DL. Gamma-glutamyl transpeptidase and its multiple forms in the tissues and sera of normal dogs. Res Vet Sci 1985;39:385–387.

121. Abdelkader SV, Hauge JG. Serum enzyme determination in the study of liver disease in dogs. Acta Vet Scand 1986;27:59–70.

122. Engelking LR. Disorders of bilirubin metabolism in small animal species. Compen Contin Educ Pract Vet 1988;10:712–722.

123. Cornelius CE. Biochemical evaluation of hepatic function in dogs. J Am Anim Hosp Assoc 1979;15:259–269.

124. Osborne CA, Stevens JB, Lees GE, et al. Clinical significance of bilirubinuria. Compen Contin Educ Pract Vet 1980;1:897–903.

125. Lees GE, Hardy RM, Stevens JB, et al. Clinical implications of feline bilirubinuria. J Am Anim Hosp Assoc 1984;20:765–771.

126. Center SA, Baldwin BH, Erb H, et al. Bile acid concentrations in the diagnosis of hepatobiliary disease in the cat. J Am Vet Med Assoc 1986;189:891–896.

127. Johnson CA, Armstrong PJ, Hauptman JG. Congenital portosystemic shunts in dogs: 46 cases (1979–1986). J Am Vet Med Assoc 1987;191:1478–1483.

128. Birchard SJ, Sherding RG. Feline portosystemic shunts. Compen Contin Educ Pract Vet 1992;14:1295–1300.

129. Center SA, Erb HN, Joseph SA. Measurement of serum bile acids concentrations for diagnosis of hepatobiliary disease in cats. J Am Vet Med Assoc 1995;207:1048–1054.

130. Center SA, ManWarren T, Slater MR, et al. Evaluation of twelve-hour preprandial and two-hour postprandial serum bile acids concentrations for diagnosis of hepatobiliary disease in dogs. J Am Vet Med Assoc 1991;199:217–226.

131. Johnson S, Rogers W, Bonagura J, et al. Determination of serum bile acids in fasting dogs with hepatobiliary disease. Am J Vet Res 1985;46:2048–2053.

132. Hauge JG, Abdelkader SV. Serum bile acids as an indicator of liver disease in dogs. Acta Vet Scand 1984;25:495–503.

133. Rutgers H, Stradley R, Johnson S. Serum bile acid analysis in dogs with experimentally induced cholestatic jaundice. Am J Vet Res 1988;49:317–320.

134. Vulgamott JC. Portosystemic shunts. Vet Clin North Am Small Anim Pract 1985;15:229–242.

135. Rothuizen J, van den Ingh TSGAM. Rectal ammonia tolerance test in the evaluation of portal circulation in dogs with liver disease. Res Vet Sci 1982;33:22–25.

136. Evans SM. The radiographic appearance of primary liver neoplasia in dogs. Vet Radiol 1987;28:192–196.

137. Kirpensteijn J, Fingland RB, Ulrich T, et al. Cholelithiasis in dogs: 29 cases (1980–1990). J Am Vet Med Assoc 1993;202:1137–1142.

138. Feeney DA, Johnston GR, Hardy RM. Two-dimensional, gray-scale ultrasonography for assessment of hepatic and splenic neoplasia in the dog and cat. J Am Vet Med Assoc 1984;184:68–81.

139. Wu J, Carlisle CH. Ultrasonographic examination of the canine liver based on recognition of hepatic and portal veins. Vet Radiol Ultrasound 1995;36:234–239.

140. Hager DA, Nyland TG, Fisher P. Ultrasound-guided biopsy of the canine liver, kidney, and prostate. Vet Radiol 1985;26:82–88.

141. Barr F. Percutaneous biopsy of abdominal organs under ultrasound guidance. J Small Anim Pract 1995;36:105–113.

142. Leveille R, Partington BP, Biller DS, et al. Complications after ultrasound-guided biopsy of abdominal structures in dogs and cats: 246 cases (1984–1991). J Am Vet Med Assoc 1993;203:413–415.

143. Spaulding KA. Gallbladder wall thickness. Vet Radiol Ultrasound 1993;34:270–272.

144. Jones BD, Hitt M, Hurst T. Hepatic biopsy. Vet Clin North Am Small Anim Pract 1985;15:39–65.

145. Feldman EC, Ettinger SJ. Percutaneous transthoracic liver biopsy in the dog. J Am Vet Med Assoc 1976;169:805–810.

146. Osborne CA, Stevens JB, Perman V. Needle biopsy of the liver. J Am Vet Med Assoc 1969;155:1605–1620.

147. Hitt M, Hanna P, Singh A. Percutaneous transabdominal hepatic needle biopsies in dogs. Am J Vet Res 1992;53:785–787.

148. Hardy RM. Liver biopsy: The percutaneous approach. Vet Med Rep 1990;2:192–194.

149. Pope ER. Liver biopsy: The surgical approach. Vet Med (Prague) 1990;2:197–198.

150. Sherding RG. Acute hepatic failure. Vet Clin North Am Small Anim Pract 1985;15:119–133.

151. Twedt DC, Grauer GF. Fluid therapy for gastrointestinal, pancreatic, and hepatic disorders. Vet Clin North Am Small Anim Pract 1982;12:463–485.

152. Laflamme DP. Dietary management of canine hepatic encephalopathy. Compen Contin Educ Pract Vet 1988;10:1258–1263.

153. Marks SL, Rogers QR, Strombeck DR. Nutritional support in hepatic disease: Part II. Dietary management of common liver disorders in dogs and cats. Compen Contin Educ Pract Vet 1994;16:1287–1295.

154. Marks SL, Rogers QR, Strombeck DR. Nutritional support in hepatic disease: Part I. Metabolic alterations and nutritional considerations in dogs and cats. Compen Contin Educ Pract Vet 1994;16:971–978.

155. Center SA. Feline liver disorders and their management. Compen Contin Educ Pract Vet 1986;8:889–903.

156. Davenport DJ. Enteral/parenteral nutrition for gastrointestinal disorders. In: August JR, ed. Consultations in Feline Internal Medicine 2. Philadelphia, WB Saunders, 1994:107–118.

157. Bright RM, Okrasinski EB, Pardo AD, et al. Percutaneous tube gastrostomy for enteral alimentation in small animals. Compen Contin Educ Pract Vet 1991;13:15–19, 22–23.

158. Sherding RG, Johnson SE. Endoscopy for foreign bodies, strictures, and gastrostomy tubes. In: Proc Waltham/OSU Symposium, Columbus, Ohio, 1993;17: 99–107.

159. Armstrong PJ, Hardie EM. Percutaneous endoscopic gastrotomy. A retrospective study of 54 clinical cases in dogs and cats. J Vet Intern Med 1990;4:202–206.

160. Mauterer JV Jr. Endoscopic and nonendoscopic percutaneous gastrostomy tube placement. In: Bonagura JD, Kirk RW, ed. Kirk's Current Veterinary Therapy XII. Philadelphia, WB Saunders, 1995:669–674.

161. Fulton RB, Dennis JS. Blind percutaneous placement of a gastrostomy tube for nutritional support in dogs and cats. J Am Vet Med Assoc 1992;201:697–700.

162. Williams JM, White RAS. Tube gastrostomy in dogs. J Small Anim Pract 1993;34:59–64.

163. Mathews KA, Binnington AG. Percutaneous incisionless placement of a gastrostomy tube utilizing a gastroscope: Preliminary observations. J Am Anim Hosp Assoc 1986;22:601–610.

164. Bright RM, Burrows CF. Percutaneous endoscopic tube gastrostomy in dogs. Am J Vet Res 1988;49:629–633.

165. Armstrong PJ, Hardie EM. Percutaneous endoscopic gastrostomy. Vet Med Rep 1989;1:404–411.

166. DeBowes LJ, Coyne B, Layton CE. Comparison of french-pezzar and Malecot catheters for percutaneously placed gastrostomy tubes in cats. J Am Vet Med Assoc 1993;202:1963–1965.

167. Hardy RM, O'Brien T, Adams LG, et al. Periportal hepatitis associated with the use of a heartworm-hookworm preventative (diethylcarbamazine-oxibendazole) in 13 dogs. J Am Vet Anim Hosp Assoc 1989;25:419–429.

168. Polzin DJ, Stowe CM, O'Leary TP, et al. Acute hepatic necrosis associated with the administration of mebendazole to dogs. J Am Vet Med Assoc 1981;179:1013–1016.

169. Bunch SE, Castleman WL, Hornbuckle WE, et al. Hepatic cirrhosis associated with long-term anticonvulsant drug therapy in dogs. J Am Vet Med Assoc 1982;181:357–362.

170. Bunch SE, Baldwin BH, Hornbuckle WE, et al. Compromised hepatic function in dogs treated with anticonvulsant drugs. J Am Vet Med Assoc 1984;184: 444–448.

171. Bunch SE, Conway MB, Center SA, et al. Toxic hepatopathy and intrahepatic cholestasis associated with phenytoin administration in combination with other anticonvulsant drugs in three dogs. J Am Vet Med Assoc 1987;190:194–198.

172. Dayrell-Hart B, Steinberg SA, Van Winkle TJ, et al. Hepatotoxicity of phenobarbital in dogs: 18 cases (1985–1989). J Am Vet Med Assoc 1991;199:1060–1066.

173. Magne ML. Pathophysiology of inflammatory bowel disease. Semin Vet Med Surg (Small Anim) 1992;7: 112–116.

174. Johnson KE. Pathophysiology of heatstroke. Compen Contin Educ Pract Vet 1982;4:141–148.

175. Gocke DJ, Preiseg R, Morris TQ, et al. Experimental viral hepatitis in the dog: Production of persistent disease in partially immune animals. J Clin Invest 1967;46:1506–1517.

176. Weiss RC. The diagnosis and clinical management of feline infectious peritonitis. Vet Med (Prague) 1991;86: 308–319.

177. Ford RB. Canine histoplasmosis. Compen Contin Educ Pract Vet 1980;2:637–644.

178. Chapman BL, Hendrick MF, Washabau RJ. Granulomatous hepatitis in dogs: Nine cases (1987–1990). J Am Vet Med Assoc 1993;203:680–684.

179. Moreland KJ. Ulcer disease of the upper gastrointestinal tract in small animals: Pathophysiology, diagnosis, and management. Compen Contin Educ Pract Vet 1988;10: 1265–1280.

180. Martin RA, Freeman LE. Identification and surgical management of portosystemic shunts in the dog and cat. Semin Vet Med Surg (Small Anim) 1987;2:302–306.

181. Martin RA. Congenital portosystemic shunts in the dog and cat. Vet Clin North Am Small Anim Pract 1993;23: 609–623.

182. Scavelli TD, Hornbuckle WE, L R, et al. Portosystemic shunts in cats: Seven cases (1976–1984). J Am Vet Med Assoc 1986;189:317–325.

183. Swalec K, Smeak DD. Partial versus complete attenuation of single portosystemic shunts. Vet Surg 1990;19: 406–411.

184. Mathews K, Gofton N. Congenital extrahepatic portosystemic shunt occlusion in the dog: Gross observations during surgical correction. J Am Anim Hosp Assoc 1988;24:387–394.

185. Bostwick DR, Twedt DC. Intrahepatic and extrahepatic portal venous anomalies in dogs: 52 cases (1982–1992). J Am Vet Med Assoc 1995;206:1181–1185.

186. VanGundy TE, Boothe HW, Wolf A. Results of surgical management of feline portosystemic shunts. J Am Anim Hosp Assoc 1990;26:55–62.

187. Payne JT, Martin RA, Constantinescu GM. The anatomy and embryology of portosystemic shunts in dogs and cats. Semin Vet Med Surg (Small Anim) 1990;5:76–82.

188. Birchard SJ. Surgical management of portosystemic shunts in dogs and cats. Compen Contin Educ Pract Vet 1984;6:795–802.

189. Breznock EM, Berger B, Pendray D, et al. Surgical manipulation of intrahepatic portocaval shunts in dogs. J Am Vet Med Assoc 1983;182:798–805.

190. Lawrence D, Bellah JR, Diaz R. Results of surgical management of portosystemic shunts in dogs: 20 cases (1985–1990). J Am Vet Med Assoc 1992;201:1750–1753.

191. Suter PF. Portal vein anomalies in the dog: Their angiographic diagnosis. J Am Vet Radiol Soc 1975;10: 84–97.

192. Taboada J. Medical management of animals with portosystemic shunts. Semin Vet Med Surg (Small Anim) 1990;5:107–119.

193. Koblik PD, Hornof WJ, Yen C, et al. Use of technetium-99m sulfur colloid to evaluate changes in reticuloendothelial function in dogs with experimentally induced chronic biliary cirrhosis and portosystemic shunting. Am J Vet Res 1995;56:688–693.

194. Komtebedde J, Forsyth SF, Breznock EM, et al. Intrahepatic portosystemic venous anomaly in the dog: Perioperative management and complications. Vet Surg 1991;20:37–42.

195. Blaxter AC, Holt PE, Pearson GR, et al. Congenital portosystemic shunts in the cat: A report of nine cases. J Small Anim Pract 1988;29:631–645.

196. Center SA, Baldwin BH, de Lahunta A, et al. Evaluation of serum bile acid concentrations for the diagnosis of portosystemic venous anomalies in the dog and cat. J Am Vet Med Assoc 1985;186:1090–1094.

197. Meyer DJ. Liver function tests in dogs with portosystemic shunts: Measurement of serum bile acid concentration. J Am Vet Med Assoc 1986;188:168–169.

198. Center SA. Liver function tests in the diagnosis of portosystemic vascular anomalies. Semin Vet Med Surg (Small Anim) 1990;5:94–99.

199. Moon ML. Diagnostic imaging of portosystemic shunts. Semin Vet Med Surg (Small Anim) 1990;5:120–126.

200. Wrigley RH, Konde LJ, Park RD, et al. Ultrasonographic diagnosis of portacaval shunts in young dogs. J Am Vet Med Assoc 1987;191:421–424.

201. Daniel GB, Bright R, Ollis P, et al. Per rectal portal scintigraphy using ^{99m}technetium pertechnetate to diagnose portosystemic shunts in dogs and cats. J Vet Intern Med 1991;5:23–27.

202. Koblik PD, Komtebedde J, Yen CD, et al. Use of transcolonic (99m)technetium-pertechnetate as a screening test for portosystemic shunts in dogs. J Am Vet Med Assoc 1990;196:925–930.

203. Daniel GB, Bright R, Monnet E, et al. Comparison of per-rectal portal scintigraphy using ^{99m}technetium pertechnetate to mesenteric injection of radioactive microspheres for quantification of portosystemic shunts in an experimental dog model. Vet Radiol 1990;31:175–181.

204. Koblik PD, Yen C, Hornof WJ, et al. Use of transcolonic ^{123}I-iodoamphetamine to diagnose spontaneous portosystemic shunts in 18 dogs. Vet Radiol 1989;30:67–73.

205. Koblik PD, Hornof WJ, Breznock EM. Quantitative hepatic scintigraphy in the dog. Vet Radiol 1983;24:226–231.

206. Wrigley RH, Park RD, Konde LJ, et al. Subtraction portal venography. Vet Radiol 1987;28:208–212.

207. Koblik PD, Hornof WJ. Transcolonic sodium pertechnetate Tc-99m scintigraphy for diagnosis of macrovascular portosystemic shunts in dogs, cats, and potbellied pigs: 176 cases (1988–1992). J Am Vet Med Assoc 1995;207:729–733.

208. Van Vechten BJ, Komtebedde J, Koblik PD. Use of transcolonic portal scintigraphy to monitor blood flow and progressive postoperative attenuation of partially ligated single extrahepatic portosystemic shunts in dogs. J Am Vet Med Assoc 1994;204:1770–1774.

209. Holt D. Critical care management of the portosystemic shunt patient. Compen Contin Educ Pract Vet 1994;16:879–892.

210. Butler LM, Fossum TW, Boothe HW. Surgical management of extrahepatic portosystemic shunts in the dog and cat. Semin Vet Med Surg (Small Anim) 1990;5:127–133.

211. Hardie EM, Kornegay JN, Cullen JM. Status epilepticus after ligation of portosystemic shunts. Vet Surg 1990;19:412–417.

212. Matushek KJ, Bjorling D, Mathews K. Generalized motor seizures after portosystemic shunt ligation in dogs: Five cases (1981–1988). J Am Vet Med Assoc 1990;196:2014–2017.

213. Smith KR, Bauer M, Monnet E. Portosystemic communications: Follow-up of 32 cases. J Small Anim Pract 1995;36:435–440.

214. Hubbard BS, Vulgamott JC. Feline hepatic lipidosis. Compen Contin Educ Pract Vet 1992;14:459–465.

215. Armstrong PJ. Hepatic lipidosis. Vet Prev 1994;1:10–11.

216. Jacobs G, Cornelius L, Allen S, et al. Treatment of idiopathic hepatic lipidosis in cats: 11 cases (1986–1987). J Am Vet Med Assoc 1989;195:635–638.

217. Biourge VC, Groff JM, Munn RJ, et al. Experimental induction of hepatic lipidosis in cats. Am J Vet Res 1994;55:1291–1302.

218. Barsanti JA, Jones BD, Spano JS, et al. Prolonged anorexia associated with hepatic lipidosis in three cats. Fel Pract 1977;1237:52–57.

219. Biourge V. Sequential findings in cats with hepatic lipidosis. Fel Pract 1993;21:25–28.

220. Dimski D, Buffington C, Johnson S, et al. Serum lipoprotein concentrations and hepatic lesions in obese cats undergoing weight loss. Am J Vet Res 1992;53:1259–1262.

221. Akol KG, Washabau RJ, Saunders HM, et al. Acute pancreatitis in cats with hepatic lipidosis. J Vet Intern Med 1993;7:205–209.

222. Biourge V, MacDonald MJ, King L. Feline hepatic lipidosis: Pathogenesis and nutritional management. Compen Contin Educ Pract Vet 1990;12:1244–1258.

223. Dimski DS. Diagnosis, treatment, and pathophysiology of feline idiopathic hepatic lipidosis. In: Proc Waltham/OSU Symposium, Columbus, Ohio, 1993;17:56-62.

224. Jacobs G, Cornelius L, Keene B, et al. Comparison of plasma, liver, and skeletal muscle carnitine concentrations in cats with idiopathic hepatic lipidosis and in healthy cats. Am J Vet Res 1990;51:1349–1351.

225. Center SA, Guida L, Zanelli MJ, et al. Ultrastructural hepatocellular features associated with severe hepatic lipidosis in cats. Am J Vet Res 1993;54:724–731.

226. Thornburg LP, Simpson S, Digilio K. Fatty liver syndrome in cats. J Am Anim Hosp Assoc 1982;18:397–400.

227. Armstrong PJ. Enteral feeding of critically ill pets: The choices and techniques. Vet Med 1992;87:900–909.

228. Hardy RM. Chronic hepatitis in dogs: A syndrome. Compen Contin Educ Pract Vet 1986;8:904–914.

229. Thornburg LP. Chronic active hepatitis. What is it and does it occur in dogs? J Am Anim Hosp Assoc 1982;18:21–22.

230. Johnson SE. Diseases of the liver. In: Ettinger SJ, Feldman EC, eds. Textbook of Veterinary Internal Medicine. Philadelphia, WB Saunders, 1995:1313–1357.

231. Andersson M, Sevelius E. Breed, sex and age distribution in dogs with chronic liver disease: A demographic study. J Small Anim Pract 1991;32:1–5.

232. Strombeck DR, Gribble D. Chronic active hepatitis in the dog. J Am Vet Med Assoc 1978;173:380–386.

233. Hardy RM. Chronic hepatitis: An emerging syndrome in dogs. Vet Clin North Am Small Anim Pract 1985;15: 135–150.

234. Bishop L, Strandberg JD, Adams RJ, et al. Chronic active hepatitis in dogs associated with Leptospires. Am J Vet Res 1979;40:839–844.

235. Weiss DJ, Armstrong PJ, Mruthyunjaya A. Anti-liver membrane protein antibodies in dogs with chronic hepatitis. J Vet Intern Med 1995;9:267–271.

236. Andersson M, Sevelius E. Circulating autoantibodies in dogs with chronic liver disease. J Small Anim Pract 1992;33:389–394.

237. Thornburg LP, Rottinghaus G, Koch J, et al. High liver copper levels in two Doberman pinschers with subacute hepatitis. J Am Anim Hosp Assoc 1984;20: 1003–1005.

238. Doige CE, Lester S. Chronic active hepatitis in dogs: A review of fourteen cases. J Am Anim Hosp Assoc 1981;17:725–730.

239. Rutgers HC, Haywood S. Chronic hepatitis in the dog. J Small Anim Pract 1988;29:679–690.

240. Strombeck DR, Miller LM, Harrold D. Effects of corticosteroid treatment on survival time in dogs with chronic hepatitis: 151 cases (1977–1985). J Am Vet Med Assoc 1988;193:1109–1113.

241. Miller E. Immunosuppressive therapy in the treatment of immune-mediated disease. J Vet Intern Med 1992;6: 206–213.

242. Rubin RA, Kowalski TE, Khandelwal M, et al. Ursodiol. Ann Intern Med 1994;121:207–218.

243. Haywood S, Rutgers HC, Christian MK. Hepatitis and copper accumulation in Skye terriers. Vet Pathol 1988; 25:408–414.

244. van den Ingh TSGAM. Lobular dissecting hepatitis in juvenile and young adult dogs. J Vet Intern Med 1994;8:217–220.

245. Bennett AM, Davies JD, Gaskell CJ, et al. Lobular dissecting hepatitis in the dog. Vet Pathol 1983;20: 179–188.

246. Jensen AL, Nielsen OL. Chronic hepatitis in three young standard poodles. J Am Vet Med Assoc 1991;38:194–197.

247. Jarrett WFH, O'Neil BW. A new transmissible agent causing acute hepatitis, chronic hepatitis and cirrhosis in dogs. Vet Rec 1985;116:629–635.

248. Jarrett WFH, O'Neil BW, Lindholm I. Persistent hepatitis and chronic fibrosis induced by canine acidophil cell hepatitis virus. Vet Rec 1987;120:234–235.

249. Center SA, Rowland PH. The cholangitis/cholangiohepatitis complex in the cat. In: Proceedings of the 12th Annual Veterinary Medicine Forum of the American College of Veterinary Internal Medicine, San Francisco, California, 1994:766–771.

250. Armstrong PJ, Gagne J, Lund LM, et al. Clinical characteristics of feline inflammatory liver disease. In: Proceedings of the 13th Annual Veterinary Medicine Forum of the American College of Veterinary Internal Medicine, Lake Buena Vista, Florida, 1995:27–29.

251. Hirsch VM, Doige CE. Suppurative cholangitis in cats. J Am Vet Med Assoc 1983;182:1223–1226.

252. Weiss DJ, Gagne JM, Armstrong PJ. Characterization of portal lymphocytic infiltrates in feline liver. Vet Clin Pathol 1995;24:91–95.

253. Prasse KW, Mahaffey EA, DeNovo R et al. Chronic lymphocytic cholangitis in three cats. Vet Pathol 1982; 19:99–108.

254. Lucke VM, Davies JD. Progressive lymphocytic cholangitis in the cat. J Small Anim Pract 1984;25:249–260.

255. Roberts S, Lavach J, Macy D, et al. Effect of ophthalmic prednisolone acetate on the canine adrenal gland and hepatic function. Am J Vet Res 1984;45:1711–1714.

256. Meyer DJ, Moriello KA, Feder BM, et al. Effect of otic medications containing glucocorticoids on liver function test results in healthy dogs. J Am Vet Med Assoc 1990;196:743–744.

257. Badylak SF, Van Vleet JF. Tissue gamma-glutamyl transpeptidase activity and hepatic ultrastructural alterations in dogs with experimentally induced glucocorticoid hepatopathy. Am J Vet Res 1982;43:649–655.

258. Dillon AR, Spano JS, Powers RD. Prednisolone induced hematologic, biochemical, and histologic changes in the dog. J Am Anim Hosp Assoc 1980;16:831–837.

259. Dillon AR, Sorjonen DC, Powers RD, et al. Effects of dexamethasone and surgical hypotension on hepatic morphologic features and enzymes of dogs. Am J Vet Res 1983;44:1996–1999.

260. Moore GE, Mahaffey EA, Hoenig M. Hematologic and serum biochemical effects of long-term administration of anti-inflammatory doses of prednisone in dogs. Am J Vet Res 1992;53:1033–1037.

261. Bunch SE. Drug-induced hepatic disease of dogs and cats. In: Kirk RW, ed. Current Veterinary Therapy X. Philadelphia, WB Saunders, 1989:878–884.

262. Bunch SE, Castleman WL, Baldwin BH, et al. Effects of long-term primidone and phenytoin administration on canine hepatic function and morphology. Am J Vet Res 1985;46:105–115.

263. Van Cauteren H, Marsboom R, Vandenberghe J, et al. Safety studies evaluating the effect of mebendazole on liver function in dogs. J Am Vet Med Assoc 1983;183: 93–98.

264. Leveille CR, Arias IM. Pathophysiology and pharmacologic modulation of hepatic fibrosis. J Vet Intern Med 1993;7:73–84.

265. Kosnovsky JE, Manfra-Marretta S, Matthiesen DT, et al. Results of partial hepatectomy in 18 dogs with hepatocellular carcinoma. J Am Anim Hosp Assoc 1989;25: 203–206.

266. Strafuss AC. Bile duct carcinoma in dogs. J Am Vet Med Assoc 1976;169:429.

267. Lawrence HJ, Erb HN, Harvey HJ. Nonlymphomatous hepatobiliary masses in cats: 41 cases (1972 to 1991). Vet Surg 1994;23:365–368.

268. Patnaik AK, Hurvitz AI, Lieberman PH. Canine hepatic neoplasms: A clinicopathologic study. Vet Pathol 1980; 17:553–564.

269. Strombeck DR. Clinicopathologic features of primary

and metastatic neoplastic disease of the liver in dogs. J Am Vet Med Assoc 1978;173:267–269.

270. Patnaik AK, Hurvitz AI, Lieberman PH, et al. Canine bile duct carcinoma. Vet Pathol 1981;18:439–444.

271. McConnell MF, Lumsden JH. Biochemical evaluation of metastatic liver disease in the dog. J Am Anim Hosp Assoc 1983;19:173–178.

272. Lowseth LA, Gillett NA, Chang I, et al. Detection of serum alpha-fetoprotein in dogs with hepatic tumors. J Am Vet Med Assoc 1991;199:735–741.

273. Twedt DC, Sternlieb I, Gilbertson SR. Clinical, morphologic, and chemical studies on copper toxicosis of Bedlington terriers. J Am Vet Med Assoc 1979;175:269–275.

274. Thornburg LP, Shaw D, Dolan M, et al. Hereditary copper toxicosis in West Highland white terriers. Vet Pathol 1986;23:148–154.

275. Herrtage ME, Seymour CA, White RAS, et al. Inherited copper toxicosis in the Bedlington terrier: The prevalence in asymptomatic dogs. J Small Anim Pract 1987;28:1141–1151.

276. Owen CA, McCall JT. Identification of the carrier of the Bedlington terrier copper disease. Am J Vet Res 1983;44:694–696.

277. Brewer GJ, Schall W, Dick R, et al. Use of 64-copper measurements to diagnose canine copper toxicosis. J Vet Intern Med 1992;6:41–43.

278. Allen K, Twedt D, Hunsaker H. Tetramine cupruretic agents: A comparison in dogs. Am J Vet Res 1987;48:28–30.

279. Brewer GJ, Dick RD, Schall W, et al. Use of zinc acetate to treat copper toxicosis in dogs. J Am Vet Med Assoc 1992;201:564–568.

280. Grooters AM, Sherding RG, Johnson SE. Hepatic abscesses in dogs. Compen Contin Educ Pract Vet 1995;17(6):833–838.

281. Konde LJ, Lebel JL, Park RD, et al. Sonographic application in the diagnosis of intraabdominal abscess in the dog. Vet Radiol 1986;27:151–154.

282. Rutgers HC, Haywood S, Kelly DF. Idiopathic hepatic fibrosis in 15 dogs. Vet Rec 1993;133:115–118.

283. Foley RH. *Platynosomum concinnum* infection in cats. Compen Contin Educ Pract Vet 1994;16:1271–1277.

284. Chung NY, Miyahara AY, Chung G. The prevalence of feline liver flukes in the city and county of Honolulu. J Am Anim Hosp Assoc 1977;13:258–262.

285. Bielsa LM, Greiner EC. Liver flukes (*Platynosomum concinnum*) in cats. J Am Anim Hosp Assoc 1985;21:269–274.

286. Brown PJ, Henderson JP, Galloway P, et al. Peliosis hepatis and telangiectasis in 18 cats. J Small Anim Pract 1994;35:73–77.

287. DiBartola SP, Tarr MJ, Webb DM, et al. Familial renal amyloidosis in Chinese shar-pei dogs. J Am Vet Med Assoc 1990;197:483–487.

288. Loeven KO. Spontaneous hepatic rupture secondary to amyloidosis in a Chinese shar-pei. J Am Anim Hosp Assoc 1994;30:577–579.

289. Loeven KO. Hepatic amyloidosis in two Chinese shar-pei dogs. J Am Vet Med Assoc 1994;204:1212–1216.

290. Jones BR, Johnstone AC, Hancock WS. Tyzzer's disease in kittens with familial primary hyperlipoproteinaemia. J Small Anim Pract 1985;26:411–419.

291. Patnaik AK, Lieberman PH, Hurvitz AI, et al. Canine hepatic carcinoids. Vet Pathol 1981;18:445–453.

292. Trout NJ, Berg RJ, McMillan MC, et al. Surgical treatment of hepatobiliary cystadenomas in cats: Five cases (1988–1993). J Am Vet Med Assoc 1995;206:505–507.

293. Phillips L, Tappe J, Lyman R. Hepatic microvascular dysplasia without demonstrable macroscopic shunts. In: Proceedings of the 11th Annual Veterinary Medicine Forum of the American College of Veterinary Internal Medicine, Washington, DC 1993;11:438–439.

294. Whiting PG, Breznock EM, Moore P, et al. Partial hepatectomy with temporary hepatic vascular occlusion in dogs with hepatic arteriovenous fistulas. Vet Surg 1986;15:171–180.

295. Bardens JW. Glycogen storage disease in puppies. VM/SAC 1966;61:1174–1176.

296. Rafiquzzaman M, Svenkerud R, Strande A, et al. Glycogenosis in the dog. Acta Vet Scand 1976;17:196–209.

297. Miller WH, Scott DW, Buerger RG, et al. Necrolytic migratory erythema in dogs: A hepatocutaneous syndrome. J Am Anim Hosp Assoc 1990;26:573–581.

298. Fossum TW, Hay WH, Boothe HW, et al. Chylous ascites in three dogs. J Am Vet Med Assoc 1992;200:70–76.

299. Cornelius L, Mahaffey M. Kinking of the intrathoracic caudal vena cava in five dogs. J Small Anim Pract 1985;26:67–80.

300. Hunt CA, Gofton N. Primary repair of a transected bile duct. J Am Anim Hosp Assoc 1984;20:57–64.

301. Watkins PE, Pearson H, Denny HR. Traumatic rupture of the bile duct in the dog: A report of seven cases. J Small Anim Pract 1983;24:731–740.

302. Parchman MB, Flanders JA. Extrahepatic biliary tract rupture: Evaluation of the relationship between site of rupture and the cause of rupture in 15 dogs. Cornell Vet 1990;80:267–272.

303. Mullowney PC, Tennant BC. Choledocholithiasis in the dog: A review and a report of a case with rupture of the common bile duct. J Small Anim Pract 1982;23:631–638.

304. Church EM, Matthiesen DT. Surgical treatment of 23 dogs with necrotizing cholecystitis. J Am Anim Hosp Assoc 1988;24:305–310.

305. Burk RL, Johnson GF. Emphysematous cholecystitis in the nondiabetic dog: Three case histories. Vet Radiol 1980;21:242–245.

306. Van Winkle TJ, Bruce E. Thrombosis of the portal vein in eleven dogs. Vet Pathol 1993;30:28–35.

307. Roy RG, Post GS, Waters DJ, et al. Portal vein thrombosis as a complication of portosystemic shunt ligation in two dogs. J Am Anim Hosp Assoc 1992;28:53–58.

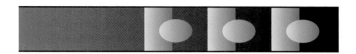

Infectious
Diseases

Chapter 35

Fever, Sepsis, and Principles of Antimicrobial Therapy

Michael R. Lappin

Fever

Fever exists when core body temperature is over 39.1°C (102.5°F). The two major differentials for elevated body temperature are fever (pyrexia) and hyperthermia. Hyperthermia results from increased muscle activity, increased environmental temperature, or increased metabolic rate (i.e., hyperthyroidism); the hypothalamic thermoregulatory set point remains unchanged. Fever develops when the thermoregulatory set point is increased, resulting in increased body temperature from physiologic mechanisms inducing endogenous heat production or heat conservation.[1] Fevers without a readily apparent cause and that persist for more than 2 weeks are classified as fevers of unknown origin.[2]

Pathophysiology

Fever results when leukocytes, particularly mononuclear cells and neutrophils, are activated. Leukocytes are generally stimulated after exposure to different antigens, including those associated with bacterial, viral, fungal, and parasitic agents; neoplasia; tissue necrosis; and primary immune-mediated diseases such as immune-mediated hemolytic anemia, immune-mediated thrombocytopenia, and systemic lupus erythematosus. These antigens are considered exogenous pyrogens.[1] Activated leukocytes release a variety of endogenous pyrogens; interleukin-1, tumor necrosis factor, and some interferons are potent stimulators of fever. Exogenous pyrogens do not cross the blood-brain barrier because of their large molecular mass. Endogenous pyrogens raise the thermoregulatory set point either directly, by entering the central nervous system at the anterior hypothalamus, or by stimulating the production of prostaglandins or cyclic adenosine monophosphate (AMP).[1] The thermoregulatory set point may also be altered by intracranial disease, including trauma and neoplasia, or by drugs such as tetracyclines. Shivering and vasoconstriction are two of the most important physiologic responses to a set-point change that result in generation and conservation of heat, respectively. Fever lower than 40.5°C (105°F) may be beneficial for the management of infectious diseases because of potentiation of phagocytosis, interferon release, and lymphocyte transformation. During chronic inflammatory conditions resulting in fever, activated mononuclear cells also sequester serum iron, decreasing bacterial replication.[1,2] Body temperatures higher than 41°C (106°F) can be detrimental because of effects on cellular metabolism.

Clinical Signs

Nonspecific signs associated with fever often include anorexia, depression, hyperpnea, reluctance to move, or stiffness. Febrile animals commonly exhibit discomfort on palpation of muscles or joints. Clinical signs or physical examination findings associated with the organ systems involved with the primary infection, tissue necrosis, neoplasia, or immune-mediated disease may be evident. In some cases, the only finding on physical examination is fever.

Diagnostic Plan

After documentation of elevated body temperature, the clinician should first try to differentiate hyperthermia from fever by determining whether the patient has been exposed recently to increased environmental temperature or has increased muscle activity due to excitement, physical exertion, or seizures. All apparently normal patients with elevated body temperature should be encouraged to lie quietly in the examination room with the client for 15 to 20 minutes, followed by repeat measurement of core body temperature. Some normal animals have persistently elevated body temperature in the clinic due to hyperthermia; these animals' core body temperature should be measured at home during periods of rest to determine whether fever is present.

After documentation of fever, a thorough history should be obtained and physical examination performed to attempt to determine the most likely source of the fever. Some drugs can induce fever—in particular, tetracycline derivatives. Prior drug administration can be excluded from the differential list based on the history. The client should be questioned concerning clinical signs involving organ systems commonly associated with fever, including the oral cavity, central nervous system, cardiopulmonary system, urogenital system, subcutaneous tissues, peritoneal cavity, and gastrointestinal tract. The clinician should ascertain whether the animal has recently been exposed to other animals, excrement, or ticks and should determine whether other animals or family members have similar clinical signs of disease, whether the patient has traveled, and whether the patient is currently undergoing vaccinations.

The oral cavity should be examined carefully for dental diseases, increased mucus, red or pale mucous membranes, petechiae, or tonsillar enlargement. The chest should be auscultated carefully for cardiac murmurs, muffled heart or lung sounds, or pulmonary crackles or wheezes. The external lymph nodes, spleen, and liver should be palpated for enlargement that may indicate immunostimulation. The muscles, long bones, and joints of animals showing clinical signs of stiffness should be palpated separately. The joints should be gently extended and flexed while the clinician evaluates for swelling, pain, or redness. The abdomen should be palpated for evidence of organomegaly, peritoneal effusion, or pain. A rectal examination should be performed to evaluate for evidence of diarrhea, masses in the anal glands, prostatic enlargement or pain, or urethral or bladder thickening. A brief neurologic examination and fundic examination should be performed to evaluate for evidence of inflammation. While performing the neurologic examination the clinician should carefully palpate the spine while watching for evidence of discomfort.

After the physical examination and history are completed, obvious causes of fever, such as subcutaneous abscessation or bite wounds, are treated appropriately. The further diagnostic plan is directed by results of the history and physical examination. A complete blood count, serum biochemical panel, and urinalysis are indicated in most animals with fever without a readily apparent cause.

The presence of neutrophilic leukocytosis, with or without a left shift, and toxic neutrophilic changes are nonspecific but may indicate an inflammatory condition. Monocytosis is commonly present with chronic inflammatory diseases such as ehrlichiosis. Eosinophilia is commonly present with type I hypersensitivity reactions and metazoan parasitisms such as dirofilariasis. Anemia may occur with some causes of fever, including primary immune-mediated hemolytic anemia, ehrlichiosis, babesiosis, hemobartonellosis, feline leukemia virus infection, and feline immunodeficiency virus infection. Hemopathology may also provide information concerning primary causes. Red cell parasites such as *Hemobartonella* spp. and *Babesia* spp. may be seen; spherocytes and microagglutination may indicate primary immune-mediated hemolytic anemia. Thrombocytopenia develops with many immune-mediated diseases (systemic lupus erythematosus), neoplastic diseases (hemangiosarcoma), and infectious diseases (ehrlichiosis).

Serum biochemical findings are usually nonspecific for the cause of fever but may provide clues for the further diagnostic plan. Azotemia with a suboptimal urine specific gravity (<1.030 in the dog and <1.035 in the cat) combined with bacteriuria and pyuria may indicate pyelonephritis. Increases in liver cytosolic enzymes (alanine aminotransferase and aspartate aminotransferase) may indicate bacterial or immune-mediated cholangiohepatitis; hepatic abscessation; primary hepatic infections, including infectious canine hepatitis, feline leukemia virus, and feline infectious peritonitis virus; or neoplastic diseases of the liver. Hyperglobulinemia occurs commonly with chronic primary immune-mediated diseases, infectious diseases, and neoplasia.

Pyuria and bacteriuria noted on urinalysis performed on urine obtained by cystocentesis indicate upper or lower urinary tract infection or prostatic inflammation. Urine culture and sensitivity should be performed in animals with pyuria or bacteriuria. Ejaculation, prostatic massage, or prostatic aspiration should be performed for cytology and culture and sensitivity in dogs with fever and evidence of prostatic disease on palpation. Proteinuria may indicate immune-complex deposition in the glomeruli from immune-mediated diseases such as systemic lupus erythematosus or chronic inflammatory infectious diseases such as ehrlichiosis or dirofilariasis. The urine protein/creatinine ratio can be used to semiquantitate protein amounts and to monitor therapy in animals with proteinuria without an inflammatory sediment (see Chap. 16).

Culture and sensitivity of body fluids, aspirates, or biopsies of tissue can be used to help confirm infectious causes of fever. Bacteremia and bacterial endocarditis can be confirmed only by blood culture. Aerobic and anaerobic bacterial cultures and fungal cultures may be indicated in some cases. Special media are required to support the growth of some organisms, such as *Mycobacterium* spp. and *Mycoplasma* spp.

Radiographs are commonly used in the search for the cause of fever; infections or neoplasia not obvious on physical examination can often thus be identified. Thoracic radiographs are indicated for coughing animals or animals with restrictive breathing patterns. Abdominal radiographs should be performed for animals with abdominal masses or pain. Thoracic and abdominal radiographs are also indicated for animals with chronic fever (>2 weeks) of inapparent cause when localizing signs are not present. Radiographs of the axial or appendicular skeleton can be used to evaluate for neoplasia or osteomyelitis. Abdominal ultrasonography may also be used to evaluate different organ systems for disease resulting in fever.

Cytologic or histologic evaluation of tissues can be used to help confirm the presence of inflammation. Animals with radiographic evidence of alveolar or bronchial lung patterns not associated with cardiac failure should be evaluated with transtracheal or bronchoalveolar wash for cytology, culture, and antimicrobial susceptibility. Enlarged peripheral lymph nodes should be aspirated to differentiate neoplastic causes from hyperplasia due to primary immune-mediated or infectious diseases. Rectal cytology is indicated for animals with fever and diarrhea; fecal culture for *Salmonella* spp. and *Campylobacter* spp. is generally indicated for the evaluation of animals with neutrophils detected on rectal cytology. Dogs and cats with hemorrhagic gastroenteritis and neutropenia can be further evaluated for the presence of parvovirus infection by fecal enzyme-linked immunosorbent assay (ELISA). Abdominal paracentesis is indicated in animals with fever and peritoneal effusion, and thoracentesis is indicated in animals with pleural effusion. Arthrocentesis can be used to confirm immune-mediated or infectious causes of polyarthritis even if joint effusion or pain is not readily apparent.

Serologic testing is indicated in some patients and the results interpreted in combination with clinical and routine laboratory findings. For example, *Ehrlichia* serology is indicated in dogs with pancytopenia, proteinuria, and previous exposure to *Rhipicephalus* ticks; feline leukemia virus and feline immunodeficiency virus serologies are indicated in cats with fever of unknown origin. Positive antibody tests indicate prior or current infection but do not prove clinical disease caused by the infectious agent. The presence of serum IgM titers or increasing IgG titers can indicate active infections. Serum antigen testing, in general, correlates with clinical disease better than does serum antibody testing because antigens document the presence of the infectious agent.

Routinely available tests for primary immune-mediated diseases include direct Coombs, antinuclear antibody, rheumatoid factor, and antimegakaryocytic antibody tests. Positive test results combined with appropriate clinical or laboratory evidence of disease may support a diagnosis of immune-mediated disease.

Bone marrow aspiration and cytology may aid in the identification of immune-mediated, infectious, or neoplastic diseases. Protein electrophoresis and immunoelectrophoresis may give indirect confirmation of some diseases associated with fever, such as feline infectious peritonitis virus infection or multiple myeloma.

Sepsis

Sepsis is the systemic response to infection by bacteria, viruses, or fungi.[3] Most cases are caused by bacteria; virus or fungal sepsis is rare. Bacteremia, the presence of bacteria in the circulating blood, can be transient, intermittent, or continuous.[4, 5] Transient bacteremia develops after a number of conditions, including routine dentistry, and is generally resolved uneventfully by the immunocompetent patient. Intermittent bacteremia often occurs in immunosuppressed or critically ill animals. The source of infection is extravascular; the urogenital tract is a common source of infection. Bacterial endocarditis is the most common cause of continuous bacteremia.[3] Septic shock is peripheral circulatory failure with hypotension caused by an infectious disease, resulting in cell death from inadequate tissue perfusion.[3, 6]

Pathophysiology

Persistence of severe infections results in stimulation of a systemic inflammatory response. This inflammatory response is induced by antigens released by the infectious agents that activate white blood cells, in particular, macrophages and neutrophils. The inflammatory response is mediated by substances released by the activated white blood cells, including tumor necrosis factor, interleukin-1, interleukin-6, platelet activating factor, nitric oxide, and eicosanoids (prostaglandins and leukotrienes).[3] Leukotrienes increase vascular permeability. Arterial vasodilation combined with increased vascular permeability causes decreased systemic vascular resistance and hypovolemia. This, combined with depressed cardiac function, results in decreased peripheral perfusion and septic shock. Failure to adequately control septic shock results in the multiple organ dysfunction syndrome.[3]

Clinical Signs

Clinical signs associated with the primary organ system infected are often noted initially in patients with bacteremia and early sepsis. The respiratory, gastrointestinal, and urogenital systems are common sources of primary infection, so cough, vomiting, diarrhea, and polyuria or pollakiuria are common presenting findings. Intermittent fever is common with bacterial endocarditis, and cardiac murmurs may be auscultated. Recent dental prophylaxis or previous infections may be reported. As sepsis and septic shock develop, tachycardia, pale mucous membranes, dehydration, and either fever or hypothermia develop. Clinical signs or physical examination abnormalities associated with multiple organ systems commonly develop. Acute renal failure with vomiting, polyuria, and polydipsia or hepatic failure with icterus is common. Dyspnea due to interstitial pulmonary edema from increased vascular permeability is frequently detected in animals with multiple organ dysfunction syndrome.

Diagnostic Plan

Animals with suspected bacteremia, sepsis, or septic shock should be evaluated for the primary infection foci, as discussed for fever. Neutrophilia or neutropenia and a left shift are often detected on complete blood cell count and may suggest bacteremia or sepsis, particularly if the left shift is "degenerative" or innappropriate. Materials for bacterial or fungal culture should be collected as soon as possible so appropriate intravenous antibiotic therapy can be initiated. At least three bacterial blood cultures over 2 hours should be collected from the jugular vein after sterile preparation of the skin in animals with life-threatening sepsis.[4]

Principles of Antimicrobial Therapy

Antimicrobial Selection

Antibiotic selection is usually based on culture and sensitivity results. However, veterinarians commonly make empiric antibiotic decisions for patients that require immediate therapy or have simple, first-time infections, or when client finances preclude the expense of culture and sensitivity. Often, the life of the patient is dependent on making an appropriate antibiotic choice. Optimal antibiotic therapy can be selected by considering the organ system involved, the most likely pathogens (gram positive, gram negative, aerobic, or anaerobic), the antimicrobial most likely to be effective against the pathogens, the most effective dose and route of administration to deliver an appropriate concentration of the antimicrobial to the affected site, the expense, the practicality of administration, and the potential toxicity.[7]

Classification of Antibiotics

Antibiotics can be classified as broad or narrow spectrum.[7] Antibiotics such as chloramphenicol, cephalosporins, and quinolones have an effect against multiple bacterial types and are considered broad spectrum. Penicillin G, macrolides such as erythromycin, lincosamides such as clindamycin, and aminoglycosides have an effect against a limited number of organisms and are considered narrow spectrum.

Antibiotics that can kill a microorganism are bacteriocidal; antibiotics that inhibit the growth and replication of a microorganism are bacteriostatic. Bacteriostatic agents may be bacteriocidal if a high tissue concentration is achieved. Tetracyclines, chloramphenicol, macrolides, lincosamides, and sulfonamides are generally bacteriostatic. Penicillins, cephalosporins, aminoglycosides, quinolones, polymyxins, and tri-methoprim-sulfonamide combinations are generally bacteriocidal. Bacteriocidal antimicrobials require organism replication to be effective, so in general they should not be administered concurrently with bacteriostatic antibiotics. Bacteriostatic agents require an intact immune system to eliminate infections, so bacteriocidal agents should be used in immunosuppressed animals.

Penicillins and cephalosporins inhibit cell wall synthesis and are usually bacteriocidal. These agents can be inhibited by the concurrent administration of bacteriostatic agents. Polymyxin B, nystatin, and amphotericin B disrupt the bacterial cell membrane, are bacteriocidal, and are not inhibited by bacteriostatic agents. Tetracyclines, chloramphenicol, macrolides (erythromycin), and lincosamides (lincomycin,

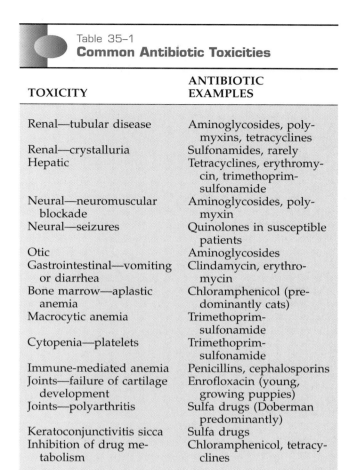

Table 35–1
Common Antibiotic Toxicities

TOXICITY	ANTIBIOTIC EXAMPLES
Renal—tubular disease	Aminoglycosides, polymyxins, tetracyclines
Renal—crystalluria	Sulfonamides, rarely
Hepatic	Tetracyclines, erythromycin, trimethoprim-sulfonamide
Neural—neuromuscular blockade	Aminoglycosides, polymyxin
Neural—seizures	Quinolones in susceptible patients
Otic	Aminoglycosides
Gastrointestinal—vomiting or diarrhea	Clindamycin, erythromycin
Bone marrow—aplastic anemia	Chloramphenicol (predominantly cats)
Macrocytic anemia	Trimethoprim-sulfonamide
Cytopenia—platelets	Trimethoprim-sulfonamide
Immune-mediated anemia	Penicillins, cephalosporins
Joints—failure of cartilage development	Enrofloxacin (young, growing puppies)
Joints—polyarthritis	Sulfa drugs (Doberman predominantly)
Keratoconjunctivitis sicca	Sulfa drugs
Inhibition of drug metabolism	Chloramphenicol, tetracyclines

clindamycin) inhibit protein synthesis and are bacteriostatic. Aminoglycosides (streptomycin, neomycin, kanamycin, gentamicin, amikacin, tobramycin) are bacteriocidal protein synthesis inhibitors. Sulfonamides, griseofulvin, and the nitrofurans are bacteriostatic examples of nucleic acid and intermediary metabolism inhibitors; trimethoprim-sulfonamide combinations and the quinolones are bacteriocidal.

Many antibiotics have potential for toxicity. Renal, hepatic, neural, bone marrow, and gastrointestinal toxicity are common (Table 35–1). Hypersensitivity reactions, including keratoconjunctivitis sicca, thrombocytopenia, immune-mediated anemia, and polyarthritis, also occur with some antibiotics.

For most clinical syndromes, the most common pathogens are generally known (Table 35–2). Antibiotics are chosen based on their distribution in tissues and spectrum of activity against the common pathogens (Table 35–3).

Antibiotic Dosage Schedule

Antibiotic dosage (Table 35–4) for individual animals is based on the suspected pathogen, the organ

Table 35–2
Bacterial Pathogens Associated With Common Clinical Syndromes

CLINICAL SYNDROME OR ORGAN SYSTEM	COMMON PATHOGENS
Bacteremia—aerobic	*Staphylococcus, Streptococcus, Escherichia coli, Klebsiella, Enterobacter, Pseudomonas*
Bacteremia—anaerobic	*Clostridium, Bacteroides* (see Chap. 36)
Bacterial endocarditis	*Staphylococcus aureus, E. coli,* β-hemolytic *Streptococcus*
Intestinal bacterial overgrowth	Gram-negative (*E. coli, Pseudomonas, Enterobacter*), anaerobes
Bite wound abscesses	*Staphylococcus aureus, Pasteurella,* anaerobes (see Chap. 36)
Hepatic	Gram-negative, anaerobes
Nervous system	Anaerobes
Orchitis	*Brucella, E. coli, Enterobacter, Klebsiella, Pseudomonas*
Osteomyelitis	*Staphylococcus, Streptococcus, E. coli, Proteus, Pseudomonas*
Peritonitis	Gram-negative (*E. coli, Pseudomonas, Enterobacter*), anaerobes (see Chap. 36)
Pneumonia—dog	*E. coli, Klebsiella* spp., *Pasteurella* spp., *Pseudomonas* spp., *Bordetella bronchiseptica, Streptococcus zooepidemicus, Mycoplasma,* anaerobes (especially in consolidated lungs)
Pneumonia—cat	*Bordetella, Pasteurella, Mycoplasma,* anaerobes (especially in consolidated lungs)
Pyothorax—dog and cat	Anaerobes, *Nocardia,* gram-negative
Prostatitis	*E. coli, Enterobacter, Klebsiella, Pseudomonas, Brucella*
Pyoderma	*Staphylococcus intermedius,* gram-negative (deep pyoderma)
Pyometra	*E. coli,* anaerobes
Rhinitis	Anaerobes (see Chap. 36), *Pasteurella, Bordetella, Mycoplasma* (rarely), *Chlamydia* (cats)
Surgical wounds (nonalimenteric)	*Staphylococcus aureus* (dogs), *Pasteurella* (cats)
Urinary tract—dogs	*E. coli, Proteus, Klebsiella, Pseudomonas, Enterobacter,* β-hemolytic *Streptococcus, Staphylococcus, Mycoplasma* (rarely)
Urinary tract—cats	*E. coli, Staphylococcus, Streptococcus*

Data from Ferguson and Lappin.[7]

system involved, and the potential for toxicity. The low end of the dose and the longest duration interval should be used in animals with potential for toxicity. In general, intracellular pathogens, anaerobic infections, and life-threatening infections including bacteremia and central nervous system infections should be treated with the high end of the dose and the shortest dosage interval.

Route of Administration

Parenteral antibiotics should be used in all animals with vomiting or regurgitation (see Table 35–4). Animals with life-threatening conditions resulting in bacteremia or sepsis should receive intravenous antibiotic therapy for the first 3 to 7 days, if possible. Oral administration of antibiotics can be initiated when vomiting, regurgitation, or life-threatening sepsis has resolved.

Duration of Therapy

Simple, non–life-threatening, first-time infections such as urinary tract infections, subcutaneous abscesses, and superficial pyoderma generally are treated for 2 weeks. Chronic infections are generally treated for a minimum of 4 weeks or for 2 to 4 weeks after resolution of clinical or radiographic signs of disease. Infection of bone or parenchymal tissues resulting in granulation tissue, including bronchopneumonia, should be treated for a minimum of 6 to 8 weeks. Diseases induced by intracellular organisms such as *Brucella canis* should be treated for a minimum of 6 weeks. See the appropriate chapters for specific recommendations concerning treatment duration for specific infectious agents.

Changing Antibiotic Therapy

Antibiotic therapy is changed if antimicrobial susceptibility reveals a more appropriate antibiotic choice or if clinical signs of disease are not resolving during the administration of the initial antibiotic. Depending on the organ system and degree of inflammation associated with the infection, positive response to therapy may not occur for several days. In general, infections resulting in fever are treated with the initial antibiotic for 72 hours before an antibiotic change is considered.

Table 35–3
Empirical Antibiotic Choices by Organ System or Infectious Agent

ORGAN SYSTEM OR INFECTIOUS AGENT	ANTIBIOTIC CHOICES
Discospondylitis	Cephalosporin (first generation) or clavamox or clindamycin
Encephalitis	Chloramphenicol or amoxicillin or trimethoprim-sulfonamide or enrofloxacin
Mastitis	Cephalosporin (first generation) or amoxicillin or clavamox
Osteomyelitis	Clavamox or clindamycin or cephalosporin (first generation) or chloramphenicol
Polyarthritis	
Bacterial	Cephalosporin (first generation) or enrofloxacin
Rocky Mountain spotted fever	Doxycycline or chloramphenicol or enrofloxacin
Ehrlichia spp.	Doxycycline or chloramphenicol
Borrelia burgdorferi	Doxycycline or amoxicillin
Pyothorax—dog and cat	Enrofloxacin and (ampicillin or amoxicillin or clindamycin or metronidazole) Chloramphenicol
Respiratory	
Upper	Amoxicillin or clindamycin or cephalosporin (first generation) or doxycyline
Lower	Enrofloxacin and (penicillin or ampicillin or amoxicillin or clindamycin or metronidazole) Chloramphenicol
Sepsis and bacterial endocarditis	Enrofloxacin and (penicillin or ampicillin or amoxicillin or clindamycin) Gentamycin or amikacin and (penicillin or ampicillin or amoxicillin or clindamycin) Cephalosporin (second or third generation) Imipenem Ticarcillin and clavulanate
Staphylococcal pyoderma	Cephalosporin (first generation) or clavamox or cloxacillin or clindamycin or oxacillin or trimethoprim-sulfonamide or erythromycin
Gram-negative pyoderma	Enrofloxacin
L-form bacteria	Doxycycline or chloramphenicol
Atypical *Mycobacterium*	Doxycycline or chloramphenicol or enrofloxacin
Nocardia or *Actinomyces*	Amoxicillin or penicillin and trimethoprim-sulfonamide
Toxoplasmosis	Clindamycin or trimethoprim-sulfonamide
Urogenital	
Aerobic	Amoxicillin or clavamox or cephalosporin (first generation) or trimethoprim-sulfonamide or enrofloxacin
Mycoplasma/Ureaplasma	Doxycycline or chloramphenicol or enrofloxacin
Prostate	Trimethoprim-sulfonamide or enrofloxacin or chloramphenicol or erythromycin or clindamycin
Pyometra	Enrofloxacin and amoxicillin or chloramphenicol
Brucella canis	Streptomycin and tetracycline derivative, or enrofloxacin or doxycycline or minocycline
Cholangiohepatitis	Amoxicillin or cephalosporin (first generation) or chloramphenicol or metronidazole

Data from Ferguson and Lappin.[7]

Often, the decision to change antibiotics is based on clinical trends. For example, if the core body temperature in an animal with fever decreases from 41°C to 39.5°C (105.5°F–103.0°F) over the first 72 hours of treatment, the same antibiotic should be continued for several more days, and the animal's temperature should be monitored. Often, clinical signs of disease secondary to organ infection may take days to weeks to resolve completely. For example, animals with consolidated lung lobes after aspiration pneumonia may continue to cough for weeks, even though an appropriate antibiotic is being administered, due to deep infection of devitalized tissue. In this case, resolution of complete blood count abnormalities; improvement in attitude, activity, and appetite; and improvement in thoracic radiographic abnormalities are used initially to monitor for positive response to therapy.

Table 35–4
Antibiotics Commonly Used for Treatment of Bacterial Infections in Dogs and Cats

DRUG	SPECIES	DOSAGE	ROUTE OF ADMINISTRATION
Amikacin	Dog and cat	5–10 mg/kg, t.i.d.	IV, IM, SC
Amoxicillin	Dog and cat	10–22 mg/kg, b.i.d.–t.i.d.	PO, SC
Amoxicillin and clavulanate	Dog	12.5–25 mg/kg, b.i.d.–t.i.d.	PO
	Cat	62.5 mg/cat, b.i.d.–t.i.d.	PO
Ampicillin sodium	Dog and cat	10–20 mg/kg, t.i.d.	SC, IM, IV
Cefadroxil*	Dog and cat	22 mg/kg, b.i.d.–t.i.d.	PO
Cefazolin*	Dog and cat	20–25 mg/kg, t.i.d.	IM, IV
Cefotaxime†	Dog and cat	25–50 mg/kg, t.i.d.	SC, IM, IV
Cefoxitin‡	Dog and cat	22 mg/kg, t.i.d.	IM, IV
Cephalexin*	Dog and cat	22 mg/kg, t.i.d.	PO
Chloramphenicol	Dog	25–50 mg/kg, t.i.d.	PO, SC, IV
	Cat	10–15 mg/kg, b.i.d.	PO, IV
Clindamycin	Dog and cat	5.5–11 mg/kg, b.i.d.	PO, SC, IM
Ciprofloxacin	Dog and cat	5–15 mg/kg, b.i.d.	PO
Doxycycline	Dog and cat	5 mg/kg, b.i.d.	PO, IV
Enrofloxacin	Dog and cat	2.5–5 mg/kg, b.i.d.	PO, IM, SC, IV
Gentamicin	Dog and cat	2–4 mg/kg, t.i.d.	IV, IM, SC
Imipenem	Dog and cat	2–5 mg/kg, t.i.d.	IV
Metronidazole	Dog	10 mg/kg, t.i.d.	PO
	Cat	10 mg/kg, b.i.d.	PO
Oxacillin	Dog and cat	22–40 mg/kg, t.i.d.	PO
Penicillin G	Dog and cat	22,000 U/kg, t.i.d.–q.i.d.	IM, IV
Tetracycline	Dog and cat	22 mg/kg, t.i.d.	PO
Ticarcillin and clavulanate	Dog	40–110 mg/kg, q.i.d.	IM, IV
Tobramycin	Dog and cat	2 mg/kg, t.i.d.	IV, IM, SC
Trimethoprim-sulfonamide	Dog and cat	15 mg/kg, b.i.d.	PO, SC

IM, intramuscular; IV, intravenous; SC, subcutaneous; PO, by mouth; b.i.d., twice per day (every 12 hours); t.i.d., three times per day (every 8 hours); q.i.d., four times per day (every 6 hours).
*First-generation cephalosporin.
†Third-generation cephalosporin.
‡Second-generation cephalosporin.

References

1. Greene CE. Fever. In: Greene CE, ed. Infectious Diseases of the Dog and Cat, 2nd ed. Philadelphia, WB Saunders, 1990:64–71.
2. Lorenz MD. Pyrexia (fever). In: Lorenz MD, Cornelius LM, eds. Small Animal Medical Diagnosis, 2nd ed. Philadelphia, JB Lippincott, 1993:15–22.
3. Kirby R. Septic shock. In: Bonagura JD, ed. Kirk's Current Veterinary Therapy XII. Philadelphia, WB Saunders, 1995:139–146.
4. Dow SW. Diagnosis of bacteremia in critically ill dogs and cats. In: Bonagura JD, ed. Kirk's Current Veterinary Therapy XII. Philadelphia, WB Saunders, 1995:137–139.
5. Nostrandt AC. Bacteremia and septicemia in small animal patients. Problems Vet Med 1990;2:348–361.
6. Weeren FR, Muir MM. Clinical aspects of septic shock and comprehensive approaches to treatment in dogs and cats. J Am Vet Med Assoc 1992;200:1859–1870.
7. Ferguson DC, Lappin MR. Antimicrobial therapy. In: Lorenz MD, Cornelius LM, Ferguson DC, eds. Small Animal Medical Therapeutics. Philadelphia, JB Lippincott, 1992:457–478.

Chapter 36

Bacterial Diseases

Michael R. Lappin

Anaerobic Infections

Pathophysiology

Etiology. *Bacteroides* spp., *Fusobacterium* spp., *Peptostreptococcus* spp., *Peptococcus* spp., *Clostridium* spp., *Actinomyces* spp., *Propionibacterium* spp., and *Eubacterium* spp. are the anaerobic bacteria most commonly associated with clinical disease (Table 36–1).[1–4] In one study of anaerobic infections in dogs and cats, *Bacteroides* spp. and *Fusobacterium* spp. were most common (30%), followed by *Clostridium* spp. (14%), *Peptostreptococcus* spp. (11%), and *Actinomyces* spp. (9%).[4] With the exception of *Actinomyces* spp., the organisms are obligate anaerobes that cannot use oxygen metabolically and die in its presence. *Actinomyces* is a facultative anaerobe that can tolerate oxygen but does not use it metabolically. The organisms die rapidly outside the host when exposed to oxygen and are generally susceptible to routine disinfectants.

Epidemiology. Anaerobic bacteria are found most frequently in areas with low oxygen tension and low oxygen-reduction potential such as the mucous membranes of the oral cavity and vagina.[1–3] Most of the body's normal flora are anaerobes.[2] Anaerobic infections are usually considered endogenous because the origin of the infection is often the animal's own flora.

Pathogenesis. Clinical anaerobic infections are most common after introduction of the anaerobic bacteria from regions where they are found as normal flora to regions with low oxygen-reduction potential, such as the subcutaneous space, pleural space, peritoneal cavity, and central nervous system. Bacteria from the oropharynx, gastrointestinal tract, and vagina are most commonly involved. The bacteria are introduced through the skin or mucous membranes, usually by bite wounds, foreign bodies, or trauma. Infection is potentiated by poor blood supply, tissue necrosis, prior infection, and immunosuppression. In humans, increased risk of anaerobic infection has been associated with diabetes mellitus, corticosteroid therapy, leukopenia, hypogammaglobulinemia, and splenectomy.[2]

Anaerobic bacteria produce a variety of factors that predispose the host to infection and clinical disease.[1, 2] Lecithinase (*C. perfringens*), collagenase (*B. melaninogenicus*), deoxyribonuclease (*B. fragilis*), and heparinase (*B. fragilis*) are examples of enzymes produced by some anaerobes that damage tissue favoring replication. Some anaerobic bacteria, including *Fusobacterium* spp., produce endotoxins. Production of leukocidin, an enzyme that destroys white blood cells, inhibition of opsonization of bacteria by *B. melaninogenicus*, production of β-lactamases that inactivate penicillins and cephalosporins, production of folate that inhibits the activity of trimethoprim-sulfonamides, and inhibition of leukocyte chemotaxis are examples of ways some anaerobic bacteria promote colonization. Synergism with aerobic bacteria can potentiate disease associated with anaerobic bacteria.[1, 2]

Clinical Signs

Anaerobic infections can develop in animals of any age, breed, or sex (Table 36–2). Historical findings, clinical signs of disease, and physical examination findings correlate with the primary tissues involved. A history of fighting or exposure to foreign bodies is common in animals with anaerobic infections. Animals with anaerobic infection of the lungs commonly have a history of aspiration. In general, anaerobic infections result in putrid, foul-smelling discharges. Anaerobic infections are associated with a diverse group of clinical conditions (see Table 36–2).

Oropharyngeal. *Fusobacterium* spp., *Peptostreptococcus* spp., and *Bacteroides* spp. are common oral cavity flora in the dog.[1] *Bacteroides* spp. were cultured from

---

Table 36–1
Characteristics of Common Anaerobic Pathogens

GENUS	GRAM STAIN	MORPHOLOGY	COMMENTS
Peptococcus	Positive	Cocci	Singles, pairs, variable groups; resembles *Staphylococcus*
Peptostreptococcus	Positive	Cocci	Pairs, chains; resembles *Streptococcus*
Actinomyces	Positive (variable)	Rods, filaments	Can form tangled mats, branching or radiating
Clostridium	Positive	Large rods	Spores rarely appear in clinical specimens
Eubacterium	Positive	Rods	Non–spore-forming
Fusobacterium	Negative	Thin bacilli	Tapered or pointed ends and cigar or needle appearance
Bacteroides	Negative	Coccobacilli	Pleomorphic, beaded or coccoid, difficult to stain

Adapted from Dow SW. Anaerobic infections. In: Greene CE, ed. Infectious Diseases of the Dog and Cat, 2nd ed. Philadelphia, WB Saunders, 1990:563.

Table 36–2
Clinical Findings Consistent With Anaerobic Infections in Dogs and Cats

FINDINGS	CLINICAL CONDITION
Signalment	**Oropharyngeal**
Any age, breed, or sex	Stomatitis
	Oropharyngeal abscess
History	Retrobulbar abscess
Fighting	
Foreign body	**Respiratory**
Vomiting or regurgitation with aspiration	Rhinitis or sinusitis
Recent surgery, open wound or fracture, or dentistry	Pneumonia with consolidated areas of lung tissue
History of immunosuppressive drugs or diseases	Pyothorax
Infection resistant to sulfonamides or aminoglycosides	
Neutrophilic inflammation with cytologically evident bacteria but	**Central Nervous System**
negative aerobic culture	Encephalitis
	Otitis media or otitis interna
Physical Examination	
Flaccid paralysis (Clostridium botulinum)	**Cutaneous**
Rigid paralysis and trismus (C. tetani)	Subcutaneous abscessation
Subcutaneous gas production	Bite wounds
Putrid odor from lesion	Puncture wounds
Serosanguineous discharge from a painful lesion	
Necrotic tissue	**Musculoskeletal**
Open wound or fracture	Osteomyelitis
High fever	Open fractures
Sulfur granules	Flaccid paralysis (C. botulinum)
Abscesses	Rigid paralysis (C. tetani)
Blackish exudate	Myonecrosis
Cytologic Findings	**Gastrointestinal**
Degenerate and nondegenerate neutrophils with mixed population	Peritonitis
of bacteria	Cholangiohepatitis
Large gram-positive rods with minimal neutrophils	Hepatic abscessation
Sulfur granules	
Branching filamentous rods (Actinomyces)	**Urogenital**
	Pyometra
	Cardiovascular
	Bacteremia

the oral cavity of 37.5% of healthy cats.[5] Stomatitis, oropharyngeal abscess, and retrobulbar abscess are commonly induced by these agents and result from direct extension of the normal flora in the oral cavity. Inappetence, halitosis, pain on opening the mouth, and exophthalmos (retrobulbar abscess) are common clinical manifestations of disease. *Actinomyces* spp. are also frequently involved with oropharyngeal abscesses associated with foreign bodies in dogs.

Respiratory. The normal flora of the nasopharynx is similar to that of the oropharynx, so the organisms associated with rhinitis or sinusitis are similar to those causing disease associated with the oral cavity. Sneezing and mucopurulent nasal discharge are the most common clinical signs. Anaerobes are most often associated with pneumonia with consolidated or devitalized areas of lung tissue. This usually results after aspiration, so oral cavity flora is often involved. Pyothorax results from penetrating wounds, foreign body

migration, rupture of infected lung tissues, or hematogenous spread of bacteria. Dogs and cats with pneumonia or pyothorax are generally presented for depression, dyspnea, and cough. Fever and abnormal lung sounds are common abnormalities found during physical examination. *Bacteroides* spp. are involved in 45% of cats with pyothorax.[5] *Actinomyces* spp. are involved in 85% of dogs with pyothorax.[6]

Central Nervous System. Depression and focal neurologic deficits without fever caused by mixed anaerobic infection of the central nervous system with *Bacteroides* spp., *Fusobacterium* spp., *Peptostreptococcus* spp., and *Eubacterium* spp. have been reported uncommonly in dogs and cats.[7] Because the oral cavity communicates with the middle ear by the auditory tube, dogs and cats with a history and physical examination findings consistent with otitis media or otitis interna should be considered infected by anaerobic bacteria.

Cutaneous. All subcutaneous abscesses induced by bite wounds, puncture wounds, or foreign bodies should be considered infected by anaerobic bacteria. Mixed infections are common. *Bacteroides* spp. can be isolated from 45% of the cats with cat-bite abscesses.[5] *Bacteroides* spp., *Fusobacterium* spp., and *Peptostreptococcus* spp. are the most common anaerobes in hunting dogs with thoracic wall or abdominal wall abscesses.[8] *Actinomyces* spp. can be isolated in 26% of these cases.[8]

Musculoskeletal. Anaerobic infection should be considered in animals with evidence of osteomyelitis, open fractures, flaccid paralysis (*C. botulinum*), rigid paralysis (*C. tetani*), and myonecrosis. Infection with *C. tetani* results in trismus and muscle rigidity due to toxin production. *C. botulinum* toxin results in lower motor neuron disease and flaccid paralysis (see Chap. 28). Detection of subcutaneous gas production combined with extreme pain and a serosanguineous discharge can be consistent with myonecrosis secondary to *Clostridium* spp. Anaerobes can be isolated from 64% of dogs and cats with osteomyelitis.[9]

Gastrointestinal. Peritonitis is often induced by migrating foreign bodies or leakage of intestinal contents, so anaerobic bacteria are common. *Bacteroides* spp., *Clostridium* spp., *Fusobacterium* spp., and anaerobic streptococci are common isolates.[1] *Clostridium* spp. and *Bacteroides* spp. should be suspected in animals with clinical, laboratory, or ultrasonographic evidence of biliary tract inflammation or hepatic abscessation.

Urogenital. Anaerobic bacteria can be isolated in 38% of the uterine infections of dogs and cats but are rare in urinary tract infections.[1]

Cardiovascular. Bacteria were cultured from 49 of 100 critically ill dogs and cats with clinical or laboratory evidence of bacteremia.[10] Anaerobic bacteria were present in 31% of the positive cultures; *Clostridium* spp. and *Bacteroides* spp. were most commonly isolated.

Laboratory and Radiographic Abnormalities. Laboratory abnormalities and radiographic abnormalities vary depending on the organ system affected. Neutrophilic leukocytosis with or without a left shift is a common complete blood count abnormality. Some animals with *Clostridium* infection have hemolysis. Serum biochemical abnormalities are variable but may show hyperbilirubinemia and increased activities of liver enzymes in animals with biliary tract infection. Proteinuria with and without pyuria or bacteriuria is often identified in dogs with pyometra. Increased numbers of neutrophils are detected in the cerebrospinal fluid of animals with central nervous system anaerobic infection.[7]

Radiographic abnormalities vary. Most subcutaneous infections appear as increased soft tissue density; radiodense foreign bodies may or may not be identified. Osteomyelitis is characterized by a combination of sclerosis and lysis at the site of infection (Fig. 36–1). Pleural effusion with or without obvious foreign bodies or consolidated lung lobes is common in animals with pyothorax (Fig. 36–2). The uterus is enlarged in animals with pyometra. There may be loss of abdominal detail with peritonitis. Ultrasound can be used to document fluid in the abdominal cavity and uterus. The liver may have a mottled echodensity or hypoechoic areas due to abscessation on ultrasound examination. Computed tomography is superior to skull radiographs for documenting brain abscessation.

Pathology

Gross pathologic appearance with most anaerobic infections includes abscessation and fibrin deposition. Histologically, necrosis with neutrophilic and mononuclear cell inflammation is most common. Myonecrosis is most common with *Clostridium* spp. Pyogranulomatous disease with fibrosis is common with *Actinomyces* spp. infection.

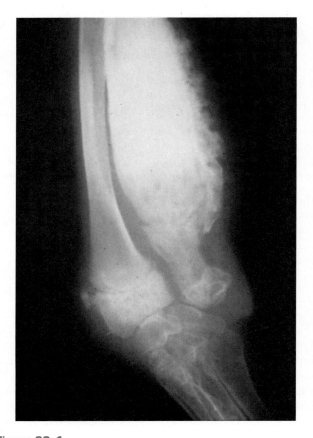

Figure 36–1
Bacterial osteomyelitis of the distal ulna in a dog. (Courtesy of Richard Park, DVM, Fort Collins, Colorado.)

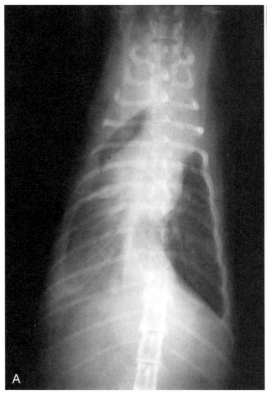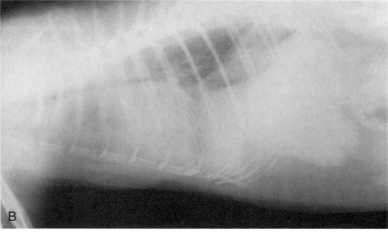

Figure 36-2
Ventrodorsal **(A)** and lateral **(B)** thoracic radiographs of a cat with pyothorax. **(A)** Widened radiopaque pleural space, collapse of lung lobes, and rounded costal phrenic angle on the right side. **(B)** Retraction of the lung lobes and fluid obscuring the ventral aspect of the cardiac silhouette.

Diagnostic Plan

Cytologic evaluation of material from animals with suspected anaerobic infection generally reveals degenerate and nondegenerate neutrophils with mixed populations of bacteria (Fig. 36–3). Some *Clostridium* spp. produce leukocidin, which lyses white blood cells. In these cases, large gram-positive rods with minimal neutrophils are noted cytologically.[1, 3] "Sulfur" granules and branching filamentous rods are common with *Actinomyces. Nocardia*, a related aerobic bacteria, can appear similarly cytologically. In general, *Nocardia* is acid-fast and *Actinomyces* is not, but culture is required to differentiate these agents definitively.[11, 12] Owing to the resident normal population of anaerobes on skin and mucosal surfaces, swabs from the surface or from draining tracts are impossible to interpret. Abscess material, fluids, or tissue from deep within the infected area should be cultured. When tissue is cultured, 1 cm^3 should be submitted.[13] If free fluid is aspirated, air should be removed, the needle capped with a rubber stopper, and the sample inoculated onto a culture medium within 10 minutes of collection, if possible. Samples with large volume (1–3 mL) may support the growth of anaerobes for up to 12 hours in a capped syringe. Transport media (Port-a-Cul) and anaerobic culterettes are available but may not be ideal for fastidious *Bacteroides* spp. and *Fusobacterium* spp. Samples can be inoculated or placed into carbon dioxide–containing vials or into commercial blood culture bottles designed to support the growth of anaerobes. Materials in transport media to be cultured for anaerobes should be stored at room temperature and should be cultured within 2 days.

Treatment and Prognosis

The primary therapy for anaerobic infections is to remove devitalized tissue to improve the blood supply to and oxygenation of the infected area, which

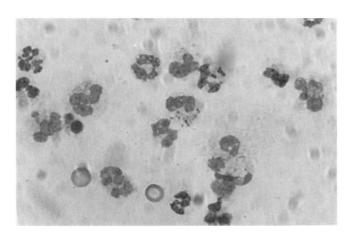

Figure 36-3
Cytology of an abdominocentesis from a dog with peritonitis. The mixed bacterial population is characteristic of anaerobic infections.

Table 36–3

Antibiotics Commonly Used for the Treatment of Anaerobic Infections in Dogs and Cats

DRUG	SPECIES	DOSAGE	ROUTE OF ADMINISTRATION
Amoxicillin	Dog and cat	10–22 mg/kg, b.i.d.–t.i.d.	PO, SC
Ampicillin sodium	Dog and cat	10–22 mg/kg, t.i.d.	SC, IM, IV
Cefadroxil*	Dog and cat	22 mg/kg, b.i.d.	PO
Cephalexin*	Dog and cat	22 mg/kg, t.i.d.	PO
Cefazolin*	Dog and cat	20–25 mg/kg, t.i.d.	IM, IV
Cefoxitin†	Dog and cat	22 mg/kg, t.i.d.	IM, IV
Cefotaxime‡	Dog and cat	25–50 mg/kg, t.i.d.	SC, IM, IV
Imipenem	Dog and cat	2–5 mg/kg, t.i.d.	IV
Chloramphenicol	Dog	25–50 mg/kg, t.i.d.	PO, SC, IV
Chloramphenicol	Cat	10–15 mg/kg, b.i.d.	PO, IV
Clindamycin	Dog and cat	5.5–11 mg/kg, b.i.d.	PO, SC, IM
Metronidazole	Dog	10 mg/kg, t.i.d.	PO
Metronidazole	Cat	10 mg/kg, b.i.d.	PO
Penicillin G	Dog and cat	22,000 U/kg, t.i.d.–q.i.d.	IM, IV
Trimethoprim-sulfonamide	Dog and cat	15 mg/kg, b.i.d.	PO, SC

IM, intramuscular; IV, intravenous; SC, subcutaneous; PO, by mouth; b.i.d., twice per day (every 12 hours); t.i.d., three times per day (every 8 hours); q.i.d., four times per day (every 6 hours).
*First-generation cephalosporin.
†Third-generation cephalosporin.
‡Second-generation cephalosporin.

will inhibit growth of the bacteria. The source of infection should be removed if possible. Pleural lavage should be performed in animals with pyothorax. Lobectomy should be performed in animals with pyothorax secondary to known pulmonary foreign bodies or those that fail to respond to pleural lavage clinically or by reinflation of consolidated lung lobes in 3 to 5 days. Peritonitis should be managed with open peritoneal lavage. Soft tissue infections and osteomyelitis should be debrided surgically. Infected uteri should be removed surgically or drained by use of prostaglandin $PGF_{2\alpha}$.

Antibiotic therapy is generally used concurrently with drainage or debridement. In general, parenteral antibiotics should be administered for several days initially, particularly in animals with pyothorax, pneumonia, peritonitis, and clinical signs consistent with bacteremia. Penicillin derivatives, clindamycin, chloramphenicol, metronidazole, and cephalosporins are commonly used for the treatment of anaerobic infections (Table 36–3).[1, 3] Many laboratories do not provide antimicrobial susceptibility for anaerobes, and treatment should be started before culture results are known; therefore, most decisions concerning treatment of anaerobic infections are made empirically. Not all anaerobic bacteria have the same antibiotic susceptibility (Table 36–4). Clinicians should estimate which organisms are most likely based on organ system involvement (see Clinical Signs) and cytology (see Table 36–1) and choose antibiotics accordingly.

Penicillin derivatives in general have excellent activity against anaerobes, with the exception of *B. fragilis*. This organism is usually resistant to first-generation cephalosporins. Whenever gram-negative coccobacilli are detected cytologically in a neutrophilic exudate, particularly if associated with the oral cavity, an alternative antibiotic should be chosen (see Table 36–4). Chloramphenicol has a broad antianaerobic spectrum and crosses the blood-brain barrier well, so it is a good choice for the treatment of central nervous system anaerobic infections. Chloramphenicol is also a good treatment choice for animals with pyometra because it also kills most isolates of *Escherichia coli*. Metronidazole and clindamycin penetrate tissue well, so they are good choices for animals with pneumonia with consolidated lung lobes and pyothorax.

Because anaerobic infections frequently coexist with aerobic bacteria, combination antimicrobial therapy is often indicated. For example, for animals with peritonitis or bacteremia secondary to intestinal tract disease, drugs such as enrofloxacin against the gram-negative coliform spectrum should be combined with a drug against the anaerobic spectrum, such as metronidazole or penicillins, and administered at high doses.

Whereas trimethoprim-sulfonamides generally work well for the treatment of anaerobes in vitro,[14] the high concentrations of folate produced in pyogenic infections may overwhelm the effect of this drug combination in vivo. Researchers have suggested that there is little indication for the combination of trimethoprim-sulfonamide with ampicillin for the treatment of bacterial infections.[15] However, this combination may be indicated in dogs or cats with suspected *Nocardia* or *Actinomyces* infection. *N. asteroides, N. brasiliensis,* and *N. caviae* have been associated with a number of clinical syndromes similar to those induced by *Actinomyces,* including chronic draining cutaneous lesions, arthritis, encephalitis, pyothorax, pneumonia, osteomyelitis, and mixed infections.[11, 12, 16, 17] The two organisms can be difficult to differentiate cytologically. While *Actinomyces* usually responds to penicillin derivations, *Nocardia* is more likely to respond to sulfonamide-containing compounds.[11, 12, 16, 17] Trimethoprim-sulfonamide and penicillin derivatives are indicated for the treatment of animals with cytologic demonstration of sulfur granules or branching filamentous rods until culture results are obtained.

The prognosis for superficial or localized anaerobic infections such as subcutaneous abscesses and pyometra can be very good if drainage, debridement, or surgical removal and appropriate antibiotic therapy are instituted rapidly. The prognosis is slightly worse for animals with pyothorax. Prognosis is guarded to grave for animals with peritonitis or central nervous system infection.

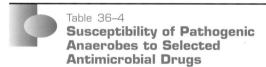

Table 36–4
Susceptibility of Pathogenic Anaerobes to Selected Antimicrobial Drugs

BACTERIA	DRUGS OF CHOICE	ALTERNATIVES
Anaerobic cocci	pen*	clin, chlor, cep,† cef‡, cefot§
Bacteroides fragilis‖	met, clin, cef	chlor, cefot, imip
Bacteroides spp.	pen, clin, met	cef, chlor
Fusobacterium spp.	pen, clin, chlor	met, cefot
Actinomyces spp.	clin, chlor, pen	cef
Clostridium perfringens	pen, cep, chlor	clin, met
Clostridium spp.	pen, chlor, met	clin, cefot

pen, penicillin; cep, cephalosporins; cef, cefoxitin; cefot, cefotaxime; chlor, chloramphenicol; clin, clindamycin; imip, imipenem; met, metronidazole.
*Penicillins include penicillin G, ampicillin, and amoxicillin.
†First-generation cephalosporin.
‡Second-generation cephalosporin.
§Third-generation cephalosporin.
‖Anaerobe most likely to be resistant to penicillin and most cephalosporins.
From Dow SW. Anaerobic infections. In: Greene CE, ed. Infectious Diseases of the Dog and Cat, 2nd ed. Philadelphia, WB Saunders, 1990:534.

Prevention

Because anaerobic bacteria live as normal flora, contact cannot be eliminated. Care should always be taken to avoid bite wounds, foreign bodies, and contamination of abraded skin or mucous membranes. All bite wounds should be thoroughly cleansed.

Zoonotic Aspects

An estimated 50% of Americans are bitten by an animal or a person at some time, and anaerobic infection occurs in approximately 33.3%.[18] *C. tetani* spores can be passed in the feces of domestic animals, but infection due to direct contact with dogs or cats seems unlikely.

Feline Plague

Pathophysiology

Etiology. The cause of feline plague is the gram-negative coccobacillus *Yersinia pestis.*[19] The organism is a facultative anaerobe that appears as small, bipolar-staining rods on cytologic evaluation. Fomite transmission is unlikely because the organism is sensitive to drying, but it can survive for weeks to months in infected carcasses and up to 1 year in infected fleas.[19]

Epidemiology. *Y. pestis* is primarily a disease of wild rodents and has been found on every continent except Australia.[19] The organism is maintained in a sylvan life cycle between rodent fleas and infected rodents, including rock squirrels, ground squirrels, and prairie dogs. Infection in people is most commonly associated with rodent flea bites but also has occurred after direct tissue contact with infected rabbits, prairie dogs, squirrels, bobcats, coyotes, and domestic cats.[19–21] Approximately 90% of the human cases have been documented in New Mexico, Arizona, and California.[19] Cats are the most susceptible domestic animal and usually die after natural and experimental infection.[21] Dogs are highly resistant to infection. Experimental infection of dogs has resulted in transient fever; clinical disease in naturally infected dogs is usually not recognized.[19, 22] Cats with clinical disease are recognized most frequently from spring through early fall, when rodents and rodent fleas are most active. Outdoor cats are most often affected.

Pathogenesis. Cats are infected after being bitten by infected rodent fleas or ingestion of bacteremic rodents. The organism replicates in the tonsils and pharyngeal lymph nodes initially, followed by the development of bacteremia.[21] After a flea bite, the incubation period is 2 to 6 days; after ingestion or inhalation of the organism, the incubation period is 1 to 3 days. *Y. pestis* replication results in a neutrophilic inflammatory response and resultant abscess formation in infected tissues, which results in the clinical signs of disease. In experimentally infected cats, the organism is most commonly found in the tonsils; anterior cervical, submandibular, and cranial thoracic lymph nodes; lungs; and spleen.[21] Outcomes in experimentally infected cats included death (6 of 16 cats, 38%), transient febrile illness with lymphadenopathy (7 of 16 cats, 44%), or inapparent infection (3 of 16 cats, 18%).[21]

Clinical Signs

Cats develop bubonic, septicemic, and pneumonic plague syndromes the way infected humans do (Table 36–5).[19] Bubonic is the most common form of disease in cats.[23, 24] Individual cats can show clinical signs of all three syndromes. Outdoor cats with a history of hunting commonly have a history of anorexia, depression, cervical swelling, dyspnea, or cough. Clinical signs of depression are generally recognized first. Fever is common and is usually over 40°C (104.0°F). Fever persisting for more than 5 days correlated well with fatality in experimentally inoculated cats.[21] Detection of enlarged tonsils, submandibular lymph nodes, and anterior cervical lymph nodes is common (bubonic form), occurring in 53% of the cats.[23] Lymph node enlargement can be either unilateral or bilateral. In contrast to cervical lymph node abscessation secondary to anaerobic infection from fighting, wounds are not noted. Cats with pneumonic plague commonly have respiratory difficulty and may have cough.

Laboratory and Radiographic Abnormalities. Abnormalities in the complete blood count are common in experimentally and naturally infected cats.[20, 21, 23] Experimentally infected cats generally develop neutrophilia by day 3 after inoculation, with the peak counts (average count, 25,000/μL) by day 6 after inoculation; lymphopenia (average count, 2800/μL) develops at the same time.[21] Neutrophilia was reported in 3 of 9 naturally infected cats tested; increased numbers of band neutrophils were reported in 8 of 9 cats.[23] Serum biochemical abnormalities included hypoalbuminemia, hyperglobulinemia, hyperglycemia, azotemia, hypokalemia, hypochloremia, hyperbilirubinemia, and increased activity of alkaline phosphatase (AP) and alanine aminotransferase (ALT).[20, 21] Results from urinalysis have not been reported. Chest radiograph abnormalities associated with the pneumonic form consist of increased alveolar and diffuse interstitial densities.

Cytologic evaluation of exudates reveals degenerate and nondegenerate neutrophils. Numerous intracellular and extracellular bipolar rods are noted.

Table 36–5
Clinical and Laboratory Findings Consistent With Feline Plague

Signalment
Any age, breed, or sex (may be more common in males)

History and Physical Examination
Outdoor cats
Hunting of rodents or exposure to rodent fleas
Depression
Dyspnea or cough
Cervical swellings, draining tracts, lymphadenopathy

Laboratory and Radiographic Evaluation
Neutrophilia
Lymphopenia
Neutrophilic exudates with bipolar rods
Serum antibody titers either negative (peracute) or positive
Interstitial and alveolar lung disease

Diagnosis
Culture of blood, exudate, tonsillar region, respiratory secretions
Fluorescent antibody identification of organism in exudates
Fourfold increase in antibody titer and appropriate clinical signs

Pathology

Histopathologic examination of tissues reveals hemorrhage and necrosis of involved tissues. Large clusters of bacteria are seen.[23] In experimentally infected cats, the organism is most commonly found in the tonsils; anterior cervical, submandibular, and cranial thoracic lymph nodes; lungs; and spleen.[21]

Diagnostic Plan

Presumptive diagnosis is based on the history of potential exposure, presence of rodent fleas, clinical signs, and cytologic demonstration of bipolar rods on cytologic examination of lymph node aspirates, exudates from draining abscesses, or transtracheal wash fluids. Antibodies against *Y. pestis* can be detected in serum 4 to 5 days after experimental inoculation.[21] However, because some cats survive infection and antibodies can be detected in serum for at least 300 days, detection of antibodies alone may indicate only exposure, not clinical infection.[22] A fourfold increase in antibody titer is consistent with recent infection.[19] Definitive diagnosis is made by culture or fluorescent antibody confirmation of *Y. pestis* in smears of the tonsilar region, lymph node aspirates, exudates from draining abscesses, or transtracheal wash fluids. Culture of blood can also be used to confirm infection; the organism was isolated from 12 of 13 clinically ill, experimentally infected cats.[21]

Treatment and Prognosis

Supportive care should be administered as indicated. Cervical abscesses should be drained and flushed with chlorhexidine.[19] Tetracycline at 20 mg/kg by mouth, three times per day (t.i.d.), for 21 days should be used for bubonic plague and for prophylaxis.[19] Streptomycin administered intramuscularly at 5 mg/kg, twice per day (b.i.d.), for 21 days or gentamicin (beware of nephrotoxicity) administered intramuscularly or intravenously at 2 to 4 mg/kg every day or b.i.d. for 21 days has been recommended for use in cats with septicemic or pneumonic plague. Chloramphenicol at 15 mg/kg, by mouth or intravenously, b.i.d., for 21 days can be used in animals with central nervous system signs.[19] In one study of naturally infected cats, 90.9% of those treated with antibiotics survived; 23.8% of untreated cats survived.[23] The prognosis is poor for cats with pneumonic or septicemic plague.

Prevention

Cats should not be allowed to hunt. Appropriate flea control should always be administered. Rodent control should be instituted if possible. When handling cats from endemic areas in the spring, summer, and early fall months showing clinical signs of bacteremia, respiratory disease, or cervical draining areas or masses, the veterinarian should wear gloves, a mask, and a gown until the diagnosis is made or ruled out. Flea control should be instituted immediately in cats with a presumptive diagnosis of plague. The areas of the hospital where infected cats are handled should be thoroughly cleaned with routine disinfectants. A killed vaccine has been administered to cats but did not protect against bacteremia or death.[19] In animals with suspected exposure, tetracycline should be administered at 20 mg/kg by mouth, t.i.d., for 7 days.[19]

Zoonotic Aspects

Clinical signs in humans are similar to those in cats and include pneumonic, septicemic, and bubonic forms. Infection occurs after contact with infected fleas or the tissues of infected animals, including cats.[25–29] Exposure is most commonly associated with exudates, pharyngeal secretions, or respiratory secretions of infected cats. However, human infection has also occurred from cat bites or scratches.[28, 29] *Y. pestis* was not cultured from the nail beds of experimentally inoculated cats on day 1 or 2 after inoculation, so the risk of this form of transmission is unknown.[21]

Lyme Disease

Pathophysiology

Etiology. *Borrelia burgdorferi* is a tick-borne spirochete identified as the etiologic agent of Lyme borreliosis.[30, 31] Koch's postulates have been fulfilled, documenting this agent as a cause of clinical illness in dogs.[32, 33] Some cats (10 of 71 in one study) had serologic evidence of exposure to *B. burgdorferi*,[34] and clinical disease was induced in a small number of cats by inoculating the organism intradermally.[35, 36] There are multiple field strains of *B. burgdorferi*. The organism has been identified in many countries around the world, but its distribution is ultimately limited to the geographic areas of the tick vector.

Epidemiology. *B. burgdorferi* has worldwide distribution that is associated with the primary tick vector, the *Ixodes ricinus* complex, a group of three host ticks with a 2- to 3-year life cycle. The organism can be transmitted to dogs during either the nymph or the adult stage of the tick.[33] In the nymph stage, the tick feeds on rodents and other small mammals early in the tick season; in the adult stage, it feeds primarily on large mammals, particularly deer. The vectors in the United States include *I. dammini* (East Coast), *I. pacificus* (West Coast), and *I. scapularis* (Atlantic Coast to Midwest). *I. dammini* is the most capable of harboring the organism. *I. dammini* and *I. scapularis* are geographic variants.[37] Other arthropods carry *B. burgdorferi*, but it appears unlikely that they transmit the organism to people or dogs.[31] Because uninfected ticks can be infected after feeding on infected dogs, dogs are considered a reservoir for the organism.[38] Transplacental transmission has been documented in dogs inoculated intradermally during gestation.[39] Other modes of transmission appear unlikely.[31] Based on seroprevalence, many dogs in endemic areas are exposed to *B. burgdorferi* or closely related spirochetes. However, because of the difficulty in making a definitive diagnosis, the true incidence of clinical disease is unknown. Correlation is poor between joint disease and positive serum antibody tests for *B. burgdorferi*.[40] Cats appear to be resistant to the development of clinical disease; there was no association with lameness and seropositivity in one study.[34]

Pathogenesis. Infection of dogs is usually subclinical. Although clinical borreliosis can be induced using both vector-borne experimental infection and intradermal inoculation, the pathogenesis of disease is largely undetermined. It is likely that disease is due to organism replication during the acute phase of infection. Persistence of the organism in synovial fluid was documented by polymerase chain reaction in most human patients who were untreated or treated with antibiotics for short periods.[41] Findings in some patients with chronic disease were negative by polymerase chain reaction, suggesting an immune-mediated pathogenesis.

Clinical Signs

Dogs of any age, breed, or sex have the potential for the development of clinical Lyme disease. Young dogs seem more likely to contract clinical disease when inoculated experimentally.[33] Clinical disease occurs almost exclusively in outdoor dogs with the chance for exposure to *Ixodes* ticks. Their history often includes tick exposure or travel to an endemic area. Most affected dogs are presented for evaluation of lameness, lethargy, and inappetence. Erythema chronicum migrans, the characteristic red circular lesion at the tick attachment site that is common in humans, is not usually noted in dogs. Dogs occasionally contract clinical disease after acute or chronic infection. Mild fever, malaise, and lymphadenomegaly can occur. Nonseptic, suppurative polyarthritis can be induced experimentally and is the most well-defined syndrome in both acute and chronic naturally occurring cases. Polyarthritis is generally intermittent, recurrent, and nonerosive. Joints can be swollen, hot, and painful on palpation or can be normal. Limited information is available concerning renal, neurologic, and cardiologic manifestations of disease in dogs. Myocarditis and atrioventricular block[42] and renal lesions[43] attributed to *B. burgdorferi* have been described in individual dogs. Local production of *B. burgdorferi*–specific antibodies has been documented in some dogs with neurologic disease, suggesting that the organism may replicate in the central nervous system tissues and occasionally induce disease.[44] Clinical signs of disease in cats are not well defined but appear to be less severe than in dogs.

Laboratory and Radiographic Abnormalities. Cytology of joint taps from infected dogs generally reveals a nonseptic exudate; most of the cells are nondegenerate neutrophils (Fig. 36–4). In acute infections, the volume of fluid obtained is often minimal. Abnormalities on complete blood count and serum biochemical profiles are inconsistent and nonspecific. Azotemia, proteinuria, hematuria, pyuria, and tubular casts in the urine occur in some dogs with renal manifestations of disease.[31, 43] Radiographs of joints occasionally reveal joint distension without erosive changes.

Pathology

Three of six experimentally infected dogs with acute lameness and clinicopathologic evidence of polyarthritis had fibrinopurulent arthritis and synovitis on histopathologic examination.[33] Nonsuppurative

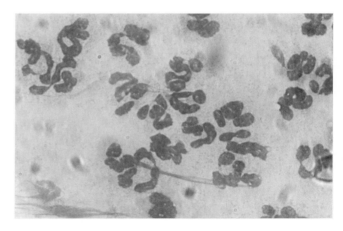

Figure 36–4
Cytology of joint fluid showing nonseptic, suppurative changes consistent with Lyme disease.

inflammation (lymphocytes and plasma cells) were noted in most of the other more mildly affected dogs. Cortical hyperplasia of lymph nodes was common in these dogs.[33] A dog with suspected Lyme carditis had infiltrates of neutrophils, macrophages, lymphocytes, and plasma cells into heart muscle.[42] Membranoproliferative glomerulonephritis, tubular necrosis, and lymphocytic interstitial nephritis have been reported in dogs with renal borreliosis.[31, 43]

Diagnostic Plan

Definitive diagnosis of Lyme borreliosis is difficult. It can be made by culture of the organism from affected joints, blood, urine, or cerebral spinal fluid or by demonstration of *Borrelia*-specific DNA in blood, synovial fluids, or tissues by polymerase chain reaction.[30–33, 39, 41] Culture requires special techniques and specimen handling, and the organism is rarely recovered. Polymerase chain reaction is not widely available clinically, and the significance of persistent *Borrelia* in canine tissues is undetermined. The organism also can be detected rarely in tissues evaluated by histopathology or immunohistochemistry.

Circulating antibodies are detected in serum by indirect immunofluorescent antibody assay, enzyme-linked immunosorbent assay (ELISA), and Western blot immunoassay.[45, 46] Both IgM and IgG antibodies against *B. burgdorferi* can be detected in canine serum. Titers considered significant vary by laboratory and assay. Both antibody classes can persist in serum for months after exposure. Cross-reactivity with other bacteria can occur depending on the antigen preparation and assay used, so a positive titer does not document exposure to *B. burgdorferi*.[46–49] Some dogs with acute Lyme disease are seronegative on initial testing; documentation of an increasing antibody titer can suggest recent exposure. Healthy dogs have the same antibody responses as clinically ill dogs, making interpretation of serum antibodies difficult. The presence of antibodies against *B. burgdorferi* antigens in serum documents only exposure to *B. burgdorferi* or an organism with similar antigens, not clinical disease. Detection of a greater concentration of antibody in cerebral spinal fluid than in serum occurs in some dogs with suspected neurologic disease secondary to Lyme disease.[44] For clinically practical purposes, a presumptive diagnosis of clinical Lyme disease in dogs can be based on appropriate clinical, historical, and laboratory evidence of disease combined with positive serologic testing and response to therapy. Positive serologic results alone do not prove the presence of clinical disease, and negative serologic findings do not definitively rule out the diagnosis.

Treatment and Prognosis

If a clinical infection is strongly suspected, several antibiotics can be used. Amoxicillin at a dosage of 10 to 22 mg/kg by mouth, b.i.d., tetracycline at a dosage of 22 mg/kg by mouth, t.i.d., or doxycycline at a dosage of 5 mg/kg by mouth, b.i.d., is commonly prescribed. Appropriate duration of therapy is unknown, but antibiotics are generally prescribed for 10 to 21 days. Amoxicillin should be used in pregnant animals. Tetracyclines are commonly associated with gastrointestinal irritation. Doxycycline penetrates the blood-brain barrier better than the other drugs do and is indicated for the treatment of dogs with suspected central nervous system disease. Several other causes of nonseptic, suppurative polyarthritis, including *Ehrlichia* spp., *Mycoplasma,* L-form bacteria, and Rocky Mountain spotted fever, also respond to doxycycline, making it a logical first choice. Aspirin can be administered at 10 to 25 mg/kg by mouth, t.i.d., for pain relief. Exercise restriction is recommended during the initial treatment period. The prognosis is good with acute-phase disease. Treatment of dogs during the acute phase of the disease may reduce the likelihood of chronic disease. Dogs with chronic disease may have a more variable response to therapy. Therapeutic effectiveness is monitored by resolution of clinical signs. Detectable antibody titers persist after treatment and so are not valuable for monitoring therapy.[46] Repeated cytology of joint taps can be performed to document resolution of inflammatory changes. Degenerative joint disease can develop as a sequela to infection. Alternative therapeutic regimens used in humans with poor response to tetracyclines or amoxicillin include penicillin G administered intravenously every 6 hours for 14 to 21 days, ceftriaxone administered intravenously for 14 days, or doxycycline administered by mouth for 30 days.

Prevention

Avoidance of exposure to the organism through tick control is an effective form of prevention. Removal of ticks from individual animals within 24 hours lessens the likelihood of infection. Owners traveling from nonendemic to endemic areas with their pets should be counseled on tick control. Giving tetracycline or amoxicillin to dogs traveling to endemic areas for short periods has been advocated. A commercial vaccine has been shown to protect vaccinates against the development of clinical disease after experimental inoculation.[50] Results of a clinical trial suggested that the vaccine did not induce significant adverse reactions and may have decreased incidence of clinical disease.[51] Limitations of the vaccine studies to date were recently reviewed.[52] Although it is unknown whether the vaccine protects against all field strains, the safety and clinical efficacy studies performed to date suggest that the vaccine may be indicated for high-risk dogs in endemic areas, especially if not previously exposed. Western blot immunoassay (available at New York State College of Veterinary Medicine Diagnostic Laboratory and other commercial laboratories) can be used to differentiate naturally exposed dogs from vaccinated dogs.[46]

Zoonotic Aspects

Although *B. burgdorferi* can be passed in urine, infection of humans from direct contact with dogs or cats is unlikely. The most significant role dogs and cats play in human exposure is through bringing ticks into the human environment.

Leptospirosis

Pathophysiology

Etiology. Leptospires are small, motile, filamentous spirochetes that infect animals and humans.[53, 54] The organisms are 0.1 to 0.2 μm wide and 6 to 12 μm long and are shed intermittently from the host.[53] There are multiple serovars in the genus *Leptospira interrogans.* Dogs are infected by *L.* serovar. *australis, L.* serovar. *autumnalis, L.* serovar. *bratislava, L.* serovar. *bataviae, L.* serovar. *canicola, L.* serovar. *grippotyphosa, L.* serovar. *icterohaemorrhagiae, L.* serovar. *pomona,* and *L.* serovar. *tarassovi* (Table 36–6).[53–59] Cats are infected by *L.* serovar. *bratislava, L.* serovar. *canicola, L.* serovar. *grippotyphosa,* and *L.* serovar. *pomona.*[53, 60] The organisms are host adapted in some species in which they act as reservoirs.[59] Exposure to non–host-adapted species commonly results in clinical illness. Leptospires are susceptible to detergents and iodine-based disinfectants.[53, 54]

Table 36–6
Common *Leptospira interrogans* Serovars Infecting Dogs

SEROVAR	PRIMARY RESERVOIR	CLINICAL DISEASE IN DOGS
L. serovar. *bataviae*	Dog, rat, mouse	Acute hepatic and renal disease, with hemorrhage
L. serovar. *bratislava*	Cow	Nephritis
L. serovar. *canicola*	Dog	Acute interstitial nephritis
		Chronic interstitial nephritis
L. serovar. *grippotyphosa*	Vole	Chronic active hepatitis
		Acute or subacute renal failure
L. serovar. *icterohaemorrhagiae*	Rat	Acute hemorrhagic disease with high fever and death
		Acute hepatic syndrome with icterus, fever, and hemorrhage
		Uremia and hemorrhagic enteritis
L. pomona	Cow, pig	Acute or subacute renal failure
L. tarassovi	Cow, pig	Acute hepatic syndrome with icterus and depression

Data from Greene and Shotts,[53] Baldwin and Atkins,[54] Renko et al.,[55] Watson,[56] Bishop et al.,[57] Mackintosh et al.[58]

Epidemiology. The organisms are most common in semitropical areas.[53] Outbreaks of clinical disease are common in the summer and early fall and have been associated with flooding in areas with neutral to alkaline soil conditions.[53] Disease occurs in dogs from both rural and suburban environments.[53–55] Transmission occurs by direct contact, bite wounds, or venereal contact; transplacentally; and by ingestion of contaminated tissues, soil, water, bedding, food, and other fomites. Urine from the infected host is the most common source of environmental contamination.[53, 54]

Pathogenesis. Leptospires enter the body through abraded skin or intact mucous membranes.[53, 54] Leptospiremia then develops rapidly, and the organism disseminates throughout the body. Whether disease occurs is dependent on host and organism factors. Hosts with pre-existing antibody titers usually eliminate the organism quickly, and clinical signs of disease do not develop. In dogs exposed to a non–host-adapted species, the organism replicates in multiple tissues; the highest levels of infection develop in the liver and kidneys. These animals develop renal or hepatic clinical syndromes with resultant recovery if an appropriate immune response develops or if therapy is instituted. Inflammation is associated with organism replication and production of toxins. Clinical disease develops approximately 7 days after exposure.[53, 54] In some animals, the infection clears 2 to 3 weeks after exposure, yet chronic active hepatitis or chronic renal disease may occur. Some animals maintain low levels of renal infection and pass the organism into the environment in urine. Animals with poor immune responses generally die. Hosts exposed to a host-adapted serovar are usually subclinically affected but develop chronic renal infection and shed the organism

into the environment intermittently. Cats are generally subclinically affected but may shed the organism into the environment for variable periods after exposure.[53]

Clinical Signs

Animals of any age, breed, or sex can be affected. Clinical manifestations relate to the host immune status and the infecting serovar (Table 36–7). The most common clinical syndromes induced by leptospirosis are nonspecific and include lethargy, anorexia, and depression. Leptospirosis should be considered a differential diagnosis for dogs with historical or physical examination findings of fever, petechiae, ecchymoses, vomiting, diarrhea, generalized hyperesthesia, anterior uveitis, coughing, respiratory distress, renal pain, renomegaly, polyuria, polydipsia, and icterus.[53, 54]

Some animals are peracutely infected and are presented for evaluation of depression, generalized muscle hyperesthesia, tachypnea, and vomiting. These animals are generally febrile and in a state of vascular collapse. Petechiae or ecchymoses and other manifestations of coagulopathy, including melena and epistaxis, may be present. Dogs with peracute infections may fail to develop significant renal or hepatic disease because of rapid progression of infection to death.[53]

Subacutely infected dogs have fever, depression, hemorrhagic syndromes, hepatic disease, renal disease, or a combination of hepatic and renal disease. Conjunctivitis, rhinitis, and tonsillitis occur in some dogs.[53] Chronic interstitial nephritis[55] and chronic active hepatitis[57] are chronic syndromes associated with leptospire infections.

Laboratory and Radiographic Abnormalities. Multiple nonspecific laboratory abnormalities occur in dogs with naturally occurring or experimentally induced leptospirosis and vary depending on the host, the serovar, and whether the disease was acute or subacute. Leukopenia develops during the leptospiremic phase of infection but progresses to leukocytosis with or without a left shift.[53, 54] Thrombocytopenia and disseminated intravascular coagulation characterized by increased fibrinogen degradation products are common and are likely to result in the hemorrhagic syndromes recognized during peracute syndromes.[53, 54] Anemia can occur and is regenerative secondary to blood loss acutely and nonregenerative secondary to renal disease and inflammation chronically.

Hyponatremia, hypokalemia, hyperphosphatemia, hypoalbuminemia, hypocalcemia, azotemia, hyperbilirubinemia, and increased activities of ALT, AP,

and aspartate aminotransferase (AST) are common serum biochemical abnormalities.[53–55] Hyponatremia and hypokalemia are probably secondary to pooling of secretions in the gastrointestinal tract or to renal loss. Azotemia, hyperphosphatemia, and hypoalbuminemia are secondary to renal inflammation. Hypocalcemia occurs secondary to the hypoalbuminemia. Hyperbilirubinemia and increased activities of ALT, AP, and AST are secondary to hepatic inflammation. Some dogs with chronic disease have hyperglobulinemia. Dogs with inflammation of muscle may have increased creatine phosphokinase. Urinalysis abnormalities include bilirubinuria, suboptimal urine specific gravity in the presence of azotemia, granular casts, and increased numbers of granulocytes and erythrocytes. The organism is not detected in the urine sediment by light microscopy.[53]

Renomegaly and hepatomegaly are common abnormalities noted on radiography or ultrasonography. Mineralization of the renal pelves and cortices can occur with chronic disease. Interstitial and alveolar infiltrates can occur in dogs with respiratory tract involvement.

Pathology

Grossly, petechiae and icterus are common on the mucous membranes and serosal surfaces. Petechiae may also be seen in the meninges. The lungs may appear edematous or have diffuse or focal areas of pneumonia. The liver and kidneys are commonly enlarged in animals with acute disease. The liver is friable, with pronounced interlobar markings. The kidneys are pale and bulge on the cut surface. Histologically, necrosis of the pulmonary, hepatic, and renal tissues is the most common lesion.[53, 54] Chronic active hepatitis, hepatic fibrosis, and mononuclear chronic interstitial nephritis occur in some animals.[53, 54]

Diagnostic Plan

Definitive diagnosis requires demonstration of the organism by urine darkfield microscopy, phase contrast microscopy, or culture. However, examination and culture of urine for leptospires are low-yield procedures. In acute disease, leptospiremia occurs for a few days to 2 weeks after infection, during which time the organism may sometimes be cultured from blood. Because of intermittent shedding, urine cultures may have to be repeated to prove leptospirosis.

Detection of serum antibodies can be used to document exposure to *Leptospira*. Antibodies are detected by microscopic agglutination test (MAT), ELISA (IgM and IgG), and microscopic microcapsular agglutination test.[53, 54, 61] The primary disadvantage of serologic testing is that it is difficult to determine

Table 36–7
Clinical and Laboratory Findings Consistent With Canine Leptospirosis

Signalment
Any age, breed, or sex

History and Physical Examination
Exposure to appropriate reservoir host or contaminated environment
Anorexia, depression, lethargy
Fever
Anterior uveitis
Hemorrhagic tendencies, including melena, epistaxis, petechiae, and ecchymoses
Vomiting, diarrhea
Muscle or meningeal pain
Renomegaly with or without renal pain
Hepatomegaly
Polyuria or polydipsia
Icterus
Coughing or respiratory distress

Laboratory Evaluation
Thrombocytopenia
Leukopenia, acutely
Leukocytosis, subacutely
Increased BUN and creatinine
Suboptimal urine concentrating ability
Pyuria and hematuria without obvious bacteriuria
Hyperbilirubinemia and bilirubinuria
Increased activities of ALT, AST, AP, and creatine phosphokinase
Interstitial to alveolar lung disease

Diagnosis
Culture of urine or tissues
Demonstration of the organism by darkfield or phase contrast microscopy
Combination of increasing antibody titer with clinical signs and response to therapy

BUN, blood urea nitrogen; ALT, alanine aminotransferase; AST, aspartate aminotransferase; AP, alkaline phosphatase.

whether positive titers are due to active infection, previous infection, or vaccination.

The IgM ELISA and microscopic microcapsular agglutination test are most likely to detect recent infection.[53, 54] Titers detected by the IgM ELISA are positive by 1 week after inoculation, peak at 14 days after inoculation, and then decline. Acutely infected dogs are often IgM ELISA positive and MAT negative. Dogs with suggestive clinical signs of disease but negative MAT results should be retested in 2 to 4 weeks; development of a positive titer confirms recent infection. Titers detected by the IgG ELISA are generally positive by 2 to 3 weeks after inoculation, with peak levels reached by 1 month after inoculation.[53]

Vaccination induces positive MAT titers. Most commercial canine bacterins contain antigens of *L.* serovar. *canicola* and *L.* serovar. *icterohaemorrhagiae*, so antibodies against other serovars may be significant. Vaccination generally leads to high IgG ELISA titers with low to negative IgM ELISA titers, so ELISA appears to be superior to MAT for differentiation of antibodies induced by natural infection from those produced after vaccination.[53]

The combination of seroconversion (negative to positive) and IgM antibodies, or a fourfold increase in antibody titers along with appropriate clinical pathologic abnormalities and clinical findings, is suggestive of clinical leptospirosis. Confirmation of the diagnosis is therefore usually not made until after treatment is begun.

Treatment and Prognosis

Supportive care should be administered as needed. Diuresis for renal involvement is required in most cases (see Chap. 16). The penicillin derivatives are reported to be the preferred drugs for elimination of leptospiremia.[53, 54] Animals with severe clinical disease should be treated with penicillin G administered intramuscularly or intravenously at 25,000 to 40,000 units/kg, b.i.d., or ampicillin administered intravenously at 22 mg/kg, t.i.d., during the initial treatment period. When the affected animal is in the recovery phase and oral medications can be used, amoxicillin at 22 mg/kg by mouth, b.i.d., should be administered for 2 weeks. Dihydrostreptomycin administered intramuscularly at 15 mg/kg, b.i.d., for 2 weeks after penicillin therapy should be used to eliminate the renal carrier phase. If the animal is still azotemic after initial therapy with penicillin derivatives, doxycycline at 2.5 to 5.0 mg/kg by mouth, b.i.d., for 2 weeks should be administered instead of streptomycin to clear the carrier state.[53]

Prevention

Reservoir hosts should be avoided or eliminated. Care should be taken to avoid infected urine or contaminated water. The veterinarian should wear gloves while handling dogs with suspected leptospirosis. Contaminated surfaces should be cleaned with detergents and disinfected with iodine-containing products. Vaccines are available for some serovars and reduce severity of disease but not the chronic carrier state. Bacterins have commonly been associated with vaccine reactions. Subunit vaccines now available that use immunogenic proteins from the outer envelope rather than the entire organism appear to have lessened these reactions. Dogs in endemic areas should receive three vaccinations 2 to 3 weeks apart. Duration of immunity is more than 1 year in dogs receiving three vaccinations.[53]

Zoonotic Aspects

All the serovars infecting mammals should be considered zoonotic to humans.[53, 54, 62] Clinical syndromes vary with the serovar but are similar to those that occur in dogs.

Streptococcosis

Pathophysiology

Etiology. Streptococci are gram-positive, nonmotile, facultative anaerobic bacteria. Streptococci are commonly grouped based on antigenic differences in the cell wall (Lancefield's groups)[63] and type of hemolysis induced in erythrocyte-containing cultures.[64] Most of the pathogenic streptococci are in the β-hemolytic group (Lancefield's groups A, B, C, E, G, L, and M) and induce total erythrocyte lysis and a resultant clear zone around colonies in culture. Lancefield's group D is usually α-hemolytic (green zone in the hemolytic area around colonies) or nonhemolytic.[64] Streptococci are susceptible to most common disinfectants.

Epidemiology. Of the many strains of streptococci, some are normal flora of the skin, gastrointestinal tract, and mucous membranes; others are pathogenic and cause disease in animals and humans (Table 36–8). Clinical disease in dogs and cats is most common with Lancefield's groups B, C, G, L, and D and groups B, C, and G, respectively.[64–68] Zoonotic transfer occasionally occurs, particularly with the group A streptococci, *Streptococcus pyogenes* and *S. pneumoniae*.[64, 69] Dogs and cats can be temporary hosts of these two species but are infected subclinically. Groups M and E are generally normal flora.

Many streptococcal infections are more common in immunosuppressed hosts, which include puppies and kittens. Infection usually occurs by direct contact with the streptococci. Any species of streptococcus can be opportunistic, leading to local infections

Table 36–8
Pathogenic Streptococcal Infections of Humans, Dogs, and Cats

STREPTOCOCCAL SPECIES	HOST SPECIES	MICROFLORAL DISTRIBUTION	DISEASE SYNDROMES
Group A			
Streptococcus pyogenes	Human	Tonsils	Tonsillitis, pharyngitis, otitis, impetigo, bacteremia, toxemia[81]
S. pneumoniae	Human	Tonsils	Pneumonia, otitis, bacteremia, polyarthritis, meningitis
	Cat	None (human reservoir)	Polyarthritis, bacteremia[80]
Group B			
S. agalactiae	Human	Anorectum, vagina	Neonate: sepsis Immunocompromised: bacteremia, meningitis, endocarditis Postparturient: metritis; septic arthritis; pharyngitis; respiratory, skin, wound infections
	Dog	Urogenital	Fatal septicemia in pups, necrotizing pneumonia, bacteremia, pyelonephritis[72,76]
	Cat	Urogenital	Peritonitis, septicemia, placentitis[73]
Group C			
S. zooepidemicus and *S. equisimilis*	Human	None (animal reservoir)	Pharyngitis, glomerulonephritis
	Dog	Skin, genitourinary tract	Septicemia, fibrinopurulent bronchopneumonia, acute death,[70] urinary tract infections[71]
Group D			
S. suis	Cat	Skin	Dermatitis, pneumonia[74]
S. faecalis	Dog, human	Intestine, feces	Normal flora, urinary tract infections[71]
Group G			
S. canis	Human	Tonsils, vagina	Pharyngitis
	Cat	Tonsils	Abscesses, neonatal sepsis, umbilical infections, arthritis[77,78]
	Dog	Tonsils, genitalia, anorectum	Otitis media, neonatal sepsis, umbilical infections, polyarthritis, abscesses, dermatitis, mastitis,[75,76] genital infections, infertility, anestrus, abortion, failure to conceive[71]
Group L	Dog	Genitalia	Abortion, fading puppy, sterility in bitch, endometritis[79]

Adapted from Greene CE. Streptococcal and other gram-positive bacterial infections. In: Greene CE, ed. Infectious Diseases of the Dog and Cat, 2nd ed. Philadelphia, WB Saunders, 1990:600.

after trauma or other sources of primary inflammation. Puppies and kittens that develop neonatal septicemia with groups B and G are probably infected by contact with vaginal secretions of the dam.[65, 68] Respiratory transmission with resultant pneumonia and septicemia can occur in racing greyhounds after exposure to group C agents.[66, 70] Urinary tract infection with group D occurs after contamination of the urinary tract with the organism that resides as normal flora in the intestinal tract.[71]

Pathogenesis. Whether disease occurs because of streptococci is determined by the strain of the

bacteria and host immune response. Disease is a manifestation of the inflammatory response against the organism or its toxins as it replicates in tissue.

Clinical Signs

Dogs or cats of any age, breed, or sex can potentially develop clinical illness secondary to streptococcal infection. Historical and physical examination findings are dependent on the organ systems affected (see Table 36–8).

Group B. *S. agalactiae* is the species that usually

causes disease in dogs and cats. It has been associated with neonatal septicemia, necrotizing pneumonia, bacteremia, and pyelonephritis in dogs[65, 72] and peritonitis, septicemia, and placentitis in cats.[73]

Group C. Weakness, cough, dyspnea, fever, hematemesis, red urine, and sudden death due to septicemia have been reported in racing greyhounds after infection with *S. zooepidemicus*.[66, 70] This group is also usually isolated from dogs with pollakiuria and hematuria due to urinary tract infection.[71]

Group D. Fibronecrotic pneumonia, necrotizing pleuropneumonia, and moist dermatitis have been associated with infection of *S. suis* in cats.[74] Overgrowth of *S. faecalis* has been associated with diarrhea in puppies. This agent is commonly isolated from dogs with clinical signs of lower urinary tract infections.[71]

Group G. Organisms in this group are common normal flora of the skin and mucosa of dogs and cats, so it is unclear whether disease in dogs is due to pathogenic strains or other predisposing conditions that allowed for overgrowth of the normal flora.[67, 68, 75, 76] *S. canis* has been cultured from dogs with a variety of clinical diseases, including cellulitis, mastitis, pharyngitis, tonsillitis, and genital infections. The organism lives in the vagina of the bitch and is associated with neonatal septicemia. The affected puppies probably are infected at birth, and the disease develops only when immunosuppression or other stresses, including lack of warmth and failure to nurse, are complicating factors.[67]

In cats, *S. canis* is most commonly associated with neonatal septicemia in kittens and cervical lymphadenitis in juvenile kittens.[68, 77] Neonatal sepsis is most common in kittens born to queens younger than 2 years of age during the first litter. Older, multiparous queens are less likely to harbor the agent in the genital tract. Kittens become clinically ill and usually die if not treated within 7 to 11 days of age. The kittens are depressed, are usually smaller than littermates, and may have a swollen umbilicus. Fever may be detected but can be transient and missed on the first physical examination. Cats with cervical lymphadenitis are usually febrile, depressed, and anorectic and have unilateral or bilateral swelling in the ventral cervical area. Arthritis with lameness and fever has also been reported in cats in a closed breeding colony. Most cats had only one affected joint and generally responded to treatment.[78]

Group L. Group L streptococci are rarely isolated from sick dogs but can induce clinical syndromes similar to those in group G.[79]

Laboratory and Radiographic Abnormalities. Neutrophilic leukocytosis with a left shift is common in animals with clinical disease secondary to streptococcal infections. Kittens with group G sepsis commonly have degenerative left shifts and may have cocci visible in neutrophils.[68] Serum biochemical abnormalities are variable based on organ system involvement. Pyuria, bacteriuria, hematuria, and proteinuria are common in dogs with streptococcal urinary tract infections.[71] Cytologic evaluation of material from animals with lymphadenitis, abscesses, polyarthritis, and pneumonia due to streptococcal infection usually reveals neutrophilic inflammation and is often septic. There is a mixed population of degenerate and nondegenerate neutrophils, and macrophages are common. Radiographic changes are dependent on the organ system involved and are characteristic of inflammation induced by bacterial infection.

Pathology

Neutrophilic and mononuclear cell inflammation with intracellular and extracellular cocci are visualized in the primary tissues infected. Dogs with group C infection often have widespread petechial and ecchymotic hemorrhages and pulmonary congestion.[66, 70]

Diagnostic Plan

Definitive diagnosis is based on culture of the organism from tissues or fluids. Documentation of single or short chains of gram-positive cocci in combination with inflammatory cells cytologically is suggestive of infection.

Treatment and Prognosis

Supportive care is administered as indicated. If abscessation is present, drainage should be established concurrently with initiation of antibiotic therapy. Penicillin derivatives, erythromycin, and chloramphenicol are generally effective (Table 36–9). Cephalosporins can be administered to animals with resistant group A infections.[64] Parenteral administration should be used initially, particularly in animals with clinical signs consistent with sepsis.

Prevention

Sanitation should be maintained, and stressful situations—including crowding and variations in environmental temperature—should be avoided. The umbilicus of newborns should be dipped in 2% tincture of iodine. Amoxicillin administered at 25 mg/kg by mouth or subcutaneously, t.i.d., for 5 to 7 days can be used to prevent group G infection at parturition in cats (queen and kittens).[68] Care should be taken to avoid contact with exudates from animals with streptococcal infections. Routine disinfectants should be used to clean contaminated surfaces.

Table 36-9
Drug Therapy for Streptococcal Infections in Dogs and Cats

DRUG	SPECIES	DOSE	ROUTE	INTERVAL (HOURS)	DURATION (DAYS)
Amoxicillin	Dog and cat	22 mg/kg	PO, IM, SC	8–12	5–7
Penicillin G	Dog and cat	10,000–20,000 U/kg	IM, SC	12–24	5–7
Penicillin V	Dog and cat	8–30 mg/kg	PO	8	5–7
Erythromycin	Dog	3–20 mg/kg	PO	8	5–7
Chloramphenicol	Dog	15–25 mg/kg	PO, IV, SC	8	5–7
	Cat	10–15 mg/kg	PO, IV, SC	12	5–7
Cephalexin	Dog and cat	10–40 mg/kg	PO	12	5–7

IM, intramuscular; IV, intravenous; SC, subcutaneous; PO, by mouth.

Adapted from Greene CE. Group A streptococcal infections of dogs and cats. In: Greene CE, ed. Infectious Diseases of the Dog and Cat, 2nd ed. Philadelphia, WB Saunders, 1990:601.

Zoonotic Aspects

Humans are the principal natural hosts for group A streptococcus.[64, 69] *S. pyogenes* (tonsillitis, pharyngitis, otitis, impetigo, bacteremia, and toxemia) and *S. pneumoniae* (pneumonia, otitis, bacteremia, polyarthritis, and meningitis) are pathogenic to people. Septicemia and septic arthritis in a cat occurred due to infection with *S. pneumoniae* after contact with an infected child.[80] Generally, dogs and cats are subclinically infected, temporary reservoirs of group A streptococcus after exposure to infected people. It is possible that infected dogs or cats could reinfect humans during the 2 to 3 weeks the organism survives in the pharynx.[64, 69, 81] Animals thought to be infected can be cultured for group A streptococci by swabbing the surface of the tonsils while the animal is sedated. Alternatively, these animals can be treated (see Table 36–9). However, owners should be counseled that another human source of the organism is more likely the cause of recurrent infection in people and that all family members should be assessed by culture or treated.

Mycoplasma and Ureaplasma

Pathophysiology

Etiology. Mycoplasma spp. and *Ureaplasma* spp. are small, free-living microorganisms that lack a rigid, protective cell wall.[82, 83] They are limited in synthetic capacity and depend on their environment for nourishment. Multiple species of *Mycoplasma* and *Ureaplasma* have been isolated from dogs and cats.[82, 84] *M. felis* and *M. gateae* are the species most commonly associated with disease in cats[83]; *M. cynos, M. spumans,* and *M. canis* are the species most commonly associated with disease in dogs.[82, 84] *Mycoplasma* spp. and *Urea-* *plasma* spp. are fragile because of the lack of cell wall and so are susceptible to routine disinfectants and rapidly die outside the host.

Epidemiology. Mycoplasma spp. are commonly isolated from the vagina (75% of dogs),[84, 85] prepuce (70% of dogs),[84, 85] pharynx (100% of dogs,[86] 35% of cats[87]), colon (33% of dogs),[84] and conjunctivae (17% of dogs,[84] 5% of cats[88]) of healthy animals. *Ureaplasma* spp. are commonly isolated from the vagina (40%) and prepuce (10%) of healthy dogs.[85] Based on these findings, *Mycoplasma* spp. and *Ureaplasma* spp. are considered part of the normal flora of mucous membranes. Puppies and kittens are first exposed to *Mycoplasma* spp. and *Ureaplasma* spp. when passing through the birth canal. When clinical disease is recognized and *Mycoplasma* spp. or *Ureaplasma* spp. are isolated, infection appears to have occurred via direct extension from a mucous membrane where the organisms are normally found.

Mycoplasma spp. are commonly isolated by transtracheal aspiration biopsy or bronchoalveolar lavage in dogs (65 of 93 dogs, 69.9%[89]; 13 of 38 dogs, 34%[86]) and cats (6 of 28, 21.4%[87]; 4 of 9 cats, 44.4%[90]) presented for clinical signs consistent with lower airway inflammation. Most dogs with pneumonia and positive lower airway *Mycoplasma* spp. cultures (58 of 65 dogs, 89.2%[89]; 8 of 13 dogs, 61.5%[86]) have concurrent isolation of other bacteria. *Mycoplasma* spp. were isolated in pure culture from the lower airways of four of six cats with pulmonary disease.[87] Respiratory tract inflammation due to *Ureaplasma* spp. infection appears to be unusual in dogs and cats.[86, 87]

Mycoplasma or *Ureaplasma* spp. were isolated from urine from 41 of 2900 dogs; 20 of the 31 dogs that had the organism isolated in pure culture also had clinical signs of urinary tract infection.[91] *Mycoplasma* spp. (95%) or *Ureaplasma* spp. (60%) were isolated from the majority of dogs with infertility or vaginitis.[85]

Whether these organisms are the cause of disease is not clear.

Pathogenesis. Although *Mycoplasma* spp. and *Ureaplasma* spp. have been isolated from dogs and cats with clinical diseases, the pathogenic potential for most species is undetermined. Disease associations have been most commonly made by documenting a higher incidence of organism isolation from tissues of clinically affected animals when compared with healthy animals.[84] It is unclear in most clinical illnesses associated with *Mycoplasma* spp. or *Ureaplasma* spp. whether the organisms are colonizing diseased tissues in an opportunistic fashion secondary to inflammation induced by other diseases or if the agents are primarily pathogenic. A variety of bacteria are often isolated concurrently with *Mycoplasma* spp. or *Ureaplasma* spp., or the affected animal has coexisting immunosuppressive conditions, making determination of the primary pathogenic mechanism difficult.[86, 89]

M. felis conjunctivitis in cats, *M. felis* upper respiratory infection in cats, *M. gatae* polyarthritis in cats, and *M. cynos* (one strain) pneumonia in dogs have been induced by experimental inoculation.[92–95] *Mycoplasma* spp. have been obtained in pure culture from some dogs with clinical signs of urinary tract inflammation and respiratory tract disease.[86, 89, 91] These findings suggest that some species may be primary pathogens.

Clinical Signs

Cats. *Mycoplasma* spp. infection should be considered in cats of any age, breed, or sex presented for evaluation of conjunctivitis, sneezing, and mucopurulent nasal discharge, coughing, dyspnea, fever, lameness with or without swollen painful joints,[94, 96] subcutaneous abscessation,[82] or abortion (Table 36–10).[97] Cats with *M. felis* infection generally have inflamed conjunctivae and a mucopurulent discharge without keratitis. Cats with respiratory tract inflammation associated with *Mycoplasma* spp. have been older, and crackles and wheezes often were auscultated in their lower airways. Chronic abscessation associated with bite wounds that respond poorly to penicillins or cephalosporins should be suspected to be caused by *Mycoplasma* spp. infections.

Dogs. *Mycoplasma* spp. infection should be considered in dogs of any age, breed, or sex presented for evaluation of coughing, dyspnea, fever, pollakiuria, hematuria, lameness with or without swollen painful joints,[98] mucopurulent vaginal discharge, or infertility (see Table 36–10). Clinical and urinalysis evidence of urinary tract inflammation with negative bacterial culture should prompt the clinician to suspect *Mycoplasma* spp. infection. *Mycoplasma* spp. are isolated

Table 36–10
Clinical Disorders With Potential Association With *Mycoplasma* or *Ureaplasma* Infections in Dogs and Cats

CANINE	FELINE
Pneumonia	Conjunctivitis
Nephritis, cystitis	Pneumonia
Reproductive diseases or infertility	Reproductive diseases or infertility
Polyarthritis	Polyarthritis
Colitis	Abscesses

from the lower airways most frequently from diseased dogs younger than 1 year of age[86] or diseased dogs older than 5 years of age[89]; there is no obvious breed or sex predisposition. Crackles and wheezes are common on thoracic auscultation. Affected dogs may have a history of other predisposing conditions, including glucocorticoid administration, hyperadrenocorticism, or aspiration.

Laboratory and Radiographic Abnormalities. The clinical laboratory abnormalities associated with *Mycoplasma* spp. and *Ureaplasma* spp. infections are similar to those associated with other bacterial infections; they are dependent on the organ system involved, the immune status of the host, and the severity of infection. Many of the laboratory changes associated with *Mycoplasma* or *Ureaplasma* infections are secondary to concurrent infection with other bacteria.

Neutrophilia and monocytosis are common in dogs with pneumonia.[89] Biochemical abnormalities are uncommon, but azotemia may occur in some dogs with pyelonephritis. Pyuria (88% of cases) was the most common abnormal urinalysis result in one study of mycoplasmal urinary tract infection.[91] Proteinuria was reported in 5 of 41 dogs.[91]

Microscopic examination of cytologic preparations made from preputial material, vaginal material, chronic draining wounds, and airway washings reveals neutrophils as the most common cell type. *Mycoplasma* spp. and *Ureaplasma* spp. are the smallest bacterial species and are not generally recognized cytologically or on urine sediment examination. Other concurrent bacteria may or may not be noted.

Dogs with lower respiratory tract disease and positive *Mycoplasma* cultures commonly show radiographic evidence of alveolar lung patterns consistent with pneumonia or aspiration pneumonia.[89] Significant thoracic radiographic differences were not noted between dogs with pure *Mycoplasma* cultures and those with mixed bacterial and *Mycoplasma* cultures.[89] Joint radiographs of animals with *Mycoplasma*-associated polyarthritis generally reveal nonerosive changes.

Pathology

Puppies inoculated with a virulent strain of *M. cynos* developed suppurative bronchitis, bronchiolitis, and alveolitis acutely, and interstitial pneumonia characterized by perivascular and peribronchial lymphocytic-plasmacytic infiltrates chronically.[84, 95] Inoculation of dogs with *M. canis* has resulted in suppurative orchitis and epididymitis in some males (2 of 4) and suppurative endometritis and cystic enlargement of endometrial glands in some females (3 of 10).[84] Glomerulonephritis can be identified histologically.[91]

Diagnostic Plan

Diagnosis of *Mycoplasma* spp. or *Ureaplasma* spp. infection is made by culture. Specimens for culture should be plated immediately or transported to the laboratory in Hayflick's broth medium, Amies medium without charcoal, or modified Stuart bacterial transport medium.[82] Specimens should be shipped on ice packs if the transport time is expected to be less than 24 hours and on dry ice if more than 24 hours.[82]

Because *Mycoplasma* spp. and *Ureaplasma* spp. are common flora and a direct disease association is difficult to make in individual animals, interpretation of positive culture results is difficult. If *Mycoplasma* spp. or *Ureaplasma* spp. are isolated in pure culture from tissues from which isolation is unusual (lower airways, uterus, joints), then the disease association may be strong. In animals with positive findings for *Mycoplasma* spp. or *Ureaplasma* spp. and other bacteria, it is impossible to determine which organism is the primary pathogen. Response to treatment with drugs with known anti-*Mycoplasma* activity may help support the diagnosis of disease induced by these agents.

Treatment and Prognosis

Commonly used drugs with known anti-*Mycoplasma* activity include tylosin, erythromycin, clindamycin, lincomycin, tetracyclines, chloramphenicol, aminoglycosides, and enrofloxacin.[82, 99, 100] I generally use doxycycline at 5 mg/kg, by mouth, b.i.d., for the treatment of *Mycoplasma* spp. or *Ureaplasma* spp. infections in animals thought to have a competent immune system. In dogs with pneumonia, clinical signs referable to bacteremia or sepsis, and positive culture results for *Mycoplasma* spp. or *Ureaplasma* spp., the combination of enrofloxacin administered at 2.5 to 5.0 mg/kg by mouth, b.i.d., and clindamycin administered at 11 mg/kg by mouth, b.i.d., is commonly used. Because these organisms are cell-wall deficient, long-term treatment (4–6 weeks) is indicated. Erythro-

mycin administered at 20 mg/kg by mouth, b.i.d. to t.i.d., or lincomycin administered at 22 mg/kg by mouth, b.i.d., should be used in pregnant animals.[82]

Prevention

Most *Mycoplasma* spp. or *Ureaplasma* spp. that infect dogs and cats cause disease by direct extension from normal mucous membrane sites to other tissues; they are not likely to be directly contagious from animal to animal. However, *M. felis* can be transmitted from cat to cat by conjunctival discharges. Whether the species associated with respiratory diseases in dogs and cats are primary pathogens that can be spread from animal to animal, as *M. pneumoniae* is in humans, is unknown, but *Mycoplasma* spp. have been isolated from multiple clinically ill dogs in the same environment.[101] Animals with conjunctivitis or respiratory tract disease should be isolated from other animals until clinical signs of disease have resolved. Care should be taken to avoid fomite transmission.

Zoonotic Aspects

Bite wound transmission of *Mycoplasma* spp. from an infected cat to the hand of a human has been reported.[102]

Tularemia

Pathophysiology

Etiology. Tularemia is a disease of animals and humans caused by *Francisella tularensis*. There are two strains of this gram-negative, rod-shaped bacterium: type A (*F. tularensis* biovar. *tularensis*) and type B (*F. tularensis* biovar. *palaearctica*).[103–105] Both types have been isolated from clinically ill cats in the United States.[103] The organism may survive for 3 to 4 months in mud, water, and decaying carcasses but is inactivated by treatment with tricresol (1%), formalin (0.1%), or chlorine (1.0 ppm) or by heating to 55° to 60°C for 10 minutes.[104]

Epidemiology. *F. tularensis* infects over 100 species of mammals, birds, fish, and reptiles.[104] Type A strains are found only in North America.[104] Type B strains are found in North America, Asia, and Europe.[104, 105] Tularemia has been documented in each state in the United States except for Hawaii; the majority of cases have been in Arkansas, Missouri, and Oklahoma (55%).[104] Infection occurs by arthropod vectors or contact with the organism in infected mammals or contaminated water. Type A is transmitted most commonly by *Dermacentor variabilis* (American dog tick), *D. andersoni* (wood tick), *Amblyomma americanum* (Lone Star tick), and *Chrysops discalis* (deerfly).[104] Infection also commonly occurs by contact with infected mammalian hosts, particularly rabbits and cats. Type B is usually transmitted by contact with infected rodents or contaminated water.[104] Infected dogs generally do not develop clinical disease. *F. tularensis* can enter the host via the arthropod vector, by inhalation, by ingestion, and by penetration of the skin or mucous membranes. The organism is passed transovarially and trans-stadially in tick vectors. Human cases peak in the summer, when the tick vectors are most prevalent, and in the winter during hunting season because of increased exposure to rabbits.[104]

Pathogenesis. In humans, the incubation period is 3 to 5 days. Fever, malaise, chills, and fatigue are the most common clinical signs.[104] Untreated type A infections in humans have a fatality rate of 5% to 7%.[105] Depending on the site of inoculation, there are five major forms of the disease—ulceroglandular, glandular, typhoidal, oculoglandular, and oropharyngeal. Inoculation of the extremities results in the ulceroglandular form of the disease (75%–85% of cases), which is characterized by ulcerated skin lesions and lymphadenopathy. The glandular form of the disease is characterized by fever and lymphadenopathy without ulceration (5%–10% of cases). Fever, prostration, and weight loss without lymphadenopathy is characteristic of the typhoidal form of disease (5%–15% of cases), which occurs after ingestion of the organism. Inoculation of the conjunctivae results in the oculoglandular form of the disease (1%–2% of cases). Occasionally, after oral inoculation, pharyngotonsillitis and cervical lymphadenopathy occur, the oropharyngeal form of the disease.

The oral cavity is likely a common route of exposure for cats after ingestion of infected rabbit; clinical signs develop 3 to 5 days later.[103, 104] Abscesses associated with bacterial replication occur in many organs, including lymph nodes, liver, spleen, and lungs, and lead to manifestation of the clinical signs of the disease. Based on serologic evidence of infection in some subclinically infected cats, it appears that not all cats develop terminal disease.[104, 106] Type B is less pathogenic than type A in humans.[105]

Clinical Signs

There have been very few documented cases of clinical feline tularemia (Table 36–11).[103, 104, 107, 108] Most involved young, male, outdoor cats with a history of hunting. Lethargy and anorexia were the most common clinical findings. Fever, dehydration, cervical lymphadenopathy, oral erosions or ulcers, and icterus were the most common abnormalities noted during physical examination. Most clinically ill cats (6 of 7) died.

Laboratory Abnormalities. Panleukopenia with toxic neutrophils, leukocytosis with a left shift, and thrombocytopenia are the most common complete blood count abnormalities in cats with tularemia (see Table 36–11).[103, 104] Hyperbilirubinemia and bilirubinuria were reported in two of three cats with tularemia.[103]

Pathology

Most infected cats have had gross evidence of small (2–10 mm) white to yellow abscesses in multiple tissues, including lymph nodes, spleen, lungs, and liver.[103, 107, 108] Enterocolitis was seen in three of three cases.[103] Oral erosions or ulcers are also common. Necrosis with neutrophilic and monocytic infiltrates are the most common histologic abnormalities. The organism is rarely identified histologically with routine stains; Warthin-Starry stain may be superior to hematoxylin and eosin, Giemsa, Gram, or GMS stain.[107]

Diagnostic Plan

Definitive diagnosis is obtained by isolation of the bacterium in a culture of blood or tissue specimens or by identification of the organism in tissue by immunofluorescence. Special culture media are required (consult your laboratory staff for their specific preference).[104] Antibodies are measured in serum by tube agglutination.[104] Cross-reactivity with *Brucella abortus* and certain strains of *Proteus vulgaris* has been documented with human serum. Time between initial exposure and development of a positive titer in cats is not known but may be as short as 2 weeks.[104] A single titer of 1:80 or higher or a fourfold rise in titer between acute and convalescent sera (3 weeks later) is presumptive evidence of infection.

Treatment and Prognosis

Successful treatment has not been reported in the cat. Supportive care should be administered as indicated. Streptomycin and gentamicin are the drugs of choice for humans.[104, 105] Chloramphenicol and tetracycline derivatives may also be successful, but recurrences may be more common.[104]

Prevention

Ectoparasites should be controlled. Exposure to lagomorphs should be avoided. Cats with fever, oral ulcer or erosions, and lymphadenopathy should be handled with care. Gloves, gown, and mask should be worn when necropsying cats that die with clinical signs of bacteremia, particularly if gross evidence of abscessation of internal organs is present. Contaminated surfaces should be cleansed with routine disinfectants.

Table 36-11
Clinical and Laboratory Abnormalities Associated With Clinical Tularemia in Seven Cats

PARAMETER	NO. OF CATS	PARAMETER	NO. OF CATS
Signalment		*Laboratory Evaluation*	
Sex		Complete blood count	
Male	1	Throbocytopenia	2
Male/castrated	5	Panleukopenia with toxic neutrophils	3
Unknown	1	Leukocytosis with left shift	1
Breed		Not tested	3
Domestic shorthair	2	Biochemical profile	
Siamese	2	Hyperbilirubinemia	2
Unknown	3	Increased activity of ALT	1
Age		Not tested	4
0–1 years	2	Urinalysis	
1–5 years	2	Bilirubinuria	2
5–10 years	1	Not tested	5
Unknown	2	Serology	
		Seropositive	2
History		Seronegative	2
Reluctance to move/lethargy	7	Not tested	3
Anorexia	5		
		Outcome	
Physical Examination		Death	6
Fever	5	Survival	1
Dehydration	5		
Lymphadenopathy	5		
Oral erosions/ulcers	4		
Icteric	2		
Hepatomegaly	1		
Splenomegaly	1		
Abdominal masses	2		
Gross Abnormalities			
Abscesses			
Lymph nodes	6		
Spleen	6		
Lungs	4		
Liver	5		
Myocardium	1		
Icterus	2		
Petechiae	1		
Enterocolitis	3		

Data from Baldwin et al.,[103] Rohrbach,[104] Rhyan et al.,[107] Gliatto et al.[108]

Tissues and blood for culture should be clearly labeled as suspected to be contaminated with *F. tularensis* to decrease laboratory worker contact. Contaminated water supplies and rodents should be avoided.

Zoonotic Aspects

At least 51 cases of cat-related tularemia have been reported.[109] Skin infections, soft tissue infections, and pneumonia are common (see Pathogenesis). Dogs are not considered a source of *F. tularensis* for infection of humans, but they may facilitate transmission of the disease to humans by bringing ticks into the human environment.

References

1. Dow SW. Anaerobic infections. In: Greene CE, ed. Infectious Diseases of the Dog and Cat, 2nd ed. Philadelphia, WB Saunders, 1990:530–537.
2. Dow SW, Jones RL. Anaerobic infections. Part I. Pathogenesis and clinical significance. Compen Contin Educ Pract Vet 1987;9:711–720.
3. Dow SW, Jones RL. Anaerobic infections. Part II. Diagnosis and treatment. Compen Contin Educ Pract Vet 1987;9:827–839.
4. Dow SW, Jones RL, Adney WS. Anaerobic bacterial infections and response to treatment in dogs and cats: 36 cases (1983–1985). J Am Vet Med Assoc 1986;189:930–934.

5. Love DN, Johnson JL, Moore LVH. *Bacteroides* species from the oral cavity and oral-associated diseases of cats. Vet Microbiol 1989;19:275–281.

6. Hardie EM, Barsanti JA. Treatment of canine actinomycosis. J Am Vet Med Assoc 1982;180:537–541.

7. Dow SW, LeCouteur RA, Henik RA, et al. Central nervous system infection associated with anaerobic bacteria in two dogs and two cats. J Vet Intern Med 1988;2:171–176.

8. Frendin J, Grekot C, Hellmen E, et al. Thoracic and abdominal wall swellings in dogs caused by foreign bodies. J Small Anim Pract 1994;35:499–508.

9. Muir P, Johnson KA. Anaerobic bacteria isolated from osteomyelitis in dogs and cats. Vet Surg 1992;21:463–466.

10. Dow SW, Curtis CR, Jones RL, et al. Bacterial culture of blood from critically ill dogs and cats: 100 cases (1985–1987). J Am Vet Med Assoc 1989;195:113–117.

11. Marino DJ, Jaggy A. Nocardiosis. A literature review with selected case reports in two dogs. J Vet Intern Med 1993;7:4–11.

12. Ackerman N, Grain E, Castleman W. Canine nocardiosis. J Am Anim Hosp Assoc 1982;18:147–153.

13. Dow SW, Jones RL, Rosychuk RAW. Bacteriologic specimens: Selection, collection, and transport for optimum results. Compen Contin Educ Pract Vet 1989;11:686–702.

14. Indiveri MC, Hirsh DC. Susceptibility of obligate anaerobes to trimethoprim-sulfamethoxazole. J Am Vet Med Assoc 1986;188:46–48.

15. Hirsh DC, Jang SS, Biberstein EL. Lack of supportive susceptibility data for use of ampicillin together with trimethoprim-sulfonamide as broad-spectrum antimicrobial treatment of bacterial disease in dogs. J Am Vet Med Assoc 1990;197:594–596.

16. Buchanan AM, Beaman BL, Pedersen NC, et al. *Nocardia asteroides* recovery from a dog with steroid and antibiotic unresponsive idiopathic polyarthritis. J Clin Microbiol 1983;18:702–708.

17. Davenport DJ, Johnson GC. Cutaneous nocardiosis in a cat. J Am Vet Med Assoc 1986;188:728–729.

18. Goldstein EJC. Bite wounds and infection. Clin Infect Dis 1992;14:633–638.

19. Macy DW, Gasper PW. Plague. In: Greene CE, ed. Infectious Diseases of the Dog and Cat, 2nd ed. Philadelphia, WB Saunders, 1990:621–627.

20. Rollag OJ, Skeels MR, Nims LJ, et al. Feline plague in New Mexico. J Am Vet Med Assoc 1981;179:1381–1383.

21. Gasper PW, Barnes AM, Quan TJ, et al. Plague (*Yersinia pestis*) in cats: Description of experimentally induced disease. J Med Entomol 1993;30:20–26.

22. Rust JH, Cavanaugh DC, O'Shita R. The role of domestic animals in the epidemiology of plague: I. Experimental infection of dogs and cats. J Infect Dis 1971;124:522–526.

23. Eidson J, Thilsted JP, Rollarg OJ. Clinical, clinicopathologic, and pathologic features of plague in cats: 119 cases (1977–1988). J Am Vet Med Assoc 1991;199:1191–1197.

24. Montman C. Feline plague in Bernadillo County, New Mexico 1980–1987. Proceedings of the Annual Meeting of the Utah Mosquito Abatement Association 1987;40:22–23.

25. Kaufmann AF, Mann JM, Gardiner TM, et al. Public health implications of plague in domestic cats. J Am Vet Med Assoc 1981;179:875–878.

26. Eidson M, Tierney LA, Rollag OJ, et al. Feline plague in New Mexico: Risk factors and transmission to humans. Am J Public Health 1988;78:1333–1335.

27. Werner SB, Weidmer CE, Nelson BC, et al. Primary plague pneumonia contracted from a domestic cat at South Lake Tahoe, California. JAMA 1984;251:929–931.

28. Thornton DJ, Tustin RC, Piennar WN, et al. Cat bite transmission of *Yersinia pestis* infection to man. J S Afr Vet Assoc 1975;46:165–169.

29. Weniger BG, Warren AJ, Forseth V. Human bubonic plague transmitted by a domestic cat scratch. J Am Vet Med Assoc 1984;251:929–931.

30. Appel MJG. Lyme disease in dogs and cats. Compen Contin Educ Pract Vet 1990;12:617–626.

31. Levy SA, Barthold SW, Dombach DM, et al. Canine Lyme borreliosis. Compen Contin Educ Pract Vet 1993;15:833–846.

32. Wasmoen TL, et al. Examination of Koch's postulates for *Borrelia burgdorferi* as the causative agent of limb/joint dysfunction in dogs with borreliosis. JAMA 1992;201:412–418.

33. Appel MJG, Allan S, Jacobson RH, et al. Experimental Lyme disease in dogs produces arthritis and persistent infection. J Infect Dis 1993;167:651–664.

34. Magnarelli LA, Anderson JF, Levine HR, et al. Tick parasitism and antibodies to *Borrelia burgdorferi* in cats. J Am Vet Med Assoc 1990;197:63–66.

35. Burgess EC. Experimentally induced infection of cats with *Borrelia burgdorferi*. Am J Vet Res 1992;53:1507–1511.

36. Gibson MD, Young CR, Omran MT, et al. *Borrelia burgdorferi* infection of cats (letter). J Am Vet Med Assoc 1993;202:1786.

37. Oliver JH, Owsley MR, Hutcheson HJ, et al. Conspecificity of the ticks *Ixodes scapularis* and *Ixodes dammini* (Acari: Ixodidae). J Med Entomol 1993;30:54–63.

38. Mather TN, Fish D, Coughlin RT. Competence of dogs as reservoirs for Lyme disease spirochetes (*Borrelia burgdorferi*). J Am Vet Med Assoc 1994;205:186–188.

39. Gustafson JM, Burgess EC, Wachal MD, et al. Intrauterine transmission of *Borrelia burgdorferi* in dogs. Am J Vet Res 1993;54:882–890.

40. Levy SA, Magnarelli LA. Relationship between development of antibodies to *Borrelia burgdorferi* in dogs and the subsequent development of limb/joint borreliosis. J Am Vet Med Assoc 1992;200:344–347.

41. Nocton JJ, Dressler F, Rutledge BJ, et al. Detection of *Borrelia burgdorferi* DNA by polymerase chain reaction in synovial fluid from patients with Lyme arthritis. N Engl J Med 1994;330:229–234.

42. Levy SA, Duray PH. Complete heart block in a dog seropositive for *Borrelia burgdorferi*: Similarity to human Lyme carditis. J Vet Intern Med 1988;2:138–144.

43. Grauer GF, Burgess EC, Cooley AJ, et al. Renal lesions associated with *Borrelia burgdorferi* infection in a dog. J Am Vet Med Assoc 1988;193:237–239.

44. Feder DM, Joseph RJ, Moroff SD, et al. *Borrelia burgdorferi* antibodies in canine cerebrospinal fluid. Proceed-

ings of the 9th Annual Veterinary Medical Forum of the American College of Veterinary Internal Medicine, New Orleans, 1991:892.

45. Lindenmayer J, Weber M, Bryant J, et al. Comparison of indirect immunofluorescent-antibody assay, enzyme-linked immunosorbent assay, and Western immunoblot for the diagnosis of Lyme disease in dogs. J Clin Microbiol 1990;28:92–96.

46. Barthold SW, Levy SA, Fikrig E, et al. Serologic responses of dogs naturally exposed to or vaccinated against *Borrelia burgdorferi* infection. J Am Vet Med Assoc 1995;207:1435–1440.

47. Schillhorn van Veen TW, Murphy AJ, Colmery B. False positive *Borrelia burgdorferi* antibody titres associated with periodontal disease in dogs. Vet Rec 1993; 132:512.

48. Shin SJ, Chang YF, Jacobson RH, et al. Cross-reactivity between *B. burgdorferi* and other spirochetes affects specificity of serotests for detection of antibodies to the Lyme disease agent in dogs. Vet Microbiol 1993;36: 161–174.

49. Sugiyama Y, Sugiyama F, Yagami K. Comparative study on cross-reaction of leptospiral antibodies in several serological tests to detect antibodies to *Borrelia burgdorferi* in dogs. J Vet Med Sci 1993;55:149–151.

50. Chu HJ, Chavez LG, Blumer BM, et al. Immunogenicity and efficacy study of a commercial *Borrelia burgdorferi* bacterin. J Am Vet Med Assoc 1992;201:403–411.

51. Levy SA, Lissman BA, Ficke CM. Performance of a *Borrelia burgdorferi* bacterin in borreliosis-endemic areas. J Am Vet Med Assoc 1993;202:1834–1838.

52. Kazmierczak JJ, Sorhage FE. Current understanding of *Borrelia burgdorferi* infection, with emphasis on its prevention in dogs. J Am Vet Med Assoc 1993;203:1524–1528.

53. Greene CE, Shotts EB. Leptospirosis. In: Greene CE, ed. Infectious Diseases of the Dog and Cat, 2nd ed. Philadelphia, WB Saunders, 1990:498–507.

54. Baldwin CJ, Atkins CE. Leptospirosis in dogs. Compen Contin Educ Pract Vet 1987;9:499–507.

55. Rentko VT, Clark N, Ross LA, et al. Canine leptospirosis. J Vet Intern Med 1992;6:235–244.

56. Watson ADJ. *Leptospira interrogans* serovar *bratislava* infection. J Am Vet Med Assoc 1991;199:1239.

57. Bishop L, Strandberg JD, Adams RJ, et al. Chronic active hepatitis in dogs associated with leptospires. Am J Vet Res 1979;40:839–844.

58. Mackintosh CG, Blackmore DK, Marshall RB. Isolation of *Leptospira interrogans* serovars *tarassovi* and *pomona* from dogs. N Z Vet J 1980;28:100.

59. Heath SE, Johnson R. Leptospirosis. J Am Vet Med Assoc 1994;205:1518–1523.

60. Batza HJ, Weiss R. Occurrence of *Leptospira* antibodies in cat serum samples. Kleintierpraxis 1987;32:171–174.

61. Arimitsu Y, Haritan K, Ishiguro N, et al. Detection of antibodies to leptospirosis in experimentally infected dogs using the microcapsule agglutination test. Br Vet J 1989;145:356–361.

62. Songer JG, Thiermann AB. Leptospirosis. J Am Vet Med Assoc 1988;193:1250–1254.

63. Lancefield RC. A serological differentiation of human and other groups of hemolytic streptococci. J Exp Med 1933;57:571–595.

64. Greene CE. Group A streptococcal infections of dogs and cats. In: Greene CE, ed. Infectious Diseases of the Dog and Cat, 2nd ed. Philadelphia, WB Saunders, 1990: 599–602.

65. Greene CE. Group B streptococcal infections of dogs and cats. In: Greene CE, ed. Infectious Diseases of the Dog and Cat. Philadelphia, WB Saunders, 1990:602.

66. Greene CE. Group C streptococcal infections of dogs and cats. In: Greene CE, ed. Infectious Diseases of the Dog and Cat, 2nd ed. Philadelphia, WB Saunders, 1990:602.

67. Greene CE. Group G streptococcal infections of dogs. In: Greene CE, ed. Infectious Diseases of the Dog and Cat. Philadelphia, WB Saunders, 1990:605.

68. Blanchard PC, Wilson DW. Group G streptococcal infections of cats. In: Greene CE, ed. Infectious Diseases of the Dog and Cat. Philadelphia, WB Saunders, 1990: 603–605.

69. Greene CE. Zoonotic aspects of group A streptococcal infection in dogs and cats. J Am Anim Hosp Assoc 1988;24:218–222.

70. Sundberg JP, Hill D, Wyand DS, et al. *Streptococcus zooepidemicus* as the cause of septicemia in racing greyhounds. Vet Med Small Anim Clin 1981;76:839–842.

71. Ling GV, Biberstein EL, Hirsh DC. Bacterial pathogens associated with urinary tract infections. Vet Clin North Am 1979;9:617–630.

72. Kornblatt AN, Adams RL, Barthold SW, et al. Canine neonatal deaths associated with group B streptococcal septicemia. J Am Vet Med Assoc 1983;183:700–701.

73. Dow SW, Jones RL, Thomas TN, et al. Group B streptococcal infection in cats. J Am Vet Med Assoc 1987;190:71–72.

74. Devriese LA, Haesebrouck F. *Streptococcus suis* infections in horses and cats. Vet Rec 1992;130:380.

75. Biberstein EL, Brown C, Smith T. Serodiagnosis and biotypes among beta-hemolytic streptococcus of canine origin. J Clin Microbiol 1980;11:558–561.

76. Davies ME, Skulski G. A study of beta-hemolytic streptococci in the fading puppy in relation to canine virus hepatitis infection in the dam. Br Vet J 1956;112: 404–410.

77. Reitmeyer JC, Steele JH. The occurrence of beta-hemolytic streptococcus in cats. Southwest Vet 1984;36: 41–42.

78. Iglauer F, Kunstyr, I, Morstedt R, et al. *Streptococcus canis* arthritis in a cat breeding colony. J Exp Anim Sci 1991;34:59–65.

79. Montovani AR, Restani D, Sciarra D, et al. Streptococcus L infection in the dog. J Small Anim Pract 1961;2: 185–194.

80. Stallings B, Ling GV, Lagenauur LA, et al. Septicemia and septic arthritis caused by *Streptococcus pneumoniae* in a cat: Possible transmission from a child. J Am Vet Med Assoc 1987;191:703–704.

81. Roos K, Lind L, Holm SE: Beta-hemolytic streptococci group A in a cat, as a possible source of repeated tonsillitis in a family. Lancet 1988;2:1072.

82. Rosendal, S. *Mycoplasma* infections. In: Greene CE, ed.

Infectious Diseases of the Dog and Cat. Philadelphia, WB Saunders, 1990:446–449.

83. Slavik MF, Beasley JN. *Mycoplasma* infections of cats. Fel Pract 1992;20:12–14.

84. Rosendal, S. Canine mycoplasmas: Their ecologic niche and role in disease. J Am Vet Med Assoc 1982;180:1212–1214.

85. Doig PA, Ruhnke HL, Bosu WTK. The genital mycoplasma and ureaplasma flora of healthy and diseased dogs. Can J Comp Med 1981;45:233–238.

86. Randolph JF, Moise NS, Scarlett JM, et al. Prevalence of mycoplasmal and ureaplasmal recovery from tracheobronchial lavages and prevalence of mycoplasmal recovery from pharyngeal swab specimens in dogs with or without pulmonary disease. Am J Vet Res 1993;54:387–391.

87. Randolph JF, Moise NS, Scarlett JM, et al. Prevalence of mycoplasmal and ureaplasmal recovery from tracheobronchial lavages and of mycoplasmal recovery from pharyngeal swab specimens in cats with or without pulmonary disease. Am J Vet Res 1993;54:897–900.

88. Campbell JH, Fox JG, Snyder SB. Ocular bacteria and mycoplasma of the clinical normal cat. Feline Pract 1973;3:10–12.

89. Jameson PH, King LA, Lappin MR, et al. Comparison of clinical signs, diagnostic findings, organisms isolated, and clinical outcome in dogs with bacterial pneumonia: 93 cases (1986–1991). J Am Vet Med Assoc 1995;206:206–209.

90. Moise NS, Wiedenkeller D, Yeager AE, et al. Clinical, radiographic, and bronchial cytologic features of cats with bronchial disease: 65 cases (1980–1986). J Am Vet Med Assoc 1989;194:1467–1473.

91. Jang SS, Ling GV, Yamamoto R, et al. *Mycoplasma* as a cause of canine urinary tract infection. J Am Vet Med Assoc 1984;185:45–47.

92. Tan RJS, Miles JAP. Incidence and significance of mycoplasmas in sick cats. Res Vet Sci 1974;16:27–34.

93. Tan RJS. Susceptibility of kittens to *Mycoplasma felis* infections. Jpn J Exp Med 1974;44:235–240.

94. Moise NS, Crissman JW, Fairbrother JF, et al. *Mycoplasma gatae* arthritis and tenosynovitis in cats: Case report and experimental reproduction of the disease. Am J Vet Res 1983;44:16–21.

95. Rosendal S. Canine mycoplasmas: Pathogenicity of mycoplasmas associated with distemper pneumonia. J Infect Dis 1978;138:203–210.

96. Hooper PT, Ireland LA, Carter A. *Mycoplasma* polyarthritis in a cat with probable severe immune deficiency. Aust Vet J 1985;62:352.

97. Tan RJS, Miles JAR. Possible role of feline T-strain mycoplasmas in cat abortion. Aust Vet J 1974;50:142.

98. Barton MD, Ireland L, Kirschner JL, et al. Isolation of *Mycoplasma spumans* from polyarthritis in a greyhound. Aust Vet J 1985;62:206.

99. Harai J, Lincoln J. Pharmacologic features of clindamycin in dogs and cats. J Am Vet Med Assoc 1989;195:124–125.

100. Boothe DM. Enrofloxacin revisited. Vet Med 1994;8:744–753.

101. Kirchner BK, Port CD, Magoc TJ, et al. Spontaneous bronchopneumonia in laboratory dogs with untyped *Mycoplasma* sp. Lab Anim Sci 1990;40:625–628.

102. McCabe SJ, Mujrray JF, Ruhnke HL, et al. *Mycoplasma* infection of the hand acquired from a cat. J Hand Surg 1987;12:1085.

103. Baldwin CJ, Panciera RJ, Morton RJ, et al. Acute tularemia in three domestic cats. J Am Vet Med Assoc 1991;199:1602–1605.

104. Rohrbach BW. Tularemia. J Am Vet Med Assoc 1988;193:428–432.

105. Markowitz LE, Hynes NA, de la Cruz P, et al. Tick-borne tularemia. JAMA 1985;254:2922–2925.

106. McKeever S, Schubert JH, Moody MD, et al. Natural occurrence of tularemia in marsupials, carnivores, lagomorphs, and large rodents in southwestern Georgia and northwestern Florida. J Infect Dis 1958;103:120–126.

107. Rhyan JC, Gahagan T, Fales WH. Tularemia in a cat. J Vet Diagn Invest 1990;2:239–241.

108. Gliatto JM, Rae JF, McDonough PL, et al. Feline tularemia on Nantucket Island, Massachusetts. J Vet Diag Invest 1994;6:102–105.

109. Capellan J, Fong IW. Tularemia from a cat bite: Case report and review of feline-associated tularemia. Clin Infect Dis 1993;16:472–475.

Chapter 37

Rickettsial Diseases

Michael R. Lappin

Rocky Mountain Spotted Fever

Pathophysiology

Etiology. Rocky Mountain spotted fever (RMSF) is caused by *Rickettsia rickettsii*, a gram-negative bacterium in the family Rickettsiaceae.[1, 2] Members of the spotted fever group are found throughout the world; infection by *R. rickettsii* is found in the Western Hemisphere. Most cases of RMSF are now recognized in the southeastern states.[3] *R. montana, R. belli,* and *R. rhipicephali* are nonpathogenic members of the genus found in the United States; infection of dogs by these species can produce false-positive antibody results in RMSF serologic tests. Infection by *R. rickettsii* causes clinical disease most commonly in humans and dogs.

Epidemiology. Ticks are the natural host, reservoir, and vector of *R. rickettsii*.[4] *Dermacentor andersoni* (American wood tick), *D. variabilis* (American dog tick), and *Amblyomma americanum* (Lone Star tick) are the principal tick vectors of *R. rickettsii*. The organism can be transmitted trans-stadially and transovarially in the tick; thus, larval and nymph stages of ticks can carry *R. rickettsii* without previously feeding. Ticks in the larval and nymph stages feed primarily on small mammals; those in the adult stage feed on large mammals. Significant rickettsemia develops in voles, ground squirrels, and chipmunks after infection, and previously uninfected ticks can acquire the organism from these species during feeding. Previously uninfected ticks generally do not acquire *R. rickettsii* from feeding on infected dogs[5] or humans because of minimal levels of rickettsemia in these species. The organism is maintained in nature by the cycle of infection in small rodents and the nymph and larval stages of the tick vectors.[4]

R. rickettsii requires an activation period; a previously unfed tick must be attached for 5 to 20 hours for infection to occur.[3] Ticks that have recently fed are capable of transmission shortly after attachment. Transmission can also occur to people when ticks harboring activated *R. rickettsii* are removed by hand, and the organism contacts conjunctivae or open wounds. It appears unlikely that humans acquire RMSF from contact with dogs, but dogs may increase human exposure to RMSF by bringing ticks into the human environment. *R. rickettsii* is susceptible to environmental factors and does not persist outside the host.[1]

Clinical disease can potentially develop in all infected humans and dogs. In humans, RMSF is most common in young, white males in a rural setting; mortality is greatest in those older than 30 years of age.[3, 6] Clinical infection is recognized almost exclusively in the spring and summer months (April to September), when the tick vectors are most active;

thus, RMSF should be considered a differential diagnosis only during this time. Untreated RMSF is fatal in approximately 20% of infected people.[3]

Pathogenesis. After infection, dogs either develop acute disease with approximately a 14-day clinical course or are subclinically infected.[1] The organism preferentially replicates in endothelial cells, leading to the development of diffuse vasculitis. Clinical disease depends on the areas most severely affected and can involve almost any body system (see Clinical Signs and Table 37–1). Disseminated intravascular coagulation is common. Fever is probably related to release of endogenous pyrogens from activated leukocytes involved in the vasculitis. Hemorrhage is

Table 37–1

Clinical Abnormalities in Humans and Dogs With Rocky Mountain Spotted Fever

CLINICAL ABNORMALITY	HUMANS (N = 262) N (%)	DOGS (N = 79) N (%)
Low fever	99 (37.8) >100°F [>37.8°C]	67 (84.8) >102.3°F [>39.2°C]
High fever	90 (34.4) >102°F [>38.9°C]	54 (68.4) >104°F [>40°C]
Headache	91 (34.7)	NR
Rash or petechiae	88 (33.6)	19 (24.1)
Myalgia or arthralgia	83 (31.7)	49 (62.0)
Anorexia	NR	51 (64.6)
Known tick exposure	67 (25.6)	52 (65.8)
Nausea or vomiting	60 (22.9)	18 (22.8)
Diarrhea	19 (7.3)	16 (20.3)
Abdominal pain	52 (19.8)	30 (38.0)
Conjunctivitis or scleral congestion	30 (11.5)	34 (43.0)
Lymphadenomegaly	27 (10.3)	43 (54.4)
Hepatomegaly	12 (4.6)	3 (3.8)
Splenomegaly	16 (6.1)	3 (3.8)
Depression or altered mental status	26 (9.9)	65 (83.0)
Vestibular deficits	18 (6.9)	41 (51.9)
Coma or unconsciousness	9 (3.4)	4 (5.1)
Seizures	8 (3.1)	10 (12.7)
Edema of face or extremities	18 (6.9)	25 (31.6)
Polyuria or polydipsia	NR	5 (6.3)
Pneumonitis, dyspnea, or cough	12 (4.6)	39 (49.4)
Icterus	9 (3.4)	4 (5.1)
Cardiac arrhythmias	7 (2.7)	8 (10.1)
Death	4 (1.5)	3 (3.8)

NR, not reported.
Data from Greene and Breitschwerdt,[1] Helmick et al.[6]

due to the combination of vasculitis, thrombocytopenia that results from consumption of platelets at sites of vasculitis, and disseminated intravascular coagulation.

Clinical Signs

Any dog not previously exposed to *R. rickettsii* can develop RMSF; many reported cases have involved purebred dogs younger than 3 years of age. RMSF in dogs has an acute or subclinical course. Owners may or may not have noted ticks on the dog. Because clinical disease is due to vasculitis, manifestations can vary greatly (see Table 37–1). Fever and depression are the most common clinical signs. Respiratory signs, including dyspnea and cough, occur in many infected dogs and are probably due to interstitial pulmonary edema secondary to vasculitis. Vomiting and diarrhea occur in some acutely infected dogs. Lymphadenopathy and splenomegaly occur in some dogs but not as often as in dogs with ehrlichiosis. Evidence of hemorrhage, including petechiae and epistaxis, is commonly noted. Subconjunctival hemorrhage, hyphema, anterior uveitis, iris hemorrhage, retinal petechiae, and retinal edema occur frequently in acutely infected dogs.[7, 8] Dermal necrosis has been rarely reported.[9] Cardiac arrhythmias and shock, pulmonary disease, acute renal failure, or severe central nervous system disease occurs in most dogs that die of RMSF. Vasculitis can induce diffuse meningoencephalitis. Clinical signs consistent with vestibular disease, including nystagmus, ataxia, and head tilt, are recognized most often.

Laboratory and Radiographic Abnormalities. Neutrophilic leukocytosis with or without a left shift is the most common leukogram abnormality and results from a demand for neutrophils at sites of vasculitis.[1, 2] Magnitude of thrombocytopenia varies but can be less than 75×10^3. Platelet counts are rarely less than 25×10^3, and because the pathogenesis is consumption, giant platelets indicating release of young platelets from normal bone marrow megakaryocytes are commonly noted on cytologic examination of peripheral blood. If anemia occurs, it is related to blood loss. Anemia is generally mild and is characterized as normocytic normochromic and nonregenerative after acute bleeding and as macrocytic hypochromic and regenerative within several days after bleeding. Some dogs show positive results on Coombs test.[1]

A variety of nonspecific biochemical abnormalities have been reported in dogs with RMSF. Increased activities of alanine aminotransferase, aspartate aminotransferase, and alkaline phosphatase are common.[1, 10] Hypoalbuminemia occurs frequently and results from blood loss or third-spacing of albumin in tissues secondary to vasculitis. The hyperglobulinemia seen with chronic-phase ehrlichiosis does not develop

in dogs with RMSF because *R. rickettsii* does not result in chronic intracellular infection. Elevated blood urea nitrogen, elevated creatinine, and metabolic acidosis are common in dogs with developing renal insufficiency. Serum sodium, chloride, and potassium concentrations may decrease in dogs with vomiting or diarrhea. Hematuria and concurrent proteinuria are common; in contrast to dogs with chronic ehrlichiosis, proteinuria without hematuria due to glomerulonephritis is unusual. Polyarthritis occurs in some dogs and is most commonly characterized by increased protein concentrations and neutrophilic pleocytosis. Cerebrospinal fluid analysis from dogs with central nervous system manifestations of disease usually reveals increased protein concentrations and neutrophilic pleocytosis.[1] Some dogs may have mononuclear cell increases in the cerebrospinal fluid or may have mixed inflammation.

No pathognomonic radiographic abnormalities are present. Dogs with respiratory signs most commonly have increased pulmonary interstitial markings. Severe vasculitis can result in hemorrhage or edema that spills into the alveoli, resulting in an alveolar pulmonary pattern in some dogs.

Pathology

Pathologic abnormalities are consistent with vasculitis and are characterized grossly primarily by the presence of petechial and ecchymotic hemorrhages in a variety of tissues. Lymphadenopathy and splenomegaly may be noted. Necrotizing vasculitis with infiltrates of neutrophils is the predominant histopathologic abnormality.

Diagnostic Plan

Definitive diagnosis of RMSF is made by documenting the infection by inoculating affected tissues or blood into susceptible laboratory animals[1] or by documenting the organism in endothelial cells using direct fluorescent antibody staining.[11] Because these techniques are not widely available, clinical diagnosis of RMSF in dogs should be based on appropriate clinical, historical, and laboratory evidence of disease combined with positive serologic testing and response to therapy.

Antibodies against *R. rickettsii* can be measured in dog serum by immunofluorescence assay (IFA), enzyme-linked immunosorbent assay (ELISA), and latex agglutination.[12] IgM and IgG antibodies against RMSF can be detected by ELISA or IFA. Latex agglutination is not antibody class–specific. Cutoffs for positive antibody titers as well as specificity and sensitivity vary by the assay. After experimental inoculation, IgM antibodies can be detected by IFA by day 9, peak by day 20, and are negative by day 80 after inoculation.[13] In dogs with clinical illness due to RMSF, IgM antibody titers are generally positive. Because of the antibodies' short duration in serum, false-negative results may occur with IgM testing. False-positive results are most common in the IgM-ELISA when compared with those of IFA and latex agglutination.[12] Positive IgG titers are detectable 20 to 25 days after infection. Serum samples with IgG titers equal to or greater than 1:64 are generally considered positive. If IgG or IgM antibodies are not detected in a patient with clinical and laboratory evidence of RMSF, a convalescent IgG titer 2 to 3 weeks later is recommended. Timing of the second titer is not critical because IgG antibody titers do not decrease until 3 to 5 months after infection.[1] Documentation of seroconversion or a fourfold increase in IgG titer is consistent with recent infection.

Serum antibodies are commonly detected in clinically normal dogs with no history of illness consistent with RMSF, suggesting that subclinical illness is common. Thus, the presence of antibodies in serum indicates only exposure, not clinical illness. Cross-reaction in the serologic tests occurs when antibodies against other nonpathogenic spotted fever group agents (e.g., *R. montana, R. rhipicephali, R. belli,* and some typhus group rickettsiae) are present, so a positive antibody titer does not definitively document exposure to *R. rickettsii*. A clinical diagnosis should be based on the combination of serologic findings, history, physical examination findings, laboratory abnormalities, and response to therapy.

Treatment and Prognosis

Supportive care for gastrointestinal tract fluid and electrolyte losses, renal disease, disseminated intravascular coagulation, and anemia is administered as indicated. Administration of intravenous fluid therapy must be monitored closely. Because of the vasculitis that commonly occurs in the pulmonary interstitium and meninges, overzealous fluid therapy may worsen respiratory or central nervous system manifestations of disease.

Successful treatment can be achieved with tetracycline derivatives, chloramphenicol, and enrofloxacin. Tetracycline at a dosage of 22 mg/kg by mouth, three times per day (t.i.d.) for 14 to 21 days, generally leads to rapid improvement of clinical signs not involving the central nervous system. Fever, depression, and thrombocytopenia often begin to resolve within days (24–48 hours) of therapy initiation. Doxycycline, a synthetic tetracycline derivative administered at 5 mg/kg by mouth, twice per day (b.i.d.) for 14 to 21 days, is an alternative to tetracycline. This drug is more lipid soluble than are other tetracycline derivatives and thus is better absorbed from the

gastrointestinal tract and penetrates the cerebrospinal fluid more readily. Chloramphenicol at a dosage of 25 mg/kg by mouth, t.i.d. for 14 days, has been used in puppies younger than 5 months of age to avoid dental staining associated with tetracyclines. Enrofloxacin administered at 3 mg/kg by mouth, b.i.d. for 7 days, is as effective as tetracycline or chloramphenicol in the treatment of RMSF.[14] The prognosis for clinical RMSF is guarded in some cases because of the severity of vasculitis, although most animals respond well to antibiotic therapy. Death was reported in 3 of 79 dogs in one report.[1]

Prevention

After recovery, dogs infected by RMSF are immune to reinfection for approximately 6 to 12 months.[1, 3] Naturally occurring RMSF has not been reported twice in the same dog, suggesting permanent immunity. Infection can be prevented only by avoiding the tick vector. Tick control in the immediate canine environment cannot eliminate RMSF totally because the tick vector maintains the rickettsial life cycle within other mammalian hosts.

Zoonotic Aspects

Dogs with RMSF are not directly infectious to people and probably do not maintain a high enough level of rickettsemia to infect previously naive ticks.[5] Dogs can be a sentinel for human RMSF because infection in dogs in a given geographic area tends to parallel infection in people. Dogs can bring ticks into the human environment, and tick removal from pets can result in infection of people if the organism makes contact with conjunctivae or abraded skin. Other animals, including birds, also may transport ticks infected with *R. rickettsii* into the human environment.

Ehrlichiosis

Pathophysiology

Etiology. Ehrlichia spp. are tick-borne, intracellular, gram-negative bacteria in the family Rickettsiaceae.[10, 15, 16] Clusters of the organism called morulae form intracellularly. Known species that infect dogs are *E. canis, E. equi, E. risticii, E. platys,* and an antigenically distinct granulocytic species recently named *E. ewingii*.[15–21] *E. canis* infects mononuclear cells, appears to be the most common *Ehrlichia* species infecting dogs, and causes the most severe clinical disease. *E. risticii,* the cause of Potomac horse fever, infects mononuclear cells but has been associated with clinical illness in naturally infected dogs only anecdotally.[19] *E. platys* infects platelets and causes infectious cyclic thrombocytopenia.[16] *E. ewingii* and *E. equi* infect granulocytes and lead to mild clinical disease syndromes, including polyarthritis.[15–17, 20, 21] *E. chaffeensis* infects mononuclear cells and causes disease in humans in the United States.[22] *Ehrlichia* spp. morulae have been detected in cells of naturally infected, clinically ill cats in Kenya, France, and the United States.[23–25]

Epidemiology. The principal vector for *E. canis* is *Rhipicephalus sanguineus* (brown dog tick). The vectors for *E. platys*, *E. ewingii*, *E. equi*, and *E. risticii* in dogs and the *Ehrlichia* spp. infecting cats in the United States are undetermined. *E. canis* is passed only trans-stadially in the tick, so unexposed ticks must feed on a rickettsemic dog to become infected and perpetuate the disease. *E. canis* is maintained in the environment by passage from ticks to dogs. Both the male and the female *Rhipicephalus* can transmit *E. canis* for approximately 155 days.[15] Ticks can be infected only by feeding on infected dogs in the acute phase of infection. *Ehrlichia* spp. can also be transmitted by blood transfusion. The organism does not survive outside the host.

Dogs seropositive for *E. canis* have been identified in most of the United States, but the majority of cases occur in areas with high concentrations of *R. sanguineus*. *E. platys* has been diagnosed most frequently in dogs in the southern states. Serum antibodies against *E. canis* and *E. platys* were detected in 20.3% and 54.2% of healthy dogs, respectively, in Louisiana.[26] Cases of suspected feline ehrlichiosis have been identified in Colorado, New Mexico, Arizona, and California. The remainder of the discussion concerns *E. canis* infection in dogs.

Clinical disease can occur in any dog, but severity varies depending on a combination of organism and host factors. Virulence of different field strains varies. Purebred dogs, particularly German shepherds, may have depressed cell-mediated immunity and acquire severe disease. Because of the variable duration of the subclinical phase of the disease, *E. canis* infection does not have a seasonal incidence, but the acute phase of the disease is recognized most frequently in the spring and summer.

Pathogenesis. *E. canis* infection causes three successive phases of infection: acute, subclinical, and chronic. During the acute phase, infected mononuclear cells marginate in small vessels or migrate into the endothelial tissue, inducing vasculitis. Replication also occurs in lymphoreticular organs, including the liver, spleen, and lymph nodes. The acute phase begins 1 to 3 weeks after infection and lasts 2 to 4 weeks.[15] Clinical signs of disease can develop before the development of detectable antibody levels. Most immunocompetent dogs survive the acute ·phase of the disease. A subclinical phase of variable duration then ensues. This phase lasts 40 to 120 days in experimentally infected dogs; it has lasted as long as 5 years in naturally infected dogs.[27] In some dogs, the organism clears during this phase. The organism persists intracellularly in most dogs because of incomplete clearance, leading to the chronic phase of infection. This phase is characterized by the development of hyperglobulinemia.

Clinical abnormalities that develop during the chronic phase of infection are usually due to immune-mediated disease. Immune complex glomerulonephritis with resultant proteinuria occurs in some dogs. Pancytopenia with resultant bleeding disorders, anemia, and secondary infections may be the result of immune-mediated damage to bone marrow stem cells. Clinical signs that develop during the chronic phase of infection may not develop until months to years after primary exposure. Clinical signs of central nervous system disease are due to mononuclear cell meningitis or hemorrhage. Polyarthritis develops in some dogs infected with *Ehrlichia* spp. Most dogs with polyarthritis from which the organism has been demonstrated have been infected with granulocytic strains, probably *E. ewingii* or *E. equi*.[28] However, immune-complex deposition in the joints may lead to suppurative polyarthritis in dogs infected with *E. canis* because of the chronic immune stimulation. If a dog dies of ehrlichiosis, it is generally because of severe anemia, hemorrhage from thrombocytopenia, or secondary infection.

Clinical Signs

The age range for dogs with clinical ehrlichiosis is 2 months to 14 years, and males are affected approximately 1.5 times more than females.[15] Clinical signs (Table 37–2) of canine ehrlichiosis vary with the phase of infection (Table 37–3).[10, 15, 16] Ticks are most commonly noted or reported on dogs during the acute phase of infection. A previous short-lived episode of malaise may be reported by some owners of dogs with chronic ehrlichiosis. Fever is more common in acute than in chronic ehrlichiosis. Petechial hemorrhage and epistaxis can occur with both acute and chronic ehrlichiosis and in the absence of thrombocytopenia. This finding is probably related to the development of vasculitis or platelet function abnormalities. Pale mucous membranes usually occur only in the chronic phase during the development of pancytopenia. Hepatomegaly, splenomegaly, and lymphadenopathy are common and are detected most frequently in dogs with chronic-phase disease. Louder-than-normal breath sounds, crackles, wheezes, or dyspnea occur in some dogs and may be due to interstitial edema secondary to vasculitis, pulmonary parenchymal hemorrhage secondary to vasculitis or thrombocytopenia, or secondary infections from neutropenia. Tortuous retinal

Table 37–2
Prevalence of Historical, Physical Examination, and Laboratory Abnormalities Associated With Canine Ehrlichiosis

CLINICAL ABNORMALITY	% (NO. OF DOGS EVALUATED)	LABORATORY ABNORMALITY	% (NO. OF DOGS EVALUATED)
Depression	64 (390)	Thrombocytopenia	86 (327)
Anorexia	56 (345)	Anemia	70 (27)
Weight loss	53 (371)	Eosinopenia	56 (120)
Fever	45 (366)	Lymphopenia	46 (74)
Pale mucous membranes	45 (204)	Increased ALT activity	41 (271)
Bleeding tendencies	42 (380)	Hypoalbuminemia	40 (295)
Lymphadenomegaly	36 (330)	Leukopenia	31 (300)
Splenomegaly	20 (345)	Hyperproteinemia	26 (299)
Vomiting	11 (265)	Increased AP activity	22 (271)
Anterior uveitis	8 (265)	Increased BUN	19 (259)
		Increased creatinine	11 (238)
		Leukocytosis	11 (300)
		Increased total bilirubin	10 (212)

ALT, alanine aminotransferase; AP, alkaline phosphatase; BUN, blood urea nitrogen.
Data from Troy and Forrester.[15]

vessels, perivascular retinal infiltrates, retinal hemorrhage, anterior uveitis, and exudative retinal detachment are noted in some dogs. Polyuria and polydipsia are reported in some dogs that develop renal insufficiency. Suppurative polyarthritis occurs in some dogs. Not all dogs with polyarthritis have swollen, painful joints; stiffness or exercise intolerance is a more common clinical manifestation. The granulocytic strains, *E. ewingii* and *E. equi,* are commonly identified in neutrophils from dogs with polyarthritis. Central nervous system signs can include depression, pain, ataxia, paresis, nystagmus, and seizures. Meningitis was reported in one dog with granulocytic ehrlichiosis.[21]

Laboratory and Radiographic Abnormalities. Mild neutropenia develops in 1 to 2 weeks after infection with *E. canis;* a rebound neutrophilic leukocytosis then occurs rapidly and may persist for weeks. Neutrophil counts tend to decrease again as the disease becomes chronic. Monocytosis or lymphocytosis (or both disorders) is often identified in dogs with subclinical and chronic ehrlichiosis. Azurophilic granules are commonly noted in mononuclear cells of dogs with ehrlichiosis and probably result from chronic immune stimulation.[29] Anemia rarely occurs in dogs with acute ehrlichiosis unless it is related to blood loss. Chronic-phase ehrlichiosis often results in a normocytic, normochromic, nonregenerative anemia owing to bone marrow suppression or anemia of chronic disease. Thrombocytopenia can occur with either acute (vasculitis) or chronic (bone marrow

suppression) ehrlichiosis but is generally more severe with chronic-phase disease. Platelet counts less than 25×10^3 probably occur only in chronic-phase disease. Thrombocytopathies with decreased platelet function are thought to occur in some cases of subclinical or chronic ehrlichiosis with hyperglobulinemia.[15] Disseminated intravascular coagulation is not common with canine ehrlichiosis compared with dogs with RMSF. Changes in bone marrow cell lines associated with ehrlichiosis vary from hypercellular to hypocellular depending on whether the disease is acute or chronic. Bone marrow plasmacytosis is common in dogs with subclinical and chronic-phase ehrlichiosis, and the disease can be confused with multiple myeloma, particularly in dogs with monoclonal gammopathies. Although classic cases of dogs with chronic ehrlichiosis involve pancytopenia, chronically infected, seropositive dogs have presented with all combinations of neutropenia, thrombocytopenia, and anemia.

Hypoalbuminemia can occur in dogs with acute or chronic ehrlichiosis. In acute-phase disease, hypoalbuminemia is probably due to third-spacing of albumin in tissues because of vasculitis, whereas in chronic-phase disease, hypoalbuminemia is due to glomerular loss. The presence of hyperglobulinemia with hypoalbuminemia is consistent with subclinical or chronic ehrlichiosis. Hyperglobulinemia associated with ehrlichiosis is almost always polyclonal, but monoclonal (IgG) gammopathies have been reported.[30] Azotemia occasionally occurs with acute or chronic disease and is usually prerenal.

Rarely, renal azotemia develops in some dogs with severe glomerulonephritis from chronic ehrlichiosis.

Lymph node aspiration of dogs with lymphadenopathy generally reveals reactive hyperplasia. Antinuclear antibody measurement, Coombs test, rheumatoid factor test, and lupus erythematosus cell preparations are positive in some dogs. Nondegenerate neutrophils are the primary cell infiltrates in dogs with polyarthritis. Cerebrospinal fluid abnormalities include increased protein and increased cell counts; ehrlichiosis generally causes mononuclear pleocytosis.

No pathognomonic radiographic signs of ehrlichiosis are present. Dogs with polyarthritis usually do not have erosive changes, as noted on joint radiographs. Radiographs of dogs with respiratory signs most commonly show increased pulmonary interstitial markings.

Pathology

Gross necropsy findings vary based on stage of disease. Dogs with vasculitis or thrombocytopenia often have petechiae on multiple organs. Bone marrow is red in acute disease and pale in chronic disease.[15] Edema may be noted in dogs with vasculitis. Splenomegaly and lymphadenopathy are common. Central nervous system histopathologic changes include mononuclear cell infiltrates in the ventral brain stem and periventricular gray matter and white matter. Perivascular infiltrates of lymphocytes and plasma

Table 37–3
Clinical and Laboratory Abnormalities Associated With *Ehrlichia canis* Infection in Dogs

STAGE OF INFECTION	CLINICAL ABNORMALITIES	LABORATORY ABNORMALITIES
Acute	Fever Serous or purulent oculonasal discharge Anorexia Weight loss Dyspnea Lymphadenopathy Tick infestation often evident	Thrombocytopenia Leukopenia initially followed by neutrophilic leukocytosis and monocytosis Morulae Low-grade, nonregenerative anemia unless hemorrhage has occurred Variable *Ehrlichia* titer
Subclinical	No clinical abnormalities Ticks often not present	Hyperglobulinemia Thrombocytopenia Neutropenia Lymphocytosis Monocytosis Positive *Ehrlichia* titer
Chronic	Ticks often not present Depression Weight loss Pale mucous membranes Abdominal pain Evidence of hemorrhage: epistaxis, retinal hemorrhage Lymphadenopathy Splenomegaly Dyspnea, increased lung sounds Ocular: perivascular retinitis, hyphema, retinal detachment, anterior uveitis, corneal edema CNS: meningeal pain, paresis, cranial nerve deficits, seizures Hepatomegaly Arrhythmias and pulse deficits Polyuria and polydipsia Stiffness and swollen, painful joints	Monocytosis Lymphocytosis Thrombocytopenia Nonregenerative anemia Hyperglobulinemia Hypocellular bone marrow Bone marrow plasmacytosis Hypoalbuminemia Proteinuria Polyclonal or IgG monoclonal gammopathy CSF mononuclear cell pleocytosis Nonseptic, suppurative polyarthritis Rare azotemia Increased ALT and AP activities Positive *Ehrlichia* titer

IgG, immunoglobulin G; CSF, cerebrospinal fluid; CNS, central nervous system; ALT, alanine aminotransferase; AP, alkaline phosphatase.

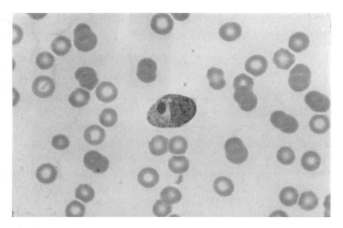

Figure 37-1
Morulae in a mononuclear cell from a dog with clinical ehrlichiosis.

cells occur in multiple tissues, including the lungs, liver, kidneys, and retinas. Lymphoid changes include lymphoreticular hyperplasia in paracortical areas of lymph nodes and splenic red pulp soon after infection. Infiltration of lymphocytes and plasma cells into tissue surrounding follicular tissues occurs chronically. Morphologic changes that develop in experimentally infected dogs are consistent with early membranoproliferative glomerulonephritis and minimal-change glomerulopathy.[31] Myelofibrosis is noted in some dogs with chronic-phase disease.

Diagnostic Plan

Definitive diagnosis of ehrlichiosis requires documentation of morulae in cells, but this occurs only rarely with *E. canis* (Fig. 37–1). Morulae are more commonly noted with the granulocytic strains, particularly in joint fluid and cerebrospinal fluid.[21] Evaluation of buffy coat smears or blood smears made from peripheral blood obtained from an ear vein may be more sensitive for the demonstration of *E. canis* morulae than peripheral blood collected from a central vein. *E. canis* can also be identified in infected dogs by inoculation of blood into susceptible dogs or by cell culture. Polymerase chain reaction can be used to detect organism-specific DNA in peripheral blood leukocytes. Polymerase chain reaction is available in some commercial laboratories (Southwest Veterinary Diagnostic Laboratory, Phoenix, Arizona). Studies correlating polymerase chain reaction results with serologic results and clinical response with therapy are ongoing (Russell Greene, personal communication, 1994).

Most cases of ehrlichiosis are diagnosed by serologic testing. Circulating antibodies against *E. canis* are detected in serum by IFA, ELISA, and Western blot immunoassay.[15, 32–34] The IFA is used by most commercial laboratories. *Ehrlichia* morulae are grown in

cell culture and coated onto IFA slides. Specific IFA slides are available for *E. equi*, *E. risticii*, *E. canis*, and *E. platys*. Some dogs infected with one species of *Ehrlichia* produce antibodies that bind to morulae from other species.[32–34] Thus, a dog seropositive for *E. canis* may actually have been infected by another ehrlichial agent. Dogs infected with *E. canis* produce antibodies with little or no cross-reaction with *R. rickettsii* or *E. platys* antigens, so specific tests must be requested for these agents.[15]

The most commonly used IFA detects IgG antibodies against *E. canis*. Antibodies can be detected as early as 7 days after experimental inoculation with *E. canis* and are usually positive by 20 days after inoculation. Antibody titers continue to increase for weeks to months after inoculation in untreated, experimentally infected dogs.[35] An *E. canis* titer of 1:10 is suspect and should be rechecked in approximately 21 days, whereas a titer of 1:20 or higher is considered diagnostic in many laboratories. Check with the reference laboratory used for titers considered significant. Because most dogs infected with *E. canis* ultimately have chronic-phase disease, all seropositive dogs should be treated even if currently subclinically affected. Titers remain increased in most untreated dogs, with the titer magnitude closely correlating with duration of infection. Positive antibody titers have been detected for up to 31 months after therapy in some naturally infected dogs.[36] Dogs with antibody titers less than 1:1024 generally revert to negative within 1 year following therapy. Dogs with antibody titers greater than 1:1024 often maintain positive antibody titers after therapy.[37] Whether these dogs are persistent carriers of the organism is undetermined.

Treatment and Prognosis

Intravenous fluid therapy is usually indicated for anorectic animals or those with vomiting or diarrhea. Tetracyclines are the primary treatment for canine ehrlichiosis. Tetracycline should be administered at a dosage of 22 mg/kg by mouth, t.i.d., for at least 14 to 21 days. Oxytetracycline is available for intravenous administration to anorectic or vomiting patients using a similar dosing schedule. The most common significant side effects of the tetracyclines include gastrointestinal irritation and induction of fever. Tetracyclines can lead to dental discoloration if used in young animals before permanent dentition eruption. Variable gastrointestinal absorption occurs with the tetracyclines. Doxycycline is a synthetic tetracycline derivative that is more fat soluble than tetracycline and leads to less gastrointestinal irritation. The greater fat solubility results in improved absorption by the gastrointestinal tract and greater penetration across the blood-brain barrier. Therefore, this drug may be superior to tetracycline for the treatment of rickettsial infections causing central nervous system signs. Doxycycline is given at a dosage of 5 mg/kg by mouth, b.i.d., for at least 14 days for the treatment of acute phase canine ehrlichiosis. In chronic cases, a dosage of 5 mg/kg by mouth, b.i.d., for at least 21 to 28 days is indicated. In some dogs treated for 21 days, ehrlichial DNA can still be detected in peripheral blood leukocytes by polymerase chain reaction (Russell Greene, personal communication, 1994). Whether this indicates incomplete clearance of the organism is being studied. Chloramphenicol administered at a dosage of 25 mg/kg by mouth, t.i.d., for 14 to 21 days has been used successfully to control the clinical signs of *E. canis* infection in dogs.

The prognosis is good for acute ehrlichiosis and variable to guarded for chronic ehrlichiosis. In acute ehrlichiosis, fever, petechiation, vomiting, diarrhea, epistaxis, and thrombocytopenia often resolve within days after initiation of therapy. The bone marrow suppression that often occurs secondary to chronic-phase ehrlichiosis may not respond for weeks to months after therapy, if at all. In general, the degree of improvement noted by 120 days after therapy reflects maximal response. Secondary myelofibrosis due to chronic ehrlichiosis is likely irreversible. Bone marrow suppression associated with chronic-phase ehrlichiosis occasionally results in a nonregenerative anemia severe enough to require blood transfusion. Anabolic steroids can be administered in an attempt to support or stimulate erythropoiesis, but the results have been disappointing.

Because the pathogenesis of ehrlichiosis may include immune-mediated events leading to the destruction of red blood cells or thrombocytes, some authors have advocated the administration of immunosuppressive doses of corticosteroids to acutely affected animals.[15] Prednisone administered at a dosage of 1.0 mg/kg by mouth, b.i.d., during the first 3 to 4 days after diagnosis may be beneficial in some cases. Generally, this therapy should be reserved for dogs showing initially poor response to tetracycline therapy alone or those in which phagocytosis of red blood cells or platelets has been demonstrated on cytologic evaluation of bone marrow aspiration. Vincristine administered at a dosage of 0.01 mg/kg intravenously, weekly, has been used to stimulate bone marrow release of platelets in severely thrombocytopenic animals. This therapy is unlikely to be effective if megakaryocytic hypoplasia is detected on cytologic evaluation of bone marrow aspirates.

Prevention

Dogs with ehrlichiosis are subject to reinfection. The organism is not passed transovarially in the tick and thus can be eliminated in the environment by tick control or by treating all dogs through a generation of ticks. If tick control is not feasible, tetracycline should be administered at a dosage of 6.6 mg/kg by mouth, daily, for at least 200 days. Blood donors should be screened serologically yearly or should be splenectomized.

Zoonotic Aspects

The cause of human ehrlichiosis in the United States was recently shown to be *E. chaffeensis*, a species separate from *E. canis*.[22] Dogs can be experimentally infected with *E. chaffeensis* and so may be a reservoir for this agent.[38] The vector has not been identified. A granulocytic strain of *Ehrlichia* has been detected in some humans in the United States.[39] Zoonotic information is lacking.

Salmon Poisoning

Pathophysiology

Etiology. Salmon disease complex is caused by *Neorickettsia helminthoeca* (salmon poisoning) and *N. elokominica* (Elokomin fluke fever), gram-negative bacteria in the family Rickettsiaceae.[40–42] These two rickettsia are probably strain variants of the same organism. Mixed infections with both organisms in the same host are common. Both *Neorickettsia* species are primary parasites of the fluke *Nanophyetus salmincola*.

Epidemiology. *Nanophyetus salmincola* is a three-host trematode. *Neorickettsia helminthoeca* and *N. elokominica* survive in the fluke through all development stages from egg to adult. The first intermediate host of the fluke is *Oxytrema silicula*, a snail that lives in fresh or brackish waters. The snail determines the geographic range of the canine disease. Clinical disease in dogs has been identified from northwestern California to southwestern Washington.[40, 41] Several cases have been identified in southern Vancouver Island, Canada.[43] Cercaria of *Nanophyetus* are released from infected snails, infecting salmonid fish, some nonsalmonid fish, and Pacific giant salamanders. *Neorickettsia*-infected metacercaria develop in many tissues of the second intermediate host but concentrate in renal tissues. Fish are infected by the fluke in fresh water, and both the fluke and the *Neorickettsia* survive in tissues for as long as 3 years. The fluke life cycle is completed by the passage of eggs in feces, when tissues of the second intermediate host are ingested by dogs, coyotes, bears, raccoons, and some birds. During completion of the fluke life cycle, the *Neorickettsia* infect the definitive host. Clinical disease has been recognized almost exclusively in dogs. Other natural modes of transmission are unknown, but the organism can be transmitted by blood transfusion.

Pathogenesis. *Neorickettsia* spp. invade intestinal epithelial cells of infected dogs and replicate in intestinal lymph tissue, leading to diarrhea.[41] The organism then disseminates in blood, with further replication in the spleen, thymus, lungs, brain, and other lymph tissues. Polysystemic clinical signs of disease are related to organism replication and resultant immune responses against the organism. Ova of *Nanophyetus* develop 5 to 8 days after ingestion of infected fish. The intestinal phase of the fluke can also cause mild enteritis.[41]

Clinical Signs

Any previously unexposed dog is susceptible to infection by both species of *Neorickettsia*. Whereas infection by *N. helminthoeca* and *N. elokominica* results in similar clinical syndromes in dogs, clinical illness is more severe with *N. helminthoeca*. Following an incubation period of 5 to 7 days, infected dogs develop fever of 40°C to 42°C (104.0°F–107.6°F) and anorexia.[40, 41] Small-bowel diarrhea begins at approximately the time of peak fever and ultimately consists of pure blood in many fatal cases. Vomiting usually occurs. Ocular discharge that progresses from serous to mucopurulent is common, and lymphadenopathy develops in most dogs. Secondary clinical syndromes include dehydration and depression. Death commonly occurs in 7 to 10 days after initial onset of clinical signs of disease. The combination of ocular discharge and severe gastrointestinal disease makes the differentiation of salmon poisoning from distemper virus infection and canine parvovirus infection difficult. The prognosis is guarded to good for treated dogs.

Clinical Laboratory Abnormalities. Neutropenia develops during peracute infection; neutrophilic leukocytosis is common in later stages. Acute lymphopenia is also common, with lymphocytosis predominating several days after onset of clinical signs.[41, 44] Severe anemia develops in some dogs because of gastrointestinal blood loss. Serum biochemical abnormalities are consistent with dehydration and gastrointestinal losses of sodium, chloride, and potassium. Whereas rickettsial bodies are almost never identified in circulating leukocytes, Giemsa-stained smears of lymph node aspirates often reveal single or multiple purple-staining rickettsial bodies within the cytoplasm of mononuclear cells.[45] Cytologic examination of lymph node aspirates is consistent with lymph node hyperplasia.

Fluke eggs are pointed at one end and have a distinct operculum at the other. Because of their density, the eggs often do not float in salt solutions with low specific gravity. Eggs are most commonly identified by direct smear, sugar (specific gravity 1.27) or sodium nitrate (specific gravity 1.33) flotation, or fecal sedimentation.

Pathology

Gross pathologic findings include generalized lymphadenopathy and hemorrhagic gastroenteritis. Lymph nodes are yellow, with cortical follicular hyperplasia. Other lymphoreticular organs, including the liver and spleen, show evidence of lymphoid hyperplasia. Histopathologic evaluation of lymph tissue reveals depletion of mature lymphocytes, hyperplasia of reticuloendothelial cells, and multiple purple-staining (Giemsa) coccoid or coccobacillary organisms in reticuloendothelial cells. If meningitis or meningoencephalitis occurs, the cellular infiltrates are generally mononuclear.[41, 46]

Diagnostic Plan

Clinical diagnosis is based on history of ingestion of potential intermediate hosts, clinical signs of disease, and documentation of fluke eggs in feces, combined with response to antirickettsial drugs. Definitive diagnosis can be made by documenting rickettsial bodies in lymphocytes and monocytes from lymph node aspiration or by laboratory animal inoculation. Complement fixation and Western blot immunoassay have been evaluated for detection of serum antibodies against *Neorickettsia helminthoeca* and *N. elokominica* but are not available for routine clinical use.[33, 47]

Treatment and Prognosis

Supportive care for severe hemorrhagic gastroenteritis, including intravenous fluid therapy and electrolyte therapy, is usually required. Therapeutic protocols are similar to those used for canine parvovirus infection (see Chap. 32). Tetracycline or its synthetic derivatives are the antibiotics of choice. Chloramphenicol and sulfonamides are alternative drugs. Intravenous therapy with oxytetracycline (7 mg/kg t.i.d.) or chloramphenicol (25 mg/kg three or four times per day) is usually required for the first several days because of vomiting. Oral therapy using tetracycline, doxycycline, or chloramphenicol at doses described for ehrlichiosis is generally continued for a minimum of 5 days. *Nanophyetus salmincola* infection can be treated with praziquantel administered at a dosage of 10 to 20 mg/kg by mouth or subcutaneously once. Alternatively, fenbendazole can be administered at a dosage of 50 mg/kg by mouth, daily, for 10 to 14 days or until trematode eggs are no longer present in feces.

Prevention

Vaccines are not available for salmon poisoning. Prevention is achieved primarily by avoiding ingestion of infected intermediate hosts. If fish products from appropriate geographic areas are to be fed to dogs, they should first be frozen at −20°C (−4°F) for 24 hours or thoroughly cooked to inactivate the rickettsia and fluke. Recovered animals are unlikely to develop clinical illness from *Neorickettsia* on second exposure but can be reinfected by *Nanophyetus*.

Zoonotic Aspects

There is no known zoonotic health risk.

References

1. Greene CE, Breitschwerdt EB. Rocky Mountain spotted fever and Q fever. In Greene CE, ed. Infectious Diseases of the Dog and Cat, 2nd ed. Philadelphia, WB Saunders, 1990:419–433.
2. Hibler SC, Hoskins JD, Greene, CE. Rickettsial infections in dogs part 1. Rocky Mountain spotted fever and *Coxiella* infections. Compen Contin Educ Pract Vet 1985; 7:856–865.
3. Greene CE. Rocky Mountain spotted fever. J Am Vet Med Assoc 1987;191:666–671.
4. McDade JE, Newhouse VF. Natural history of *Rickettsia rickettsii*. Annu Rev Microbiol 1986;40:287–309.
5. Norment BR, Burgdorfer W. Susceptibility and reservoir potential of the dog to spotted fever-group rickettsiae. Am J Vet Res 1984;45:1706–1710.
6. Helmick CG, Bernard KW, D'Angelo LJ. Rocky Mountain spotted fever: Clinical, laboratory, and epidemiological features of 262 cases. J Infect Dis 1984;150:480–488.
7. Davidson MG, Breitschwerdt EB, Walker DH, et al. Vascular permeability and coagulation during *Rickettsia rickettsii* infection in dogs. Am J Vet Res 1990;51:165–170.
8. Davidson MG, Breitschwerdt EB, Naisse MP, et al. Ocular manifestations of Rocky Mountain spotted fever in dogs. J Am Vet Med Assoc 1989;194:777–781.
9. Weiser IB, Greene CE. Dermal necrosis associated with Rocky Mountain spotted fever in four dogs. J Am Vet Med Assoc 1989;195:1756–1758.
10. Greene CE, Burgdorfer W, Cavagnolo R, et al. Rocky Mountain spotted fever in dogs and its differentiation from canine ehrlichiosis. J Am Vet Med Assoc 1985;186: 465–472.
11. Davidson MG, Breitschwerdt EB, Walker DH, et al. Identification of Rickettsiae in cutaneous biopsy specimens from dogs with experimental Rocky Mountain spotted fever. J Vet Intern Med 1989;3:8–11.
12. Greene CE, Marks MA, Lappin MR, et al. Comparison of latex agglutination, indirect immunofluorescent antibody, and enzyme immunoassay methods for serodiagnosis of Rocky Mountain spotted fever in dogs. Am J Vet Res 1993;54:20–28.
13. Breitschwerdt EB. Laboratory diagnosis of tick-transmitted diseases in the dog. In: Kirk RW, Bonagura JD, eds. Current Veterinary Therapy XI. Philadelphia, WB Saunders, 1992:252–255.
14. Breitschwerdt EB, Davidson MG, Aucoin DP, et al. Efficacy of chloramphenicol, enrofloxacin, and tetracycline for treatment of experimental Rocky Mountain spotted fever in dogs. Antimicrob Agents Chemother 1991;35:2375–2381.
15. Troy GC, Forrester SD. Canine Ehrlichiosis. In: Greene CE, ed. Infectious Diseases of the Dog and Cat, 2nd ed. Philadelphia, WB Saunders, 1990:404–418.
16. Hibler SC, Hoskins JD, Greene CE. Rickettsial infections in dogs part II. Ehrlichiosis and infectious cyclic thrombocytopenia. Compen Contin Educ Pract Vet 1986; 8:106–114.
17. Lewis GE, Huxsoll DL, Ristic M, et al. Experimentally induced infection of dogs, cats, and nonhuman primates with *Ehrlichia equi*, etiologic agent of equine ehrlichiosis. J Am Vet Med Assoc 1975;36:85–88.
18. Ristic M, Dawson J, Holland CJ, et al. Susceptibility of dogs to infection with *Ehrlichia risticii*, causative agent of equine monocytic ehrlichiosis (Potomac horse fever). Am J Vet Res 1988;49:1497–1500.
19. Kakoma I, Hansen R, Lui L, et al. Serologically atypical canine ehrlichiosis associated with *Ehrlichia risticii* "infection." J Am Vet Med Assoc 1991;199:1120.
20. Anderson BE, et al. *Ehrlichia ewingii* sp. nov., the etiologic agent of canine granulocytic ehrlichiosis. Int J Syst Bacteriol 1992;42:299–302.
21. Maretzki CH, Fisher DJ, Greene CE. Granulocytic ehrlichiosis and meningitis in a dog. J Am Vet Med Assoc 1994;205:1554–1556.
22. Anderson BE, et al. *Ehrlichia chaffeensis*, a new species associated with human ehrlichiosis. J Clin Microbiol 1991;29:2838–2842.
23. Buoro IBJ, Atwell RB, Kiptoon J, et al. Feline anaemia associated with ehrlichia-like bodies in three domestic short-haired cats. Vet Rec 1989;125:434–436.
24. Charpentier F, Groulade P. Probable case of ehrlichiosis in a cat. Bull Academ Vet Fr 1986;59:287–290.
25. Bouloy RP, Lappin MR, Holland CH, et al. Clinical ehrlichiosis in a cat. J Am Vet Med Assoc 1994;204:1475–1478.
26. Hoskins JD, Breitschwerdt EB, Gaunt SD, et al. Antibodies to *Ehrlichia canis*, *Ehrlichia platys*, and spotted fever group *Rickettsia* in Louisiana dogs. J Vet Intern Med 1988;2:55–59.
27. Codner EC, Farris-Smith LL. Characterization of the subclinical phase of ehrlichiosis in dogs. J Am Vet Med Assoc 1986;189:47–50.
28. Stockham SL, Schmidt DA, Curtis KS, et al. Evaluation of granulocytic ehrlichiosis in dogs of Missouri, including serologic status to *Ehrlichia canis*, *Ehrlichia equi*, and *Borrelia burgdorferi*. Am J Vet Res 1992;53:63–68.
29. Weiser MG, Thrall MA, Fulton R, et al. Granular lymphocytosis and hyperproteinemia in dogs with chronic ehrlichiosis. J Am Anim Hosp Assoc 1991;27:84–88.
30. Breischtwerdt EB, Woody BJ, Zerbe CA, et al. Monoclonal gammopathy associated with naturally occurring canine ehrlichiosis. J Vet Intern Med 1987;1:2–9.
31. Codner EC, Caceci T, Saunders GK, et al. Investigation of

glomerular lesions in dogs with acute experimentally induced *Ehrlichia canis* infection. Am J Vet Res 1992;53: 2286–2291.

32. Brouqui P, Dumler JS, Raoult D, et al. Antigenic characterization of ehrlichia: Protein immunoblotting of *Ehrlichia canis, Ehrlichia sennetsu,* and *Ehrlichia risticii.* J Clin Microbiol 1992;30:1062–1066.

33. Rikihisa Y. Cross-reacting antigens between *Neorickettsia helminthoeca* and *Ehrlichia* species, shown by immunofluorescence and Western immunoblotting. J Clin Microbiol 1991;29:2024–2029.

34. Shankarappa B, Dutta SK, Mattingly-Napier BL. Antigenic and genomic relatedness among *Ehrlichia risticii, Ehrlichia sennetsu,* and *Ehrlichia canis.* Int J Syst Bacteriol 1992;42:127–132.

35. Buhles WC, Huxsoll DL, Ristic M. Tropical canine pancytopenia: Clinical, hematologic, and serologic responses of dogs to *Ehrlichia canis* infection, tetracycline therapy, and challenge inoculation. J Infect Dis 1974;130: 357–367.

36. Perille AL, Matus RE. Canine ehrlichiosis in six dogs with persistently increased antibody titers. J Vet Intern Med 1991;5:195–198.

37. Greene RT, Bartsch RC. Antibody titers after treatment in canine ehrlichiosis. Proceedings of the 11th Annual Veterinary Medical Forum, American College of Veterinary Internal Medicine, Washington, DC, May 1993:951.

38. Dawson JE, Ewing SA. Susceptibility of dogs to infection with *Ehrlichia chaffeensis,* causative agent of human ehrlichiosis. Am J Vet Res 1992;53:1322–1327.

39. Chen SM, Dumler JS, Bakken JS, et al. Identification of a granulocytic *Ehrlichia* species as the etiologic agent of human disease. J Clin Microbiol 1994;32:589–595.

40. Hibler SC, Hoskins JD, Greene CE. Rickettsial infections in dogs part III. Salmon disease complex and Haemobartonellosis. Compen Contin Educ Pract Vet 1986; 8:251–256.

41. Gorham JR, Foreyt WJ. Salmon poisoning disease. In: Greene CE, ed. Infectious Diseases of the Dog and Cat, 2nd ed. Philadelphia, WB Saunders, 1990:397–403.

42. Campbell RSF. Pathogenesis and pathology of the complex rickettsial infections. Vet Bull 1994;64:1–24.

43. Booth AJ, Stogdale L, Grigor JA. Salmon poisoning disease in dogs on southern Vancouver Island. Can Vet J 1984;25:2–6.

44. Schalm OW. Leukocyte counts and lymph node cytology in salmon poisoning of dogs. Canine Pract 1978;5:59–63.

45. Farrell RK, Ott RL, Gorham JR. The clinical laboratory diagnosis of salmon poisoning. J Am Vet Med Assoc 1955;127:241–244.

46. Hadlow WJ. Neuropathology of experimental salmon poisoning in dogs. Am J Vet Res 1957;18:898–908.

47. Sakawa H, Farrel RK, Mori M. Differentiation of salmon poisoning disease and Elokomin fluke fever: Complement fixation. Am J Vet Res 1973;34:923–925.

Chapter 38

Viral Diseases

Michael R. Lappin

Canine Distemper Virus

Pathophysiology

Etiology. Canine distemper virus (CDV) is in the family Paramyxoviridae, genus *Morbillivirus*.[1, 2] This single-stranded RNA virus is closely related to the human measles virus. The virus has a lipoprotein envelope and is capable of incorporating into the host cell membrane. The natural disease occurs predominantly in terrestrial carnivores. Disease due to canine distemper virus or a similar virus occurs in other species, including seals, ferrets, porpoises, exotic Felidae, and a nonhuman primate.[1, 2] Experimentally inoculated domestic cats contract subclinical, self-limited infection.

Epidemiology. The virus is shed in respiratory exudates, feces, saliva, urine, and conjunctival exudates for up to 60 to 90 days after natural infection. The principal route of transmission is from aerosolization of respiratory exudates.[1, 2] There are multiple field strains of the virus with different degrees of pathogenicity.[1-3] Up to 75% of infected dogs are estimated to have subclinical, self-limited infection.[1] Clinical illness is most common in puppies between 3 and 6 months of age. However, nonimmune dogs of any age are susceptible. The virus is maintained in nature by transfer from infected to susceptible dogs.[1, 2]

Pathogenesis. The virus is lymphotropic, neurotropic, and epitheliotropic. After aerosol transmission to the respiratory epithelium, the virus is engulfed by macrophages. Within 24 hours, it is carried by lymphatics to tonsillar, pharyngeal, and bronchial lymph nodes. Viral numbers increase over the next 2 to 6 days while being disseminated to other lymphoid organs, including the spleen, Kupffer cells of the liver, lamina propria of the stomach and small intestine, and mesenteric lymph nodes. Spread to central nervous system (CNS) and epithelial tissue occurs hematogenously from 8 to 14 days after infection.[1, 2, 4] This stage of infection is dependent on the degree of humoral and cell-mediated immune responses (Fig. 38–1).

Fever and leukopenia characterized by lymphopenia occur during the initial replication in lymphoid tissues. Animals with virus-neutralizing antibody titers less than 1:100 by day 14 after infection have massive viral replication in the epithelial cells of the respiratory tract, gastrointestinal system, and genitourinary system and usually die of polysystemic

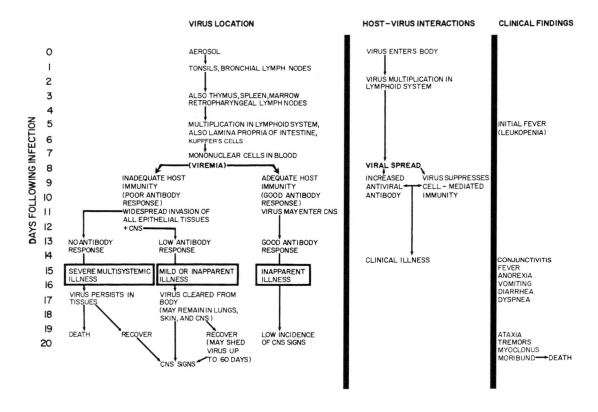

Figure 38–1

Pathogenesis of canine distemper virus infection. (From Greene CE, Appel MJ. Canine distemper. In: Greene CE, ed. Infectious Diseases of the Dog and Cat, 2nd ed. Philadelphia, WB Saunders, 1990:228.)

Table 38–1
Clinical Manifestations of Canine Distemper Virus Infection

In Utero Infection
Stillbirth
Abortion
Fading puppy syndrome in the neonatal period
Central nervous system signs at birth

Polysystemic Disease

Gastrointestinal tract disease	Vomiting
	Small-bowel diarrhea
Respiratory tract	Mucoid to mucopurulent nasal discharge
	Sneezing
	Coughing with increased bronchovesicular sounds or crackles on auscultation
	Dyspnea
Miscellaneous	Fever
	Anorexia
	Tonsillar enlargement
	Dehydration
	Pustular dermatosis
	Hyperkeratosis of the nose and footpads
	Enamel hypoplasia in surviving puppies
	Retinochoroiditis, medallion lesions, optic neuritis
	Keratoconjunctivitis sicca
	Mucopurulent ocular discharge

Neurologic Disease

Spinal cord disease	Paresis and ataxia
Central vestibular disease	Head tilt, nystagmus, other cranial nerve and conscious proprioception deficits
Cerebellar disease	Ataxia, head bobbing, hypermetria
Cerebral disease	Generalized or partial seizures (chewing gum fits)
	Depression
	Unilateral or bilateral blindness
Chorea myoclonus	Rhythmic jerking of single muscles or muscle groups

disease.[1, 4] Animals with virus-neutralizing antibody titers greater than 1:100 clear the virus from most tissues and may not be clinically affected. Potential for clinical illness also varies depending on the age of the infected dog and the strain of the virus.

CNS infection probably occurs in most infected dogs but is most commonly associated with clinical signs in dogs with low or no antibody responses to envelope proteins.[2] The CNS is thought to be infected by free virus or cell-associated virus at the vascular endothelial cells of the meninges, choroid plexus epithelial cells of the fourth ventricle, and ependymal cells lining the ventricular system.[2, 5] Acute demyelination results from restrictive infection of oligodendrogliocytes and subsequent necrosis.[5] Chronic demyelination develops in dogs surviving acute encephalitis. Immune-mediated mechanisms, including antimyelin antibodies[2] and macrophage-induced disease secondary to CDV immune complexes,[5] appear to induce the demyelination associated with CDV infection. These immune-mediated events seem to develop during virus clearance.[5] The pathogenesis of old dog encephalitis, a chronic progressive panencephalitis in dogs older than 6 years of age, is unknown but results in microglial proliferation and neuronal degeneration in the cerebral cortex.[1]

Clinical Signs

Clinically affected dogs tend to be puppies between 3 and 6 months of age, but any nonimmune dog is susceptible (Table 38–1). Affected dogs tend to be unvaccinated, have not received colostrum from an immune bitch, have been inappropriately vaccinated, or have been immunosuppressed. History of exposure to infected animals (pet store, humane shelter, pound) is common. Clients most commonly present affected animals for evaluation of respiratory tract, gastrointestinal tract, or CNS signs of disease. Clinical signs of disease of the gastrointestinal and respiratory systems often are partially due to secondary bacterial disease but can result from viral disease alone.

Mild depression, malaise, oculonasal discharge, and cough are common in many partially immune dogs. Some dogs are presumptively diagnosed as having infectious tracheobronchitis. Dogs with poor immune responses generally progress rapidly from having mild upper respiratory signs and abnormalities noted on physical examination to anorexia, lethargy, dyspnea, abnormal lower respiratory sounds, vomiting, diarrhea, and CNS disease.[1, 2] Physical examination findings vary based on immune responses and virus virulence. Dehydration, tonsillar enlargement, increased bronchial sounds (including crackles and wheezes), depression, and mucopurulent oculonasal discharge are common. Ocular abnormalities include anterior uveitis, optic neuritis with resultant blindness and dilated pupils, and retinochoroiditis. Dogs with chronic infection can contract keratoconjunctivitis sicca and often have hyperreflective retinal scars called medallion lesions (see Fig. 19–8). Dogs infected before the development of permanent dentition will acquire enamel hypoplasia. Hyperkeratosis of the nose and foot pads and pustular dermatitis are common dermatologic abnormalities. Transplacentally infected puppies may be stillborn, aborted, or born with CNS disease or present as fading puppies.[1, 2, 6] Immune responses against CDV have been implicated as a cause of rheumatoid arthritis in dogs, but this problem is probably rare.[7] Cardiac necrosis occurs in puppies experimentally infected at 5 to 7 days of age but not in puppies infected at 10 or 21 days of age.[8]

CNS signs of CDV infection generally occur within 21 days after recovery from systemic disease but may not develop for months to years. Neurologic manifestations can be acute or chronic, are generally progressive, and are dependent on the areas of the CNS involved. Hyperesthesia, seizures, cerebellar or vestibular disease, paresis, and chorea myoclonus are common (see Table 38–1).[1, 2, 9, 10] Concurrent retinochoroiditis was detected in 9 of 22 dogs with encephalitis in one study.[10] Approximately 30% of dogs with CDV infection do not have recognizable systemic infection before the development of CNS disease.[9] Cerebral dysfunction characterized by depression, circling, head pressing, and visual deficits is common in dogs with old dog encephalitis, which may be caused by prior CDV infection.[1]

Laboratory Abnormalities. Lymphopenia and thrombocytopenia are consistent but nonspecific hematologic abnormalities associated with CDV infection.[1, 2, 11] Serum biochemical and urinalysis abnormalities are also nonspecific. Viral inclusions can sometimes be found in erythrocytes, leukocytes, and leukocyte precursors of infected dogs.[1, 2] Examination of thin smears made from buffy coat or bone marrow aspiration may be more likely to demonstrate inclusions than blood smears.[2] Mononuclear cell pleocytosis and increased protein levels are common cerebrospinal fluid (CSF) abnormalities; however, some dogs have normal CSF.[1, 2, 9, 10]

Radiographic and Electroencephalographic Abnormalities. Thoracic radiographic findings vary from those consistent with interstitial pneumonia to those consistent with bronchopneumonia (alveolar pattern) because of secondary bacterial invaders such as *Bordetella bronchiseptica.* Electroencephalograms show evidence of diffuse encephalitis but are not specific for CDV-induced disease.[2, 10]

Pathology

Thymic atrophy is a consistent finding in puppies infected in utero and in the immediate postnatal period. Inflammation of the lungs, eyes, intestines, airways, and nose is evident grossly in dogs with polysystemic disease. Hyperkeratosis of foot pads is noted in some dogs and most commonly is seen in dogs with CNS. disease. Gross lesions are variable in dogs with CNS disease but may include dilated ventricles and meningeal congestion. Characteristic histopathologic findings have been reviewed[2, 10, 12]; polioencephalopathy and leukoencephalomyelopathy are common. Nonsuppurative encephalomyelitis with segmental internodal primary demyelination is the characteristic finding in dogs with chronic encephalitis. Perivascular infiltrates of mononuclear cells develop over time (see Chap. 24).

Diagnostic Plan

Definitive diagnosis of canine distemper virus infection requires demonstration of viral inclusions by cytologic examination, direct fluorescent antibody staining of cytologic or histopathologic specimens, or histopathologic evaluation. Immunohistochemical documentation of CDV antigen in tissues was superior to histopathologic examination for inclusion bodies in one study.[13] In acute canine distemper, immunofluorescence of epithelial cells from the tonsils, respiratory tree, or urinary tract or conjunctiva scrapings and cells from the cerebrospinal fluid can document infection.[1, 2, 14, 15] Fluorescence can be detected 5 to 21 days after infection. Antigen is present in buffy coat smears for only 2 to 9 days after infection; therefore, inclusions are often inapparent when clinical signs occur.[2]

A presumptive diagnosis of polysystemic CDV infection can be made on the basis of appropriate signalment (young age), history (nonvaccinated, appropriate exposure, immunosuppression), and physical examination findings. CSF and serum immunoglobulin (Ig) antibodies against canine distemper virus can be measured by serum virus neutralization, immunofluorescence assay (IFA), or enzyme-linked immunosorbent assay (ELISA).[2] Serum IgM antibodies can be measured by ELISA.[16, 17] Detection of serum IgG antibodies is of minimal diagnostic value because a positive titer could develop secondary to vaccination or previous exposure. A fourfold increase in serum IgG titer over a 3 to 4 week period is suggestive of recent infection or recent vaccination. Detection of IgM antibodies in serum is consistent with recent infection or recent vaccination but not clinical disease.[16, 17]

CSF antibodies to CDV are increased in some dogs subsequently diagnosed by histopathologic examination as having distemper encephalitis.[1, 2, 7, 9, 10, 12] False-positive results can occur in CSF samples contaminated with blood. Concurrent measurement of serum antibody levels can be helpful; if CSF levels are greater than serum levels, the antibody in CSF had to have been produced locally and is consistent with CNS distemper virus infection. A presumptive diagnosis of CDV encephalitis can be made if increased CSF protein and lymphocytic pleocytosis are present with CSF antibodies against CDV in a sample not contaminated with peripheral blood.

Treatment and Prognosis

Treatment for canine distemper virus infection is nonspecific. In dogs with polysystemic signs of disease, dehydration should be managed and secondary infections treated with broad-spectrum antibiotics. Because *B. bronchiseptica* is a common secondary invader, antibiotics should be those with known anti-*Bordetella* activity, such as tetracycline derivatives, chloramphenicol, enrofloxacin, and clindamycin. Tetracyclines and enrofloxacin should be avoided in puppies.

Anticonvulsants are administered as needed to control seizures (see Chap. 24). There is no known effective treatment for chorea myoclonus. Glucocorticoids are administered to some dogs with CNS disease from CDV infection but are contraindicated in acutely infected dogs because of the potential for virus activation. The prognosis is poor for dogs with CNS distemper.

Prevention

The CDV cannot survive for long periods in the environment. It probably survives in exudates for only approximately 20 minutes. The virus is susceptible to most routine hospital disinfections, including 0.3% quaternary ammonium compounds and 0.75% phenolics. In-house hospital prevention should include routine disinfection and isolation of clinically ill dogs to avoid aerosolization to susceptible populations.[1, 2]

Vaccination against CDV can result in long-term immunity. All animals should receive at least two immunizations at a time when they can respond (i.e., after maternal immunity has waned) because one immunization provides immunity for only 10 months.[2] Modified live vaccines should be used; killed products are not as effective. Immunity wanes with time, so yearly boosters are indicated. Vaccination is not as effective if the body temperature is 39.8°C (103.8°F) or greater. The use of modified live CDV vaccines is questionable in immunosuppressed animals, especially those with suspected parvovirus infection, because of possible vaccine-associated encephalitis.[18] Puppies should be vaccinated at 6 to 8 weeks of age and receive boosters every 3 weeks until at least 14 weeks of age.[19]

Maternal antibodies against CDV can block the effect of CDV vaccination. Measles virus vaccines are available to induce heterologous antibodies and protect puppies against CDV as maternal antibodies wane. Measles vaccine should not be given before 6 weeks or after 12 weeks of age. Measles vaccination can be given concurrently with modified live distemper vaccine. At least two distemper boosters should be given after the initial measles vaccine.

CNS disease attributed to CDV infection has occurred in some vaccinated dogs.[1, 2, 20, 21] Rarely, disease has been attributed to modified live virus vaccination.[18, 22, 23] Clinical disease in vaccinated dogs may also develop if the host was immunocompromised, infected with the virus before vaccination, had vaccine-suppressive levels of maternal antibodies, or was incompletely vaccinated.[1, 2] Alternatively, the vaccine may have been inactivated by improper handling or may not have protected against all field strains of CDV. Distemper virus encephalitis has developed after modified live vaccination of dogs coinfected with canine parvovirus.[18] Although the incidence of this phenomenon in the field is unknown, administration of modified live CDV vaccines should be delayed in dogs showing clinical signs of disease consistent with parvovirus infection. Thrombocytopenia is associated with canine distemper virus infection as well as with modified CDV vaccination.[11, 23] Although petechial hemorrhage and other clinical signs of bleeding are rare, routine surgery should be delayed for at least 21 days after vaccination.

Zoonotic Aspects

There is no direct evidence that dogs infected with CDV are a public health risk. Multiple sclerosis[2, 24] and Paget disease[25] in people have been epidemiologally linked to dog ownership. However, it now appears that multiple sclerosis is not associated with the canine paramyxovirus.[26]

Infectious Canine Hepatitis

Pathophysiology

Etiology. Infectious canine hepatitis is caused by canine adenovirus-1 (CAV-1), a DNA virus with

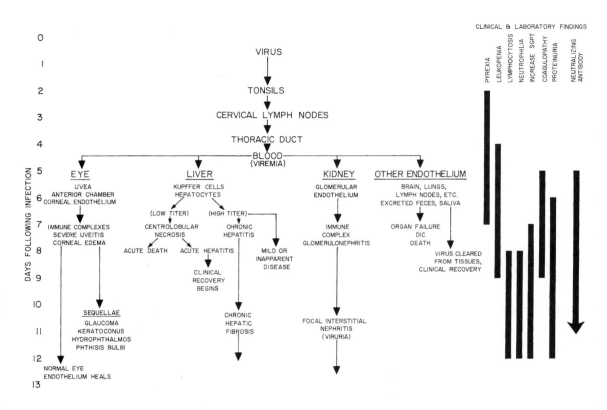

Figure 38–2

Pathogenesis of canine adenovirus-1 infection. The solid vertical bars at the right margin correspond to the chronologic occurrence and the duration of the respective clinical or laboratory findings associated with canine adenovirus-1 infection. (From Greene CE. Infectious canine hepatitis and canine acidophil cell hepatitis. In: Greene CE, ed. Infectious Diseases of the Dog and Cat, 2nd ed. Philadelphia, WB Saunders, 1990:243.)

worldwide distribution. The organism is distinct from CAV-2, a virus resulting in upper respiratory clinical signs of disease.[27] Dogs infected with CAV-2 commonly acquire a clinical respiratory syndrome consistent with infectious tracheobronchitis.

Epidemiology. CAV-1 causes clinical disease in Canidae and Ursidae.[28] Seroprevalence studies suggest that the organism is widespread in the dog population. During the acute stage of the disease, the organism is passed in all body secretions. The organism is isolated to the kidneys by 10 to 14 days after infection and is passed in urine of infected dogs for 6 to 9 months. Aerosol transmission does not seem to occur. Transmission is by direct contact with infected animals or contaminated fomites. The organism is environmentally resistant and survives for days to months under appropriate conditions.[28]

Pathogenesis. Pathogenesis of CAV-1 has been extensively detailed (Fig. 38–2). After oronasal exposure, the virus localizes in the tonsils and spreads to the blood stream via local lymphatics and the thoracic ducts. The organism preferentially replicates in endothelial cells and hepatic parenchymal cells, leading to vasculitis and hepatitis, respectively. Vasculitis results in petechial hemorrhages noted on physical examination and necropsy. During the viremic stage (4–8 days), the organism is shed in urine, saliva, and feces. In animals that survive viremia, the organism is localized to the kidneys and shed in urine. Clinical signs of disease are primarily due to tissue damage related to virus replication. Dogs with poor humoral immunity generally die from centrilobular to panlobular hepatic necrosis.[28, 29] Dogs with partial humoral immunity contract chronic active hepatitis and hepatic fibrosis. Dogs with sufficient humoral immunity are generally subclinically infected. Although the virus is harbored in renal tissues for months, chronic renal insufficiency does not occur as a result of infection.[30] Corneal edema and uveitis develop initially due to replication of the virus in corneal endothelial cells and then are potentiated by deposition of immune complexes. Complications secondary to infection include predisposition to pyelonephritis, disseminated intravascular coagulation secondary to vasculitis, hepatic insufficiency secondary to hepatitis, and glaucoma secondary to uveitis.[28]

Clinical Signs

Dogs of any age, breed, or sex can be infected by CAV-1 if not previously exposed or vaccinated. Clinical disease is recognized most commonly in puppies because of lack of prior exposure. Clinically affected puppies generally have a history of exposure to other dogs. Disease syndromes can be peracute or acute. Peracutely affected dogs can die within hours of infection. Clinical signs of acutely infected dogs include vomiting; diarrhea; depression; anorexia; coughing; petechial or ecchymotic hemorrhage; epistaxis; abdominal distension; and CNS signs, including seizures, depression, and coma.[28] Physical examination abnormalities include fever, hepatomegaly, cervical lymphadenopathy, tonsillar hyperemia and enlargement, subcutaneous edema, abdominal pain, petechial or ecchymotic hemorrhage, crackles or wheezes in the pulmonary parenchyma due to pneumonia, epistaxis, and depression. Ocular manifestations generally develop during the recovery phase of acute infection. Corneal edema, ocular pain manifested by blepharospasm and photophobia, and secondary corneal ulceration or glaucoma are common.

Laboratory and Radiographic Abnormalities. Although not pathognomonic for CAV-1 infection, multiple clinical pathologic abnormalities occur during acute infection (Table 38–2). Radiographic abnormalities can include hepatomegaly, loss of abdominal detail from abdominal effusion, and both interstitial and alveolar lung patterns.

Pathology

Dogs with acute infectious canine hepatitis have multiple gross necropsy abnormalities.[28] Subcutaneous edema and diffuse hemorrhage of serosal surfaces and superficial lymph nodes are common findings. The liver is generally enlarged, dark, mottled in appearance, and coated with a fibrinous exudate. Serosanguineous fluid and fibrin tags are commonly found in the abdominal cavity. Splenomegaly and intraluminal gastrointestinal hemorrhage are common. Multifocal hemorrhagic renal cortical infarcts and multiple areas of pulmonary consolidation are frequently found. Hemorrhage of CNS tissues is occasionally noted.

Table 38–2
Clinical Pathologic Abnormalities Associated With Canine Adenovirus-1 Infection in Dogs

PARAMETER	ABNORMALITY
Hematology	
Acute phase	Neutropenia
	Lymphopenia
	Thrombocytopenia
Recovery phase	Neutrophilia
	Lymphocytosis
Coagulogram	Thrombocytopenia
	Increased activated clotting time, prothrombin time, thrombin time due to disseminated intravascular coagulation or decreased hepatic synthesis of coagulation factors
	Increased fibrin degradation product because of disseminated intravascular coagulation
Biochemical panel	Variable increases in alanine aminotransferase and alkaline phosphatase activities dependent on sample timing. Activities generally decreased after 14 days unless chronic active hepatitis develops.
	Hyperbilirubinemia is rare
	Hypoglycemia in terminal phase
	Transient increase in α_2-globulins on serum electrophoresis
Urinalysis	Bilirubinuria
Abdominal paracentesis	
Acute phase	Exudate
Chronic active hepatitis	Transudate
Cerebrospinal fluid	Increased protein levels
	Mononuclear pleocytosis
Aqueous humor	Increased protein levels
	Increased inflammatory cells (predominantly neutrophils)

Data from Greene.[28]

Corneal opacity and cloudiness of the aqueous humor are common.

Chronic infectious canine hepatitis generally results in a small, firm, nodular liver. Chronic renal changes consist of small, white fibrotic foci that extend from the renal pelvis to the cortex. Ocular changes, including glaucoma and phthisis bulbi, occur with chronic inflammation. Histologic findings of infectious canine hepatitis have been reviewed.[28] The principal findings associated with acute hepatitis are centrilobular to panlobular necrosis; dogs with subacute to chronic hepatitis have sporadic foci of necrosis containing neutrophils, lymphocytes, and plasma cells.

Diagnostic Plan

Definitive diagnosis is made by detecting the virus in secretions, aqueous humor, CSF, or tissues by virus isolation, demonstration of characteristic viral inclusions, or immunofluorescent and immunoperoxidase techniques.[28, 31] A presumptive diagnosis can be made by combining clinical signs of disease and clinical pathologic abnormalities with serologic demonstration of antibodies against CAV-1. Antibodies can be detected by indirect hemagglutination, complement fixation, immunodiffusion, and ELISA.[28, 32] Most vaccinated dogs have detectable serum antibodies against CAV-1; titer amounts detected by ELISA are greater after natural infection than after vaccination.[28, 32] Documentation of a fourfold increase in serum antibody titer is consistent with recent infection.

Treatment and Prognosis

There is no specific treatment for infectious canine hepatitis. Supportive care to correct dehydration and control of secondary bacterial infections is indicated. Glucose should be administered parenterally to hypoglycemic animals. Plasma transfusions and heparin therapy may be required in some dogs with disseminated intravascular coagulation. Specific treatment for hepatic encephalopathy is indicated in dogs with CNS signs of disease and hyperammonemia (see Chap. 34). Ocular inflammation can be partially controlled with topical administration of glucocorticoids if corneal ulceration is not present (see Chap. 19). Glaucoma is managed with standard protocols.[33]

Prevention

CAV-1 persists in the environment for days to months depending on conditions. The organism is resistant to many chemical disinfectants. Iodine, phenol, and sodium hydroxide can be successful for killing the virus. Steam cleaning is also effective.[28]

Maternal antibodies against CAV-1 begin to decline at 5 to 7 weeks of age; negligible concentrations are present by 14 to 16 weeks of age. Vaccination with modified live or killed CAV-2 cross-protects against CAV-1 but is not associated with development of corneal edema, a frequent side effect of CAV-1 vaccines.[28, 34] The vaccine should first be administered to puppies 6 to 8 weeks of age, with boosters at 10 to 12 weeks and 14 to 16 weeks of age. Annual immunization is recommended.[19] Clinical signs of upper respiratory infection can develop if modified live CAV-2 vaccine is aerosolized and reaches the upper airway mucosa.

Zoonotic Aspects

No public health risks are associated with CAV-1 infection.

Canine Herpesvirus

Pathophysiology

Etiology. Several herpesviruses have been isolated in dogs. Classic canine herpesvirus (CHV) infection as discussed here was first identified as a cause of neonatal mortality in puppies in 1965.[35] Herpesviruses antigenically and biochemically similar to feline herpesvirus-1 but dissimilar to CHV have been isolated from some dogs with clinical disease.[36–38] Whether these viruses are pathogenic in dogs is controversial. CHV is a double-stranded DNA virus that replicates in the host nucleus.

Epidemiology. CHV infects only Canidae and grows only in canine cell cultures.[39] The virus has been identified in many countries throughout the world and has widespread distribution in the United States. Seroprevalence has been estimated; 6% of dogs tested in eastern Washington had antibodies against CHV in serum.[40] Because of the relatively short duration of antibodies in the serum of infected dogs, seroprevalence studies probably underestimate the true prevalence of infection.

Routes of infection include venereal (in adult dogs), transplacental, and ingestion or inhalation of the organism.[39] Infected animals pass the organism in respiratory and genital tract secretions. The organism does not survive for long periods in the environment, so most cases of postnatal infection are probably from direct contact with the organism in secretions from infected dogs or contact with contaminated fomites. Neonatal puppies are most commonly infected as they pass through the reproductive tract, from contact with infected littermates, or from oronasal secretions of the bitch. Clinical illness occurs in young and adult dogs but is usually severe only in neonates. The virus is maintained in nature by transfer from infected dogs to susceptible dogs.

Table 38–3
Clinical Manifestations of Canine Herpesvirus Infections

INFECTION STAGE	CLINICAL MANIFESTATIONS
In utero infection	Normal, latently infected puppies Prenatal death resulting in stillbirth, abortion fetal resorption, or mummification Neonatal death due to viremia within 1 week after birth
Neonatal infection	Normal, latently infected puppies Viremia with resultant death Mild upper respiratory signs Vesicular and papular disease on genitalia or skin Delayed-onset central nervous system disease Panuveitis, retinal atrophy, retinal necrosis, optic neuritis
Adult infection	Subclinical, latent carriers Mild upper respiratory disease Vesicular disease of vestibule, prepuce, or base of penis
Latent infection	Subclinical Recrudescence of genital disease Variable transplacental infection of puppies

Pathogenesis. Depending on the stage of gestation in which infection occurs, CHV can induce infertility or prenatal death, resulting in stillbirth, fetal reabsorption, or abortion.[39, 41, 42] Some puppies survive transplacental infection and are inapparent carriers of the virus; others acquire clinical disease in the neonatal period.

CHV replicates in nasal epithelial cells and tonsils after oronasal exposure. The organism disseminates in infected macrophages within 24 hours after infection. Widespread tissue infection occurs in 3 to 4 days; virus concentrations are greatest in the adrenals, kidneys, lungs, spleen, and liver.[39] Lymphoid hyperplasia, necrosis, and hemorrhage of affected organs are common. Hemorrhage is secondary to thrombocytopenia, disseminated intravascular coagulation, vascular endothelial damage, and tissue necrosis. Subclinical or clinical meningoencephalitis occurs in some infected puppies.[39, 43] Severity of clinical disease lessens in puppies older than 1 to 2 weeks of age; this finding has been attributed to maturation of temperature regulation and immune responses.[44, 45] Replication of CHV is optimal at body temperatures maintained by neonatal puppies, that is, 35°C to 36°C (95°F–96.8°F). Puppies born to seropositive bitches generally are subclinically infected, suggesting that lactogenic passage of antibodies or sensitized lymphocytes are protective.[45]

Venereal transmission is probably rare but can lead to papulovesicular lesions on the base of the penis or in the prepuce, vestibule, or vagina.[39, 41, 46] Hyperplasia of lymphoid follicles and hyperemia can occur, and clinical signs may recur.

Oronasal infection of adult dogs has a pathogenesis similar to that of neonatal puppies. However, because of the higher normal body temperature of adult dogs and mature immune responses, infection is limited to the oronasal tissues. Although studies had suggested clinical upper respiratory disease in some dogs, it is now thought that infection of older dogs is subclinical unless the animal is coinfected with other pathogens.[47]

Infected dogs can be latently infected.[48] Recurrence of viral shedding can be induced by immunosuppression. Some dogs infected with CHV are likely to shed virus repeatedly after a period of stress, including that associated with pregnancy.[39]

Clinical Signs

Clinical syndromes associated with CHV are summarized in Table 38–3. Although clinical illness can occur in any dog, disease manifestations are most severe in puppies younger than 3 weeks of age; the bitch may or may not have a history of previous problems. Bitches giving birth to infected puppies rarely have clinically affected puppies on subsequent litters.[49]

In utero infection resulting in stillbirth, abortion, or neonatal death within 1 week is the most common manifestation of CHV infection. Neonatal infection is most severe in puppies infected within 1 to 2 weeks after birth and commonly results in death. Infected puppies become depressed and anorectic, pass yellow-green diarrhea, have pain on abdominal palpation, appear bloated, and cry incessantly. Petechial hemorrhages on mucous membranes and vesicular or papular lesions in the oral cavity, ventral integument, and genital tract occur in some puppies.

Neurologic signs culminating in death are common. Some puppies that survive the initial infection acquire neurologic disease characterized by ataxia, blindness, and cerebellar signs. Ocular CHV infection has been associated with panuveitis and resultant keratitis, synechiae, and cataracts as well as retinal atrophy, retinal dysplasia, retinal necrosis, and optic neuritis.[50] Infection of adult dogs usually is subclinical; vesicular lesions on the base of the penis or in the prepuce, vestibule, or vagina with or without concurrent inflammation may occur rarely.

Laboratory and Radiographic Abnormalities. Although thrombocytopenia and increased serum activity of alanine aminotransferase are common in infected puppies, no pathognomonic clinical pathologic abnormalities are associated with CHV infection. Radiographic findings are nonspecific.

Pathology

The most consistent gross necropsy finding of CHV infection in puppies is multifocal hemorrhage of many organs, particularly the liver, kidney, lung, adrenal glands, and serosal surfaces of the intestines (Fig. 38–3). Serosanguineous peritoneal and pleural effusion, icterus, splenomegaly, and lymphadenopathy also occur in some animals. Disseminated foci of perivascular necrosis in the lung, liver, kidney, spleen, and brain are characteristic histopathologic findings that have been reviewed elsewhere.[35, 39, 42, 43, 51] Vesicles with marked acantholysis are found in affected cutaneous tissues. Intranuclear inclusions usually occur singly.

Diagnostic Plan

Definitive diagnosis of CHV infection is based on demonstration of the organism by electron microscopy, virus isolation, or immunofluorescent antibody techniques or by demonstration of characteristic histopathologic abnormalities and basophilic or acidophilic cell inclusions in tissues. Genital tract or respiratory secretions can be collected on sterile swabs and submitted for virus isolation.

Clinical diagnosis of CHV infection is based on appropriate signalment, history, and clinical signs of disease. Gross necropsy demonstration of diffuse hemorrhage on the kidneys, liver, lungs, and intestinal serosal surfaces is strongly suggestive of herpesvirus infection in neonatal puppies (see Fig. 38–3). Several methods are available for the detection of CHV antibodies[39, 52]; most laboratories use serum neutralization techniques. The presence of serum antibody against CHV strengthens the presumptive diagnosis if clinical disease is present. However, low neutralizing antibody titers can be detected in serum for at least 2

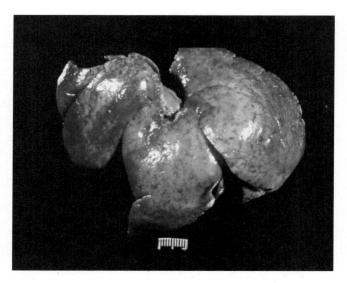

Figure 38–3
Characteristic multifocal hemorrhages on the liver of a puppy that died of neonatal herpesvirus infection. (Courtesy of David Getzy, DVM, Fort Collins, Colorado.)

years,[39] so the presence of serum antibodies alone does not prove clinical disease due to CHV. Serum antibody titers can be negative in latently infected and peracutely infected dogs.

Puppies with appropriate clinical signs of disease should be assumed to have CHV infection and managed as described in Treatment and Prognosis. Gross necropsy should be performed immediately in any case of neonatal mortality so that the presumptive diagnosis can be strengthened by characteristic findings. Virus isolation and serologic techniques help confirm presence of CHV in an individual breeding animal. However, because not all infected animals spread the organism, individual animals do not necessarily have to be removed from a breeding program (see Prevention).

Treatment and Prognosis

Because little information concerning efficacy of antiviral treatment is available,[39] supportive care is the primary treatment for CHV infection. Puppies should be housed in an environment with an ambient temperature of 36.6°C to 37.7°C (97°F–100°F) to attempt to maintain a core body temperature over 38.4°C (101°F), which inhibits viral replication. Hydration should be maintained by intravenous, intraperitoneal, or intraosseous administration of fluids. Tube feeding should be attempted. Intraperitoneal administration of 1 to 2 mL of hyperimmune serum collected from bitches with known CHV infection to puppies with a presumptive diagnosis of CHV infection may decrease mortality if administered before systemic infection occurs. The prognosis is guarded to poor for clinically affected puppies infected in utero or within 1 to 3 weeks after whelping. Genital infection in adult dogs resolves spontaneously, and treatment is rarely required.

Prevention

Because latent, seronegative carriers are probably common, serologic testing of breeding animals to attempt to develop a CHV-negative breeding colony is not useful. Bitches that whelp infected puppies once only rarely whelp infected puppies on subsequent litters, so culling, artificial insemination, or cesarean section is not indicated. Physical examination of the dog and bitch for characteristic genital lesions prior to breeding should be performed. Clinically affected dogs should not be bred until lesions resolve.

Puppies should be maintained in a warm environment. Animals with known CHV infection should be isolated from puppies for at least the first 3 weeks of life. If neonatal CHV infection is suspected in a litter, the puppies should be separated from the bitch and raised on milk replacement to prevent further exposure from the bitch. Clinically affected puppies should be housed separately from normal puppies. Prophylactic intraperitoneal administration of hyperimmune serum (1–2 mL per pup) to newborn puppies may be indicated in kennels with recurrent CHV infection. No effective commercial vaccine is currently available.

CHV does not persist in the environment. Infection generally results from direct contact with secretions from actively shedding animals or contaminated fomites. The organism is inactivated by most disinfectants, including a 1:30 chlorine bleach solution, quaternary ammonium compounds, and phenolics.[39, 49]

Zoonotic Aspects

No public health risks are associated with CHV infection.

Feline Coronavirus Infections

Pathophysiology

Etiology. There are multiple antigenically related coronaviruses that infect mammals. Cats can be experimentally infected with feline infectious peritonitis virus (FIPV), feline enteric coronavirus (FECV), porcine transmissible gastroenteritis virus, and canine coronavirus. Naturally occurring clinical disease in cats is thought to be most commonly associated with FIPV and FECV.[53] Infection with FECV results in self-limited fever and gastrointestinal signs of disease. Infection with FIPV can be subclinical or result in polysystemic signs of feline infectious peritonitis (FIP). There are multiple field strains of FECV and FIPV with varying degrees of virulence.[53, 54] Some field isolates of feline coronavirus are capable of inducing systemic FIP and enteric disease.[55] It is possible that all feline coronaviruses are descendants of a single strain. Some experts hypothesize that FIPV strains are mutated or recombinant strains of FECV that develop in the gastrointestinal tract of infected cats.[56, 57]

Epidemiology. Prevalence of coronavirus infections in cats is based primarily on seroprevalence studies; it is impossible to determine from serum antibodies which coronavirus a cat has been exposed to. Coronavirus antibodies are commonly detected in serum of more than 80% of cats housed in catteries and between 16% and 67% of the general cat population.[58] An estimated 5% to 12% of seropositive cats ultimately acquire fatal FIP.[59] The incidence of FIP in the general cat population has been estimated at less than 1%.[58, 60] Most cases of FIP develop in multicat households or in catteries.

Coronaviruses are shed in feces and oronasal secretions. Infection is thought to occur primarily from ingestion or inhalation of virus. Coronaviruses could be transmitted by biting or oral contact.[56] The incidence of transplacental transmission is unknown; one epidemiologic study suggests that this mode of transmission is unlikely.[61] After experimental inoculation, FIPV can be recovered from infected cats for approximately 14 days. There is no direct evidence of a latent carrier state in cats, but results of an epidemiologic study suggest that approximately 30% of seropositive adult cats actively excrete virus.[59] Most cats infected by a coronavirus are exposed as kittens. Kittens that are allowed to interact with adult cats other than their mothers are more likely to become exposed to a coronavirus.[59] Fulminant FIP can occur in cats of any age but is generally recognized in cats younger than 5 years of age; most are younger than 1 year of age.[58] An increased incidence of FIP is also recognized in cats older than 10 years of age.

Pathogenesis. After oronasal exposure to coronaviruses, replication first occurs in the tonsils and epithelial cells of the pharynx, respiratory mucosa, and small intestine.[62] With FECV, replication is limited to the apical columnar epithelial cells in the small intestine. Clinical disease due to FECV is related to inflammation associated with viral replication in the epithelial cells of the ileum and jejunum.[60] These changes are likely to result in the self-limited fever, vomiting, and mucoid diarrhea occasionally associated with FECV.

The ability of FIPV to induce polysystemic

disease has been attributed to the ability to infect monocytes, resulting in viremia and spread of the virus throughout the body.[53] Infected monocytes persist in reticuloendothelial organs and in many tissues perivascularly, resulting in vasculitis. Cats with poor cell-mediated immune responses acquire the effusive form of the disease, which is basically an immune complex vasculitis characterized by leakage of protein-rich fluid into the pleural space, peritoneal cavity, pericardial space, and subcapsular space of the kidneys. Cats with partial cell-mediated immunity acquire the noneffusive form of the disease, which is characterized by pyogranulomatous lesions in multiple tissues, particularly the eyes, brain, kidneys, and liver. Cats that acquire strong cell-mediated immune responses do not contract the disease.

Clinical disease associated with FIPV may be influenced by a number of factors, including the virulence of the strain, dose of the virus, route of infection, immune status of the host, genetically determined host factors, presence of other concurrent infections, and previous exposure to a coronavirus. Some experts hypothesize that most coronaviruses induce a state of immunologic tolerance after oral infection.[56] In this circumstance, mucosal immunity, but not systemic immunity, is induced. If variants that lead to polysystemic infection develop, or if the virus is introduced to the systemic immune responses by cat bites or in utero infection, oral tolerance is circumvented, leading to polysystemic immune responses resulting in vasculitis and FIP.

Clinical FIP is recognized commonly in pure-bred cats. This may be related only to increased risk of exposure. Alternatively, some hypothesize that decreased variability in the major histocompatibility complex in inbred cats may predispose them to FIPV infection of macrophages.[63]

Concurrent respiratory tract infection or feline leukemia virus infection results in a higher incidence of FIP.[60] These findings suggest that the immune status of the host is important in determining the development of FIP.

After exposure to FIPV, kittens with serologic evidence of previous infection by a coronavirus acquired accelerated FIP when compared with seronegative kittens. This was apparently a result of antibody-dependent enhancement of virus infectivity. Cells are more effectively infected by virus complexed with antibody than by virus alone.[64]

Clinical Signs

Clinical FIP is a disease of young cats; most are younger than 1 year of age when presented. There is no sex or breed predisposition other than that associated with purebred animals.

Owner complaints are generally nonspecific; anorexia, weight loss, and general malaise are common (Table 38–4).[65] In multicat households, usually only one or two kittens in a litter are clinically affected. Occasionally, multiple cats are affected; in this case, the FIPV probably was introduced for the first time.[65] Many cats have a history of self-limited, mild respiratory disease or gastrointestinal disease, which probably correlates to initial infection and dissemination of the virus.[59] Occasionally, the owner notices icterus, ocular inflammation, abdominal distension, dyspnea, or CNS abnormalities.

Elevated body temperature and weight loss are common with both the effusive and the noneffusive forms of disease. Pale mucous membranes or petechiation are noted in some cats. Cats with the effusive form commonly have dyspnea and a restrictive breathing pattern (shallow and rapid) noted on physical examination, secondary to pleural or peritoneal effusions. Heart and lung sounds may be muffled. Abdominal distension is common, and a fluid wave can often be ballotted. Some cats with the effusive form of the disease have renal enlargement due to subcapsular effusion. Male cats sometimes have scrotal enlargement due to fluid accumulation. Ocular abnormalities, including anterior uveitis and chorioretinitis, are often present, particularly with the noneffusive form of the disease. Pale or icteric mucous membranes are common. FIP is one of the most common causes of icterus in cats younger than 2 years of age.[65] Occasionally, cats with the noneffusive form of the disease have palpable, pyogranulomatous lesions in the omentum and mesentery. CNS signs associated with the noneffusive form of the disease can vary; pyogranulomatous disease can develop anywhere in the CNS. Depression, ataxia, paresis, head tilt, seizures, and nystagmus are common neurologic manifestations of disease.[66] In one study, ophthalmic disease occurred in 5 of 19 cats (26.3%) with CNS involvement.[66]

Feline coronaviruses have been suggested as a cause of failure to conceive, abortion, stillbirth, and congenital defects as well as the fading kitten syndrome (kitten mortality complex). However, a 1993 epidemiologic study failed to link feline coronavirus with reproductive failure or neonatal kitten mortality.[61]

Hematologic, Biochemical, and Urinalysis Abnormalities. No pathognomonic changes are noted on hematologic examination, and abnormalities are similar between the effusive and noneffusive forms of the disease.[67, 68] Normocytic, normochromic, nonregenerative anemia occurs in approximately 50% of affected cats,[65] particularly if the animals are coinfected by *Haemobartonella felis* or feline leukemia virus. Neutrophilic leukocytosis and lymphopenia are commonly

Table 38-4
Clinical Findings Suggestive of Feline Infectious Peritonitis in Cats

Signalment and History

Cats younger than 5 years of age or older than 10 years of age
Purebred cat
Purchase from a cattery or multicat household
History of a mild, self-limited gastrointestinal or respiratory disease
Serologic evidence of infection by feline leukemia virus
Nonspecific signs of anorexia, weight loss, or depression
Seizures, nystagmus, or ataxia
Acute, fulminant course in effusive cats
Chronic, intermittent course in noneffusive cats
Reproductive failure or kitten mortality complex

Physical Examination

Fever
Weight loss
Pale mucous membranes with or without petechiae
Dyspnea with a restrictive breathing pattern
Muffled heart or lung sounds
Abdominal distension with a fluid wave with or without scrotal swelling
Icterus with or without hepatomegaly
Chorioretinitis or iridocyclitis
Multifocal neurologic abnormalities
Irregularly marginated kidneys with or without renomegaly
Mesenteric lymphadenopathy
Splenomegaly

Laboratory Abnormalities

Nonregenerative anemia
Neutrophilic leukocytosis with or without a left shift
Lymphopenia
Hyperglobulinemia characterized as a polyclonal gammopathy with increases in α_2- and γ-globulins
Nonseptic, pyogranulomatous exudate in pleural space, peritoneal cavity, or pericardial space
Increased protein concentrations and neutrophilic pleocytosis in cerebrospinal fluid
Positive coronavirus antibody titer
Pyogranulomatous or granulomatous inflammation in perivascular location on histologic examination of tissues
Positive results of immunofluorescence or polymerase chain reaction performed on pleural or peritoneal exudate

observed. Thrombocytopenia occurs in some cats, with concurrent disseminated intravascular coagulation. Elevated plasma protein levels are common.

Serum biochemical changes are nonspecific and dependent on the organ system involved. Hyperproteinemia with or without hypoalbuminemia can occur. Hyperbilirubinemia occurs in some cats. Variable increases in alanine aminotransferase activity and alkaline phosphatase activity occur.[67] Increases in lipase and amylase activities often are detected in cats with pancreatic involvement. Azotemia is variable and can be prerenal or renal depending on renal involvement. Cats with renal involvement commonly have suboptimal urine concentrating ability (<1.035) in the presence of dehydration or azotemia. Proteinuria due to tubular or glomerular disease occurs in some cats.

CSF Abnormalities. Protein concentrations in the CSF are consistently elevated (>30 mg/dL). In one study, nucleated cell counts varied from 69 to 2000 cells/μL; neutrophils predominated in most cases.[66]

Serum Protein Electrophoresis. Hyperproteinemia occurs in some cats with either effusive or noneffusive disease; combined increases in α_2-globulins and γ-globulins are most commonly detected.[67, 68] Polyclonal gammopathies are most common; monoclonal gammopathies are rare. These findings are consistent with chronic inflammation and do not denote FIP.

Assessment of Effusions. Effusions from cats with FIP are sterile, are colorless to straw colored, may contain fibrin strands, and may clot when exposed to air. Protein concentration on fluid analysis varies in individual reports but commonly ranges from 3.5 to 12 g/dL. Mixed inflammatory cell populations of lymphocytes, macrophages, and neutrophils occur most commonly; nondegenerate neutrophils predominate in most cases. Globulin concentrations, γ-globulin concentrations, and the ratio of γ-globulins to albumin determined by electrophoresis in effusions have been assessed for diagnostic value.[68, 69] If the albumin/globulin ratio is greater than 0.81, or the albumin component is greater than 48% of the total protein concentration, FIP is unlikely.[69] If the γ-globulin concentration is greater than 32% of the total protein concentration, FIP is likely.[69] The finding of total protein concentration greater than 3.5 g/dL and globulin component greater than 50% of the total is highly predictive of a diagnosis of FIP.[68]

Radiographic Abnormalities. Radiographic abnormalities are nonspecific. Characteristic changes noted with pleural, pericardial, or peritoneal effusions are most common. Hepatomegaly or renomegaly may be detected in some cats. Mass lesions resulting from lymphadenopathy may be detected in the mesenteric root of some cats. Ultrasound helps confirm fluid in cats with minimal fluid volumes. In one study, multifocal or diffuse hyperechoic disease was detected in the kidneys of two cats.[70] FIP appeared to be the cause in 17% of the 66 total cases, with pericardial effusion diagnosed by echocardiography in one study.[71]

Pathology

The characteristic fluid associated with the effusive form of FIP is commonly found in the pleural space, peritoneal cavity, and pericardial sac. The pleura, peritoneum, and omentum are usually thickened, appear coated with plaques or nodules (0.5–2 mm), and usually have adherent fibrin strands (Fig. 38–4). Pyogranulomatous vasculitis is the principal histopathologic lesion associated with the effusive form of the disease.[60] Mesenteric lymph nodes are often enlarged in effusive and noneffusive FIP. Noneffusive disease induces perivascular granulomas in multiple body tissues, particularly the CNS, ocular tissues, mesenteric lymph nodes, renal tissue, liver, and pancreas. Some cats with primarily noneffusive disease also have minimal fluid production and pyogranulomatous lesions.

Diagnostic Plan

Antemortem diagnosis of FIP is difficult. Serum antibodies against coronaviruses can be detected in feline serum by IFA and ELISA. Antibody to coronavirus indicates prior exposure to a coronavirus in the FIP antigenic group; enteric coronaviruses cause cross-reacting antibodies. Some cats have antibodies in serum against bovine serum products that result from vaccination; these antibodies can cause false-positive results in some coronavirus antibody tests.[58] Maternal antibodies decline to undetectable concentrations by 4 to 6 weeks of age. If kittens are infected in the postnatal

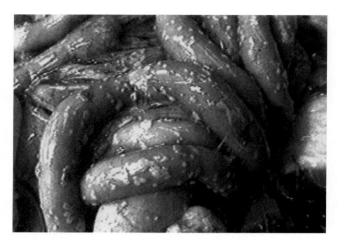

Figure 38–4
Fibrinous exudate on the surface of the small intestines in a cat with effusive feline infectious peritonitis. (Courtesy of David Getzy, DVM, Fort Collins, Colorado.)

period, antibodies can be detected again at 8 to 14 weeks of age. A positive antibody titer does not indicate a diagnosis of FIP, protect against disease, or predict when a cat may acquire clinical FIP. However, virus appears to be secreted by approximately 30% of antibody-positive, healthy cats,[59] so serologic testing is indicated for use as a screening procedure in breeding colonies that are coronavirus antibody negative. Cats with FIP are occasionally serologically negative because of rapidly progressive disease, with a delayed rise in titers, disappearance of antibody in terminal stages of the disease, or immune complex formation. Coronavirus antibody titers are therefore of limited utility for the diagnosis of FIP in individual clinically ill cats.

Direct immunofluorescence performed on cytocentrifuged pleural and peritoneal effusions documented coronavirus in 20 of 21 (95.2%) cats with histopathologically confirmed FIP.[72] Epithelial cells collected from the nictitating membrane of cats infected with coronaviruses are consistently positive for coronavirus on immunofluorescent staining (M3-test); however, the assay cannot distinguish between enteric coronavirus and FIPV.[73] Immunofluorescent techniques can also be used to identify coronavirus antigen in tissues.

Polymerase chain reaction has been used to detect coronavirus in feces, plasma, tissues, and effusions of cats.[74] A biotinylated cDNA probe has also been used successfully to detect FIPV in cell culture and peripheral blood mononuclear cells from experimentally infected cats.[75] A coronavirus-specific polymerase chain reaction is available commercially (Professional Animal Laboratory, Inc., Irvine, California).

Whether these techniques can effectively differentiate multiple field strains of FIPV from nonpathogenic FECV is being studied further. The predictive value of the polymerase chain reaction is greater with effusions than plasma; coronavirus has been detected in the plasma of some cats with enteric coronavirus infections.[74]

Definitive diagnosis of FIP is based on detection of characteristic histopathologic findings (pyogranulomatous vasculitis), virus isolation, or demonstration of the virus in pleural or peritoneal effusions by immunofluorescence[72] or polymerase chain reaction.[74] Virus isolation is not practical clinically. A presumptive diagnosis is usually based on the combination of clinical and laboratory findings. The positive and negative predictive values of individual and combinations of laboratory tests have recently been reported.[68] The combination of lymphopenia, coronavirus antibody titer 1:160 or greater, and hyperglobulinemia gave the highest predictive value of a positive test (88.9%).[68]

Treatment and Prognosis

Supportive care including correction of electrolyte and fluid balance abnormalities should be administered to cats with FIP as indicated.[76] Optimal treatment for FIP would combine virus elimination with suppression of B-lymphocyte function and stimulation of T-lymphocyte function. However, the efficacy of treatment with antiviral drugs and immunomodulating agents has been inconsistent.[77] Antiviral drugs such as ribavirin are toxic, with inconsistent effectiveness, and therefore are not currently recommended.[77] Administration of the immunomodulating drug interferon-α (Roferon-A) early in the course of disease may be effective in some cats (see Feline Leukemia Virus).[78]

Because disease due to FIP is secondary to immune-mediated reactions against the organism, modulation of the inflammatory reaction is the principal form of palliative treatment. Administration of glucocorticoids, cytotoxic drugs, and antibiotics to cats with systemic FIP have all been reported.[78] Antibiotics are not likely to have primary antiviral effects but may be indicated for the treatment of secondary bacterial infection. Although ampicillin has been used most frequently, amoxicillin may be preferred because of its superior bioavailability. Prednisone is generally administered by mouth at 50 to 100 mg/m² per day. Concurrent administration of cyclophosphamide (50 mg/m² by mouth, every 24 hours, 4 days per week), melphalan (0.5 mg per cat by mouth, every 48 hours), or chlorambucil (20 mg/m² by mouth, every 2–3 weeks) have been recommended most frequently.[76, 78] Cyclophosphamide may be the best choice based on its

lytic effect on B lymphocytes and its alleged potentiation of delayed hypersensitivity reactions.[78] Anabolic steroids (stanozolol, 1 mg by mouth, every 12 hours), aspirin (10 mg/kg by mouth, every 48–72 hours), and ascorbic acid (125 mg by mouth, every 12 hours) have also been recommended. Cytotoxic treatment should not be administered to anorectic cats.

Most cats with systemic clinical signs of FIP die or require euthanasia within days to months after diagnosis. The effusive form of the disease carries a grave prognosis, and most cats fail to respond to any treatment. Depending on the organ system involved and the severity of polysystemic clinical signs, cats with noneffusive disease have a variable survival time. Cats with ocular FIP may respond to topical, oral, or parenteral glucocorticoid treatment (see Chap. 19) or enucleation of the affected eye (or both eyes) and have a better prognosis than cats with systemic FIP.

It is difficult to assess the results of studies reporting successful treatment of FIP because of the difficulty in making a definitive antemortem diagnosis. In addition, spontaneous remission occurs in a small percentage of cats, adding to the confusion concerning response to treatment.

Prevention

Prevention of coronavirus infection is best accomplished by avoiding exposure to the virus. Although viral particles of FIPV can survive in dried secretions for up to 7 weeks, routine disinfectants inactivate the virus.[58] It would be best to maintain a coronavirus-seronegative household and not allow contact with other cats. Epidemiologic studies suggest the following:

Some healthy, coronavirus-seropositive cats shed the virus.
Seronegative cats are unlikely to shed the virus.
Kittens can be infected by seropositive queens.
Maternally derived coronavirus antibodies wane by 5 to 6 weeks of age.
Coronavirus antibodies resulting from natural infection develop by 10 weeks of age.[59, 79]

These findings have led to the recommendations that kittens born in a breeding situation with coronavirus-seropositive cats should be weaned early, isolated from seropositive cats until sold, and tested for coronavirus antibodies at 10 weeks of age.[79] Not all seropositive cats develop FIP, and most cats become seronegative after a few months.[79]

A temperature-sensitive mutant strain of coronavirus that replicates only on mucosal surfaces after intranasal administration has been developed for use as a vaccine.[80] This strain does not induce FIP, and backpassage studies have failed to show reversion to a strain capable of polysystemic replication. Stimulation of the membrane-associated immune responses by the vaccine blocks dissemination of coronaviruses contacted during the immune period. The vaccine appears to be safe; in one study, most cats in which abnormalities developed after vaccination exhibited only mild signs associated with placement of liquid in the nares.[81] Antibody-dependent enhancement of virus infectivity has occurred in some vaccinated cats after challenge with the virus[82, 83] but this seems unlikely to occur in the field.[84] The vaccine appears to be effective in at least some cats.[80–85] Whether the vaccine protects against all field strains is unknown. Vaccination induces serum antibody titers, making the interpretation of serologic test results difficult in vaccinated cats with clinical signs of FIP. The greatest benefit from the vaccine is recognized in cats entering environments with many cats for the first time.[85, 86] Vaccination of low-risk cats (those in households with few indoor cats) is not strongly recommended.[86]

Zoonotic Aspects

There is no known zoonotic transfer of FIPV or FECV to humans.

Feline Leukemia Virus

Pathophysiology

Etiology. Feline leukemia virus (FeLV) is in the family Retroviridae, subfamily Oncovirinae. Other members of this subfamily include feline sarcoma virus, RD-114, and endogenous FeLV-related sequences. It is a single-stranded RNA virus that produces reverse transcriptase enzyme.[87]

FeLV virus is made up of several core and envelope proteins; p15e, gp70, and p27 have the most clinical significance. The envelope protein p15e is associated with the development of immunosuppression.[88] The core protein p27 is present in the cytoplasm of infected cells as well as in the peripheral blood, saliva, and tears of infected cats; detection of p27 is the basis of testing with IFA and ELISA for FeLV. The envelope glycoprotein 70 (gp70) contains subgroup antigen A, B, or C.[87, 89] The subgroups are associated with the infectivity, virulence, and disease caused by individual strains of the virus. Exposure to gp70 results in the production of neutralizing antibodies in some cats. Feline oncornavirus cell membrane antigen (FOCMA) is an FeLV-induced antigen expressed on the surface of cells with virus-induced malignant transformation. Antibodies formed against this antigen can be detected in some cats.

Epidemiology. FeLV infects domestic cats and some exotic cats. The principal route of infection is prolonged contact with infected cat saliva and nasal secretions.[90, 91] Casual contact among cats from grooming or sharing common water or food sources effectively results in infection; biting is not required. Fomite and aerosol transmission is unlikely because of poor survival of the organism in the environment.[90, 92] The organism does not survive well in urine or feces.[90, 93] Transplacental infection and transmission by milk occur but are less important than casual contact.[94] FeLV has been detected in semen and vaginal epithelium, so venereal transmission is possible.

FeLV infection has worldwide distribution. Prevalence varies by region and by the testing procedure used. The seroprevalence of FeLV infection in the United States determined by ELISA in clinically normal and clinically ill cats is 6.8% and 21.1%, respectively.[95] Most FeLV-positive cats are between 1 and 6 years of age. An increased risk of infection is apparent for outdoor cats and male cats. Coinfection with FeLV and feline immunodeficiency virus may occur in 1.5% of cats.[95]

Pathogenesis. The steps of infection in a susceptible cat after oronasal exposure to an infective dose of FeLV are outlined in Table 38–5.[96, 97] Whether infection occurs after natural exposure to FeLV is determined by the virus subtype or strain, the virus dose, the age of the cat when exposed, and the cat's immune responses. There are four recognized outcomes to FeLV exposure (Table 38–6).[90] Most cats with persistent viremia die of an FeLV-related illness within 2 to 3 years. Most cats with self-limited infection are subclinically affected. Approximately 30% of the cats with self-limited infection have provirus (latent infection), which can be associated with p27-negative lymphoma and possible reactivation to persistent viremia.[97] Cats with latent infection also have evidence of immunosuppression.[97, 98] Latent infection in some cats can be activated by the administration of glucocorticoids or other immunosuppressive drugs.[90, 99] Most cats with transient viremia are subclinically affected. The primary problem with this category is that the transiently positive result on ELISA may be misinterpreted by the clinician as consistent with persistent infection, resulting in euthanasia of the affected cat. Atypical or sequestered (localized) infection occurs in up to 26% of cats exposed to FeLV; the bone marrow, spleen, lymph node, and small intestine are the most commonly involved tissues.[90, 100] It is unknown what percentage of these cats acquire clinical disease, but some cats transmit the virus to offspring.[94]

The age of the cat when exposed to FeLV is the most important host factor related to establishment of persistent infection. In experimental studies, 100% of neonatal kittens, 70% to 85% of weanling kittens, and 15% to 30% of cats older than 4 months of age were

Table 38-5
Stages of Feline Leukemia Virus Infection With Corresponding Test Results

STAGE	ORGANISM LOCALIZATION	DURATION	IFA RESULT	ELISA RESULT
I	Replication in local lymphoid tissues (tonsillar and pharyngeal with oronasal exposure)	2–12 d	Negative	Negative
II	Dissemination in circulating lymphocytes and monocytes	2–12 d	Negative	Positive
III	Replication in the spleen, distant lymph nodes, and gut-associated lymphoid tissue	2–12 d	Negative	Positive
IV	Replication in bone marrow cells and intestinal epithelial crypts	2–6 wk	Negative	Positive
V	Peripheral viremia, dissemination via infected bone marrow derived neutrophils and platelets	4–6 wk	Positive	Positive
VI	Disseminated epithelial cell infection with virus secretion in saliva and tears	4–6 wk	Positive	Positive

IFA, immunofluorescent assay; ELISA, enzyme-linked immunosorbent assay.
Data from Rojko et al.,[96] Rojko and Kociba.[97]

infected when exposed.[97] The immune status of the host is also important. Administration of glucocorticoids and concurrent infections with other agents potentiates infectivity by FeLV.[90, 97]

The dose of FeLV, the route of administration, and the subtype or field strain of the virus influence infectivity and disease. Parenteral administration of FeLV is more likely to result in persistent viremia than alimenteric administration, so cats infected by biting may be more susceptible.[97] Different field isolates vary greatly in ability to infect cats or induce disease. Strains

of FeLV that rapidly induce immunodeficiency syndromes in cats have been isolated[101] and cloned.[102]

The pathogenesis of various syndromes induced by FeLV is complex and is reviewed elsewhere.[90, 97] Induction of lymphoma has been ascribed to activation of oncogenes by the virus or insertion of provirus into the genome of lymphoid precursors.[90] Researchers have proposed that the ability of subgroup C to induce aplastic anemia is due to the tropism of this subgroup for macrophages, resulting in increased secretion of tumor necrosis factor-α.[103] Immunodefi-

Table 38-6
Outcomes of Feline Leukemia Virus Infection in Cats

PARAMETER	CATEGORY			
	Persistent Infection	Self-limited Infection	Transient Infection*	Localized Infection†
p27 ELISA	Positive	Negative	Positive	Positive or negative
p27 IFA	Positive	Negative	Usually negative	Usually negative
Neutralizing Ab	Negative	Positive	Positive or negative	Positive or negative
FOCMA Ab	Positive or negative	Positive	Positive or negative	Positive
Virus isolation	Positive	Positive or negative	Positive or negative	Positive
Virus shedding	Positive	Negative	Negative	Usually negative
Frequency	30%	60%	30%‡	5%–26%
Outcome	FeLV-related disease	Usually subclinical§	Usually subclinical	Subclinical or FeLV-related disease‖

ELISA, enzyme-linked immunosorbent assay; IFA, immunofluorescent assay; Ab, antibody; FOCMA, feline oncornavirus cell membrane antigen; FeLV, feline leukemia virus.
*Approximately 30% to 40% of the self-limited category is transiently antigenemic or viremic initially after exposure.
†Atypical or sequestered infection. Virus is isolated most readily from the spleen, lymph nodes, intestines, and bone marrow.
§Approximately 30% of this category are latently infected and may acquire persistent viremia or FeLV-negative neoplasia.
‡This represents 30% of the self-limited category.
‖This state is unstable and usually eventually converts to persistent infection or self-limited infection.
Data from Hoover and Mullins,[90] Hayes et al.[100]

ciency syndromes are likely to occur secondary to T-lymphocyte depletion (both CD4+ and CD8+ lymphocytes) or dysfunction and either neutropenia or neutrophil function deficits.[98, 104–108] Myeloproliferative diseases probably develop from viral induction of bone marrow growth-promoting substances.[109]

Clinical Signs

Although cats of any age, sex, or breed can develop FeLV infection, most are male cats between 1 and 6 years of age. Owners generally present FeLV-infected cats for evaluation of nonspecific signs such as anorexia, weight loss, and depression or for evaluation of abnormalities associated with specific organ systems. Of FeLV-infected cats evaluated at necropsy, 23% have evidence of neoplasia (96% lymphoma-leukemia complex), and the remainder die of non-neoplastic diseases.[110] Of the non-neoplastic diseases, nonregenerative anemia and recurrent or chronic infection such as recurrent cutaneous abscesses, nonhealing wounds, or chronic respiratory disease are common. Many of the non-neoplastic diseases have been attributed to secondary invaders after immunosuppression induced by FeLV infection. Many of the clinical syndromes diagnosed in FeLV-seropositive cats also occur in FeLV-seronegative cats and do not require immunosuppression to induce disease. The clinician must be careful not to ascribe all clinical diseases in FeLV-infected cats to the virus. A positive FeLV test result does not correlate directly with immunodeficiency or disease directly related to FeLV.

Gastrointestinal Abnormalities. Stomatitis and halitosis occur in some FeLV-infected cats. It has been hypothesized that inflammation may be secondary to overgrowth of normal bacterial flora or persistent calicivirus infection secondary to immunosuppression. However, in one study, FeLV infection did not correlate with increased prevalence of chronic carriage of feline calicivirus in the oral cavity of affected cats.[111]

Vomiting and diarrhea occur in some FeLV-infected cats and may be due to opportunistic infections such as salmonellosis, giardiasis, or cryptosporidiosis.[112] A distinct form of enteritis clinically and histopathologically resembling panleukopenia but apparently related to FeLV infection has been described[110, 113] and is possibly secondary to enteric coronavirus infection.[110] Cats with alimenteric lymphosarcoma also are commonly presented for evaluation of vomiting and diarrhea.

Icterus. Icterus occurs in some FeLV-infected cats. Prehepatic icterus is related to immune-mediated destruction of red blood cells induced by FeLV or secondary infection by *H. felis*.[87] Hepatic icterus is

related to hepatic lymphoma, hepatic lipidosis, and focal liver necrosis.[110] Posthepatic icterus may occur because of alimenteric lymphoma. Some cats with icterus may be concurrently infected by FIPV or *Toxoplasma gondii*.

Respiratory Abnormalities. Sneezing and nasal discharge occur in some FeLV-infected cats, which may result from secondary infection with herpesvirus 1 or calicivirus.[114] Pneumonia, bronchitis, and pyothorax resulting in cough or dyspnea occur in some FeLV-infected cats. Dyspnea and restrictive breathing pattern with muffled heart or lung sounds are common in cats with thymic lymphoma. These cats are generally younger than 3 years of age; decreased cranial chest compliance may be noted on palpation.[90] Heart sounds may be displaced caudodorsally. Neoplastic cells can be documented cytologically in pleural effusions from some cats.[87]

Lymphadenopathy. Lymphadenopathy due to lymphoma or hyperplasia of lymphoid tissues occurs in FeLV-infected cats.[115] FeLV may be the cause of lymphoid hyperplasia in 50% of adult cats and up to 67% of immature cats.[110]

Neoplasia. Thymic, multicentric, and alimenteric lymphomas are the most common neoplasms associated with FeLV.[87, 90] Most cats with lymphoma are presented for evaluation of anorexia, weight loss, or depression. Cats with thymic lymphoma most commonly are presented with dyspnea or a restrictive breathing pattern. Cats with multicentric lymphoma generally are presented with nonspecific signs of anorexia and weight loss. Clinical illness is related to infiltration of various organs by malignant lymphocytes. Enlarged lymph nodes or organomegaly is often noted on physical examination. Uveitis due to intraocular tumor may be present. Alimenteric lymphoma most commonly involves the small intestines, mesenteric lymph nodes, kidneys, and liver of older cats. Owners often report vomiting, diarrhea, and icterus. Hepatomegaly, renomegaly, and abdominal masses are often noted on palpation.

Fibrosarcomas occasionally develop in young cats coinfected with FeLV and feline sarcoma virus. The feline sarcoma virus is replication defective and requires coinfection by FeLV.[87, 90] Cats are usually presented for evaluation of multiple firm, cutaneous or subcutaneous mass lesions.

Lymphocytic, myelogenous, erythroid, and megakaryocytic leukemias all are reported secondary to FeLV infection; erythroid leukemia and myelomonocytic leukemia are the most common.[87, 90] History and physical examination findings are nonspecific. Many cats have pale mucous membranes due to anemia and may have petechiae due to thrombocytopenia. Hepatosplenomegaly is common, and some cats have clinical evidence of secondary infections.

Urinary Tract Abnormalities. Urinary tract problems most frequently associated with FeLV-infected cats are urinary incontinence and renal failure. Clinical signs of renal failure include polyuria, polydipsia, weight loss, and hyporexia during the last stages of disease (see Chap. 16). Urinary incontinence has been predominantly associated with a small bladder and nocturnal incontinence that appears to be caused by either sphincter incompetence or detrusor hyperactivity.[116, 117] Renal failure is generally secondary to renal lymphoma; one or both kidneys are usually enlarged, with irregular margins noted on physical examination. Glomerulonephritis may be induced by FeLV infection[87] but is not common.[110]

Ocular Abnormalities. Intraocular lymphoma induces uveitis and glaucoma in some cats. Cats are generally presented for miosis, blepharospasm, or cloudy eyes. Aqueous flare, mass lesions, keratic precipitates, lens luxations, and glaucoma are often found on ocular examination. It is unlikely that FeLV induces uveitis without lymphoma.[118] Uveitis from *T. gondii* infection occurs in some cats with FeLV-induced immunodeficiency but seems to be more common in cats with feline immunodeficiency virus infection.[119]

Reproductive Abnormalities. FeLV-infected queens may be presented for abortion, stillbirth, or infertility.[120] Breeding can be successful, but fetal death often occurs within the first month of gestation. Reabsorption of the fetuses gives the appearance of infertility. Kittens that are infected in utero but survive to parturition generally acquire accelerated FeLV syndromes or die as a part of the kitten mortality complex.

Neurologic Abnormalities. Anisocoria, ataxia, weakness, behavior change, and urinary incontinence are the most common neurologic abnormalities reported in FeLV-infected cats.[90, 121] Nervous system disease is likely to develop because of polyneuropathy or lymphoma. In cats with FeLV-induced neurologic disease, neurologic examination commonly reveals tetraparesis or paraparesis and decreased conscious proprioception. Leukemic cells were detected in the bone marrow of 69% of a group of cats with spinal lymphoma.[122] Neurologic abnormalities are occasionally secondary to other infectious agents, such as FIPV or *T. gondii*.

Secondary Infections. Concurrent infections by viral, bacterial, fungal, rickettsial, and parasitic agents are commonly detected in FeLV-seropositive cats; it is difficult clinically to determine which are primary and which are secondary to FeLV-induced immunosuppression. A strong association exists between FeLV and

FIPV and *H. felis.*[87] Secondary infections may be more difficult to treat in FeLV-infected cats that are immunosuppressed.

Musculoskeletal Abnormalities. Some FeLV-seropositive cats are presented for lameness or weakness. Multiple cartilaginous exostoses occur in some cats and may be FeLV related. Polyarthritis with resultant stiffness and lameness with or without swollen, hot, and painful joints occurs in some cats and has been attributed to immune complex deposition.[87]

Hematologic, Biochemical, and Urinalysis Abnormalities. Anemia is common in FeLV-infected cats. Nonregenerative anemia occurs alone or in combination with decreases in lymphocytes, neutrophils, and platelets. Evidence of abnormal red blood cell release from the bone marrow characterized by increased numbers of circulating nucleated red blood cells without an appropriate reticulocytosis is common. Examination of bone marrow often documents a maturation arrest in the erythroid line. Regenerative anemia is detected in some cats with immune-mediated destruction of erythrocytes induced by FeLV or in some cats coinfected with *H. felis.* Microagglutination of erythrocytes or a positive direct Coombs test result occurs in some cats. *H. felis* is identified in an epicellular location on erythrocytes in some cats. Neutropenia occurs in some FeLV-infected cats because of bone marrow suppression or immune-mediated destruction. Some FeLV-infected cats acquire a syndrome characterized by neutropenia and gastrointestinal tract signs that is difficult to differentiate from panleukopenia virus infection. Usually, cats with FeLV-induced panleukopenia-like syndrome also have anemia and thrombocytopenia, abnormalities rarely associated with panleukopenia virus infection.

Prerenal azotemia is common in anorectic FeLV-infected cats. Renal azotemia occurs in cats with renal lymphoma. Hyperbilirubinemia occurs because of prehepatic hemolytic anemia or hepatic disease associated with lymphosarcoma. Elevated liver enzymes develop secondary to hepatic lipidosis or hepatic lymphosarcoma. Electrolyte abnormalities develop in cats with anorexia or gastrointestinal signs. Proteinuria occurs in some FeLV-infected cats secondary to glomerulonephritis. Pyuria and bacteriuria occur in some cats with secondary urinary tract infections.

Radiographic Abnormalities. Mediastinal or cranial thoracic masses can be detected in cats with mediastinal or thymic lymphoma. Diffuse hepatomegaly or renomegaly is detected in cats with hepatic or renal lymphoma, respectively. Ultrasound evaluation of tissues with lymphoma generally reveals mottled increased densities.[70] Alimenteric lymphoma can result in obstruction of the gastrointestinal system, resulting in an obstructive gas pattern and characteristic signs of obstruction on evaluation of a barium series. Spinal lymphoma can lead to a compressive lesion, which is noted on myelography.

Cytologic Abnormalities. Malignant lymphocytes characteristic of FeLV-induced lymphosarcoma are easily identified cytologically. Cats with mediastinal masses, lymphadenomegaly, renomegaly, hepatomegaly, splenomegaly, and intestinal masses should be evaluated by cytology of fine-needle aspirates for lymphosarcoma prior to surgical intervention. Malignant lymphocytes are also occasionally identified in peripheral blood smears and in CSF.

Pathology

Gross pathologic findings vary with the organ system involved. Tissues are often pale because of anemia. Renomegaly, lymphadenomegaly, hepatomegaly, intestinal masses, mediastinal masses, and spinal cord masses are common with lymphosarcoma. Pleural effusion is often detected in cats with thymic lymphoma. Histopathologic abnormalities vary by syndrome and organ system involved.[87]

Diagnostic Plan

Detection of FeLV antigens in neutrophils and platelets by IFA or in whole blood, plasma, serum, saliva, or tears by ELISA are most commonly used clinically to document infection by FeLV. Antibody titers to FeLV envelope antigens (neutralizing antibody) and against virus-transformed tumor cells (FOCMA antibody) are available in some research laboratories (Retrovirus Research Laboratory, Department of Pathology, College of Veterinary Medicine and Biomedical Sciences, Colorado State University, Fort Collins, Colorado).

Results of IFA and ELISA during the dissemination of FeLV are listed in Table 38–5. The ELISA can detect p27 antigen prior to infection of bone marrow and release of infected neutrophils and platelets and thus can be positive in some cats during early stages of infection or during self-limited infection even though IFA results are negative. Positive serum test results occur between 2 and 30 weeks (generally 2 to 8 weeks) after infection occurs. Infection of systemic epithelial tissue (including salivary glands and tear glands) occurs after bone marrow infection. There is usually a delay of 1 to 2 weeks after the onset of viremia before ELISA tear and saliva results become positive.

Because p27 can be detected by ELISA in cats that are acquiring self-limited infection, all positive serum ELISA results should be confirmed immediately by IFA, or the cats should be isolated and retested by ELISA in 4 to 6 weeks. Some cats with ELISA-positive

results that revert to negative have become latently infected. Most latently infected cats have negative ELISA and IFA results, but the virus can be isolated from the bone marrow.[90] False-positive ELISA results can develop secondary to poor laboratory technique. False-negative ELISA results with tears or saliva occur during early stages of infection.

IFA results are accurate 98.3% of the time.[123] False-negative reactions can occur when leukopenia or thrombocytopenia prevents evaluation of an adequate number of cells. False-positive reactions can occur if the blood smears submitted for evaluation are too thick. A positive IFA result indicates that the cat is viremic and contagious. The viremia is sustained for life in 90% to 97% of cats with positive IFA results.[123]

Virtually all IFA-positive cats are also ELISA positive. The rare combination of IFA-positive and ELISA-negative results suggests technique-related artifact. Negative ELISA results correlate well with negative IFA results and an inability to isolate FeLV. Results that are ELISA positive and IFA negative are termed discordant results; these are usually due to false-positive ELISA results, false-negative IFA results, or self-limited infection. Cats with positive ELISA results and negative IFA results are probably not contagious at the time, but they should be isolated until retested 4 to 6 weeks later because their condition may be progressing to persistent viremia and epithelial cell infection.[124]

Virus isolation and polymerase chain reaction (available at the Retrovirus Research Laboratory) are the only reliable means of identifying local or latent FeLV infections. The clinical significance of locally or latently infected cats is unclear. It is unlikely that the cats pass the virus horizontally, but infected queens may pass the virus to kittens during gestation, during parturition, or in milk.[94] Neutrophil function defects have been detected in some latently infected cats, so some may be immunocompromised.[98] A latently infected cat may become viremic (IFA and ELISA positive) after administration of corticosteroids or after extreme stress.[99] Alternatively, the infection may be cleared.

Positive test results do not document immunodeficiency or disease induced by FeLV; many virus-positive cats have disease manifestations that were induced by secondary invaders. Potential for immunodeficiency can be evaluated in some research laboratories by assessment of delayed hypersensitivity reactions[125] and measurement of CD4+ lymphocyte numbers (Retrovirus Research Laboratory).

Treatment and Prognosis

Treatment for retroviral infections such as FeLV is limited. The reverse transcriptase inhibitor, 3'-azido-

Table 38–7

Current Drug Treatment Regimens for Use in the Persistently Viremic, Clinically Ill Cat With Feline Leukemia Virus Infection

THERAPEUTIC AGENT	PROPOSED MECHANISM OF ACTION	ADMINISTRATION
Antiviral Drug AZT (zidovudine, Retrovir)	Reverse transcriptase inhibition	20 mg/kg by mouth, three times per day, daily for 7 days and then 10 mg/kg, by mouth, three times per day, daily. Cats should be monitored for development of anemia.
Immunotherapy Interferon-α (Roferon-A)	Prevents release of budding virions	Dilute 1.5×10^6 units of interferon-α into 500 mL sterile saline and freeze in 1-mL aliquots. This solution is stable for years if frozen. A concentration of 30 units/mL is made by diluting 1 mL with 100 mL saline. This solution is stable for several months if refrigerated. 30 units (1 mL) by mouth, once daily, for 7 days, with treatment administered every other week until the cat is clinically normal.
Staphylococcus A	B-lymphocyte and T-lymphocyte activation, immune-complex binding, interferon induction, and immunoglobulin Fc binding.	Dissolve a 5-mg vial in 3 mL sterile water and add to 500 mL sterile saline to give 10 µg/mL. Freeze in 5-mL aliquots. 1 mL/kg, intraperitoneally, twice weekly for 10 weeks, followed by 1 mL/kg, intraperitoneally, twice weekly, every fourth week for life.
Propionibacterium acnes	Activation of macrophages and natural killer cells. Increased production of interferon, tumor necrosis factor, and interleukin 1.	0.5 mL, intravenously, twice weekly, for 2 weeks followed by 0.5 mL, intravenously weekly for 20 weeks or until p27 antigen is no longer detected in serum.
Acemannan	Enhanced release of tumor necrosis factor, prostaglandin E_2, and interleukin 1-α by macrophages.	2 mg/kg, intraperitoneally, intravenously, or subcutaneously once weekly for 6 weeks.

Data from McCaw.[126]

3'-deoxythymidine (AZT, or zidovudine [Retrovir]) has been studied the most. Unfortunately, AZT must be administered before infection by the FeLV to give significant results. AZT does not appear to clear viremia in most persistently viremic cats.[126]

Immunotherapy seems to be the most effective therapy for clinically ill, persistently viremic cats. Although no drug is able to consistently clear viremia, interferon-α, *Staphylococcus* protein A, *Propionibacterium acnes,* or Acemannan (Table 38–7) improves clinical signs of disease in some cats.[126] Immunotherapy generally requires 4 to 6 weeks to achieve maximal effect. In cats with severe clinical illness not likely to survive 4 to 6 weeks, AZT may be indicated initially. Immunotherapy or AZT should not be used alone in cats with FeLV-associated neoplasia or true leukemia; chemotherapy also is indicated for these cats.

Many cats with FeLV infection have secondary infections due to immunosuppression induced by the virus or its products.[87] Antibiotic treatment is often indicated. The duration of treatment is generally longer than for FeLV-negative cats because of possible immunosuppression by the virus. Rhinitis, stomatitis, and pyothorax should be treated with antibiotics with an anaerobic spectrum, such as the penicillin derivatives, metronidazole, or clindamycin hydrochloride.

Anorectic cats should be given maintenance fluids subcutaneously or intravenously. Enteral nutrition can be supplied via force-feeding or nasogastric, pharyngostomy, gastrostomy (see Chap. 34), or jejunostomy tube placement.

When concurrent *H. felis* infection exists, doxycycline administered at a dosage of 5 mg/kg by mouth, two times per day, for 14 to 21 days is indicated. Supportive treatment with hematinic agents, vitamin B_{12}, folic acid, and anabolic steroids generally has been unsuccessful in the management of the nonregenerative anemia. Immunosuppressive therapy may be required in the management of hemolytic anemia (see Chap. 41). Blood transfusions are required in some cases. Information concerning immunosuppressive therapy for the treatment of other hematologic abnormalities is limited, and this form of treatment may be contraindicated because of the potential for virus activation. Prophylactic antibiotic treatment may be indicated in cats with severe neutropenia (<2000 cells/μL). Whether recombinant erythropoietin is beneficial for the treatment of nonregenerative anemia has not been extensively studied. The prognosis for persistently viremic cats is guarded; most die within 2 to 3 years.

Prevention

Avoidance of exposure is the best form of FeLV prevention. Because the virus is easily transmitted by casual contact, all contact between infected and noninfected cats should be avoided. Although FeLV is inactivated after a short time out of the host and is easily inactivated by routine disinfectants, fomite transmission through common food and water dishes is common. Test and removal of seropositive cats can result in virus-free catteries and multiple-cat households but is not practical for the cat population as a whole.[87, 127]

Multiple FeLV vaccines have been developed and licensed in the last several years. Because of variation in challenge study methods and the difficulty in assessing the preventable fraction of a disease with a relatively low infection rate, a long subclinical phase, and multiple field strains, efficacy of individual vaccines continues to be in question.[128] Vaccination of cats not previously exposed to FeLV should be considered for cats at high risk (i.e., having contact with other cats). Owners should be warned of the potential efficacy of less than 100% and should be counseled concerning housing cats indoors. Uncommonly, soft tissue sarcomas may develop at the vaccination site in some cats receiving certain vaccines.[129]

FeLV-infected cats should be housed indoors to avoid infecting other cats and to avoid exposure to opportunistic agents. Flea control should be maintained to avoid exposure to *H. felis*. FeLV-infected cats should not be allowed to hunt or to eat undercooked meats so as to avoid infection by *T. gondii.*

Zoonotic Aspects

Although FeLV grows in some human cell cultures, antigens of FeLV have not been documented in the serum of humans, suggesting that this virus is species specific.

Feline Immunodeficiency Virus

Pathophysiology

Etiology. The feline immunodeficiency virus (FIV) is a member of the virus family Retroviridae, subfamily Lentivirinae.[130–132] The virus is morphologically similar to the human immunodeficiency virus but antigenically distinct. The virus is an exogenous, single-stranded RNA virus similar to FeLV but more complex. FIV produces reverse transcriptase enzyme to catalyze the insertion of viral RNA into the host genome.[130–132] FIV comprises multiple field strains that vary genetically and have different biologic properties.[133–136]

Epidemiology. Aggressive biting behavior is thought to be the primary route of transmission of FIV.[137] The chance for exposure increases over time. Thus, older male, outdoor cats are the group most commonly infected.[95, 137] Casual contact, including grooming and sharing of common dishes and litterboxes, has been reported but is less likely than biting to result in transmission of infection among cats housed in the same environment.[138] Postnatal transmission from FIV-infected queens to kittens in milk has been documented.[139] Transplacental infection is thought to occur rarely. The virus has been isolated from the semen of infected toms, but the epidemiologic significance of venereal transmission is relatively unknown.[140] The role of blood-sucking arthropods in the transmission of FIV is largely unknown but is likely of minimal importance.

FIV infection of cats has worldwide distribution.[132] Antibodies against FIV have been detected in serum of cats stored since 1968.[141] In the United States, seroprevalence of infection varies from 1.2% to 4.0% in clinically normal or low-risk cats and from 11.6% to 14% in clinically ill or high-risk cats.[95, 137] The number of FIV-seropositive cats increases with age; most are older than 6 years of age.[95, 137] An increased risk of infection is apparent for outdoor cats and male cats because of increased potential for biting behavior. Detection of antibodies against FIV in the serum of cats documents exposure and correlates well with persistent infection but does not correlate with disease induced by the virus.

Pathogenesis. FIV has been documented to replicate in a number of white blood cells and astrocytes.[132, 133, 142] After exposure, a primary phase of infection occurs during which the virus disseminates throughout the body, initially leading to low-grade fever, neutropenia, and generalized lymphadenopathy.[131] A subclinical, latent period of variable length develops after the primary phase of infection; the duration depends on the strain of virus and the age of

Table 38–8
Clinical Stages of Feline Immunodeficiency Virus Infection

STAGE	HIV CORRELATE	CLINICAL MANIFESTATIONS	DURATION
1	Acute or primary	Fever, neutropenia, generalized lymphadenopathy.	2–9 months
2	Asymptomatic	Clinically normal, but early suppression of immune responses can be detected within 18–24 months following infection.	Months–years
3	Persistent, generalized lymphadenopathy	Vague clinical disease not obviously caused by secondary or opportunistic agents. Fever, anemia, lymphadenopathy, anorexia, weight loss, and behavioral changes.	Months–years
4	AIDS-related complex	Chronic secondary bacterial infections of the mouth, skin, respiratory tract, gastrointestinal tract, and urinary tract.	Months–years
5	AIDS	Chronic weight loss and opportunistic infections. Severe anemia and leukopenia.	1–6 months

HIV, human immunodeficiency virus; AIDS, acquired immunodeficiency syndrome.
Data from Pedersen and Barlough.[132]

the animal.[130, 131, 136, 143] The first strain of FIV isolated, the Petaluma strain, induces laboratory evidence of immunodeficiency within 14 months after infection. However, cats experimentally infected with this strain of virus have remained clinically normal for years after primary infection. The median ages of healthy naturally infected cats and clinically ill naturally infected cats are approximately 3 years and 10 years, respectively, suggesting a latent period of years for most strains of FIV.[132, 144] Chronic experimental[136, 145–147] and naturally occurring infection[148–151] results in a slow decline in CD4+ lymphocyte numbers, response to mitogens, and decreased production of interleukin-2.[132] Humoral immune responses, neutrophil function, and natural killer cell function are also affected.[152, 153] What stimulates the induction of the immune deficiency stage of FIV infection is unknown. Coinfection with FeLV potentiates the primary and immune deficiency phases of FIV.[154] Coinfection with *H. felis, T. gondii,* feline herpesvirus 1, and feline calicivirus as well as immunization failed to potentiate FIV-associated immunodeficiency.[155, 156]

Clinical Signs

Older male cats are most commonly infected with FIV. They are presented for evaluation of nonspecific signs such as anorexia, weight loss, and depression or for evaluation of abnormalities associated with specific organ systems. Clinical signs resulting from FIV infection are diverse and may be due to direct viral effects or secondary infections that develop after the development of immunodeficiency. Stages of FIV infection that correlate with those associated with human immunodeficiency virus infection have been proposed (Table 38–8).[132] Although many clinical syndromes are

diagnosed in FIV-seropositive cats,[132, 137, 157] most also occur in FIV-naive cats and do not require immunodeficiency to induce disease. The clinician must be careful not to ascribe all clinical diseases in FIV-infected cats to the virus; many conditions are secondary, and primary treatment is given (Table 38–9). Although the presence of antibodies against FIV in serum correlate well with persistent infection, they do not correlate directly with immunodeficiency or disease directly related to FIV. Coinfection by FIV and FeLV results in a greater chance for clinical disease than infection by either agent alone.[132]

Gastrointestinal Abnormalities. Stomatitis and gingivitis are commonly detected in FIV-infected cats, possibly from overgrowth of normal bacterial flora secondary to immunodeficiency induced by the virus. Cats coinfected with feline calicivirus and FIV have a high prevalence of severe oral lesions.[111] Chronic diarrhea can occur in FIV-infected cats as a primary viral effect[157] or may be secondary to opportunistic infections (see Table 38–9).

Dermatologic Abnormalities. Recurrent bacterial skin infections; chronic, poorly responsive abscesses; and otitis externa occur in some FIV-infected cats. Cats with generalized demodectic mange, notoedric mange, poxvirus, dermatophytosis, and atypical mycobacteriosis have also been reported.[157]

Respiratory Tract Abnormalities. Upper respiratory tract infection, pneumonia, herpesvirus 1, pyothorax, cryptococcosis, and pulmonic toxoplasmosis occur in some FIV-infected cats. Many of the adult cats that die of pulmonic toxoplasmosis are immunosuppressed by FIV infection (Lappin MR, unpublished data; see Chap. 40 for further discussion).

Table 38–9

Clinical Syndromes Associated With FIV Infection and Possible Opportunistic Agents

CLINICAL SYNDROME	AGENT
Stomatitis	Calicivirus; overgrowth of bacteria flora; candidiasis
Diarrhea*	*Cryptosporidium* spp.; *Isospora* spp.; *Giardia* spp.; *Salmonella* spp.; *Campylobacter jejuni*
Upper respiratory tract	Feline herpesvirus 1; overgrowth of bacterial flora; *Cryptococcus neoformans*
Pyothorax	Bacterial
Pneumonia, pneumonitis	Bacterial; *Toxoplasma gondii*; *C. neoformans*
Dermatologic	Bacterial; atypical *Mycobacterium*; *Otodectes cynotis*; *Demodex cati*; *Notoedres cati*; dermatophytosis; *C. neoformans*
Hematologic*	*H. felis*; FeLV
Neurologic*	*T. gondii*; *C. neoformans*; feline infectious peritonitis virus; FeLV
Neoplasia*	FeLV
Urinary tract infection	Bacterial
Glomerulonephritis*	Secondary infections
Renal failure*	Secondary infections
Ocular*	*T. gondii*; feline infectious peritonitis virus; *C. neoformans*

FIV, feline immunodeficiency virus; FeLV, feline leukemia virus.
*Syndrome also associated primarily with FIV.

Urinary Tract Abnormalities. Whether urinary tract infections including cystourethritis and pyelonephritis occur more frequently in FIV-infected cats than in FIV-naive cats is unknown. Renal disease has been ascribed to a primary viral effect.[158] Glomerulonephritis may occur more commonly in cats infected with FIV than in cats infected with FIPV or FeLV.[159]

Ophthalmic Abnormalities. Intraocular inflammation has been detected in FIV-infected cats.[136, 160] Pars planitis, an infiltrate in the anterior portion of the vitreous humor, is a common manifestation and may be an immune-mediated, direct viral effect. Serologic evidence of coinfection with *T. gondii* is commonly detected in FIV-infected cats with uveitis.[161, 162] Demonstration of local production of *T. gondii*–specific antibody in aqueous humor can support the diagnosis of ocular toxoplasmosis (see Chap. 40).[162]

Neurologic Abnormalities. Neurologic manifestations of disease occur in approximately 5% of FIV-infected cats; microscopic evidence of viral disease occurs much more frequently.[132, 133, 157] Most of the reported neurologic signs in FIV-infected cats have been behavioral; dementia, hiding, rage, inappropriate elimination, and roaming are common. Occasionally, seizures, nystagmus, ataxia, and peripheral nerve abnormalities occur. Primary viral disease is thought to be more likely than opportunistic infections, but cryptococcosis, toxoplasmosis, and FIPV are associated with neurologic disease in some FIV-infected cats.

Neoplasia. Lymphoid malignancies, myeloproliferative diseases, and several carcinomas and sarcomas have been detected in some FIV-infected, FeLV-naive cats, suggesting a potential association between FIV and malignancy.[132, 141, 163] Lymphoid neoplasia in FIV-infected cats is most frequently extranodal, and FIV-infected cats are older (mean, 8.7 years of age) than FeLV-infected cats with lymphoid neoplasia.[141]

Lymphatic and Immunologic Abnormalities. Lymphadenopathy is common in FIV-infected cats and is often a direct viral effect.[131] Polyarthritis occurs in some FIV-infected cats and may be an immune-mediated manifestation of the disease.

Hematologic, Biochemical, and Urinalysis Abnormalities. Neutropenia, thrombocytopenia, and nonregenerative anemia are the most common hematologic abnormalities associated with FIV infection in cats.[132, 164] Regenerative anemia and positive direct Coombs test results occurs in some cats, particularly those coinfected with *H. felis*. Monocytosis and lymphocytosis occur in some cats and may be due to the virus or to chronic infection with opportunistic pathogens. Cytologic examination of bone marrow aspirates may reveal maturation arrest in some cats with nonregenerative anemia or hyperplasia in others with leukemia or myeloproliferative disease. None of the hematologic changes are pathognomonic for FIV infection. Some laboratories can enumerate T-lymphocyte subsets from naturally or experimentally infected cats (Retrovirus Research Laboratory). A progressive decline in CD4+ lymphocytes, a plateau or progressive increase in CD8+ lymphocytes, and an inversion of the CD4+/CD8+ ratio occurs in experimentally infected cats over time.[132]

Different biochemical abnormalities occur depending on the stage of disease and secondary infections. Renal azotemia (urine specific gravity <1.035) and hyperglobulinemia may be due to direct viral effects.[158] The hyperglobulinemia is generally polyclonal. Evidence of secondary infection characterized by pyuria or bacteriuria may also be noted.

Radiographic Abnormalities. Abnormalities associated with FIV infection result from secondary conditions such as pulmonic toxoplasmosis or pyothorax.

Pathology

Hyperplasia of lymphoid tissues is common in FIV-infected cats.[165, 166] Nonspecific signs of wasting are present in most cats with chronic infection. Pathologic evidence of opportunistic agents may be present. Characteristic changes associated with lymphoid neoplasia may be found in some cats.

Diagnostic Plan

Infection by FIV can be confirmed by virus isolation or polymerase chain reaction,[132, 167] which are not practical clinically. Antibodies against FIV are detected in serum by ELISA, IFA, Western blot immunoassay, and radioimmunoprecipitation.[132, 168] Seropositive cats are probably infected with FIV for life. Seroconversion occurs 2 to 4 weeks after inoculation. The virus can be isolated from some seronegative cats[138]; however, false-negative reactions are more common during peracute infection. False-positive reactions are common with ELISA and therefore should be confirmed using Western blot immunoassay or IFA, especially if the positive cat is healthy or from a low-risk population. Kittens can have detectable colostrum-derived antibodies until 12 to 14 weeks of age, so they should not be tested until they are older than 14 weeks of age.

Presence of antibody in serum confirms only FIV infection, not clinical illness. However, seropositive cats with secondary or opportunistic infections probably have FIV-induced immunodeficiency. Enumeration of CD4+ lymphocytes is available (Retrovirus Research Laboratory) but has not been evaluated extensively as an indicator of prognosis in naturally infected cats.

Treatment and Prognosis

An extensive search for secondary infections should be performed on clinically ill, FIV-seropositive cats. Supportive care and treatment of secondary infections are key. Secondary infections of the skin, oral cavity, ears, urinary tract, and gastrointestinal tract are managed as discussed elsewhere in this text. The major difference in the management of bacterial infections in FIV-infected cats is that immunosuppression dictates long-term treatment or multiple treatment periods for the management of recurrent disease. Clinical feline toxoplasmosis occurs frequently as a sequela of immunodeficiency induced by FIV infection. Treatment with clindamycin hydrochloride, as discussed in Chapter 40, has been successful in some cases, but clinical signs are more difficult to control than in cats that are not immunosuppressed.

The prognosis with FIV-infected cats is variable. Supportive care and control of secondary infections has extended the lifespan of some cats considerably.

Administration of antiviral agents such as the reverse transcriptase inhibitor AZT (see Feline Leukemia Virus) has had little success in the treatment of FIV.[169] Immunostimulators such as interleukin-2 or interferons may ultimately be useful, but information is still lacking.

Prevention

Prevention of FIV infection is best achieved by avoidance of fighting. Housing cats indoors and testing new cats before introduction to an FIV-seronegative, multiple-cat household prevents most cases of FIV. FIV-naive cats housed in the same environment as FIV-infected cats are not likely to become infected unless fighting or aggressive playing occurs. Because the virus is not easily transmitted by casual contact, transmission by fomites is unusual. FIV is susceptible to most routine disinfectants and dies when out of the host for minutes to hours, especially when dried. Litterboxes and dishes shared among cats should be cleaned with scalding water and detergent to inactivate the virus. FIV-infected cats should be housed indoors at all times to lessen their chance of acquiring an opportunistic infection and to protect FIV-naive cats from exposure. To avoid infection by *T. gondii*, FIV-infected cats should not be allowed to hunt or to eat undercooked meat products.

To avoid transmission by ingestion of milk, kittens queened by FIV-infected cats should not be allowed to nurse. These kittens should be shown to be serologically negative at 14 weeks of age to document failure of lactogenic or transplacental transmission prior to leaving the mother.

Possible vaccines for the prevention of FIV infection are being evaluated.[170] However, because multiple strains of the virus exist and could potentially mutate to vaccine-resistant strains, it is unlikely that an effective vaccine will be available in the near future.

Zoonotic Aspects

Although FIV is morphologically similar to the human immunodeficiency virus, the viruses are antigenically distinct. Antibodies against FIV have not been documented in the serum of humans even after accidental exposure to virus-containing material, suggesting that this virus is species specific.[132, 137]

References

1. Shell LG. Canine distemper. Compen Contin Educ Pract Vet 1990;12:173–179.
2. Greene CE, Appel MJ. Canine distemper. In: Greene CE, ed. Infectious Diseases of the Dog and Cat, 2nd ed. Philadelphia, WB Saunders, 1990:226–241.
3. Evans MB, Bunn TO, Hill HT, et al. Comparison of in vitro replication and cytopathology caused by strains of canine distemper virus of vaccine and field origin. J Vet Diagn Invest 1991;3:127–132.
4. Appel M. Pathogenesis of canine distemper. Am J Vet Res 1969;30:1167–1182.
5. Zurbriggen A, Vandevelde M. The pathogenesis of nervous distemper. Prog Vet Neurol 1994;5:109–116.
6. Krakowka S, Hoover EA, Koestner A, et al. Experimental and naturally occurring transplacental transmission of canine distemper virus. Am J Vet Res 1977;38:919–922.
7. Bell SC, Carter SD, Bennett D. Canine distemper viral antigens and antibodies in dogs with rheumatoid arthritis. Res Vet Sci 1991;50:64–68.
8. Higgins RJ, Krakowka S, Metzler AE, et al. Canine distemper virus-associated cardiac necrosis in the dog. Vet Pathol 1981;18:472–486.
9. Tipold A, Vandevelde M, Jaggy A. Neurological manifestations of canine distemper virus infection. J Small Anim Pract 1992;33:466–470.
10. Thomas WB, Sorjonen DC, Steiss JE. A retrospective evaluation of 38 cases of canine distemper encephalomyelitis. J Am Anim Hosp Assoc 1993;29:129–133.
11. Axthelm MK, Krakowka S. Canine distemper virus-induced thrombocytopenia. Am J Vet Res 1987;48:1269–1275.
12. Sorjonen DC, Cox NR, Swango LJ. Electrophoretic determination of albumin and gamma globulin concentrations in the cerebrospinal fluid of dogs with encephalomyelitis attributable to canine distemper virus infection: 13 cases (1980–1987). J Am Vet Med Assoc 1989;195:977–980.
13. Palmer DO, Huxtable CRR, Thomas JB. Immunohistochemical demonstration of canine distemper virus antigen as an aid in the diagnosis of canine distemper encephalomyelitis. Res Vet Sci 1990;49:177–181.
14. Simon-Valencia MC, Garcia-Sanchez J, Girones-Punet O, et al. Contribution to the study of canine distemper. 1. Direct immunofluorescence and detection of inclusion bodies in live animal smears. Medicina Veterinaria 1987;4:211–218.
15. Brown RAL, Morrow A, Heron I, et al. Immunocytological confirmation of a diagnosis of canine distemper using cells in urine. J Small Anim Pract 1987;28:845–851.
16. Blixenkrone-Moller M, Pedersen IR, Appel MJ, et al. Detection of IgM antibodies against canine distemper virus in dog and mink sera employing enzyme-linked immunosorbent assay (ELISA). J Vet Diagn Invest 1991;3:3–9.
17. Noon KF, Rogul M, Binn LN, et al. Enzyme-linked immunosorbent assay for evaluation of antibody to canine distemper virus. Am J Vet Res 1980;41:605–609.
18. Krawkowka S, Olsen RG, Axthelm M, et al. Canine parvoviruses potentiate canine distemper encephalitis attributable to modified live-virus vaccine. J Am Vet Med Assoc 1982;180:137–139.
19. Canine and feline immunization guidelines. J Am Vet Med Assoc 1989;195:314–317.
20. Raw ME, Pearson GR, Brown PJ, et al. Canine distemper infection associated with acute nervous signs in dogs. Vet Rec 1992;130:291–293.
21. Harder TC, Kuczka A, Dubberke M, et al. An outbreak of canine distemper in a dogs home with vaccinated population of dogs. Kleintierpraxis 1991;36:305–314.
22. McCandlish IAP, Cornwell HJC, Thompson H, et al. Distemper encephalitis in pups after vaccination of the dam. Vet Rec 1992;130:27–30.
23. Tizard I. Risks associated with use of live vaccines. J Am Vet Med Assoc 1990;196:1851–1858.
24. Cook SD, Blumberg B, Dowling PC, et al. Multiple sclerosis and canine distemper on Key West, Florida. Lancet 1987;1:1426–1427.
25. Cartwright EJ, Gordon MT, Freemont AJ, et al. Paramyxoviruses and Paget's disease. J Med Virol 1993;40:133–141.
26. McStreet GH, Elkunk RB, Latiwonk QI. Investigations of environmental conditions during cluster indicate probable vectors of unknown exogenous agent(s) of multiple sclerosis. Comp Immun Microbiol Infect 1992;15:75–77.
27. Assaf R, Marsolais G, Yelle J, et al. Unambiguous typing of canine adenovirus isolates by deoxyribonucleic acid restriction-endonuclease analysis. Can J Comp Med 1983;47:460–463.
28. Greene CE. Infectious canine hepatitis and canine acidophil cell hepatitis. In: Greene CE, ed. Infectious Diseases of the Dog and Cat, 2nd ed. Philadelphia, WB Saunders, 1990:242–251.
29. Gocke DJ, Morris TQ, Bradley SE. Chronic hepatitis in the dog: The role of immune factors. J Am Vet Med Assoc 1970;156:1700–1705.
30. Wright NG. Canine adenovirus: Its role in renal and ocular disease; a review. J Small Anim Pract 1976;17:25–33.
31. Rakich PM, Prasse KW, Lukert PD, et al. Immunohistochemical detection of canine adenovirus in paraffin sections of liver. Vet Pathol 1986;23:478–484.
32. Noon KF, Rogul M, Binn LN, et al. An enzyme-linked immunosorbent assay for the detection of canine antibodies to canine adenoviruses. Lab Anim Sci 1979;29:603–609.
33. Pentlarge VW. External ophthalmic diseases and glaucoma. In: Lorenz MD, Cornelius LM, Ferguson DC, eds. Small Animal Medical Therapeutics. Philadelphia, JB Lippincott, 1992:446–456.
34. Curran JM, Cunningham CK. Efficacy of an inactivated canine adenovirus-type 2 vaccine. Vet Med Small Anim Clin 1983;78:51–59.
35. Carmichael LE, Squire RA, Krook L. Clinical and pathologic features of a fatal viral disease of newborn pups. Am J Vet Res 1965;26:803–814.
36. Rota PA, Maes RK. Homology between feline herpesvirus-1 and canine herpesvirus. Archives Virol 1990;115:139–145.

37. Evermann JF, McKeirnan AJ, Ott RL, et al. Diarrheal condition in dogs associated with viruses antigenically related to feline herpesvirus. Cornell Vet 1982;72: 285–291.

38. Kramer JW, Evermann JF, Leathers CW, et al. Experimental infection of two dogs with a canine isolate of feline herpesvirus type I. Vet Pathol 1991;28: 338–340.

39. Carmichael LE, Greene CE. Canine herpesvirus infection. In: Greene CE, ed. Infectious Diseases of the Dog and Cat, 2nd ed. Philadelphia, WB Saunders, 1990: 252–258.

40. Fulton RW, Ott RL, Duenwald JC, et al. Serum antibodies against canine respiratory viruses: Prevalence among dogs of eastern Washington. J Am Vet Med Assoc 1974;35:853–855.

41. Poste G, King N. Isolation of a herpesvirus from the canine genital tract: Association with infertility, abortion, and stillbirths. Vet Rec 1971;88:229–233.

42. Hashimoto A, Hirai K, Yamaguchi T, et al. Experimental transplacental infection of pregnant dogs with canine herpesvirus. Am J Vet Res 1982;43:844–850.

43. Percy DH, Munnel JF, Olander HJ, et al. Pathogenesis of canine herpesvirus encephalitis. Am J Vet Res 1970;31: 145–156.

44. Carmichael LE, Barnes FD, Percy DH. Temperature as a factor in resistance of young puppies to canine herpesvirus. J Infect Dis 1969;120:669–678.

45. Carmichael LE. *Herpesvirus canis:* Aspects of pathogenesis and immune response. J Am Vet Med Assoc 1970;156:1714–1721.

46. Hill H, Mare CJ. Genital disease in dogs caused by canine herpesvirus. Am J Vet Res 1974;35:669–672.

47. Kraft S, Evermann JF, McKeirnan AJ, et al. The role of neonatal canine herpesvirus infection mixed infection in older dogs. Compen Contin Educ Pract Vet 1986;8: 688–696.

48. Okuda Y, Ishida K, Hashimoto A, et al. Virus reactivation in bitches with a medical history of herpesvirus infection. Am J Vet Res 1993;54:551–554.

49. Anvik JO. Clinical considerations of canine herpesvirus infection. Vet Med 1991;86:394–403.

50. Albert DM, Lahav M, Carmichael L, et al. Canine herpes-induced retinal dysplasia and associated ocular anomalies. Invest Ophthalmol 1976;15:267–278.

51. Percy DH, Carmichael LE, Albert DM, et al. Lesions in puppies surviving infection with canine herpesvirus. Vet Pathol 1971;8:37–53.

52. Takumi A, Kusanagi K, Tuchiya K, et al. Serodiagnosis of canine herpesvirus infection—Development of an enzyme-linked immunosorbent assay and its comparison with two improved methods of serum neutralization test. Jpn J Vet Sci 1990;52:241–250.

53. Pedersen NC. An overview of feline enteric coronavirus and infectious peritonitis virus infections. Feline Pract 1995;23:7–20.

54. Pedersen NC, Floyd K. Experimental studies with three new strains of feline infectious peritonitis virus: FIPV-UCD2, FIPV-UCD3, and FIPV-UCD4. Compen Contin Educ Pract Vet 1985;7:1001–1010.

55. Hayashi T, Watabe, Y, Nakayama H, et al. Enteritis due to feline infectious peritonitis virus. Jpn J Vet Sci 1982;44:97–106.

56. Evermann JF, McKeirnan AJ, Ott RL. Perspectives on the epizootiology of feline enteric coronavirus and the pathogenesis of feline infectious peritonitis. Vet Microbiol 1991;28:243–255.

57. Pedersen NC, Boyle JF, Floyd K, et al. An enteric coronavirus infection of cats and its relationship to feline infectious peritonitis. Am J Vet Res 1981;42: 368–377.

58. Scott FW. Feline infectious peritonitis: Transmission and epidemiology. In: Proceedings of the Symposium: New Perspectives on Prevention of Feline Infectious Peritonitis. January 11, 1991, Orlando, Florida, 1991:8–13.

59. Addie DD, Jarrett O. A study of naturally occurring feline coronavirus infections in kittens. Vet Rec 1992; 130:133–137.

60. Pederson NC. Feline infectious peritonitis. In: Pederson NC, ed. Feline Infectious Diseases. Goleta, California, American Veterinary Publications, 1988:45–59.

61. Addie DD, Toth S. Feline coronavirus is not a major cause of neonatal kitten mortality. Feline Pract 1993;21: 13–18.

62. Stoddart ME, Gaskell RM, Harbour DA, et al. The sites of early viral replication in feline infectious peritonitis. Vet Microbiol 1988;18:259–271.

63. O'Brien Sj, Roelke M, Marker L, et al. Genetic basis of the species vulnerability in the cheetah. Science 1985; 227:1428–1434.

64. Scott FW, Olsen CW, Corapi WV. Antibody-dependent enhancement of feline infectious peritonitis virus infection. Feline Pract 1995;23:77–80.

65. Weiss RC. The diagnosis and clinical management of feline infectious peritonitis. Vet Med 1991;86:308–319.

66. Baroni M, Heinold Y. A review of the clinical diagnosis of feline infectious peritonitis viral meningoencephalitis. Prog Vet Neurol 1995;6:88–94.

67. Sparkes AH, Gruffydd-Jones TJ, Harbour DA. Feline infectious peritonitis: A review of clinicopathological changes in 65 cases, and a critical assessment of their diagnostic value. Vet Rec 1991;129:209–212.

68. Sparkes AH, Gruffydd-Jones TJ, Harbour DA. An appraisal of the value of laboratory tests in the diagnosis of feline infectious peritonitis. J Am Anim Hosp Assoc 1994;30:345–350.

69. Shelly SM, Scarlett-Kranz J, Blue, JT. Protein electrophoresis in effusions from cats as a diagnostic test for feline infectious peritonitis. J Am Anim Hosp Assoc 1988;24:495–500.

70. Walter PA, Johnston GR, Feeney DA, et al. Applications of ultrasonography in the diagnosis of parenchymal kidney disease in cats: 24 cases (1981–1986). J Am Vet Med Assoc 1988;192:92–98.

71. Rush JE, Keene BW, Fox PR. Pericardial disease in the cat: A retrospective evaluation of 66 cases. J Am Anim Hosp Assoc 1990;26:39–46.

72. Parodi MC, Cammarata G, Paltrinieri S, et al. Using direct immunofluorescence to detect coronaviruses in peritoneal and pleural effusions. J Small Anim Pract 1993;34:609–613.

73. Thoresen SI. Feline infectious peritonitis-FIP. New

diagnostic method for FIP (feline coronavirus) infections. Norsk Veterinaertidsskrift 1990;102:661–667.

74. Herrewegh AAPM, Egberink HF, Horzinek MC, et al. Polymerase chain reaction (PCR) for the diagnosis of naturally occurring feline coronavirus infections. Feline Pract 1995;23:56–60.

75. Martinez ML, Weiss RC. Detection of feline infectious pertonitis virus infection in cell cultures and peripheral blood mononuclear leukocytes of experimentally infected cats using a biotinylated cDNA probe. Vet Microbiol 1993;34:259–271.

76. Sherding RG. Feline infectious peritonitis: Clinical manifestations and treatment. In: Proceedings of the Symposium: New Perspectives on Prevention of Feline Infectious Peritonitis. January 11, 1991. Orlando, Florida, 1991:18–23.

77. Weiss RC. Treatment of feline infectious peritonitis with immunomodulating agents and antiviral drugs: A review. Feline Pract 1995;23:103–106.

78. Weiss RC. Feline infectious peritonitis virus: Advances in therapy and control. In: August JR, ed. Consultations in Feline Internal Medicine, 2nd ed. Philadelphia, WB Saunders, 1994:3–12.

79. Addie DD, Jarrett O. Control of feline coronavirus infection breeding catteries by serotesting, isolation, and early weaning. Feline Pract 1995;23:92–95.

80. Gerber JD, Ingersoll JD, Gast AM, et al. Protection against feline infectious peritonitis by intranasal inoculation of a temperature-sensitive FIPV vaccine. Vaccine 1990;8:536–542.

81. Postorino-Reeves NC, Pollock RVH, Thurber ET. Long-term follow-up study of cats vaccinated with a temperature-sensitive feline infectious peritonitis vaccine. Cornell Vet 1992;82:117–123.

82. Scott FW, Corapi WV, Olsen CW. Independent evaluation of a modified live FIPV vaccine under experimental conditions (Cornell experience). Feline Pract 1995;23:74–76.

83. McArdle F, Tennant B, Bennett M, et al. Independent evaluation of a modified live FIPV vaccine under experimental conditions (University of Liverpool experience). Feline Pract 1995;23:67–71.

84. Fehr D, Holznagel E, Bolla S, et al. Evaluation of the safety and efficacy of a modified live FIPV vaccine under field conditions. Feline Pract 1995;23:83–88.

85. Postorino-Reeves, N. Vaccination against naturally occurring FIP in a single large cat shelter. Feline Pract 1995;23:81–82.

86. Pedersen NC, Addie D, Wolf A. Recommendations from working groups of the international enteric coronavirus and feline infectious peritonitis workshop. Feline Pract 1995;23:108–111.

87. Cotter SM. Feline leukemia virus infection. In: Greene CE, ed. Infectious Diseases of the Dog and Cat, 2nd ed. Philadelphia, WB Saunders, 1990:316–333.

88. Mathes LE, Olsen RG, Hebebrand LC, et al. Immunosuppressive properties of a virion polypeptide, a 15,000-dalton protein, from feline leukemia virus. Cancer Res 1979;39:950–955.

89. Sarma PS, Log T. Viral envelope antigens of the viruses of feline leukemia-sarcoma complex. Bibl Haematol 1973;39:113–124.

90. Hoover EA, Mullins JI. Feline leukemia virus infection and diseases. J Am Vet Med Assoc 1991;199:1287–1297.

91. Hardy WD Jr, Old LJ, Hess PW, et al. Horizontal transmission of feline leukaemia virus. Nature 1973;27:266–299.

92. Francis DP, Essex M, Hardy WD Jr. Excretion of feline leukaemia virus by naturally infected pet cats. Nature 1977;269:252–254.

93. Hoover EA, Olsen RG, Hardy WD Jr, et al. Horizontal transmission of feline leukemia virus under experimental conditions. J Natl Cancer Inst 1977;58:443–444.

94. Pacitti AM, Jarrett O, Hay D. Transmission of feline leukemia virus in the milk of a non-viraemic cat. Vet Rec 1986;118:381–384.

95. O'Connor TP, Tonelli QJ, Scarlett JM. Report of the national FeLV/FIV awareness project. J Am Vet Med Assoc 1991;199:1348–1353.

96. Rojko JL, Hoover EA, Mathes LE, et al. Pathogenesis of experimental feline leukemia virus infection. J Natl Cancer Inst 1979;63:759–768.

97. Rojko JL, Kociba GJ. Pathogenesis of infection by the feline leukemia virus. J Am Vet Med Assoc 1991;199:1305–1310.

98. Lafrado LJ, Dezzutti CS, Lewis MG, et al. Immunodeficiency in latent feline leukemia virus infections. Vet Immunol Immunopathol 1989;21:39–46.

99. Rojko JL, Hoover EA, Quackenbush SL, et al. Reactivation of latent feline leukaemia virus infection. Nature 1982;298:385–388.

100. Hayes KA, Rojko JL, Mathes LE. Incidence of localized feline leukemia virus infection in cats. Am J Vet Res 1992;53:604–607.

101. Hoover EA, Mullins JI, Quackenbush SL, et al. Experimental transmission and pathogenesis of immunodeficiency syndrome in cats. Blood 1987;70:1880–1892.

102. Overbaugh J, Bonahue PR, Quackenbush SL, et al. Molecular cloning of a feline leukemia virus that induces fatal immunodeficiency disease in cats. Science 1988;239:906–910.

103. Khan KN, Kociba GJ, Wellman ML. Macrophage tropism of feline leukemia virus (FeLV) of subgroup-C and increased production of tumor necrosis factor-alpha by FeLV-infected macrophages. Blood 1993;81:2585–2590.

104. Tompkins MB, Nelson PD, English RV, et al. Early events in the immunopathogenesis of feline retrovirus infections. J Am Vet Med Assoc 1991;199:1305–1310.

105. Tompkins MB, Ogilvie GD, Gast AM, et al. Interleukin-2 suppression in cats naturally infected with feline leukemia virus. J Biol Resp Mod 1989;8:86–96.

106. Ogilvie GK, Tompkins MB, Tompkins WAF. Clinical and immunologic aspects of FeLV-induced immunosuppression. Vet Microbiol 1988;17:287–296.

107. Pardi D, Hoover EA, Quackenbush SL, et al. Selective impairment of humoral immunity in feline leukemia virus-induced immunodeficiency. Vet Immunol Immunopathol 1991;28:183–200.

108. Kiehl AR, Fettman MJ, Quackenbush SL, et al. Effects of feline leukemia virus infection on neutrophil chemotaxis in vitro. Am J Vet Res 1987;48:76–80.

109. Linenberger ML, Abkowitz JL. In vivo infection of marrow stromal fibroblasts by feline leukemia virus. Exp Hematol 1992;20:1022–1027.

110. Reinacher M. Diseases associated with spontaneous feline leukemia virus (FeLV) infection in cats. Vet Immunol Immunopathol 1989;21:85–95.

111. Tenorio AP, Franti CE, Madewell BR, et al. Chronic oral infections of cats and their relationship to persistent oral carriage of feline calici-, immunodeficiency, or leukemia viruses. Vet Immunol Immunopathol 1991;29:1–14.

112. Madewell BR, Holmberg CA, Ackerman N. Lymphosarcoma and cryptococcosis in a cat. J Am Vet Med Assoc 1979;175:65–68.

113. Reinacher M. Feline leukemia virus associated enteritis-a condition with features of feline panleukopenia. Vet Path 1987;24:1–4.

114. Bech-Nielsen S, Fulton RW, Downing MM, et al. Feline infectious peritonitis and viral respiratory diseases in feline leukemia virus infected cats. J Am Anim Hosp Assoc 1981;17:759–765.

115. Moore FM, Emerson WE, Cotter SM, et al. Distinctive peripheral lymph node hyperplasia of young cats. Vet Pathol 1986;23:386–391.

116. Barsanti JA, Downey R. Urinary incontinence in cats. J Am Anim Hosp Assoc 1984;20:979–982.

117. Lappin MR, Barsanti JA. Urinary incontinence secondary to idiopathic detrusor instability: Cystometrographic diagnosis and pharmacologic management in 2 dogs and a cat. J Am Vet Med Assoc 1987;191:1439–1442.

118. Brightman AH, Ogilvie GK, Tompkins M. Ocular disease in FeLV positive cats: 11 cases (1981–1986). J Am Vet Med Assoc 1991;198:1049–1051.

119. Lappin MR, Marks A, Greene CE, et al. Serologic prevalence of selected infectious diseases in cats with uveitis. J Am Vet Med Assoc 1992;201:1005–1009.

120. Hardy WD Jr. Feline leukemia virus non-neoplastic disorders. J Am Anim Hosp Assoc 1981;17:941–949.

121. Haffer KN, Sharpee RL, Beckenhauer W, et al. Is feline leukemia virus responsible for neurologic conditions in cats? Vet Med 1987;82:802–805.

122. Spodnick GJ, Berg J, Moore FM, et al. Spinal lymphoma in cats: 21 cases (1977–1989). J Am Vet Med Assoc 1992;200:373–376.

123. Hardy WD Jr, Zuckerman EE. Development of the immunofluorescent antibody test for detection of feline leukemia virus infection in cats. J Am Vet Med Assoc 1991;199:1327–1335.

124. Hardy WD Jr, Zuckerman EE. Ten-year study comparing enzyme-linked immunosorbent assay with the immunofluorescent antibody test for detection of feline leukemia virus infection in cats. J Am Vet Med Assoc 1991;199:1365–1373.

125. Otto CM, Brown CA, Lindl PA, Dawe DL. Delayed hypersensitivity testing as a clinical measure of cell-mediated immunity in the cat. Vet Immunol Immunopathol 1993;38:91–102.

126. McCaw DL. Advances in therapy for retroviral infections. In: August JR, ed. Consultations in Feline Internal Medicine, 2nd ed. Philadelphia, WB Saunders, 1994: 21–25.

127. Hardy WD Jr, McClelland AJ, Zuckerman EE, et al. Prevention of the contagious spread of feline leukaemia virus and the development of leukaemia in pet cats. Nature 1976;263:326–328.

128. Macy DW. Vaccination against feline retroviruses. In:

August JR, ed. Consultations in Feline Internal Medicine, 2nd ed. Philadelphia, WB Saunders, 1994:33–39.

129. Kass PH, Barnes WG, Spangler WL, et al. Epidemiologic evidence for a causal relationship between vaccination and fibrosarcoma tumorigenesis in cats. J Am Vet Med Assoc 1993;203:396–405.

130. Pederson NC, Ho EW, Brown ML, et al. Isolation of a T-lymphotrophic virus from domestic cats with an immunodeficiency-like syndrome. Science 1987;235:790–793.

131. Yamamoto JK, Sparger E, Ho EW, et al. Pathogenesis of experimentally induced feline immunodeficiency virus infection in cats. Am J Vet Res 1988;49:1246–1258.

132. Pedersen NC, Barlough JE. Clinical overview of feline immunodeficiency virus. J Am Vet Med Assoc 1991;199:1298–1305.

133. Dow SW, Poss ML, Hoover EA. Feline immunodeficiency virus: A neurotropic lentivirus. J Acquir Immune Defic Syndr 1990;3:658–668.

134. Miyazawa T, Fukasawa M, Hasegawa A, et al. Molecular cloning of a novel isolate of feline immunodeficiency virus biologically and genetically different from the original U.S. isolate. J Virol 1991;65:1572–1577.

135. Miyazawa T, Furuya T, Itagaki S, et al. Preliminary comparisons of the biological properties of two strains of feline immunodeficiency virus (FIV) isolated in Japan with FIV Petaluma strain isolated in the United States. Arch Virol 1989;108:59–68.

136. Tompkins MB, Nelson PN, English RV, et al. Early events in the immunopathogenesis of feline retrovirus infections. J Am Vet Med Assoc 1991;199:1311–1315.

137. Yamamoto JK, Hanson H, Ho EW, et al. Epidemiologic and clinical aspects of feline immunodeficiency virus infections in cats from the continental United States and Canada and possible mode of transmission. J Am Vet Med Assoc 1989;194:213–220.

138. Dandekar S, Beebe AM, Barlough J, et al. Detection of feline immunodeficiency virus (FIV) nucleic acids in FIV-seronegative cats. J Virol 1992;66:4040–4049.

139. Sellon R, Jordan H, Kennedy-Stoskopf S, et al. The NCSU₁ isolate of FIV is transmitted postnatally via milk International Symposium on Feline Retrovirus Research, Research Triangle Park, North Carolina, October 1993:16.

140. Jordan H, Howard J, Kennedy-Stoskopf S, et al. Feline immunodeficiency virus is present in cat semen. Proceedings of the 12th American College of Veterinary Internal Medicine Forum, San Francisco, May 1994: 1005.

141. Shelton GH, Grant CK, Cotter SM, et al. Feline immunodeficiency virus and feline leukemia virus infections and their relationships to lymphoid malignancies in cats: A retrospective study (1968–1988). J Acquir Immune Defic Syndr 1990;3:623–630.

142. English RV, Johnson CM, Gebhard DH, et al. In vivo lymphocyte tropism of feline immunodeficiency virus. J Virol 1993;67:5175–5186.

143. George JW, Pedersen NC, Higgins J. The effect of age on the course of experimental feline immunodeficiency virus infection in cats. AIDS Res Hum Retroviruses 1993;9:897–905.

144. Shelton GH, Waltier RM, Connor SC, et al. Prevalence of

feline immunodeficiency virus and feline leukemia virus infections in pet cats. J Am Anim Hosp Assoc 1989;25:7–12.

145. Ackley CD, Yamamoto JK, Levy N, et al. Immunologic abnormalities in pathogen-free cats experimentally infected with feline immunodeficiency virus. J Virol 1990;64:5652–5655.

146. Torten M, Fanichi M, Barlough JE, et al. Progressive immune dysfunction in cats experimentally infected with feline immunodeficiency virus. J Virol 1991;65:2225–2230.

147. Barlough JE, Ackley CD, George JW, et al. Acquired immune dysfunction in cats with experimentally induced feline immunodeficiency virus infection: Comparison of short-term and long-term infections. J Acqir Immune Defic Syndr 1991;4:219–227.

148. Novotney C, English RV, Housman J, et al. Lymphocyte population changes in cats naturally infected with feline immunodeficiency virus. AIDS 1990;4:1213–1218.

149. Hoffman-Fezer G, Thum J, Ackley C, et al. Decline in CD4+ cell numbers in cats with naturally acquired feline immunodeficiency virus infection. J Virol 1992;66:1484–1488.

150. Hara Y, Ishida T, Ejima H, et al. Decrease in mitogen-induced lymphocyte proliferative responses in cats infected with feline immunodeficiency virus. Jpn J Vet Sci 1990;52:573–579.

151. Taniguchi A, Ishida T, Konno A, et al. Altered mitogen response of peripheral blood lymphocytes in different stages of feline immunodeficiency virus infection. Jpn J Vet Sci 1990;52:513–518.

152. Taniguchi A, Ishida T, Washizu T, et al. Humoral immune response to T cell dependent and independent antigens in cats infected with feline immunodeficiency virus. J Vet Med Sci 1991;53:333–335.

153. Hanlon MA, Marr JM, Hayes KA, et al. Loss of neutrophil and natural killer cell function following feline immunodeficiency virus infection. Viral Immunol 1993;6:119–124.

154. Pedersen NC, Torten M, Rideout B, et al. Feline leukemia virus infection as a potentiating cofactor for the primary and secondary stages of experimentally induced feline immunodeficiency virus infection. J Virol 1990;64:598–606.

155. Reubel G, Dean G, Barlough J, et al. Immunizations and incidental infections do not accelerate immunologic abnormalities occurring in experimentally FIV-infected cats. International Symposium on Feline Retrovirus Research, Research Triangle Park, North Carolina, October 1993:16.

156. Lappin MR, George JW, Pedersen NC, et al. Experimental induction of toxoplasmosis in cats chronically infected with feline immunodeficiency virus. First International Conference of Feline Immunodeficiency Virus Researchers, Davis, California, September 1991:29.

157. Shelton GH. Clinical manifestations of feline immunodeficiency virus infection. Feline Pract 1991;19:14–20.

158. Poli A, Abramo F, Taccini, et al. Renal involvement in feline immunodeficiency virus infection: A clinicopathological study. Nephron 1993;64:282–288.

159. Reinacher M, Frese K. Glomerulonephritis in dogs and cats. Tierarztliche-Praxis 1991;2:175–180.

160. English R, Davidson M, Nasisse M. Preliminary report of the ocular manifestations of feline immunodeficiency virus infections. J Am Vet Med Assoc 1990;196:1116–1119.

161. Chavkin MJ, Lappin MR, Powell CC. Seroepidemiologic and clinical observations of 93 cases of uveitis in cats. Prog Vet Comp Ophthalmol 1992;2:29–36.

162. Lappin MR, Roberts SM, Davidson MG, et al. Enzyme-linked immunosorbent assays for the detection of *Toxoplasma gondii*-specific antibodies and antigens in the aqueous humor of cats. J Am Vet Med Assoc 1992;201:1010–1016.

163. Hutson CA, Rideout BA, Pedersen NC. Neoplasia associated with feline immunodeficiency virus infection in cats of Southern California. J Am Vet Med Assoc 1991;199:1357–1362.

164. Shelton GH, Linenberger ML, Abkowitz JL. Hematologic abnormalities in cats seropositive for feline immunodeficiency virus. J Am Vet Med Assoc 1991;199:1353–1357.

165. Brown PJ, Hopper CD, Harbour DA. Pathological features of lymphoid tissues in cats with natural feline immunodeficiency virus infection. J Comp Pathol 1991;104:345–355.

166. Rideout BA, Lowenstine LJ, Huston CA, et al. Characterization of morphologic changes and lymphocyte subset distribution in lymph nodes from cats with naturally acquired feline immunodeficiency virus infection. Vet Pathol 1992;29:391–399.

167. Matteucci D, Baldinotti F, Mazzetti P, et al. Detection of feline immunodeficiency virus in saliva and plasma by cultivation and polymerase chain reaction. J Clin Microbiol 1993;31:494–501.

168. Egberink HF, Lutz H, Horzinek MC. Use of Western blot and radioimmunoprecipitation for diagnosis of feline leukemia and feline immunodeficiency virus infections. J Am Vet Med Assoc 1991;199:1339–1342.

169. Shelton GH. Management of the feline immunodeficiency virus-positive patient. In: August JR, ed. Consultations in Feline Internal Medicine, 2nd ed. Philadelphia, WB Saunders, 1994:27–31.

170. Yamamoto JK, Okuda T, Ackley CD, et al. Experimental vaccine protection against feline immunodeficiency virus. AIDS Res Hum Retroviruses 1991;7:911–922.

Chapter 39

Fungal Diseases

Michael R. Lappin

Cryptococcosis

Pathophysiology

Etiology. *Cryptococcus neoformans* is a small yeastlike organism (3.5–7.0 μm in diameter) with a thick polysaccharide capsule that reproduces by narrow-based budding (Table 39–1).[1] Both *C. neoformans* var. *neoformans* and *C. neoformans* var. *gatti* have been shown to cause disease in cats.[2] The organism can survive in moist, shaded areas for up to 2 years.

Epidemiology. *C. neoformans* has worldwide distribution. Infections in humans and domestic animals are more common in some areas, including southern California and the eastern coast of Australia.[2, 3] Increased concentrations of *Cryptococcus* spp. in the environment are associated with bird excrement (*C. neoformans* var. *neoformans*) or eucalyptus trees (*C. neoformans* var. *gatti*).[1, 2] The organism is commonly associated with pigeon droppings, but birds rarely become clinically ill because their high body temperature inhibits replication.[1]

Cryptococcosis is the most common systemic fungal infection of cats. Approximately one half of clinically affected humans are immunosuppressed.[1] Potentially immunosuppressive conditions have also been documented in some infected cats[1–3] and dogs.[4–7] The route of transmission is unknown but is suspected to be secondary to airborne inhalation of the organism.[1] The organism is not transmitted horizontally.

Pathogenesis. After inhalation of the organism, the nasal cavity or lower airways and alveoli become infected. In one study, granulomatous pneumonia developed in one intranasally inoculated cat, suggesting that inhalation is the route of infection in animals with pneumonic cryptococcosis.[8] Hematogenous spread is the likely pathogenesis in animals with disease outside the respiratory system. The central nervous system is infected by direct extension across the cribriform plate or by hematogenous spread.

Infection stimulates cell-mediated immune responses. Human T lymphocytes and natural killer cells inhibit the growth of *C. neoformans*.[9] If the cell-mediated immune responses are incomplete and fail to result in complete removal of the organism, granulomatous lesions result. The polysaccharide capsule of the organism potentiates establishment of infection by inhibiting plasma cell function, phagocytosis, leukocyte migration, and opsonization.[1]

Clinical Signs

In three retrospective studies[2, 3, 10] of cats (29, 48, and 35 cats, respectively) with cryptococcosis, affected cats ranged from 6 months to 16 years of age, and male cats were overrepresented. Clinical disease in the cat most commonly involves the respiratory tract, skin, eyes, and central nervous system (Table 39–2). Mycotic rhinitis with resultant sneezing and nasal discharge are the most common client complaints (56.3%–83.0%).[2, 3, 10] Lesions on the nasal planum are often ulcerated (Fig. 39–1). Granulomatous lesions can be seen extruding from the external nares in many cats and are sometimes associated with facial deformity over the bridge of the nose. Nasal disease can be either unilateral or bilateral; discharges vary from serous to mucopurulent and occasionally contain blood.

Cutaneous or subcutaneous masses (31.4%–55.0%) are the next most common clinical complaint or physical examination finding.[2, 3, 10] Masses are generally smaller than 1 cm, can be single or multiple, are firm or fluctuant, and, if ulcerated, pass a serous discharge.[11] Lymphadenopathy (12.5%), intraocular inflammation (10.4%), and central nervous system disease (6.3%) are detected frequently.[3] Most cats with nasal disease have submandibular lymphadenopathy.

Cats with intraocular inflammation can have anterior uveitis, chorioretinitis, or optic neuritis.[1, 12, 13] Chorioretinitis is punctate or large, leading to suppurative retinal detachment. Inflammation can result in

Table 39–1
Cytologic Appearance of the Systemic Canine and Feline Fungal Diseases

AGENT	CYTOLOGIC APPEARANCE
Cryptococcus neoformans	Extracellular yeast, 3.5–7.0 μm in diameter, thick unstained capsule, thin-based bud, violet with light red capsule with Gram stain, unstained capsule with India ink
Blastomyces dermatitidis	Extracellular yeast, 5–20 μm in diameter, thick, refractile double contoured wall, broad-based bud, routine stains adequate
Histoplasma capsulatum	Intracellular yeast in mononuclear phagocytes, 2–4 μm in diameter, basophilic center with lighter body with Wright stain
Coccidioides immitis	Extracellular spherules (20–200 μm in diameter) containing endospores, deep red to purple double outer wall with bright red endospores with periodic acid–Schiff stain

Table 39–2
Manifestations of the Systemic Canine and Feline Fungal Diseases

CLINICAL MANIFESTATION	*Cryptococcus neoformans*	*Blastomyces dermatitidis*	*Histoplasma capsulatum*	*Coccidioides immitis*
Cardiac disease	—	—	—	Dog
Central nervous system disease	Dog and cat	Dog and cat	Dog	Dog and cat
Dermatologic disease	Dog and cat	Dog and cat	Dog and cat	Dog and cat
Gastrointestinal disease	—	Cat	Dog and cat	—
Hepatic disease	—	—	Dog and cat	—
Lymphatic disease	Dog and cat	Dog and cat	Dog and cat	—
Orchitis or prostatitis	—	Dog	—	Dog
Ocular disease	Dog and cat	Dog and cat	Dog and cat	Dog and cat
Osteomyelitis	Dog	Dog	Dog and cat	Dog and cat
Pleural or peritoneal effusion	—	Cat	Dog	Dog
Pulmonary disease	Dog and cat	Dog and cat	Dog and cat	Dog and cat
Upper respiratory disease	Dog and cat	—	—	—
Urinary tract disease	—	Cat	—	—

lens luxations and glaucoma. Central nervous system signs of disease are diverse and depend on the location of the lesion and whether diffuse meningoencephalitis or a focal granuloma is occurring. Depression, behavioral change, seizures, blindness, circling, ataxia, loss of sense of smell, and paresis occur.[1] Anorexia (10.4%) and weight loss (20.8%) occur in many cats; fever is rare (12.5%) and mild when it occurs.[3]

Cryptococcosis is diagnosed most commonly (79%) in dogs 1 to 7 years of age.[4] Disease is rare in dogs younger than 1 and older than 10 years of age. Purebred dogs are slightly more likely than mixed

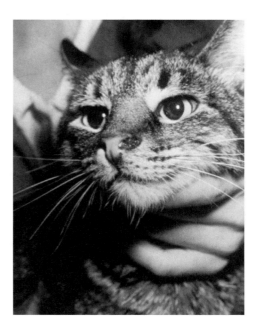

Figure 39–1
Characteristic nasal lesion of a cat with cryptococcosis.

breed dogs to acquire cryptococcosis. The American cocker spaniel appears to be at increased risk.[4] Common clinical manifestations in canine cases include extraneural head lesions (69%), disseminated disease (68%), central nervous system disease (68%), disease of the orbit or eye (47%), skin lesions (24%), nasal cavity disease (24%), and lymph node involvement (21%).[4] Potentially immunosuppressive conditions are identified in less than 10% of dogs with cryptococcosis. For example, corticosteroids, ehrlichiosis, heartworm disease, and neoplasia may predispose dogs to clinical cryptococcosis.[4, 5–7]

Clinical history and physical examination findings are dependent on the organ systems involved and are similar to those that occur in the cat. Most dogs with central nervous system disease have seizures, ataxia, central vestibular syndrome, deficits in one or more of cranial nerves V to XII, or clinical signs of cerebellar disease.[4]

Laboratory and Radiographic Abnormalities. Hematologic abnormalities potentially related to cryptococcosis in cats include nonregenerative anemia (45%) and monocytosis (66%).[2] Neutrophil counts are generally normal (73%), but neutrophilia or neutropenia may be noted.[2] Serum biochemical changes are unusual. Serologic evidence of coinfection with feline immunodeficiency virus (0%,[3] 5.7%,[10] and 28%[2]) or with feline leukemia virus (0%,[2] 8.8%,[3] and 11.4%[10]) occurs in some cats with cryptococcosis. In one study, the prevalence of cryptococcosis was greater in FIV-seropositive cats than in FIV-seronegative cats, suggesting that retroviral infection may predispose cats to cryptococcosis but is not required.[14] No pathognomonic changes are noted on hematologic or biochemical testing or urinalysis in dogs.

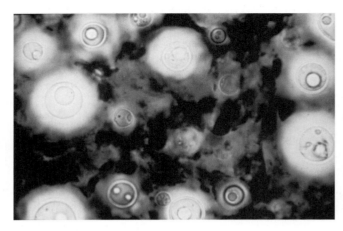

Figure 39-2

Cytologic appearance of *Cryptococcus neoformans*. The organism is 3.5 to 7.0 μm in diameter and has a thick polysaccharide capsule. (Courtesy of Dennis Macy, DVM, Fort Collins, Colorado.)

The cryptococcal organism is evident cytologically in cerebrospinal fluid (CSF) (92.6%) and by culture of CSF (75%) in most dogs with neurologic involvement.[15] In most dogs with neurologic cryptococcosis, abnormalities are noted on CSF cytology. Protein concentrations in CSF vary from normal to 500 mg/dL (normal, <25 mg/dL), and cell counts vary from normal to 4640/μL (normal, <5/μL).[15] The predominant cells in CSF are neutrophils (35%), mononuclear cells (24%), a 50% mixture of neutrophils and mononuclear cells (12%), or eosinophils (30%).[15]

Cytologic analysis is often positive (Fig. 39-2) because there are usually numerous yeasts in affected tissues (nasal lesions, cutaneous lesions, lymph nodes, CSF, and bronchoalvelolar lavage fluid).[16] Gram staining or India ink should be used (see Table 39-1). Lymphocytes, fat droplets, and ink particles may resemble the organism if India ink is used and budding is absent.

Radiographic changes are most common with the nasal cavity and lungs. Increased soft tissue density due to fungal granuloma formation or lytic changes, and nasal bone deformity due to fungal invasion are common in animals with nasal disease. Thoracic radiographic changes are often absent in cats (zero of nine cats evaluated).[10] If thoracic radiographic abnormalities are present in affected dogs and cats, hilar lymphadenopathy and diffuse to miliary interstitial patterns are most common. Radiography of dogs with central nervous system cryptococcosis may show discontinuity of the cribriform plate.[17]

Pathology

Lesions associated with cryptococcosis generally appear as masses. Hydrocephalus occurs in some dogs with central nervous system disease.[15] Histologically, numerous organisms are seen; the primary cellular responses are macrophages and giant cells. Lymphocytes and plasma cells occur in low numbers, and neutrophilic inflammation is rare.[1]

Diagnostic Plan

Definitive diagnosis of cryptococcosis is based on demonstration of the organism by cytology, histopathology, or culture.

Measurement of antibodies against *C. neoformans* is not clinically useful. Cryptococcal antigen is detected in serum, aqueous humor, or CSF using latex agglutination (LA). Serum antigen tests are positive in most cats (13 of 14[3] and 19 of 20[18]) and dogs (14 of 16) with cryptococcosis.[15] Negative serum LA titers may occur in early disease or uncommonly in chronic low-grade infections, chemotherapy-induced remission, or nondisseminated disease. The specificity of the serum LA may be 100%.[18] The LA was positive using CSF in 100% of dogs with central nervous system cryptococcosis.[15] A titer greater than 1:1 in serum or CSF is positive; very high titers are commonly detected. Cryptococcal encephalitis may cause a positive CSF LA titer despite a negative serum LA. Serum and CSF LA antigen titers diminish with therapy and can be used to monitor response.

Treatment and Prognosis

The primary drugs used for the treatment of cryptococcosis in dogs and cats include amphotericin B, ketoconazole, itraconazole, fluconazole, and 5-flucytosine (Table 39-3).[19] Most cases of feline cryptococcosis have been treated with ketoconazole alone or in combination with 5-flucytosine, itraconazole alone, or fluconazole alone.[2, 3, 10, 17, 20-23] Success rates for the treatment of cryptococcosis in cats have been reported in case series using fluconazole (96.6%),[2] ketoconazole (34.6%),[3] and itraconazole (57.1%).[10] Ketoconazole commonly leads to inappetence, vomiting, diarrhea, weight loss, and elevation of liver enzymes[8, 19, 22, 23]; the triazoles itraconazole and fluconazole are less toxic.[19] Cats treated with 100 mg/day of itraconazole occasionally (7 of 21 cats) exhibited anorexia, depression, and increased activity of alanine aminotransferase; only 1 of 13 cats receiving 50 mg/day developed toxicity.[10] Cats showing signs of toxicity normalized after stopping the drug and tolerated one half the original dose for the duration of therapy. Inappetence in a few cats was the only side effect attributed to fluconazole.[2]

Cases of canine cryptococcosis have been treated with amphotericin B, ketoconazole, 5-flucytosine, itraconazole, and fluconazole alone and in varying combinations.[15, 17, 24-26] Amphotericin B is no

Table 39–3

Antifungal Drugs Used in the Management of the Systemic Canine and Feline Fungal Diseases

DRUG	SPECIES	DOSAGE*	ORGANISM†
Amphotericin B	Dog	0.5 mg/kg IV, 3 times per week‡	B, H, Cr, Co
	Cat	0.25 mg/kg IV, 3 times per week§	B, H, Cr, Co
Fluconazole	Cat	50 mg PO, b.i.d.	Cr
Flucytosine	Dog and cat	50 mg/kg PO, q.i.d.	Cr
Ketoconazole	Dog and cat	10 mg/kg PO, daily	B, H, Cr, Co
Itraconazole	Dog	5 mg/kg PO, b.i.d., for 4 days and then 5 mg/kg PO, daily	B, Cr, H
	Cat	5 mg/kg PO, b.i.d.	B, Cr, H

*IV, intravenous; PO, by mouth; b.i.d., twice per day; q.i.d., four times per day.

†B, *Blastomyces*; H, *Histoplasma*; Cr, *Cryptococcus*; Co, *Coccidioides*.

‡In dogs with normal renal function, dilute in 60–120 mL 5% dextrose and administer IV over 15 min; in dogs with renal insufficiency but blood urea nitrogen <50 mg/dL, dilute in 500 mL–1 L 5% dextrose and administer IV over 3–6 h. Cumulative dose of 8–10 mg/kg if used alone or 4–6 mg/kg if combined with another antifungal drug.

§In cats with normal renal function, dilute in 50–100 mL 5% dextrose and administer IV over 3–6 h.

longer indicated unless life-threatening disseminated disease requires rapid response to therapy (see Blastomycosis). Ketoconazole is cheaper than itraconazole and fluconazole but has more significant side effects, including anorexia, vomiting, hepatic toxicosis, and suppression of testosterone and cortisol production.[19] Hepatic toxicosis occurs in 5% of the dogs receiving the daily dose of itraconazole (5 mg/kg by mouth). Ulcerative dermatitis and limb edema occurred in approximately 10% of the dogs receiving itraconazole at 5 mg/kg by mouth, twice per day (b.i.d.), but it did not occur in any dogs receiving 5 mg/kg by mouth daily.[19]

Flucytosine crosses the blood-brain barrier better than ketoconazole or amphotericin B and so has been used for the treatment of central nervous system cryptococcosis.[1, 15] The drug, however, has to be used in combination with other antifungal drugs and has many side effects, including vomiting, diarrhea, hepatotoxicity, cutaneous reactions, and bone marrow suppression. Because fluconazole and itraconazole are lipid soluble, they are successful in the treatment of central nervous system disease. Itraconazole and fluconazole should be considered the drugs of choice for the treatment of canine and feline cryptococcosis because of their superior success and fewer side effects than other drugs.[19, 27]

The prognosis for cryptococcosis is good for the nasal and cutaneous forms of disease. Coinfection with feline immunodeficiency virus did not appear to affect the prognosis in one study.[2] Central nervous system disease and ocular disease are the clinical manifestations least likely to respond to treatment. Treatment should continue for at least 1 to 2 months beyond the resolution of clinical disease. Optimally, cases should be treated until LA antigen test on serum or CSF is negative.[19] However, some animals have had long-term clinical resolution of disease even though the antigen test is still positive.[3]

Prevention

Because *C. neoformans* is a saprophyte that lives in soil, with worldwide distribution, prevention is difficult. Avoiding areas with high concentrations of pigeon droppings is indicated. Hydrated lime solution (40 g/L of water) applied at 1.36 L/m² can reduce the numbers of organism in contaminated areas.[1]

Zoonotic Aspects

The yeastlike phase of the organism found in tissues is not generally transmissible to humans, so the zoonotic risk of transmission is low. However, humans and animals can have the same environmental exposure. The organism also grows as a yeast in culture and thus is not as dangerous as are other systemic fungi in the laboratory.

Blastomycosis

Pathophysiology

Etiology. Blastomyces dermatitidis is a dimorphic, saprophytic yeast found in several regions of the United States. The organism is an extracellular yeast (5–20 μm in diameter) with a thick, refractile, double-contoured wall (Fig. 39–3) in the vertebrate host (see Table 39–1). When budding occurs it is broad based, in

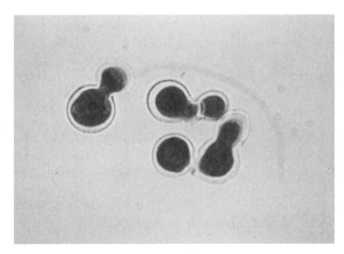

Figure 39-3
Cytologic appearance of the budding yeast *Blastomyces dermatitidis*. The organism is 5 to 20 µm in diameter and has a thick, refractile double contoured wall. (Courtesy of Dennis Macy, DVM, Fort Collins, Colorado.)

contrast to the narrow-based bud found with *C. neoformans*. The mycelial phase occurs in the soil and in culture.[28]

Epidemiology. *B. dermatitidis* survives optimally in sandy, acid soils near bodies of water, which explains the common occurrence of blastomycosis in the Mississippi, Missouri, and Ohio river valleys, the mid-Atlantic states, and southern Canada.[28, 29] High humidity and fog are thought to increase the chance of aerosolizing spores from the environment and may also partially explain the geographic distribution.[29] Infection in humans and animals is not equally distributed throughout an endemic area.[28] Frequently, infections are associated with a "point source" from which several cases occur. In 22% of households affected, several clinically affected dogs are diagnosed.[30] Unlike with histoplasmosis, subclinical infection is uncommon in dogs.[28] Most cases of blastomycosis in dogs are diagnosed in the autumn.[29] The route of transmission is thought to be primarily from inhalation of spores from the environment.[28] Also, some cases may occur after contamination of open wounds with the organism, leading to localized skin disease.[31] Horizontal transmission from domestic animals to other animals or humans is unlikely because the yeast phase is not as infectious as the mycelial phase.

Pathogenesis. After inhalation of spores, the organism is proposed to replicate in the lungs, with distant dissemination to other tissues. Multiple tissues are infected, including the skin and subcutaneous tissues, eyes, bones, lymph nodes, external nares, brain, testes, mouth, nasal passages, prostate, liver, mammary

glands, vulva, and heart.[28] There are differences in the virulence of field isolates.[28] Inoculum dose also affects the progression of the infection. Many animals with blastomycosis are probably immunosuppressed.[28] Posterior-segment ophthalmic disease is attributed to local organism replication. Anterior uveitis is thought to be due to diffusion of soluble inflammatory mediators from the posterior segment.[32] Immunity is primarily cell mediated, and antibody is not protective. Incomplete clearance of the organism results in pyogranulomatous inflammation in affected organs, which ultimately results in the clinical signs of disease.

Clinical Signs

Large-breed sporting dogs are infected most commonly; this is attributed to increased chance for exposure to the organism.[28, 29] The group at highest risk may be sexually intact male dogs, 2 to 4 years of age, weighing 22.7 to 34.1 kg.[29] Dogs are presented most frequently for evaluation of anorexia, cough, dyspnea, exercise intolerance, weight loss, ocular disease, skin disease, depression, or lameness.

Physical examination findings vary depending on the organ systems involved (see Table 39-2). Low-grade fever (39.5°C, 103.0°F) occurs in approximately 40% of affected dogs.[28] Thoracic auscultation usually reveals dry, harsh lung sounds; dyspnea occurs in severely affected dogs. Hypertrophic osteopathy can occur secondary to thoracic masses.[33]

Ocular involvement occurs in 31% (40 of 131) of dogs with blastomycosis.[32] Ocular manifestations can be divided into three groups: anterior uveitis (30%), endophthalmitis (26%), and posterior segment disease (44%). Optic neuritis occurs in 10% of the dogs and is commonly associated with central nervous system infection. Central nervous system involvement can be diffuse or multifocal; common manifestations include depression and seizures.[28]

Cutaneous ulcers with a serosanguineous or purulent fluid, nodules, subcutaneous abscesses, or plaques occur in 20% to 40% of the infected dogs.[11, 28] Lymphadenomegaly is common. Lesions are most common on the nasal planum, face, and nail beds.[11, 28]

Up to 30% of the dogs with blastomycosis are presented for evaluation of lameness. Fungal osteomyelitis most frequently involves the spine or appendicular skeleton; most of the lesions are single and occur distal to the stifle and elbow.[28] Some dogs have genitourinary tract involvement; however, infection of the testes, prostate,[34] urinary bladder, and kidneys rarely occurs.[28]

Clinical blastomycosis has been recognized in cats ranging from 6 months to 18 years of age; most are 4 years of age or older.[31] Male cats are more commonly infected than female cats. Most infected cats are seronegative for exposure to feline leukemia virus or feline immunodeficiency virus.

Cats most often have respiratory tract disease (70%), central nervous system disease (30%), regional lymphadenopathy (30%), dermatologic disease (30%), ocular disease (36%), gastrointestinal tract disease (21%), and urinary tract disease (9%).[31] Pleural or peritoneal effusion resulting in dyspnea or abdominal distention occurs in some cats (21%).[31] Ocular disease usually involves the posterior segment; in one study, central blindness occurred in 3 of 23 cats.[31]

Laboratory and Radiographic Abnormalities. Normocytic, normochromic, nonregenerative anemia is the most common clinical laboratory abnormality noted. Lymphopenia and neutrophilic leukocytosis with or without a left shift also occur frequently. Hypoalbuminemia and hyperglobulinemia are common serum biochemical abnormalities. The hyperglobulinemia is due to chronic inflammation and is polyclonal on protein electrophoresis. Hypercalcemia occurs in some dogs; most have been hyperphosphatemic as well.[28, 35]

Pulmonary changes in dogs with respiratory tract infection are usually diffuse but occasionally appear as single masses. Most dogs have a diffuse miliary to nodular interstitial pattern or a bronchointerstitial pattern. Osteomyelitis secondary to blastomycosis appears lytic radiographically, with a secondary periosteal reaction and soft tissue swelling.[28]

Nonregenerative anemia and degenerative left shift with lymphopenia are the most common complete blood count abnormalities in cats with blastomycosis; each occurs in 25% of cases.[31] Mild elevations in plasma proteins are also noted in affected cats.[31]

Cats with pulmonary involvement have radiographic changes similar to those found in dogs and consist primarily of interstitial lung densities.[31, 36] Pleural effusion may be noted.[31, 36] Loss of intraabdominal contrast is evident on abdominal radiographs of cats with peritoneal effusion.

Pathology

Histopathologic lesions of blastomycosis in affected tissues consist of granulomatous and pyogranulomatous inflammation. The yeast phase of the organism is generally easy to identify; special stains such as periodic acid–Schiff (PAS) are superior to hematoxylin and eosin. Rarely, the mycelial phase of the organism is seen.[28]

Diagnostic Plan

Definitive diagnosis requires identification of the yeast by cytology, histopathology, or fungal culture. Impression smears from skin lesions and aspirates from enlarged lymph nodes frequently reveal organisms; recovery of organisms from transtracheal aspiration, pulmonary aspiration biopsy, or urine is less consistent. Bronchoalveolar lavage was more sensitive (five of seven dogs) than transtracheal wash (three of seven dogs) for the cytologic demonstration of the organism.[37] Culture requires 10 to 14 days and has a lower yield than cytology or biopsy.

Circulating serum antibodies are detected in serum by agar gel immunodiffusion (AGID), counterimmunoelectrophoresis, and enzyme-linked immunosorbent assay (ELISA).[28] Results from AGID testing are occasionally positive but are more commonly negative in cats with blastomycosis.[31, 36] False-negative results can occur in animals with peracute infection or in advanced cases that overwhelm the immune system. In addition, antibody titers do not always revert to negative after successful treatment. However, because diffuse nodular pulmonary interstitial lung disease and hilar lymphadenopathy are commonly seen on thoracic radiographs, positive serologic results combined with appropriate clinical signs and radiographic abnormalities allow presumptive diagnosis if the organism cannot be demonstrated.

Treatment and Prognosis

Amphotericin B, ketoconazole, amphotericin B with ketoconazole, and itraconazole alone have been evaluated for the treatment of blastomycosis in dogs.[19, 28, 38] If amphotericin B alone is used (see Table 39–3), the cumulative dose should be 8 to 9 mg/kg. Therapy should be discontinued if the blood urea nitrogen exceeds 50 mg/dL. The animal should be well hydrated with 0.9% NaCl prior to treatment; the addition of 0.5 g/kg of mannitol to the drip lessens nephrotoxicity.[28] If amphotericin B is combined with ketoconazole for the treatment of severe lung or neurologic disease, the cumulative dose of amphotericin B should be 4 to 6 mg/kg. Itraconazole alone is likely to be as effective as amphotericin B or ketoconazole alone or in combination and has fewer side effects (see treatment and prognosis in Cryptococcosis). Itraconazole should be administered to dogs at 5 mg/kg by mouth, b.i.d., for 4 days and then 5 mg/kg by mouth daily in dogs and 5 mg/kg by mouth, b.i.d., in cats (Table 39–3). Treatment should be continued for 60 to 90 days.[19]

Approximately 80% of the canine cases respond to therapy. Relapses occur in 20% to 25% of treated dogs. If relapse occurs, a complete course of therapy should be reinitiated.[28] Disease associated with the prostate may be more likely to recur.[38] Posterior segment ocular disease responds well to itraconazole (76%), but most animals with anterior uveitis (64.7%) require enucleation of the affected eye. In one study, euthanasia (53.5%) or enucleation (33.3%) was required in many dogs with endophthalmitis.[32] In cats with blastomycosis, 4 of 23 survived after treatment; 2 were treated with amphotericin B and ketoconazole, 1 was treated with amputation, and 1 was treated with potassium iodide.[31]

Prevention

There is no vaccine for the prevention of blastomycosis. Avoiding lakes and creeks in endemic areas may decrease the chance for exposure.

Zoonotic Aspects

The yeast phase of *B. dermatitidis* is not usually transmitted from infected animals to humans. One veterinarian was infected after material from a pulmonary aspirate from an infected dog was injected intramuscularly[39]; another acquired disease after being bitten by an infected dog.[40] The mycelial phase of the organism is infectious, so culturing the fungus should be done with care. Humans and animals can have the same environmental exposure; there have been several reports of canine and human blastomycosis occurring in the same environment.[30, 41, 42]

Histoplasmosis

Pathophysiology

Etiology. *Histoplasma capsulatum* is a saprophytic dimorphic fungus. A mycelial phase that produces microconidia (2–4 μm in diameter) and macroconidia (5–18 μm in diameter) occurs in the environment. In the vertebrate host, the organism is found as a 2- to 4-μm-diameter intracellular yeast in mononuclear phagocytes (Fig. 39–4; see Table 39–1).[43, 44]

Epidemiology. *H. capsulatum* can be found in the soil in all regions with tropical and subtropical climates.[43, 44] Histoplasmosis is diagnosed most frequently in the Mississippi, Missouri, and Ohio river valleys and the mid-Atlantic states. The organism is concentrated most heavily in soil contaminated with bird or bat excrement. There are point sources for infection within endemic areas.[43] Occasionally, multiple cases are recognized in dogs and humans; 2 dogs and 20 humans contracted pulmonary histoplasmosis after removal of a tree that had served as a bird roost.[45] Infection is by ingestion or inhalation of microconidia from the environment. Inhalation is the proposed route of transmission for cats.[46] Most of the infections are resolved by the immune system and remain subclinical. Although up to 36% of the dogs in endemic areas are exposed, only approximately 60 of 100,000 cases of histoplasmosis are diagnosed at veterinary teaching

hospitals in these areas.[44] Most cases occur in young dogs and cats, so immunosuppression may predispose these animals to clinical infection.[43, 44, 46–48] Corticosteroids may have contributed to disease in some dogs.[47, 49]

Pathogenesis. After inhalation or ingestion, the organism is engulfed by mononuclear phagocytes, is transformed to the yeast phase, and is transported intracellularly throughout the body in the blood and lymph.[43, 44] Infection is limited by immune responses most of the time. Granulomatous inflammation results in persistently infected organs (see Table 39–2). Monocytes, lymphocytes, macrophages, and plasma cells are the primary infiltrating cells.[43, 44] Granuloma formation disrupts normal organ function, resulting in clinical signs of disease. The immunologic reaction against the organism, particularly cytokines such as interleukin-1 and tumor necrosis factor, result in systemic signs of disease, such as fever, anorexia, and wasting.[44]

Clinical Signs

In dogs, subclinical infection, pulmonary infection, and disseminated infection are recognized.[44] Most of the dogs with clinical illness are younger than 7 years of age.[43, 44, 47] Larger outdoor or sporting dogs, such as pointers and spaniels, may have a predisposition for disease[44] but also may be more commonly infected because of increased chance of exposure. There is no obvious gender predisposition.

Most dogs with clinical disease are presented for evaluation of anorexia, fever, depression, weight loss, coughing, dyspnea, or diarrhea (see Table

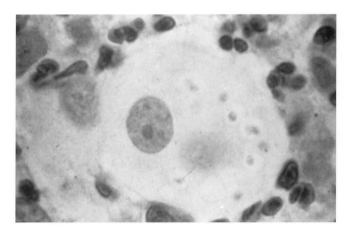

Figure 39–4
Cytologic appearance of *Histoplasma capsulatum*. The organism is 2 to 4 μm in diameter. There are small, dark areas with pale halos in the central area of a mononuclear cell. (Courtesy of Dennis Macy, DVM, Fort Collins, Colorado.)

39–2).[43, 44, 47, 49–51] Diarrhea usually contains blood and mucus and is consistent with large-bowel diarrhea, but infection of the small bowel results in watery stool and protein-losing enteropathy in some dogs.[43, 44] Common abnormal findings on physical examination include depression, increased lung sounds, fever, evidence of diarrhea, and pale mucous membranes.[43, 44]

Hepatomegaly, splenomegaly, icterus, ascites, and intra-abdominal lymph node enlargement develop in some dogs.[43, 44] Lameness, peripheral lymphadenopathy, ocular inflammation, central nervous system disease, and vomiting are more rare abnormal findings in the history and physical examination.[43, 44, 52] Polyarthritis and chorioretinitis resulting in retinal detachment may occur rarely in dogs with systemic histoplasmosis.[52] Skin lesions are found less often than with cryptococcosis and blastomycosis. Subcutaneous nodules that rarely drain or ulcerate are the most common. The organism is usually recognized cytologically in aspirates of these nodules or in the serosanguineous discharge that occasionally develops.[11, 43, 44]

Infected cats can be subclinically affected or can acquire disseminated disease.[43, 46, 48, 53] Most clinically affected cats are younger than 4 years of age; there is no obvious breed or sex predilection. Coinfection by feline leukemia virus occurs in some cats (3 of 15)[48, 53] but is not required for the development of histoplasmosis.

Most cats are presented for evaluation of depression, weight loss, anorexia, lameness, or dyspnea (see Table 39–2).[43, 46, 48, 53] Weight loss can be dramatic and occur in as little as 2 weeks.[46] Physical examination may reveal fever (39.5°–40.5°C, 103.1°–105.0°F), pale mucous membranes, abnormal lung sounds, oral erosions or ulcers, peripheral or visceral lymphadenomegaly, icterus, hepatomegaly, soft tissue swelling around osseous lesions, hepatomegaly, skin nodules, and (rarely) splenomegaly.[43, 46, 48, 53]

In most cats with osseous histoplasmosis, bones of the appendicular skeleton are involved distal to the stifle or elbow joints. Disease may be evident on one or more limbs. Pain on palpation is common. Regional lymphadenopathy and draining tracts occur in some affected cats.[53]

Cats with ocular histoplasmosis have conjunctivitis, chorioretinitis, retinal detachment, or optic neuritis and may develop glaucoma and blindness.[46, 48, 53] The organism is found in the brain of some cats, but central nervous system clinical signs other than nonspecific depression appear to be uncommon.[46]

Laboratory and Radiographic Abnormalities. Normocytic, normochromic, nonregenerative anemia secondary to chronic inflammation, bone marrow invasion by the organism, and intestinal blood loss is the most common abnormality found on laboratory analysis in both dogs and cats.[43, 44, 46] Neutrophil counts can be normal, increased, or decreased. The organism may be noted most commonly in circulating mononuclear cells but may occasionally be noted in neutrophils or eosinophils as well.[43, 44, 49] Thrombocytopenia occurs in approximately 50% of dogs[50] and some cats (4 of 12).[48] Mechanisms include consumption by disseminated intravascular coagulation and microangiopathic destruction.[50] Some affected cats acquire pancytopenia.[46, 48] Hypoalbuminemia occurs in many cats with disseminated disease.[46] Hyperglobulinemia may occur as a result of chronic inflammation. Dogs often contract panhypoproteinemia secondary to protein-losing enteropathy.[43, 44] Increased activities of alkaline phosphatase and alanine transaminase may occur in some animals with hepatic involvement. Urinalyses are usually normal.[43]

Osteolytic lesions predominate in animals with osseous involvement; periosteal and endosteal new bone production occurs in some animals.[53] In those with pulmonary involvement, diffuse interstitial or miliary to nodular interstitial lung changes are most commonly noted on radiographs.[43, 44] Alveolar lung disease, tracheobronchial lymphadenomegaly, and calcified lymph nodes are uncommon in cats.[54] Dogs often develop hilar lymphadenopathy, and some have calcified pulmonary parenchyma due to chronic disease.[43] Pleural or peritoneal effusion occurs rarely in dogs. Nonspecific abdominal radiographic findings, including hepatomegaly, splenomegaly, and excessive gas or fluid in the intestines, are common. Gross lesions noted during colonoscopic examination of infected dogs include increased mucosal granularity, friability, ulceration, and thickness.[55]

Pathology

Grossly, lesions appear as small masses in affected organs (see Table 39–2). The primary histologic abnormality associated with histoplasmosis is granulomatous inflammation. The organism is usually intracellular but is occasionally noted outside cells. With routine hematoxylin and eosin staining, the organism may be missed. The organism is stained better with PAS, Gomori methenamine silver, or Gridley's fungal stain.[43]

Diagnostic Plan

Definitive diagnosis requires demonstration of the organism by cytology, biopsy, or culture. Cytologic examination of rectal scrapings in dogs with signs of large-bowel diarrhea with disseminated histoplasmosis is often diagnostic.[43, 44, 47] Organisms are usually apparent on bone marrow cytology from cats with systemic histoplasmosis.[43, 46, 48] The organism is often found in other infected organs, including lymph nodes, lung, spleen, liver, and skin nodules and in pleural and peritoneal effusions[51] or CSF.[52]

Circulating antibodies are detected in serum by complement fixation (CF) and AGID. The CF test has poor sensitivity and specificity, and it cross-reacts with antibodies to other fungi and undetermined antigens. AGID has questionable clinical usefulness because titers persist more than 1 year after resolution of disease in some animals. Serologic diagnosis is unreliable in dogs and cats[44, 46] and is used only to establish a presumptive diagnosis when the organism cannot be demonstrated by cytology, histopathology, or culture and when clinical signs are suggestive of the disease.

Treatment and Prognosis

Historically, most cases of histoplasmosis in dogs or cats have been treated with amphotericin B or ketoconazole alone or in combination.[43, 44, 46, 48, 56] However, because of its effectiveness and minimal toxicity, itraconazole is the initial drug of choice for treatment of histoplasmosis.[19] Cats should be given 5 mg/kg by mouth, b.i.d., for 60 to 90 days or until clinical illness has been resolved for at least 1 month. Dogs should be given 5 mg/kg by mouth, b.i.d., for 90 days or until clinical illness has been resolved for at least 1 month. In dogs with poor response to itraconazole initially or with severe intestinal disease potentially inhibiting absorption of itraconazole from the intestinal tract, amphotericin B can be administered at 0.5 mg/kg intravenously, 3 days per week for 4 to 5 treatments, followed by itraconazole.[19] Ketoconazole can be administered to pets of owners who cannot afford itraconazole (see Table 39–3), but toxicity is more common with ketoconazole (see treatment and prognosis in Cryptococcosis). Fluconazole (see Table 39–3) is effective for the treatment of experimental histoplasmosis in mice and has been used for the treatment of disseminated histoplasmosis in AIDS patients.[27] The overall success rate for the treatment of histoplasmosis in cats is 33%.[46] Pulmonic disease in dogs has a fair to good prognosis, whereas disseminated disease in both cats and dogs has a poor prognosis.[43]

Prevention

Avoiding potentially contaminated soil, particularly that mixed with bird or bat excrement in endemic areas, may lessen the chance for exposure. A focal area of contamination can be treated with 3% formalin to reduce organism numbers.[43] There is no vaccine for the prevention of histoplasmosis.

Zoonotic Aspects

The yeast phase of *H. capsulatum* is not usually transmitted from infected animals to humans. The mycelial phase of the organism is infectious, so culturing the fungus should be done with care. Humans and animals can have the same environmental exposure.[45, 57]

Coccidioidomycosis

Pathophysiology

Etiology. *Coccidioides immitis* is a soil fungus that exists in the environment in the mycelial phase. The organism produces arthrospores (2–4 μm wide, 3–10 μm long) that are released and dispersed by the wind. Arthrospores enter the vertebrate host by inhalation or wound contamination and form spherules (20–200 μm in diameter). Spherules contain endospores (see Table 39–1) that are released by cleavage and produce new spherules.[58, 59]

Epidemiology. *C. immitis* survives in sandy alkaline soils in regions with low elevation, low rainfall, and high environmental temperatures. The organism is found in the southwestern United States, California, Mexico, Central America, and South America. Most cases of coccidioidomycosis in the United States are diagnosed in California, Arizona, New Mexico, Utah, Nevada, and southwest Texas.[58, 59] The organism survives deep in the soil and returns to the surface after periods of rainfall, when large numbers of arthrospores are released into the environment. The number of cases increases in years that follow high rainfall.[58–60] Most humans and animals in endemic areas are exposed to the organism. Humans are more resistant to infection than dogs or cats and acquire asymptomatic infection or mild, transient respiratory signs.[58] Dogs and cats are usually subclinically affected but can acquire severe respiratory and disseminated disease.[58, 59, 61] Most animals are infected by inhalation of arthrospores, but local infection of wounds can occur.[58, 59, 61] A seasonal occurrence has been recognized in cats; most cases (67%) are diagnosed between December and May.[61]

Pathogenesis. Arthrospores are inhaled and enter the alveoli and peribronchiolar tissues. Neutrophilic inflammation develops first, followed by increased numbers of monocytes, lymphocytes, and plasma cells.[58] Humoral immune responses develop in most infected animals, but cell-mediated immunity is more important for elimination of infection. Disseminated infection initially involves the mediastinal and tracheobronchial lymph nodes, followed by the bones and joints, the visceral organs (liver, spleen, and kidneys), heart and pericardium, testicles, eyes, brain, and spinal cord (see Table 39–2).[58] Respiratory signs generally develop 1 to 3 weeks after exposure.[58] Clinical signs of disseminated disease generally develop 4 months after pulmonary signs.[58]

Clinical Signs

Clinical disease in dogs occurs most commonly in those younger than 7 years of age (mean, 3.4 years of age).[59] Males are more likely than females to have disseminated disease.[58, 59] Dogs are usually presented for evaluation of cough or dyspnea, anorexia, weakness, weight loss, lymphadenomegaly, lameness, clinical signs of ocular inflammation, or diarrhea.[58, 59, 62] Examination of the respiratory tract may reveal louder than normal breath sounds or crackles, wheezing secondary to compression of the carina by enlarged tracheobronchial lymph nodes, or dyspnea due to severe pulmonary parenchymal disease or pleural effusion.

Lameness is due to appendicular skeletal involvement approximately 90% of the time.[58] Affected bones and joints are usually swollen and painful. The distal diaphysis, epiphysis, and metaphysis of long bones are most commonly involved. One or more bones may be involved. Subcutaneous abscesses, nodules, ulcers, and draining tracts occur in some dogs, generally over affected bones.[11, 58, 59]

On physical examination, findings in some dogs are consistent with right- or left-sided heart failure because of myocardial dysfunction resulting from invasion of the organism into the myocardium. Icterus is found in some dogs. Renomegaly, splenomegaly, or hepatomegaly may be found on palpation. The most common manifestations of ocular inflammation are keratitis (49% of dogs with ocular disease), iritis (43% of dogs), granulomatous uveitis (31% of dogs), and glaucoma (31% of dogs).[62] Occasionally, central nervous system infection can result in depression, seizures, ataxia, and behavioral changes.[58] Orchitis and epididymitis occur in some dogs.[59]

Cats with coccidioidomycosis range from 1 to 15 years of age (median, 5 years of age).[61] There is no obvious sex or breed predilection. Most of the cats have been clinically ill for less than 4 weeks (82%) when presented. The cats are usually presented for evaluation of skin disease (56%), respiratory disease (25%), musculoskeletal disease (19%), and either ophthalmic or neurologic disease (19%).[61] Clinical signs and physical examination findings are summarized in Table 39–4.

Laboratory and Radiographic Abnormalities. Clinical laboratory findings are nonspecific. Some dogs and cats (20%) develop normocytic, normochromic, nonregenerative anemia secondary to chronic inflammatory disease.[58, 59, 61] In one study, leukocytosis or leukopenia occurred in 5 of 12 (42%) cats tested.[61] Leukocytosis with or without a left shift and monocytosis occur in some dogs.[58, 59] Hyperproteinemia due to a polyclonal gammopathy is common in dogs[59] and cats (10 of 19 cats; 52%).[61] Hypoalbuminemia, renal azotemia, and proteinuria occur in dogs with renal involvement. Coinfection with feline leukemia virus (0 of 39 cats) or

Table 39–4

Clinical and Laboratory Findings in 48 Cats With Coccidioidomycosis

FINDING	NUMBER AFFECTED/ REPORTED (%)
Dermatologic disease	27/48 (56)
Draining skin lesions	16/27 (59)
Subcutaneous masses	9/27 (33)
Localized lymphadenomegaly	8/27 (30)
Abscesses	7/27 (26)
Fever	15/48 (31)
Inappetence	10/48 (21)
Weight loss	9/48 (19)
Respiratory disease	12/48 (25)
Dyspnea	11/12 (92)
Musculoskeletal disease	9/48 (19)
Retinal detachment, uveitis, iritis	6/48 (13)
Hyperesthesia, posterior paresis, seizure, incoordination	3/48 (6)

Data from Greene and Troy.[61]

feline immunodeficiency virus (1 of 21 cats) is unusual.[61]

Radiographically, dogs with pulmonary involvement most commonly have diffuse interstitial lung infiltrates.[58, 59, 63] Bronchovascular, miliary to nodular interstitial disease, and alveolar disease are sequentially less common.[58] Pleural effusion secondary to pleuritis, right-sided heart failure, or constrictive pericarditis can occur (18 of 38 cases).[63] Hilar lymphadenopathy is common in dogs (up to 75%)[59] and cats; sternal lymphadenopathy or calcification of lymph nodes is not.[58] Bony lesions are more proliferative than lytic lesions (Fig. 39–5).[58]

Pathology

Gross lesions are most common in the lungs and bones. The lesions can be diffuse or nodular, miliary to tumorous, and firm to liquefactive. Bones appear enlarged. Tracheobronchial lymph nodes are often large and firm. Granulomatous lesions may be noted in the brain, eyes, pericardium, and myocardium. Microscopically, the lesions are granulomatous, pyogranulomatous, or suppurative.[58]

Diagnostic Plan

Definitive diagnosis requires demonstration of the organism on smears, aspirates, histopathologic evaluation, or culture; however, the organism is often difficult to demonstrate by cytology. Transtracheal aspiration or bronchoalveolar lavage is often negative.[37] Spherules are more likely to be found in lymph node aspirates, draining masses, and pericardial fluid.[58] Wet-mount examination of unstained smears

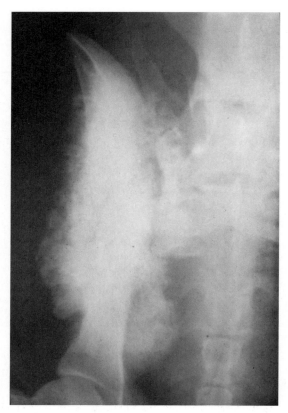

Figure 39–5
Typical osteomyelitis associated with coccidioidomycosis in the ilium of a dog. (Courtesy of Richard Park, DVM, Fort Collins, Colorado.)

or PAS-stained smears is more suitable than is dry-mount examination, which may distort the spherules.[58] In one study, the organism was identified by cytology, histopathology, and culture in 10, 17, and 11 of 48 cats, respectively.[61]

Circulating antibodies are detected in serum by CF, AGID, and tube precipitin (TP) tests. TP detects immunoglobulin M antibodies; CF and AGID detect immunoglobulin G antibodies.[58, 59] False-negative results in the TP test occur in early infections (less than 2 weeks), chronic infection, rapidly progressive acute infection, and primary cutaneous coccidioidomycosis. False-positive results in the CF test occur as a result of anticomplementary serum, which may be due to bacterial contaminants or immune complexes. Cross-reactions in patients with histoplasmosis and blastomycosis can occur with all tests. For clinically practical purposes, the combination of positive serologic tests and radiographic signs of interstitial lung disease, dermatologic disease, or osteomyelitis in animals from endemic areas can be used to make a tentative diagnosis if the organism cannot be demonstrated. Positive serologic test results were detected in all 39

cats tested in one study.[61] After resolution of disease, CF titers decrease over weeks to months but can remain positive (e.g., 1:32) for months to years.

Treatment and Prognosis

Ketoconazole is the drug of choice for treatment of coccidioidomycosis in dogs (see Table 39–3).[58, 64, 65] In animals with poor response or severe toxicity with ketoconazole, amphotericin B can be used. If amphotericin B is used alone, a cumulative dose of 8 to 11 mg/kg should be given. If ketoconazole and amphotericin B are used together, a cumulative dose of 4 to 6 mg/kg of amphotericin B should be given.[58] The use of itraconazole does not seem advantageous.[19] Because of its superior penetration into the central nervous system, fluconazole should be considered for the treatment of meningoencephalitis.[1, 27] Approximately 90% of treated dogs show improvement, but cure is less likely with osseous involvement.[58] Repeated treatments are often required in dogs with bone lesions.

Ketoconazole, itraconazole, and fluconazole have been used to treat coccidioidomycosis in cats.[61] Of the treated cats, 32 of 44 were asymptomatic during or after treatment. Relapse occurred in 11 cats during or after treatment.

Prevention

A spherule-derived vaccine for use in humans has been evaluated but is not available.[66] Vaccines are not available for domestic animals. The disease can be prevented only by avoiding endemic areas.

Zoonotic Aspects

There is little risk for direct transmission of coccidioidomycosis from infected animals to people. However, the mycelial phase may grow on fomites such as bandage material.[59] Care must be taken while handling the mycelial phase in culture.

References

1. Medleau L, Barsanti JA. Cryptococcosis. In: Greene CE, ed. Infectious Diseases of the Dog and Cat, 2nd ed. Philadelphia, WB Saunders, 1990:687–695.
2. Malik R, Wigney DI, Muir DB, et al. Cryptococcosis in cats: Clinical and mycological assessment of 29 cases and evaluation of treatment using orally administered fluconazole. J Med Vet Mycol 1992;30:133–144.
3. Flatland B, Greene RT, Lappin MR. Clinical response and serologic findings of 52 cats with cryptococcosis. J Am Vet Med Assoc 1996 (in press).
4. Berthelin CF, Bailey CS, Kass PH, et al. Cryptococcosis of the nervous system in dogs, part 1: Epidemiologic,

clinical, and neuropathological features. Prog Vet Neurol 1994;5:88–97.

5. Hodgin EC, Corstvet RE, Blakewood BW. Cryptococcosis in a pup. J Am Vet Med Assoc 1987;191:697–698.

6. Collett MG, Doyle AS, Reyers F, et al. Fatal disseminated cryptococcosis and concurrent ehrlichiosis in a dog. J S Afr Vet Assoc 1987;58:197–202.

7. Kock ND, Lane EP, Rowbotham F, et al. Concurrent systemic cryptococcosis and haemangiosarcoma in a dog. J Comp Pathol 1991;104:117–120.

8. Medleau L, Greene CE, Rakich PM. Evaluation of ketoconazole and itraconazole for treatment of disseminated cryptococcosis in cats. Am J Vet Res 1990;51:1454–1458.

9. Levitz SM, Dupont MP, Smail EH. Direct activity of human T lymphocytes and natural killer cells against *Cryptococcus neoformans*. Infect Immun 1994;64:194–202.

10. Medleau L, Jacobs GJ, Marks MA. Itraconazole for the treatment of cryptococcosis in cats. J Vet Intern Med 1995;9:39–42.

11. Rosychuk RAW, White SD. Systemic infectious diseases and infestations that cause cutaneous lesions. Vet Med 1991;164–181.

12. Crispin SM. Uveitis associated with systemic disease in cats. Feline Pract 1987;17:16–19.

13. Rosenthal JJ, Heidgerd J, Peiffer RL. Ocular and systemic cryptococcosis in a cat. J Am Anim Hosp Assoc 1981;17:307–310.

14. Mancianti F, Giannelli C, Bendinelli M, et al. Mycological findings in feline immunodeficiency virus–infected cats. J Med Vet Mycol 1992;30:257–259.

15. Berthelin CF, Legendre AM, Bailey CS, et al. Cryptococcosis of the nervous system in dogs, part 2: Diagnosis, treatment, monitoring, and prognosis. Prog Vet Neurol 1994;5:136–146.

16. Hamilton TA, Hawkins EC, DeNicola DB. Bronchoalveolar lavage and tracheal wash to determine lung involvement in a cat with cryptococcosis. J Am Vet Med Assoc 1991;198:655–656.

17. Cook JR, Evinger JV, Wagner LA. Successful combination chemotherapy for canine cryptococcal meningoencephalitis. J Am Anim Hosp Assoc 1991;27:61–64.

18. Medleau L, Marks MA, Brown J, et al. Clinical evaluation of a cryptococcal antigen latex agglutination test for diagnosis of cryptococcosis in cats. J Am Vet Med Assoc 1990;196:1470–1473.

19. Legendre AM. Antimycotic drug therapy. In: Bonagura JD, Kirk RW, eds. Kirk's Current Veterinary Therapy XII. Philadelphia, WB Saunders, 1995:327–331.

20. Mikiciuk MG, Fales WH, Schmidt DA. Successful treatment of feline cryptococcosis with ketoconazole and flucytosine. J Am Anim Hosp Assoc 1990;26:199–202.

21. Shaw SE. Successful treatment of 11 cases of feline cryptococcosis. Aust Vet Pract 1988;18:135–139.

22. Emms SG. Ketoconazole in the treatment of cryptococcosis in cats. Aust Vet J 1987;64:276–277.

23. Pentlarge VW, Martin RA. Treatment of cryptococcosis in three cats, using ketoconazole. J Am Vet Med Assoc 1986;188:536–538.

24. Mason GD, Labato MA, Bachrach A. Ketoconazole therapy in a dog with systemic cryptococcosis. J Am Vet Med Assoc 1989;195:954–956.

25. Faggi E, Gargani G, Pizzirani C, et al. Cryptococcosis in domestic mammals. Mycoses 1993;36:165–170.

26. Stampley AR, Barsanti JA. Disseminated cryptococcosis in a dog. J Am Anim Hosp Assoc 1988;24:17–21.

27. Como JA, Dismukes WE. Oral azole drugs as systemic antifungal therapy. N Engl J Med 1994;330:263–272.

28. Legendre AM. Blastomycosis. In: Greene CE, ed. Infectious Diseases of the Dog and Cat, 2nd ed. Philadelphia, WB Saunders, 1990:669–678.

29. Rudmann DG, Coolman BR, Perez CM, et al. Evaluation of risks factors for blastomycosis in dogs: 857 cases (1980–1990). J Am Vet Med Assoc 1992;201:1754–1759.

30. Archer JR, Trainer DO, Schnell RF. Epidemiologic study of canine blastomycosis in Wisconsin. J Am Vet Med Assoc 1987;190:1292–1295.

31. Miller PE, Miller LM, Schoster JV. Feline blastomycosis: A report of three cases and literature review (1961 to 1988). J Am Anim Hosp Assoc 1990;26:417–424.

32. Brooks DE, Legendre AM, Gum GG, et al. The treatment of canine ocular blastomycosis with systemically administered itraconazole. Prog Vet Comp Ophthalmol 1991;1:263–268.

33. Brockus CW, Hathcock JT. Hypertrophic osteopathy associated with pulmonary blastomycosis in a dog. Vet Radiol 1988;4:184–188.

34. Hastings J, Payton C, Backmon M. Treating prostatitis caused by *Blastomyces dermatitidis*. Vet Med 1987;82:1236–1237.

35. Dow SW, Legendre AM, Stiff M, et al. Hypercalcemia associated with blastomycosis in dogs. J Am Vet Med Assoc 1986;188:706–709.

36. Breider MA, Walker TL, Legendre AM, et al. Blastomycosis in cats: Five cases (1979–1986). J Am Vet Med Assoc 1988;193:570–572.

37. Hawkins EC, DeNicola DB. Cytologic analysis of tracheal wash specimens and bronchoalveolar lavage fluid in the diagnosis of mycotic infections in dogs. J Am Vet Med Assoc 1990;197:79–83.

38. Legendre AM, Selcer BA, Edwards DF, et al. Treatment of canine blastomycosis with amphotericin B and ketoconazole. J Am Vet Med Assoc 1984;185:1249–1254.

39. Ramsey DT. Blastomycosis in a veterinarian. J Am Vet Med Assoc 1994;205:968.

40. Gnann JW, Bressler GS, Bodet CA. Human blastomycosis after a dog bite. Ann Intern Med 1983;98:48–49.

41. Baumgardner DJ, Burdick JS. An outbreak of human and canine blastomycosis. Rev Infect Dis 1991;13:898–905.

42. McCune MB. A blastomycosis field investigation: Canine outbreak suggests risk to human health. J Environ Health 1988;51:22–23.

43. Wolf AM. Histoplasmosis. In: Greene CE, ed. Infectious Diseases of the Dog and Cat, 2nd ed. Philadelphia, WB Saunders, 1990:679–686.

44. Clinkenbeard IKD, Wolf AM, Cowell RL, et al. Canine disseminated histoplasmosis. Compen Contin Educ Pract Vet 1989;11:1347–1360.

45. Ward JI, Weeks M, Allen D, et al. Acute histoplasmosis: Clinical, epidemiologic and serologic finding of an

outbreak associated with exposure to a fallen tree. Am J Med 1979:66:587–595.

46. Clinkenbeard KD, Wolf AM, Cowell RL, et al. Feline disseminated histoplasmosis. Compen Contin Educ Pract Vet 1989;11:1223–1233.

47. Clinkenbeard KD, Cowell RL, Tyler RD. Disseminated histoplasmosis in dogs: 12 cases (1981–1986). JAMA 1988;193:1443–1447.

48. Clinkenbeard KD, Cowell RL, Tyler RD. Disseminated histoplasmosis in cats: 12 cases (1981–1986). JAMA 1987;190:1445–1448.

49. Clinkenbeard KD, Cowell RL, Tyler RD. Identification of *Histoplasma* organisms in circulating eosinophils of a dog. J Am Vet Med Assoc 1988;192:217–218.

50. Clinkenbeard KD, Tyler RD, Cowell RL. Thrombocytopenia associated with disseminated histoplasmosis in dogs. Compen Contin Educ Pract Vet 1989;11:301–306.

51. Kowalewich N, Hawkins EC, Skowronek AJ, et al. Identification of *Histoplasma capsulatum* organisms in the pleural and peritoneal effusions of a dog. J Am Vet Med Assoc 1993;202:423–426.

52. Meadows RL, MacWilliams PS, Dzata G, et al. Diagnosis of histoplasmosis in a dog by cytologic examination of CSF. Vet Clin Pathol 1992;21:122–125.

53. Wolf AM. *Histoplasma capsulatum* osteomyelitis in the cat. J Vet Intern Med 1987;1:158–162.

54. Wolf AM, Green RW. The radiographic appearance of pulmonary histoplasmosis in the cat. Vet Radiol 1987;28:34–37.

55. Leib MS. Codner EC, Monroe WE. Common colonoscopic findings in dogs with chronic large bowel diarrhea. Vet Med 1991:913–921.

56. Wolf AM. Successful treatment of disseminated histo-

plasmosis with osseous involvement in two cats. J Am Anim Hosp Assoc 1988;24:511–516.

57. Davies SF, Colbert RL. Concurrent human and canine histoplasmosis from cutting decayed wood. Ann Intern Med 1990;113:252–253.

58. Barsanti JA, Jeffery KL. Coccidioidomycosis. In: Greene CE, ed. Infectious Diseases of the Dog and Cat, 2nd ed. Philadelphia, WB Saunders, 1990:696–706.

59. Armstrong PJ, DiBartola SP. Canine coccidioidomycosis: A literature review and report of 8 cases. J Am Anim Hosp Assoc 1983;19:937–945.

60. Coccidioidomycosis—United States, 1991–1992. Morb Mortal Wkly Rep 1993;42:21–24.

61. Greene RT, Troy GC. Coccidioidomycosis in 48 cats: A retrospective study (1984–1993). J Vet Intern Med 1995;9:86–91.

62. Angell JA, Merideth RE, Shively JN, et al. Ocular lesions associated with coccidioidomycosis in dogs: 35 cases (1980–1985). J Am Vet Med Assoc 1987;190:1319–1322.

63. Millman TM, O'Brien TR, Suter PF, et al. Coccidioidomycosis in the dog; its radiographic diagnosis. J Am Vet Radiol Soc 1979;20:50–65.

64. Jackson JA, Mauldin RA, Bauman DS, et al. Treatment of canine coccidioidomycosis with ketoconazole: Serological aspects of a case study. J Am Anim Hosp Assoc 1985;21:572–578.

65. Hinsch BG. Ketoconazole treatment of disseminated coccidioidomycosis in a dog. Mod Vet Pract 1988;69:161–162.

66. Pappagianis D. Evaluation of the protective efficacy of the killed *Coccidioides immitis* spherule vaccine in humans. Valley Fever Vaccine Study Group. Am Rev Respir Dis 1993;148:656–660.

Chapter 40

Polysystemic Protozoal Diseases

Michael R. Lappin

Toxoplasmosis

Pathophysiology

Etiology. *Toxoplasma gondii* is an obligate intracellular coccidian parasite with worldwide distribution.[1] The organism has three life stages and possesses a group of organelles that enables it to penetrate all cell types. Tachyzoites are the rapidly dividing stage of the parasite and occasionally are found in tissues or disseminating in blood or lymph during active infection. Bradyzoites are present in the slowly dividing tissue stage of the parasite and can be found in most extraintestinal tissues of infected hosts. Sporozoites develop in oocysts passed in feces of infected cats after 1 to 5 days of exposure to oxygen and appropriate environmental temperature and humidity.[1]

Epidemiology. *T. gondii* is one of the most prevalent parasites and can infect all vertebrates. The tissue stage of *T. gondii* is likely to persist for the life of the host. Seroprevalence studies suggest that approximately 30% to 40% of cats and humans and approximately 20% of dogs in the United States are infected.[1]

Cats are the only known species that can complete the enteroepithelial phase of toxoplasmosis resulting in passage of environmentally resistant oocysts in feces. All other vertebrates, including dogs, are intermediate hosts that harbor the tissue stages of the organism. Infection occurs primarily after ingestion of the organism during any of its three life stages or transplacentally.[1] Rarely, the organism is transmitted by organ transplantation.

Because cats are not coprophagic, most are exposed to *T. gondii* bradyzoites during carnivorous feeding. After ingestion of an infected intermediate host by a previously *Toxoplasma*-naive cat, bradyzoites are released from tissue cysts and penetrate the epithelial cells of the intestines, initiating the enteroepithelial cycle (Fig. 40–1). The enteroepithelial cycle results in the formation of unsporulated oocysts that are released into the intestinal lumen and are passed with feces.[1] After sporulation for 1 to 5 days, sporulated oocysts contain two sporocysts, each with four infective sporozoites (Fig. 40–2). Oocysts can usually be found in feces within 3 days after ingestion of tissue cysts. After ingestion of sporulated oocysts, the onset of oocyst shedding may be delayed for 3 weeks or more. Oocyst shedding is generally completed within 1 to 2 weeks after tissue cyst ingestion and within several weeks after sporulated oocyst ingestion. More oocysts are shed after tissue cyst ingestion than after sporulated oocyst ingestion.[1]

An extraintestinal phase of infection occurs in all vertebrates exposed to *T. gondii.* After ingestion of sporulated oocysts or tissue cysts, sporozoites or bradyzoites, respectively, are released in the intestinal lumen. After penetrating the lamina propria of the intestine, the organism disseminates in the blood and lymph as tachyzoites. Tachyzoites can penetrate most cells of the body and replicate intracellularly until the infected cell is destroyed. A combination of humoral and cell-mediated immune responses in immunocompetent hosts attenuates replication, leading to the development of tissue cysts containing bradyzoites. Bradyzoites are generally not associated with inflammation and may persist in tissues for the life of the host. Tissue cysts form most readily in the central nervous system (CNS), muscles, and visceral organs.[1]

Sporulated oocysts can survive in the environment for months to years and are resistant to most disinfectants. Tissue cysts are infective for days to weeks in meat stored at room temperature or 4°C (39°F). Freezing meat at –20°C (–4°F) inactivates some but not all tissue cysts. Cooking meat to medium well–done (66°C [150°F] for 20 minutes) inactivates tissue cysts. Tachyzoites are readily inactivated outside the host by routine disinfectants and by gastric secretions if ingested.[1, 2]

Pathogenesis. *T. gondii* is a well-adapted parasite, and clinical disease is much less common in dogs and cats than is serologic evidence of infection. The enteroepithelial cycle rarely leads to gastrointestinal tract signs in infected cats. Clinical disease is most often associated with the extraintestinal phase of infection and can occur in dogs or cats.[1–16]

Clinical toxoplasmosis due to the extraintestinal stage of infection has been attributed to cell destruction secondary to tachyzoite replication, *T. gondii*–containing immune complex formation and deposition in tissues, delayed hypersensitivity reactions against *T. gondii* antigens, and rarely, tissue cyst rupture.[1, 2, 17] Bradyzoites in tissue cysts can be reactivated when the host is immunosuppressed, as occurs with acquired immunodeficiency syndrome (AIDS)[18] or administration of high doses of glucocorticoids,[19] leading to repeated dissemination of tachyzoites and rupture of tissue cells, resulting in clinical disease. It has been hypothesized that coinfection of cats with immunosuppression-inducing viruses, including feline leukemia virus and feline immunodeficiency virus (FIV), increases the incidence of clinical toxoplasmosis in cats.[7, 8] Recurrent antigenemia has been documented in healthy, experimentally infected cats for up to 1 year after inoculation.[20] This has been attributed to antigen release from tissue cysts. The circulating antigens form immune complexes with *T. gondii*–specific antibodies. Immune complexes have been hypothesized to play a role in the development of toxoplasmic uveitis in cats.[17]

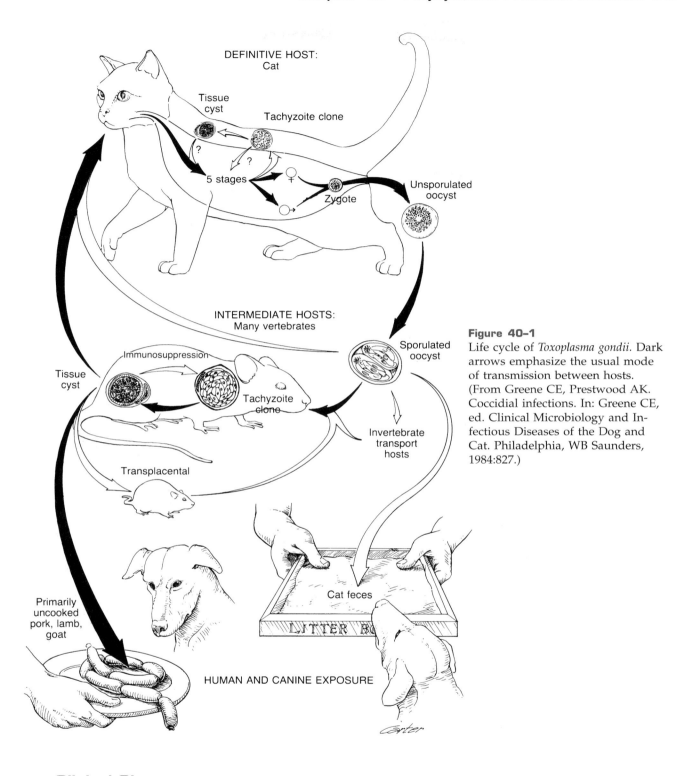

DEFINITIVE HOST:
Cat

Tissue cyst

Tachyzoite clone

5 stages

Zygote

Unsporulated oocyst

INTERMEDIATE HOSTS:
Many vertebrates

Immunosuppression

Tissue cyst

Tachyzoite clone

Sporulated oocyst

Invertebrate transport hosts

Transplacental

Primarily uncooked pork, lamb, goat

Cat feces

LITTER BOX

HUMAN AND CANINE EXPOSURE

Figure 40–1
Life cycle of *Toxoplasma gondii*. Dark arrows emphasize the usual mode of transmission between hosts. (From Greene CE, Prestwood AK. Coccidial infections. In: Greene CE, ed. Clinical Microbiology and Infectious Diseases of the Dog and Cat. Philadelphia, WB Saunders, 1984:827.)

Clinical Signs

Cats rarely develop clinical signs of gastrointestinal disease during the enteroepithelial cycle. Documentation of oocyst shedding in clinically ill cats has not been studied extensively but may occur in some cats.[13] Inflammatory bowel disease suspected to be related to *T. gondii* was reported in two cats.[14]

Extraintestinal toxoplasmosis can lead to clinical signs of disease in all vertebrates. In cats, transplacentally infected kittens develop the most severe signs of toxoplasmosis and generally die of pulmonic or hepatic disease.[1, 15, 16, 21] Pulmonic toxoplasmosis has been recognized in some neonatal kittens.[15, 16] Clinical feline toxoplasmosis can occur in cats of any age and

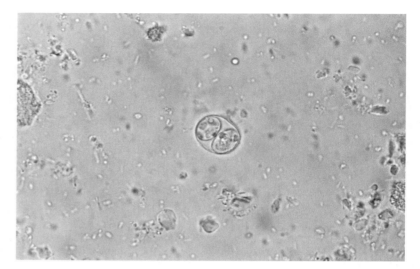

Figure 40–2
Sporulated oocyst of *Toxoplasma gondii*. The oocyst is 10×12 µm.

can be acute or chronic.[1, 7–16] In most published cases of clinical feline toxoplasmosis, diagnosis was made at necropsy and appeared to be associated with organism replication in tissues, resulting in natural death or euthanasia. A number of sublethal syndromes in cats, possibly from infection by *T. gondii*, have been identified (Fig. 40–3). Common clinical signs include anterior uveitis, posterior uveitis, fever, muscle hyperesthesia, weight loss, anorexia, seizures, ataxia, icterus, diarrhea, and vomiting associated with pancreatitis.[1, 7–12, 14] Toxoplasmosis appears to be a common infectious cause of uveitis and chorioretinitis in cats (Fig. 40–4).[7, 9–11] Clinical toxoplasmosis may be more severe in cats coinfected with FIV.[7, 8]

In dogs, clinical signs generally involve the respiratory, gastrointestinal, or neuromuscular system.[2] Fever, vomiting, diarrhea, dyspnea, and icterus occur in generalized toxoplasmosis. Myocardial dysfunction may also occur. Neurologic signs occur in some dogs. Signs are dependent on lesion localization but have included ataxia, seizures, tremors, cranial nerve deficits, paresis, and paralysis.[5] Dogs with myositis can have weakness, stiff gait, or muscle wasting.[6] Rapid progression to tetraparesis and paralysis with lower motor neuron dysfunction can occur. Some cases thought to be neuromuscular canine toxoplasmosis were probably neosporosis (see Neosporosis). Retinitis, anterior uveitis, iridocyclitis, and optic neuritis can occur in dogs with toxoplasmosis but seem less common than in the cat.[2]

Hematologic, Biochemical, and Urinalysis Abnormalities. A multitude of clinical pathologic abnormalities have been described in cats and dogs with clinical toxoplasmosis due to extraintestinal infection.[2, 7, 8, 16] Nonregenerative anemia, neutrophilic leukocytosis, lymphocytosis, monocytosis, neutropenia, and eosinophilia have been described in some cats.[7, 8, 16] Increased

serum proteins, creatinine kinase activity, bilirubin, alanine aminotransferase activity, alkaline phosphatase activity, and lipase activity can develop depending on the organ system involved. Proteinuria and bilirubinuria are detected by urinalysis in some cats.[16] None of the clinical laboratory changes are pathognomonic for toxoplasmosis.

Radiographic Abnormalities. Pulmonic toxoplasmosis most commonly causes diffuse interstitial or alveolar patterns. Pleural effusion may develop in some cases. Abdominal radiographic findings may include homogeneous increased density due to peritoneal effusion, hepatomegaly, lymphadenopathy, intestinal masses, or loss of contrast in the cranial right quadrant of the abdomen due to pancreatitis. Rarely, radiographic changes in the brain or spinal cord have been reported.[12] Radiographic abnormalities do not occur in subclinically ill dogs or cats or in cats undergoing the enteroepithelial cycle.

Cytologic and Cerebrospinal Fluid Analyses. Protein levels ranging from normal to 149 mg/dL and nucleated cell counts ranging from fewer than 5 to 28 cells/mm³ were detected in a series of cats with suspected CNS toxoplasmosis[12]; the predominant white blood cells were small mononuclear cells. Mixed inflammatory cell infiltrates occur in dogs with CNS toxoplasmosis.[2, 5] Tachyzoites are rarely found in blood, cerebrospinal fluid (CSF), transtracheal wash fluids, peritoneal effusions, and pleural effusions from clinically ill animals.

Fecal Examination. Demonstration of oocysts in feline feces can be made after flotation using solutions with a specific gravity of at least 1.18 (all standard fecal flotation solutions).[1] Oocysts of *T. gondii* are 10×12 µm. Focusing on only one plane may result in oocysts' being overlooked. The oocysts cannot be distinguished grossly from *Hammondia hammondi* or *Besnoitia darlingi,* which are nonpathogenic coccidians infecting cats. A definitive diagnosis of *T. gondii* can be made only with laboratory animal inoculation. Because oocyst shedding has rarely been documented in cats with sublethal clinical toxoplasmosis, the diagnostic utility of fecal examination is limited. However, the feces of cats with clinical signs referable to *T. gondii* should be evaluated because of the potential zoonotic risks, but failure to find oocysts does not eliminate the risk. Because oocysts passed in feces are unsporulated and noninfectious, working with fresh feline feces passed within 24 hours is not a risk for veterinary health care personnel. Feline fecal samples containing oocysts 10×12 μm should be incinerated. Using currently available techniques, it is impossible to predict when a cat has shed oocysts in the past or whether a seropositive cat will shed oocysts again in the future.

Demonstration of* T. gondii *in Tissues. Demonstration of *T. gondii* tachyzoites or bradyzoites in tissue biopsy sections can be made using hematoxylin and eosin or immunohistochemical staining procedures.[1] The latter procedures have the advantage of being specific for *T. gondii.* Histopathology is not a beneficial technique for the diagnosis of toxoplasmosis in sub-

Cat	Gender	Age (years)	Breed	Abscess	Anorexia	Arthritis	Ataxia	Anterior uveitis	Blindness	Behavioural change	Cystitis	Diarrhoea	Fever	Glaucoma	Gingivitis	Lethargy	Lens luxation	Muscle pain	Optic nerve atrophy	Pars planitis	Respiratory tract disease	Retinal atrophy	Retinochoroiditis	Retinal haemorrhage	Seizures	Urinary incontinence	Weight loss	
1	FS	10	DSH			■		■						■										■	■			1
2	FS	2	Siamese			■		■						■														2
3	FS	7	DSH			■																	■	■				3
4	MC	6	DSH		■	■		■				■															■	4
5	FS	8	DLH			■		■				■											■					5
6	FS	5	DSH			■																		■			■	6
7	MC	12	DLH			■													■						■			7
8	MC	9	DSH		■																							8
9*	MC	9	DSH		■		■																				■	9
10*	MC	10	DSH	■	■								■							■							■	10
11*	MC	7	DSH			■																	■					11
12*	MC	12	DSH			■																	■					12
13*	M	16	DSH	■	■				■					■													■	13
14*	FS	7	DSH			■																						14
15*	M	9	DSH								■								■				■					15
16*	MC	11	DLH		■						■			■	■								■					16
17*	M	11	DSH								■			■								■	■					17
18	MC	3	DLH		■							■		■	■												■	18
19	FS	7	DLH		■																						■	19
20	MC	14	DLH		■	■										■	■										■	20
21	F	10	DSH							■															■			21
22	MC	10	Tonkonese			■						■					■			■								22
23	F	4	DLH			■	■					■					■		■	■								23
24	MC	6	DSH			■																						24
25	F	8	Persian			■																						25
26	MC	3	DSH									■							■									26
27	MC	5	DSH				■					■							■									27
28	MC	4	ABY			■						■											■	■				28

Gender: FS – Female spayed MC – Male castrated
Breed: DSH – Domestic short hair DLH – Domestic long hair ABY – Abyssinian

*Cats 9–17 are FIV Seropositive

Figure 40–3
Signalment, history, and initial physical examination findings from 28 cats with suspected sublethal clinical toxoplasmosis. (From Lappin MR. Feline toxoplasmosis. Waltham Focus 1994;4:2–8.)

clinically infected animals. It may be difficult to document the organism in the tissues of some clinically ill animals because of the small sections of tissue evaluated histopathologically and because the pathogenesis of disease in some animals may be immune mediated. This appears to be particularly true for the ophthalmic form of the disease in cats. Histopathologic studies of ocular tissues from cats with uveitis rarely document the presence of *T. gondii* organisms.[16, 22] However, many cats with uveitis are serologically positive for toxoplasmosis[7, 9–11] and often improve after receiving clindamycin hydrochloride (Antirobe), a drug with anti-*Toxoplasma* activity.[7, 10, 11] Fresh tissue suspensions (tachyzoites or bradyzoites) can be inoculated into mice or onto tissue cultures. Demonstration of *T. gondii* in tissue does not confirm clinical disease unless the organism is associated with inflammation.

Serology. In cats, *T. gondii*–specific antibodies,[1, 2, 23] antigens,[20] and immune complexes[17] can be detected in serum, aqueous humor, and CSF. *T. gondii*–specific antibodies and antigens can be detected in the serum, aqueous humor, and CSF of dogs.

Antibodies against *T. gondii* can be detected with multiple techniques including enzyme-linked immunosorbent assay (ELISA), immunofluorescent antibody (IFA) test, Western blot immunoassay, Sabin Feldman dye test, and a variety of agglutination tests.[1, 2, 23–25] Agglutination tests, IFA, and ELISA are available in most commercial laboratories for use with dog and cat sera.

T. gondii–specific IgM is detectable in serum by ELISA in approximately 80% of healthy, experimentally infected cats within 2 to 4 weeks after inoculation with *T. gondii*; these IgM titers generally are negative within 16 weeks after infection. IgM titers greater than 1:256 have been detected only within the first 12 weeks after experimental induction of toxoplasmosis.[23] Detectable IgM titers were present in the serum of 93.3% of the cats in one report on clinical toxoplasmosis; IgG titers were detected in 60%.[7] Some clinically ill cats have IgM titers greater than 1:256 that persist longer than 12 weeks. Persistent IgM titers (that persist longer than 16 weeks) have been documented often in cats coinfected with FIV and in cats with ocular toxoplasmosis. After another inoculation with *T. gondii*,[26] primary inoculation with the Petaluma isolate of FIV,[27] and administration of glucocorticoids,[28] some cats with chronic toxoplasmosis have short-term recurrence of detectable IgM titers. Healthy and clinically ill dogs occasionally develop detectable IgM titers. The temporal appearance of serum IgM titers after infection of dogs is unknown.

After experimental induction of infection in healthy cats, *T. gondii*–specific IgG can be detected by ELISA in serum in most cats in 3 to 4 weeks after

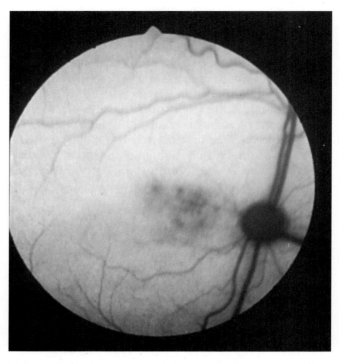

Figure 40–4
Chorioretinitis due to *Toxoplasma gondii*.

infection.[23] Positive IgG antibody titers generally last for years after infection. It has been suggested that single, high IgG titers suggest recent or active infection. I have demonstrated IgG antibody titers greater than 1:16,384 in healthy cats up to 5 years after experimental induction of toxoplasmosis. Thus, the presence of a positive IgG antibody titer in a single serum sample indicates only exposure, not recent or active disease. Demonstration of an increasing IgG titer can document recent or active disease. Unfortunately, in experimentally infected cats, the time span from the first detectable positive IgG titer to the maximal IgG titer is approximately 2 to 3 weeks, leaving little time for the documentation of an increasing titer value. Many cats with clinical toxoplasmosis have chronic low-grade clinical signs and may not be evaluated serologically until their IgG antibody titers have reached maximal values. In humans with reactivation of chronic toxoplasmosis, IgG titers only rarely increase. This seems to occur in cats as well.

Several agglutination tests have been evaluated using cat serum. A latex agglutination assay and an indirect hemagglutination assay are available commercially. These assays can be used with sera from multiple species and can potentially detect all classes of immunoglobulin directed against *T. gondii*. However, these assays rarely detect antibody in feline serum samples that are positive only for IgM as determined by ELISA.[29]

Antigen and Immune Complex Testing. T. gondii–specific antigens and immune complexes can be detected in body fluids from cats and dogs using ELISA.[11, 17, 20] After experimental induction of toxoplasmosis, most subclinically infected cats develop circulating antigenemia and immune complexes transiently after inoculation. Circulating antigens and immune complexes can be detected intermittently in some cats for months to years after infection and result from intermittent release of antigen from tissue cysts. Occasionally, cats with clinical feline toxoplasmosis develop antigenemia or immune complexes without the presence of serum antibodies.[7]

Aqueous Humor and CSF Antibody Measurement. Local production of T. gondii–specific antibodies in CSF[30] and aqueous humor[26] has been documented in experimentally inoculated, healthy cats and in cats[11, 12] and dogs (MR Lappin, 1996) with clinical signs of disease referable to toxoplasmosis. Most cats with uveitis and evidence of local production of T. gondii–specific antibodies in aqueous humor have responded to the administration of anti-*Toxoplasma* drugs, suggesting that aqueous humor antibody testing can aid in the diagnosis of clinical ocular toxoplasmosis in cats.[11] Local production of IgG occurs in aqueous humor of healthy cats[26] or cats with uveitis[11]; IgM has been detected only in cats with uveitis.[11]

Pathology

Gross necropsy findings generally include necrosis in CNS tissues, pulmonary parenchyma, liver, and mesenteric lymph nodes. Necrotic foci can be present in the pancreas, kidneys, and spleen. Animals with acute cases of myositis generally have pale, flaccid muscles, whereas those with chronic disease have gross evidence of fibrosis. Principal histopathologic abnormalities include necrosis and mixed inflammatory cell infiltrates. Tachyzoites and clones of tachyzoites are usually noted in fatal cases. Immunohistochemistry can be used to differentiate. T. gondii from *Neospora caninum* and is available in some laboratories. The organism is found in ocular tissue from approximately 45% of the cats with ocular and systemic toxoplasmosis.[16] Infiltrates of lymphocytes and plasma cells are commonly detected in the iris and ciliary body of cats with suspected immune-mediated pathogenesis of uveitis.

Diagnostic Plan

Antemortem definitive diagnosis of clinical feline toxoplasmosis has rarely been made by demonstrating bradyzoites or tachyzoites in tissues or effusions. Because T. gondii–specific antibodies, antigens, and immune complexes can be detected in the serum, CSF, and aqueous humor of normal animals as well as those with clinical signs of disease, it is impossible to make an antemortem diagnosis of clinical toxoplasmosis based on these tests alone. The antemortem diagnosis of clinical toxoplasmosis can be tentatively based on the combination of the following:

Demonstration of antibodies, antigens, or immune complexes in serum, aqueous humor, or CSF that document exposure to T. gondii

Demonstration of an IgM titer greater than 1:64, a fourfold or greater increase in IgG titer, the presence of T. gondii–specific antigens without antibodies in serum, or documentation of local antibody production in aqueous humor or CSF that suggests recent or active infection

Clinical signs of disease referable to toxoplasmosis

Exclusion of other common causes

Positive response to appropriate treatment

Treatment and Prognosis

Animals thought to have clinical toxoplasmosis should be given supportive care as needed. Clindamycin hydrochloride has been used in the management of many cases.[7, 10–12] It is administered at a dosage of 25 mg/kg by mouth, divided into doses for administration twice per day (b.i.d.) or three times per day (t.i.d.), for 4 weeks. Clinical signs not involving the eyes or the CNS usually resolve within the first 2 or 3 days of drug administration. Recurrence of clinical signs may be more common in animals treated for less than 4 weeks. There is no evidence to suggest that this drug can totally clear the body of the organism. Ocular and CNS toxoplasmosis respond more slowly to therapy. Clindamycin hydrochloride can be detected in the CNS tissues of cats[31] and has been used successfully in a limited number of cats thought to have CNS toxoplasmosis.[12] Some animals also respond to trimethoprim-sulfonamide at a dosage of 15 mg/kg by mouth, b.i.d., for 4 weeks. Pyrimethamine combined with sulfa drugs has been recommended for the treatment of clinical feline toxoplasmosis but commonly results in toxicity.

Animals with anterior uveitis should be treated with clindamycin hydrochloride in combination with topical (1% prednisolone acetate), oral, or parenteral corticosteroids to avoid secondary damage to the eye induced by inflammation; glaucoma and lens luxations are common.[4, 9, 10] Topical corticosteroids administered every 4 to 6 hours are generally used initially. If uveitis is still present after 2 or 3 days, oral or parenteral corticosteroids should be considered. If oral corticosteroids are needed, prednisone is given at 0.22 to 1.1 mg/kg per day for 5 to 7 days, then reduced by 50% for

5 days, then given every other day for 5 to 10 days (see also Chap. 19). Chorioretinitis often responds rapidly to clindamycin hydrochloride alone. Recurrence of ocular inflammation is common with anterior uveitis and unusual with chorioretinitis. Occasionally, anterior uveitis initially worsens after clindamycin hydrochloride administration. It has been hypothesized that this is due to increased release of antigen from tissue cysts, leading to magnification of immune-mediated disease. It is more difficult to induce clinical remission in cats with concurrent FIV infection, and recurrences of clinical disease are more common than in FIV-naive cats.

Zoonotic Aspects and Prevention

Infection of the human fetus transplacentally during gestation can lead to clinical toxoplasmosis.[1] CNS disease and ocular disease are the two most common clinical manifestations. *T. gondii* is the most common infectious cause of CNS disease in AIDS patients, approximately 10% of whom die of activated cerebral toxoplasmosis.[18] Primary infection in immunocompetent individuals can cause fever, malaise, and lymphadenopathy.[1]

The role of the cat in human infection is primarily related to producing oocysts and perpetuating the disease in the environment and food chain. Individual adult cats generally shed oocysts for only days to several weeks after primary inoculation.[1, 23, 26] Inoculation of cats with *T. gondii* 8 and 16 months after primary inoculation did not result in repeat oocyst shedding.[26, 32] Inoculation of cats 6 years after primary inoculation resulted in repeated oocyst shedding in four of nine cats; each cat was seropositive.[33] It is unknown how many naturally infected cats repeat oocyst shedding on exposure to *T. gondii*. Oocyst shedding in cats with chronic toxoplasmosis can be induced with extremely high doses of glucocorticoids.[19] Doses of glucocorticoids typically used clinically failed to induce oocyst shedding in recently or chronically infected cats.[28] Although oocyst production in the intestines can occur, most cats with clinical toxoplasmosis do not shed oocysts.[13] Coinfection with FIV[32] or feline leukemia virus[34] does not lead to prolonged periods of oocyst shedding. Primary-phase FIV infection failed to induce oocyst shedding in cats with chronic toxoplasmosis.[27]

Infection of humans by direct contact with oocyst-shedding cats is extremely unlikely. Because of the short oocyst shedding period, it may not be necessary to remove cats from the home environment of pregnant or immunosuppressed individuals.[35] Because oocysts have to sporulate to be infectious, contact with fresh feces cannot cause infection. Cats are fastidious and usually do not allow feces to remain on

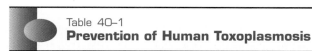

Table 40–1
Prevention of Human Toxoplasmosis

Prevention of Oocyst Ingestion
Avoid feeding cats undercooked meats.
Do not allow cats to hunt.
Clean the litterbox daily and incinerate or flush the feces.
Clean the litterbox daily with scalding water or use a litterbox liner.
Wear gloves when working with soil.
Wash hands thoroughly with soap and hot water after gardening.
Wash fresh vegetables well before ingestion.
Keep children's sandboxes covered.
Boil drinking water that has been obtained from the general environment.
Control potential transport hosts.
Treat oocyst-shedding cats with anti-*Toxoplasma* drugs.

Prevention of Tissue Cyst Ingestion
Cook all meat products to 66°C (150°F).
Wear gloves when handling meats.
Wash hands thoroughly with soap and hot water after handling meats.
Freeze all meat for a minimum of 3 days before cooking.

their skin long enough to lead to oocyst sporulation. Increased risk of acquired toxoplasmosis was not associated with cat ownership in individuals with AIDS.[36] However, because some cats shed oocysts repeatedly, feces should always be handled carefully. Oocysts can survive in the environment for months to years.[1] Human contact with sporulated oocysts probably occurs most frequently via geophagia when people work with soil or drink contaminated water. Oocyst induction of infection is rarely confirmed but has been implicated as the source of at least two outbreaks of clinical toxoplasmosis.[37, 38] Accidental hosts, including filth flies, cockroaches, earthworms, and dung beetles, have been shown to transport *T. gondii* oocysts and may be a source of infection for cats housed indoors. Recommendations for prevention of toxoplasmosis are summarized in Table 40–1.

Some species of *Hammondia* and *Besnoitia*, two nonpathogenic protozoans, lead to the shedding of oocysts in cat feces that are indistinguishable microscopically from those of *T. gondii*. Because of public health risks, if a fecal sample from a cat is shown to contain oocysts measuring 10 × 12 μm, it should be assumed that the organism is *T. gondii*. The feces should be collected and incinerated daily until the oocyst shedding period is completed. Administration of clindamycin (25 mg/kg by mouth, daily) can reduce levels of oocyst shedding.[2]

Humans are commonly infected after ingesting

tissue cysts in undercooked meats. In the United States, pork products have the highest incidence of *Toxoplasma* cysts.[1] Meat should be cooked to an internal temperature of at least 66°C (150.8°F) for 20 minutes.[1] Gloves should be worn when handling raw meats (including field dressing) for cooking, or hands should be cleansed thoroughly afterward. Freezing meat at −20°C (−4°F) for several days greatly reduces tissue cyst viability.

AIDS patients, other immunosuppressed people, and pregnant women commonly question their veterinarians concerning the likelihood of individual cats to shed *T. gondii* oocysts in their environment. Fecal examination is an adequate procedure for determining when cats are actively shedding oocysts but is not helpful for determining when a cat shed oocysts in the past. No serologic assay accurately predicts when a cat shed *T. gondii* oocysts in the past, and most cats currently shedding oocysts are seronegative. There is no way to determine whether an owner acquired toxoplasmosis from contact with individual cats. Owners who think they may have toxoplasmosis should consult their physicians.

A mutant strain of *T. gondii* that does not lead to oocyst formation has been identified and is being evaluated for use as a vaccine for cats.[39] After vaccination with *T. gondii* clone T-263, oocyst shedding after challenge with oocyst-forming strains of *T. gondii* is blocked. There is no vaccine for the prevention of clinical toxoplasmosis in dogs or cats.

Neosporosis

Pathophysiology

Etiology. *N. caninum* is a tissue protozoan morphologically similar to but antigenically distinct from *T. gondii*. The life stages identified include a rapidly dividing stage (tachyzoite) and a slowly dividing stage (bradyzoite) that exists in tissue cysts.[40–45]

Epidemiology. The life cycle of *N. caninum* has not been determined. Tissue cysts have been found in naturally infected dogs, calves, and lambs and a foal.[41, 44, 45] Infected calves can be aborted or stillborn, and neuromuscular disease is common.[46–48] Dogs, cats, sheep, goats, fox, mice, and macaques can be experimentally infected.[44, 49–53] Encephalomyelitis and myositis develop in experimentally infected kittens.[50] Clinical disease in naturally infected cats has not been reported. Because of similarities with *T. gondii*, it is proposed that the sexual cycle is completed in a carnivore. However, oocysts have not been documented in infected dogs, cats, or raccoons. Transplacental infection occurs experimentally in dogs, cattle, sheep, mice, macaques, and cats.[41, 42, 44, 45, 48, 49, 54] Dams that give

birth to transplacentally infectedoffspring can do so again in subsequent pregnancies.

Canine neosporosis has been reported in Norway, Sweden, Finland, the Netherlands, Germany, France, Hungary, Belgium, Scandinavia, Switzerland, the United Kingdom, Ireland, Australia, New Zealand, South Africa, Canada, Japan, and the United States.[44, 45] Prevalence of disease in dogs is largely undetermined, but the seroprevalence of infection was estimated at 2% and 12.9% in populations of subclinically affected dogs in Kansas and England, respectively.[41, 55] There is no known sex predisposition. Although many cases have involved large-breed dogs, clinical disease has also been identified in small- to medium-sized breeds.[40–42, 44, 45, 56–61]

Pathogenesis. *N. caninum* tachyzoites replicate intracellularly in most tissue cells until the infected cells are destroyed. Infection of CNS structures is accompanied by mononuclear cell infiltrates, suggesting an immune-mediated component to the pathogenesis of disease. Similar to *T. gondii* infection, intact tissue cysts in neural structures are generally not associated with inflammation. However, ruptured tissue cysts induce inflammation. Untreated disease usually results in death.

Clinical Signs

Congenital infection of puppies results in ascending paralysis. Hind limbs are generally more severely affected, and hyperextension of the limbs is common. Many canine neuromuscular cases previously reported to be caused by toxoplasmosis were probably caused by neosporosis.[41] Muscle atrophy occurs in some animals. Polymyositis and multifocal CNS disease can occur alone or in combination. Myocarditis, dysphagia, ulcerative dermatitis, pneumonia, and hepatitis occur in some dogs. Clinical signs can be evident soon after birth or may be delayed for several weeks. Neonatal death is common. Although disease tends to be most severe in congenitally infected puppies, dogs as old as 15 years of age have been clinically affected.[40, 45] It is unknown whether clinical disease in older dogs is due to acute primary infection or exacerbation of chronic infection. Administration of glucocorticoids may activate bradyzoites in tissue cysts, resulting in clinical illness.[52, 60]

Laboratory Abnormalities. Hematologic and biochemical findings are nonspecific. Increased creatine kinase and aspartate aminotransferase activity may occur as a result of muscle inflammation. CSF abnormalities include increased protein levels (20–50 mg/dL) and a mild, mixed inflammatory cell pleocytosis (10–50 cells/dL) consisting of monocytes, lymphocytes, neutrophils, and (rarely) eosinophils.[42, 45] Tachyzoites are rarely identified on cytologic examination of CSF, imprints of dermatologic lesions, or bronchoalveolar lavage.

Pathology

Principal pathologic lesions include nonsuppurative polyradiculoneuritis, encephalomyelitis, myositis, and myofibrosis.

Diagnostic Plan

Definitive diagnosis is based on demonstration of the organism in CSF or tissues. Tachyzoites of *N. caninum* cannot be distinguished from those of *T. gondii* under the light microscope. *N. caninum* tissue cysts have a wall larger than 1 μm; *T. gondii* tissue cysts have a wall smaller than 1 μm. The organism can be differentiated from *T. gondii* by electron microscopic examination and immunohistochemistry.[62]

Circulating antibodies against *N. caninum* are detected in serum by IFA assay. IgG antibody titers 1:200 or greater have been detected in all dogs with clinical neosporosis; minimal serologic cross-reactivity occurs with *T. gondii* at titers 1:50 or greater.[45] The presence of antibodies against *N. caninum* in serum documents only infection, not clinical disease due to infection. A presumptive diagnosis of neosporosis can be made by combining appropriate clinical signs of disease and positive serology or the presence of antibodies in CSF, excluding other causes that induce similar clinical syndromes, particularly *T. gondii*. Bitches that whelp clinically affected puppies can have subsequent litters with transplacentally infected puppies and thus should not be bred.

Treatment and Prognosis

Although several drugs inhibit the replication of *N. caninum* in vitro,[41, 63] minimal information concerning treatment of neosporosis in dogs is available. Treatment of mice with sulfadiazine reduces the severity of clinical disease.[41] Several dogs survived infection after treatment with trimethoprim-sulfadiazine combined with pyrimethamine; sequential treatment with clindamycin hydrochloride, trimethoprim-sulfadiazine, and pyrimethamine; or clindamycin alone.[45] Administration of trimethoprim-sulfadiazine at 15 mg/kg by mouth for 4 weeks, with pyrimethamine at 1 mg/kg by mouth daily for 4 weeks, or clindamycin at 10 mg/kg by mouth t.i.d. for 4 weeks is currently recommended for the treatment of canine neosporosis.[45] Treatment of clinically affected dogs should be initiated prior to the development of extensor rigidity if possible. The prognosis for dogs with severe neurologic involvement is grave.

Zoonotic Aspects and Prevention

There is no known zoonotic risk associated with *N. caninum*.

Until the definitive host is identified, final recommendations concerning prevention cannot be made. Bitches that whelp clinically affected puppies should not be bred. Glucocorticoids should not be administered to seropositive animals if possible because of the potential for activation of infection.[41, 52]

References

1. Dubey JP, Beattie CP. Toxoplasmosis of Animals and Man. Boca Raton, Florida, CRC Press, 1988:1–220.
2. Dubey JP, Greene CE, Lappin MR. Toxoplasmosis and neosporosis. In: Greene CE, ed. Infectious Diseases of the Dog and Cat, 2nd ed. Philadelphia, WB Saunders, 1990:818–834.
3. Dubey JP, Carpenter JL, Topper MJ, et al. Fatal toxoplasmosis in dogs. J Am Anim Hosp Assoc 1989;25:659–664.
4. Averill DR, de Lahunta A. Toxoplasmosis of the canine nervous system: Clinicopathologic findings in four cases. J Am Vet Med Assoc 1971;159:1134–1141.
5. Hass JA, Shell L, Saunders G. Neurological manifestations of toxoplasmosis: A literature review and case summary. J Am Anim Hosp Assoc 1989;25:253–260.
6. Braund KG, Blagburn BL, Toivio-Kinnucan M, et al. *Toxoplasma* polymyositis/polyneuropathy—A new clinical variant in two mature dogs. J Am Anim Hosp Assoc 1988;24:93–97.
7. Lappin MR, Greene CE, Winston S, et al. Clinical feline toxoplasmosis: Serologic diagnosis and therapeutic management of 15 cases. J Vet Intern Med 1989;3:139–143.
8. O'Neil SA, Lappin MR, Reif JS, et al. Clinical and epidemiological aspects of feline immunodeficiency virus and *Toxoplasma gondii* coinfections in cats. J Am Anim Hosp Assoc 1991;27:211–220.
9. Lappin MR, Marks A, Greene CE, et al. Serologic prevalence of select infectious diseases in cats with uveitis. J Am Vet Med Assoc 1992;201:1005–1010.
10. Chavkin MJ, Lappin MR, Powell CC, et al. Seroepidemiologic and clinical observations of 93 cases of uveitis in cats. Prog Vet Comp Ophthalmol 1992;2:29–36.
11. Lappin MR, Roberts SM, Davidson MG, et al. Enzyme-linked immunosorbent assays for the detection of *Toxoplasma gondii*-specific antibodies and antigens in the aqueous humor of cats. J Am Vet Med Assoc 1992;201: 1010–1016.
12. Hertzel L, Lappin MR. Feline central nervous system toxoplasmosis: Clinical manifestations, serologic diagnosis and therapeutic management of 8 cases. In preparation, Prog Vet Neurol, 1996.
13. Dubey JP, Zajac A, Osofsky SA, et al. Acute primary toxoplasmic hepatitis in an adult cat shedding *Toxoplasma gondii* oocysts. J Am Vet Med Assoc 1990;197:1616–1618.
14. Peterson JL, Willard MD, Lees GE, et al. Toxoplasmosis in two cats with inflammatory intestinal disease. J Am Vet Med Assoc 1991;199:473–476.

15. Dubey JP, Carpenter JL. Neonatal toxoplasmosis in littermate cats. J Am Vet Med Assoc 1993;203:1546–1549.
16. Dubey JP, Carpenter JL. Histologically confirmed clinical toxoplasmosis in cats: 100 cases (1952–1990). J Am Vet Med Assoc 1993;203:1556–1566.
17. Lappin MR, Cayatte S, Powell CC, et al. Demonstration of *Toxoplasma gondii*–antigen containing immune complexes in the serum of cats. Am J Vet Res 1993;54:415–419.
18. Porter SB, Sande MA. Toxoplasmosis of the central nervous system in the acquired immunodeficiency syndrome. N Engl J Med 1992;327:1643–1648.
19. Dubey JP, Frenkel JK. Immunity to feline toxoplasmosis: Modification by administration of corticosteroids. Vet Pathol 1974;11:350–379.
20. Lappin MR, Greene CE, Prestwood AK, et al. Enzyme-linked immunosorbent assay for the detection of circulating antigens of *Toxoplasma gondii* in the serum of cats. Am J Vet Res 1989;50:1586–1590.
21. Dubey JP, Lappin MR, Thulliez P. Diagnosis of transplacentally induced toxoplasmosis in cats. J Am Vet Med Assoc 1995;207:179–185.
22. Peiffer RL, Wilcock BP. Histopathologic study of uveitis in cats: 139 cases (1978–1988). J Am Vet Med Assoc 1991;198:135–138.
23. Lappin MR, Greene CE, Prestwood AK, et al. Diagnosis of recent *Toxoplasma gondii* infection in cats by use of an enzyme-linked immunosorbent assay for immunoglobulin M. Am J Vet Res 1989;50:1580–1585.
24. Dubey JP, Thulliez P. Serologic diagnosis of toxoplasmosis in cats fed *Toxoplasma gondii* tissue cysts. J Am Vet Med Assoc 1989;194:1297–1299.
25. Lappin MR, Bush DJ, Reduker DW. Feline serum antibody responses to *Toxoplasma gondii* and characterization of target antigens. J Parasitol 1994;80:73–80.
26. Chavkin MJ, Lappin MR, Powell CC, et al. *Toxoplasma gondii*–specific antibodies in the aqueous humor of cats with toxoplasmosis. Am J Vet Res 1994;55:1244–1249.
27. Lappin MR, Gasper PW, Rose BJ, et al. Effect of primary phase feline immunodeficiency virus infection on cats with chronic toxoplasmosis. Vet Immunol Immunopathol 1992;35:121–131.
28. Lappin MR, Dawe DL, Lindl PA, et al. The effect of glucocorticoid administration on oocyst shedding, serology, and cell-mediated immune responses of cats with recent or chronic toxoplasmosis. J Am Anim Hosp Assoc 1992;27:625–632.
29. Lappin MR, Powell CC. Comparison of latex agglutination, indirect hemagglutination, and ELISA techniques for the detection of *Toxoplasma gondii*–specific antibodies in the serum of cats. J Vet Intern Med 1991;5:299–301.
30. Munana KR, Lappin MR, Powell CC, et al. Sequential measurement of *Toxoplasma gondii*–specific antibodies in the cerebrospinal fluid of cats with experimentally induced toxoplasmosis. Prog Vet Neurol 1995;6:27–31.
31. Brown SA, Zaya MJ, Dieringer TM, et al. Tissue concentrations of clindamycin after multiple oral doses in normal cats. J Vet Pharmacol Ther 1990;13:270–277.
32. Lappin MR, George JW, Pedersen NC, et al. Experimental induction of toxoplasmosis in cats chronically infected with feline immunodeficiency virus. Proceedings of the First International Conference of Feline Immunodeficiency Virus Researchers, 1991:29.
33. Dubey JP. Toxoplasmosis. J Am Vet Med Assoc 1994;205:1593–1598.
34. Patton S, Legendre AM, McGavin MD, et al. Concurrent infection with *Toxoplasma gondii* and feline leukemia virus. J Vet Intern Med 1991;5:199–201.
35. Angulo FJ, Glaser CA, Juranek DD, et al. Caring for pets of immunocompromised persons. J Am Vet Med Assoc 1994;205:1711–1718.
36. Wallace MR, Rossetti RJ, Olson PE. Cats and toxoplasmosis risk in HIV-infected adults. J Am Med Assoc 1993;269:76–77.
37. Beneson MW, et al. Oocyst-transmitted toxoplasmosis associated with ingestion of contaminated water. N Engl J Med 1982;307:666–669.
38. Teutsch SM, et al. Epidemic toxoplasmosis associated with infected cats. N Engl J Med 1979;300:695–699.
39. Fishback JL. Prospective vaccines to prevent feline shedding of *Toxoplasma* oocysts. Compen Contin Educ Pract Vet 1990;12:643–648.
40. Dubey PJ, Carpenter JL, Speer CA, et al. Newly recognized fatal protozoan disease of dogs. J Am Vet Med Assoc 1988;192:1269–1285.
41. Dubey JP. *Neospora caninum:* A look at a new *Toxoplasma*-like parasite of dogs and other animals. Compen Contin Educ Pract Vet 1990;12:653–665.
42. Dubey JP, Greene CE, Lappin MR. Toxoplasmosis and neosporosis. In: Greene CE, ed. Infectious Diseases of the Dog and Cat, 2nd ed. Philadelphia, WB Saunders, 1990:830–835.
43. Dubey JP, Hattel AL, Lindsay DS, et al. Neonatal *Neospora caninum* infection in dogs: Isolation of the causative agent and experimental transmission. J Am Vet Med Assoc 1988;193:1259–1263.
44. Dubey JP. Neosporosis. Proceedings of the Eleventh Annual Veterinary Medical Forum, American College of Veterinary Internal Medicine, Washington DC, May 1993:710–712.
45. Ruehlmann D, Podell M, Oglesbee M, et al. Canine neosporosis: A case report and literature review. J Am Anim Hosp Assoc 1995;31:174–183.
46. Thilsted JP, Dubey JP. Neosporosis-like abortions in a herd of dairy cattle. J Vet Diagn Invest 1989;1:205–209.
47. Dubey JP, Leathers CW, Lindsay DS. *Neospora caninum*–like protozoon associated with fatal myelitis in newborn calves. J Parasitol 1989;75:146–148.
48. Barr DC, Conrad PC, Breitmeyer R, et al. Congenital *Neospora* infection in calves born from cows that had previously aborted *Neospora*-infected fetuses: Four cases (1990–1992). J Am Vet Med Assoc 1993;202:113–117.
49. Dubey JP, Lindsay DS. Transplacental *Neospora caninum* infection in cats. J Parasitol 1989;75:765–771.
50. Dubey JP, Lindsay DS. Fatal *Neospora caninum* infection in kittens. J Parasitol 1989;75:148–151.
51. Dubey JP, Lindsay DS, Lipscomb TP. Neosporosis in cats. Vet Pathol 1990;27:335–339.
52. Dubey JP, Lindsay DS. Neosporosis in dogs. Vet Parasitol 1990;36:147–151.
53. Barr BD, Conrad PA, Sverlow KW, et al. Experimental

fetal and transplacental *Neospora* infection in the nonhuman primate. Lab Invest 1994;71:236–242.

54. Dubey JP, Koestner A, Piper RC. Repeated transplacental transmission of *Neospora caninum* in dogs. J Am Vet Med Assoc 1990;197:857–860.

55. Trees AJ, Guy F, Tennant BJ, et al. Prevalence of antibodies to *Neospora caninum* in a population of urban dogs in England. Vet Rec 1993;132:125–126.

56. Jacobson LS, Jardine JE. *Neospora caninum* infection in three Labrador littermates. J S Afr Vet Assoc 1993;64:47–51.

57. Odin M, Dubey JP. Sudden death associated with *Neospora caninum* myocarditis in a dog. J Am Vet Med Assoc 1993;203:831–833.

58. Cuddon P, Lin DS, Bowman DD, et al. *Neospora caninum* infection in English Springer spaniel littermates: Diagnostic evaluation and organism isolation. J Vet Intern Med 1992;6:325–332.

59. Hay WH, Shell LG, Lindsay DS, et al. Diagnosis and treatment of *Neospora caninum* infection in a dog. J Am Vet Med Assoc 1990;197:87–89.

60. Hoskins JD, Bunge MM, Dubey JP, et al. Disseminated infection with *Neospora caninum* in a ten-year-old-dog. Cornell Vet 1991;81:329–334.

61. Greig B, Rossow KD, Collins JE, et al. *Neospora caninum* pneumonia in an adult dog. J Am Vet Med Assoc 1995;206:1000–1001.

62. Lindsay DS, Dubey JP. Immunohistochemical diagnosis of *Neospora caninum* in tissue sections. Am J Vet Res 1989;50:1981–1983.

63. Lindsay DS, Dubey JP. Evaluation of anti-coccidial drug inhibition of *Neospora caninum* development in cell cultures. J Parasitol 1989;175:990–992.

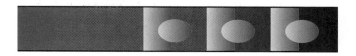

Hemic and Lymphatic Diseases

Chapter 41

Erythrocyte Diseases

Rafael Ruiz de Gopegui
Bernard F. Feldman

Anatomy

Normal erythrocytes have no nucleus. Canine erythrocytes have a marked biconcave discoid shape, causing them to have distinctive central pallor in blood smears. In the cat, the biconcave shape is shallow and the zone of central pallor is less obvious, a fact that often precludes the observation of feline spherocytes.

Erythrocyte production occurs in bone marrow. The maturation and proliferation sequence, stimulated by erythropoietin, is as follows: burst-forming unit–erythrocyte, colony-forming unit–erythrocyte, rubriblast, prorubricyte, basophilic rubricyte, polychromatophilic rubricyte, metarubricyte, reticulocyte, and erythrocyte.[1] Morphologic differentiation of erythrocyte precursors (rubriblasts to mature red blood cells [RBCs]) is based on the gradual shrinkage of the nucleus and gradual maturation of the cytoplasm as hemoglobin (Hb) is produced. The cytoplasmic staining pattern varies from basophilic, early protein production or RNA activity, to gray-blue as Hb is produced. Mitotic activity is restricted to the rubriblast, prorubricyte, and basophilic rubricyte. The nucleus is extruded at the end of metarubricyte maturation.[2]

Physiology

The production of RBCs is an extravascular process in mammals. Erythrocyte production occurs in bone marrow. The liver, kidneys, gastrointestinal tract, and mononuclear phagocyte system, however, are all involved.

The liver synthesizes or stores vitamin B_{12}, folate, iron, bone marrow colony-stimulating factors, and the α_2-globulin precursor of erythropoietin, all of which play an important role in Hb synthesis or erythropoiesis. In addition, Hb catabolism occurs in the liver.[3] The kidney synthesizes erythropoietin and excretes degraded Hb, iron, and bilirubin.

Gastric mucosa releases iron from organic molecules through the action of hydrochloric acid. For absorption, vitamin B_{12} must be bound to a protein intrinsic factor in gastric secretions. Intrinsic factor is an alkali-stable, thermolabile glycoprotein with a high affinity for vitamin B_{12}. In humans, it is thought to be derived from the fundus and body of the stomach. The intestinal mucosa regulates absorption of iron, folate, and vitamin B_{12}.[4]

The spleen is a reservoir of erythrocytes, destroys abnormal or senescent erythrocytes, degrades Hb, stores iron, and removes Heinz bodies and parasites from erythrocytes and nuclei from metarubricytes. The spleen also retains its embryologic potential for hematopoiesis.

The mononuclear phagocyte system degrades Hb and stores iron.[1] Within macrophages, the erythrocyte membrane is broken and Hb iron is oxidized, forming methemoglobin. Heme and globin dissociate. Iron is retained in storage pools—ferritin and hemosiderin. Globin is reduced to component amino acids for further protein production. The protoporphyrin ring of heme is broken and the opened tetrapyrrole (bilirubin) is carried by plasma albumin to the liver, where it is conjugated to form glucuronide and excreted through bile as bilirubin glucuronide.

Erythropoiesis is induced by interleukin-3 (synthesized by activated T lymphocytes), granulocyte-macrophage colony-stimulating factor, and erythropoietin (an α-globulin precursor is produced in the liver but most erythropoietin synthesis occurs in interstitial renal cells, induced by decreased oxygen tension at the cellular level).[5] Other substances such as interleukin-9, prostaglandins, erythroblast-enhancing factor, erythropoietic stimulating cofactor, androgens, glucocorticoids, growth hormone, thyroxine, and cobalt have been described as stimulators of erythropoiesis.[1, 6] Estrogens, lithium, suppressor T lymphocytes, and other as yet undetermined factors are inhibitors of erythropoiesis.[1]

Erythropoiesis begins when the primitive stem cell in bone marrow, committed to the erythroid line, differentiates into an erythrocyte precursor, a burst-forming unit–erythrocyte. This is a process regulated by interleukin-3 and granulocyte-macrophage colony-stimulating factor.

The major function of the RBCs is to carry oxygen to tissues. Hb in the RBC binds oxygen in the oxygen-rich environment of the lungs and releases it in the relatively oxygen-poor environment of metabolically active tissues.

The metabolic activity of the mature red cell is mostly restricted to anaerobic glucose catabolism, which maintains cell integrity and the ability to transport oxygen. Phosphofructokinase and pyruvate kinase are enzymes that produce ATP, which is necessary for red cell membrane plasticity. Deficiency of these enzymes in particular results in increased red cell fragility and shortened lifespan.

The integrity and oxygen transport capability of Hb depend on the methemoglobin reductase pathway, glutathione reductase and peroxidase, and the Luebering-Rapoport pathway, which regulates the oxygen affinity of Hb by regulating the concentration of 2,3-diphosphoglycerate (2,3-DPG). Increased 2,3-DPG concentration may compensate for anemia by decreasing the Hb oxygen affinity and thereby facilitating tissue oxygenation at a low packed cell volume (PCV) of RBCs.[7] An increase in 2,3-DPG concentration results in an increase in oxygen liberation. Canine erythrocytes have a longer lifespan (110 days) than feline erythrocytes (70 days).[2]

Problem Identification

Anemia

Anemia may be defined as a reduction in the oxygen-carrying capacity of blood, characterized by a reduced PCV, RBC count, or Hb concentration. Anemia is a sign of disease, not a disease per se.

Pathophysiology

Anemia results in reduced delivery of oxygen to tissues. Heart and respiratory rate and depth increase in an attempt to compensate for the reduction in oxygen-carrying capacity of the blood. The erythrocyte concentration of 2,3-DPG is increased in anemic animals and shows a close correlation with the degree of anemia. An increased 2,3-DPG concentration causes RBC Hb to release oxygen more readily to tissues.

Anemias are either hypoproliferative (nonresponsive or nonregenerative) or hyperproliferative (responsive or regenerative). The regenerative anemias are caused by destruction of RBCs, most often by immune-mediated attack, RBC parasites, or blood loss. The hypoproliferative anemias broadly include lack of marrow production, iron deficiency, inflammation, the early stages of acute hemorrhage or hemolysis, and the diseases characterized by decreased erythropoietin production. The latter include renal disease, hypothyroidism, and hypoadrenocorticism. It is suggested that increased parathyroid hormone concentration may have a direct negative effect on the production, function, or metabolism of erythropoietin in the genesis of the anemia of chronic terminal renal dysfunction in dogs.[7-9]

The anemia of inflammatory disease (the so-called anemia of chronic disease) is induced by iron sequestration, a nonspecific host response against infection. The intestinal absorption of iron is decreased, but ferritin concentration and macrophage iron—hemosiderin—increase.[1, 10, 11]

Clinical Signs

The common clinical signs of anemia may include mucosal membrane pallor, tachycardia, tachypnea, weakness, exercise intolerance, pica, anemic cardiac murmur, and depression.[1, 10]

Infectious hemolytic anemias may present with fever, organomegaly, and particular features of the underlying disease. Tubular lesions and subsequent renal disease may occur in severe hemolytic anemias as a result of the toxic effects of free Hb. Hemostatic dysfunction is another feature of hemolytic anemias. Fragmentation of lipid-filled RBC membranes releases phospholipid (thromboplastin), which stimulates and catalyzes secondary hemostasis, coagulation. Disseminated intravascular coagulation is often a

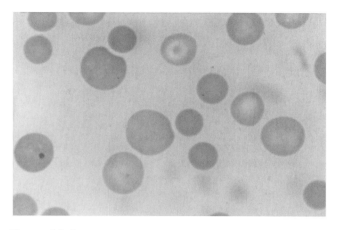

Figure 41–1
Blood smear showing spherocytes and small red blood cells lacking zones of central pallor.

major complicating problem in hemolytic anemias. Neurologic and gastrointestinal signs may appear in toxin-induced anemias (lead poisoning is an example, but anemia is not a pathognomonic feature of this intoxication). In systemic inflammatory and neoplasic diseases, anemia is consistently among the clinical features of the primary disease.

Diagnostic Plan

It is necessary to differentiate a relative anemia (hemodilution), which can be present after fluid therapy, from absolute anemia. When absolute anemia is observed, the differential diagnosis is based on clinical history, physical examination, and laboratory findings. The first diagnostic approach is to ascertain whether the anemia is regenerative. This is based on reticulocyte numbers, the reticulocyte production index (RPI), and the morphologic features of the RBCs (see Diagnostic Procedures).

By definition, regenerative anemia is characterized by an RPI greater than 2, increased mean corpuscular volume (MCV), and decreased mean corpuscular hemoglobin concentration (MCHC) (see Diagnostic Procedures). The two possible causes of regenerative anemias are hemolysis and hemorrhage. Hemorrhage is characterized by decreasing total protein, variable platelet counts, clinical signs of hypovolemia, and often readily apparent hemorrhage. When hemolysis is the cause of anemia, hemoglobinemia, hemoglobinuria, and increased serum bilirubin may be observed.

Hemolyis may be caused by parasitism as in haemobartonellosis, babesiosis, or cytauxzoonosis; by intravascular fragmentation induced by vascular diseases (i.e., disseminated intravascular coagulation); and by immune attack.

With immune hemolytic anemia (IHA), spherocytosis (Fig. 41–1), stomatocytosis, and bowl-shaped

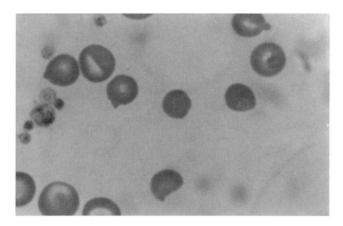

Figure 41-2
Blood smear showing Heinz bodies and refractile masses protruding from the red blood cell membrane.

red cells are observed. The antiglobulin (Coombs') test theoretically should be positive. True autoimmune hemolysis is probably a relatively infrequent event: immune activity directed against self-RBCs recognized as nonself antigens. Secondary immune-mediated hemolysis is the result of infectious processes, neoplasia, and often drug therapy.

Infectious hemolysis may be diagnosed by observing parasites on RBCs in the blood smear. Respective enzyme-linked immunoassay or indirect immunofluoresence tests may be positive. Other etiologic agents may induce hemolysis in small animals as a secondary feature of the primary septic process. These include *Leptospira, Fusobacterium necrophorum*,[12] *Streptococcus*, and *Pseudomonas* spp.

Heinz body anemia is often recognized by the finding of Heinz bodies on RBCs in the blood smear (Fig. 41-2). A history of ingestion of oxidant substances such as onions or zinc (pennies or some hardware) or drug therapy such as with vitamin K, acetaminophen (especially in cats), propylene glycol in semimoist foods, or methylene blue is often suggestive. Numerous drugs cause Heinz body formation in cats.

Other uncommon causes of hemolysis include congenital diseases that result in increased osmotic fragility. Often these are associated with younger animals (see Uncommon Erythrocyte Diseases).

Acute hemorrhage induces regenerative anemia. Chronic hemorrhage may develop into a nonregenerative anemia related to iron depletion. Blood-sucking parasites may induce nonregenerative anemia, also through iron depletion.[13, 14] External blood loss is more severe than internal hemorrhage, because reutilization of plasma proteins, Hb, and other blood components is not possible. Marked external blood loss carries the risk of hypovolemic shock. Trauma, gastrointestinal ulceration, and hemostatic

disorders are associated with marked external blood loss.

Laboratory findings associated with acute hemorrhage include reduced red cell count, Hb concentration, PCV (with appropriate RBC indices, at least in the early stages), and plasma proteins. The platelet count is often altered and characterized by modest thrombocytopenia. Neutrophilia may also be observed. These laboratory findings are consistent for at least 48 hours after hemorrhage. Compensatory mechanisms such as interstitial fluid mobilization into the circulation (plasma expansion), splenic contraction, and bone marrow activity change most of these hematologic analytes. If hemorrhage is ongoing, prolonged reticulocytosis, thrombocytosis, and activated platelets (platelet degranulation, platelet clumps, platelet shape change) may be observed.

When the laboratory signs point to blood loss as the cause of anemia without visible signs of blood loss, a rectal examination should be performed to assess the presence of melena or hematochezia. Internal blood loss may be manifest by abdominal distention or dyspnea from hemothorax. If bleeding into a body cavity is suspected and free fluid is noted on radiographs, thoracentesis or abdominocentesis is indicated to confirm internal bleeding.

By definition, nonregenerative anemia in the dog has an RPI less than 2. The causes of nonregenerative anemia include iron deficiency, marrow damage, the early stages of hemorrhage and hemolysis, anemia of inflammatory disease (chronic disease), and the diseases involving decreased erythropoietin including renal disease, hypothyroidism, and hypoadrenocorticism. A good approach to the differential diagnosis of mild to moderate nonregenerative anemias is first to consider whether the history, abnormalities on physical examination, and routine laboratory evaluation indicate the presence of chronic inflammatory disease, renal failure, hypoadrenocorticism, or hypothyroidism. Anemia associated with all inflammatory processes, specifically neoplasia in all animals and feline leukemia virus (FeLV) infections in cats, is characterized by iron sequestration and involves a mild to modest anemia, normocytosis, and normochromia. If hypoadrenocorticism is suspected, an adrenocorticotropic hormone response test is indicated (Chap. 46), and tests of thyroid function such as simultaneous resting plasma thyroxine and thyroid-stimulating hormone concentrations are indicated in patients suspected of being hypothyroid (Chap. 47).

Animals with moderate to severe nonregenerative anemia for which there is no apparent cause based on the history, physical examination, or routine laboratory evaluation or hormonal testing should have a bone marrow examination. Marrow damage caused by leukemias (myeloproliferative diseases) or by feline infectious panleukopenia is often characterized by hypercellular bone marrows with increased myeloid/erythroid ratios. Often the leukocyte and platelet counts in peripheral blood are significantly abnormal. This includes both cytopenias and cytoses. The associated anemia is characterized by normocytosis and normochromia. Other examples of marrow damage include the initial phases of hyperestrogenism—often observed because of the misuse of estrogen-containing preparations to prevent mismating or in some testicular neoplasias in male dogs; copper poisoning; and lead poisoning. Lead poisoning is characterized by normal to modestly anemic RBC numbers, increased metarubricytosis, basophilic stippling of both adult and immature red cells (including nucleated red cells), and, eventually, microcytosis and hypochromia. Another cause of microcytosis and hypochromia associated with bone marrow damage is iron deficiency. Hepatic fibrosis and lack of sufficient iron storage may initially be manifest with microcytosis and hypochromia noted on examination of peripheral blood smears and the associated hemogram.

In cats, myeloproliferative diseases, specifically erythroleukemia and erythremic myelosis, often associated with FeLV infection, involve nonregenerative anemias characterized as macrocytic and normochromic. This finding is often pathognomonic for these myeloproliferative diseases in cats. Pure RBC aplasia is characterized by severe peripheral anemia, appropriate red cell indices, normocellular bone marrow without appropriate erythropoiesis, and increased myeloid/erythroid ratios.

Several other anemias are characterized by hypocellular bone marrow, appropriate RBC indices, and decreased leukocyte and platelet counts. This is appropriately called aplastic pancytopenia. Aplastic anemia is a misnomer. Causes include toxins such as estrogen; radiation; and drugs such as phenylbutazone, chloramphenicol, cyclophosphamide, sulfonamides, phenytoin, azathioprine, gold salts, and D-penicillamine. Numerous other drugs are implicated in aplastic pancytopenia. Myelofibrosis and myeloproliferative diseases inducing myelophthisis are similarly characterized. Infectious causes include canine ehrlichiosis and parvoviral infection and feline panleukopenia and FeLV infection.

Erythrocytosis (Polycythemia)

Erythrocytosis is an increase of PCV, Hb, or RBCs (RBC $>10^7$/μL, PCV $>60\%$–70%, Hb >22 mg/dL).

Pathophysiology

Relative erythrocytosis represents an increase in RBC concentration without a real increase in total RBC mass. It is a consequence of hemoconcentration resulting from dehydration or splenic contraction. Splenic contraction is related to exercise, excitement, and fear. Relative erythrocytosis associated with hypovolemic states is most often caused by diarrhea, vomiting, or polyuria.

The cause of absolute erythrocytosis is not well described. It can be secondary to diseases that lead to increased erythropoietin production or occur as a primary disorder (primary erythrocytosis, polycythemia rubra vera) with low or normal plasma concentration of erythropoietin.

Primary erythrocytosis (polycythemia rubra vera) is a myeloproliferative disease. In this disease excessive red cell production occurs without regulation. Increased production of RBCs without dehydration, hypoxia, or increased erythropoietin concentration (concentration is usually normal or low) is observed. No other cell lines (leukocytes and platelets) proliferate in canine primary erythrocytosis. This is unlike the situation in human polycythemia rubra vera.[15]

Secondary erythrocytosis results from increased erythropoietin production. Increased erythropoietin secretion may be due to hypoxia (moderate increases in serum erythropoietin concentration) or erythropoietin-secreting neoplasia (marked elevations in serum erythropoietin concentration; a paraneoplastic syndrome). Hypoxia is related to environmental conditions (high altitude) or circulatory and respiratory diseases. Patients with tissue hypoxia (low partial pressure of arterial oxygen [Pao_2]) may have localized disease (renal artery compression or stenosis, ureteral obstruction), leading to hypoxia localized to renal tissues, or generalized disease associated with the lungs, heart, or abnormal Hb concentration. Liver, kidney, adrenal, and cerebellar neoplasias have been found to induce secondary erythrocytosis by producing erythropoietin excessively.

Clinical Signs

In relative erythrocytosis clinical signs are related to dehydration. Absolute erythrocytosis produces remarkably few clinical signs. Marked erythrocytosis results in darker mucous membranes and larger retinal blood vessels, and if oxygen delivery is compromised, cyanosis may develop. At hematocrit concentrations exceeding 60%, whole blood viscosity increases, especially at the low flow rates encountered in microvasculature. This represents a threat to tissue oxygenation. Cerebral circulation and oxygen supply are significantly affected, and lactate concentrations in exercising individuals are inappropriately increased. Extremely high hematocrit values are associated with malaise, fatigue, depression, and sometimes seizure activity. Congestive heart failure may result from increased cardiac output related to hypervolemia. Patients so affected are predisposed to thrombotic complications.

Diagnostic Plan

Erythrocytosis is thought to be relative when there is volume depletion resulting from dehydration or evidence of stress or fear likely to produce splenic contraction. Erythrocytosis is considered absolute in normovolemic patients.

Laboratory changes associated with relative erythrocytosis resulting from dehydration include increased RBC, PCV, and Hb concentration associated with increased total protein and, if severe, other analytes such as urea, creatinine, and sodium. If fluid administration to correct dehydration also corrects erythrocytosis, it was probably relative rather than absolute. Splenic contraction (which does not increase total plasma protein concentration) induces moderate and transient PCV, RBC, and Hb increases.

Absolute erythrocytosis is diagnosed when patients have marked elevations in red cell analytes and no clinical or laboratory evidence of hypovolemia. Diagnosis is dependent on Pao_2 and on serum erythropoietin concentration. If Pao_2 is low, secondary erythrocytosis is diagnosed. If Pao_2 is appropriate, serum erythropoietin concentration should be determined. In patients with appropriate Pao_2 and elevated serum erythropoietin concentration (appropriate values are laboratory dependent), paraneoplastic syndrome is diagnosed. Evaluation of the patient for neoplasia is required, with thoracic and abdominal radiographs or abdominal ultrasonography. If the Pao_2 is appropriate and serum erythropoietin concentration is normal to low, primary erythrocytosis, a myeloproliferative disease, is diagnosed.

Diagnostic Procedures

Routine Hematologic Testing

Routine hematologic testing is performed using ethylenediaminetetra-acetic acid (EDTA)–anticoagulated venous blood. Included in a routine hemogram examination of the RBCs are the PCV, Hb concentration, RBC count, RBC indices (MCV, MCHC, and mean corpuscular hemoglobin [MCH]), comments on reticulocyte and nucleated RBC numbers and RBC morphology, and total plasma protein.

The RBC count represents the erythrocyte concentration in peripheral blood. Hb concentration indicates the oxygen-carrying capacity of blood. PCV is the volume percentage of erythrocytes in blood. This can differ slightly from the hematocrit, which is calculated based on the volume of red cells in plasma.

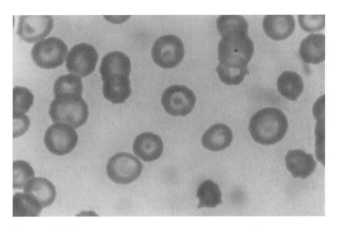

Figure 41–3
Blood smear showing rouleau formation by red blood cells. The cells are stacked like coins.

The RBC or erythrocyte indices include MCV, MCHC, and MCH. The MCV is the relation between PCV and RBC count. It allows differentiation of macrocytic, normocytic, and microcytic anemias. The MCH is the ratio between Hb and RBC count and reflects the weight of Hb within the RBC. MCH differentiates hypochromic and normochromic anemias. The MCHC is the ratio between Hb and PCV and is a more accurate indicator of whether the anemia is hypochromic or normochromic. The MCHC reflects the percentage of Hb in the RBCs.

Blood smear examination allows observation of erythrocyte distribution, morphology, and staining properties. Some etiologic agents may also be observed. Alterations in erythrocyte distribution include rouleau formation and RBC agglutination. In rouleau formation, groups of erythrocytes are observed forming "coin stacks" (Fig. 41–3). Increased rouleau formation is associated with systemic inflammatory states. Erythrocyte agglutination is described as groups of erythrocytes forming clumps or grape-like clusters (Fig. 41–4). Erythrocyte agglutination is associated with increased RBC membrane immunoglobulin concentrations observed in immune-mediated hemolysis.

Erythrocyte morphologic alterations include altered size, shape, and staining pattern. Altered RBC size includes macrocytes, which have increased cell volume, and microcytes, which have decreased cell volume. Normocytes have appropriate cell volume. Anisocytosis describes the presence of macro- or microcytes among normocytes, that is, variability of size within a given RBC population (Fig. 41–5).

Erythrocytes with altered shape are called poikilocytes. Poikilocytes include dacryocytes, which have teardrop shapes and are associated with bone marrow diseases; acanthocytes, which have spiked sufaces and are associated with hepatic diseases; fragmentocytes or schistocytes (Fig. 41–6), which are

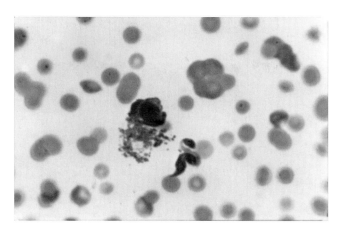

Figure 41-4
Blood smear showing erythrocyte agglutination.

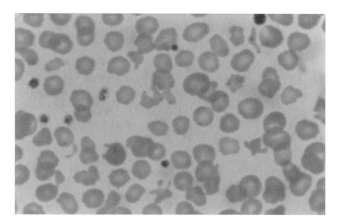

Figure 41-6
Blood smear demonstrating schistocytes and fragmented red blood cells.

cells fractured by intravascular fibrin (such as may occur with disseminated intravascular coagulation) or phagocytic attack; and spherocytes, which are microcytes without biconcavity reflecting decreased membrane with appropriate internal volume and are associated with immune-mediated hemolysis (see Fig. 41-1). Other RBCs with altered shapes include echinocytes, which have spiculated surfaces and are also associated with hepatic diseases and phagocytic attack; stomatocytes, which are RBCs with central pallor with a noncircular shape also associated with immune-mediated attack; and codocytes or target cells (see Fig. 41-3), cells with a stained central area encircled by normal pallor. Target cells are also associated with hepatic disease.

Altered erythrocyte staining patterns include hypochromia, which is decreased stain intensity; polychromasia, which is variation of color among normal RBCs; basophilic stippling, which represents residual ribosomal RNA and is observed in responsive anemia (especially in cats) and in lead toxicity; Howell-Jolly

bodies, which represent DNA residues forming a conspicuous discrete round spot in Romanowsky (Wright-based) stains; and Heinz bodies, which are refractile round structures representing crystallization of oxidized Hb in the RBC membrane (see Fig. 41-2). Heinz bodies represent oxidative attack on RBCs.

Reticulocyte Count and Reticulocyte Production Index

The reticulocyte count is performed to determine the percentage of RBCs that are immature, which is an indication that anemia is regenerative. Once reticulocyte numbers have been determined, adjustments may be made to determine whether reticulocyte production is appropriate. Normal individuals are expected to have a reticulocyte percentage of 1% of the total RBC population (0.4%-1.7%). This percentage increases in regenerative anemia. The reticulocyte count must be corrected to be considered a true reflection of RBC production (e.g., the RPI). The first factor of the RPI is the ratio between the patient's PCV or Hb and the normal PCV or Hb. The second factor is related to the time of reticulocyte release from the bone marrow—increased erythropoietin production reduces the reticulocyte maturation time. These factors, in the dog, may be applied in a ratio[16]:

- PCV 45% correction factor = 1
- PCV 35% to 44% correction factor = 1.5
- PCV 25% to 34% correction factor = 2
- PCV 15% to 24% correction factor = 2.5

RPI equals reticulocyte percentage multiplied by the patient's PCV or Hb divided by the mean of the reference interval (midpoint of the normal range) for PCV or Hb. The result is then divided by the correction factor. An RPI greater than 2.0 is considered regenerative. This reticuloycte production index is seldom used in feline anemia.

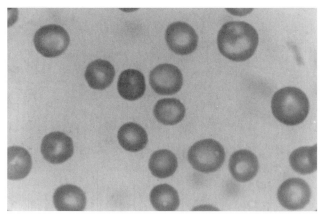

Figure 41-5
Blood smear with anisocytosis showing variation in size of red blood cells.

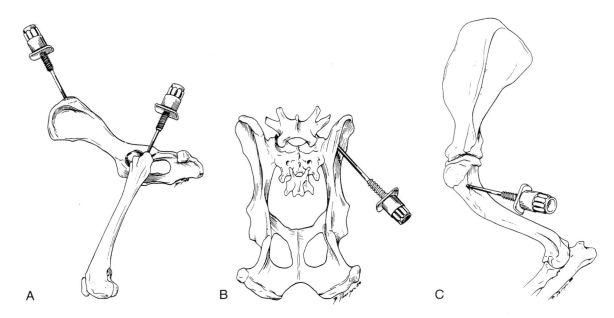

Figure 41-7
Sites for bone marrow aspiration. **(A)** Dorsal crest of the ilium and proximal femur.
(B) Transilial approach. **(C)** Lateral approach to the proximal humerus. (From Grindem
CB: Bone marrow biopsy and evaluation. Vet Clin North Am 1989;19:673.)

Bone Marrow Examination

Bone marrow examination may give useful information on nonregenerative anemias. Bone marrow examination is indicated to examine any unexplained cytopenia, to stage neoplasia, to investigate unusual cells observed in peripheral blood, and to determine iron storage. Bone marrow biopsy is useful in determining marrow architecture, myelofibrosis, or myelophthisis.

Bone marrow aspiration in small animal practice is performed at one of several sites. These include the humeral crest, trochanteric fossa, or the wing of the ilium (Fig. 41–7). It is preferable to perform bone marrow aspiration with the animal sedated and using systemic analgesics or, particularly for cats, general anesthesia. The site should be clipped and surgically scrubbed. After cutaneous and periosteal anesthesia is achieved using a local anesthetic in animals that are not under general anesthesia, a small "stab" incision is made in the skin. The tip of a 16- to 18-gauge bone marrow needle with stylet in place is introduced through the skin incision and into the pericortical bone. With a gentle back-and-forth screwing motion and firm pressure, the marrow needle penetrates the marrow cavity. The operator may feel a momentary release of resistance. The needle stylet is removed and a 10- to 12-mL syringe that contains 0.5 mL of 10% EDTA solution (15% edetate disodium diluted to a 10%

solution with 0.9% NaCl) is attached, and the syringe plunger is pulled back to collect 0.5 to 1.0 mL of marrow, which will include blood contamination. The marrow can then be placed in an EDTA tube for the laboratory to make smears, or smears can be made immediately by placing some of the marrow in a Petri dish and tilting it to allow blood to run away from a marrow spicule. The spicule is then retrieved using a capillary tube, blown onto a microscope slide, and smeared with a second slide using the "squash" method. Alternatively, to reduce the effects of blood contamination on cytologic examination, a drop of marrow with blood can be placed on one end of a microscope slide and the slide tilted to allow the blood to run to the other end, away from the marrow spicule. A second slide is then placed over the spicule, perpendicular to the first slide, and a smear is made by pressing the second slide to the first and drawing it away, perpendicular to the first slide, while maintaining gentle pressure on the spicule between the two slides. Alternatively, if EDTA solution is not available, just enough marrow to be seen in the hub can be aspirated into a dry syringe, which is then immediately squirted onto a microscope slide and smeared with a second slide. When not using EDTA, there is no use in collecting several milliliters of marrow because it is markedly diluted with blood and clots very rapidly, precluding cytologic examination without blood contamination.

The marrow slide preparations are submitted with a simultaneously obtained hemogram. Because the marrow contents are referable to the hemogram and because of diurnal variation of all cell numbers, the hemogram should be obtained *at the same time* as the bone marrow aspirate.

Tests of Iron Metabolism

Tests of iron metabolism include serum or plasma iron, total iron-binding capacity (transferrin concentration), and examination of bone marrow storage iron.[16, 17] Samples must be collected in trace mineral–free tubes and into anticoagulants free of iron. These tubes may be obtained from most hospital supply sources or are provided by veterinary clinical laboratories. Serum or plasma iron is the quantity of free iron (iron freed from the carrier molecule, transferrin, at a low pH). Serum iron is low in true iron deficiency and in anemia of inflammatory disease. Total iron-binding capacity (transferrin) is a measure of serum transferrin and is determined after saturation of the patient's transferrin with excess iron. Transferrin saturation is the ratio between plasma iron and total iron-binding capacity expressed as a percentage. This percentage may be increased in true iron deficiency and decreased in the anemia of inflammatory disease. Examination of bone marrow hemosiderin (iron) is also a measure of body iron storage. This is accomplished with special stains—the Prussian blue stain is an example—on marrow smear preparations.

Common Erythrocyte Diseases

Immune-Mediated Hemolytic Anemia

IHA is the most common cause of canine hemolytic disease.[18] The term immune-mediated indicates that the presence of antibody on the red cells is the cause of their elimination. Hemolysis may be intravascular or extravascular (macrophages), with splenomegaly and spherocytosis as well as other RBC morphologic changes (see earlier).[19] Dogs with IHA range in age from 1 to 13 years, with a mean age of 6.4 ± 3.4 years. An increased seasonal incidence was observed during May and June.[20] Breed (cocker spaniel) and sex (female) predispositions are also suggested but not defined. The etiology of IHA is not as yet defined, but the influence of infectious agents, drugs, and genetic predisposition or autoimmune mechanisms[21] has been proposed.

Pathophysiology

Hemolytic anemias are characterized by a marked decrease in erythrocyte lifespan. Erythrocyte destruction may be intravascular or extravascular. Intravascular hemolysis tends to be acute to peracute. Extravascular hemolysis tends to be more chronic. Destruction of RBCs is an antibody- or complement-mediated type II immune reaction. The complement system and phagocytic cells contribute to the destruction of RBCs. Antibody is bound to the RBC surface with the Fab region, leaving the Fc region available for the interaction with the Fc receptor on phagocytic cells or with the first component of the complement system (C1). In this position the antibody acts as a marker for elimination. Until elimination happens, the cell is considered sensitized. A sensitized cell may be eliminated by phagocytic attack or by complement-mediated lysis.

Clinical Signs

Clinical findings are variable. Jaundice may be present. Hepatomegaly, splenomegaly, jaundice, petechiae, lymphadenopathy, lameness, and skin lesions (cold agglutinin disease, acrocyanosis) may appear in addition to signs related to anemia (pale mucous membranes, weakness, depression, tachycardia).[22]

Diagnostic Plan

Commonly observed laboratory changes include reduced RBC count and PCV, hemoglobinemia, hyperbilirubinemia, and reticulocytosis. Clinical presentations, however, are variable. Intravascular hemolysis results in hemoglobinemia. Extravascular hemolysis generally results in hyperbilirubinemia, with jaundiced plasma. Increased total protein and liver enzymes are often observed. Hemoglobinuria and possibly signs of azotemia (tubule damage) may be present.

Autoagglutination may be observed in a small percentage of cases. Agglutination can be observed in glass syringes, glass test tubes, or blood smears prepared on glass slides (see Fig. 41–4). When autoagglutination is present, the direct antiglobulin test (Coombs test) is not necessary. Many dogs presented are positive for IgG antibodies without complement (C') as detected by the direct antiglobulin test and have severe anemia, spherocytosis (see Fig. 41–1), and marked bilirubinuria. Hemoglobinemia and hemoglobinuria are less common. Concomitant mild to severe thrombocytopenia is also observed frequently.[20] Nonregenerative IHA has also been described but is infrequently observed except in the early stages of disease.[23] Lack of RBC regeneration in later stages of this disease is considered a poor prognostic sign.

Diagnosis of IHA is based on the presence of hemolytic anemia with spherocytosis, a positive direct (and in some cases indirect) antiglobulin test, and bone marrow examination revealing marked erythroid activity. However, if the reticulocyte response is appropriate, bone marrow examination is unnecessary.

Treatment

Immunosuppression is generally accomplished with glucocorticoid administration (prednisone, 1–2 mg/kg b.i.d.). Although it is widely accepted by most authorities that high doses of corticosteroids (prednisone at 1–2 mg/kg b.i.d.) are necessary, we believe low-dose glucocorticoid therapy (1 mg/kg s.i.d. by mouth) is equally effective. The addition of a second immunosuppressive drug is recommended early in the therapeutic protocol if evidence of RBC response and stabilization of the RBC mass is not obtained. A number of drugs are used in conjunction with glucocorticoid therapy. We recommend the use of azathioprine (2 mg/kg by mouth every day) (not recommended for cats) along with glucocorticoid. These drugs are always administered in tandem and reduced in tandem. There is a scientific mythology not supported by the veterinary literature that suggests that azathioprine takes several weeks to become effective. That has not been noted in our practice.

Therapy is continued until the PCV increases into the normal range and remains there for 1 to 2 weeks. Drugs are then withdrawn slowly by reducing the dose or doses by 25% every 1 to 2 weeks, eventually to every other day and complete withdrawal with monitoring of the PCV. Some animals require immunosuppressive therapy indefinitely.

Other immunosuppressive drugs (not generally recommended by us) include cyclophosphamide, cyclosporine, and vincristine. To date, no original veterinary articles specifically suggest that these drugs are useful in the treatment of immune-mediated hemolytic anemia. The use of danazol has been suggested, but we do not recommend it.[23]

Splenectomy may be considered in refractory canine cases. Splenectomy may also be considered when the dosages and side effects of drug therapy endanger the patient.

When autoagglutination is evident, we advocate the prophylactic use of low-dose heparin therapy (5–10 IU/kg subcutaneously t.i.d.). This dose is always tapered through a minimum of 48 hours. If there is clinical and laboratory evidence for disseminated intravascular hemolysis, plasma transfusion (see Chap. 44) is used in conjunction with heparin therapy.

Feline IHA may be treated with higher doses of prednisone (2–4 mg/kg b.i.d.). Chlorambucil (4–6 mg per cat once weekly) may also be administered.[24]

In severe cases of IHA (PCV <15% in dogs and <10% in cats) (or when IHA is observed with concomitant thrombocytopenia), rapid and aggressive supportive transfusion therapy may be required. Transfusion

of washed packed RBCs dog erythrocyte antigen (DEA) 1.1, 1.2, and 7 negative (canine universal donor) is recommended.[22] At present, no studies in veterinary medicine suggest that transfusion of RBCs aggravates the hemolytic process. Transfusion of RBCs certainly ameliorates hypoxic injury to cells or organs.

Transfusion Therapy

Blood typing of canine and feline donors and recipients is always recommended. Commercially available cards are now available for in-house blood typing of dogs and cats (Rapid Vet-H Feline and Rapid Vet-H Canine). The procedure can be accomplished in minutes. Cross-matching patient's and donor's blood minimizes transfusion reactions, allows compatible donor RBCs longer viability, and avoids burdening a patient already in difficulty.

Cats have three blood groups: A (most frequent), B, and AB (rare). Severe transfusion reactions may be expected in 70% of type B cats receiving non–type B blood.[25] Transfusion of non–type A blood to type A cats results in almost immediate loss of the transfused RBCs in all transfused patients. Transfusion reaction may occur in more than 70% of the recipient patients.[25]

Dogs have eight blood groups. Severe transfusion reactions are expected with incompatible transfusion of blood from donors positive for DEA 1.1 and 1.2. Dogs negative for DEA 1.1, 1.2, and 7 are considered universal donors; however, cross-matching is recomended before transfusion.[26] Canine patients negative for DEA 1.1 can have an anamnestic transfusion reaction if transfused repeatedly with DEA 1.1–positive RBCs.[27]

Transfusion therapy with whole blood or packed RBCs may be indicated for anemic patients to restore blood oxygen-carrying capacity. Use of whole blood is generally relegated to patients with severe blood loss. We recommend that whole blood or packed RBCs be used when there is clinical evidence that the patient needs increased oxygen-carrying capacity. Clinical signs include tachypnea and dyspnea. Anemic patients that require handling for either diagnosis or therapy may require additional RBCs. We do not recommend a specific hematocrit, RBC count, or Hb concentration below which transfusion is required. However, patients with an inappropriately low RBC mass require transfusion. Normovolemic patients with depressed RBC mass should receive packed RBCs. More blood may be administered without causing potential volume overload, and the remaining plasma products can be used in other needful patients. Clinical signs indicate a patient's poor general condition, ongoing blood loss, and severity of anemia (low PCV may be considered a sufficient but not necessary condition for transfusion, e.g., a PCV less than 20%

with acute anemia or less than 15% with subacute to chronic anemia). A patient exhibiting clinical signs referable to anemia (exercise intolerance, polypnea, dyspnea) should receive RBCs. The required dosage of blood products may be calculated in relation to PCV: total needed volume = kg body weight × 90 mL/kg (dog) or 70 mL/kg (cat) × (desired PCV − patient's PCV)/donor PCV.

Packed RBCs have a PCV between 60% and 80%. It is recommended that warmed sterile saline—never water or lactated Ringer's solution—be added to the packed RBC unit before administration, unless there has been addition of another type of diluent. This is done to reduce the viscosity of the administered product.[28] Administration of packed RBCs is recommended for anemic patients unless hypovolemia or ongoing hemorrhage is observed.[29] IHA, primary bone marrow disease, gastrointestinal tract blood loss, and renal failure have been considered the most common indications for administration of packed RBCs in canine practice.[30] Although feline patients may survive profound anemias, transfusion of packed RBCs is indicated, especially if the patient exhibits depression or cachexia or if the anemia is nonregenerative.[31] In general, ill canine and feline patients with anemia, even modest anemia, exhibit clinical improvement and become more responsive to other forms of therapy if RBCs are administered.

Prognosis

Mortality is significantly higher in dogs without marked reticulocytosis, in those with lower PCV, and in those with a serum bilirubin concentration of 10 mg/dL or greater.[20] In one large institutional study, IHA was associated with a 43% mortality rate.[19] Cocker spaniels, terriers, schnauzers, Doberman pinschers, Old English sheepdogs, and German shepherds had mortality rates exceeding 60%.[19]

Babesiosis

Babesiosis is a tick-borne disease caused by protozoa of the genus *Babesia*. Dogs are affected by several species: *B. canis*, *B. vogeli*, and *B. gibsoni*.[32] Cats are affected by *B. felis*. *B. canis* produces severe anemia in dogs. Transmitted by ticks, *B. canis* is often accompanied by *Ehrlichia canis* as well as other organisms. The incidence in North America is relatively low, with some regionality; the incidence is higher in the southwestern United States. Dogs of all ages and either sex are affected. Clinical signs are often present acutely.

Pathophysiology

Hemolysis is intravascular, caused by trophozoites escaping from infected RBCs. Splenic macrophages may also phagocytize infected erythrocytes, releasing trophozoites into the circulation.

Clinical Signs

Typical signs of anemia such as pale mucous membranes, weakness, and tachycardia along with hemoglobinemia, hemoglobinuria, hyperbilirubinemia, bilirubinuria, thrombocytopenia, and hyperthermia may be observed in the acute phase of the disease. Hepatomegaly and splenomegaly may also be seen. Complications such as disseminated intravascular coagulation are anticipated in severe cases.

Diagnostic Plan

Anemia with babesiosis is generally regenerative; the reticulocyte count is increased. However, in chronic forms of babesiosis, nonregenerative anemia may develop. Babesiosis may be diagnosed by direct observation of the blood smear—the organisms may be easily recognized in the RBCs but only when parasitemia is at its peak and by indirect immunofluorescence.[33] Obtaining capillary blood by pricking the ear with a lancet is suggested to obtain a higher concentration of parasitized RBCs. Indirect immunofluorescence is available through specialized laboratories. Generally the organisms are large teardrop-shaped structures approximately one quarter to one third the size of an RBC (Fig. 41–8). Organisms are often paired. It is usual to see two organisms per cell. Less often, four or even eight organisms may be observed.

Treatment

Administration of imidocarb dipropionate (5 mg/kg intramuscularly, single dose) or diminazene aceturate (3 mg/kg intramuscularly for 3 days) is

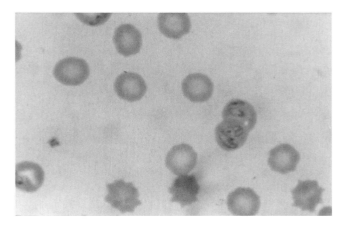

Figure 41–8
Canine blood smear infected with *Babesia* showing teardrop-shaped organisms in red blood cells.

indicated for dogs, but complete elimination of the protozoal infection is difficult to achieve.[1, 34] However, in most cases the drugs are sufficiently effective to allow the patient a good quality of life. Imidocarb dipropionate is not available for use in small animals in North America. However, the drug is available for use in large domestic species. Use of this drug in nonapproved species requires notification of the client.

Prognosis

The prognosis for successful treatment of babesiosis is good. Concurrent *Ehrlichia* infections do not worsen the prognosis. Re-examination and retreatment may be required.

Haemobartonellosis

Haemobartonellosis is a rickettsial infection caused by *Haemobartonella canis* and *H. felis.* The number of *H. felis* cases diagnosed throughout North America appears to have dropped dramatically. The reasons for this apparent decrease are not known. FeLV-infected cats appear to have a higher risk of infection.[35]

Pathophysiology

Infected erythrocytes have increased osmotic fragility and are readily phagocytized by macrophages, leading to extravascular hemolysis. Erythrophagocytosis is observed in peripheral blood smears and in bone marrow preparations. *H. felis* is the etiologic agent of feline infectious anemia.

Clinical Signs

Canine haemobartonellosis may be subclinical but otherwise may present as a hemolytic anemia with fever, hyperbilirubinemia, and leukocytosis. Canine haemobartonellosis is rarely encountered in clinical settings except in functionally asplenic patients. *H. canis* may complicate canine babesiosis. Clinical signs of feline haemobartonellosis may include anorexia, depression, splenomegaly, fever, pale mucous membranes, and icterus.

Diagnostic Plan

Acridine orange or May-Grünwald-Giemsa staining of blood smears may reveal the organism.[35] The organisms appear attached to the erythrocyte surface membrane (Fig. 41–9). Direct immunofluorescence may increase the sensitivity for identifying the organism. RBC agglutination noted after refrigerating the patient's EDTA-anticoagulated blood for 8 to 10 hours is suggestive of infection with *Haemobartonella.*

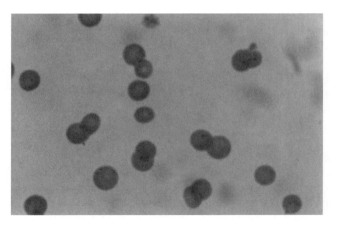

Figure 41–9
Feline blood infected with *Haemobartonella felis,* which is seen as dark spots on the surface (often periphery) of red blood cells.

Treatment

Therapy is based on administration of tetracycline (22 mg/kg by mouth t.i.d. for 21 days) or chloramphenicol (15–20 mg/kg by mouth t.i.d. for 21 days). Doxycycline (5–10 mg/kg by mouth s.i.d. or b.i.d.) is preferable for cats as it does not seem to cause fever or anorexia. It should be noted that chloramphenicol therapy has a potential for marked hematotoxicity. At best, chloramphenicol therapy suppresses hematopoiesis. Baseline hematologic data should be used as a reference. Transfusion of whole blood or packed RBCs may be indicated when PCV is less than 10% (see Transfusion Therapy in the section on IHA). The administration of glucocorticoids for this infection is most controversial. We do not recommend the use of glucocorticoids in the treatment of this infection.

Prognosis

The prognosis depends on whether the infection is secondary to another process. Primary *Haemobartonella* infections are treated successfully in the majority of patients. It is possible that some forms of the organism (originating in Africa) may be refractory to treatment. When haemobartonellosis is thought to be a secondary infection (i.e., to FeLV), the prognosis is based on the primary disease.

Uncommon Erythrocyte Diseases

Pure Red Blood Cell Aplasia

Pure RBC aplasia has been described as an acquired process[10] and as congenital pure RBC aplasia with similarities to human Diamond-Blackfan anemia.

It is an infrequently encountered disease that appears as a severe normochromic, normocytic anemia. The diagnosis is based on histologic studies of liver, spleen, and bone marrow.[36]

Feline Cytauxzoonosis

Feline cytauxzoonosis is a severe protozoal tick-borne infection caused by *Cytauxzoon felis*. Clinical findings are related to anemia caused by hemolysis. Hemorrhagic complications may be observed. Diagnosis may be achieved by observation of protozoa in RBCs in blood smears. Effective therapy has not yet been described.[1, 10]

Zinc-Induced Hemolysis

Zinc poisoning induces marked hemolytic anemia with spherocytosis.[37] Acute zinc toxicosis resulting from the ingestion of zinc-based coins was diagnosed in dogs with hemolytic anemia characterized by Heinz body formation.[38]

Heinz Body Anemia

Heinz body anemia is uncommon in the dog. Ingestion of onions, methylene blue, acetaminophen, zinc, benzocaine, excessive doses of vitamin K, and phenylhydrazine may induce Heinz body anemia in the dog.[39] Onions consumed by dogs oxidize erythrocyte glutathione with resultant Heinz body formation and subsequent hemolytic anemia. The anemia is more severe in potassium- and glutathione-depleted dogs.[40] The feline Hb molecule seems more susceptible to oxidation. Heinz body formation is frequently observed in cats. Cat foods containing propylene glycol induce Heinz body formation in feline erythrocytes.[41] There is a strong correlation between diabetes mellitus, hyperthyroidism, and lymphoma and Heinz body formation. Diabetic cats, in particular, consistently have pronounced Heinz body formation. Polychromasia and numbers of punctate reticulocytes are slightly increased in cats with Heinz body formation.[42] Administration of methylene blue has been observed to induce Heinz body anemia in cats.[43]

Erythrocyte Pyruvate Kinase Deficiency

Erythrocyte pyruvate kinase deficiency has been described in beagle, basenji,[44] cairn terrier, and West Highland white terrier.[45] Clinical and laboratory features are exercise intolerance, persistent severe and highly regenerative anemia, splenomegaly, and progressive myelofibrosis and osteosclerosis.[46] Treatment by splenectomy followed by desferoxamine, insulin, and fludrocortisone acetate has been proposed.[47]

Phosphofructokinase Deficiency

Phosphofructokinase deficiency causing hemolytic anemia has been described in English springer spaniels. Erythrocytes had lower 2,3-DPG concentrations, had higher ATP concentrations, and were more fragile in an alkaline milieu than normal canine erythrocytes. Reticulocytes from a phosphofructokinase-deficient dog had nearly three times the ATP concentration of normal canine erythrocytes and had 2,3-DPG concentrations similar to those of normal canine erythrocytes. Phosphofructokinase-deficient reticulocytes are not fragile in an alkaline milieu.[10, 48, 49]

Erythrocyte Methemoglobin Reductase Deficiency

Erythrocyte methemoglobin reductase deficiency has been described in a toy American Eskimo dog, a miniature poodle, and a cocker-poodle crossbreed. Blood methemoglobin contents ranged from 19% to 36% of total Hb, with methemoglobin reductase values between 13% and 33% of normal. Oral riboflavin therapy was not effective in reducing the blood methemoglobin content in deficient dogs.[50]

Hereditary Stomatocytosis

Stomatocytosis has been associated with dwarfism in Alaskan malamutes.[10] Stomatocytosis and macrocytosis were found, but there was no evidence of shortened erythrocyte survival based on lack of regenerative anemia. However, shortened erythrocyte survival cannot be ruled out.[51]

Hereditary Nonspherocytic Hemolytic Anemia

Hereditary nonspherocytic hemolytic anemia of poodles is an uncommon autosomally inherited macrocytic, hypochromic anemia.[1]

Primary Erythrocytosis, Polycythemia Vera

Primary erythrocytosis is considered a myeloproliferative disorder. Increased production of RBCs without dehydration, hypoxia, or abnormal erythropoietin concentration is observed. No other cell lines (leukocytes and platelets) proliferate in canine primary erythrocytosis. This is unlike the situation in human polycythemia rubra vera.[15] In therapy of primary (absolute) erythrocytosis the clinical signs and blood counts may be stabilized through phlebotomy or chemotherapeutic agents. Hydroxyurea (Hydrea, 30 mg/kg by mouth s.i.d.) is administered for 7 to 10 days; subsequently the dose and the interval of administration may be adjusted.[52]

References

1. Jain NC. Essentials of Veterinary Hematology. Philadelphia, Lea & Febiger, 1993:133–221.
2. Duncan JR, Prasse KW. Veterinary Laboratory Medicine Clinical Pathology. Ames, Iowa, Iowa State University Press, 1986:3–30.
3. Rothuizen J, Van den Brom WE, Fevery J. The origins and kinetics of dogs with hepatobiliary and haemolytic diseases. J Hepatol 1992;15:17–24.
4. Conrad ME, Umbreit JN, Moore EG. Regulation of iron absorption: Proteins involved in duodenal mucose uptake and transport. J Am Coll Nutr 1993;12:720–728.
5. Hammond WP, Boone TC, Donahue RE, et al. A comparison of treatment of canine cyclic hematopoiesis with recombinant human granulocyte-macrophage colony-stimulating factor (GM-CSF), G-CSF, interleukin-3, and canine G-CSF. Blood 1990;76:523–532.
6. Ogilvie GK. Hematopoietic growth factors: Tools for a revolution in veterinary oncology and hematology. Compen Contin Educ Pract Vet 1993;15:851–854.
7. King LG, Giger U, Diserens D, et al. Anemia of chronic renal failure in dogs. J Vet Intern Med 1992;6:264–270.
8. Henry PA. Human recombinant erythropoietin used to treat a cat with anemia caused by chronic renal failure. Can Vet J 1994;35:370–375.
9. Petrites-Murphy MB, Pierce KR, Lowry SR, et al. Role of parathyroid hormone in the anemia of chronic terminal renal dysfunction in dogs. Am J Vet Res 1989;50:1898–1905.
10. Tvedten H. Erythrocyte disorders. In: Willard MD, Tvedten H, Turnwald GH, eds. Small Animal Clinical Diagnosis by Laboratory Methods. Philadelphia, WB Saunders, 1989:36–56.
11. Weiss DJ, Murtaugh M. Neutrophil-induced erythrocyte injury: A potential cause of erythrocyte destruction in the anemia of inflammatory disease. Vet Clin Pathol 1989;18:1–13.
12. Amoako KK, Goto Y, Shinjo T. Studies on the factors affecting the hemolytic activity of *Fusobacterium necrophorum*. Vet Microbiol 1994;41:11–18.
13. King JM. Clinical exposures: Hook worm anemia. Vet Med 1989;84:476–478.
14. Dryden MW, Gaafar SM. Blood consumption by the cat flea, *Ctenocephalides felis (Siphonaptera pulicidae)*. J Med Entomol 1991;28:394–400.
15. Hoffman R, Wasserman LR. Natural history and management of polycythemia vera. Adv Intern Med 1979;24:255–285.
16. Hillman RS, Finch CA. Red Cell Manual, 5th ed. Philadelphia, FA Davis, 1985:33–55.
17. Smith JE. Irom metabolism and its diseases. In: Kaneko JJ, ed. Clinical Biochemistry of Domestic Animals, 4th ed. San Diego, Academic Press, 1989:263–268.
18. Klaq AR. Hemolytic anemia in dogs. Compen Contin Educ Pract Vet 1992;14:1090–1095.
19. Stewart AF, Feldman BF. Immune-mediated hemolytic anemia. Part I. An overview. Compen Contin Educ Pract Vet 1993;15:372–381.
20. Klaq AR, Giger U, Shofer FS. Idiopathic immune mediated hemolytic anemia in dogs: 42 cases (1986–1990). J Am Vet Med Assoc 1993;202:783–788.
21. Barker RN, Gruffydd-Jones TJ, Stokes CR, et al. Identification of autoantigens in canine autoimmune haemolytic anaemia. Clin Exp Immunol 1991;85:33–40.
22. Stewart AF, Feldman BF. Immune mediated hemolytic anemia. Part II. Clinical entity, diagnosis, and treatment theory. Compen Contin Educ Pract Vet 1993;15:1479–1491.
23. Holloway SA, Meyer DJ, Mannella C. Prednisolone and danazol for treatment of immune-mediated anemia, thrombocytopenia, and ineffective erythroid regeneration in a dog. J Am Vet Med Assoc 1990;197:1046–1048.
24. Couto CG. Anemia in the cat. Proceedings of the North American Veterinary Conference, Orlando, Florida, 1992:172–174.
25. Giger U. Feline blood groups and incompatibility reactions. Proceedings of the Eighth ACVIM Forum, Washington, DC, 1990:319–321.
26. Authement IM, Wolfsheimer KJ. Canine blood component therapy: Product preparation, storage and administration. J Am Anim Hosp Assoc 1987;23:483–493.
27. Giger U, Gelens CJ, Callan MB, et al. An acute hemolytic transfusion reaction caused by dog erythrocyte antigen 1.1 incompatibility in a previously sensitized dog. J Am Vet Med Assoc 1995;206:1358–1362.
28. Kristensen AT, Feldman BF. Blood banking and transfusion medicine. In: Ettinger SJ, Feldman EC, eds. Textbook of Veterinary Internal Medicine, 4th ed. Philadelphia, WB Saunders, 1995:347–360.
29. Medinger TL, Williams DA, Druyette DS. Severe gastrointestinal tract hemorrhage in three dogs with hypoadrenocorticism. J Am Vet Med Assoc 1993;202:1869–1872.
30. Stone E, Badner D, Cotter SM. Trends in transfusion medicine in dogs at a veterinary school clinic: 515 cases (1986–1989). J Am Vet Med Assoc 1992;200:1000–1004.
31. Norsworthy GD. Clinical aspects of feline blood transfusions. Compen Contin Educ Pract Vet 1992;14:469–475.
32. Murase T, Hashimoto T, Ueda T, et al. Multiplication of *Babesia gibsoni* in in vitro culture and its relation to hemolysis of infected erythrocytes. J Vet Med Sci 1991;53:759–760.
33. Morishige T, Takahashi K, Abe S, et al. Detection of circulating immune complex in dogs infected with *Babesia gibsoni*. J Coll Dairying 1988; 12:443–452.
34. Freeman MJ, Kirby BM, Panciera DL, et al. Hypotensive shock syndrome associated with acute *Babesia canis* infection in a dog. J Am Vet Med Assoc 1994;204:94–96.
35. Boujon CE, Scharer V, Bestetti GE. Haemobartonellen-Nachweis im Katzenblutausstrich. Schweiz Arch Tierheilkd 1991;133:135–136.
36. Moore AH, Day MJ, Graham MWA. Congenital pure red blood cell aplasia (Diamond-Blackfan anaemia) in a dog. Vet Rec 1993;132:414–415.
37. Latimer KS, Jain AV, Inglesby HB, et al. Zinc-induced hemolytic anemia caused by ingestion of pennies by a pup. J Am Vet Med Assoc 1989;195:77–80.
38. Luttgen PJ, Whitney MS, Wolf AM, et al. Heinz body hemolytic anemia associated with high plasma zinc

concentration in a dog. J Am Vet Med Assoc 1990;197: 1347–1350.

39. Houston DM, Myers SL. A review of Heinz-body anemia in the dog induced by toxins. Vet Hum Toxicol 1993; 35:158–161.

40. Yamoto O, Maede Y. Susceptibility to onion-induced hemolysis in dogs with hereditary high erythrocyte reduced glutathione and potassium concentrations. Am J Vet Res 1992;53:134–137.

41. Bauer MC, Weiss DJ, Perman V. Hematologic alterations in adult cats fed 6 or 12% propylene glycol. Am J Vet Res 1992;53:69–72.

42. Christopher MM. Relation of endogenous Heinz bodies to disease and anemia in cats: 120 cases (1978–1987). J Am Vet Med Assoc 1989;194:1089–1095.

43. Quinley JW. Heinz body anemia induced by methylene blue in a cat. Calif Vet 1987;41:11–13.

44. Giger U, Noble NA. Determination of erythrocyte pyruvate kinase deficiency in Basenjis with chronic hemolytic anemia. J Am Vet Med Assoc 1991;198:1755–1761.

45. Chapman BL, Giger U. Inherited erythrocyte pyruvate kinase deficiency in the West Highland white terrier. J Small Anim Pract 1990;31:610–616.

46. Giger U, Wang P, Mason GD. Inherited erythrocyte

47. Schaer M, Harvey JW, Calderwood-Mays M, et al. Pyruvate kinase deficiency causing hemolytic anemia with secondary hemochromatosis in a cairn terrier. J Am Anim Hosp Assoc 1992;28:233–239.

48. Giger U, Harvey JW, Yamaguchi RA, et al. Inherited phosphofructokinase deficiency in dogs with hyperventilation induced hemolysis. Increased in vitro and in vivo alkaline fragility of erythrocytes. Blood 1985;65:345–348.

49. Harvey JW, Sussman WA, Pate MG. Effect of 2,3-diphosphoglycerate concentration on the alkaline fragility of phosphofructokinase-deficient canine erythrocytes. Comp Biochem Physiol 1988;89:105–109.

50. Harvey JW, King RR, Berry CR, et al. Methaemoglobin reductase deficiency in dogs. Comp Haematol Int 1991; 1:55–59.

51. Brown DE, Weiser MG, Thrall MA, et al. Erythrocyte indices and volume distribution in a dog with stomatocytosis. Vet Pathol 1994;31:247–250.

52. Smith M, Turrel JM. Radiophosphorus (^{32}P) treatment of bone marrow disorders in dogs: 11 cases (1970–1987). J Am Vet Med Assoc 1989;194:98–102.

pyruvate kinase deficiency in a beagle dog. Vet Clin Pathol 1991;20:83–86.

Chapter 42

Diseases of Nonlymphocytic Leukocytes

Rafael Ruiz de Gopegui
Bernard F. Feldman

Anatomy

Granulopoiesis occurs in the bone marrow. Regulation of granulopoiesis depends on interleukin-3, granulocyte-macrophage colony-stimulating factor, and granulocyte colony-stimulating factor.[1] Other interleukins such as interleukin-2 and tumor necrosis factor induce granulocyte maturation and activation.[2]

The myeloid maturation developmental stem cell sequence consists of the granulocyte-macrophage colony-forming unit (or the eosinophil or basophil colony-forming unit), followed by the granulocyte colony-forming unit.

The myeloid maturation developmental sequence for cells that can be identified morphologically is as follows: myeloblast; progranulocyte (promyelocyte), characterized by the presence of azurophilic primary cytoplasmic granules; myelocyte, characterized by the presence of specific or secondary granules (neutrophilic, eosinophilic, or basophilic); metamyelocyte (neutrophilic, eosinophilic, or basophilic); band (neutrophilic, eosinophilic, or basophilic); and adult granulocyte (neutrophilic, eosinophilic, or basophilic).

The cells of the mitotic pool are the myeloblast, progranulocyte, and myelocyte. The cells of the postmitotic developmental pool are the metamyelocyte and band. The basic differences among the myelocyte, metamyelocyte, band, and adult granulocytes are the nuclear configuration, nuclear chromatin condensation, and maturation of the cytoplasm. The myelocyte has an essentially round nucleus, the metamyelocyte a bean-shaped nucleus, and the band a nucleus with essentially parallel sides. The nucleus of the adult cell is segmented. Cytoplasmic basophilia is most notable in the myelocyte, whereas the adult granulocyte has a clear to neutral color. The only cytoplasmic color in these cells is associated with the specific granules of the neutrophil, eosinophil, or basophil.

Neutrophil. The neutrophil is a cell with pale cytoplasm and inconspicuous (neutral-colored) granules. Nuclear segmentation increases with maturation. Immature neutrophils have less segmentation than adult cells and less condensed chromatin. Cell volume decreases with maturation, although volume changes among late-stage cells (metamyelocyte and band forms) are negligible.

Monocyte. The monocyte represents the circulating precursor of the tissue macrophage. The monocyte has an oval or ameboid-appearing, nonsegmented (bilobulated or trilobulated) nucleus and a pale gray-blue cytoplasm that is frequently vacuolated.

Eosinophil. The eosinophil has a lobulated, segmented nucleus and red or eosinophilic cytoplasmic granules. Canine eosinophils have bigger, more variable, and less numerous granules than feline eosinophils.

Basophil. Canine basophils have purple cytoplasmic granulation. The staining pattern of feline basophils is blue-gray. Because of the variability in feline basophil staining—numerous light-staining granules and a few dark-staining granules—the staining pattern is termed metachromatic.

Lymphocytes. Mature lymphocytes have round nuclei and sparse light blue to basophilic cytoplasm. Activated lymphocytes are larger and have intense basophilic cytoplasm with a pale perinuclear zone (Golgi apparatus).

Plasma Cells. Plasma cells are rarely observed in peripheral blood preparations. Plasma cells have eccentric nuclei with variably condensed chromatin often described as "clock faced" or "wagon wheel." The cytoplasm is plentiful, is basophilic, and has a pale perinuclear zone.

Physiology

Neutrophil. Neutrophil function is involved in host defense against microorganisms. Neutrophils participate in the initiation of the inflammatory response, are phagocytic cells, and are also involved in iron metabolism and hemostasis.[3]

Monocyte. Monocyte functions include phagocytosis of larger organisms or substances, substances too large for neutrophil phagocytosis. Monocytes participate in the initiation of inflammation, the immune response (antigen processing), and hemostasis.

Eosinophil. The functions of eosinophils include participation in host defense against parasites and activation and regulation of the inflammatory response, hemostasis, and complement.[3] Eosinophils participate in hemostasis through activation of tumor necrosis factor and activation of coagulation proteins leading to fibrin formation. The eosinophil is a participant in hypersensitivity reactions.

Basophils. Basophil (and, to a certain extent, mast cell) function is related to inflammation, hemostasis, and lipid metabolism through mechanisms similar to those of eosinophils. The basophil is a participant in hypersensitivity reactions.

Diagnostic Procedures

Leukogram

The number of white blood cells represents the balance between bone marrow production and tissue

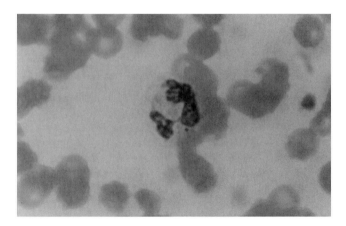

Figure 42–1
Canine neutrophil with Döhle bodies.

demand. This is reflected in the distribution of the various leukocytes in plasma.[4]

The white blood cell (WBC) count is the determination of the total leukocyte numbers in peripheral blood per microliter. The presence of nucleated red blood cells (RBCs) falsely elevates the WBC count. If large numbers of nucleated RBCs are present, the WBC count must be corrected. The correction formula is

$$\frac{\text{Corrected}}{\text{WBC}} = \frac{100}{100 + \text{number of nucleated RBCs}} \times \frac{\text{measured}}{\text{WBC}}$$

The differential leukocyte count is the determination of the numbers of neutrophils and their precursors as well as of lymphocytes, monocytes, eosinophils, and basophils/μL in peripheral blood. It is expressed as relative distribution (percentage) and absolute (concentration) number of leukocytes. From a diagnostic standpoint, *only* absolute numbers are used. The presence of immature cells or unusual cells must be reported as an addendum to the differential leukocyte count. The presence of damaged cells must also be reported.

Blood Smear

Toxic alterations of neutrophil morphology on blood smears include general indications of toxicity such as Döhle bodies (basophilic inclusions within neutrophil cytoplasm), cytoplasmic vacuolation, cytoplasmic granulation, and changes in the configuration of neutrophil nuclear patterns. Döhle bodies are formed from free ribosomes or ribosomes attached to endoplasmic reticulum and represent asynchronous cytoplasmic maturation (Fig. 42–1). Cytoplasmic vacuolation often results from the autodigestion of neutrophil cytoplasm after endogenous release of enzymes from lysosomes.

When there is cytoplasmic toxic granulation (abnormal size and staining pattern of neutrophil

cytoplasmic granules), azurophilic granules are visible in the normally neutral-staining neutrophil cytoplasm (Fig. 42–2). Toxic granulation occurs with severe inflammation.

Karyorrhexis and karyolysis are terms that describe neutrophil nuclear changes. Karyorrhexis indicates fragmentation of neutrophil nuclei. Karyolysis indicates swelling and vacuolation of neutrophil nuclei. Nuclear hypersegmentation, with more than five nuclear lobes, may also be a sign of neutrophil toxicity. Intracytoplasmic inclusions of canine distemper virus are occasionally seen in association with active canine distemper infections. Cytoplasmic inclusions may also be observed with equine *Ehrlichia* infections of canine neutrophils.

Alterations of monocyte morphology include erythrophagocytosis and platelet phagocytosis. Activated monocytes have granular and vacuolated cytoplasm. Because monocytes vacuolate swiftly in a test tube, blood smears should be made immediately after obtaining blood samples.

Lymphocyte morphologic alterations include the presence of Rieder's cells, reactive lymphocytes with irregular, cleft shapes. Rieder's cells are not specifically associated with any disease process.

Other lymphocyte morphologic changes include the presence of immunocytes, activated lymphocytes characterized by large cell size, and cytoplasmic basophilia. Immunocytes are commonly observed in younger animals and animals exposed to "new" antigens.

Buffy Coat

Buffy coat examination allows observation of concentrated leukocytes and platelet numbers. Abnormal leukocytes, leukocyte dysplasia, and parasitized leukocytes (or platelets) may be more readily observed than in the blood smear.

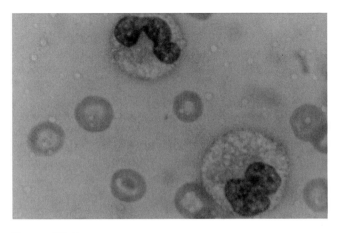

Figure 42–2
Canine neutrophils with toxic cytoplasmic granulation.

Bone Marrow Cytology

The reader is directed to Chapter 41 for a description of bone marrow examination procedures. Bone marrow examination reveals mitotic and maturation activity. It is indicated whenever an unexplained cytopenia is present or abnormal cells are observed in peripheral blood. Bone marrow aspiration allows the observation of quantitative cell production in terms of aplasia, hypoplasia, normoplasia, or hyperplasia of all cell lines. These findings are compared with hemogram results. These comparisons allow the diagnosis of ineffective hematopoiesis. Complete bone marrow examination includes determination of the maturation index (correlation between mature cells and precursors), of cell morphology, of the myeloid/erythroid ratio, and of the presence of cellular atypia, dysplasia, or inappropriate numbers. Bone marrow biopsy may be necessary to diagnose severe generalized marrow alterations such as myelofibrosis.

Cytochemical Staining

The major usage of cytochemical staining is for the identification of cells in leukemia.[3, 5, 6] Cytochemical staining is available only at specialized referral centers. Fresh air-dried blood or bone marrow smears may be submitted for cell identification at these centers.

Problem Identification

Neutropenia

Neutropenia is a reduction in the absolute number of circulating neutrophils. Reference intervals are dependent on individual laboratories.

Pathophysiology

Leukopenia is most often caused by neutropenia. Neutropenia may be the result of overwhelming inflammatory processes that shorten the survival of circulating neutrophils, especially when myelopoiesis, neutrophil production specifically, is ineffective or when there is myelosuppression. Infection of myeloid cells with feline leukemia virus (FeLV), feline immunodeficiency virus (FIV), and canine or feline parvoviruses is often involved in the pathogenesis of cytopenias.[7] Cytopenias associated with ehrlichiosis are also associated with infection of myeloid cells. Cytopenias associated with leukemia or other bone marrow neoplasia, such as myeloma, are the result of myelophthisis, reduction of blood cell precursors in bone marrow resulting from neoplastic infiltration.

Clinical Signs

In neutropenic patients with absolute neutrophil counts less than 1000 cells/µL, susceptibility to infection and clinical signs of infection such as fever may be present.

Diagnostic Plan

When neutropenia is observed, repetition of the test is necessary to confirm that the condition is a trend rather than a single exclusive finding. If neutropenia is confirmed, the rest of the white cell differential and white cell morphology should be examined.

If the animal is receiving drugs with known potential for marrow suppression, such as the chemotherapeutic agents cyclophosphamide, mitoxantrone, and doxorubicin (Adriamycin) or antibiotics such as griseofulvin, chloramphenicol, or cephalosporin, therapy should be stopped for several days with monitoring of the hemogram (complete blood count) for a response.

Griseofulvin administration has been associated with the development of absolute neutropenia in cats. This is especially apparent in cats infected with FIV.[8] Cephalosporin administration may induce bone marrow suppression in dogs, with ineffective erythropoiesis and granulopoiesis.[9] Administration of zidovudine (dose 30 mg/kg/per day) to cats resulted in dose-dependent progressive anemia and neutropenia.[10]

Neutropenia and toxic morphologic alterations of neutrophils may be anticipated in gram-negative sepsis and endotoxemia.[5] The presence of fewer mature neutrophils than immature cell forms is regarded as a degenerative left shift. Degenerative left shifts may appear with neutrophilia or neutropenia and indicate an inappropriate and deficient bone marrow response.[11] Increased neutrophil margination, adherence of neutrophils to microvascular endothelium (pseudoneutropenia), may result from endotoxemia and anaphylactic reactions.[4]

Viral infections, rickettsial infections, a wide variety of drugs and environmental toxins, and neoplasia (especially during chemotherapy) may induce severe neutropenia and potentially affect other cell lines in a similar manner. If evidence of primary disease that would explain neutropenia is not apparent from the clinical signs or routine laboratory evaluation (for *Salmonella* or parvoviral gastroenteritis), FeLV and FIV testing should be performed in cats and rickettsial titers (for *Ehrlichia* and Rocky Mountain spotted fever) should be measured in dogs. If these tests are negative, a bone marrow examination should be performed (see Diagnostic Procedures in Chap. 41). If the patient is a cat, immunofluorescent antibody testing for FeLV should be performed on a marrow smear in addition to routine cytology. Occasionally, latently infected cats are negative for FeLV in peripheral blood, yet positive in bone marrow. Routine bone marrow cytology should rule out or confirm infiltrative diseases such as neoplasia as a cause of neutropenia.

FIV infection is characterized by moderate to severe leukopenia, neutropenia and often lymphopenia, and eosinopenia. Appropriate myeloid activity or mild bone marrow myeloid hyperplasia with a left shift in peripheral blood to progranulocytes often accompanies the neutropenia. Chronic infection is characterized by intermittent neutropenia and lymphopenia.[12–14]

Neutrophilia

Neutrophilia is an increase in the absolute number of circulating neutrophils. Reference intervals are dependent on individual laboratories. The most marked leukocytosis may be observed in some forms of infection and in some forms of myeloproliferative disease.

Pathophysiology

Leukocytosis is frequently caused by neutrophilia in small animals. Mild to moderate neutrophilia may appear in physiologic conditions such as fear, exercise, or excitement, particularly in cats. Physiologic neutrophilia represents mobilization of the marginal pool of neutrophils and is often accompanied by marked lymphocytosis.[5] Glucocorticoid administration, hyperadrenocorticism, and stress induce neutrophilia, accompanied by monocytosis (in the dog), lymphopenia, and eosinopenia. Glucocorticoid administration reduces neutrophil adherence to endothelial cells (the neutrophil marginal pool) and thus increases circulating neutrophil numbers. Hypersegmentation may be observed as neutrophils age in the circulation, glucocorticoids inhibit cell margination and extravascular migration (diapedesis). The phagocytic and microbiocidal activity of canine neutrophils so mobilized may also be diminished.[15]

Diagnostic Plan

Neutrophil numbers above the upper end of the reference interval are caused by inflammation or stress. Stress-induced neutrophilia (15,000 to 25,000 cells/µL) is more modest than neutrophilia induced by inflammation and is accompanied by other changes in the leukogram associated with stress: lymphopenia, monocytosis, and eosinopenia. Neutrophilia caused by inflammation is associated with marked increases in neutrophil counts (25,000 to >40,000 cells/µL) and the presence of a left shift. Toxic changes in neutrophils and other white cells may be observed.

Neutrophilia is frequent and intense in young cats, possibly as a result of release of neutrophils from the large marginal neutrophil pool observed in cats. Neutrophilia is frequently observed in acute septic and nonseptic inflammatory processes. Examples include canine pyometra,[16] pancreatitis,[17] Lyme disease,[18] immune-mediated disease, and neoplastic processes. Left-shift neutrophilia (increased band neutrophils or more immature forms) appears in active inflammatory processes—the tissue demand for neutrophils increases the rate of bone marrow neutrophil release. With chronic inflammation, neutrophilia is not often accompanied by a left shift. Instead, monocytosis may occur. If mature neutrophils are more numerous than immature forms, the left shift is considered regenerative.

If the cause of neutrophilia is not apparent from the clinical signs, a serum chemistry profile and urinalysis should be obtained. Evidence for pancreatitis, hepatitis, or pyelonephritis may be apparent in the serum chemistry values, explaining neutrophilia. Changes in the urinary sediment such as pyuria and cylindruria (see Chap. 16) indicate that a urinary tract infection such as pyelonephritis may be the cause of neutrophilia. If routine laboratory evaluation does not reveal a cause for neutrophilia, thoracic and abdominal radiographs or ultrasonography may identify the presence of pyothorax, pneumonia, pulmonary foreign bodies, tumors, abscesses, peritonitis, or pyometra as a cause of neutrophilia. Fine-needle aspiration of masses or body cavity fluids may then be indicated in order to make a definitive diagnosis.

Monocytosis

Monocytosis is present when monocyte numbers are increased above the upper end of the reference interval. Reference intervals are dependent on individual laboratories. The highest monocyte counts are associated with significant tissue breakdown. Examples occur with trauma, neoplastic metastasis, and fungal infection. Monocytosis is observed in processes characterized by tissue destruction, including suppuration, necrosis, neoplasia, hemorrhage, hemolysis, and immune-mediated and granulomatous diseases.[5, 19] Monocytosis may be induced by glucocorticoids in dogs and may be observed in infectious processes associated with neutrophilia or associated with eosinophilia in parasitism.[19, 20]

Lymphocytosis

Lymphocytosis is defined as lymphocyte numbers in excess of the upper end of the laboratory reference interval. Lymphocytosis may be observed with physiologic neutrophilia or in chronic stages of infection with an associated hypergammaglobulinemia.[5] Cats may experience marked physiologic lymphocytosis without neutrophilia in peracute stress associated with epinephrine release. Persistent lymphocytosis may be expected in chronic infection and with immune-mediated disease.[4]

Lymphopenia

Lymphopenia is defined as absolute lymphocyte numbers below the lower end of the laboratory reference interval. Many patients with lymphopenia have some component of stress, such as that associated with systemic infection or inflammation, and may have been treated with glucocorticoids. Other causes of lymphopenia include primary immunodeficiency, lymphangiectasia, and granulomatous or neoplastic diseases of the lymphoid system. Lymphopenia is a feature of viral infections such as feline infectious peritonitis, FeLV infection, FIV infection, infectious canine hepatitis (or canine adenovirus), distemper (or canine paramyxovirus), canine parvovirus, and canine coronavirus.[21]

FIV is tropic for feline T-lymphoblastoid cells.[22] Anemia, lymphopenia, neutropenia, and thrombocytopenia may appear in FIV-seropositive cats.[23–25] FeLV and FIV may induce lymphopenia as a result of T-lymphocyte infection.[26] Cytologic evaluation of bone marrow aspirates may reveal appropriate cellular morphology, maturation, and myeloid/erythroid ratio. However, significant inhibition of progenitors derived from granulocyte-macrophage colony-forming units was observed when marrow cells were cultured in the presence of autologous serum, suggesting the presence of a humoral inhibitory substance directed specifically at the granulocyte-macrophage lineage.[9] This may be responsible for bone marrow myelosuppression.

Eosinophilia

Eosinophilia is defined as absolute eosinophil numbers in excess of the upper end of the laboratory reference interval. Eosinophilia is related to hypersensitivity reactions—antigen-antibody allergic interactions—such as occur with parasitism (e.g., heartworm infection). Eosinophilia is generally related to processes involving epithelial surfaces of the pulmonary tree, the gastrointestinal tract, and the genitourinary tract, as well as superficial skin surfaces. Viruses, fungi, and other infectious agents may also induce an eosinophilic response. Eosinophilia is most frequently observed in cats with flea allergy dermatitis, eosinophilic granuloma complex, asthma, chronic upper respiratory infections, and gastrointestinal disease.[27] Hypereosinophilia (marked and unexplained eosinophilia) has been described in the cat in feline hypereosinophilic syndrome and eosinophilic leukemia and as a paraneoplastic syndrome in lymphosarcoma and transitional cell carcinoma of the urinary bladder.[28]

Mast cell neoplasia in dogs may induce eosinophilia[4] as well as basophilia.[29] Eosinophilia has also been described in dogs with rectal adenomatous polyps. Eosinophilia may be associated with extreme neutrophilic leukocytosis and monocytosis.[30]

Basophilia

Basophils are rarely observed in blood smears. Thus, the presence of even one or two basophils in a differential count constitutes basophilia. Basophilia may be observed in association with eosinophilia and is often induced by the same processes (e.g., heartworm infection). However, basophilia without eosinophilia has been observed in dogs with altered lipid metabolism and is related to systemic mastocytosis.[4, 29]

Leukemoid Reaction

A leukemoid reaction may appear in severe purulent inflammation or as a paraneoplastic syndrome, characterized by marked leukocytosis (>50,000–100,000 WBCs/μL, the range of true leukemias) with a neutrophilic left shift to myelocytes or even earlier myeloid precursors.[5] A leukemoid reaction involving lymphocytes has been described in salmon poisoning disease in dogs.[31] An eosinophilic leukemoid reaction without apparent cause has been reported in the dog.[32]

Leukoerythroblastic Reaction

A leukoerythroblastic reaction is characterized by the presence of nucleated erythrocyte precursors (normoblastemia) and increased immature leukocytes in peripheral blood. Leukoerythroblastic reactions have been observed in neoplasia, myelodysplastic syndromes, immune-mediated hemolytic anemia or thrombocytopenia, and some forms of trauma.[33]

Treatment

Recombinant canine granulocyte colony-stimulating factor has been observed to be effective in stimulating myelopoiesis in normal and neutropenic dogs at a dose of 2.5 μg/kg b.i.d. as needed.[34] It has been used successfully to treat myelosuppression induced by the chemotherapeutic agent mitoxantrone.[1]

Myeloproliferative Diseases (Leukemias)

Leukemias are uncommon neoplastic diseases originating in hematopoietic tissues that may include myeloproliferative disorders and lymphoproliferative disorders. Leukocytosis and abnormal blast cells (dysplastic or neoplastic blast cells) may be found in

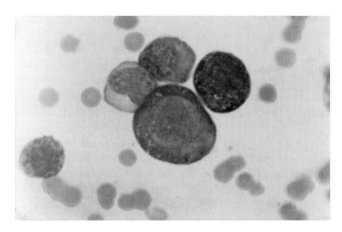

Figure 42-3
Bone marrow smear of a cat with acute myelogenous leukemia.

peripheral blood. However, leukopenia and absence of neoplastic cells (aleukemic leukemia) or presence of neoplastic cells without leukocytosis (subleukemic leukemia) may also be observed in peripheral blood smears. Acute myeloid leukemias (undifferentiated, blastic leukemia cells; Figs. 42–3 and 42–4) are seen more frequently in young patients; chronic forms (leukemic cells, relatively well differentiated) are expected in older patients.[35]

Eosinophilic leukemia has been described in cats with marked eosinophilia. Mature and immature eosinophils are observed in peripheral blood, and there is often marked organ infiltration with eosinophils, both mature and immature. Differentiation between eosinophilic leukemia and feline hypereosinophilic syndrome is difficult. Basophilic leukemia is rare. It has been described in FeLV-positive cats.

Myelomonocytic leukemias are frequently en-

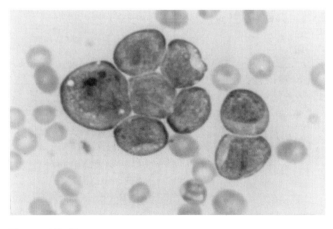

Figure 42-4
Blood film of a dog with an acute blastic crisis during chronic granulocytic leukemia.

countered in dogs.[6, 36, 37] This form of leukemia has also been described in FeLV-positive cats.

Monocytic leukemia has been described in dogs and FeLV-positive cats as an uncommon form of leukemia with marked monocytosis and the presence of monocyte precursors in peripheral blood. Severe bone marrow infiltration has also been described.[6, 36, 37]

Acute undifferentiated leukemia (formerly called Di Guglielmo syndrome or reticuloendotheliosis) has been described in cats. Erythroleukemia and erythremic myelosis have also been described predominantly in cats. Megakaryoblastic leukemia has been described in cats and dogs. Myelodysplastic syndrome has been described in cats in association with cytopenias and FeLV infection. This syndrome has been infrequently described in dogs. Myelogenous leukemia (granulocytic leukemia) has been described in both cats and dogs.

Clinical Signs

Clinical signs of leukemia may include general manifestations such as anorexia, depression, weight loss, anemia, thrombocytopenia, recurrent infections, and hemorrhage or disseminated intravascular coagulation. Osteolysis, dyspnea, renal failure, or neurologic signs may also be observed.[36, 37] These signs are referable to invasion of leukemic cells in the respective tissues.

Diagnostic Plan

The diagnosis of leukemia requires blood and bone marrow examinations using specific staining procedures, cytochemistry, and immunocytochemistry in order to identify and quantify the predominant cell types. The grade of maturation and differentiation of the neoplastic cell that is proliferating contributes to the subclassification of leukemia. When the leukemic cells are undifferentiated, the leukemia is classified as acute. When cells are differentiated, it is classified as chronic. Estimation of the myeloid/erythroid ratio of the bone marrow is also necessary to characterize the myeloproliferative disorder. The presence of leukemic cells in extramedullary tissues confirms the diagnosis of leukemia. The diagnosis of leukemia is difficult unless there is a singular monomorphic population of cells within the bone marrow or in peripheral blood. Cytochemical changes may definitively diagnose many leukemias.

The following classification of leukemias, reported by the Animal Leukemia Study Group, is derived from the French-American-British group and National Cancer Institute of the United States for classification of acute myeloid leukemias in humans.[31] Classification of chronic leukemias in small animals has not, as yet, been completely defined.

Acute Myeloid Leukemias

In acute myeloid leukemias, bone marrow examination reveals an erythroid population less than 50% and blast cell population greater than 30% of the total nucleated cell population.

Acute Undifferentiated Leukemia

Acute undifferentiated leukemia, described in cats, is characterized by marked to moderate infiltration of neoplastic cells in spleen, liver, and lymph nodes. A blast cell population predominates in bone marrow.[31, 35]

Myelomonocytic Leukemia

Myelomonocytic leukemia has been described in FeLV-positive cats and in dogs. Myeloblasts and monoblasts predominate in marrow (greater than 30%); mature granulocytes and monocytes make up less than 20% of the total nucleated cell population.[31, 35–37] The proportions of monocytes and neutrophils as well as the maturity of the neoplastic cells may change during the disease.[6, 36, 37]

Monocytic Leukemia

Monocytic leukemia has been described in FeLV-positive cats. Monoblasts and promonocytes predominate in the bone marrow (greater than 30% to less than 80%), with the mature granulocyte population being less than 20% of the total nucleated cell population.[31, 35–37]

Erythroleukemia and Erythremic Myelosis

Erythroleukemia and erythremic myelosis in cats often present with severe nonregenerative anemia and increased nucleated RBCs in peripheral blood. Slight infiltration of lymph nodes, spleen, and liver has also been described in this myeloproliferative process. In erythroleukemia, the erythroid population is greater than 50% of the total nucleated cell population in bone marrow examinations of affected patients. Myeloblasts and monoblasts are less than 30%. By definition, erythremic myelosis is present when myeloblasts and monoblasts are greater than 30% or when the blast cell count, including rubriblasts, is greater than 30% of the total nucleated cell population. Erythroleukemia and erythremic myelosis have been described predominantly in cats. Evolution from erythroleukemia to erythremic myelosis and, indeed, to myeloblastic leukemia can occur.[31, 35]

Megakaryoblastic Leukemia

In megakaryoblastic leukemia, megakaryoblasts constitute more than 30% of the nucleated bone marrow cell population. If megakaryoblasts are less than 30% and megakaryocytes predominate, essential thrombocythemia is the suggested diagnosis.[31] Megakaryoblastic leukemia has been described in cats and dogs.

Myelodysplastic Syndrome (Preleukemia, Smoldering Leukemia)

On bone marrow examination of patients with the myelodysplastic syndrome, erythroid, myeloid, or megakaryocytic cell lines are dysplastic. The developing erythroid, myeloid, and megakaryocytic cells are morphologically atypical, usually large cells with atypical nuclear configurations. Blast cell populations are less than 30% and erythroid cells less than 50% of the total nucleated cell population of the marrow.[31, 35, 38]

Chronic Myeloid Leukemias

Chronic myeloid leukemias are characterized by increased immature myeloid cells in the bone marrow; erythroid cells in bone marrow make up less than 50% of the total nucleated cell population. Blast cells are less than 30% of the total nucleated cell population in the bone marrow, and dysplastic changes are not often observed. Mature leukocytes predominate in both peripheral blood and marrow. Chronic leukemias may have a longer clinical course.

The classification of chronic myeloid leukemias includes chronic myelogenous leukemia, chronic eosinophilic leukemia, chronic basophilic leukemia, chronic monocytic leukemia, and chronic myelomonocytic leukemia.[31]

Marked leukocytosis in peripheral blood and an insidious presentation of the disease are often observed.[35] Myelogenous leukemia (granulocytic leukemia) has been described in cats and dogs with nonregenerative anemia, thrombocytopenia, and persistent severe leukocytosis (with a shift to metamyelocytes) in peripheral blood. Extramedullary hematopoiesis and organ infiltration have been described.[5, 31, 36, 37]

It can be difficult to distinguish the findings in chronic myelogenous leukemia from a severe inflammatory leukogram. However, leukemic neutrophils are quantitatively different from normal neutrophils with respect to enzyme activities.[39] Finding severe leukocytosis without the presence of other inciting causes may be the most practical criterion for diagnosis.

Diagnosis of eosinophilic leukemia is based on eosinophil numbers, which, in reported cases, exceeded 100,000 eosinophils/μL.[6]

Leukemic forms of mast cell neoplasia may be difficult to distinguish from basophilic leukemia with currently available techniques,[4, 6] although basophilic leukemia is much more rare.

Pathophysiology

The etiology of leukemias has not been completely defined. A higher incidence of leukemia in cats and especially in FeLV-positive cats has been observed.[6] Myelophthisis may often occur, leading to cytopenias. Leukemic cells also infiltrate other tissues, leading to dysfunction depending on the tissue invaded.

Treatment

Treatment of leukemic patients has been problematic in clinical veterinary medicine. Treatment is dependent on the type and grade of leukemia. Treatment of chronic myelogenous leukemia may include splenectomy, chemotherapy, antibiotic therapy, and blood transfusions. The recommended chemotherapeutic agent for chronic myelogenous leukemia is hydroxyurea, 50 mg/kg by mouth every day for 14 days. If remission is achieved, the dosing interval is reduced to 2-day and then 3-day intervals.[40] Chemotherapy for acute myelogenous leukemia has been unrewarding.

Prognosis

Acute leukemias generally have a short clinical course (less than 6 months without treatment). Chronic leukemias have a better prognosis but may evolve to acute forms. Blast crisis (see Fig. 42–4), the sudden and unexpected presence of immature cells in the peripheral blood of patients treated for chronic leukemias, is associated with increased mortality.[6]

Uncommon Diseases of Nonlymphocytic Leukocytes

Feline Hypereosinophilic Syndrome

Feline hypereosinophilic syndrome is considered an idiopathic disorder. Hypereosinophilia and mature eosinophilic infiltration of tissues such as skin, liver, spleen, lymph nodes, bone marrow, and digestive tract may be present. The differential diagnosis between this process and eosinophilic leukemia is difficult. Therapy for these processes using glucocorticoids or hydroxyurea has been attempted, but results are not predictable.[41, 42]

Cyclic Neutropenia

Cyclic neutropenia (grey collie syndrome, canine cyclic hematopoiesis) is an inherited disease in grey collies characterized by recurrent episodes of neutropenia lasting 12 to 14 days. Diagnosis is supported by repeated hemogram analysis. Thrombocytopenia and anemia may accompany cyclic neutropenia. Neutrophil functions are also impaired, and

therefore frequent infections may be anticipated.[43] Affected dogs that were given low-dose recombinant canine granulocyte colony-stimulating factor continued to have neutropenic cycles, but the neutropenia and associated clinical signs were ameliorated.[34] Cyclic hematopoiesis has been described in the cat as an acquired disease possibly related to FeLV infection.[4]

Chronic Idiopathic Neutropenia Syndrome

Persistent neutropenia described in the cat resembles chronic idiopathic neutropenia syndrome of humans. Decreased numbers of mature granulocytic cells and granulocyte-macrophage colony-forming units have been observed in the bone marrow and in bone marrow culture, respectively.[44]

Pelger-Huët Anomaly

This anomaly is an inherited defect observed in dogs and cats as well as many other species. Mature neutrophils of affected individuals have nuclear hyposegmentation and, possibly, moderate dysfunction, such as diminished migration capability. Pseudo–Pelger-Huët anomaly has been also described as an acquired defect.[45, 46] The acquired form of Pelger-Huët anomaly has been described in cattle in association with an inflammatory process characterized by a moderate or marked left shift.

The Pelger-Huët anomaly may not have associated clinical signs. It can, however, be problematic for the clinician, as persistent and inappropriate neutrophil left shifts to bands and metamyelocytes may be reported. When marked left shifts are observed when not anticipated, Pelger-Huët anomaly must be considered.

Other Leukocyte Dysfunctional Processes

Other leukocyte dysfunctions described in small animals include Chédiak-Higashi syndrome (see hemostatic disorders in Chap. 44), canine granulocytopathy,[47] and defective neutrophil function of the Doberman pinscher.[48] Neutrophil dysfunctions may also be associated with complement or immunoglobulin deficiencies. Defective humoral immune components include specific IgA deficiency of the German shepherd,[49] beagle,[50] and Chinese shar-pei[51] as well as others; IgM deficiency of the Doberman pinscher[52]; C3 deficiency of the Brittany spaniel[53]; and possible IgG deficiency of the weimaraner.[54]

References

1. Ogilvie GK, Obradovich JE, Cooper MF, et al. Use of recombinant canine granulocyte colony-stimulating fac-

tor to decrease myelosuppression associated with the administration of mitoxantrone in the dog. J Vet Intern Med 1992;6:44–47.

2. Tompkins MB, Novotney C, Grindem CB, et al. Human recombinant interleukin-2 induces maturation and activation signals for feline eosinophils in vivo. J Leukoc Biol 1990;48:531–540.

3. Van der Poll T, Van Deventer, Hack CE, et al. Effects of leukocytes following injection of tumor necrosis factor in healthy humans. Blood 1992;79:693–698.

4. Tvedten H. Leukocyte disorders. In: Willard MD, Tvedten H, Turnwald GH, eds. Small Animal Diagnosis by Laboratory Methods. Philadelphia, WB Saunders, 1989:57–85.

5. Duncan JR, Prasse KW. Veterinary Laboratory Medicine. Ames, Iowa, Iowa State University Press, 1986:31–87.

6. Latimer KS. Leukocytes in health and disease. In: Ettinger SJ, Feldman EC, eds. Textbook of Veterinary Internal Medicine, 4th ed. Philadelphia, WB Saunders, 1995:1892–1929.

7. Mandell CP, Sparger EE, Pedersen NC, et al. Long-term haematological changes in cats experimentally infected with feline immunodeficiency virus (FIV). Comp Haematol Int 1992;2:8–17.

8. Shelton GH, Grant CK, Linenberger ML, et al. Severe neutropenia associated with griseofulvin therapy in cats with feline immunodeficiency virus infection. J Vet Intern Med 1990;4:317–319.

9. Deldar A, Lewis H, Bloom J, et al. Cephalosporin-induced changes in the ultrastructure of canine bone marrow. Vet Pathol 1988;25:211–218.

10. Haschek WM, Weigel RM, Scherba G, et al. Zidovudine toxicity to cats infected with feline leukemia virus. Fundam Appl Toxicol 1990;14:764–775.

11. Jain NC. Essentials of Veterinary Hematology. Philadelphia, Lea & Febiger, 1993:295–306.

12. Linenberger ML, Shelton GH, Persik MT, et al. Hematopoiesis in asymptomatic cats infected with feline immunodeficiency virus. Blood 1991;78:1963–1968.

13. Fleming EJ, McCaw DL, Smith JA, et al. Clinical, hematologic, and survival data from cats infected with feline immunodeficiency virus: 42 cases (1983–1988). J Am Vet Med Assoc 1991;199:913–916.

14. Shelton GH, Linenberger ML, Abkowitz JL. Hematologic abnormalities in cats seropositive for feline immunodeficiency virus. J Am Vet Med Assoc 1991;199:1353–1357.

15. Molina JM, Garrido A, Anguiano A, et al. Experimental study of the effect of 6-methyl-prednisolone on ingestion-microbicidal function activity in dog neutrophils. Comp Immunol Microbiol Infect Dis 1991;14:21–29.

16. Gandotra VK, Singla VK, Kochhar HPS, et al. Haematological and bacteriological studies in canine pyometra. Indian Vet J 1994;71:816–818.

17. Hill RC, Van Winkle TJ. Acute necrotizing pancreatitis and acute suppurative pancreatitis in the cat: A retrospective study of 40 cases (1976–1989). J Vet Intern Med 1993;7:25–33.

18. May C, Bennett D, Carter SD. Lyme disease in the dog. Vet Rec 1990;126:293–295.

19. Villalba EJ, Garrido A, Molina JM, et al. El hemograma en brucelosis canina. Med Vet 1990;9:99–100.

20. Mason KV. Haematological and cerebrospinal fluid findings in canine neural angiostrongylosis. Aust Vet J 1989;66:152–154.

21. Sparkes AH, Gruffydd Jones TJ, Harbour DA. Feline infectious peritonitis: A review of clinicopathological changes in 65 cases, and a critical assessment of their diagnostic value. Vet Rec 1991;129:209–212.

22. Yamamoto JK, Sparger E, Ho EW, et al. Pathogenesis of experimentally induced feline immunodeficiency virus infection in cats. Am J Vet Res 1988;49:1246–1258.

23. Shelton GH, Linenberger ML, Grant CK, et al. Hematologic manifestations of feline immunodeficiency virus infection. Blood 1990;76:1104–1109.

24. Reubel GH, George JW, Barlough JE, et al. Interaction of acute feline herpesvirus-1 and chronic feline immunodeficiency virus infections in experimentally infected specific pathogen free cats. Vet Immunol Immunopathol 1992;35:95–119.

25. Teng CS. Induction of feline immunodeficiency syndrome by feline leukemia virus: Pituitary and adrenocortical dysfunctions. AIDS 1990;4:1219–1224.

26. Tompkins MB, Nelson PD, English RV, et al. Early events in the immunopathogenesis of feline retrovirus infections. J Am Vet Med Assoc 1991;199:1311–1315.

27. Center SA, Randolph JF, Erb HN, et al. Eosinophilia in the cat: A retrospective study of 312 cases (1975 to 1986). J Am Anim Hosp Assoc 1990;26:349–358.

28. Sellon RK, Rottman JB, Jordan HL, et al. Hypereosinophilia associated with transitional cell carcinoma in a cat. J Am Vet Med Assoc 1992;201:591–593.

29. O'Keefe DA, Couto CG, Burke-Schwartz C, et al. Systemic mastocytosis in 16 dogs. J Vet Intern Med 1987;1:75–80.

30. Thompson JP, Christopher MM, Ellison GW, et al. Paraneoplastic leukocytosis associated with a rectal adenomatous polyp in a dog. J Am Vet Med Assoc 1992;201:737–738.

31. Jain NC, Blue JT, Grindem CB, et al. Proposed criteria for classification of acute myeloid leukemia in dogs and cats. Vet Clin Pathol 1991;20:63–82.

32. Jensen AL, Nielsen OL. Eosinophilic leukaemoid reaction in a dog. J Small Anim Pract 1992;33:337–340.

33. Mandell CP, Jain NC, Farver TB. The significance of normoblastemia and leukoerythroblastic reaction in the dog. J Am Anim Hosp Assoc 1989;25:665–672.

34. Mishu L, Callahan G, Allebban Z, et al. Effects of recombinant canine granulocyte colony-stimulating factor on white blood cell production in clinically normal and neutropenic dogs. J Am Vet Med Assoc 1992;200:1957–1964.

35. Jain NC. Essentials of Veterinary Hematology. Philadelphia, Lea & Febiger, 1993:307–348.

36. Grindem CB, Perman V, Stevens JB. Morphological classification and pathologic characteristics of spontaneous leukemia in 17 dogs. J Am Anim Hosp Assoc 1985;21:219–226.

37. Grindem CB, Stevens JB, Perman V. Morphological classification and pathologic characteristics of spontaneous leukemia in 10 cats. J Am Anim Hosp Assoc 1985;21:227–236.

38. Blue JT. Myelofibrosis in cats with myelodysplastic

syndrome and acute myelogenous leukemia. Vet Pathol 1988;25:154–160.

39. Thomsen MK, Jensen AL, Skak-Nielsen T, et al. Enhanced granulocyte function in a case of chronic granulocytic leukemia in a dog. Vet Immunol Immunopathol 1991;28: 143–156.

40. Grindem CB, Stevens JB, Brobst DR, et al. Chronic myelogenous leukaemia with meningeal infiltration in a dog. Comp Haematol Int 1992;2:170–174.

41. Hendrick M. A spectrum of hypereosinophilic syndromes. Vet Pathol 1981;18:188–200.

42. Harvey RG. Feline hypereosinophilia with cutaneous lesions. J Small Anim Pract 1990;31:453–456.

43. Lund JE, Padget GA, Oh RL. Cyclic neutropenia in gray collie dogs. Blood 1967;29:452–461.

44. Swenson CL, Kociba GJ, Arnold P. Chronic idiopathic neutropenia in a cat. J Vet Intern Med 1988;2:100–102.

45. Shrull RM, Powell D. Acquired hyposegmentation of granulocytes (pseudo-Pelger-Huët anomaly) in a dog. Cornell Vet 1979;69:241–247.

46. Feldman BF, Ramans AV. The Pelger-Huët anomaly of granulocyte leucocytes. Canine Pract 1976;3:5–10.

47. Renshaw HW, Davis WC. Canine granulocytopathy syndrome. Am J Pathol 1979;95:731–744.

48. Breitschwerdt EB, Brown TT, De Buysscher, et al. Rhinitis, pneumonia and defective neutrophil function in the Doberman pinscher. Am J Vet Res 1987;48:1054–1062.

49. Withbread TJ, Batt RM, Garthwaite G. Relative deficiency of serum IgA in the German shepherd dog: A breed abnormality. Res Vet Sci 1984;37:350–352.

50. Felsburg PJ, Glickman LT, Jezyk PF. Selective IgA deficiency in the dog. Clin Immunol Immunopathol 1985;36:297–305.

51. Moroff SD, Hurvitz AI, Peterson ME et al. IgA deficiency in shar pei dogs. Vet Immunol Immunopathol 1986;13: 181–188.

52. Plechner AJ. IgM deficiency in 2 Doberman pinschers. Mod Vet Pract 1979;60:150.

53. Winkelstein JA, Cork LC, Griffin DE. Genetically determined deficiency of the third component of complement in the dog. Science 1981;212:1169–1170.

54. Hansen P, Clercx C, Henroteaux M et al. Neutrophil phagocyte dysfunction in a weimaraner with recurrent infections. J Small Anim Pract 1995;36:128–131.

Chapter 43

Lymphatic Diseases

Rafael Ruiz de Gopegui
Bernard F. Feldman

Anatomy

The organs of the mononuclear phagocyte (reticuloendothelial) system include lymph nodes, spleen, thymus, bone marrow, liver, tonsils, Peyer's patches of the small intestine, and other minor areas of lymphoid and lymphopoietic tissue. In this chapter, the anatomy and physiology of only the spleen and lymph nodes are discussed.

Mandibular, prescapular, inguinal, and popliteal lymph nodes are palpable in healthy small animals. Axillary, cervical, femoral, and retropharyngeal lymph nodes are often palpated only in disease.[1] Hepatic, renal, pancreatic, splenic, mesenteric, lumbar, colonic, medial iliac, hypogastric, and sacral lymph nodes may be examined (but not easily) by ultrasonography.[2]

Each lymph node consists of a cortex and a medulla. Lymphatic fluid drains into the regional nodes via afferent channels. Lymphatic fluid exits from the lymph node via efferent channels that connect to larger lymphatic vessels. A connective tissue capsule surrounds each node, which is divided into cortex and medulla by connective tissue trabeculae.

The cortex of a lymph node contains primary follicles appearing as nodules of small lymphocytes; secondary follicles or germinal centers, which appear as loosely arranged nodules of medium to large lymphocytes surrounded by a rim of packed lymphocytes; and paracortical lymphocytes, which occur between the primary and secondary nodules. The B-lymphocyte domain (the domain of antibody-producing cells) is in the cortical follicles. The T-lymphocyte domain (the domain of lymphoid humoral activity) is the paracortical area. Each domain contains monocyte-macrophage cells. The medulla of the lymph node consists of sinusoidal channels composed of phagocytic reticular cells.

Beneath the connective tissue capsule of each lymph node is a network of lymphatic sinus channels. The trabeculae that divide the node into cortex and medulla are surrounded by lymphatic channel extensions of the subcapsular lymphatic sinus. Thus, the lymphatic fluid enters the lymph node through afferent lymphatic channels into the subcapsular lymphatic space and drains into the medullary sinuses via the peritrabecular channels. The arterial and venous blood supply of each lymph node is located in the hilum adjacent to the medulla. These vessels also serve as a place for lymphocytes to exit and enter the lymph node.

The spleen consists of red pulp and white pulp with an intermediate marginal zone. The white pulp of the spleen is composed of lymphocytes and follicles with surrounding lymphoid tissue. The white pulp surrounds central arterioles. The red pulp is composed of a reticular meshwork and the splenic sinuses. The splenic B-lymphocyte domain is present in the white pulp. The T-lymphocyte domain is located at the periarteriolar sheath. The splenic artery enters at the hilum and divides and branches following the trabeculae, becoming trabecular arteries. These arteries leave the trabeculae and become surrounded with small lymphocytes, a structure referred to as the periarteriolar sheath.

Physiology

Lymph nodes are a major site of immunologic recognition. Cells of lymph nodes respond to diverse insults or etiologic agents such as viruses, bacteria, parasites, fungi, immune complexes, or neoplastic cells and represent the first line of defense against systemic spread of disease via the lymphatic system.

The functions of the spleen are diverse. The spleen functions in lymphopoiesis, hematopoiesis, expansion of blood volume, reutilization of iron from red blood cells degraded by splenic histiocytic phagocytes, removal of senescent and abnormal erythrocytes and of erythrocyte inclusions, phagocytosis of foreign antigens, accumulation of lymphocytes, pooling of platelets, and immune functions including B-lymphocyte transformation into plasma cells with immunoglobulin production.

The splenic sinuses in dogs, lined with phagocytic endothelial cells, are important for filtration. This ensures that only deformable red blood cells and leukocytes can enter the lumen. In addition, macrophages associated with the subendothelial adventitia serve as phagocytes.

The spleen is a major component of the mononuclear phagocyte system. Splenic anatomy and physiology are slightly different in dogs and cats. The canine spleen has greater red blood cell storage capacity and more capacity to phagocytize abnormal cells than does the feline spleen. The feline spleen, in marked contrast to the canine spleen, is considered nonsinusoidal, meaning that cells filtering through the feline spleen do not come into intimate contact with phagocytes. In general, the spleen acts as a reservoir for red blood cells and platelets; as a red blood cell filter for determining maturation of reticulocytes and removing membrane and cytoplasmic inclusions; and as a site of macrophage phagocytic activity, cellular and humoral immunity, iron metabolism and storage, and factor VIII storage.

Problem Identification

Lymphadenopathy

Lymphadenopathy is a clinical sign of disease characterized by enlargement of single lymph nodes or regional lymph nodes or a generalized pattern of lymph node enlargement. Lymphadenopathy may be benign or malignant. Benign lymphadenopathy includes reactive follicular hyperplasia (as in rheumatoid arthritis, systemic lupus erythematosus, and acquired immunodeficiency); paracortical hyperplasia (as in dermatopathic lymphadenopathy, viral lymphadenopathy, and postvaccinal lymphadenopathy); sinusoidal proliferations (such as occur with extramedullary hematopoiesis); mixed proliferations (toxoplasmosis is the only example); granulomatous inflammation (as in fungal or mycobacterial infections); necrotizing lymphadenopathies (such as occur with most other infectious etiologies); and a small group of miscellaneous lymphadenopathies (amyloidosis is the best example).

Pathophysiology

Lymph node enlargement is a common clinical sign that may be induced by inflammation or by infiltrative diseases. Thus, lymphadenopathy may be one sign of the primary process (e.g., vaccine reaction, systemic infection) or, less frequently, a primary disease itself (e.g., lymphoma). Non-neoplastic infiltrative lymphadenopathy includes invasion of lymph nodes by eosinophils in feline hypereosinophilic syndrome.

Metastatic neoplasias may infiltrate lymph nodes. More common neoplasms that metastasize to lymph nodes include mast cell neoplasia, melanoma, squamous cell carcinoma, many sarcomas, and apocrine gland adenocarcinomas of the anal sac.

Clinical Signs

Clinical signs of lymphadenopathy vary depending on the underlying disease process but often include fever, depression, lethargy, anorexia, and reluctance to move. Physical examination shows enlargement of one or more lymph nodes. However, the size of the lymph nodes does not necessarily correlate with either cytologic or histologic findings. Enlarged lymph nodes are often painful on palpation.

Diagnostic Plan

The etiology of lymphadenopathy is extensive.[1] Diagnosis related to the etiology of lymphadenopathy is based on clinical history, clinical signs, and supporting studies (laboratory analysis, radiology, ultrasonography, cytology, biopsy). Lymphadenopathy may have a sudden or progressive clinical onset depending on the geographic and seasonal prevalence of diseases. Leishmaniasis and rickettsial diseases often cause marked generalized lymphadenopathy. These diseases are often seasonal (occurring in summer) or observed throughout the year in subtropical and tropical environments. A history of previous diseases or previous

therapy must be considered. Clinical signs such as general manifestations of primary disease, regional lesions, and palpation of abnormal lymph nodes are valuable in the diagnosis. The consistency and degree of lymph node enlargement, the presence of pain and hyperthermia, and the extent of the lymphadenopathy (solitary, regional, or generalized lymphadenopathy) are determined by clinical examination. Laboratory analysis to ascertain the etiology of generalized or secondary lymphadenopathy may include hematology, biochemistry, immunologic tests reflecting specific infectious processes, and bone marrow examination (see Chap. 41). Radiology and ultrasonography may also be indicated to more thoroughly examine thoracic and abdominal lymph nodes and related structures or organs, to determine which lymph nodes to aspirate, and to aid in obtaining samples for cytology or histopathology.

Fine-needle aspiration of abnormal lymph nodes is well established (see Diagnostic Procedures) and distinguishes among reactive, inflammatory, and infiltrative lymphadenopathy, based on the predominant cell subpopulation and morphology. Fine-needle aspiration is most diagnostically rewarding if several affected lymph nodes are aspirated.

Depending on the degree of inflammation (reactivity, hyperplasia), increased numbers of plasma cells, monocyte-macrophages, mast cells, eosinophils, neutrophils, and immature lymphoid cells are observed in lymph node aspirates. For example, aspiration of the lymph nodes of young, small animals is notable for the number of plasma cells observed as these individuals are beginning to recognize foreign antigens. Lymph nodes responding to purulent disease processes have markedly increased numbers of neutrophils. Rickettsial and fungal diseases are notable for the increased number of monocyte-macrophages. Eosinophil and mast cell numbers in lymph nodes reflect hypersensitivity states and may reflect peripheral blood eosinophilia.

Metastatic neoplasias may infiltrate lymph nodes. Metastatic lymph node disease can vary from a few unusual cells in the lymph node, such as fibrocytes and fibroblasts in fibroma or fibrosarcoma, to clumps of epithelioid cells in various carcinomas. Melanoma, mast cell neoplasia, and squamous cell carcinoma often appear to obliterate the normal cellular composition of the lymph node. Metastasis has been observed with adenocarcinoma of the apocrine glands of the anal sac,[3] mast cell neoplasia, melanoma, sarcoma, and many other forms of neoplasia.[1]

The principal indication of malignancy of lymphoid tissue is the appearance of increased numbers of prolymphocytes and lymphoblasts. Often these cells are uniform in appearance. Most notable is the virtual absence of cells of inflammation—neutrophils, monocyte-macrophages, eosinophils, mast cells, or plasma cells. Primary neoplasia of lymph nodes includes lymphocytic lymphoproliferative disorders, namely the various types of lymphoma. Lymphoma is common in small animal practice. When glucocorticoids have been administered before cytologic sampling of the lymph node, identification of lymphoid neoplasia becomes problematic. If glucocorticoids have been administered, this should be noted on the submission form. The presence of glucocorticoids must be taken into account by the consulting cytologist.

Reactive lymphadenopathy may be secondary to inflammatory processes—infectious or immune mediated (e.g., postvaccinal reactions)—or may be idiopathic.[4] Reactive lymphadenopathy is characterized by moderate but general lymph node enlargement and an increase of normal cellular constituents without abnormal nodal architecture. Diagnosis must be directed to the primary process (protozoal or rickettsial diseases, feline viral diseases) via culture or serology.[5–8]

Lymphadenitis represents inflammatory disease of the lymph node induced by bacteria, fungi, rickettsiae, algae (*Prototheca* spp.), protozoa, and metazoa. Lymphadenitis may be characterized by regional to solitary lymphadenopathy with painful, hyperthermic lymph nodes with variable palpable consistency (soft to fluctuant in purulent lymphadenitis and hard in granulomatous lymphadenitis). Cytologic examination may reveal an increased population of specific cells of the lymph node (e.g., neutrophils or macrophages) and give a definitive diagnosis by direct observation of such diverse etiologic agents as *Mycobacterium avium*,[9] *Cryptococcus neoformans*,[10] *Yersinia pestis*,[11] or *Aspergillus deflectus*.[12]

Canine juvenile cellulitis may present with mandibular, prescapular, or generalized suppurative lymphadenopathy; vesiculopustular dermatitis (edema, pustules, papules, or crusts) around the mouth and eyes, chin or muzzle, and ears; suppurative arthritis; and general signs including fever, depression, and anorexia.[13] Cytology of the affected lymph nodes may suggest nonseptic lymphadenitis.

Non-neoplastic infiltrative lymphadenopathy includes feline hypereosinophilic syndrome (see Uncommon Lymphatic Diseases).

Cytology does not always provide a diagnosis of the cause of lymphadenopathy. If the cause is not apparent from cytology combined with the clinical and routine laboratory signs or specific serologic testing for systemic infectious or immune-mediated diseases, biopsy of abnormal lymph nodes may be necessary to assess altered organ structure. The definitive diagnosis of primary lymphadenopathy (i.e., lymphoma) and several secondary lymphadenopathies (e.g., protozoal, rickettsial, or fungal diseases, mast cell neoplasia) may be resolved by biopsy.

Peripheral Edema

Peripheral edema is defined as the accumulation of extracellular, extravascular fluid in tissues.

Pathophysiology

Edema fluid accumulates in tissues as a result of four pathologic processes. Because the major factor in maintaining the oncotic pressure of plasma is albumin, edema occurs when the plasma albumin concentration is low (usually <1.0–1.5 g/dL) and hence plasma oncotic pressure is reduced, favoring net movement of fluid out of vessels. Increased venous pressure resulting from vessel occlusion or an arteriovenous shunt leads to edema caused by increased intravenous fluid pressure as compared with interstitial pressure. Lymphatic obstruction leads to edema by reducing the flow of lymphatic fluid. Vasculitis causes excessive permeability or leaking of vessels, resulting in the movement out of vessels of more fluid than can be carried away by the lymphatic system.

Clinical Signs

The primary clinical sign of edema is nonpainful swelling of tissues in which "pits" remain for a few seconds after pressure is applied to the region for several seconds with the fingers. Peripheral edema is most readily apparent in the extremities (i.e., between the toes, between the flexor carpi tendons and the radius, and between the Achilles tendon and the tibia). If edema becomes severe, discomfort and a stiff gait may be apparent. Other clinical signs are usually related to the underlying disease process.

Diagnostic Plan

The distribution and extent of edema should be determined in the physical examination. Edema involving the front and rear limbs implies a general or "central" process. Edema involving only the front or rear limbs or a single limb implies a local process.

Animals with generalized edema should be examined carefully for evidence of generalized venous hypertension. Jugular vein distention is often present with right-sided heart failure or pericardial disease. A murmur may be present with right-sided heart failure resulting from primary valvular disease or heartworm disease. Ascites is also often present with generalized venous hypertension. A test for heartworms should be accomplished in these cases. With pericardial disease the heart sounds are often muffled.

When the physical examination does not identify the cause of generalized edema, a hemogram (complete blood count), serum chemistry profile, and urinalysis should be obtained. As a minimum, the serum albumin concentration should be measured. If albumin is reduced below 1.0 to 1.5 g/dL, hypoalbuminemia may be the cause. See Chapter 34 for further discussion of hypoalbuminemia.

If the albumin is appropriate, generalized vasculitis may be a cause of edema. In these cases animals often exhibit systemic signs of the underlying disease such as anorexia, lethargy, and fever. Vasculitis is also often associated with thrombocytopenia. If edema and thrombocytopenia are seen, serologic tests for rickettsial diseases such as ehrlichiosis and Rocky Mountain spotted fever should be performed. Immune-mediated causes of vasculitis can be pursued by testing for antinuclear antibody and possibly by skin biopsy.

When edema is localized to the front or rear limbs or a single limb, evidence for localized venous hypertension should be sought. Arteriovenous shunts are uncommon but may be associated with a history of injury to the limb. In addition, a bruit may be heard on auscultation of the affected limb. A venogram may demonstrate local venous obstruction in cases of localized edema. If venography is negative, the case should be referred to a veterinary center capable of performing lymphangiography to evaluate obstructive lymphatic disease.

Splenomegaly

Splenomegaly is defined as splenic enlargement.

Pathophysiology

Congestive splenomegaly is secondary to portal hypertension often associated with gastric dilatation and volvulus. Hemolytic splenomegaly is associated with hemolytic anemia. Splenomegaly can be seen with extramedullary hematopoiesis, hypereosinophilic syndrome, and amyloidosis. Splenomegaly may be the result of infiltrative diseases including the leukemias, malignant histiocytosis, lymphoma, and myeloma. Granulomatous splenomegaly is observed with histoplasmosis, leishmaniasis, and mycobacterial infections.

Lymphoplasmacytic splenomegaly (splenitis) is associated with chronic canine hepatitis, ehrlichiosis, and numerous other infectious etiologies.

Clinical Signs

Splenomegaly is often associated with abdominal distention. The spleen may be palpated in the left anterior to middle abdominal quadrant.

Diagnostic Plan

Palpation, radiology, and especially ultrasonography may reveal splenic masses, abnormal splenic shape, or abnormal splenic structure. Fine-needle aspiration of the spleen or a splenic mass may be diagnostic. Splenic biopsy carries a high risk of hemorrhage when performed percutaneously[14]; it is safer and may be diagnostic more commonly when performed at laparotomy via partial or complete splenectomy.

Congestive splenomegaly is a consequence of circulatory diseases (congestive cardiopathy and portal hypertension), anesthesia (halothane), or administration of barbiturate derivatives.[15] Splenic torsion and subsequent congestive splenomegaly are frequently observed with gastric volvulus and dilatation and rarely seen as primary splenic pedicle torsion (see Uncommon Lymphatic Diseases). The clinical signs usually identify these causes of splenomegaly. In some cases, ultrasonography is required to identify portal hypertension as a cause of splenomegaly.

Splenic lymphoreticular hyperplasia and splenic lymphoplasmacytic splenitis or hyperplasia may cause generalized splenomegaly and be caused by the same etiologic agents that induce reactive lymphadenopathy. Examples include *Leishmania* spp., *Borrelia burgdorferi*,[16] *Babesia canis*,[17] hemolytic anemias, and other immune-mediated diseases. Eosinophilic splenitis and infiltration have also been described (see Feline Hypereosinophilic Syndrome in Chap. 42) with generalized splenomegaly. Cytology often shows the cause of diffuse, generalized splenomegaly.

Splenic hematomas and hemangiosarcomas appear as cavitary lesions on ultrasonography. Splenic hematomas have been related to hyperplastic lymphoid nodules. Splenic hematoma may also be induced by compression of splenic vasculature.[18] Cytology may not differentiate hematomas from hemangiosarcomas, so biopsy may be necessary. Hemangiosarcoma is often associated with episodes of abdominal hemorrhage.

Granulomatous splenitis has been observed in association with numerous systemic mycoses such as coccidioidomycosis,[19] histoplasmosis, *Acremonium* spp. infections,[20] mycobacterial infections, and feline infectious peritonitis.[15] Cytology is expected to be diagnostic.

Extramedullary hematopoiesis is frequently found in splenomegaly associated with immune hemolytic anemia, hemangiosarcoma, and bone marrow hypoplasia.[21] Myeloproliferative disorders, lymphoproliferative disorders, and other splenic neoplasias including leiomyosarcoma, mesothelioma, fibrosarcoma, myxosarcoma, and myelolipoma as well as other metastatic neoplasms have been observed in the spleen.[18, 22] The appearance of the spleen in these disorders with ultrasonography is usually nodular. Cytology is expected to be diagnostic.

Diagnostic Procedures

Routine Laboratory Evaluation

Routine laboratory tests such as complete blood count, serum chemistry profiles, and urinalysis are useful in lymphatic diseases to help define the general health of the animal and to clinically stage malignant processes.

Lymph Node Aspiration and Cytology

Fine-needle aspiration of abnormal lymph nodes is well established and distinguishes among reactive, inflammatory, and infiltrative lymphadenopathies based on the predominant cell subpopulation and morphology. Fine-needle aspiration is most diagnostically rewarding if several affected lymph nodes are aspirated. The submandibular lymph node is almost always a poor choice to aspirate because it drains the oral cavity and is often reactive—so reactive that neoplasia is often difficult to ascertain. Fine-needle aspiration is accomplished by surgically preparing a small area over the affected lymph node. A small-gauge needle (22 gauge or smaller) is introduced into the node. We have found through experience that simply redirecting the needle, without removing it from the lymph node, accumulates more than sufficient cell numbers for cytologic examination. After being redirected three to five times, the needle is removed from the lymph node and removed from the syringe. Several milliliters of air are aspirated into the syringe, the needle is then replaced on the syringe, and the luminal contents are flushed onto several slides. Aspiration of enlarged lymph nodes by creating a vacuum within the attached syringe most often results in marked blood dilution and insufficient numbers of lymphoid elements to be diagnostic. Staining lymph node aspirations can be problematic. Allowing the stained preparation prolonged time in the buffer solution results in superior cell staining quality.

The lymphocytes of normal lymphoid tissue are predominantly mature small and large lymphocytes. In a normal node these lymphocytes constitute 70% to 95% of the nucleated cells. The remaining cells can be varied. Plasma cells may be numerous in nodes draining the digestive tract. Immature lymphocytes (prolymphocytes and lymphoblasts) are present in normal nodes, but the numbers are relatively low, depending to a large extent on the degree of antigenic stimulation within the node. Monocyte-macrophages are present in normal lymph nodes. The numbers reflect the degree of phagocytic activity. Mast cells are also found in normal lymph nodes; approximately one mast cell is observed per low-power microscopic field. Eosinophils are rare in normal lymph nodes. Red blood cells and neutrophils are also rare in normal lymph nodes.

Bone Marrow Aspiration Cytology and Biopsy

Bone marrow aspiration and biopsy (see Chap. 41 for a description of the procedure) are often necessary to diagnose lymphoid diseases such as lymphoma or myeloma. This procedure is also often necessary for clinical staging of neoplastic disease.

Serum Protein Electrophoresis

Serum protein electrophoresis is useful in differentiating monoclonal from polyclonal gammopathies. Monoclonal gammopathies are most commonly associated with lymphoid malignancies such as myeloma or some forms of lymphoma but may also be seen with infectious peritonitis in cats or ehrlichiosis in dogs (see Diagnostic Plan under Myeloma). For a gammopathy to be considered monoclonal, the gamma peak should be no wider than the albumin peak. Serum is harvested and sent to the laboratory with no special sample handling requirements. Many commercial laboratories offer this test.

Common Lymphatic Diseases

Lymphoma

Lymphoma (lymphosarcoma, malignant lymphoma, malignant lymphosarcoma) is defined as neoplasia originating in lymphoid organs and is thus differentiated from lymphatic neoplasias originating in the bone marrow (e.g., lymphocytic leukemia). In the cat, lymphomas are the most frequent hematopoietic neoplasms.

Lymphoma may develop in a variety of sites. With mediastinal lymphoma the primary tumor develops in mediastinal lymph nodes. The primary tumor may also develop in the digestive tract, mesenteric lymph nodes, liver, or spleen. Multicentric lymphoma is possibly the most frequent form of canine lymphoma.[23] Extranodal lymphoma, occurring in kidneys, central nervous system, eyes, and cutaneous sites (perhaps the most common extranodal site), is also encountered in the dog. Lymphoma in the cat is more commonly associated with the alimentary tract or with mediastinal sites than with multicentric or extranodal sites. Mediastinal lymphoma is considered the most frequent form of lymphoma in the cat.

Although most dogs that develop lymphoma are middle aged, the tumor can be seen in dogs of all ages. The average age of cats with lymphoma that are positive for feline leukemia virus (FeLV) is 3 years, and that of cats with lymphoma that are negative for FeLV is 7 years.[24]

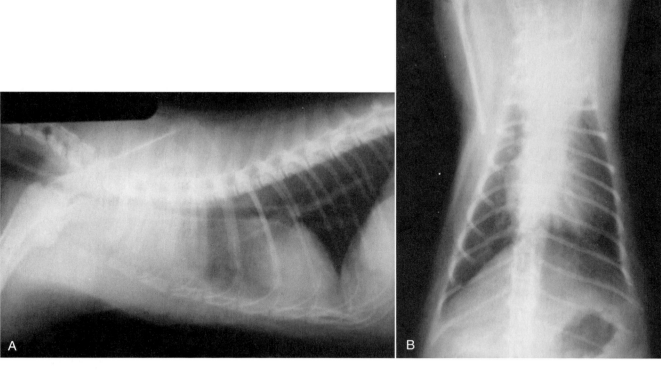

Figure 43–1
(A) Lateral thoracic radiograph of a cat with mediastinal lymphoma showing elevation of the trachea and a soft tissue mass cranial to the heart. **(B)** Ventrodorsal view of the cat in **A** showing a widened cranial mediastinum. (Courtesy of Martha L. Moon, DVM, MS, Blacksburg, Virginia.)

Lymphoma may be classified from a cytologic standpoint as well-differentiated lymphoma, prolymphocytic lymphoma, lymphoblastic lymphoma, and histiocytic-type lymphoma (possibly Hodgkin-like lymphoma).

Pathophysiology

Etiologically, feline lymphoma is most commonly related to FeLV. About 70% of lymphomatous cats are FeLV positive.[25] Feline lymphoma induced by feline immunodeficiency virus (FIV) infection has been reported in both natural and experimental infections (B-cell lymphoma).[26–28]

Toxins such as 2,4-dichlorophenoxyacetic acid herbicide are associated with a higher incidence of canine, feline, and human lymphoma.[29] No definitive single agent has thus far been described as causing canine lymphoma.

Carbohydrate metabolism is altered in dogs with lymphoma; many of these alterations parallel those observed in human patients with cancer cachexia.[30]

Clinical Signs

With mediastinal lymphoma (Fig. 43–1), compression and displacement of the trachea (with signs of dyspnea), the esophagus (with signs of regurgitation), and the lungs (coughing, dyspnea) are observed. Thoracic effusions may lead to dyspnea with muffled heart and breath sounds on auscultation.

The primary lymphoid tumor may develop in the digestive tract,[31] mesenteric lymph nodes, spleen, liver, or kidneys.[32] Associated clinical signs may include vomiting, diarrhea, and abdominal distention resulting from organomegaly and, probably, abdominal effusion.

Multicentric lymphoma is associated with generalized infiltrative lymphadenopathy and possible infiltration of the liver and the spleen. Palpation most commonly reveals painless and severely swollen lymph nodes.

There are several miscellaneous forms of lymphoma. Clinical signs are usually referable to the neoplastic site. Primary tumors have been encountered in several atypical locations such as within the eye or associated with the optic nerve,[33] central nervous

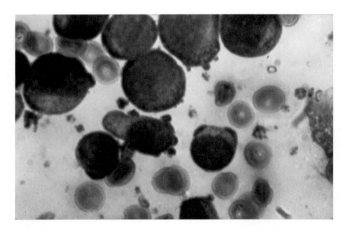

Figure 43–2
Cytologic preparation of a lymph node aspirate from a dog with lymphosarcoma.

system (dura mater),[34] skin,[35–38] myocardium,[39, 40] kidney,[26] bone tissue,[41, 42] prostate,[43] and stifle.[44]

General clinical signs of lymphoma include progressive depression, anorexia, and weight loss. Development of cancer cachexia is an important sign to consider in the diagnosis (when neoplasia is suspected) and in the the prognosis for lymphoma. Thereafter, depending on the anatomic location, variable clinical signs may be anticipated in lymphoma.

Diagnostic Plan

Diagnosis of lymphoma is based on clinical history, clinical signs, and supporting laboratory, ultrasonographic, and radiographic data. A definitive diagnosis requires cytologic examination of tissue aspirates or biopsies (see Diagnostic Plan under Lymphadenopathy for the cytologic description of lymphoma).

The hemogram may reveal nonregenerative, normocytic, normochromic anemia. Plasma proteins and leukocyte counts are variable. Paraneoplastic syndromes such as hypercalcemia (observed primarily in dogs), monoclonal gammopathy,[45] and leukocytosis—characterized most often by lymphocytosis—have also been described. Cytologic examination of thoracic or abdominal effusions may also reveal neoplastic lymphoid cells (Fig. 43–2).[27, 46]

Enzyme-linked immunosorbent assays for FeLV and FIV and immunofluorescent antibody tests for FeLV infection are an essential part of the minimum database for cats diagnosed with or suspected of having lymphoma. Occasionally, cats with lymphoma that are negative for FeLV antigen in peripheral blood are positive using immunofluorescent antibody tests on bone marrow smears. Finding neoplastic lymphoid cells in the bone marrow or finding marrow elements positive for FeLV or FIV is important for clinical staging of the neoplasm.[1]

Radiology and especially ultrasonography may indicate the presence of abnormal organs or masses.[24] Cytologic examination and biopsy of these sites may give a definitive diagnosis.

Staging of lymphoma is important both diagnostically and prognostically. One staging system, derived from the World Health Organization's system for humans, has been routinely used for dogs and cats. Stage I is characterized by involvement of a solitary lymph node. In stage II, more than one lymph node is involved but affected nodes are on one side of the diaphragm. Stage III indicates generalized lymph node involvement. Stage IV is the same as stage III but with hepatomegaly, splenomegaly, or both. Stage V has the same characteristics as any of the other stages plus bone marrow (see Chap. 41 for a description of bone marrow examination) or extranodal involvement. Prognostically, these stages may not always correlate well with survival times.[1]

Treatment

Treatment of lymphoproliferative disorders may include surgical debulking procedures, radiotherapy,[47, 48] and chemotherapy. For most cases other than those involving only a single node, chemotherapy is the modality used most frequently, because lymphoma is one of the most chemotherapy-responsive tumors in veterinary medicine.

Chemotherapy of canine and feline lymphoma using single agents or combined protocols has been extensively described. Prior treatment with glucocorticoids may adversely affect both tumor response and survival rates.[49] Staging this form of neoplasia is necessary to help decide on treatment while considering potential undesirable effects of chemotherapy.[39] Chemotherapy may be divided into several phases: induction of remission, maintenance, and reinduction of remission when relapse occurs. A number of chemotherapeutic protocols have been suggested for treating lymphoma. We recommend the cyclophosphamide, vincristine (Oncovin), prednisolone, and cytosine arabinoside (COAP) protocol (discussed later) to induce remission. Several protocols are outlined here. In areas in which we have had personal clinical experience, drug dosages are indicated. They are not indicated in areas in which we have not had personal clinical experience.

The COP protocol includes cyclophosphamide (Cytoxan), vincristine (Oncovin), and prednisone. Cyclophosphamide is administered as 50 mg/m² of body surface area (BSA) by mouth for 4 days a week. Vincristine is administered at 0.5 mg/m² BSA intravenously once a week (care must be taken to ensure that this drug is not given perivascularly, as significant vascular and perivascular tissue sloughing occurs). Prednisone is administered at 50 mg/m^2 BSA by mouth once a day for 1 week, then reduced to 25 mg/m^2 BSA by mouth every other day. Induction therapy is continued for 8 weeks for dogs and 6 weeks for cats.

The COAP protocol is similar to the COP protocol but also includes cytosine arabinoside (Cytosar-U). The dosage of cytosine arabinoside is 100 mg/m^2 BSA per day for the first 4 days of induction in dogs and for the first 2 days of induction in cats[49] and is given intravenously or subcutaneously. If intensification is required we recommend one dose of L-asparaginase (Elspar), 10,000 to 20,000 IU/m^2 BSA subcutaneously.

For maintenance we recommend the LMP protocol: chlorambucil (Leukeran) administered at 20 mg/m^2 BSA by mouth every 2 weeks, methotrexate (Methotrexate) at 2.5 mg/m^2 BSA by mouth two or three times per week, and prednisone at 20 mg/m^2 by mouth q.o.d.[48, 50]

For rescue at the first relapse we recommend the COAP protocol. For the second relapse in dogs we recommend the ADIC protocol. This consists of doxorubicin (Adriamycin; see Chap. 55) at 30 mg/m^2 BSA (day 1) intravenously and dacarbazine (DTIC) at 1000 mg/m^2 BSA (also day 1) through intravenous infusion over 6 to 8 hours. Both drugs are given once every 3 weeks for three cycles. Toxicity associated with ADIC treatment (severe neutropenia) was acceptable and did not exceed that seen when doxorubicin was given as a single agent.[51]

For the second rescue in cats we recommend the CHOP 21-day cycle. This consists of cyclophosphamide, 200 to 300 mg/m^2 intravenously on day 10; doxorubicin, 20 to 25 mg/m^2 intravenously on day 1; vincristine, 0.5 mg/m^2 intravenously on days 8 and 15; and prednisone, 20 to 25 mg/m^2 by mouth.[50–55]

Prognosis

Although the response to chemotherapy of dogs with lymphoma may be affected by the clinical stage or histologic grade of the tumor, results of studies conflict. In general, with the COP protocol, 70% of dogs achieve complete remission that lasts for a median of 130 days, with remission lasting in some cases for as long as 640 days.[24] The prognosis for cats may be related to clinical stage, with about 90% with stage I disease showing complete remission in response to chemotherapy and 40% to 50% with higher stages responding. Duration of remission in cats also seems to be affected by the stage: 7 to 8 months for

stages I and II and 2 to 3 months for stages III, IV, and V.[24]

Myeloma (Multiple Myeloma, Myelomatosis, Plasma Cell Neoplasia)

Myeloma is a clonal neoplasm of B lymphocytes characterized by proliferation of malignant plasma cells and production of monoclonal immunoglobulin.

Pathophysiology

The unrestricted proliferation of plasma cells and the elaboration of monoclonal immunoglobulin, a paraprotein, are directly responsible for the clinical consequences. This disorder represents a derangement arising early in B-lymphocyte development. The most common presenting feature of myeloma is bone destruction, which is often responsible for chronic pain, pathologic fractures, neurologic signs, and hypercalcemia. Bone destruction is apparently mediated by bone reabsorption related to excessive osteolytic activity. The substance mediating bone reabsorption, osteoclast activating factor, is distinctly different from other substances involved in bone metabolism such as parathyroid hormone, prostaglandin E, and vitamin D. This substance and its bone-reabsorbing properties are not found in other hematologic disorders not associated with bone lesions or hypercalcemia. Bone-reabsorbing activity has been found, however, in other neoplasms, particularly in lymphoma.[56, 57] Associated problems are diverse and may include renal disease, neurologic disease, signs associated with hyperviscosity, and signs associated with hypercalcemia.

Clinical Signs

The more general clinical signs of myeloma in dogs and cats include anorexia, depression, weight loss, and hemorrhage (epistaxis, gingival petechiae or bleeding, and hematuria). The clinical syndrome of elevated whole blood or serum viscosity, often resulting from intense monoclonal immunoglobulin production, involves spontaneous bleeding from mucosal sites. The most common presenting feature of myeloma is bone destruction, which is often responsible for chronic pain, pathologic fractures, neurologic signs, and hypercalcemia.

Many canine patients with myeloma are susceptible to infection, with bacterial sepsis, pneumonia, pyelonephritis, meningitis, and septic arthritis. Infection probably results from failure of immune surveillance.[56]

Neurologic complications may result from pathologic fractures of the spine, specific invasion of the nervous system by neoplastic plasma cells, hyper-

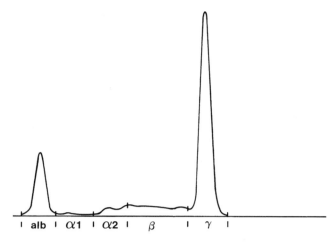

Figure 43–3
Serum electrophoretogram of a cat with myeloma showing a typical monoclonal gammopathy. (From Forrester SD, Greco DS, Relford RL. Serum hyperviscosity syndrome associated with multiple myeloma in two cats. J Am Vet Med Assoc 1992;200:79–82.)

calcemia, hyperviscosity, amyloid-induced neuropathy, or neural infectious processes.

Diagnostic Plan

Diagnosis of myeloma is based on the following criteria: osteolytic lesions caused by clones of aberrant plasma cells (lytic sites should be sampled for cytologic diagnosis), monoclonal gammopathy (Fig. 43–3), Bence Jones proteinuria (often difficult to diagnose in nonhuman animal species), and plasma cell infiltration of bone marrow (Fig. 43–4). The liver, spleen, lymph nodes, and kidneys may also be infiltrated.

Monoclonal gammopathy related to myeloma must be differentiated from that seen with benign idiopathic gammopathy, ehrlichiosis in dogs, and feline infectious peritonitis in cats. Significant monoclonality is rare in feline patients with infectious peritonitis or dogs with ehrlichiosis. The distinction may be made with survey radiographs of the skeleton, fine-needle aspiration cytology or biopsy of bone marrow or lytic lesions, and *Ehrlichia* spp. titers. Immunoelectrophoresis of serum and urine or radial immunodiffusion may show that the monoclonal spike is caused by a single immunoglobulin class, which would indicate myeloma as the cause of the gammopathy. Whereas the other processes usually present as polyclonal gammopathy, myeloma rarely does.

Laboratory findings may include nonregenerative anemia, thrombocytopenia, and abnormal bleeding times and coagulation tests. Renal disease is present in almost 50% of small animal (especially canine) myeloma patients. The most specific effects of

the paraproteinemia may range from simple proteinuria to deposition of amyloid.[56, 57]

Treatment

Treatment with melphalan (0.1 mg/kg by mouth every day for 10 days, then 0.05 mg/kg every day indefinitely) and prednisone (0.5 mg/kg every day for 10 days, then 0.5 mg/kg every 48 hours for 30–60 days or indefinitely) has been used with some success.[55, 56]

Prognosis

Our clinical impression is that remission and good quality of life for years can be achieved with chemotherapy in the dog. Approximately 90% of canine cases respond to therapy, with a median survival time of 540 days.[57] In contrast, 40% of cats respond, with a median survival of 170 days.[58]

Splenic Hemangiosarcoma

Hemangiosarcoma is a malignant tumor arising from vascular endothelium. It is considered the most frequent splenic neoplasia. High prevalence of this neoplasm has been observed in German shepherds.

Pathophysiology

Clinical disease is caused by infiltration of tissues by tumor and hemorrhage associated with rupture of neoplastic tissues.

Clinical Signs

Clinical signs are often nonspecific. The most common clinical signs are weakness, often to the point of collapse; tachycardia and pale mucous membranes resulting from anemia; and hypovolemia associated

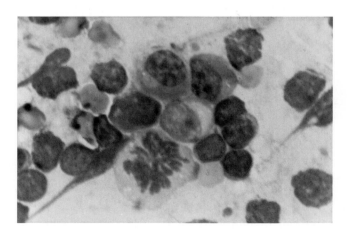

Figure 43–4
Cytology of a bone marrow preparation from a dog with myeloma.

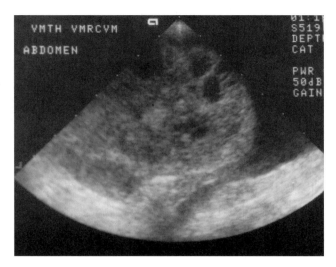

Figure 43-5
Abdominal ultrasonogram of a dog wth a complex cavitating mass in the spleen surrounded by free abdominal fluid (blood). (Courtesy of Martha L. Moon, DVM, MS, Blacksburg, Virginia.)

with acute abdominal hemorrhage on rupture of neoplastic tissues. The signs are often episodic. The hemorrhage may stop, followed by rapid reabsorption of blood from the peritoneal cavity within 1 to 3 days, with subsequent recurrence of hemorrhage and clinical signs. Splenomegaly or splenic masses may be palpated.

Diagnostic Plan

Hemogram findings may include regenerative anemia, normoblastemia, thrombocytopenia, and neutrophilia. Abdominal radiography or ultrasonography often shows splenomegaly and abdominal fluid. Abdominocentesis produces blood that rarely contains neoplastic cells that are apparent cytologically. Ultrasonography may reveal images suggestive of hemangiosarcoma or hematoma, which are cavitary masses within the spleen (Fig. 43-5). Cytology and biopsy may give the definitive diagnosis,[15, 18] although it is uncommon to be able to make a definitive diagnosis cytologically. Because 25% of dogs with splenic hemangiosarcoma also have hemangiosarcoma involving the right atrium, it is important to perform echocardiography before therapy.[59]

Treatment

Treatment includes surgery followed by adjunct chemotherapy with cyclophosphamide, methotrexate, doxorubicin, and vincristine. Surgical excision followed by doxorubicin (30 mg/m² BSA every 3 weeks for up to five cycles), as well as other chemotherapy protocols, may prolong survival (see Chap. 55).[59]

Prognosis

The prognosis for hemangiosarcoma is poor. Splenic rupture, disseminated intravascular coagulation, or metastasis may develop.[60, 61] The effects of chemotherapy on survival have been difficult to ascertain. Surgery followed by doxorubicin as described in the preceding paragraph was associated with an average survival of 267 days in dogs in which all visible disease had been resected and with an average survival of 67 days for dogs in which resection was incomplete.[59]

Uncommon Lymphatic Diseases

Acute Lymphoblastic Leukemia

Acute lymphoblastic leukemia has been described in cats as a leukemic form of lymphoma[62] with or without the presence of primary tumors. Clinical signs are nonspecific, as described for lymphoma. Anemia and leukopenia or marked lymphocytosis may occur. Bone marrow examination reveals marrow hyperplasia (often associated with neoplastic T lymphocytes). Definitive diagnosis of this and other forms of leukemia requires specific histochemical stains or immunohistochemical techniques. We suggest consulting with specialized laboratories that regularly use these techniques. Two such laboratories are the Clinical Hematology Laboratory at the School of Veterinary Medicine, University of California at Davis, Davis, California, and the Clinical Hematology Laboratory at the College of Veterinary Medicine, Ohio State University, Columbus, Ohio.

Lymphocytic Leukemia

Lymphocytic leukemia has been described in dogs. A breed predisposition for both lymphoma and lymphocytic leukemia has been observed in female German shepherds.[63] Acute forms of this leukemia occur more frequently in younger dogs. Clinical onset is sudden, and prognosis is poor.[64] Clinical signs may include depression, vomiting, weight loss, and organomegaly. The hemogram may reveal nonregenerative anemia and severe lymphocytosis. Bone marrow examination shows lymphoblastic hyperplasia. Chronic forms of this leukemia are related to mature B-lymphocyte proliferation.

Waldenström Macroglobulinemia

This form of plasma cell lymphoproliferative disease has been described in the dog. Clinical signs may include lymphadenopathy, splenomegaly, nonspecific neurologic signs, congestive heart failure, renal failure, and hemorrhage. Laboratory findings include monoclonal gammopathy (associated with IgM) and plasmacytoid infiltration of bone marrow without leukemia. Therapy may include chemotherapy, plasmapheresis, and transfusion.[65]

Malignant Histiocytosis

This progressive neoplastic disorder has been well described in Bernese mountain dogs but does occur in other canine breeds. Malignant histiocytosis is characterized by multisystemic infiltration of neoplastic histiocytes.

Clinical signs include anorexia, lethargy, weight loss, weakness, pale mucous membranes, fever, vomiting, and lymphadenopathy. Infiltration of lymph nodes, spleen, lung, liver, kidneys, and bone marrow may be observed.[66]

Lymphedema

Lymphedema is characterized by an abnormal accumulation of interstitial lymph. Lymphedema may be congenital or acquired (through trauma, infection, or surgery) and has a chronic and progressive clinical onset. The affected limb initially exhibits pitting and painless edema. Fibrosis, cellulitis, and lameness may develop. Diagnosis is based on lymphangiography and lymphangioscintigraphy.[67, 68]

Lymphangiosarcoma

Lymphangiosarcoma is an infrequently encountered malignant neoplasm. Clinical signs are related to subcutaneous edema, effusion, and metastasis.[69] Clinical and laboratory findings include hypovolemia, hyponatremia, and hyperkalemia and may be related to isotonic fluid loss and a transient defect in renal potassium excretion.[70] Clinical signs are related to the location of this neoplasm. It is most often observed in the cranial mediastinum, mesentery, or omentum.[71]

Lymphangiectasia

Lymphangiectasia is an obstructive disorder of the lymphatic system that may affect the intestinal tract[72, 73] as well as the mesentery and peritoneum, thorax,[74] and skin.[75] The etiology is not completely defined, but it may be related to congenital malformation, trauma, neoplasia, or infection. Clinical signs include chylous effusions and pitting edema. Other signs are related to the anatomic location of lymphangiectasia and affect the respiratory tract or the gastrointestinal tract.[76–78]

Primary Hypersplenism

Primary hypersplenism has been described in the dog with recurrent moderate anemia and leukopenia associated with anorexia, febrile syndromes, and splenomegaly. Clinical signs are often ameliorated after treatment with antibacterial drugs and glucocorticoids. Clinical signs disappear after splenectomy. In one study, histopathologic examination of the affected spleen revealed congestion and moderate hemosiderosis.[79]

Splenic Pedicle Torsion

Abdominal distention with acute abdominal signs and a palpably enlarged, firm spleen are typical features of acute splenic torsion. Hemolysis and subsequent disseminated intravascular coagulation may be anticipated. Diagnosis is based on radiographic and ultrasonographic examination. Surgery is indicated.[80, 81]

References

1. Rogers KS, Barton CL, Landis M. Canine and feline lymph nodes. Part II. Diagnostic evaluation of lymphadenopathy. Compen Contin Educ Pract Vet 1993;15: 1493–1503.
2. Mattoon JS, Nyland TG. Ultrasonography of the general abdomen. In: Nyland TG, Mattoon JS, eds. Veterinary Diagnostic Ultrasound. Philadelphia, WB Saunders, 1995:43–51.
3. Ross JT, Scavelli TD, Matthieson DT, et al. Adenocarcinoma of the apocrine glands of the anal sac in dogs: A review of 32 cases. J Am Anim Hosp Assoc 1991;27: 349–355.
4. Kirkpatrick GE, Moore FM, Patnaik AK, et al. Argyrophilic, intracellular bacteria in some cats with idiopathic peripheral lymphadenopathy. J Comp Pathol 1989;101: 341–349.
5. Comer KM. Rocky Mountain spotted fever. Vet Clin North Am Small Anim Pract 1991;21:27–44.
6. Theaker AJ, Rest JR. Lupoid dermatosis in a German short haired pointer. Vet Rec 1992;131:495.
7. Barr SC, Gossett KA, Klei TR. Clinical, clinicopathologic, and parasitologic observations of trypanosomiasis in dogs infected with North American *Trypanosoma cruzi* isolates. Am J Vet Res 1991;52:954–960.
8. Baker JL, Craig TM, Barton CCL, et al. *Hepatozoon canis* infection in a dog with oral pyogranulomas and neurological disease. Cornell Vet 1988;78:179–183.
9. Jordan HL, Cohn LA, Armstrong, PJ. Disseminated *Mycobacterium avium* complex infection in three Siamese cats. J Am Vet Med Assoc 1994;204:90–93.
10. Ferrer L, Romas JA, Bonavia R, et al. Cryptococcosis in two cats seropositive for feline immunodeficiency virus. Vet Rec 1992;131:393–394.
11. Eidson M, Thilsted JP, Rollag OJ. Clinical, clinicopathologic, and pathologic features of plague in cats: 119 cases (1977–1988). J Am Vet Med Assoc 1991;199:1191–1197.
12. Kahler JS, Leach MW, Jang S, et al. Disseminated aspergillosis attributable to *Aspergillus deflectus* in a springer spaniel. J Am Vet Med Assoc 1990;197:871–874.
13. Jeffers JG, Duclos DD, Goldschmidt MH. A dermatosis

resembling juvenile cellulitis in an adult dog. J Am Anim Hosp Assoc 1995;31:204–208.

14. Nyland TG, Mattoon JS, Wisner ER. Ultrasound guided biopsy. In: Nyland TG, Mattoon JS, eds. Veterinary Diagnostic Ultrasound. Philadelphia, WB Saunders, 1995:30–42.

15. Couto,CG. A diagnostic approach to splenomegaly in cats and dogs. Vet Med 1990;85:220–238.

16. Font A, Closa JM, Mascort J. Lyme disease in dogs in Spain. Vet Rec 1992;130:227–228.

17. Abdullahi SU, Mohammed AA, Trimnell AR, et al. Clinical and haematological findings in 70 naturally occurring cases of canine babesiosis. J Small Anim Pract 1990;31:145–147.

18. Spangler WL, Culbertson MR. Prevalence, type, and importance of splenic diseases in dogs: 1,480 cases (1985–1989). J Am Vet Med Assoc 1992;200:829–834.

19. Brunnberg L, Hart S, Tobias R, et al. Disseminierte Kokzidioidomykose bei einem Hund. I. Klinische Befunde. Kleintierpraxis 1993;38:83–88.

20. Simpson KW, Khan KNM, Podell M. Systemic mycosis caused by *Acremonium* sp in a dog. J Am Vet Med Assoc 1993;203:1296–1302.

21. O'Keefe DA, Couto CG. Fine-needle aspiration of the spleen as an aid in the diagnosis of splenomegaly. J Vet Intern Med 1987;1:102–109.

22. Spangler WL, Culbertson MR. Prevalence and type of splenic diseases in cats: 455 cases (1985–1991). J Am Vet Med Assoc 1992;201:773–776.

23. Roccabianca P, Caniatti M, Scanziani E, et al. Linfoma multicentrico nel cane. 1a parte: Approcio clinico. Summa 1994;11:7–10.

24. Ogilvie GK, Moore AS. Lymphoma. In: Managing the Veterinary Cancer Patient. Trenton, New Jersey: Veterinary Learning Systems, 1995:228–259.

25. Matsumoto Y, Tsujimoto H, Fukasawa M, et al. Molecular cloning of feline leukemia provirus genomes integrated in the feline large granular lymphoma cells. Arch Virol 1990;111:177–185.

26. Poli A, Abramo F, Baldinotti F, et al. Malignant lymphoma associated with experimentally induced feline immunodeficiency virus infection. J Comp Pathol 1994; 110:319–328.

27. Buracco P, Guglielmino R, Abate O, et al. Large granular lymphoma in a FIV-positive and FeLV-negative cat. J Small Anim Pract 1992;33:297–284.

28. Feder BM, Hurvitz AI. Feline immunodeficiency virus infection in 100 cats and association with lymphoma. J Vet Intern Med 1990;4:110–112.

29. Hayes HM, Tarone RE, Cantor KP, et al. Case-control study of canine malignant lymphoma: Positive association with dog owner's use of 2,4-dichloro- phenoxyacetic acid herbicides. J Natl Cancer Inst 1991;83: 1226–1231.

30. Vail DM, Ogilvie GK, Wheeler SL, et al. Alterations in carbohydrate metabolism in canine lymphoma. J Vet Intern Med 1990;4:8–11.

31. Grooters AM, Biller DS, Ward H, et al. Ultrasonographic appearance of feline alimentary lymphoma. Vet Radiol Ultrasound 1994;35:468–472.

32. Podell M, DiBartola SP, Rosol TJ. Polycystic kidney disease and renal lymphoma in a cat. J Am Vet Med Assoc 1992;201:906–909.

33. García GA, Pineda F, Alcaraz AL. Informe de un caso clínico de linfoma linfoblástico generalizado concomitante a neuritis y atrofia del nervio óptico: Estudio clínico histopatológico. Vet Mex 1990;21:315–318.

34. Dargent FJ, Fox LE, Anderson WI. Neoplastic angioendotheliomatosis in a dog: An angiotropic lymphoma. Cornell Vet 1988;78:253–262.

35. Moore F, Olivry T, Naydan D. Canine cutaneous epitheliotropic lymphoma (mycoides fungoides) is a proliferative disorder of $CD8^+$ T cells. Am J Pathol 1994;144: 421–429.

36. Tobey JC, Houston DM, Breur GJ, et al. Cutaneous T-cell lymphoma in a cat. J Am Vet Med Assoc 1994;204: 606–609.

37. Brain PH. An unusual presentation of cutaneous lymphoma in a cat. Aust Vet Pract 1991;21:182–184.

38. Doe R, Zackheim HS, Hill JR. Canine epidermotropic cutaneous lymphoma. Am J Dermatopathol 1988;10: 80–86.

39. Teske E, Vos JP de, Egberink HF, et al. Clustering in canine malignant lymphoma. Vet Q 1994;16:134–136.

40. Brummer DG, Moise NS. Infiltrative cardiomyopathy responsive to combination chemotherapy in a cat with lymphoma. J Am Vet Med Assoc 1989;195:1116–1119.

41. Turner JL, Luttgen PJ, VanGundy TE, et al. Multicentric osseous lymphoma with spinal extradural involvement in a dog. J Am Vet Med Assoc 1992;200:196–198.

42. Hosgood G, Davidson J, Blevins WE. Pathologic pelvic fractures secondary to malignant lymphoma in a dog. Aust Vet Pract 1991;21:70–73.

43. Mainwaring CJ. Primary lymphoma of the prostate in a dog. J Small Anim Pract 1990;31:617–619.

44. Somer T, Sittnikow K, Henriksson K, et al. Pigmented villonodular synovitis and plasmacytoid lymphoma in a dog. J Am Vet Med Assoc 1990;197:877–879.

45. Rosenberg MP, Hohenhaus AE, Matus RE. Monoclonal gammopathy and lymphoma in a cat infected with feline immunodeficiency virus. J Am Anim Hosp Assoc 1991; 27:335–337.

46. Madewell BR, Jain NC, Padrid P, et al. Bizarre lymphoid cells in serous effusion of a dog with mediastinal lymphoma. J Comp Pathol 1988;99:229–233.

47. Laing EJ, Fitzpatrick PJ, Binnington AG, et al. Half-body radiotherapy in the treatment of canine lymphoma. J Vet Intern Med 1989;3:102–108.

48. Giger U, Evans SM, Hendrick MJ, et al. Orthovoltage radiotherapy of primary lymphoma of bone in a dog. J Am Vet Med Assoc 1989;195:627–630.

49. Dobson JM, Gorman NT. Canine multicentric lymphoma. 2: Comparison of response to two chemotherapeutic protocols. J Small Anim Pract 1994;35:9–15.

50. Couto CG, Hammer AS. Diseases of the lymph nodes and the spleen. In: Ettinger SJ, Feldman EC, eds. Textbook of Veterinary Internal Medicine, 4th ed. Philadelphia, WB Saunders, 1995:1930–1945.

51. Van Vechten M, Helfand SC, Jeglum KA, et al. Treatment of relapsed canine lymphoma with doxorubicin and dacarbazine. J Vet Intern Med 1990;4:187–191.

52. Shimoda T. Clinicopathological findings in 12 cases of

feline thymic lymphoma. J Jpn Vet Med Assoc 1993;46:227–230.

53. Hahn KA, Richardson RC, Teclaw RF, et al. Is maintenance chemotherapy appropriate for the management of canine malignant lymphoma? J Vet Intern Med 1992;6:3–10.

54. Carter RF, Harris CK, Withrow SJ, et al. Chemotherapy of canine lymphoma with histopathological correlation: Doxorubicin alone compared to COP as first treatment regimen. J Am Anim Hosp Assoc 1987;23:587–596.

55. MacEwen EG, Rosenthal RC, Fox LE, et al. Evaluation of L-asparaginase: Polyethylene glycol conjugate versus native L-asparaginase combined with chemotherapy: A randomized double-blind study in canine lymphoma. J Vet Intern Med 1992;6:230–234.

56. Ruiz de Gopegui R, Espada Y, Vilafranca M, et al. Paraprotein-induced defective haemostasis in a dog with IgA (kappa-light chain) forming myeloma. Vet Clin Pathol 1994;23:70–71.

57. Matus RE, Leifer CE, MacEwen EG, et al. Prognostic factors for multiple myeloma in the dog. J Am Vet Med Assoc 1986;188:1288–1292.

58. Ogilvie GK, Moore AS. Plasma cell tumors. In: Managing the Veterinary Cancer Patient. Trenton, New Jersey: Veterinary Learning Systems, 1995:280–290.

59. Ogilvie GK, Moore AS. Hemangiosarcoma. In: Managing the Veterinary Cancer Patient. Trenton, New Jersey: Veterinary Learning Systems, 1995:367–380.

60. Rishniw M, Lewis DC. Localized consumptive coagulopathy associated with cutaneous hemangiosarcoma in a dog. J Am Anim Hosp Assoc 1994;30:261–264.

61. Hargis AM, Feldman BF. Evaluation of hemostatic defects secondary to vascular tumors in dogs: 11 cases (1983–1988). J Am Vet Med Assoc 1991;198:891–894.

62. Jarplid B, Feldman BF. Large granular lymphoma with toxoplasmosis in a cat. Comp Haematol Int 1993;3:241–243.

63. Rallis T, Koutinas A, Lekkas S, et al. Lymphoma (malignant lymphoma, lymphosarcoma) in the dog. J Small Anim Pract 1992;33:590–596.

64. Morris JS, Dunn JK, Dobson JM. Canine lymphoid leukaemia and lymphoma with bone marrow involvement: A review of 24 cases. J Small Anim Pract 1993;34:72–79.

65. González M, Caballero MO. Macrogobulinemia de Waldenström. In: López Borasca A, ed. Enciclopedia Iberoamericana de Hematología. Salamanca, Spain, Universidad de Salamanca, 1992:557–567.

66. Kohn B, Arnold P, Kaser-Hotz B, et al. Maligne Histiozytose beim Hund: 26 Falle (1989–1992). Kleintierpraxis 1993;38:409–424.

67. Fossum TW, King LA, Miller MW, et al. Lymphedema: Clinical signs, diagnosis, and treatment. J Vet Intern Med 1992;6:312–319.

68. Knight KR, Collopy PA, McCann JJ, et al. Protein metabolism and fibrosis in experimental canine obstructive lymphedema. J Lab Clin Med 1987;110:558–566.

69. Rudd RG, Veatch JK, Whitehair JG, et al. Lymphangiosarcoma in dogs. J Am Anim Hosp Assoc 1989;25:695–698.

70. Lamb WA, Muir P. Lymphangiosarcoma associated with hyponatraemia and hyperkalaemia in a dog. J Small Anim Pract 1994;35:374–376.

71. Stobie D, Carpenter JL. Lymphangiosarcoma of the mediastinum, mesentery, and omentum in a cat with chylothorax. J Am Anim Hosp Assoc 1993;29:78–80.

72. van der Gaag I, Happe RP. The histological appearance of peroral small intestinal biopsies in clinically healthy dogs and dogs with chronic diarrhea. J Vet Med Ser A 1990;37:401–416.

73. Kaup FJ, Drommer W, Kersten U, et al. Ultrastrukturelle Untersuchungen bei einem Fall von intestinaler Lymphangiektasie. Kleintierpraxis 1988;33:81–86.

74. Kerpsack SJ, McLoughlin MA, Birchard SJ, et al. Evaluation of mesenteric lymphangiography and thoracic duct ligation in cats with chylothorax: 19 cases (1987–1992). J Am Vet Med Assoc 1994;205:711–715.

75. White SD, Thalhammer JG, Pavletic M, et al. Acquired cutaneous lymphangiectasis in a dog. J Am Vet Med Assoc 1988;193:1093–1094.

76. Fossum TW, Hodges CC, Scruggs DW, et al. Generalized lymphangiectasis in a dog with subcutaneous chyle and lymphangioma. J Am Vet Med Assoc 1990;197:231–236.

77. Erickson SL. Dietary management of canine lymphangiectasia. Vet Med 1988;83:282–286.

78. Birchard SJ, Smeak DD, Fossum TW. Results of thoracic duct ligation in dogs with chylothorax. J Am Vet Med Assoc 1988;193:68–71.

79. Sawasima K, Shitaka H, Sawasima Y, et al. Primary hypersplenism in a dog. J Jpn Vet Med Assoc 1990;43:203–206.

80. Konde LJ, Wrigley RH, Lebel JL, et al. Sonographic and radiographic changes associated with splenic torsion in the dog. Vet Radiol 1989;30:41–45.

81. Hurley RE, Stone MS. Isolated torsion of the splenic pedicle in a dog. J Am Anim Hosp Assoc 1994;30:119–122.

Chapter 44

Hemostatic Diseases

Rafael Ruiz de Gopegui
Bernard F. Feldman

Anatomy

Vascular endothelial cells are the lining cells of all blood vessels. They play an important role in hemostasis.

The circulating platelet is a small anuclear discoid cell (1.0–3.0 μm) that arises from megakaryocytes with a maturation time of 4 to 5 days and a circulating lifespan of 9 to 10 days. Platelets, along with endothelial cells, modulate the initial hemostatic phase (the vascular and platelet reaction—primary hemostasis). The platelet has an extensive invagination of the surface membrane that results in an open canalicular system that forms an interconnecting network within the cell and allows substances within platelet granules to be released readily into the exterior plasma. The platelet has three types of granules: lysosomes, alpha granules, and dense granules. When platelets are activated, the granules fuse with the canalicular system, and granule contents are released. Lysosomal granules contain lysosomal enzymes; alpha granules contain fibrinogen; and dense granules contain adenine nucleotides, serotonin, catecholamines, and platelet factor 4, which is involved in the activation of heparin.

Physiology

The hemostatic response could be considered a defensive function: it prevents or avoids blood loss from damaged vasculature (hemorrhage) and ensures adequate blood flow, keeping the vascular tree free of obstruction (thrombosis). Procoagulant activity (inactive hemostatic proteins) is modulated or inhibited by several mechanisms involving the vascular endothelium. Endothelial cells play a key role in the control of these functions. Adequate equilibrium between activation and inhibition of hemostasis depends on interactions between endothelial cells, platelets, other circulating blood cells, coagulation activators, and inhibitors.

When vessels are damaged, local vasoconstriction occurs. Platelets adhere to damaged endothelium (or subendothelial collagen); degranulate, activating other platelets and coagulation; and aggregate, forming the hemostatic plug. The surface of the platelet aggregate activates coagulation with subsequent fibrin formation (coagulation or secondary hemostasis). Finally, the fibrinolytic system inhibits thrombus formation and lyses or removes the hemostatic plug through enzymatic action (fibrinolysis or tertiary hemostasis).

Platelet adhesion to the subendothelium is mediated by von Willebrand's factor (vWF), the major adhesion protein, which binds to the platelet surface. Platelet activation is stimulated by collagen, adenosine diphosphate (ADP), epinephrine, platelet-activating factor, thrombin, and arachidonic acid. After the adhesion stimulus, platelet morphology and biochemistry are altered, with resultant degranulation (release of platelet granule contents) and platelet aggregation. Platelet aggregation requires fibrinogen binding. Finally, the activated platelets expose platelet factor 3, which binds coagulation factors V, VIII:C (factor VIII coagulant), and X, accelerating thrombin formation.[1]

The contact coagulation system (part of the intrinsic pathway; Fig. 44–1) includes factors XII and XI and the kinins. Activation of the contact system occurs through contact with negatively charged surfaces (collagen, exposed by endothelial damage).[2] The activation of the two contact factors, factors XII and XI, is modulated by complement. Coagulation factors VII and XI are activated by activated factor XII.

A factor called tissue factor (factor III) activates factor VII (part of the extrinsic pathway; see Fig. 44–1). Tissue factor is a glycoprotein complexed to phospholipids from cell membranes and from cytoplasmic contents of damaged cells. Endothelial cells and monocytes may express tissue factor by adsorbing the factor to their surfaces or releasing the factor when endothelial cells are damaged.[3] The formation of factor VII–tissue factor complexes induces factor X and factor IX activation. This activation is inhibited by tissue factor pathway inhibitor.

Factor X is also activated by factor IXa (factor VIIIa accelerates the reaction), and factor Xa activates prothrombin; the presence of factor Va accelerates thrombin activation as well.

There are two main inhibitors of coagulation factors: antithrombin III (ATIII) and protein C. Heparin cofactor II (formerly called antithrombin II) is also an important thrombin inhibitor. The major inhibitor of

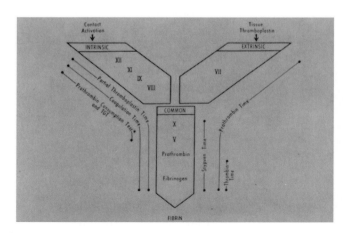

Figure 44–1

Diagram of the coagulation cascade (intrinsic, extrinsic, and common pathways), showing the portions of the pathways evaluated by various coagulation tests.

thrombin and factor Xa, however, is ATIII. Thrombin activates protein C and results in feedback inhibition of thrombin (thrombin loses its coagulant effect).[3–5]

Thrombin activates factor V, factor VIII:C, and factor XIII (FXIII) and cleaves fibrinopeptides A and B from fibrinogen to yield fibrin monomers. The monomers polymerize into fibrin clots stabilized by factor XIIIa.[6] Thrombin also binds irreversibly to platelets, promoting platelet adhesion to endothelial cells and platelet aggregation, and induces secretory release of platelet alpha granule and dense granule contents.[7] ADP and thromboxane A_2 release from platelets further accelerates platelet aggregation, causing amplification of coagulation processes and thrombin generation.

Plasmin functions to control hemostasis through fibrinolysis and removal of the hemostatic plug (tertiary hemostasis). It is generated by the enzymatic conversion of circulating plasminogen (a proenzyme synthesized by kidneys, liver, and eosinophils). Tissue plasminogen activator is secreted by endothelium and macrophages, and contact system activation contributes to plasmin generation as well. Plasmin is capable of hydrolyzing not only fibrin and fibrinogen but also other proteins such as factors V, VIII, IX, and XI, insulin, adrenocorticotropic hormone, casein, and gelatin.[6, 8] Digestion of fibrinogen by plasmin results in fibrin(ogen) degradation products (FDPs).[6] FDPs in the circulation interfere with fibrin monomer polymerization (basically by inhibiting fibrin polymerization and blocking the receptor sites of fibrinogen on thrombin), causing further amplification of fibrinolysis, impairment of hemostasis, and resultant hemorrhage.[6, 7, 9] Some FDPs have high affinity for platelet membranes, inducing platelet dysfunction through platelet granule release and platelet aggregation inhibition.[10]

The inflammatory response has important interactions with hemostasis; it may activate or impair hemostasis. Inflammation activates hemostasis through neutrophil activation (inducing platelet aggregation), monocyte expression of tissue factor, complement activation (inducing platelet procoagulant activity), and cytokine release (which induces endothelial tissue factor expression and endothelial changes more receptive to coagulation).[3, 11, 12]

Problem Identification

Clinical Bleeding

Hemostatic disorders vary from too much hemostasis (thrombosis) to too little hemostasis (bleeding). Hemostatic problems can be hereditary or acquired. Acquired hemostatic problems are clinically more numerous than hereditary problems.

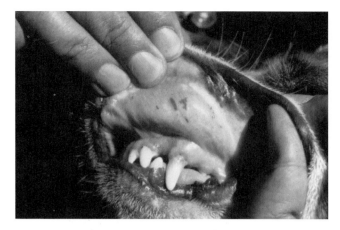

Figure 44–2
A dog with severe thrombocytopenia with petechiae (small pinpoint hemorrhages) and ecchymoses (larger hemorrhages) in the buccal mucosa.

Pathophysiology

Hemorrhagic hemostatic problems can be primary, involving damage or dysfunction of endothelial cells, too few platelets (thrombocytopenia), too many platelets (thrombocytosis), or dysfunctional platelets (thrombocytopathy). Hemorrhagic hemostatic problems can also be secondary, with too little fibrin formation (coagulation deficits), or rarely tertiary, with excess fibrinolysis.

Thrombocytopathia (platelet dysfunction) can be secondary to a number of disease processes. In hepatic disease, platelet surface glycoprotein Ib (GPIb) can be reduced[13] and FDPs such as D-dimer and E fragments increased, interfering with platelet aggregation. Platelet aggregation is impaired in nephropathies with uremia because there is an imbalance between prostacyclin and thromboxane synthesis; platelet adhesion is also diminished.[13] Paraproteins in dysproteinemias produced in lymphoproliferative disorders can, in theory, coat circulating platelets and impair their adhesiveness and aggregating capability.[14] Rickettsiaceae infections (see Chap. 37) appear to impair platelet function as well as platelet production. Canine patients with rickettsia-induced thrombocytopenia often hemorrhage excessively because of rickettsia-induced thrombocytopathia. When hemorrhage occurs, thrombocytopenia is often not severe.

Clinical Signs

Hemostatic disorders may induce spontaneous or prolonged hemorrhage. Clinical signs may include petechiae (Fig. 44–2), purpura (Fig. 44–3), hematoma (Fig. 44–4), hemarthrosis, epistaxis (Fig. 44–5), hematemesis, hemoptysis, hematuria, melena, and hematochezia, as well as other forms of external hemorrhage

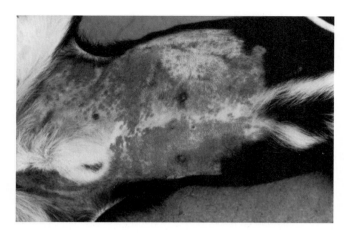

Figure 44-3
Purpura in a dog with severe thrombocytopenia.

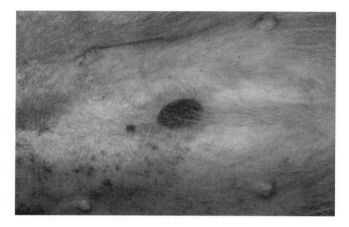

Figure 44-4
A thrombocytopenic dog with a subcutaneous hematoma at the site of needle puncture for cystocentesis.

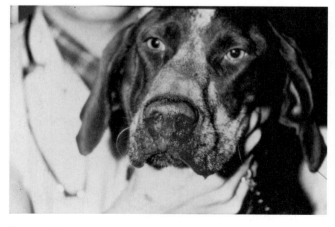

Figure 44-5
A dog with epistaxis.

that may be associated with depression, anorexia, hyperthermia, and pallor.

Diagnostic Plan

The clinical history must determine whether the disorder is acquired or congenital to identify the possible etiology (e.g., anti–vitamin K intoxication, drug administration, infection). Hemostatic dysfunction is likely if there is hemorrhage from more than one site, if the amount of hemorrhage is excessive for the amount of trauma, if the hemorrhage appears to be spontaneous, if there is a history of hemorrhage in the patient or in the patient's family, or if there is a history of recent trauma or the possibility of toxin exposure. The presence of a primary disease such as liver disease, nephrotic syndrome, infection, or neoplasia must be ruled out. To aid in this, a complete blood count, serum biochemistry profile, and urinalysis are indicated.

Initial work-up for an animal suspected of bleeding resulting from hemostatic dysfunction in which an underlying primary disorder has not been identified should include a platelet count, prothrombin time (PT), activated partial thromboplastin time (APTT), and assay for FDPs (see Diagnostic Procedures). If the platelet count is less than 50,000/μL, hemorrhage is probably due to thrombocytopenia (see Thrombocytopenia). If the platelet count is greater than 50,000/μL, hemorrhage is more likely to be caused by vascular disease, platelet dysfunction, a coagulation defect, or a combination of the three. When thrombocytopenia is present, rickettsial titers (Rocky Mountain spotted fever and *Ehrlichia*) are indicated because they cause bleeding, thrombocytopenia, platelet dysfunction, and vasculitis.

If the platelet count is reduced (<100,000/μL) with prolongation of the PT, APTT, or both, often with increased FDPs, disseminated intravascular coagulation (DIC) is likely. There is always an underlying disorder apparent from clinical signs and routine laboratory evaluation (see Disseminated Intravascular Coagulation).

When the platelet count is normal and the APTT and PT are prolonged, the owner should be questioned again about vitamin K antagonist intoxicants. With this disorder the PT may be prolonged before the APTT becomes abnormal. If the APTT and the PT are prolonged, vitamin K rodenticide intoxication should be suspected, even when there is no known history of exposure. In these cases, blood should be sent for assay for coumarin derivatives, and therapy should be started with vitamin K (see Vitamin K–Dependent Coagulopathy). When vitamin K antagonist intoxication has been ruled out either by lack of response to therapy or by negative blood test results, inherited or acquired factor deficiencies or dysfunction should be considered (see Uncommon Hemostatic Diseases). Samples should be sent for specific factor analysis (see Diagnostic Procedures).

If the platelet count is greater than 50,000/µL and the PT and APTT are normal, bleeding could be due to vascular disease or platelet dysfunction. The buccal mucosa bleeding time (BMBT; see Diagnostic Procedures) should be determined in these cases. The BMBT is prolonged with vascular disease (see Primary Hemostasis) or platelet dysfunction. If the BMBT is prolonged, a sample should be sent for assay for the concentration of vWF (see Diagnostic Procedures). In addition, the chemistry profile should be reviewed for the presence of hyperglobulinemia caused by a paraprotein (myeloma; see Chap. 43) that may be inhibiting platelet function. With vasculitis, the platelet count is often mildly reduced (50,000–100,000/µL) because of increased consumption. Vascular disease other than that caused by rickettsial diseases can be difficult to diagnose without a biopsy. In general, hemorrhage associated with vascular disease alone consists primarily of petechiae or ecchymoses rather than bleeding into body cavities or epistaxis. Other causes of hemostatic dysfunction are usually pursued and ruled out before a biopsy is performed.

Drug-induced thrombocytopathia (platelet dysfunction) may be commonly encountered clinically. Antithrombotic therapy includes platelet antiaggregants such as nonsteroidal anti-inflammatory drugs (e.g., acetylsalicylic acid, ibuprofen, phenylbutazone [Butazolidin]) and anticoagulants with platelet inhibitory effects such as standard heparin.[15] It should be noted that acetaminophen does not have antithrombotic effects. Administration of high-molecular-weight dextran to dogs impairs hemostasis by inducing a diminution of vWF and factor VIII:C.[16]

Thrombocytopenia

Thrombocytopenia is the most common acquired hemostatic defect in small animal medicine, especially in dogs. Thrombocytopenia is identified by determining platelet numbers. A platelet number below the laboratory reference interval is considered thrombocytopenia. Reference intervals vary depending on the laboratory, but a platelet count less than 100,000/µL is considered reduced.

Pathophysiology

Platelets are reduced because of lack of production, consumption, destruction, or sequestration in the liver or spleen with hepatomegaly or splenomegaly, respectively. The mechanism of thrombocytopenia with ehrlichiosis depends on the stage of the disease: platelets are consumed or sequestered during the acute phase of the disease, and platelet production is decreased in the chronic phase. Immune-mediated thrombocytopenia (IMT) causes destruction of platelets. Myeloproliferative disorders lead to thrombocytopenia through decreased production related to myelophthisis. With vasculitis resulting from rickettsial or immune-mediated disease, as well as with DIC, the mechanism of thrombocytopenia is consumption.

Clinical Signs

The clinical signs of thrombocytopenia cannot be separated from those of vascular disorders or platelet dysfunction. Most commonly, petechiae (see Fig. 44–2) or ecchymoses are observed. These are specific signs of primary hemostatic defects. Other commonly observed signs such as epistaxis and hematuria are not specific for primary hemostatic defects.

Platelet sequestration is related to splenomegaly; hepatomegaly may also induce thrombocytopenia as a result of sequestration. However, sequestration usually does not result in a platelet count less than 100,000/µL.

Renal disease, vasculitis, neoplasia, and DIC may induce thrombocytopenia, thrombopathy, and coagulopathy. There are often clinical signs of the primary disorder when thrombocytopenia is secondary to a systemic disease.

Diagnostic Plan

When it has been determined that platelet numbers are reduced, the cause of thrombocytopenia should be diagnosed. Severe hemorrhage alone reduces platelet numbers but seldom below 75,000/µL. Sequestration of platelets related to hepatomegaly or splenomegaly rarely reduces platelet counts below 100,000/µL. When the platelet count is reduced below 30,000/µL, the differential diagnosis includes immune-mediated platelet damage, bone marrow productive defects, and DIC. Other forms of platelet damage are exceedingly rare. Immune-mediated platelet damage is most common.

Rickettsial titers should be determined in patients with thrombocytopenia, particularly if other clinical signs of rickettsial disease are present. Canine ehrlichiosis can reduce the number of platelets as well as the number of white and red blood cells (see Chap. 37).[17, 18] In affected dogs, a prolonged BMBT is frequently observed owing to platelet dysfunction even when platelet numbers are only modestly reduced.[19] Clinically, noninfectious thrombocytopenia usually does not have significant anemia as an associated process. Thrombocytopathy, in addition to thrombocytopenia, may be suspected when anemia is found with modest thrombocytopenia (50,000–100,000/µL).

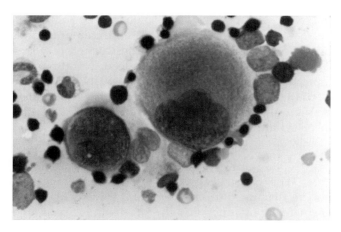

Figure 44–6
Bone marrow cytology with active megakaryocytes.

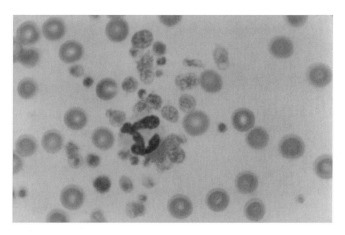

Figure 44–7
Blood smear from a dog with large, immature circulating platelets.

Rocky Mountain spotted fever causes signs of primary hemostatic dysfunction: petechiae, purpura, and ecchymoses. Other clinical signs include fever, lethargy, and neurologic signs including vestibular signs, stupor, confusion, paresis, upper respiratory signs such as cough and exercise intolerance, and lymphadenopathy. Diagnosis is based on clinical signs, thrombocytopenia, and an increased serologic titer.

Viral diseases and, potentially, vaccination with modified live virus may induce thrombocytopenia or thrombocytopathia in small animals. Bone marrow thrombopoiesis (as well as erythropoiesis and myelopoiesis) may be decreased.

The APTT, PT, and FDPs should be determined in patients with thrombocytopenia. Patients with DIC often have a prolonged APTT or PT and increased FDPs. DIC is secondary to a primary problem, most often significant systemic inflammation.

If there is no evidence of infectious thrombocytopenia or DIC, bone marrow examination should be performed. Bone marrow platelet production deficits are almost always accompanied by another cytopenia, such as anemia, neutropenia, or both.

Thrombocytopenia that is immune mediated may be caused by infection or drugs or can be autoimmune. IMT is diagnosed by ruling out other causes, with evidence of normal or increased platelet production, active bone marrow megakaryocytes (Fig. 44–6), or giant circulating platelets (Fig. 44–7). Immunofluorescence testing of bone marrow for antiplatelet or antimegakaryocyte antibody confirms the diagnosis, but therapy must usually be initiated before these test results are available, and practical availability is limited.

Drug-induced thrombocytopenia is a frequent undesirable effect of drug therapy; just how frequent is as yet undetermined. Impaired platelet production or increased platelet consumption may be induced by drugs. Administration of estrogen and antibiotic, antimicrobial, antithrombotic, and chemotherapeutic agents has been associated with thrombocytopenia.[20]

The diagnosis of drug-induced thrombocytopenia may be based on clinical history—drug administration, unexplained thrombocytopenia, and return of the platelet count toward the reference interval after the drug in question is discontinued (unless irreversible myelosuppression has occurred). Furthermore, thrombocytopenia should recur after re-exposure to the same drug. Immediate discontinuation of the suspected drug is the first goal of treatment. Glucocorticoid therapy or blood product administration may be considered if hemorrhage is ongoing.[21]

Diagnostic Procedures

Primary Hemostasis

Platelet Count

Assessment of primary hemostasis involves the evaluation of endothelial cell function and platelet quality and quantity. Primary hemostasis may be partially assessed by determining platelet numbers. Thrombocytopenia may be readily determined from the platelet count. Blood for a platelet count should be drawn into a tube containing ethylenediaminetetraacetic acid and submitted to the laboratory for testing within 12 hours.

Bone Marrow Examination and Immunofluorescence

Bone marrow megakaryocyte examination (see Chap. 41) helps to determine whether platelet production is adequate (see Fig. 44–6). Bone marrow examination is always indicated if the cause of thrombocytopenia is uncertain and certainly if other cell lines are also reduced in number (anemia or neutropenia). Bone marrow examination also allows detection of anti-megakaryocyte antibody. Antiplatelet antibody detection and bone marrow direct immunofluorescence are used in the diagnosis of IMT. This test is available in a number of veterinary laboratories. We recommend the Clinical Laboratory of the School of Veterinary Medicine, University of California at Davis.

Buccal Mucosa Bleeding Time

If appropriate platelet numbers are present (>100,000/µL), a bleeding time test may further determine the adequacy of the vascular response and platelet function. A prolonged bleeding time in this clinical setting suggests thrombocytopathia or vascular dysfunction—endothelial cell dysfunction. Thrombocytopathia can be determined by several tests. The best test of platelet function is the BMBT. The BMBT should be performed using a standard device (Simplate II). The buccal mucosa is exposed by folding the lip back. A site in the mucosa that is free of protruding vessels should be selected, with access for unobstructed ventral drainage. The Simplate II is placed gently over the site on the buccal mucosa, and the trigger is released and timing begun. Using the edge of filter paper or gauze, blood should be absorbed as it flows ventrally, without touching the incisions. Timing is stopped when the flow of blood has stopped and blood is no longer absorbed into the filter paper or gauze. The operator should note the time taken for each cut to stop bleeding, and calculate the average. The normal range for bleeding time is 1.7 to 4.2 minutes; more than 5 minutes is definitely abnormal. If the platelet count is depressed (<100,000/µL), the BMBT is prolonged even though platelet function is normal.

von Willebrand's Factor Assay

When the BMBT is prolonged with a normal platelet count, platelet dysfunction (thrombocytopathia) may be caused by von Willebrand's disease (see von Willebrand's Disease). The activity of vWF can be measured by specialized laboratories (Clinical Laboratory, School of Veterinary Medicine, University of California at Davis, Davis, California; New York State Department of Health, Albany, New York) that are capable of determining the concentration of vWF with several different types of testing modalities. Nonhemolyzed plasma obtained from nonstressed canine patients is obtained from citrated (3.8% trisodium citrate) blood taken in plastic syringes with 0.4 mL of citrate solution per 4 mL of blood. The blood is placed in a plastic tube and immediately centrifuged for 15 minutes. The plasma is removed with a plastic pipette, placed in a plastic tube with a plastic stopper, and

frozen immediately at −20° C (typical household freezer temperature) or lower. The sample should be packed in dry ice and sent by overnight courier so that it arrives at the laboratory frozen. Hemolyzed plasma can falsely lower concentrations of vWF.[22] In addition, hypoadrenocorticism, estrus, parturition, and other stresses may alter the circulating concentration of vWF.

Secondary Hemostasis— Fibrin Formation (Coagulation Times)

Prothrombin Time

The PT evaluates the extrinsic and common pathways (factor VII in the extrinsic pathway and factors X, V, II, and I [fibrinogen] in the common pathway) (see Fig. 44–1). Blood should be drawn into citrate tubes and centrifuged immediately. Plasma should be withdrawn within 30 minutes and refrigerated until assayed. The test should be performed within 4 hours of drawing the blood if possible. If the test cannot be performed within 4 hours, the sample should be frozen until it can be sent to the laboratory on dry ice in order to arrive frozen. Sending a sample from a normal dog as a control is recommended to detect errors in sample handling.

Activated Partial Thromboplastin Time

The APTT evaluates the intrinsic pathway (factors XII, XI, IX, and VIII) and the common pathway (see Fig. 44–1) (see Prothrombin Time for sample handling).

Thrombin Time

The thrombin time (TT; also called the thrombin clotting time) evaluates fibrinogen—factor I—both quantitatively and qualitatively (see Fig. 44–1) (see Prothrombin Time for sample handling).

Fibrinogen

Fibrinogen may be quantified by heat precipitation.

Specific Coagulation Factor Activity

Specific coagulation factor activity may be quantified using specific factor–depleted plasma. This test does require a specialized laboratory (Clinical Laboratory, School of Veterinary Medicine, University of California at Davis, Davis, California; New York State Department of Health, Albany, New York). Samples should be obtained and handled in the manner described earlier for measuring vWF.

Acquired Inhibitors of Coagulation

Acquired inhibitors may be assessed by combination—a mixing study—and incubation of the problem plasma with control plasma to differentiate between factor deficiency and inhibitors. If the prolonged coagulation time observed is due to a factor deficiency, the addition of equal parts of normal plasma corrects the prolonged time. If an acquired inhibitor is present, the combination generally does not correct the test, or the test is initially corrected but the time becomes prolonged within 1 to 2 hours.

Antithrombin III

The coagulation inhibitor ATIII may be quantitated. A decrease in this analyte is associated with thrombotic tendencies. Currently, ATIII quantitation is available in only a few veterinary laboratories (e.g., Clinical Laboratory, School of Veterinary Medicine, University of California at Davis). Decreases in ATIII are associated with protein-losing gastroenteropathies and nephropathies. A decreased ATIII concentration is the hallmark of DIC.

Tertiary Hemostasis

Fibrin Degradation Products

Tertiary hemostasis involves fibrinolysis. Tests for tertiary hemostasis are not well elucidated in veterinary clinical medicine. One test of fibrinolysis, determination of general FDPs, is considered a more traditional test in veterinary clinical medicine. Elevation of FDPs is caused by thrombotic processes, and the highest concentrations are observed with major vascular thrombosis. However, increased amounts of FDPs (>10 and <40 µg/mL) are considered to be a feature of DIC. Unfortunately, increased FDPs are not a feature of all patients with DIC.

Common Hemostatic Diseases

Immune-Mediated Thrombocytopenia

IMT is a clinical disorder characterized by severe thrombocytopenia caused by destruction of platelets by the patient's own immune system. As veterinary scientists improve their ability to detect infectious etiologies, IMT may be revealed to be a rare process.

Pathophysiology

In IMT, the platelet lifespan is markedly decreased. Antiplatelet antibodies attach to the platelet surface and induce destruction by the mononuclear phagocyte system. The etiology of primary IMT remains unclear, but the presence of antiplatelet antibodies has been related to neoplasia, infection, drugs, and autoimmune diseases.[23] Thrombopoiesis is increased in most cases of IMT. However, antibody-mediated megakaryocyte damage or megakaryocytic hypoplasia may occur, worsening the prognosis.[24] The hemorrhagic tendency observed in IMT is related to both decreased platelet numbers and platelet dysfunction. The in vitro addition of serum from patients with IMT has been observed to impair aggregation of platelets from normal dogs.[25] In immune-mediated thrombopathia, antiplatelet antibodies may damage platelet membranes and cause release of platelet granule contents, affecting platelet function, specifically platelet aggregation.[26]

Clinical Signs

Clinical signs of IMT are identical to those of other forms of primary hemostatic dysfunction and other forms of thrombocytopenia: petechiae, purpura, and ecchymoses (see Figs. 44–2 and 44–3).

Diagnostic Plan

IMT may be definitively diagnosed by the antimegakaryocyte antibody test (see Diagnostic Procedures). This test, using immunofluorescent-tagged anti-antibodies, determines the immunofluorescence of bone marrow megakaryocytes in a patient's bone marrow aspirate.

If the laboratory can determine mean platelet volume (most new hematology instruments can do so), early in the course of IMT, microthrombocytes are present in 55% of cases and mean platelet volume is reduced.[27] For practical purposes, however, the diagnosis of IMT is usually based on exclusion: unexplained severe thrombocytopenia (often <20,000 platelets/µL) without evidence of DIC (see Disseminated Intravascular Coagulation), infectious diseases (particularly rickettsial diseases; see diagnostic plan under Clinical Bleeding), or production failure resulting from bone marrow disease. The confirmation of antiplatelet antibodies may be attempted indirectly or directly by enzyme-linked immunosorbent assay, radioimmunoassay, or indirect fluorescent antibody techniques, but the immunoassay techniques have not received widespread acceptance.[28–30] None of these techniques is routinely available to practitioners. Bone marrow examination may reveal megakaryocyte damage (megakaryocyte vacuolation) if antibodies are directed toward megakaryocytes as well as platelets, or normal megakaryocytes (see Fig. 44–6), usually in normal or increased numbers. The suggestion of megakaryocyte damage may be confirmed by a direct or indirect fluorescent antibody test (see Diagnostic

Procedures). The release of large immature platelets into the circulation usually indicates active marrow production of platelets in response to an increased demand related to destruction (see Fig. 44–7).

Treatment

In dogs, immunosuppressive therapy with glucocorticoids (prednisone, 1 mg/kg per day) combined with azathioprine (1 mg/kg per day) is indicated. Both drugs should be given on the same day. These drugs are administered and their dosage reduced in tandem. We recommend 2 to 3 weeks of initial therapy. If the platelet count has increased (>75,000/µL), the two drugs are reduced simultaneously. Platelet count is monitored and the doses are reduced by 25% every 2 weeks, as long as the platelet count remains stable. When the doses of both drugs approach 0.25 mg/kg, the dosing interval is lengthened (i.e., every other day, then every third day, and so on) until the lowest dose that maintains the platelet count at or above 75,000/µL is attained.

Transfusion therapy in the form of whole blood or platelet-rich plasma is not indicated unless used just before performing splenectomy or any other surgical procedure to prevent bleeding during surgery. In our experience, splenectomy in IMT is not particularly successful. Platelet transfusions are often ineffectual, as transfused platelets are usually quickly destroyed. In addition, many units of platelets may be required for the same patient, and the risk of developing platelet alloantibodies can be enhanced.[31]

Administration of an anabolic steroid as well as glucocorticoids and fresh whole blood has been described in dogs with IMT and nonregenerative anemia.[32, 33] We consider the use of anabolic steroids (e.g., danazol) ineffectual.

Prognosis

Uncomplicated acute thrombocytopenia, thrombocytopenia that normalizes rapidly with or without treatment in 7 to 10 days, has a good prognosis and the chance of relapse is small. Uncomplicated chronic thrombocytopenia, thrombocytopenia that is refractory to treatment or responds slowly, also has a good prognosis. However, chronic canine thrombocytopenias almost always require some form of continuous therapy that may well span the life of the patient. Clinical success is evident when the platelet count is maintained in excess of 75,000/µL. Transient increases in platelet counts to counts within or above the reference interval are just that, transient. The platelet counts of these patients virtually always return to baseline numbers that are below the reference interval.

Vitamin K–Dependent Coagulopathy

Vitamin K antagonism is a common acquired problem resulting from intoxication with coumarin-based rodenticides, which prevent vitamin K activation of inactive precursor proteins.

Pathophysiology

Vitamin K functions as an essential cofactor for the synthesis of the coagulation proteins, factors II, VII, IX, and X and protein C. Factors II, VII, IX, and X and protein C are synthesized in the liver but require the presence of vitamin K (in a reduced oxidative state) to become functional.

Vitamin K deficiency may appear as a result of impaired dietary intake with malabsorption and potentially after long-term broad-spectrum antibiotherapy, but in veterinary medicine vitamin K deficiency is most frequently induced by rodenticide intoxication. Anticoagulant rodenticides are hydroxycoumarin derivatives that represent a heterogeneous group of widely used toxins. Second-generation rodenticides (e.g., brodifacoum, bromadialone, the indandiones) are a major hazard because of their long-acting effects and potential for secondary poisoning by ingestion of anticoagulant-poisoned rodents.[34]

Clinical Signs

Clinical signs of vitamin K antagonism are often nonspecific and vague. Often, gross bleeding is not observed. Hemorrhage is observed in association with injection sites and minor trauma and can be severe in the retroperitoneal area. Clinical signs are related to hemorrhage (internal or external): depression, weakness, anorexia, fever, pallor, dyspnea resulting from hemothorax or pulmonary parenchymal hemorrhage, or neurologic signs resulting from cerebral or spinal cord bleeding.

Diagnostic Plan

Diagnosis of vitamin K deficiency should be based on the clinical history with the identification and, if possible, quantification of the toxin ingested. Methods of toxicologic analysis such as high-performance chromatography may be used to detect specific coumarins.[35]

Laboratory diagnosis is based on the presence of carboxy-vitamin K–dependent coagulation factors, the so-called proteins induced by vitamin K absence or antagonism (PIVKA). The PIVKA test is prolonged before the PT. The PIVKA test is not routinely available, however, in commercial veterinary laboratories. The PT tends to be more prolonged and abnormal sooner after the ingestion of toxin than the APTT because the halflife of factor VII is shorter.

Treatment

Therapy consists of vitamin K_1 administration. The route of administration may be oral, when possible, or subcutaneous. Intravenous or intramuscular administration is not recommended. Vitamin K_1 is administered at a dose of 1.0 to 2.5 mg/kg divided every 8 hours. Warfarin intoxication is successfully treated by administering vitamin K_1 for 5 consecutive days. The second-generation rodenticides generally require continuous therapy for at least 21 days at a dose of 2.0 to 5.0 mg/kg divided every 8 hours; the lower dose is preferred. If the rodenticide is unknown, suggested treatment is for 5 consecutive days. A PT or PIVKA is determined 3 hours after the last vitamin K administration—on the fifth day—and is considered the baseline. The tests are repeated 48 and again 96 hours after baseline. Any prolongation of the test suggests reintroduction of the toxin or intoxication with a second-generation rodenticide. If the latter is probable, the patient must be treated for 21 days. At the end of that period, baseline and 48- and 96-hour testing must be done. Any prolongation of the tests at this time has the same meaning as previously stated. Second-generation rodenticide intoxication may require many months of therapy.

If a patient is hemorrhaging, the blood product of choice is fresh frozen plasma (separated from red cells and frozen within 8 hours of drawing the blood; stored frozen for up to 1 year) or stored plasma (separated from red cells and frozen within 8–10 hours of drawing the blood; stored frozen for up to 1 year). Cross-matched whole blood can also be administered.[36]

Prognosis

When vitamin K antagonism is recognized and treated appropriately, the prognosis is excellent. The prognosis is imperiled when therapy is not appropriate in terms of dosage or duration. Excessive use of vitamin K_1 is contraindicated for the dog and cat as it can result in hemoglobin oxidation, causing rapid fulminant hemolysis.

Disseminated Intravascular Coagulation

DIC is always a secondary event complicating a primary systemic inflammatory state (Table 44–1). There is a higher association of DIC with certain disease processes. However, DIC is often a severe complicating event that is unexpected.

Table 44–1
Conditions Associated With Disseminated Intravascular Coagulation

Intravascular hemolysis
  Hemolytic transfusion reactions
  Hemolytic anemia
Septicemia (see Table 44–2)
  Gram-negative (endotoxin)
  Gram-positive (bacterial coat mucopolysaccharide)
Viremia (see Table 44–2)
Parasitic infections
  Protozoal infection
  Metazoal infection
Obstetric complications
Miscellaneous
  Gastric dilatation or volvulus
  Diabetes mellitus

Malignancy (see Table 44–3)
Massive tissue injury
  Trauma
  Burns
  Surgical procedures
  Heatstroke
Venoms and toxins
  Snake bite
  Bee or insect sting
  Aflatoxin
Liver disease
Pancreatitis

Pathophysiology

DIC is associated with numerous clinical conditions (Tables 44–2 and 44–3; see Table 44–1). Depending on the activation rate of the hemostatic system, DIC may occur as an acute and life-threatening event or as a chronic form without severe thrombosis and hemorrhage. DIC may be initiated by a single cause or by multiple causes occurring sequentially or simultaneously. Pathologic processes that may cause DIC include intravascular hemolysis,[37] infectious etiologies,[38–40] obstetric complications,[40] gastric dilatation or volvulus,[41] diabetes mellitus,[37] neoplasia,[42] traumatic shock,[43] heatstroke,[41] severe hepatopathy,[44] snake and arthropod enven-

Table 44–2
Bacteria and Viruses Incriminated in Disseminated Intravascular Coagulation

BACTERIA	VIRUSES
Gram-negative bacteria	Infectious canine hepatitis
Escherichia coli	Canine distemper
Pasteurella haemolytica	Canine herpesvirus
Pasteurella multocida	Feline infectious peritonitis
Salmonella species	Feline panleukopenia
Gram-positive bacteria	
Staphylococcus species	
Streptococcus species	
Clostridium species	
Mycobacterium species	

Table 44–3

Mechanisms That Incite Disseminated Intravascular Coagulation in Cancer Patients

Stimulation of the coagulation cascade
  Cancer cells induce platelet activation and aggregation.
  Cancer cells release thromboplastin and/or other procoagulant factors that enhance coagulation.
  Cancer cells stimulate macrophages and monocytes to release procoagulant factors.
  Some cancer cells release a specific factor X activator.
Vascular damage by neoplastic growth or vascular damage of vessels within neoplastic tissues—might lead to exposure of subendothelial collagen
Enhancement of the hemostatic system by complications of malignancy such as surgery, chemotherapy, and sepsis
Decreased hepatic synthesis of antithrombin III and protein C in metastatic cancer
Activation of the fibrinolytic cascade by a plasminogen activator released from some tumor cells

omation,[10, 45] and pancreatitis,[46] to mention a few of the more common etiologies.

DIC may be considered an uncontrolled burst of thrombin generation and activity. This massive activation overwhelms hemostatic inhibitors, depletes procoagulants and platelets, induces thrombosis, and as a final result severely damages tissues. Thrombus formation and subsequent ischemia and necrosis may activate an enhanced fibrinolytic response that impairs platelet function and depletes coagulation factors.[47]

Clinical Signs

A primary inciting event causing DIC may have associated evidence of excessive hemorrhage or lack of specific organ perfusion. The clinical signs of DIC are often subtle and not fulminant. These include evidence of modest hemorrhage at injection sites or at sites of surgical or accidental trauma. Bleeding can include petechiae, purpura, ecchymoses, hematoma formation (see Figs. 44–2 through 44–4), and bleeding into synovial joints (hemarthrosis).

Although the classic presentation of DIC may include fever, acidosis, hypoxemia, proteinuria, bleeding, shock, and evidence of multiple organ failure,[37] it is essential to note that there is considerable variability in clinical findings. DIC can be acute or chronic, depending on whether the underlying illness is acute (decompensated DIC) or chronic (compensated DIC).[48]

Diagnostic Plan

Laboratory results vary according to the underlying cause of DIC and the evolution of the process and may include schistocyte (see Fig. 41–4) or fragmentocyte formation[48]; thrombocytopenia or thrombopathia[6, 37]; prolonged PT, APTT, and TT[9]; decreased fibrinogen; and elevated FDP concentrations.[9, 48] For clinical purposes, DIC is diagnosed when there is an underlying disease process that could be causative (see Tables 44–1 and 44–2) and some combination of the following: abnormal bleeding, otherwise unexplained organ failure, thrombocytopenia, schistocytes, prolonged APTT or PT, decreased fibrinogen concentration, and increased FDPs.

Treatment

The treatment for acute DIC should be sequential and have a logical strategy. The most important therapeutic modality is removal of the inciting cause. Fluid therapy is indicated to correct hypovolemia, prevent or alleviate vascular stasis, and dilute thrombin, FDPs, and activators of fibrinolysis.[49] Use of coagulation inhibitors is indicated.

Transfusion of fresh (or fresh frozen) plasma (10–20 mL/kg, repeated in 12 to 24 hours if needed) provides ATIII and other serine protease inhibitors and coagulation factors, and subsequent administration of low doses of heparin may sustain appropriate hemostasis.[50, 51] The initial heparin dose (100 IU/kg) should be added to the container of thawed, fresh frozen plasma and incubated at room temperature for 30 minutes to ensure a continuous infusion of activated ATIII and avoid ATIII depletion.[52] Subsequently, heparin is given subcutaneously at a dose of 100 IU/kg 8 hours after the first dose, 50 IU/kg every 8 hours for two doses, and then 25 IU/kg three times per day (t.i.d.).

For effective therapy for DIC and to avoid complicating the existing condition, therapy should be monitored every 12 to 24 hours. The return of fibrinogen concentration, platelet numbers, and PT and APTT toward reference intervals is among the most consistent signals of therapeutic success. It should be noted that this statement is in direct opposition to the myth of prolonging the universal tests of coagulation (PT and APTT) toward some predetermined time. If DIC appears to be worsening, administration of plasma should be repeated and the dose of heparin maintained at the higher level (50–100 IU/kg t.i.d.). If improvement is noted, heparin should be continued at a dose of 25 to 50 IU/kg t.i.d. until the underlying disease process has been corrected, then reduced slowly (no more often than every 16 to 24 hours) from 50 to 25 to 10 IU/kg and then eliminated.

Additional blood product therapy must be considered. The severity of blood loss, thrombocytopenia, hypofibrinogenemia, and coagulopathy dictates the selection of blood products. Packed red cells, fresh frozen plasma, cryoprecipitate, or fresh whole blood may be considered.[53] In patients that are not moderately to severely anemic, administration of fresh or stored frozen plasma or cryoprecipitate may be sufficient. DIC may be the result of the use of incompatible blood or blood products. Blood typing and cross-matching are considered essential, especially for patients at risk for complications such as DIC.[53]

Prognosis

When DIC is severe, the prognosis for survival is grave, particularly if the underlying disease is not readily identifiable or treatable. If DIC is mild to moderate and the underlying condition is corrected quickly, before major organ failures occur, the prognosis is fair to poor.

Von Willebrand's Disease

Von Willebrand's disease is the most frequent inherited bleeding disorder in dogs. Patients with von Willebrand's disease have a reduced quantity of functional vWF. This deficiency produces impaired platelet adhesion to damaged endothelium.

Pathophysiology

vWF is necessary for normal platelet function. When vWF is severely reduced, platelet adhesion to damaged endothelial cells is impaired, resulting in dysfunction of primary hemostasis and clinical bleeding.

Factor VIII:C circulates bound to vWF in plasma. The halflife of this factor is shorter without vWF. In von Willebrand's disease, a reduction of FVIII:C concentration (under 50%) is observed. It is therefore potentially possible to observe moderate APTT prolongation. However, this is clinically unusual in small animal practice.

Von Willebrand's disease has been described in humans and dogs as an acquired defect secondary to endocrine disorders such as hypothyroidism.[54, 55] Subsequent studies appear to refute these findings.[56] Parturition and other stresses, estrus, and hypoadrenocorticism may alter the circulating concentrations of vWF but not severely enough to cause clinically apparent hemostatic dysfunction.

Clinical Signs

The clinical signs of von Willebrand's disease can be mild to severe and are for the most part confined to mucosal hemorrhage, hemorrhage at venipuncture sites, and hemorrhage associated with surgery. Clinical signs are associated with defects in primary hemostasis, petechiae, purpura, and ecchymosis (see Figs. 44–2 through 44–4). Abnormal bleeding is usually not apparent unless there is a secondary factor such as estrus, hypoadrenocorticism, parturition, or other stresses that may alter the circulating concentration of vWF.

Diagnostic Plan

The BMBT (see Diagnostic Procedures) of affected dogs is prolonged. These canine patients do not have other clinical signs and have appropriate platelet numbers unless there has been recent, severe hemorrhage. If a patient is suspected of having von Willebrand's disease and breeding is considered, determination of the vWF antigen is essential (see Diagnostic Procedures). Definitive diagnosis of von Willebrand's disease must be supported by a specific determination of the concentration (with a result lower than 49% compared with the reference pool, considered to be 100%). Hemolyzed plasma can falsely lower concentrations of vWF.[22] Parturition and other stresses, estrus, and hypoadrenocorticism may alter the circulating concentration of vWF.

Treatment

Treatment of vWF deficiency is indicated only when clinical hemorrhage is deemed excessive. Presurgical treatment of von Willebrand's disease is recommended. Administration of the antidiuretic hormone analog desamino-8-D-arginine vasopressin (DDAVP, 1 µg/kg subcutaneously) is recommended, although the results of this therapy in the dog are less predictable than in humans. Transfusion therapy, specifically with cryoprecipitate because vWF is concentrated in this blood product, may be indicated if there is evidence of excessive hemorrhage. The advantage of cryoprecipitate is the low volume needed to infuse a large quantity of vWF (1 unit per 10 kg body weight as needed). If cryoprecipitate is not available, fresh frozen plasma (6–10 mL/kg body weight twice per day [b.i.d.] or t.i.d. as needed to stop hemorrhage) or fresh whole blood (12–25 mL/kg per day) is indicated, especially if marked hemorrhage has occurred.[57–59]

Prognosis

Von Willebrand's disease is most often a minor problem. When excessive hemorrhage is encountered, treatment as just described is often successful in ameliorating clinical signs.

Vascular Dysfunction and Vasculitis

Vascular dysfunction is not commonly diagnosed because, at this time, most vasculitides require a histopathologic diagnosis. Vascular dysfunction is probably a far more common event than has heretofore been realized. Disorders of the blood vessels without demonstrable defects in platelet number or function are most often observed in conjunction with systemic disease.

Pathophysiology

The most common vascular lesion producing hemorrhage is vascular damage secondary to trauma, immune-mediated damage, or neoplasia. Gastrointestinal ulceration is a common sequela of vascular pathology.[60] Gastrointestinal ulceration also can induce vascular pathology. In severe cases of hypoadrenocorticism, gastrointestinal hemorrhage has also been described.[61, 62] Ecchymosis may also occur with hypoadrenocorticism, probably as a result of diminished muscular support of the vascular tree.

Acquired vascular purpuras in small animals are generally related to endothelial inflammation; vasculitis, caused by infection by Rickettsiaceae, *Leishmania* spp., or *Dirofilaria immitis;* or endotoxins. Vascular purpuras may have an immune-mediated etiology. Hemostasis is altered when vasculitis is present with either hemorrhagic or thrombotic sequelae.[63–65]

Canine juvenile polyarteritis syndrome has been described as a vasculitis and perivasculitis of unknown etiology. However, a potential immune-mediated mechanism has been suggested. [66]

Rocky Mountain spotted fever, caused by *Rickettsia rickettsii*, affects host endothelial cells and causes necrotizing vasculitis (see Chap. 37), which results in compromised hemostasis. The altered endothelium induces platelet and fibrinolytic activation, causing thrombocytopenia, petechiae, and even consumption coagulopathy (DIC).

Clinical Signs

Vascular dysfunction may present clinically similarly to other primary hemostatic defects, with petechiae, purpura, and ecchymoses (see Figs. 44–2 through 44–4).

Diagnostic Plan

The diagnosis of vascular dysfunction may be made from clinical signs and from a prolonged BMBT (see Diagnostic Procedures) with appropriate platelet numbers. Vascular dysfunction can be an inherited structural defect or, most commonly, the result of immune or infectious etiologies. Therefore, the diagnosis of vascular dysfunction most often relies on histopathology.

Treatment

Treatment of vascular disorders depends on the etiology. If the primary inciting process can be eliminated or modulated, most vascular disorders do not have to be treated specifically and the lesions are ameliorated. If DIC is present, transfusion therapy must be considered.[67–70]

Prognosis

The prognosis for vascular disease depends on the underlying cause. If it can be corrected and if major organ damage has not been caused by thrombosis and hemorrhage (i.e., renal or hepatic necrosis or failure), the prognosis is good.

Uncommon Hemostatic Diseases

Estrogen Toxicity

Severe side effects of estrogen therapy may occur. Pancytopenia is often encountered, with severe thrombocytopenia, anemia, and leukopenia. Clinical signs include mucosal petechiae, ecchymoses, pale mucous membranes, and hemorrhagic diarrhea. The prognosis is poor if thrombocytopenia lasts more than 2 weeks. Although anemia and thrombocytopenia often may be treated, death caused by leukopenia (neutropenia) is common. Treatment with nonestrogenic anabolic steroids, lithium, and blood transfusion is recommended.[71, 72]

Platelet Function Disorders

Inherited Thrombopathia

Chédiak-Higashi syndrome is an autosomal recessive disease reported in cats (and other animals including cattle, rat, mink, and fox). Collagen, ADP, and epinephrine-induced platelet aggregation are markedly impaired. Some patients are deficient in constituents of platelet dense granules. The defect may include partial ocular albinism and enhanced susceptibility to bacterial infection caused by neutrophil dysfunction.[73] Cats with the syndrome have platelet storage pool deficiency and have prolonged bleeding times because of a platelet abnormality (which platelet transfusion can effectively correct). The halflife of donor platelets in cats with Chédiak-Higashi syndrome was 3.5 days. Current treatments for storage pool deficiency are DDAVP, cryoprecipitate, bone marrow transplantation, and platelet transfusion.[74]

Platelet storage pool disease has been described in American cocker spaniels. Platelet aggregation and secretion were impaired. The hemorrhagic tendency was severe and required platelet transfusions.[75]

Basset hound hereditary thrombopathia is an autosomal inherited trait. Affected dogs may have different clinical presentations depending on the degree of severity. Platelet aggregation is impaired. Thrombin-induced aggregation is diminished but not absent, and quantitatively normal platelet surface glycoproteins are present, resulting in appropriate fibrinogen binding and clot retraction. Appropriate fibrinogen binding and clot retraction differentiates this defect from human Glanzmann thrombasthenia. Topical use of thrombin has been proposed to control posttraumatic cutaneous hemorrhage.[13, 76]

Canine thrombasthenic thrombopathia is an autosomal inherited disorder described in otter hounds. This defect resembles Bernard-Soulier syndrome (there is a significant subpopulation of giant platelets with impaired platelet adhesion) and human Glanzmann thrombasthenia (reduction or absence of GPIIb-IIIa complex with subsequent impairment of clot retraction).[13, 76]

Acquired Bleeding Disorders of Cats

Acquired bleeding disorders of cats are more frequently related to hepatic failure; rodenticide intoxication with vitamin K antagonists is unusual. Bleeding cats are also anemic, so generally fresh whole blood is indicated. Fresh frozen plasma can be administered to cats with an initial dose of 10 mL/kg.[36]

Hepatic Disease

The liver is the most important site for the synthesis of noncellular components of hemostasis; the majority of coagulation factors and coagulation inhibitors are produced in this organ. The liver is responsible for clearance of metabolites of coagulation activation and inhibition; for example, the metabolites of the fibrinolytic system can interfere with hemostasis as a result of abnormal hepatic function.[77]

In fact, the liver is related to all components of hemostasis: splenic platelet sequestration may result from hepatomegaly, and platelet function can be impaired as well. As most of the hemostatic proteins are produced in the liver, production may be compro-

mised in liver disease. Liver disease, in general, is associated with an increased hemorrhagic tendency (see Chap. 34).[78, 79]

Nephrotic Syndrome

Nephrotic syndrome has been associated with a potential hypercoagulable state (an increased risk of thrombotic disease) in both human and veterinary medicine. Nephrotic syndrome in dogs can result in a significantly decreased ATIII concentration, increased platelet count, and coagulation factor activity (factors V, VII, VIII:C, IX, X, and fibrinogen). Factor X activity is decreased in human renal amyloidosis, but this has been not observed in the dog.[80]

Acquired Inhibitors of Coagulation

There are few reports of acquired inhibitors in veterinary medicine. Pathologic inhibitors of coagulation are acquired inhibitors that are described as circulating anticoagulants. The first report of such inhibitors was a specific factor XI inhibitor in a 5-year-old male cat.[81]

A lupus anticoagulant was described in a 3-year-old Chesapeake Bay retriever. SLE was diagnosed.[82]

A 12-year-old German shepherd was diagnosed with IgA-forming multiple myeloma. The paraprotein inhibited coagulation factors (especially VIII:C) and affected primary hemostasis (a prolonged bleeding time with modest thrombocytopenia was observed).[14]

Mast Cell Neoplasia

Coagulation abnormalities such as prolonged PT and APTT have been reported in canine systemic mastocytosis. This has been related to increased heparin secretion by the neoplastic mast cells.[83]

Thrombotic Disorders

Canine hyperadrenocorticism and diabetes mellitus and, especially, feline cardiomyopathy have been suggested to induce thrombosis. However, the real incidence and effective therapy have not yet been defined in veterinary medicine.[84–86]

Inherited Coagulation Disorders[87–90]

Hypofibrinogenemia

Hypofibrinogenemia has been described in Saint Bernards and possibly in vizslas and borzois. PT, APTT, and TT are prolonged, and fibrinogen determination reveals a concentration below the reference interval. Transfusion of cryoprecipitate or fresh frozen plasma may be required.

Dysfibrinogenemia

Dysfibrinogenemia is an autosomal inherited defect described in the collie and borzoi with mild hemorrhagic tendency. Diagnosis of such a defect requires a comparison between functional fibrinogen (von Clauss method) and total fibrinogen (heat precipitation).[15] PT, APTT, and TT may be prolonged in this defect.

Prothrombin Deficiency

Prothrombin deficiency has been described in boxers and cocker spaniels. The hemorrhagic tendency may be severe. PT is prolonged, TT remains normal, and APTT may be slightly prolonged. Administration of fresh frozen plasma may be indicated.

Factor VII Deficiency

Factor VII deficiency has been described in the beagle, Alaskan malamute, miniature schnauzer, boxer, and English bulldog. PT is prolonged with normal APTT and TT. The hemorrhagic tendency may be subclinical to moderate, and therapy is not usually required.

Hemophilia A

Hemophilia A or factor VIII:C deficiency is the second most common inherited hemostatic defect of dogs (von Willebrand's disease is first). Hemophilia A has been described in numerous breeds of dogs and in mixed breed dogs, with higher frequency in the German shepherd. It has been described in British shorthair, Siamese, American domestic shorthair, and Himalayan cats as well. Hemophilia A has a sex-linked inheritance pattern, with female dogs being heterozygotes and clinically asymptomatic. The APTT is prolonged with normal PT and TT. Male dogs may present with severe, moderate, or mild deficiency. The severity correlates with the degree of factor VIII:C activity. Therapy is therefore dependent on the degree of deficiency. Factor concentrations must be determined individually for affected patients. The best therapeutic choice for normovolemic, nonanemic individuals is cryoprecipitate to avoid potential hypervolemia, but fresh frozen plasma (5–8 mL/kg b.i.d. or t.i.d. for 3 days), fresh whole blood, and DDAVP (1 µg/kg) subcutaneously may also be considered.[36] Acquired factor VIII:C inhibitor may be a potential complicating consequence of this therapy. Anti–factor VIII antibody activity is frequently observed in humans with hemophilia.

Hemophilia B

Deficiency of factor IX has a sex-linked recessive inheritance pattern. It has been described in several canine breeds (Cairn terrier, black-and-tan coonhound, Saint Bernard, Alaskan malamute, cocker spaniel, Scottish terrier, and German shepherd) and in several feline breeds (British shorthair, Siamese, American domestic shorthair, and Himalayan). The hemorrhagic tendency of affected males can be severe. APTT is prolonged; PT and TT tend to be normal. Stored plasma, fresh frozen plasma, or fresh whole blood may be administered (see Hemophilia A).[36, 91]

Hemophilia AB

Hemophilia AB has been described in a female French bulldog. Affected and carrier dogs with both defects have been reported in this family.

Factor X Deficiency

Factor X deficiency has been described in two canine breeds: cocker spaniel and Jack Russell terrier. Inheritance is autosomal dominant and the hemorrhagic tendency is variable. APTT and PT are prolonged, and TT is normal. Transfusion of fresh frozen or stored plasma may be indicated (see Hemophilia A).[92]

Hemophilia C (Factor XI Deficiency)

Hemophilia C, or factor XI deficiency, has an autosomal recessive inheritance pattern. It has been described in the springer spaniel, Great Pyrenees, Kerry blue terrier, and weimaraner. The hemorrhagic tendency tends to be moderate. APTT is prolonged; PT and TT remain normal.

Factor XII (Hageman Factor) Deficiency

Factor XII deficiency has been described in cats and several canine breeds—poodle and German shorthaired pointer. The inheritance pattern is autosomal recessive. This deficiency does not induce a bleeding tendency. A diagnosis is often made after evaluation of screening hemostatic tests. Deficiency in factor XII has been associated with a thrombotic tendency in humans. APTT is prolonged, with normal PT and TT.

Vitamin K–Responsive Coagulopathy

Vitamin K–responsive coagulopathy has been described in Devon rex cats. Affected individuals are deficient in vitamin K–dependent coagulation factors (factors II, VII, IX, and X). This defect has been observed in male and female cats. Therapy is based on vitamin K_1 supplementation, but transfusion therapy must be considered if severe hemorrhage is present.[93, 94]

References

1. Laposata M, Connor AM, Hicks DG, et al. The Clinical Hemostasis Handbook. Chicago, Year Book Medical Publishers, 1989:19–21.

2. Wachtfogel YT, de la Cadena R, Colman R. Structural biology, cellular interactions and pathophysiology of the contact system. Thromb Res 1993;72:1–21.

3. Esmond CT. Possible involvement of cytokines in diffuse intravascular coagulation and thrombosis. Baillieres Clin Haematol 1994;7:453–468.

4. Alcaraz A, España F, Sánches-Cuenca J, et al. Activation of the protein C pathway in acute sepsis. Thromb Res 1995;79:83–93.

5. Walsh LJ, Trincheri G, Waldorf HA, et al. Human dermal mast cells contain and release tumor necrosis factor α, which induces endothelial leukocyte adhesion molecule E. Proc Natl Acad Sci USA 1991;88:4220–4224.

6. Muller BG. Pathophysiologic and biochemical events in disseminated intravascular coagulation: Dysregulation of procoagulant and anticoagulant pathways. Semin Thromb Hemost 1989;15:58–87.

7. Venturini CM, Kaplan JE. Thrombin induces platelet adhesion to endothelial cells. Semin Thromb Hemost 1992;18:275–283.

8. Jandl JH. Blood: Pathophysiology. Boston, Blackwell Scientific Publications, 1991:510–533.

9. Feldman BF. Disseminated intravascular coagulation. Compen Contin Educ Pract Vet 1981;3:45–52.

10. Wintrobe MW, Lee GR, Boggs DR, et al. Clinical Hematology. Philadelphia, Lea & Febiger, 1981:104–162.

11. Wu HF, Lundblad RL, Church FC. Neutralization of heparin activity by neutrophil lactoferrin. Blood 1995;85:421–428.

12. Nguyen P, Petitfrere E, Potron G. Mechanisms of the platelet aggregation induced by activated neutrophils and inhibitory effect of specific PAF receptor agonists. Thromb Res 1995;78:33–42.

13. Catafalmo JL, Dodds WJ. Hereditary and acquired thrombopathias. Vet Clin North Am Small Anim Pract 1988;18:185–194.

14. Ruiz de Gopegui R, Espada Y, Vilafranca M, et al. Paraprotein-induced defective hemostasis in a dog with IgA (kappa-light chain) forming myeloma. Vet Clin Pathol 1994;23:70–71.

15. Ruiz de Gopegui R. Estudio experimental de las alteraciones de la hemostasia en el conejo según distintos fármacos antitrombóticos. PhD Thesis, Universidad Autónoma de Barcelona, 1994.

16. Concannon KT, Haskins SC, Feldman BF. Hemostatic defects associated with two infusion rates of dextran 70 in dogs. Am J Vet Res 1992;53:1369–1375.

17. Van Heerden J. Canine ehrlichiosis. In: Fivaz B, Petney T, Horak I, eds. Tick Vector Biology: Medical and Veterinary Aspects. Berlin, Springer-Verlag, 1992:109.

18. Iqbal Z, Rikhhsa Y. Reisolation of Ehrlichia canis from blood and tissues of dogs after doxycycline treatment. J Clin Microbiol 1994;32:1644–1649.

19. Woody BJ, Hoskins JD. Ehrlichial diseases of dogs. Vet Clin North Am Small Anim Pract 1991;21:75–98.

20. Handagama P, Feldman BF. Thrombocytopenia and drugs. Vet Clin North Am Small Anim Pract 1988;18:51–66.

21. Hargis AM, Feldman BF. Evaluation of hemostatic defects secondary to vascular tumors in dogs: 11 cases (1983–1988). J Am Vet Med Assoc 1991;198:891–894.

22. O'Neill SL, Feldman BF. Hemolysis as a factor in clinical chemistry and hematology of the dog. Vet Clin Pathol 1989;18:58–68.

23. Mackin A. Canine immune-mediated thrombocytopenia. Part I. Compen Contin Educ Pract Vet 1995;17:353–364.

24. Joshi BC, Jain NC. Detection of antiplatelet antibody in serum and on megakaryocytes of dogs with autoimmune thrombocytopenia. Am J Vet Res 1976;37:681–685.

25. Kristensen AT, Weiss DJ, Klausner JS. Platelet dysfunction associated with immune-mediated thrombocytopenia in dogs. J Vet Intern Med 1994;8:323–327.

26. Feldman BF. Platelet disorders. Proceedings of American Animal Hospital Association, Boston, 1994:385.

27. Northern J, Tvedten HW. Diagnosis of microthrombocytosis and immune-mediated thrombocytopenia in dogs with thrombocytopenia: 68 cases (1987–1989). J Am Vet Med Assoc 1992;200:368–371.

28. Campbell KL, Wright GJ, Greene CE. Application of the enzyme-linked immunosorbent assay for the detection of platelet antibodies in dogs. Am J Vet Res 1984;45:2561–2564.

29. Thiem PA, Abbot DL, Moroff S, et al. Preliminary findings on the comparison of flow cytometric and solid-phase radioimmunoassay techniques for the detection of platelet antibodies in dogs. Vet Clin Pathol 1991;20:18.

30. Jain NC, Kono CS. The platelet factor-3 for detection of canine antiplatelet antibody. Vet Clin Pathol 1980;9:10–14.

31. Kristensen AM, Feldman BF. Blood banking and transfusion medicine. In: Ettinger SJ, Feldman EC, eds. Textbook of Veterinary Internal Medicine, 4th ed. Philadelphia, WB Saunders, 1995:347–360.

32. Holloway SA, Meyer DJ, Mannella C. Prednisolone and danazol for treatment of immune-mediated anemia, thrombocytopenia, and ineffective erythroid regeneration in a dog. J Am Vet Med Assoc 1990;197:1045–1048.

33. Nolte I, Niemann C, Failing K, et al. Untersuchung zur Wirsamkeit der kombinierten Behandlung thrombozytarer hamorrhagischer Diathesen des Hundes mit Prednisolon und Bluttransfusion am Beispiel einer durch Aspirin hervorgerufenen Thrombozytopathie. Tierarztl Prax 1988;16:417–422.

34. Mount ME. Diagnosis and therapy of anticoagulant rodenticide intoxications. Vet Clin North Am Small Anim Pract 1988;18:115–130.

35. Shearer MJ. High-performance liquid chromatography

of K vitamins and the antagonists. Adv Chromatogr 1983;21:243–301.

36. Hohenhaus AE. Canine blood transfusions. Probl Vet Med 1992;4:612–624.

37. Bick RL. Disorders of Hemostasis and Thrombosis. New York, Thieme 1985:157–204.

38. Ellison GW, King RR, Calderwood MM. Medical and surgical management of multiple organ infarctions secondary to bacterial endocarditis in a dog. J Am Vet Med Assoc 1988;193:1289–1291.

39. Suliman HB, Feldman BF. Pathogenesis and aetiology of anaemia in trypanosomiasis with special reference to *T. brucei* and *T. evansi*. Vet Bull 1989;59:99–107.

40. Dillon AR, Braund KG. Distal polyneuropathy after canine heartworm disease therapy complicated by disseminated intravascular coagulation. J Am Vet Med Assoc 1982;181:239–242.

41. Drazner FH. Clinical implication of disseminated intravascular coagulation. Compen Contin Educ Pract Vet 1982;4:974–981.

42. Madewell BR, Feldman BF. Characterization of anemias associated with neoplasia in small animals. J Am Vet Med Assoc 1980;176:419–425.

43. Hardaway RM. Prediction of survival or death of patients in a state of severe shock. Surg Gynecol Obstet 1981;152:200–206.

44. Green RA. Hemostatic disorders: Coagulopathies and thrombotic disorders. In: Ettinger SJ, ed. Textbook of Veterinary Internal Medicine, 3rd ed. Philadelphia, WB Saunders, 1989:2246–2264.

45. Cowell AK, Cowell RL, Tyler RD, et al. Severe systemic reactions to Hymenoptera stings in three dogs. J Am Vet Med Assoc 1991;198:1014–1416.

46. Axelsson L, Bergenfeldt M, Bjork P, et al. Release of immunoreactive canine leukocyte elastase normally and in endotoxin and pancreatitis shock. Scand J Clin Lab Invest 1990;50:35–42.

47. Schrier SL. Disorders of hemostasis and coagulation. In: Rubinstein E, Federman DD, eds. Scientific American Medicine, vol 5. New York, Scientific American, 1993:1–59.

48. Slappendel RJ. Disseminated intravascular coagulation. Vet Clin North Am Small Anim Pract 1988;18:169–184.

49. Ruehl W, Mills C, Feldman BF. Rational therapy in disseminated intravascular coagulation. J Am Vet Med Assoc 1982;181:76–78.

50. Wisecarver JL, Haire WD. Disseminated intravascular coagulation with multiple arterial thromboses responding to antithrombin-III concentrate infusion. Thromb Res 1989;54:709–717.

51. Welch RD, Watkins JP, Taylor TS, et al. Disseminated intravascular coagulation associated with colic in 23 horses (1984–1989). J Vet Intern Med 1992;6:29–35.

52. Feldman BF. Disseminated intravascular coagulation (DIC) disseminated intravascular thrombosis (DIT) consumption coagulopathy (CC). Proceedings of Second International Veterinary Emergency and Critical Care Symposium, San Antonio, Texas, 1990.

53. Hardaway RM, McKay DG, Wahle GH, et al. Pathologic study of intravascular coagulation following incompatible blood transfusion in dogs. Am J Surg 1956;91:24.

54. Avgeris S, Lothrop CD, McDonald TP. Plasma von Willebrand factor concentration and thyroid function in dogs. J Am Vet Med Assoc 1989;196:921–924.

55. Dalton RG, Dewar MS, Savidge GF, et al. Hypothyroidism as a cause of acquired von Willebrand's disease. Lancet 1987;1:1007–1009.

56. Lumsden JH, O'Grady MR, Johnstone IB, et al. Prevalence of hypothyroidism and von Willebrand's disease in Doberman pinschers and the observed relationship between thyroid, von Willebrand and cardiac status. Proc Am Coll Vet Intern Med Forum 1993;11:928.

57. Brooks M. Management of canine von Willebrand's disease. Probl Vet Med 1992;4:636–646.

58. Dodds WJ. HEMOPET: A national non-profit animal blood bank program. Canine Pract 1992;17:12–16.

59. Kraus KN, Turrentine MA, Jergens AE, et al. Effect of desmopressin acetate on bleeding times and plasma von Willebrand factor in Doberman pinscher dogs with von Willebrand's disease. Vet Surg 1989;18:59.

60. Van Pelt DR, Miller E, Martin LG, et al. Hematologic emergencies. Vet Clin North Am Small Anim Pract 1994;24:1139–1172.

61. Medinger TL, Williams DA, Bruyette DS. Severe gastrointestinal tract hemorrhage in three dogs with hypoadrenocorticism. J Am Vet Med Assoc 1993;202:1869–1872.

62. Malik R, Dowden M, Allan GS. Acute mediastinal haemorrhage and haemothorax in young dogs—two suspected cases. Aust Vet Pract 1993;23:134–138.

63. Busch DS, Noxon JO. Pneumothorax in a dog infected with *Dirofilaria immitis*. J Am Vet Med Assoc 1992;201:1893.

64. Pumarola M, Brevik L, Badiola J, et al. Canine leishmaniasis associated with systemic vasculitis in two dogs. J Comp Pathol 1991;105:279–286.

65. Scott-Moncrieff JCR, Snyder PW, Glickman LT, et al. Systemic necrotizing vasculitis in nine young beagles. J Am Vet Med Assoc 1992;201:1553–1558.

66. Synder PW, Kazacos EA, Scott-Moncrieff, et al. Pathologic features of naturally occurring juvenile polyarteritis in beagle dogs. Vet Pathol 1995;32:337–345.

67. Comer KM: Rocky mountain spotted fever. Vet Clin North Am Small Anim Pract 1991;21:27–44.

68. Davidson MG, Breitschwerdt EB, Walker DH, et al. Vascular permeability and coagulation during *Rickettsia rickettsii* infection in dogs. Am J Vet Res 1990;51:165–170.

69. Barnett KC, Cottrell BD. Ehlers-Danlos syndrome in a dog. J Small Anim Pract 1987;28:941–946.

70. Weir JAM, Yager JA. Familial cutaneous vasculopathy of German shepherd dogs. Vet Dermatol 1993;4:41–42.

71. Castellan E, Burgat-Sacaze V, Petit C, et al. Toxicite iatrogene des estrogenes chez le chien. Rev Med Vet 1993;144:285–289.

72. Merchier D, De Cock I, De Schepper J. Een geval van ernstige oestrogeenintoxicatie met volledig herstel bij de hond. Vlaams Diergeneeskd Tijdschr 1989;58:127–129.

73. Hardistry RM, Hutton RA. Bleeding tendency associated

with "new" abnormality of platelet behaviour. Lancet 1967;1:983–985.

74. Cowles BE, Meyers KM, Wardrop KJ, et al. Prolonged bleeding time of Chédiak-Higashi cats corrected by platelet transfusion. Thromb Haemost 1992;67:708–711.

75. Callan MB, Giger U, Bennet JS, et al. Platelet storage pool disease in American cocker spaniels. Proc Am Coll Vet Intern Med Forum 1993;11:940.

76. Patterson WR, Estry DW, Schwartz KA, et al. Absent platelet aggregation with normal fibrinogen binding in basset hound hereditary thrombopathy. Thromb Haemost 1989;62:1011–1015.

77. Dial SM. Clinicopathologic evaluation of the liver. Vet Clin North Am Small Anim Pract 1995;25:257–273.

78. Hughes D, King LG. The diagnosis and management of acute liver failure in dogs and cats. Vet Clin North Am Small Anim Pract 1995;25:437–460.

79. Pichler ME, Turnwald GH. Blood transfusion in the dog and cat: Part I. Physiology, collection, storage, and indications for whole blood therapy. Compen Contin Educ Pract Vet 1985;7:64–71.

80. Rasedee A, Feldman BF, Washabau R. Naturally occurring nephrotic syndrome is a potentially hypercoagulable state. Acta Vet Scand 1986;27:369–377.

81. Feldman BF, Soares CJ, Kitchell BE, et al. Hemorrhage in a cat caused by inhibition of factor XI (plasma thromboplastin antecedent). J Am Vet Med Assoc 1983;182:589–591.

82. Stone MS, Johnstone IB, Brooks M, et al. Lupus-type "anticoagulant" in a dog with hemolysis and thrombosis. J Vet Intern Med 1994;8:57–61.

83. Hottendorf GH, Nielsen SW, Kenyon AJ. Canine mastocytoma. I. Blood coagulation in dogs with mastocytoma. Pathol Vet 1965;2:129–141.

84. Feldman BF, Rasedee A. Haemostatic abnormalities in canine Cushing's syndrome. Res Vet Sci 1986;41:228–230.

85. Pion PD. Feline aortic thromboemboli and the potential utility of thrombolytic therapy with tissue plasminogen activator. Vet Clin North Am Small Anim Pract 1988;18:79–86.

86. Couto CG. Disorders of hemostasis. In: Nelson RW, Couto CG, eds. Essentials of Small Animal Internal Medicine. St. Louis, Mosby, 1992;940.

87. Dodds, WJ. Bleeding disorders. In: August JR, ed. Consultations in Feline Internal Medicine. Philadelphia, WB Saunders, 1991:383–388.

88. Foch JM, Foch IT. Inherited coagulation disorders. Vet Clin North Am Small Anim Pract 1988;18:231–244.

89. Hoskins JD. Congenital defects of the cat. In: Ettinger SJ, Feldman EC, eds. Textbook of Veterinary Internal Medicine, 4th ed. Philadelphia, WB Saunders, 1995:2106–2114.

90. Hoskins JD. Congenital defects of the dog. In: Ettinger SJ, Feldman EC, eds. Textbook of Veterinary Internal Medicine, 4th ed. Philadelphia, WB Saunders, 1995:2115–2129.

91. Feldman DG, Brooks MB, Dodds WJ. Hemophilia B (factor IX deficiency) in a family of German shepherd dogs. J Am Vet Med Assoc 1995;206:1901–1905.

92. Cook AK, Werner LL, O'Neill LO, et al. Factor X deficiency in a Jack Russel terrier. Vet Clin Pathol 1993;22:68–71.

93. Soute BAM, Ulrich MMW, Watson DJ, et al. Congenital deficiency of all vitamin K–dependent blood coagulation factors due to a defective vitamin K–dependent carboxylase in Devon Rex cats. Thromb Haemost 1992;68:521–525.

94. Littlewood JD, Shaw SC, Coombes LM. Vitamin K–dependent coagulopathy in a British Devon rex cat. J Small Anim Pract 1995;36:115–118.

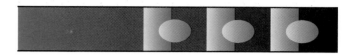

Endocrine
and Metabolic
Diseases

Chapter 45

Diseases of the Pituitary Gland

William E. Monroe

Anatomy

The pituitary gland is a small gland that adjoins the base of the diencephalon, just caudal to the optic chiasm. It is composed of an anterior portion, termed the adenohypophysis, which is made up of the pars distalis and pars intermedia, and a posterior portion, termed the neurohypophysis or pars nervosa.[1, 2]

The hypophyseal portal system is a venous portal system that transports regulatory hormones from the hypothalamus to the anterior pituitary gland. Arterioles carry blood to capillaries within the lower hypothalamus, where the hypothalamic hormones are absorbed. The capillaries drain into portal veins that course to the anterior pituitary gland (primarily the pars distalis), where they again arborize into capillaries so that the hypothalamic hormones can diffuse into the pituitary gland.[1]

Physiology

The pars distalis contains cells that produce growth hormone (GH, also called somatotropin), adrenocorticotrophic hormone (ACTH), and thyroid-stimulating hormone (TSH, also called thyrotropin). The pars distalis also produces hormones involved with lactation and gonadal function: prolactin (PRL), follicle-stimulating hormone (FSH), and luteinizing hormone (see Chap. 21).[3]

Secretion of the hormones of the anterior pituitary is under the control of the hypothalamus. Hormones of the hypothalamus (corticotropin-releasing hormone, thyrotropin-releasing hormone, gonadotropin-releasing hormone, growth hormone–releasing hormone, and somatostatin) are secreted and carried to the adenohypophysis by way of the hypophyseal portal vessels. The hormones of the adenohypophysis have negative feedback on the hypothalamus to inhibit secretion of hypothalamic hormones.[3]

The hormones of the adenohypophysis have tropic effects on their target endocrine glands; that is, TSH stimulates release of thyroid hormones from the thyroid gland, ACTH stimulates release of glucocorticoids from the adrenal cortices, and GH stimulates production of somatomedins (which are responsible for the anabolic functions of GH) from the liver.[3]

The pars nervosa contains neurons whose cell bodies originate in the hypothalamus and produce oxytocin (see Chap. 23) and vasopressin (antidiuretic hormone [ADH]). These hormones are stored in the cells in the pars nervosa and are secreted into the blood stream. Osmoreceptors in the hypothalamus detect changes in plasma osmolality, stimulate secretion of ADH when plasma osmolality increases, and inhibit ADH secretion when osmolality decreases. Vascular baroreceptors and stretch receptors, which detect changes in blood pressure and volume, respectively, also affect ADH release, stimulating its release when blood pressure or volume is reduced. The ADH, in turn, makes renal tubular cells permeable to water, allowing water to be reabsorbed in times of need, with resulting increased concentration of urine.[3]

Problem Identification

Failure to Grow and Thrive

Occasionally, a puppy or kitten may fail to keep up with its littermates in terms of growth and development, and may fail to thrive and put on weight normally. The condition can be caused by acquired disease such as severe parasitism or chronic infectious diseases, or it may be caused by an inborn anatomic or metabolic defect.

Pathophysiology

Some causes of failure to grow and thrive in puppies and kittens are listed in Table 45–1. Young animals with congenital or acquired swallowing disorders, such as those caused by a cleft palate, megaesophagus, or a vascular ring anomaly, fail to grow because of an inability to take in sufficient nutrients. A poor or inadequate diet also leads to growth failure from insufficient consumption of nutrients. Puppies with pancreatic exocrine insufficiency fail to digest nutrients, so they are not absorbed or utilized. Severely parasitized animals may fail to absorb sufficient nutrients to supply the needs of a growing animal (with hookworm or roundworm infestation) or may

Table 45–1
Causes of Failure to Grow and Thrive in Puppies and Kittens

Excessive competition for food
Inadequate diet
Swallowing disorders

  Dysphagia (cleft palate)
  Regurgitation

    Megaesophagus
    Vascular ring anomaly
    Esophageal foreign body

Gastrointestinal parasites
Pancreatic exocrine insufficiency (puppies)
Congenital heart defects or heart failure
Renal dysplasia or failure
Hepatic portosystemic shunt
Juvenile diabetes mellitus
Congenital hypothyroidism
Pituitary dwarfism
Chronic infection e.g., feline leukemia virus, feline
  infectious peritonitis

become severely anemic from blood loss (with hookworm infestation). Chronic infectious diseases such as feline infectious peritonitis (FIP) and feline leukemia virus (FeLV) increase the metabolic demand on an animal and often cause a reduced appetite. Animals with anatomic or metabolic defects that prevent normal utilization of nutrients (e.g., portosystemic shunt) or cause accumulation of metabolic waste products (e.g., renal dysplasia) also fail to grow normally. Animals with cardiac defects that result in poor oxygenation of tissues use nutrients inefficiently and lose weight or fail to grow properly. Congenital deficiencies of hormones such as GH, thyroxine, and insulin all lead to failure of normal growth and maturation.

Clinical Signs

The clinical signs vary depending on the underlying cause. Puppies and kittens lag behind littermates in terms of stature, physical ability, and body weight. Animals with cleft palates have dysphagia and nasal discharge, often with milk running out the nose during nursing. Those with esophageal diseases such as megaesophagus or vascular ring anomalies regurgitate food shortly after eating, beginning at the time of weaning, when the puppy or kitten begins consuming solid food. Animals with gastrointestinal parasites often have diarrhea, anemia, or both. Older puppies with pancreatic exocrine insufficiency usually have soft, voluminous, fetid stools or outright diarrhea, often with polyphagia. These patients also frequently have excessive borborygmus and flatulence.

Animals with chronic infectious diseases may have signs of the underlying condition. Kittens with FIP may have a distended abdomen or dyspnea from pleural effusion with the "wet" form, or perhaps just poor appetite and lethargy, often with uveitis with the "dry" form. Kittens with FeLV may have anemia or tumors (e.g., lymphoma, often of the mediastinum) causing pleural effusion and dyspnea, or chronic recurring respiratory, oral, gastrointestinal, or skin infections.

In addition to poor growth, puppies with portosystemic shunts often have polyuria and polydipsia (PU/PD), are difficult to housebreak, and may be presented for dementia from hepatoencephalopathy (see Chap. 34). Animals with congenital renal dysplasia also often have PU/PD and may have a poor appetite with vomiting. Diabetic animals also have PU/PD and may initially have a voracious appetite, followed by anorexia and vomiting if severe ketoacidosis ensues. Patients with cardiac defects usually have murmurs and may develop signs of heart failure, such as coughing, tachypnea, or ascites (see Chap. 14). Animals with pituitary dwarfism usually have a proportionate reduction in stature, whereas hypothyroid dwarves have disproportionate reduction in the length of the limbs. In both disorders, there are often hair coat abnormalities such as failure to develop primary hairs and alopecia.

Diagnostic Plan

If a puppy or kitten is failing to grow and thrive normally, the diagnosis may be apparent from the history and physical examination. Questioning of the owner about diet or excessive competition for teats or food with excessively large litters, particularly if the puppy or kitten was smaller and weaker at birth than its siblings, may determine that inadequate dietary intake or a poor diet is the cause for failure to grow. Very young puppies with cleft palates may have a history of dysphagia and nasal discharge, often including milk or food. The cleft palate is apparent on the physical examination. Puppies with a history of regurgitation should have thoracic radiographs and possibly an esophagram to identify a megaesophagus, vascular ring anomaly, or esophageal foreign body. Young animals with heart murmurs should have thoracic radiography, electrocardiography, and echocardiography performed if available (see Chap. 14). Young puppies or kittens with a history of diarrhea and possibly also a distended abdomen or pale mucous membranes may have gastrointestinal parasites and should have fecal examinations performed.

If the clinical signs do not lead to a diagnosis or direct the work-up to the specific diagnostic procedures discussed, the next step is to do fecal examinations for gastrointestinal parasitism and deworm the animal with a safe, broad-spectrum anthelmintic such as pyrantel pamoate. Older puppies with persistent soft stools, excessive flatulence, and often polyphagia should have serum trypsin–like immunoreactivity (STLI) measured in order to rule out pancreatic exocrine insufficiency.

If other signs are present, or if fecal examinations or response to deworming and STLI are negative, a complete blood count (including a platelet count), serum chemistry profile, urinalysis, and test for FeLV in kittens should be done to help identify chronic infectious diseases, diabetes mellitus, renal dysplasia, or portosystemic shunts. If there are any signs of liver failure in the biochemistry profile, such as hypoalbuminemia, reduced blood urea nitrogen (BUN), or ammonium biurate crystals in the urine sediment, bile acids should be measured after fasting and 2 hours after feeding (see Chap. 34). If PU/PD is present with apparently normal routine laboratory testing results, serum bile acids should also be tested to rule out a portosystemic shunt. Animals with pituitary dwarfism may have hypoglycemia evident on the chemistry profile, and it may occasionally be severe enough to cause clinical signs.

If the diagnosis is still not apparent, the serum thyroxine and TSH concentrations should be measured (see Chap. 47). Hypothyroidism causes reduction of serum GH concentration. Hypothyroid dwarves usually have primary hypothyroidism (disease of the thyroid gland) and are usually disproportionate, so they are often distinguishable from pituitary dwarves on the basis of the clinical signs. Hypothyroid dwarves are expected to have a low thyroxine concentration with a high TSH concentration. Pituitary dwarves may have panhypopituitarism, so they have GH deficiency as well as secondary hypothyroidism and hypoadrenocorticism. In these cases, the serum thyroxine is expected to be reduced or normal, with a low TSH concentration. Patients with these parameters suggestive of pituitary dwarfism should also have plasma endogenous ACTH measured and an ACTH response test performed. There is no available assay for GH in dogs and cats, so an indirect assessment of GH production, serum somatomedin C concentration, should be measured (see Special Laboratory Tests). Diagnosis of pituitary dwarfism is based on clinical signs, ruling out of other diseases, a low somatomedin C concentration, and, in some cases, finding other defects of pituitary function such as secondary hypothyroidism or hypoadrenocorticism.

Polyuria and Polydipsia

PU/PD can occur in association with many diseases (see Chap. 16). Pituitary diseases such as acromegaly and central diabetes insipidus also cause PU/PD. In the case of central diabetes insipidus, PU/PD is profound in 100% of patients, usually with no other clinical signs. With acromegaly, PU/PD is just one of many signs such as soft tissue proliferation of the head, neck, and extremities, inspiratory stridor, increased interdental spaces, hepatomegaly, heart failure (cats), and poorly controlled diabetes mellitus.

Diagnostic Procedures

Routine Laboratory Evaluation

Routine laboratory tests are usually not specific for diseases of the pituitary gland, but nonspecific changes may be present, such hyperglycemia and elevated liver enzymes with acromegaly. The urine specific gravity (USG) is hyposthenuric in patients with diabetes insipidus. Routine laboratory tests are the most useful for ruling in or ruling out other diseases.

Radiography

For most pituitary diseases, radiography is of little value other than to rule in or rule out other diseases. With acromegaly in cats, there may be an increase in the size of the mandible and thickening of the calvarial ridges.[4] In addition, there may be increased soft tissue in the oropharyngeal area, with soft tissue swelling in the limbs and head, particularly in dogs.[5] Cardiomegaly, hepatomegaly, and renomegaly may also be present in cats, as well as pulmonary edema and pleural effusion from heart failure.[4] Although usually available only at referral centers, computed tomography is extremely useful to identify pituitary tumors.[4]

Special Laboratory Tests

Growth Hormone

Measurement of GH is useful to identify hyposomatotropism (pituitary dwarfism)[6, 7] or acromegaly,[5] but no validated assay is presently available for use with dog or cat sera. Basal values in canine patients with hyposomatotropism overlap with those of normal animals, so stimulation testing is necessary.[6] Secretion of GH is stimulated by xylazine or clonidine,[6, 8] which is useful in identifying hyposomatotropism. Although in most dogs and cats with acromegaly the basal plasma GH concentration is clearly above normal, suppression testing may be necessary to absolutely confirm the diagnosis.[9] The administration of glucose suppresses the GH concentration of normal dogs, but not those with acromegaly.[5]

Somatomedin C

Because there is no valid GH assay available for use with dogs and cats, measurement of somatomedin C (now called insulin-like growth factor I, or IGF-I) has been useful to identify abnormalities of GH secretion. GH stimulates production of somatomedins, which in turn are responsible for the anabolic effects of GH. Somatomedin C concentration is high in dogs[10] and cats[11, 12] with acromegaly. Somatomedin C concentration in canine patients with hyposomatotropism is reduced.[6, 7] The test is commercially available as a radioimmunoassay and has been validated for use in dogs,[13] but not cats, at the Animal Health Diagnostic Laboratory, Michigan State University, East Lansing, Michigan. Normal values have been established in this laboratory for dogs.

Endogenous ACTH Concentration

Because patients with pituitary disease may have secondary hypoadrenocorticism, measurement of the endogenous ACTH concentration may be useful. It should always be interpreted in view of cortisol concentration, measured at the 0 hour of an ACTH stimulation test (see Chap. 46).

Modified Water Deprivation Test

Before a modified water deprivation test is performed, all other differential diagnoses for PU/PD except CDI, idiopathic or congenital nephrogenic diabetes insipidus (NDI), and psychogenic polydipsia should have been ruled out (see Chap. 16). Results of the test can be confusing in patients with hyperadrenocorticism, appearing similar to results in those with partial CDI[14, 15] or psychogenic polydipsia,[14] and it is dangerous to deprive patients with renal or liver disease of water.

Food is withheld overnight (12 hours) before and also during the water deprivation phase of the test, so that the determination of dehydration based on loss of body weight reflects loss of body water and not changes associated with food consumption or defecation. The bladder is emptied by catheterization or by allowing the animal to void. The USG is determined, and a sample is saved for osmolality. Water is withheld and the bladder is emptied hourly (by catheter or by voiding if the patient cooperates), with the patient carefully weighed afterward. Placement of an indwelling catheter facilitates the test and is usually necessary for cats. Because these animals often feel quite well, however, the catheter can be difficult to maintain. USG should be measured hourly. Mental attitude and clinical hydration should also be assessed hourly. Ideally, the BUN (measured by Azostix) should be monitored periodically during water deprivation. If azotemia occurs (BUN >30 mg/dL), the test should be terminated. If the animal is presented clinically dehydrated (loss of ≥6% body weight), the water deprivation phase is not necessary and exogenous vasopressin (ADH) is given with monitoring of the response, as outlined in the next paragraph.[14]

After the patient has lost 5% of its body weight (or is obviously dehydrated; that is, loss of ≥6% body weight), a urine sample is saved to determine the osmolality and USG. Most patients with severe CDI or NDI lose 5% of their body weight within 3 to 10 hours of water deprivation.[14, 15] Normal dogs require more than 24 hours of water deprivation to lose 5% of their body weight. If USG is greater than 1.030 (osmolality >1100 mOsm/kg) when the patient has lost 5% body weight, renal concentrating ability is normal,[14] and the diagnosis is likely to be psychogenic polydipsia. If the USG is less than 1.030, the animal is given 0.55 U/kg (up to a total of 5 U) of aqueous vasopressin intramuscularly. The bladder is emptied at 30, 60, and 90 minutes after the injection, while water deprivation is

continued. The USG is determined in urine samples obtained at these times, and samples are refrigerated to be sent out for determination of osmolality in case the results of the test using USG are equivocal. Osmolality is more accurate than USG,[14] but it is more expensive to determine (about $20 per sample). For practical purposes, osmolality needs be determined only in urine samples taken before water deprivation, at the end of water deprivation, and 90 minutes after injection of ADH. At the end of the test, water should be offered in small amounts every 15 to 30 minutes to prevent overhydration or vomiting caused by rapid consumption of a large volume.[14]

If the USG is less than 1.006 (or osmolality is <290–310 mOsm/kg, the normal osmolality of plasma) at the end of the water deprivation phase, and USG increases to more than 1.010 (or osmolality increases 50% to 600%) in response to exogenous ADH, the probable diagnosis is severe CDI (Fig. 45–1). If the USG at the end of water deprivation is less than 1.006 (osmolality <290–310 mOsm/kg) and it is still less than 1.006 after administration of ADH (or if osmolality increases by <10%), the probable diagnosis is NDI. If the USG is between 1.008 and 1.020 (osmolality >290–310 mOsm/kg) after water deprivation and increases by more than 0.002 to 0.003 (or osmolality increases by 10%–50% or more), the animal may have a partial deficiency of ADH (partial CDI) or hyperadrenocorticism.[14, 15]

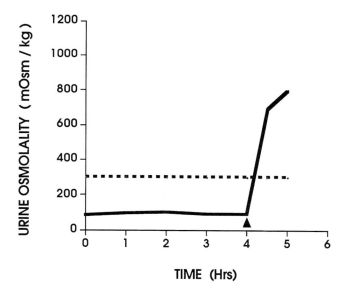

Figure 45–1
Graphic results of a modified water deprivation test from a 4-month-old female Shetland sheepdog with central diabetes insipidus. The dashed horizontal line represents normal plasma osmolality, 300 mOsm/kg. The arrowhead indicates the time when 5% body weight was lost and antidiuretic hormone was administered.

If the results of the modified water deprivation test indicate possible psychogenic polydipsia with renal medullary solute washout from prolonged polyuria (i.e., the USG after the water deprivation phase is between 1.012 and 1.030, or the osmolality is between 290 and 1100 mOsm/kg) and there is no response to exogenous ADH (no more than a 0.001–0.002 increase in USG or a 10% increase in osmolality), the test should be repeated after reinstatement of the renal medullary solute. Renal medullary solute is replaced by supplementing the diet with salt and by partially restricting water consumption for 3 days before the test is conducted. Consumption is restricted to 120 to 150 mL/kg the first day, 90 mL/kg the second day, and 60 mL/kg the day before the water deprivation test begins.[14] This procedure of partial water deprivation to reinstate renal medullary solute can be used in all cases for which a water deprivation test is performed, in order to make the results easier to interpret. However, partial restriction of water from animals with severe NDI or CDI for 3 days could lead to severe morbidity and perhaps death from dehydration, so the animal should be carefully evaluated. In addition, this procedure does not replace much of the medullary solute in patients with severe CDI or NDI.[14]

Desmopressin (DDAVP) Response Test

A more practical yet less accurate test is to treat an animal with PU/PD with synthetic vasopressin (DDAVP) and note the response. The owner should measure water consumption for 2 or 3 days and collect a urine sample at the same time every day for determinations of USG. DDAVP is given at a dose of 1 to 4 drops in the conjunctival sac twice daily for 5 to 7 days. The owner should continue to measure water consumption and collect urine for USG on days 5 through 7. If water consumption decreases and urine concentration increases markedly (>50%), the diagnosis of CDI is likely. Animals with NDI do not respond to DDAVP, and those with primary or psychogenic polydipsia may have only a mild reduction in water intake and urine output.[14]

Central Diabetes Insipidus

CDI leads to a primary polyuria with secondary polydipsia, caused by a partial or complete deficiency of ADH. There is no apparent sex or breed predisposition in dogs or cats. The disease can occur at any age, but most dogs are between 2 and 6 years of age at diagnosis. The average age in cats is 1.5 years.[14]

Pathophysiology

The metabolic defect with CDI is a partial or complete deficiency of ADH. Although most patients have idiopathic disease, known causes include head trauma, neoplasia, pituitary malformation, inflammation,[14, 16] and congenital, possibly familial disease.[17] Without ADH, the cells of the distal renal tubules and collecting ducts remain impermeable to water, and hypotonic urine is excreted, leading to primary polyuria. Polydipsia occurs to compensate for excessive urinary water loss. In patients with CDI caused by pituitary tumors, neurologic signs may occur from compression of other brain structures.

Clinical Signs

Clinical signs of CDI are primarily those of PU/PD. Some animals may be presented for what the owners believe is incontinence. Weight loss may occur in some patients because the desire to eat is reduced as a result of continuous water consumption. Some animals may vomit water after consuming large quantities. Patients with CDI caused by pituitary lesions such as tumors may have neurologic signs such as dementia, stupor, ataxia, seizures, and blindness (see Chaps. 24 and 25).[14, 16] Dehydration, sometimes severe, may be present if the animal's access to water has been limited.

Diagnostic Plan

The complete blood count and serum chemistries are usually unremarkable in cases of CDI. Some animals may have a reduced BUN value because of chronic polyuria. If the animal has not had access to sufficient water, azotemia may be present (increased BUN and creatinine), and serum sodium concentration may be elevated.[14, 16] USG is almost always hyposthenuric, often as low as 1.001 to 1.002.

The definitive diagnosis is based on failure to concentrate urine more than plasma (USG usually <1.006; osmolality <290–310 mOsm/kg) with water deprivation, with concentration (USG >1.010; increase in urine osmolality of 50% to 600%)[14] after exogenous administration of vasopressin (see Fig. 45–1). Animals with partial CDI have a USG of 1.008 to 1.020 after water deprivation (osmolality >290–310 mOsm/kg), with an increase in USG of 0.002 to 0.003 or more (10%–50% or greater increase in osmolality) after the administration of ADH.

Alternatively, the diagnosis of CDI is made by noting a marked reduction in urine volume and water consumption after 5 to 7 days of DDAVP administration in the conjunctival sac. Computed tomography of the skull may identify pituitary masses that are causing CDI.

Treatment

Replacement of ADH by administration of the synthetic vasopressin analog DDAVP has been used successfully in dogs and cats.[14, 18, 19] The dose is 1 to 4 drops (1.5–4.0 µg/drop) in the conjunctival sac twice daily. The dose may need to be as high as 20 µg twice daily in dogs to effectively reduce water consumption.[18] To prevent overhydration, it is suggested that access to water be limited for the first few hours after administration of the drug, because there may be a lag between the time urine begins to be concentrated and the time thirst is reduced. Also to prevent overhydration, it is recommended that the dose not be repeated on a regular schedule, but rather be repeated after mild PU/PD returns. This is to prevent accumulation with resultant overdosing of the drug, because the duration of activity may vary among patients. Most clients, however, are unwilling to follow those instructions and give the medication on a set schedule, without apparent problems.

For those dogs with pituitary masses identified on computed tomography, referral for radiation therapy may be indicated.[20]

Prognosis

The prognosis for animals with idiopathic or congenital disease is excellent for long-term survival with a normal lifespan as long as the owner is willing to manage the disease and can afford the expense of DDAVP. The expense of therapy is usually the most important prognostic factor. Patients with an expanding pituitary mass often develop neurologic signs within 0.5 to 5 months of diagnosis and die or are euthanized.[14, 16] Radiation therapy for these patients could potentially prolong life,[20] but the expense makes it prohibitive for most clients.

Uncommon Diseases of the Pituitary Gland

Psychogenic Polydipsia

Psychogenic or primary polydipsia is considered an uncommon behavioral disorder that has been recognized in dogs. The patients are often hyperactive, large dogs with a recent change in their environment such that exercise or human or animal contact is restricted. With water deprivation, they concentrate urine normally unless polydipsia is of sufficient duration to cause renal medullary solute washout. They have little response to ADH in the modified water deprivation test or to DDAVP in the desmopressin response test. If renal medullary solute washout is

suspected because they partially concentrated urine during a water deprivation test, the test can be repeated after partial water restriction for 3 days and addition of salt to the diet (see Diagnostic Procedures). Therapy includes gradual restriction of water intake, increasing exercise, adding another dog to the environment if the patient is alone, or keeping the dog in an environment where there is more human contact.[14]

Nephrogenic Diabetes Insipidus

Patients with NDI have PU/PD from a failure of the renal tubules to respond to ADH. It commonly occurs as an acquired disorder in dogs and cats as a result of pyometra, hyperadrenocorticism, hypoadrenocorticism, hypercalcemia, hypokalemia, hepatic insufficiency, pyelonephritis, hyperthyroidism, or acromegaly.[14] Rarely, NDI can occur as an idiopathic or congenital condition in dogs.[14, 21, 22] Most cases of acquired NDI can be diagnosed on the basis of the clinical signs, routine or special laboratory test results, and radiography or ultrasonography; these animals should not, therefore, be subjected to water deprivation testing. Animals with NDI do not respond to DDAVP in the desmopressin response test (see Diagnostic Procedures). These animals do not concentrate urine with water deprivation or when given exogenous ADH at the end of the water deprivation phase. Treating the underlying condition alleviates PU/PD in acquired cases. Therapy with chlorothiazide diuretics (20–40 mg/kg twice daily), along with salt restriction, paradoxically reduces polyuria in dogs with congenital NDI[21] by reducing renal sodium excretion.

Congenital Pituitary Dwarfism

Pituitary dwarfism occurs in dogs and cats as a result of malformation and dysfunction of the adenohypophysis. It occurs most frequently in German shepherds.[6, 9, 23–25] Deficiencies of ACTH, TSH, and gonadotropins also may occur concurrent with GH deficiency. Puppies and kittens often are normal until 3 to 4 months of age, when they lag behind littermates. They develop a "proportionate" reduction in size compared with the breed standard.[6, 9, 23–25]

Because of failure to develop primary hairs, pituitary dwarves retain a puppy hair coat, which with time is worn off, with resultant alopecia of the neck, trunk, and proximal limbs. Signs of secondary hypothyroidism and secondary hypoadrenocorticism may also develop. Diagnosis is based on signalment, clinical signs, ruling out of other causes of failure to grow and thrive (see previous discussion), and documentation of low basal GH concentration, with no response to stimulators of its release (e.g., clonidine, xylazine; see Diagnostic Procedures). Because there is presently no canine-specific GH assay available, measurement of somatomedin C (IGF-I) may be a useful alternative (see Diagnostic Procedures). Assay for endogenous ACTH, an ACTH stimulation test, and assay for thyroxine should all be performed to diagnose concurrent secondary hypoadrenocorticism, hypothyroidism, or both.

Therapy for pituitary dwarfism should include bovine or human synthetic GH, 0.1 IU/kg subcutaneously three times per week for 4 to 6 weeks.[9] Dogs may develop antibodies to human GH, which may limit its usefulness.[26] GH is extremely difficult to obtain. It may be obtained by contacting Dr. A.F. Parlow, Harbor-UCLA Medical Center, 1000 West Carson Street, Torrance, CA 90509.[27] Supplementation with thyroxine and cortisol is recommended for those patients with hypothyroidism and hypoadrenocorticism (see Chaps. 46 and 47).[9, 23–25]

Canine Acromegaly

Acromegaly occurs in dogs as a result of excessive GH secretion caused by hyperprogesteronemia in older bitches in the luteal phase of the estrus cycle, or as a result of exogenous administration of progesterones.[5, 28, 29] Most patients are females, 4 to 11 years old, presented for inspiratory stridor from excessive soft tissue in the oropharyngeal area, PU/PD, fatigue, abdominal enlargement, excessive skin folds, mammary tumors, or vaginal discharge. Increased interdental spaces may also be noted. There may be elevation of serum alkaline phosphatase and hyperglycemia that can progress to diabetes mellitus. Diagnosis is based on signalment and clinical signs and demonstration of increased serum values of somatomedin C (IGF-I; see Diagnostic Procedures).[10] For therapy, intact bitches should be spayed or administration of progesterone withdrawn. Patients with blood glucose concentrations consistently higher than 200 mg/dL should begin receiving insulin therapy. The need for treatment with insulin is often transient. Prognosis for recovery from the other signs of acromegaly is good once the source of excess progesterone is eliminated.[5, 9, 29]

Feline Acromegaly

Cats may rarely develop acromegaly from a GH-producing pituitary tumor. Most patients are males, 8 to 14 years old, and have insulin-resistant diabetes mellitus. Clinical signs commonly include PU/PD, cardiomegaly, hepatomegaly, heart murmur, renomegaly, renal failure, an enlarged head, weight gain, and an enlarged abdomen. Radiographs often reveal pleural effusion from heart failure, spondylosis, arthritis, and, rarely, mandibular enlargement. With routine laboratory testing, all patients are shown to have hyperglycemia. Hyperproteinemia, azotemia, hyperphosphatemia, hypercholesterolemia, and erythrocytosis are frequently present.[4, 11, 12] Diagnosis is based on clinical and routine laboratory signs, persistent increase in body size in spite of poorly controlled diabetes mellitus, ruling out of hyperadrenocorticism by an ACTH response test (see Chap. 46),[9] and documentation of an increased serum concentration of somatomedin C. (Published normal values for cats in two reports were 170–438 U/L and 510–610 U/L; see Diagnostic Procedures).[11, 12] Documentation of the presence of a pituitary mass by computed tomography of the skull also helps to make the diagnosis more certain. Radiation therapy may[9] or may not[30] be successful, but it is expensive. Palliative therapy includes large doses of insulin, often 20 to 130 U/day, and diuretics for heart failure. Without specific therapy for the tumor, the long-term prognosis is poor; however, with medical management cats live 4 to 42 months, with a mean of 22 months.[30]

Pituitary Neoplasia

Neoplasia of the pituitary gland occurs uncommonly in small animals, with the exception of ACTH-producing tumors in dogs, which cause pituitary-dependent hyperadrenocorticism (see Chap. 46).[31] Most pituitary tumors are chromophobe adenomas, but adenomas of acidophils and basophils also may occur. Nonfunctional primary tumors include craniopharyngiomas and astrocytomas, and metastatic tumors include mammary carcinomas, lymphosarcomas, and malignant melanomas.[32] Clinical signs include those caused by excess production of hormone in the case of chromophobe adenomas (hyperadrenocorticism), or by lack of hormone secretion (hypopituitarism) resulting from destruction of normal tissue, and neurologic signs such as behavioral changes, dementia, tetraparesis, nystagmus, seizures, facial paralysis, trigeminal paralysis, and blindness.[20, 33, 34] Response to radiation therapy is good with chromophobe adenomas.[20] Palliative therapy may include replacement of deficient hormones (i.e., cortisol, thyroxine, and ADH).

References

1. Hullinger RL. The endocrine system. In: Evans HE, ed. Miller's Anatomy of the Dog, 3rd ed. Philadelphia. WB Saunders, 1993:574–579.
2. Peterson ME, Randolph JF, Mooney CT. Endocrine diseases. In: Sherding RG, ed. The Cat: Diseases and Clinical Management, 2nd ed, vol 2. New York, Churchill Livingstone, 1994:1479–1481.

3. Stabenfeldt GH. The endocrine system. In: Cunningham, JG, ed. Textbook of Veterinary Physiology. Philadelphia, WB Saunders, 1992:378–386.

4. Peterson ME, Taylor RS, Greco DS, et al. Acromegaly in 14 cats. J Vet Intern Med 1990;4:192–201.

5. Eigenmann JE, Venker-van Haagen A. Progestagen-induced and spontaneous canine acromegaly due to reversible growth hormone overproduction: Clinical picture and prognosis. J Am Anim Hosp Assoc 1981;17:813–822.

6. Eigenmann JE, Zanesco S, Arnold U, et al. Growth hormone and insulin-like growth factor I in German shepherd dwarf dogs. Acta Endocrinol 1984;105:289–293.

7. Rijnberk A, van Herpen H, Mol JA, et al. Disturbed release of growth hormone in mature dogs: A comparison with congenital growth hormone deficiency. Vet Rec 1993;133:542–545.

8. Hampshire J, Altszuler N. Clonidine or xylazine as provocative tests for growth hormone secretion in the dog. Am J Vet Res 1981;42:1073–1076.

9. Feldman EC, Nelson RW. Disorders of growth hormone. In: Feldman EC, Nelson RW, eds. Canine and Feline Endocrinology and Reproduction, 2nd ed. Philadelphia, WB Saunders, 1996:38–66.

10. Eigenmann JE, Patterson DF, Zapf J, et al. Insulin-like growth factor I in the dog: A study in different dog breeds and in dogs with growth hormone elevation. Acta Endocrinol 1984;105:294–301.

11. Abrams-Ogg ACG, Holmberg DL, Stewart WA, et al. Acromegaly in a cat: Diagnsosis by magnetic resonance imaging and treatment by cryohypophysectomy. Can Vet J 1993;34:682–685.

12. Middleton DJ, Culvenor JA, Vasak E, et al. Growth hormone-producing pituitary adenoma, elevated serum somatomedin C concentration and diabetes mellitus in a cat. Can Vet J 1985;26:169–171.

13. Randolph JF, Miller CL, Cummings JF, et al. Delayed growth in two German shepherd dog littermates with normal serum concentrations of growth hormone, thyroxine, and cortisol. J Am Vet Med Assoc 1990;196:77–83.

14. Feldman EC, Nelson RW. Water metabolism and diabetes insipidus. In: Feldman EC, Nelson RW, eds. Canine and Feline Endocrinology and Reproduction, 2nd ed. Philadelphia, WB Saunders, 1996:2–37.

15. Mulnix JA, Rijnberk A, Hendriks HJ. Evaluation of a modified water-deprivation test for diagnosis of polyuric disorders in dogs. J Am Vet Med Assoc 1976;169:1327–1330.

16. Harb M, Nelson R, Feldman E, et al. Central diabetes insipidus (CDI) in 20 dogs. J Vet Intern Med 1994;8:161 (abstract).

17. Post K, McNeill JRJ, Clark EG, et al. Congenital central diabetes insipidus in two sibling Afghan hound pups. J Am Vet Med Assoc 1989;194:1086–1088.

18. Greene CE, Wong PL, Finco DR. Diagnosis and treatment of diabetes insipidus in two dogs using two synthetic analogs of antidiuretic hormone. J Am Anim Hosp Assoc 1979;15:371–377.

19. Kraus KH. The use of desmopressin in diagnosis and treatment of diabetes insipidus in cats. Compen Contin Educ Pract Vet 1987;9:751–758.

20. Dow SW, LeCouteur RA, Rosychuk RAW, et al. Response of dogs with functional pituitary macroadenomas and macrocarcinomas to radiation. J Small Anim Pract 1990;31:287–294.

21. Breitschwerdt EB, Verlander JW, Hribernik TN. Nephrogenic diabetes insipidus in three dogs. J Am Vet Med Assoc 1981;179:235–238.

22. Joles JA, Gruys E. Nephrogenic diabetes insipidus in a dog with renal medullary lesions. J Am Vet Med Assoc 1979;174:830–834.

23. DeBowes LJ. Pituitary dwarfism in a German shepherd puppy. Compen Contin Educ Pract Vet 1987;9:931–937.

24. Eigenmann JE. Diagnosis and treatment of dwarfism in a German shepherd dog. J Am Anim Hosp Assoc 1981;17:798–804.

25. Scott DW, Kirk RW, Hampshire J, et al. Clinicopathological findings in a German shepherd with a pituitary dwarfism. J Am Anim Hosp Assoc 1978;14:183–191.

26. Van Herpen H, Rijnberk A, Mol JA. Production of antibodies to biosynthetic human growth hormone in the dog. Vet Rec 1994;134:171.

27. Schmeitzel LP, Lothrop CD, Rosenkrantz WS. Congenital adrenal hyperplasia-like syndrome. In: Bonagura JD, ed. Kirk's Current Veterinary Therapy XII. Philadelphia, WB Saunders, 1995:600–604.

28. Rutteman GR, Stolp R, Rijnberk A, et al. Medroxyprogesterone acetate administration to ovariohysterectomized, oestradiol-primed beagle bitches: Effect on secretion of growth hormone, prolactin and cortisol. Acta Endocrinol 1987;114:275–282.

29. Rijnberk A, Eigenmann JE, Belshaw BE, et al. Acromagaly associated with transient overproduction of growth hormone in a dog. J Am Vet Med Assoc 1980;177:534–537.

30. Peterson M, Taylor R, Greco D, et al. Acromegaly in 14 cats. J Vet Intern Med 1990;4:192–201.

31. Nelson RW, Ihle SL, Feldman EC. Pituitary macroadenomas and macroadenocarcinomas in dogs treated with mitotane for pituitary-dependent hyperadrenocorticism: 13 cases (1981–1986). J Am Vet Med Assoc 1989;194:1612–1617.

32. Nichols R, Thompson L. Pituitary-hypothalamic disease. In: Ettinger SJ, Feldman EC, eds. Textbook of Veterinary Internal Medicine, 4th ed. Philadelphia, WB Saunders, 1995:1422–1436.

33. Allison RMM, Watson ADJ, Church DB. Pituitary tumor causing neurological and endocrine disturbances in a dog. J Small Anim Pract 1983;24:229–236.

34. Sarfaty D, Carrillo JM, Peterson ME. Neurologic, endocrinologic, and pathologic findings associated with large pituitary tumors in dogs: Eight cases (1976–1984). J Am Vet Med Assoc 1988;193:854–856.

Chapter 46

Diseases of the Adrenal Gland

William E. Monroe

Anatomy

The adrenal glands are two small, bilaterally symmetrical, tan to yellow organs located cranial to the kidneys in the retroperitoneal space.[1, 2] They are divided into a cortex and a medulla, which produce different hormones and function independently. The width of the gland is made up mostly of the cortex,[2] which comprises three layers, or zones: the outer layer, zona glomerulosa, produces mineralocorticoids; the middle layer, zona fasciculata, is the major producer of glucocorticoids; and the innermost layer, zona reticularis, is a minor producer of glucocorticoids and weak or minor sex hormones.[1, 2] The zona glomerulosa is also referred to as the zona arcuata in carnivores because the cells are arranged in arcades or curved cords.[3] The adrenal medulla is composed of modified neuronal cells that are analogous to postganglionic neurons and secrete catecholamines.[4]

The left adrenal gland is adjacent to the aorta, and the right is bounded medially by the caudal vena cava. Each gland is bisected ventrally by its respective phrenicoabdominal vein. Caudally, each gland is adjacent to its respective renal artery. Because of the proximity to these blood vessels and the fact that there is usually ample fat surrounding the glands, surgical resection of the adrenal glands is a challenge.[2, 5]

Physiology

Corticosteroids are a product of cholesterol metabolism. They are metabolized and conjugated in the liver and probably excreted primarily in urine in dogs[6] and in bile in cats.[2]

The major glucocorticoid secreted in the body is cortisol (hydrocortisone); lesser amounts of corticosterone are secreted. These two hormones primarily have glucocorticoid activity but also have a small amount of mineralocorticoid action. Glucocorticoids have multiple effects on metabolism. They increase gluconeogenesis in liver, with a net increase in hepatic glycogen. In addition, glucocorticoids decrease peripheral utilization of glucose, antagonizing the effects of insulin. Glucocorticoids cause protein catabolism by increasing amino acid mobilization from all cells except those of the liver and brain. This provides a ready supply for gluconeogenesis yet leads to a negative nitrogen balance and muscle wasting in conditions of glucocorticoid excess. The effects of glucocorticoids on lipid metabolism are to increase lipolysis and to mobilize fatty acids.

Glucocorticoids are very important for allowing an animal to cope with almost any form of stress.[1, 6] How glucocorticoids aid in stress is unknown. One supposition is that their enhancement of gluconeogenesis, glycogenolysis, and lipolysis increases energy and

protein substrate for damaged cells. Their permissive effects, which enhance certain humoral immune responses and increase the pressor activities of vasoactive substances such as norepinephrine, may also be involved.[7] Glucocorticoids increase renal excretion of water by inhibiting secretion of antidiuretic hormone; by enhancing the production, secretion, and activity of atrial natriuretic factor; and by increasing glomerular filtration.[7]

The major stimulus for glucocorticoid secretion is the release of adrenocorticotropic hormone (ACTH) from the anterior pituitary gland in response to secretion of corticotropin-releasing hormone (CRH) from the hypothalamus. CRH is released in response to almost any type of physical or emotional stress. Cortisol secretion is controlled by a classic negative feedback effect of cortisol on the hypothalamus and by a direct effect on the pituitary gland to inhibit the secretions of CRH and ACTH, respectively.[1, 6] Although ACTH and cortisol concentrations fluctuate throughout the day in dogs[8] and cats,[2, 9] there does not appear to be a circadian rhythm, as there is in humans.

The major mineralocorticoid secreted is aldosterone, although cortisol and corticosterone also account for a small amount of mineralocorticoid activity. The major functions of aldosterone are to maintain electrolyte balance and extracellular water volume. Aldosterone increases renal retention of sodium and increases potassium secretion. It also has a minor effect of increasing renal tubular hydrogen ion secretion.[1, 6] Aldosterone has similar effects on sweat and salivary glands and increases sodium absorption from the intestines, particularly the colon.[6]

In contrast to glucocorticoids, aldosterone secretion is not under the primary regulation of the pituitary gland and ACTH. The major stimuli for aldosterone secretion are increased extracellular fluid potassium ion concentration by a direct effect on the adrenal cortex and decreased blood pressure through the renin-angiotensin system. In response to decreased blood pressure, the juxtaglomerular cells in the kidney produce renin, an enzyme that acts on the circulating protein angiotensinogen to produce angiotensin I. Angiotensin I is further metabolized by angiotensin-converting enzyme to angiotensin II, which stimulates the adrenal gland to produce aldosterone and is a powerful vasopressor, causing peripheral vasoconstriction (see Chap. 16). A minor stimulus for aldosterone secretion is a reduced extracellular sodium ion concentration, which leads to an increase in renin secretion by the juxtaglomerular apparatus and subsequent increase in aldosterone secretion through the renin-angiotensin system.[1, 6] Physiologic concentrations of ACTH have a very minor stimulatory effect on the adrenal gland to increase mineralocorticoid secretion.[6]

Sympathetic preganglionic neurons originating from the spinal cord synapse directly on the adrenal medullary cells, stimulating them to secrete norepinephrine (20%) and epinephrine (80%) directly into the blood stream. Secretion from the adrenal medulla results in a prolonged (5–10 minutes) sympathetic-like effect, including constriction of most blood vessels, increased strength and rate of cardiac contraction, gastrointestinal (GI) inhibition, mydriasis, and increased metabolic rate.[4]

Problem Identification

Bilaterally Symmetrical Alopecia

Bilateral alopecia is partial or complete loss of hair in a generalized manner so that both sides of the body are affected equally. For the sake of this discussion, it is more narrowly defined to include only those cases in which alopecia is acquired and occurs as the initial problem without evidence of pruritus or other secondary or primary lesions such as pustules, crusts, excoriations, or bullae that could have led to hair loss as a secondary event.

Pathophysiology

In cats, bilateral alopecia without evidence of self-induced trauma to the skin can be associated with the cat's chewing or licking the hair off. Because cats are such private animals, chewing of fur may go unnoticed by the owner. In dogs, if alopecia is secondary to chewing or pruritus there almost always are lesions evident on the skin consistent with self-induced trauma, such as erythema, excoriations, and broken hairs, or at least historical information from the owner to indicate that the dog is pruritic.

Common endocrine disorders such as hypothyroidism and hyperadrenocorticism lead to alopecia by their effects on metabolism and alterations in the hair cycle. Typically, follicular atrophy is observed histologically in skin biopsies from animals with endocrine alopecias.[10] Adult-onset hyposomatotropism and sex steroid imbalances (e.g., hyperestrogenism in male dogs with Sertoli cell tumors, adrenal sex steroid imbalance) lead to alopecia by similar mechanisms. Animals with inherited alopecias such as pattern baldness or follicular dysplasia have alopecia from a defect in or failure of the formation of the hair follicles.

Clinical Signs

Dogs and cats with bilateral alopecia may be presented early, when there is thinning of the coat with an unkempt or rough, dry, lusterless appearance. As disease progresses, there may be a complete loss of hair, which for most causes of bilateral alopecia is most severe on the trunk, sparing the head and extremities.[10] Hyperpigmentation may occur secondary to hair loss because of greater exposure to light, or it may be associated with the cause of alopecia.[11] Some causes of alopecia may also predispose to lichenification, seborrhea, and secondary infections that may lead to pruritus. Depending on the cause, other clinical signs may also be apparent (see next section).

Diagnostic Plan

The history is very important when attempting to solve the problem of bilaterally symmetrical alopecia. It should be determined whether alopecia occurred without or at least before the onset of pruritus or evidence of infection such as pyoderma or excoriations. In general, acquired alopecia without pruritus that is not secondary to inflammatory lesions is caused by an endocrinopathy. The signalment is very important. Naturally occurring hyperadrenocorticism usually is seen in late middle-aged or older dogs. Hypothyroidism is most common in middle-aged to older dogs as well. Uncommon disorders such as adult-onset hyposomatotropism and adrenal sex hormone imbalance usually begin when the dog is 1 to 2 years of age. These two syndromes (if they are different syndromes) are also most common in the Pomeranian, chow chow, keeshond, and Samoyed breeds.[10]

The distribution of the alopecia should also be considered. Hyperadrenocorticism and hypothyroidism usually cause alopecia that begins at pressure points (e.g., lateral thighs) and progresses to the trunk, including the abdomen and dorsum. Alopecia from sex hormonal imbalances often begins around the perineum and may progress to the flanks and trunk. Changes in the genitalia (e.g., testicular mass, pendulous prepuce, enlarged nipples) are also seen with alopecia caused by Sertoli cell tumor in the male dog.[10]

Because cats with bilaterally symmetrical alopecia can be chewing off the hair without the owner's knowledge and without other apparent lesions in the skin itself, it is important to roll the skin between the fingers to observe for short hairs. If a normal number of hairs are present but are broken off very close to the skin, the cause is probably self-induced trauma rather than an endocrine or metabolic disorder (which would cause hairs to fall out), and psychogenic alopecia should be considered. Hairs shed or plucked from the affected areas should also be examined under a microscope to look for evidence of breakage where they were chewed or licked off (see Chap. 1).[12]

Because parasites such as *Demodex* or dermatophytosis can also cause alopecia (although usually not bilaterally symmetrical alopecia) with few other lesions, it is important to perform skin scrapings, Wood lamp examination, and dermatophyte cultures (see

Chap. 1). If these are negative, the other clinical signs should be considered and a routine laboratory database obtained, including a complete blood count (CBC), chemistry profile, and urinalysis. A dog with alopecia as well as polyuria and polydipsia (PU/PD) and a pendulous abdomen most likely has hyperadrenocorticism.[13] Changes in the laboratory data, such as a stress leukogram, elevated alkaline phosphatase (AP), and hyposthenuria, further suggest hyperadrenocorticism as the cause. With these signs present, the next step is to do an adrenal function test (i.e., ACTH stimulation testing; see Diagnostic Procedures). A dog with alopecia, lethargy, and mild anemia with hypercholesterolemia is more likely to have hypothyroidism. A resting thyroxine test, an endogenous thyroid-stimulating hormone (TSH) test, or best of all, a TSH stimulation test would be indicated in such a patient to confirm hypothyroidism.

If clinical signs, routine laboratory testing, and tests of adrenal and thyroid function are normal, the less common causes of bilateral alopecia, such as sex steroid imbalances and adult-onset hyposomatotropism (adrenal sex steroid imbalance), should be considered. Skin biopsy at this time may be helpful but may only suggest an endocrine dermatosis. Inherited conditions such as follicular dysplasia are diagnosed by skin biopsy.[14] Because growth hormone assays are not available and measurement of sex steroid hormones is not often helpful in diagnosing most sex steroid imbalances as the cause of alopecia, a presumptive clinical diagnosis may be the best the clinician can do, taking into account the history, signalment, other clinical signs, and exclusion of adrenal and thyroid disease.

Hyponatremia

Hyponatremia is a reduction of the serum or plasma concentration of sodium below the reference range for the laboratory used (usually <140 mEq/L).

Pathophysiology

Hyponatremia can occur if an animal's ability to excrete water in excess of solute such as sodium (free water) is reduced; if water containing sodium is lost from the body by urinary, insensible (panting), or GI routes; or by a combination of these two mechanisms. If fluid losses are replaced by ingested or parenteral fluid with a relatively lower sodium concentration than that which was lost, hyponatremia is exacerbated. Hyponatremia can therefore occur with an increased, decreased, or normal total body sodium content.[15]

Pseudohyponatremia is caused by the presence of substances that displace the aqueous portion of plasma (i.e., lipid or protein). Because sodium exists only in the aqueous phase of serum or plasma, analytic

methods (e.g., flame photometry, indirect potentiometry) that measure sodium in the whole sample rather than in the aqueous phase underestimate the sodium concentration.[15]

Hyponatremia associated with a high concentration of another osmotically active substance (as in hyperglycemia or administration of mannitol) is caused by fluid shifting into the vascular space. The concentration of sodium is diluted by the movement of water into the intravascular compartment.[15]

The multiple other "pathologic" causes of hyponatremia involve excess consumption (i.e., psychogenic polydipsia) or administration of hypotonic fluids, failure of the kidney to excrete sufficient free water, or a combination of excessive loss of sodium with reduced renal excretion of free water.

If hyponatremia is present in association with congestive heart failure or the nephrotic syndrome, the effective circulating vascular volume is reduced. This stimulates ADH secretion, which causes retention of (or failure to excrete) free water by the kidneys, which, in turn, dilutes the plasma sodium concentration even though there is a whole-body sodium excess. In addition, the renin-angiotensin system is stimulated, which increases the proportion of sodium and water in the glomerular filtrate that is reabsorbed in the proximal portion of the renal tubules. This, along with a decrease in renal perfusion, which reduces glomerular filtration rate, leads to a reduced amount of sodium and water that reaches the distal renal tubules, where solute normally is reabsorbed in excess of water. When less sodium and water reach the distal nephron, less free water can be formed and excreted. Hyponatremia may occur in severe renal failure because of a severe reduction in glomerular filtration, which leads to an absolute reduction in the volume of water available for excretion that actually reaches the distal diluting tubule, in combination with tubular failure to reabsorb sodium.[15]

Diseases that are associated with fluid and electrolyte loss, such as GI disease (i.e., vomiting and diarrhea) or hypoadrenocorticism, lead to hyponatremia because hypovolemia stimulates the mechanisms just described that occur from reduction of the effective circulating intravascular volume. Loss of sodium from the body in these conditions also contributes to hyponatremia.[15]

Clinical Signs

The clinical signs of hyponatremia depend on the speed of onset and the underlying cause. If the condition develops slowly, particularly in those cases associated with excessive sodium loss, there may be no clinical signs other than those caused by hypovolemia and dehydration (i.e., decreased skin turgor, enophthalmos, cool extremities, and eventually shock). If hyponatremia occurs abruptly, as in acute water intoxication, cerebral edema can occur, resulting in lethargy, nausea, vomiting, coma, and death.[15] For those cases associated with increased vascular volume (e.g., severe liver disease, heart failure), clinical signs may include ascites, pleural effusion, pulmonary edema, or peripheral edema. Because multiple diseases may lead to hyponatremia, there may be other signs consistent with the underlying disorder.

Diagnostic Plan

If hyponatremia is noted on a serum chemistry profile, the first thing to do is to determine whether lipemia was noted on the report or is evident in the sample. If either case is true, the hyponatremia may be factitious if the assay was performed with the use of flame photometry or indirect potentiometry. The next step is to consider the history. Infusion of mannitol causes hyponatremia by fluid shifting and displacement, with a high plasma osmolality if measured. Psychogenic polydipsia, administration of hypotonic fluids, or use of diuretics may lead to hyponatremia. A history of vomiting or diarrhea may explain hyponatremia by excessive loss. Consideration of the physical examination may then make third-space causes of fluid loss leading to hyponatremia apparent—that is, pancreatitis, peritonitis, uroabdomen, or congestive heart failure.[15]

Further evaluation of the serum chemistry profile may elucidate other causes of hyponatremia. Severe hyperglycemia can cause hyponatremia by fluid shifting. The sodium can be "corrected" by adding 1.6 mEq/L to the measured value for every 100 mg/dL the glucose exceeds normal.[15] Severe hyperproteinemia (>10 g/dL)[15] can cause pseudohyponatremia with some methods of analyzing sodium (as with lipemia, already discussed). Increases in blood urea nitrogen (BUN) and creatinine with inadequate urinary concentration (see Chap. 16) and possibly pyuria or cylindruria on the urinalysis may rule in advanced renal failure as the cause of hyponatremia.[15] If hyperkalemia is present along with hyponatremia such that the sodium/potassium ratio is less than 27:1, often with evidence of azotemia, hypoadrenocorticism should be considered and confirmed with an ACTH response test (see Diagnostic Procedures). If the albumin is decreased, a urinalysis and possibly a urinary protein/creatinine ratio should be evaluated to ascertain the presence of protein-losing nephropathy and the nephrotic syndrome as a cause of hyponatremia. With nephrotic syndrome, peripheral edema and elevation of serum cholesterol also often occur. Hypoalbuminemia and hyponatremia may be caused by protein-losing nephropathy or by panhypoproteine-

mia and diarrhea, which may indicate protein-losing enteropathy as the cause.

Hyperkalemia

Hyperkalemia is an increase in the serum or plasma potassium concentration above the reference range for the laboratory. In general it is a value greater than 5 mEq/L.

Pathophysiology

Most potassium in the body exists intracellularly. The primary route of excretion for potassium is renal, and it is under the control of aldosterone, which increases renal tubular secretion.[16] Serum potassium can be "pathologically" increased by excessive intake (usually iatrogenic); by decreased renal excretion, as with anuric renal failure or postrenal azotemia; by hypoaldosteronism or a failure of the renal tubules to respond to aldosterone; or by a shifting of potassium from the intracellular to the extracellular space as a result of acidosis.[17]

The deleterious effects of hyperkalemia are mediated by an increase in resting membrane potential. This reduces the strength of the action potential, slowing conduction and thereby reducing neuromuscular activity throughout the body, particularly the heart.[17]

Clinical Signs

The primary clinical signs of hyperkalemia (usually not present until potassium concentration is >7.5 mEq/L) are muscular weakness, reduced cardiac output, and cardiac arrhythmias.[17] If the potassium concentration exceeds 6.5 mEq/L, the T waves on the electrocardiogram become peaked. As the potassium concentration increases, the P waves are reduced and eventually disappear, the P-R interval becomes prolonged, the QRS complex is prolonged or widened, the R-wave amplitude is reduced, and bradycardia (often profound) occurs frequently.[17, 18]

Diagnostic Plan

The initial step when presented with an animal with hyperkalemia is to make sure that the laboratory value is not factitious. If clinical signs are not consistent with hyperkalemia, the analysis should be repeated before therapy or further diagnostic steps are undertaken. An electrocardiogram (ECG) can help determine if hyperkalemia is truly present (see previous discussion), but the ECG changes are not always present. With dry chemistry methods, hemolysis can artifactually increase measured potassium concentration.[19] Extreme leukocytosis (>100,000 cells/μL) or thrombocytosis (>600,000–1,000,000 cells/μL) may artifactually increase the measured serum potassium.[17, 20] Factitious hyperkalemia can occur in samples from Akitas if the serum or plasma is not removed promptly from the red blood cells (RBCs), because these dogs have higher potassium concentrations than other breeds in their RBCs, and the potassium may leak out with time.[21]

If factitious hyperkalemia is ruled out, the clinician should carefully review the history to rule out iatrogenic causes such as overadministration in parenteral fluids or the use of other drugs that may lead to hyperkalemia (e.g., potassium citrate, potassium-sparing diuretics).[17] A history of trauma or dysuria may suggest postrenal azotemia as the cause of the hyperkalemia. Physical evidence of postrenal azotemia includes a distended abdomen with a ballotable fluid wave, a large, distended bladder, and calculi or other swellings in the urethra externally or on rectal palpation. If azotemia is severe and urine output is poor or absent after rehydration, anuric or oliguric renal failure may be the cause.

Further evaluation of the blood chemistry results may help to determine the cause of hyperkalemia. If there is evidence of severe acidosis such as decreased bicarbonate or carbon dioxide, it may cause hyperkalemia as a result of shifting of potassium out of cells as hydrogen ions move in. However, the most common causes of acidosis in animals, those involving an increased anion gap (i.e., ketoacidosis, lactic acidosis) or renal failure, rarely cause shifting of potassium severe enough to significantly increase the plasma concentration.[17] If hyperkalemia occurs with low sodium (with or without mild to moderate azotemia) and the sodium/potassium ratio is less than 27:1, hypoadrenocorticism (Addison's disease) or primary GI diseases such as parvoviral diarrhea, whipworms, salmonellosis, or ruptured duodenal ulcers should be considered as the cause of hyperkalemia. Vomiting and diarrhea are usually much more prominent with primary GI disorders than with hypoadrenocorticism.[22] An ACTH response test is then indicated to rule out other causes and rule in hypoadrenocorticism.

Episodic Weakness or Collapse

Weakness is very common with hypoadrenocorticism. It can be episodic initially, or it can appear to be episodic if the animal is treated with steroids or fluids (or both) at each occurrence. Other causes of episodic weakness include metabolic disorders such as hypoglycemia (which may also play a role in the episodic weakness of hypoadrenocorticism), cardiac arrhythmias or failure, neuromuscular disorders such as myasthenia gravis, and periodic internal hemorrhage from a vascular tumor such as hemangiosarcoma. A more complete discussion of weakness is found in Chapters 9 and 28.

Azotemia

Azotemia from hypoadrenocorticism is usually mild but can be moderate to severe. Because the mechanism of azotemia with Addison's disease is prerenal (hypovolemia), the urine specific gravity is expected to be concentrated (>1.035 in dogs; >1.045 in cats). However, some dogs with hypoadrenocorticism have urine specific gravities in the range of minimal concentration (<1.035),[23] creating the appearance of renal failure. With hormonal therapy, their ability to concentrate urine returns. Dogs with azotemia secondary to hypoadrenocorticism respond to fluid therapy rapidly (1–2 days), but azotemia recurs within a few days after withdrawal of therapy. Dogs with recurrent azotemia that responds readily to fluid therapy should be suspected of having hypoadrenocorticism.[24] See Chapter 16 for a complete discussion of azotemia.

Bradycardia

Because severe hyperkalemia of any cause, including that associated with hypoadrenocorticism, alters resting membrane potential and neuromuscular conduction, bradycardia, other arrhythmias, and ECG changes are often noted.[6] The ECG changes usually do not occur until the potassium concentration is greater than 6.5 mEq/L, and they progressively worsen as the concentration increases.[17] The ECG abnormalities include reduced P waves that eventually disappear, prolonged P-R interval, widened QRS complexes, reduced R-wave amplitude, bradycardia, and all degrees of heart block (see bradyarrhythmias in Chap. 10).[18, 24]

Polyuria and Polydipsia

PU/PD occurs in 85%[25–29] of dogs with hyperadrenocorticism and in about 25% of those with hypoadrenocorticism.[23, 24, 30, 31] Many other disorders can also lead to PU/PD, many of which are more common than adrenal disease (see Chap. 16). Among the other causes of PU/PD are renal failure, diabetes mellitus, liver disease, pyometra, hyperthyroidism, hypercalcemia, psychogenic polydipsia, central diabetes insipidus, nephrogenic diabetes insipidus, and hypokalemia.

Polyphagia

Owners seldom present animals for polyphagia itself, but it may become apparent during the history. Dogs with hyperadrenocorticism have polyphagia with weight gain, primarily in the abdomen with muscle wasting elsewhere. Polyphagia with weight gain may also occur in otherwise healthy animals because of gluttonous eating. Most other causes of polyphagia are associated with weight loss in spite of an increased appetite; these include GI parasites, pancreatic exocrine insufficiency, diabetes mellitus, hyperthyroidism, and less commonly, infiltrative bowel disease (see Chap. 47).

Increased Panting (Heat Intolerance)

Increased panting and heat intolerance can be a historical problem in dogs with hyperadrenocorticism. It may occur because of abdominal distention from the typical fat deposition and hepatomegaly often present with hyperadrenocorticism (which applies pressure on the thorax, thereby reducing compliance) or from a direct effect of excessive steroids on the brain. Uncommonly, dogs with hyperadrenocorticism are presented in acute respiratory distress from pulmonary thromboembolism.[13]

Elevated Serum Alkaline Phosphatase

Serum AP is elevated in 86% of dogs with hyperadrenocorticism.[27] The steroid-induced isoenzyme produced by the liver makes up the majority of the increased AP. The increase is usually severe. Although bone disease can lead to increases in serum AP, it is usually mild in comparison. Biliary stasis can cause elevations of AP (see Chap. 34) similar to those seen with hyperadrenocorticism, as can therapy with anticonvulsants such as phenobarbital or primidone.[32]

Diagnostic Procedures

Routine Laboratory Evaluation

With hyperadrenocorticism in dogs, there may be a stress leukogram (mature neutrophilia, lymphopenia, eosinopenia, and monocytosis); with hypoadrenocorticism, there may be no stress leukogram when one would be expected.

The serum chemistry profile is usually what makes the clinician initially suspect hypoadrenocorticism; it reveals hyponatremia, hyperkalemia (sodium/potassium ratio <27:1), and azotemia. Moderate to severe elevation of serum AP is commonly seen with hyperadrenocorticism, as is hypercholesterolemia.

The urinalysis (particularly specific gravity) is always helpful to sort out causes of azotemia (as seen with hypoadrenocorticism). Changes in the sediment (e.g., casts) may be more consistent with renal disease than adrenal disease, but proteinuria and pyuria may be seen often with hyperadrenocorticism, perhaps secondary to urinary tract infection from immunosuppression.

Radiography

Thoracic and abdominal radiographs may be useful for diagnosing adrenal gland disease in dogs and cats. Abdominal radiography may reveal he-patomegaly or an adrenal mass (often calcified) in dogs with hyperadrenocorticism. Nonspecific changes in thoracic radiographic anatomy may also be noted with hypoadrenocorticism (microcardia and small great vessels) or hyperadrenocorticism (bronchial wall mineralization). Abdominal ultrasound can be very useful to help identify adrenal tumors or, if both glands can be imaged, the bilateral hyperplasia seen with pituitary-dependent hyperadrenocorticism (PDH). For further discussion, see the section on clinical signs for each disease.

Specific Tests of Adrenal Function

Basal concentration of cortisol can be elevated in up to 35% of dogs with nonadrenal illness[33] and normal in dogs with hyperadrenocorticism.[33, 34] Stimulation or suppression tests are therefore always necessary to evaluate adrenal gland function. In general, all tests of adrenal function should start at a standard time in the morning, such as between 8 and 10 AM, unless the case circumstances dictate otherwise (e.g., hypoadrenal crisis). No other procedures should be done during adrenal function testing, and handling should be kept to a minimum.

ACTH Stimulation Test (Dogs)

The ACTH stimulation test is useful for evaluating adrenal gland function to diagnose hypoadrenocorticism and hyperadrenocorticism, whether iatrogenic or naturally occurring. It is also useful to monitor response to therapy in cases of hyperadrenocorticism. Although it is not the most sensitive test to identify hyperadrenocorticism, it is the most specific, meaning that it produces the fewest false-positive results in dogs with nonadrenal disease.[33, 35]

The ACTH stimulation test is positive (exaggerated response after ACTH) in about 85% of dogs with PDH[34] and in 33% to 60% of dogs with functional adrenal tumors (adrenal-dependent hyperadrenocorticism, or ADH).[34, 36–39] Because pituitary-dependent disease represents 85% of all cases of hyperadrenocorticism, the overall positive rate for dogs with hyperadrenocorticism is about 83%. Most dogs with hypoadrenocorticism have a low basal plasma cortisol concentration, with no response to exogenous ACTH administration. A normal basal concentration with a response to ACTH that is less than the reference range can be indicative of early or impending hypoadrenocorticism.[24]

Although several protocols have been described (Table 46–1),[38, 40] I prefer to draw a basal blood sample for cortisol concentration by radioimmunoassay (RIA) after the animal has been fasted for 12 hours, and to give 2.2 U/kg of porcine ACTH extract (H.P. Acthar Gel) intramuscularly, with a second blood sample

Table 46–1
Protocols for ACTH Stimulation Testing

PRODUCT	ROUTE	DOSE	SAMPLING TIMES
ACTH gel*	Intramuscular	2.2 U/kg	0 and 120 min
ACTH gel	Intramuscular	20 U/dog	0 and 120 min
Cortrosyn†	Intramuscular	0.25 mg/ dog	0 and 60 min

*Porcine ACTH extract (H.P. Acthar Gel).
†Synthetic ACTH (Cortrosyn).
Data from references 38 and 40.

taken at 2 hours after the injection. Blood samples can be placed in a clot tube, heparin tube, or ethylenediaminetetra-acetic acid (EDTA) tube, and serum or plasma withdrawn after centrifugation. The clinician should follow the protocol that the laboratory used to establish a reference range, including product used (porcine ACTH extract or synthetic ACTH [Cortrosyn]), route of administration, timing of samples, and type of tube for the blood sample. Cortisol appears to be stable even at room temperature for a few days,[41] so unless samples are to be mailed with a delivery time of several days, they do not need to be sent on ice.

Interpretation of results should be based on the reference ranges established by the laboratory for the species being tested and the protocol they recommend. Only laboratories that have established their own reference ranges should be used for hormonal testing. Because basal cortisol concentrations of normal dogs, dogs with hyperadrenocorticism, and those with nonadrenal disease overlap, the basal concentration is of little value other than to document that the animal actually received and absorbed the ACTH and to provide a check on the whole testing procedure.

Corticosteroid therapy (including topical steroid administration) affects the results of the ACTH stimulation test, depending on the dose and duration, but usually suppresses the cortisol response to ACTH as well as the basal concentration below the lower limits of the reference range.[42–44] Some exogenous steroids such as prednisolone are measured by the cortisol assay, so the basal cortisol concentration may be elevated if the drug has not been withdrawn for 24 to 48 hours before testing.

Dexamethasone Screening Test (Dogs)

The dexamethasone screening test (low-dose dexamethasone suppression test) has been used exten-

sively for the diagnosis of hyperadrenocorticism in dogs. It is of no value in the evaluation of iatrogenic hyperadrenocorticism or in monitoring of therapy for naturally occurring hyperadrenocorticism. Although it is more sensitive (85%–95%)[27, 34, 45] than the ACTH response test for diagnosing hyperadrenocorticism, it is less specific (44%–85%).[34, 45] In other words, it is positive for a greater number of patients that truly have hyperadrenocorticism than the ACTH stimulation test is, but it is falsely positive in a higher number of patients that do not have hyperadrenocorticism.

The protocol involves fasting the dog for 12 hours, drawing a blood sample for cortisol concentration (0 hour), then giving dexamethasone (sodium phosphate or in propylene glycol) at a dose of 0.01 mg/kg intravenously or 0.015 mg/kg intravenously or intramuscularly. Samples are then taken at 3 to 4 hours and at 8 hours after dexamethasone administration, the 8-hour sample being most important. The clinician should follow the recommended protocol that the laboratory used to establish the reference range for normal dogs.

A test result is considered positive if the cortisol concentration at 8 hours is not suppressed below the level considered normal by the laboratory. In general, this level is 1.0 to 1.4 mg/dL. The 3- to 4-hour sample is useful in some cases to distinguish PDH from ADH. As many as 30% to 50% of dogs with PDH may have the cortisol concentration at 3 to 4 hours suppressed to less than 50% of the baseline concentration,[27, 46] with a rebound by 8 hours, whereas only rarely will the cortisol concentration of those with ADH be so suppressed.[27, 45, 46]

Urinary Cortisol/Creatinine Ratio

The urinary cortisol/creatinine ratio has been used as a convenient, inexpensive, and practical screening test for the presence of hyperadrenocorticism.[45, 47–49] Although it is a very sensitive test, it lacks specificity and may frequently be falsely positive in dogs with PU/PD[47] or other moderate to severe nonadrenal diseases.[47, 48] However, if cases are selected for testing strictly on the basis of the presence of clinical signs of hyperadrenocorticism, without clinical signs of nonadrenal disease, the specificity may be acceptable.[45] Yet, because the urinary cortisol/creatinine ratio is a screening test, requiring further adrenal function testing to definitively diagnose hyperadrenocorticism, and because an ACTH stimulation test is only moderately more expensive and time-consuming, has greater specificity, and is valuable to have as a baseline before starting therapy for hyperadrenocorticism, I prefer to use the ACTH stimulation test for initial evaluation of adrenal function.

Tests to Differentiate Pituitary-Dependent From Adrenal-Dependent Hyperadrenocorticism

High-Dose Dexamethasone Suppression Test

The high-dose dexamethasone suppression test differentiates PDH from ADH in most cases. The negative feedback threshold of glucocorticoid on the hypothalamus and pituitary is increased in PDH, and, in most cases, a low dose of dexamethasone is not sufficient to suppress endogenous cortisol production. A high dose of dexamethasone exceeds that threshold level in most cases by enough so that the endogenous cortisol concentration is reduced. About 85% of dogs with PDH have their endogenous cortisol suppressed after administration of high-dose dexamethasone,[27, 50, 51] but virtually no dogs with adrenal tumors do so.[27, 50, 51] However, because 15% of dogs with PDH do not have their cortisol suppressed by high-dose dexamethasone, failure to suppress is inconclusive.

The most reliable definition of suppression is controversial, but my preference is to use suppression to less than 50% of the basal concentration as the criterion.[50, 51] If the clinician chooses to use an absolute value to define suppression, he or she should use the value determined by the laboratory that performs the cortisol testing.[27]

Although one should follow the protocol suggested by the laboratory doing the testing, it usually involves fasting the animal for 12 hours, taking a blood sample for basal cortisol, and then administering 0.1 mg/kg dexamethasone intravenously.[50] Samples for serum or plasma cortisol are taken at 3 to 4 and at 8 hours after the administration of dexamethasone. These times are suggested because some dogs have their cortisol reduced at 3 to 4 hours, with escape from suppression at 8 hours, and others have their cortisol suppressed to its lowest at 8 hours.[27]

Endogenous ACTH Concentration

Although published reports describe the endogenous ACTH concentration as the most reliable test to discriminate PDH from ADH,[50, 51] I have not found it to be as reliable as reported. It is also less practical because it is generally considered to require special handling of the samples. Before ACTH is administered for an ACTH stimulation test, or dexamethasone for a dexamethasone screening test, a sample is taken in a siliconized EDTA tube or heparinized polypropylene plastic tube and centrifuged immediately (preferably in a refrigerated centrifuge). The plasma sample should be removed from the RBCs immediately after centrifugation, placed in a polypropylene plastic tube, frozen, and shipped overnight on dry ice.

The Endocrine Diagnostic Laboratory at Auburn University (P.O. Box 2148, Auburn, Alabama) offers an assay for endogenous ACTH using a special preservative (aprotinin), which is provided in "ACTH submission kits," that reduces the need for special handling other than centrifuging and removing the plasma from the red cells, freezing the plasma sample, and sending it on ice packs in an insulated container (also provided in the kit) by overnight mail.

It is best to use the criteria established by the laboratory that performs the assay to determine the conclusions of the test. Published criteria are as follows: endogenous ACTH less than 20 pg/mL indicates ADH, ACTH less than 40 pg/mL but greater than 20 pg/mL is inconclusive, and ACTH higher than 40 pg/mL indicates PDH.[50]

Combined Dexamethasone Suppression/ACTH Stimulation Test

A combined dexamethasone suppression/ACTH stimulation test has been used to diagnose the presence of hyperadrenocorticism and differentiate between PDH and ADH with a single test procedure.[52] I prefer to use individual tests, separated by at least 3 days, because the individual components of the combined test may not be as sensitive as when the tests are performed alone.[51, 53] Also, administration of dexamethasone may variably affect the results of ACTH testing, depending on the dose given and the time elapsed between dexamethasone administration and ACTH testing.[54, 55]

Common Diseases of the Adrenal Gland

Canine Hyperadrenocorticism

Hyperadrenocorticism is overproduction (or exogenous administration) of glucocorticoids such that a clinical syndrome produced by the deleterious effects of excessive glucocorticoids is apparent. Cushing's disease in humans is defined as hyperadrenocorticism associated with a pituitary tumor. The spectrum of clinical signs caused by the effects of excessive glucocorticoids is termed Cushing's syndrome, no matter the cause.[13] About 80% to 85% of canine patients with naturally occurring hyperadrenocorticism are pituitary dependent (PDH, overproduction of ACTH), and 15% to 20% of cases of hyperadrenocorticism are caused by functional adrenal tumors (ADH). Iatrogenic hyperadrenocorticism is also seen commonly.

Hyperadrenocorticism is one of the most common endocrinopathies diagnosed in dogs. It is considered to occur frequently,[13] although the prevalence in dogs admitted to veterinary institutions for all reasons may be only 0.1%.[56]

Hyperadrenocorticism is most commonly seen in older dogs. The majority (90%) of patients with either PDH or ADH are between 4 and 14 years old, with the peak of occurrence at ages 7 to 9 years.[29, 56, 57] Dogs with ADH tend to be slightly older, with a mean age of about 11 years.[38, 39, 58] Although there is no difference in the overall incidence of hyperadrenocorticism between males and females, females are more likely to have ADH (63%–68% of patients are female).[38, 39, 58]

Hyperadrenocorticism in general is seen most commonly in small breeds (miniature poodle, dachshund, Boston terrier, silky terrier),[29, 56, 57] although almost any breed can be affected. A higher proportion (about 50%) of dogs with ADH than those with PDH weigh more than 20 kg.[38, 39, 58] Hyperadrenocorticism is rare in cats (see Uncommon Diseases of the Adrenal Gland).

Pathophysiology

Many cases of hyperadrenocorticism or Cushing's syndrome are iatrogenically caused by overadministration of glucocorticoids. Naturally occurring cases are caused by endogenous overproduction of glucocorticoids. Although the basal cortisol concentration at any time is often not in excess of that in normal dogs, dogs with hyperadrenocorticism may not have the normal fluctuations in secretion, and their total daily secretion of cortisol is in excess compared to that of normal dogs.[59] The majority of naturally occurring cases (80%–85%)[25, 26, 50] are caused by overproduction of ACTH, with resultant bilateral adrenal hyperplasia and excessive production of cortisol. Most of these PDH patients (85%–90%) have a functional pituitary tumor,[60, 61] although some tumors may arise secondary to pituitary corticotrophic hyperplasia as a result of excessive stimulation from the hypothalamus.[61] This mechanism of excessive stimulation of the pituitary, possibly from a failure of negative feedback, is the theorized cause of the other naturally occurring 15% to 20% of cases of PDH.

This 15% to 20% of cases of naturally occurring hyperadrenocorticism are ADH, caused by a functional adrenocortical tumor.[25, 26, 50] Sixty percent of functional adrenocortical tumors are adenocarcinoma, and 40% are adenoma.[36, 38, 39, 58] Almost all adrenal tumors are unilateral,[39] with atrophy of the contralateral adrenal cortex from negative feedback on ACTH secretion. Rarely, bilateral adrenocortical neoplasia is seen.[39, 62]

The presence of excessive glucocorticoids has multiple effects on the body. Glucocorticoids lead to diuresis and polyuria, with a resultant polydipsia because they inhibit the actions of vasopressin on renal tubules and increase the glomerular filtration rate.[1] The protein catabolic effect of glucocorticoids is responsible for muscle wasting and weakness[1, 6] and probably contributes to the pendulous abdomen seen in cases of hyperadrenocorticism from weakening of the abdominal muscles.

Glucocorticoids have profound effects on glucose metabolism. They cause increased gluconeogenesis and deposition of glycogen in the liver,[1, 6] which often leads to hepatomegaly, that can be profound and may contribute to the pendulous abdomen. Dogs with hyperadrenocorticism have insulin resistance as well as increased hepatic production of glucose,[63] which is responsible for the hyperglycemia that is noted in some cases. Cortisol-induced insulin resistance is the reason for difficult control of hyperglycemia in the rare case in which diabetes mellitus and hyperadrenocorticism occur together.[64] Glucocorticoids lead to lipolysis from fatty acid mobilization,[1, 6] which may contribute to loss of peripheral body mass and hypercholesterolemia. Although lipolysis is stimulated, there often is excess abdominal fat in dogs with hyperadrenocorticism. This is probably caused by excessive food intake secondary to central stimulation by the excess cortisol, so that fat generation in some tissues exceeds the rate of fat mobilization.[6]

Excess glucocorticoids inhibit inflammation and immune function.[6, 65] This explains the high incidence of bacteriuria and other secondary infections, such as pyoderma, that are often seen in patients with hyperadrenocorticism.

Clinical Signs

The most common clinical signs of hyperadrenocorticism include PU/PD, bilaterally symmetrical nonpruritic alopecia, pendulous abdomen, hepatomegaly, and polyphagia (Table 46–2; Figs. 46–1 and 46–2).[27, 29, 57] Many other clinical signs are seen with a lesser frequency, occasionally including severe dyspnea from pulmonary thrombosis.[66] Dogs with large pituitary tumors may have neurologic signs including behavior changes, lethargy, pacing, circling, wandering, weakness, tetraparesis, stupor, seizures, rotary nystagmus, visual deficits, and strabismus.[67, 68] The onset of these signs often is after treatment has begun with mitotane (o,p'-DDD).[67]

Diagnostic Plan

The most common hemogram findings noted with hyperadrenocorticism include absolute eosinopenia, lymphopenia, and a mature neutrophilia (steroid leukogram), although these changes are not universally present (Table 46–3).[27, 29, 57] The most common serum biochemical changes include increased AP, hypercholesterolemia, elevated alanine aminotransferase, and mild to moderate elevations of glucose.[27, 29, 57] Although serum AP concentration is elevated in a high proportion of cases, the steroid-induced isoenzyme of AP may not be specific enough

Table 46–2
Clinical Signs in Dogs With Naturally Occurring Hyperadrenocorticism

CLINICAL SIGN	FREQUENCY	
Polyuria and polydipsia	419/492	(85%)
Pendulous abdomen	304/435	(70%)
Hair loss or alopecia	343/492	(70%)
Hepatomegaly	290/487	(60%)
Lethargy	234/435	(54%)
Polyphagia	237/435	(54%)
Anestrus	37/69	(54%)
Muscle weakness	199/435	(46%)
Obesity	191/417	(46%)
Muscle atrophy	149/357	(42%)
Testicular atrophy	49/147	(33%)
Pyoderma	19/57	(33%)
Spinal osteoporosis	9/27	(33%)
Comedones	140/435	(32%)
Increased panting	93/300	(31%)
Cutaneous hyperpigmentation	116/435	(27%)
Clitoral enlargement	3/13	(23%)
Corneal ulcers	10/57	(18%)
Calcinosis cutis	66/492	(13%)
Facial palsy	21/300	(7%)

Data from references 25–29.

to be used as a screening test that is any more useful than the spectrum of typical clinical signs.[69–71]

On the urinalysis, proteinuria is common (67%),[29, 57] as is bacteriuria (43%),[29] often without pyuria. Urine specific gravity may be consistent with hyposthenuria and is often in the range of minimal concentration (<1.035), but it is extremely variable (<1.010–1.056).[29]

The most common abnormality (75%–90% of

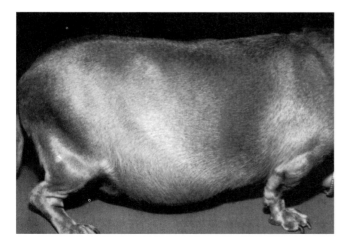

Figure 46–1
Dachshund with hyperadrenocorticism with hair loss and a pendulous abdomen.

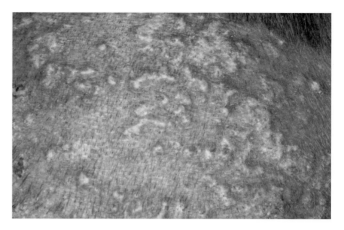

Figure 46–2
Calcinosis cutis lesions in a dog with hyperadrenocorticism.

cases) on survey abdominal radiographs of dogs with either PDH or ADH is hepatomegaly (Fig. 46–3).[72, 73] Calcinosis cutis is apparent in 17% to 18% of dogs,[72, 73] and dystrophic mineralization of internal tissues (including the renal pelves, gastric mucosa, and liver) can be seen in 18% of dogs.[72] About 15% of dogs with hyperadrenocorticism have osteoporosis, which is particularly visible in the bodies of the vertebrae.[72, 73] Cystic calculi, with or without clinical signs, may be noted in a small number of cases,[72] perhaps secondary to hypercalciuria (calcium oxalate) associated with excess glucocorticoids.

Among dogs with ADH, in 20%[73] to 50%[72] a soft tissue adrenal mass is apparent on survey abdominal

Table 46–3
Hematologic and Serum Biochemical Abnormalities in Dogs With Naturally Occurring Hyperadrenocorticism

LABORATORY ABNORMALITY	FREQUENCY	
Hematologic Changes		
Eosinopenia	429/519	(83%)
Lymphopenia	169/474	(36%)
Mature neutrophilia	166/474	(35%)
Erythrocytosis	51/300	(17%)
Biochemical Changes		
Elevated serum alkaline phosphatase	399/479	(83%)
Hypercholesterolemia	237/406	(58%)
Elevated alanine aminotransferase	267/466	(57%)
Hyperglycemia*	241/485	(50%)
Hypokalemia	25/52	(48%)
Hypophosphatemia	114/300	(38%)
Elevated total carbon dioxide	99/300	(33%)

*Mild to moderate elevation.
Data from references 25–29.

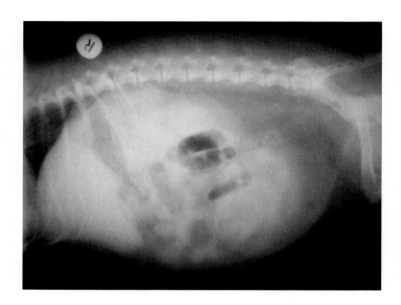

Figure 46–3
Abdominal radiograph of a dog with hyperadrenocorticism with hepatomegaly, pendulous abdomen,
and distended bladder (perhaps secondary to
chronic polyuria and polydipsia).

radiographs medial, craniomedial, or dorsomedial to the kidney. Ten percent[72] to 50%[73] of adrenal tumors in dogs are seen radiographically as a unilateral (rarely bilateral) area of mineralization in the area of the affected adrenal gland.

Rarely, dogs with hyperadrenocorticism with acute signs of pulmonary thrombosis can have pleural effusion, enlargement and blunting of pulmonary arteries, decreased perfusion of the obstructed pulmonary vessels, overperfusion of the unaffected vasculature, or normal radiographic appearance.[66] Ultrasonography of the adrenal glands may help identify an adrenal mass in those cases in which tests to differentiate PDH from ADH are equivocal.[74] This is particularly important because 15% of dogs with PDH do not have suppression of cortisol with a high-dose dexamethasone suppression test, the most commonly used test to differentiate the two common forms of the disease. Ultrasonography is also useful (perhaps 60% of the time) to determine which gland is affected by an adrenal tumor.[75] This is important if the flank approach is to be used for adrenalectomy. Failure to visualize one or more of the adrenal glands by ultrasonography does not have particular meaning, because in normal dogs the left gland can be visualized only 70% to 90% of the time and the right only 50% to 70% of the time.[76, 77] If both glands are visualized on abdominal ultrasound, and they are both large or normal in size in a dog confirmed to have hyperadrenocorticism by clinical and laboratory signs as well as adrenal function tests, it is strong evidence for the presence of pituitary-dependent disease.

Definitive diagnosis of hyperadrenocorticism requires the presence of typical clinical signs and a positive ACTH stimulation or low-dose dexamethasone suppression test. Other severe diseases (e.g., uncontrolled diabetes mellitus, liver disease, renal disease[35]) can also be associated with abnormally high values on adrenal function tests. In addition, therapy with the antiepileptic drugs phenobarbitol and primidone can lead to clinical signs that are commonly seen with hyperadrenocorticism (e.g., PU/PD, polyphagia, elevated serum AP) and produce abnormally high values on adrenal function tests as well.[78, 79]

Because therapy differs depending on the form of the disease, after the diagnosis of hyperadrenocorticism has been made, a high-dose dexamethasone suppression test, a determination of endogenous ACTH concentration, or abdominal radiographs or ultrasound (to demonstrate the presence of an adrenal mass) should be carried out to determine which form is present (see Diagnostic Procedures). My preference for a discriminatory test is the high-dose dexamethasone suppression test because of its practicality, low cost, and sensitivity. If cortisol is suppressed after administration of high-dose dexamethasone, results are definitive, indicating the presence of PDH. If cortisol is not suppressed, results are equivocal, because 15% of dogs with PDH do not show suppression of cortisol after administration of high-dose dexamethasone. Although virtually no dogs with ADH have serum cortisol suppression after high-dose dexamethasone, dogs with ADH represent only 15% of all cases of hyperadrenocorticism; therefore, the probability of ADH or PDH is 50% if the cortisol fails to suppress. In these cases, another test is required. I prefer to use radiography or ultrasonography of the abdomen next. If an adrenal mass is present, the diagnosis of ADH is made. If both adrenal glands can be imaged on ultrasound examination and are normal in size or bilaterally enlarged, it is strong evidence for the presence of pituitary-dependent disease. If one or both of those procedures fail to make the differentiation, an endogenous ACTH test or repeat of the high-dose dexamethasone suppression test is indicated. Measuring the endogenous ACTH more than one time appears to improve its accuracy.[50]

Treatment

Pituitary-Dependent Hyperadrenocorticism

In the United States, PDH is usually treated medically with the adrenocorticolytic drug mitotane (o,p'-DDD).[26, 57, 59, 80] Before therapy begins, the prognosis should be discussed with the owner, and it should be made clear that the disease will not be cured but only managed by continuous medication that requires frequent monitoring. The cost of monitoring and follow-up therapy can be high, depending on the complications that occur, which can be frequent and disturbing.[80]

Although multiple protocols have been recommended, I prefer to have the owner administer induction therapy at home, without the use of concurrent steroid therapy.[59] If it has not been done as part of the diagnostic work-up, it is useful to perform an ACTH stimulation test to use as a baseline for response to therapy. The owner is then asked to measure daily water consumption and appetite and note the approximate amount of time required for the dog to consume each meal at home for 2 or 3 consecutive days. Mitotane is given at a dosage of 50 mg/kg daily, divided into at least two doses; they are given after a meal because absorption of the drug is enhanced by food. Because the drug is not evenly distributed throughout the tablet, accurate dosing is not possible if portions of a tablet are administered. It is therefore recommended for any dog small enough to require partial tablets (one-fourth tablet or less) at each dose that the tablet be crushed and mixed into a liquid suspension (e.g., Ora-Plus, methylcellulose gel), so that dosing will be more accurate.

During the induction phase, the dog should be fed one half of its usual amount of food, divided into two meals daily, in order to make changes in appetite more noticeable. If there is any reduction in appetite or noticeable increase in time required to eat a meal, or if the dog's water consumption is 66 mL/kg per day or less, the daily dosing with mitotane is stopped and the dog is returned for an ACTH stimulation test. The consequences of o,p'-DDD overdosage are very serious, and determination of an accurate end point is critical to prevent overdosage. Beginning on the second day of therapy, the veterinarian or a technician should call the client daily to ask about the dog's appetite, the specific amount of daily water consumption, and the general attitude and well-being of the dog.

Most dogs show a clinical response within the first 5 to 9 days of therapy.[59] If there has not been a clinical response by 9 days of treatment, the dog should be returned for a physical examination and an ACTH stimulation test. Mitotane should be discontinued while the results of the test are awaited. The desired end point that seems to coincide with the best reduction or elimination of clinical signs is for both the resting and post-ACTH stimulated cortisol to be within the normal resting or basal reference range.[59, 80] If the post-ACTH stimulated cortisol is above the normal reference range for resting or basal cortisol, mitotane should be continued daily for 3 to 7 more days, depending on the clinical response and the cortisol values. The ACTH stimulation test should be repeated every 7 days or until a clinical response is noted, or until the dog has received 21 days of induction therapy.

If there appears to be no response to induction therapy with mitotane after 21 days, the following should be considered: (1) the dog may not have hyperadrenocorticism (normal dogs are relatively resistant to mitotane's effects); (2) the dog may actually have an adrenal tumor rather than PDH; (3) the drug may be expired and therefore not potent; (4) the owners may not be getting the drug into the dog or may not be giving it with a meal; (5) the dog may be one of a small proportion that needs 30 to 60 days of consecutive treatment or a much higher dose (100–150 mg/kg daily) to get a response; or (6) the dog may have iatrogenic Cushing's syndrome.[59] The latter diagnostic error can be avoided by using the ACTH stimulation test as the initial screening test for hyperadrenocorticism.

After the desired cortisol response is achieved, the dog should be treated with 50 mg/kg of mitotane weekly by mouth, in two or three divided doses. An ACTH stimulation test and physical examination should be performed after 1 month of maintenance therapy and every 3 months thereafter. If the post-ACTH cortisol level is increasing toward the upper limit of the resting reference range, the maintenance dose should be increased by 25% to 50% and the ACTH stimulation test repeated in 30 days. If the post-ACTH cortisol level is much higher than the resting reference range, treatment with 50 mg/kg per day of mitotane for 3 to 5 days is usually required to bring it back to the desired value. An ACTH stimulation test should be performed at the end of this daily treatment, then in 1 month and every 3 months thereafter.

If the cortisol levels before and after ACTH are below the normal basal reference range after a clinical response is noted, maintenance therapy with mitotane is delayed until the cortisol levels have increased to within the basal reference range. An ACTH stimulation test should be performed in 1 month and then every 3 months, depending on the clinical signs.

I do not recommend that the owner give oral

prednisolone concurrently with mitotane during the induction phase of therapy, because it may make the therapeutic end point more difficult to ascertain. However, it is recommended that prednisolone be dispensed and that the client keep it on hand to be given in case the dog shows signs of mitotane overdosage (i.e., lethargy, anorexia, weakness, vomiting, or diarrhea). The signs of a direct toxicity from mitotane, as opposed to an actual overdose with resultant hypoadrenocorticism, are seen in only a few patients. The signs of direct toxicity from mitotane are the same as those seen with overdosage except that direct toxicity usually occurs within the first 1 to 3 days of therapy. If lethargy, anorexia, weakness, vomiting, or diarrhea occurs, mitotane should be stopped and prednisolone given at a dose of 0.5 to 1.0 mg/kg initially. If the clinical signs resolve within 1 to 4 hours, mitotane overdosage with resultant hypoadrenocorticism is likely, rather than direct toxicity. Prednisolone should then be given at 0.5 to 1.0 mg/kg per day in two doses, tapered over 7 days and then stopped. An ACTH stimulation test should be performed 2 to 3 days after prednisolone is stopped. If the adverse clinical signs seem to be a direct toxic effect of the mitotane, it can be reinstituted by further dividing the daily dose into smaller, more frequent doses.

Overdosage of mitotane during the maintenance phase of therapy is common (30%).[59, 80] Only rarely is it severe enough to require replacement therapy with mineralocorticoids as well as glucocorticoids.[59, 80, 81] Recurrence of the signs of hyperadrenocorticism is also common during the maintenance phase (40%–58%).[59, 80]

The antifungal drug ketoconazole effectively reduces cortisol concentration in 80% of dogs with hyperadrenocorticism (PDH or ADH) by enzymatic inhibition of cortisol synthesis.[59, 82] Therapy should be initiated at a dose of 5 mg/kg every 12 hours for 7 days. If there are no untoward side effects (e.g., anorexia, vomiting, icterus), the dose is increased to 10 mg/kg every 12 hours for 14 days. At that time, the clinical status of the dog should be assessed and an ACTH stimulation test performed. If the clinical signs are resolving and the plasma cortisol concentrations before and after ACTH are within the normal resting reference range, this dose is continued indefinitely. If the desired response is not noted, the dose is increased to 15 mg/kg every 12 hours, and the clinical evaluation and ACTH stimulation test are repeated in 14 days. If there is good response at that time, therapy is continued at this dosage indefinitely. If response at that time is poor, ketoconazole should be discontinued and other forms of therapy tried.

Compared to mitotane, ketoconazole is expensive, is not always efficacious, and must be given twice daily for an indefinite period. It is potentially useful to treat dogs that cannot tolerate mitotane, to improve the clinical condition of dogs with adrenal tumors before surgery, or as the sole therapy for dogs with ADH. In addition, because the effects of ketoconazole are quickly and completely reversible when the drug is withdrawn, it is useful as a diagnostic aid in cases in which the diagnosis is still questionable after appropriate work-up.[59]

Adrenal-Dependent Hyperadrenocorticism

The preferred therapy for dogs with ADH is surgical removal of the affected gland. Surgery has the potential to cure as many as half of the patients with adrenal tumors. Presurgical thoracic radiographs are indicated, because a few dogs with adrenal carcinomas have evidence of pulmonary metastases,[59] which means that surgery will not be beneficial. Abdominal ultrasonography may also be helpful to detect local invasion of other tissues or metastasis to the liver in dogs with carcinomas. Presurgical therapy with ketoconazole may be indicated to improve the clinical condition of the dog and potentially decrease the risk of surgery. Because of the difficulty of the procedure, it is recommended that candidates for adrenalectomy be referred to a veterinary surgical specialist. Because the contralateral gland is atrophied, these patients must be treated during and temporarily after surgery with glucocorticoids, and some need mineralocorticoids as well.[59] For those patients for which surgery is not curative or indicated (e.g., those with metastatic or invasive adenocarcinoma), medical therapy with ketoconazole or mitotane may reduce clinical signs and prolong life.

Mitotane can be used to treat dogs with ADH, but these patients usually require higher doses for successful induction and maintenance therapy than patients with PDH. The protocol is similar to that for PDH, but if there is no response or a poor response after the initial 7 to 14 days of induction therapy, the dose of mitotane is progressively increased until a response or toxicity is noted.[59, 83, 84] The maintenance dose required for many dogs is at least 100 mg/kg per week.[84]

Prognosis

With mitotane therapy, PDH is never cured, only managed. Almost all dogs with PDH that are treated with mitotane show a clinical response; improvement in clinical signs is good to excellent in 83% and fair in 16%.[80] Average survival time is approximately 2 years,[59, 80] and most dogs (90%) die of problems unrelated to hyperadrenocorticism.[80] A more practical assessment is to consider that 70% of treated dogs are alive at 1 year, 50% at 2 years, 20% at 4 years, 8% at 6 years, and about 1.5% at 8 years.[80]

Prognosis for dogs with ADH treated surgically depends on the tumor type present (i.e., adenoma versus adenocarcinoma). Surgery has the potential to cure those 40% of dogs with adenomas and perhaps as many as half of those dogs with adenocarcinomas, because the proportion of patients that have inoperable tumors (metastasis or invasion of critical tissues) appears to be about 50%,[39] although reports vary from 0[85] to 70%.[86] Survival past the immediate postsurgical period may depend on the surgical approach (flank versus ventral), but 60% to 100% of dogs with adenoma and 20% to 100% of those with adenocarcinoma have been reported to survive, usually longer than 8 months.[85, 86]

It is not expected that medical therapy for ADH can be curative in any patients, but clinical response to mitotane is good to fair, with more than 60% of dogs having a good to excellent response and with an average survival of 16 months.[84] Ketoconazole can also be effective in eliminating the clinical signs of hyperadrenocorticism in 80% of dogs with ADH (see previous discussion of treatment of PDH). Those dogs that respond to ketoconazole do well clinically, and side effects are uncommon. Dogs that die usually do so as a result of tumor invasion or metastasis.[82]

Canine Hypoadrenocorticism

This section includes a discussion of canine hypoadrenocorticism only. The feline disease is discussed in the section on uncommon diseases. Hypoadrenocorticism is the clinical syndrome caused by a lack of the hormones produced by the adrenal cortices—usually a deficiency of both glucocorticoids and mineralocorticoids, but sometimes of glucocorticoids only. Most commonly, it results from destruction of the adrenal cortices (primary hypoadrenocorticism, or Addison's disease), but glucocorticoid deficiency can occasionally occur as a result of ACTH deficiency from pituitary disease (secondary hypoadrenocorticism). The true incidence is unknown. It occurs uncommonly in dogs yet is a disease most small animal practitioners see. Hypoadrenocorticism is rare in cats.[87] The majority of dogs with hypoadrenocorticism are young adults, with an age range of 3 months to 14 years and an average age of 4 to 4.5 years.[23, 24, 30, 88, 89] Half of the dogs are between 2.5 and 6.5 years old, and 75% to 85% are younger than 6 to 7 years of age.[23, 24] Female dogs are more commonly affected (62%–70% of cases).[23, 24, 30, 88, 89] Sexually intact females have a greater risk of developing the disease than spayed females, but sexually intact males have a lower risk than neutered males.[24] Any breed can be affected,[23, 30, 88, 89] but the Portuguese water dog, Great Dane, West Highland white terrier, standard poodle, wheaten terrier, rottweiler, springer spaniel, German short-haired pointer, and basset hound breeds are at increased risk, whereas the golden retriever, Yorkshire terrier, Lhasa apso, Chihuahua, schnauzer, cocker spaniel, and pit bull terrier breeds have a decreased risk of developing hypoadrenocorticism.[24]

Pathophysiology

Hypoadrenocorticism in dogs most commonly is caused by destruction of the adrenal cortices (primary hypoadrenocorticism, or Addison's disease). The most common lesion is idiopathic atrophy,[90] which may be caused by an immune-mediated mechanism.[91] The pathophysiologic defect is a deficiency of glucocorticoids and, in most cases, of mineralocorticoids. Occasional cases of primary hypoadrenocorticism are seen in which only glucocorticoids appear to be deficient initially (i.e., electrolytes are normal), with subsequent loss of mineralocorticoid production, presumably from progressive destruction of the adrenal cortices to include the zona glomerulosa.[24] Other less common causes of adrenal cortical destruction include granulomatous inflammation from systemic fungal infection, infarction, amyloidosis, metastatic neoplasia,[90] and iatrogenically overdosing with mitotane.[31, 81] Occasionally, hypoadrenocorticism can be seen associated with loss of pituitary production of ACTH (secondary hypoadrenocorticism), with only glucocorticoid deficiency.[24, 88]

Lack of both mineralocorticoids and glucocorticoids leads to multisystemic dysfunction, including electrolyte and water imbalances. Glucocorticoid deficiency would be expected to cause weakness and lethargy because of a lack of ability to deal with stress or because of hypoglycemia, or both. The clinical signs of pure glucocorticoid deficiency, however, are often vague and nonspecific. Because glucocorticoids have profound effects on glucose metabolism, increasing gluconeogenesis[1, 6] and inhibiting insulin activity,[92] dogs with hypoadrenocorticism may not be able to increase their plasma glucose in times of need, resulting in mild to severe hypoglycemia.

Mineralocorticoid deficiency leads to severe loss of sodium from excess renal excretion, which in turn leads to severe hypovolemia.[1, 6] Mineralocorticoids also have mild effects on GI epithelium (particularly the colon) to reduce secretion of sodium.[6] Excessive colonic sodium loss with obligatory water loss may therefore be the mechanism of diarrhea seen with hypoadrenocorticism.

Dogs with hypoadrenocorticism retain potassium because of the lack of the direct influence of mineralocorticoids on renal tubular secretion of potassium as well as because of the reduced glomerular filtration rate expected from hypovolemia and the lack of influence of glucocorticoids.[1, 6] Hyperkalemia leads

Table 46–4
Clinical Signs in Dogs With Naturally Occurring Hypoadrenocorticism

CLINICAL SIGN	FREQUENCY
Anorexia or poor appetite	263/298 (88%)
Lethargy	236/275 (86%)
Vomiting	221/298 (74%)
Weakness	217/298 (71%)
Weight loss	141/298 (47%)
Waxing and waning course*	97/225 (43%)
Dehydration	12/262 (43%)
Diarrhea	109/298 (37%)
Hypothermia	76/225 (34%)
Shock	83/248 (33%)
Emaciation	12/37 (32%)
Polyuria and polydipsia	76/298 (26%)
Shaking	68/262 (26%)
Melena	34/225 (15%)
Sensitive abdomen	3/37 (8%)

*These patients usually were treated with fluids and in some cases steroids with rapid improvement, followed by recurrence of clinical signs in a few days.
Data from references 23, 24, 30, and 31.

to decreased strength of cardiac contraction and to the arrhythmias that are often noted (see Hyperkalemia).[6] Because mineralocorticoids increase tubular secretion of hydrogen ions, deficiency can lead to metabolic acidosis.[6]

Clinical Signs

The most common clinical signs are anorexia, lethargy or depression, vomiting, bradycardia, and dehydration, with collapse and shock in the more severe cases (Table 46–4).[23, 24, 30, 88, 89] Melena from GI hemorrhage is seen in some cases[24, 93] and can be severe.[94]

Diagnostic Plan

Hematologic abnormalities observed in dogs with hypoadrenocorticism are variable (Table 46–5) but may include a relative lymphocytosis and eosinophilia, or lack of a stress leukogram when one would be expected by the severity of clinical signs.[23, 24, 30, 93] Mild, nonregenerative anemia can be present in some patients, but it is not a consistent finding at presentation[23, 24, 30] and becomes apparent more commonly after rehydration.[93]

Common biochemical changes (see Table 46–5) include prerenal azotemia, mild to moderate hypercalcemia,[95] and, characteristically, hyponatremia with hyperkalemia such that the sodium/potassium ratio is less than 27:1, although these electrolyte abnormalities are not pathognomonic for hypoadrenocorticism[20, 22]

and are not always present.[95] Because dogs with secondary hypoadrenocorticism have ACTH deficiency leading to glucocorticoid deficiency without mineralocorticoid deficiency, they do not have the typical electrolyte changes,[88] although hyponatremia may be present.[24] Some dogs with primary hypoadrenocorticism may initially have normal electrolytes that become abnormal later.[24, 96] These dogs may initially have destruction of the glucocorticoid-producing areas of the adrenal gland only, with progression to affect mineralocorticoid production. Hypoglycemia is seen in some cases, but hyperglycemia may also be present.[23, 24, 30, 88, 89] Occasionally, hypoglycemia is severe enough to cause seizures.[97] The clinician should suspect hypoadrenocorticism in dogs with azotemia that responds quickly to fluid therapy but that relapse in a few days.[24]

Electrocardiographic (ECG) changes are primarily caused by hyperkalemia but are not always present (Fig. 46–4). Changes in the ECG include bradycardia,

Table 46–5
Selected Hematologic and Serum Biochemical Abnormalities in Dogs With Naturally Occurring Hypoadrenocorticism

LABORATORY ABNORMALITY	FREQUENCY
Hematologic Changes	
Mature neutrophilia	71/225 (32%)
Monocytopenia	72/225 (32%)
Decreased packed cell volume	72/285 (25%)
Eosinopenia	67/285 (24%)
Eosinophilia	56/285 (20%)
Increased packed cell volume	35/262 (13%)
Lymphocytosis	32/285 (11%)
Lymphopenia	30/285 (11%)
Biochemical Changes	
Sodium/potassium <27:1	252/262 (96%)
Hyperkalemia	266/285 (93%)
Increased blood urea nitrogen	246/285 (86%)
Hyponatremia	239/285 (84%)
Hyperphosphatemia	153/225 (68%)
Increased creatinine	147/225 (65%)
Hypochloremia	91/225 (40%)
Decreased total carbon dioxide	81/225 (36%)
Elevated serum alkaline phosphatase*	68/225 (30%)
Hypercalcemia	82/285 (29%)
Elevated alanine aminotransferase	62/225 (28%)
Hyperbilirubinemia	48/225 (21%)
Hyperglycemia	49/285 (17%)
Hypoglycemia	40/285 (14%)
Hypocalcemia	33/285 (12%)

*Most of these patients had been treated with steroids long enough before evaluation that values could have been increased from steroid therapy.
Data from references 23, 24, and 30.

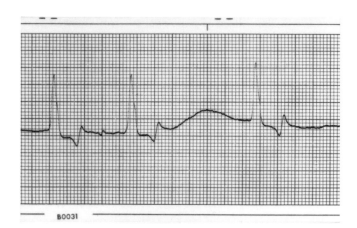

Figure 46-4
Electrocardiogram from a dog with hyperkalemia (serum potassium, 8.7 mEq/L) caused by hypoadrenocorticism. Note the absence of P waves and prolongation of the QRS complexes.

peaked T waves, decreased R-wave amplitude, decreased P-wave amplitude with eventual disappearance of P waves,[23] increased QRS duration, increased P-R interval, and ultimately ventricular asystole or fibrillation.[88] All degrees of heart block may also be noted.[24]

Thoracic radiographs of dogs with hypoadrenocorticism may show a small heart and great vessels caused by hypovolemia.[24, 88] Transient megaesophagus may also be seen.[24, 98]

If the tentative diagnosis is hypoadrenocorticism based on clinical signs or routine laboratory test abnormalities (particularly a low sodium/potassium ratio), it is prudent to begin therapy before making a definitive diagnosis, because death is imminent in dogs that are presented in a severe crisis (see Treatment). After the dog is out of imminent danger, an ACTH stimulation test (see Diagnostic Procedures) should be done to confirm the diagnosis. This test usually can be started during fluid therapy after shock has been resolved.

Differential diagnoses for primary hypoadrenocorticism include acute oliguric or anuric renal failure, postrenal uremia, GI disease, severe metabolic acidosis from diabetes or liver disease, massive tissue injury, pseudohyperkalemia (in Akitas), primary polydipsia, and congestive heart failure. A definitive diagnosis is made based on a low basal plasma cortisol concentration, with little (less than the reference range for normal dogs) or no response to exogenous ACTH administration. A normal basal concentration with a response to ACTH that is less than the reference range can be indicative of early or impending hypoadrenocorticism. If no electrolyte abnormalities are present, particularly if serum potassium concentration is not elevated, the only way to

differentiate primary from secondary hypoadrenocorticism is to measure endogenous ACTH concentration (see Diagnostic Procedures). The sample must be taken before any steroid therapy is given, or the value will be affected (suppressed).[24] It is important to differentiate secondary hypoadrenocorticism from early primary disease in which destruction of the adrenal cortex has yet to involve the mineralocorticoid-producing areas, because dogs with early primary disease usually develop mineralocorticoid deficiency and eventually the consequent electrolyte abnormalities and will require mineralocorticoid supplementation at that time.

Treatment

A dog presented in an apparent hypoadrenal crisis needs to be treated vigorously before definitive diagnosis. If the dog appears to be in hypovolemic shock or if shock is imminent, vascular volume should be replaced by the intravenous (IV) administration of 0.9% saline solution at an initial rate of 90 mL/kg per hour until improvement is noted (i.e., capillary refill time <1 second, extremities warm). Although the fluid of choice is 0.9% saline, lactated Ringer's solution is acceptable if it is the only fluid available or when it is used to treat dehydration in an animal before suspicion of hypoadrenocorticism. Because lactated Ringer's solution contains a lower concentration of potassium than that usually seen in the plasma of a dog with hypoadrenocorticism, and because it expands vascular volume and increases urinary output, serum potassium is usually reduced with administration of that fluid.[99] The remaining fluid deficit should be made up over the next 6 to 12 hours (quickly because the animals are usually azotemic), and then fluids are administered at a rate that provides maintenance plus an amount required to make up for ongoing losses (see Chap. 31). If a dog is presented dehydrated but not in shock, with only mild azotemia, fluid deficit should be made up within 12 to 24 hours. A few dogs with hypoadrenocorticism are hypoglycemic enough to have clinical signs, and dextrose should be added to the fluids to a concentration of 2.5% to 5% for those dogs. If urine output is questionable, a urethral catheter should be placed so that output can be monitored.[99] An ACTH stimulation test (see Diagnostic Procedures) should be started as soon as clinical signs of shock have been eliminated, and in most cases at the time fluid therapy is initiated.

If the cardiac rhythm is severely affected because of severe hyperkalemia and it is believed death is impending, more aggressive measures to reduce hyperkalemia can be taken. IV sodium bicarbonate, 0.5 to 1.0 mEq/kg, or IV 10% calcium gluconate, 0.5 mL/kg (not to exceed 10–15 mL regardless of weight), rapidly reduces serum potassium concentration or its effects. Either of these should be given slowly, over several minutes, with monitoring of the ECG. Administration of glucose intravenously as a 10% solution, 0.5 to 1 g/kg over 30 minutes, also quickly reduces the serum potassium concentration.[99] Administration of glucose leads to endogenous insulin secretion and hence glucose transport into cells. Because potassium moves inside cells along with glucose, extracellular potassium is shifted intracellularly. Some clinicians also administer insulin along with the glucose, but this is not necessary and may lead to hypoglycemia in a dog whose ability to correct hypoglycemia is reduced (i.e., with glucocorticoid deficiency). None of these aggressive measures is usually necessary, because rapid IV infusion of saline solution usually reduces serum potassium sufficiently to improve cardiac function.

In most cases, replacement of glucocorticoids can wait for the 1 to 2 hours needed to complete the ACTH response test. If the animal's condition dictates that glucocorticoids be given sooner, it is recommended that dexamethasone or dexamethasone sodium phosphate be given intravenously at a dose of 0.5 mg/kg, because it is not measured in the cortisol assay and therefore does not interfere with the ACTH stimulation test. After the initial crisis has been averted, dexamethasone can be used for maintenance glucocorticoid replacement at a dosage of 0.08 to 0.2 mg/kg per day given in the IV fluids, although it is not needed if hydrocortisone is used (see later discussion).[99]

After the ACTH response test is completed, replacement therapy with mineralocorticoids is begun. Because desoxycorticosterone acetate (DOCA) is no longer available, the present drug of choice for the dog in an acute adrenal crisis is hydrocortisone. Hydrocortisone has primarily glucocorticoid activity but also has enough mineralocorticoid activity to correct electrolyte imbalances in an acute crisis if given with fluid therapy. It is given as the succinate salt (Solu-Cortef) or as hydrocortisone sodium phosphate (Hydrocortone Phosphate) intravenously at a dose of 1.25 mg/kg initially, then 1 mg/kg every 6 hours the first day and 0.5 mg/kg every 6 hours the second day, tapering to 0.25 mg/kg intravenously or intramuscularly every 6 hours until the dog is eating and can be started on oral medication. Administration of hydrocortisone is recommended whether or not dexamethasone was given initially. Serum sodium, serum potassium, and BUN should be monitored daily during the first 2 to 3 days of therapy. All dogs should be kept on nothing by mouth for the first 24 hours and then offered water, followed by small amounts of bland food frequently if water is tolerated without vomiting for 12 to 24 hours.[99, 100]

After the dog can tolerate oral medications, it should be started on oral fludrocortisone (Florinef Acetate) at a dosage of 0.1 mg per 5 kg, divided into two doses or given once daily. Prednisolone, 0.5 mg/kg divided into two daily doses, is also given initially for glucocorticoid replacement. After the dog is stabilized (1–2 weeks), the dose of prednisolone is tapered over a period of 1 to 2 weeks and withdrawn. At least 50% of the dogs remain stable on fludrocortisone alone, because it does have a small amount of glucocorticoid activity. Some dogs may require continuous therapy with small doses of glucocorticoid (prednisolone) if they become weak and lethargic while receiving only fludrocortisone. This should be titrated to the smallest possible dose that keeps the dog feeling well. Often this is 0.2 mg/kg or less per day, or every second or third day. Owners should always have oral prednisolone on hand in case the dog has a stressful incident or becomes weak in an apparent hypoadrenal crisis.[99, 100]

The serum sodium, serum potassium, and BUN should be monitored daily for the first 2 to 3 days of fludrocortisone therapy, because the dose may need to be adjusted in order to keep electrolyte balance normal. The dog should be sent home and rechecked once weekly for the first 2 to 3 weeks to monitor serum sodium, serum potassium, and BUN and adjust the fludrocortisone dose as needed. Rechecks are then recommended every 3 to 4 months during the first year of therapy, depending on the stability of the patient, in order to take a history, perform a physical examination, and measure serum sodium, serum potassium, and BUN, as a minimum. Many dogs need the dose of fludrocortisone adjusted within the first 6 to 18 months of therapy.[99, 100] After the first year of therapy, rechecks should occur every 3 to 6 months. The dose of fludrocortisone should be that which maintains the serum potassium in the high-normal range and prevents clinical signs of hypoadrenocorticism. In large dogs, cost can be several dollars per day.[99]

In some cases, fludrocortisone at high enough doses to maintain normal serum potassium can be associated with PU/PD. In these cases, oral hydrocortisone (Cortef), given at a dosage of 0.125 mg/kg per day divided so that three fourths of the daily dose is given in the morning and one fourth in the evening, may allow the dose of fludrocortisone to be reduced to 0.05 mg per 5 kg per day in order to maintain potassium in the normal range and reduce PU/PD.[99]

The mineralocorticoid desoxycorticosterone pivalate (DOCP) has recently been made available to practitioners as part of an ongoing clinical trial.[89, 101] At present, it can be obtained only directly from the manufacturer (CIBA Animal Health, P.O. Box 18300, Greensboro, NC 27419-1180) by request. The advantages of DOCP over oral fludrocortisone are that it is given as an intramuscular or subcutaneous injection every 25 to 30 days instead of daily and it has less of a tendency to cause PU/PD at doses that control electrolyte balance. With DOCP, glucocorticoid therapy may also be needed, as described above in conjunction with oral fludrocortisone. The initial dosage of DOCP is 2.2 mg/kg every 25 days. For the first 2 to 3 months of therapy, dogs should have serum sodium, serum potassium, and BUN concentration rechecked 2 weeks after each injection and on the day of the next injection. If the parameters are normal at 2 weeks, the dose is adequate. If the parameters are normal on the day of the next injection, the interval between injections can be extended by 5 days. This is because the duration of activity of the drug varies from dog to dog. If on the day of the next injection the sodium and potassium are abnormal (low sodium, high potassium), the interval between injections should be shortened to 21 days.[89, 99, 101, 102] A very few dogs require the injections as frequently as every 14 days.[99]

Disadvantages of DOCP are that the dog must be returned every 25 to 30 days for an injection unless the owners can be taught to give the injections reliably, and the dose cannot be adjusted quickly because it is a repositol-type drug. If the owner is giving the injections, the dog should still be re-evaluated by the veterinarian at least every 3 to 4 months.

Some dogs require oral salt supplementation to maintain normal serum sodium concentration without inordinately large doses of mineralocorticoid. The dose of salt is empiric. I usually have owners add salt to the food, and then I monitor the sodium concentration at the usual rechecks. The amount of salt can be adjusted as needed as long as the dose of mineralocorticoid is adequate to maintain serum potassium within the normal range. If hyponatremia is mild with normal serum potassium concentration, it is not necessary to attempt to raise the serum sodium concentration into the normal range unless there are associated clinical signs of hyponatremia.

Prognosis

Dogs with hypoadrenocorticism have an excellent prognosis for long-term survival with medical management after the crisis is over, and most dogs survive the crisis if recognized and treated aggressively. Patients are not cured but are managed, usually to a point at which they lead normal lives. However, these patients can decompensate and go into a crisis at almost any time, particularly if the dog does not receive its medication. The owner should therefore be instructed to keep a constant vigil for problems such as vomiting in the pet and to seek veterinary attention should problems occur. The owner should understand

that compliance with recommended therapy is imperative. Cost of therapy can become prohibitive in large dogs.

Uncommon Diseases of the Adrenal Gland

Feline Hyperadrenocorticism

Hyperadrenocorticism occurs rarely in cats.[100, 103, 104] The clinical signs are similar to those seen in dogs, except that diabetes mellitus occurs in almost all affected cats, elevation of serum AP is uncommon,[104] and extremely fragile skin that tears with normal manipulation such as grooming may be fairly common.[104, 105] Most cats (perhaps 80%) have pituitary-dependent disease.[103, 104] Because results of dexamethasone suppression testing have been inconsistent,[106–109] the ACTH stimulation test may be the best to use. Time to peak cortisol response to ACTH is variable; it is prudent to measure cortisol at 30 and 60 minutes after intramuscular administration of 0.125 mg per cat of synthetic ACTH, cosyntropin (Cortrosyn),[108] or at 60 and 120 minutes after intramuscular administration of 2.2 U/kg of ACTH gel (H.P. Acthar Gel).[109] Cats appear to be relatively unresponsive to mitotane[104, 105] and ketoconazole,[110] although some cats may respond.[111] Bilateral adrenalectomy appears to be the most effective mode of therapy for PDH,[103] although the enzyme inhibitor metyrapone may be useful for medical management.[112]

Feline Hypoadrenocorticism

Hypoadrenocorticism occurs rarely in cats.[87, 99, 113] Clinical signs and therapy are similar to those of dogs, but cats do not respond as quickly; lethargy and weakness continue for 3 to 5 days after initiation of therapy.[87, 99] (See the previous section for ACTH stimulation testing protocol.)

Primary Hyperaldosteronism

Primary hyperaldosteronism occurs rarely in dogs and cats.[73, 114] Clinical signs are weakness, profound hypokalemia with normal to elevated serum sodium concentration, and reduced packed cell volume, presumably from fluid retention secondary to sodium retention leading to dilution of RBC mass. The disease is caused by a functional adrenocortical mass (adenoma or adenocarcinoma).

Pheochromocytoma

Pheochromocytomas are tumors that produce catecholamines and arise from neuroectodermal chromaffin cells. They usually arise from the adrenal medulla but may occur at extra-adrenal sites.[115] They occur in older dogs, comprising 0.1% to 0.01% of all tumors,[115] and very rarely in cats. Because the clinical signs are vague and nonspecific, pheochromocytomas are often detected incidentally at necropsy. The clinical effects of the tumor are from excessive and often episodic release of catecholamines or from tumor invasion, often of the caudal vena cava, which can lead to ascites or edema of the rear limbs. The clinical signs are often episodic and include tachycardia, panting, weakness, collapse, weight loss, anorexia, and flushing or blanching of mucous membranes.[115–117] The tumors may be visible on abdominal radiographs or, more commonly, apparent on abdominal ultrasound.[115] Definitive diagnosis requires measurement of urinary catecholamines or their metabolites, and surgical removal is the treatment of choice,[117] although the tumors often metastasize.[115]

References

1. Stabenfeldt GH. Endocrine glands and their function. In: Cunningham JG, ed. Textbook of Veterinary Physiology. Philadelphia, WB Saunders, 1992:396–404.
2. Peterson ME, Randolph JF, Mooney CT. Endocrine diseases. In: Sherding RG, ed. The Cat: Diseases and Clinical Management, 2nd ed, vol 2. New York, Churchill Livingstone, 1994:1479–1481.
3. Banks WJ. Applied Veterinary Histology, 3rd ed. St Louis, Mosby–Year Book, 1993:408–428.
4. Guyton AC, Hall JE. The autonomic nervous system: The adrenal medulla. In: Guyton AC, Hall JE, eds. Textbook of Medical Physiology, 9th ed. Philadelphia, WB Saunders, 1996:769–782.
5. Hullinger RL. The endocrine system. In: Evans HE, ed. Miller's Anatomy of the Dog, 3rd ed. Philadelphia, WB Saunders, 1993:574–579.
6. Guyton AC, Hall JE. The adrenocortical hormones. In: Guyton AC, Hall JE, eds. Textbook of Medical Physiology, 9th ed. Philadelphia, WB Saunders, 1996:957–970.
7. Munck A, Naray-Fejes-Toth A. Glucocorticoid action physiology. In: DeGroot LJ, ed. Endocrinology, 3rd ed, vol 2. Philadelphia, WB Saunders, 1995:1642–1656.
8. Orth DN, Peterson ME, Drucker WD. Plasma immunoreactive proopiomelanocortin peptides and cortisol in normal dogs and dogs with Cushing's syndrome: Diurnal rhythm and responses to various stimuli. Endocrinology 1988;122:1250–1262.
9. Johnston S, Mather E. Feline plasma cortisol (hydrocortisone) measured by radioimmunoassay. Am J Vet Res 1979;40:190–192.
10. Scott DW, Miller WH, Griffin CE. Endocrine and metabolic diseases. In: Scott DW, Miller WH, Griffin CE, eds. Muller and Kirk's Small Animal Dermatology, 5th ed. Philadelphia, WB Saunders, 1995:627–719.
11. Scott DW, Miller WH, Griffin CE. Pigmentary abnormalities. In: Scott DW, Miller WH, Griffin CE, eds. Muller and Kirk's Small Animal Dermatology, 5th ed. Philadelphia, WB Saunders, 1995:806–823.
12. Scott DW, Miller WH, Griffin CE. Acquired alopecias. In: Scott DW, Miller WH, Griffin CE, eds. Muller and Kirk's Small Animal Dermatology, 5th ed. Philadelphia, WB Saunders, 1995:720–735.
13. Chastain CB, Ganjam VK. Clinical Endocrinology of Companion Animals. Philadelphia, Lea & Febiger, 1986.
14. Scott DW, Miller WH, Griffin CE. Congenital and hereditary defects. In: Scott DW, Miller WH, Griffin CE, eds. Muller and Kirk's Small Animal Dermatology, 5th ed. Philadelphia, WB Saunders, 1995:736–805.
15. DiBartola SP. Hyponatremia. Vet Clin North Am Small Anim Pract 1989;19:215–230.
16. Guyton AC, Hall JE. Integration of renal mechanisms for control of blood volume and extracellular fluid volume; and renal regulation of potassium, calcium, phosphate, and magnesium. In: Guyton AC, Hall JE, eds. Textbook of Medical Physiology, 9th ed. Philadelphia, WB Saunders, 1996:367–383.
17. Willard MD. Disorders of potassium homeostasis. Vet Clin North Am Small Anim Pract 1989;19:241–263.
18. Tilley L. Essentials of Canine and Feline Electrocardiography, 3rd ed. Philadelphia, Lea & Febiger, 1992:182–183.
19. Kodak Ektachem Clinical Chemistry Products. Test Methodologies: Operational Manual. Rochester, New York, Eastman Kodak, 1990.
20. Reimann KA, Knowlen GG, Tvedten HW. Factitious hyperkalemia in dogs with thrombocytosis: The effect of platelets on serum potassium concentration. J Vet Intern Med 1989;3:47–52.
21. Degen M. Pseudohyperkalemia in Akitas. J Am Vet Med Assoc 1987;190:541–543.
22. DiBartola SP, Johnson SE, Davenport DJ, et al. Clinicopathologic findings resembling hypoadrenocorticism in dogs with primary gastrointestinal disease. J Am Vet Med Assoc 1985;187:60–63.
23. Willard MD, Schall WD, McCaw, DE, et. al. Canine hypoadrenocorticism: Report of 37 cases and review of 39 previously reported cases. J Am Vet Med Assoc 1982;180:59–62.
24. Peterson ME, Kintzer PP, Kass PH. Pretreatment clinical and laboratory findings in dogs with hypoadrenocorticism: 225 cases (1979–1993). J Am Vet Med Assoc 1996;208:85–91.
25. Siegel ET, Kelly DF, Berg P. Cushing's syndrome in the dog. J Am Vet Med Assoc 1970;157:2081–2090.
26. Schechter RD, Stabenfeldt GH, Gribble DH, et al. Treatment of Cushing's syndrome in the dog with an adrenocorticolytic agent (o,p'-DDD). J Am Vet Med Assoc 1973; 162:629–639.
27. Peterson ME. Hyperadrenocorticism. Vet Clin North Am Small Anim Pract 1984;14:731–749.
28. Lorenz M. Diagnosis and medical management of canine Cushing's syndrome: A study of 57 consecutive cases. J Am Anim Hosp Assoc 1982;18:707–716.

29. Ling GV, Stabenfeldt GH, Comer KM, et al. Canine hyperadrenocorticism: Pretreatment clinical and laboratory evaluation of 117 cases. J Am Vet Med Assoc 1979;174:1211–1215.

30. Rakich PM, Lorenz MD. Clinical signs and laboratory abnormalities in 23 dogs with spontaneous hypoadrenocorticism. J Am Anim Hosp Assoc 1984;20: 647–649.

31. Schaer M, Chen CL. A clinical survey of 48 dogs with adrenocortical hypofunction. J Am Anim Hosp Assoc 1983;19:443–452.

32. Willard MD, Twedt DC. Gastrointestinal, pancreatic, and hepatic disorders. In: Willard MD, Tvedten H, Turnwald GH, eds. Small Animal Clinical Diagnosis by Laboratory Methods, 2nd ed. Philadelphia, WB Saunders, 1994:179–218.

33. Kaplan AJ, Peterson ME, Kemppainen RJ. Effects of disease on the results of diagnostic tests for use in detecting hyperadrenocorticism in dogs. J Am Vet Med Assoc 1995;207:445–451.

34. Feldman E. Comparison of ACTH response and dexamethasone suppression as screening tests in canine hyperadrenocorticism. J Am Vet Med Assoc 1983;182: 506–510.

35. Chastain C, Franklin R, Ganjam V, et al. Evaluation of the hypothalamic pituitary-adrenal axis in clinically stressed dogs. J Am Anim Hosp Assoc 1986;22:435–442.

36. Feldman EC. Effect of functional adrenocortical tumors on plasma cortisol and corticotropin concentrations in dogs. J Am Vet Med Assoc 1981;178:823–826.

37. Meijer JC, Lubberink A, Rijnberk A, et al. Adrenocortical function tests in dogs with hyperfunctioning adrenocortical tumours. J Endocrinol 1979;80:315–319.

38. Peterson M, Gilbertson S, Drucker W. Plasma cortisol response to exogenous ACTH in 22 dogs with hyperadrenocorticism caused by adrenocortical neoplasia. J Am Vet Med Assoc 1982;180:542–544.

39. Reusch CE, Feldman EC. Canine hyperadrenocorticism due to adrenocortical neoplasia: Pretreatment evaluation of 41 dogs. J Vet Intern Med 1991;5:3–10.

40. Feldman EC, Stabenfeldt GH, Farver TB, et al. Comparison of aqueous porcine ACTH with synthetic ACTH in adrenal stimulation tests of the female dog. Am J Vet Res 1982;43:522–524.

41. Olson PN, Bowen RA, Husted PW, et al. Effects of storage on concentration of hydrocortisone (cortisol) in canine serum and plasma. Am J Vet Res 1981;42:1618–1620.

42. Eichenbaum JD, Macy DW, Severin GA, et al. Effect in large dogs of ophthalmic prednisolone acetate on adrenal gland and hepatic function. J Am Anim Hosp Assoc 1988;24:705–709.

43. Moriello K, Fehrer-Sawyer S, Meyer D, et al. Adrenocortical suppression associated with topical otic administration of glucocorticoids in dogs. J Am Vet Med Assoc 1988;193:329–332.

44. Zenoble RD, Kemppainen RJ. Adrenocortical suppression by topically applied corticosteroids in healthy dogs. J Am Vet Med Assoc 1987;191:685–688.

45. Rijnberk A, van Wees A, Mol JA. Assessment of two tests for the diagnosis of canine hyperadrenocorticism. Vet Rec 1988;122:178–180.

46. Mack RE, Feldman EC. Comparison of two low-dose dexamethasone suppression protocols as screening and discrimination tests in dogs with hyperadrenocorticism. J Am Vet Med Assoc 1990;197:1603–1606.

47. Feldman EC, Mack RE. Urine cortisol:creatinine ratio as a screening test for hyperadrenocorticism in dogs. J Am Vet Med Assoc 1992;200:1637–1641.

48. Smiley LE, Peterson ME. Evaluation of a urine cortisol:creatinine ratio as a screening test for hyperadrenocorticism in dogs. J Vet Intern Med 1993;7:163–168.

49. Stolp R, Rijnberk A, Meijer JC, et al. Urinary corticoids in the diagnosis of canine hyperadrenocorticism. Res Vet Sci 1983;34:141–144.

50. Feldman E. Distinguishing dogs with functioning adrenocortical tumors from dogs with pituitary-dependent hyperadrenocorticism. J Am Vet Med Assoc 1983;183:195–200.

51. Feldman EC. Evaluation of a combined dexamethasone suppression/ACTH stimulation test in dogs with hyperadrenocorticism. J Am Vet Med Assoc 1985;187: 49–53.

52. Eiler H, Oliver J. Combined dexamethasone suppression and cosyntropin (synthetic ACTH) stimulation test in the dog: New approach to testing of adrenal gland function. Am J Vet Res 1980;41:1243–1246.

53. Feldman EC. Evaluation of a six-hour combined dexamethasone suppression/ACTH stimulation test in dogs with hyperadrenocorticism. J Am Vet Med Assoc 1986;189:1562–1566.

54. Kemppainen R, Thompson F, Lorenz M. Effects of dexamethasone infusion on the plasma cortisol response to cosyntropin (synthetic ACTH) injection in normal dogs. Res Vet Sci 1982;32:181–183.

55. Kemppainen RJ, Sartin JL, Peterson ME. Effects of single intravenously administered doses of dexamethasone on response to the adrenocorticotropic hormone stimulation test in dogs. Am J Vet Res 1989;50:1914–1917.

56. Willeberg P, Priester WA. Epidemiological aspects of clinical hyperadrenocorticism in dogs (canine Cushing's syndrome). J Am Anim Hosp Assoc 1982;18: 717–724.

57. Lorenz MD, Scott DW. Treatment of canine Cushing's disease with o,p'-DDD: A summary. J Am Anim Hosp Assoc 1972;8:388–389.

58. Scavelli TD, Peterson ME, Matthiesen DT. Results of surgical treatment for hyperadrenocorticism caused by adrenocortical neoplasia in the dog: 25 cases (1980–1984). J Am Vet Med Assoc 1986;189:1360–1364.

59. Feldman EC. Hyperadrenocorticism. In: Ettinger SJ, Feldman EC, eds. Textbook of Veterinary Internal Medicine, 4th ed, vol 2. Philadelphia, WB Saunders, 1995:1538–1578.

60. Peterson ME, Krieger DT, Drucker WD, et al. Immunocytochemical study of the hypophysis in 25 dogs with pituitary-dependent hyperadrenocorticism. Acta Endocrinol (Copenh) 1982;101:15–24.

61. McNicol AM, Thomson H, Stewart C. The corticotrophic cells of the canine pituitary gland in pituitary-dependent hyperadrenocorticism. J Endocrinol 1983;96:303–309.

62. Ford SL, Feldman EC, Nelson RW. Hyperadrenocorticism caused by bilateral adrenocortical neoplasia in dogs: Four cases (1983–1988). J Am Vet Med Assoc 1993;202:789–792.

63. Peterson ME, Winkler B, Kintzer PP, et al. Effect of spontaneous hyperadrenocorticism on endogenous production and utilization of glucose in the dog. Domest Anim Endocrinol 1986;3:117–125.

64. Peterson M, Nesbitt G, Schaer M. Diagnosis and management of concurrent diabetes mellitus and hyperadrenocorticism in thirty dogs. J Am Vet Med Assoc 1981;178:66–69.

65. Cohn LA. The influence of corticosteroids on host defense mechanisms. J Vet Intern Med 1991;5:95–104.

66. Burns M, Kelley S, Hornof W, et al. Pulmonary artery thrombosis in three dogs with hyperadrenocorticism. J Am Vet Med Assoc 1981;178:388–393.

67. Nelson RW, Ihle SL, Feldman EC. Pituitary macroadenomas and macroadenocarcinomas in dogs treated with mitotane for pituitary-dependent hyperadrenocorticism: 13 cases (1981–1986). J Am Vet Med Assoc 1989;194:1612–1617.

68. Sarfaty D, Carrillo JM, Peterson ME. Neurologic, endocrinologic, and pathologic findings associated with large pituitary tumors in dogs: Eight cases (1976–1984). J Am Vet Med Assoc 1988;193:854–856.

69. Solter PF, Hoffman WE, Hungerford LL, et al. Assessment of corticosteroid-induced alkaline phosphatase isoenzyme as a screening test for hyperadrenocorticism in dogs. J Am Vet Med Assoc 1993;203:534–538.

70. Jensen AL, Poulsen JSD. Preliminary experience with the diagnostic value of the canine corticosteroid-induced alkaline phosphatase isoenzyme in hypercorticism and diabetes mellitus. J Vet Med 1992;39A:342–348.

71. Teske E, Rothuizen J, Bruijne JD, et al. Corticosteroid-induced alkaline phosphatase isoenzyme in the diagnosis of canine hypercorticism. Vet Rec 1989;125:12–14.

72. Huntley K, Frazer J, Gibbs C, et al. The radiological features of canine Cushing's syndrome: A review of forty-eight cases. J Small Anim Pract 1982;23:369–380.

73. Penninck DG, Feldman EC, Nyland TG. Radiographic features of canine hyperadrenocorticism caused by autonomously functioning adrenocortical tumors: 23 cases (1978–1986). J Am Vet Med Assoc 1988;192:1604–1608.

74. Schelling CG. Ultrasonography of the adrenal gland. Probl Vet Med 1991;3:604–617.

75. Kantrowitz B, Nyland T, Feldman E. Adrenal ultrasonography in the dog: Detection of tumors and hyperplasia in hyperadrenocorticism. Vet Radiol 1986;27:91–96.

76. Grooters AM, Biller DS, Miyabayashi T, et al. Evaluation of routine abdominal ultrasonography as a technique for imaging the canine adrenal glands. J Am Anim Hosp Assoc 1994;30:457–462.

77. Voorhout G. X-ray–computed tomography, nephrotomography, and ultrasonography of the adrenal glands of healthy dogs. Am J Vet Res 1990;51:625–631.

78. Feldman EC, Nelson RW. Hyperadrenocorticism. In: Feldman EC, Nelson RW, eds. Canine and Feline Endocrinology and Reproduction. Philadelphia, WB Saunders, 1987:137–194.

79. Chauvet AE, Feldman EC, Kass PH. Effects of phenobarbital administration on results of serum biochemical analyses and adrenocortical function tests in epileptic dogs. J Am Vet Med Assoc 1995;207:1305–1307.

80. Kintzer PP, Peterson ME. Mitotane (o,p'-DDD) treatment of 200 dogs with pituitary-dependent hyperadrenocorticism. J Vet Intern Med 1991;5:182–190.

81. Willard MD, Schall WD, Nachreiner RF, et al. Hypoadrenocorticism following therapy with o,p'-DDD [mitotane] for hyperadrenocorticism in four dogs. J Am Vet Med Assoc 1982;180:638–641.

82. Feldman EC, Bruyette DS, Nelson RW, et al. Plasma cortisol response to ketoconazole administration in dogs with hyperadrenocorticism. J Am Vet Med Assoc 1990;197:71–78.

83. Feldman EC, Nelson RW, Feldman MS, et al. Comparison of mitotane treatment for adrenal tumor versus pituitary-dependent hyperadrenocorticism in dogs. J Am Vet Med Assoc 1992;200:1642–1647.

84. Kintzer PP, Peterson ME. Mitotane treatment of 32 dogs with cortisol-secreting adrenocortical neoplasms. J Am Vet Med Assoc 1994;205:54–62.

85. Emms S, Jognstom D, Eigenmann J, et al. Adrenalectomy in the management of canine hyperadrenocorticism. J Am Anim Hosp Assoc 1987;23:557–564.

86. Scavelli TD, Peterson ME, Matthiesen DT. Results of surgical treatment for hyperadrenocorticism caused by adrenocortical neoplasia in the dog; 25 cases (1980–1984). J Am Vet Med Assoc 1986;189:1360–1364.

87. Peterson ME, Greco DS, Orth DN. Primary hypoadrenocorticism in ten cats. J Vet Intern Med 1989;3:55–58.

88. Feldman EC, Nelson RW. Hypoadrenocorticism. In: Feldman EC, Nelson RW, eds. Canine and Feline Endocrinology and Reproduction. Philadelphia, WB Saunders, 1987:195–217.

89. Lynn R, Feldman E. Treatment of canine hypoadrenocorticism with microcrystalline desoxycorticosterone pivalate. Br Vet J 1991;147:478–483.

90. Capen CC, Belshaw BE, Martin SL. Endocrine disorders. In: Ettinger SJ, ed. Textbook of Veterinary Internal Medicine: Diseases of the Dog and Cat. Philadelphia, WB Saunders, 1975:1351–1452.

91. Schaer MR, Buergelt WJ, Bowen CD, et al. Autoimmunity and Addison's disease in the dog. J Am Anim Hosp Assoc 1986;22:789–794.

92. Peterson ME, Altszuler N, Nichols CE. Decreased insulin sensitivity and glucose tolerance in spontaneous canine hyperadrenocorticism. Res Vet Sci 1984;36:177–182.

93. Chastain CB, Ganjam VK. Clinical Endocrinology of Companion Animals. Philadelphia, Lea & Febiger, 1986:395–408.

94. Medinger TL, Williams DA, Bruyette DS. Severe gastrointestinal tract hemorrhage in three dogs with hypoadrenocorticism. J Am Vet Med Assoc 1993;202:1869–1872.

95. Peterson ME, Feinman BS. Hypercalcemia associated with hypoadrenocorticism in sixteen dogs. J Am Vet Med Assoc 1982;181:802–804.

96. Rogers W, Straus J, Chew D. Atypical hypoadrenocorticism in three dogs. J Am Vet Med Assoc 1981;179:155–158.

97. Levy JK. Hypoglycemic seizures attributable to hypoadrenocorticism in a dog. J Am Vet Med Assoc 1994;204:526–530.

98. Burrows C. Reversible mega-oesophagus in a dog with hypoadrenocorticism. J Small Anim Pract 1987;28:1073–1078.

99. Hardy RM. Hypoadrenal gland disease. In: Ettinger SJ, Feldman EC, eds. Textbook of Veterinary Internal Medicine, 4th ed, vol 2. Philadelphia, WB Saunders, 1995:1579–1593.

100. Feldman EC. Adrenal gland disease. In: Ettinger SJ, ed. Textbook of Veterinary Internal Medicine, 3rd ed, vol 2. Philadelphia, WB Saunders, 1989:1721–1774.

101. Lynn RC, Feldman EC, Nelson RW, et al. Efficacy of microcrystalline desoxycorticosterone pivalate for treatment of hypoadrenocorticism in dogs. J Am Vet Med Assoc 1993;202:392–396.

102. Feldman EC, Nelson RW, Lynn RC. Desoxycorticosterone pivalate (DOCP) treatment of canine and feline hypoadrenocorticism. In: Kirk RW, Bonagura JD, eds. Kirk's Current Veterinary Therapy XI. Philadelphia, WB Saunders, 1992:353–355.

103. Duesberg C, Nelson R, Feldman E, et al. Adrenalectomy for treatment of feline hyperadrenocorticism. Proc Annu Meet Am Coll Vet Intern Med Forum 1993;11:926.

104. Nelson R, Feldman E, Smith M. Hyperadrenocorticism in cats: Seven cases (1978–1987). J Am Vet Med Assoc 1988;193:245–250.

105. Zerbe C, Nachreiner R, Dunstan R, et al. Hyperadrenocorticism in a cat. J Am Vet Med Assoc 1987;190:559–563.

106. Medleau L, Cowan L, Cornelius L, et al. Adrenal function testing in the cat: The effect of low dose intravenous dexamethasone administration. Res Vet Sci 1987;42:260–261.

107. Peterson M, Graves T. Effects of low dosages of intravenous dexamethasone on serum cortisol concentrations in the normal cat. Res Vet Sci 1988;44:38–40.

108. Smith M, Feldman E. Plasma endogenous ACTH concentrations and plasma cortisol response to synthetic ACTH and dexamethasone sodium phosphate in healthy cats. Am J Vet Res 1987;48:1710–1724.

109. Zerbe CA, Refsal KR, Peterson ME, et al. Effect of nonadrenal illness on adrenal function in the cat. Am J Vet Res 1987;48:451–454.

110. Willard MD, Nachreiner RF, Howard VC, et al. Effect of long-term administration of ketoconazole in cats. Am J Vet Res 1986;47:2510–2513.

111. Nelson RW, Feldman EC. Hyperadrenocorticism. In: August JR, ed. Consultations in Feline Internal Medicine. Philadelphia, WB Saunders, 1991:267–270.

112. Daley CA, Zerbe CA, Schick RO, et al. Use of metyrapone to treat pituitary-dependent hyperadrenocorticism in a cat with large cutaneous wounds. J Am Vet Med Assoc 1993;202:956–960.

113. Greco DS, Peterson ME. Feline hypoadrenocorticism. In: Kirk RW, ed. Current Veterinary Therapy X. Philadelphia, WB Saunders, 1989:1042–1045.

114. Eger C, Robinson W, Huxtable C. Primary aldosteronism (Conn's syndrome) in a cat: A case report and review of comparative aspects. J Small Anim Pract 1983;24:293–307.

115. Gilson SD, Withrow SJ, Wheeler SL, et al. Pheochromocytoma in 50 dogs. J Vet Intern Med 1994;8:228–232.

116. Bouayad H, Feeney DA, Caywood DD, et al. Pheochromocytoma in dogs: 13 cases (1980–1985). J Am Vet Med Assoc 1987;191:1610–1615.

117. Twedt D, Tilley L, et al. Pheochromocytoma in the canine. J Am Anim Hosp Assoc 1975;11:491–496.

Chapter 47

Diseases of
the Thyroid Gland

S. Dru Forrester
William E. Monroe

Anatomy

The thyroid gland consists of paired lobes located on the ventrolateral surface of the proximal trachea. In addition, cats may have accessory thyroid tissue in the neck and thorax.[1] The size of the gland varies with body weight. In adult medium-sized dogs, a lobe of the thyroid gland is approximately 5 cm in length, 1.5 cm in width, and 0.5 cm in thickness.[2] In normal cats, a thyroid lobe is approximately 2 cm in length, 0.3 cm in width, and 0.5 cm in thickness.[1] The cranial and caudal thyroid arteries arise from the common carotid artery and brachiocephalic trunk, respectively, to supply the thyroid gland in dogs; in cats, the cranial thyroid artery supplies the thyroid gland. The thyroid nerve, which arises from the cranial laryngeal nerve, innervates the thyroid gland. The external parathyroid glands lie on the surface of the thyroid lobes, whereas the internal parathyroid glands are embedded within thyroid tissue.[1, 2]

Microscopically, the thyroid gland is composed of spheric follicles that are lined by epithelial cells. The epithelial cells produce colloid, a gel-like glycoprotein, which is stored within thyroid follicles. Colloid contains thyroglobulin, the precursor for synthesis of thyroid hormones.

Physiology

Synthesis of thyroid hormone requires iodine, which is absorbed from the small intestine, converted to iodide, bound to plasma proteins, and transported to the thyroid gland. Iodide is actively transported into the thyroid gland, where it is oxidized and incorporated into the thyroglobulin molecule as tyrosine residues. Iodinated tyrosine residues then combine to form either thyroxine (T_4) or triiodothyronine (T_3), which are stored extracellularly. In order for thyroid hormone to be secreted into the blood, thyroglobulin must re-enter the follicular cell. Within the follicular epithelial cell, thyroglobulin undergoes proteolysis to produce T_4 and T_3, which are subsequently released from the base of follicular cells into the blood stream.

In circulation, thyroid hormones are highly bound to plasma proteins, so that less than 1% of T_3 and T_4 is free. Only the free or unbound hormone is capable of exerting metabolic effects, including negative feedback on the pituitary gland. The large fraction of protein-bound thyroid hormone serves as a reservoir from which thyroid hormone is obtained when needed.

Most hormone produced by the thyroid gland is T_4; however, it is metabolized in the tissues to form either T_3, which is metabolically active, or reverse T_3 (rT_3), which is inactive. Thyroid hormones affect virtually every tissue in the body. With few exceptions,

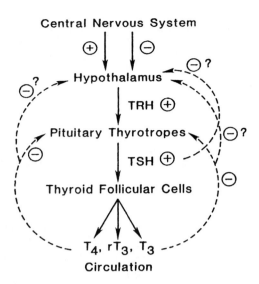

Figure 47–1
Schematic representation of the hypothalamic-pituitary-thyroid axis. The hypothalamus releases thyrotropin-releasing hormone (TRH), which causes the pituitary gland to release thyrotropin or thyroid-stimulating hormone (TSH). TSH increases production and release of thyroxine (T_4), triiodothyronine (T_3), and reverse T_3 (rT_3) from the thyroid gland. Increased serum T_4 is the major factor that inhibits further release of TSH from the pituitary gland. +, stimulation; –, inhibition. (From Feldman EC, Nelson RW, eds. Canine and Feline Endocrinology and Reproduction, 2nd ed. Philadelphia, WB Saunders 1996:70.)

thyroid hormones increase overall metabolic rate. They are important for normal fetal development, especially of the nervous system and skeleton. Thyroid hormones stimulate calorigenesis, protein synthesis and breakdown, carbohydrate metabolism, and fat utilization. Activities of many enzymes also are affected by thyroid hormones. Other effects of thyroid hormones include stimulation of erythropoiesis, formation and reabsorption of bone, increased mitochondrial oxygen consumption, and cardiac effects, including increased heart rate and strength of contraction.

Thyroid hormone secretion is regulated by the pituitary gland and the hypothalamus (Fig. 47–1). Thyroid-stimulating hormone (TSH), or thyrotropin, released from the pituitary gland exerts the most influence on thyroid hormone secretion. Increased amounts of TSH cause increased release of thyroid hormone from the thyroid gland. Increased serum concentrations of thyroid hormone, in turn, cause negative feedback on the pituitary gland to decrease release of TSH. Other hormones, including glucocorticoids, growth hormone, and androgens, also decrease secretion of TSH. Activity of the pituitary-thyroid axis is further modulated by thyrotropin-releasing hormone (TRH), which is secreted from the hypothalamus. The primary action of TRH is to stimulate release of TSH from the pituitary gland. Increased thyroid hormone concentrations may exert negative feedback on hypothalamic release of TRH.

Problem Identification

Polyphagia With Weight Loss

Polyphagia is voracious or excessive consumption of food, which can be the result of a physiologic response to increased energy demand or can be caused by a disease state.

Pathophysiology

Polyphagia with weight loss is caused by a small number of disorders that lead to a negative nutrient balance from excessive metabolic demand or a catabolic state from failure to assimilate or utilize nutrients (Table 47–1). The actual pathophysiologic mechanisms vary depending on the cause. An animal with hyperthyroidism has an absolute increased demand for nutrients that may be too great to be compensated by increased food consumption. Animals eating poor-quality diets and those with malabsorptive disorders such as gastrointestinal parasites, pancreatic exocrine insufficiency (PEI), or infiltrative bowel disease have a relative increased nutrient demand caused by loss of or failure to assimilate nutrients. Animals with diabetes mellitus fail to utilize absorbed nutrients because of a deficiency of the major anabolic hormone, insulin.

Clinical Signs

Patients that are polyphagic and losing weight because of a diet that contains insufficient metaboliz-

Table 47–1
Causes of Polyphagia With Weight Loss in Dogs and Cats

Poor-quality diet
Endocrine disorders
  Hyperthyroidism
  Diabetes mellitus
Gastrointestinal malabsorptive disorders
  Parasitism
  Pancreatic exocrine insufficiency
  Infiltrative bowel disease
    Inflammatory bowel disease
    Lymphoma
    Histoplasmosis

able nutrients to prevent weight loss in spite of high consumption have a history of being fed a poor-quality diet. Otherwise, the clinical signs associated with polyphagia with weight loss are those associated with the underlying disease. Hyperthyroid cats often present with polyuria and polydipsia (PU/PD), large fecal volume, hyperactivity, and unusually strong cardiac apex beats and peripheral pulses. A mass also may be palpable in the cervical region.

Animals with diabetes mellitus are almost always polydipsic and polyuric, may have a recent onset of bilateral cataracts (dogs), and often have moderate to severe hepatomegaly from hepatic lipid deposition. Animals with malassimilation diseases such as PEI, gastrointestinal parasites, or infiltrative bowel disease usually have small bowel diarrhea (see Chap. 32).

Diagnostic Plan

The first step in evaluating dogs and cats with polyphagia and concomitant weight loss is to determine whether the diet is adequate. Next, gastrointestinal parasitism should be ruled out on three fecal flotations. If fecal flotations are negative, a minimum database, including complete blood count (CBC), serum chemistries, and urinalysis, should be obtained. Results of these tests indicate whether diabetes mellitus is present. In cats, serum T_4 concentration (see Diagnostic Procedures) should be measured to rule out hyperthyroidism. If the diagnosis is not apparent from the results of these tests, dogs with diarrhea should have serum trypsin–like immunoreactivity measured (see Chap. 33) in order to rule out PEI. If the diagnosis still is not apparent, animals with diarrhea and perhaps serum chemistry changes such as panhypoproteinemia consistent with a protein-losing enteropathy should have biopsies of the small intestine taken by endoscopy or by laparotomy to rule out infiltrative bowel diseases such as inflammatory bowel disease, lymphoma, and fungal diseases such as histoplasmosis. However, dogs and cats with infiltrative bowel disease usually do not have good appetites.

Cervical Mass

A cervical mass is an abnormal swelling or enlargement of tissue located in the skin or subcutaneous tissue of the neck.

Pathophysiology

A mass in the cervical area may be caused by a granuloma, tumor, cyst, abscess, hematoma, or enlarged lymph node (Table 47–2). Granulomas may result from immune-mediated processes or foreign body reactions. Tumors result from new cell growth

Table 47–2
Causes of Cervical Masses in Dogs and Cats

Granuloma
  Foreign body reaction
  Eosinophilic granuloma
Neoplasia
  Thyroid carcinoma
  Cutaneous neoplasm
    Basal cell tumor
Mandibular lymph node enlargement
  Primary hematopoietic neoplasia
    Lymphoma
    Leukemia
  Metastatic neoplasia
    Carcinoma
    Melanoma
    Mast cell tumor
Salivary mucocele
Abscess
Hematoma
  Jugular venipuncture
  Thrombocytopenia
  von Willebrand's disease
  Hemophilia
  Disseminated intravascular coagulation

and may be malignant or benign. A cyst is caused by accumulation of fluid, which often is produced by epithelial cells (e.g., salivary mucocele, cystic adenocarcinoma). Abscesses most often result from localized bacterial infections and less often from other infectious disorders (e.g., fungal infection) or sterile processes (e.g., foreign body). Hematomas result from bleeding into the subcutaneous tissues, as a result of either trauma or coagulopathy. Enlarged lymph nodes are caused by infectious diseases, inflammatory disorders, or neoplasia.

Clinical Signs

The most common clinical sign associated with a cervical mass is an abnormal swelling, which may be detected by owners or found on physical examination. Other clinical signs depend on the cause of the mass. Most dogs with salivary mucoceles do not have signs other than a swelling in the cervical area. Patients with infectious, inflammatory, or neoplastic disease may have fever. Respiratory distress or cough may be present in dogs with thyroid carcinoma if the tumor is compressing the trachea or has metastasized to cause pulmonary infiltrates or pleural effusion. Regurgitation also may occur in dogs with esophageal compres-

sion caused by thyroid carcinoma. Patients with a hematoma may have evidence of bleeding elsewhere, such as hematuria, melena, epistaxis, lameness due to hemarthrosis, or petechial or ecchymotic hemorrhages. A single, enlarged lymph node in the cervical area suggests a localized disease, such as an abscess or tumor that has metastasized from the head or neck area, whereas patients with generalized lymphadenopathy usually have systemic infectious or inflammatory disease or primary hematopoietic neoplasia, most often lymphoma.

Diagnostic Plan

Initial examination of patients with a cervical mass includes evaluation of the characteristics of the mass. A fluid-filled mass is most likely a cyst, abscess, or hematoma, whereas a firm and solid mass is a tumor, granuloma, or enlarged lymph node. In general, masses that adhere to underlying tissues tend to be malignant tumors, whereas benign masses are freely moveable within the dermis or subcutaneous tissue. Except for abscesses and some rapidly growing tumors, most cervical masses do not cause pain.

Selection of diagnostic tests is made on the basis of history and physical examination findings. If a hematoma is suspected (e.g., evidence of hemorrhage elsewhere), coagulation studies are indicated, including measurement of platelet count, prothrombin time, and activated partial thromboplastin time (see Chap. 44). Other cervical masses are best evaluated by fine-needle aspiration for cytologic evaluation. Mucoceles are characterized by clear or blood-tinged, viscous fluid that looks like saliva. Degenerate neutrophils and bacteria are typical of abscesses. Granulomas are characterized by nondegenerate neutrophils and macrophages. Epithelial tumors (e.g., adenocarcinomas) and round cell tumors (e.g., mast cell tumors) exfoliate well; however, connective tissue tumors (e.g., fibrosarcoma) usually are difficult to diagnose by aspiration cytology. One epithelial tumor that often does not show many characteristics of malignancy is thyroid carcinoma. Because these tumors are well vascularized, it is common to obtain only blood on aspiration of a thyroid tumor. Results of lymph node aspiration cytology are variable, depending on the cause of lymphadenopathy. A finding of more than 90% lymphoblasts is diagnostic of lymphoma, whereas metastatic tumors are diagnosed by finding neoplastic cells in the lymph node that drains an area with a primary tumor, most often a carcinoma, melanoma, or mast cell tumor. A diagnosis of benign growth can never be made on the basis of cytologic findings alone. If cytologic evaluation of a mass does not reveal a definitive diagnosis, tissue samples should be collected for histologic evaluation.

Alopecia

Alopecia, which is loss of hair, may be a primary lesion, or it may occur secondary to disorders that cause pruritus. Dogs with endocrine disorders such as hyperadrenocorticism and hypothyroidism usually have bilaterally symmetrical alopecia of the trunk. Pruritus usually is absent unless there is concomitant disease such as pyoderma. If pruritus does exist in dogs with endocrine disease, it usually begins after the onset of alopecia. Other dermatologic findings consistent with endocrine disorders include generalized thinning of hair, hyperpigmentation, seborrhea, and secondary pyoderma.[3] In contrast to dogs with endocrine alopecia, some cats with hyperthyroidism may have patchy areas of alopecia that result from excessive licking or grooming behavior.[4, 5] If bilaterally symmetrical alopecia is observed in a middle-aged or older dog with hyperpigmentation, lethargy, depression, or obesity, a minimum database, including CBC, serum chemistries, urinalysis, and baseline T_4 concentration, should be obtained to screen for hypothyroidism. For a complete discussion of alopecia, see Chapter 1.

Vomiting

Vomiting results from primary gastrointestinal disorders or is secondary to systemic disorders such as renal failure, hepatic failure, diabetic ketoacidosis, hypoadrenocorticism, hyperthyroidism, hypercalcemia, or pancreatitis. Chronic vomiting occurs in about 50% of cats with hyperthyroidism; however, the exact mechanism is unclear.[4, 6] It is possible that excess thyroid hormone stimulates the chemoreceptor trigger zone or that rapid overeating causes gastric distention and vomiting. If chronic vomiting is observed in an older cat with a history of PU/PD, polyphagia, or weight loss, measurement of serum T_4 concentration is indicated to rule out hyperthyroidism. For a complete discussion of vomiting, see Chapter 31.

Diarrhea

Diarrhea results from disorders that affect the small or large bowel. Approximately 15% to 30% of cats with hyperthyroidism have signs of chronic small bowel diarrhea characterized by increased frequency of defecation and fecal volume.[4, 6] Diarrhea in hyperthyroid cats may result from intestinal hypermotility, reversible pancreatic exocrine insufficiency, or increased fat intake with secondary steatorrhea.[4, 5] If chronic diarrhea is observed in an older cat with a history of PU/PD, polyphagia, weight loss, or chronic vomiting, serum T_4 concentration should be measured to rule out hyperthyroidism. For a complete discussion of diarrhea, see Chapter 32.

Polyuria and Polydipsia

Polyuria (urine volume >50 mL/kg per day) and polydipsia (water consumption >100 mL/kg per day) most often result from chronic renal disease, pyometra, and endocrine disorders such as hyperadrenocorticism, diabetes mellitus, or hyperthyroidism. Polyuria with polydipsia is reported in approximately 35% to 60% of cats with hyperthyroidism.[4, 6] Potential mechanisms include increased renal medullary blood flow with subsequent medullary washout, psychogenic polydipsia, and concomitant renal disease. If an older cat is presented for evaluation of PU/PD, serum T_4 concentration should be measured to rule out hyperthyroidism, especially if there is a history of polyphagia, weight loss, or chronic vomiting or diarrhea. For a complete discussion of PU/PD, see Chapter 16.

Tachycardia

Tachycardia is an increased heart rate above normal, usually 160 beats/minute (bpm) in dogs and 240 bpm in cats. Tachycardia may be physiologic (e.g., exercise) or pathologic (e.g., congestive heart failure), and on the basis of electrocardiographic (ECG) findings it may be classified as ventricular or supraventricular; supraventricular tachycardia includes sinus, atrial, or junctional rhythms. Approximately 40% to 65% of hyperthyroid cats have tachycardia.[4, 6, 7] Other physical examination findings suggestive of cardiac disease in hyperthyroid cats include murmurs and gallop rhythms. In addition to sinus tachycardia, the most common ECG abnormality in hyperthyroid cats is increased R-wave amplitude, consistent with left ventricular enlargement.[4, 7–9] The most common echocardiographic finding is left ventricular hypertrophy.[10]

The cardiac effects of hyperthyroidism are presumed to result from effects of excessive thyroid hormone on cardiac muscle, interaction with the sympathetic nervous system, and decreased peripheral vascular resistance.[11] The end result seems to be a high cardiac output state associated with decreased peripheral vascular resistance. If any signs of cardiac disease, such as tachycardia, a murmur, or a gallop rhythm, are detected in an older cat with PU/PD, weight loss, or polyphagia, serum T_4 concentration should be measured to rule out hyperthyroidism. For a complete discussion of tachycardia, see Chapter 10.

Hypercholesterolemia

Hypercholesterolemia is increased serum cholesterol above the reference range of the laboratory.

Pathophysiology

Hypercholesterolemia can result from consumption of a high-fat diet, but most often it occurs in patients with protein-losing glomerular diseases; endocrine disorders such as hyperadrenocorticism, hypothyroidism, and diabetes mellitus; and liver diseases. Hypercholesterolemia in patients with glomerular disease may result from increased synthesis or decreased clearance of cholesterol. Although the stimulus is unknown, there appears to be an inverse relation between serum cholesterol and albumin concentration.[12] Glucocorticoid excess in dogs with hyperadrenocorticism stimulates lipolysis, which leads to increased cholesterol in the blood. In hypothyroidism, degradation of lipids is depressed because of inadequate concentration of thyroid hormones; this causes increased concentrations of plasma lipids, including cholesterol.[5] Pathogenesis of hypercholesterolemia in animals with diabetes mellitus is poorly understood. Liver disease can cause hypercholesterolemia as a result of cholestasis and increased hepatic synthesis.

Clinical Signs

Clinical signs in dogs and cats with hypercholesterolemia almost always result from the underlying cause. Protein-losing glomerular diseases may cause severe hypoalbuminemia and renal failure, which may cause inappetence, PU/PD, weight loss, and, infrequently, peripheral edema or ascites. PU/PD, bilaterally symmetrical alopecia, or hyperpigmentation may be observed in dogs with hyperadrenocorticism or hypothyroidism. Dogs and cats with diabetes mellitus also may have PU/PD. Increased appetite occurs in patients with hyperadrenocorticism or diabetes mellitus. In addition, dogs and cats with diabetes mellitus often have concomitant weight loss and can develop cataracts. Animals with liver disease may have icterus, ascites, hepatomegaly, and encephalopathy.

Diagnostic Plan

If hypercholesterolemia is identified, the first step is to determine whether the patient was fasted. If there is any doubt, the measurement of serum cholesterol should be repeated after a 12-hour fast. Also, the owner should be asked about the pet's diet to rule out high fat intake as a cause of hypercholesterolemia. After dietary causes of hypercholesterolemia have been eliminated, results of CBC, serum chemistries, and urinalysis should be evaluated. Diabetes mellitus can be ruled out by finding normal serum glucose and absence of glucosuria. Dogs with hypothyroidism often have a nonregenerative anemia, whereas hyperadrenocorticism often is associated with a normal or slightly increased hematocrit. A stress leukogram, characterized by mature neutrophilia, lymphopenia, eosinopenia, and monocytosis, is often observed in dogs with hyperadrenocorticism. Increased hepatic

enzyme concentrations, especially alkaline phosphatase, often occur in dogs with hyperadrenocorticism. Protein-losing glomerular diseases are characterized by hypoalbuminemia, severe proteinuria, and, in some cases, azotemia. Animals with liver disease may have elevated serum enzymes, hypoalbuminemia, hyperbilirubinemia, or low blood urea nitrogen.

Depending on results of clinical findings and initial laboratory evaluation, additional diagnostic tests may be indicated. Dogs with PU/PD, bilaterally symmetrical alopecia, hyperpigmentation, and increased serum alkaline phosphatase most likely have hyperadrenocorticism, and an adrenocorticotropic hormone (ACTH) response test or low-dose dexamethasone suppression test should be done (see Chap. 46). Dogs with lethargy, obesity, bilaterally symmetrical alopecia, hyperpigmentation, and nonregenerative anemia should be screened for hypothyroidism by measurement of serum T_4 concentration initially; if results are low, additional testing is indicated to more definitively diagnose hypothyroidism (see Diagnostic Procedures). If hypoalbuminemia and proteinuria are present, a urine protein/creatinine ratio should be done to determine the significance of the proteinuria (see Chap. 16 for a more complete discussion). If liver disease is suspected, hepatic ultrasound, liver function tests, and biopsy may be indicated (see Chap. 34).

Diagnostic Procedures

Routine Laboratory Evaluation

If thyroid disease is suspected on the basis of history and physical examination findings, routine laboratory evaluation, including CBC, serum chemistries, and urinalysis, is indicated. The most common laboratory findings in dogs with hypothyroidism are nonregenerative anemia, hypercholesterolemia, and hypertriglyceridemia.[5] Laboratory findings that are reported most often in cats with hyperthyroidism include erythrocytosis, stress leukogram (leukocytosis, mature neutrophilia, lymphopenia, eosinopenia, and monocytosis), increased hepatic enzyme concentrations, azotemia, and hyperphosphatemia.[4–6] Although laboratory changes often are nonspecific, they are helpful for increasing the index of suspicion for thyroid disease and recommending further testing.

Radiography

Thoracic radiography is most useful for evaluation of cats with suspected cardiac disease, which may be associated with hyperthyroidism. Findings may include generalized cardiomegaly, signs of pulmonary edema, and pleural effusion.[8, 9] Thoracic radiographs also are indicated to detect signs of metastasis in dogs with a thyroid carcinoma.

Electrocardiography and Echocardiography

Additional evaluation for cardiac disease is indicated if the physical examination reveals tachycardia, arrhythmias, gallop rhythm, or cardiac murmurs; if hyperthyroidism has been diagnosed; or if thoracic radiographs reveal cardiomegaly or pleural effusion. ECG is most useful for evaluating patients with abnormal rhythms but also provides information about cardiac chamber size. The most common ECG changes in cats with hyperthyroidism are sinus tachycardia (rate ≥240 bpm) and increased R-wave amplitude (≥0.9 mV), which suggest left ventricular enlargement.[7, 8] Echocardiography is indicated for evaluation of cardiac contractility and ventricular thickness. Hyperthyroid cats may have cardiomyopathy characterized by left ventricular hypertrophy, atrial enlargement, and increased contractility.[10] For a complete discussion of these tests, see Chapters 10 and 12.

Baseline Thyroid Hormone Concentrations

The most useful screening test for initial evaluation of dogs with suspected hypothyroidism or cats with suspected hyperthyroidism is measurement of baseline serum T_4 concentration. Currently, radioimmunoassay is the most accurate and widely used method for measuring total serum T_4 in dogs and cats.[13, 14] Although T_4 is very stable in blood, plasma, or serum, samples of serum or plasma should be refrigerated or frozen and sent to the laboratory on cold packs.[5, 15]

Interpretation of serum T_4 concentration values should be done with knowledge of the laboratory's established reference ranges. Finding a T_4 concentration greater than normal in a cat is consistent with a diagnosis of hyperthyroidism, especially if clinical signs exist. Because T_4 values may fluctuate during the day, approximately 2% to 13% of hyperthyroid cats have normal T_4 values.[6, 16, 17] In addition, presence of concomitant disease such as chronic renal failure, diabetes mellitus, congestive heart failure, hepatic disease, immune-mediated disease, or neoplasia may be associated with normal T_4 concentrations in cats with hyperthyroidism.[2, 17, 18] Therefore, if T_4 concentration is normal and hyperthyroidism is still suspected, the test should be repeated once or twice before additional tests are pursued and before hyperthyroidism is ruled out definitively.

Interpretation of T_4 concentrations in dogs with suspected hypothyroidism is not as straightforward, because there is considerable overlap between T_4 concentrations in normal dogs and in hypothyroid dogs. In addition, many disorders, including hyperadrenocorticism, hypoadrenocorticism, diabetes mellitus, renal failure, hepatic failure, hospitalization, surgical procedures, and chronic weight loss, are associated with suppressed serum T_4 concentration in the absence of hypothyroidism (i.e., euthyroid sick syndrome).[19–22] Therefore, additional testing (e.g., TSH response test) often is necessary to differentiate dogs with hypothyroidism from those that are euthyroid.

Administration of some drugs, including corticosteroids, anticonvulsants, and sulfonamides, may be associated with decreased serum thyroid hormone concentration in dogs; many other drugs cause decreased thyroid hormone concentrations in humans and may have similar effects in dogs and cats.[21, 23, 24] Because of all the extrathyroidal factors that can affect baseline thyroid hormone concentrations, it is important to interpret results together with findings from clinical and other laboratory evaluations. Despite all the disadvantages of using baseline T_4 values, some helpful generalizations can be made. It is unlikely that hypothyroidism exists in a dog with a normal T_4 concentration. Dogs with very low T_4 concentrations probably are hypothyroid, especially if clinical signs of hypothyroidism exist and concomitant systemic illness is absent.

With few exceptions, measurement of other hormones, such as T_3, rT_3, free T_4, or free T_3, does not provide clinically useful information compared with that obtained from baseline T_4 concentrations and the TSH response test.[25]

Thyroid Hormone Autoantibodies

Infrequently, measurement of T_3 or T_4 autoantibodies may be helpful.[26] Approximately 5% of canine serum samples submitted for measurement of thyroid hormone have autoantibodies; T_3 autoantibodies are more common than T_4 autoantibodies.[27] These autoantibodies may be associated with lymphocytic thyroiditis, which is presumed to be an immune-mediated disorder that causes hypothyroidism in some dogs. The importance of autoantibodies is that they may interfere with measurement of thyroid hormones by radioimmunoassay, resulting in either a falsely high or a falsely low value. If unexpected findings are observed when thyroid hormone is measured (e.g., extremely high T_4 concentration in a dog with suspected hypothyroidism), measurement of autoantibodies is indicated. Finding thyroid hormone autoantibodies in a dog with clinical signs and laboratory findings typical of hypothyroidism is suggestive of hypothyroidism caused by lymphocytic thyroiditis.[5] It is not known whether euthyroid dogs with thyroid hormone autoantibodies eventually develop hypothyroidism.

Basal TSH Concentration

When commercially available, a valid assay for measurement of basal canine TSH will be invaluable for diagnosis of hypothyroidism in dogs. Preliminary results show that dogs with primary hypothyroidism have increased concentrations of TSH.[28, 29] As expected, TSH is increased because thyroid hormone is not available to cause negative feedback on the pituitary gland. Apparently, TSH increases early in the course of primary hypothyroidism, even before there is a decline in serum thyroid hormone concentrations.

TSH Response Test

At present, the TSH response test is the best method for confirming a diagnosis of hypothyroidism in dogs and for differentiating this condition from nonthyroidal illnesses that suppress baseline T_4 concentration. Unfortunately, availability of TSH is often limited, and it is too expensive for some clients. However, obtaining a definitive diagnosis on the basis of a TSH response test result may be less expensive than long-term administration of thyroid hormone.

There are numerous protocols for performing a TSH response test. It is preferable to use a protocol recommended by the laboratory where samples are to be sent for analysis. Because thyroid hormone supplementation causes atrophy of the thyroid gland and decreased responsiveness to TSH, administration of thyroid hormones should be discontinued for 6 to 8 weeks before the TSH response test is performed.[30] Immediately before administration of TSH, blood is collected for measurement of baseline T_4 concentration. We prefer to administer bovine TSH (Dermathycin) at 0.1 IU/kg (maximum of 5 units per dog) intravenously and to collect blood 6 hours later for measurement of post-TSH T_4. As mentioned, T_4 is very stable in blood or serum; however, it is preferable to remove serum or plasma and freeze or refrigerate samples before sending them on a cold pack to the laboratory. Reconstituted TSH that is not used can be refrigerated for 3 weeks (4°C) or frozen for at least 3 months (−20°C) without loss of activity.[31, 32]

Interpretation of TSH response test results is done by comparing pre- and post-TSH concentrations of T_4. Euthyroid dogs have a normal baseline T_4 concentration, and post-TSH T_4 concentration increases above the normal range for the laboratory. Dogs with euthyroid sick syndrome (i.e., those with systemic illness) often have low baseline T_4 concentrations but respond to TSH, although the response may be suppressed compared with normal dogs. Dogs with concomitant hyperadrenocorticism and dogs receiving

corticosteroids may have TSH response test results similar to those of dogs with euthyroid sick syndrome.[19, 24, 33] In contrast, dogs with primary hypothyroidism usually do not respond to TSH; the post-TSH T_4 concentration is similar to or lower than the baseline T_4 concentration. Because thyroid function declines gradually, some dogs with early hypothyroidism have TSH response test results that are similar to those of dogs with euthyroid sick syndrome. In these cases, results should be interpreted together with clinical signs and other laboratory findings. A second TSH response test 3 to 6 months later may reveal results that are consistent with hypothyroidism.

T₃ Suppression Test

If hyperthyroidism is suspected in a cat with repeatedly normal serum T_4 concentrations, a T_3 suppression test can be done. This test is based on the principle that administration of exogenous T_3 should suppress secretion of T_4 in normal cats but not in cats with hyperthyroidism. Before the test begins, blood is collected for measurement of baseline T_3 and T_4 concentrations. Then the owner administers sodium liothyronine (Cytobin) orally at a dose of 25 μg per cat three times per day (t.i.d.) for 2 days.[34] On the morning of the third day, the owner should give another 25-μg dose and bring the cat to the clinic so that blood can be collected 2 to 4 hours later. Serum is submitted for measurement of baseline and posttreatment T_3 and T_4 concentrations. Normal cats have a marked reduction in T_4 concentration after treatment with T_3, whereas hyperthyroid cats do not.[34, 35] Serum T_3 concentrations are evaluated to determine whether the cat was successfully treated, as evidenced by an increase in serum T_3 concentration compared with baseline in normal and hyperthyroid cats.

Nuclear Scintigraphy

Radionuclide scans, available mostly at referral centers, provide very useful information in dogs and cats with hyperthyroidism or thyroid neoplasia. In dogs with thyroid tumors, radionuclide scanning helps to determine the extent of tumor involvement and aids in selection of the most appropriate treatment.[36] In hyperthyroid cats, thyroid imaging helps to objectively determine whether there is unilateral or bilateral disease (Fig. 47–2).[37, 38] Ectopic thyroid tissue (e.g., mediastinal) also can readily be identified in dogs and cats with hyperthyroidism or thyroid neoplasia with the use of thyroid imaging.[36, 39]

Thyroid Biopsy

Collection of thyroid tissue for cytologic or histologic evaluation is indicated for patients with suspected thyroid malignancy. Although lymphocytic

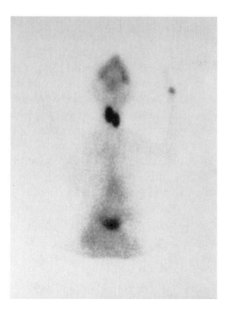

Figure 47–2
Radionuclide scan of a cat with hyperthyroidism. Note bilateral enlargement of the thyroid gland. There also is uptake of radioactive iodine in the salivary glands and gastric mucosa. (Courtesy of Don Barber, DVM, MS, Blacksburg, Virginia.)

thyroiditis and thyroid atrophy may be diagnosed, other less invasive tests should be used in dogs with suspected hypothyroidism. Initial evaluation of dogs with a potentially malignant thyroid mass includes aspiration of the mass for cytologic evaluation. The most common findings in dogs with thyroid carcinoma are numerous red blood cells and, in some cases, clusters of well-differentiated epithelial cells. If a diagnosis cannot be made on the basis of cytologic findings, histologic evaluation is indicated. Samples for histologic evaluation can be collected with a biopsy needle, using a closed technique, or by exposing the mass and excising a wedge of tissue. Regardless of the procedure used, the most common complication of thyroid biopsy is hemorrhage, which can be severe and difficult to control in some patients. Samples of thyroid tissue should be placed in formalin or in another medium, as directed by the laboratory, and sent for histologic evaluation.

Common Diseases of the Thyroid Gland

Canine Hypothyroidism

Hypothyroidism is characterized by lack of thyroid hormone production by the thyroid gland with subsequent development of clinical signs. It is the most common disorder affecting the thyroid gland in dogs and is rare in cats. Clinical signs most often develop in middle-aged dogs that are medium to large in size.[3, 40] Breeds that are often affected include the golden retriever, Doberman pinscher, Labrador retriever, cocker spaniel, Irish setter, boxer, miniature schnauzer, dachshund, Shetland sheepdog, Airedale terrier, Great Dane, and poodle.[3, 5, 40–42] It is possible that some of these breeds may be genetically predisposed to development of hypothyroidism; however, some may be overrepresented because of breed popularity. There does not appear to be a sex predisposition, although neutered dogs may have an increased risk for development of hypothyroidism.[41]

Pathophysiology

Almost all dogs with hypothyroidism have primary disease of the thyroid gland, either lymphocytic thyroiditis or thyroid atrophy. Lymphocytic thyroiditis is believed to be an immune-mediated disease, although the inciting cause is unknown.[26, 35, 43] The cause of thyroid atrophy is unknown in dogs. Regardless of which process occurs, the end result is destruction of the thyroid gland with inability to produce and secrete thyroid hormones. Secondary hypothyroidism caused by decreased pituitary production of TSH and subsequent lack of thyroid hormone secretion is very uncommon in dogs. However, excessive cortisol associated with either administration of glucocorticoids or naturally occurring hyperadrenocorticism often causes reversible, secondary hypothyroidism.[19, 24] Because thyroid hormones affect almost every organ in the body, clinical signs of systemic disease are common.

Clinical Signs

Clinical signs observed in dogs with hypothyroidism often are nonspecific and occur so gradually that many owners do not recognize a problem. Lethargy, depression, and obesity despite appropriate caloric intake often are reported.[3, 41] Dermatologic abnormalities such as bilaterally symmetrical truncal alopecia, seborrhea, dry skin, dull hair coat, hyperpigmentation, or pyoderma are observed in up to 60% of dogs (Fig. 47–3).[3, 41] Signs of neuromuscular disease such as facial paralysis, peripheral vestibular disease, generalized neuromuscular weakness, megaesophagus, and laryngeal paralysis also may be observed in dogs with hypothyroidism; however, it is not known whether these findings are due to thyroid hormone deficiency.[41, 44] Lastly, there may be reproductive abnormalities associated with hypothyroidism, such as infertility, prolonged interestrus intervals, silent estrus, or failure to cycle in females and testicular atrophy, decreased libido, and deficient sperm production in males.[5]

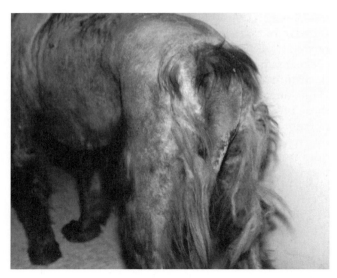

Figure 47-3
Hypothyroid dog with characteristic dermatologic signs including bilaterally symmetrical alopecia, hyperpigmentation, and "rat-tail" appearance. These changes were completely reversed after treatment for several months with levothyroxine.

Diagnostic Plan

If clinical findings are suggestive of hypothyroidism, initial screening tests, including CBC, serum chemistries, and baseline T_4, should be done. The most common laboratory abnormalities are hypercholesterolemia, which occurs in almost 75% of hypothyroid dogs, and normocytic, normochromic, nonregenerative anemia, which is identified in about 33% of patients.[41] Serum concentration of T_4 is almost always decreased below normal in dogs with hypothyroidism. Low serum T_4 is not specific for hypothyroidism, however, because other illnesses also can suppress T_4 secretion. Therefore, a dog with a low serum T_4 concentration requires further evaluation (i.e., TSH response test or measurement of basal TSH) to make a definitive diagnosis. For a complete discussion of tests used to diagnose hypothyroidism, see Diagnostic Procedures.

Treatment

Thyroid hormone supplementation is indicated for dogs with definitively diagnosed hypothyroidism or when response to treatment is used as a diagnostic test in dogs with clinical and laboratory findings of hypothyroidism, including a low baseline T_4 concentration. The drug of choice is synthetic L-levothyroxine (e.g., Synthroid) administered at a dose of 0.02 mg/kg orally twice per day (b.i.d.). In general, twice-daily administration of levothyroxine is more likely to result in serum T_4 concentrations that are within the normal range, compared with once-daily treatment.[45] Because of higher serum concentrations with brand-name veterinary products, it is probably best to administer a brand-name levothyroxine preparation initially instead of generic products or human preparations.[45] This is especially critical if response to treatment is being used as a diagnostic test. Also, the initial dosage regimen may need to be individualized. Dogs with concomitant illness, especially cardiac disease, may be best treated with a lower dose of levothyroxine (0.005 mg/kg per day) initially, with a gradually increasing dose over a period of 3 to 4 weeks.[5]

Efficacy of levothyroxine should not be evaluated until 4 to 6 weeks after treatment has begun. Although changes in mentation improve after treatment for several days and resolution of laboratory abnormalities occurs within the first month, dermatologic lesions and neurologic signs may not improve for several months.[5] Reproductive problems are the last to be corrected, sometimes requiring up to 1 year of appropriate treatment with levothyroxine. After clinical signs resolve, frequency of administering levothyroxine may be changed to once daily; however, if signs recur, twice-daily treatment is indicated.

If the patient does not seem to respond as expected, several possibilities should be considered. It is possible that hypothyroidism was incorrectly diagnosed, especially if response to treatment is being used as a diagnostic test. Another potential cause of treatment failure is inadequate absorption of levothyroxine or another factor that results in decreased serum T_4 concentration. Changing to a different levothyroxine product may be all that is necessary to alleviate this problem, especially if a generic or human drug is being used.[45] Because of individual differences in metabolism of levothyroxine, some dogs may require a change in the dosage regimen to produce adequate serum T_4 concentrations; measurement of post-pill T_4 concentration may be helpful in these cases.[5] Ideally, this should be done 2 to 4 weeks after beginning treatment or making a dosage change. Samples for measurement of T_4 should be collected just before dosing and 4 to 6 hours after treatment with levothyroxine. An appropriate dosage regimen should result in pre- and post-pill serum T_4 concentrations that are within or slightly above the reference range of the laboratory. A low pre-pill serum T_4 concentration indicates a need to increase the dose or the frequency of administration.

Potential complications of excessive levothyroxine supplementation are similar to signs of thyrotoxicosis and include PU/PD, polyphagia, weight loss, hyperactivity, and tachycardia. Serum T_4 can be measured to further support a diagnosis of thyrotoxicosis; however, dogs with signs of thyrotoxicosis can have normal T_4 concentrations, and dogs without signs of thyrotoxicosis can have increased serum T_4 concentrations.[5] If signs of thyrotoxicosis occur, thyroid hormone supplementation should be discontinued; after signs resolve, usually within 1 to 3 days, treatment should be reinstituted at a lower dose.[5] Re-evaluation, including history, physical examination, and measurement of serum T_4, should be done 2 to 4 weeks later.

Prognosis

The prognosis for dogs with hypothyroidism is good to excellent. Clinical signs and laboratory abnormalities are reversible with appropriate treatment, although neuromuscular and reproductive problems may take up to 1 year to resolve.

Feline Hyperthyroidism

Hyperthyroidism is a disorder characterized by excessive production of thyroid hormone, which results in clinical signs of thyrotoxicosis. This disease was virtually unheard of 20 years ago when the first cases were diagnosed, but now hyperthyroidism is commonly seen in cats.[6, 46, 47] Ages of cats with hyperthyroidism range from 4 to 22 years, with a mean age of approximately 13 years.[4-6, 48] There appear to be no breed or sex predispositions.[4, 6]

Pathophysiology

Hyperthyroidism in cats almost always results from excessive production of thyroid hormones by a functional adenoma of the thyroid gland and rarely from thyroid carcinoma.[4-6, 39, 46, 47] The inciting cause of thyroid adenomas or carcinomas is unknown.

Regardless of the inciting cause of hyperthyroidism, excessive serum concentrations of thyroid hormones are responsible for clinical signs and laboratory findings in hyperthyroid cats. In general, thyrotoxicosis causes an overall increase in the metabolic rate of tissues, which increases calorigenesis and leads to weight loss despite increased food intake. Excess thyroid hormone also causes polyuria, possibly because of increased blood flow through the vasa recta in the renal medulla, which causes medullary washout and decreased ability to concentrate urine. Polydipsia most likely is a compensatory response. Although the cause of gastrointestinal signs is unknown, it is possible that vomiting is mediated centrally through stimulation of the chemoreceptor trigger zone by excess thyroid hormone or is caused by gastric distention associated with overeating. Diarrhea in hyperthyroid cats may result from increased intestinal transit time or from inhibition of pancreatic enzyme secretion by excessive thyroid hormone. Hyperactivity and nervousness in hyperthyroid cats are probably direct effects of thyroid hormone on the nervous system. Thyroid hormone may act directly on cardiac muscle to stimulate hypertrophy and increase heart rate, or these effects may be mediated in part by interaction with the sympathetic nervous system.

Clinical Signs

Clinical signs in cats with hyperthyroidism are gradual in onset and often are not noticed by owners for 6 to 12 months.[5] Weight loss is reported in more than 90% of hyperthyroid cats. Polyphagia occurs in more than half of cats and may be extreme in some cases. Owners may report unusual eating behavior in some hyperthyroid cats, such as a cat's consuming an entire loaf of bread or pacing around the table while the family is eating a meal. In contrast, a small percentage of hyperthyroid cats, approximately 6% to 7%, are inappetent.[5, 6] Other common clinical signs include an unkempt hair coat, patchy areas of alopecia, PU/PD, hyperactivity or irritability, vomiting, and diarrhea.[4-6, 48] Less frequently, signs of weakness, decreased activity, tremors, panting, increased fecal volume, and dyspnea are observed.[5, 6]

Hyperthyroid cats most often are very thin and may be difficult to examine because of hyperactivity. A thyroid nodule can be palpated in 80% to 90% of cats with hyperthyroidism; approximately 65% to 70% of cats have bilaterally enlarged thyroid lobes, and the remainder have unilateral disease.[4-6] Some thyroid nodules may slip into the thoracic inlet and not be detected. It is best for the examiner to extend the cat's neck and place the forefinger and thumb over the trachea near the thoracic inlet, then gently slide them forward to feel the thyroid nodule slip under the finger and thumb. Other findings of hyperthyroidism include tachycardia, cardiac murmur, small kidneys, and a gallop rhythm.

Diagnostic Plan

Hyperthyroidism should be suspected in an older cat that is presented for evaluation of weight loss, polyphagia, hyperexcitability, or PU/PD or if a thyroid nodule is identified. Hyperthyroidism is often diagnosed after serum T_4 concentration is found to be increased on routine screening of older cats. Laboratory evaluation, including CBC, serum chemistries, and urinalysis, is indicated to detect findings consistent with hyperthyroidism and to identify other disorders of older cats such as renal disease, hepatic disease, and diabetes mellitus. The most common laboratory abnormalities in cats with hyperthyroidism are increased serum concentrations of alanine aminotransferase and alkaline phosphatase, erythrocytosis, azotemia, and hyperphosphatemia. Results of urinalysis may not be as helpful for localizing the cause of azotemia, because hyperthyroidism can interfere with urine concentrating ability. In addition, it is not uncommon for hyperthyroid cats to have concomitant renal failure.[49, 50]

Measurement of baseline serum T_4 concentration is indicated if hyperthyroidism is suspected on the basis of history, physical examination, or laboratory findings. A serum T_4 concentration that is increased above normal is diagnostic of hyperthyroidism. Some hyperthyroid cats, especially those with concomitant illness, have a normal T_4 concentration. In these cases, additional evaluation (e.g., T_3 suppression test) is indicated before hyperthyroidism can be excluded. For a more complete discussion of these tests, see Diagnostic Procedures.

Cats with hyperthyroidism should be evaluated for cardiac disease, especially if physical examination reveals tachycardia, a cardiac murmur, gallop rhythm, or signs of congestive heart failure such as respiratory distress, muffled heart sounds, or jugular pulses. The most common ECG changes that may be observed in hyperthyroid cats are sinus tachycardia and increased amplitude of R waves.[7] Thoracic radiographs are helpful for identifying cardiomegaly, pleural effusion, and signs of pulmonary edema. If available, echocardiography is the preferred diagnostic test for evaluation of hyperthyroid cats. The most common abnormalities identified include left ventricular hypertrophy, thickening of the interventricular septum, and left atrial and ventricular dilatation.[8, 10] Occasionally, hyperthyroid cats have congestive heart failure associated with dilated cardiomyopathy.[51]

Treatment

Cats with hyperthyroidism may be treated by administration of an antithyroid drug or radioactive iodine, or by surgical excision of the thyroid gland. There are advantages and disadvantages of each treatment, and it is important to consider these when selecting a protocol for an individual patient. In addition to management of hyperthyroidism, some cats require treatment for concomitant disorders such as chronic renal failure, cardiomyopathy, and congestive heart failure.

Antithyroid Drugs

Methimazole (Tapazole) is the antithyroid drug of choice for treatment of feline hyperthyroidism. It inhibits the synthesis of thyroid hormones, an effect that is reversible after the drug is discontinued. Methimazole is indicated for long-term control of hyperthyroidism or for stabilization of cats before thyroidectomy or treatment with radioactive iodine. It is relatively inexpensive and readily available, and owners can administer it at home. Another advantage of methimazole is that its antithyroid effect is reversible, which makes it an ideal treatment for cats with concomitant renal disease. Because correction of hyperthyroidism may worsen renal function, hyperthyroid cats with azotemia should be treated with methimazole initially before more permanent treatment is undertaken.[49, 50]

Despite its convenience, treatment with methimazole does have some disadvantages. Some owners may find it difficult to administer oral medication several times daily to a cat for the rest of its life. Another disadvantage is that approximately 15% of cats experience side effects, which may include lethargy, inappetence, vomiting, thrombocytopenia with bleeding, leukopenia, increased hepatic enzyme activities, icterus, or excoriation of the face and neck.[5, 52] Complications of methimazole therapy are most likely to occur during the first 2 to 3 months after initiation of treatment; however, some cats have a delayed reaction. If side effects occur, treatment with methimazole should be discontinued. If only mild complications such as lethargy, inappetence, or vomiting occur, treatment can be restarted at a lower dose after side effects resolve. If serious or life-threatening complications occur, other treatment of hyperthyroidism is indicated.

Many clinicians initiate treatment with 5 mg methimazole per cat b.i.d. However, to decrease occurrence of side effects some recommend starting with a low dose of methimazole and then gradually increasing to a maintenance protocol.[5] An initial oral dose of 2.5 mg per cat b.i.d. should be administered for 2 weeks, and then the cat should be re-evaluated. If the owner reports no problems and the results of physical examination, CBC, platelet count, and serum chemistries are normal compared with baseline values, the dose of methimazole is increased to 2.5 mg per cat orally t.i.d. for another 2 weeks. At that time, a similar re-evaluation should be done, as well as measurement of serum T_4 in a sample obtained 4 to 6 hours after dosing. If serum T_4 is within the reference range, methimazole treatment is continued as before. If hyperthyroidism still exists, the daily dose is increased by 2.5 mg per cat every 2 weeks until a normal serum T_4 is obtained. Although serum T_4 may return to normal after the first few weeks of treatment, clinical improvement does not occur for another 2 to 6 weeks.[5] Most cats can be controlled by administration of 10 to 12.5 mg/day; rarely, a cat requires up to 20 mg/day to control hyperthyroidism. If a cat requires a high dose of methimazole to control hyperthyroidism, inability of the owner to administer the pill should be suspected. After good control is achieved, an attempt can be made to administer the daily dose in one or two treatments, which is more convenient for owners who elect long-term methimazole treatment. Most cats require twice-daily treatment, although some may be managed by once-daily treatment.

Because side effects are most likely to occur

during the first 2 to 3 months of treatment, it is ideal to re-evaluate the cat by performing CBC, platelet count, and serum chemistries every 2 weeks during this time. Some cats have side effects after prolonged treatment, however, and owners should be instructed to call the veterinarian if any signs of methimazole toxicity are observed. If possible, cats should be monitored for side effects by re-evaluation every 3 to 6 months as long as methimazole is administered.

Surgery

Thyroidectomy is another readily available method of effectively treating cats with hyperthyroidism. Potential disadvantages of surgical treatment of hyperthyroidism are the risks of anesthesia in older cats that often have concomitant problems such as renal or cardiac disease and the potential for development of postoperative hypocalcemia owing to excision of the parathyroid glands or disruption of their vascular supply. Other complications of thyroidectomy include damage to the recurrent laryngeal nerve and hypothyroidism. Cats with ectopic or metastatic thyroid tissue (e.g., mediastinal) may best be treated with modalities other than surgery.

Before surgery, it is preferable to stabilize the cat by administration of methimazole for 3 to 4 weeks to control hyperthyroidism so that the serum T_4 concentration is normal and clinical signs of hyperthyroidism are resolving. Treatment of concomitant diseases such as hypertrophic cardiomyopathy also is indicated and may require a longer period of stabilization before surgery. For a complete discussion of treatment of cardiac disorders associated with hyperthyroidism, see Chapter 12.

Because of concomitant diseases (e.g., renal failure, cardiac disease), anesthetic management of hyperthyroid cats should be done carefully. If an anticholinergic is necessary, glycopyrrolate (Robinul) should be used at a dose of 0.02 mg/kg subcutaneously 10 to 15 minutes before induction. It is preferable to avoid ketamine in cats with renal or cardiac disease. In addition, xylazine (Rompun) should be avoided because of its cardiotoxic effects. Thiobarbiturates such as thiopental (Pentothal; 15 mg/kg intravenously) may be administered to effect to allow endotracheal intubation. Isoflurane is the preferred inhalational agent for maintenance of anesthesia. Ideally, ECG monitoring should be done to detect arrhythmias. A balanced electrolyte solution (e.g., lactated Ringer's solution) should be administered throughout surgery at a rate of 10 mL/kg per hour. In cats with renal disease, intravenous fluids should be continued until the cat is eating and drinking well enough to maintain hydration.

A variety of surgical techniques have been described for thyroidectomy; however, the goals of all

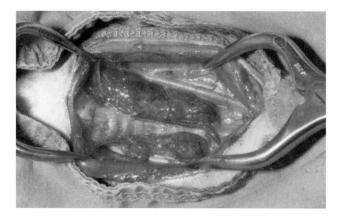

Figure 47–4
Enlargement of both thyroid lobes in a hyperthyroid cat. Although one lobe appears smaller, both should be removed.

techniques are to remove all abnormal thyroid tissue and to preserve function of at least one parathyroid gland.[53–55] A modified extracapsular technique may be associated with fewer recurrences and side effects such as hypocalcemia.[53] Results of a radionuclide scan done before surgery are helpful for objectively distinguishing between unilateral and bilateral thyroid involvement. All tissue that appears to be functional on the basis of a radionuclide scan should be surgically excised. If a radionuclide scan is not done, the surgeon must decide which gland or glands to remove on the basis of gross appearance. Obviously if both glands are enlarged, they should be removed (Fig. 47–4). However, this decision may not be so clear if one gland is obviously enlarged and the other is not. In general, if only one lobe is affected, the other lobe will be atrophied and barely visible, in which case unilateral excision is indicated. If, however, one lobe is enlarged and the other is of normal size or slightly enlarged, it is best to perform bilateral thyroidectomy.

After surgery, cats should be monitored closely for hypocalcemia or signs of hypoparathyroidism, including weakness, restlessness, muscle tremors, or seizures.[56] If the cat cannot be watched for signs of hypocalcemia 24 hours per day, it may be best to send the cat home with the owners after it is eating and drinking and have them monitor the cat. If the cat is hospitalized, an intravenous catheter can be maintained for 3 days postoperatively in case emergency administration of calcium is necessary.[53] Ideally, serum calcium should be measured daily for 4 to 7 days after surgery, especially if bilateral thyroidectomy is performed. Although approximately 20% to 30% of cats have hypocalcemia after bilateral thyroidectomy, only 5% to 10% actually have clinical signs that require treatment.[55] For a complete discussion of treatment of hypocalcemia caused by hypoparathyroidism, see Chapter 49. Most cats require only short-term treatment for hypocalcemia after thyroidectomy. If results of serum calcium concentration cannot be obtained quickly, the ECG should be monitored and calcium therapy initiated when there is lengthening of the Q-T interval.

Hypothyroidism is a potential complication of bilateral thyroidectomy. Although serum T_4 concentrations may be very low postoperatively, clinical signs of hypothyroidism after thyroidectomy are rare in cats.[55] If signs of hypothyroidism occur (e.g., lethargy, obesity, alopecia), synthetic thyroid hormone (e.g., Soloxine) can be supplemented at a dose of 0.1 mg per cat orally once or twice daily. With time, these cats may recover the ability to produce thyroid hormone; therefore, an attempt can be made to gradually discontinue supplementation after 1 to 3 months.

Perhaps of more concern to owners is the possibility of recurrent hyperthyroidism after thyroidectomy. Approximately 10% of hyperthyroid cats have recurrence of hyperthyroidism 1 to 3 years after surgery.[55, 57] Monitoring of the serum T_4 concentration every 6 to 12 months after thyroidectomy is helpful for detecting recurrent hyperthyroidism. These cats may best be treated by either long-term methimazole or radioactive iodine, because the occurrence of complications is higher after a second surgery.[55]

Radioactive Iodine

Administration of radioactive iodine (^{131}I) is an excellent treatment for hyperthyroidism in cats.[58–61] There are no significant side effects, and the only disadvantages are that cats must be referred to a special facility and, depending on state laws, cats must be hospitalized for 1 to 4 weeks after treatment. This treatment is effective because the thyroid gland takes up ^{131}I as it would regular iodine. Within the thyroid gland, ^{131}I emits radiation, which causes death of functioning adenomatous cells. Normal thyroid tissue is atrophied in hyperthyroid cats and is not affected by ^{131}I. Parathyroid tissue also is not affected, because the emitted radiation travels only a short distance within the thyroid gland. Serum T_4 concentration returns to normal in most cats within 1 month of treatment.[58] Fewer than 5% of hyperthyroid cats have persistent or recurrent hyperthyroidism after treatment with ^{131}I.[60, 62] Recurrence may be more common among cats with very high serum T_4 concentrations and greatly enlarged thyroid glands; these cats usually respond to a second dose of ^{131}I.[60] Depending on therapeutic protocol, 2% to 10% of hyperthyroid cats have low serum T_4 concentrations after administration of ^{131}I; most of these cats do not have clinical signs of hypothyroidism, however.[60–62] If clinical signs of hypothyroidism occur, supplementation with levothy-roxine may be given at a dose of 0.1 mg per cat orally once or twice daily.

Prognosis

Prognosis for most cats with hyperthyroidism is good to excellent. A cure can be achieved in most hyperthyroid cats treated by thyroidectomy or by administration of ^{131}I. Clinical signs can be well controlled in cats by administration of methimazole, although a cure does not result. Although the prognosis for hyperthyroid cats may be excellent, the median survival time is only 2 years.[60] This can be explained by the fact that hyperthyroid cats often are already at the end of their lifespan when diagnosed. It is often the presence of concomitant disorders such as congestive heart failure, renal failure, and malignant neoplasia that limits prognosis in hyperthyroid cats.[60, 62]

Thyroid Neoplasia

Thyroid neoplasia is abnormal growth of thyroid cells that may be benign or malignant. Clinically important thyroid tumors are almost always malignant and most often affect dogs; malignant thyroid tumors are rare in cats.[39, 63–69] Thyroid tumors are most common in middle-aged to older dogs; the average age is about 10 years.[5, 63–69] In the United States, beagles are at increased risk for thyroid carcinoma.[64, 66, 69] Boxers, golden retrievers, dachshunds, Labrador retrievers, and German shepherds often are affected; however, this may be a result of breed popularity.[5] There is no sex predisposition.[63–65, 67–69]

Pathophysiology

As with most neoplasms, the inciting cause of thyroid neoplasia is unknown. The clinical signs of thyroid tumors result from local invasion into the ventral cervical area and pulmonary metastases.

Clinical Signs

Clinical signs in dogs with thyroid tumors include ventral cervical swelling, dyspnea, coughing, dysphagia, or an altered voice; some dogs have no clinical signs. Physical examination most often reveals a firm, nonpainful mass in the laryngeal area that is adhered to adjacent tissues. Fewer than 10% of dogs have functional thyroid tumors that may be associated with clinical signs of hyperthyroidism, including weight loss, cachexia, polyphagia, restlessness, and PU/PD.[5]

Diagnostic Plan

Thyroid neoplasia should be suspected in any dog with a ventral cervical mass. Results of laboratory evaluation, including CBC, serum chemistries, and urinalysis, often are nonspecific. Serum T_4 concentrations usually are normal or decreased in dogs with thyroid neoplasia; however, measurement is indicated if clinical signs of hyperthyroidism exist. Thoracic radiographs with three views (i.e., left lateral, right lateral, and ventrodorsal or dorsoventral) are indicated in dogs with a suspected thyroid mass to detect signs of distant metastasis, which occurs in 40% to 50% of cases.[5, 64] Radionuclide scans usually are abnormal in dogs with thyroid tumors, even though the tumors are most often nonfunctional.[36]

A definitive diagnosis of thyroid neoplasia is made after cytologic or histologic examination of thyroid tissue. Because malignant thyroid tumors are so difficult to treat, all masses in the ventral cervical area of dogs should be thoroughly evaluated, including histologic examination if necessary. Fine-needle aspiration of a cervical mass is indicated for initial evaluation; results are diagnostic in up to 50% of dogs with thyroid tumors.[64] Cytologic evaluation often reveals numerous red blood cells and, in some cases, clusters of well-differentiated epithelial cells, which are typical of thyroid carcinoma. If there is any question about the diagnosis, histologic evaluation should be done, ideally before surgical treatment (see Diagnostic Procedures). Malignant thyroid tumors are extremely vascular, and severe hemorrhage can result from a biopsy; therefore, it is advisable to be prepared to manage a patient that may have this complication.

Treatment

Therapeutic options that are most often used for dogs with malignant thyroid tumors include surgical debulking and chemotherapy. Because of the biologic behavior of thyroid carcinomas, most dogs cannot be cured. If there is no evidence of distant metastasis, surgical debulking of the tumor is the initial treatment of choice. An exception would be an extremely invasive or enlarged thyroid mass, in which case excessive hemorrhage at surgery could be life-threatening. Because of their vascular nature, invasion around vital structures, and tendency to bleed excessively, surgical excision of thyroid masses requires an experienced surgeon. In some situations, it may be best to refer these cases for surgical management.

Chemotherapy is indicated in most patients, because surgical excision usually is incomplete and thyroid tumors usually have metastasized by the time of diagnosis, even if metastases cannot be detected by radiography. The efficacy of chemotherapy for treatment of thyroid carcinoma in dogs is questionable, however. Although no complete remissions have occurred, regression of thyroid carcinoma occurs in some dogs treated with doxorubicin (Adriamycin) at 30

mg/m^2 intravenously once every 3 weeks.[70] Because of cardiotoxicity, it is usually recommended that no more than six treatments of doxorubicin be administered.

Prognosis

Most dogs with thyroid carcinoma eventually die from their disease. Dogs with freely moveable tumors and no evidence of metastasis may live 2 years or more after surgical excision.[63] Dogs with evidence of metastasis, however, have a grave prognosis. Dogs treated with chemotherapy (doxorubicin) with or without surgical excision have a median survival time of 9 months.[70]

Uncommon Diseases of the Thyroid Gland

Canine Hyperthyroidism

Hyperthyroidism occurs rarely in dogs with functional thyroid tumors and in those supplemented with excessive doses of synthetic thyroid hormone. Almost all thyroid tumors are malignant; however, benign functioning tumors may occur.[5, 71] Clinical signs are similar to those of cats with hyperthyroidism and include PU/PD, polyphagia, weight loss, restlessness, hyperactivity, and tachycardia. Diagnosis is made by finding a serum T_4 concentration that is increased above the reference range for the laboratory. Surgical excision of functioning thyroid tumors is the treatment of choice. Administration of radioactive iodine after surgery may prolong survival time, but this therapy has not been evaluated in a large number of dogs.[72]

Feline Hypothyroidism

Hypothyroidism in cats is most often caused by treatment of hyperthyroidism, either bilateral thyroidectomy or administration of radioactive iodine. Naturally occurring cases of congenital or adult-onset hypothyroidism are rare in cats.[5, 73, 74] Congenital hypothyroidism, however, has been observed more commonly. Kittens appear normal until 6 to 8 weeks of age, when they manifest skeletal signs of disproportionate dwarfism, including failure to grow, enlarged head, short and broad neck, and short limbs. Serum T_4 concentrations are below the reference range of the laboratory. Because nonthyroidal factors may cause a low serum T_4 concentration, a TSH response test is better for assessing thyroid function. Administration of synthetic levothyroxine at a dose of 0.1 mg per cat orally once or twice daily is the treatment of choice for feline hypothyroidism.

References

1. Peterson ME, Randolph JF, Mooney CT. Endocrine diseases. In: Sherding RG, ed. The Cat: Diseases and Clinical Management, 2nd ed. New York, Churchill Livingstone, 1994:1403–1506.
2. Hullinger RL. The endocrine system. In: Evans HE, Christensen GC, eds. Miller's Anatomy of the Dog, 2nd ed. Philadelphia, WB Saunders, 1979:602–631.
3. Nesbitt GH, Izzo J, Peterson L, et al. Canine hypothyroidism: A retrospective study of 108 cases. J Am Vet Med Assoc 1980;177:1117–1122.
4. Peterson ME, Kinter PB, Cavanagh PG, et al. Feline hyperthyroidism: Pretreatment clinical and laboratory evaluation of 131 cases. J Am Vet Med Assoc 1983;183: 103–110.
5. Feldman EC, Nelson RW. The thyroid gland. In: Feldman EC, Nelson RW, eds. Canine and Feline Endocrinology and Reproduction, 2nd ed. Philadelphia, WB Saunders, 1996:68–185.
6. Broussard JD, Peterson ME, Fox PR. Changes in clinical and laboratory findings in cats with hyperthyroidism from 1983–1993. J Am Vet Med Assoc 1995;206:302–305.
7. Peterson ME, Keene B, Ferguson DC, et al. Electrocardiographic findings in 45 cats with hyperthyroidism. J Am Vet Med Assoc 1982;180:934–937.
8. Moise NS, Dietze AE. Echocardiographic, electrocardiographic, and radiographic detection of cardiomegaly in hyperthyroid cats. Am J Vet Res 1986;147:1487–1494.
9. Liu S, Peterson ME, Fox PR. Hypertrophic cardiomyopathy and hyperthyroidism in the cat. J Am Vet Med Assoc 1984;185:52–57.
10. Bond BR, Fox PR, Peterson ME, et al. Echocardiographic findings in 103 cats with hyperthyroidism. J Am Vet Med Assoc 1988;192:1546–1550.
11. Woeber KA. Thyrotoxicosis and the heart. N Engl J Med 1992;327:94–98.
12. Appel GB, Blum CB, Chien S, et al. The hyperlipidemia of the nephrotic syndrome. N Engl J Med 1985;312:1544–1548.
13. Reimers TJ, Cowan RG, Davidson HP, et al. Validation of radioimmunoassays for triiodothyronine, thyroxine, and hydrocortisone (cortisol) in canine, feline, and equine sera. Am J Vet Res 1981;42:2016–2021.
14. Reimers TJ. Radioimmunoassays and diagnostic tests for thyroid and adrenal disorders. Compen Contin Educ Pract Vet 1982;4:65–76.
15. Reimers T, McCann JP, Cowan RG, et al. Effects of storage, hemolysis, and freezing and thawing on concentrations of thyroxine, cortisol, and insulin in blood samples. Proc Soc Exp Biol Med 1982;170:509–516.
16. Peterson ME, Graves TK, Cavanagh I. Serum thyroid hormone concentrations fluctuate in cats with hyperthyroidism. J Vet Intern Med 1987;1:142–146.
17. McLoughlin MA, DiBartola SP, Birchard SJ, et al. Influence of systemic nonthyroidal illness on serum concentration of thyroxine in hyperthyroid cats. J Am Anim Hosp Assoc 1993;29:227–234.
18. Peterson ME, Gamble DA. Effect of nonthyroidal illness on serum thyroxine concentrations in cats: 494 cases (1988). J Am Vet Med Assoc 1990;197:1203–1208.
19. Peterson ME, Ferguson DC, Kintzer PP, et al. Effects of spontaneous hyperadrenocorticism on serum thyroid hormone concentrations in the dog. Am J Vet Res 1984;45:2034–2038.
20. Vail DM, Panciera DL, Ogilvie GK. Thyroid hormone concentrations in dogs with chronic weight loss, with special reference to cancer cachexia. J Vet Intern Med 1994;8:122–127.
21. Ferguson DC. The effect of nonthyroidal factors on thyroid function tests in dogs. Compen Contin Educ Pract Vet 1988;10:1365–1377.
22. Elliot DA, King LG, Zerbe CA. Thyroid hormone concentrations in critically ill canine intensive care patients. J Vet Emerg Crit Care 1995;5:17–23.
23. Hall IA, Campbell KL, Chambers MD, et al. Effect of trimethoprim/sulfamethoxazole on thyroid function in dogs with pyometra. J Am Vet Med Assoc 1993;202:1959–1962.
24. Torres SMF, McKeever PJ, Johnston SD. Effect of oral administration of prednisolone on thyroid function in dogs. Am J Vet Res 1991;52:416–421.
25. Nelson RW, Ihle SL, Feldman EC, et al. Serum free thyroxine concentration in healthy dogs, dogs with hypothyroidism, and euthyroid dogs with concurrent illness. J Am Vet Med Assoc 1991;198:1401–1407.
26. Thacker EL, Refsal KR, Bull RW. Prevalence of autoantibodies to thyroglobulin, thyroxine, or triiodothyronine and relationship of autoantibodies and serum concentrations of iodothyronines in dogs. Am J Vet Res 1992;53:449–453.
27. Nachreiner RF, Refsal KR, Thacker EL, et al. Incidence of T_3 and T_4 autoantibodies in dogs using a sensitive binding assay. J Vet Intern Med 1990;4:114.
28. Williams DA, Scott-Moncrieff JC, Bruner J. Canine serum thyroid-stimulating hormone following induction of hypothyroidism. J Vet Intern Med 1995;9:184.
29. Nachreiner RF, Forsberg M, Johnson CA, et al. Validation of an assay for canine TSH (cTSH). J Vet Intern Med 1995;9:184.
30. Panciera DL, MacEwen EG, Atkins CE, et al. Thyroid function tests in euthyroid dogs treated with L-thyroxine. Am J Vet Res 1989;51:22–26.
31. Kobayashi DL, Nichols R, Peterson ME. Serum thyroid hormone concentrations in clinically normal dogs after administration of freshly reconstituted vs previously frozen and stored thyrotropin. J Am Vet Med Assoc 1990;197:597–600.
32. Bruyette DS, Nelson RW, Bottoms GD. Effect of thyrotropin storage on thyroid-stimulating hormone response testing in normal dogs. J Vet Intern Med 1987;1:91–94.
33. Kemppainen RJ, Thompson FN, Lorenz MD, et al. Effects of prednisone on thyroid and gonadal endocrine function in dogs. J Endocrinol 1983;96:293–302.
34. Peterson ME, Graves TK, Gamble DA. Triiodothyronine (T_3) suppression test. J Vet Intern Med 1990;4:233–238.
35. Refsal KR, Nachreiner RF, Stein BE, et al. Use of the triiodothyronine suppression test for diagnosis of hyperthyroidism in ill cats that have serum concentrations of iodothyronines within normal range. J Am Vet Med Assoc 1991;199:1594–1601.
36. Marks SL, Koblik PD, Hornof WJ, et al. ^{99m}Tc-

pertechnetate imaging of thyroid tumors in dogs: 29 cases (1980–1992). J Am Vet Med Assoc 1994;204:756–760.

37. Peterson ME, Becker DV. Radionuclide thyroid imaging in 135 cats with hyperthyroidism. Vet Radiol 1984;25:23–27.

38. Mooney CT, Thoday KL, Nicoll JJ, et al. Qualitative and quantitative thyroid imaging in feline hyperthyroidism using technetium-99m as pertechnetate. Vet Radiol 1992;33:313–320.

39. Turrel JM, Feldman EC, Nelson RW, et al. Thyroid carcinoma causing hyperthyroidism in cats: 14 cases (1981–1986). J Am Vet Med Assoc 1988;193:359–364.

40. Milne KL, Hayes HM. Epidemiologic features of canine hypothyroidism. Cornell Vet 1981;71:3–14.

41. Panciera DL. Hypothyroidism in dogs: 66 cases (1987–1992). J Am Vet Med Assoc 1994;204:761–767.

42. Chastain CB. Canine hypothyroidism. J Am Vet Med Assoc 1982;181:349–353.

43. Jaggy A, Oliver JE, Ferguson DC, et al. Neurological manifestations of hypothyroidism: A retrospective study of 29 dogs. J Vet Intern Med 1994;8:328–336.

44. Beale KM, Halliwell REW, Chen CL. Prevalence of antithyroglobulin antibodies detected by enzyme-linked immunosorbent assay of canine serum. J Am Vet Med Assoc 1990;196:745–748.

45. Nachreiner RF, Refsal KR. Radioimmunoassay monitoring of thyroid hormone concentrations in dogs on thyroid replacement therapy: 2,674 cases (1985–1987). J Am Vet Med Assoc 1992;201:623–629.

46. Peterson ME, Johnson GF, Andrews LK. Spontaneous hyperthyroidism in the cat. Proc Am Coll Vet Int Med 1979;108 (abstract).

47. Holzworth J, Theran P, Carpenter JL, et al. Hyperthyroidism in the cat: Ten cases. J Am Vet Med Assoc 1980;176:345–353.

48. Thoday KL, Mooney CT. Historical, clinical and laboratory features of 126 hyperthyroid cats. Vet Rec 1992;131:257–264.

49. DiBartola SP, Broome MR, Stein BS, et al. Effect of treatment of hyperthyroidism on renal function in cats. J Am Vet Med Assoc 1996;208:875–878.

50. Graves TK, Olivier NB, Nachreiner RF, et al. Changes in renal function associated with treatment of hyperthyroidism in cats. Am J Vet Res 1994;55:1745–1749.

51. Jacobs G, Hutson C, Dougherty J, et al. Congestive heart failure associated with hyperthyroidism in cats. J Am Vet Med Assoc 1986;188:52–56.

52. Peterson ME, Kintzer PP, Hurvitz AI. Methimazole treatment of 262 cats with hyperthyroidism. J Vet Intern Med 1988;2:150–157.

53. Salisbury SK. Hyperthyroidism in cats. Compen Contin Educ Pract Vet 1991;13:1399–1410.

54. Flanders JA, Harvey HJ, Erb HN. Feline thyroidectomy: A comparison of postoperative hypocalcemia associated with three different surgical techniques. Vet Surg 1987;16:362–366.

55. Welches CD, Scavelli TD, Matthiesen DT, et al. Occurrence of problems after three techniques of bilateral thyroidectomy in cats. Vet Surg 1989;18:392–396.

56. Peterson ME. Hypoparathyroidism and other causes of hypocalcemia in cats. In: Kirk RW, Bonagura JD, eds. Kirk's Current Veterinary Therapy XI. Philadelphia, WB Saunders, 1992:376–379.

57. Swalec KM, Birchard SJ. Recurrence of hyperthyroidism after thyroidectomy in cats. J Am Anim Hosp Assoc 1990;26:433–438.

58. Meric SM, Hawkins EC, Washabau RJ, et al. Serum thyroxine concentrations after radioactive iodine therapy in cats with hyperthyroidism. J Am Vet Med Assoc 1986;188:1038–1040.

59. Meric SM, Rubin SI. Serum thyroxine concentrations following fixed-dose radioactive iodine treatment in hyperthyroid cats: 62 cases (1986–1989). J Am Vet Med Assoc 1990;197:621–624.

60. Peterson ME, Becker DV. Radioiodine treatment of 524 cats with hyperthyroidism. J Am Vet Med Assoc 1995;207:1422–1428.

61. Theon AP, Van Vechten MK, Feldman E. Prospective randomized comparison of intravenous versus subcutaneous administration of radioiodine for treatment of hyperthyroidism in cats. Am J Vet Res 1994;55:1734–1738.

62. Slater MR, Komkov A, Robinson LE, et al. Long-term follow-up of hyperthyroid cats treated with iodine-131. Vet Radiol 1994;35:204–209.

63. Klein MK, Powers BE, Withrow SJ, et al. Treatment of thyroid carcinoma in dogs by surgical resection alone: 20 cases (1981–1989). J Am Vet Med Assoc 1995;206:1007–1009.

64. Harari J, Patterson JS, Rosenthal RC. Clinical and pathologic features of thyroid tumors in 26 dogs. J Am Vet Med Assoc 1986;188:1160–1164.

65. Sullivan M, Cox F, Pead MJ, et al. Thyroid tumors in the dog. J Small Anim Pract 1987;28:505–512.

66. Haley PJ, Hahn FF, Muggenburg BA, et al. Thyroid neoplasms in a colony of beagle dogs. Vet Pathol 1989;26:438–441.

67. Birchard SJ, Roesel OF. Neoplasia of the thyroid gland in the dog: A retrospective study of 16 cases. J Am Anim Hosp Assoc 1981;17:369–372.

68. Carver JR, Kapatkin A, Patnaik AK. A comparison of medullary thyroid carcinoma and thyroid adenocarcinoma in dogs: A retrospective study of 38 cases. Vet Surg 1995;24:315–319.

69. Mitchell M, Hurov LI, Troy GC. Canine thyroid carcinomas: Clinical occurrence, staging by means of scintiscans, and therapy of 15 cases. Vet Surg 1979;8:112–118.

70. Jeglum KA, Whereat A. Chemotherapy of canine thyroid carcinoma. Compen Contin Educ Pract Vet 1983;5:96–98.

71. Lawrence D, Thompson J, Layton AW, et al. Hyperthyroidism associated with a thyroid adenoma in a dog. J Am Vet Med Assoc 1991;199:81–84.

72. Adams WH, Walker MA, Daniel GB, et al. Treatment of differentiated thyroid carcinoma in 7 dogs utilizing [131]I. Vet Radiol 1995;36:417–424.

73. Rand JS, Levine J, Best SJ, et al. Spontaneous adult-onset hypothyroidism in a cat. J Vet Intern Med 1993;7:272–276.

74. Jones B, Gruffyd-Jones TJ, Sparkes AH, et al. Preliminary studies on congenital hypothyroidism in a family of Abyssinian cats. Vet Rec 1992;131:145–148.

Chapter 48

Diseases of the Endocrine Pancreas

William E. Monroe

Anatomy

The endocrine pancreas is composed of groups of cells in islets, the islets of Langerhans, dispersed throughout the exocrine tissue of the organ. These islets contain four types of cells, which produce different hormones. The β-cells are the most numerous cells in the islets; they produce insulin. The α-cells produce glucagon, the D-cells produce somatostatin, and the F- or PP-cells produce pancreatic polypeptide.[1] The venous drainage from the pancreas is through the hepatic portal vein,[2, 3] so the majority of a pancreatic hormone's influence is on the liver. See Chapter 33 for a complete description of the anatomy of the pancreas.

Physiology

Postprandially, after glucose and other nutrients are absorbed from the gastrointestinal (GI) tract, insulin release is stimulated by an increased blood glucose or amino acid concentration, or by GI hormones. During this phase, insulin increases movement of glucose into cells for metabolism for energy and formation of glycogen and fat,[1] with a net effect of reducing blood glucose concentration and facilitating storage of fat and protein production. During this time of nutrient absorption, glucagon is also secreted in response to an increased blood amino acid concentration. Glucagon inhibits insulin secretion and increases glycogenolysis and gluconeogenesis, with a net effect of increasing blood glucose concentration. This dual secretion of insulin and glucagon is beneficial to prevent hypoglycemia when an animal consumes a meal that is particularly high in protein and low in carbohydrate.

The increased blood glucose concentration that occurs in response to glucagon secretion has a negative feedback effect on the α-cells of the pancreatic islets, suppressing the secretion of glucagon. Insulin is necessary, however, for glucose to enter into the α-cells in order to suppress glucagon secretion.[1] This may explain why blood glucagon concentration is increased in diabetic animals with an absolute insulin deficiency, despite the presence of hyperglycemia.

During the postabsorptive state (several hours after eating, after the majority of nutrients from the meal, including glucose, have been absorbed from the GI tract), the blood glucose concentration begins to drop. In response to a decreasing blood glucose concentration, insulin secretion is reduced and glucagon secretion is increased. This leads to an increase in production of glucose from glycogenolysis and gluconeogenesis to compensate for the lack of glucose being absorbed from the GI tract, in order to maintain the blood glucose concentration in the normal range. The major stimulus for secretion of glucagon is hypoglycemia.[1]

Insulin is the major hormone that facilitates fatty acid storage in fat cells, and glucagon stimulates fatty acid mobilization. During prolonged periods of fasting or insulin deficiency (i.e., diabetes), fatty acids are mobilized because blood glucagon concentration is increased whereas blood insulin concentration is low. These fatty acids can be used directly by some cells for energy production, but most are converted by the liver to ketones, which may also be used as an energy source.[1]

Glucose serves as the primary source of energy for several tissues in the body, including nervous tissue.[4] Because nerves can store only a few minutes' supply of glucose (as glycogen), the blood glucose concentration must be maintained in the normal range.[5] If the blood glucose concentration drops substantially below the normal range, glucagon secretion is increased rapidly, as is epinephrine production. This response depends not only on the magnitude of the reduction in blood glucose concentration but also on the rate. Epinephrine inhibits insulin secretion and increases glucose production by stimulating gluconeogenesis and glycogenolysis. If the blood glucose concentration is low, glucocorticoids and growth hormone are also secreted, leading to increased glucose production and decreased peripheral utilization. These latter two hormones are released after glucagon and epinephrine, whose effects last about 30 minutes. The effects of cortisol and growth hormone last for hours.[6] These mechanisms are necessary to prevent severe hypoglycemia, in order to provide a constant supply of glucose to the brain.[4, 6–9]

Problem Identification

Hypoglycemia

Hypoglycemia is defined as a reduction in blood glucose concentration below the lower limit of normal. In general, a value below 50 to 60 mg/dL is considered hypoglycemia.[7, 8, 10] Some restrict use of the term to those cases in which the reduction is severe enough to cause clinical signs. The value at which clinical signs occur depends on the animal's adaptation to the presence of low blood glucose and the rate at which the glucose dropped.

Pathophysiology

Hypoglycemia may occur as the result of increased use of glucose, as occurs with insulin-producing tumors[11–15]; reduced production of glucose, as occurs with severe hepatic disease,[8] hypoadrenocorticism,[16] or juvenile transient hypoglycemia[17]; or a combination of these two mechanisms, which may occur with sepsis.[18]

The clinical signs of hypoglycemia are the result of brain dysfunction (neuroglycopenia). The brain requires glucose for energy production and can store only a small supply.[4, 6, 9] Before the glucose concentration drops to the point of brain dysfunction, glucose sensors in the hypothalamus detect a low glucose concentration and stimulate increased sympathetic activity.[19] Sympathetic stimulation may prevent severe hypoglycemia from developing by increasing glucose production through glycogenolysis and gluconeogenesis and inhibiting insulin secretion.[1] However, this increased sympathoadrenal activity also results in some of the clinical signs of hypoglycemia such as tachycardia, nervousness, panting, and tremor.[4, 19]

Chronic hypoglycemia leads to metabolic adaptations in the brain that allow it to take up glucose more efficiently. This reduces the threshold concentration at which the patient becomes aware of hypoglycemia, and clinical signs of hypoglycemic brain dysfunction occur.[19] If profound hypoglycemia is present for several hours, cerebral damage occurs,[4] with residual clinical signs such as seizures, coma, stupor, and blindness even after hypoglycemia is corrected.

Hypoglycemia can occur artifactually if the serum or plasma being tested is not separated from the red blood cells (RBCs) within a short period (30–60 min). The RBCs continue to metabolize glucose in the sample unless the blood is placed in a sodium fluoride tube. In general, the glucose is reduced by 10% for every 1 hour the serum or plasma remains in contact with the RBCs.[20]

Clinical Signs

The clinical signs of hypoglycemia are those of sympathoadrenal stimulation and neuroglycopenic brain dysfunction.[6] The severity of signs is affected by the rate of reduction and the duration of hypoglycemia more than by the actual concentration of glucose.[7] Clinical signs are usually not evident until the glucose concentration is less than 45 mg/dL,[21] and some dogs do not show signs even if their blood glucose is 30 mg/dL or lower.[8] Tachycardia, nervousness, trembling, and panting occur first as a result of sympathetic stimulation; this is followed by signs of brain dysfunction such as behavioral changes (often bizarre), weakness, dementia, dullness, collapse, ataxia, hysteria, seizures, stupor, and coma.[7, 12, 13, 15] Very young animals (<30 days old) do not have the sympathetic response of older animals and therefore usually demonstrate only the effects of brain dysfunction.

Diagnostic Plan

If hypoglycemia is noted on a serum biochemistry panel, the patient's clinical signs should be assessed to determine whether they are consistent with low blood glucose. If hypoglycemia is profound without clinical signs, artifact may be the cause, and the measurement of blood glucose should be repeated, paying careful attention to sample handling. After artifact has been ruled out, the clinician should determine whether there is a history of insulin administration, exposure to oral hypoglycemic drugs, or extreme, vigorous exercise, as is the case with so-called hunting dog hypoglycemia. After drug-related causes and severe, vigorous exercise have been eliminated, the clinical signs should be considered along with the results of a complete blood count (CBC) to determine whether sepsis (inflammatory leukogram) could be the cause of hypoglycemia.[18] Although sepsis is a common cause of hypoglycemia in clinical practice, the clinical signs for which the animal is presented are usually those of the septic condition (i.e., fever, shock, and signs associated with the organ or organs primarily affected) and not those of hypoglycemia, even though it may be fairly severe.

If clinical signs of hypoglycemia are present (historically or on physical examination), the signalment should be considered. Neonatal puppies (<6 weeks of age) often become hypoglycemic from any cause of disease or distress such as diarrhea, hypothermia, starvation, parasitism, or septicemia.[9] These puppies benefit from supplementation with glucose and from diagnosis and treatment of the underlying problem. In puppies, particularly toy breeds, older than 6 weeks but younger than 3 to 6 months, hypoglycemia with clinical signs (transient juvenile hypoglycemia) may be precipitated by starvation, cold, or GI disease.[9, 22] The precipitating event is often so mild that the owner would not suspect it as a cause (e.g., it has been seen in puppies merely left for 4–6 hours without food). These animals respond to administration of glucose, 1 mL/kg of body weight of intravenous (IV) 50% dextrose diluted with an equal volume of physiologic saline (see sections on treatment of specific diseases), with no residual disease unless hypoglycemia was present long enough to cause cerebral damage.

Dogs younger than 1 year of age with hypoglycemia and evidence of liver failure on the serum chemistry profile—such as hypoalbuminemia, low blood urea nitrogen (BUN), and, occasionally, elevated liver enzymes—may have a portosystemic shunt and should have abdominal radiographs to evaluate liver size (small with shunts) and a liver function test (e.g., bile acids, fasting blood ammonia; see Chap. 34). Likewise, adult dogs with similar laboratory abnormalities may have severe liver disease (portosystemic shunts or cirrhosis) as a cause of hypoglycemia from failure to produce adequate glucose.[8]

If there are changes in the biochemistry profile such as hyponatremia, hyperkalemia (with a sodium/

potassium ratio <27:1), azotemia, and hypercalcemia, hypoadrenocorticism may be the cause of the hypoglycemia.[16] In these cases, an ACTH response test (see Chap. 46) should be performed to make a definitive diagnosis.

If changes in the CBC, serum biochemical profile, and urinalysis are not specific for the presence of one of the diseases already mentioned as causes of hypoglycemia in adult or young adult animals, one should carefully repeat abdominal palpation and perform abdominal radiography or ultrasonography to rule out large, abdominal, nonpancreatic tumors[23, 24] as a cause of hypoglycemia. After other causes are ruled out, hypoglycemia in adult dogs may be the result of an insulin-producing pancreatic tumor (insulinoma). Dogs with insulinomas may have elevations of liver enzymes, so liver disease must be ruled out with liver function tests such as bile acids. After other causes are ruled out, serum insulin concentration should be measured by radioimmunoassay at a time when blood glucose concentration is low (fast with observation and measurement of glucose hourly; see Special Laboratory Tests) in order to justify exploratory abdominal surgery to diagnose and treat insulinoma.[11–15]

Polyuria and Polydipsia

Dogs and cats with diabetes mellitus have an osmotic diuresis from loss of excess glucose in the urine, leading to polyuria with secondary polydipsia (PU/PD). There are many other causes of PU/PD in dogs and cats (see Chap. 16). Diabetes mellitus should be suspected if PU/PD occurs along with weight loss in spite of a good to excessive appetite, or with the acute onset of bilateral cataracts in dogs.

Weight Loss With a Good Appetite

Weight loss in spite of a good appetite can be caused by diabetes mellitus or by GI parasites, pancreatic exocrine insufficiency (in dogs), hyperthyroidism (in cats), or, occasionally, infiltrative bowel disease. A more thorough discussion of this problem can be found in Chapter 47. Dogs and cats with weight loss associated with diabetes mellitus also often have PU/PD, fasting hyperglycemia, and glucosuria.

Vomiting

Dogs or cats with diabetic ketoacidosis (DKA) may be presented with vomiting. There are many other causes of vomiting in small animals, including other metabolic causes and primary GI disease (see Chap. 31). DKA should be suspected as a cause of vomiting if the dog or cat has a history of PU/PD, weight loss in spite of a good appetite, and hyper-

glycemia, glucosuria, and ketonuria on routine laboratory tests.

Diagnostic Procedures

Routine Laboratory Evaluation

Serum chemistries and urinalysis to detect abnormalities in plasma glucose concentration or glucosuria, respectively, are imperative to diagnose disorders of the endocrine pancreas. Other values in serum or plasma chemistry profiles, and results of CBCs and complete urinalysis, are useful primarily to identify associated electrolyte or acid-base disturbances or the presence of concomitant diseases that may complicate management of diseases such as diabetes mellitus.

Radiography

Thoracic and abdominal radiographs typically are not useful to diagnose diseases of the endocrine pancreas. However, radiography may be useful to identify complicating disorders such as neoplasia, cardiac disease, pancreatitis, or pyometra that may affect management of diabetes mellitus, and it can help rule out other diseases (e.g., nonpancreatic tumors) as a cause of hypoglycemia.[23–25] Emphysematous cystitis may be noted on abdominal radiographs of dogs with diabetes mellitus.

Ultrasonography

Abdominal ultrasound examination may be useful for identifying concomitant or complicating diseases such as pancreatitis (see Chap. 33) or neoplasia in patients with diabetes mellitus.[26] It does not usually identify insulin-producing islet cell tumors, but metastasis of such tumors to the liver or lymph nodes may be apparent.[27]

Specific Laboratory Tests

Analysis of plasma insulin concentration by radioimmunoassay simultaneously with measurement of plasma glucose concentration is often useful to confirm the diagnosis of insulinoma, or at least make the diagnosis sufficiently likely to justify exploratory surgery to confirm the diagnosis. If the blood glucose concentration is not below the reference range in a dog suspected of having an insulin-producing islet cell tumor, the patient should cautiously be fasted, starting in the morning after its usual postprandial period, with monitoring of the dog's clinical signs in the hospital and measurement of blood glucose hourly. This can be done practically by using reagent strips and a reflectance colorimeter (see discussion of management of uncomplicated diabetes). If blood glucose drops below 40 to 50 mg/dL, as indicated by reagent strips with a reflectance colorimeter to measure blood glucose concentration, hypoglycemia should be confirmed by plasma or serum glucose determination in a clinical pathology laboratory. If the plasma or serum glucose concentration is confirmed to be less than normal (<60–70 mg/dL), plasma insulin concentration should be measured for the same sample.[12, 27, 28]

An insulin concentration that is increased in the presence of hypoglycemia is inappropriate, and insulinoma is highly likely. A high-normal insulin concentration in the presence of hypoglycemia may also be inappropriate. However, there has not been a clear definition of what concentration of insulin is indicative of the presence of an insulinoma when the insulin concentration is in the normal range with concurrent hypoglycemia.[27] It has been stated that if the insulin concentration is in approximately the upper 50% of the reference range, insulinoma is likely.[28]

Because 25% to 35% of patients with insulinoma have an insulin concentration in the normal range with concomitant hypoglycemia, making the diagnosis uncertain, insulin/glucose ratios have been used in an attempt to better define what insulin concentration is appropriate and to find a more sensitive marker to identify those patients with insulinoma that have a normal insulin concentration. The amended insulin/glucose ratio (AIGR) is calculated as follows: (insulin concentration × 100)/ (plasma glucose − 30). If glucose is less than 30 mg/dL, the denominator should be 1. This calculation increases the sensitivity of testing to identify the presence of insulinoma (normal = <30).[11–13] Unfortunately, the test is not very specific, because dogs with hypoglycemia from causes other than insulinoma (e.g., sepsis or large, non–islet cell tumors) may also have an increased AIGR.[13, 18] For cases in which an insulinoma is suspected and yet insulin concentration is not elevated in the presence of hypoglycemia, the glucose-insulin pair can be repeated if other causes of hypoglycemia cannot reasonably be ruled out.

Common Diseases of the Endocrine Pancreas

Diabetes Mellitus

Diabetes mellitus is a persistent abnormality of carbohydrate metabolism caused by an absolute or relative deficiency of insulin such that persistent hyperglycemia occurs. Virtually all dogs and 50% to 70% of cats with diabetes mellitus are insulin dependent and require insulin therapy for glycemic control.[26]

Diabetes mellitus is one of the most common

endocrinopathies in dogs, occurring in approximately 2 dogs out of every 1000 seen once in a year by a veterinarian for all reasons.[29] It is more common in females (64% to 77% of cases),[29–31] and castrated males may have a greater risk of developing the disease than intact males.[29] The disease can occur at almost any age (<1 to >15 years), but 70% of all patients are 7 years of age or older at the time of diagnosis, with the peak occurrence between 7 and 11 years.[29, 31, 32] Breeds at increased risk for development of diabetes mellitus include dachshunds, poodles, cairn terriers, keeshonds, Alaskan malamutes, schipperkes, Finnish spitzes, Manchester terriers, miniature schnauzers, English springer spaniels, and miniature pinschers.[29–31] Breeds that uncommonly develop the disease or are at a reduced risk include cocker spaniels, German shepherds, collies, Pekingese, and boxers.[29]

Diabetes mellitus is also one of the most common endocrinopathies seen in cats, occurring in approximately 2.5 cats for every 1000 seen once in a year by a veterinarian for all reasons.[33] Although diabetes mellitus can be seen in cats of all ages, the majority of patients are 10 years of age or older,[33–36] and 76% of patients are older than 7 years at the time of diagnosis.[33] Males are 1.5 times more likely to become diabetic than females, and neutering increases the risk of developing the disease by a factor of 2 for either sex.[33] In addition, obesity tends to increase the risk for developing diabetes in cats.[33, 35] There does not appear to be a breed predilection.[33, 36]

Pathophysiology

Most canine patients with diabetes mellitus have what has been termed type I or insulin-dependent diabetes mellitus (IDDM), caused by primary destruction of the β-cells.[26, 37] Although not well understood or documented in dogs, this destruction may be caused by immune-mediated processes.[37–39] The development of diabetes mellitus probably depends on the combination of genetic susceptibility, environmental or infectious damage of β-cells followed by continuous immune destruction resulting in severe insulin deficiency,[37] and perhaps concurrent endocrine factors causing insulin resistance that contributes to β-cell exhaustion.[26]

Most feline patients with diabetes mellitus, from the standpoint of pathogenetic mechanism, may have what is known in human medicine as type II or adult-onset, usually non–insulin-dependent diabetes mellitus (NIDDM).[35, 40–42] Type II diabetes arises from a combination of insulin resistance and abnormal insulin secretion.[40, 43, 44] Although much of what is known about NIDDM comes from the study of human patients, cats have abnormalities such as the development of islet amyloid that are very similar to those found in the human disorder.[41, 45–47] Probably because diabetes is usually not diagnosed in cats until late in the course of disease, β-cell function has been lost to the point that 50% to 70% of feline diabetic patients require insulin therapy.[35]

Diabetes mellitus can also be seen as a secondary disease caused by another endocrinopathy that causes insulin resistance. This is probably the mechanism in cats with hyperadrenocorticism (90% have overt diabetes mellitus),[48–50] in those feline cases occurring in association with megestrol acetate therapy,[51] and in dogs with hyperadrenocorticism[52, 53] or progesterone-induced hypersomatotropism.[54]

The relative or absolute deficiency of insulin in diabetic patients leads to hyperglycemia, because glucose is unable to move into cells of many tissues, and gluconeogenesis and glycogenolysis proceed unchecked. Because insulin appears to be necessary for glucose to move inside pancreatic islet α-cells,[4, 55] plasma glucagon concentration is increased.[45, 56] Without the presence of insulin, the α-cells cannot respond to hyperglycemia, which usually suppresses glucagon secretion. The resulting elevated glucagon concentration worsens hyperglycemia. In addition, the lack of the anabolic effect on protein metabolism normally provided by insulin leads to an increased release of amino acids from tissues, which in turn are used in gluconeogenesis. When the glucose concentration exceeds the renal threshold, glycosuria occurs, leading to an osmotic diuresis and polyuria, with compensatory polydipsia. Because tissues that cannot use glucose without the actions of insulin are starving for energy, and because the animal lacks the insulin to facilitate deposition of fatty acids in tissues as fat, fatty acids are mobilized at an increased rate. Although some tissues can use fatty acids for energy, the bulk of the fatty acids are metabolized in the liver to ketoacids, which may also serve as an energy source for many tissues. The rate of ketone production exceeds the rate of metabolism, leading to acidosis and renal excretion, contributing to the osmotic diuresis.[26] Osmotic diuresis contributes to renal sodium and potassium loss, which may lead to hyponatremia or hypokalemia, respectively, and to a total body potassium deficit. In addition, hyponatremia may be associated with a dilutional effect from the hyperosmolality caused by hyperglycemia and ketosis.

Because the body is in a catabolic state, and because without insulin the brain fails to respond to the satiety signal of hyperglycemia, polyphagia may ensue. Weight loss occurs in spite of a normal to increased appetite as a result of a general anabolic failure caused by lack of insulin action.[26]

For the development of the very ill DKA syndrome, intercurrent disease that leads to increases

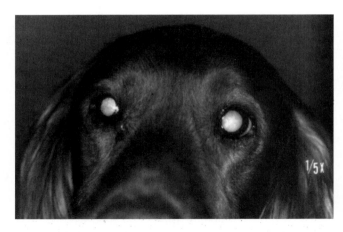

Figure 48–1
Dog with bilateral cataracts from diabetes mellitus. (Courtesy of J. Phillip Pickett, DVM, Blacksburg, Virginia.)

of insulin-antagonistic hormones such as glucagon, cortisol, and growth hormone probably is necessary. Any cause of reduced food or water intake leads to dehydration and stress, which worsen hyperglycemia and ketosis. Complicating diseases in the dog include urinary tract infection, pancreatitis, hyperadrenocorticism or exogenous administration of corticosteroids, otitis, pyometra, neoplasia, renal failure, estrus or pregnancy, exocrine pancreatic insufficiency, and respiratory disease.[31, 57, 58] Intercurrent diseases in cats include renal disease, inflammatory bowel disease, asthma, urinary tract infection, pancreatitis, hyperthyroidism, heart disease, neoplasia, and administration of corticosteroids.[59] Anorexia and vomiting in the DKA patient worsen total body sodium and potassium deficits, leading to hyponatremia and occasionally to hypokalemia on admission to a veterinary hospital. However, because intracellular buffering of acidosis leads to shifting of potassium out of cells, normokalemia or hyperkalemia may be noted at presentation, before rehydration. Whole body phosphorus deficits occur for reasons similar to those causing potassium deficiency. Serum phosphorus may be normal or elevated, because dehydration often leads to reduced glomerular filtration rate and prerenal azotemia. Because the glucose transport mechanism stimulated by insulin tends to move phosphorus and potassium inside cells as well, and because fluid and insulin therapy decreases acidosis and increases the glomerular filtration rate, hypokalemia and hypophosphatemia may occur within hours of beginning therapy. Hypokalemia occurs commonly, and severe hypophosphatemia uncommonly.

Severe dehydration in DKA often leads to prerenal azotemia. That, along with acidosis and hyperosmolality, contributes to lethargy, anorexia, vomiting, and cardiovascular dysfunction.[59, 60]

Clinical Signs

Uncomplicated Diabetes Mellitus

The classic clinical signs of uncomplicated diabetes mellitus in dogs and cats are polydipsia, polyuria, and weight loss despite polyphagia.[26, 30–32, 34, 36] Dogs often (26%–67% of cases) have cataracts bilaterally (Fig. 48–1) that have developed or have begun to develop at the time of presentation, often rapidly over a few days.[30–32] Hepatomegaly is common in dogs and cats on physical examination.[26, 30–32, 34, 36] Although some patients are obese at the time of presentation,[31, 34, 35] at least one half have lost weight recently.[26, 30–32, 34, 36] Almost 50% of patients are thin with apparent muscle wasting.[61] A small proportion of cats (perhaps 8%) have a plantigrade stance (Fig. 48–2), presumably caused by distal polyneuropathy,[61–63] but this sign is only rarely seen in dogs.[61] Cats frequently have an unkempt hair coat,[63] and dogs may often (20 of 56 cases) have dermatologic changes such as generalized or local alopecia, pyoderma, seborrhea, and hyperkeratosis.[32]

Diabetic Ketoacidosis

The complication of ketoacidosis leads to severe metabolic derangements, morbidity, and sometimes death. Although most dogs (75%–84%)[30–32] and about one half of cats presented with diabetes mellitus have ketonuria,[34, 36, 64] they are not considered to have DKA requiring aggressive treatment unless ketoacidosis is severe enough to cause anorexia, lethargy, vomiting and dehydration, and occasionally recumbence, semicoma, and shock.[31, 36, 57, 63] Dogs and cats with DKA have clinical signs of uncomplicated diabetes (or at least a history of them), often profound, before developing the signs of ketoacidosis.[26, 61] About 33% of

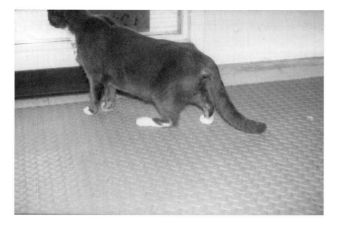

Figure 48–2
Cat with plantigrade stance typical of that seen in some cases of diabetes mellitus from presumed peripheral neuropathy. (Courtesy of Linda G. Shell, DVM, Blacksburg, Virginia.)

cats[36, 63] and 14% of dogs[57] may be icteric. Other signs that may be seen include abdominal pain, hypothermia, hyperthermia,[57] and diarrhea.[29, 32, 64] Evidence of intercurrent disease that may have contributed to the development of the severe ketoacidotic state is often present. Intercurrent diseases in dogs include urinary tract infection, pancreatitis, hyperadrenocorticism or exogenous administration of corticosteroids, otitis, pyometra, neoplasia, renal failure, estrus or pregnancy, exocrine pancreatic insufficiency, and respiratory disease.[31, 57, 58]

Diagnostic Plan

Uncomplicated Diabetes Mellitus

The diagnosis of uncomplicated diabetes mellitus is made by finding typical clinical signs and moderate to severe (>300 mg/dL) fasting hyperglycemia and glucosuria. The most important criterion is that hyperglycemia is persistent. This criterion can be documented by repeating the test a few days later, but that is not necessary if persistence is documented by the presence of the typical clinical signs. Because cats can often have severe hyperglycemia from the stress of phlebotomy, it is important to document the persistence of hyperglycemia by the presence of at least three of the typical clinical signs[65] (polyuria, polydipsia, weight loss, and polyphagia) or by repeating the test—on a sample taken through an IV catheter (after 24 hours to relax from catheter placement), by repeated venipuncture after 24 hours of acclimation to the hospital environment, or by having the owner collect urine for glucose testing to document glucosuria.

In order to evaluate for the presence of concurrent disease that may affect diabetic management or affect the owner's decision about proceeding with therapy, all diabetic dogs and cats should have a CBC, a serum chemistry profile including amylase and lipase, and a urinalysis and culture (sample taken by cystocentesis). Radiographs of the thorax and abdomen or abdominal ultrasound are also suggested.

Glucosuria is present in all dogs and cats with diabetes mellitus.[31, 36, 64] Ketones are present in the urine in 60% of cats[36, 64] and in 75% to 84% of dogs.[30–32] Other changes in the urinalysis are also noted, such as proteinuria and pyuria,[31, 64] particularly when urinary tract infection is also present, which occurs commonly in dogs. Fasting lipemia is present in at least 50% of dogs with diabetes mellitus,[31] and hypercholesterolemia is present in 83% of cats[64] and 61% of dogs.[30]

Diabetic Ketoacidosis

Dogs and cats with DKA have all of the clinical signs and laboratory abnormalities that patients with uncomplicated disease have, plus those associated with acidosis and the consequent metabolic changes.

As stated previously, many dogs and cats with diabetes are ketotic (i.e., have acetone, acetoacetic acid, and β-hydroxybutyric acid in urine and serum) but are not considered ketoacidotic for therapy purposes because they lack the severe clinical signs of ketoacidosis (see Clinical Signs).

Ketones can be measured in urine or blood using nitroprusside-impregnated strips (Ketostix, Labstix, Multistix) or tablets (Acetest Reagent tablets). Nitroprusside primarily detects acetone and acetoacetic acid but does not detect β-hydroxybutyric acid, which is the predominant ketoacid produced in animals with DKA. After severe dehydration leads to poor tissue perfusion and decreased oxygen tension, the proportion of β-hydroxybutyric acid increases drastically; therefore, severe ketosis can be present with only a trace of ketones or no ketones detected in urine or blood by methods utilizing nitroprusside.[66, 67]

Because there is a high incidence of urinary tract infections in patients with DKA, pyuria is often present. There is often leukocytosis with an inflammatory leukogram, and mild anemia or hemoconcentration may be present.[31, 64]

Elevations of alanine aminotransferase are common in both dogs (50%–80%)[30, 68] and cats (86%).[36] Serum alkaline phosphatase is elevated commonly in dogs (76%–86%)[30, 68] and less commonly in cats (28%).[36] Hyperbilirubinemia is present in 50% of cats[36, 64] but is less common in dogs. Hyponatremia is present in about 50% of cases,[36, 57] and potassium may be normal, elevated, or reduced at presentation.[36, 57, 58] Correction of acidosis causes shifting of extracellular potassium intracellularly, as does insulin therapy, because potassium is transported into cells along with glucose. Because of this intracellular shifting of potassium, and because there is usually a total body potassium deficit from anorexia, vomiting, and diuresis, potassium concentration often drops markedly during therapy.[26, 60] Phosphorus may be low at presentation,[64, 69] or it may be reduced after the first few hours to days of therapy.[60, 69, 70]

Many cats and dogs with DKA have prerenal azotemia, leading to elevation of BUN and creatinine.[30, 31, 36, 57, 63] Serum amylase and lipase may be elevated in those animals with concurrent pancreatitis or dehydration.[31, 63] Most dogs have a reduced level of total carbon dioxide.[57]

About 50% of dogs[57] and almost all cats[60] that are severely ill from diabetes mellitus to the point of anorexia, lethargy, and dehydration have hyperosmolality (plasma osmolality >350 mOsm/kg). If laboratory assay for osmolality is not practically available, the effective osmolality can be estimated from serum or plasma chemistry values by the following formula: serum osmolality in mOsm/kg = 2(sodium) + glucose/18 + BUN/2.8.[60]

Treatment

Uncompliated Canine Diabetes Mellitus

Managing the diabetic dog can be very rewarding or very frustrating. The regimen must be practical for the client and not prevent the client from living a normal life. Many diabetic dogs are euthanized after the clients realize they cannot provide the care needed. The number of euthanasias can be minimized if the clinician tailors the protocol to the lifestyle of the client. Often, we have to be satisfied with a degree of glycemic control that would be considered unacceptable for a human with diabetes. As long as the dog is eating well, is not losing weight, is not drinking more than 66 mL/kg per day because of polyuria, is not having accidents in the house, and does not have episodes of hypoglycemia or ketoacidosis, diabetic control is usually adequate.

For the dog that is eating and drinking and therefore does not require intensive therapy for ketoacidosis, the mainstay of management of diabetes has been the use of intermediate-acting insulin injections—those lasting 6 to 24 hours in the dog[26] (Table 48–1). My first choice in most cases is neutral protamine Hagedorn (NPH) insulin. The species source of the insulin product (beef/pork, recombinant human, or purified pork) is of lesser importance to the kinetics than is the type of insulin (regular, semilente, NPH, lente, or ultralente). However, purified pork and human recombinant insulins may have a earlier onset and peak of activity and shorter duration than beef/pork insulin.[26]

Insulins have been classified as short-, intermediate-, or long-acting based on their duration of activity in human patients. The intermediate- and long-acting products are formulated so that they are absorbed slowly from the subcutaneous injection site in order to extend the duration of activity for most or all of a day. There is a large amount of variation and overlap in the kinetics of the intermediate- and long-acting products in dogs and cats. All of the extended-duration insulin products (lente, NPH, and ultralente) are suspensions that must be thoroughly mixed before administration. Mixing should be done gently, by rolling the bottle between the palms, to prevent formation of a stable foam that makes accurate dosing impossible.

There is no set dose of insulin; the dose must be determined for each individual dog by giving insulin and monitoring the response. In the past, we have assumed that each dog would respond to an insulin preparation in a uniform manner in terms of peak and duration of effect. The response to insulin was monitored by measuring the glucose concentration of urine and adjusting the dose accordingly. We have since come to realize that there is a great deal of variation

Table 48–1
Properties of Beef/Pork Insulin Preparations Used in Dogs and Cats*

TYPE OF INSULIN	ROUTE OF ADMINISTRATION	ONSET OF EFFECT	TIME TO MAXIMUM EFFECT (h)		DURATION OF EFFECT (h)	
			Dog	Cat	Dog	Cat
Regular, semilente	Intramuscular	10–30 min	1–4	1–4	3–8	3–8
	Subcutaneous	10–30 min	1–5	1–5	4–10	4–10
NPH (isophane)†	Subcutaneous	0.5–3 h	2–10	2–8	6–24	4–12
PZI§	Subcutaneous	1–4 h	4–14	3–12	6–28	6–24
Lente†	Subcutaneous	<1 h	2 peaks, 2–4 and 6–12	2–8	8–24	6–14
Ultralente‡	Subcutaneous	2–8 h	4–16	4–16	8–28	8–24

NPH, neutral protamine Hagedorn; PZI, protamine zinc insulin.
*Purified pork and recombinant human insulins appear to be more potent, act faster, and have a shorter duration of action than beef/pork insulins.
†Initial insulin of choice for the diabetic dog.
‡Initial insulin of choice for the diabetic cat.
§Not commercially available.
Modified from Nelson RW. Diabetes mellitus. In: Ettinger SJ, Feldman EC, eds. Textbook of Veterinary Internal Medicine, 4th ed. Philadelphia, WB Saunders, 1995, 1510–1537.

among dogs in response to an insulin preparation.[71] It has also become apparent from monitoring blood glucose concentrations that urine glucose evaluation does not provide an adequate assessment of glucose control. This is attributable partly to the variation in responses to insulin among dogs and also to variations in the renal threshold for glucose from dog to dog. Other factors, such as urine specific gravity, time since last voiding, severity of hyperglycemia, and duration of hyperglycemia, affect urine glucose concentration.[72] Determination of the appropriate dose of insulin should be based on measurement of blood glucose rather than urine glucose.

After the diagnosis of diabetes mellitus has been made, the patient should be evaluated for other problems that may affect the management. For this a CBC, biochemical profile, urinalysis, and urine culture are indicated. Injections of intermediate-acting insulin are started in the morning, at a time that fits the owner's schedule.

The dog is fed one fourth to one half of its caloric requirements within 30 minutes of the injection of insulin. Whether to feed before or after the injection of insulin is somewhat controversial. Each method has its advantages and disadvantages. Feeding before giving insulin, with instructions to withhold the insulin injection if the dog does not eat, is advantageous to help prevent hypoglycemia. However, it may lead to or worsen the hyperglycemia that is often present in the morning just before the insulin injection and after feeding because glucose is absorbed before insulin. In addition, I have managed some finicky dogs that

would not have received insulin as much as 75% of the time had the owner been instructed to withhold the insulin injection if the dog did not eat within 30 minutes of feeding. Feeding after the insulin injection may match the absorption of glucose more closely with the onset of insulin activity and therefore improve glycemic control. Initially, the remainder of the caloric needs are fed approximately 8 hours after the insulin injection, at a time that is practical for the owner.

High-fiber diets have been shown to decrease the postprandial and fasting glucose concentrations and reduce the insulin requirement when compared with low-fiber diets.[73–75] Prescription diets such as Prescription Diet w/d or r/d are high in fiber and therefore may be good choices for diabetic dogs if they will eat them consistently. Prescription Diet r/d may not have a high enough caloric density to prevent weight loss in small dogs. Soft, moist diets should be avoided because they are high in simple sugars and lead to wide fluctuations in blood glucose concentration.[76]

Because a dog's response to an insulin preparation may change after receiving it for a few days, it is recommended to start with a modest dose of insulin (0.5 U/kg), check the blood glucose when it is expected to be the lowest (4–8 hours after insulin administration) to make sure the dog will not become hypoglycemic, then send the dog home or keep it in the hospital without close monitoring of blood glucose on this regimen for 3 to 4 days. This usually keeps the dog from becoming severely ketoacidotic, but it is not adequate for optimal control of blood glucose.

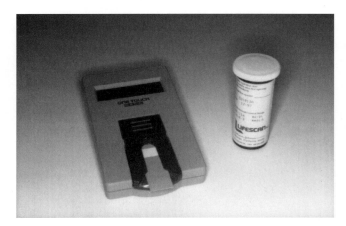

Figure 48–3
One Touch test strips and meter used to measure blood glucose in cats and dogs for glucose curves.

After 3 to 4 days of insulin therapy, the dog is returned to determine a glucose response curve to the insulin. To do this, the animal is given insulin at the dose of 0.5 U/kg and fed its morning meal, and blood glucose is measured every 2 hours for at least 12 hours and ideally 24 hours, starting just before injection of the insulin. Blood glucose can be measured repeatedly by obtaining a drop of blood with a 26-gauge or smaller needle, or from an indwelling venous catheter, and using glucose reagent strips such as Glucostix or Chemstrip bG. These are accurate enough to provide the information needed. Accuracy can be improved by using a reflectance colorimeter such as a Glucometer II, Accu-Chek II, or One Touch with the appropriate reagent strips (Fig. 48–3).

The animal should be fed its afternoon meal to determine the peak and duration of insulin activity accurately. Knowing the peak and duration of insulin activity allows the clinician (1) to measure the blood glucose at an appropriate time to evaluate and adjust the dose of insulin, (2) to determine whether one injection of intermediate-acting insulin would be adequate to provide glucose control for 24 hours, and (3) to determine the optimum time to feed the dog its afternoon meal. After the response to insulin has been determined, the dog is fed 25% of its food in the morning and, ideally, 75% 1 to 2 hours before the peak of insulin effect when using NPH insulin. It is important, however, that the dog be fed on a schedule that is feasible for the client and can be maintained constantly.

With the use of lente insulin once daily, it is usually better to feed the majority of the total daily calories at the time of the insulin injection, with a smaller meal later in the day. Lente insulin is a combination of 30% semilente (short-acting) and 70% ultralente (long-acting) insulins. This product usually provides two peaks of insulin activity, the larger of which occurs 2 to 4 hours and the smaller 6 to 12 hours after the injection.

Insulin dose is adjusted by measuring the blood glucose concentration just before the insulin injection and again at the time when glucose is expected to be at its lowest based on the glucose response curve. The dose is adjusted by 1 to 4 units per day to achieve a lowest glucose concentration between 80 and 120 mg/dL and, ideally, a peak glucose concentration of less than 200 mg/dL. Many times a peak of 300 mg/dL or less is the best that can be achieved, which is adequate if the dog is not glycosuric long enough to cause polydipsia. This is usually the case if the blood glucose is maintained below 200 mg/dL for at least 18 hours per day. In order to accurately determine the duration of action of insulin, the glucose curve should be repeated after the dose that is required to reduce the blood glucose to 80 to 120 mg/dL has been reached. For clinical purposes, the duration of action of insulin is defined as that time after the injection of insulin when the blood glucose exceeds 250 mg/dL after the glucose nadir (80–120 mg/dL) has occurred.[26]

After the appropriate dose of insulin has been determined, the dog is sent home with a fixed dose and fed the same amount and brand of food at the same times daily. Exercise is maintained as constant as possible. Initially, the dog is rechecked weekly to determine a 12- to 24-hour blood glucose curve. The owner is asked to monitor water consumption, which should be less than 66 mL/kg per day, as well as the dog's attitude, appetite, and weight. If the dog is eating, acts normally, is not losing weight, and is not polydipsic, diabetic control is usually adequate. I do not have owners routinely monitor urine glucose, but many do so by their own choice. Monitoring once weekly for urinary ketones, however, is probably a good idea. Owners who monitor urine glucose should *not* adjust the insulin dose based on the urine glucose concentration but merely record the result to monitor for trends and alert the clinician if there are consistent changes in urine glucose concentration or if ketones appear for 2 to 3 days in a row. The urine glucose in a patient with well-controlled diabetes will be 0 to 2+ in the morning before the insulin injection and 0 in the afternoon in many cases, but not in all.

If the diabetes appears to be well controlled at the first two rechecks and the insulin requirement does not appear to have changed at home, rechecks are scheduled at less frequent intervals (30 days, then 60 days, then every 3 to 4 months) as long as the dog is doing well. If the results of the blood glucose curve indicate that diabetic control is not good (i.e., blood glucose is too high for a large part of the day), yet the owner's home-monitoring reveals good control, the home-monitoring results should be considered correct. The stress of hospitalization causes some dogs to have high blood glucose concentrations for the whole day of the glucose curve. For some of these dogs, a more accurate curve can be determined on an outpatient basis.

If the duration of intermediate-acting insulin (NPH or lente) is shorter than 14 hours, it should be given twice daily. The injections should be given at times that are convenient for the owner, approximately 12 hours apart. Ideally, four small meals should be given, each within 30 minutes of the injection of insulin and 1 to 2 hours before the peak of insulin activity. This is not practical for most clients, however, so an adequate compromise is to feed two equal meals within 30 minutes of each insulin injection. Insulin dose is then adjusted as previously described.

If intermediate-acting insulin does not provide a satisfactory duration of activity, a long-acting insulin (ultralente) may be tried. These preparations may be useful for the client who cannot give two insulin injections per day. When I have used ultralente insulin by itself, it has often had an unacceptably delayed onset of activity. A mixture of 1 part regular insulin and 3 parts ultralente insulin can be used for patients that require twice-daily injections of intermediate-acting insulin and whose owners have requested that no more than one injection be given daily.[77] The insulins are mixed in a sterile vial, ideally in a bacteriologic hood, and then allowed to equilibrate for 24 hours before use. This is done because some of the regular insulin may combine with excess zinc in the ultralente insulin, altering the mixture.[78] After 24 hours, the mixture will be stable for 60 days if refrigerated. Regular insulins containing phosphate buffer (Humulin BR or Velosulin) should not be mixed with lente insulins because the phosphate causes precipitation and loss of potency.[78] If the clinician does not wish to mix insulins in a sterile vial for long-term use, the insulins can be drawn up in the same syringe at the time of injection, always drawing up the regular insulin first. When the appropriate dosing protocol has been established in the hospital, the owner must use the same mixture at home. These mixtures usually provide a peak of activity at 1 to 3 hours and another, much lower peak at 10 to 14 hours.[79] The dog is fed one half to two thirds of its caloric needs within 30 minutes of the insulin injection, and the rest of its food 1 to 2 hours before the second peak of insulin activity. The proportions of food can be altered depending on how the dog responds to the insulin. One injection per day of this mixture has provided reasonable 24-hour glucose control in dogs that previously had required two injections per day of NPH insulin.[77]

Although lente insulin is generally considered to be an intermediate-acting insulin, it is a 30% semilente (short-acting) and 70% ultralente (long-acting) mixture. In most dogs, it acts like a double-peak insulin. This preparation may be tried for dogs that require NPH twice a day whose owners cannot give two doses of insulin per day, in place of the mixture of regular and ultralente insulins just described. In my experience, however, the proportion of short-acting insulin is too large to allow for good glycemic control late in the day; that is, 70% ultralente is not enough when the dose is low enough to prevent an unacceptably low glucose nadir at the first peak of insulin activity.

Measurements of glycosylated hemoglobin (GHb) and fructosamine (FRA) have been used for long-term monitoring of glycemic control in human diabetic patients, and their utility for such monitoring has been evaluated for use in dogs and cats.[80–85] Although these two parameters may be valuable to help monitor glycemic control in patients whose owners are unreliable, they are probably not as valuable as a reliable owner's assessment of diabetic control based on the pet's daily water consumption, urination habits, attitude and appetite, and periodic 12-hour blood glucose curves. The validity of GHb depends greatly on the method used,[72] and values for both GHb and FRA in diabetic dogs and cats overlap with those of normal animals.[80–85] For these reasons, I do not recommend the use of GHb and FRA for monitoring of glycemic control in diabetic animals.

The most serious complication of diabetic management is hypoglycemia. The client should be warned of this. If the client finds the dog seizing, weak, disoriented, or comatose, the client should assume that the dog is hypoglycemic and should rub corn syrup or honey on the gums until the dog revives. The animal should be fed its meal, and then the client should call the veterinarian. The blood glucose should be checked and the dog observed for the rest of the day or until the management protocol has been evaluated and adjusted if needed. If the dog refuses to eat its meal after receiving insulin, it should be watched carefully by the owner or veterinarian. If the dog vomits, it also should be watched carefully by the owner or checked by the veterinarian to determine the cause and monitor for hypoglycemia. It is usually better to skip a dose of insulin than to cause hypoglycemia. If a client makes a mistake or if the dog moves during the injection so that it does not receive its full dose of insulin, the client should *not* try to estimate the deficit and replace it. The dog should be fed normally and the usual dose given at the next regularly scheduled time. If an owner gives an overdose and becomes aware of it immediately, the dog should be monitored at the veterinarian's hospital for the day.

Uncomplicated Feline Diabetes

Only about 25% to 30% of diabetic cats have NIDDM and therefore respond well to dietary management and oral hypoglycemic therapy.[35] There is no good way at present to differentiate cats that have NIDDM from those with IDDM, even with a glucagon or glucose tolerance test and measurement of the insulin response.[35] Candidates for oral hypoglycemic therapy are selected based on their clinical presentation. Those that are not severely ill or debilitated, are eating and drinking well, and have no or only slight ketonuria are considered candidates for a trial with the oral hypoglycemic drug glipizide (Glucotrol).[35, 86] Glipizide is given at a dosage of 5 mg per cat, two or three times daily, with a meal. Cats should be rechecked every 1 to 2 weeks for a history, physical examination including body weight, urinalysis (glucose and ketones), and fasting and 2- to 3-hour postprandial serum or blood glucose measurement. Cats that can respond to the drug usually do so by 1 to 2 months of therapy. Cats that have a worsening of clinical signs, become ketoacidotic, or continue to have blood glucose values over 300 mg/dL and those whose owners do not believe the clinical signs to be controlled should be started on insulin therapy.[35]

Approximately 25% to 30% of cats may respond to glipizide with resolution of clinical signs and blood glucose concentrations consistently below 200 mg/dL. About 33% of cats may have resolution of or reduction in the severity of clinical signs, with blood glucose concentrations reduced but still consistently higher than 200 mg/dL, and owners that are satisfied with the response. The remaining cats do not respond at all and must be placed on insulin.[35] For a cat that becomes euglycemic or hypoglycemic, the drug can be discontinued and the cat rechecked in 1 to 2 weeks. If the cat and its blood glucose values remain normal, the drug need not be reinstated. If hyperglycemia recurs, therapy is reinstated and the dose adjusted to that which controls hyperglycemia without causing hypoglycemia. A few cats remain normoglycemic after withdrawal of glipizide once ideal body weight has been reached, and dietary management with a high-fiber diet is continued.[35]

The most frequent side effects of glipizide in cats are vomiting and hypoglycemia. A few cats have elevation of alanine aminotransferase or hyperbilirubinemia. These conditions usually resolve after withdrawal of the drug. In a few cases, these side effects have resolved in spite of uninterrupted treatment.[35]

High-fiber diets may improve glycemic control in diabetic cats, as in dogs.[74] Prescription diets such as Prescription Diet w/d or r/d and Science Diet Feline Maintenance Light are high in fiber and therefore may be good choices for diabetic (NIDDM or IDDM) cats if they eat them consistently. Prescription Diet r/d may not have a high enough caloric density to prevent weight loss, although for the obese cat this is desirable. If the cat is obese, it should be fed the amount needed to achieve its ideal body weight, but cats should not lose weight too quickly, because of the potential for developing hepatic lipidosis.

For the cat that is eating and drinking and therefore not so severely ketoacidotic that intensive therapy is required, the mainstay of management of diabetes has been subcutaneous injections of a long-acting insulin, most commonly protamine zinc insulin (PZI), or one of the intermediate acting insulins (NPH or lente; see Table 48–1). NPH insulin, however, often causes fairly large daily fluctuations in serum glucose concentration, with a duration of action in many cats that would require two, and in some cases three, daily injections to achieve adequate glycemic control.[34] Recently, PZI has been removed from the market, although it may be returned in the near future by Anpro Pharm.[87] It is therefore recommended that cats be started on once-daily injections of the long-acting insulin, ultralente.

There is no set dose of insulin, and a great deal of variation among cats in their response to an insulin preparation occurs[88]; therefore, the dose, peak, and duration of activity must be determined for each individual cat and each insulin product by giving insulin and monitoring the response. As stated in the section on managing canine diabetes, urine glucose concentration is of little value for monitoring glycemic control and adjusting insulin dose in cats. It is also logistically difficult for most owners to consistently obtain a urine sample from their cats. Therefore, determination of the appropriate dose of insulin should be based on blood glucose measurement rather than on urine glucose concentration.

Injections of ultralente insulin (Humulin U Ultralente, the only product presently available, is a recombinant DNA human source insulin) are started in the morning at a time that fits the owner's schedule. Cats that are usually portion-fed, at which time all food is consumed within a few minutes, are fed one half of their caloric requirements at the time of the injection and the remainder of their caloric needs 8 to 10 hours later, at a time that is practical for the owner. Cats that are used to having food left out for them to nibble all day long are allowed to continue this feeding pattern. Because a cat's response to an insulin preparation may change after receiving it for a few days, I do not monitor the response to insulin closely during the first few days of therapy. Therapy is initiated with a modest dose of insulin, 1 to 3 units per cat once daily, and the blood glucose concentration is checked when it is expected to be the lowest, 4 to 8 hours after administration of insulin, for 1 to 2 days to make sure the cat will not become hypoglycemic.

After 4 to 5 days of insulin therapy at home or in the hospital, a glucose response curve is determined as for dogs. It may be preferable for the owner to feed the cat before bringing it to the hospital, because some cats will not eat their usual amount in a strange environment. The cat should be fed its afternoon meal in order to determine the duration of insulin activity accurately. The duration of insulin activity is the elapsed time from the injection until the blood glucose concentration exceeds 250 mg/dL. To accurately determine the duration of insulin activity, the dose of insulin should be high enough so the blood glucose nadir is 80 to 120 mg/dL. A glucose nadir of less than 80 mg/dL may also cause duration of insulin activity to be measured inaccurately because of possible rebound hyperglycemia,[89] which can last for 48 hours or longer in the cat. See the section on management of uncomplicated canine diabetes for a discussion of the value of a glucose curve.

After the response to insulin has been determined, the cat is fed one half of its food in the morning and one half 1 to 2 hours before the peak insulin effect. The feeding schedule, however, must be practical for the owner so that it can remain constant. The cat is sent home with a fixed dose of insulin and is fed the same amount and brand of food at the same times daily. The patient is rechecked every 1 to 2 weeks and the blood glucose concentration is determined every 1 to 2 hours for an 8- to 12-hour period after the owner has fed the cat in the morning and given the insulin. Glucose monitoring should begin within 1 hour of the insulin injection. The dose is adjusted by 0.5 to 1 units each weekly or biweekly visit to achieve a lowest blood glucose value between 80 and 120 mg/dL and, ideally, a peak glucose concentration of less than 200 mg/dL. Many times, a peak of 300 mg/dL or less is the best that can be achieved, and this is adequate if the cat is not glycosuric enough to develop polydipsia. The owner is asked to monitor water consumption, attitude, and appetite. If the cat is eating, acts normally, is not losing weight (unless desirable to do so and fed at a level to achieve weight loss), and is not polydipsic, diabetic control is adequate. If the diabetes appears to be well controlled at the first two rechecks and the insulin requirement does not seem to have changed at home, rechecks are scheduled at less frequent intervals (30 days, then 60 days, then every 2–4 months) as long as the cat is doing well.

If the duration of insulin activity is less than or equal to 12 hours, it should be given twice daily in equal doses (50%–75% of cats need ultralente insulin twice daily).[89, 90] The injections should be given at times that are convenient for the owner, approximately 12 hours apart. Ideally, four small meals should be given, one each at the time of each injection of insulin and 1 to 2 hours before the peak of insulin activity. This is not practical for most clients, so an adequate compromise is to feed two equal meals 0 to 30 minutes after each insulin injection. Insulin dose is then adjusted as previously described.

If the duration of insulin activity with ultralente insulin is greater than 12 hours but the cat is still polyuric and polydipsic and losing weight, insulin may need to be given twice daily at a 12-hour interval with a reduced dose. Blood glucose should be monitored carefully for the first 5 to 7 days in this circumstance to ensure that insulin does not accumulate and lead to hypoglycemia.[89] An alternative would be to try an intermediate-acting insulin such as NPH or lente,[91] given twice daily. Cats for which ultralente insulin does not provide adequate control of blood glucose because of delayed onset or lack of absorption from subcutaneous sites can be switched to lente or NPH insulin (Lente Iletin I, NPH Iletin I).

To facilitate drawing up and injecting such small doses of insulin, U 100 insulin can be diluted 1:10 to a final concentration of 10 U/mL, using the specific diluting fluid for each type of insulin, available from the manufacturer. It is also suggested that the owners use low-dose syringes (0.3 or 0.5 mL capacity, Monoject). For example, to administer 3 U of a 1:10 dilution of U 100 insulin with a U 100 syringe, the owner needs to draw up 30 U on the syringe.

Diabetic Ketoacidosis

Management of the ketoacidotic patient is a medical emergency because of the severe metabolic abnormalities present. The patient is severely ill and exhibits anorexia and lethargy. The goals of therapy should include correction of dehydration and electrolyte and acid-base imbalances, reduction of blood glucose, and identification of concurrent precipitating diseases.[60] Initially a CBC, a serum chemistry profile that includes bicarbonate or total carbon dioxide, a urinalysis, and urine culture should be performed in order to assess the patient. Because diabetic patients are immunocompromised,[92, 93] urethral catheterization should be avoided. Urine samples should be taken by cystocentesis after the skin is clipped and scrubbed. After the patient is through the crisis (i.e., rehydrated and not azotemic), serum amylase and lipase, abdominal radiography or abdominal ultrasonography, and thoracic radiography should be performed in order to identify potential underlying precipitating diseases.

Fluid therapy is important to reduce hyperosmolality and restore renal perfusion and glomerular filtration.[67] The initial fluid of choice is 0.9% sodium chloride.[60, 67] Although lactated Ringer's solution may be used, it is less ideal because it may not restore sodium concentration as well. In addition, lactate may not be metabolized to bicarbonate under conditions of ketoacidosis, and it would therefore be excreted in urine, adding to loss of cations such as sodium and potassium.[60, 67] After insulin therapy has reduced the blood glucose level to less than 250 mg/dL, dextrose is added to the fluids in order to make a 2.5% or 5% concentration, depending on the insulin therapy protocol used.

Because these patients are severely dehydrated, fluids should be given intravenously, preferably by a central venous catheter so that blood can be taken easily for monitoring. To obtain blood samples, the catheter is flushed with 0.5 to 1 mL of heparinized saline solution (10 U heparin/mL), followed by aspiration of 2 mL of blood into the flush syringe. The blood sample for testing is then aspirated into a second syringe. The original syringe that was used to flush and purge the catheter, which contains 2 mL of the animal's blood, is then used to flush the catheter, returning to the patient the blood that is not to be used for testing.[60] This method helps prevent iatrogenic anemia. As long as the fluids do not contain glucose, these samples can be used for measurement of blood glucose.

The rate of fluid administration depends on severity. Animals in shock should receive fluids at a rate of 90 mL/kg per hour. Although suggested rates of rehydration vary,[26, 60, 67] once perfusion is adequate, as evidenced by normal capillary refill, reduced heart rate, and warming extremities, I prefer to reduce the rate in order to replace the estimated deficit over a period of 12 hours in dogs, 24 hours in cats. For animals that have severe hyperosmolality (plasma osmolality >350 mOsm/kg; see Diagnostic Plan for a formula to calculate an estimate of osmolality), shock-rate fluid administration should be avoided because correcting hyperosmolality too quickly can lead to cerebral edema.[60] Calculation of total fluid volume in 24 hours should consider the fluid deficit, maintenance requirements (66 mL/kg per day), and continuing losses (see treatment of gastritis in Chap. 31).

Because many patients with DKA are azotemic and may occasionally develop acute oliguric renal failure, it is important to monitor urine output.[26] Because diabetic animals are immunocompromised,[92, 93] I prefer to assess urine output initially by repeated bladder palpation, avoiding urethral catheterization if possible. If, after the first 6 to 12 hours of fluid administration, urine output is in doubt, a urethral catheter should be placed in order to accurately monitor urine production. If the patient fails to produce at least 1 mL/kg per hour of urine after rehydration, steps should be taken to initiate urine production (see treatment of acute renal failure in Chap. 16).

Although serum potassium concentration may be normal or increased at presentation, it often is reduced below normal within a few hours of beginning

therapy as potassium shifts intracellularly (see Diagnostic Plan).[58, 60, 67, 94] Development of severe hypokalemia is associated with increased mortality.[94] As long as urine output is adequate (>1 mL/kg per hour), potassium should be supplemented according to the serum potassium concentration (see Table 31–7). If serum potassium concentration cannot be measured, 20 to 40 mEq/L can usually be added safely after the first 4 hours of fluid therapy.[57, 67] Ideally, serum potassium should be monitored every 12 to 24 hours. If it cannot be monitored, the electrocardiogram may be useful to identify hypokalemia. With hypokalemia, a prolonged Q-T interval, biphasic T waves, and tachycardia or bradycardia occur. If the Q-T interval lengthens after a few hours of fluid and insulin therapy (>0.22 second in dogs; >0.18 second in cats), the potassium supplementation in fluids should be increased and the serum potassium concentration measured.

In rare cases, after a few hours of fluid and insulin therapy, phosphorus can become dangerously low. Possible clinical abnormalities associated with hypophosphatemia include coma, hemolysis, rhabdomyolysis, cardiomyopathy, and decreased oxygen-carrying capacity of blood.[60, 67, 69, 70] Serum phosphorus should therefore be monitored every 12 to 24 hours if possible. Although routine supplementation of phosphorus is probably not necessary or suggested,[95] potassium phosphate (4.4 mEq/mL of potassium and 3 mmol/mL of phosphorus) can be used to prevent hypophosphatemia (as one fourth of the potassium supplement). If phosphorus drops below 1 to 1.2 mg/dL, supplementation at a rate of 0.01 to 0.03 mmol/kg of phosphorus per hour should be given intravenously for 6 hours, and then the phosphorus concentration should be rechecked.[60, 67, 69] Because phosphorus supplementation can lead to hypocalcemia,[69] it is wise to monitor calcium concentration during phosphate therapy.

The use of bicarbonate therapy to correct acidosis in DKA is controversial. Suppression of ketone formation with insulin therapy and correction of hypovolemia with the consequent improvement in renal function and reduction of lactic acidosis often are adequate to correct the acidemic state. If acidosis is severe (pH is ≤7.1 or bicarbonate [total carbon dioxide] is <12), bicarbonate therapy may be indicated.[44, 47] A conservative approach is to give a dose determined by the following formula: base deficit (24 − measured bicarbonate) × 0.1 × body weight in kilograms. This dose is given over a period of 2 hours and is followed by a recheck of the blood pH, the concentration of bicarbonate or total carbon dioxide, or both.[60] The clinician should beware of paradoxical cerebral acidosis and alkalosis, which may cause decreased oxygen delivery to tissues.

Insulin therapy decreases glucose concentration, stops the mobilization of free fatty acids, and helps decrease glucagon concentration. Because of the decrease in fatty acid production and glucagon concentration, ketosis is decreased. Insulin should be short acting (regular insulin) for good control, and it should be given intramuscularly or intravenously, because patients that are hypovolemic, dehydrated, or in shock cannot absorb the insulin from subcutaneous sites. IV therapy is perhaps ideal,[96] and in some situations it is practical (i.e., in a well-equipped emergency facility). The low-dose, intramuscular method, however, generally provides adequate, safe, and more clinically practical control,[26, 58, 60, 66, 67] so it is the method recommended for most situations. Advantages of low-dose intramuscular insulin therapy include ease of performance, accurate dosing, and low risk of hypoglycemia and hypokalemia.

Most cats with severe illness from diabetes mellitus, whether ketoacidosis is present or not, have severe hyperosmolality (plasma osmolality >350 mOsm/kg[60]; see formula to calculate an estimate of osmolality in Diagnostic Plan). Insulin therapy should be delayed until fluids have been administered for 2 to 6 hours in cats that have a plasma osmolality greater than 350 mOsm/kg, because too-rapid reduction of blood glucose could lead to cerebral edema.

Using the intramuscular method, animals are given 0.2 U/kg of regular crystalline insulin intramuscularly initially, followed by 0.1 U/kg hourly.[26, 60, 67] To facilitate measurement and administration of small doses, U 100 insulin should be diluted 1:10 with 0.9% saline solution or with special diluent obtained from the manufacturer. If saline is used, a fresh solution should be made up every 24 hours. Blood glucose levels should be measured hourly before each dose of insulin. When blood glucose is lower than 250 mg/dL, hourly intramuscular dosing with insulin is stopped and dextrose is added to the IV fluids in order to make a 5% solution. The average time required to reduce the blood glucose concentration to less than 250 mg/dL in dogs is 4 hours, with a range of 2 to 7 hours. If the blood glucose level is higher than 150 mg/dL, regular insulin is administered subcutaneously at a dose of 0.1 to 0.5 U/kg every 6 to 8 hours if the animal is well hydrated, or intramuscularly every 4 to 6 hours if not. If blood glucose is less than 150 mg/dL, no insulin is given until it is above that level when checked 2 to 4 hours later. The subcutaneous or intramuscular dose of regular insulin is changed by 1 to 2 U to maintain blood glucose at 2 to 4 hours after the last injection between 100 and 200 mg/dL. Intermediate- or long-acting insulin can be started in the morning after hydration is normal and the animal has begun eating and drinking sufficiently to maintain water balance.

Using the low-dose, continuous intravenous method of insulin therapy, 2.2 U/kg of regular crystalline insulin for dogs, or 1.1 U/kg for cats, is added to 250 mL of 0.9% sodium chloride solution in a separate infusion set from that used for fluid therapy. A fresh insulin infusion solution should be made up every 24 hours; because some insulin binds to plastic tubing, 50 mL of the solution should be discarded by allowing it to run through the infusion set to occupy the binding sites so that the concentration of the insulin solution infused remains constant. The rate of insulin infusion depends on the blood glucose concentration: 10 mL/hour if it is greater than 250 mg/dL, 7 mL/hour if it is 200 to 250 mg/dL, or 5 mL/hour if it is 100 to 200 mg/dL. The average time required for the blood glucose to be reduced to less than 250 mg/dL is 10 hours in dogs (range, 4–24 hours) and 16 hours in cats (range, 4–48 hours).[57, 60] The insulin infusion should be stopped if the blood glucose concentration is less than 100 mg/dL. Blood glucose should be monitored every 1 to 2 hours. The content of the fluid therapy solution is changed depending on the blood glucose concentration. When treating dogs, 0.45% saline with 2.5% glucose is administered when the blood glucose concentration is between 150 and 250 mg/dL, and 0.45% sodium chloride with 5% glucose when it is less than 150 mg/dL.[57, 60]

Because most cats with severe illness from diabetes mellitus, whether ketoacidosis is present or not, have severe hyperosmolality (plasma osmolality >350 mOsm/kg[60]; see formula to calculate osmolality in Diagnostic Plan), the fluid for cats should be 0.9% saline. Glucose should be added to make a 2.5% or 5% solution, depending on the blood glucose concentration as suggested for dogs.[60] The use of 0.45% saline solution may reduce hyperosmolality too quickly, resulting in cerebral edema. For the same reason, insulin therapy should be delayed until fluids have been administered for 2 to 6 hours in cats that have severe hyperosmolality.

If insulin is administered by the intravenous method, the volume of fluid administered as the insulin infusion should be included as part of the fluid therapy needed to meet the total daily requirement. For small dogs and cats, the volume infused as insulin solution may account for a large proportion of the fluid need. For most animals, additional fluids must be delivered through a second IV catheter or piggy-backed through the catheter used for insulin infusion if two infusion pumps are available. If necessary to meet electrolyte and glucose needs, potassium chloride and dextrose can be added to the insulin infusion solution.

Insulin infusion is continued intravenously until the urine ketones are negative and the patient is eating (range, 8–120 hours). After the animal is eating and drinking adequately to maintain water balance, intermediate- or long-acting insulin is begun as for the uncomplicated diabetic patient.

The Difficult or Brittle Diabetic

The brittle or difficult diabetic is one that seems to have frequent episodes of hypoglycemia or hyperglycemia despite seemingly good diabetic management. The problem may be attributable to poor owner compliance or to physiologic or pathologic conditions in the patient. Hormonally mediated physiologic mechanisms prevent hypoglycemia by counteracting the effects of insulin.[6, 97] Certain disease states can stimulate excessive production or release of insulin-antagonistic hormones, causing insulin resistance and poor diabetic control.[51, 54, 98–106]

To determine why a patient's diabetes is poorly controlled, a careful history is first required. Although routine urine testing is not recommended, if urine glucose is monitored by the client, the veterinarian must be sure that testing reagents are used correctly and not outdated. The insulin must be handled and given properly. Outdated or unrefrigerated insulin may be inactive. Mixing of insulin should be performed adequately but gently (see discussion of treatment of uncomplicated diabetes). The client's injection technique should also be observed. I often ask the owner to bring the patient, insulin, and syringes to the hospital so that the client can be observed drawing up the insulin and injecting it. The insulin preparation must be the proper concentration, and the syringes must match the insulin; U 100 syringes are used with U 100 of insulin. The same brand of syringe should always be used. Diet type, brand, amount, and times of feedings must remain constant. Insulin must be given at the proper times. The amount of exercise, which tends to decrease insulin requirement, should be kept constant. The owner should be asked about any recent medications, estrus or pregnancy if the pet is not spayed, and any recent stress.[97]

If a thorough history has not revealed a reason for poor diabetic control, the patient should receive a physical examination. Evidence of inflammation, infection, obesity, organ failure, or other endocrinopathies may explain poor glucose control caused by insulin resistance. If no abnormalities are apparent, the patient should be hospitalized so that the blood glucose response to insulin can be determined.

To determine the animal's glucose response to insulin, it should be fed and given insulin identically to the owner's protocol, using the owner's insulin and food, and a blood glucose curve should then be obtained (see discussion of management of uncomplicated diabetes). Animals may have a desired response to insulin or one of a few undesirable responses that can be associated with poor diabetic control; these in-

clude the transient response, the transient response with hypoglycemia and rebound hyperglycemia (Somogyi overswing), delayed response, and insulin resistance.[107]

Patients that have a transient response to intermediate-acting insulins have a blood glucose concentration that is reduced to a normal, desirable concentration (80–120 mg/dL), but the duration of the response is inadequate to prevent considerable hyperglycemia (>200 mg/dL) for a large part of the day.[108] This leads to glycosuria, polyuria, polydipsia, and possibly weight loss. If the duration of NPH or lente insulin activity is less than 18 hours but longer than 12 to 14 hours, long-acting insulin may be tried. If the duration of activity is 12 to 14 hours or less, NPH or lente insulin may be given twice daily.

The Somogyi effect occurs when the blood glucose is reduced below normal (<60 mg/dL) for a short period of time, followed by moderate to severe hyperglycemia (often >300 mg/dL), usually within 12 hours of the insulin injection. Catecholamines, glucagon, growth hormone, and corticosteroids are released in response to hypoglycemia. These hormones are insulin antagonistic and tend to increase blood glucose. The catecholamine and glucagon responses are short lived, but the actions of growth hormone and cortisol persist for many hours and occur unopposed after exogenous insulin has been metabolized, causing a rebound hyperglycemia.[109–111] One of the reasons it is no longer recommended to adjust the insulin dose based on morning urine glucose is that doing so can contribute to the occurrence of the Somogyi overswing. Because these patients consistently have severe glycosuria, an owner who is adjusting the insulin dose based on morning urine glucose may continue to increase the dose, which worsens hypoglycemia and subsequent hyperglycemia. The animal may show signs of hypoglycemia (e.g., weakness, restlessness, seizures, coma) in the afternoon but have severe glycosuria the next morning. In these cases, the owner should stop adjusting the insulin dose on the basis of morning urine glucose. The insulin dose should be reduced by 50% to 75% to prevent hypoglycemia. In dogs, the duration of NPH or lente insulin may then be adequate so that a single daily injection provides reasonable control. The insulin dose then needs to be adjusted using blood glucose concentrations. In some cases of the Somogyi overswing, a single injection of NPH or lente insulin does not provide good control for 24 hours after the dose is reduced. Ultralente insulin once or twice daily (often required twice daily in cats), or NPH or lente insulin twice daily may be needed to achieve adequate control for 24 hours in these patients. After the appropriate insulin dosage has been determined, it should remain constant and not be adjusted by the owner.

Some dogs and cats receiving intermediate- or long-acting insulin may have a response that is delayed, in which the blood glucose remains elevated for several hours after the injection but drops to an acceptable concentration late in the day. NPH or lente insulin given twice daily may provide adequate control for these patients. Mixtures or combinations of short-acting insulin and intermediate- or long-acting insulins may be necessary to control diabetes in these patients. The patient's diabetes should be regulated using the mixture protocol that is to be used by the owner at home.

Some dogs and cats are resistant to insulin, with blood glucose remaining higher than 300 mg/dL throughout the day despite doses of insulin that approach or exceed 2.0 U/kg per dose, the level considered consistent with insulin resistance.[26, 107, 112] A thorough search for the cause of insulin resistance is important to achieve proper control. In some animals, insulin resistance may be caused by destruction or binding of insulin at the subcutaneous site. To determine whether this is the problem, a modest dose of regular insulin (0.25–0.5 U/kg) is given intravenously, followed by hourly blood glucose measurement. If the glucose drops below 200 mg/dL, there is probably a subcutaneous problem rather than true insulin resistance. These patients may respond to a switch in insulin preparations (e.g., from ultralente or NPH to lente insulin, or from ultralente to NPH).[97]

Although anti-insulin antibodies occur commonly in dogs treated with beef/pork insulin, they rarely cause significant insulin resistance. This diagnosis is made by excluding all other causes of insulin resistance. Because anti-insulin antibodies interfere with some radioimmunoassays for insulin by falsely elevating the concentration, finding a markedly elevated serum insulin concentration (often >400 µU/mL) 24 hours after the last dose raises suspicion for anti-insulin antibodies.[113] Dogs that are insulin resistant because of anti-insulin antibodies may have their diabetes controlled with the use of purified porcine insulin products,[114] and cats may respond to beef insulin.[113]

Obesity in dogs[102] and cats[115] causes insulin resistance. Weight reduction reduces insulin resistance and improves glycemic control.

A large number of infectious or inflammatory diseases, organ failures, and other endocrinopathies can cause insulin resistance by production of increased amounts of insulin-antagonistic hormones.[51, 54, 98–106] Any animal with insulin resistance should have a urinalysis and urine culture performed on a sample obtained by cystocentesis. A CBC, serum chemistry profile, and radiographs of the thorax and abdomen may help identify an occult infection or neoplasm. Cats should be tested for the presence of feline leukemia virus or feline immunodeficiency virus infection.

Major organ disease or failure also may lead to excess production of insulin-antagonistic hormones. Renal failure, heart failure, acute pancreatitis, and liver disease all are possible causes of insulin resistance.[97] Endocrinopathies or therapy with hormones that are insulin antagonistic also lead to insulin resistance.[51, 54, 100, 103] Glucocorticoids are well-known insulin antagonists. Dogs with diabetes mellitus concurrent with hyperadrenocorticism often have severe insulin resistance that improves after the hyperadrenocorticism is controlled.[52] Hyperthyroidism can create insulin resistance in cats,[100, 101] making diabetic management difficult.

Recent estrus or pregnancy can cause a patient with previously well-controlled diabetes to become insulin resistant because of the antagonistic effects of estrogen and progesterone.[105] All intact female diabetic patients should be spayed. A bitch can gradually be brought out of heat with the use of mibolerone (Cheque drops) and then kept out of heat until it is safe to spay her.[66] Therapeutic progestogens also cause insulin resistance, making diabetic management difficult.[51, 103, 106, 116]

Other sex steroid imbalances may also lead to insulin resistance and poor diabetic control. Excess estrogen produced by a Sertoli cell tumor in a male dog can lead to insulin resistance. Castration of diabetic dogs may be well advised.[97]

Prognosis

The length of survival of diabetic patients depends to a great extent on the commitment and perseverance of the owner. A large proportion of the patients that do not survive are euthanized because the owner cannot or will not provide the care needed. Most dogs and cats with uncomplicated diabetes mellitus, however, can survive for several years with insulin therapy. Most dogs eventually develop diabetic cataracts (38 of 39 survivors in one study).[31] Although the success rate for management of patients with DKA varies,[57, 58] as many as 25% to 30% may not survive the crisis.[60] Many of the nonsurvivors, however, die from their underlying disease rather than from ketoacidosis.[57]

Insulin-Secreting Islet Cell Tumors (Insulinomas)

Insulinomas are insulin-secreting islet cell tumors (Fig. 48–4) that often produce other pancreatic hormones besides insulin.[117] The predominating clini-

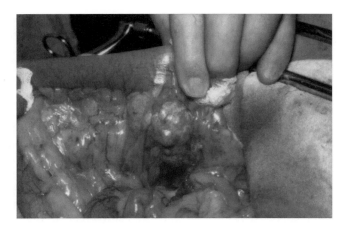

Figure 48–4
Insulin-secreting islet cell tumor in the pancreas of a dog.

cal signs are those associated with adult-onset hypoglycemia from hyperinsulinism. The true incidence of insulinoma is unknown, but it is considered uncommon in dogs[27] and is rare in cats. The mean age of dogs presented with insulinoma is 9 years, with a range of 3 to 14 years.[11–15, 27, 118, 119] Distribution of cases by sex is about equal: males, 45% and females, 55%.[11, 13, 27, 119] Boxers, Irish setters, German shorthaired pointers, and weimaraners may be predisposed to the development of insulin-secreting islet cell tumors.[27]

Pathophysiology

The cause of insulin-secreting islet cell tumors is not known. Although these tumors produce other pancreatic hormones besides insulin,[117, 120] the clinical signs caused by insulinomas are primarily the result of excess insulin leading to hypoglycemia. The clinical signs of hypoglycemia include those associated with dysfunction of the central nervous system from lack of energy substrate (glucose) as well as those caused by the sympathetic nervous response that occurs as a physiologic attempt to correct hypoglycemia.[4,6,9] Release of epinephrine contributes to muscle fasciculation, trembling, anxiety, hyperactivity, and tachycardia. However, because patients can adapt to chronically low blood glucose concentrations,[19] they often appear normal in spite of very low glucose levels. Clinical signs such as vomiting, anorexia, and diarrhea that are occasionally noted in dogs with insulinoma may be associated with production of other peptides (e.g., gastrin).[117, 120]

Virtually all insulin-producing islet cell tumors are malignant, eventually recurring from invasion of tissues locally or metastasizing,[15] most commonly to the liver and local lymph nodes.[11, 13–15] Some of the clinical signs such as vomiting or icterus that are seen in a few cases may be caused by metastatic tumor infiltration of tissues.[121]

Clinical Signs

The clinical signs in dogs with insulinoma are generally those associated with hypoglycemia, including central nervous system dysfunction and the sympathetic nervous system response to hypoglycemia. Often, clinical signs are episodic and occur some hours after eating, or they may be initiated by exercise. The most common clinical sign is seizures, which occur in 65% of cases; they manifest most commonly as generalized or focal (often facial) seizures, or occasionally an animal is presented in status epilepticus.[11–15, 27, 118, 119, 121–123] Other clinical signs that occur with less frequency include generalized weakness, rear limb weakness, collapse, ataxia, muscle fasciculation, disorientation, lethargy and depression, and bizarre behavior (Table 48–2).[11–15, 27, 118, 119, 121–123] Occasionally, vomiting, diarrhea, anorexia, and head tilt may also be noted.

Diagnostic Plan

The only consistent abnormality in routine clinical laboratory test results is hypoglycemia.[12, 13] Occasionally, hypokalemia is noted.[13] Some dogs may have elevations of serum alkaline phosphatase,[12, 121, 122] serum alanine aminotransferase, or both.[12, 122] Occasionally icterus may be noted,[121, 122] particularly if liver metastasis has occurred.[121]

Radiographs of the thorax do not show evidence of lung metastasis,[11, 12] and in fact the tumor rarely metastasizes to lung. The primary tumor usually cannot be imaged with abdominal ultrasonography,

Table 48–2
Clinical Signs in Dogs With Insulin-Producing Islet Cell Neoplasms

CLINICAL SIGN	FREQUENCY
Seizures	65% (183/281)
Generalized weakness	36% (102/281)
Collapse	34% (77/229)
Caudal weakness	34% (65/191)
Muscle fasciculation	27% (48/181)
Disorientation	25% (19/76)
Ataxia	22% (61/275)
Depression/lethargy	19% (42/222)
Bizarre behavior	17% (33/199)
Blindness	14% (6/42)
Polyphagia	12% (25/202)
Shaking/trembling	11% (22/203)
Exercise intolerance	11% (24/226)
Polyuria/polydipsia	10% (21/202)
Stupor	9% (3/35)
Hyperactivity/anxiety	8% (6/78)
Weight gain	8% (14/167)

Data from references 11–15, 27, 118–122.

although metastases to liver or other abdominal sites may be apparent.[27]

To confirm that hypoglycemia is the cause of clinical signs, the clinician could attempt to see if the signs satisfy Whipple's triad: (1) presence of neurologic signs typical of hypoglycemia, (2) documentation of low blood glucose concentration at the time signs are occurring, and (3) resolution of clinical signs with administration of glucose to correct the low blood glucose concentration.[27, 122] Verification of these points, however, does not confirm insulinoma; it merely confirms that hypoglycemia is the cause of the clinical signs.

Confirmation of the diagnosis of insulinoma requires surgical exploration of the pancreas and histologic documentation of islet cell tumor. Documentation of an elevated plasma insulin concentration with concurrent hypoglycemia is strong enough evidence, along with appropriate clinical and laboratory signs, to justify exploratory surgery.

If the blood glucose concentration is not below the reference range when first measured in a dog suspected of having an insulin-producing islet cell tumor, the patient should cautiously be fasted, starting in the morning after its usual postprandial period, while its clinical signs are monitored in the hospital and blood glucose is measured hourly. The protocol for withholding food in order to measure plasma insulin at the time when the dog is hypoglycemic is described in detail in the section on specific laboratory tests.

Most dogs (66%–76%) with insulinoma have an elevated plasma insulin concentration in the presence of hypoglycemia.[11-13, 28] Virtually no dog with insulinoma has an insulin concentration lower than normal when blood glucose is low. Because 25% to 35% of patients with insulinoma have an insulin concentration in the normal range with concomitant hypoglycemia, insulin/glucose ratios (e.g., AIGR) have been used to attempt to find a more sensitive means of identifying those patients with insulinoma that have a normal insulin concentration. The AIGR increases the sensitivity of testing to identify the presence of insulinoma[11-13] (see Specific Laboratory Tests). The AIGR is not very specific, however, because dogs with hypoglycemia associated with sepsis or with large non–islet cell tumors may also have an increased AIGR.[13, 18] For cases in which an insulinoma is suspected but insulin concentration is not elevated in the presence of hypoglycemia, the insulin-glucose pair can be repeated, at which time the insulin concentration may be elevated, making insulinoma likely. Perhaps more practically, other causes of hypoglycemia can be ruled out by a review of the physical examination, history, routine laboratory results, and abdominal radiography or ultrasonography (see Hypoglycemia). For most other causes of hypoglycemia, changes are apparent in one or more of these parameters. Dogs with sepsis are expected to have readily apparent clinical and laboratory signs of sepsis,[18] and virtually all other non–islet cell tumors associated with hypoglycemia can be palpated, are visibly apparent, or are easily demonstrated with abdominal radiography.[23–25]

Treatment

If an animal is showing clinical signs of hypoglycemia, IV glucose (50% dextrose, drawn up 1 mL/kg, then diluted with an equal volume of 0.9% saline or sterile water) should be given slowly over 30 to 60 seconds to effect. After the animal responds, it should be fed a small meal of a diet with high protein, high complex carbohydrates, and low simple sugars. If feeding multiple small meals does not prevent clinical signs, the dog can be maintained on a continuous infusion of 5% dextrose at a rate (1.5–2 times maintenance)[28] that prevents clinical signs. If signs such as seizures, dementia, stupor, or coma occur after hypoglycemia has been corrected by administration of dextrose, it should be assumed that cerebral damage with edema has occurred, and therapy for cerebral edema and seizure control should be initiated (see Chap. 24).[27, 28]

Although surgical therapy may be considered controversial by some,[28] it is usually recommended to remove what are most commonly (about 85% of cases)[11, 14] solitary nodules within the pancreas (see Fig. 48–4). About 45% of patients have evidence of metastasis, most often to liver or lymph nodes, at the time of surgery.[11, 13–15] If evidence of metastasis is found, surgical debulking can reduce or eliminate clinical signs for a variable period.[11, 13–15] Readers are directed to surgical texts for a description of the surgical procedures.

In order to fast the animal for anesthesia before surgery, 5% dextrose should be infused intravenously continuously, as previously described. Postoperative complications include pancreatitis (about 33% of cases), persistence of hypoglycemic clinical signs (25%–33% of cases), and hyperglycemia (persistent in 10%–15% of all surgical cases).[11–14] For dogs in which hyperglycemia persists for 5 or more days, insulin therapy is recommended (see discussion of treatment of uncomplicated diabetes).

Medical management for patients that do not undergo surgery or have had surgery followed by continued or recurrent signs of hypoglycemia initially should consist of multiple small feedings of diets low in simple sugars. If that does not prevent signs, prednisone at a dose of 0.25 mg/kg can be given twice daily, with gradual increases in the dose to 2.0 to 3.0 mg/kg twice daily, as needed to control clinical signs.[27, 28]

If corticosteroids cease to be effective or the side effects become unacceptable, diazoxide can be used. Diazoxide is a benzothiadiazide diuretic that increases blood glucose levels, primarily by inhibiting insulin secretion and to a lesser extent by increasing gluconeogenesis, glycogenolysis, and inhibition of peripheral glucose use through stimulation of the adrenergic system and release of epinephrine.[124] The initial dose is 5 mg/kg twice daily, which can gradually be increased to a maximum of 30 mg/kg twice daily. The most common adverse effects, vomiting, diarrhea, and anorexia, can be reduced by giving the drug with food.[27, 28] About 60% to 65% of dogs treated with diazoxide show an improvement in clinical signs.[13, 14] Among these, the average duration of response is about 6 months, with a range of 2 to 15 months.[14]

Dogs being medically managed may have recurrences of clinical signs periodically. The owner should be prepared for this, with instructions to rub corn syrup or honey on the dog's buccal mucosa, taking care not to be bitten by a seizing animal, until it revives enough to eat a meal. Foods high in simple sugars should be avoided because they may contribute to recurrence of hypoglycemic signs within 1 to 2 hours of eating.[28]

Prognosis

The histologic appearance of insulin-producing islet cell tumors may vary,[12] and the morphologic appearance of endocrine tumors in general is unreliable to determine malignant behavior.[27] The number of mitotic figures noted in insulinomas, however, may be negatively correlated with survival time.[121] Almost all insulinomas in dogs recur or metastasize, eventually leading to recurrence of clinical signs unless death occurs from intervening disease, regardless of the histologic appearance.[11, 13, 15]

With surgery and concurrent medical management or medical therapy after recurrence of clinical signs postsurgically, the average life span is 10 to 14 months, with a range of 1 month to more than 40 months.[11–15, 121] Dogs without evidence of metastasis at surgery, and those with metastases that are surgically removable, appear to survive longer than dogs with nonresectable metastases.[11, 14] The type of surgical procedure performed may also affect survival time; animals receiving local excision of just the abnormal-appearing tissue survive an average of 12 months, and those receiving partial pancreatectomies survive an average of 18 months.[14] In addition, the preoperative plasma insulin concentration may be negatively correlated with survival time.[11]

Transient Juvenile Hypoglycemia

Transient juvenile hypoglycemia is a common disorder that affects primarily miniature and toy breeds of dogs between 6 weeks and 6 months of age. Puppies present with signs of hypoglycemia but usually outgrow the tendency to develop low blood glucose by 6 months of age, and often within 4 weeks of presentation.[6, 9]

Pathophysiology

Puppies have a large brain/liver ratio (the brain requires relatively large amounts of glucose for energy) and immature gluconeogenic and glycogenolytic enzyme systems, as well as small muscle mass and minimal fat stores, which are needed to provide a substrate for gluconeogenesis and fatty acid mobilization, respectively. If small puppies are not fed frequent meals throughout the day or if there is an increased demand for energy (e.g., exertion, cold stress, GI disease, severe parasitism), they may not be able to mobilize glucose fast enough to prevent hypoglycemia and its associated clinical signs.[17]

Clinical Signs

Clinical signs are those typical of hypoglycemia, with puppies most commonly presenting with severe depression, stupor or coma, and twitching of facial muscles. Cold environmental stress, starvation, heavy parasite loads, or other GI diseases are often predisposing factors.[6, 9]

Diagnostic Plan

The diagnosis is based on the clinical signs and documenting hypoglycemia. Therapy should be initiated, however, as soon as blood samples are taken, in order to prevent permanent brain damage. Blood glucose values are usually less than 30 mg/dL.[6, 125] Glucose can be measured quickly and practically with reagent strips; accuracy is increased by use of a colorimeter made for that type of reagent strip (see Fig. 48–3 and the section on treatment of uncomplicated diabetes mellitus). Hypoglycemia should be confirmed by simultaneous measurement of plasma glucose by a clinical pathology laboratory.

Treatment

Treatment should begin immediately after hypoglycemia is suspected and blood has been drawn for analysis. A solution of 1 to 2 mL/kg of 50% dextrose, diluted with an equal volume of 0.9% saline or sterile water for injection to make a 25% solution of dextrose, is given intravenously over 30 to 60 seconds. If a vein cannot be accessed, 50% dextrose can be rubbed on the buccal mucosa, or dextrose can be given intramedullary by inserting an 18-gauge hypodermic or bone marrow needle into the proximal tibia from the medial aspect. Once revived, the puppy should be fed a high-protein, high–complex carbohydrate meal (i.e., avoiding soft, moist diets) and then be fed multiple small meals throughout the day to prevent recurrence. Some puppies require continuous infusions of 10% glucose at a rate of 5 to 10 mL/kg per hour for 24 to 48 hours to prevent recurrence until they can eat sufficiently to maintain euglycemia. Because this solution is hypertonic, it is best administered through a central vein such as the jugular, if possible.[6] To prevent hyperglycemia and consequent osmotic diuresis and dehydration, the rate of glucose administration should be no greater than perhaps 8 mg/kg per minute. If the puppy is not eating, potassium should be added to the fluids at a concentration of 20 mEq/L as long as urine output is adequate. If serum potassium concentration is monitored, supplementation should be according to Table 31–7.

If, after hypoglycemia is corrected, the puppy continues to show neurologic signs such as seizures, dementia, stupor, or coma, it should be assumed that cerebral damage with edema has occurred, and therapy for cerebral edema and seizure control should be initiated (see Chap. 24).[6, 125]

After the crisis is past, feeding of multiple small meals and identification and elimination of the precipitating problem usually serve to prevent recurrence until the puppy outgrows the tendency to develop hypoglycemia.

Prognosis

As long as severe cerebral damage from prolonged hypoglycemia has not occurred, the prognosis is excellent. Most puppies outgrow the tendency to develop hypoglycemia within a few weeks to months, usually by 5 to 6 months of age.[9, 22]

Uncommon Diseases of the Endocrine Pancreas

Hunting Dog Hypoglycemia

Hunting dog hypoglycemia is seen in nervous, eager hunting dogs after about 1 to 2 hours of vigorous exercise. They usually recover rapidly without therapy, but their ability to hunt is severely limited for the rest of the day.[9] The condition can be prevented by frequent (hourly) feeding of small meals (100 to 200 Kcal) during the hunt, or by giving 2.5 to 5 mg of prednisolone 2 to 4 hours before the hunt.

Hyperosmolar, Nonketotic Diabetes Mellitus

Animals with diabetic hyperosmolar, nonketotic syndrome present with severe mental depression from hyperosmolarity. This form of diabetes mellitus appears to be rare in dogs, but many cats that are severely ill with diabetes mellitus have severe hyper-

osmolality with concurrent neurologic signs, often with concomitant ketosis.[60] These animals have the typical signs of diabetes mellitus such as PU/PD and weight loss followed by those of a precipitating event such as is seen with DKA. These patients have severe hyperglycemia (usually >600 mg/dL), severe dehydration, and hyperosmolarity (serum osmolality >350 mOSm/kg), have a normal acid-base status or are only mildly acidotic, and lack ketonuria and ketonemia.[26, 61] Effective serum osmolality can be calculated from the formula stated in the section on diagnosis of DKA.

Pathogenesis of hyperosmolar, nonketotic diabetic syndrome is poorly understood. It may involve impaired central nervous system recognition of hyperosmolality along with the presence of enough insulin production to prevent ketogenesis and a lack of the typical increases of ketogenic hormones (e.g., glucagon, growth hormone, cortisol) seen with DKA.[26] These patients should be treated similarly to DKA patients except that fluid and insulin therapy should be given more cautiously to avoid a rapid drop in osmolality that could lead to cerebral edema.[60, 67] Insulin therapy should be delayed until fluids have been administered for 2 to 6 hours, and the insulin dose using the low-dose intravenous method should be reduced to 1.1 U/kg every 24 hours.[60]

References

1. Stabenfeldt GH. The endocrine system. In: Cunningham JG, ed. Textbook of Veterinary Physiology. Philadelphia, WB Saunders, 1992:378–386.
2. Evans HE. The digestive apparatus and abdomen. In: Evans HE, ed. Miller's Anatomy of the Dog, 3rd ed. Philadelphia, WB Saunders, 1993:385–395.
3. Evans HE. The veins. In: Evans HE, ed. Miller's Anatomy of the Dog, 3rd ed. Philadelphia, WB Saunders, 1993:682–716.
4. Guyton AC, Hall JE. Insulin, glucagon, and diabetes mellitus. In: Guyton AC, Hall JE, eds. Textbook of Medical Physiology, 9th ed. Philadelphia, WB Saunders, 1996:971–983.
5. Guyton AC, Hall JE. Cerebral blood flow, the cerebrospinal fluid, and brain metabolism. In: Guyton AC, Hall JE, eds. Textbook of Medical Physiology, 9th ed. Philadelphia, WB Saunders, 1996:783–789.
6. Atkins CE. Disorders of glucose homeostasis in neonatal and juvenile dogs: Hypoglycemia, part I. Compen Contin Educ Pract Vet 1984;6:197–208.
7. Morgan RV. Endocrine and metabolic emergencies: Part II. Compen Contin Educ Pract Vet 1982;4:814–820.
8. Walters PC. Hypoglycemia. Compen Contin Educ Pract Vet 1992;14:1150–1158.
9. Turnwald GH, Troy GC. Hypoglycemia: Part II. Clinical aspects. Compen Contin Educ Pract Vet 1984;6:115–124.
10. Turnwald GH, Troy GC. Hypoglycemia. Part I. Carbohydrate metabolism and laboratory evaluation. Compen Contin Educ Pract Vet 1983;5:931–938.

11. Caywood DD, Klausner JS, O'Leary TP, et al. Pancreatic insulin-secreting neoplasms: Clinical, diagnostic, and prognostic features in 73 dogs. J Am Anim Hosp Assoc 1988;24:577–584.

12. Kruth SA, Feldman EC, Kennedy PC. Insulin-secreting islet cell tumors: Establishing a diagnosis and the clinical course in 25 dogs. J Am Vet Med Assoc 1982;181:54–58.

13. Leifer CE, Peterson ME, Matus RE. Insulin secreting tumor: Diagnosis and medical and surgical management in 55 dogs. J Am Vet Med Assoc 1986;188:60–64.

14. Mehlhaff CJ, Peterson ME, Patnaik AK, et al. Insulin-producing islet cell neoplasms: Surgical considerations and general management in 35 dogs. J Am Anim Hosp Assoc 1985;21:607–612.

15. Steinberg HS. Insulin secreting pancreatic tumors in the dog. J Am Anim Hosp Assoc 1980;16:695–698.

16. Levy JK. Hypoglycemic seizures attributable to hypoadrenocorticism in a dog. J Am Vet Med Assoc 1994; 204:526–530.

17. van Toor AJ, van der Linde-Sipman JS, van den Ingh TSGAM, et al. Experimental induction of fasting hypoglycaemia and fatty liver syndrome in three Yorkshire terrier pups. Vet Q 1991;13:16–23.

18. Breitschwerdt EB, Loar AS, Hribernik TN, et al. Hypoglycemia in four dogs with sepsis. J Am Vet Med Assoc 1981;178:1072–1076.

19. Boyle PJ, Kempers SF, O'Connor AM, et al. Brain glucose uptake and unawareness of hypoglycemia in patients with insulin-dependent diabetes mellitus. N Engl J Med 1995;333:1726–1731.

20. Nelson RW, Turnwald GH, Willard MD. Endocrine, metabolic, and lipid disorders. In: Willard MD, Tvedten H, Turnwald GH, eds. Small Animal Clinical Diagnosis by Laboratory Methods, 2nd ed. Philadelphia, WB Saunders, 1994:147–178.

21. Leifer CE, Peterson ME. Hypoglycemia. Vet Clin North Am Small Anim Pract 1984;14:873–889.

22. Strombeck DR, Rogers Q, Freedland R, et al. Fasting hypoglycemia in a pup. J Am Vet Med Assoc 1978;173: 299–305.

23. Bagley RS, Levy JK, Malarkey DE. Hypoglycemia associated with intra-abdominal leiomyoma and leiomyosarcoma in six dogs. J Am Vet Med Assoc 1996;208: 69–71.

24. Leifer CE, Peterson ME, Matus RE, et al. Hypoglycemia associated with nonislet cell tumor in 13 dogs. J Am Vet Med Assoc 1985;186:53–55.

25. Beaudry D, Knapp DW, Montgomery T, et al. Hypoglycemia in four dogs with smooth muscle tumors. J Vet Intern Med 1995;9:415–418.

26. Nelson RW. Diabetes mellitus. In: Ettinger SJ, Feldman EC, eds. Textbook of Veterinary Internal Medicine, 4th ed, vol 2. Philadelphia, WB Saunders, 1995:1510–1537.

27. Steiner JM, Bruyette DS. Canine insulinoma. Compen Contin Educ Pract Vet 1996;18:13–24.

28. Nelson RW. Insulin-secreting islet cell neoplasia. In: Ettinger SJ, Feldman EC, eds. Textbook of Veterinary Internal Medicine, 4 ed, vol 2. Philadelphia, WB Saunders, 1995:1501–1509.

29. Marmor M, Willeberg P, Glickman LT, et al. Epizootiologic patterns of diabetes mellitus in dogs. Am J Vet Res 1982;43:465–470.

30. Doxey DL, Milne EM, Mackenzie CP. Canine diabetes mellitus: A retrospective survey. J Small Anim Pract 1985;26:555–561.

31. Ling GV, Lowenstine LJ, Pulley LT, et al. Diabetes mellitus in dogs: A review of initial evaluation, immediate and long-term management, and outcome. J Am Vet Med Assoc 1977;170:521–530.

32. Wilkinson JS. Spontaneous diabetes mellitus. Vet Rec 1960;72:548–555.

33. Panciera D, Thomas C, Eicker S, et al. Epizootiologic patterns of diabetes mellitus in cats: 333 cases (1980–1986). J Am Vet Med Assoc 1990;197:1504–1508.

34. Moise N, Reimers T. Insulin therapy in cats with diabetes mellitus. J Am Vet Med Assoc 1983;182: 158–164.

35. Nelson RW, Feldman EC, Ford SL, et al. Effect of an orally administered sulfonylurea, glipizide, for treatment of diabetes mellitus in cats. J Am Vet Med Assoc 1993;203:821–827.

36. Schaer M. A clinical survey of thirty cats with diabetes mellitus. J Am Anim Hosp Assoc 1977;13:23–27.

37. Hoenig M. Pathophysiology of canine diabetes. Vet Clin North Am Small Anim Pract 1995;25:553–561.

38. Alejandro R, Feldman EC, Shienvold, FL, et al. Advances in canine diabetes mellitus research: Etiopathology and results of islet transplantation. J Am Vet Med Assoc 1988;193:1050–1056.

39. Haines D, Penhale W. Autoantibodies to pancreatic islet cells in canine diabetes mellitus. Vet Immunol Immunopathol 1985;8:149–156.

40. Lutz TA, Rand JS. Pathogenesis of feline diabetes mellitus. Vet Clin North Am Small Anim Pract 1995;25: 527–552.

41. Johnson KH, O'Brien TD, Betsholtz C, et al. Islet amyloid, islet-amyloid polypeptide, and diabetes mellitus. N Engl J Med 1989;321:513–518.

42. Nelson RW, Feldman EC. Non–insulin-dependent diabetes mellitus in cats. Waltham/OSU Symposium for the Treatment of Small Animal Diseases: Endocrinology. California, Waltham USA. 1992;15:81–85.

43. Polonsky KS, Given BD, Hirsch LJ, et al. Abnormal patterns of insulin secretion in non–insulin-dependent diabetes mellitus. N Engl J Med 1988;318: 1231–1239.

44. Mitrakou A, Kelley D, Mokan M, et al. Role of reduced suppression of glucose production and diminished insulin release in impaired glucose tolerance. N Engl J Med 1992;326:22–29.

45. O'Brien TD, Hayden DW, Johnson KH, et al. High dose intravenous glucose tolerance test and serum insulin and glucagon levels in diabetic and non-diabetic cats: Relationships to insular amyloidosis. Vet Pathol 1985; 22:250–261.

46. Johnson KH, O'Brien TD, Jordan K, et al. Impaired glucose tolerance is associated with increased islet amyloid polypeptide (IAPP) immunoreactivity in pancreatic beta cells. Am J Pathol 1989;135:245–250.

47. Johnson KH, O'Brien TD, Betsholtz C, et al. Islet amyloid polypeptide: Mechanisms of amyloidogenesis in the pancreatic islets and potential roles in diabetes mellitus. Lab Invest 1992;66:522–35.

48. Duesberg CA, Nelson RW, Feldman EC, et al. Adrenalectomy for treatment of feline hyperadrenocorticism: 10 cases (1988–1992). J Am Vet Med Assoc 1995;207: 1066–1070.

49. Feldman EC. Adrenal gland disease. In: Ettinger SJ ed. Textbook of Veterinary Internal Medicine, 3rd ed, vol 2. Philadelphia, WB Saunders, 1989:1721–1774.

50. Nelson R, Feldman E, Smith M. Hyperadrenocorticism in cats: Seven cases (1978–1987). J Am Vet Med Assoc 1988;193:245–250.

51. Peterson ME. Effects of megestrol acetate on glucose tolerance and growth hormone secretion in the cat. Res Vet Sci 1987;42:354–357.

52. Peterson M, Nesbitt G, Schaer M. Diagnosis and management of concurrent diabetes mellitus and hyperadrenocorticism in thirty dogs. J Am Vet Med Assoc 1981;178:66–69.

53. Peterson ME, Altszuler N, Nichols CE. Decreased insulin sensitivity and glucose tolerance in spontaneous canine hyperadrenocorticism. Res Vet Sci 1984;36: 177–182.

54. Eigenmann J. Diabetes mellitus in elderly female dogs: Recent findings on pathogenesis and clinical implications. J Am Anim Hosp Assoc 1981;17:805–812.

55. Stabenfeldt GH. Endocrine glands and their function. In: Cunningham JG, ed. Textbook of Veterinary Physiology. Philadelphia, WB Saunders, 1992:396–404.

56. Manns JG, Martin CL. Plasma insulin, glucagon, and nonesterified fatty acids in dogs with diabetes mellitus. Am J Vet Res 1972;33:981–985.

57. Macintire DK. Treatment of diabetic ketoacidosis in dogs by continuous low-dose intravenous infusion of insulin. J Am Vet Med Assoc 1993;202:1266–1272.

58. Chastain C, Nichols C. Low-dose intramuscular insulin therapy for diabetic ketoacidosis in dogs. J Am Vet Med Assoc 1981;178:561–564.

59. Nichols R, Crenshaw KL. Complications and concurrent disease associated with diabetic ketoacidosis and other severe forms of diabetes mellitus. In: Bonagura JD, ed. Kirk's Current Veterinary Therapy XII. Philadelphia, WB Saunders, 1995:384–387.

60. Macintire DK. Emergency therapy of diabetic crises: Insulin overdose, diabetic ketoacidosis, and hyperosmolar coma. Vet Clin North Am Small Anim Pract 1995;25:639–650.

61. Plotnick AN, Greco DS. Diagnosis of diabetes mellitus in dogs and cats. Vet Clin North Am Small Anim Pract 1995;25:563–570.

62. Kramek BA, Moise S, Cooper B, et al. Neuropathy associated with diabetes mellitus in the cat. J Am Vet Med Assoc 1984;184:42–45.

63. Peterson ME. Endocrine diseases. In: Sherding RG, ed. The Cat: Diseases and Clinical Management, 2nd ed, vol 2. New York, Churchill Livingstone, 1994:1465–1479.

64. Peterson ME, Randolph JF, Mooney CT. Endocrine diseases. In: Sherding RG, ed. The Cat: Diseases and Clinical Management, 2nd ed, vol 2. New York, Churchill Livingstone, 1994:1479–1481.

65. Feldman EC, Nelson RW. Advances in feline diabetes mellitus. Proc Annu Meet Am Coll Vet Intern Med 1991;9:759–760.

66. Chastain C. Intensive care of dogs and cats with diabetic ketoacidosis. J Am Vet Med Assoc 1981;179:972–978.

67. Wheeler S. Emergency management of the diabetic patient. Semin Vet Med Surg 1988;3:265–273.

68. Ling GV, Stabenfeldt GH, Comer KM, et al. Canine hyperadrenocorticism: Pretreatment clinical and laboratory evaluation of 117 cases. J Am Vet Med Assoc 1979;174:1211–1215.

69. Willard MD, Zerbe CA, Schall WD, et al. Severe hypophosphatemia associated with diabetes mellitus in six dogs and one cat. J Am Vet Med Assoc 1987;190: 1007–1010.

70. Adams LG, Hardy RM, Weiss DJ, et al. Hypophosphatemia and hemolytic anemia associated with diabetes mellitus and hepatic lipidosis in cats. J Vet Intern Med 1993;7:266–271.

71. Church DB. The blood glucose response to three prolonged duration insulins in canine diabetes mellitus. J Small Anim Pract 1981;22:301–310.

72. Chastain CB. Monitoring long-term control in the diabetic patient. In: Bonagura JD, ed. Kirk's Current Veterinary Therapy XII. Philadelphia, WB Saunders, 1995:403–406.

73. Nelson RW. Dietary therapy for diabetes mellitus. Compen Contin Educ Pract Vet 1988;10:1387–1392.

74. Nelson R, Lewis L. Nutritional management of diabetes mellitus. Semin Vet Med Surg 1990;5:178–186.

75. Nelson RW, Ihle SL, Lewis LD, et al. Effects of dietary fiber supplementation on glycemic control in dogs with alloxan-induced diabetes mellitus. Am J Vet Res 1991; 52:2060–2066.

76. Holste LC, Nelson RW, Feldman EC, et al. Effect of dry, soft moist, and canned dog foods on postprandial blood glucose and insulin concentrations in healthy dogs. Am J Vet Res 1989;50:984–989.

77. Monroe WE. The use of insulin mixtures to achieve better control of diabetes mellitus. Proc Annu Meet Am Coll Vet Intern Med 1990;8:197.

78. Skyler JS. Insulin pharmacology. Med Clin North Am 1988;72:1337–1354.

79. Matz ME, Monroe WE. Plasma concentrations and effects of ultralente alone, and in combination with regular insulin, in the normal dog. Proc Annu Meet Am Coll Vet Intern Med 1990;8:1117.

80. Mahaffey EA, Cornelius LM. Glycosylated hemoglobin in diabetic and nondiabetic dogs. J Am Vet Med Assoc 1982;180:635–637.

81. Akol KG, Waddle JR, Wilding P. Glycated hemoglobin and fructosamine in diabetic and nondiabetic cats. J Am Anim Hosp Assoc 1992;28:227–231.

82. DeLack JB, Stogdale L. Glycosylated hemoglobin measurement in dogs and cats: Implications for its utility in diabetic monitoring. Can Vet J 1983;24:308–311.

83. Kaneko JJ, Kawamoto M, Heusner AA, et al. Evaluation of serum fructosamine concentration as an index of

blood glucose control in cats with diabetes mellitus. Am J Vet Res 1992;53:1797–1801.

84. Reusch CE, Liehs MR, Hoyer M, et al. Fructosamine: A new parameter for diagnosis and metabolic control in diabetic dogs and cats. J Vet Intern Med 1993;7: 177–182.

85. Wood PA, Smith JE. Glycosylated hemoglobin and canine diabetes mellitus. J Am Vet Med Assoc 1980;176: 1267–1268.

86. Miller AB, Nelson RW, Compen CA, et al. Effect of glipizide on serum insulin and glucose concentrations in healthy cats. Res Vet Sci 1992;52:177–181.

87. Greco DS, Broussard JD, Peterson ME. Insulin therapy. Vet Clin North Am Small Anim Pract 1995;25:677–689.

88. Broussard JD, Peterson ME. Comparison of two ultralente insulin preparations with protamine zinc insulin in clinically normal cats. Am J Vet Res 1994;55: 127–131.

89. Nelson RW, Feldman EC. Treatment of feline diabetes mellitus. In: Kirk RW, Bonagura JD eds. Kirk's Current Veterinary Therapy XI. Philadelphia, WB Saunders, 1992:364–367.

90. Nelson R, Feldman E, DeVries S. Use of ultralente insulin in cats with diabetes mellitus. J Am Vet Med Assoc 1992;200:1828–1829.

91. Bertoy E, Nelson R, Feldman E. Lente insulin for the treatment of feline diabetes mellitus. Proc Annu Meet Am Coll Vet Intern Med 1993;11:925.

92. Latimer K, Mahaffey E. Neutophil adherence and movement in poorly and well-controlled diabetic dogs. Am J Vet Res 1984;45:1498–1500.

93. Stickle JE, Tredten HW, Schall WD, et al. Adherence of neutrophils from dogs with diabetes mellitus. Am J Vet Res 1986;47:541–544.

94. Cotton RB, Cornelius LM, Theran P. Diabetes mellitus in the dog: A clinicopathologic study. J Am Vet Med Assoc 1971;159:863–870.

95. Wilson HK, Keuer SP, Lea AS, et al. Phosphate therapy in diabetic ketoacidosis. Arch Intern Med 1982;142: 517–520.

96. Kitabchi AE, Murphy MB. Diabetic ketoacidosis and hyperosmolar hyperglycemic nonketotic coma. Med Clin North Am 1988;72:1545–1563.

97. Monroe WE. Managing the difficult or "brittle" diabetic dog. Canine Pract 1990;15:7–16.

98. Mahaffey MB, Anderson N. Effect of staphylococcal alpha-toxin pancreatitis on glucose tolerance in the dog. Am J Vet Res 1976;37:947–952.

99. Eigler N, Sacca L, Sherwin RS. Synergistic interactions of physiologic increments of glucagon, epinephrine, and cortisol in the dog: A model for stress-induced hyperglycemia. J Clin Invest 1979;63:114–123.

100. Hoenig M, Ferguson DC. Impairment of glucose tolerance in hyperthyroid cats. J Endocrinol 1989;121: 249–251.

101. Hoenig M, Peterson ME, Ferguson DC. Glucose tolerance and insulin secretion in spontaneously hyperthyroid cats. Res Vet Sci 1992;53:338–341.

102. Mattheeuws D, Rottiers MD, Kaneko JJ, et al. Diabetes mellitus in dogs: Relationship of obesity to glucose

tolerance and insulin response. Am J Vet Res 1984;45: 98–103.

103. McCann JP, Altszuler N, Hampshire J, et al. Growth hormone, insulin, glucose, cortisol, luteinizing hormone, and diabetes in beagle bitches treated with medroxyprogesterone acetate. Acta Endocrinol 1987; 116:73–80.

104. Rayfield E, Curnow RT, George DT, et al. Impaired carbohydrate metabolism during a mild viral illness. N Engl J Med 289:618–621.

105. Tischler S. The effects of the estrous cycle on diabetes mellitus in the dog. J Am Anim Hosp Assoc 1974;10: 122–125.

106. Selman PJ, Rutteman GR, Rijnberk A. Progestin treatment in the dog: I. Effects on growth hormone, insulin-like growth factor I and glucose homeostasis. Europ J Endocrinol 1994;131:413–421.

107. Chastain CB, Ganjam VK. Clinical Endocrinology of Companion Animals. Philadelphia, Lea & Febiger, 1986.

108. Schaer M. Transient insulin responses in dogs and cats with diabetes mellitus. J Am Vet Med Assoc 1976;168: 417–418.

109. Wilson DE. Excessive insulin therapy: Biochemical effects and clinical repercussions current concepts of counterregulation in type I diabetes. Ann Intern Med 1983;98:219–227.

110. Feldman E, Nelson R. Insulin-induced hyperglycemia in diabetic dogs. J Am Vet Med Assoc 1982;180:1432–1437.

111. McMillan FD, Feldman EC. Rebound hyperglycemia following overdosing of insulin in cats with diabetes mellitus. J Am Vet Med Assoc 1986;188:1426–1431.

112. Nelson R, Feldman E. Complications of insulin therapy in canine diabetes mellitus. J Am Vet Med Assoc 1983;182:1321–1325.

113. Nelson RW. Insulin resistance in diabetic dogs and cats. In: Bonagura JD, ed. Kirk's Current Veterinary Therapy XII. Philadelphia, WB Saunders, 1995.

114. Feldman EC, Nelson RW, Karam JH. Reduced immunogenicity of pork insulin in dogs with spontaneous insulin-dependent diabetes mellitus. Diabetes 1983; 32(Suppl 1):153A.

115. Nelson RW, Himsel CA, Feldman EC, et al. Glucose tolerance and insulin response in normal-weight and obese cats. Am J Vet Res 1990;51:1357–1362.

116. Church DB, Watson ADJ, Emslie DR, et al. Effects of proligestone and megestrol on plasma adrenocorticotrophic hormone, insulin and insulin-like growth factor-1 concentrations in cats. Res Vet Sci 1994;56: 175–178.

117. O'Brien TD, Hayden DW, O'Leary TP, et al. Canine pancreatic endocrine tumors: Immunohistochemical analysis of hormone content and amyloid. Vet Pathol 1987;24:308–314.

118. Caywood DD, Wilson JW, Hardy RM, et al. Pancreatic islet cell adenocarcinoma: Clinical and diagnostic features of six cases. J Am Vet Med Assoc 1979;174: 714–717.

119. Chrisman CL. Postoperative results and complications of insulinomas in dogs. J Am Anim Hosp Assoc 1980;16:677–684.

120. Hawkins KL, Summers BA, Kuhajda FP, et al. Immunocytochemistry of normal pancreatic islets and spontaneous islet cell tumors in dogs. Vet Pathol 1987;24:170–179.
121. Dunn JK, Bostock DE, Herrtage ME, et al. Insulin-secreting tumours of the canine pancreas: Clinical and pathological features of 11 cases. J Small Anim Pract 1993;34:325–331.
122. Rogers KS, Luttgen PJ. Hyperinsulinism. Compen Contin Educ Pract Vet 1985;7:829–840.
123. Wilson JW, Caywood DD. Functional tumors of the pancreatic beta cells. Compen Contin Educ Pract Vet 1981;3:458–464.
124. Feldman EC, Nelson RW. Hypoglycemia. In: Feldman EC, Nelson RW, eds. Canine and Feline Endocrinology and Reproduction. Philadelphia, WB Saunders, 1987:304–327.
125. Johnson RK, Atkins CE. Non-neoplastic causes of canine hypoglycemia. In: Kirk RW, ed. Current Veterinary Therapy VII. Philadelphia, WB Saunders, 1980:1023–1027.

Chapter 49

Diseases of the Parathyroid Glands

William E. Monroe

Anatomy

In dogs and cats, two pairs of parathyroid glands are associated with the thyroid glands. The external parathyroids are located at the craniolateral poles of the thyroid glands, and the caudal glands (internal parathyroids) are located within the thyroid gland, usually at the medial surface, at about the midpoint on the long axis.[1] The secretory cells of the parathyroid gland (chief cells) are arranged in clusters, cords, sheets, strands, or rosettes, with supporting reticular stroma and many capillaries.[2] The C cells (parafollicular cells) of the thyroid glands produce calcitonin.[1] They occur interspersed between and adjacent to the thyroid follicles.[2]

Physiology

Parathyroid hormone (PTH), produced by the chief cells of the parathyroid glands, is a peptide hormone primarily responsible for the minute-to-minute control of the concentration of ionized calcium in the blood. If calcium concentration is decreased, PTH secretion increases. The acute effects of PTH are to increase calcium release from the labile bone pool, which is made up of amorphous crystals and soluble calcium bound between osteoblasts and osteoclasts and is the source of calcium ions for rapid movement into the blood. Additional acute effects of PTH are to increase renal reabsorption of calcium in the distal convoluted tubules and to increase phosphorus excretion from the proximal renal tubules. Long-term effects of PTH include mobilization of calcium and phosphorus by reabsorption of hydroxyapatite crystals from bone matrix (stable bone) and increased absorption of calcium and phosphorus from the gastrointestinal tract indirectly by stimulation of the production of the active form of vitamin D in the kidneys.[1] Because the renal effects of PTH seem to be quantitatively more important,[3] the net effects of PTH activity are to increase plasma calcium concentration and decrease the concentration of phosphorus. Hypercalcemia inhibits secretion of PTH.[1]

Calcitonin is a peptide hormone produced by the parafollicular or C cells in the thyroid glands. Calcitonin probably is not involved with minute-to-minute control of calcium concentration, but it functions in hypercalcemia to lower the calcium concentration. Its secretion is stimulated by hypercalcemia and inhibited by hypocalcemia. The primary effects are to decrease calcium and phosphorus mobilization from bone and to increase movement of phosphate into bone from extracellular fluid. Calcitonin also increases renal excretion of calcium and phosphorus.[1]

Vitamin D is produced in the skin from 7-dehydrocholesterol during exposure to ultraviolet light. To be biologically active, it is hydroxylated at C-25 in the liver and at C-1 in the renal tubules to form 1,25-vitamin D (calcitriol, or 1,25-dihydroxycholecalciferol).[1] The last activation step is PTH dependent. The major effects of vitamin D are to increase absorption of calcium and phosphorus from the gastrointestinal tract. It also promotes movement of calcium and phosphorus from bone into extracellular fluid by movement of calcium from the labile pool, by bone resorption, and by enhancing the effects of PTH on bone metabolism.[1] The net effects of vitamin D on plasma mineral concentrations are to increase calcium and phosphorus.

Problem Identification

Hypercalcemia

Hypercalcemia is defined as a serum or plasma total calcium concentration exceeding the normal interval. Although reference ranges for normal dogs and cats vary by laboratory, a serum calcium concentration higher than 13 mg/dL is usually considered to be a clinically important elevation.[3] Young dogs (<1 year) have higher serum calcium concentrations than adults, but usually not greater than 13 mg/dL. The calcium concentration reported in routine chemistry profiles is total calcium, which is composed of 50% ionized calcium (the metabolically active form), 40% protein-bound calcium (most is bound to albumin), and 10% calcium complexes.[4] In dogs, the serum calcium concentration should be adjusted for alterations in albumin concentration by subtracting the latter (in g/dL) from the former (in mg/dL) and adding 3.5; this formula yields a corrected serum calcium concentration in mg/dL.[5] The formula does not appear to be accurate for correcting feline serum calcium concentration.[6] Lipemia or hemolysis can cause severe artifactual elevation of serum calcium concentration, depending on the methodology used to measure calcium.[3]

Pathophysiology

Table 49–1 lists the more common causes of hypercalcemia. The pathogenesis of hypercalcemia caused by primary hyperparathyroidism is excessive secretion of PTH. The pathogenesis of hypercalcemia of malignancy can vary depending on the tumor type and location. Tumors that often involve bone, such as myeloma, may produce local osteoclast-activating factors that lead to calcium mobilization.[3, 7] Lymphomas and other solid tumors may produce a peptide called parathyroid hormone–related protein (PTHrP) that acts much like PTH but is not measured by assays that measure the intact PTH peptide.[3, 8, 9] Hypercalcemia results from vitamin D intoxication because of excessive absorption of calcium from the gastrointestinal tract.[10]

Table 49-1
Common Causes of Hypercalcemia

Growth (puppies)
Hypercalcemia of malignancy
  Lymphoma
  Anal sac adenocarcinoma
  Myeloma
  Other solid tumor
Renal failure
Hypoadrenocorticism
Primary hyperparathyroidism
Hypervitaminosis D
Hemoconcentration

The pathogenesis of other causes of hypercalcemia is less well understood. In the uncommon case in which renal failure is associated with hypercalcemia, renal secondary hyperparathyroidism may become "autonomous."[3] Other factors, such as decreased renal calcium excretion, hemoconcentration, and an increase in calcium complexes, may also play a role.[7] The pathogenesis of the hypercalcemia seen with hypoadrenocorticism is unknown[7]; however, it is of little consequence in that disorder because it is generally mild and may not be associated with increased concentration of ionized calcium.

The fraction of serum calcium that is important for physiologic and pathophysiologic function is the ionized calcium. An increased concentration of ionized calcium has negative effects on cell function because it affects membrane activity and permeability and can result in cell death.[7] The principal deleterious effects of hypercalcemia are neuromuscular, cardiovascular, and kidney dysfunction. Gastrointestinal function may also be altered because of decreased excitability of smooth muscle or direct central nervous system effects.[7]

Mineralization of soft tissues may occur, particularly if the serum calcium concentration is sufficiently elevated such that the product of the calcium concentration and the concentration of serum phosphorus (calcium × phosphorus) is greater than 60.[7] Of particular importance is mineralization of the heart or kidneys, which can lead to cardiac rhythm disturbances or renal failure, respectively.[7] Before the development of renal failure from soft tissue mineralization, hypercalcemia can cause defects in renal concentrating ability by inhibiting the action of antidiuretic hormone (ADH) on renal tubular cells.[3]

Clinical Signs

Often there are few clinical signs associated with hypercalcemia, and a high calcium level is often discovered during evaluation of a serum chemistry profile. The serum calcium concentration is usually greater than 15 mg/dL before signs attributable to hypercalcemia itself occur.[7] Signs associated with hypercalcemia include polyuria and polydipsia (PU/PD), anorexia or hyporexia, lethargy, weakness, and cardiac arrhythmias such as ventricular premature depolarizations or ventricular fibrillation. Uncommonly, neurologic signs such as seizures or muscle twitching may be noted.[7]

The clinical signs of the underlying cause of hypercalcemia are often more readily apparent than those caused by hypercalcemia. These may include lymphadenomegaly with lymphoma; bone pain, lameness, or neurologic dysfunction with myeloma; vomiting with renal failure or vitamin D intoxication; or hematuria, pollakiuria, and palpable urinary calculi with primary hyperparathyroidism.

Diagnostic Plan

After hypercalcemia has been documented by repeating the serum biochemical evaluation and correcting the value for changes in albumin (by the formula previously described), the history should aid in ruling in or out causes such as vitamin D intoxication. The clinician should ask the owner again about the possibility of exposure to vitamin D–containing rodenticides or house plants (e.g., day-blooming jessamine). If the animal is dehydrated on physical examination, mild increases in calcium concentration (12–13 mg/dL) may be caused by hemoconcentration, which is rapidly corrected by rehydration.[7] In these cases, the "corrected" calcium may be normal.

Further examination of the biochemical profile should allow the clinician to decide whether hypoadrenocorticism is a possible diagnosis. If the calcium, phosphorus, blood urea nitrogen (BUN), creatinine, and potassium levels are elevated, with a low sodium concentration and a sodium/potassium ratio of less than 27:1, hypoadrenocorticism is likely and an adrenocorticotropic hormone (ACTH) response test should be performed (see Chap. 46). If hypercalcemia is associated with hyperphosphatemia and azotemia, without changes in sodium and potassium, primary renal failure,[11, 12] vitamin D intoxication, or renal failure secondary to chronic, severe hypercalcemia are the most likely causes. Renal failure secondary to hypercalcemia can be difficult to differentiate from renal failure as a primary cause of hypercalcemia. However, renal failure secondary to hypercalcemia is uncommon at the time of clinical presentation and is often milder than renal failure that is a primary cause of hypercalcemia. Also, hypercalcemia from renal failure is usually accompanied by moderate to severe hyperphosphatemia and other signs, such as nonregenerative anemia and small, irregular kidneys. Measurement of the concentration of ionized calcium (see Diagnostic Procedures) helps to separate renal failure as a cause of hypercalcemia from hypercalcemia that has led to renal failure. With primary hyperparathyroidism or hypercalcemia of malignancy, the ionized calcium is elevated.[3] Only 10% of dogs with renal failure have an elevated ionized calcium.[11]

If the calcium is elevated and the phosphorus level is normal or low, without azotemia, major differential diagnoses include hypercalcemia of malignancy and primary hyperparathyroidism. Another careful physical examination with particular attention to the lymphoid organs may identify lymphosarcoma as a possible cause of hypercalcemia.[13, 14] Attention should also be paid to the anal sacs, including a rectal examination, because anal sac adenocarcinoma is second to lymphosarcoma as the most common cause of hypercalcemia of malignancy in adult dogs.[15, 16] The mammary glands and testicles should also be palpated for tumors. Tumors in these organs have been associated with hypercalcemia, either caused by metastases to bone or as a paraneoplastic-type syndrome.[7] The bones should be palpated for pain that may be associated with myeloma. Elevation of the serum globulin with a monoclonal peak on electrophoresis is suggestive of myeloma as a possible cause of hypercalcemia.

If, after evaluation of the biochemistry profile and repetition of the physical examination, the clinician still cannot differentiate primary hyperparathyroidism from hypercalcemia of malignancy, a more extensive search for occult neoplasia should be performed. This should include thoracic radiographs to look for mediastinal or pulmonary masses and abdominal radiographs or ultrasonography to evaluate for lymph node enlargement or infiltration of liver or spleen with neoplasms. A lymph node aspirate and cytologic analysis are also indicated at this time.

If tumors are not found and the animal is not azotemic, evaluation of serum PTH concentration (see Diagnostic Procedures) simultaneously with serum calcium measurement is indicated. If the calcium concentration is high with a mid-normal or increased concentration of PTH in an animal in which primary renal failure has been ruled out as the cause of hypercalcemia, primary hyperparathyroidism is likely, and cervical exploration to find and remove a parathyroid adenoma is indicated. Cervical ultrasonography may identify parathyroid masses,[3, 17] providing further evidence that cervical surgery is indicated.

If the calcium concentration is high and the PTH concentration is low, hypercalcemia is probably caused by occult malignancy. Some tumors that cause hypercalcemia may be associated with an elevated serum concentration of PTHrP,[8, 9] which should be measured if PTH is low (see Diagnostic Procedures). Further diagnostic procedures in search of neoplasia (usually lymphosarcoma) should include lymph node biopsy and bone marrow aspiration or biopsy.

Aggressive therapy for hypercalcemia is indicated if the animal is showing clinical signs attributable to hypercalcemia or is dehydrated or azotemic, if the calcium × phosphorus product is greater than 70, or if the calcium level is greater than 16 mg/dL even without clinical signs (see Primary Hyperparathyroidism).

Hypocalcemia

Hypocalcemia is defined as a reduction in the serum or plasma calcium concentration below the normal range. Clinical signs are usually not apparent unless the concentration of total serum calcium is below 6 to 7 mg/dL. However, the value at which an animal shows signs varies, because physiologic function is dependent on the concentration of ionized calcium, not on total calcium.[18] The proportion of total calcium that exists in the ionized state varies with the acid-base status. In conditions of acidosis, more of the total calcium is in the ionized state.

Pathophysiology

The pathophysiologic cause of clinically apparent hypocalcemia depends on the initiating disorder (Table 49–2). With primary hypoparathyroidism, a deficiency of PTH leads to reduced calcium concentration from failure to reabsorb calcium in the renal tubules, from reduced mobilization from bone, and, indirectly, from reduced gastrointestinal absorption because of the dependence of vitamin D activation on PTH. In puerperal tetany, the demand for calcium for lactation or for rapid skeletal mineralization of fetal puppies in the last trimester in pregnant bitches is greater than can be met by either dietary absorption or mobilization from skeletal reserves (see Chap. 23).

Because calcium precipitates in the presence of excess phosphate, hyperphosphatemia of any cause can lead to hypocalcemia. This is the cause of hypocalcemia in acute renal failure and after excessive administration of phosphate parenterally or in the form of phosphate enemas (Fleet Enemas).[19] Ethylene glycol toxicosis can lead to hypocalcemia because calcium complexes with metabolites of the toxin and

Table 49–2
Common Causes of Hypocalcemia

Hypoalbuminemia
Chronic or acute renal failure
Ethylene glycol intoxication
Puerperal tetany
Acute pancreatitis
Hypoparathyroidism
Phosphate enema

also as a result of hyperphosphatemia from acute renal failure. It is uncommon for chronic renal failure to be associated with clinically apparent hypocalcemia because of compensatory secondary hyperparathyroidism and because patients in renal failure are acidotic, which increases the proportion of calcium that is in the ionized state.[20]

The cause of the hypocalcemia seen with acute pancreatitis is poorly understood. It is classically thought to occur from saponification of calcium with peripancreatic fatty acids.[3] Failure to absorb sufficient calcium from the gastrointestinal tract is the mechanism of hypocalcemia in some of the more uncommon causes, such as malabsorption syndromes, dietary imbalance, and vitamin D deficiency.[20]

The clinical manifestations of hypocalcemia are primarily neuromuscular because a sufficient concentration of ionized calcium is necessary for the release of neurotransmitters such as acetylcholine, for muscle contraction, and for stabilization of nerve cell membranes by decreasing the permeability of sodium.[18]

Clinical Signs

Animals with hypocalcemia are often restless or anxious and exhibit tremors, seizures, muscle fasciculations, weakness, poor appetite or anorexia, ataxia or a stiff gait, lethargy, aggressive behavior, facial rubbing, and panting. Tachyarrhythmias or bradycardia and a weak pulse may be detected, and the abdomen may be tense on palpation.[3]

Diagnostic Plan

Animals presented with signs of hypocalcemia and a history consistent with a hypocalcemic disorder (e.g., week 3 to 4 of lactation) should have blood drawn for a serum biochemical profile and then be treated for acute hypocalcemia (see Primary Hypoparathyroidism). If hypocalcemia is noted serendipitously on a serum chemistry profile, the value should be confirmed by repeating the measurement. Because about 40% of measured serum calcium is bound to protein, particularly albumin, the serum calcium concentration should be corrected for alterations in albumin concentration using the following formula: measured Ca mg/dL − albumin in g/dL + 3.5 = corrected Ca in mg/dL.[5] If not part of the original database, a complete blood count (CBC), urinalysis, and biochemical profile including amylase/lipase should be obtained for all animals for which hypocalcemia is confirmed.

If hypocalcemia is present along with vomiting, abdominal pain, an inflammatory leukogram, pyrexia, and elevation of serum amylase/lipase, acute pancreatitis is likely (see Chap. 33). If hyperphosphatemia and elevated BUN and creatinine are present, particu-

Table 49–3
Common Causes of Hyperphosphatemia

Growth (puppies and kittens)
Azotemia

  Prerenal
  Acute or chronic renal failure
  Postrenal (urethral obstruction)

Primary hypoparathyroidism
Vitamin D intoxication
Phosphate administration

  Intravenous supplementation
  Phosphate enema

larly in an animal that may have been exposed to ethylene glycol, acute renal failure from ethylene glycol toxicosis should be suspected. The presence of severe oxaluria or a positive assay for ethylene glycol in the blood of such patients would confirm antifreeze poisoning (see Chap. 16) and the likely cause of hypocalcemia. Hypocalcemia may also occasionally be seen with chronic renal failure.[11, 21]

If hypocalcemia is present with concurrent hyperphosphatemia, without azotemia and without clinical signs of other diseases, primary hypoparathyroidism is likely. In these cases serum magnesium should be measured, because severe hypomagnesemia may uncommonly lead to PTH resistance or functional hypoparathyroidism.[22] If serum magnesium concentration is normal, the serum concentration of intact PTH should be determined (see Diagnostic Procedures) to confirm the diagnosis of primary hypoparathyroidism.

Hyperphosphatemia

Hyperphosphatemia is defined as an increase in the serum phosphorus concentration above normal. Serum phosphorus exists in three forms: $H_2PO_4^-$, HPO_4^{-2}, and PO_4^{-3}. The distribution among the three depends on the pH. The actual reference range varies by laboratory, but adult dogs and cats usually have total serum phosphorus concentrations in the range of 3.0 to 6.0 mg/dL. Because of osteoblastic activity associated with bone growth, young animals (<1 year) often have higher values (dogs, 4–9 mg/dL; cats, 4–8 mg/dL).[4]

Pathophysiology

The common or clinically important causes of hyperphosphatemia are listed in Table 49–3. Serum phosphorus becomes increased because it is absorbed in excess from the diet (e.g., with hypervitaminosis

D), because renal excretion is reduced with azotemia of any cause (e.g., prerenal, renal, or postrenal), or because of primary hypoparathyroidism.[4] Serum phosphorus concentration may also be elevated from excessive intravenous (IV) administration or from the use of phosphate enemas.[19] Hyperphosphatemia itself causes few or no clinical signs, but because phosphate precipitates with calcium, hyperphosphatemia can lead to hypocalcemia. Chronically, hypocalcemia secondary to hyperphosphatemia is compensated by increased secretion of PTH (secondary hyperparathyroidism).

Clinical Signs

There are no clinical signs of hyperphosphatemia other than those associated with the underlying cause, unless it is accompanied by severe hypocalcemia. Typically, hypocalcemia leads to nervousness, tremors, weakness, and seizures. Renal failure, the most common cause of hyperphosphatemia in sick animals,[20] usually is associated with vomiting, anorexia, and lethargy (see Chap. 16).

Diagnostic Plan

Usually, hyperphosphatemia is found serendipitously on a serum biochemistry profile. If the elevation is mild (≤9 mg/dL), often with a mild elevation of serum calcium concentration (≤12 mg/dL), and the animal is younger than 1 year of age, hyperphosphatemia is probably associated with bone growth and is inconsequential. If there is concurrent azotemia with severe elevation of calcium, the owner should be questioned carefully to determine possible exposure to vitamin D rodenticides. If there is no history of exposure yet the biochemistry profile is typical of vitamin D intoxication, serum should be sent to be assayed for vitamin D concentration (see Diagnostic Procedures).

If hyperphosphatemia is present with concurrent azotemia and a normal, low-normal, mildly reduced, or mildly elevated calcium concentration, it is probably caused by renal failure. Some cases of acute renal failure, particularly those caused by ethylene glycol intoxication, may have concurrent moderate to severe hypocalcemia as well. Further diagnostic work-up in these cases should be directed toward determining the cause of renal failure (see Chap. 16).

If hyperphosphatemia is present along with hypocalcemia that is often severe enough to cause clinical signs, without azotemia, primary hypoparathyroidism is likely. Because severe hypomagnesemia can sometimes lead to signs of hypoparathyroidism by inhibiting release or activity of PTH,[22] the serum magnesium concentration should be determined. If the magnesium concentration is normal, serum should be

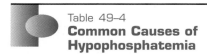

Table 49–4
Common Causes of Hypophosphatemia

Hypercalcemia of malignancy
Diabetic ketoacidosis (during therapy)
Enteral nutrition (anorexic cats)
Primary hyperparathyroidism

sent for simultaneous measurement of ionized calcium and intact PTH concentrations (see Diagnostic Procedures). If the PTH concentration is low or not detectable, with a concurrently low ionized calcium concentration, the concentration of PTH is inappropriate, indicating the presence of primary hypoparathyroidism.

Other clinically uncommon or insignificant causes of hyperphosphatemia, such as tissue trauma or necrosis, fracture healing, phosphate enema administration, IV phosphate therapy, hemolysis, and laboratory error,[3] are usually apparent from the history, from notation on the laboratory profile report, or on repetition of the phosphorus assay.

Hypophosphatemia

Table 49–4 lists the clinically important causes of hypophosphatemia. Hypophosphatemia occurs as a result of increased urinary loss or excretion or failure of absorption (or lack of intake) from the gastrointestinal tract. Serum phosphorus may also be reduced because of translocational shifts from the extracellular to the intracellular space when there is also a whole-body phosphorus deficit, as occurs when insulin and fluid therapy are initiated in severely ketoacidotic diabetics. It is rare for hypophosphatemia itself to lead to clinical signs. It is often seen concurrently with severe hypercalcemia associated with malignancy or primary hyperparathyroidism (see Hypercalcemia). Mild hypophosphatemia may also be seen with hyperadrenocorticism (see Chap. 46). In these cases, treatment of the underlying disease is indicated, whereas phosphate therapy generally is not. The phosphorus concentration usually must be lower than 2 mg/dL for it to be associated with dysfunction.[20] Clinical disorders that may occur as a result of severe hypophosphatemia include hemolysis, rhabdomyolysis, coma, and cardiomyopathy.[23] Occasionally, animals treated for ketoacidotic diabetes mellitus (see Chap. 48) or anorexic cats with a variety of underlying diseases treated with enteral nutrition develop hypophosphatemia severe enough to cause clinical signs and require phosphate supplementation.[24–26]

Diagnostic Procedures

Routine Laboratory Evaluation

Serum chemistry profiles are essential for diagnosis of parathyroid diseases, and disorders of calcium and phosphorus balance are often noted serendipitously. It is important to always evaluate changes in calcium concentration in view of any changes in phosphorus concentration, and vice versa, and to correct the calcium concentration for alterations in the albumin concentration (see Hypocalcemia and Hypercalcemia). Other values in the profile, such as BUN, creatinine, amylase/lipase, serum protein, and magnesium, are useful to aid in the diagnosis of nonparathyroid causes of calcium and phosphorus imbalance.

The CBC is usually normal with parathyroid disease, but it is useful to help rule out other causes of calcium-phosphorus disturbances. Abnormalities are often present with diseases such as pancreatitis (inflammatory leukogram), lymphoma (circulating neoplastic cells and anemia), and chronic renal failure (anemia).

The urinalysis is often normal in patients with parathyroid diseases, except that the urine specific gravity (USG) is usually reduced, often to the level of isosthenuria or hyposthenuria, in animals that have hypercalcemia caused by hyperparathyroidism. As many as 90% of dogs with primary hyperparathyroidism have a USG lower than 1.028, and about 80% have a USG lower than 1.015.[3] Dogs with calcium-containing uroliths secondary to hypercalcemia may have hematuria, pyuria, bacteriuria, or crystalluria.[3] The urinalysis may also be useful to rule out nonparathyroid causes of calcium-phosphorus imbalance, such as acute renal failure from ethylene glycol intoxication, in which oxalate crystals are often present (see Chap. 16).

Radiography

Radiography is unremarkable in many cases of parathyroid disease. In primary hyperparathyroidism in dogs, there may be generalized skeletal demineralization in a very few cases,[3, 27–29] or calcium uroliths may be present on abdominal radiographs in as many as 30% of dogs.[3, 27, 30] For evaluating diseases of the parathyroid glands, radiography of the thorax or abdomen is most useful for ruling out or in other causes of calcium-phosphorus imbalance, such as hypercalcemia of malignancy or hypocalcemia from pancreatitis. Radiography of the skeleton may help identify causes of hypercalcemia associated with bone lysis (e.g., myeloma).

Ultrasonography

With cervical ultrasonography, parathyroid adenomas or hyperplasia may be detected in perhaps as many as 70% of canine patients with primary hyperparathyroidism.[3, 17] Ultrasonography may also be useful in cats with suspected hyperparathyroidism.

Special Laboratory Tests

Parathyroid Hormone Assay

Measurement of serum PTH concentration in patients with hypercalcemia or hypocalcemia suspected of having primary hyperparathyroidism or hypoparathyroidism, respectively, has been very useful to make definitive diagnoses. The two-site assay (Allegro Intact PTH, Nichols Institute), which measures the intact PTH molecule, has been validated for use in dogs and cats[31, 32] and seems to give the most reliable assessment of parathyroid function.[33, 34] It is important to measure the ionized calcium (or at least the total calcium) simultaneously, so that the PTH concentration can be interpreted in view of the calcium concentration. If PTH concentration is elevated or in the upper 50% of the normal range while the calcium concentration is simultaneously increased, the PTH level is inappropriate, strongly indicating the presence of primary hyperparathyroidism. Patients with hypercalcemia of malignancy usually have serum concentrations of PTH that are low or in the mid-normal to low-normal range.[33] Patients with renal failure also have increased serum concentrations of PTH. Ruling out renal failure as a cause of hypercalcemia therefore depends on other factors (see Hypercalcemia). The serum PTH concentration in animals with primary hypoparathyroidism is lower than normal or undetectable, with concomitant hypocalcemia.[3, 31, 33]

To measure PTH concentration, the blood sample should be taken after an overnight fast and allowed to clot at room temperature, and the serum should be removed within 1 hour. The serum sample should be frozen until it is shipped to the laboratory on ice by overnight delivery. Many commercial laboratories offer a PTH assay. The Animal Health Diagnostic Laboratory, Michigan State University, has validated the assay and established reference ranges for animals.

Serum Ionized Calcium

Because the ionized calcium concentration is the biologically active form, it provides the most useful information about calcium-phosphorus balance.[11, 35] Although special sample handling may be required,[36, 37] some commercial laboratories offer an assay for ionized calcium. The laboratory should be contacted for sample requirements. It may be best to avoid using siliconized separator tubes, because calcium may be released from the silicone gel. It is important to have the test run at a laboratory that has established normal reference ranges for the target species. One such laboratory is the Animal Health Diagnostic Laboratory,

Michigan State University. Sample and sample handling requirements for serum ionized calcium at this laboratory are the same as those for measurement of PTH.

Parathyroid Hormone-Related Peptide

PTHrP, a peptide similar in structure and function to PTH, has been detected in some cases of hypercalcemia of malignancy in dogs.[8, 9] It is different enough that it is not measured in assays for PTH. It may be useful to aid in diagnosing patients suspected of having occult neoplasia on the basis of hypercalcemia with normal or low phosphorus concentrations and concurrent low to low-normal PTH concentration. Although many commercial laboratories designed to test samples from humans may offer the test, it is best to have it run by a laboratory that has established normal reference ranges for the species of animal whose blood is being tested. The Animal Health Diagnostic Laboratory, Michigan State University, is one such laboratory; sample handling requirements are the same as for measurement of PTH.

Vitamin D

Measurement of the serum vitamin D concentration may be useful to identify cases of intoxication if it cannot be confirmed historically.[35] The Animal Health Diagnostic Laboratory, Michigan State University, offers an assay for 25-hydroxyvitamin D. The sample should be handled the same as for measurement of PTH.

Diseases of the Parathyroid Glands

Primary Hyperparathyroidism

Primary hyperparathyroidism is overproduction of PTH as a result of disease in the parathyroid glands themselves, as opposed to a response to chronic reductions in serum ionized calcium (e.g., renal or nutritional secondary hyperparathyroidism). The true incidence is unknown, but it occurs uncommonly in dogs and rarely in cats.

The age at onset in dogs ranges from 5 to 15 years, with an average of about 10 years[3, 27]; in cats, the mean age is 13 years, with a range of 8 to 15 years.[38] In dogs, there is no sex predilection, and keeshonds may be overrepresented.[3, 27] In cats, females and the Siamese breed may be predisposed.[38]

Pathophysiology

The usual cause of primary hyperparathyroidism is an adenoma (Fig. 49–1), but adenocarci-

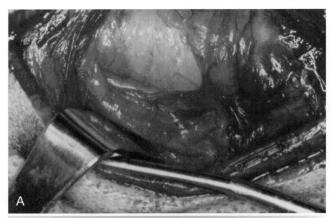

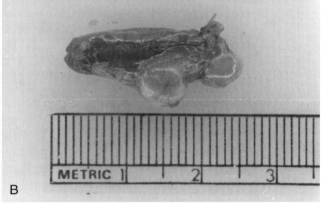

Figure 49–1
(A) Intraoperative appearance of a parathyroid adenoma involving the external (cranial) parathyroid gland in a dog with primary hyperparathyroidism. **(B)** Excised thyroid/parathyroid gland from the dog in **A** that has been sectioned longitudinally.

noma[3, 27, 38] and idiopathic[39] or congenital[28] hyperplasia have also been described.

Clinical derangement is almost exclusively the result of hypercalcemia. The fraction of serum calcium important for physiologic and pathophysiologic function is the ionized calcium. An elevated ionized calcium concentration has negative effects on cell function because it adversely affects membrane activity and permeability, perhaps resulting in cell death.[7] The main deleterious effects of hypercalcemia are neuromuscular, cardiovascular, and kidney dysfunction. Gastrointestinal function may also be reduced because of decreased excitability of smooth muscle or direct central nervous system effects.[7]

Mineralization of soft tissues may occur, particularly if the serum calcium concentration is sufficiently elevated such that the calcium × phosphorus product is greater than 60.[7] In addition to mineralization, which leads to defects in renal concentrating ability because of renal failure, hypercalcemia can directly inhibit the action of ADH on renal tubular cells.[3]

Clinical Signs

The clinical signs of primary hyperparathyroidism are caused mainly by hypercalcemia. In dogs, signs are often subtle. Many times, hypercalcemia is noted serendipitously on a serum biochemistry profile. The most common clinical signs are PU/PD, lethargy, urinary incontinence, weakness, poor appetite, and signs of lower urinary tract disease, such as pollakiuria, stranguria, and hematuria. Uncommonly, the dog may shiver or have muscle wasting, vomiting, constipation, or a stiff gait.[3, 27] Urinary calculi may be palpable in the bladder. Occasionally, skeletal demineralization may lead to soft, flexible bones, particularly those of the skull ("rubber jaw"; Fig. 49–2). Parathyroid masses usually cannot be palpated in canine patients.

The most common signs in cats with primary hyperparathyroidism are anorexia and lethargy, with vomiting, PU/PD, weakness, and weight loss occurring less commonly. A cervical mass may be palpated in the upper third of the neck.[38]

Diagnostic Plan

The diagnosis is based on the presence of typical biochemical changes, ruling out of other causes of hypercalcemia with normal or low phosphorus concentration (i.e., hypercalcemia of malignancy), measurement of serum PTH concentration, and cervical surgery with biopsy. The CBC is typically normal. On serum biochemistries, the calcium is elevated (dogs, 12.1–23 mg/dL; cats, 13.3–22.8 mg/dL), and the phosphorus is low to normal (dogs, 1.6–3.8 mg/dL; cats, 1.8–3.4 mg/dL) in most cases. If azotemia is present, there may be mild elevation of phosphorus.[3, 27, 38] Some patients may have mild elevations of BUN and creatinine, usually from renal mineralization (hypercalcemic nephropathy). Patients with primary hyperparathyroidism that are presented with azotemia (about 10% of all canine cases) can be hard to differentiate from those with primary renal failure with secondary hypercalcemia. However, patients with renal failure usually have milder hypercalcemia and relatively more severe azotemia and hyperphosphatemia than those with primary hyperparathyroidism (see Hypercalcemia). Serum alkaline phosphatase concentrations are mildly elevated in about 25% of canine and feline patients with primary hyperparathyroidism.[3, 27, 38]

Urinalyses often show low USG; almost all dogs have USG lower than 1.028, and about 80% are lower than 1.015.[3, 27] Cats have USGs lower than 1.028, and most are isosthenuric.[38] Dogs with uroliths often have hematuria, pyuria, and crystalluria, and some have bacteriuria, even without the presence of calculi.[3]

On radiographs, there may be generalized skeletal demineralization in a few cases,[3, 27–29] and calcium uroliths may be present on abdominal radiographs in as many as 30% of dogs.[3, 27, 30] Ultrasonography of the cervical region, using a 10-MHz transducer, may detect parathyroid adenomas or hyperplasia in as many as 70% of canine patients with primary hyperparathyroidism.[3, 17]

Serum PTH concentration is high or in the upper half of the normal range in virtually all dogs. A PTH concentration in this range, concurrent with hypercalcemia, is inappropriate and indicates the probability of primary hyperparathyroidism if primary renal failure has been ruled out.

Before serum PTH is measured in hypercalcemic animals, a reasonable search for malignancy that may be the cause is prudent. Diagnostic testing should include thoracic and abdominal radiography or abdominal ultrasonography, or both, and aspiration for cytology of any suspicious lymph nodes.

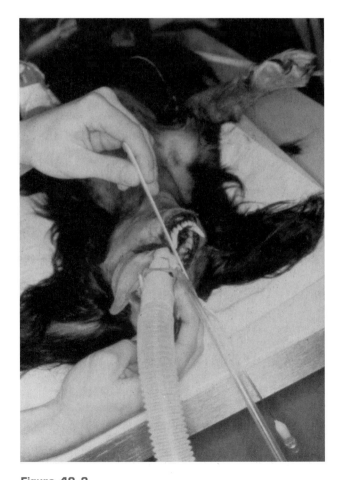

Figure 49–2
A dog with "rubber jaw" caused by skeletal demineralization from primary hyperparathyroidism.

Treatment

Definitive therapy for primary hyperparathyroidism is surgical removal of the adenoma (see Fig. 49–1) or adenocarcinoma or at least three of four hyperplastic glands if the cause is idiopathic hyperplasia. The surgical procedure has been described elsewhere.[27, 40]

Medical therapy to reduce hypercalcemia while awaiting surgery is indicated in most cases. Aggressive therapy is indicated if the calcium concentration is higher than 16 mg/dL; if neurologic signs, cardiac arrhythmias, azotemia, or dehydration is present; or if the calcium × phosphorus product is greater than 60 to 70. In these cases, normal saline solution should be given intravenously at a rate to correct dehydration in 6 hours (see Chap. 31). Thereafter, saline diuresis should occur at a rate equal to two to three times maintenance (132–198 mL/kg per day). Once the animal is rehydrated, diuretics such as furosemide (2 mg/kg intravenously, subcutaneously, or orally, twice per day [b.i.d.] or three times per day [t.i.d.]) also increase calcium excretion. Thiazide diuretics should not be used because they reduce calcium excretion.

In most cases, the calcium concentration is reduced to normal or near-normal levels with fluid and diuretic therapy alone. Some refractory cases may require additional, more aggressive therapy. For those cases, prednisolone (2 mg/kg, orally or subcutaneously b.i.d.) can be used. Corticosteroids reduce the serum calcium concentration by inhibiting intestinal calcium absorption, increasing renal excretion of calcium, and decreasing resorption of calcium from bone.[41] In patients with lymphoma, corticosteroids also reduce calcium concentration by their cytotoxic effects on neoplastic lymphocytes. Therefore, steroid therapy may alter lymph node cytology, making diagnosis of lymphoma difficult if that is the cause of hypercalcemia.

If corticosteroids fail to lower the calcium concentration within 24 hours, calcitonin (4–6 IU/kg subcutaneously or intramuscularly every 8–12 hours) is usually successful. The expense of calcitonin may limit its use.

Maintenance medical therapy for patients not amenable to surgery can include furosemide, 2 mg/kg orally every 8 to 12 hours, or prednisolone, 2 mg/kg orally b.i.d., or both. Calcitonin may also be used long-term, and in some cases the dosing interval can be increased to as much as 3 days and still maintain the calcium concentration within, or just above, the normal range.

Prolonged, severe hypercalcemia caused by a solitary parathyroid tumor suppresses the function of the other normal glands, causing them to atrophy. Removal of the hyperfunctioning tumor causes sudden hypoparathyroidism, which may lead to hypocalcemia 12 hours to 5 days after surgery. If the serum calcium concentration is less than 14 mg/dL before surgery, it should be monitored daily in the hospital for 5 days after surgery. If it drops below 8.5 mg/dL, with or without clinical signs, vitamin D and calcium therapy should be initiated (see Primary Hypoparathyroidism). If the presurgical serum calcium concentration is greater than 14 mg/dL, vitamin D and calcium therapy should be initiated at the time of surgery. The goal of therapy is to maintain calcium concentration in the range of 8 to 10 mg/dL.[3] Serum calcium should be rechecked every 1 to 2 weeks. If hypercalcemia occurs, all medications should be stopped until calcium concentration is <8.5 mg/dL. After the calcium concentration has stabilized between 8 and 10 mg/dL for 2 to 4 weeks, vitamin D therapy is gradually withdrawn at a rate of 25% every 1 to 2 weeks, while serum calcium concentration is still monitored. Vitamin D therapy can usually be withdrawn by 8 to 16 weeks after surgery.

Prognosis

Prognosis is good with surgery for patients that are not in renal failure when the cause is adenoma or idiopathic hyperplasia. About 35% may show signs of hypocalcemia after surgery. The presence of azotemia worsens the prognosis.[3]

Primary Hypoparathyroidism

Primary hypoparathyroidism is the clinical syndrome caused by an absolute deficiency of PTH as a result of iatrogenic or naturally occurring destruction, failure in development, or functional failure of the parathyroid glands. It is rare in dogs and is observed even less frequently in cats. It can occur at any age, but the average age at occurrence in dogs is about 5 years,[3, 42–44] and in cats about 2 to 3 years.[45] Hypoparathyroidism has been identified in many breeds of dogs.

Pathophysiology

The most common cause of hypoparathyroidism in cats is damage to the blood supply or removal of the parathyroid glands during thyroidectomy for hyperthyroidism. The frequency of occurrence of hypocalcemia as a result of hypoparathyroidism after thyroidectomy depends on the surgical technique (see Chap. 47).[46, 47] Hypoparathyroidism can also occur iatrogenically in dogs after surgical removal of a parathyroid adenoma to treat primary hyperparathyroidism. Because the remaining glands have atrophied from prolonged hypercalcemia, the animal is hypoparathyroid until the glands recover. Naturally occurring cases of hypoparathyroidism are associated with apparent immune destruction and atrophy in dogs[42, 44] and with idiopathic atrophy in cats.[45] Failure of complete development or genetic predisposition to atrophy or immune destruction may be involved in some cases, especially if young animals of a breed are overrepresented.[43]

The clinical manifestations of hypoparathyroidism result from hypocalcemia. Clinical abnormalities are primarily neuromuscular, because a sufficient concentration of ionized calcium is necessary for the release of neurotransmitters such as acetylcholine, for muscle contraction, and for stabilization of nerve cell membranes by decreasing the sodium permeability. The vast majority of clinical signs in dogs and cats are the result of the latter mechanism.

Clinical Signs

All the clinical signs of primary hypoparathyroidism are the result of hypocalcemia. Signs appear abruptly and are often episodic, often brought on by excitement. Panting may lead to a relative respiratory alkalosis, reducing the proportion of ionized calcium below the threshold for development of clinical signs.

Commonly observed signs include nervousness, seizures, muscle fasciculations or tremors, ataxia or a stiff gait, weakness, muscle cramping or pain, hyperthermia, lethargy, poor appetite or anorexia, and pruritus, often affecting the face in dogs. Seizures often begin with focal muscle twitching with progression to generalized seizures. Dogs may exhibit aggressive behavior, and cats may have ptyalism or dysphagia. A few dogs may have PU/PD. Cardiac rhythm disturbances may include tachyarrhythmias or bradycardia in dogs and bradycardia in cats. Dogs often appear tense, with abdominal splinting when palpated.[3, 42–45] Small lenticular cataracts can be seen in dogs and cats.[3, 43–45]

Diagnostic Plan

All dogs and cats with primary hypoparathyroidism have a severely reduced serum calcium concentration (dogs, range 2.7–6.4 mg/dL, mean 4.5; cats, range 2.8–4.2 mg/dL, mean 3.8)[42, 44, 45] In most cases, the phosphorus is elevated (dogs, 4.7–10.9 mg/dL; cats, 5.2–19 mg/dL). Other biochemical parameters are unremarkable. The concentration of serum magnesium should be determined, because severe hypomagnesemia can inhibit PTH secretion and function.[22] Animals with primary hypoparathyroidism usually have normal[42, 44] or only mildly reduced serum magnesium concentrations.[43, 44] Results of other routine laboratory tests are unremarkable. Electrocardiography (ECG) may reveal a prolonged Q-T interval and often bradycardia.[3, 45]

The clinical diagnosis of primary hypoparathy-

roidism can be made based on the presence of typical clinical signs of hypocalcemia, severe hypocalcemia on the biochemical profile with hyperphosphatemia, normal magnesium concentration, and a lack of azotemia. Definitive diagnosis is made by measuring the concentration of PTH (see Diagnostic Procedures). Most patients have a PTH concentration below normal, or in the mid-normal to low-normal range.[43–45] A low or low-normal PTH concentration in the presence of hypocalcemia is inappropriate.

Treatment

Therapy for Hypocalcemic Tetany

For the patient with clinical signs of hypocalcemia, 10% calcium gluconate (9.3 mg elemental calcium/mL) should be infused intravenously at a dose of 5 to 15 mg/kg of elemental calcium, diluted in 25 to 50 mL of 5% dextrose, slowly over 20 to 30 minutes to effect. The ECG should be monitored (alternatively, the heart should be auscultated frequently) for bradycardia, shortening of the Q-T interval, or S-T segment elevation. Infusion should be stopped if they occur. After tetany is controlled, calcium should be given by continuous IV infusion or subcutaneously to prevent clinical signs by keeping the serum calcium concentration between 8 and 10 mg/dL until oral vitamin D and calcium supplementation can be effective. The intravenous dosage is approximately 20 mg/kg of elemental calcium over 6 to 8 hours,[48] diluted in a maintenance volume of 5% dextrose in water. Perhaps a more practical alternative is to give the dose of 10% calcium gluconate that was required to stop tetany, subcutaneously every 6 to 8 hours (calcium gluconate should be diluted in an equal volume of normal saline solution).[3] The use of calcium chloride in place of calcium gluconate (even for IV infusion) is strongly discouraged because it is very irritating, causing tissue sloughing if it is accidentally or intentionally administered subcutaneously.[3] Parenteral calcium supplementation can usually be stopped in 1 to 5 days of the beginning of oral therapy.

Maintenance Therapy

After the animal is capable of taking medications orally, it should be started on a vitamin D preparation and calcium supplementation. Vitamin D preparations (vitamin D_2, dihydrotachysterol, or calcitriol) vary in time to onset, time to maximal effect, and time required for the effects of overdosage to subside. With vitamin D_2, the time to maximal effect is 5 to 21 days, and toxicity from overdose subsides in 1 to 18 weeks. The dosage is initially 4000 to 6000 U/kg orally per day until the calcium concentration is higher than 8 mg/dL. The dose is then reduced to 1000 to 2000 U/kg every 1 to 7 days to maintain serum calcium between 8 and 10 mg/dL.

With dihydrotachysterol (Hytakeral), the time to maximal effect is 1 to 7 days. Toxicity subsides in 1 to 3 weeks. The dosage is 0.03 mg/kg per day orally for 2 days, then 0.02 mg/kg per day for 2 days, then 0.01 mg/kg every 24 to 48 hours, adjusted as needed to maintain the serum calcium concentration between 8 and 10 mg/dL. The dosage of calcitriol (Rocaltrol) is 0.03 to 0.06 µg/kg per day orally. The maximal effect occurs in 1 to 4 days, and toxicity subsides within 1 day to 2 weeks. Vitamin D (or its analogs) can usually be withdrawn after 8 to 16 weeks for hypoparathyroidism secondary to thyroid or parathyroid surgery.

Oral calcium supplementation can be given in the form of carbonate (40% Ca), gluconate (9.3% Ca), lactate (13% Ca), or acetate (25% Ca) salts. Carbonate is preferred because it has the highest proportion of elemental calcium, is readily available in inexpensive over-the-counter preparations, and also acts as a phosphate binder to reduce hyperphosphatemia that may persist on vitamin D therapy. The oral dose of elemental calcium is 50 to 75 mg/kg per day in two to three divided doses. Calcium supplementation can usually be tapered and withdrawn as vitamin D reaches maximal effect.

Because vitamin D increases absorption of phosphorus as well as calcium from the gastrointestinal tract, animals treated for hypoparathyroidism with vitamin D may remain or become hyperphosphatemic. It is important to maintain the calcium × phosphorus product below 70 to prevent soft tissue mineralization. Low-phosphorus diets (kidney diets, Prescription Diet k/d) are recommended. If the calcium × phosphorus product remains higher than 70 on low-phosphorus diets, oral phosphate binders should be included in the management of these patients (see Chap. 16). Calcium acetate (PhosLo, Phos-Ex) and calcium carbonate (Rolaids, Tums) are good phosphorus binders and good calcium supplements, although less calcium is absorbed with calcium acetate. Animals receiving these calcium supplements may not require additional phosphate binder therapy. Animals that maintain their serum calcium concentration in the range of 8 to 10 mg/dL without calcium supplements, and those patients receiving calcium carbonate or calcium acetate that continue to have hyperphosphatemia, should receive a phosphate binder that does not contain calcium, such as aluminum hydroxide. The initial dose of aluminum hydroxide is 100 mg/kg per day in divided doses, with or before meals. The dose should be adjusted every 10 to 14 days until serum phosphorus concentration is normal.

Therapeutic Monitoring

Serum calcium should be monitored daily until it has stabilized (8–10 mg/dL) for several days, then weekly until vitamin D and calcium therapy is regulated. The serum calcium concentration should then be rechecked every 1 to 3 months indefinitely, or until therapy is no longer needed in iatrogenic cases.

Serum phosphorus should be measured weekly until it is normal or until the serum calcium × phosphorus product remains lower than 70. Phosphorus concentration should then be monitored every 1 to 3 months at the time calcium is measured.

The owner should be advised to monitor for PU/PD as a sign of hypercalcemia. If hypercalcemia develops, medications should be withdrawn until the calcium concentration is normal for 2 to 3 days. Vitamin D therapy should then be reinitiated at a lower dose. Hypercalcemia should be treated aggressively if it is severe (>16 mg/dL) or if clinical signs are present, as described for therapy of hyperparathyroidism.

Prognosis

With proper medical management, the prognosis for long-term survival with a near-normal life expectancy is good for animals with primary hypoparathyroidism. A small proportion may die during the initial hypocalcemic crisis. After that, survival is determined primarily by the owner's willingness and financial ability to continue lifelong medical management.[3, 44]

Vitamin D Intoxication

Intoxication from rodenticides containing vitamin D occasionally occurs in dogs and cats. However, the use of vitamin D as a rodenticide has decreased because it is not as effective as anticoagulant rodenticides. Clinical signs of vitamin D intoxication in dogs and cats include lethargy, anorexia, vomiting (sometimes hematemesis), and shock. Serum calcium and phosphorus concentrations are elevated, with concomitant moderate to severe azotemia. Therapy includes IV fluids, furosemide, and calcitonin (see therapy for hypercalcemia with primary hyperparathyroidism).[10, 49–51]

References

1. Stabenfeldt GH. Endocrine glands and their function. In: Cunningham JG, ed. Textbook of Veterinary Physiology. Philadelphia, WB Saunders, 1992:396–404.
2. Banks WJ. Applied Veterinary Histology, 3rd ed. St Louis, Mosby–Year Book, 1993.

3. Feldman EC. Disorders of the parathyroid glands. In: Ettinger SJ, Feldman EC, eds. Textbook of Veterinary Internal Medicine, 4th ed. Philadelphia, WB Saunders, 1995:1437–1465.

4. Nelson RW, Turnwald GH, Willard MD. Endocrine, metabolic, and lipid disorders. In: Willard MD, Tvedten H, Turnwald GH, eds. Small Animal Clinical Diagnosis by Laboratory Methods, 2nd ed. Philadelphia, WB Saunders, 1994:147–178.

5. Meuten DJ, Chew DJ, Capen CC, et al. Relationship of serum total calcium to albumin and total protein in dogs. J Am Vet Med Assoc 1982;180:63–67.

6. Flanders JA, Scarlett JM, Blue JT, et al. Adjustment of total serum calcium concentration for binding to albumin and protein in cats: 291 cases (1986–1987). J Am Vet Med Assoc 1989;194:1609–1611.

7. Chew DJ, Carothers M. Hypercalcemia. Vet Clin North Am Small Anim Pract 1989;19:265–287.

8. Grone A, Werkmeister JR, Steinmeyer CL, et al. Parathyroid hormone–related protein in normal and neoplastic canine tissues: Immunohistochemical localization and biochemical extraction. Vet Pathol 1994;31:308–315.

9. Rosol TJ, Nagode LA, Couto CG, et al. Parathyroid hormone (PTH)–related protein, PTH, and 1,25-dihydroxyvitamin D in dogs with cancer-associated hypercalcemia. Endocrinology 1992;131:1157–1164.

10. MacKenzie CP, Burnie AG, Heads KW. Poisoning in four dogs by a compound containing warfarin and calciferol. J Small Anim Pract 1987;28:433–445.

11. Chew DJ, Nagode LA. Renal secondary hyperparathyroidism. In: Proceedings of the Annual Meeting of The Society for Comparative Endocrinology 1990;4:17–26.

12. Finco DR, Rowland GN. Hypercalcemia secondary to chronic renal failure in the dog: A report of four cases. J Am Vet Med Assoc 1978;173:990–994.

13. Elliot J, Dobson JM, Dunn JK, et al. Hypercalcaemia in the dog: A study of 40 cases. J Small Anim Pract 1991;32:564–571.

14. Weller RE, Holmberg CA, Theilen GH, et al. Canine lymphosarcoma and hypercalcaemia: Clinical, laboratory and pathologic evaluation of twenty-four cases. J Small Anim Pract 1982;23:649–658.

15. Hause WR, Stevenson S, Meuten DJ, et al. Pseudohyperparathyroidism associated with adenocarcinomas of anal sac origin in four dogs. J Am Anim Hosp Assoc 1981;17:373–379.

16. Ross JT, Scavelli TD, Matthiesen DT, et al. Adenocarcinoma of the apocrine glands of the anal sac in dogs: A review of 32 cases. J Am Anim Hosp Assoc 1991;27:349–355.

17. Wisner ER, Nyland TG, Feldman EC, et al. Ultrasonographic evaluation of the parathyroid glands in hypercalcemic dogs. Vet Radiol Ultrasound 1993;34:108–111.

18. Kornegay JN. Hypocalcemia in dogs. Compen Contin Educ Pract Vet 1982;4:103–110.

19. Jorgensen LS, Center SA, Randolph JF, et al. Electrolyte abnormalities induced by hypertonic phosphate enemas in two cats. J Am Vet Med Assoc 1985;187:1367–1368.

20. Chew DJ, Meuten DJ. Disorders of calcium and phosphorus metabolism. Vet Clin North Am Small Anim Pract 1982;411–438.

21. Finco DR. Interpretations of serum calcium concentration in the dog. Compen Contin Educ Pract Vet 1983;5:778–787.

22. Levi J, Massry SG, Coburn JW, et al. Hypocalcemia in magnesium-depleted dogs: Evidence for reduced responsiveness to parathyroid hormone and relative failure of parathyroid gland function. Metabolism 1974;23:323–335.

23. Forrester SD, Moreland KJ. Hypophosphatemia: Causes and clinical consequences. J Vet Intern Med 1989;3:149–159.

24. Justin RB, Hohenhaus AE. Hypophosphatemia associated with enteral alimentation in cats. J Vet Intern Med 1995;9:228–233.

25. Adams LG, Hardy RM, Weiss DJ, et al. Hypophosphatemia and hemolytic anemia associated with diabetes mellitus and hepatic lipidosis in cats. J Vet Intern Med 1993;7:266–271.

26. Willard MD, Zerbe CA, Schall WD, et al. Severe hypophosphatemia associated with diabetes mellitus in six dogs and one cat. J Am Vet Med Assoc 1987;190:1007–1010.

27. Berger B DVM, Feldman EC DVM. Primary hyperparathyroidism in dogs: 21 cases (1976–1986). J Am Vet Med Assoc 1987;191:350–356.

28. Thompson KG, Jones LP, Smylie WA, et al. Primary hyperparathyroidism in German shepherd dogs: A disorder of probable genetic origin. Vet Pathol 1984;12:370–376.

29. Weller RE, Cullen J, Dagle GE. Hyperparathyroid disorders in the dog: Primary, secondary and cancer-associated (pseudo). J Small Anim Pract 1985;26:329–341.

30. Klausner JS, O'Leary TP, Osborne CA. Calcium urolithiasis in two dogs with parathyroid adenomas. J Am Vet Med Assoc 1987;191:1423–1426.

31. Barber PJ, Elliot J, Torrance AG. Measurement of feline intact parathyroid hormone: Assay validation and sample handling studies. J Small Anim Pract 1993;34:614–620.

32. Torrance AG, Nachreiner R. Human-parathormone assay for use in dogs: Validation, sample handling studies, and parathyroid function testing. Am J Vet Res 1989;50:1123–1127.

33. Torrance AG, Nachreiner R. Intact parathyroid hormone assay and total calcium concentration in the diagnosis of disorders of calcium metabolism in dogs. J Vet Intern Med 1989;3:86–89.

34. Blind E, Schmidt-Gayd H, Scharla S, et al. Two-site assay of intact parathyroid hormone in the investigation of primary hyperparathyroidism and other disorders of calcium metabolism compared with a midregion assay. J Clin Endocrinol Metab 1988;67:353–360.

35. Nachreiner RF, Refsal KR. The use of parathormone, ionized calcium and 25-hydroxyvitamin D assays to diagnose calcium disorders in dogs. In: Proceedings of the Annual Meeting of The Society for Comparative Endocrinology 1990;4:27–30.

36. Schenk PA, Chew DJ, Brooks CL. Effects of storage on

serum ionized calcium and pH values in clinically normal dogs. Am J Vet Res 1995;56:304–307.

37. Szenci O, Brydl E, Bajcsy CA. Effect of storage on measurement of ionized calcium and acid-base variables in equine, bovine, and canine venous blood. J Am Vet Med Assoc 1991;199:1167–1169.

38. Kallet AJ, Richter KP, Feldman EC, et al. Primary hyperparathyroidism in cats: Seven cases (1984–1989). J Am Vet Med Assoc 1991;199:1767–1771.

39. DeVries SE, Feldman EC, Nelson RW, et al. Primary parathyroid gland hyperplasia in dogs: Six cases (1982–1991). J Am Vet Med Assoc 1993;202:1132–1136.

40. Black AP, Peterson ME. Thyroid biopsy and thyroidectomy. In: Bojrab MJ, ed. Current Techniques in Small Animal Surgery, 2nd ed. Philadelphia, Lea & Febiger, 1983:388.

41. Feldman EC, Nelson RW. Hypercalcemia and primary hyperparathyroidism. In: Feldman EC, Nelson RW, eds. Canine and Feline Endocrinology and Reproduction, 2nd ed. Philadelphia, WB Saunders, 1996:455–496.

42. Sherding RG, Meuten DJ, Chew DJ, et al. Primary hypoparathyroidism in the dog. J Am Vet Med Assoc 1980;176:439–444.

43. Jones BR, Alley MR. Primary idiopathic hypoparathyroidism in St. Bernard dogs. N Z Vet J 1985;33:94–97.

44. Bruyette DS, Feldman EC. Primary hypoparathyroidism in the dog: Report of 15 cases and review of 13 previously reported cases. J Vet Intern Med 1988;2:7–14.

45. Peterson ME, James KM, Wallace M, et al. Idiopathic hypoparathyroidism in five cats. J Vet Intern Med 1991;5:47–51.

46. Flanders J, Harvey H, Erb H. Feline thyroidectomy: A comparison of postoperative hypocalcemia associated with three different surgical techniques. Vet Surg 1987; 16:362–366.

47. Welches CD, Scavelli TD, Matthiesen DT, et al. Occurrence of problems after three techniques of bilateral thyroidectomy in cats. Vet Surg 1989;18:392–396.

48. Peterson ME. Treatment of canine and feline hypoparathyroidism. J Am Vet Med Assoc 1982;181:1434–1436.

49. Gunther R, Felice LJ, Nelson RK, et al. Toxicity of a vitamin D3 rodenticide to dogs. J Am Vet Med Assoc 1988;193:211–214.

50. Livezey KL, Dorman DC, Hooser SB, et al. Hypercalcemia induced by vitamin D_3 toxicosis in two dogs. Canine Pract 1991;16:26–32.

51. Moore FM, Kudisch M, Richter K, et al. Hypercalcemia associated with rodenticide poisoning in three cats. J Am Vet Med Assoc 1988;193:1099–1100.

Chapter 50

Diseases of Lipid Metabolism

William E. Monroe

Anatomy

Most lipid absorbed from the gastrointestinal tract is absorbed by the lacteals (small intestinal lymphatic capillaries) and transported to the blood vascular system by way of the cisterna chyli in the abdomen, through the thoracic duct in the thorax, to drain at variable locations into the jugular vein.

Physiology

Lipids, primarily triglycerides and cholesterol, are transported in blood in the form of lipoproteins. Lipoproteins have a central core of nonpolar lipid surrounded by a "shell" of polar phospholipid and a special protein called apolipoprotein. The major classes of lipoproteins are chylomicrons, very-low-density lipoproteins (VLDLs), low-density lipoproteins (LDLs), and high-density lipoproteins (HDLs). The classes of lipoproteins differ in size, density, and lipid content, with the chylomicrons being the largest and least dense and the HDLs the smallest and most dense. Chylomicrons and VLDLs contain primarily triglycerides, whereas LDLs and HDLs contain mostly cholesterol. The various classes also contain different apolipoproteins. The phospholipid shell makes the lipoproteins miscible in plasma, and the apolipoproteins direct metabolism by binding to enzymes or transport proteins.[1, 2]

Chylomicrons are formed by the intestinal epithelial cells and function primarily to transport dietary lipid (exogenous lipid) to tissues such as fat, muscle, and liver for metabolism or storage (see Chaps. 32 and 34). The VLDLs are produced by the liver and are responsible for transport of lipid from the liver (endogenous lipid) to adipose tissue and striated muscle. The remnants of VLDLs, after most of the triglyceride has been "extracted" by peripheral tissues, are metabolized by the liver to form LDLs, which may function primarily to carry cholesterol to tissues actively producing steroid hormones or cells that are rapidly dividing and have a high need for cholesterol for membrane synthesis. The HDLs are secreted into the blood stream by the liver and intestine and function primarily to collect excess cholesterol from peripheral tissues and transport it back to the liver for excretion as bile acids or for redistribution.[2] Thyroxine stimulates the excretion of cholesterol by the liver.[2, 3]

The enzyme lipoprotein lipase is bound to endothelial cells in capillary beds of striated muscle and adipose tissue. It hydrolyzes the triglycerides in chylomicrons and VLDLs so that it can be absorbed and then resynthesized into fat for storage in fat cells or metabolized for energy by striated muscle cells. Hepatic lipase performs this same function in the liver.[2] Certain hormones such as insulin and thyroxine stimulate the activity of lipoprotein lipase.[1, 4]

Enzymes at the cellular level alternately increase or reduce lipid hydrolysis and mobilization into the blood stream. Certain hormones influence these enzyme systems (hormone-sensitive lipase). Insulin stimulates lipid formation and storage and inhibits its mobilization from fat cells.[5] The net effects of thyroxine appear to be to decrease circulating lipid,[3] and cortisol increases peripheral lipolysis, increasing the circulating lipid in blood.[4, 6]

Problem Identification

Lipemia (Hypertriglyceridemia)

Hyperlipidemia is an increase in lipid content—either triglyceride (hypertriglyceridemia) or cholesterol (hypercholesterolemia)—in the blood. Because lipid occurs in blood in the form of lipoproteins, hyperlipidemia is also referred to as hyperlipoproteinemia. Lipid particles (lipoproteins) refract light, and if the concentration in serum is very high, the serum takes on a lactescent appearance and can appear almost white (Fig. 50–1). Lactescent serum is termed lipemic. The lipid responsible for lipemia is triglyceride; cholesterol has little or no effect on the appearance of the serum. Hypertriglyceridemia, therefore, is detected if serum samples are visibly lipemic or if an increased triglyceride concentration is noted in a serum biochemistry profile. For a discussion of hypercholesterolemia, see Chapter 47.

Pathophysiology

Lipemia or hyperlipidemia begins about 1 hour after eating, peaks at 2 to 6 hours, and lasts for 3 to 10 hours.[1, 2] If hyperlipidemia persists longer than 12 hours after eating, it is considered abnormal. Fasting

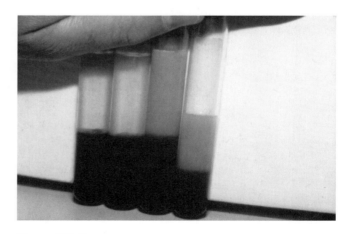

Figure 50–1
Blood samples with lipemic serum (two tubes on the right). The serum has a pink, lactescent appearance from excessive triglyceride and hemoglobin. Lipemia increases red cell fragility and hemolysis in vitro.

Table 50–1
Common Causes of Hyperlipidemia in Dogs and Cats

Physiologic
    Postprandial
Secondary hyperlipidemia
    Diabetes mellitus
    Hyperadrenocorticism
    Hypothyroidism
    Nephrotic syndrome
    Pancreatitis
Primary hyperlipidemia
    Idiopathic canine hyperlipidemia
    Familial feline hyperchylomicronemia

hyperlipidemia in small animals is usually secondary to diseases that lead to a defect in lipid transport or metabolism. Much less commonly, hyperlipidemia may be caused by an inborn (primary) defect in lipid metabolism (Table 50–1).

Diabetes mellitus causes hypertriglyceridemia because a low concentration of insulin leads to reduced lipoprotein lipase activity, slowing clearance of triglyceride from blood.[1, 4] In addition, the lack of insulin results in mobilization of fatty acids from adipose tissue, because insulin normally stimulates deposition of fat and inhibits its hydrolysis in fat cells.[5]

The hypertriglyceridemia seen with hypothyroidism may be caused by a combination of decreased lipoprotein lipase activity and a net formation of lipid.[3, 4] Hyperadrenocorticism may cause hypertriglyceridemia by increasing peripheral mobilization of lipid.[4, 6] It is unclear whether lipemia seen in association with acute pancreatitis is the cause or the result of that disease.[4]

The underlying cause of primary hyperlipidemia is not known for most cases in dogs.[7] Some cats have an inherited defect in lipoprotein lipase activity, leading to a failure of transport of triglyceride to adipose and muscle tissues.[8]

Severe hypertriglyceridemia (>500 mg/dL) may lead to pancreatitis or a pancreatitis-like syndrome; to neurologic manifestations such as seizures,[1, 7] perhaps caused by increased viscosity leading to local ischemia; or to xanthomata (lipid deposits in tissues, often with granulomatous inflammation in response to the lipid) that cause dysfunction by their physical presence. Xanthomata may form in areas of trauma from extravasation of lipid with blood during small hemorrhages. They occur primarily in cats in areas of constant minor trauma such as the spinal nerves, the sciatic nerve where it traverses the ischiatic notch, and over bony prominences.[9] Pressure from the xanthomata in cats leads to nerve dysfunction.[8]

Lipemia retinalis is caused by the lactescent appearance of blood in retinal vessels; it occurs when the triglyceride concentration is greater than 1000 mg/dL. It is of no clinical consequence other than to indicate the presence of hyperlipidemia.[9]

Hyperlipidemia interferes with colorimetric or spectrophotometric chemical analyses of serum or plasma. Because of this, calcium and bilirubin are often artifactually elevated. Dry chemistry methods are affected very little by hyperlipidemia.

Clinical Signs

The clinical signs of severe hypertriglyceridemia in dogs are usually episodic and include abdominal pain, vomiting, diarrhea, abdominal distention, and seizures.[1]

Cats with severe hypertriglyceridemia may have cutaneous nodules (xanthomata) and lipemia retinalis. They also have neurologic dysfunction depending on the location of xanthomata that apply pressure to peripheral nerves. Common signs include Horner's syndrome (see Chap. 26) and tibial and radial nerve paralyses (see Chap. 28).

Diagnostic Plan

Hypertriglyceridemia or lipemia is usually detected when blood is taken for serum biochemical analysis. The first step is to make sure the animal was fasted for a sufficient amount of time before the blood was drawn to exclude postprandial hyperlipidemia. To ensure this, the analysis should be repeated after food has been withheld for 12 hours. If postprandial hyperlipidemia is eliminated, fasting hypertriglyceridemia is usually secondary to another condition. The clinical signs, serum chemistry profile, complete blood count, and urinalysis should help identify causes such as diabetes mellitus (see Chap. 48), hyperadrenocorticism (see Chap. 46), or hypothyroidism (see Chap. 47). Specific hormonal function testing may be indicated, depending on the other signs.

If no underlying cause of secondary hyperlipidemia is found, it is assumed that hypertriglyceridemia is caused by a primary defect of lipid metabolism. The chylomicron test (see Diagnostic Procedures) may be useful to characterize the disorder, but it usually does not alter the management of the case. The most common syndromes in dogs and cats are associated with hyperchylomicronemia.[7, 8]

Hypolipidemia

Hypolipidemia is uncommon in small animals. It is usually associated with severe protein-losing enteropathy such as that seen with intestinal lymphangiectasia (see Chap. 32). Other clinical and laboratory signs in such cases usually predominate and may include diarrhea, weight loss, hypoproteinemia (albumin and globulin), peripheral edema, or ascites.

Diagnostic Procedures

Routine Laboratory Evaluation

Serum triglyceride is routinely measured in biochemical profiles. Because lactescent (lipemic) serum (see Fig. 50–1) can cause artifactual alterations of other components being analyzed in the sample, some laboratories "clear" lipemic samples by ultracentrifugation before analysis. In order to obtain a true assessment of the degree of hyperlipidemia, the sample should be analyzed with and without "clearing." Routine laboratory testing is very useful to identify what usually is a secondary cause of hypertriglyceridemia.

Chylomicron Test

The chylomicron test is performed by letting serum that has been separated from red blood cells stand refrigerated for 6 to 10 hours. If the hyperlipidemia is caused by hyperchylomicronemia, there will be a creamy white layer on top of a more clear, lower layer of serum termed the infranatant. If some of the hyperlipidemia is caused by an increase in VLDLs, the infranatant will be cloudy. If hyperlipidemia is a result solely of increased triglyceride in VLDLs, there will be no "cream layer," and the lactescence will remain diffusely dispersed in the serum.[1]

Lipoprotein Electrophoresis and Ultracentrifugation

Lipoprotein electrophoresis and the use of ultracentrifugation to separate and determine the specific lipid content of the various lipoprotein classes have not been sufficiently standardized for use in veterinary patients to be practically available or useful. Certain methodologies have been adapted and validated for specifically quantitating each lipoprotein class in dog serum samples,[10] but they are not routinely commercially available.

Diseases of Lipid Metabolism

Idiopathic Canine Hyperchylomicronemia

Severe primary hyperlipidemia is seen uncommonly in dogs, predominately in the miniature schnauzer breed, but other breeds may also be affected. Patients are usually older than 4 years of age when the condition is detected. Fasting serum triglyceride is severely increased (often >1000 mg/dL; range, 500–8000 mg/dL) with moderate elevations of cholesterol.[1, 11] The chylomicron test is positive (see Diagnostic Procedures). The serum is obviously lipemic (see Fig. 50–1), and clinical signs, which are usually episodic, include abdominal pain, vomiting, diarrhea, abdominal distention, and seizures.[1, 7] Patients are also at risk for development of pancreatitis. Diagnosis is made by finding triglyceride concentrations higher than 500 mg/dL in uncleared serum (see Diagnostic Procedures) and ruling out causes of secondary hyperlipidemia. The metabolic defect is unknown, but most of the excess lipid may be contained in chylomicrons (hyperchylomicronemia)[1] or in chylomicrons and VLDLs.[12] Therapy is mainly reduction of dietary fat (no more than 8%–12% fat on a dry matter basis; suitable diets are Prescription Diet r/d or w/d, Waltham Veterinarian Canine Low Fat Diet, Purina CNM OM-Formula Canine Veterinary Diet, and Eukanuba Lite).[13] The goal is to reduce the triglyceride concentration in uncleared serum to less than 500 mg/dL. Low-fat diets should be fed for life. If dietary therapy does not reduce hypertriglyceridemia, dogs can be treated with clofibrate, niacin, gemfibrozil (150–300 mg per dog every 12 hours orally),[13] or n-3 polyunsaturated fatty acids (DermCaps), but doses and therapeutic guidelines have not been clearly substantiated.[1] Dogs that are vomiting should be treated with intravenous fluids (see discussion of acute gastritis in Chap. 31). Those with confirmed pancreatitis should also receive intravenous fluids and be given nothing by mouth until there is a clinical response (see Acute Pancreatitis in Dogs in Chap. 33). Prognosis is good for those dogs that recover from or never get pancreatitis, as long as the triglyceride concentration can be reduced and maintained below 500 mg/dL.

Familial Feline Hyperchylomicronemia

Familial primary hyperlipidemia associated with severe elevations of fasting serum triglyceride concentration (mean, 900 mg/dL) and moderate elevations of cholesterol (mean, 255 mg/dL) is seen uncommonly in cats. The cats in most reports have been related, and in one group the disorder was probably inherited as an autosomal recessive trait.[14] Various breeds are represented, and clinical signs are usually apparent at an early age (3 weeks to 8 months). Clinical signs include lipemia retinalis (triglyceride >1000 mg/dL), cutaneous xanthomata (lipid deposition leading to granulomatous subcutaneous swellings), neurologic deficits such as Horner's syndrome (see Chap. 26), and tibial and radial nerve paralyses (see Chap. 28) caused by pressure of xanthomata on peripheral nerves. The metabolic defect appears to be a deficiency in lipoprotein lipase activity. Diagnosis is made on the basis of clinical signs and severe hypertriglyceridemia with a positive chylomicron test (see Diagnostic Procedures). Therapy is reduction of dietary fat (Prescription Diet r/d or w/d, Purina CNM OM-Formula Feline Veterinary Diet, Eukanuba Lite).[13] Affected kittens should be weaned. For cats whose serum lipid concentrations are not reduced to the normal or near-normal range by dietary fat reduction, medium-chain triglyceride oil (0.5 ml/kg per day) can be considered as an alternative source of dietary lipid in a homemade diet,[8, 9, 13] or gemfibrozil (7.5 mg/kg twice daily by mouth) may be effective.[9] If triglyceride concentration is reduced to normal or near-normal, peripheral nerve function will return within 2 to 3 months.[8, 9]

References

1. Ford RB. Canine hyperlipidemia. In: Ettinger SJ, Feldman EC, eds. Textbook of Veterinary Internal Medicine, 4th ed. Philadelphia, WB Saunders, 1995:1414–1419.
2. Watson TDG, Barrie J. Lipoprotein metabolism and hyperlipidaemia in the dog and cat: A review. J Small Anim Pract 1993;34:479–487.
3. Guyton AC, Hall JE. The thyroid metabolic hormones. In: Guyton AC, Hall JE, eds. Textbook of Medical Physiology, 9th ed. Philadelphia, WB Saunders, 1996:945–956.
4. DeBowes LJ. Lipid metabolism and hyperlipidemia in dogs. Compend Contin Educ Pract Vet 1987;9:727–734.
5. Guyton AC, Hall JE. Insulin, glucagon, and diabetes mellitus. In: Guyton AC, Hall JE, ed. Textbook of Medical Physiology, 9th ed. Philadelphia, WB Saunders, 1996:971–983.
6. Guyton AC, Hall JE. The adrenocorticol hormones. In: Guyton AC, Hall JE, eds. Textbook of Medical Physiology, 9th ed. Philadelphia, WB Saunders, 1996:957–970.
7. Ford RB. Idiopathic hyperchylomicronaemia in miniature schnauzers. J Small Anim Pract 1993;34:488–492.
8. Jones BR. Inherited hyperchylomicronaemia in the cat. J Small Anim Pract 1993;34:493–499.
9. Jones BR. Feline hyperlipidemia. In: Ettinger SJ, Feldman EC, eds. Textbook of Veterinary Internal Medicine, 4th ed. Philadelphia, WB Saunders, 1995:1410–1414.
10. Barrie J, Nash AS, Watson TDG. Quantitative analysis of canine plasma lipoproteins. J Small Anim Pract 1993;34:226–231.
11. Armstrong PJ, Ford RB. Hyperlipidemia. In: Kirk RW, Bonagura JD, eds. Current Veterinary Therapy X. Philadelphia, WB Saunders, 1989:1046–1050.
12. Whitney MS, Boon GD, Rebar AH, et al. Ultracentrifugal and electrophoretic characteristics of the plasma lipoproteins of miniature schnauzer dogs with idiopathic hyperlipoproteinemia. J Vet Intern Med 1993;7:252–260.
13. Barrie J, Watson TDG. Hyperlipidemia. In: Bonagura JD, Kirk RW, eds. Kirk's Current Veterinary Therapy XII. Philadelphia, WB Saunders, 1995:430–434.
14. Jones BR, Johnstone AC, Cahill JI, et al. Peripheral neuropathy in cats with inherited primary hyperchylomicronaemia. Vet Rec 1986;119:268–272.

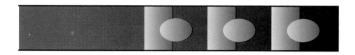

Respiratory
Diseases

Chapter 51

Diseases of the Nasal Cavity

Alice M. Wolf

Anatomy and Physiology

The nasal cavity is the entry and exit point for air passing through the respiratory system. The bony framework of the nasal cavity consists of the nasal bones dorsally, the premaxillae and maxillae laterally, and the vomer and palatine bones and palatine processes of the premaxillae and maxillae ventrally (hard palate). Anteriorly the external nares are defined by the flexible rhinarium, which is supported by nasal cartilages that extend from the nasal bones. The ethmoid bones form the posterior limit of the nasal cavity, the cribriform plate, and support the internal (posterior) nares.

The nasal cavity is divided along the midline into two separate chambers by a bony and cartilaginous septum. Each side is further divided into several longitudinal channels by the nasal turbinates (conchae). The turbinate structures are composed of thin, scroll-like bones or cartilage covered with secretory mucosa and respiratory epithelial cells that greatly increase the surface area of the nasal cavity. The dorsal nasoturbinates (dorsal nasal conchae) and maxilloturbinates (ventral nasal conchae) are in the anterior portion of the nasal cavity. The dorsal nasal meatus passes between the dorsal nasoturbinates and the nasal bones; the middle nasal meatus lies between the dorsal nasoturbinates and maxilloturbinates; and the ventral nasal meatus lies between the maxilloturbinates and the hard palate. The ethmoturbinates (ethmoidal conchae) arise from the ethmoid bone, fill the posterior nasal cavity, and extend dorsally into the frontal sinuses.

As air moves through the nasal cavity, it passes through the turbinate system. The extensive capillary network in the turbinate system warms and humidifies inspired air and recovers heat and moisture from expired air. The nasal cavity is also the first line of defense for the respiratory system. Invading organisms and particulate matter are trapped by mucus secreted by the respiratory epithelium. Ciliated nasal epithelial cells transport mucus-entrapped materials to the external nares or nasopharynx, where they are expelled by sneezing or swallowing. Immunoglobulin A in nasal secretions also acts to neutralize invading organisms and prevent penetration of the epithelial surface.

Modified neuroepithelium in the mucous membrane of the ethmoturbinates and maxilloturbinates is responsible for olfaction. Sensory information is transmitted via the olfactory nerve to the brain.

Air passes from the internal nares into the nasopharynx above the soft palate. The dorsal walls of the nasopharynx contain lymphoid follicles; the auditory (eustachian) tube openings are on the lateral nasopharyngeal walls.

Paranasal sinuses are diverticula of the nasal cavity in both dogs and cats. These sinuses are lined by mucus-secreting glands and ciliary epithelium. Although their function is unclear, paranasal sinuses are often secondarily involved in processes that affect the nasal cavity. The frontal sinuses are dorsal to the nasal cavity and directly connected to it by a well-defined ostium. In brachycephalic breeds, these sinuses may be very attenuated or absent. Dogs also have maxillary sinuses below the eye; cats have small sphenoid sinuses dorsal to the hard palate.

Problem Identification

Sneezing

Sneezing is acute, explosive retrograde expulsion of air and debris from the nasal passages.

Pathophysiology

Sneezing is caused by irritation or inflammation, usually in the anterior portion of the nasal cavity.

Clinical Signs

Inhaled foreign bodies routinely cause acute paroxysmal episodes of sneezing until the object is expelled or becomes lodged deeper in the nasal cavity. Other disorders usually cause chronic, intermittent sneezing that may be accompanied by expulsion of nasal exudate or blood or stertorous breathing efforts.

Diagnostic Plan

Occasional sneezing with no accompanying clinical signs may be a normal finding associated with clearing the nasal passages of routinely accumulated debris. More frequent or paroxysmal sneezing and sneezing accompanied by significant nasal discharge or other evidence of intranasal disease indicate a need for further diagnostic evaluation including nasal cavity examination, radiography, and biopsy.

Nasal Discharge

The mucous membranes of the nasal cavity normally produce small amounts of seromucoid secretions that cover and protect the epithelium of the nasal cavity. A minimal amount of serous discharge from the external nares is normal for most animals.

Pathophysiology

Nasal secretions increase and exit the nares in abnormal amounts in response to allergic, inflammatory, infectious, or traumatic stimuli. The character of the nasal discharge may help define the disease process in the nasal cavity, and its appearance may change over the course of the disease.

Clinical Signs

Viral upper respiratory diseases, allergic rhinitis, and early parasitic infections typically produce serous discharge early in the disease, but the discharge becomes mucopurulent when secondary bacterial invasion occurs. Mucoid or mucopurulent discharge is more common with chronic disorders such as bacterial rhinosinusitis, lymphoplasmacytic rhinitis, neoplasia, or fungal infection. Fresh blood may intermittently be mixed with the discharge, particularly in the latter two disorders.[1] Discharge of frank blood from the nasal cavity (epistaxis) is discussed later.

Unilateral discharge from the nasal cavity suggests a focal problem such as a nasal tumor, fungal infection, chronic foreign body, or tooth root abscess. Bilateral discharge may also occur with fungal and neoplastic rhinitis as these diseases worsen over time. Allergic rhinitis, viral and bacterial rhinosinusitis, lymphoplasmacytic rhinitis, and parasitic rhinitis usually cause bilateral discharge.

Diagnostic Plan

The history of duration, location, appearance, and progression of the nasal discharge may help localize the affected side of the nasal cavity. Acute onset of nasal discharge in conjunction with systemic signs of illness is most likely associated with viral upper respiratory disease. Serous discharge with sneezing may be due to allergic rhinitis. When discharge becomes chronic or contains fresh blood, further evaluation is warranted. Cytologic examination of material that has exited the external nares is rarely rewarding because of secondary contamination with bacteria and debris. Further diagnostic steps include radiography, nasal cavity examination, and cytology or biopsy of affected tissue.

Epistaxis

Frank hemorrhage (epistaxis) from the nasal cavity is usually the result of trauma (e.g., direct trauma, acute foreign body inhalation) or a bleeding or vascular disorder (e.g., coagulation factor deficiency, disseminated intravascular coagulation, thrombocytopenia, vasculitis).[1]

Pathophysiology

The turbinate structures contain a rich capillary network that is easily disrupted by trauma. Even normal day-to-day irritations may cause severe bleeding if there are abnormalities of the intrinsic or extrinsic coagulation system. Vascular disorders such as immune-mediated vasculitis or rickettsial diseases may also result in frank hemorrhage from the nasal cavity. Rarely, neoplastic or fungal diseases may erode through blood vessels in this area, resulting in a severe hemorrhagic event.

Clinical Signs

Bleeding may be triggered by a sneezing episode or may appear spontaneously. Blood, sometimes mixed with clots, may drip intermittently or continuously from the external nares. The patient should be examined carefully for other evidence of a systemic bleeding disorder. Signs suggesting a major factor deficiency include suffusion or ecchymotic hemorrhages and hemorrhage into body cavities or internal organs. Vascular or platelet disorders are more likely to be associated with less internal hemorrhage, but cutaneous petechiation may be observed. Other physical evidence of trauma is usually present in patients with traumatic nasal damage.

Diagnostic Plan

Inhaled foreign bodies causing acute hemorrhage should be suspected if paroxysmal sneezing and nasal discomfort are observed on physical examination. Patients with physical trauma and associated nasal hemorrhage should be evaluated for shock and other traumatic injuries. Evaluation of patients with suspected coagulation defects should include a coagulation profile consisting of a prothrombin time, partial thromboplastin time, and platelet count. Fibrin degradation products should also be measured in patients with suspected disseminated intravascular coagulation. If a systemic coagulopathy can be ruled out, further evaluation should include nasal inspection, followed, if necessary, by radiography and biopsy, as described for other disorders.

Distortion or Destruction of the Nasal Cavity

Pathophysiology

Internal distortion or destruction of the turbinates occurs because of lysis related to a chronic inflammatory or infectious process (e.g., herpesvirus rhinitis, chronic bacterial rhinosinusitis) and results from the effects of lysosomal enzymes and swelling of affected tissues. Expansion of a mass lesion (e.g., fungal granuloma, neoplasm, nasal polyp) also causes internal nasal destruction that may involve deviation or destruction of portions of the nasal septum. Lysis of the bones of the skull (e.g., maxillary, facial, nasal bones) is almost always the result of an aggressive expansile disease such as a fungal infection or tumor[1] (Fig. 51–1). Damage to the internal or external bones of the nasal cavity may also result from trauma.

Clinical Signs

Clinical signs of internal nasal cavity damage may be limited to nasal discharge and reduced airflow through the nasal passages. Destruction of the overlying bony structure of the nasal cavity can result in external facial or maxillary swelling or distortion, swelling of tissues overlying the nasal cavity, draining wounds on the face, and exophthalmos or periorbital swelling.

Diagnostic Plan

The history of the patient in conjunction with the physical findings should lead to the nasal cavity as the primary site of the problem. Acute traumatic damage to the nasal cavity is usually obvious because of the history and other physical evidence of trauma. If a soft tissue mass is present, particularly if a bony defect of the nasal cavity is palpable, fine-needle aspiration cytology may yield a diagnosis. Radiography is helpful in assessing the extent and location of the damage and determining the best site for biopsy procedures. The oral cavity, nasal cavity, posterior nares, and nasopharynx should be examined carefully for lesions. Biopsy procedures should be performed as previously described.

Stertor or Stridor

Stertor or stridor is defined as increased noise associated with respiratory efforts.

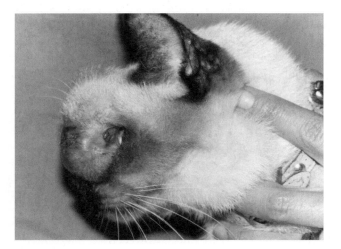

Figure 51-1
A large mass distorting the face is present in this 4-year-old Siamese cat with feline leukemia virus–negative nasal lymphosarcoma.

Pathophysiology

These abnormal sounds may originate in the nasal cavity or nasopharynx (see Chap. 52) as a result of obstruction to airflow. Intranasal obstruction is most commonly caused by the presence of soft tissue swelling, exudate or blood, or mass lesions.

Clinical Signs

In addition to the noise noted on respiration, nasal obstruction may prolong the inspiratory phase of respiration if the mouth is closed. Bilateral nasal cavity obstruction may result in open-mouth breathing or panting, during which increased nasal sounds do not occur. Stertor or stridor originating in the nasal cavity may be accompanied by nasal discharge, sneezing, snorting, gagging, or reverse sneezing. All of these are indications for further diagnostic evaluation of the nasal cavity.

Diagnostic Plan

It may be possible to isolate the source of the increased sounds by careful listening with a stethoscope over the nasal chambers, pharynx, larynx, and trachea. For stridor originating in the nasal cavity, radiography, inspection, and biopsy are recommended.

Other Signs

Central nervous system (CNS) signs may rarely occur with an intranasal disease because of direct extension of the process through the cribriform plate into the brain.[2] These diseases tend to be aggressive and destructive, such as fungal infections or neoplasia. Occasionally, the signs of brain derangement (e.g., seizures, behavioral changes, ataxia, depression, gait abnormalities) may occur without obvious evidence of intranasal disease.[2] Pain originating in or noticed on palpation of the nasal cavity is usually associated with erosive or expanding mass lesions. Foreign bodies or allergic rhinitis may cause a patient to paw at its face or rub its muzzle. Exophthalmos suggests extension of the problem into the retrobulbar space; ocular discharge may be associated with the primary disease (e.g., viral rhinitis) or be caused by obstruction of the nasolacrimal system (Fig. 51–2). Exudate draining into the nasopharynx, nasopharyngeal foreign bodies, or polyps may cause gagging. Finally, lesions that erode or disrupt the hard or soft palate may result in expulsion of food or water from the nose and difficulty in eating or drinking. The diagnostic approach previously described should lead to a diagnosis in these patients.

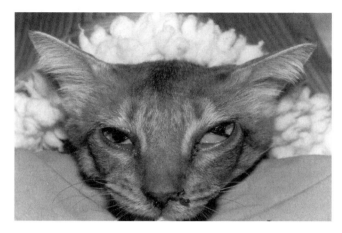

Figure 51-2
This 8-year-old domestic shorthair cat exhibits exophthalmos and deviation of the globe secondary to nasal aspergillosis.

Diagnostic Procedures

Radiography and Special Imaging

Radiographs of the nasal cavity should be taken before invasive examination or diagnostic procedures are performed. Lateral, ventrodorsal open-mouth, and skyline frontal sinus views are taken with the patient under deep general anesthesia[3] (Fig. 51–3). Fine-detail, rare-earth intensifying screen-film combinations provide the best detail of intranasal structures.[3] Additional views that are helpful in selected patients include the intraoral dorsoventral view on nonscreen film, oblique views of the dental arcades, and spot dental radiographs.

The radiographic appearance of increased fluid density in the nasal cavity or sinus may be caused by the accumulation of exudate or blood or by the presence of a soft tissue mass. Destruction or distortion of the turbinate bones and nasal septum may be caused by a chronic inflammatory process but is more likely the result of fungal or neoplastic disease. Destruction of bones of the external nasal cavity is highly suggestive of neoplasia but may also occur with some fungal diseases.

Computed tomography and magnetic resonance imaging are extremely sensitive tools for evaluating subtle changes in the nasal cavity and distinguishing between fluid accumulation and mass lesions and may be available at referral centers.[4, 5]

Microbiologic Culture

Sterile prepackaged and guarded swabs may be used to obtain material from the nasal cavity for bacteriologic and fungal culture. Specimens should be obtained by passing the swab through a sterile nasal

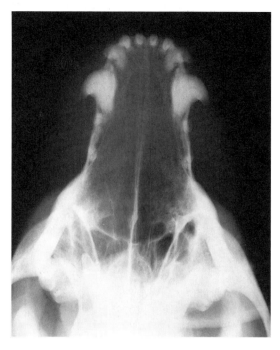

Figure 51-3
Increased density in the posterior portion of the right side of the nasal cavity is seen in this ventrodorsal, open-mouth view of the nasal cavity in a 4-year-old golden retriever with lymphoplasmacytic rhinitis.

speculum under direct observation to avoid contamination with superficial debris. Unfortunately, because the nasal cavity has such a mixed and varied normal flora, interpreting the results of these cultures is difficult.[6] Many organisms that are potential bacterial pathogens are normal commensal residents of the nasal cavity. Fungal cultures of nasal exudate may be falsely positive for *Aspergillus* and *Penicillium* species because these organisms are ubiquitous in the environment.[7] Conversely, false-negative fungal cultures may occur if an inadequate sample is submitted. Fungal culture of tissue biopsy specimens is more likely to be rewarding than culture of swab or wash specimens alone.

Rhinoscopy

Rhinoscopy should be performed while the patient is still under general anesthesia after radiographic examination. Anterior rhinoscopy may be performed with an otoscope, nasal speculum, fiberscope, or arthroscope (the last two are preferred).[4] The patient should be positioned in ventral recumbence with the head tipped slightly downward to facilitate drainage of material from the nasal cavity. The cuff of the endotracheal tube should be checked for adequate inflation to avoid aspiration during the procedure.

Superficial debris can be removed from the nasal cavity prior to endoscopy by gentle irrigation with normal saline solution. The scope should enter the naris angled toward the midline and then be moved slowly laterally and guided gently into the nasal cavity. Irrigation through the biopsy channel of the instrument with normal saline keeps the lens clear of debris and allows better observation of important structures. The size of the patient, the size of the endoscopic instrument, radiographic findings, and observation during the procedure determine the depth to which the instrument can or should be passed into the nasal cavity. Biopsy specimens can be obtained through the biopsy channel of some instruments under direct visualization.

The posterior nasopharynx can be visualized by retracting the soft palate with an ovariectomy hook and examining the area with a dental mirror, nasopharyngeal illuminator, or fiberscope (preferred).[4] Care should be taken during these examinations to avoid excessive hemorrhage, which significantly limits visualization of important structures.

Nasal Lavage

With the patient under general anesthesia with endotracheal intubation, the nasopharynx is packed with gauze sponges, and the nasal cavity is vigorously lavaged with saline via a soft rubber or latex catheter. Refluxed fluid can be recovered from the nares. Mucus, tissue fragments, or foreign materials are often found on the gauze sponges in the nasopharynx. The recovered fluid can be examined directly or centrifuged to prepare concentrated samples for cytologic examination. Tissue fragments are placed on slides and prepared for cytologic examination. Culture of bacteria from nasal lavage specimens is rarely useful. Nasal lavage is less invasive than a core biopsy and is rarely associated with excessive hemorrhage or complications. Unfortunately, specimens recovered with this technique are rarely diagnostic.

Nasal Cavity Biopsy and Cytology

Tissue or brush biopsy specimens can be obtained during rhinoscopy for cytologic analysis, histopathologic examination, or culture. Hemorrhage is expected when nasal biopsies are performed. A platelet count and other tests of bleeding status should be evaluated if the presence of a coagulation abnormality is suspected. A long-bladed, clamshell-type biopsy instrument is ideal for collecting biopsy specimens from the nasal cavity. Alternatively, biopsy specimens can be collected by a nasal core procedure.[8] To perform this procedure, the patient is prepared as for

nasal lavage with the nasopharynx packed with gauze sponges. The biopsy specimen is collected with an 8- to 18-gauge polypropylene urinary catheter cut at a 45° angle about 12 to 15 cm from the end that is attached to a syringe. The distance from the external naris to the medial canthus of the eye is marked on the catheter because this approximates the distance to the cribriform plate. A 12-mL syringe is attached to the catheter. The catheter is advanced quickly into the affected tissue, with care taken not to exceed the depth marked on the catheter that indicates the location of the cribriform plate.[8] Suction is applied to the syringe after penetration and a core of tissue is withdrawn. If a good core is not obtained with a single penetration into the nasal cavity, several brisk advances should be performed to dislodge tissue before removing the catheter. Saline can be flushed into the nasal cavity after removal of the catheter to flush out blood and debris and to dislodge and collect loose tissue fragments from the external naris or nasopharynx. Biopsy specimens can also be taken with biopsy forceps passed through the biopsy channel of a flexible endoscope during the endoscopic examination of the nasal cavity.

Biopsy specimens from the nasal cavity can be submitted for fungal culture, and smears of small tissue fragments can be prepared for cytologic examination.[4] Because the specimens are small, they may become disrupted during transport or lost during histopathologic processing. To help keep specimens intact, they should be placed firmly on a piece of surgical hemostatic foam, paper towel, or thin plastic foam sponge before being placed in formalin. Some bleeding from the nasal cavity after biopsy is expected, but this usually subsides in 30 to 60 minutes.[4] If bleeding is profuse or prolonged, the cavity can be packed with cotton-tipped swabs that have been dipped in dilute (1:10,000) epinephrine solution.

Exploratory Rhinotomy

Exploratory rhinotomy may be required if the cause of the nasal cavity signs has not been determined by one or more of the aforementioned procedures[4] (Fig. 51–4). Rhinotomy is a very invasive procedure but has the advantage of allowing thorough examination of the nasal cavity and access to the sinuses for both additional diagnostic evaluation and potential correction of the problem (e.g., removal of a deep-seated foreign body). A surgical textbook should be consulted for a complete description of this procedure. Culture and biopsy specimens can be collected during rhinotomy and are handled as previously described.

Common Diseases of the Nasal Cavity

Feline Viral Rhinosinusitis

Feline herpesvirus and calicivirus are the most common causes of upper respiratory infection in cats.[9] These viruses, as single agents or in combination, cause approximately 90% of feline upper respiratory disease. Infection with herpesvirus or calicivirus is most common among purebred cattery cats and cats raised in multiple-cat households, animal shelters, or other environments where endemic virus carriers are likely to reside.

Pathophysiology

These viral agents damage the respiratory epithelium and may cause distortion of the nasal turbinates, particularly in young animals. Bacterial colonization is secondary to epithelial damage and causes the change in the nasal discharge from serous to mucopurulent. Affected cats may become chronic virus carriers, with calicivirus being shed continuously and herpesvirus shed intermittently for months to years after infection. Cats that shed virus chronically are commonly found in catteries and multiple-cat households and are a source of infection for young, susceptible cats introduced into these environments.

Clinical Signs

These viruses produce sneezing, ocular discharge, and bilateral serous nasal discharge that becomes mucopurulent after secondary bacterial invasion as the disease progresses. Systemic signs of illness, including malaise, fever, and inappetence, are also usually present. Ulceration of the tongue or hard palate occurs in some cats.[9] Dendritic corneal ulceration is typical of herpesvirus (see Chap. 19). Infection with either or both of these viruses at a young age may cause permanent damage to the nasal mucosa and turbinates, predisposing to chronic bacterial rhinosinusitis that may persist for life.

Diagnostic Plan

Diagnosis is usually based on history and clinical signs. Hematologic evaluation may reveal a neutrophilic leukocytosis or may be normal. Biochemistry profiles and urinalyses may show evidence of dehydration but are usually normal. Virus can be isolated from pharyngeal swab specimens if a definitive diagnosis is required. Indirect fluorescent antibody or polymerase chain reaction testing of conjunctival scrapings may also be used to identify the agent causing respiratory disease.

Treatment

Treatment of acute feline viral upper respiratory disease includes correcting dehydration and maintaining the cat's hydration status, removing nasal and ocular exudates, providing nutritional support, and treating secondary bacterial infection. Most bacterial invaders are part of the normal flora, and a broad-spectrum antibiotic such as a protected penicillin or cephalosporin or potentiated sulfa is a good first choice. Specific treatment with an antiviral ophthalmic preparation is indicated if herpetic ulcers are present.

Prognosis

The prognosis for recovery depends on the age and immunologic status of the cat but is usually excellent with good nursing care. Most cats recover completely from the signs of acute disease in 10 to 14 days. Of these cats, a variable number become chronic carriers of the viruses and shed infectious virus. Clinical signs of disease are usually not present in chronic carriers, although a few intermittently show signs of oculonasal discharge or corneal ulceration. Permanent nasal turbinate or mucosal damage may result from feline viral upper respiratory disease, particularly in cats that acquire the infection early in life. These cats may be predisposed to develop chronic bacterial rhinosinusitis (chronic snufflers) that may persist for life.

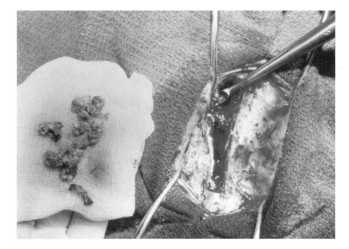

Figure 51–4
Granulomatous debris is being removed from the nasal cavity during exploratory rhinotomy in this 7-year-old Doberman pinscher with nasal aspergillosis.

Prevention

Vaccines are available to protect against both of these viral illnesses. The parenteral vaccines usually provide excellent protection against severe disease but do not completely protect against infection. Intranasal vaccines may provide better protection against infection, particularly if they are given before natural exposure to the virulent strains of virus has occurred.[9]

Canine Viral Rhinosinusitis

Canine morbillivirus (paramyxovirus, canine distemper) infection can cause severe upper respiratory involvement in affected dogs. (See Chap. 24 for a complete discussion of canine distemper virus infection.) The virus is highly contagious, and disease is most common among young dogs that are housed in groups. Poor husbandry and poor sanitation also contribute to the development of disease.

Pathophysiology

Canine morbillivirus affects all epithelial tissues. Viral damage to the epithelium permits secondary bacterial infection and produces the typical mucopurulent oculonasal discharge and secondary bacterial pneumonia seen with this disease. Gastrointestinal epithelial damage results in vomiting and diarrhea. Infection when the dental enamel epithelium is forming produces irregular tooth enamel surfaces and discolored teeth. Retinal epithelial damage results in chorioretinitis. Infection of the CNS causes more insidious signs that may not appear for months to years after infection. Progressive paresis or paralysis results from demyelination and myoclonus caused by damage to inhibitory interneurons in the spinal cord.

Clinical Signs

Signs include mild sneezing and copious bilateral mucopurulent oculonasal discharge. Fever, anorexia, and lethargy accompany the respiratory signs. In most dogs, lower respiratory tract involvement is present, beginning as an interstitial pneumonia and progressing to secondary bacterial bronchopneumonia. Neurologic signs, including myoclonus, seizures, paresis, or paralysis, occur in approximately 25% of affected dogs. Gastrointestinal signs are not common, but some patients may exhibit vomiting and diarrhea. Chorioretinitis, hypoplasia of dental enamel, and hyperkeratosis of the nasal planum and foot pads may be present in some patients.

Diagnostic Plan

A clinical diagnosis is usually made on the basis of history and clinical signs. Evidence of chorioretinitis in the presence of typical signs of upper respiratory infection is highly suggestive of canine distemper virus infection. Hematologic studies may reveal leukocytosis and lymphopenia. Biochemistry profiles and urinalyses are usually normal. Immunofluorescent antibody testing of conjunctival scrapings or foot pad biopsy specimens may confirm the diagnosis. Distemper antibody titers in serum cannot be used alone for diagnosis, but they are sometimes measured in patients with neurologic symptoms for comparison with titers in the cerebrospinal fluid to determine whether active antibody production is occurring in the CNS.

Treatment

Treatment includes supportive care and treatment of secondary bacterial complications. Broad-spectrum antibiotics are given to prevent secondary infection of affected epithelial tissues. Fluid therapy and nutritional support aid in recovery. CNS infection is generally progressive and irreversible. Anticonvulsant agents may be used to attempt to control distemper-associated seizures, but the prognosis for patients with CNS disease is grave.

Prognosis

Recovery from acute disease occurs in about 50% of affected dogs and is dependent on their age, their immunologic status, and the presence of concurrent problems such as intestinal parasitism. However, neurologic signs, dental enamel hypoplasia, or hyperkeratosis of the foot pads or nasal planum may be late-developing complications following the initial apparent recovery from illness.

Prevention

Modified live canine distemper vaccines are highly effective in preventing infection and disease if given prior to exposure to virulent virus.

Chlamydia Infection

Chlamydia psittaci is an obligate intracellular organism more closely related to bacteria than to viruses. It accounts for approximately 5% to 10% of the feline respiratory disease seen in the United States but is a more common upper respiratory pathogen in other countries. Disease caused by *Chlamydia* occurs most commonly in cats housed in groups in catteries, shelters, or pet stores. The organism is transmitted horizontally by symptomatic or asymptomatic carrier cats. Kittens are usually infected early in life and may become chronic carriers of the organism.

Pathophysiology

Chlamydia infection usually causes mild upper respiratory and conjunctival epithelial damage that is self-limited. Occasionally, other bacterial invaders may complicate the infection, resulting in more severe signs of disease. Lower respiratory or systemic infection with *Chlamydia* is rare. Chronic carrier cats may have intermittent recrudescences of mild upper respiratory signs, particularly if they are stressed.

Clinical Signs

C. psittaci usually causes mild symptoms of sneezing, bilateral serous oculonasal discharge, and conjunctival chemosis in cats.[9] Systemic signs of illness (e.g., fever, anorexia) are not usually present or are very mild. Early infection of young kittens, before 10 to 14 days of age, may result in the accumulation of purulent exudate beneath the sealed eyelids, causing apparent bulging of the lids and periorbital swelling.

Diagnostic Plan

The diagnosis may be confirmed by finding intracytoplasmic chlamydial inclusions on cytologic examination of a conjunctival scraping.[9]

Treatment

Treatment includes removing exudate from the eyes and applying tetracycline ophthalmic ointment several times daily to prevent corneal erosions or conjunctival adhesions. Kittens affected before their eyelids open naturally should have the lids forcibly opened manually so that the eyes can be treated aggressively. The accumulation of exudate and lysosomal enzymes beneath the lids may cause severe damage to ocular tissues and may result in blindness. Systemic treatment with tetracycline or doxycycline may be used for selected patients with more severe disease.

Prognosis

Recovery from acute *Chlamydia* infection usually occurs in 10 to 14 days. Chronic carrier cats may have intermittent exacerbation of clinical signs associated with stress or corticosteroid administration. Cats with a foreshortened facial conformation (e.g., Persian-type cats) may develop chronic dacryocystitis resulting in chronic epiphora.

Prevention

Chlamydial antigen is available in combination with some of the multivalent feline viral vaccines. Protection is reported to last less than 1 year with vaccines that are currently available. Because *Chlamydia* infection accounts for little feline respiratory disease in household cats, clinicians must decide whether the additional cost of adding this antigen to a vaccination program is justified for their clientele.

Chronic Bacterial Rhinosinusitis

Chronic secondary bacterial rhinosinusitis in cats is a common sequela of infection with feline herpesvirus or calicivirus early in life.[10] Damage to the turbinates and nasal mucosa produces an environment conducive to secondary bacterial colonization and makes effective treatment difficult.

Pathophysiology

Chronic bacterial rhinosinusitis is usually a consequence of turbinate and respiratory mucosal distortion and damage caused by viral upper respiratory infection that occurs early in life. Occasionally, an older cat also develops chronic rhinitis after acute respiratory viral infection. Respiratory clearance mechanisms do not function well in this abnormal environment. Mucus and debris accumulate and the normal bacterial flora of the nasal cavity proliferates, causing inflammation, additional mucosal swelling, and mucus secretion. The epithelium of the frontal sinuses may be similarly affected, or the frontal sinuses may be secondarily involved because swelling within the nasal cavity blocks drainage from the sinuses.

Clinical Signs

Clinical signs include a previous history of upper respiratory viral infection (often at an early age), chronic sneezing, stertor, and mucopurulent to occasionally mucohemorrhagic nasal discharge. Signs may be unilateral but are usually bilateral. Epiphora may be present because of blockage of the nasolacrimal system by mucosal swelling or mucus obstruction. Systemic signs of illness are usually absent in this chronic stage, and these cats usually eat well, are active, and are otherwise normal in appearance.

Diagnostic Plan

The diagnosis is assisted by a history of previous viral respiratory disease and is made by ruling out other more specific and serious disorders. Routine laboratory studies are usually normal. Testing for feline leukemia virus (FeLV) and feline immunodeficiency virus (FIV) should be performed to rule out immunosuppression as an underlying cause of chronic infection. Radiographs reveal variable degrees of increased density in the nasal passages and sinuses.[10] Radiographic evidence of turbinate destruction may be present in severe cases, but destruction of the overlying bones of the nasal cavity should not occur. The frontal sinuses may appear opaque because of inflamed mucosa or accumulation of mucus. Examination of the nasal cavity reveals inflamed, swollen nasal mucosa; cytology and biopsies demonstrate purulent inflammation with bacteria present and with thickening and distortion of the nasal turbinates.

Treatment

Treatment is palliative and supportive. The owner should be advised that cure is unlikely and that intermittent therapy will be required for many cats.[10] Antibiotic therapy may help reduce numbers of bacteria, topical decongestants may provide temporary relief of nasal congestion, and humidification with a vaporizer or nebulizer may help the cat expel inspissated secretions from the nasal passages. Surgical exploration with removal of the turbinates and drainage of the frontal sinuses (possibly followed by fat graft or polymethyl methacrylate implantation) has been recommended by some clinicians to improve respiration.[10, 11] However, this surgery is traumatic, and chronic serosanguineous nasal discharge may persist afterward.

Prognosis

A cat with chronic bacterial rhinosinusitis often has a normal lifespan if the owner does not become discouraged and remove the cat from the household because of contamination of the environment with debris from the chronic nasal discharge. The prognosis for controlling the condition is guarded because the underlying turbinate and mucosal damage is permanent and the abnormal intranasal environment is a persistent problem.

Aspergillosis and Penicilliosis

Aspergillus and *Penicillium* spp. are ubiquitous saprophytic hyphal fungi. *Aspergillus* is by far the more common infection; however, because both agents appear to cause the same clinical syndrome, these infections are discussed as a single disorder.[7] Fungal colonization of the nasal passages occurs after inhalation of fungal spores from the environment. Aspergillosis is more common in immunosuppressed human beings, but an underlying immunosuppressive problem has rarely been identified in affected dogs or cats.

Nasal aspergillosis is most common in young to middle-aged dogs with a dolichocephalic (long-nosed) conformation.[7] Golden retrievers and German shepherds may be at greater risk of infection; males are more commonly affected than females. Cats are rarely affected by either fungus.

Pathophysiology

It is not clear why *Aspergillus* and *Penicillium* spp. seem able to colonize the nasal respiratory epithelium in some animals with apparently intact immune systems. Undiagnosed minor intranasal trauma or disruption of the nasal epithelium may permit these organisms to gain a foothold and begin to proliferate in these patients. Bone lysis results from direct pressure from the expanding fungal granuloma and toxins secreted by the fungal organisms. Secondary bacterial infection often accompanies fungal rhinitis because of the abnormal environment created by the fungal mass.

Clinical Signs

Clinical signs include sneezing, stertor, and mucopurulent, sanguinopurulent, or hemorrhagic nasal discharge.[7] Discharge is usually unilateral initially but becomes bilateral over time. Ulceration of the external nares may occur because of chronic irritation by the accumulated nasal exudate. Pain may be evident on palpation over the bridge of the nose on physical examination or may be evidenced by face pawing or rubbing by the patient.

Diagnostic Plan

Routine hematologic studies are usually unremarkable; peripheral eosinophilia and lymphopenia have been described in a few patients. *Aspergillus* organisms or toxins destroy the nasal turbinates, producing increased lucency in the rostral part of the nasal cavity on radiographs. Classic aspergillosis lesions include punctate lysis of the vomer or frontal bones. A granulomatous mass or mat of fungal growth may accumulate in the posterior portion of the nasal cavity, producing increased radiographic density mixed with osteolysis in this area (Fig. 51–5). Frontal sinuses may be radiodense because of accumulated mucus due to poor drainage or may be involved with the fungal infection (Fig. 51–6). Rhinoscopic examination may reveal edematous nasal mucosa with yellow-green to gray-black fungal colonies.[4, 7] Material should be collected for cytologic study and histopathology, as previously described. Special stains for fungi should be requested, as these improve detection if few organisms are present in the specimens. Agar gel double-diffusion and other immunologic tests to detect serum antibodies against *Aspergillus* spp. can be used to support the diagnosis.[7] Antibodies are not usually present in patients with only surface contamination; therefore, a systemic response suggests more invasive disease. Cross-reactivity with *Penicillium* spp. occurs, and false-positive rates for these tests are 5% to 15%. Therefore, serologic findings should always be correlated with the clinical picture and the results of other diagnostic studies.

Treatment

Topical antifungal therapy is currently the most effective approach to the treatment of nasal aspergillosis. Clotrimazole (1 g/100 mL polyethylene glycol) can be used to irrigate the nasal chambers through indwelling nasal catheters twice daily for 7 to 10 days or as a single 1-hour treatment at nasal exploratory surgery[12] (Fig. 51–7). Enilconazole (Imaverol) is also effective when used in the twice-daily irrigation protocol at a

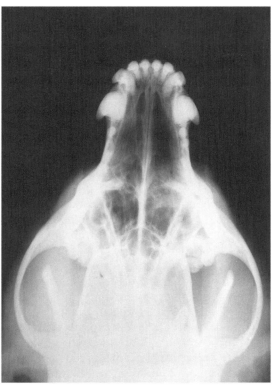

Figure 51-5
Ventrodorsal, open-mouth radiograph of the nasal cavity of a 5-year-old Brittany spaniel with nasal aspergillosis. The left side of the nasal cavity demonstrates increased lucency rostrally due to destruction of bone and increased density in the posterior nasal cavity secondary to the presence of a fungal granuloma.

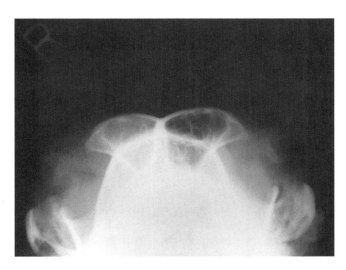

Figure 51-6
Skyline rostrocaudal radiograph of the frontal sinuses of the patient in Figure 51–4 demonstrating increased fluid density in the right frontal sinus secondary to the presence of an aspergillus granuloma.

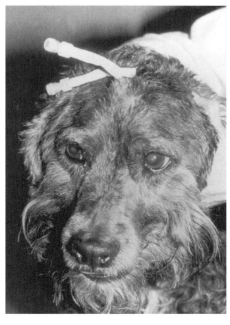

Figure 51-7
Bilateral indwelling catheters have been placed through the frontal sinuses into the nasal cavity in this 5-year-old mixed breed dog with nasal aspergillosis. These tubes are well tolerated by most dogs. Topical antifungal treatment is administered through the tubes twice daily for 10 days.

dilution of 10 mg/kg per treatment.[7] Enilconazole is diluted 1:1 with water to facilitate passage through the indwelling catheters. Both clotrimazole and enilconazole are bitter; patients may salivate profusely after intranasal instillation of the drugs and may physically resist being treated after exposure to the drug for several days. Both clotrimazole and enilconazole protocols produce cure rates of approximately 90%. Treatment with oral antifungals including ketoconazole (10 mg/kg by mouth every 12 hours) or itraconazole (10 mg/kg by mouth every 24 hours) has been about 50% effective in eliminating nasal *Aspergillus* infection.[7] Oral antifungal treatment may be needed for 6 to 8 months to effect cure.

Prognosis

With appropriate treatment, the prognosis for recovery for most patients with nasal aspergillosis is good. Relapse rates are about 10% following topical therapy and about 50% with oral antifungal treatment. Because residual intranasal damage may account for some nasal discharge persisting after treatment, reexamination and biopsy should be performed to confirm relapse before antifungal therapy is reinitiated.

Cryptococcosis

Cryptococcus neoformans is a saprophytic yeastlike fungus with a worldwide distribution. Infection of

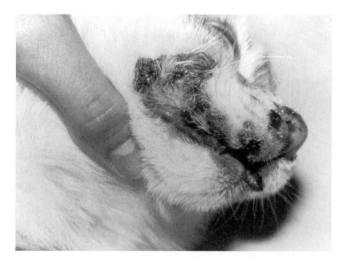

Figure 51–8
Perioral cutaneous and nasal planum involvement is present in this 3-year-old domestic shorthair cat with nasal cryptococcosis.

the nasal cavity probably occurs by inhalation of the organism from the environment. However, preferential localization in the nasal cavity following intravenous inoculation has been demonstrated for some strains of *Cryptococcus*. Nasal cryptococcosis occurs most commonly in cats and is a rare infection of dogs.[13, 14] There is no apparent age, breed, or sex predilection. Concurrent retrovirus infection (FeLV or FIV) does not predispose to the infection, but cats with either of these immunosuppressive diseases are likely to have more disseminated disease and are more resistant to treatment.

Pathophysiology

The expansion of the pyogranulomatous reaction to the fungal organisms causes both soft tissue and bone destruction within the nasal cavity. Secondary bacterial infection is often superimposed on the fungal disease. The development of subretinal cryptococcal granulomas causes elevation of the retinal epithelium (serous retinal detachment) and chorioretinitis. Further systemic dissemination of the organism is more common in cats that have concurrent retrovirus infection or have been treated with corticosteroids. Fungal granulomas can be found in the lymph nodes, skin, lung, CNS, or other organs in these patients.

Clinical Signs

Clinical signs of infection include unilateral or bilateral, mucopurulent to hemorrhagic nasal discharge and sneezing.[13] Fever is usually absent. Systemic signs of illness may include anorexia, weight loss, and lethargy. Regional lymphadenopathy and skin granulomas are present in about 30% of affected patients (Fig. 51–8). Ocular involvement including chorioretinitis, optic neuritis, retinal detachment, and anterior uveitis occurs in some animals (see Chap. 19). CNS spread of the organism can result in seizures, ataxia, circling, paresis, paralysis, or amaurotic blindness (see Chaps. 24 and 39). Disseminated disease with involvement of the lung, bone, and kidney is found in a few patients.

Diagnostic Plan

Routine hematologic studies and urinalyses are usually normal. Biochemistry profiles may reveal hyperglobulinemia consistent with chronic antigenic stimulation but are usually otherwise normal. In patients with CNS involvement, cerebrospinal fluid analysis demonstrates increased cellularity, neutrophilia, and an elevated protein content. FeLV antigen and FIV antibody tests are usually negative for cats with only nasal cavity involvement; cats with disseminated cryptococcosis are more likely to have concurrent retrovirus infection.[13] Radiographic studies usually reveal evidence of unilateral or bilateral soft tissue density in the nasal cavity early in the course of infection. Destruction of the nasal turbinates and overlying nasal bones may result from expansion of the fungal granulomas as the disease progresses. The diagnosis can be confirmed by identifying the *Cryptococcus* organisms in cytologic or biopsy specimens. Organisms are usually numerous in cytologic specimens and are easily detected with routine Wright or Giemsa hematologic stains. Special fungal stains may be required to find organisms in histologic specimens. The latex cryptococcal antigen test is a sensitive method for detecting the polysaccharide cryptococcal capsular antigen in serum and other body fluids. The test is 95% sensitive and 100% specific and can be used to confirm the diagnosis as well as monitor the efficacy of therapy.[15]

Treatment

Itraconazole (10 mg/kg by mouth every 24 hours) and fluconazole (2.5–5.0 mg/kg by mouth every 12 to 24 hours) are very effective in eliminating nasal cryptococcal infection in most affected patients.[13, 14] Ketoconazole (10 mg/kg by mouth every 12 hours) is also effective; however, side effects including anorexia and hepatic dysfunction often limit its use in cats.[14] Treatment may be required for 2 to 12 months, depending on the severity and extent of disease. Cryptococcal antigen titers can be followed to monitor the progress of treatment.[15] A progressively decreasing titer after 1 to 2 months of treatment is considered good evidence of improvement. Cryptococcal antigen titers may remain positive at a low level for long periods of time despite successful treatment. Good clinical resolution of disease should be a factor in determining when antifungal treatment can and should be discontinued. Fluconazole is the drug of choice for patients with CNS involvement because of its excellent penetration into the cerebrospinal fluid. However, the prognosis for recovery from this form of infection is guarded.

Prognosis

The prognosis for nasal cryptococcosis in patients without retrovirus infection is good with appropriate treatment. The prognosis for patients with concurrent retrovirus infection or CNS cryptococcosis is guarded to grave.

Nasopharyngeal Polyps

Nasopharyngeal inflammatory polyps are an unusual, predominantly feline disorder.[16–18] These masses originate in the middle ear and extend through the auditory tube into the nasopharynx. The initiating cause of the polyps is unknown, but calicivirus has been isolated from some cats.[18] Affected cats are usually younger than 6 years of age; there is no breed or sex predilection.[16]

Pathophysiology

Nasal stertor and stridor are caused by obstruction of airflow by the polyp in the nasopharynx. In some patients, the polyp may be sufficiently large or hang ventrally far enough to partially occlude the esophageal opening or larynx. This results in gagging, difficulty in swallowing (dysphagia; see Chap. 29), or forceful and severely compromised inspiratory efforts.

Clinical Signs

Clinical signs include stertor, stridor, occasional sneezing, and occasional serous or mucoid nasal discharge. Difficulty in swallowing and a change in voice occur in some patients. Anorexia, weight loss, and malaise may result from difficulty in eating and drinking.

Diagnostic Plan

Laboratory parameters and examination of the nasal cavity are usually normal.[16] A nasopharyngeal mass can be seen on radiographs or during examination of the nasopharynx. Radiographic examination of the tympanic bullae may reveal increased soft tissue density on the side associated with the polyp.[16, 17]

Treatment

Surgical removal of the polyp from the nasopharynx by blunt dissection and gentle traction alleviates signs of respiratory obstruction and may be curative.[16, 18] Because the inflammatory process originates from the middle ear, exploration and curettage of the tympanic bulla may be necessary to prevent recurrence in some patients.[16, 18]

Lymphoplasmacytic Rhinitis

Although this condition has not been well defined, the lymphoid and plasma cell infiltrates that characterize lymphoplasmacytic rhinitis suggest that there is an immune-mediated basis for this disorder.[19] Adult dogs are most commonly affected.

Pathophysiology

Mucosal swelling caused by lymphocyte and plasma cell accumulation results in obstruction of airflow and stimulation of mucus secretion. Secondary bacterial infection is often superimposed on the immunologic disorder because of altered clearance mechanisms within the nasal cavity, which produces the typical mucopurulent discharge seen in this disease. The mucosal infiltrates also render the tissue more friable than usual, and spontaneous hemorrhage can occur with mild trauma or sneezing.

Clinical Signs

Clinical signs include sneezing, stertor, nasal congestion, and unilateral or bilateral nasal discharge. The nasal discharge is usually mucopurulent; however, serous, mucoid, and hemorrhagic discharge has been reported in patients with this condition.

Diagnostic Plan

Routine laboratory studies are unremarkable. Radiographs demonstrate increased fluid density, usually confined to the rostral half of the nasal cavity. Lysis of the turbinates, the vomer, or both is present in some patients. Examination of the nasal cavity may be apparently normal or may reveal mucosal edema, erythema, or ulceration.[19] Cytologic examination usually demonstrates secondary bacterial infection. Biopsies reveal lymphoplasmacytic infiltration into the nasal mucosa and submucosa. It is important to collect adequate and representative biopsy specimens because a lymphoplasmacytic infiltration has also been reported in association with nasal aspergillosis and nasal tumors.

Treatment

Immunosuppressive doses of corticosteroids (e.g., oral prednisone at a dose of 2.2–4.4 mg/kg per day) are the initial treatment of choice for idiopathic lymphoplasmacytic rhinitis. High-dose corticosteroid therapy should be maintained for at least 2 to 4 weeks until significant improvement is obtained. The dose can then be tapered slowly by halving it every 2 to 3 weeks to maintain remission of clinical signs. Ultimately, the corticosteroid dose should be reduced to an alternate-day schedule to minimize side effects.

Prognosis

The prognosis for improvement of patients with lymphoplasmacytic rhinitis is fair; treatment may be needed for months to years.[19]

Allergic Rhinitis

Allergic rhinitis is a poorly described entity in dogs and cats. Allergy usually develops in middle-aged to older animals; however, allergic rhinitis may occur in a patient of any age. The onset of clinical signs may be acute if there is an abrupt environmental change (e.g., new rugs, household cleaners, change of location). More commonly, signs develop slowly over time. Intermittent, seasonal occurrence is present in some affected patients.

Pathophysiology

Inhalant allergens are the most common cause of allergic rhinitis, although food allergens have also been implicated in this disease. Mucosal swelling and eosinophilic cellular infiltration produce upper respiratory obstruction, sneezing, and serous nasal discharge. If secondary bacterial infection is present, clinical signs are usually more severe and the nasal discharge is mucopurulent.

Clinical Signs

Clinical signs are usually similar to those of bilateral chronic bacterial rhinosinusitis; however, epistaxis without chronic discharge has been described.[20, 21] Concurrent dermatologic signs of allergy, including pruritus and face rubbing or pawing, occur in some individuals.

Diagnostic Plan

Peripheral eosinophilia has been observed occasionally, but laboratory studies are usually unremarkable. Radiographic changes include variable degrees of increased fluid density in the nasal cavities. There is usually no evidence of nasal turbinate destruction unless the condition is chronic. Cytologic and biopsy findings are usually similar to those for chronic rhinosinusitis; however, eosinophils may be the predominant cell type.

Treatment

An attempt should be made to discover the sensitizing environmental allergen. If there is a history of an environmental change, it may be possible to remove the potentially offending object or chemical from the environment to observe whether the patient's clinical signs improve. The accuracy of feline intradermal skin tests or serum enzyme-linked immunosorbent assay tests for identifying sensitizing inhalant allergens is controversial. Skin or blood testing for dietary allergens is not reliable, and the diagnosis of food allergy requires a response to limited antigen diet trials. Depending on the allergens suspected of causing hypersensitivity, treatment for allergic rhinitis might include an elimination diet trial, skin testing with possible hyposensitization, or corticosteroid therapy with prednisone at a tapering dose, as previously described for lymphoplasmacytic rhinitis.

Neoplastic Disease

Nasal tumors occur most commonly in middle-aged to older animals. Epithelial tumors (carcinoma, adenocarcinoma) are the most common neoplasms of the nasal cavity of dogs and cats.[22–24] Mesenchymal tumors (sarcomas) are uncommon with the exception of lymphosarcoma, which is occasionally found in cats. This form of lymphoma is often restricted to the nasal cavity in cats but may involve regional lymphoid tissue or distant organs or lymph nodes. Rare tumors of the nasal cavity include transmissible venereal tumor and mast cell tumor.

Pathophysiology

Neoplastic diseases exert their destructive effects on the nasal cavity by direct involvement, invasion, or compression of tissues of the nasal cavity and surrounding anatomic structures. Extranasal signs and deformation of the face may also result from compression by the expanding tumor mass or extension of the tumor into extranasal structures.

Clinical Signs

The clinical signs associated with nasal neoplasms are similar to those of chronic rhinosinusitis. Signs are often initially unilateral but progress to involve both sides of the nasal cavity over time. The nasal discharge is often mucopurulent because of secondary bacterial infection and occasionally contains fresh blood. There may be erosion of the tumor

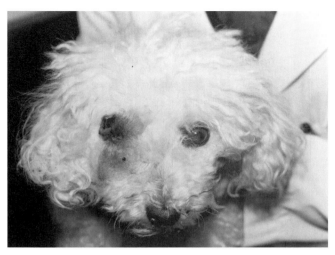

Figure 51–9
Right-sided facial distortion, exophthalmos, and periorbital swelling are present in this 11-year-old miniature poodle with an adenocarcinoma of the nasal cavity.

through the facial bones, distortion of the face, exophthalmos, or pain on opening the mouth, depending on the duration, location, and extent of tumor invasion (Fig. 51–9).

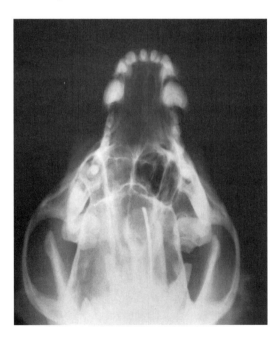

Figure 51–10
A ventrodorsal, open-mouth radiograph of the nasal cavity of a 12-year-old mixed breed dog with nasal undifferentiated carcinoma demonstrates bone destruction on the right side of the anterior nasal cavity with destruction of the posterior portion of the nasal septum. Increased density, most likely associated with a portion of the tumor mass, is seen in the posterior portion of the right nasal cavity.

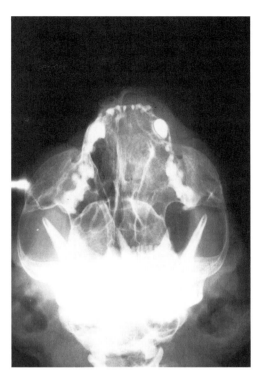

Figure 51–11
A ventrodorsal, open-mouth radiograph of the nasal cavity of a 13-year-old domestic shorthair cat with nasal adenocarcinoma demonstrates a bony destructive mass lesion in the left nasal cavity that has caused deviation of the nasal septum and expansion into the right nasal cavity. The left dental arcade has also been distorted by the expanding mass, and soft tissue swelling is also present.

Diagnostic Plan

Routine laboratory studies are often unremarkable. FeLV antigen or FIV antibody tests may be positive in cats with lymphoma.[23] Radiographs usually demonstrate varying degrees of increased intranasal density accompanied by bone destruction, distortion, or erosion (Figs. 51–10 and 51–11). Computed tomography and magnetic resonance imaging, if available, are sensitive tools for evaluating the true extent of tumor involvement.[5, 23] Examination of the anterior nasal cavity may demonstrate a tissue mass obstructing the nasal passage. Posterior rhinoscopy, as previously described, may demonstrate a mass lesion in the posterior nasopharyngeal region. Exfoliative cytology and biopsy are often diagnostic for neoplastic lesions. However, because inflammation is often associated with the neoplasm, a sufficiently large and representative sample of tissue must be examined before a diagnosis of neoplasia can be confirmed or excluded. Exploratory rhinotomy and biopsy may be required to make a definitive diagnosis of neoplasia in some patients. Although metastasis from nasal neoplasms is usually slow, aspiration cytology or biopsy should be performed on lymph nodes draining the affected area, and thoracic radiographs are recommended prior to initiating therapy.[25]

Treatment

The efficacy of treatment for nasal neoplasms is variable and depends on the tumor type; the extent of involvement of the nasal cavity, sinuses, retrobulbar space, and overlying bone; the presence of regional or distant metastases; and the presence of concurrent diseases (e.g., retroviral infection in cats).[22] Unfortunately, because of the slow development of clinical signs and the limitations of early recognition, nasal neoplasms are usually in an advanced stage of locally invasive disease by the time of diagnosis.[23] Generally, surgical excision alone is unlikely to provide a substantial increase in survival time. Surgical debulking followed by orthovoltage or megavoltage radiation therapy or ^{192}Ir brachytherapy with or without surgery cannot be expected to cure disease but may improve survival and quality of life with substantial temporary relief of clinical signs.[22, 24–27] Radiotherapy appears to provide a longer disease-free interval for mesenchymal tumors than epithelial tumors.[23, 24] Lymphoma is very radiosensitive, and excellent long-term control of disease may be achieved by radiation therapy alone. Complications of radiotherapy include radiation-induced ocular, dermal, and CNS damage.[22, 24] These effects are usually not severe and are easily managed. Brachytherapy may be associated with necrosis of the soft tissues, hard palate, or nasal bones.[26] Chemotherapy has not been uniformly successful for the treatment of nonhematopoietic neoplasms of the nasal cavity but may be effective for nasal lymphoma.[28] Permanent tracheostomy has been used as temporary palliative therapy to improve respiration and quality of life in some dogs with untreated or untreatable nasal tumors.

Prognosis

Survival times for patients with nasal tumors that are not treated or receive only surgical debulking, cryosurgery, or immunotherapy average from 3 to 5 months.[28] Approximate median survival times for dogs and cats with nasal tumors that receive radiation therapy are 23 and 20 months, respectively.[22–25, 28]

Nasal Foreign Body

Various plant and foreign materials have been found lodged in the nasal cavity. These most commonly include plant awns, seeds, twigs, and grass blades.

Pathophysiology

Acutely inhaled foreign bodies cause direct trauma to and irritation of the nasal mucosa. If not expelled by sneezing or removed, the foreign body usually lodges deeper in the nasal chambers. Depending on the size and location of the foreign body, pressure necrosis of soft tissue or bone may occur. Chronic irritation and inflammation cause continued intermittent episodes of sneezing and discomfort and provide an environment conducive to secondary bacterial infection.

Clinical Signs

Clinical signs are caused by trauma and irritation by the foreign material and include acute paroxysms of sneezing, snorting, face rubbing, and unilateral nasal discharge or epistaxis. Grass blades extending into the nasopharynx may also cause sporadic gagging or choking. As the foreign body becomes lodged deeper in the nasal cavity, signs become more intermittent and secondary bacterial infection results from mucosal damage and inflammation.

Diagnostic Plan

Routine laboratory parameters are usually normal. Radiographs may be normal, demonstrate a metallic foreign body, or demonstrate unilateral increased soft tissue density. The diagnosis is made by ruling out other disorders and by locating and removing the nasal foreign body. The posterior nasopharynx should be examined thoroughly because grass blades may be discovered above the soft palate in this area. Occasionally, exploratory surgery is required to diagnose and remove deeply lodged foreign bodies.

Prognosis

Removal of the foreign body is curative, but secondary infections associated with chronic intranasal damage may persist.

Nasal Trauma

Nasal trauma is most commonly associated with vehicular accidents or falling from a height ("high-rise syndrome").[29, 30]

Pathophysiology

Blunt trauma usually causes superficial tearing of the nasal mucosa or minor disruption of turbinates. The small superficial mucosal vessels bleed profusely, but clots form quickly if coagulation is normal. Local subcutaneous emphysema is produced by air dissecting into the subcutaneous tissues from the nasal cavity through fractures in the overlying bones.

Clinical Signs

The primary clinical sign is epistaxis, which may be associated with obvious facial damage and maxillary or hard palate fractures. Signs of traumatic injury to other organs or systems may be present in some patients. Concurrent pneumothorax is a common finding in animals that have fallen from a height. Fractures of the nasal or frontal bones may produce local subcutaneous emphysema.

Diagnostic Plan

Routine laboratory studies and nasal radiography are not usually necessary because the cause of the nasal hemorrhage is obvious.

Treatment

Epistaxis resulting from trauma is usually self-limited and treatment is not usually necessary. In patients with severe or uncontrollable hemorrhage, cotton-tipped swabs dipped in dilute epinephrine solution (see Nasal Cavity Biopsy and Cytology) can be applied to the nasal mucosa, or the nasal cavity can be packed with sterile gauze. Acepromazine (0.05–0.10 mg/kg intravenously) can also be used to assist in reducing acute hemorrhage. However, because the mechanism of action of this drug is to reduce blood pressure, it should not be used in trauma patients that already have or may develop significant hypotension.

Prognosis

The prognosis for patients with traumatic nasal injury is excellent. Hard palate fractures usually seal without intervention, but surgical correction may be required if an oronasal fistula persists after healing.[29]

Dental Disease

Oronasal fistulae, severe periodontitis, and apical abscesses may cause chronic nasal discharge.[31] Older animals and small-breed dogs are more commonly affected.

Pathophysiology

Disruption of the periodontal attachments allows bacteria to colonize along the tooth root and create an abscess pocket at the tooth root apex. Pressure necrosis and lysosomal enzymes in the expanding abscess cause bone lysis and drainage of exudate into the nasal cavity. Naturally occurring loss or veterinary extraction of affected teeth may leave a permanent stoma between the oral cavity and nasal chambers (oronasal fistula; see Chap. 29), creating a pathway for food debris and bacteria to enter the nasal cavity.

Clinical Signs

Clinical signs include chronic unilateral or bilateral nasal discharge that may be serous, mucopurulent, or hemorrhagic. Patients with large oronasal fistulae may have food particles mixed with the nasal exudate. A fetid odor may be noticed around the mouth or nasal cavity. Epiphora and swelling below the eye are occasionally present in dogs with an apical abscess of the fourth upper premolar. Oral examination may reveal an obvious dental or periodontal problem. However, small oronasal fistulae, apical abscesses, or retained tooth roots may not be identified on gross inspection of the oral cavity.[31]

Diagnostic Plan

There are no specific laboratory findings for this disorder, and results are usually consistent with the patient's age. Routine nasal radiographs may demonstrate rhinitis, but oblique views or dental radiographs may be needed for thorough evaluation of the dental arcades for apical abscesses, retained tooth roots, or bone lysis. Nonscreen No. 4 intraoral film provides exquisite detail for these studies. Nasal biopsy helps rule out more serious diseases if radiographs and careful oral cavity examination are equivocal for dental disease.

Treatment

Treatment involves dental prophylaxis and specific treatment for apical abscesses. Apical abscesses may be treated by extraction of the affected tooth, periapical curettage, or standard endodontic drainage followed by packing of the root canal with gutta-percha. Broad-spectrum antibiotic therapy should be administered for several weeks after these procedures. Pre-existing oronasal fistulae or those created by dental extraction should be surgically closed by primary closure or sliding flap technique to eliminate communication of the oral cavity with the nasal chambers.

Prognosis

The prognosis for most patients with nasal disease secondary to dental disease is very good with appropriate treatment. Patients with large or chronic oronasal fistulae have a more guarded prognosis, and it may be difficult to completely eliminate signs of nasal disease.

Anatomic Abnormalities

Stenotic nares are common in brachycephalic breeds of dogs, and the condition is often associated with an elongated soft palate (see Chap. 52). This problem is also seen occasionally in Persian and Persian-crossbreed cats. The stenosis results in noisy respiration and mouth breathing. Surgical correction by removal of the dorsolateral nasal cartilages is curative.

Anatomic abnormalities of the hard palate (e.g., cleft palate) or soft palate (e.g., unilateral or bilateral hypoplasia) can result in nasal discharge and food or waters being expelled from the nares. These defects are more common in dogs, and signs are usually present from an early age. Careful examination of the oral cavity usually reveals the abnormality. Laboratory and radiographic studies are not usually performed in these patients. Treatment consists of surgical correction of the anatomic abnormality.

Uncommon Diseases of the Nasal Cavity

Rhinosporidiosis

Rhinosporidiosis is a rare infection of the canine nasal cavity with the soil-borne fungus *Rhinosporidium seeberi*.[13] Damage to the nasal mucosa may predispose to infection after inhalation of the fungal spores from dust or stagnant water. Young to middle-aged, male, large-breed dogs living in warm, humid environments are more frequently affected. The disease has not been reported in cats. Clinical signs include sneezing, stertor, snoring, and unilateral mucopurulent, serosanguineous, or hemorrhagic nasal discharge. The fungal polyps frequently develop in the anterior part of the nasal cavity and may protrude from the naris. Rhinosporidiosis is limited to the nasal cavity, and systemic signs of illness are not present. Routine laboratory studies are usually normal. Radiography is usually not performed because the nasal mass is often readily apparent on nasal examination. Cytologic and biopsy specimens reveal a mixed population of inflammatory cells and unique fungal spores or sporangia. Complete surgical excision is the treatment of choice and is usually curative. Dapsone (diaminodiphenylsulfone) has also been used effectively at 1 mg/kg by mouth every 12 hours; however, the adverse effects of this drug can be serious and include hemolytic anemia, methemoglobinemia, and bone marrow suppression.[13] The prognosis with successful surgical removal of the fungal polyp is excellent.

Other Fungal and Algal Nasal Infections

Other unusual fungi including *Exophiala spinifera*, *Alternaria alternata*, *Trichosporon*, *Histoplasma*, *Blas-*

tomyces, and *Prototheca* have occasionally been associated with nasal granulomas in dogs or cats.[13] Signs are similar to those of other previously described nasal mycoses.

Parasitic Rhinitis

Pneumonyssus caninum, *Linguatula serrata*, *Capillaria aerophila*, and *Eucoleus bohemi* are occasional parasites of the canine nasal cavity.[32] *Cuterebra* spp. larvae have been reported in the nasal cavity of cats. Clinical signs include sneezing and unilateral or bilateral, serous to mucopurulent nasal discharge. Facial pruritus resulting in self-trauma has also been reported in some cases of *Pneumonyssoides* infestation. Bacterial secondary infection is often associated with parasitic disease. Systemic signs of illness are absent, and laboratory findings are unremarkable. Radiographs may reveal apparently normal nasal passages or increased fluid density in one or both sides of the nasal cavity. Rhinoscopy may be apparently normal; occasionally mites, *Capillaria* spp. larvae, or *Cuterebra* spp. larvae may be seen on nasal examination. Nasal cytology or flushing may reveal *Pneumonyssoides* mites or eggs or *E. bohemi* or *Capillaria* spp. eggs (Fig. 51–12). Other rhinoscopic findings are similar to those for chronic rhinosinusitis. *Capillaria* spp. or *E. bohemi* eggs may

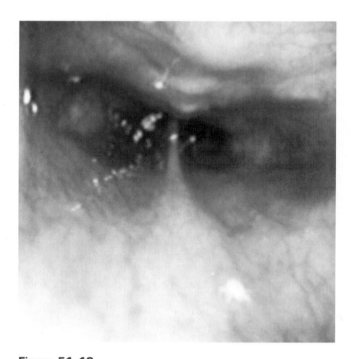

Figure 51–12
Endoscopic examination of the nasopharynx demonstrates nasal mites (*Pneumonyssoides*) as the cause of chronic sneezing and nasal discharge in this 7-year-old mixed breed dog. The mites are seen as whitish specks trapped in mucus draining from the posterior nares.

also be found on fecal flotation.[32] *Pneumonyssoides* and *Capillaria* spp. infections have been successfully treated with a single ivermectin dose of 200 µg/kg. Manual removal of *Cuterebra* spp. larvae is curative; surgical exploration may be required for diagnosis and removal of *L. serrata*.

Primary Ciliary Dyskinesia

Primary ciliary dyskinesia is a rare disorder resulting from congenital structural abnormalities of ciliated cells.[33–35] Because the cilia move in an uncoordinated fashion, the respiratory mucosal epithelium cannot perform its protective clearance function. Affected patients are usually identified early in life because of recurring upper and lower respiratory infections.[33] The predominant clinical sign of upper respiratory involvement is bilateral mucopurulent nasal discharge. The discharge may respond temporarily to antibiotic therapy but recurs when treatment is discontinued. Clinical signs of concurrent bronchopneumonia are often present. Hearing loss and otitis media have been reported in some patients. Hematologic studies may be normal or demonstrate neutrophilia caused by the secondary infections.[34] Biochemistry profiles and urinalyses are usually normal. Radiographs of the nasal cavity are consistent with rhinosinusitis. Radiographs of the thorax may reveal the presence of bronchopneumonia. Situs inversus (reversed positioning of the intrathoracic organs) is also observed in some patients (Kartagener syndrome).[33, 34] The diagnosis of primary ciliary dyskinesia should be suspected on the basis of chronic, recurring respiratory infections in a young patient. The diagnosis is confirmed by electron microscopic examination of ciliated cells that demonstrates structural abnormalities of the ciliary microtubules.[33, 34] Because the ciliary abnormalities cannot be corrected, the treatment for this disorder is symptomatic and supportive. Chronic antibiotic administration and pulmonary therapy may help control secondary infections and improve respiration. The long-term prognosis for these patients is fair if secondary infections are treated appropriately.[35] Because the condition is believed to be inheritable, affected individuals should not be bred.[33]

References

1. Dhupa N, Littman M. Epistaxis. Compen Contin Educ Pract Vet 1992;14:1033–1042.
2. Smith MO, Turrel JM, Bailey CS, et al. Neurologic abnormalities as the predominant signs of neoplasia of the nasal cavity in dogs and cats: Seven cases (1973–1986). J Am Vet Med Assoc 1989;195:242–246.
3. Miyabayashi T, Biller DS, Haider PR, et al. Radiographic appearances of the nasal conchae in dogs using different screen-film systems: A postmortem study. J Am Anim Hosp Assoc 1994;30:382–388.
4. Forbes Lent SE, Hawkins EC. Evaluation of rhinoscopy and rhinoscopy-assisted mucosal biopsy in diagnosis of nasal disease in dogs: 119 cases (1985–1989). J Am Vet Med Assoc 1992;201:1425–1429.
5. Park RD, Beck ER, LeCouteur RA. Comparison of computed tomography and radiography for detecting changes induced by malignant nasal neoplasia in dogs. J Am Vet Med Assoc 1992;201:1720–1724.
6. Abramson AL, D'Amato RF, Senberg HD, et al. Microbiology of the canine nasal cavities. Ann Otol Rhinol Laryngol 1976;85:394–397.
7. Sharp NJH, Sullivan M, Harvey CE, et al. Treatment of nasal aspergillosis with enilconazole. J Vet Intern Med 1994;7:40–43.
8. Withrow SJ, Susaneck SJ, Macy DW, et al. Aspiration and punch biopsy techniques for nasal tumors. J Am Anim Hosp Assoc 1985;21:551–554.
9. Gaskell RM. Upper respiratory disease in the cat (including *Chlamydia*): Control and prevention. Feline Pract 1993;21:29–34.
10. Cape L. Feline idiopathic chronic rhinosinusitis: A retrospective study of 30 cases. J Am Anim Hosp Assoc 1992;28:149–155.
11. Norsworthy GD. Surgical treatment of chronic nasal discharge in 17 cats. Vet Med 1993;88:526–537.
12. Davidson A, Komtebedde J, Pappagianis D, et al. Treatment of nasal aspergillosis with topical clotrimazole. Proc Am Coll Vet Intern Med Forum 1992;10:807.
13. Wolf AM. Fungal diseases of the nasal cavity of the dog and cat. Vet Clin North Am Small Anim Pract 1992;22:1119–1132.
14. Medleau L, Greene CE, Rakich PM. Evaluation of ketoconazole and itraconazole for treatment of disseminated cryptococcosis in cats. Am J Vet Res 1990;51:1454–1457.
15. Medleau L, Marks A, Brown J, et al. Clinical evaluation of a cryptococcal antigen latex agglutination test for diagnosis of cryptococcosis in cats. J Am Vet Med Assoc 1990;196:1470–1473.
16. Kapatkin AS, Matthiesen DT, Noone KE, et al. Results of surgery and long-term follow-up in 31 cats with nasopharyngeal polyps. J Am Anim Hosp Assoc 1990;26:387–392.
17. Faulkner JE, Budsberg SC. Results of ventral bulla osteotomy for treatment of middle ear polyps in cats. J Am Anim Hosp Assoc 1990;26:496–499.
18. Schmidt JF, Kapatkin A. Nasopharyngeal and ear canal polyps in the cat. Feline Pract 1990;18(4):16–19.
19. Burgener DC, Slocombe RF, Zerbe CA. Lymphoplasmacytic rhinitis in five dogs. J Am Anim Hosp Assoc 1987;23:565–568.
20. McCarthy TC, McDermaid SL. Rhinoscopy. Vet Clin North Am Small Anim Pract 1990;20:1265–1290.
21. McDougal BJ. Allergic rhinitis—a cause of recurrent epistaxis. J Am Vet Med Assoc 1977;171:545–546.
22. Theon AP, Peaston AE, Madewell BR, et al. Irradiation of nonlymphoproliferative neoplasms of the nasal cavity

and paranasal sinuses in 16 cats. J Am Vet Med Assoc 1994;204:78–83.

23. Cox NR, Brawner WR Jr, Powers RD, et al. Tumors of the nose and paranasal sinuses in cats: 32 cases with comparison to a national database (1977–1987). J Am Anim Hosp Assoc 1991;27:339–347.

24. Theon AP, Madewell BR, Harb MF, et al. Megavoltage irradiation of neoplasms of the nasal and paranasal cavities in 77 dogs. J Am Vet Med Assoc 1993;202:1469–1475.

25. Evans SM, Goldschmidt M, McKee LJ, et al. Prognostic factors and survival after radiotherapy for intranasal neoplasms in dogs: 70 cases (1974–1985). J Am Vet Med Assoc 1989;194:1460–1463.

26. Thompson JP, Ackerman N, Bellah JR, et al. [192]Iridium brachytherapy, using an intracavitary afterload device, for treatment of intranasal neoplasms in dogs. Am J Vet Res 1992;53:617–622.

27. Straw RC, Withrow SJ, Gillette EL, et al. Use of radiotherapy for the treatment of intranasal tumors in cats: Six cases (1980–1985). J Am Vet Med Assoc 1986;189:927–929.

28. Hahn KA, Knapp DW, Richardson RC, et al. Clinical response of nasal adenocarcinoma to cisplatin chemotherapy in 11 dogs. J Am Vet Med Assoc 1992;200:355-357.

29. Whitney WO, Mehlhaff CJ. High-rise syndrome in cats. J Am Vet Med Assoc 1987;191:1399–1403.

30. Gordon LE, Thacher C, Kapatkin A. High-rise syndrome in dogs: 81 cases (1985–1991). J Am Vet Med Assoc 1993;202:118–122.

31. Marretta SM. Chronic rhinitis and dental disease. Vet Clin North Am Small Anim Pract 1992;22:1101–1131.

32. Campbell BG, Little MD. Identification of the effects of a nematode (*Eucoleus boehmi*) from the nasal mucosa of North American dogs. J Am Vet Med Assoc 1991;198:1520–1523.

33. Vaden SL, Breitschwerdt EB, Henrikson CK, et al. Primary ciliary dyskinesia in Bichon Frise litter mates. J Am Anim Hosp Assoc 1991;27:633–640.

34. Morrison WB, Wilsman, NJ, Fox LE, et al. Primary ciliary dyskinesia in the dog. J Vet Intern Med 1987;1:67–74.

35. Crager CS. Canine primary ciliary dyskinesia. Compen Contin Educ Pract Vet 1992;11:1440–1445.

Chapter 52

Diseases of the Nasopharynx, Larynx, and Trachea

S. Dru Forrester

Anatomy

The upper airway consists of the nasopharynx, larynx, and trachea. The nasopharynx is the area between the caudal aspect of the nasal passages and the larynx. The larynx, a musculocartilaginous organ that is suspended by the hyoid apparatus, is composed of the epiglottis, thyroid, cricoid, and paired arytenoid cartilages.[1] The paired vocal folds are located caudomedially to the arytenoid cartilages (Fig. 52–1). Laryngeal saccules or ventricles are located on both sides of the larynx, between the arytenoid cartilages and vocal folds. The intrinsic muscles of the larynx are innervated by branches of the vagus nerve, including the recurrent laryngeal nerve and the spinal accessory nerve. Cough receptors are located in the laryngeal mucosa and respond to irritant stimuli. The cricoid cartilage of the larynx is connected to the trachea, a flexible tube composed of cartilaginous rings that are joined dorsally by the trachealis muscle. The trachea is lined by a mucociliary system consisting of secretory and ciliated epithelial cells and is supplied by secretory bronchial glands.[2] Smooth muscle in the walls of the trachea forms a band on the dorsal surface of the trachea.

Physiology

The upper airway passages serve as conduits for movement of air to the lower respiratory passages and lungs. After air traverses the nasal passages, it enters the nasopharyngeal and laryngeal area. During inspi-

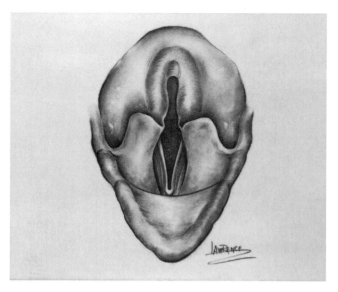

Figure 52–1
Appearance of the larynx during inspiration as viewed from the oral cavity. Note the abduction of arytenoid cartilages and vocal folds away from the midline.

ration, the arytenoid cartilages and vocal folds of the larynx abduct (i.e., move away from the midline), allowing movement of air into the trachea. During swallowing, the arytenoid cartilages and vocal folds close tightly, and the epiglottis covers the laryngeal opening to prevent aspiration into the air passages.[1] In addition to movement of air, the trachea also transports mucus and extraneous material away from the lower airways. Cilia of the epithelial lining of the trachea beat in a coordinated motion, which serves to move substances from the lower airways and lungs up the tracheobronchial tree to the larynx. Mucus and extraneous material are then coughed up into the pharynx and swallowed.

Problem Identification

Stertorous Respiration

Stertorous respiration, also referred to as respiratory stridor, is noisy breathing.

Pathophysiology

Stertorous respiration results from obstruction of the upper airways, which include the nasal passages, nasopharynx, larynx, and extrathoracic trachea. Disorders that most often cause stertorous respiration in dogs and cats include stenotic nares, nasal neoplasia, fungal rhinitis, chronic upper respiratory tract infection in cats, nasopharyngeal polyps, elongated soft palate, laryngeal paralysis, collapsing trachea, and pharyngeal and tracheal foreign bodies. In general, airway diameter must be compromised by more than 50% to cause stertorous respiration; this explains why unilateral laryngeal paralysis usually is not associated with clinical signs in dogs.

Clinical Signs

In addition to noisy respiration, patients often have other problems suggestive of upper respiratory disease. Respiratory distress often accompanies stertorous respiration, especially if airway obstruction is severe. In addition to respiratory stridor, the hallmark of upper airway obstruction is dyspnea characterized by prolonged inspiration. Nasal discharge usually is present when stertorous respiration is caused by nasal disease. Facial swelling may be observed in dogs or cats with fungal rhinitis, although it tends to be more common with nasal neoplasia. Cats with nasopharyngeal polyps most often have nasal discharge in addition to stertorous respiration but may have signs of peripheral vestibular disease, including circling, rolling, spontaneous nystagmus, and head tilt.[3–6] Dogs with laryngeal paralysis may have a change in voice or bark. Most dogs with collapsing trachea usually have a "goose-honk" cough precipitated by excitement, whereas dogs with laryngeal paralysis frequently have coughing or gagging that is often associated with eating or drinking. If concomitant neurologic disease is present, laryngeal paralysis may be accompanied by other abnormalities, such as dysphagia, regurgitation, weakness, and ataxia.[7, 8]

Diagnostic Plan

Because stertorous respiration localizes disease to the upper airways, diagnostic evaluation should focus on this part of the respiratory tract. Information from the signalment, history, and thorough physical examination are helpful for further localizing the cause of stertorous respiration. Some disorders are more common in certain breeds or species. Cats with nasopharyngeal polyps usually are young (1–3 years of age) and have unilateral nasal discharge.[3–5, 9] Except for nasal disease (i.e., fungal rhinitis, viral infections, and nasopharyngeal polyps), upper airway disorders are less common in cats than dogs. Brachycephalic (short-headed) dogs are predisposed to upper airway obstruction caused by stenotic nares, elongated soft palate, laryngeal collapse, and hypoplastic trachea. Nasal neoplasia is more common in dogs with long noses (i.e., dolichocephalic breeds) and occurs infrequently in brachycephalic breeds. Congenital laryngeal paralysis occurs in the Siberian husky, bull terrier, Dalmatian, and Bouvier des Flandres, whereas acquired laryngeal paralysis is most common in older large-breed dogs such as the Labrador retriever, golden retriever, Great Dane, Doberman pinscher, and Saint Bernard.[7, 8, 10–15] A change in the patient's voice or bark suggests laryngeal disease. Clinical signs of collapsing trachea almost always occur in middle-aged to older toy or small-breed dogs; it is not uncommon for these dogs to also be overweight. Although stertorous respiration occurs in dogs with collapsing trachea, most owners notice coughing or collapse that is exacerbated by exercise, excitement, eating, or drinking.

Physical examination findings of patients with stertorous respiration depend on the underlying cause. Patients with nasal disease often have nasal discharge, nasal or facial deformity, or ocular discharge. Infrequently, a patient with clinically important nasal disease may have no obvious clinical signs, either because the patient keeps the discharge cleaned by continued licking or because the discharge drains caudally into the nasopharynx. The clinician must determine whether air is moving through both nares. This can be easily accomplished by holding the patient's nose next to a metal examination table or holding a glass slide in front of the nose and looking for condensation on both sides during expiration. Palpa-

tion of the trachea frequently elicits a cough in dogs with collapsing trachea. Thoracic auscultation in patients with stertorous respiration usually reveals referred upper airway sounds.

After obtaining the history and performing the physical examination, the clinician usually uses additional diagnostic tests to determine the cause of stertorous respiration. The least invasive tests, which do not require sedation or anesthesia, should be done first. Cytologic evaluation of nasal discharge may be diagnostic of nasal cryptococcosis in cats; it rarely is useful for diagnosis of other nasal disorders. Nasal cryptococcosis also may be diagnosed by the presence of an increased cryptococcal antigen titer in serum. Additional evaluation of patients with suspected nasal disease (see Chap. 51) includes nasal and skull radiographs and collection of tissue for cytologic and preferably histologic examination. Plain thoracic and cervical radiographs show hypoplastic trachea. Comparison of inspiratory and expiratory films may be diagnostic of collapsing trachea. If plain films are not diagnostic, however, collapsing trachea cannot be ruled out until more definitive tests, such as fluoroscopy or tracheoscopy, have been done.

Diagnosis of other causes of stertorous respiration usually requires sedation or anesthesia for direct examination of the nasopharyngeal or laryngeal area (see Examination of the Nasopharynx and Larynx). If these procedures do not reveal a cause for stertorous respiration, tracheoscopy should be done next. Dyspneic patients should be handled carefully, and the clinician should be prepared to correct potential causes of upper airway obstruction at the time diagnostic tests are done. If definitive treatment is not possible and the patient is in respiratory distress, a tracheostomy often is necessary to relieve clinical signs and stabilize the patient prior to referral for surgical management.

Dyspnea

Dyspnea, or respiratory distress, is an inappropriate degree of respiratory effort as assessed by respiratory rate, rhythm, and character.

Pathophysiology

Dyspnea (see Chap. 9) results from systemic, respiratory, or cardiovascular disease (Table 52–1). It usually occurs secondary to disorders that interfere with pulmonary gas exchange including decreased red blood cells (i.e., anemia) or hemoglobin-carrying capacity (e.g., methemoglobinemia), airway obstruction or compression (e.g., laryngeal paralysis), pulmonary infiltrative disease (e.g., neoplasia, pneumonia), cardiac dysfunction (causing pulmonary edema or pleural effusion) (see Chaps. 53 and 54), or inadequate blood flow to the lungs (e.g., thromboembolism). Dyspnea infrequently results from weakness of the respiratory muscles resulting from neuromuscular disease (e.g., polyradiculoneuritis, severe hypokalemia) or as a compensatory response in patients with hyperthermia or severe metabolic acidosis.

Clinical Signs

In addition to respiratory distress, patients may exhibit other clinical signs, including stertorous respiration, nasal discharge, cyanosis, and coughing. Patients with anemia severe enough to cause dyspnea usually have pale mucous membranes, whereas patients with methemoglobinemia often have brown mucous membranes. In most patients with cardiovascular disease, findings on physical examination may include abnormalities such as arrhythmias, pulse deficits, gallop rhythm, tachycardia, cardiac murmurs, jugular pulses or distended jugular veins, weak peripheral pulses, ascites, muffled heart sounds, or crackles on thoracic auscultation. Patients with pneumothorax may have decreased breath sounds, whereas those with pleural effusion have muffled heart sounds, decreased breath sounds ventrally, and increased breath sounds dorsally. The cranial thorax may be difficult to compress in cats with mediastinal masses.

Diagnostic Plan

Before any diagnostic tests are performed, the patient should be evaluated for severity of respiratory distress; some patients may require emergency treatment (e.g., oxygen supplementation, thoracentesis, tracheal intubation) or supportive care first. If there is any possibility that pleural effusion or pneumothorax exists, thoracentesis should be done prior to stressful diagnostic procedures such as thoracic radiography. This is especially true of cats because they often do not show severe clinical signs and may become severely distressed during positioning for radiography.

Once the patient's condition is stable, the first diagnostic step is to rule out systemic and metabolic disorders that may cause dyspnea. The most common systemic or metabolic cause of dyspnea is anemia, which usually is suspected if pale mucous membranes are noted. Packed cell volume or hematocrit should be measured to diagnose anemia. The clinician should ask owners if they have administered any medications such as acetaminophen (Tylenol) within the past week. Cats with acetaminophen toxicosis may have brown mucous membranes as a result of methemoglobinemia. Other systemic and metabolic disorders are uncommon causes of dyspnea, and in patients with these disorders, other abnormalities are usually found on physical examination (e.g., generalized muscle weak-

Table 52–2
Causes of Dyspnea in Dogs and Cats

Systemic and Metabolic Disorders
  Hypoxemia
    Anemia
    Methemoglobinemia (acetaminophen toxicosis)
  Hyperthermia
  Metabolic acidosis (compensatory response)
  Neuromuscular weakness
  Severe hypokalemia (potassium <2 mmol/L)

Respiratory Disorders
Upper airway
  Nasopharyngeal disease
    Stenotic nares
    Neoplasia
    Fungal rhinitis
    Nasopharyngeal polyps
    Tonsillar neoplasia (lymphoma, squamous cell carcinoma, metastatic melanoma)
  Laryngeal disease
    Paralysis
    Laryngeal collapse
    Neoplasia
    Trauma
  Tracheal disease
    Collapsing trachea
    Hypoplastic trachea
    Neoplasia (extraluminal and intraluminal)
Lower airway
  Hilar lymphadenopathy (lymphoma, fungal pneumonia)
  Chronic bronchitis
  Feline asthma
  Pulmonary infiltrates with eosinophilia
  Pneumonia
    Aspiration
    Bacterial
    Fungal (blastomycosis, histoplasmosis, coccidioidomycosis)
    Parasitic (aelurostrongylosis, paragonimiasis)
    Viral (feline infectious peritonitis, canine distemper virus)
    Protozoal (toxoplasmosis)
  Pulmonary contusions, hemorrhage
  Pulmonary edema
  Neoplasia
    Primary (adenocarcinoma)
    Metastatic (osteosarcoma, thyroid/mammary carcinoma, hemangiosarcoma, others)
Pleural and mediastinal
  Pleural effusion
  Pneumothorax
  Diaphragmatic hernia
  Mediastinal or heart base masses
    Lymphoma
    Thymoma

Table 52–2
Causes of Dyspnea in Dogs and Cats
Continued

Cardiovascular Disorders
  Congestive heart failure
    Congenital defects
    Valvular insufficiency (mitral insufficiency)
    Myocardial disease (cardiomyopathy)
  Heartworm disease
  Pulmonary thromboembolism

ness) or laboratory evaluation (e.g., metabolic acidosis, severe hypokalemia).

After systemic and metabolic disorders have been excluded, the next step is to distinguish between cardiac (see Chap. 9) and primary respiratory disease as the cause of dyspnea. Information from the signalment and history is often helpful. Younger patients are more likely to have congenital defects (e.g., patent ductus arteriosus, congenital laryngeal paralysis), whereas older patients are more likely to have acquired disorders (e.g., mitral valvular insufficiency, pulmonary neoplasia, acquired laryngeal paralysis). As discussed earlier, some upper respiratory disorders are more common in certain species and breeds. Ask the owner about pre-existing medical conditions (e.g., cardiac murmur, vomiting, or regurgitation), vaccination and heartworm prevention status, environment and travel history, and possible exposure to trauma. Some disorders are more common in animals that live outdoors; these include all trauma-induced disorders such as hemothorax, pulmonary contusions, traumatic myocarditis, and diaphragmatic hernia, and infectious diseases such as heartworm disease, aelurostrongylosis, paragonimiasis, toxoplasmosis, and fungal infections. Dogs and cats that live in or travel to certain geographic areas are more likely to develop fungal pneumonia or heartworm disease (see Chaps. 13, 39, and 40 for a more complete discussion of heartworm, fungal, and protozoal diseases, respectively).

A thorough physical examination should be performed, with special emphasis on the cardiopulmonary system. The most common cardiac diseases that cause respiratory distress are congestive heart failure due to mitral insufficiency or cardiomyopathy and heartworm disease associated with pulmonary thromboembolism. Most patients with dyspnea due to cardiac disease have some abnormal finding on physical examination (see Clinical Signs). If no signs of cardiac disease are noted on physical examination, respiratory disease should be suspected as the cause of dyspnea. One useful finding for distinguishing be-

tween upper and lower respiratory disease is the patient's pattern of ventilation. Dyspneic patients with a prolonged phase of inspiration usually have upper airway obstruction; other signs may be present, such as stertorous respiration or a change in voice or bark. A prolonged expiratory phase is characteristic of lower airway obstruction resulting from disorders such as feline asthma, chronic bronchitis, or pulmonary edema. A restrictive respiratory pattern, characterized by rapid, shallow respirations, often is observed in patients with pleural space disease (e.g., effusion, pneumothorax), fractured ribs, or diaphragmatic hernia. However, there are exceptions to these general rules, and every patient must be evaluated individually.

Although it usually is possible to determine whether dyspnea is due to systemic or metabolic, cardiovascular, or respiratory disease on the basis of history and physical examination findings, a definitive diagnosis usually requires additional diagnostic tests. Once systemic and metabolic disorders and upper airway obstruction have been excluded, thoracic radiography is the most useful and cost-effective diagnostic test for evaluation of dyspneic patients. First, look for signs of trauma, such as fractured ribs, diaphragmatic hernia, pleural effusion, or a pulmonary alveolar pattern consistent with contusions. Next, look for signs consistent with cardiac disease, such as cardiomegaly. Right heart enlargement; enlarged or dilated and tortuous pulmonary arteries; and patchy, pulmonary interstitial infiltrates are highly suggestive of heartworm disease. An alveolar pattern is consistent with bacterial pneumonia, pulmonary edema, pulmonary contusions, or atelectasis. A diffuse, miliary to nodular interstitial pattern suggests fungal pneumonia or metastatic neoplasia, whereas a single pulmonary nodule suggests primary pulmonary neoplasia. Radiographs may be normal in cats with asthma or may reveal a bronchial pattern, sometimes with collapse of the right middle lung lobe. Other possible findings in animals with dyspnea include megaesophagus and aspiration pneumonia, pleural effusion, pneumothorax, hilar lymphadenopathy, and mediastinal masses, which usually are due to lymphoma.

Additional diagnostic tests may be indicated depending on the patient's clinical signs (see Stertorous Respiration for diagnostic tests for patients with suspected upper airway disorders). Thoracentesis should be performed if pleural effusion or pneumothorax is diagnosed. Pleural fluid analysis is one of the most useful diagnostic tests for evaluation of patients with pleural effusion (see Chap. 53). Transtracheal wash, bronchial brushings, and bronchoalveolar lavage (see Chap. 54) are useful for obtaining specimens for cytologic examination and bacterial culture in patients with suspected bronchial or alveolar diseases (e.g., asthma, bronchitis, pneumonia). Cytologic evaluation of pulmonary aspirates is useful for patients with a diffuse interstitial pattern or with pulmonary masses or consolidation near the rib cage (see Chap. 54). Thoracic ultrasonography prior to removal of all pleural fluid may help identify mediastinal masses, other intrathoracic masses, and diaphragmatic hernia. Echocardiography is extremely useful for patients with suspected cardiac disease (see Chap. 9).

Cough

Cough (see Chaps. 9 and 54) is a protective mechanism that clears extraneous material from the respiratory passages; it results from either cardiac or respiratory disease. The most common upper respiratory disorders that cause cough are collapsing trachea and laryngeal disease. Dogs with collapsing trachea usually have a goose honk cough that is exacerbated by exercise, excitement, eating, or drinking. Laryngeal paralysis causes inspirator stridor and sometimes is associated with coughing and gagging that most often occurs after eating.

Inappetence and Weight Loss

Inappetence and weight loss (see Chaps. 45 and 47) are nonspecific signs that infrequently occur in patients with upper airway obstruction. Dogs with laryngeal paralysis are more concerned with breathing than eating, and it is not uncommon for large-breed dogs to lose 5 to 10 kg of body weight in a short time. Except for laryngeal paralysis, upper airway disorders usually do not cause changes in appetite or body weight.

Diagnostic Procedures

Routine Laboratory Evaluation

A minimum database, including serum chemistry analyses, complete blood count (CBC), urinalysis, and fecal flotation, infrequently reveals abnormal findings in animals with upper airway disease. Serum chemistry analyses may reveal severe hypokalemia (serum potassium <2 mmol/L), which is a rare cause of respiratory distress. A CBC is helpful for identifying anemia, a potential cause of dyspnea. Urinalysis adds to the minimum database and is necessary to interpret serum chemistry analyses. Some animals with respiratory distress become dehydrated and develop azotemia; a urine specific gravity greater than 1.030 in dogs and 1.040 in cats indicates prerenal azotemia and rules out renal failure. Fecal flotation using zinc sulfate or the Baermann technique may reveal ovae or larvae of *Oslerus osleri,* parasites that rarely affect the trachea in dogs.[16]

Examination of the Nasopharynx and Larynx

Examination of the nasopharynx is indicated for cats thought to have nasopharyngeal polyps. Heavy sedation or general anesthesia usually is needed for adequate examination. A dental mirror and focused light source are helpful for evaluating the nasopharynx after the soft palate is retracted with a spay hook. Alternatively, a flexible endoscope can be retroflexed into the nasopharyngeal area for evaluation. Most cats have unilateral disease; however, both sides should be examined because bilateral involvement sometimes occurs.

The larynx should be evaluated when stertorous respiration or dyspnea characterized by prolonged inspiration is present and no other obvious cause for clinical signs can be easily identified. To accurately assess laryngeal function, the larynx should be examined with the patient lightly anesthetized so that spontaneous breathing continues. Short-acting barbiturates such as sodium thiopental (Pentothal) are ideal agents for evaluation of laryngeal function. Administer an initial dose of 2 to 4 mg/kg; additional boluses up to a total dose of 10 mg/kg may be needed. Alternatively, a combination of ketamine (Ketaset) at 10 mg/kg and diazepam (Valium) at 0.5 mg/kg can be administered intravenously. After the patient is sedated, examine the larynx using a laryngoscope or other focused light source while an assistant watches the thoracic wall and indicates when the animal inhales. This allows the clinician evaluating the larynx to determine whether the arytenoid cartilages and vocal folds abduct (move away from the midline) during inspiration. Most dogs with clinical signs of laryngeal paralysis have bilateral disease, and both arytenoid cartilages remain in a neutral position—neither abducted nor adducted—during inspiration. After evaluation of laryngeal function, the nasopharyngeal and laryngeal area should be thoroughly examined for other abnormalities (e.g., masses, foreign bodies), especially if a cause for clinical signs has not been identified.

Radiography

Radiography is useful for evaluating some upper respiratory tract disorders. Cats with nasopharyngeal polyps have soft tissue density in the nasopharyngeal area; however, this finding is nonspecific, and direct visualization of the polyp is probably more cost-effective. Radiography of the cervical and thoracic trachea is indicated when collapsing trachea is suspected. A lateral radiograph of the cervical and thoracic trachea should be obtained during inspiration and another during expiration. The veterinarian must be careful when positioning the patient because overextension of the neck may cause collapse of the trachea in a normal dog. A narrowed lumen during inspiration

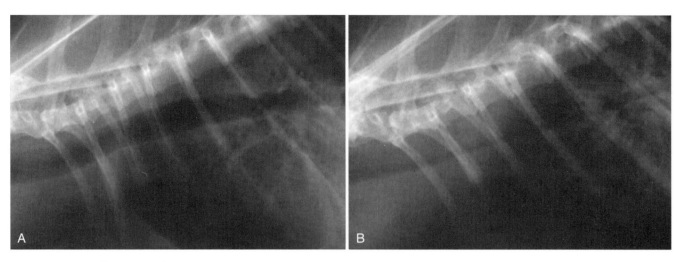

Figure 52-2
(A) Lateral thoracic radiograph of a dog with a collapsing trachea taken during inspiration. **(B)** Lateral thoracic radiograph of the same dog taken during expiration. Note the severe collapse of the intrathoracic trachea that occurs during expiration.

is characteristic of extrathoracic tracheal collapse, whereas during expiration, intrathoracic tracheal collapse occurs (Fig. 52–2). If collapsing trachea is not diagnosed by plain films, however, additional evaluation with fluoroscopy or tracheoscopy is indicated to make a definitive diagnosis.

Tracheal Wash

Tracheal wash (see Diagnostic Procedures in Chap. 54) is indicated for evaluation of patients with chronic cough or evidence of pulmonary parenchymal disease, although it also may provide useful information in patients thought to have tracheobronchitis.[17]

Tracheoscopy

For patients thought to have upper airway disease, endoscopic evaluation of the trachea is indicated when less invasive tests fail to yield a diagnosis. This procedure is most often performed to confirm presence of collapsing trachea and determine its location and severity. In addition, tracheoscopy also is useful for identifying tracheal masses, foreign bodies, and parasites. (For a complete discussion on tracheobronchoscopy, see Diagnostic Plan in Chap. 54.)

Common Diseases of the Nasopharynx, Larynx, and Trachea

Brachycephalic Airway Syndrome

Brachycephalic airway syndrome is characterized by upper airway obstruction resulting from one or more disorders, including stenotic nares, elongated soft palate, everted laryngeal saccules, and hypoplastic trachea; laryngeal collapse may occur secondary to chronic or severe upper airway obstruction. Brachycephalic airway syndrome occurs to some extent in all brachycephalic breeds. No brachycephalic dog has normal respiratory function.[18] All brachycephalic breeds, including the Boston terrier, Pekingese, boxer, shih tzu, Lhasa apso, and pug, are affected; however, the English bulldog appears to be the most severely affected.[19] Although all components of brachycephalic airway syndrome can occur in all brachycephalic breeds, hypoplastic trachea occurs most often in English bulldogs and Boston terriers.[19, 20] Some breeds of cats, such as Persians and Himalayans, are brachycephalic; however, they represent a minority of animals that present with clinical signs of brachycephalic airway syndrome.[18]

Clinical Signs

The most common clinical signs of brachycephalic airway syndrome are characteristic of upper airway obstruction and include stertorous respiration, inspiratory dyspnea, cyanosis, and episodes of collapse. Other signs that may occur include dysphagia, coughing, gagging, inappetence, weight loss, and exercise intolerance. Brachycephalic dogs may present with chronic signs that worsen progressively over time, or owners may report acute respiratory distress and cyanosis. It is not uncommon for brachycephalic dogs with chronic, stable respiratory disease to rapidly decompensate. Physical examination usually reveals stenotic nares, and occasionally, hypoplastic trachea may be noted on palpation. Dogs in respiratory distress usually have marked respira-

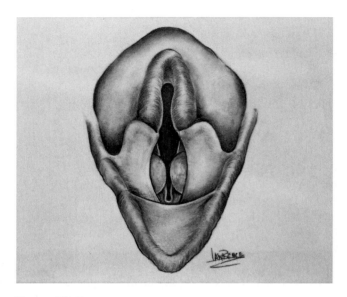

Figure 52–3
Appearance of larynx in a dog with everted laryngeal saccules, which usually appear as whitish nodules located cranial to the vocal folds.

tory stertor and cyanosis; hyperthermia also may occur.

Diagnostic Plan

Most disorders that cause brachycephalic airway syndrome are diagnosed by direct examination. Stenotic nares can be identified on physical examination; palpation sometimes reveals hypoplastic trachea. Cervical and thoracic radiographs should be obtained to confirm the presence of hypoplastic trachea. Elongated soft palate and laryngeal disease are best diagnosed while the animal is anesthetized; oropharyngeal examination in a nonanesthetized patient often is not diagnostic and may increase respiratory distress. Because all brachycephalic dogs have the potential to rapidly decompensate, they should be handled with extreme caution. Anesthesia carries greater risks in brachycephalic dogs; therefore, the clinician should be prepared to surgically correct any abnormalities at the time of diagnostic evaluation. In nonbrachycephalic dogs, the soft palate just overlaps the epiglottis during inspiration. In brachycephalic dogs, the soft palate often extends over the epiglottis and may even occlude the laryngeal area during inspiration. The laryngeal area should be evaluated for swelling and the ability of the vocal folds and arytenoid cartilages to abduct during inspiration. Everted laryngeal saccules appear as whitish nodules in the ventral area of the glottis, just cranial to the vocal folds (Fig. 52–3).[21] Laryngeal collapse is characterized by collapse of the arytenoid cartilages into the laryngeal lumen. Laryngeal collapse should not be confused with laryngeal paralysis, which is characterized by arytenoid cartilages that remain in a neutral position and fail to move away from the midline during inspiration.

Pathophysiology

The inciting cause of brachycephalic airway syndrome is abnormal conformation of the skull and external nares, which leads to chronic upper airway obstruction and compromised respiration. Increased negative pressure generated by the accentuated effort to inspire causes airway collapse and subsequent thickening of the mucous membranes (e.g., elongated soft palate) and soft tissue edema. In addition, the increased negative pressure at the glottis during inspiration causes eversion of laryngeal saccules, which further compromises respiration. Over time, upper airway obstruction eventually causes laryngeal collapse.[1] Additional abnormalities, such as hypoplastic trachea, may further increase the severity of clinical signs.

Because of the conformation of upper respiratory passages in brachycephalic dogs, several factors should be remembered. Brachycephalic dogs cannot deal effectively with increased environmental temperature or humidity and are highly susceptible to hyperthermia and heatstroke, even at room temperature. Respiratory distress can be precipitated by even mild exercise, especially in humid conditions. Also, particular caution should be taken with brachycephalic dogs that are sedated or anesthetized. Sedation or anesthesia causes relaxation of the pharyngeal muscles, which invariably results in upper airway obstruction. To ensure a patent airway and to prevent hypoxia, all brachycephalic dogs that are sedated or anesthetized should be intubated. In addition, oxygenation before and during the procedure is recommended. The endotracheal tube should not be removed until the clinician is certain the dog can maintain a patent airway. After sedation or anesthesia, all brachycephalic dogs should remain under constant observation until they have been extubated. Because of the severity of the disease in English bulldogs, these animals should not be extubated until they are standing.

Treatment

As stated earlier, it is best to perform surgical correction of stenotic nares, elongated soft palate, and everted laryngeal saccules at the time of diagnosis, while the patient is still anesthetized. However, if this is not possible, the patient should be treated with drugs and stabilized prior to referral for surgical management. Parenteral administration of corticosteroids such as prednisolone sodium succinate (Solu-Cortef) (10–20 mg/kg intravenously), methylprednisolone sodium succinate (Solu-Medrol) at 30 mg/kg intravenously initially, followed by 15 mg/kg intravenously in 2 to 4 hours, or dexamethasone (Azium or Azium-SP) at 2 to 4 mg/kg intravenously is indicated to decrease pharyngeal and laryngeal edema.[18, 22] The patient should be placed in a cool environment and handled as little as possible. These measures often result in marked improvement; however, if severe dyspnea persists, a temporary tracheostomy should be done.

Surgical techniques for correction of brachycephalic airway syndrome have been described.[19, 23, 24] Correction of stenotic nares is easily accomplished by removing a section from the wing of each nostril.[23] With an oral approach, excessive soft palate is excised so that the palate just overlaps the open epiglottis. The clinician must be sure not to excise too much of the soft palate because this could predispose the patient to dysphagia and aspiration of food into the nasal passages. Everted laryngeal saccules can be removed easily using an oral approach by grasping the saccule with forceps and excising it with scissors. After surgery, corticosteroids are administered to control edema (dosages listed earlier), which commonly occurs as a result of surgical manipulation.

Prognosis

The prognosis for dogs with brachycephalic airway syndrome depends on the severity and chronicity of upper airway obstruction. Many brachycephalic dogs treated by surgical correction improve markedly. Their improvement appears to be greater when laryngeal surgery is not necessary, when correction of stenotic nares is done concomitantly with soft palate resection, and when soft palate resection is done in dogs younger than 2 years of age.[19] It seems reasonable that patients treated early, before the condition can progress, have a better prognosis. Patients with laryngeal collapse have a poorer prognosis

because this condition results from chronic airway obstruction and indicates end-stage disease. Last, patients with moderate to severe hypoplastic trachea also have a more guarded prognosis because this condition has no effective treatment and may predispose patients to complications such as pneumonia.

Nasopharyngeal Polyps

Nasopharyngeal polyps are inflammatory growths that originate from the eustachian tube or middle ear. Approximately 50 cases have been reported in the veterinary literature.[3–6, 9] These polyps most often affect cats younger than 3 years of age, although older cats have been affected infrequently.

Clinical Signs

The most common clinical signs are sneezing, stertorous respiration, dyspnea characterized by prolonged inspiration, and mucopurulent nasal discharge, which most often is unilateral.[3–6, 9] Less frequent signs include otic discharge, Horner's syndrome, head tilt, circling, and rolling.[4, 6, 9]

Diagnostic Plan

A cat thought to have a nasopharyngeal should be anesthetized for examination of the nasopharyngeal area. A spay hook is useful for retracting the soft palate and increasing visualization of the affected area (Fig. 52–4). Both sides of the nasopharynx should be examined because bilateral involvement occurs in some cases. While the animal is anesthetized, skull radiographs should be obtained to look for evidence of otitis media, such as thickening of the osseous bulla, increased density within the tympanic cavity, and sclerosis of the petrous-temporal bone (Fig. 52–5).[5] Radiographic evidence of otitis media is noted in

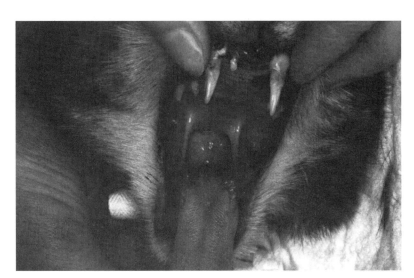

Figure 52–4
Direct examination of nasopharynx of a cat with a nasopharyngeal polyp.

approximately 65% to 85% of cats with nasopharyngeal polyps.[3–6] Radiographs of the pharyngeal area are nonspecific but reveal a soft tissue density in the region of the soft palate in most of these cats.[5] A definitive diagnosis is made on the basis of histologic examination of the polyp.

Pathophysiology

The inciting cause of nasopharyngeal polyps is unknown. They are believed to originate in the mucosa of either the eustachian tube or the middle ear and to grow down the auditory tube into the pharynx.[6] They occur secondary to inflammation such as otitis media; however, it is not known whether otitis is a primary or secondary factor in the pathogenesis of nasopharyngeal polyps.[5]

Treatment

The treatment of choice for nasopharyngeal polyps is surgical excision. In cats with radiographic evidence of otitis media, a ventral bulla osteotomy should be performed to remove inflammatory tissue in the auditory canal associated with the polyp. The remainder of the polyp is then removed through the oral

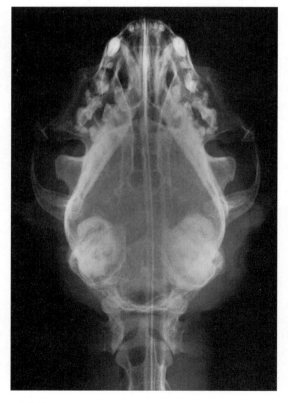

Figure 52-5
Ventrodorsal skull radiograph of a cat with a left-sided nasopharyngeal polyp. Note the marked thickening and increased fluid density of the right osseous bulla.

cavity. Because of the potential for recurrence if the entire polyp is not removed, it may be preferable to also perform bulla osteotomy in cats with normal skull radiographs.[5] The excised polyp should be submitted for histologic evaluation to confirm that it is an inflammatory mass and to distinguish it from other disorders, such as neoplasia.

Prognosis

The prognosis for cats after surgical excision of nasopharyngeal polyps is good to excellent. Regrowth of the polyp occurs infrequently, usually within 8 months of initial surgical excision, most commonly in cats that did not undergo a bulla osteotomy.[5] If regrowth occurs, the polyp can be successfully treated by a second surgical excision and a bulla osteotomy.

Laryngeal Paralysis

Laryngeal paralysis is a condition in which the arytenoid cartilages of the larynx do not move away from the midline during inspiration. It is common in dogs but rarely occurs in cats.[7, 8, 10–15, 25–27] In approximately 20% to 25% of cases the condition is congenital, whereas 75% to 80% of dogs with laryngeal paralysis have the acquired form.[13] Dogs with congenital laryngeal paralysis usually are younger than 1 year of age and may present with the condition at 4 to 6 months of age.[8, 10, 13] Although dogs of any breed can have congenital laryngeal paralysis, it is most common in the Bouvier des Flandres, Siberian husky, bull terrier, and Dalmatian.[7, 8, 10, 11, 28] Acquired laryngeal paralysis most often affects large-breed dogs (e.g., Labrador retriever, golden retriever, Siberian husky, Irish setter, Saint Bernard) at an average of 10 to 12 years of age.[11–15, 27] Laryngeal paralysis appears to be more common in male dogs.[10, 12, 13, 15, 26, 27]

Clinical Signs

The most common clinical signs of laryngeal paralysis are inspiratory dyspnea, exercise intolerance, and respiratory stridor. Coughing or gagging may occur and often is associated with eating or drinking.[12, 14, 15, 25–27] Some dogs may have a hoarse bark or be unable to bark. Systemic neurologic signs such as weakness and ataxia may occur in some dogs.[7, 8] Regurgitation due to megaesophagus occurs infrequently.[8]

Diagnostic Plan

Laryngeal paralysis is suspected on the basis of signalment and clinical signs and is definitively diagnosed by direct examination of the larynx (see Examination of the Nasopharynx and Larynx). The arytenoid

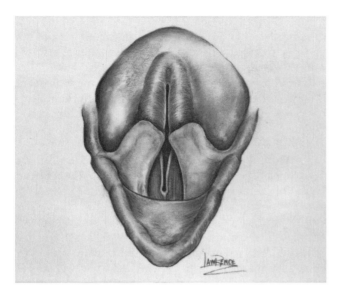

Figure 52–6
Larynx of a dog with bilateral laryngeal paralysis. Note failure of the arytenoid cartilages and vocal folds to abduct during inspiration.

cartilages and vocal folds in dogs and cats with laryngeal paralysis remain in a neutral position during inspiration and fail to abduct (Fig. 52–6). Almost all affected patients have bilateral disease; unilateral laryngeal paralysis rarely causes clinical signs.

Additional diagnostic tests may be indicated for patients with laryngeal paralysis. Thoracic radiographs should be obtained if concomitant pulmonary disease cannot be excluded. Some dogs with laryngeal paralysis develop secondary pulmonary edema, presumably due to decreased intrathoracic pressure.[29] Aspiration pneumonia may occur in patients with concomitant megaesophagus. If hypothyroidism is suspected, a thyroid-stimulating hormone response test should be performed; alternatively, baseline serum thyroid hormone concentration should be measured.

Pathophysiology

With few exceptions, the cause of laryngeal paralysis is unknown, and most cases are idiopathic. In the Bouvier des Flandres, laryngeal paralysis is an inherited disorder characterized by degeneration of recurrent laryngeal nerves.[10] In the Dalmatian, congenital laryngeal paralysis is associated with a diffuse polyneuropathy that affects recurrent laryngeal and appendicular peripheral nerves.[8] In other dogs, laryngeal paralysis may be only one sign of a more diffuse polyneuropathy.[7] Acquired laryngeal paralysis has been associated with hypothyroidism; however, a cause-and-effect relationship remains to be proved.[7, 12, 30] Other infrequent causes of laryngeal

paralysis in dogs and cats include trauma, abscesses, and neoplasia that affect laryngeal innervation.[13]

Treatment

Surgical correction is indicated for dogs and cats with clinical signs caused by laryngeal paralysis. Several procedures with excellent results have been described; selection of technique depends on the surgeon's preference and skill.[14, 15, 25, 31] Unilateral arytenoid lateralization, or laryngeal tieback, is accomplished via a paramedian incision through the subcutaneous tissue over the larynx. A suture is passed through the muscular process of the arytenoid cartilage and then through the caudodorsal portion of the thyroid cartilage.[13] For castellated laryngofissure, a midline ventral incision is made over the larynx, and a castellated or stepped incision is made through the thyroid cartilage so that it can be separated, resulting in widening of the laryngeal opening.[31] In some cases, the vocal folds are removed also, to further relieve airway obstruction. Depending on the severity of clinical signs and the surgical procedure performed, a temporary tracheostomy may be indicated during the initial postoperative period. Medical management consisting of anti-inflammatory doses of corticosteroids helps stabilize the patient prior to surgery and is indicated to decrease swelling associated with surgical manipulation (see Brachycephalic Airway Syndrome for dosage regimens).

Prognosis

The prognosis for patients with idiopathic laryngeal paralysis is good to excellent after surgical correction in 90% to 100% of dogs and cats.[13–15, 25, 27, 32] In contrast to idiopathic laryngeal paralysis, dogs with concomitant disorders such as polyneuropathies, megaesophagus, and aspiration pneumonia often do not respond favorably.[8]

Infectious Tracheobronchitis (Kennel Cough)

Infectious tracheobronchitis, also called kennel cough, is a contagious disorder characterized by inflammation of the upper airways caused by infection with a variety of organisms. The disorder is common in dogs, most often affecting young dogs or those that are exposed to affected dogs (e.g., at boarding kennels or dog shows). There is no breed or sex predisposition.

Clinical Signs

The most common clinical sign in dogs with infectious tracheobronchitis is the acute onset of paroxysmal coughing that is exacerbated by excitement or exercise. Coughing often is severe and may sound as if the dog is trying to dislodge a foreign body. Systemic signs such as inappetence, depression, and fever are not present unless secondary bacterial infection is present, especially in the lungs. Clinical signs usually develop within 1 week of exposure to affected dogs. Infections are self-limited, and clinical signs usually resolve within 2 weeks. Physical examination findings usually are normal, except for a dry, hacking cough on tracheal palpation.

Diagnostic Plan

A tentative diagnosis of infectious tracheobronchitis is made on the basis of history and physical examination findings. Results of CBC, serum chemistry analyses, and thoracic radiography are normal unless secondary pneumonia is present.

Pathophysiology

Infectious tracheobronchitis is caused by several organisms. Although *Bordetella bronchiseptica* and parainfluenza virus are most commonly isolated from dogs with infectious tracheobronchitis, other organisms—such as canine adenovirus types 1 and 2, canine herpesvirus, canine distemper virus, and mycoplasmas—also may be involved.[33, 34] The disorder is transmitted by aerosol exposure and is highly contagious. Dogs most often become infected by contact with other dogs (e.g., at boarding kennels or dog shows). Clinical signs most often begin 2 to 10 days after exposure.

Treatment and Prevention

Treatment of dogs with infectious tracheobronchitis is mostly supportive. The disorder usually is self-limited, and clinical signs often resolve within 1 to 2 weeks regardless of treatment. Antimicrobials may not be necessary for all patients, although they often are used to treat potential infection with *B. bronchiseptica.* Tetracycline (22 mg/kg by mouth, three times per day [t.i.d.], for 7 to 10 days) or trimethoprim-sulfadiazine (Tribrissen) (15 mg/kg by mouth, twice per day [b.i.d.], for 7 days) may be used.[34, 35] Selection of antimicrobials for dogs with secondary pneumonia should be based on results of tracheal wash and bacterial culture. Short-term administration of corticosteroids such as prednisone (0.25 to 0.5 mg/kg by mouth, b.i.d., for 5 to 7 days) is helpful for treatment of cough in dogs with uncomplicated tracheobronchitis; however, corticosteroids are contraindicated for dogs with concomitant pneumonia.[34, 36] Antimicrobials and corticosteroids seem to cause improvement in clinical signs, although they probably

do not shorten the course of infection. Cough suppressants should be considered if the dog does not respond to corticosteroids; however, these suppressants have the potential to compromise ventilation and increase accumulation of lower airway secretions.[34] Hydrocodone (Hycodan) and codeine may be the most effective substances for controlling severe cough in dogs with infectious tracheobronchitis (Table 52–2).

Vaccination is effective for decreasing the prevalence and severity of infectious tracheobronchitis.[37] Parenteral vaccines, including *B. bronchiseptica,* canine parainfluenza virus, canine adenovirus type 2, and canine distemper virus, should be administered. Puppies should receive at least two vaccinations, given 2 to 4 weeks apart; to avoid interference by maternal antibody, the last vaccine should be given when the puppy is at least 4 months of age. Parenteral vaccines should be repeated annually. Intranasal vaccines containing a combination of *B. bronchiseptica* and modified live canine parainfluenza virus are indicated when rapid onset of protection is required (e.g., prior to boarding at a kennel or attending a dog show). Ideally, parenteral vaccines should be given 7 days before anticipated exposure and should be boostered annually.[37]

Table 52–2
Drugs Used to Treat Dogs With Collapsing Trachea

DRUG	TRADE NAME	DOSAGE REGIMEN (BY MOUTH)
Bronchodilators		
Aminophylline		10 mg/kg b.i.d.
Theophylline	Theo-Dur	20 mg/kg b.i.d.
	Slo-Bid	20–25 mg/kg b.i.d.
	Choledyl	25–30 mg/kg b.i.d.
Terbutaline	Brethine	1.25–5.0 mg/dog b.i.d. or t.i.d.
Cough Suppressants		
Butorphanol	Torbutrol	0.4 mg/kg b.i.d.–q.i.d.
Codeine		0.1–0.3 mg/kg t.i.d. or q.i.d.
Hydrocodone	Hycodan	0.22 mg/kg t.i.d. or q.i.d.
Dextromethorphan	Robitussin-DM	1–2 mg/kg t.i.d. or q.i.d.
Corticosteroids		
Prednisone		0.5–1.0 mg/kg every day

b.i.d., two times per day; t.i.d., three times per day; q.i.d., four times per day.

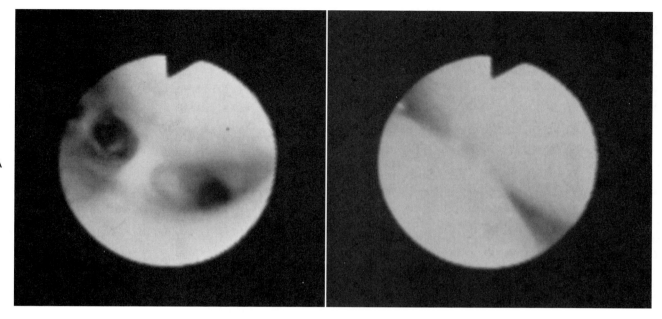

Figure 52-7
(A) Endoscopic picture of the distal trachea, cranial to the tracheal bifurcation, taken during inspiration. **(B)** Endoscopic picture from same dog showing severe tracheal collapse during expiration.

Prognosis

The prognosis for recovery from uncomplicated infectious tracheobronchitis is excellent. In most dogs, clinical signs resolve within 2 weeks. Dogs with concomitant disorders such as collapsing trachea or chronic bronchitis may be at increased risk for developing complications from infectious tracheobronchitis.[34]

Collapsing Trachea

Collapsing trachea is characterized by failure of the trachea to maintain its rigidity; weakness of the tracheal rings results in dorsoventral collapse. This common disorder most often affects toy breeds of dogs (e.g., Yorkshire terrier, Pomeranian, miniature poodle); cats rarely are affected. Although collapsing trachea may occur in young dogs, it most often is diagnosed in middle-aged to older dogs. There is no sex predilection.

Clinical Signs

Dogs with collapsing trachea most often have a dry, hacking cough, often described as a goose-honk cough, that is exacerbated by exercise, excitement, eating, or drinking. Cyanosis and collapse may be observed during periods of severe cough. Tracheal palpation usually elicits the characteristic cough. Other physical examination findings may include obesity, hepatomegaly, cardiac murmurs, and harsh breath sounds referred from the upper airways.

Diagnostic Plan

Collapsing trachea may be confirmed by radiographic studies or tracheoscopy. Comparison of a lateral thoracic or cervical radiograph on inspiration versus expiration may demonstrate collapse of the extrathoracic trachea on inspiration and collapse of the intrathoracic trachea during expiration. If plain films are not diagnostic, fluoroscopy is indicated to show dynamic tracheal collapse. Alternatively, a tracheoscopy may be performed to demonstrate dorsoventral flattening of the trachea and collapse of the dorsal tracheal membrane. Endoscopy of the airways also allows evaluation of the lower airways, which often are affected in dogs with collapsing trachea (Fig. 52–7). Results of cytologic evaluation and bacterial culture of tracheal wash specimens often are nonspecific; however, some dogs may improve when antimicrobials are used to treat secondary infections. Other diagnostic tests, such as thoracic radiographs, bronchoscopy, and cardiac evaluation, may be indicated if lower airway disease or cardiac disease is suspected as a cause of clinical signs.

Pathophysiology

The cause of collapsing trachea is unknown. There may be a congenital defect in the cartilage of the tracheal and bronchial rings that causes them to lose their rigidity, leading to subsequent airway collapse.[38] Collapse of the extrathoracic trachea occurs during inspiration, causing signs typical of upper airway obstruction, such as inspiratory dyspnea and stertorous respiration. Collapse of the intrathoracic trachea occurs during expiration and is characterized by expiratory dyspnea and wheezes. Collapse of the intrathoracic and extrathoracic trachea as well as collapse of the mainstem bronchi is not uncommon in dogs.

Treatment

Most dogs with collapsing trachea are managed by supportive care and medical treatment (see Table 52–2). Weight loss in overweight patients may be helpful for reducing the severity of clinical signs. Bronchodilators seem to be helpful, possibly because of concomitant lower airway disease, such as chronic bronchitis or small airway collapse. Cough suppressants such as hydrocodone, codeine, and butorphanol (Torbutrol) often are used to decrease the severity and frequency of coughing in dogs with collapsing trachea. Hydrocodone and codeine may be more effective, but sedation is a side effect of both drugs. Over-the-counter cough suppressants containing dextromethorphan (Robitussin-DM) also may be useful. Cough suppressants should be used with caution in patients with concomitant bronchial or pulmonary disease because coughing is a defense mechanism that helps clear the lower airways. Anti-inflammatory doses of corticosteroids may help decrease inflammation and coughing associated with collapsing trachea. Corticosteroids should be administered only when there is no response to other treatments and should not be used for longer than 5 days.[39] Antimicrobials have been used to treat patients with collapsing trachea on the premise that secondary bacterial infection is present; they are not routinely indicated unless a culture reveals bacterial growth.

Selected patients with collapsing trachea may benefit from surgical treatment. Several techniques have been described; most involve placement of prosthetic rings.[40, 41] Only dogs without lower airway disease (e.g., collapse of mainstem bronchi, chronic bronchitis), as determined by thorough bronchoscopic evaluation, should be considered for surgical treatment. Although surgery is recommended for dogs with chronic severe collapsing trachea, it may be better to offer this option to owners early in the course of disease.[39] Dogs with extrathoracic collapse only may be better candidates for surgery, although intrathoracic placement of prosthetic rings also has been successful.[41]

Prognosis

Prognosis for patients with collapsing trachea depends on the severity of collapse and the presence of concomitant abnormalities. Most patients with mild to moderate collapse can be managed successfully with medical treatment; periodic exacerbation of clinical signs may require adjustment in treatment, however. Dogs with severe collapsing trachea have a guarded to poor prognosis.

Uncommon Diseases of the Nasopharynx, Larynx, and Trachea

Laryngeal Neoplasia

Tumors of the larynx occur infrequently in dogs and cats. A variety of tumors, including leiomyoma, rhabdomyosarcoma, and squamous cell carcinoma, have been reported in dogs; however, lymphoma is the most common laryngeal tumor in cats.[42, 43] Clinical signs are similar to those described for laryngeal paralysis. Diagnosis is confirmed by direct visualization of the tumor during laryngeal examination and subsequent histologic evaluation. Small tumors can be surgically excised; however, most laryngeal tumors are malignant and locally invasive and cannot be completely removed without complete laryngectomy, which requires a permanent tracheostomy. Unless there is severe obstruction, lymphoma affecting the larynx should be treated by chemotherapy.

Laryngeal Trauma

Laryngeal trauma occasionally occurs in dogs and cats as a result of blunt trauma or bite wounds. It usually requires only supportive care, including cage rest and anti-inflammatory doses of corticosteroids. Severe trauma may require tracheostomy.

Tracheal Foreign Bodies

Inhalation of foreign bodies into the tracheobronchial tree seems to be most common in dogs.[44] Grass awns, or foxtails, are the most commonly reported tracheal foreign body.[44] Clinical signs begin acutely after inhalation of the foreign body and include coughing, wheezing, and respiratory distress. Diagnosis is confirmed by identification of the foreign body during tracheobronchoscopic examination; it may be easier to identify the foreign body if endoscopy is done within 2 weeks of foreign body inhalation.[44] The treatment of choice is removal of the foreign body via endoscopy.

Tracheal Neoplasia

Neoplasia of the trachea sometimes occurs in dogs and cats.[17, 45] A variety of tumors have been reported in dogs, whereas adenocarcinoma and lymphoma are most common in cats.[17, 45] Clinical signs may include coughing, wheezing, and respiratory distress. Radiography may reveal a soft tissue density in the trachea. The diagnosis is confirmed by identification of a tumor during tracheoscopy and subsequent histologic evaluation. The treatment of choice is surgical excision of the tumor.

Tracheal Trauma

Trauma affecting the trachea most often results from blunt force injury or bite wounds. Clinical signs may include respiratory distress, coughing, or subcutaneous emphysema. Diagnosis usually is established on the basis of history and physical examination findings. Treatment is primarily supportive and includes cage rest and oxygen administration. Depending on the cause, tracheal lacerations often are repaired surgically.

Tracheal Parasites

O. osleri, previously called *Filaroides osleri,* is a nematode that in rare cases affects dogs, usually those younger than 1 year of age. The parasite lives in nodules within the tracheal mucosa, most often near the tracheal bifurcation. Clinical signs include inspiratory wheezing, chronic cough, and respiratory distress. Plain radiographs may reveal thickened tracheal mucosa and soft tissue densities within the tracheal lumen. Ovae or larvae may be identified in specimens of tracheal wash fluid and sometimes on fecal flotation using zinc sulfate or the Baermann technique.[16] Tracheoscopy allows direct visualization of the nodules within the tracheal mucosa and collection of samples for cytologic or histologic evaluation. Albendazole (Valbazen) at 25 mg/kg by mouth, b.i.d., for 5 days, repeated in 2 weeks, or ivermectin (Ivomec) at 0.4 mg/kg subcutaneously, once, have been used to treat infection with *O. osleri.*[16]

References

1. Wykes PM. Canine laryngeal diseases. Part I. Anatomy and disease syndromes. Compen Contin Educ Pract Vet 1983;5:8–15.
2. Robinson NE. Airway physiology. Vet Clin North Am 1992;22:1043–1064.
3. Bradley RL, Noone KE, Saunders GK, et al. Nasopharyngeal and middle ear polypoid masses in five cats. Vet Surg 1985;14:141–144.
4. Lane JG, Orr CM, Lucke VM, et al. Nasopharyngeal polyps arising in the middle ear of the cat. J Small Anim Pract 1981;22:511–522.
5. Kapatkin AS. Results of surgery and long-term follow-up in 31 cats with nasopharyngeal polyps. J Am Anim Hosp Assoc 1990;26:387–392.
6. Parker NR, Binnington AG. Nasopharyngeal polyps in cats: Three case reports and a review of the literature. J Am Anim Hosp Assoc 1985;21:473–478.
7. Braund KG. Laryngeal paralysis in immature and mature dogs as one sign of a more diffuse polyneuropathy. J Am Vet Med Assoc 1989;194:1735–1740.
8. Braund KG, Shores A, Cochrane S, et al. Laryngeal paralysis-polyneuropathy complex in young Dalmations. Am J Vet Res 1994;55:534–542.
9. Harvey CE, Goldschmidt MH. Inflammatory polypoid growths in the ear canal of cats. J Small Anim Pract 1978;19:669–677.
10. Venker-van Haagen AJ, Hartman W, Goedegebuure SA. Spontaneous laryngeal paralysis in young Bouviers. J Am Anim Hosp Assoc 1978;14:714-720.
11. Harvey CE, O'Brien JA. Treatment of laryngeal paralysis in dogs by partial laryngectomy. J Am Anim Hosp Assoc 1982;18:551–556.
12. Gaber CE, Amis TC, LeCouteur RA. Laryngeal paralysis in dogs: A review of 23 cases. J Am Vet Med Assoc 1985;186:377–380.
13. Greenfield CL. Canine laryngeal paralysis. Compen Contin Educ Pract Vet 1987;9:1011–1020.
14. LaHue TR. Treatment of laryngeal paralysis in dogs by unilateral cricoarytenoid laryngoplasty. J Am Anim Hosp Assoc 1989;25:317–324.
15. Trout NJ, Harpster NK, Berg J, et al. Long-term results of unilateral ventriculocordectomy and partial arytenoidectomy for the treatment of laryngeal paralysis in 60 dogs. J Am Anim Hosp Assoc 1994;30:401–407.
16. Reinemeyer CR. Parasites of the respiratory system. In: Bonagura JD, ed. Kirk's Current Veterinary Therapy XII. Philadelphia, WB Saunders, 1995:895–898.
17. Ettinger SJ, Ticer JW. Diseases of the trachea. In: Ettinger SJ, ed. Textbook of Veterinary Internal Medicine, 3rd ed. Philadelphia, WB Saunders, 1989:795–815.
18. Hendricks JC. Brachycephalic airway syndrome. Vet Clin North Am Small Anim Pract 1992;22:1145–1153.
19. Harvey CE. Soft palate resection in brachycephalic dogs. J Am Anim Hosp Assoc 1982;18:538–544.
20. Coyne BE, Finland RB. Hypoplasia of the trachea in dogs: 103 cases (1974–1990). J Am Vet Med Assoc 1992;201:768–772.
21. Aron DN, Crowe DT. Upper airway obstruction. Vet Clin North Am Small Anim Pract 1985;15:891–917.
22. Wykes PM. Canine laryngeal diseases. Part II. Diagnosis and treatment. Compen Contin Educ Pract Vet 1983;5:105–113.
23. Harvey CE. Stenotic nares surgery in brachycephalic dogs. J Am Anim Hosp Assoc 1982;18:535–537.
24. Harvey CE. Everted laryngeal saccule surgery in brachycephalic dogs. J Am Anim Hosp Assoc 1982;18:545–547.
25. Holt D, Harvey C. Idiopathic laryngeal paralysis: Results of treatment by bilateral vocal fold resection in 40 dogs. J Am Anim Hosp Assoc 1994;30:389–395.
26. Ross JT, Matthiesen DT, Noone KE, et al. Complications and long-term results after partial laryngectomy for treatment of idiopathic laryngeal paralysis in 45 dogs. Vet Surg 1991;20:169–173.
27. White RAS. Unilateral arytenoid lateralization: An as-

sessment of technique and long term results in 62 dogs with laryngeal paralysis. J Small Anim Pract 1989; 30: 543–549.

28. Venker-van Haagen AJ, Bouw J, Hartman W. Hereditary transmission of laryngeal paralysis in Bouviers. J Am Anim Hosp Assoc 1981;17:75–76.

29. Kerr LY. Pulmonary edema secondary to upper airway obstruction in the dog: A review of nine cases. J Am Anim Hosp Assoc 1989;25:207–212.

30. Harvey H, Irby NL, Watrous BJ. Laryngeal paralysis in hypothyroid dogs. In: Kirk RW, ed. Current Veterinary Therapy VIII, Philadelphia, WB Saunders, 1983:694–697.

31. Gourley IM, Paul H, Gregory C. Castellated laryngofissure and vocal fold resection for the treatment of laryngeal paralysis in the dog. J Am Vet Med Assoc 1983;182:1084–1086.

32. Hardie EM, Kolata RJ, Stone EA, et al. Laryngeal paralysis in three cats. J Am Vet Med Assoc 1981;179: 879–882.

33. Ford RB, Vaden SL. Canine infectious tracheobronchitis. In: Greene CE, ed. Infectious Diseases of the Dog and Cat. Philadelphia, WB Saunders, 1990:259–265.

34. Ford RB. Infectious tracheobronchitis. In: Bonagura JD, ed. Kirk's Current Veterinary Therapy XII. Philadelphia, WB Saunders, 1995:905–908.

35. Bemis DA. Bordetella and mycoplasma respiratory infections in dogs and cats. Vet Clin North Am Small Anim Pract 1992;22:1173–1186.

36. Ford RB. Concurrent use of corticosteroids and antimicrobial drugs in the treatment of infectious diseases in small animals. J Am Vet Med Assoc 1984;185: 1142–1144.

37. Konter EJ, Wegrzyn RJ, Goodnow RA. Canine infectious tracheobronchitis: Effects of an intranasal live canine parainfluenza-*Bordetella bronchiseptica* vaccine on viral shedding and clinical tracheobronchitis (kennel cough). Am J Vet Res 1981;42:1694–1698.

38. Dallman MJ, McClure RC, Brown EM. Histochemical study of normal and collapsed tracheas in dogs. Am J Vet Res 1988;49:2117–2125.

39. Padrid P, Amis TC. Chronic tracheobronchial disease in the dog. Vet Clin North Am Small Anim Pract 1992;22: 1203–1229.

40. Hobson HP. Total ring prosthesis for the surgical correction of collapsed trachea. J Am Anim Hosp Assoc 1976;12:822–828.

41. Fingland RB, DeHoff WD, Birchard SJ. Surgical management of cervical and thoracic tracheal collapse in dogs using extraluminal spiral prostheses: Results in seven cases. J Am Anim Hosp Assoc 1987;23:173–181.

42. Venker-van Haagen AJ. Diseases of the larynx. Vet Clin North Am Small Anim Pract 1992;22:1155–1172.

43. Saik JE, Toll SL, Diters RW, et al. Canine and feline laryngeal neoplasia: A 10-year survey. J Am Anim Hosp Assoc 1986;22:359–365.

44. Lotti U, Niebauer GW. Tracheobronchial foreign bodies of plant origin in 153 hunting dogs. Compen Contin Educ Pract Vet 1992;14:900–905.

45. Neer TM, Zeman D. Tracheal adenocarcinoma in a cat and review of the literature. J Am Anim Hosp Assoc 1987;23:377–380.

Chapter 53

Diseases of the Pleural Space and Mediastinum

Alice M. Wolf

Anatomy and Physiology

The pleural cavity is a potential space between the chest wall and thoracic viscera. The thoracic wall, mediastinum, and diaphragm are covered by a single layer of mesothelial cells (the parietal pleura) that joins the mesothelial layer covering the lung surfaces (the visceral pleura) at the hilum. Fenestrations in the mediastinal pleura allow communication between the right hemithorax and left hemithorax in most companion animals. The pleural space normally contains only a few milliliters of a low-protein, serous fluid that lubricates the pleural surfaces and prevents friction during respiratory motion. There is continuous turnover of fluid as a result of the hydrostatic and oncotic forces in the systemic and pleural circulatory and lymphatic systems. Disorders that affect the regional circulatory or lymphatic flow and alterations in plasma oncotic pressure, capillary permeability, or surface area cause a disturbance of this fragile fluid balance. These disturbances usually result in excessive fluid accumulation in the pleural space.

The mediastinum is the space created by the central, bilateral reflections of the parietal pleural epithelium. The mediastinum extends cranially to the thoracic inlet and communicates with the fascial planes and perivascular, peritracheal, and periesophageal sheaths in the cervical region. Caudally the mediastinum extends to the diaphragm and communicates with the retroperitoneal space through the aortic hilus. This space normally contains the thymus (in young animals), trachea, esophagus, heart, aorta, and vena cava, as well as additional smaller blood vessels, lymph channels, nerves, airways, and lymph nodes.

Problem Identification

Dyspnea

Dyspnea, difficult or labored breathing, is the most common sign of pleural effusion or pneumothorax. More focal pleural disorders or mediastinal disorders (e.g., masses) may not cause observable changes in the respiratory efforts. Dyspnea can also be caused by metabolic, cardiovascular, and upper and lower airway disorders. (See Chaps. 9 and 52 for a further discussion of dyspnea.)

Pathophysiology

Dyspnea caused by pleural disease usually occurs when fluid or air in the pleural space compresses lung tissue and restricts normal lung expansion and oxygen exchange.

Clinical Signs

The onset of noticeable dyspnea may be acute, as when caused by traumatic intrathoracic hemorrhage or pneumothorax, but is more often slowly progressive, as when associated with pleural effusion. The animal may seem to be uncomfortable and unable to rest. It may prefer a sitting or sternal position and avoid lateral recumbence. The excursions of the chest wall and diaphragm during respiration are more pronounced. Breathing may be more rapid and shallow or may appear to have an abdominal component because of diaphragmatic efforts. Patients with dyspnea related to tension pneumothorax may have little movement of the chest wall and may have pronounced diaphragmatic motion. Exercise intolerance may be noticed in dogs; open-mouth breathing is a serious sign of extreme dyspnea, particularly in cats. Cyanosis of the oral mucous membranes in patients with dyspnea indicates severe compromise of oxygen exchange.

Diagnostic Plan

Significant dyspnea is always a sign that requires immediate and thorough diagnostic investigation. Auscultation and percussion may reveal dullness or hyperresonance of the thoracic cavity, which indicates the presence of fluid or air, respectively. Thoracic radiographs should be taken if the patient's condition is stable. Thoracentesis for diagnosis and treatment may be performed before or after radiography, depending on the physical examination or radiographic findings. Ultrasound evaluation of the thorax may be useful for patients with underlying mass lesions or cardiac disease. Fine-needle aspiration cytology of mass lesions can also be performed on the basis of the radiographic findings or with ultrasound guidance.

Pleural Effusion

Pleural effusion is the accumulation of a greater than normal amount of fluid in the pleural space. It occurs commonly in dogs and cats.

Pathophysiology

Fluid exchange within the normal pleural space is a well-balanced system. Normally, there is a 1-cm water gradient between the parietal pleura and visceral pleura that favors fluid absorption from the pleural space and keeps the small volume of pleural fluid relatively constant.[1] Changes in systemic or pulmonary capillary hydrostatic pressure, oncotic pressure, capillary permeability, or lymph flow upset the fluid balance by causing excessive fluid transudation into or decreased fluid absorption from the pleural space. Blood can accumulate in the pleural space as the result of rupture of intrathoracic blood vessels secondary to trauma, tissue necrosis, or tumor erosion and to hemostatic defects or disorders of coagulation. Fluid accumulating in the pleural space is modified over time by the body's immunologic response and the presence or absence of infectious agents. Common causes of pleural effusion in dogs and cats include hypoalbuminemia, right-sided congestive heart failure, intrathoracic neoplasia, pyothorax, feline infectious peritonitis, hemothorax, and chylous effusion.

Clinical Signs

Dyspnea is the primary clinical sign of pleural effusion. The duration of illness is particularly difficult to ascertain in the cat because of this species' propensity to moderate its activity in response to reduced breathing capacity. Thus, the onset of dyspnea may appear to be acute to the cat's owner when in reality the problem has been present for days or weeks. Exercise intolerance is more likely to be noticed sooner in dogs.

The severity of dyspnea is related to the volume of pleural fluid that is present, adhesions on the lung or between the lung and pleural surface, and the presence of chronic lung collapse. Concurrent problems, including anemia, pulmonary parenchymal disease, mediastinal disease, or cardiovascular disease, may contribute to the apparent respiratory distress.

Other clinical signs occasionally associated with pleural disease include cough, fever, and pleuritic pain. With the exception of chylous effusion, coughing in association with primary pleural effusion is more common in the dog than the cat.

Physical examination of animals with pleural disorders may reveal dyspnea with a pronounced diaphragmatic lift in the respiratory pattern. Patients with a large volume of pleural fluid may have an apparent bulging of one or both hemithoraces. Thoracic auscultation can reveal muffled heart sounds and decreased lung sounds in the ventral thorax. Thoracic wall percussion may reveal dullness ventrally when the animal is in an upright or sternal position. Mucous membranes may be pale or cyanotic because of poor oxygen exchange capacity. Cardiac arrhythmias or murmurs may be present in patients with cardiovascular disease, severe anemia, fever, or trauma. Fever is most commonly associated with infectious lesions but may occur with other disorders. Pleuritic pain can be elicited in a few animals by firm palpation of the intercostal spaces. Cats with an anterior mediastinal mass may have an incompressible anterior thorax.

Diagnostic Plan

Thoracentesis for diagnosis or treatment should be performed as the first step when historical and clinical signs suggest pleural effusion as the cause of dyspnea. The fluid should be examined cytologically and submitted for microbiologic culture if appropriate. With severely dyspneic animals, radiography should not be performed until their condition has stabilized, and it is more likely to be diagnostic when most of the pleural fluid volume has been removed by aspiration.

Cough

Coughing is only occasionally a primary feature of pleural or mediastinal disease but may occur because of pulmonary or cardiac disorders that subsequently lead to pleural involvement. (See Chaps. 9 and 54.) Chylothorax or pleuritis associated with foreign body penetration is more likely than other pleural disorders to produce a cough.

Pathophysiology

Mediastinal masses may cause coughing because of compression or irritation of the trachea. Similarly, enlarged mediastinal lymph nodes at the hilus of the lung may cause coughing because of compression of adjacent airways. Pulmonary bullae or blebs may rupture during the coughing efforts, causing pneumothorax.[2] Coughing may occur with primary bacterial or foreign body pneumonia, and pyothorax may result from extension of the infection. Coughing associated with pleural effusion caused by cardiac disease is usually the result of pulmonary edema or the compressive effects of enlarged cardiac chambers on major airways. Chylous effusion is the most common primary type of effusion associated with coughing, most likely because of the irritating effects of chyle on the pleural surfaces.[3]

Diagnostic Plan

The patient's history and physical examination findings should help localize the suspected source of the cough to the upper or lower airways or heart. The diagnostic investigation should then specifically focus on these areas. For suspected lower airway, pulmonary, or cardiac disorders, thoracic radiography should be the first diagnostic step. The investigation can then proceed to include, as appropriate, ultrasound examination of the thorax or heart, electrocardiography, thoracentesis, tracheal or bronchial endoscopy, transtracheal wash or bronchoalveolar lavage, and fine-needle aspiration or lung biopsy.

Mediastinal Mass

Most mediastinal mass lesions arise in the anterior mediastinum, because there are more vascular, lymphoid, and visceral structures there that may become pathologic than in the posterior mediastinum.

Pathophysiology

Abnormalities of any of the normal structures, infection or hemorrhage in the mediastinal space, or abnormal structures may be detected as a mass lesion of the mediastinum. An enlarging anterior mediastinal mass may impinge on the trachea, produce pleural effusion, or become large enough to cause displacement and collapse of the anterior lung lobes, resulting in coughing or dyspnea. Compression of the esophagus can cause regurgitation and the development of secondary megaesophagus. Invasion of intrathoracic nervous tissue may produce Horner's syndrome. Rarely, thymoma in dogs may be associated with myasthenia gravis, which can cause megaesophagus and generalized muscular weakness.

Diagnostic Plan

Radiographic examination and ultrasonography are helpful in delineating the size and nature of the anterior mediastinal mass. Fine-needle aspiration or core biopsy can be used for definitive diagnosis. Exploratory surgery may occasionally be needed for diagnosis as well as treatment.

Fever

True fever is an elevation of body temperature that is caused by dysregulation of the hypothalamic thermoregulatory center and resetting of the hypothalamic thermostat to a higher setting. (See Chap. 35.)

Pathophysiology

Body temperature elevation is caused by interleukin compounds released from inflammatory cells in response to infectious, inflammatory, and immunologic stimuli. The hypothalamic neural effects are mediated by prostaglandin E and result in an elevation of body temperature and resetting of the hypothalamic thermostat to a higher set point. Fever in patients with primary pleural or mediastinal disease is most often caused by infectious processes such as bacterial, viral, or fungal infection. Neoplasia, particularly of the lymphoid system, may also induce fever.

Clinical Signs

Patients with fever have a persistent or fluctuating body temperature above the normal range. Lethargy and inappetence are common associated findings. Other signs of pleural or mediastinal disease (e.g., dyspnea, pleural effusion, cough) are often present.

Diagnostic Plan

Fever generally signals the presence of an infectious or inflammatory disease. The diagnostic evaluation discussed for the particular disease should be used to evaluate this problem.

Ascites

Ascites is the presence of excess fluid in the peritoneal cavity. (See Chap. 34.) The causes of fluid accumulation in this space are similar to those described for pleural effusion. Ascites is a rare accompanying problem in patients with pleural or mediastinal disease.[4]

Pathophysiology

Altered hemodynamics in right-sided heart failure, widely metastatic inflammatory tumors, and feline infectious peritonitis (FIP) may produce fluid accumulation in both the pleural and peritoneal spaces. Patients with low serum oncotic pressure caused by hypoalbuminemia may have ascites, pleural effusion, and occasionally peripheral edema. Lymphatic obstruction secondary to neoplasia or inflammation may cause lymph or chyle to accumulate in both the pleural and the peritoneal cavities. Trauma or bleeding disorders may cause hemorrhage into more than one body cavity and from external body orifices. Diaphragmatic herniation with strangulation of the liver or other viscera may be associated with both thoracic and intra-abdominal effusions.

Clinical Signs

In addition to signs associated with pleural or mediastinal disease, the abdomen appears distended and a fluid wave may be detected with abdominal percussion. Organomegaly may be present; however, the fluid accumulation may make abdominal palpation difficult. Pale mucous membranes, thready pulses, or cardiac murmurs may be found in patients with significant intracavitary hemorrhage. Muffled heart sounds, arrhythmias, and poor pulse quality may be present in patients with cardiac disease. Fever (persistent or undulating) is often present in cats with FIP-associated effusion and patients with septic peritonitis.

Diagnostic Plan

Because ascites is often much less immediately life threatening than pleural effusion, the major diagnostic effort is usually directed at diagnosis and treatment of the pleural disorder. Diagnostic studies used to evaluate patients with ascites include abdominal radiography (often of little value if significant effusion is present), abdominal or thoracic ultrasonography, and abdominocentesis with cytologic or biochemical fluid evaluation and microbiologic culture. Additional organ- and system-specific diagnostic studies may be selected after this initial evaluation has been completed.

Diagnostic Procedures

Auscultation and Percussion

Thoracic auscultation or percussion should be performed in a quiet room in order to assess the patient adequately for subtle changes in lung sounds and thoracic resonance. Changes are usually present bilaterally, although unilateral involvement may occur in a few animals. Pleural effusion muffles heart and lung sounds in the ventral thorax. A line demarcating the interface of the pleural fluid and air-filled lung in the chest may be detected with the animal in a standing position. Thoracic wall percussion may also demonstrate the fluid line in the chest. Patients with pneumothorax usually have reduced sounds in all lung fields because of collapse and retraction of lung lobes away from the chest wall. Heart sounds may be louder than normal. Pneumothorax may also cause hyperresonance on thoracic wall percussion.

Animals with only pleural masses or mediastinal disease may not have detectable abnormalities on thoracic auscultation or percussion. Abnormalities, if noticed, may be localized to a focal region of the chest.

Radiography and Ultrasonography

The decision to perform radiographic or ultrasonographic examination of a dyspneic patient should

be made carefully. Cats, in particular, are often at the limit of their respiratory reserve capacity at the time their disease is recognized and they are brought to a veterinarian for examination. The stress of radiographic positioning may cause severely dyspneic patients to decompensate and develop respiratory arrest. It is often better to perform thoracentesis if pleural effusion or pneumothorax is suspected on the basis of the history and physical examination. Thoracentesis not only confirms the diagnosis but immediately improves oxygenation by removal of the fluid or air. In addition, the diagnostic quality of radiographs is enhanced by removal of pleural fluid before radiography.

If a severely dyspneic animal must be examined radiographically, it should be stabilized as much as possible by reducing stress and supplementing oxygen with an oxygen cage or nasal oxygen delivery system before the procedure is performed. Dorsoventral and standing (or sternal) lateral views are recommended, and minimal restraint should be used. An oxygen source should be available to provide support during the procedure.

Radiographic findings suggestive of pleural effusion include rounding of the costophrenic angles, apparent widening of the mediastinum, observable pleural fissure lines, blurring or loss of the cardiac silhouette, separation of the lung margins from the thoracic wall, and leafing of the lung margins above the sternum[1] (Fig. 53–1A, B). Pneumothorax causes retraction or collapse of lung lobes, increased intrathoracic

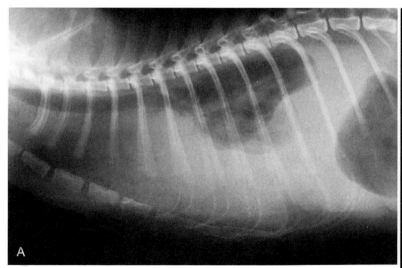

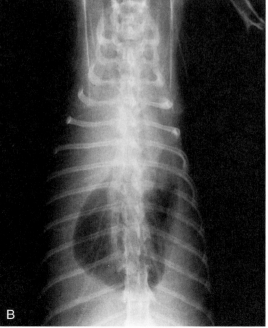

Figure 53–1
(A) Lateral and **(B)** dorsoventral radiographs of a 7-year-old domestic shorthair cat with a large volume of chylous pleural effusion. Note the small amount of functional lung tissue remaining to exchange air. This cat should have had thoracentesis to improve respiration before radiography.

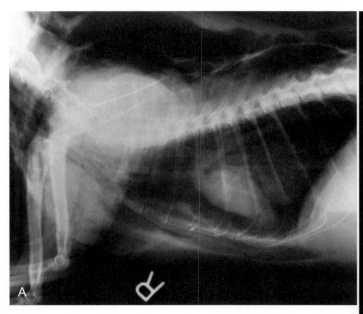
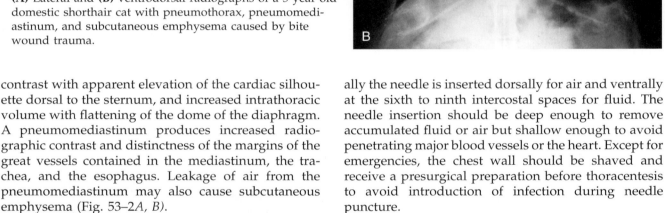

Figure 53–2

(A) Lateral and **(B)** ventrodorsal radiographs of a 5-year-old domestic shorthair cat with pneumothorax, pneumomediastinum, and subcutaneous emphysema caused by bite wound trauma.

contrast with apparent elevation of the cardiac silhouette dorsal to the sternum, and increased intrathoracic volume with flattening of the dome of the diaphragm. A pneumomediastinum produces increased radiographic contrast and distinctness of the margins of the great vessels contained in the mediastinum, the trachea, and the esophagus. Leakage of air from the pneumomediastinum may also cause subcutaneous emphysema (Fig. 53–2*A, B*).

In addition to its utility for evaluating cardiac performance, ultrasonography may detect the presence of fluid in the pleural or pericardial space, fluid or masses in the mediastinum, and herniation of abdominal viscera through the diaphragm. Because air in the lung tends to scatter ultrasonic waves, ultrasonography is generally less helpful for assessing generalized diffuse changes in the pulmonary parenchyma than for evaluating consolidated areas or mass lesions. Ultrasonography can also be used effectively to guide fine-needle aspiration and biopsy of intrathoracic structures.

Thoracentesis

Thoracentesis is used for diagnosis and treatment of fluid or air accumulations in the pleural space. The site selected for needle introduction depends on the location (as judged by physical examination and radiographic or ultrasonographic findings) and the type of material expected in the pleural space. Gener-

ally the needle is inserted dorsally for air and ventrally at the sixth to ninth intercostal spaces for fluid. The needle insertion should be deep enough to remove accumulated fluid or air but shallow enough to avoid penetrating major blood vessels or the heart. Except for emergencies, the chest wall should be shaved and receive a presurgical preparation before thoracentesis to avoid introduction of infection during needle puncture.

Sedation or local anesthesia may be required in order to perform thoracentesis in some patients. A syringe with attached needle can be used for emergency situations; however, for routine thoracentesis, a 21- or 23-gauge butterfly-type needle with attached extension tube is recommended. After penetration of the pleural space, the butterfly attachment is used to stabilize the needle against the chest wall to avoid lung laceration. A two- or three-way stopcock and syringe are attached to the extension tube to perform the aspiration. The needle can be repositioned to perform aspiration from multiple sites if necessary.

Placement of an indwelling chest tube is recommended for patients that require repeated pleural aspiration. The technique for this is described later in this chapter.

Laboratory Analysis of Fluid

If fluid is aspirated, a portion of the sample should be saved for further analysis. Fresh, air-dried smears should be made immediately and submitted with a fluid sample in an ethylenediaminetetra-acetic acid (EDTA) tube for protein analysis, nucleated cell count, and cytologic evaluation. Cytologic examination should take place as soon as possible after collection because the cells in fluid deteriorate rapidly. A second specimen should be collected in a sterile tube for bacteriologic evaluation. A third specimen may be saved in a tube without anticoagulant for possible biochemical analysis.

Effusion fluids are classically categorized on the basis of their protein concentration, cell counts, and cell types as transudates, modified transudates, and exudates.[1, 5, 6] However, because pleural fluid exchange is dynamic and cell types change over time, these categorizations are generally too broad.[1] Cytologic examination and identification of specific cell types (e.g., neoplastic cells, eosinophils) and of infectious agents (e.g., bacteria, fungi) and, occasionally, biochemical analysis of fluid are critical to definitive diagnosis of the cause of the effusion. The following discussion uses a modified classification scheme employing the general categories and more specific definitions of fluid types based on their cytologic, bacteriologic, and biochemical characteristics.

Other Diagnostic Tests

Other laboratory tests may be helpful in evaluating the patient. A basic laboratory database consisting of a complete blood count, serum biochemistry profile with electrolyte analysis, and urinalysis is suggested for all patients. These tests may be helpful in assessing the patient for an underlying cause of the effusion such as generalized systemic diseases (e.g., FIP, histoplasmosis), hypoproteinemia, and coagulopathies. Cats should be tested for the feline leukemia virus (FeLV) antigen and feline immunodeficiency virus (FIV) antibody. Additional diagnostic tests or procedures can then be selected depending on the suspected etiology of pleural air or fluid accumulation (see specific disorders).

Diseases of the Pleural Space

Pleural effusions are described on the basis of their cytologic and etiologic characteristics.

Transudate

A pure transudate is classically a water-clear, low-protein (<2.5 g/dL) fluid with a low cell count (<1000 nucleated cells/μL).[1] It is usually associated with hypoalbuminemia (often <1.0 g/dL).

Pathophysiology

The most common causes of thoracic transudate accumulation are conditions of overhydration or vascular volume overload (e.g., iatrogenic fluid overload) or reduced plasma oncotic pressure caused by low-protein states such as end-stage hepatic disease (see Chap. 34) or protein-losing disorders (e.g., glomerular diseases [see Chap. 16], protein-losing enteropathies [see Chap. 32]) that result in hypoproteinemia with hypoalbuminemia.

The occurrence of pure transudates is rare. However, because of the reaction of the pleura to fluid accumulation, the transudate changes gradually over time, generally increasing in protein content and cell count. Therefore, by the time of diagnosis, some effusions that may have been pure transudates initially have become modified transudates.

Clinical Signs

If the transudate results from iatrogenic fluid overload, the onset of dyspnea is often acute. Pulmonary edema may be present as a complicating feature in these patients. Other signs depend on the primary condition under treatment. Transudates secondary to protein-losing conditions are usually slower to accumulate, and other signs of the underlying disease such as weight loss, malaise, anorexia, polyuria or polydipsia, or diarrhea are generally present. Ascites may accompany the pleural effusion in fluid overload or protein-losing conditions.

Diagnostic Plan

The diagnosis of the effusion as a transudate is made by fluid analysis. Further evaluation of the patient focuses on identifying the underlying cause of fluid overload, poor protein production, or excessive protein loss. The biochemistry profile and urinalysis may reveal the site of production failure or pathologic protein loss. Further organ-specific diagnostic tests are directed at identifying the specific cause of the disorder. Hepatic function testing may be needed to identify some patients with end-stage liver disease or shunting lesions.

Treatment

As in all patients with pleural effusion, the initial therapeutic effort should focus on stabilization of the patient's respiration. Thoracentesis may be necessary if dyspnea is severe. In early cases of fluid overload, a reduction in the fluid infusion rate and treatment with an appropriate diuretic drug (e.g., furosemide) are often sufficient to improve breathing and clear the pleural space. Diuretics may also be used for temporary removal of pleural fluid accumulation in patients with hypoalbuminemia. Plasma volume expanders such as plasma or hetastarch may also be useful on a short-term basis. However, the long-term treatment of such patients should be directed at increasing serum protein levels by managing the cause of the protein loss or decreased production.

Prognosis

Patients with iatrogenic fluid overload can usually be managed successfully through their acute episode of effusion if the problem is recognized early. Management of patients with severe hypoalbuminemia is often difficult because the primary underlying condition is often well advanced and may not be reversible by the time of diagnosis.

Obstructive Effusion: Modified Transudate

A modified transudate is a serous to serosanguineous fluid with a moderate protein level (>2.5 g/dL) and cell content (<5000 nucleated cells/µL).[1]

Pathophysiology

Accumulation of a modified transudate usually results from increased venous pressure causing transudation of fluid from the lymphatic or vascular bed into the pleural space. A modified transudate is most often associated with cardiac disease (particularly cardiomyopathy in cats), diaphragmatic hernias with organ strangulation, intrathoracic neoplasms that do not exfoliate cells into the fluid, or pericardial effusion.[6, 7]

Clinical Signs

In addition to dyspnea, the clinical signs in patients with modified transudates depend on the underlying condition causing the effusion. Cardiac failure may cause lethargy, cough, anorexia, tachycardia, and arrhythmias. Diaphragmatic hernia may also cause icterus, vomiting or regurgitation, and a reduction in abdominal contents on palpation. Heart sounds are muffled and jugular pulses may be present in patients with pericardial effusion. Patients with pancreatitis may vomit and have abdominal pain.

Diagnostic Plan

The diagnosis of modified transudate is based on fluid analysis. Cytologic examination demonstrates a mixed population with variable numbers of nondegenerate neutrophils, lymphocytes, macrophages, red blood cells (RBCs), and mesothelial cells. Eosinophilia in the effusion suggests neoplasia, allergic lung disease, or parasitic infection.[8, 9]

Further studies should be directed at identifying the inciting cause of the effusion. Thoracic radiography and ultrasonography may be helpful in identifying patients with cardiac or pericardial disease or diaphragmatic herniation. Evaluation of both right and left lateral thoracic radiographic views may facilitate the discovery of lung or mediastinal masses. The presence of other extrarespiratory signs may assist in focusing the diagnostic investigation.

Treatment and Prognosis

Treatment is directed at managing or eliminating the primary cause of the effusion. The prognosis is dependent on the nature of the underlying disease process.

Septic Exudate

A septic exudate is a high-protein (>2.5 g/dL), turbid fluid with a high cell content (>5000 nucleated cells/µL) consisting predominantly of neutrophils in various stages of degeneration.[1] Bacteria are usually present but may or may not be observed on fluid examination.

Pathophysiology

Septic effusion (pyothorax) results from the introduction of bacteria into the pleural space via an external penetrating wound or foreign body or by extension from an internal organ (e.g., ruptured lung abscess, esophageal perforation with mediastinitis). Pyothorax is more common in the cat than the dog and is suspected to result from bite wound trauma, although evidence of the original injury is rarely found.[10] Septic pleuritis in dogs is more likely to result from aspiration or thoracic wall penetration by foreign bodies such as grass awns or extension from pneumonic lung.[11]

Clinical Signs

Clinical signs in animals with pyothorax are due to both the effusion accumulation and the presence of bacterial toxins and leukocyte byproducts in the fluid.[12] Typical signs include fever, malaise, and anorexia. Pleuritic pain or cough may be present in some patients. Regurgitation may precede signs associated with pyothorax in patients with esophageal perforation by foreign bodies. Patients with penetrating pleural foreign bodies may have a wound on the exterior of the thoracic cavity.

Diagnostic Plan

Septic exudates may be yellow or red to brown and turbid with high protein content and specific gravity. There may be large amounts of fibrin and

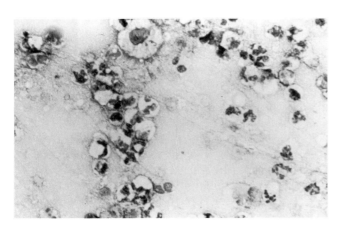

Figure 53-3
Cytologic preparation of pleural fluid from a 3-year-old
Siamese cat with pyothorax. Degenerate neutrophils and
occasional macrophages are surrounded by a granular
background of proteinaceous debris (×1000).

debris, and the fluid is often foul smelling. Cytologic
examination reveals high cell counts, and the predominant cell type is the neutrophil in various stages of
degeneration.[10] Variable numbers of macrophages or
mesothelial cells are also present along with lesser
numbers of RBCs and lymphocytes (Fig. 53-3). Bacteria
may or may not be seen within neutrophils or free in
the exudate. A bacteriologic culture (aerobic and
anaerobic) and sensitivity test should be performed on
the fluid. Cultures may be negative despite the direct
observation of bacteria on cytology, because the observed bacteria are dead or fail to grow with routine
aerobic culture techniques. The agents associated with
feline pyothorax are often anaerobes, most commonly
Bacteroides and *Fusobacterium* spp. *Pasteurella* spp. is the
most common aerobic isolate.[6, 10] *Actinomyces*, *Nocardia*, and *Bacteroides* spp. and other anaerobes are the
most common isolates from canine patients with septic
pleuritis.[11, 13]

The complete blood count frequently reveals an
inflammatory leukogram. The presence of a degenerative left shift is considered by some clinicians to be a
poor prognostic sign. FeLV and FIV are not known to
predispose a cat to develop pyothorax; however,
infection with either of these viruses may make
successful treatment more difficult. The biochemistry
profile and urinalysis are not usually helpful in
diagnosis but may reveal other conditions that require
concurrent treatment.

Radiography of the thorax after drainage may
be useful in identifying radiopaque foreign bodies,
collapsed lung lobes, or pockets of loculated exudate.
Ultrasound examination also helps determine the
extent of loculation of fluid and fibrosis and can be
used to detect intrathoracic abscesses that may require
surgical intervention to allow drainage.

Treatment

The initial treatment for pyothorax includes
closed chest-tube drainage and pleural lavage.[10, 12] A
large-bore, soft rubber or polyethylene indwelling
chest tube is placed in one or both sides of the chest to
facilitate pleural aspiration several times daily. Placement of an indwelling drain tube requires general
anesthesia or heavy sedation and local anesthesia. With
the patient in lateral recumbence, the lateral thorax is
clipped and prepared for aseptic surgery. A small skin
incision is made over the 10th to 12th intercostal spaces
just above the costochondral rib junction. A large
hemostat is used to create a subcutaneous tunnel
directed cranially to the eighth or ninth intercostal
space. Alternatively, the skin incision can be advanced
by sliding the skin forward over the eighth to ninth
intercostal space before tube insertion. The subcutaneous tunnel thus created helps to prevent air leakage
around the tube into the pleural space. The distal end
of the chest tube is then carried in the jaws of the
hemostat and inserted sharply through the intercostal
musculature at the level of the eighth to ninth
intercostal space. The hemostat is then used to advance
the tube cranioventrally into the pleural space. A
polyethylene or Silastic catheter with an indwelling
trocar can be used in similar fashion to create the
subcutaneous tunnel and to penetrate the chest wall
forcefully instead of carrying the tube in hemostats.
The catheter is then advanced off the trocar into the
chest cavity. A C-clamp is closed around the indwelling catheter and a three-way stopcock is used to seal
the open proximal end of the tube. The chest tube
should be sutured to the skin with a Chinese finger trap
type of suture or through a "butterfly" of tape secured
on the tube next to the skin. The C-clamp can then be
removed or left on the tube to ensure that it remains
closed when not being used for aspiration of thoracic
fluid. Antibiotic or antiseptic ointment is applied
around the site of tube entry, and a chest bandage may
be used to secure the tube further and reduce the
likelihood of its being dislodged by the patient.
Intermittent aspiration is effective in clearing the
pleural space and alleviating dyspnea in most patients.
Continuous pleural suction (Pleur-Evac) has also been
used to keep inflammatory exudates from accumulating in the pleural space.[11] The cellularity and character
of the aspirated fluid should be evaluated frequently to
monitor the progress of therapy.

Pleural lavage with warmed Ringer's lactate or
0.9% saline solution may help reduce pleural irritation
and facilitate the removal of tenacious exudate. After
aspiration of residual exudate, a volume of lavage
solution of approximately 10 mL/kg is instilled slowly
into the pleural cavity through the indwelling tube.
The patient should be observed carefully for signs of

respiratory embarrassment during the lavage procedure. After fluid instillation, the patient is moved gently to help distribute the lavage fluid, and then as much fluid as possible is aspirated. Three volumes of fluid should be exchanged during each lavage procedure, twice daily. The amount of lavage fluid recovered can be somewhat less than the amount instilled; the residual isotonic solution is rapidly absorbed by the pleural surface. Some clinicians recommend the addition of antibiotics or antiseptics to the pleural lavage solution; however, no controlled studies have shown that these additives improve clinical recovery over that achieved with isotonic electrolyte solutions used alone. Pleural lavage may be discontinued after 3 to 5 days as the fluid becomes less tenacious and voluminous. The indwelling chest tube should be removed when intermittent aspiration recovers less fluid than about 2 mL/kg every 8 to 12 hours, because irritation from the chest tube alone can account for this amount of fluid accumulation. In addition, the neutrophil count and the number of degenerate neutrophils should decrease, and bacteria should not be visible microscopically.

Additional management of patients with pyothorax includes fluid and nutritional support. Systemic antibiotics should be selected on the basis of microbiologic culture and sensitivity testing of pleural fluid. If no growth is observed in bacteriologic culture, broad-spectrum antibiotics effective against aerobic and anaerobic organisms should be used, such as a penicillin (ampicillin, 11–22 mg/kg three times per day [t.i.d.] or four times per day [q.i.d.] intravenously [IV], intramuscularly [IM], or subcutaneously [SC]) or cephalosporin (cefazolin, 20–25 mg/kg t.i.d. or q.i.d. IV or IM), in combination with an aminoglycoside (gentamicin, 2–4 mg/kg t.i.d. IV, IM, or SC) or quinolone (enrofloxacin, 2.5 mg/kg twice per day [b.i.d.] IM). Except for aminoglycosides, which should not be used for more than 7 days, antibiotic therapy should be continued for at least 6 weeks. After the clinical condition improves, antibiotics should be administered orally. Treatment of *Nocardia* or *Actinomyces* infections may be required for 6 to 12 months. Radiographs can be used to evaluate clearing of the effusion and to assess for residual pulmonary disease and scarring.

If the effusion recurs or is inadequately controlled with this protocol, exploratory thoracic surgery may be required to clear residual pockets of walled-off infection or remove a foreign body.

Prognosis

The prognosis for most cats with pyothorax is good with aggressive management.[10] Dogs are more likely to have a foreign body as the initiating cause and to have infection with resistant organisms, and they may be more difficult to manage.[11] Complications of pyothorax include fibrinous pleuritis; walled-off abscesses in the lung, mediastinum, and pleura; pneumothorax from thoracentesis or tearing of lung adhesions; chronic lung lobe atelectasis; and lung lobe torsion.[12]

Pyogranulomatous Exudate

Pyogranulomatous pleural effusion in cats is usually the result of infection with FIP coronavirus[6] (see Chap. 38). The effusion fluid is usually yellow-tinged, high in protein, and modestly cellular, with a pleocellular cytologic appearance. Rarely, pyogranulomatous effusions may occur in both dogs and cats secondary to fungal pneumonia.

Pathophysiology

FIP coronavirus infection is an immune-mediated disease. Virus-antibody immune complexes are trapped in small blood vessels or capillary beds and incite a pyogranulomatous inflammatory reaction in the surrounding tissue. High-protein fluid leaks from damaged blood vessels and accumulates in body cavities.

Clinical Signs

Approximately 10% of cats with the effusive form of FIP have only pleural effusion without ascites; in others pleural effusion may accompany ascitic fluid accumulation. Cats with pleural effusion show the signs previously described. Other clinical signs of FIP can be variable and include fluctuating antibiotic-unresponsive fever, malaise, depression, anorexia, weight loss, anterior uveitis, chorioretinitis, and central nervous system dysfunction.

Diagnostic Plan

Classic FIP pyogranulomatous effusion is usually a straw to yellow color, clear to slightly cloudy, with moderate cellularity and high protein content and specific gravity. The predominant cell types are nondegenerate neutrophils and macrophages.[1] Variable numbers of lymphocytes, plasma cells, mesothelial cells, and RBCs are also present (Fig. 53–4). A granular, proteinaceous background material is often seen on the slides. Bacteria are not seen, and bacteriologic cultures are negative. Electrophoresis of the effusion fluid demonstrates a high level of globulins. A fluid albumin/globulin ratio greater than 0.81 is highly predictive in ruling out FIP as a cause of the fluid accumulation. Alternatively, a gamma globulin fraction of 32% or greater is highly predictive in indicating that the effusion is due to FIP.[6]

The diagnosis is usually based on finding a classic FIP-type effusion along with the historical and

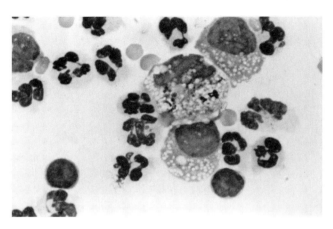

Figure 53–4
Cytologic preparation of pyogranulomatous pleural fluid from a 10-year-old domestic shorthair cat with feline infectious peritonitis. The pleocellular exudate contains non-degenerate neutrophils, macrophages, and occasional lymphocytes and red blood cells (×1000).

physical findings. Additional laboratory findings in FIP-infected cats can include neutrophilic leukocytosis, lymphopenia, and low-grade, normocytic, normochromic anemia. Hyperproteinemia with hyperglobulinemia and occasionally evidence of abdominal organ system dysfunction (e.g., elevated liver enzyme values) is found in biochemical profiles. Serum coronavirus serology and blood or fluid polymerase chain reaction testing are not specific for FIP, and although they support a diagnosis of FIP if positive, they cannot definitively confirm this diagnosis. Histopathology or indirect fluorescent antibody examination of tissue specimens for coronavirus is required for definitive diagnosis.

Treatment and Prognosis

In most cats, the course of FIP is slowly progressive and ultimately fatal. Combined chemotherapy with immunosuppressive drugs may provide temporary symptomatic relief for some patients. Granulomatous pneumonia may be present in addition to pleural fluid in some FIP-infected cats, making even symptomatic relief difficult to maintain.

Hemorrhagic Effusion

Hemothorax is a collection of blood in the pleural space. Cytologically and biochemically, its constituents are identical to those of peripheral blood.

Pathophysiology

Hemorrhage into the pleural space is usually the result of trauma to the lung or great vessels in the thorax. Other causes include coagulation disorders (most commonly ingestion of anticoagulant rodenticides) and neoplasms that rupture or erode vascular structures. Rarely, pleural hemorrhage may result from lung lobe torsion, pulmonary infarction, and rapid thymic involution.[14, 15]

Clinical Signs

Clinical signs in patients with hemothorax depend on the primary cause of bleeding and other lesions associated with that cause (e.g., trauma, lung lobe torsion, coagulopathy), the volume of blood extravasated into the pleural space, and the rate of accumulation of blood. Generally, in addition to dyspnea and tachypnea, there is evidence of shock with pale mucous membranes, weakness, tachycardia, and poor pulse quality.

Diagnostic Plan

Blood exposed to pleural surfaces clots and defibrinates rapidly.[1] Therefore, unless there is continued bleeding, hemorrhagic effusion fluid should not clot when removed from the chest. Hemorrhagic effusion has the same cellular and protein characteristics as peripheral blood except that it lacks fibrinogen and platelets. If bleeding has occurred over several days, there may also be evidence of erythrophagocytosis on cytologic examination. If bleeding is the result of an eroding tumor, neoplastic cells may be present in the fluid.

History, physical examination, and thoracic radiographs may provide sufficient evidence for the diagnosis of trauma as the cause of the effusion. Laboratory evaluation may or may not be helpful in diagnosis, depending on the underlying cause of the effusion. A complete blood count is often normal if bleeding is acute. With long-standing, slow hemorrhage, evidence of a low-grade, mildly regenerative anemia may be detected. Increased numbers of nucleated RBCs in the absence of significant anemia and reticulocytosis may suggest the presence of hemangiosarcoma. A platelet count and coagulation profile should reveal evidence for anticoagulant rodenticide intoxication or disseminated intravascular coagulation. The biochemical profile may reveal hepatic enzyme elevations that might be associated with acute or chronic disseminated intravascular coagulation. A *Dirofilaria* antigen test should be performed if pulmonary embolism related to heartworms is suspected.

Thoracic radiographs and ultrasonography may be helpful in determining whether a pulmonary mass, mediastinal mass, lung lobe torsion, or pulmonary embolism is present.

Treatment

If the pleural hemorrhage is due to trauma, the primary treatment effort should be directed at reversal of shock and overall stabilization of the patient. Some blood may be removed by needle aspiration from the pleural space if needed to improve respiration; however, fluid pressure in the pleural space may be helpful in terminating the hemorrhage. An indwelling chest tube is not placed in most patients because pleural hemorrhage is usually self-limited and the accumulated blood is rapidly reabsorbed from the pleural space. It is important to remember that trauma sufficient to cause pleural space hemorrhage is likely to cause pulmonary contusions. Therefore, some of the increased respiratory effort may be due to intrapulmonary hemorrhage. Providing an oxygen-enriched environment with an oxygen cage or nasal oxygen catheter may markedly improve oxygenation and reduce distress in these patients. If pleural hemorrhage continues despite good conservative management, an exploratory thoracotomy may be performed in an attempt to locate and ligate bleeding vessels. Unfortunately, such procedures are rarely productive.

If pleural hemorrhage is secondary to a coagulation disorder or bleeding neoplasm, the patient should be stabilized and treatment should then be directed at correcting the primary cause. Therapy for coagulation disorders may include transfusion with whole blood or plasma, administration of vitamin K_1 (1.0–2.5 mg/kg SC every 12 hours) for anticoagulant rodenticide intoxication, or administration of heparin (50–150 U/kg SC or IV every 6 hours) if disseminated intravascular coagulation is suspected (see Chap. 44). Bleeding neoplasms or significant bleeding associated with thymic involution may require surgical excision to terminate hemorrhage.[15]

Chylous Effusion

Chylothorax is the presence of intestinal lymph (chyle) in the pleural space.[3]

Pathophysiology

Chylous effusion results from the leakage of intestinal lymph into the pleural space from disrupted, obstructed, or abnormal thoracic lymph channels.[3] Occult traumatic thoracic duct rupture is often suspected as the underlying cause of chylothorax. However, lymphangiography has been used to demonstrate that many patients with chylothorax have lymphangiectasia of the anterior mediastinal portion of the thoracic duct secondary to obstruction of thoracic duct flow into the anterior vena cava.[16, 17] Intrathoracic neoplasms (particularly anterior mediastinal lymphoma), cardiac disorders (dirofilariasis, cardiomyop-

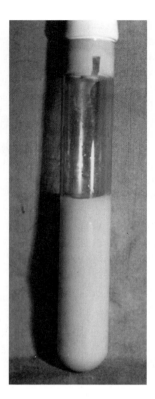

Figure 53–5
Specimen of chylous effusion exhibiting the milky appearance typical of this type of fluid.

athy), hyperthyroidism, and anterior vena cava thrombosis may also cause chylous pleural effusion. Weight loss and low peripheral lymphocyte counts occur because the high-fat chyle and lymphocytes returning from the gut-associated lymphoid tissue are deposited in the pleural space rather than being channeled into the systemic vascular circulation.

Clinical Signs

Clinical signs usually develop gradually because of the slow accumulation of the fluid. In addition to respiratory distress, cough is more likely to occur with chylothorax than with other types of pleural effusion.[18] Additional clinical signs include weight loss, fatigue, and polydipsia.[18, 19] Afghan hounds[19, 20] and Siamese cats[18, 20] appear to be predisposed to the development of chylothorax.

Diagnostic Plan

Fluid analysis is usually sufficient to confirm the diagnosis of chylothorax. Chyle has a characteristic opaque, milky-white appearance (Fig. 53–5). Initially, cellularity is moderate, with small lymphocytes predominating. There may also be variable numbers of RBCs and macrophages and mesothelial cells containing fat vacuoles. Chyle is irritating to the pleura, and over time more RBCs and inflammatory cells are present in the fluid. If refrigerated or centrifuged, chyle may form a "cream layer" on the surface of the sample. A Sudan III–stained sample may demonstrate chylomicrons. Triglyceride levels in chyle are often quite high, and the fluid cholesterol/triglyceride ratio should be less than 1.[21] Other suggestive laboratory findings include a low circulating lymphocyte count, low serum protein level, and negative intestinal fat absorption test. Occasional patients with chylothorax have hyponatremia and hyperkalemia (pseudohypoadrenocorticism).[22]

After confirming that the fluid is chylous, further diagnostic efforts should be directed at attempting to identify a specific cause of the effusion. Plain film radiographs usually demonstrate bilateral pleural effusion; however, unilateral disease may occasionally be present. Radiography and thoracic or cardiac ultrasonography may also help to identify evidence of occult trauma, underlying cardiac or neoplastic disease, or diaphragmatic hernia. Lymphangiography or lymphoscintigraphy can be performed at some university and specialist veterinary hospitals to identify anterior mediastinal lymphangiectasia.[16, 17, 20, 23] A test for adult *Dirofilaria* antigen should be performed in patients residing in areas where heartworm is endemic. A serum thyroxine measurement should be obtained in cats older than 6 years of age.

Treatment

Treatment should be aggressive, because chyle is extremely irritating to pleural surfaces and chronic chylothorax can lead to fibrotic pleuritis with severe respiratory compromise despite elimination of chyle accumulation.[24] If an underlying disease is identified, treatment should be directed at that specific cause. For the remaining patients with idiopathic chylothorax, a number of treatment strategies have been suggested. Conservative medical management consists of removal of the chylous fluid intermittently as needed for 4 to 6 weeks to improve respiration and allow any suspected lymphatic leak to seal. Although chyle is believed to inhibit bacterial growth, pyothorax has been an occasional complication of frequent pleural aspiration in patients with chylothorax. Therefore, strict aseptic technique should be followed during pleural aspiration to avoid introducing infectious materials into the pleural space. Pleurodesis with tetracycline compounds and other sclerosing agents has also been variably successful in resolving chronic recurrent chylous effusion.[25–27]

Surgical approaches to primary therapy include ligation of the thoracic duct, cyanoacrylate obstruction of the cisterna chyli, circumaortic ligation of the cisterna chyli, mesh fenestration of the diaphragm, and installation of a pleurovenous or pleural-peritoneal shunt.[16, 20, 28–31] These procedures are reasonably difficult to perform, are associated with a high complication rate, and generally result in poor long-term management of the problem.[18, 29] Surgical intervention to improve lung expansion by lung decortication in patients with chronic fibrosing pleuritis secondary to chronic chylothorax has been similarly unsuccessful.[32]

A medical approach to the treatment of chylothorax using a commercially available benzopyrone compound is currently under study. Benzopyrone compounds increase proteolysis by tissue macrophages, thus aiding in removal of proteinaceous fluids. The reduction in protein content allows better reabsorption of fluid and reduces inflammation and fibrosis in the surrounding tissue. In controlled trials in humans, 5,6-benzo-[α]-pyrone (1,2-benzopyrone) was effective in reducing chronic lymphedema of the limbs.[33] We are currently using the benzopyrone compound rutin at 50 mg/kg by mouth every 8 hours in both dogs and cats with chylothorax. The compound is apparently tasteless and can be easily mixed with food. Preliminary results suggest that this compound may resolve some cases of chylothorax and reduce the rate of chyle accumulation in others. In one benzopyrone-treated patient with unresolved disease that subsequently underwent thoracic duct ligation, the fibrosing pleuritis usually seen with chronic chylous effusion was absent.

Dietary management with a low-fat diet supplemented with medium-chain triglyceride oil has been considered an important adjunct to both medical and surgical treatment of patients with chylothorax. However, experimental studies in dogs demonstrate that the fat content of the diet does not affect the rate of production of thoracic duct chyle and that medium-chain triglyceride oil is absorbed by intestinal lymphatics and appears in thoracic duct lymph.[34] Therefore, because of the weight loss frequently associated with this condition, our current recommendation is to feed a nutritionally balanced, high-quality diet that the patient eats readily.

Prognosis

The prognosis for patients with secondary chylothorax depends on accurate identification of the underlying cause of the effusion and whether it can be managed successfully. For patients with idiopathic chylothorax, the prognosis is fair to guarded, depending on the success of medical or surgical management strategies. Once fibrosing pleuritis has developed, the prognosis is poor.

Neoplastic Effusion

A neoplastic effusion may have characteristics of an obstructive, chylous, or hemorrhagic effusion with neoplastic cells present among the other cell types on cytologic examination. However, not all neoplasms exfoliate cells into pleural fluid, so the absence of neoplastic cells does not rule out neoplasia as the underlying cause of the effusion.

Pathophysiology

Tumors produce effusion by obstruction or invasion of vascular or lymphatic channels. Some types of carcinomas incite a pronounced inflammatory response causing increased pleural vascular permeability. These tumors often exfoliate neoplastic cells readily into the fluid. Anterior mediastinal lymphosarcoma is the most common cause of neoplastic pleural effusion in the cat (see later discussion). Other neoplastic effusions in both dogs and cats are usually caused by intrathoracic epithelial tissue tumors, including primary lung tumors or metastatic tumors from mammary or intra-abdominal carcinomas or adenocarcinomas. Mesothelioma is an occasional cause of neoplastic pleural effusion.[35, 36] Mesenchymal tumors (osteosarcoma, fibrosarcoma) rarely produce a pleural effusion.

Clinical Signs

In addition to dyspnea, the clinical signs of neoplastic effusion are related to the primary tumor causing the effusion. In some patients with anterior mediastinal lymphoma, the mediastinal mass makes the anterior thorax stiff and incompressible on palpation.[6] In a few, the mass may impinge on the esophagus, causing regurgitation or, rarely, compressing the trachea and causing a cough or further respiratory distress. The degree of pulmonary compromise caused by primary and metastatic lung tumors depends on their type, location, and size. Coughing as a result of pulmonary or mediastinal neoplasia may be present in some patients. Obvious extrathoracic neoplastic masses such as thoracic wall masses or mammary tumors may be observed in some animals. In others, the primary neoplasm may be small and cause no obvious clinical signs, making it difficult to locate. Concurrent peritoneal effusion may be found in some animals with neoplastic disease.[37]

Diagnostic Plan

The cytologic preparation should be scanned carefully for neoplastic cells if neoplasia is suspected. Eosinophilia of the fluid is suggestive of neoplasia and should prompt a thorough search for tumor cells.[8] Large, abnormal lymphoblasts with a basophilic cytoplasm are characteristic of anterior mediastinal lymphoma (Fig. 53–6). Carcinomas and adenocarcinoma cells may exfoliate in large clusters, which may sometimes be seen grossly as granular material settling out in the specimen tube[4] (Fig. 53–7). When a cytologic preparation is made, these larger clumps may be pushed to the feathered edge of the smear. One should be cautious when evaluating cells for malignant characteristics, because all types of pleural inflammation incite exfoliation of reactive mesothelial cells into pleural fluid and it is tempting to interpret these active mesothelial cells as neoplastic ones.[35]

Thoracic radiography should be performed with two lateral views to fully evaluate the lung fields for mass lesions indicative of primary or metastatic neoplasia. Ultrasonography is most helpful in evaluating the anterior mediastinum or pericardium, heart, and great vessels for abnormalities. Abdominal radiographs and ultrasonography may be used to survey intra-abdominal organs for neoplasia.

Laboratory testing may be helpful in locating the site of an occult primary neoplasm. A complete blood count may reveal unsuspected blood loss or anemia of chronic inflammation. An increased number of nucleated RBCs without an obvious regenerative reticulocyte response in a patient with a hemorrhagic effusion should raise the possibility of hemangiosarcoma. A coagulation profile may also demonstrate evidence of low-grade disseminated intravascular coagulation in these patients. Many cats with anterior mediastinal lymphoma have FeLV antigenemia and may show evidence of severe anemia or other hematologic effects of this viral infection.

Biochemical profiles may suggest hepatic or other organ system involvement. Additional aspiration cytology or biopsy specimens can be taken from other obvious masses or those detected with radiography

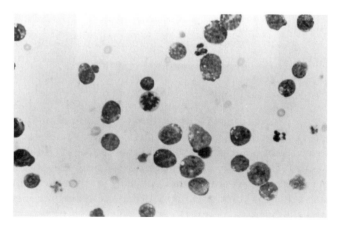

Figure 53–6
Cytologic preparation of neoplastic pleural effusion from a 2-year-old domestic longhair cat with anterior mediastinal lymphoma. The predominant cell type is the large lymphoblast. A mitotic figure can be seen in the center of the field (×1000).

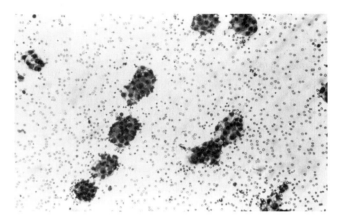

Figure 53–7
Cytologic preparation of neoplastic pleural effusion from a
12-year-old Burmese cat with pulmonary adenocarcinoma.
Large clusters of neoplastic carcinoma cells are present
in a background of red blood cells and occasional neutrophils, macrophages, and lymphocytes (×250).

and ultrasonography to try to better define the origin
of the effusion.

Treatment and Prognosis

The treatment and prognosis for patients with
neoplastic effusions depend on the tumor type and size
and the extent of intrathoracic and extrathoracic
involvement. Both radiation and chemotherapy have
been used to obtain long-term remissions in cats with
anterior mediastinal lymphoma. Pleural metastasis is
widespread by the time neoplastic effusion is recognized in patients with carcinomas, adenocarcinomas,
or mesotheliomas. However, intrapleural administration of radioactive colloids or cisplatin alone or
combined with systemic chemotherapy, surgical debulking, or pleurodesis has produced prolonged
symptom-free remissions in some patients with neoplastic disease.[38, 39] Mast cell neoplasia may respond to
combined systemic chemotherapy. Hemangiosarcomas respond poorly to any type of intervention, and
because of respiratory compromise and the debilitating
effects of repeated episodes of bleeding, the long-term
prognosis for these patients is poor.

Pneumothorax

Pneumothorax is defined as the accumulation
of air or gas in the pleural space. In most patients
air accumulates in both hemithoraces, but the accumulation may occasionally be unilateral.[40] Traumatic
pneumothorax occurs with similar frequency in cats
and dogs. Pneumothorax secondary to pulmonary or
pleural disease is most common in middle-aged,
deep-chested dogs of large breeds and occurs rarely
in cats.[40]

Pathophysiology

The most common cause of pneumothorax is
thoracic trauma with or without penetration of the
thoracic wall.[2, 41, 42] Pneumothorax may also be due to
tracheal trauma, the presence of a bronchopleural
fistula, spontaneous rupture of a pulmonary bulla or
bleb, or an intrapulmonary or pleural diagnostic or
surgical procedure.[43, 44] Air may be introduced into the
pleural space after rupture of a pulmonary abscess or
may be secondary to bacterial, parasitic, or granulomatous pneumonia, neoplasia, or dirofilariasis.[44, 45]
Occasionally, pneumothorax may appear spontaneously without any obvious underlying cause.[40, 41]

Clinical Signs

The primary clinical sign of pneumothorax is
dyspnea. Experimental studies have suggested that
pulmonary distress may not become evident until the
volume of pneumothorax is greater than 150% of the
total lung volume.[46] Dyspnea may be acute or slowly
progressive, depending on the rate of air accumulation
in the thorax.[43] Patients with tension pneumothorax
may appear to have a distended thoracic cage, but little
thoracic wall motion is noted during breathing efforts.[40] Other clinical signs and evidence of injury may
be present in traumatized patients.[41] A history of cough
or prior evaluation for a primary pulmonary or pleural
disease may be present when pneumothorax results
from these disorders.

Diagnostic Plan

Thoracic radiographic examination demonstrates retraction of the lung borders from the chest
wall and increased lucency in the pleural space.[41] The
cardiac silhouette often appears to be elevated off the
sternum in the lateral radiographic view. Other signs of
thoracic trauma, such as pulmonary contusions or rib
fractures, may also be present[42] (Fig. 53–8). The
airways and pulmonary parenchyma should be examined carefully for lesions that may be the underlying
cause of the development of pneumothorax; however,
pulmonary bullae may be small and difficult to
visualize[40] (Fig. 53–9). Needle thoracentesis confirms
the presence of air in the pleural space and should
significantly alleviate dyspnea.

Treatment

Intermittent aspiration of air from the pleural
space is often all that is required to treat pneumothorax
related to blunt trauma in most patients. Most of these
traumatically induced lesions heal spontaneously in a
short period of time.[42] If penetrating wounds are
present, they should be cleaned and the thoracic wall
sealed by skin coverage and bandaging until the

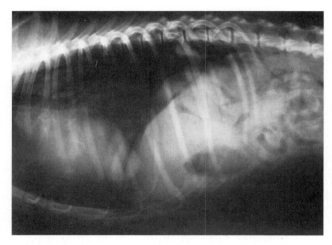

Figure 53-8
Lateral radiograph of a 4-year-old mixed breed dog with pneumothorax and diaphragmatic hernia caused by vehicular trauma. A loop of intestine can be seen in the posterior thorax overlying the heart and diaphragm.

patient is stable and definitive repair can be performed. If significant pleural air accumulation continues after 24 to 48 hours of intermittent aspiration, an indwelling chest tube and continuous pleural drainage system should be used to maintain the patient comfortably and provide an opportunity for healing of the air leak.[42] If air accumulation continues after an additional 24 to 48 hours, surgical exploration of the thorax to discover and correct the source of the leak should be considered.[2, 40]

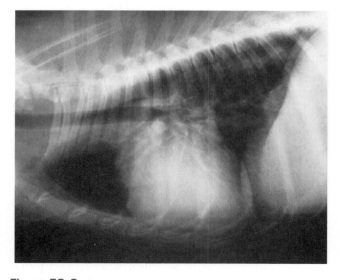

Figure 53-9
Lateral radiograph of a 5-year-old terrier with pulmonary bullae.

Prognosis

The prognosis for most patients with traumatic and spontaneous pneumothorax without underlying disease is excellent.[46] The prognosis for patients with pneumothorax secondary to a primary pulmonary or pleural disease depends on the ability to control the primary disorder adequately.

Diaphragmatic Hernia

The most frequent cause of a soft tissue mass in the pleural space is traumatically induced diaphragmatic hernia.[47] Congenital diaphragmatic hernias also occur occasionally.[48]

Some or most of the abdominal contents may be displaced into the pleural space, depending on the size of the tear in the diaphragm and the nature of the trauma (Fig. 53–10).

Pathophysiology

Blunt trauma to the abdomen or lower thorax produces an acute, dramatic increase in intra-abdominal pressure. This results in diaphragmatic rupture with herniation of intra-abdominal organs into the pleural space. The lateral sides of the diaphragm seem to be most susceptible to tearing. The size and location of the tear determine which abdominal organs herniate into the pleural space. Dyspnea occurs because of displacement of lung by the herniated organs. Other signs develop depending on the extent of herniation and the organs involved.

Clinical Signs

Clinical signs associated with a diaphragmatic hernia depend on the type and volume of the herniated organ, the amount of associated trauma, and the secondary effects of the herniation. In acute cases, external signs of trauma are usually present and the herniation may be recognized because of evaluation of the traumatized patient for dyspnea. If dyspnea is not present initially, diaphragmatic herniation may not be recognized until this or other signs appear. Herniation of the stomach or intestines may cause regurgitation, vomiting, or signs of intestinal obstruction. Herniation of the liver may produce vomiting or icterus and pleural effusion. If strangulation of the herniated organs occurs, severe signs of dysfunction may appear acutely even though the herniation may be of long standing. Physical examination usually reveals dyspnea with dullness unilaterally or bilaterally in the ventral thorax. Cardiac sounds may be muffled or shifted in position, and borborygmi may be auscultated in the thorax. Abdominal palpation may be unremarkable or the abdomen may seem relatively

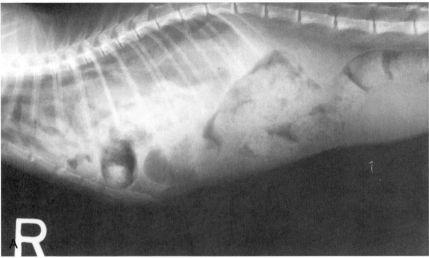

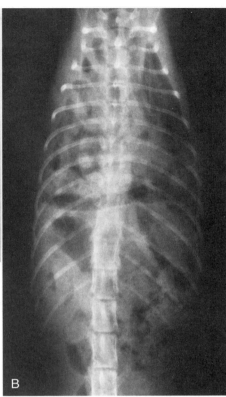

Figure 53–10
(A) Lateral and **(B)** dorsoventral radiographs of a 4-year-old domestic short-hair cat with a traumatically induced diaphragmatic hernia. Note that most of the abdominal viscera have been displaced into the thoracic cavity.

empty of contents, depending on the amount and type of organ displacement.

Diagnostic Plan

The patient with a diaphragmatic hernia usually has a history or physical evidence of trauma. The results of hematologic and biochemical studies are nonspecific and reflect the effects of trauma and associated organ or system damage caused by the herniation. Urinalyses are usually unremarkable. Thoracic radiographs demonstrate lack of definition of the diaphragmatic shadow with increased soft tissue density in one or both sides of the pleural space. The presence of gas pockets within the density suggests displacement of the stomach or intestine, and this can be confirmed by contrast gastrointestinal radiography.[47, 49] Ultrasonography can be also used to determine the nature of the soft tissue density within the pleural space.[50]

Treatment

Surgery is required to replace the herniated organs and close the tear in the diaphragm. Repair of a diaphragmatic hernia is usually done by an abdominal approach unless the hernia is of long standing and extensive intrathoracic adhesions are present. Unless dyspnea is itself life threatening or there is another reason to explore the abdomen (e.g., suspected splenic rupture, renal avulsion), the patient with acute diaphragmatic herniation should be stabilized before surgical intervention.[47] Supportive care for these patients includes avoiding stress and handling, maintenance fluid administration, treatment for associated traumatic injuries, and improvement of oxygenation by providing supplemental oxygen with an oxygen cage or nasal oxygen catheter.

Prognosis

Depending on the extent of other traumatic injuries, most patients with diaphragmatic hernia have an excellent prognosis after surgical correction of the defect.

Less Common Space-Occupying Masses of the Pleural Space

Masses arising from or on the chest wall may expand into the pleural space. These masses include tumors of the chest wall (chondrosarcoma, osteosarcoma, hemangiosarcoma), benign bone lesions (osteochondroma), osteomyelitis (coccidioidomycosis, blastomycosis), abscesses, and foreign body granulomas. These masses may occasionally erode into the pleural space or rupture, causing pleural effusion that may mask their presence. These lesions are diagnosed by radiography, fine-needle aspiration, or biopsy.

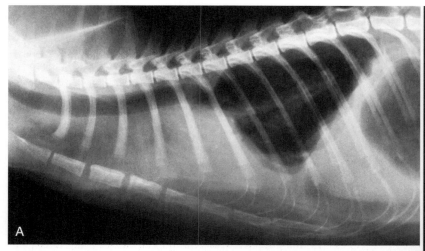

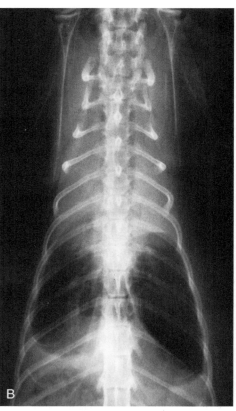

Figure 53–11
(A) Lateral and **(B)** dorsoventral radiographs of a 2-year-old domestic shorthair cat with anterior mediastinal lymphoma and pleural effusion.

Diseases of the Mediastinum

Anterior Mediastinal Lymphosarcoma

Anterior mediastinal lymphosarcoma is one of the most common forms of lymphoma in the cat, with cats younger than 3 years of age more commonly affected.[51] The mediastinal mass in cats is usually accompanied by malignant pleural effusion[51, 52] (Fig. 53–11). In dogs, the thymus and anterior mediastinal lymph nodes are rarely the primary site of lymphosarcoma, but these structures may be involved in patients with multicentric lymphoma.

Pathophysiology

Anterior mediastinal lymphosarcoma often results from malignant transformation of the thymus, although both anterior or posterior mediastinal lymph nodes may be involved. This form of lymphoma is found predominantly in young animals in which the thymus has not yet involuted, and the majority of these tumors are of the T lymphocyte type. FeLV apparently triggers the malignant lymphoid transformation in many patients, and more than 80% of cats with this form of lymphosarcoma have positive blood or serum tests for FeLV antigen. The physical effects of the tumor depend on the size of the tumor, the presence and amount of associated pleural fluid, and the systemic impact of FeLV infection on other body systems. Larger tumors are more likely to compress adjacent mediastinal structures such as the trachea and esophagus and extend laterally and posteriorly, compressing lung parenchyma. A smaller tumor may be associated with a large volume of pleural fluid, causing equally severe signs of respiratory distress.

Clinical Signs

Clinical signs are variable and depend on the size of the anterior mediastinal mass and the presence of pleural effusion.[51] Dyspnea and tachypnea are the most common signs, but cough may also be present because of compression of the trachea. Occasional patients exhibit regurgitation because of compression of the esophagus. Horner's syndrome is a rare sign. Additional nonspecific findings include lethargy, anorexia, and weight loss. Auscultation usually reveals a pleural fluid line, and the heart sounds may be dulled and displaced dorsocaudally. The anterior thorax may be incompressible. Perihilar and sternal lymphadenopathy is present in some patients; however, peripheral lymph nodes are usually not involved in this form of lymphoma.

Diagnostic Plan

Most cats with anterior mediastinal lymphosarcoma have concurrent FeLV infection.[51] Because of this, laboratory findings are variable and may reflect the effects of the virus rather than the neoplastic disease. The most common hematologic finding is normocytic, normochromic, nonresponsive anemia. Biochemical profiles are often normal unless the neoplastic effusion is chylous in type. Urinalyses are usually unremarkable.

Thoracentesis usually reveals an obstructive type of effusion containing predominantly large neoplastic lymphoblasts. Other cell types include a variable number of RBCs, a few small lymphocytes, and occasional macrophages and neutrophils. An occasional patient with anterior mediastinal lymphoma has a chylous effusion.[52] Neoplastic lymphocytes are usually present in fluid from patients with lymphoma, whereas in patients with the more usual chylous effusion, small lymphocytes predominate.

Thoracic radiographs taken after fluid removal demonstrate an anterior mediastinal mass of variable size that may displace the trachea dorsally and the heart and lungs caudally. If fluid cytology does not confirm the diagnosis, fine-needle aspiration may be performed on the mediastinal mass. Ultrasonography may further characterize the mass and direct biopsy efforts.[50] "Blind" core needle biopsies are not recommended in this area because of the presence of a number of large vascular structures.

Treatment

Many different combination chemotherapy protocols have been described for cats with anterior mediastinal lymphoma. The most commonly used regimen consists of cyclophosphamide (50 mg/m^2 by mouth every 48 hours), vincristine (0.7 mg/m^2 IV every 7 days), cytosine arabinoside (50 mg/m^2 SC b.i.d. for 2 days), and prednisone (50 mg/m^2 by mouth once a day for 1 week, then 25 mg/m^2 every 48 hours) with or without the addition of L-asparaginase.[53, 54] External beam radiation therapy is a useful adjunct to chemotherapy in these patients, because this type of lymphoma is quite radiosensitive, and rapid reduction in tumor size and significant improvement in respiration can be achieved after only one or two radiation treatments.[54]

Prognosis

The long-term prognosis for all patients with anterior mediastinal lymphoma is grave because the disease is ultimately fatal. Extended remissions have been achieved with combination chemotherapy and radiation. Cats with concurrent FeLV infection may develop other manifestations of FeLV-related disease (e.g., nonresponsive anemia, chronic infections) during the course of therapy that complicate successful treatment.

Thymoma

Thymomas are usually benign neoplasms arising from the thymic epithelial cells in dogs and cats.[55–57] This tumor occurs most commonly in middle-aged to older animals. In dogs, females and large breeds predominate.[55, 56]

Pathophysiology

Thymomas arise from any of the epithelial components of the thymus gland. Most thymomas are benign and do not metastasize to distant sites. Clinical signs arise because the tumors surround, invade, or displace other important intramediastinal structures. Myasthenia gravis may develop concurrently with thymoma in humans, dogs, and cats and may be the primary cause of clinical signs in these patients. It has been suggested that this occurs because the neoplastic thymus is producing high levels of antibodies against acetylcholine receptors.[58]

Clinical Signs

Clinical signs are usually related to the presence of an anterior mediastinal mass and associated disorders including pleural effusion; invasion of or impingement on the great vessels, nerves, or other structures in the anterior mediastinum; and myasthenia gravis. Typical signs include dyspnea, cough, anorexia, regurgitation, dysphagia, lethargy, and dysphonia. Patients with concurrent myasthenia gravis may exhibit regurgitation and generalized muscular weakness.[58] Animals with anterior mediastinal vascular invasion may exhibit edema of the head, neck, and forelimbs.[55] The apex cardiac sound may be shifted to the right side of the chest on auscultation. Patients with pleural effusion may have muffled cardiac and lung sounds in the ventral thorax.[59]

Diagnostic Plan

Hematologic and biochemical findings and urinalysis are nonspecific and usually reflect the age of the animal. Hypercalcemia has been reported in a few patients. FeLV and FIV tests are usually negative in affected cats.[55, 59] Thoracic radiographs reveal a variable-sized mass in the anterior mediastinum. Megaesophagus may be present in some patients. Ultrasonography may demonstrate a lobulated solid or partially cystic mass. Fine-needle aspirates from a thymoma contain a mixed population of thymic epithelial cells that may be accompanied by small lymphocytes, occasional mast cells, and RBCs.[59] Because of the variation of cell types within the mass, malignancy cannot be accurately assessed by fine-needle aspiration cytology. Ultrasound-guided core biopsy or surgical biopsy may be required for diagnosis in some patients and can be used to evaluate the tumor for malignant characteristics. Patients with myasthenia gravis as an associated disorder usually have high serum concentrations of antibodies against acetylcholine receptors (see Chap. 28).[58]

Treatment

Surgical removal is the treatment of choice for thymomas and may be curative. However, complete excision is difficult because even benign masses may be quite locally invasive.[59] Regional lymph nodes should be removed at the time of surgery and assessed for the presence of metastasis. Radiation therapy has been used alone or as an adjunct to surgical treatment either to reduce the size of the thymic mass before surgery or as a follow-up after incomplete surgical removal. Myasthenia gravis may resolve spontaneously after removal of the thymoma. Corticosteroids and cholinesterase inhibitors have been used to treat patients with concurrent myasthenia gravis before surgery, and this therapy is continued for patients in which myasthenia persists.[58]

Prognosis

The prognosis for patients with an uncomplicated thymoma that can be completely removed surgically is good, because most of these tumors are benign and do not recur after complete removal. If the thymoma is highly invasive, the prognosis is poor because complete excision is rarely possible. Adjunctive radiation therapy after surgery prolongs survival and improves the prognosis to fair for these patients. Animals with persistent myasthenia gravis are more difficult to manage, and the prognosis for these patients is guarded.

Mediastinal Hemorrhage

Spontaneous hemorrhage into the mediastinum is rare. Mediastinal hemorrhage is usually secondary to trauma or a generalized systemic bleeding disorder.[1, 60, 61]

Pathophysiology

Hemorrhage into the mediastinum most commonly is caused by thoracic trauma with rupture of intramediastinal blood vessels or is secondary to systemic bleeding disorders including anticoagulant rodenticide intoxication.[1] Less common causes include neoplastic erosion of blood vessels, intrathoracic surgery, and spontaneous, rapid thymic involution.[15]

Because the pleural membranes forming the mediastinal space are thin, blood often escapes from this space, resulting in hemothorax.

Clinical Signs

Dyspnea, pale mucous membranes, and hypovolemic shock are common signs in patients with significant acute mediastinal hemorrhage. Hemothorax and pulmonary hemorrhage are often associated findings and magnify dyspnea by further respiratory compromise.[15] Obvious external signs of trauma may be present in some patients. Hemorrhage into other body cavities or from external body orifices may be present in patients with coagulopathies. Other clinical signs are variable and depend on the primary disease process underlying mediastinal hemorrhage.

Diagnostic Plan

Thoracic auscultation and percussion may demonstrate dullness in the anterior ventral thorax, compatible with pleural fluid or an anterior mediastinal mass. Ultrasonography may reveal free fluid or blood clots within the mediastinal space. Aspiration with cytologic examination of the recovered fluid produces blood that does not clot if hemorrhage has been present for at least several hours. Coagulation studies should be performed for patients with suspected generalized bleeding disorders.

Treatment

Most patients with traumatic mediastinal hemorrhage can be treated conservatively with rest, fluid administration, and supplemental oxygen if required. If bleeding has been severe, transfusion may be necessary to stabilize the patient. If the cause of mediastinal hemorrhage can be corrected (e.g., trauma, coagulopathies), bleeding stops and surgical intervention is not required. Traumatic rupture of larger blood vessels, bleeding tumors, and a rapidly involuting thymus may require surgical exploration and ligation or mass removal to stop the hemorrhage.[15] Blood remaining in the mediastinal space is usually rapidly reabsorbed into the systemic circulation.

Prognosis

If the underlying cause of bleeding can be discovered and corrected, the prognosis for patients with mediastinal hemorrhage is excellent.

Uncommon Mediastinal Masses

Lymph nodes in the mediastinum may be involved in primary malignant (e.g., lymphoma) or metastatic neoplastic processes. Carcinomas of the head and neck frequently metastasize to this area.

Mediastinal nodes may be enlarged secondary to immunologic stimulation or invasion by infectious organisms from the lung, particularly the systemic mycotic agents. Lymph nodes may also be enlarged in association with noninfectious inflammatory pulmonary disorders such as eosinophilic granulomatosis or lymphoid granulomatosis. Pyogenic infection limited to the mediastinum (mediastinitis) is rare and usually occurs after introduction of infectious materials via tracheal or esophageal perforation. Thyroid carcinomas and chemodectomas are occasionally found in the mediastinal space; other tumors are rare in this location. Benign cysts of pleural, branchial, lymphatic, bronchogenic, or thymic origin may also rarely occur in the mediastinum.

Pneumomediastinum

Pneumomediastinum is defined as the presence of air within the mediastinal space.[62]

Pathophysiology

The most common causes of pneumomediastinum are thoracic trauma and cervical trauma, particularly related to bite wounds.[62] Air may escape into the mediastinum from the trachea, after esophageal rupture, or after rupture of alveoli or bronchi. Subcutaneous and retroperitoneal emphysema frequently accompanies pneumomediastinum caused by cervical lacerations, bite wounds, or tracheal rupture. Iatrogenic pneumomediastinum may be associated with accidental tracheal perforation during venipuncture, transtracheal aspiration, tracheal surgery, endotracheal intubation (with overinflation of the endotracheal tube cuff), overinflation of the lung during positive pressure ventilation, esophageal endoscopy, foreign body removal, or surgery.[62] Spontaneous pneumomediastinum has been reported after severe episodes of sneezing, coughing, vomiting, or exercise and in association with the rupture of pulmonary cysts, blebs, abscesses, granulomas, or neoplasms. Rare causes include infection with gas-forming organisms, respiratory distress, and idiopathic causes.

Clinical Signs

Clinical signs of pneumomediastinum are frequently absent unless secondary disorders (e.g., pneumothorax, pleural effusion, lung contusion, mediastinitis resulting from esophageal perforation, bronchoesophageal fistula) are present.

Diagnostic Plan

Findings on physical examination that suggest the presence of pneumomediastinum include subcutaneous emphysema and the presence of cervical lacerations. Thoracic radiography confirms the diagnosis. Pneumomediastinum is best visualized in the lateral radiographic view; the key to recognition is that structures not normally seen on thoracic radiographs can be well visualized because the air surrounding them provides contrast with these water-dense structures[62] (see Fig. 53–2B). With pneumomediastium the esophagus, aortic branches, central vena cava, and azygos vein can often be well delineated.[63] In addition, both the internal and external surfaces of the tracheal walls, peribronchial lymph nodes, and sternal lymph nodes may be well outlined. Radiographs may also demonstrate the extent of subcutaneous emphysema or pneumoretroperitoneum.[63]

Treatment

Treatment for pneumomediastinum secondary to trauma is not necessary; however, associated problems (shock, pulmonary contusion, pneumothorax, tracheal rupture, cervical lacerations) should be managed appropriately. Other causes (e.g., gas-forming infections, esophageal perforations) also require specific treatment.

Prognosis

The prognosis for patients with uncomplicated traumatic pneumomediastinum is excellent, and most cases resolve spontaneously in 10 to 14 days. The prognosis for patients with pneumomediastinum secondary to other diseases depends on the ability to control the primary disorder underlying pneumomediastinum.

References

1. Forrester SD, Troy GC, Fossum TW. Pleural effusions: Pathophysiology and diagnostic considerations. Compen Contin Educ Pract Vet 1988;10:121–135.
2. Yoshioka MM. Management of spontaneous pneumothorax in twelve dogs. J Am Anim Hosp Assoc 1982;18:57–62.
3. Fossum TW. Feline chylothorax. Compen Contin Educ Pract Vet 1993;15:549–567.
4. Steyn PF, Wittum TE. Radiographic, epidemiologic, and clinical aspects of simultaneous pleural and peritoneal effusions in dogs and cats. J Am Vet Med Assoc 1993;202:307–312.
5. Meyer DJ, Franks PT. Effusion: Classification and cytologic examination. Compen Contin Educ Pract Vet 1987;9:123–128.
6. Forrester SD. The categories and causes of pleural effusion in cats. Vet Med 1988;83:894–906.
7. Montgomery RD, Henderson RA, Powers RD, et al. Retrospective study of 26 primary tumors of the osseous thoracic wall in dogs. J Am Anim Hosp Assoc 1993;29:68–72.
8. Fossum TW, Wellman M, Relford RL, et al. Eosinophilic pleural or peritoneal effusion in dogs and cats: 14 cases (1986–1992). J Am Vet Med Assoc 1993;202:1873–1876.

9. Cantwell HD, Rebar AH, Allen AR. Pleural effusion in the dog: Principles for diagnosis. J Am Anim Hosp Assoc 1983;19:227–232.

10. Fooshee SK. Managing the cat with septic pleural effusion. Vet Med 1988;83:907–913.

11. Turner WD, Breznock EM. Continuous suction drainage for management of canine pyothorax—A retrospective study. J Am Anim Hosp Assoc 1988;24:485–496.

12. Withrow SJ. Closed chest tube drainage and lavage for treatment of pyothorax in the cat. J Am Anim Hosp Assoc 1975;11:90–94.

13. Marino DJ, Jaggy A. Nocardiosis: A literature review with selected case reports in two dogs. J Vet Intern Med 1993;7:4–11.

14. Johnston GR, Feeney DA, O'Brien TD, et al. Recurring lung lobe torsion in three Afghan hounds. J Am Vet Med Assoc 1984;184:842–845.

15. Klopfer U, Perl S, Yokobson B, et al. Spontaneous fatal hemorrhage in the involuting thymus in dogs. J Am Anim Hosp Assoc 1985;21:261–264.

16. Birchard SJ, Cantwell HD, Bright RM. Lymphangiography and ligation of the canine thoracic duct: A study in normal dogs and three dogs with chylothorax. J Am Anim Hosp Assoc 1982;18:769–777.

17. Hodges CC, Fossum TW, Komkov A, et al. Lymphoscintigraphy in healthy dogs and dogs with experimentally created thoracic duct abnormalities. Am J Vet Res 1992;53:1048–1053.

18. Fossum TW, Forrester SD, Swenson CL, et al. Chylothorax in cats: 37 cases (1969–1989). J Am Vet Med Assoc 1991;198:672–678.

19. Fossum TW, Birchard SJ, Jacobs RM. Chylothorax in 34 dogs. J Am Vet Med Assoc 1986;188:1315–1318.

20. Birchard SJ, Smeak DD, Fossum TW. Results of thoracic duct ligation in dogs with chylothorax. J Am Vet Med Assoc 1988;193:68–71.

21. Fossum TW, Jacobs RM, Birchard SJ. Evaluation of cholesterol and triglyceride concentrations in differentiating chylous and nonchylous pleural effusions in dogs and cats. J Am Vet Med Assoc 1986;188:49–51.

22. Willard MD, Fossum TW, Torrance A, et al. Hyponatremia and hyperkalemia associated with idiopathic or experimentally induced chylothorax in four dogs. J Am Vet Med Assoc 1991;199:353–358.

23. Fossum TW, Birchard SJ. Lymphangiographic evaluation of experimentally induced chylothorax after ligation of the cranial vena cava in dogs. Am J Vet Res 1986;47:967–971.

24. Seuss RP, Flanders JA, Beck KA, et al. Constrictive pleuritis in cats with chylothorax: 10 cases (1983–1991). J Am Anim Hosp Assoc 1994;30:70–77.

25. Laing EJ, Norris AM. Pleurodesis as a treatment for pleural effusion in the dog. J Am Anim Hosp Assoc 1986;22:193–196.

26. Gallagher LA, Birchard SJ, Weisbrode SE. Effects of tetracycline hydrochloride in dogs with induced pleural effusion. Am J Vet Res 1990;51:1682–1687.

27. Birchard SJ, Gallagher L. Use of pleurodesis in treating selected pleural diseases. Compen Contin Educ Pract Vet 1988;10:826–832.

28. Pardo AD. Thoracic duct embolization: Use in canine chylothorax. Vet Med Rep 1989;1:394–398.

29. Rigg DL, Riedesel EA. Circumaortic cysterna chyli ligation. Vet Radiol 1985;26:70–72.

30. Peterson SL, Pion PD, Breznock EM. Passive pleuroperitoneal drainage for management of chylothorax in two cats. J Am Anim Hosp Assoc 1989;25:569–572.

31. Willauer CC, Breznock EM. Pleurovenous shunting technique for treatment of chylothorax in three dogs. J Am Vet Med Assoc 1987;191:1106–1109.

32. Fossum TW, Evering WN, Miller MW, et al. Severe bilateral fibrosing pleuritis associated with chronic chylothorax in five cats and two dogs. J Am Vet Med Assoc 1992;201:317–324.

33. Casley-Smith JR, Morgan RG, Piller NB. Treatment of lymphedema of the arms and legs with 5,6-benzo-[α]-pyrone. N Engl J Med 1993;329:1158–1163.

34. Sikkema DA, McLoughlin MA, Birchard SJ. Effect of dietary fat on thoracic duct lymph volume and composition in dogs. J Vet Intern Med 1993;7:119 (abstract).

35. Morrison WB, Trigo FJ. Clinical characterization of pleural mesothelioma in seven dogs. Compen Contin Educ Pract Vet 1984;6:342–348.

36. Dubielzig RR. Sclerosing mesothelioma in five dogs. J Am Anim Hosp Assoc 1979;15:745–748.

37. Clinkenbeard KD. Diagnostic cytology: Carcinomas in pleural effusions. Compen Contin Educ Pract Vet 1992;14:187–194.

38. Croll MN, Brady LW. Intracavitary uses of colloids. Semin Nucl Med 1979;9:108–113.

39. Moore AS, Kirk C, Cardona A. Intracavitary cisplatin chemotherapy experience with six dogs. J Vet Intern Med 1991;5:227–231.

40. Holtsinger RH, Ellison GW. Spontaneous pneumothorax. Compen Contin Educ Pract Vet 1975;17:197–210.

41. Aron DN, Kornegay JN. The clinical significance of traumatic lung cysts and associated pulmonary abnormalities in the dog and cat. J Am Anim Hosp Assoc 1983;19:903–913.

42. McKiernan BC, Adams WM, Huse DC. Thoracic bite wounds and associated internal injury in 11 dogs and 1 cat. J Am Vet Med Assoc 1984;184:959–964.

43. Waters DJ, Sweet DC. Role of surgery in the management of dogs with pathologic conditions of the thorax. Part I. Compen Contin Educ Pract Vet 1991;13:1545–1550.

44. Dallman MJ, Martin RA, Roth L. Pneumothorax as the primary problem in two cases of bronchoalveolar carcinoma in the dog. J Am Anim Hosp Assoc 1988;24:710–714.

45. Schaer M, Gamble D, Spencer C. Spontaneous pneumothorax associated with bacterial pneumonia in the dog. Two case reports. J Am Anim Hosp Assoc 1981;17:783–788.

46. Bennett RA, Orton EC, Tucker A, et al. Cardiopulmonary changes in conscious dogs with induced progressive pneumothorax. Am J Vet Res 1989;50:280–284.

47. Boudrieau RJ, Muir WW. Pathophysiology of traumatic diaphragmatic hernia in dogs. Compen Contin Educ Pract Vet 1987;9:379–386.

48. Valentine BA, Cooper BJ, Dietze AE, et al. Canine

congenital diaphragmatic hernia. J Vet Intern Med 1988;2:109–112.

49. Stickle RL. Positive contrast celiography (peritoneography) for the diagnosis of diaphragmatic hernia in dogs and cats. J Am Vet Med Assoc 1984;185:295–298.

50. Stowater JL, Lamb CR. Ultrasound of noncardiac thoracic diseases in small animals. J Am Vet Med Assoc 1989;195:514–520.

51. Gruffydd-Jones T, Gaskell CJ, Gibbs C. Clinical and radiological features of anterior mediastinal lymphosarcoma in the cat: A review of 30 cases. Vet Rec 1979;104:304–307.

52. Forrester SD, Fossum TW, Rogers KS. Diagnosis and treatment of chylothorax associated with lymphoblastic lymphosarcoma in four cats. J Am Vet Med Assoc 1991;198:291–294.

53. Cotter SM. Treatment of lymphoma and leukemia with cyclophosphamide, vincristine, and prednisone. II. Treatment of cats. J Am Anim Hosp Assoc 1983;19:166–172.

54. Cuoto GC, Hammer AS. Oncology. In: Sherding RG, ed. The Cat: Diseases and Clinical Management, 2nd ed. New York, Churchill Livingstone, 1994:778–789.

55. Aronson MG, Shunk KL, Carpenter JL, et al. Clinical and pathological features of thymomas in 15 dogs. J Am Vet Med Assoc 1984;184:1355–1362.

56. Bellah JR, Stiff ME, Russell RG. Thymoma in the dog. Two case reports and review of 20 additional cases. J Am Vet Med Assoc 1983;183:306–311.

57. Carpenter JL, Holzworth J. Thymoma in 11 cats. J Am Vet Med Assoc 1982;181:248–251.

58. Kebanow ER. Thymoma and acquired myasthenia gravis in the dog: A case report and review of 13 additional cases. J Am Anim Hosp Assoc 1992;28:63–69.

59. Gores BR, Berg J, Carpenter JL, et al. Surgical treatment of thymoma in cats: 12 cases (1987–1992). J Am Vet Med Assoc 1994;204:1782–1785.

60. Morgan RV. Respiratory emergencies. Part II. Compen Contin Educ Pract Vet 1983;5:305–310.

61. Spackman CJ, Caywood DD, Feeney DA, et al. Thoracic wall and pulmonary trauma in dogs sustaining fractures as a result of motor vehicle accidents. J Am Vet Med Assoc 1984;185:975–977.

62. Fagin BD. A radiographic approach to diagnosing pneumomediastinum. Vet Med 1988;83:571–577.

63. Thrall DE. Dyspnea in the cat: Part II—Radiographic aspects of intrathoracic causes involving the mediastinum. Feline Pract 1978;8:47–57.

Chapter 54

Diseases of the Lower Airways and Lungs

S. Dru Forrester
Martha L. Moon

Anatomy

The lower respiratory passages begin where the trachea bifurcates into the left and right principal (mainstem) bronchi, which divide into lobar bronchi on entering the lung.[1, 2] Each lobar bronchus supplies an individual lung lobe. In dogs and cats, the left lung includes a cranial and a caudal lobe; the cranial lobe is further divided into cranial and caudal parts (Fig. 54–1). The right lung is divided into cranial, middle, caudal, and accessory lobes (Figs. 54–2 and 54–3. Lobar bronchi give rise to numerous segmental bronchi within the pulmonary parenchyma, which further divide into bronchioles. Terminal bronchioles branch to form respiratory bronchioles, which give rise to alveoli, the gas-exchanging units of the lungs. Bronchi are supported by cartilage, whereas bronchioles lack rigidity and are completely surrounded by smooth muscle. The entire tracheobronchial tree is lined by ciliated epithelium, secretory epithelial cells, and submucosal glands. The glands, blood vessels, and smooth muscle of the lower airways are supplied by the sympathetic and parasympathetic branches of the autonomic nervous system.

Physiology

Mucociliary clearance and coughing are protective mechanisms that remove foreign material and secretions from the lower airways and lungs. Cilia of epithelial cells lining the airways beat in a coordinated fashion, moving mucus, particulate matter, and bacteria from the lungs and lower airways toward the pharynx. Sensory receptors located beneath the epithelium in the airways, primarily the larynx, trachea, and bronchi, respond to mechanical, thermal, and chemical stimuli.[3, 4] Afferent nerve fibers from cough receptors enter the vagus and glossopharyngeal nerves, which supply the cough center in the medulla. Efferent fibers of the cough reflex are carried through the vagus, phrenic, recurrent laryngeal, and some spinal nerves to the larynx, diaphragm, tracheobronchial tree, and expiratory muscles. Coughing begins with a deep inspiration, closure of the glottis, and active contraction of expiratory muscles. The glottis opens suddenly, followed by a forceful expiratory phase, which removes extraneous substances from the lower airways.[3, 4]

The lower airways function primarily to transport air to the alveoli, where exchange of carbon dioxide and oxygen between blood and air occurs. Movement of air is controlled by airway diameter. In normal animals, parasympathetic discharge, characterized by release of acetylcholine and stimulation of muscarinic receptors, maintains resting bronchial tone in a slightly constricted state. In contrast, sympathetic stimulation of β-adrenergic receptors, primarily β₂-receptors, causes bronchodilation.

In the alveoli, oxygen moves by passive diffusion from inspired air into the pulmonary capillaries and blood stream, whereas carbon dioxide moves passively from the pulmonary capillaries into alveoli. Diffusion of gases is a passive process; oxygen and carbon dioxide move from areas with relatively high partial pressures to areas with relatively low partial pressures. Compensatory mechanisms in the lungs result in an overall balance between ventilation of alveoli and perfusion of pulmonary capillaries.[5] When alveoli are underventilated (e.g., in pulmonary edema), the reduced alveolar oxygen concentration causes arteriolar constriction, and blood is shunted to other areas of the lungs for ventilation. Conversely, when perfusion is decreased (e.g., in pulmonary thromboembolism), bronchoconstriction occurs, and ventilation is shifted

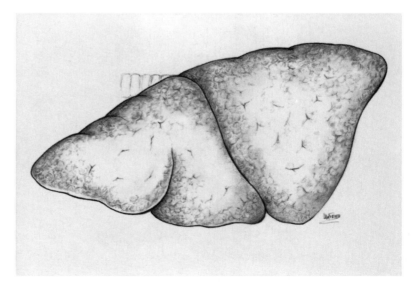

Figure 54–1
Diagram of left lateral view of canine lung showing the cranial and caudal lobes. The cranial lobe consists of cranial and caudal parts. The dog's head is on the reader's left.

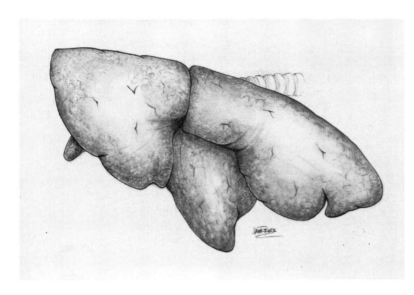

Figure 54–2
Diagram of right lateral view of canine lung showing the cranial, middle, and caudal lobes. The edge of the accessory lobe is seen behind the caudal lobe. The dog's head is on the reader's right.

to other areas of the lungs that are adequately perfused.

After blood is oxygenated in the lungs, it is transported through the systemic circulation to the tissues. The presence of hemoglobin greatly enhances the ability of red blood cells to carry oxygen. In the tissues, dissociation of oxygen from hemoglobin is favored by the lower partial pressure of oxygen. Other factors that increase release of oxygen from hemoglobin to tissues include decreased pH, increased partial pressure of carbon dioxide, and increased temperature. After releasing oxygen, hemoglobin serves as a buffer for hydrogen ions that are produced when carbon dioxide is converted to bicarbonate.

The lungs play an important role in maintenance of acid-base homeostasis.[5] In metabolic acidosis, characterized by decreased bicarbonate and pH, alveolar ventilation is increased to reduce the partial pressure of carbon dioxide, which increases the pH toward normal. In metabolic alkalosis, characterized by increased bicarbonate and pH, alveolar ventilation decreases to retain carbon dioxide, which lowers the pH toward normal. Whereas compensatory responses occur in metabolic acid-base disturbances, pulmonary disorders may cause alterations in acid-base status. Alveolar hypoventilation results in increased carbon dioxide retention, which causes decreased pH and respiratory acidosis. In contrast, hyperventilation leads to decreased carbon dioxide and increased pH and respiratory alkalosis.

Problem Identification

Nasal Discharge

Nasal discharge usually results from intranasal diseases; however, it occurs infrequently in patients with lower respiratory disorders when exudate moves up the tracheobronchial tree to the nasal passages. Bilateral, mucopurulent exudate may occur in patients with pneumonia; however, these patients almost always have other signs such as fever, coughing, respiratory distress, and crackles. Patients with fulminant pulmonary edema sometimes have a pink, frothy

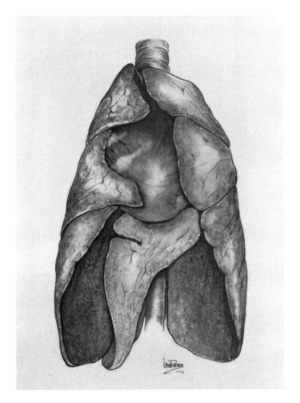

Figure 54–3
Diagram of ventral view of canine lungs showing the accessory lobe located caudal to the heart.

Table 54–1
Common Causes of Coughing in Dogs and Cats

UPPER AIRWAY	LOWER AIRWAY	CARDIAC
Tracheal foreign body	Canine chronic bronchitis	Left-sided heart failure
Collapsing trachea	Feline bronchial disease	Mitral valve insufficiency
Tracheobronchitis	Bronchial foreign body	Cardiomyopathy
	Pulmonary infiltrates with eosinophilia	Left atrial enlargement
	Pneumonia	Heartworm disease
	Aspiration	Pulmonary thromboembolism
	Bacterial	
	Fungal	
	Parasitic	
	Hilar lymphadenopathy	
	Neoplasia	
	Primary	
	Metastatic	

nasal exudate. For a complete discussion of nasal discharge, see Chapter 51.

Cough

A cough is a sudden expulsion of air from the respiratory passages. It serves as a pulmonary defense mechanism because it helps remove extraneous material from the respiratory tract.

Pathophysiology

A cough is initiated by chemical, thermal, or mechanical stimulation of cough receptors. Although cough receptors are located in nearly all areas of the respiratory tract, stimulation of receptors in the larynx, trachea, and bronchi is most likely to cause coughing. Coughing results from either respiratory or cardiac diseases (Table 54–1). Almost any disorder of the respiratory system can cause coughing by stimulation of cough receptors. Left-sided heart failure causes pulmonary edema, which causes coughing. Left atrial enlargement, often associated with mitral valve insufficiency, physically compresses the left mainstem bronchus and causes coughing.

Clinical Signs

Clinical signs vary depending on the underlying cause of the cough. It is not uncommon for dogs and cats with cough to be dyspneic and have exercise intolerance. In general, coughing is much less common in cats than dogs. Coughing that occurs after eating suggests upper airway disorders such as laryngeal disease or collapsing trachea, although it also occurs in patients with megaesophagus and aspiration pneumonia. A dry, hacking cough occurs with disorders of the

trachea such as tracheitis, collapsing trachea, and compression of the left mainstem bronchus secondary to left atrial enlargement. Dogs with collapsing trachea have a characteristic goose-honk cough that is precipitated by exercise or excitement. Palpation of the trachea in dogs with tracheitis, infectious tracheobronchitis, and collapsing trachea often results in a coughing episode. Dogs with tracheobronchial diseases such as infectious tracheobronchitis and chronic bronchitis often have a productive cough, which may end with retching and gagging. Cats with bronchial disease often have episodes of coughing characterized by expiratory wheezes and dyspnea. Hemoptysis, or coughing up blood, occurs with pulmonary disorders such as neoplasia, heartworm disease, thromboembolism, fungal pneumonia, foreign bodies, and coagulopathies such as thrombocytopenia and disseminated intravascular coagulation. Coughing associated with congestive heart failure is often productive and is usually found in patients with signs of cardiac disease, especially murmurs. For a more complete discussion of coughing associated with cardiac diseases, see Chapter 9.

Diagnostic Plan

The initial step in evaluating patients with cough is to distinguish between respiratory and cardiac disease. Often this distinction can be made on the basis of signalment, history, and physical examination findings. If physical examination reveals a murmur, arrhythmia, jugular pulses, pulse deficits, gallop rhythm, or tachycardia, cardiac disease should be suspected. If there are no signs of cardiac disease, respiratory disease is the most likely cause of cough. If the patient has signs of upper airway disease such as

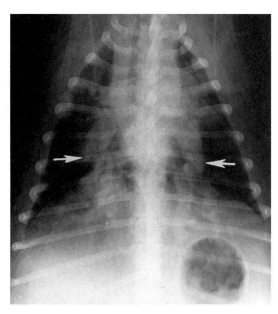

Figure 54–4
Dorsoventral thoracic radiograph of a dog with heartworm disease. Note the dilated and tortuous right and left caudal lobar arteries *(arrows)*. Enlargement of the right side of the heart and pulmonary trunk is also noted, along with a small volume of pleural effusion.

stertorous respiration, inspiratory dyspnea, or coughing and gagging after eating, diagnostic evaluation of the upper respiratory tract should be done first (see Chap. 52).

Thoracic radiography is one of the most useful tests for evaluating patients with cough. Finding left-sided cardiomegaly, an interstitial or alveolar pattern with a dorsal or hilar distribution consistent with pulmonary edema, or pulmonary venous congestion suggests that cough is due to cardiac disease. Heartworm disease with pulmonary thromboembolism is often associated with enlargement of the right side of the heart, enlarged tortuous and blunted pulmonary arteries, and a patchy, interstitial infiltrate, especially in the caudal lung fields (Fig. 54–4). Finding an alveolar, bronchial, or nodular interstitial pattern indicates a lower airway or pulmonary cause of coughing such as bacterial pneumonia, asthma, bronchitis, pulmonary infiltrates with eosinophilia (PIE), fungal pneumonia, or metastatic neoplasia. A single discrete pulmonary mass is highly suggestive of primary pulmonary neoplasia. Hilar lymphadenopathy most often occurs with neoplasia, especially lymphoma, and fungal pneumonia (Fig. 54–5). Normal thoracic radiographs suggest that coughing is not due to lower airway disease, although some dogs and cats with bronchial disease may not have radiographic abnormalities.

Additional diagnostic tests may be necessary to determine the specific cause of the cough. If cardiac disease is suspected, electrocardiography and echocardiography are indicated. An occult heartworm test should be done to rule out heartworm disease. Additional tests for patients with suspected upper airway disease may include comparison of inspiratory and expiratory cervical and thoracic radiographs, laryngeal examination, and tracheoscopy (see Chap. 52). Tracheal wash, bronchoscopy, or fine-needle aspiration of the lung is indicated for patients with suspected bronchial or pulmonary diseases. Fecal flotation is indicated to rule out parasitic infections with *Aelurostrongylus abstrusus* and *Paragonimus kellicotti*. The Baermann technique may facilitate identification of *A. abstrusus* larvae.

Dyspnea

Dyspnea is an inappropriate degree of respiratory effort that results from metabolic, respiratory, or cardiac disease. Disorders of the lower airways and lungs are often associated with dyspnea. Lower airway disorders such as feline bronchial disease and chronic bronchitis in dogs often cause additional signs such as coughing, wheezing, and prolonged expiration. Thoracic auscultation may reveal crackles and wheezes; however, these findings are not specific for lower airway disorders. Patients with pneumonia usually have other signs such as fever and cough; regurgitation is often present in patients with aspiration pneumonia and esophageal diseases. Patients with congestive

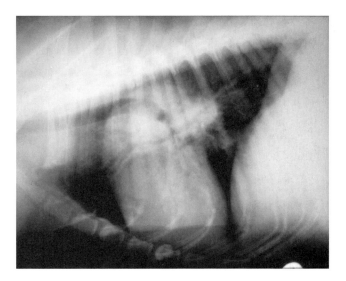

Figure 54–5
Lateral thoracic radiograph of a dog with multicentric lymphoma. Soft tissue nodular densities clustered around the tracheal bifurcation are consistent with hilar lymphadenopathy. Cranial mediastinal lymphadenopathy is also noted.

heart failure often have a history of cough, cardiac murmur, arrhythmia, gallop rhythm, or crackles on thoracic auscultation. Patients with pleural space disorders may have rapid, shallow respirations and muffled cardiac sounds. Breath sounds tend to be decreased ventrally and increased dorsally in dogs and cats with pleural effusion, and pneumothorax is often associated with decreased breath sounds. A thorough evaluation including history, physical examination, and diagnostic tests such as thoracic radiography usually helps distinguish among disorders that cause dyspnea. For a complete discussion of dyspnea, see Problem Identification in Chapters 9 and 52.

Inappetence and Weight Loss

Inappetence and weight loss may occur in dogs and cats with some pulmonary disorders. Patients with dyspnea of any cause are more concerned with breathing than eating, resulting in inappetence and weight loss. This is more likely to occur when dyspnea has been present for more than 1 week. Primary or metastatic pulmonary neoplasia may cause cancer cachexia, which results in significant weight loss. Other clinical signs such as chronic cough and respiratory distress often occur in these patients and suggest pulmonary involvement. Other respiratory disorders that are likely to be associated with dyspnea and weight loss include aspiration, bacterial, or fungal pneumonia; congestive heart failure; and disorders of the pleural space such as pleural effusion or spontaneous pneumothorax. For a more complete discussion of weight loss, see Chapter 47.

Diagnostic Procedures

Auscultation

Thoracic auscultation of normal dogs and cats reveals vesicular and bronchial breath sounds during inspiration and expiration.[6] Vesicular sounds are faint rustling sounds heard as air moves through small airways such as alveoli; they are loudest on inspiration. Bronchial sounds are heard as air moves through larger airways such as bronchi and the trachea; they are loudest on expiration. Breath sounds that are louder than normal may result from increased ventilation in panting animals, obstructive lung diseases such as bronchitis or asthma, or airway consolidation as in pneumonia. Decreased or absent breath sounds may occur in patients with severe airway consolidation or atelectasis, space-occupying masses such as neoplasia, diaphragmatic hernia, pleural effusion, pneumothorax, or emphysema. Normal animals may appear to have decreased or absent breath sounds if their respirations are shallow, especially if auscultation is done in noisy surroundings.

Adventitial sounds are heard in addition to normal breath sounds and include crackles and wheezes. Although the presence of adventitous sounds is not specific for certain disorders, it helps to localize disease to the respiratory tract. Crackles are short and explosive discontinuous sounds that are described as clicking, popping, or bubbling.[6, 7] Crackles may be produced by bursting bubbles of airway secretions or sudden opening of airways during inspiration.[6] Disorders that cause crackles include pulmonary edema, pneumonia, interstitial diseases such as PIE and neoplasia, and bronchitis. Wheezes are continuous musical or whistling sounds produced by the passage of air through a narrowed airway. Inspiratory wheezes are due to upper airway obstruction, whereas expiratory wheezes are due to intrathoracic airway obstruction. Disorders that cause expiratory wheezes include collapsing trachea, chronic bronchitis, feline asthma, pneumonia, neoplasia, foreign bodies, and hilar lymphadenopathy.[6]

Routine Laboratory Evaluation

Laboratory evaluation is sometimes helpful for patients with diseases of the lower airways and lungs. A complete blood count may reveal leukocytosis and a left shift associated with bacterial pneumonia, aspiration pneumonia, or eosinophilia in patients with asthma, bronchitis, PIE, heartworm disease, and parasitic infection. Serum chemistry values may reveal azotemia related to dehydration, hypercalcemia associated with blastomycosis or mediastinal lymphoma, or increased total carbon dioxide consistent with respiratory acidosis and compensatory metabolic alkalosis. Serologic tests are useful for diagnosis of some infectious disorders including occult heartworm disease, coccidioidomycosis, and toxoplasmosis (see Chaps. 13, 39, and 40 for additional information on these disorders).

Zinc sulfate fecal flotation (see Chap. 32) may identify ova or larvae of *A. abstrusus* or *P. kellicotti*. The Baermann technique may facilitate identification of *A. abstrusus* larvae.[8] Equipment for performing the Baermann technique includes a glass funnel connected to a rubber tube that is clamped at the bottom. The glass funnel should be supported by a ring stand. Alternatively, a disposable wine or champagne glass with a hollow stem can be used. The operator should place 10 g of feces in a piece of double-layer cheesecloth and gather the cheesecloth around the sample so that it is completely enclosed. Then the cheesecloth should be placed on a wire mesh or sieve so that it is suspended in the funnel or glass. The operator should fill the funnel or glass with lukewarm tap water and

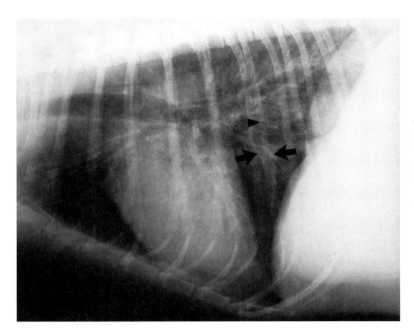

Figure 54–6
Lateral thoracic radiograph of a dog with chronic bronchitis. Note the thickened bronchial walls, which appear like railroad tracks when seen longitudinally *(arrows)* and doughnuts when seen end on *(arrowhead).*

allow the sample to sit at least 8 hours, preferably overnight. The clamp on the rubber tube should be loosened and the first three or four drops of water collected onto a microscope slide. Alternatively, one should collect the first 10 mL of water, centrifuge it for several minutes, and then place several drops of the sediment on a microscope slide. If a disposable glass is used, the operator should remove the fecal sample and collect the material at the bottom of the hollow stem using a pipette. One should examine slides under the microscope at 10× and look for larvae of *A. abstrusus*, which are characterized by a kinked tail with an accessory spine.

Radiography

Thoracic radiography is one of the most useful diagnostic procedures for evaluation of patients with diseases of the lower airways and lungs. In most cases a ventrodorsal and a lateral view are sufficient; however, both a left and a right lateral view should be obtained if metastasis is suspected. Try to determine whether the predominant pattern is bronchial, alveolar, interstitial, or vascular. A bronchial pattern is observed in dogs with chronic bronchitis and cats with bronchial disease such as asthma (Fig. 54–6). Collapse of the right middle lung lobe occurs in about 10% of cats with chronic or severe bronchial disease.[9] Bronchiectasis, or dilation of airways, is a chronic change that may result from chronic bronchial diseases. PIE causes a diffuse bronchial and alveolar pattern (Fig. 54–7). Fungal pneumonia and metastatic neoplasia cause a diffuse miliary to nodular interstitial pattern (Fig. 54–8). Primary pulmonary neoplasia is associated with a discrete pulmonary mass; however, metastatic

lesions that are smaller may be observed in the same lobe or other lobes (Fig. 54–9). An alveolar pattern occurs when air in alveoli is replaced by blood, purulent exudate, or transudate as a result of pulmonary contusions or coagulopathies, bacterial pneumonia, or pulmonary edema, respectively (Fig. 54–10). Atelectasis also causes an alveolar pattern, although there is also a loss of lung volume. Enlarged and tortuous pulmonary arteries are almost always associated with heartworm disease (see Chap. 13), which may cause an interstitial or alveolar pattern, especially with thromboembolic disease.

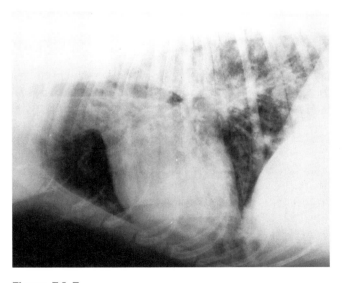

Figure 54–7
Lateral thoracic radiograph of a dog with pulmonary infiltrates with eosinophilia. Patchy alveolar, interstitial, and bronchial infiltrate is noted in the dorsal lung fields.

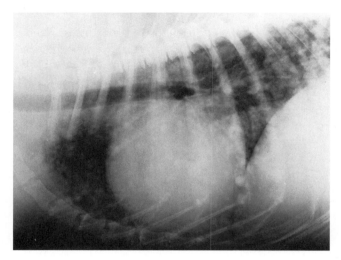

Figure 54-8
Lateral thoracic radiograph of a dog with metastatic hemangiosarcoma. Multiple soft tissue nodules are noted throughout the pulmonary parenchyma. Generalized heart enlargement is also present, consistent with pericardial effusion.

Ultrasonography

Ultrasonography is occasionally used to evaluate pulmonary masses located in peripheral areas of the lungs. It is most useful for detecting mediastinal masses (see Chap. 53). Echocardiography is indicated for patients with suspected cardiac disease (see Chap. 9).

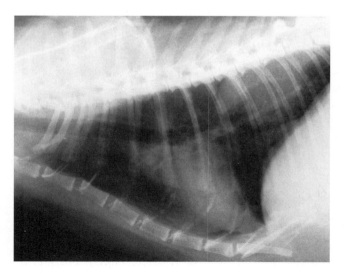

Figure 54-9
Lateral thoracic radiograph of a cat with primary pulmonary adenocarcinoma. A large soft tissue density mass is present in a caudal lung lobe.

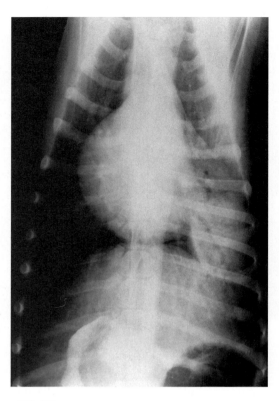

Figure 54-10
Dorsoventral thoracic radiograph of a dog with bacterial pneumonia. Note the alveolar infiltrate characterized by air bronchograms in the left caudal lung lobe. (From Little SE, Forrester SD. Challenging cases in internal medicine, what's your diagnosis? Vet Med 1995;90:742.)

Tracheal Wash

Tracheal wash is indicated for evaluation of patients with chronic cough or diffuse pulmonary disease with a bronchial or an alveolar pattern on radiography. Although results from tracheal wash may provide useful information on patients with interstitial pulmonary disease, other procedures such as fine-needle aspiration may be more diagnostic. Tracheal wash should be done only after other, less invasive tests (e.g., radiography) have been performed. Two methods are used to perform tracheal wash: the transtracheal approach and the endotracheal approach. Complications of tracheal wash are minimal but include tracheal laceration, pneumomediastinum, and subcutaneous emphysema. These side effects are more likely to occur with the transtracheal technique.

Selection of technique depends on the clinician's preference and ability to perform them adequately and safely. Although either procedure can be done with any patient, it is generally safer to use the endotracheal technique for cats and very small dogs. The endotracheal approach may also be more appropriate for fractious dogs and cats. Sedation is usually not needed for the transtracheal approach unless the animal is difficult to restrain. If sedation is used, a regimen that provides a light plane of sedation is preferred because the cough reflex must remain intact to obtain adequate samples from the lower airways. Protocols that meet this criterion include acepromazine at 0.02 to 0.05 mg/kg intravenously (IV) or subcutaneously (SC) or oxymorphone (Numorphan) at 0.02 to 0.05 mg/kg IV, SC, or intramuscularly (IM). For the endotracheal technique, general anesthesia with a short-acting agent administered intravenously is sufficient. Thiopental (2–4 mg/kg IV boluses to effect) or propofol (Diprivan) at 6 to 8 mg/kg IV to effect may be used in dogs. A combination of ketamine (10 mg/kg IV) and either diazepam (0.5 mg/kg IV) or acepromazine (0.02–0.05 mg/kg IV) is adequate for cats.

For the transtracheal technique, the patient should be restrained, the head held, and the neck extended so that the nose is tilted slightly upward. The patient may sit or stand, whichever seems more comfortable. The cricothyroid ligament should be located by palpating for the raised cricoid cartilage that forms a band around the trachea. The cricothyroid ligament is the triangular depression cranial to the cricoid cartilage and caudal to the thyroid cartilage. The hair over this area should be shaved and the skin prepared aseptically using either a povidone-iodine (Betadine) or chlorhexidine (Nolvasan) scrub followed by alcohol wipes. Before the final scrub, the subcutaneous area over the cricothyroid ligament should be infiltrated with a small amount (<1 mL) of 2% lidocaine. The person performing the procedure should wear sterile gloves. The person should stabilize the trachea by grasping it with one hand and pulling it away from the patient slightly. With the opposite hand, the cricothyroid ligament is located, and the tip of needle from a jugular catheter (e.g., through the needle catheter with an 18- or 20-gauge needle) is placed through the skin with the bevel down so that it is angled slightly ventrally. Then the needle is inserted through the cricothyroid ligament into the trachea. The needle is advanced slightly; then the hand that was stabilizing the trachea is used to advance the jugular catheter through the needle and down the trachea. If the needle is in the tracheal lumen, the catheter should advance easily; most patients cough as the catheter is advanced. The operator should not pull back on the catheter once it is advanced through the needle because the catheter could be severed and enter the airway. The operator should hold the needle firmly against the neck until the catheter is advanced, ideally no farther than the tracheal bifurcation, which usually corresponds to the fourth or fifth intercostal space. Then the needle is withdrawn from the skin and the needle guard is placed around it; an assistant should hold the needle guard against the patient's neck. The

operator should attach a previously prepared 12-mL syringe containing sterile saline to the catheter and inject 2 to 4 mL of saline. As the patient coughs, the operator should quickly aspirate back into the syringe. If only air is obtained, the operator should empty the syringe of air and try again. The injection and aspiration procedure should be repeated until there is 1 to 2 mL of fluid for evaluation; this usually requires a minimum of two or three washes. The operator should not be overly concerned about causing side effects by injecting saline into the airways because much of the saline is quickly absorbed by the bronchial mucosa; as a guideline, the operator can safely inject 1.5 mL of saline/kg of body weight.[10] The aspirated sample should be turbid or contain flecks of mucus and cellular material.

After an adequate sample has been collected, the operator should carefully withdraw the catheter from the patient and maintain pressure over the cricothyroid ligament for several minutes using a sterile 4 × 4 inch gauze pad. Alternatively, the operator could place an antibacterial ointment such as povidone-iodine on the gauze pad and hold it in place using a bandage for several hours.

For the endotracheal technique, a sterile endotracheal tube is placed into the trachea, avoiding contact with structures in the oral cavity. A sterile 3.5 Fr male polypropylene urinary catheter is passed through the tube into the trachea using sterile technique. Tracheal wash is performed as described for the transtracheal approach.

Samples that have been collected should be processed quickly for cytologic examination and bacterial culture. Several drops of fluid should be placed on a culture swab and submitted for aerobic bacterial culture. From the remainder of the fluid, the operator should prepare several direct smears on microscope slides for cytologic evaluation. The operator should centrifuge any remaining fluid, pour off the supernatant, and use the resuspended button of cells from the bottom of the tube to make additional slides. Flecks of material should be placed on a glass slide so that squash preparations can be made for cytologic evaluation. If slides are to be sent out for evaluation, the operator must ask the laboratory how to prepare the slides before submission.

Normal animals have some respiratory epithelial cells, macrophages, and occasional nondegenerate neutrophils in tracheal wash fluid.[11] Relatively large numbers of eosinophils are observed in patients with presumed hypersensitivity disorders (e.g., bronchitis, asthma, PIE) and parasitic infections (e.g., heartworm disease, aelurostrongylosis).[10-12] Increased numbers of neutrophils may be observed in patients with infectious tracheobronchitis, asthma, chronic bronchitis, neoplasia, and other infectious or inflammatory disorders; degenerate neutrophils suggest bacterial infection or aspiration, especially if bacteria are observed concomitantly. Increased mucus is a nonspecific finding that occurs with many inflammatory disorders including asthma and bronchitis. Parasitic infections such as aelurostrongylosis and paragonimiasis can be diagnosed by finding ova or larvae in tracheal wash specimens.[13] Fungal organisms are sometimes recovered from patients with blastomycosis and histoplasmosis.[14] Neoplastic cells are rarely, if ever, observed in tracheal wash specimens; any neoplastic-appearing cells should be interpreted with caution because inflammation causes dysplastic changes that may be mistaken for malignancy.

Results of bacterial cultures from tracheal wash specimens should be interpreted with other diagnostic findings because the trachea and lower airways of normal dogs and cats may be inhabited by bacteria.[15, 16] This means that a positive culture does not necessarily indicate bacterial infection. In contrast, if other signs of infection exist (e.g., fever, leukocytosis, pulmonary alveolar pattern), if a pure culture (i.e., a single organism) is obtained from a primary culture plate, or if cytologic evaluation shows degenerate neutrophils and phagocytized bacteria, respiratory infection probably exists.[17]

Tracheobronchoscopy

Indications for tracheobronchoscopy are similar to those for tracheal wash. In addition to collection of samples for cytologic evaluation and bacterial culture, however, endoscopy of the airways allows visual inspection of abnormalities such as neoplasms, parasites, foreign bodies, collapsing trachea, and collapse of the mainstem bronchi or smaller airways. Other advantages of tracheobronchoscopy are that it allows collection of specimens from the lower airways and removal of foreign bodies.

Tracheobronchoscopy requires general anesthesia, which can be accomplished with inhalation anesthetics or injectable agents. When inhalation anesthesia is used there is always potential for exposure of the endoscopist or other personnel in the room to anesthetic gases; this risk can be minimized by placing a Y-shaped adapter on the end of the endotracheal tube, which has a self-sealing port for passage of the endoscope. Only medium-sized to large dogs that require an endotracheal tube with an inside diameter greater than 7.5 mm can be evaluated by placing the endoscope through the endotracheal tube. Tracheobronchoscopy in cats and small dogs must be done using injectable anesthetic agents. We prefer to use injectable agents to maintain general anesthesia in all patients for tracheobronchoscopy because the risks to personnel are minimized and endoscopy can be done

without using an endotracheal tube, which can interfere with evaluation of the upper airways and prevent maximal insertion of the endoscope into the lower airways of large dogs.

For injectable anesthesia, an indwelling intravenous catheter is placed, and premedications are administered, including glycopyrrolate (Robinul) at 0.01 mg/kg IV and oxymorphone (Numorphan) at 0.1 to 0.2 mg/kg IV (do not exceed a total dose of 4 mg regardless of body weight). The patient should be preoxygenated by administration of oxygen (3–5 L per minute) via a well-fitting facemask for 3 to 5 minutes before induction. Drugs that may be used to induce and maintain anesthesia in dogs and cats include ketamine (Ketaset) and diazepam (Valium), thiopental (Pentothal), or propofol (Diprivan)[18] (Table 54–2). It is important to administer the smallest amount of anesthetic agent that maintains adequate anesthesia; the operator should begin with the lowest possible dose and administer incremental doses only as necessary. Thiobarbiturates such as thiopental are more likely to cause laryngospasm in cats; therefore, a combination of ketamine and diazepam may be preferable. Propofol may be more likely to cause apnea during the procedure, and this drug is more expensive than the other agents. Regardless of the protocol selected, it is important to administer oxygen via a tracheal catheter (e.g., flexible rubber tube) or via the biopsy channel of the endoscope.

Once the patient is anesthetized, the endoscope is passed through the larynx into the proximal trachea. It is advanced toward the carina and into the right mainstem bronchus, which usually appears as a direct continuation of the trachea.[19–21] Each lung lobe is systematically evaluated by moving the endoscope through the numerous segmental bronchi of each lobe until it can no longer be advanced; any abnormalities and their locations are noted and recorded. The entrance to the lobar bronchus of the right cranial lung

---

Table 54–2

Injectable Anesthetic Regimens for Tracheobronchoscopy in Dogs and Cats

ANESTHETIC AGENT	DOSAGE* (INTRAVENOUS)
1. Thiopental (Pentothal)	10–20 mg/kg
2. Ketamine (Ketaset) and	5–10 mg/kg
Diazepam (Valium)	0.2–0.5 mg/kg
3. Propofol (Diprivan)	4–8 mg/kg

*Begin with the least amount that provides an adequate plane of anesthesia; inject additional drug in small increments as needed to maintain anesthesia.

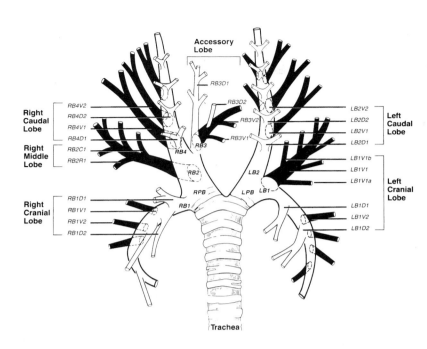

Right Caudal Lobe
RB4V2
RB4D2
RB4V1
RB4D1

Right Middle Lobe
RB2C1
RB2R1

Right Cranial Lobe
RB1D1
RB1V1
RB1V2
RB1D2

Accessory Lobe
RB3D1
RB3D2
RB3V2
RB3V1

RB3
RB4
RB2
RPB
LPB
RB1

Trachea

Left Caudal Lobe
LB2V2
LB2D2
LB2V1
LB2D1

Left Cranial Lobe
LB1V1b
LB1V1
LB1V1a
LB1D1
LB1V2
LB1D2

LB2
LB1

Figure 54–11
Diagrammatic representation of normal bronchial anatomy in dogs. Each lobar bronchus is subdivided into segmental bronchi, such that V1 = first ventral segmental bronchus, V2 = second ventral segmental bronchus, D1 = first dorsal segmental bronchus, D2 = second dorsal segmental bronchus, C1 = first caudal segmental bronchus, and R1 = first rostral segmental bronchus. Segmental bronchi are subdivided into subsegmental bronchi, such that V1a = first subsegmental bronchus and V1b = second subsegmental bronchus. LB1, lobar bronchus of left cranial lung lobe; LB2, lobar bronchus of left caudal lung lobe; LPB, left mainstem bronchus; RB1, lobar bronchus of right cranial lung lobe; RB2, lobar bronchus of right middle lung lobe; RB3, lobar bronchus of accessory lobe; RB4, lobar bronchus of right caudal lung lobe; RPB, right mainstem bronchus. (From Amis TC, McKiernan BC. Systematic identification of endobronchial anatomy during bronchoscopy in the dog. Am J Vet Res 1986;47: 2649–2658.)

lobe is encountered first; it is located in the lateral wall of the right mainstem bronchus, directly across from the carina (Fig. 54–11). After examining the right cranial lobe, the examiner should return to the right mainstem bronchus and enter the lobar bronchus of the right middle lung lobe, which originates on the ventral floor of the right mainstem bronchus between the 6 and 8 o'clock positions. The lobar bronchus of the accessory lobe is entered next; it originates from the ventromedial to the medial aspect of the right mainstem bronchus, just distal to the origin of the bronchus to the right middle lobe. The continuation of the right mainstem bronchus distal to the accessory lobe becomes the lobar bronchus of the right caudal lung lobe. After the right side is evaluated, the endoscope is retracted to the carina and enters the left mainstem bronchus. The lobar bronchus of the left cranial lung lobe originates from the ventrolateral to the lateral aspect of the left mainstem bronchus, just distal to the carina. Beyond the origin of the left cranial lobar bronchus, the left mainstem bronchus becomes the lobar bronchus to the left caudal lung lobe. It may be difficult to identify and evaluate each lobar bronchus; however, many pulmonary diseases are diffuse, and collection of samples from multiple areas often yields diagnostic specimens.

Samples of any abnormal lesions may be collected for cytologic, histologic, or microbiologic evaluation during bronchoscopy. Because of potential for contamination as the endoscope passes through the oropharynx, specimens for bacteriologic culture are best collected by tracheal wash through a sterile endotracheal tube before introducing the endoscope. Specimens for cytologic evaluation may be collected by inserting a cytology brush through the biopsy channel of the endoscope and rubbing it against the bronchial walls; these samples are superior to those collected during tracheal wash because they are obtained from the deeper airways. Material from the brush is gently rolled from the bristles and placed on a glass slide, which is stained before microscopic examination. Masses can also be brushed for cytologic evaluation. Samples of masses can be collected using a biopsy instrument through the endoscope; they should be placed in formalin and submitted for histologic evaluation.

Another technique for obtaining samples from the deeper airways and alveoli is bronchoalveolar lavage. Because of the size of the endoscope, this is most easily done in dogs. Bronchoalveolar lavage is accomplished by passing the endoscope into a segmental bronchus so that the lumen of the bronchus is completely occluded. A 25-mL aliquot of warm, sterile 0.9% saline is injected through the instrumentation channel of the endoscope, and the lavage fluid is immediately aspirated; this procedure is repeated using another 25-mL aliquot of saline. The two samples are pooled and submitted for evaluation. Bronchoalveolar lavage can be done on multiple lobes to increase the chances of obtaining a diagnostic sample. In cats and small dogs, samples of lavage fluid may be obtained without an endoscope.[22] The patient is anesthetized using an injectable agent (see Table 54–2), and an endotracheal tube is placed so that it does not extend beyond the carina. The patient is placed in lateral recumbence, preferably with the affected side down. The cuff on the endotracheal tube is inflated, and a syringe adapter is placed on the end of the endotracheal tube. Using a 35-mL syringe, warm saline (5 mL/kg) is injected into the endotracheal tube. Immediately after instillation of saline, suction is applied to remove as much fluid as possible. After several positive pressure ventilations are applied, the procedure is repeated until a total of three aliquots of saline has been used.

Lavage specimens should be evaluated soon after collection, preferably within 30 minutes.[23] Several drops of lavage fluid are placed on a culture swab and submitted for aerobic culture. A total nucleated cell count of the fluid is done using a hemocytometer. Some of the fluid is placed on a microscope slide and stained so that a differential cell count can be done. Although results depend on the technique used, most dogs and cats have total nucleated cell counts less than 500 cells/μL; in pulmonary disease, counts may be greater than 1500 cells/μL.[23, 24] In normal dogs, differential cell counts in bronchoalveolar lavage fluid reveal approximately 75% to 80% macrophages, 5% to 10% lymphocytes, 5% to 7% neutrophils, 5% eosinophils, and occasional mast cells and epithelial cells; some normal dogs can have up to 20% eosinophils.[23, 24] Differential cell counts in normal cats range from approximately 70% to 90% macrophages, 1% to 5% neutrophils, 10% to 25% eosinophils, and 1% to 5% lymphocytes; infrequently, eosinophils may account for up to 80% of nucleated cells in cats.[16, 25, 26]

Neutrophilic inflammation occurs with bacterial and fungal infection, neoplasia, and other inflammatory disorders such as aspiration pneumonia, feline bronchial disease, and chronic bronchitis in dogs. Fungal organisms may be identified in dogs with histoplasmosis and blastomycosis; fungal infection may also be characterized by increased macrophages.[14] Eosinophilic inflammation occurs with parasitic infections such as heartworm disease, aelurostrongylosis, and paragonimiasis and with hypersensitivity disorders such as asthma, chronic bronchitis, and PIE. Because normal dogs and cats can have large numbers of eosinophils in lavage fluid, however, a diagnosis of parasitic or hypersensitivity disorders should be made on the basis of additional findings including history, physical examination, and results of thoracic radiography and fecal flotation. Some neoplasms such as lymphoma and carcinoma can be diagnosed by finding lymphoblasts and malignant epithelial cells, respectively, on cytologic evaluation.[23, 27] The operator must be careful when interpreting cytologic criteria of malignancy when concomitant inflammation exists,

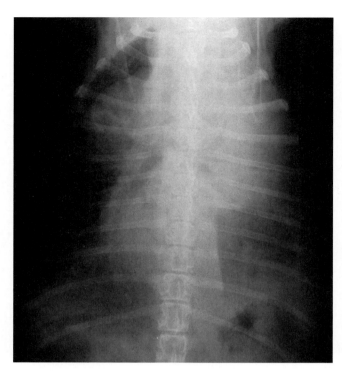

Figure 54–12
Dorsoventral thoracic radiograph of a dog with a primary pulmonary adenocarcinoma. A large soft tissue mass is present in the left cranial lung lobe.

because dysplastic epithelial changes can be mistaken for malignancy.

Transthoracic Pulmonary Aspiration

Transthoracic aspiration of the lungs is indicated when other, less invasive tests such as tracheal wash and bronchoalveolar lavage have not yielded a diagnosis.[28, 29] It is the preferred test for evaluating consolidated areas or masses located in the periphery of the lungs near the thoracic wall (Fig. 54–12). It may also be used for evaluation of patients with a diffuse interstitial pattern on thoracic radiography suggestive of metastatic neoplasia or fungal pneumonia. Transthoracic aspiration can be used to obtain samples for bacterial culture when pneumonia is suspected. Needle aspiration should not be done in patients that are fractious or have bleeding disorders or pulmonary cysts. Transthoracic pulmonary aspiration is relatively contraindicated in patients that are dyspneic, although it may be the safest diagnostic test for evaluation of these patients.

The site for aspiration is determined after obtaining lateral and ventrodorsal or dorsoventral thoracic radiographs. The operator should count the ribs to determine the ideal intercostal space for introducing the needle. If there is diffuse disease, the aspirate should be obtained from the caudal lung fields by inserting the needle through the seventh, eighth, or ninth intercostal space, above the costochondral junction.[28] The hair over the area is shaved and the skin prepared using an antiseptic scrub such as povidone-iodine (Betadine) or chlorhexidine (Nolvasan). The skin and subcutaneous tissues down to the pleura may be infiltrated with a small amount of 2% lidocaine. The person performing the aspiration should wear sterile gloves. A 23- or 25-gauge, 1- to 1.5-inch needle is sufficient for cats and small dogs. Large dogs or obese patients require a longer needle to reach the lungs; a 2.5- to 3.5-inch spinal needle with the stylet removed is ideal. The patient should be restrained by an assistant in a comfortable position, either standing or in sternal or lateral recumbence. The needle is attached to a 12-mL syringe and inserted through the skin and subcutaneous tissue into the lung to an appropriate depth as determined by evaluating a ventrodorsal or dorsoventral radiograph. A device that holds the syringe (Aspergun) is useful for stabilizing the needle during aspiration (Fig. 54–13). Once the needle is introduced, an assistant should occlude the nares so that three or four aspirates can be obtained between inspiration and expiration to minimize chances of lacerating the lung. The operator should release negative pressure, remove the needle from the patient, and separate it from the syringe. Air is then aspirated into the syringe and used to force the material in the hub of the needle onto glass slides for cytologic evaluation or the tip of a culture swab for bacterial culture. It usually requires two to four attempts to obtain adequate samples for evaluation. The patient should be monitored for complications such as pneumothorax and hemorrhage, which are most likely to occur within 1 hour.[29] If respiratory distress occurs,

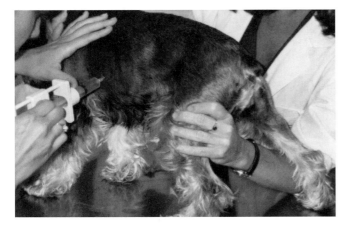

Figure 54–13
Aspiration of the consolidated pulmonary mass of the dog in Figure 54–12 using a device to stabilize the needle and syringe.

thoracic radiographs should be obtained to detect pneumothorax. Although pneumothorax occurs in up to 30% of dogs after transthoracic pulmonary aspiration, few dogs require thoracic drainage of air.[29]

Open Lung Biopsy

A thoracotomy for open lung biopsy is reserved for cases in which a diagnosis cannot be established by any other means. Ideally, it is used when the lesion appears to be resectable, such as a primary pulmonary tumor, bulla, abscess, or aspirated foreign body. In patients with suspected pulmonary neoplasia, samples of lymph node should be collected. Samples of tissue obtained at surgery should be submitted for histologic evaluation and, in some cases, bacterial culture.

Common Diseases of the Lower Airways and Lungs

Chronic Bronchitis

Chronic bronchitis is an inflammatory disorder that affects the lower airways of dogs. It is characterized by a chronic cough of at least 2 months' duration and absence of other identifiable disease on diagnostic evaluation. Chronic bronchitis is a common disorder in dogs, although there are few reports of naturally occurring disease.[30, 31] It is most common in older dogs, usually older than 6 to 8 years.[31] There seems to be no breed or sex predisposition.[31]

Pathophysiology

The cause of chronic bronchitis is unknown; a variety of factors such as environmental pollutants, allergens, cigarette smoke, or immune-mediated disease may play of role, although this remains unproved. Whatever the inciting cause, the end result is airway inflammation, hypertrophy of epithelial and goblet cells, and increased amounts of mucus. These changes stimulate bronchial cough receptors and interfere with air exchange. Collapse of small airways may occur during expiration, causing increased expiratory effort. Chronic inflammation may cause weakening of the airway walls, which subsequently causes bronchiectasis, an irreversible dilation of bronchi (Fig. 54–14). Bronchiectasis predisposes to secondary infection because it interferes with mucociliary clearance from the lower airways.

Clinical Signs

The most common signs of chronic bronchitis are chronic cough, exercise intolerance, and audible wheezes.[31] The cough is usually harsh and may be productive; it may end in a retching and gagging

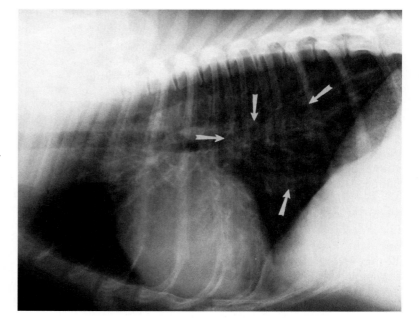

Figure 54–14
Lateral thoracic radiograph of a dog with bronchiectasis. Note the large number of dilated bronchial structures *(arrows)*.

episode. Thoracic auscultation often reveals expiratory wheezes and inspiratory or expiratory crackles. In advanced cases there may be a prolonged expiratory phase of respiration. Most dogs with chronic bronchitis are usually otherwise healthy and appear bright and alert on physical examination.

Diagnostic Plan

Chronic bronchitis is diagnosed by ruling out all other causes of chronic cough in dogs. Thoracic radiographs of most dogs with chronic bronchitis reveal a bronchial pattern characterized by "doughnuts" and "railroad tracks," which represents peribronchial inflammation and thickened bronchial walls (Fig. 54–15). Tracheal wash fluid from dogs with chronic bronchitis usually reveals a predominance of nondegenerate neutrophils and lesser numbers of lymphocytes, eosinophils, and epithelial cells; increased amounts of mucus are common.[12] Cultures of tracheal wash fluid may reveal growth of bacteria; however, their importance is unknown. These bacteria may represent colonization of the airways, which occurs in normal dogs, or secondary infection.[15, 32] Bacteria are rarely cultured from bronchial washings of dogs with chronic bronchitis; however, their growth should probably be considered significant in dogs with an acute exacerbation of chronic bronchitis, when there are signs of infection such as fever, mucopurulent nasal discharge, or leukocytosis and regenerative left shift, or when there are radiographic changes such as an alveolar pattern or bronchiectasis.[12, 31] Bronchoscopy is indicated when disease other than chronic bronchitis is suspected or when response to treatment is not as expected. Most dogs with chronic bronchitis have

erythematous airways with a roughened surface and increased mucus. There may also be collapse of mainstem bronchi or segmental bronchi during expiration.[31] Cytologic evaluation of bronchial brushings usually reveals excessive mucus and a predominance of nondegenerate neutrophils; small numbers of lymphocytes, eosinophils, ciliated cells, and epithelial cells are also present.[31]

Treatment

Administration of short-acting corticosteroids is the primary treatment for dogs with chronic bronchitis.

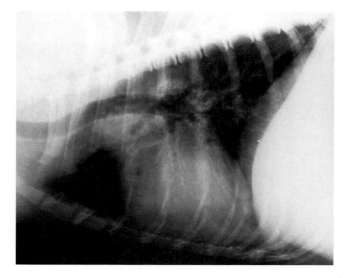

Figure 54–15
Lateral thoracic radiograph of a dog with chronic bronchitis. Multiple thickened bronchial walls are present.

Marked improvement usually occurs when prednisone is administered at 1.0 mg/kg by mouth twice per day (b.i.d.) for 5 days, followed by 0.5 mg/kg by mouth b.i.d. for another 5 days.[17] Then prednisone is administered on alternate days, and gradually, over 1 to 2 months, the dose is decreased. At this point, treatment may be discontinued; however, a maintenance dose of 0.25 mg/kg by mouth b.i.d. every 2 to 3 days may be needed in some dogs.

If response to corticosteroids is inadequate, bronchodilators may be helpful (see Table 52–2 for dosages). Another bronchodilator that has been effective in some dogs with chronic bronchitis is the β_2-agonist albuterol (Ventolin), which is available as a palatable syrup; the initial dose is 0.02 mg/kg by mouth b.i.d.[17, 31] As with most bronchodilators, potential side effects of albuterol are muscle tremors and restlessness. If a response is not noted after 5 days and no side effects have been observed, the dose of albuterol may be increased to 0.05 mg/kg by mouth b.i.d. or three times per day (t.i.d.).

Additional treatment is sometimes necessary for dogs with chronic bronchitis. For obese dogs, weight loss may be helpful in reducing the severity of clinical signs. If coughing is severe or excessive, a cough suppressant may be helpful (see Table 52–2 for dosages of common cough suppressants). Hydrocodone and codeine may be the most effective agents; however, products containing dextromethorphan are convenient because they are available over-the-counter. Because coughing is one of the pulmonary defense mechanisms that helps clear the lower airways, cough suppressants can be harmful. Ideally, they should be used for as short a time as possible and only for patients with nonproductive coughing. The goal of using cough suppressants is not to eliminate cough but to reduce its severity and frequency. Antimicrobials are not routinely used for treatment of chronic bronchitis unless there are signs of infection, such as fever, depression, inappetence, or alveolar radiographic pattern, or unless bacteria are cultured from tracheal or bronchial washings. Selection of antimicrobials ideally is based on results of bacterial culture and susceptibility. Chloramphenicol (50 mg/kg by mouth t.i.d. for 7–10 days) has been recommended because of its spectrum of activity and ability to penetrate bronchial tissue.[17]

Prognosis

Chronic bronchitis is usually not a curable disorder; however, most patients respond favorably to medical treatment. Dogs may have periods of exacerbation that require adjustments in treatment. Bronchiectasis is a potential irreversible complication of chronic bronchitis that may complicate management; affected dogs are more susceptible to secondary infections and worsening of clinical signs. Dogs that have collapse of airways during expiration appear to respond less favorably to treatment and may have a more guarded prognosis.[12]

Feline Bronchial Disease

Feline bronchial disease is characterized by inflammation of the lower airways in the absence of an identifiable cause. Bronchial diseases of cats have been called a variety of names including feline asthma, acute bronchitis, chronic bronchitis, and allergic lung disease. Asthma implies reversible airway disease characterized by intermittent bouts of clinical signs. Although this occurs in many cats, it is not clear if all cats with bronchial disease have asthma. Bronchial disease is a common cause of coughing and respiratory distress in cats, although there are few clinical reports.[9, 33] Young to middle-aged cats are most often affected. Although any breed may be affected, Siamese cats appear to be overrepresented.[9]

Pathophysiology

Although clinical signs of feline bronchial diseases are similar, clinicopathologic features suggest that multiple factors play a role in their pathogenesis. As with canine chronic bronchitis, environmental pollutants, irritants, or allergens may incite feline bronchial disease. Whatever the cause, feline bronchial disease is characterized by intrathoracic airway obstruction, which may be due to bronchial smooth muscle hypertrophy, increased mucus production, bronchial inflammation and edema, or bronchoconstriction. Bronchial obstruction prevents movement of air out of the lower airways during expiration, which can lead to air trapping and subsequent emphysema. These changes are associated with severe clinical signs that often do not respond to treatment.

Clinical Signs

The most common clinical signs in cats with bronchial disease are respiratory distress characterized by prolonged expiration, paroxysms of coughing, and wheezing.[9] Retching and vomiting may occur at the end of a coughing episode. Cats may present with a history of chronic, intermittent signs or, in severe, acute respiratory distress, with cyanosis and open-mouth breathing. Physical examination of cats with bronchial disease may yield normal results between episodes, although most cats have expiratory wheezes on thoracic auscultation. In severe cases, no breath sounds may be heard because intrathoracic airway obstruction prevents air movement.

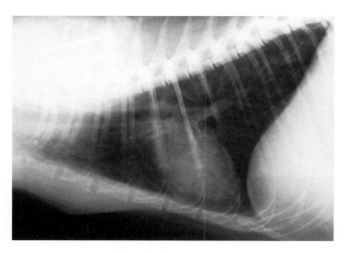

Figure 54–16
Lateral thoracic radiograph of a cat with chronic bronchitis. Thickened bronchial walls are noted in all lung fields.

Diagnostic Plan

Feline bronchial disease is diagnosed by ruling out other causes of cough and respiratory distress. It is important to distinguish between cardiac and respiratory disease because of differences in emergency treatment. Most cats with dyspnea related to cardiac disease do not have a history of cough, and a cardiac murmur or gallop rhythm is usually detected on physical examination. Thoracentesis should be done if pleural effusion is suspected (e.g., on the basis of dyspnea, muffled cardiac sounds, decreased compressibility of cranial thorax). Bronchial disease is confirmed by the results of a complete blood count, fecal flotation, thoracic radiography, and either tracheal wash or bronchoalveolar lavage. Eosinophilia is identified in approximately 20% of cats with bronchial disease.[9] Zinc sulfate fecal flotation or the Baermann technique is indicated to rule out paragonimiasis or aelurostrongylosis, respectively. These parasitic infections may cause clinical signs and diagnostic test results similar to those in bronchial disease. An occult heartworm test should be done if the cat lives in an area endemic for heartworm disease.

Thoracic radiographs of cats with bronchial disease usually show a bronchial pattern, although an interstitial or patchy alveolar pattern or a mixed pattern also may be seen[9] (Fig. 54–16). Collapse of the right middle lung lobe occurs in about 10% of cats with bronchial disease; collapse of the caudal portion of the left cranial lung lobe may occur concomitantly.[9] Other radiographic findings include aerophagia, flattening and caudal displacement of the diaphragm, and increased radiolucency of the lungs.[9]

Bronchial washes in cats with bronchial disease reveal an inflammatory response characterized by a predominance of nondegenerate neutrophils, eosinophils, or macrophages; some cats have a mixed population of cells with no single type predominating.[9] Bacteria are cultured from bronchial washes in approximately 25% of cats with bronchial disease. It is not known whether these organisms represent normal flora or indicate infection.[16]

Treatment

Cats presented in severe respiratory distress require emergency treatment. All stressful procedures such as restraint for injections or radiographs should be avoided until the cat is stable. Thoracentesis should be done to rule out pleural effusion, especially if a diagnosis has not been established. Oxygen should be administered using an oxygen cage if possible. A rapid-acting corticosteroid such as dexamethasone sodium phosphate (Azium-SP) or prednisolone sodium succinate (Solu-Delta-Cortef) or a bronchodilator such as terbutaline sulfate (Brethine) should be given (Table 54–3). Subcutaneous injection may be less stressful than other routes of administration. If the cat tolerates it, a bronchodilator can be given orally; most bronchodilators are rapidly absorbed after oral administration and reach peak concentrations within 30 to 90 minutes.[34] If there is no improvement within 5 to 10 minutes of initial treatment, the bronchodilator may be administered again.[34] Alternatively, treatment with a single dose of an anticholinergic such as atropine or glycopyrrolate (Robinul) causes bronchodilation and may provide short-term relief of respiratory distress. Long-term use of anticholinergics is not advised, however, because these agents increase the thickness of respiratory secretions, which decreases their clearance from the lower airways.

Maintenance treatment is indicated for cats with frequent bouts of coughing or respiratory distress; bronchodilators and corticosteroids are used most often (see Table 54–3). Whereas some cats may experience control of clinical signs with bronchodilators alone, others require treatment with corticosteroids. Concomitant use of a bronchodilator and a corticosteroid may lower the dose of corticosteroid necessary to control clinical signs. Ideally, the dose of corticosteroids should be tapered over a 2- to 4-week period to the lowest dose that is effective. In cats that cannot be medicated orally, injection of repositol corticosteroids such as methylprednisolone acetate (Depo-Medrol) may be used.

Prognosis

Most cats with bronchial disease respond to treatment, although adjustments may be necessary when there is exacerbation of clinical signs. About 50% of cats require maintenance treatment to control their

Table 54–3
Drugs Used to Treat Cats With Bronchial Disease

DRUG	TRADE NAME	DOSAGE REGIMEN
Emergency Treatment		
Prednisolone sodium succinate	Solu-Delta-Cortef	50–100 mg per cat IV, IM
Dexamethasone sodium phosphate	Azium-SP	1–2 mg/kg IV, IM, SC
Terbutaline	Brethine	0.01 mg/kg SC once
		0.625 mg per cat PO b.i.d.
Atropine		0.02–0.04 mg/kg SC, IM, IV
Glycopyrrolate	Robinul	0.01–0.02 mg/kg SC, IM, IV
Maintenance Treatment		
Aminophylline (immediate release)		5 mg/kg PO b.i.d. or t.i.d.
Theophylline (sustained release)	Theo-Dur	25 mg/kg s.i.d. (in evening)
	Slo-bid	25 mg/kg s.i.d. (in evening)
Terbutaline	Brethine	.625 mg per cat PO b.i.d.
Prednisone or prednisolone		0.5–1 mg/kg PO b.i.d. initially
Methylprednisolone acetate	Depo-Medrol	2–4 mg/kg IM every 2–4 wk

IM, intramuscularly; IV, intravenously; PO, by mouth; SC, subcutaneously; b.i.d., twice per day; t.i.d.; three times per day; s.i.d., every day.

clinical signs; other cats do not need treatment because their clinical signs are mild or infrequent.[9]

Pulmonary Infiltrates With Eosinophilia

PIE is an inflammatory disorder of dogs characterized primarily by interstitial involvement of the lungs. Although there are few reports of PIE, it seems to occur with some frequency.[35–38] There appears to be no breed or sex predilection, although medium-sized to large dogs that live outdoors in areas in which heartworm disease is endemic and that are not receiving heartworm preventative are more likely to be affected.[35]

Pathophysiology

The cause of PIE is presumed to be a hypersensitivity reaction. In dogs with heartworm disease, immune-mediated destruction of microfilaria in pulmonary capillaries may incite an eosinophilic inflammatory response. However, this does not explain the pathogenesis of PIE in dogs with no evidence of heartworm disease.

Clinical Signs

The most common clinical signs in dogs with PIE are coughing, exercise intolerance, and respiratory distress; some dogs may experience inappetence and weight loss.[35–38] Physical examination usually reveals diffuse crackles bilaterally; in dogs with heartworm disease, the caudal lung fields may be more severely affected.

Diagnostic Plan

A diagnosis of PIE is made on the basis of clinical and radiographic findings and results of cytologic evaluation of tracheal wash fluid, bronchial brushings, bronchoalveolar lavage fluid, or fine-needle aspirates. Thoracic radiographs may reveal a diffuse bronchial, alveolar, or interstitial pattern or a mixed pattern[38] (Fig. 54–17). Dogs with heartworm disease often have an alveolar pattern in the caudal lung lobes; other radiographic signs of heartworm disease such as enlarged and tortuous pulmonary arteries often exist (see Chap. 13). Cytologic evaluation of specimens from the lower airways reveals inflammation characterized by a predominance of eosinophils, with lesser numbers of nondegenerate neutrophils and macrophages. An occult heartworm test should be done for all dogs with PIE.

Treatment

Treatment of choice for dogs with PIE is administration of corticosteroids such as prednisone at 1 to 2 mg/kg by mouth per day. Most dogs have a marked response within 3 to 5 days, including decreased severity of clinical signs and less infiltrate on thoracic radiographs (Fig. 54–18). If there is improvement, the dose of corticosteroids can be gradually tapered over 2 to 4 weeks. Heartworm disease should be treated when clinical improvement occurs (see Chap. 13). Some dogs without heartworm disease may require long-term treatment with anti-inflammatory doses of prednisone when there is exacerbation of clinical signs.

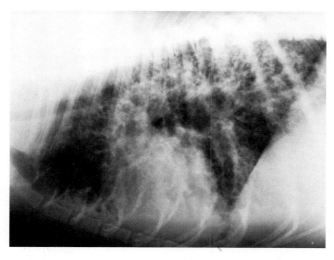

Figure 54–17
Lateral thoracic radiograph of a dog with pulmonary infiltrates with eosinophilia. A mixed alveolar, interstitial, and bronchial infiltrate is noted diffusely.

Prognosis

Most dogs with PIE respond dramatically to treatment with corticosteroids.[38] About half of dogs require continuous or intermittent treatment to control clinical signs.[38] The prognosis may also depend on the severity of the underlying heartworm disease, if present, and the patient's response to adulticide treatment.

Pulmonary Contusions

Pulmonary contusions are characterized by hemorrhage into the lungs as a result of traumatic

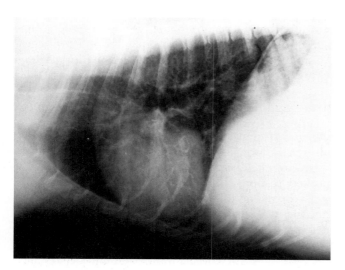

Figure 54–18
Lateral thoracic radiograph of the dog in Figure 54–17 taken 7 days after the beginning of treatment with prednisone.

injury. They occur frequently in dogs and cats that experience blunt-force trauma such as being hit by a car. Although there are no breed or sex predilections, dogs and cats that live outdoors are obviously predisposed.

Pathophysiology

Pulmonary contusions are caused by blunt-force trauma, which damages pulmonary capillary integrity, causing pulmonary edema and hemorrhage into the interstitium and alveolar spaces. Contusions are most often secondary to vehicular trauma, although penetrating injuries such as gunshot wounds and bite wounds also cause pulmonary contusions.

Clinical Signs

The most common clinical signs in patients with pulmonary contusions are dyspnea and tachypnea, which usually begin acutely after a traumatic event. Some patients do not show clinical signs until several hours after trauma, however. Thoracic auscultation often reveals crackles that may be localized to certain areas of the thorax. There may be decreased breath sounds in patients with concomitant pneumothorax. Muffled heart sounds should prompt suspicion of diaphragmatic hernia or pleural effusion such as hemothorax. Patients should be thoroughly evaluated for other injuries such as rib and long-bone fractures and penetrating wounds.

Diagnostic Plan

Pulmonary contusions should be suspected when respiratory signs exist in patients that have been traumatized within the previous 24 hours. Approximately 50% of dogs and cats that sustain fractures secondary to vehicular trauma also have pulmonary contusions.[39] Interestingly, pulmonary contusions are just as likely to occur in patients with hindlimb injuries as those with forelimb injuries.[39] Thoracic radiographs often show a localized interstitial or alveolar pattern; changes may not be evident until several hours after the traumatic incident[40] (Fig. 54–19).

Treatment

Patients with pulmonary contusions are managed primarily with supportive care. Oxygen is supplemented if signs of respiratory distress exist. Shock is treated by fluid therapy and administration of appropriate doses of corticosteroids (see Chap. 31). When the patient is stable, excessive fluid administration should be avoided; it could lead to worsening of pulmonary edema. Cage rest is indicated until signs of respiratory distress resolve. Administration of bronchodilators may help in patients that do not respond to

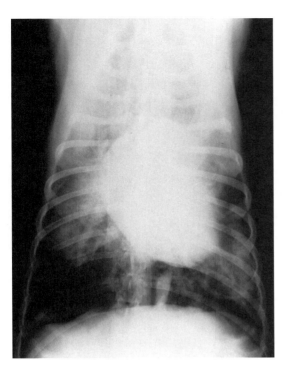

Figure 54–19
Dorsoventral thoracic radiograph of a dog with pulmonary contusions caused by vehicular trauma. Patchy alveolar infiltrate is present in all lung lobes.

conservative treatment (see Table 52–2). Fractured ribs usually do not require treatment; however, a bandage around the thorax is indicated to stabilize ribs with multiple fractures that cause flail chest or displaced fractures that can further damage lungs. Even if there are no signs of respiratory disease, patients that have sustained trauma should be monitored for 24 hours to detect deterioration in their condition.

Prognosis

The prognosis for patients with pulmonary contusions depends on the severity of underlying injuries. Most patients with only pulmonary contusions respond to treatment and show marked improvement during the first 24 hours.

Pulmonary Edema

Pulmonary edema is the accumulation of excessive fluid within the interstitial or alveolar spaces of the lungs. It commonly occurs in dogs and cats, most often associated with left-sided heart failure. Depending on its cause, pulmonary edema may be more common in dogs and cats of certain breeds and ages. Cardiogenic pulmonary edema is more likely to occur in dogs that have either mitral valve insufficiency or cardiomyopathy (see Chap. 9). Dogs and cats with pulmonary

edema secondary to electric cord bites usually are less than 1 year of age.[41]

Pathophysiology

Pulmonary edema generally results from increased hydrostatic pressure, decreased plasma oncotic pressure, increased capillary membrane permeability, lymphatic dysfunction, or increased negative intrapleural pressure. For practical purposes, most dogs and cats develop pulmonary edema as a result of increased hydrostatic pressure associated with left-sided congestive heart failure. Noncardiogenic pulmonary edema occurs infrequently in dogs and cats.[41–43] Decreased plasma oncotic pressure associated with hypoalbuminemia, usually less than 1.5 g/dL, occasionally causes pulmonary edema, ascites, pleural effusion, or peripheral edema. In most cases, patients that develop edema or effusions associated with hypoalbuminemia have concomitant abnormalities such as overzealous administration of fluids, cardiac disease, or renal disease. Upper airway obstruction resulting from brachycephalic airway syndrome or laryngeal disease may cause pulmonary edema, presumably because of increased permeability of pulmonary capillaries and increased negative intrapleural pressure.[42] Noncardiogenic pulmonary edema has also been reported in association with cranial trauma and seizures; edema in these cases is thought to result from increased sympathetic stimulation, which causes vasoconstriction and a shift of blood from the systemic circulation to the pulmonary circulation.[43] For a more complete discussion of the pathogenesis of pulmonary edema, see Chapter 9.

Clinical Signs

Clinical signs in dogs and cats with pulmonary edema depend on the severity of edema, its underlying cause, and how rapidly it develops. Some patients have signs such as exercise intolerance and cough that progressively worsen over time, whereas others have an acute onset of severe respiratory distress and cyanosis. Disorders that cause acute onset of clinical signs related to pulmonary edema include electric cord bite, cranial trauma, and ruptured chordae tendineae associated with chronic mitral insufficiency.[41] Because cardiac disease is the most common cause of pulmonary edema, physical examination of patients often reveals a murmur or gallop rhythm. It is important to evaluate patients carefully for other signs of cardiac disease such as distended jugular veins, tachycardia, pulse deficits, or cardiac arrhythmias. Thoracic auscultation may reveal crackles; however, it is not uncommon for breath sounds to be normal. Patients with noncardiogenic pulmonary edema usually have other signs to suggest the underlying cause, such as sterto-

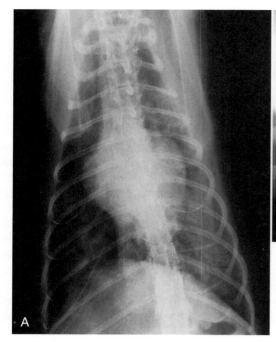
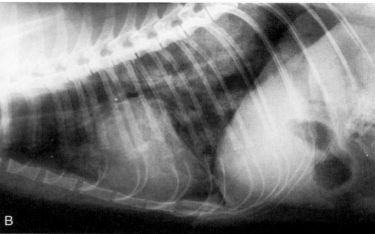

Figure 54–20

Lateral and dorsoventral thoracic radiographs of a cat with hypertrophic cardiomyopathy and pulmonary edema. **(A)** Note the elongated heart. **(B)** The patchy alveolar infiltrate in the dorsal and ventral lung lobes represents pulmonary edema. Note that in cats there is no consistent distribution for cardiogenic pulmonary edema as there is in dogs.

rous respiration and inspiratory dyspnea associated with upper airway obstruction, altered mental status or seizures related to cranial trauma, or wounds in the mouth related to electric cord bite.

Diagnostic Plan

Pulmonary edema is suspected on the basis of history and physical examination. Thoracic radiographs of patients with pulmonary edema initially reveal an interstitial pattern, which progresses to an alveolar pattern (Fig. 54–20). Dogs and cats with cardiogenic pulmonary edema often have cardiomegaly and pulmonary venous congestion. In dogs, cardiogenic edema is most prominent in the perihilar region. In cats, pulmonary edema may be asymmetrical and multifocal. Patients with noncardiogenic edema almost always have an alveolar pattern that affects the dorsocaudal lung fields most severely.[41–43] Additional evaluation, such as with echocardiography, is indicated for patients with suspected cardiac disease (see Chap. 9). Pulmonary edema secondary to hypoalbuminemia may also be associated with pleural effusion and ascites, and analysis of pleural or abdominal fluid is indicated in these cases. If hypoalbuminemia is identified, additional diagnostic tests are indicated to determine its cause (see Chap. 34).

Treatment

Noncardiogenic pulmonary edema usually responds to correction of the underlying cause (e.g., correction of upper airway obstruction, treatment of

cranial trauma) and supportive care including cage rest, oxygen supplementation, and administration of furosemide (Lasix) at 2 to 4 mg/kg IV as needed to control clinical signs. For a complete discussion of treatment of patients with cardiogenic pulmonary edema, see Chapter 11.

Prognosis

The prognosis for patients with pulmonary edema depends on the underlying cause and its severity. Patients with noncardiogenic pulmonary edema related to cranial trauma or electric cord bite may have a better prognosis than patients with upper airway obstruction or seizures.[41]

Aspiration Pneumonia

Aspiration pneumonia is inflammation of the lungs caused by inhalation of food, gastric contents, or foreign material from the oropharynx. Aspiration pneumonia is a common disorder that affects dogs more often than cats. There have been no reported breed or sex predilections; however, breeds of dogs most often affected with laryngeal disease, brachycephalic airway syndrome, or any cause of regurgitation, such as idiopathic megaesophagus, vascular ring anomaly, or myasthenia gravis, are more likely to develop aspiration pneumonia.

Pathophysiology

Aspiration pneumonia may be iatrogenic or result from compromised airway defenses. Iatrogenic causes include administration of diagnostic or therapeutic agents (e.g., barium, medications, activated charcoal, electrolyte lavage solutions) or food through an incorrectly placed nasogastric, pharyngostomy, or stomach tube. Disorders or conditions that interfere with pharyngeal, laryngeal, or esophageal function (e.g., cleft palate, laryngeal paralysis, megaesophagus, neurologic dysfunction, anesthesia, or sedation) predispose to aspiration pneumonia. Aspiration of foreign material into the lower airways and lungs may interfere with normal pulmonary function by several mechanisms. The physical presence of some materials may cause obstruction, most often of smaller airways. Aspiration of acidic gastric contents may damage airway epithelium and incite an inflammatory response of the lungs, which leads to edema and necrosis. These changes predispose to development of secondary infection by bacteria that are aspirated from the oropharynx.

Clinical Signs

Clinical signs of aspiration pneumonia often include regurgitation, cough, exercise intolerance, respiratory distress, nasal discharge, and cyanosis. Signs may be chronic (e.g., in some dogs with megaesophagus) or acute (e.g., aspiration after recovery from anesthesia). It is common for dogs with chronic aspiration pneumonia to have an acute exacerbation of clinical signs. Depending on the underlying cause, additional signs may include weakness, regurgitation,

stertorous respiration, or inspiratory dyspnea. Physical examination may reveal fever, tachypnea, or crackles on auscultation.

Diagnostic Plan

If aspiration pneumonia is suspected on the basis of history and physical examination, additional evaluation is indicated. A complete blood count often reveals neutrophilic leukocytosis and a left shift, although results may be normal in chronic cases. Thoracic radiographs reveal an interstitial to alveolar pattern that often affects the cranioventral lung lobes, although other lobes may be affected (Fig. 54–21). Radiographic changes may not be apparent for up to 24 hours after aspiration. Radiographs should be carefully examined for evidence of megaesophagus, vascular ring anomaly, or esophageal foreign body, which may predispose to the development of aspiration pneumonia. Samples for cytologic evaluation and bacterial culture should be obtained by tracheal wash. Alternatively, if an affected lobe is located near the thoracic wall, a transthoracic pulmonary aspirate may yield diagnostic samples (Fig. 54–22). Cytologic evaluation most often reveals neutrophilic inflammation, with or without bacteria. Although not all patients with aspiration pneumonia have bacterial infection, more than 90% of dogs with megaesophagus and a clinical diagnosis of aspiration pneumonia had positive cultures in one study.[44]

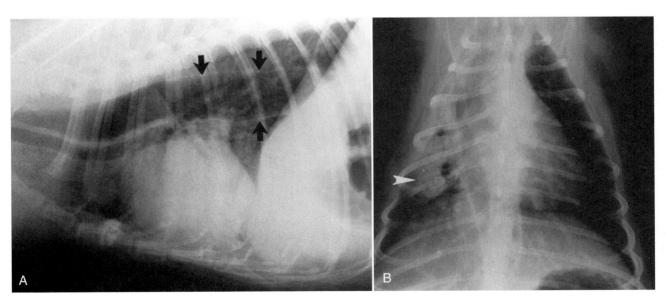

Figure 54–21
Lateral and dorsoventral thoracic radiographs of a dog with megaesophagus and aspiration pneumonia. **(A)** The esophagus is dilated and air filled *(arrows)*. **(B)** Alveolar infiltrate is present in the right middle lung lobe *(arrowhead)*.

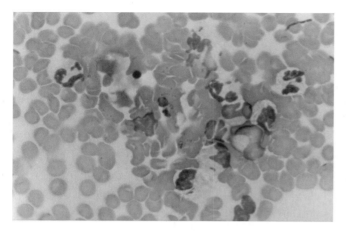

Figure 54-22
Cytologic evaluation of material obtained by transthoracic aspiration of a consolidated lung lobe in a dog with aspiration pneumonia. Note the presence of degenerate neutrophils. A hemolytic *Streptococcus* organism was cultured from the aspirated specimen (×100).

Treatment

Supportive care is an important part of treating patients with aspiration pneumonia. Patients with respiratory distress should receive oxygen supplementation, which can be given by oxygen cage or nasal catheter[45, 46] (Table 54–4 and Fig. 54–23). If oxygen is administered for more than 24 hours, it should be humidified; this can be accomplished by running the oxygen line through a humidifier before it reaches the patient. It is important to maintain hydration because this facilitates mucociliary clearance, an important defense mechanism for removing foreign material from the lungs and lower airways. One must be careful to avoid overhydration, which could cause pulmonary edema and worsening of clinical signs. For patients that receive oxygen therapy, nebulization should be done for 15 to 30 minutes two to three times daily to moisten the airways. Nebulization is accomplished by connecting the oxygen source to a commercially available nebulizer that contains sterile saline. Oxygen flows through the nebulizer and a fog of saline droplets is produced. The nebulizer may be connected to a facemask or an oxygen tent or cage so that the patient breathes the nebulized saline droplets. Because microorganisms can grow in nebulization equipment, the nebulizer and its attachments should be sterilized before each use and changed every 24 to 48 hours.[47] Physical activity and coupage are useful for loosening viscid airway secretions so that they can be more easily removed by mucociliary clearance. Coupage is accomplished by striking the rib cage over the lung fields with the palm of a cupped hand; this should be done for 10 minutes three to four times daily. Coupage may be more effective if it is done immediately after nebulization. Animals that are recumbent should be moved to a different position every 2 hours to prevent consolidation of the down lung.

Administration of antimicrobial agents may be indicated for treatment of patients with aspiration pneumonia. Aspiration does not necessarily imply that infection exists; however, it may be difficult to determine this because inflammation associated with aspiration of foreign material, especially acidic gastric contents, causes the same clinical signs as infection (e.g., fever, cough, respiratory distress, leukocytosis). We prefer to administer antimicrobial agents to patients with aspiration pneumonia that have systemic signs such as depression, inappetence, fever, or respiratory distress or that have septic inflammation on cytologic evaluation of tracheal wash fluid. For a detailed description of antimicrobial treatment of aspiration pneumonia, see the section in this chapter on treatment of bacterial pneumonia.

Prognosis

The prognosis for patients with aspiration pneumonia depends on the amount or character of material aspirated, the patient's status before aspiration, and the underlying cause.[48] Aspirated gastric contents may cause more severe inflammation than other substances. Patients with mild clinical signs that have aspirated a small amount of material probably have a better prognosis than patients with severe clinical signs or those that have aspirated a large amount of material. Dogs with idiopathic megaesophagus have a poor prognosis because this disorder responds poorly to treatment, and aspiration is a common recurring problem (see Chap. 30).

Bacterial Pneumonia

Bacterial pneumonia is infection of the lungs with bacteria; it is a common cause of respiratory disease in dogs but occurs infrequently in cats. Sporting breeds, working dogs, and hounds may be predisposed.[49] Pneumonia caused by *Bordetella bronchiseptica* is more common in dogs younger than 1 year of age.[50]

Pathophysiology

Bacterial infection of the lungs may become established by hematogenous spread during septicemia; however, it is more common for opportunistic organisms to cause infection after pulmonary defense mechanisms are compromised. Many of the bacteria isolated from patients with pneumonia are normal flora of the trachea and lower airways; therefore, it is likely that aspiration of foreign material, chronic bronchial disease, foreign bodies, viral infections, or

Table 54-4
Procedure for Nasal Administration of Oxygen

1. Apply topical anesthetic into one nostril, tip the patient's nose toward the ceiling, and wait 1–2 min before proceeding.
2. Select a 5 to 8 Fr infant feeding tube or red rubber catheter and mark the catheter at a point equal to the distance from patient's external nares to the medial canthus of the eye.
3. Place a small amount of water-soluble lubricant on the catheter tip and insert it into the nares in a dorsomedial direction to an initial depth of about 0.5–1 cm. Then direct the tip ventromedially and pass the catheter into the ventral nasal meatus until it is inserted to the point marked previously.
4. Position the catheter in the alar fold so that it fits snugly, and suture it to the skin next to the nares. Place the catheter over the midline of the nose so that it travels between the eyes and suture it to the skin of the forehead and the skin overlying the occipital protuberance.
5. Connect the catheter to oxygen tubing, which is connected to an anesthetic machine or bulk oxygen source with flow meter.
6. Administer oxygen, through a humidifier, at 50–100 mL/kg per minute to achieve 40%–50% inspired oxygen fraction; avoid higher inspired oxygen fractions, which may cause oxygen toxicosis, especially with prolonged administration (>18–24 h).

any other respiratory disease allows infection to become established. Canine distemper virus replicates in respiratory epithelium and causes interstitial pneumonia, which is often complicated by secondary bacterial infection.[51] Canine adenovirus, one of the

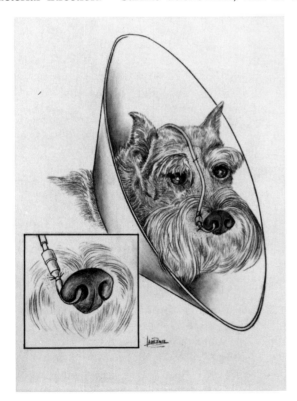

Figure 54-23
Diagram showing placement of a nasal catheter for administration of oxygen. The catheter is secured to the patient using sutures. An Elizabethan collar may be necessary to prevent the patient from removing the catheter. Pulling the catheter into the alar fold helps to secure it and to prevent removal (*inset*).

causative organisms of infectious tracheobronchitis (kennel cough) in dogs, also replicates in the respiratory epithelium and predisposes to development of secondary bacterial infections, especially with *B. bronchiseptica*. Complete suppression of coughing in dogs with uncomplicated kennel cough may prevent effective clearing of bacteria from the lungs, resulting in pneumonia.

In dogs, gram-negative organisms that cause pneumonia include *Pseudomonas*, *Escherichia coli*, and *Klebsiella* spp.; gram-positive bacteria isolated from dogs with pneumonia include *Pasteurella multocida*, *Streptococcus* spp., and *Staphylococcus* spp.[49, 52] It is not uncommon for pneumonia to be caused by multiple organisms in the same patient.[49, 52] Unvaccinated dogs are more likely to develop pneumonia related to infection with *B. bronchiseptica*, which is a component of infectious tracheobronchitis.[50]

Clinical Signs

The most common clinical signs in dogs with bacterial pneumonia are cough, depression, inappetence, and dyspnea.[49] Although the cough is usually productive, some dogs with bacterial pneumonia have a dry, nonproductive cough. Cats are more likely to be dyspneic and have nonspecific signs such as depression and inappetence. Physical examination may reveal fever, increased breath sounds and crackles, dyspnea, and nasal discharge; however, fewer than 50% of dogs with bacterial pneumonia have one or more of these abnormalities.[49]

Diagnostic Plan

A diagnosis of bacterial pneumonia is made on the basis of findings from a complete blood count, thoracic radiography, and cytologic evaluation and culture of samples obtained by tracheal wash or transthoracic pulmonary aspiration. The complete blood count in patients with bacterial pneumonia most often reveals leukocytosis, mature neutrophilia, a left shift, and monocytosis; increased plasma protein and packed cell volume may occur secondary to dehydration. However, some dogs may not have all these abnormalities.[49] Thoracic radiography may reveal an interstitial pattern early in the disease, which usually progresses to become an alveolar pattern. Cytologic evaluation of tracheal wash fluid usually reveals inflammation characterized by degenerate or nondegenerate neutrophils, although in 20% of cases inflammation may not be evident.[49] Bacteria are observed in 30% to 50% of tracheal washes from dogs with bacterial pneumonia.[49, 53] Samples of fluid should be submitted for bacterial culture, regardless of cytologic findings. Transthoracic aspiration of a consolidated area of lung near the thoracic wall often yields adequate specimens and should be done when a tracheal wash is not diagnostic.

Treatment

Patients with bacterial pneumonia should receive supportive care as described for aspiration pneumonia. Initial selection of antimicrobial agents can be based on cytologic findings after tracheal wash or transthoracic pulmonary aspiration (Table 54–5). If bacterial rods are identified, they almost always indicate gram-negative bacteria, whereas cocci are most likely streptococci or staphylococci.[53] Most gram-negative bacteria that cause pneumonia are susceptible to chloramphenicol, trimethoprim-sulfadiazine (Tribrissen), ceftiofur (Naxcel), gentamicin (Gentocin), amikacin (Amiglyde-V), and fluoroquinolones such as enrofloxacin (Baytril).[54, 55] *Pseudomonas* is resistant to enrofloxacin at the standard dose of 2.5 mg/kg but is susceptible to a dose of 11 mg/kg.[54] Antimicrobials that are effective against *B. bronchiseptica* include chloramphenicol, gentamicin, amikacin, amoxicillin clavulanate (Clavamox), tetracyline, and trimethoprim-sulfamethoxazole (Bactrim).[50, 54] Most gram-positive bacteria are susceptible to ampicillin, amoxicillin, chloramphenicol, trimethoprim-sulfonamides, gentamicin, and cephalosporins such as cephalexin (Keflex), cefazolin (Ancef), and cefadroxil (Cefa-Tabs).[51, 54, 55] If bacteria are not identified on cytologic evaluation, antimicrobial agents that provide coverage against gram-negative, gram-positive, and anaerobic organisms should be administered until results of culture and susceptibility are available. Potential regimens include penicillin and an aminoglycoside such as gentamicin. Because of potential nephrotoxicosis caused by aminoglyco-

Table 54–5

Dosage Regimens for Antimicrobial Agents Used to Treat Bacterial Pneumonia

DRUG	TRADE NAME	DOSAGE
Amikacin	Amiglyde-V	10 mg/kg IV t.i.d.
Ampicillin		22 mg/kg IV, PO t.i.d. or q.i.d.
Amoxicillin	Amoxil	22 mg/kg PO, SC t.i.d.
Amoxicillin/ clavulanate	Clavamox	12.5–25 mg/kg PO b.i.d.
Cefadroxil	Cefa-Tabs	22 mg/kg PO b.i.d.
Cefazolin	Ancef	20-25 mg/kg IV t.i.d. or q.i.d.
Ceftiofur	Naxcel	4.4 mg/kg SC b.i.d.
Cephalexin	Keflex	10–30 mg/kg PO b.i.d. to q.i.d.
Chloramphen-icol		40–50 mg/kg IV, SC, PO t.i.d (dogs) 50 mg per cat IV, SC, PO t.i.d. (cats)
Ciprofloxacin	Cipro	5–15 mg/kg PO b.i.d.
Enrofloxacin	Baytril	2.5 mg/kg PO, IM, IV b.i.d.*
Gentamicin	Gentocin	2.2 mg/kg IV, SC, IM t.i.d.†
Norfloxacin	Noroxin	22 mg/kg PO b.i.d.
Penicillin G		20,000–40,000 U/kg IV t.i.d. or q.i.d.
Tetracycline		15–20 mg/kg PO t.i.d or q.i.d.
Trimethoprim-sulfadiazine	Tribrissen	15 mg/kg PO b.i.d.

*Dose of 11 mg/kg necessary for treatment for *Pseudomonas*.
†Dose of 6.6 mg/kg IV, SC per day may be less nephrotoxic.
IM, intramuscularly; IV, intravenously; PO, by mouth; SC, subcutaneously; b.i.d., twice per day; t.i.d., three times per day; q.i.d., four times per day.

sides, however, administration of another drug such as enrofloxacin may be preferable, especially in dehydrated patients. Although enrofloxacin is not labeled for intravenous use, it has been used safely by being diluted with an equal volume of saline and being administered over several minutes. Another alternative is chloramphenicol, which provides broad-spectrum coverage and is effective against most respiratory pathogens. In patients with severe clinical signs or suspected sepsis, antimicrobial agents should be administered intravenously for the first 3 to 7 days. Oral administration is adequate for stable patients or those with a history of chronic aspiration pneumonia. Antimicrobials should be administered for a total of 4 to 8 weeks, ideally for 1 to 2 weeks beyond resolution of clinical and radiographic signs of pneumonia.

Prognosis

More than 70% of patients with bacterial pneumonia respond favorably to appropriate treatment.[49] Dogs that are treated on the basis of culture and susceptibility results are more likely to recover than those treated with antimicrobials selected empirically.[49] The presence of some concomitant conditions such as overwhelming sepsis or an underlying disorder that predisposes to recurrent pneumonia such as megaesophagus may worsen the prognosis.

Fungal Pneumonia

Pneumonia may occur secondary to systemic fungal infections in dogs and cats, most often with *Blastomyces dermatitidis*, *Histoplasma capsulatum*, or *Coccidioides immitis*.[56-60] Histoplasmosis affects dogs and cats, whereas blastomycosis and coccidioidomycosis are most often diagnosed in dogs. For more specific information on these fungal infections, see Chapter 39.

Pathophysiology

Dogs and cats become infected by inhaling fungal spores, which transform into a yeast at body temperature. After inhalation, pulmonary infection occurs; however, most infections do not cause clinical signs. Although some dogs and cats have only pulmonary involvement, others have dissemination of infection to other tissues. Growth of fungal organisms in the lungs stimulates an inflammatory response, which is responsible for clinical signs, including cough and dyspnea.

Clinical Signs

The most common respiratory signs in dogs and cats with fungal pneumonia are cough and dyspnea.

Other signs are nonspecific and include inappetence, weight loss, exercise intolerance, and lameness. Physical examination may reveal fever, increased breath sounds, crackles, lymphadenopathy, draining skin lesions, and ophthalmic lesions such as anterior uveitis and granulomatous chorioretinitis.

Diagnostic Plan

Thoracic radiography in dogs and cats with fungal pneumonia most often reveals a diffuse miliary to nodular interstitial pattern; other findings include hilar lymphadenopathy and, rarely, pleural effusion (Fig. 54–24). A diagnosis may be confirmed by identifying characteristic organisms in affected tissues such as enlarged peripheral lymph nodes or draining skin lesions. Cytologic evaluation of fluid obtained by transtracheal wash or bronchoalveolar lavage may reveal organisms in some patients with fungal pneumonia.[14] Because of its potential for causing pneumothorax, transthoracic pulmonary aspiration should be used only after less invasive tests have failed to yield a diagnosis (Fig. 54–25). In some cases, especially with cats, obtaining a pulmonary aspirate may be less stressful than performing tracheal wash or bronchoalveolar lavage. If the patient is in severe respiratory distress, it may be preferable to administer an antifungal drug orally and wait until the patient is stable before pursuing a definitive diagnosis. For a more complete discussion of methods used to diagnose systemic fungal infections, see Chapter 39.

Treatment

Treatment of dogs and cats with fungal pneumonia includes supportive care and administration of antifungal agents. Depending on the severity of clinical signs, supplemental oxygen and cage rest may also be

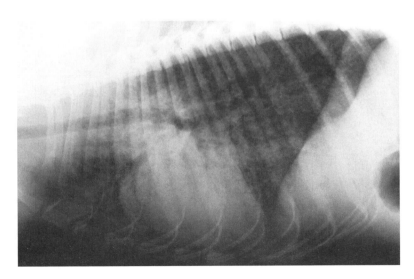

Figure 54–24
Lateral thoracic radiograph of a dog with *Blastomyces* infection. A diffuse miliary interstitial nodular pattern is present.

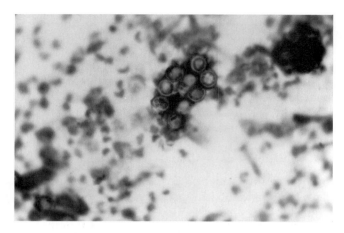

Figure 54–25
Cytologic evaluation of material obtained by transthoracic pulmonary aspiration from a dog with fungal pneumonia caused by *Blastomyces*. Note round organisms approximately 20 μm in diameter with a double cell wall (×100).

necessary. For a complete discussion of administration of antifungal agents see Chapter 39.

Prognosis

Dogs and cats with severe respiratory distress caused by fungal pneumonia have a guarded prognosis. If the patient survives the first week of treatment, chances for recovery are good, although long-term treatment is necessary in some cases.

Parasitic Pneumonia

Pneumonia is infrequently due to parasitic infection of the lower airways and lungs in dogs and cats. Organisms that most often cause parasitic pneumonia are *A. abstrusus* in cats and *P. kellicotti* in dogs and cats. *A. abstrusus*, also called the feline lungworm, lives in terminal bronchioles and alveoli of cats. *P. kellicotti* is a fluke that resides in cysts in the pulmonary parenchyma of cats and dogs.

Pathophysiology

Cats become infected with *A. abstrusus* by ingesting rodents, birds, or mollusks that have fed on infected snails or slugs.[13] First-stage larvae are coughed up, swallowed, and then passed in feces, approximately 4 to 6 weeks after infection. *A. abstrusus* lives primarily in terminal bronchioles and alveoli; it may incite an inflammatory response, which is responsible for clinical signs. Dogs and cats become infected with *P. kellicotti* by ingesting a crayfish, which serves as an intermediate host; eggs are produced beginning 4 to 5 weeks after infection.[13] *P. kellicotti* lives in the lower airways and alveoli in cysts. The presence of the parasite incites an inflammatory response, which may

cause clinical signs. Rupture of cysts causes pneumothorax and respiratory distress.

Clinical Signs

Most dogs and cats with parasitic infections of the respiratory system do not show clinical signs. When clinical signs do occur they most often include coughing and wheezing; dyspnea is present infrequently.

Diagnostic Plan

In cats with aelurostrongylosis, thoracic radiographs may be normal or may show poorly defined, diffuse nodular densities that affect the caudal lobes most severely; there may be a bronchial pattern in some cats caused by secondary inflammation. A hemogram may reveal eosinophilia. Cytologic evaluation of tracheal wash fluid may show eosinophils; first-stage larvae are identified infrequently. Finding larvae on fecal flotation using zinc sulfate or the Baermann technique is the easiest method for confirming a diagnosis.

Thoracic radiographs of dogs and cats with paragonimiasis may be normal or may show air-filled cysts or radiographic densities of soft tissue, approximately 1 cm in diameter (Fig. 54–26). There may be a bronchial, an interstitial, or an alveolar pattern related to inflammation; pneumothorax may occur if cysts rupture. A hemogram may show eosinophilia. Cytologic evaluation of tracheal wash fluid may reveal eosinophilic inflammation or ova. The most practical method for confirming a diagnosis is to identify operculated ova by zinc sulfate fecal flotation.

Treatment

Many dogs and cats do not require treatment because they either do not have clinical signs or have spontaneous resolution of signs. For patients with moderate to severe signs of infection, administration of parasiticidal agents is indicated. Aelurostrongylosis may be treated with fenbendazole (Panacur) at 20 mg/kg by mouth per day for 5 days, which should be repeated in 5 days. Although not approved for use in cats, ivermectin (Ivomec) at 0.4 mg/kg SC once may be effective.[13, 61, 62] Paragonimiasis may be treated with fenbendazole (50 mg/kg by mouth per day for 14 days), albendazole (Valbazen) at 25 mg/kg by mouth b.i.d. for 14 days, or praziquantel (Droncit) 23 mg/kg by mouth t.i.d. for 3 days.[13, 63]

Prognosis

Most dogs and cats with parasitic pneumonia are asymptomatic or have mild clinical signs, and spontaneous recovery is common. The prognosis for patients that require treatment is usually good.

Pulmonary Neoplasia

Pulmonary neoplasia is an abnormal proliferation of cells that originate with the lungs or metastasize from primary tumors elsewhere in the body. Although primary pulmonary tumors occur in dogs and cats, metastatic pulmonary neoplasia is more common. There appears to be no breed or sex predisposition; however, most primary and metastatic pulmonary tumors, except lymphoma, are more common in older patients.

Pathophysiology

Most primary tumors of the lungs are malignant and often metastasize to other areas of the lung. Primary pulmonary tumors in dogs and cats are either carcinomas or adenocarcinomas.[64, 65] Tumors that often metastasize to the lungs include thyroid carcinoma, mammary carcinoma, osteosarcoma, hemangiosarcoma, fibrosarcoma, and melanoma. Although lymphoma often affects hilar and mediastinal lymph nodes, it may also cause a mild interstitial pattern in

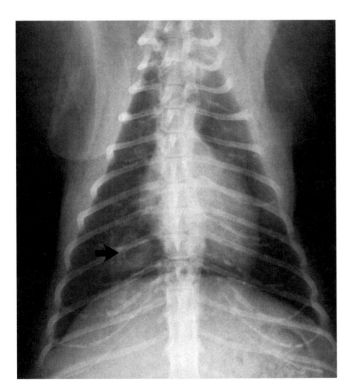

Figure 54–26
Dorsoventral thoracic radiograph of a cat with parasitic pneumonia caused by *Paragonimus kellicotti*. A soft tissue cavitated mass is present in the right caudal lung lobe (*arrow*).

the lungs. Except for lymphoma in cats, which is caused by feline leukemia virus infection, the inciting cause of most pulmonary neoplasms is unknown.

Clinical Signs

Clinical signs in patients with pulmonary neoplasia include exercise intolerance, inappetence, weight loss, cough, and respiratory distress. Dogs and cats with metastatic pulmonary neoplasia may have signs related to the primary tumor, such as lameness. Physical examination may reveal nonspecific findings such as emaciation, increased breath sounds, crackles, and increased respiratory rate.

Diagnostic Plan

Thoracic radiography is indicated for all patients with suspected neoplasia; it is important to obtain a dorsoventral view and left and right lateral views in all patients (Fig. 54–27). Patients with primary pulmonary neoplasia usually have a single, discrete nodule or consolidated lung lobe, although metastasis of primary tumors to other lobes often occurs (Fig. 54–28). Metastatic pulmonary neoplasia is characterized by a diffuse nodular interstitial pattern. Hilar lymphadenopathy may occur in patients with either primary or metastatic pulmonary neoplasia; pneumothorax occurs infrequently. Lymphoma often causes a mild diffuse, linear interstitial pattern in the lungs.

A diagnosis of metastatic neoplasia is best made by collecting samples from the primary tumor for cytologic or histologic evaluation. The patient should be carefully palpated for cutaneous or subcutaneous tumors or mammary, thyroid, or abdominal masses. A rectal examination is indicated in male dogs to detect prostatic masses. A thorough orthopedic examination should be performed in patients with lameness. Ultrasonography should be done to detect abdominal masses, especially in the liver and spleen.

Primary pulmonary tumors located near the thoracic cage can be diagnosed by cytologic evaluation of samples obtained by transthoracic aspiration. Tracheal wash and bronchoalveolar lavage occasionally allow a definitive diagnosis. However, in many cases, especially with primary neoplasia, a definitive diagnosis can be obtained only by open lung biopsy via a thoracotomy.

Treatment

Primary pulmonary neoplasia is best treated by surgical excision of the affected lobe. Samples of tissue should also be collected from thoracic lymph nodes to stage the tumor. If the tumor cannot be completely excised, if there is lymph node involvement, or if the owner wishes not to have surgery done, chemotherapy

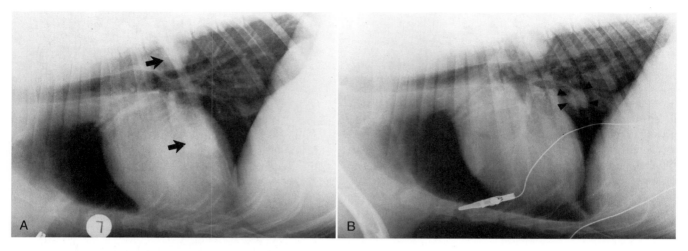

Figure 54–27
(A) Left lateral thoracic radiograph and **(B)** right lateral thoracic radiograph of a dog with transitional cell carcinoma of the urinary bladder and pulmonary metastasis. Note multiple soft tissue nodular densities in the pulmonary parenchyma *(arrows)*. One lesion is more apparent on the right lateral view *(arrowheads)*.

may be considered. However, there is no consistently reliable protocol for inducing remission in dogs and cats with primary pulmonary neoplasia.

There is no curative treatment for metastatic pulmonary neoplasia. Some tumors such as hemangiosarcoma may respond to a combination of vincristine, doxorubicin, and cyclophosphamide; however, this protocol is myelosuppressive and is associated with side effects in more than 70% of patients.[66] Surgical resection of metastatic pulmonary nodules, when less than three are present, may prolong survival in dogs with metastatic osteosarcoma.[67]

Prognosis

Patients with malignant pulmonary neoplasia have a grave prognosis and usually die as a result of their disease. Dogs with primary pulmonary tumors have a better prognosis if the tumor involves only one lobe and lymph nodes are not enlarged.[68] Median survival time of all dogs with primary pulmonary tumors treated by surgical excision is 120 days, whereas dogs that have no gross evidence of tumor after surgery, including lymph nodes, have a median survival of almost 1 year.[68]

Pulmonary Thromboembolism

Pulmonary thromboembolism is obstruction of pulmonary arteries because of the development of thrombi within the arteries or lodging of emboli that originate elsewhere. Pulmonary thromboembolism is most common in dogs with heartworm disease (see Chap. 13). Although it may be a common disorder in dogs and cats, it is not diagnosed frequently. It is

recognized most often in dogs, and there appears to be no breed or sex predisposition. Most reported cases have been middle-aged to older dogs.[69, 70]

Pathophysiology

Disorders that may predispose to development of pulmonary thromboembolism in dogs include heartworm disease, hyperadrenocorticism, protein-

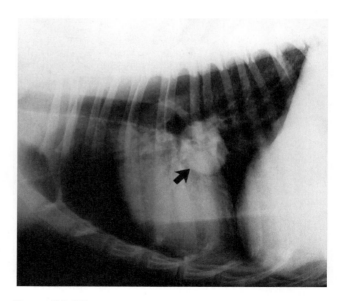

Figure 54–28
Lateral thoracic radiograph of a dog with primary pulmonary adenocarcinoma. A solitary soft tissue mass is present superimposed over the base of the heart *(arrow)*.

losing glomerular disease, immune-mediated hemo-lytic anemia, sepsis, bacterial endocarditis, other cardiac diseases, malignant neoplasia, and disseminated intravascular coagulation.[69–77] It is common for dogs with pulmonary thromboembolism to have multiple predisposing conditions at the same time.[69] The exact mechanisms by which these disorders cause pulmonary thromboembolism is unknown; it is likely that a combination of factors, such as a hypercoagulable state, vascular stasis, or disruption of vascular endothelium, is involved. Hyperadrenocorticism may cause a hypercoagulable state by increasing concentrations of clotting factors. Glomerular diseases also predispose to a hypercoagulable state because of urinary loss of antithrombin, platelet hypersensitivity associated with hypoalbuminemia, and decreased fibrinolysis.[75–78] Hemolytic anemia may cause release of thromboplastic substances from red blood cells, which leads to formation of thromboemboli.[70] Abnormal blood flow and vascular stasis in hearts of patients with dilated cardiomyopathy or valvular insufficiency may lead to formation of thrombi. Malignant neoplasms often have abnormal vascular endothelial surfaces, which can cause vascular stasis or activation of the coagulation cascade, leading to development of thrombi. Disseminated intravascular coagulation is associated with widespread formation of thrombi, which may affect any organ system, including the lungs.

Clinical Signs

Pulmonary thromboembolism is characterized by an acute onset of severe respiratory distress and tachypnea; cough and hemoptysis are observed infrequently.[69, 70] In addition to dyspnea, physical examination may reveal tachycardia, a split second heart sound, and crackles. Other than heartworm disease, the most common conditions associated with pulmonary thromboembolism are immune-mediated hemolytic anemia, cardiac diseases (e.g., cardiomyopathy, valvular insufficiency, bacterial endocarditis), malignant neoplasia, hyperadrenocorticism, disseminated intravascular coagulation, and sepsis.[69–71] Clinical signs depend on which of these conditions exists but may include pale mucous membranes, tachycardia, gallop rhythm, polyuria, polydipsia, abdominal distention, epistaxis, bleeding from venipuncture sites, petechiae and ecchymoses, or fever.

Diagnostic Plan

Initial diagnostic evaluation should include a complete blood count, serum chemistry assays, urinalysis, heartworm test, and thoracic radiographs. Regenerative anemia, spherocytosis, and autoagglutination suggest hemolytic anemia; leukocytosis and concomitant thrombocytopenia may exist.[70] Thrombo-

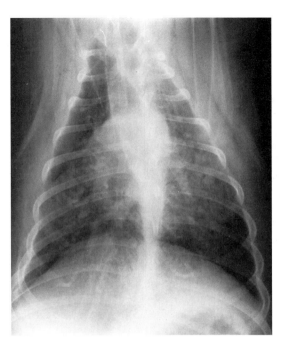

Figure 54–29
Dorsoventral thoracic radiograph of a dog with pulmonary thromboembolism. Alveolar infiltrate is present in the left and right lung lobes.

cytopenia and prolonged coagulation times occur in patients with disseminated intravascular coagulation. Hyperbilirubinemia is often observed in patients with hemolytic anemia. A stress leukogram and increased hepatic enzyme activities may be observed in dogs with hyperadrenocorticism. Dogs with pulmonary thromboembolism related to heartworm disease have thoracic radiographic changes such as right-sided heart enlargement, enlarged and tortuous pulmonary arteries, and a patchy infiltrate or alveolar pattern in the caudal lung fields. Thoracic radiographs of dogs with pulmonary thromboembolism of other causes may be normal or may show mild right-sided heart enlargement, slight pleural effusion, or an interstitial or alveolar infiltrate[70–72] (Fig. 54–29). A tentative diagnosis of pulmonary thromboembolism is made on the basis of clinical, laboratory, and radiographic findings. Pulmonary thromboembolism should be strongly suspected in dogs with severe dyspnea and no obvious cause. A definitive diagnosis requires contrast radiography, which may require sedation and special technical expertise.

Treatment

Treatment for patients with suspected or confirmed pulmonary thromboembolism includes correction of any predisposing causes, supportive care, and administration of heparin. Oxygen supplementation is indicated for most patients. Intravenous fluids should be given to maintain hydration and help improve microvascular circulation. Heparin is administered on the premise that it prevents thrombus growth and allows the fibrinolytic system to help resolve thrombi.[73] An initial dose of heparin (100–200 U/kg IV) followed in 2 hours by administration of heparin at 200 U/kg SC t.i.d. or q.i.d. is recommended.[73] Heparin dosage should be adjusted to maintain the patient's activated partial thromboplastin time by 1.5 times control values. Alternatively, activated clotting time may be monitored, with a goal of prolonging this value by 15 to 20 seconds above normal. Blood specimens should be obtained for monitoring coagulation times 2 hours after treatment or halfway between doses.[73] Length of treatment has not been established; however, it seems reasonable to continue heparin therapy until clinical signs resolve. Treatment with heparin should be discontinued gradually over several days by tapering the dose and decreasing the frequency of administration.

Prognosis

Except for heartworm disease, the prognosis for patients with pulmonary thromboembolism is guarded to grave. Despite aggressive medical treatment, many patients die from either pulmonary thromboembolism or life-threatening associated conditions.

Uncommon Diseases of the Lower Airways and Lungs

Primary Ciliary Dyskinesia

This disorder, a rare condition affecting young dogs, causes respiratory signs including mucopurulent nasal discharge and chronic cough.[79, 80] It is caused by a defect in cilia of the respiratory tract that prevents them from functioning adequately. This results in ineffective mucociliary clearance of the lower airways and predisposes to development of bronchopneumonia and bronchiectasis. It is diagnosed by electron microscopic evaluation of the nasal, tracheal, or pulmonary epithelium. Treatment is primarily supportive and includes management of any secondary infections.

Eosinophilic Granulomatosis

Eosinophilic granulomatosis is a disorder of dogs that causes multiple pulmonary nodules. The most common clinical sign is chronic cough. Thoracic radiographs reveal multiple pulmonary nodules and hilar lymphadenopathy, similar to findings in metastatic neoplasia. Tracheal wash may reveal a predominance of neutrophils or eosinophils. Approximately

50% to 80% of dogs have concomitant heartworm disease.[81, 82] Although this disorder may be suspected on the basis of these findings, a definitive diagnosis requires histologic evaluation of pulmonary tissue obtained during thoracotomy. Treatment includes administration of immunosuppressive drugs such as prednisone and cyclophosphamide; however, most dogs do not respond favorably.[82]

Lymphomatoid Granulomatosis

Lymphomatoid granulomatosis is an uncommon disorder of dogs that causes multiple, discrete pulmonary nodules that appear similar to those in metastatic neoplasia. Clinical signs include cough, dyspnea, exercise intolerance, and weight loss.[83, 84] Thoracic radiography reveals multiple pulmonary nodules and hilar lymphadenopathy. Diagnosis is confirmed by histologic evaluation of lung obtained by thoracotomy. Treatment with immunosuppressive drugs including prednisone and cyclophosphamide causes remission in about half of patients.[83, 84]

Viral Pneumonia

Infection with canine distemper virus or feline infectious peritonitis virus may cause pneumonia in dogs or cats, respectively. It is likely that canine distemper virus causes a pulmonary infection that becomes complicated by secondary bacterial pneumonia. Occasionally, cats with feline infectious peritonitis have a granulomatous pneumonia characterized radiographically by a diffuse, miliary pattern. Both viral diseases are more likely to have other signs that suggest the cause of the patient's problems (see Chaps. 24 and 38 for a complete discussion of canine distemper and feline infectious peritonitis).

Protozoal Pneumonia

Toxoplasmosis causes interstitial pneumonia in about one third of cats with toxoplasmosis.[85] The most common respiratory sign is dyspnea. Other signs of toxoplasmosis such as fever, anterior uveitis, hyperesthesia, and weight loss are usually present. Thoracic radiographs of cats with respiratory signs may reveal an interstitial pattern. For more details of diagnosis and treatment of toxoplasmosis, see Chapter 40.

References

1. Evans HE, Christensen GC. The respiratory apparatus. In: Evans HE, Christensen GC, eds. Miller's Anatomy of the Dog, 2nd ed. Philadelphia, WB Saunders, 1979:507–543.
2. Schummer A, Nickel R, Sack WO. Respiratory System. In: Schummer A, Nickel R, Sack WO, eds. The Viscera of the

Domestic Animals, 2nd ed. New York, Springer-Verlag, 1979:211–281.

3. Roudebush P. Antitussive therapy in small companion animals. J Am Vet Med Assoc 1982;180:1105–1107.

4. Irwin RS, Rosen MJ, Braman SS. Cough: A comprehensive review. Arch Intern Med 1977;137:1186–1191.

5. Steffey EP, Robinson NW. Respiratory system physiology and pathophysiology In: Ettinger SJ, ed. Textbook of Veterinary Internal Medicine, 2nd ed. Philadelphia, WB Saunders, 1983:673–691.

6. Roudebush P. Lung sounds. J Am Vet Med Assoc 1982;181:122–126.

7. Kotlikoff MI, Gillespie JR. Lung sounds in veterinary medicine. Part II. Deriving clinical information from lung sounds. Compen Contin Educ Pract Vet 1984;6:462–468.

8. Zajac AM. Fecal examination in the diagnosis of parasitism In: Sloss MW, Kemp RL, Zajac AM, eds. Veterinary Clinical Parasitology, 6th ed. Ames, Iowa, Iowa State University, 1994:3–93.

9. Moise NS. Clinical, radiographic, and bronchial cytologic features of cats with bronchial disease: 65 cases (1980–1986). J Am Vet Med Assoc 1989;194:1467–1474.

10. Ettinger SJ, Ticer JW. Diseases of the trachea In: Ettinger SJ, ed. Textbook of Veterinary Internal Medicine, 3rd ed. Philadelphia, WB Saunders, 1989:795–815.

11. Creighton SR, Wilkins RJ. Transtracheal aspiration biopsy: Technique and cytologic evaluation. J Am Anim Hosp Assoc 1974;10:219–226.

12. Padrid P, Amis TC. Chronic tracheobronchial disease in the dog. Vet Clin North Am Small Anim Pract 1992;22:1203–1229.

13. Reinemeyer CR. Parasites of the respiratory system In: Bonagura JD, ed. Kirk's Current Veterinary Therapy XII. Philadelphia, WB Saunders, 1995:895–898.

14. Hawkins EC, DeNicola DB. Cytologic analysis of tracheal wash specimens and bronchoalveolar lavage fluid in the diagnosis of mycotic infections in dogs. J Am Vet Med Assoc 1990;197:79–84.

15. McKiernan BC, Smith AR, Kissil M. Bacterial isolates from the lower trachea of clinically healthy dogs. J Am Anim Hosp Assoc 1984;20:139–142.

16. Padrid PA, Feldman BF, Funk K, et al. Cytologic, microbiologic, and biochemical analysis of bronchoalveolar lavage fluid obtained from 24 healthy cats. Am J Vet Res 1991;52:1300–1307.

17. Padrid P. Diagnosis and therapy of canine chronic bronchitis In: Bonagura JD, ed. Kirk's Current Veterinary Therapy XII. Philadelphia, WB Saunders, 1995:908–915.

18. Jacobson JD, Hartsfield SM, Haskins SC, et al. Anesthesia and respiratory disease In: Jacobson JD, ed. Introduction to Veterinary Anesthesiology. Blacksburg, Virginia, Brush Mountain Publishing, 1995:247–258.

19. Roudebush P. Tracheobronchoscopy. Vet Clin North Am 1990;20:1297–1314.

20. Amis TC, McKiernan BC. Systematic identification of endobronchial anatomy during bronchoscopy in the dog. Am J Vet Res 1986;47:2649–2658.

21. Venker-van Haagen AJ. Bronchoscopy of the normal and abnormal canine. J Am Anim Hosp Assoc 1979;15:397–410.

22. Hawkins EC, DeNicola DB. Collection of bronchoalveolar lavage fluid in cats, using an endotracheal tube. Am J Vet Res 1989;50:855–959.

23. Hawkins EC, DeNicola DB, Kuehn NF. Bronchoalveolar lavage in the evaluation of pulmonary disease in the dog and cat. J Vet Intern Med 1990;4:267–274.

24. Rebar AH, DeNicola DB, Muggenburg RA. Bronchopulmonary lavage cytology in the dog: normal findings. Vet Pathol 1980;17:294–304.

25. McCarthy GM, Quinn PJ. Bronchoalveolar lavage in the cat: cytologic findings. Can J Vet Res 1989;53:259–263.

26. Hawkins EC, Kennedy-Stoskopf S, Levy J, et al. Cytologic characterization of bronchoalveolar lavage fluid collected through an endotracheal tube in cats. Am J Vet Res 1994;55:795–802.

27. Hawkins EC, Morrison WB, DeNicola DB, et al. Cytologic analysis of bronchoalveolar lavage fluid from 47 dogs with multicentric malignant lymphoma. J Am Vet Med Assoc 1993;203:1418–1425.

28. Roudebush P, Green RA, Digilio KM. Percutaneous fine-needle aspiration biopsy of the lung in disseminated pulmonary disease. J Am Anim Hosp Assoc 1981;17:109–116.

29. Teske E, Stockhof AA, Wolvekamp WTC, et al. Transthoracic needle aspiration biopsy of the lung in dogs with pulmonic diseases. J Am Anim Hosp Assoc 1991;27:289–294.

30. Pirie HM, Wheeldon EB. Chronic bronchitis in the dog. Adv Vet Sci Comp Med 1976;20:253–276.

31. Padrid PA, Hornof WJ, Kurpershoek CJ, et al. Canine chronic bronchitis. J Vet Intern Med 1990;4:172–180.

32. Lindsey JO, Pierce AK. An examination of the microbiologic flora of normal lung of the dog. Am Rev Respir Dis 1978;117:501–505.

33. Moses BL, Spaulding GL. Chronic bronchial disease of the cat. Vet Clin North Am 1985;15:929–948.

34. Dye JA, Moise NS. Feline bronchial disease In: Kirk RW, Bonagura JD, eds. Kirk's Current Veterinary Therapy XI. Philadelphia, WB Saunders, 1992:803–811.

35. Rawlings CA, Calvert CA. Heartworm disease In: Ettinger SJ, Feldman EC, eds. Textbook of Veterinary Internal Medicine, 4th ed. Philadelphia, WB Saunders, 1995:1046–1068.

36. Calvert CA, Losonsky JM. Pneumonitis associated with occult heartworm disease in dogs. J Am Vet Med Assoc 1985;186:1097–1098.

37. Moon M. Pulmonary infiltrates with eosinophilia. J Small Anim Pract 1992;33:19–23.

38. Corcoran BM, Thoday KL, Henfrey JI, et al. Pulmonary infiltration with eosinophils in 14 dogs. J Small Anim Pract 1991;32:494–502.

39. Tamas PM, Paddleford RR, Krahwinkel DJ. Thoracic trauma in dogs and cats presented for limb fractures. J Am Anim Hosp Assoc 1985;21:161–166.

40. Crowe DT. Traumatic pulmonary contusions, hematomas, pseudocysts, and acute respiratory distress syndrome: An update—part I. Compen Contin Educ Pract Vet 1983;5:396–404.

41. Drobatz KJ, Saunders HM, Pugh CR, et al. Noncardiogenic pulmonary edema in dogs and cats: 26 cases (1987–1993). J Am Vet Med Assoc 1995;206:1732–1736.

42. Kerr LY. Pulmonary edema secondary to upper airway

obstruction in the dog: A review of nine cases. J Am Anim Hosp Assoc 1989;25:207–212.

43. Lord PF. Neurogenic pulmonary edema in the dog. J Am Anim Hosp Assoc 1975;11:778–782.

44. Hawkins EC. Aspiration pneumonia In: Bonagura JD, ed. Kirk's Current Veterinary Therapy XII. Philadelphia, WB Saunders, 1995:915–919.

45. Fitzpatrick RK, Crowe DT. Nasal oxygen administration in dogs and cats: Experimental and clinical investigations. J Am Anim Hosp Assoc 1986;22:293–300.

46. Jacobson JD, Hartsfield SM, Haskins SC, et al. Nasal oxygen therapy In: Jacobson JD, ed. Introduction to Veterinary Anesthesiology. Blacksburg, Virginia, Brush Mountain Publishing, 1995:305–307.

47. Haskins SC. Physical therapeutics for respiratory disease. Semin Vet Med Surg (Small Anim) 1986;1:276–288.

48. Hawkins EC. Diseases of the lower respiratory system In: Ettinger SJ, Feldman EC, eds. Textbook of Veterinary Internal Medicine, 4th ed. Philadelphia, WB Saunders, 1995:767–811.

49. Thayer GW, Robinson SK. Bacterial bronchopneumonia in the dog: A review of 42 cases. J Am Anim Hosp Assoc 1984;20:731–735.

50. Roudebush P, Fales WH. Antibacterial susceptibility of Bordetella bronchiseptica isolates from small companion animals with respiratory disease. J Am Anim Hosp Assoc 1981;17:793–797.

51. Roudebush P. Infectious pneumonia In: Kirk RW and Bonagura JD, eds. Kirk's Current Veterinary Therapy XII. Philadelphia, WB Saunders, 1992:228–236.

52. Jameson PH, King LA, Lappin MR, et al. Comparison of clinical signs, diagnostic findings, organisms isolated, and clinical outcome in dogs with bacterial pneumonia: 93 cases (1986–1991). J Am Vet Med Assoc 1995;206:206–209.

53. Hirsch DC. Bacteriology of the lower respiratory tract In: Kirk RW, ed. Current Veterinary Therapy IX. Philadelphia, WB Saunders, 1986:247–250.

54. Hirsch DC, Jang SS. Antimicrobial susceptibility of selected infectious bacterial agents obtained from dogs. J Am Anim Hosp Assoc 1994;30:487–494.

55. Roudebush P. Bacterial infections of the respiratory system In: Greene CE, ed. Infectious Diseases of the Dog and Cat. Philadelphia, WB Saunders, 1992:114–124.

56. Greene RT, Troy GC. Coccidioidomycosis in 48 cats: A retrospective study. J Vet Intern Med 1995;9:86–91.

57. Clinkenbeard KD, Cowell RL, Tyler RD. Disseminated histoplasmosis in cats: 12 cases (1981–1986). J Am Vet Med Assoc 1987;190:1445–1448.

58. Clinkenbeard KD, Cowell RL, Tyler RD. Disseminated histoplasmosis in dogs: 12 cases (1981–1986). J Am Vet Med Assoc 1988;193:1443–1447.

59. Breider MA. Blastomycosis in cats: Five cases (1979–1986). J Am Vet Med Assoc 1988;193:570–572.

60. Legendre AM, Walker M, Buyukmihci N, et al. Canine blastomycosis: A review of 47 clinical cases. J Am Vet Med Assoc 1981;178:1163–1168.

61. Kirkpatrick CE, Magella C. Use of ivermectin in treatment of Aelurostrongylus abstrusus and Toxacara cati infections in the cat. J Am Vet Med Assoc 1987;190:1309–1310.

62. Vig MM, Murray PA. Successful treatment of Aelurostrongylus abstrusus with fenbendazole. Compen Contin Educ Pract Vet 1986;8:214–222.

63. Bowman DD, Frongillo MK, Johnson RC, et al. Evaluation of praziquantel for treatment of experimentally induced paragonimiasis in dogs and cats. Am J Vet Res 1991;52:68–71.

64. Ogilvie GK. Classification of primary lung tumors in dogs: 210 cases (1975–1985). J Am Vet Med Assoc 1989;195:106–108.

65. Moore AS, Middleton DJ. Pulmonary adenocarcinoma in three cats with non-respiratory signs only. J Small Anim Pract 1982;23:501–509.

66. Hammer AS, Couto CG, Filppi J, et al. Efficacy and toxicity of VAC chemotherapy (vincristine, doxorubicin, and cyclophosphamide) in dogs with hemangiosarcoma. J Vet Intern Med 1991;5:160–166.

67. O'Brien MG. Resection of pulmonary metastases in canine osteosarcoma: 36 cases (1983–1992). Vet Surg 1993;22:105–109.

68. Ogilvie GK. Prognostic factors for tumor remission and survival in dogs after surgery for primary lung tumor: 76 cases (1975–1989). J Am Vet Med Assoc 1989;195:109–112.

69. LaRue MJ, Murtaugh RJ. Pulmonary thromboembolism in dogs: 47 cases (1986–1987). J Am Vet Med Assoc 1990;197:1368–1372.

70. Klein MK, Dow SW, Rosychuk RAW. Pulmonary thromboembolism associated with immune-mediated hemolytic anemia in dogs: Ten cases (1982–1987). J Am Vet Med Assoc 1989;195:246–250.

71. Burns MG, Kelly AB, Hornof WJ, et al. Pulmonary artery thrombosis in three dogs with hyperadrenocorticism. J Am Vet Med Assoc 1981;178:388–393.

72. Fluckiger MA, Gomez JA. Radiographic findings in dogs with spontaneous pulmonary thrombosis or embolism. Vet Radiol 1984;25:124–131.

73. Baty CJ, Hardie EM. Pulmonary thromboembolism: Diagnosis and management In: Kirk RW, Bonagura JD, eds. Kirk's Current Veterinary Therapy XI. Philadelphia, WB Saunders, 1992:137–142.

74. Slauson DO, Gribble DH. Thrombosis complicating renal amyloidosis in dogs. Vet Pathol 1971;8:352–363.

75. Green RA, Russo EA. Hypoalbuminemia-related platelet hypersensitivity in two dogs with nephrotic syndrome. J Am Vet Med Assoc 1985;186:485–488.

76. Green RA. Clinical implications of antithrombin III deficiency in animal diseases. Compen Contin Educ Pract Vet 1984;6:537–546.

77. Green RA, Kabel AL. Hypercoagulable state in three dogs with nephrotic syndrome: Role of acquired antithrombin III deficiency. J Am Vet Med Assoc 1982;181:914–917.

78. Relford RL, Green RA. Coagulation disorders in glomerular diseases In: Kirk RW, Bonagura JD, eds. Kirk's Current Veterinary Therapy XI. Philadelphia, WB Saunders, 1992:827–829.

79. Morrison WB, Wilsman NJ, Fox LE, et al. Primary ciliary dyskinesia in the dog. J Vet Intern Med 1987;1:67–74.

80. Edwards DF, Patton CS, Bemis DA, et al. Immotile cilia syndrome in three dogs from a litter. J Am Vet Med Assoc 1983;183:667–672.

81. Neer TM, Waldron DR, Miller RI. Eosinophilic pulmo-

nary granulomatosis in two dogs and literature review. J Am Anim Hosp Assoc 1986;22:593–599.

82. Calvert CA. Pulmonary and disseminated eosinophilic granulomatosis in dogs. J Am Anim Hosp Assoc 1988; 24:311–320.

83. Berry CR, Moore PF, Thomas WP, et al. Pulmonary lymphomatoid granulomatosis in seven dogs (1976–1987). J Vet Intern Med 1990;4:157–166.

84. Postorino NC. A syndrome resembling lymphomatoid granulomatosis in the dog. J Vet Intern Med 1989;3:15–19.

85. Lappin MR, Greene CE, Winston S, et al. Clinical feline toxoplasmosis. J Vet Intern Med 1989;3:139–143.

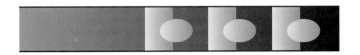

Skeletal
Diseases

Chapter 55

Joint and Skeletal Diseases

Spencer A. Johnston

Anatomy

The musculoskeletal system is a smoothly integrated system consisting of muscles acting on a rigid framework of bone. The mechanical arrangement of soft tissue attachment to bone and joint design allow ambulation. The anatomy of this system is similar for dogs and cats.

Bone anatomy is quite variable, and bones are generally classified into five general forms.[1] These are the long bones, such as the humerus, radius, femur, and tibia; the short bones, such as the carpals and metacarpals; the sesamoid bones, such as the patella; the flat bones, such as the cranial bones and pelvis; and the irregular bones, such as the vertebral column. All of these bones can be associated with disease processes.

In addition to the classification based on shape, bones can be classified according to structure. In the mature animal, bone is either cortical or cancellous. Cortical bone is dense and is mainly responsible for providing rigidity to the skeleton. It makes up the major portion of the long bones. Cancellous bone consists of bony trabeculae that contain numerous osteocytes and hematopoietic elements. It is found near the ends of long bones, in the vertebrae, and between the cortical walls of flat bones.

Each long bone is divided into regions. Identification of the various regions depends on whether the animal is growing or has reached skeletal maturity. In the growing animal, the end of each long bone is referred to as the epiphysis. The epiphysis is composed mostly of cancellous bone. A portion of the epiphysis is covered with hyaline cartilage and contributes to the formation of a joint. The metaphysis is adjacent to the epiphysis and separates the epiphysis from the diaphysis, which is the main shaft of the bone. In the growing animal, the metaphysis is separated from the epiphysis by the cartilaginous physeal growth plate (physis). The physis is a region of chondrocyte division and progressive differentiation necessary for longitudinal bone growth. The physis closes as the animal approaches maturity. Once the physis closes, the distinction between the epiphysis and metaphysis ceases to exist, and the entire region is referred to as the metaphysis and is composed primarily of cancellous bone.[2] The metaphysis joins the diaphysis, which is composed primarily of cortical bone. The interior of this rigid cortical tube is the diaphyseal medullary cavity. Bone marrow, consisting of both hematopoietic elements and fat cells, is found within the medullary cavity. The internal and external surfaces of the diaphysis and metaphysis, with the exception of the articular surface, are covered by endosteum and periosteum, respectively.

A joint is a junction between two or more bones. Joints are typically classified according to the type of connective tissue present or how much motion occurs at the junction.[3, 4] Fibrous joints, such as the cranial sutures, allow virtually no movement. Cartilaginous joints, such as occur between the vertebrae and at the pubic symphysis, allow only slight motion. The major motion joints of the body, such as the shoulder, elbow, hip, and stifle, are synovial joints. These joints consist of adjacent bone ends covered by hyaline cartilage and are connected by ligaments and a joint capsule. The joints typically affected by injury or disease are the synovial joints, although cartilaginous joints, such as the vertebral joints and their associated intervertebral discs, are frequently associated with significant morbidity.

Hyaline cartilage (the type of cartilage found on the joint surface) is a unique substance that consists of mostly water, collagen, proteoglycans, and ground substance. Cartilage is avascular, aneural, and alymphatic and receives nutrition from the synovial fluid. Chondrocytes (cartilage cells) and collagen within hyaline cartilage are oriented to provide the greatest strength and smoothest function of this tissue.

A joint capsule surrounds the synovial joint and defines the articular space. This capsule consists of two layers. The cells of the inner layer, or synovial membrane, function in phagocytosis and produce synovial fluid. The outer layer, or fibrous joint capsule, is composed of dense connective tissue and serves a more mechanical function. The joint capsule is richly innervated with mechanoreceptors and nociceptors. Mechanoreceptors provide information regarding spatial position and pressure, and nociceptor stimulation leads to the perception of pain.

Joints are supported by ligaments, tendons, and muscle.[4, 5] Ligaments are bundles of parallel collagen fibers that are anatomically located to provide the greatest stability to the joint. Muscles contribute to joint stability through their bulk and their ability to contract and exert force. The force generated by each muscle mass is transmitted to bone through tendons. Tendon insertions on bone maximize both mechanical advantage and joint stability. Muscles provide great stability to the large proximal joints of the body, such as the shoulder and hip.[4] When large muscle groups are absent, as around smaller joints like the carpus and interphalangeal joints, ligamentous support has a more important function.

Physiology

Joints distribute and disperse force associated with movement.[6] The joint capsule, ligaments, associated muscles, and tendons play an important role in controlling excessive joint motion and distributing the force over the articular surface. The collagen portion of hyaline cartilage acts as a sponge to absorb and distribute force over the underlying subchondral bone.

Table 55–1
Common Synovial Fluid Findings by Disease

SYNOVIAL FLUID (SF) FINDING	NORMAL JOINT	NONINFLAMMATORY		INFLAMMATORY			
		Degenerative Joint Disease	Hemarthrosis	Rheumatoid Arthritis	Lupus Arthropathy	Neoplastic Joint Disease	Septic Arthritis
Color	C	PY	R	YBT	YBT	YBT	CCS
Turbidity	*	†	‡	§	§	§	‡
Viscosity	Normal	Normal	Reduced	Reduced	Reduced	Reduced	Reduced
Mucin clot	Good	Good	Fair	Poor	Fair	Good	Poor
RBCs	None	Few	Many	Moderate	Moderate	Moderate	Moderate
WBCs × 10³/μL	0.25–3	1–5	3–10	8–38	4.4–371	3–10	40–267
% PMNS	0–6	0–12	60–75	20–80	15–95	15–75	90–99
% Mononuclear cells	94–100	88–100	25–40	20–80	5–85	25–85	1–10
Ragocytes	–	–	–	+	–	–	–
LE cells	–	–	–	–	+	–	–
Neoplastic cells	–	–	–	–	–	+	–
Microorganisms	–	–	–	–	–	–	+
SF glucose (% of blood glucose)	100	80–100	100	50–80	50–80	50–80	<50

C, colorless; PY, pale yellow; R, red; YBT, yellow to blood tinged; CCS, cream colored to sanguineous.
*Not turbid; †, slight turbidity; ‡, marked turbidity; §, moderate turbidity.
**–, absent; +, present.
From Toombs JP, Widmer WR. Bone, joint, and periskeletal enlargement. In: Lorenz MD, Cornelius LM, eds. Small Animal Medical Diagnosis, 2nd ed. Philadelphia, JB Lippincott, 1993:409.

Healthy articular cartilage and synovial fluid allow nearly frictionless movement between joint surfaces. Periarticular soft tissues provide the greatest resistance to movement, as the energy required to stretch the soft tissues surrounding the joint is nearly 100 times greater than that required to overcome the resistance produced between two healthy articular surfaces.[7]

Normal chondrocytes are metabolically active cells that serve both an anabolic and a catabolic function. They are able to synthesize collagen and proteoglycans, which make up a large portion of the extracellular matrix of cartilage. They are also sensitive to injury to this extracellular matrix and respond by producing degradative enzymes such as collagenase and proteases, in addition to altering the production of collagen and proteoglycan. Normal cartilage homeostasis can be altered in response to mechanical injury or biochemical changes associated with disease states.

Normal synovium is responsible for the production of synovial fluid and the phagocytosis of cellular debris and particulate matter from the joint cavity.[8] Synoviocytes can also produce various biochemical mediators, such as cytokines and prostaglandins. These substances play an important role in the pathogenesis of both immune-mediated arthritis and osteoarthritis (arthritis secondary to injury).

Synovial fluid is produced as an ultrafiltrate of plasma. It is composed primarily of hyaluronan but also contains some proteoglycan, white blood cells, and other biochemical mediators. It is normally clear, colorless or pale yellow, and viscous, and it has relatively few cells (the majority of which are mononuclear cells). The normal joint maintains a delicate homeostasis between cartilage anabolism and catabolism, and the synovial fluid content of various cells and biochemical mediators can be used as an indication of disease (Table 55–1).

Synovial fluid serves primarily to lubricate the joint and provide nutrition to chondrocytes. It lubricates the joint by providing a physical separation between the adjoining articular surfaces so that direct contact and subsequent wear are minimized. Synovial fluid, specifically the hyaluronan portion, also provides boundary lubrication, which allows smooth movement between the joint and the surrounding periarticular tissues.

Problem Identification

Lameness

Lameness is defined as an abnormal gait and may be due to injury, maldevelopment, or disease. Single-limb lameness is most easily identified, as it results in an asymmetrical gait that can be detected visually. Bilaterally symmetrical lameness is more difficult to detect; it occurs frequently in diseases such as hip dysplasia and immune-mediated arthropathies. Lameness is characterized by joint stiffness, a shortened stride, and altered weight bearing. Single-limb lameness is an extremely common problem in small animal patients. Fortunately, single-limb lameness is often due to minor strains or sprains that are usually self-limited and resolve with rest within 1 to 3 days of onset. When the problem is severe or persists for longer periods, further diagnostic work-up is warranted.

Pathophysiology

Lameness may be due to mechanical causes, an attempt to decrease limb loading in response to pain, or both. Mechanical lameness includes conditions such as malunion of a fracture and angular limb deformity associated with growth plate injury. Lameness in response to pain occurs in conditions such as immune-mediated arthritis, panosteitis, neoplasia, or septic arthritis. Most frequently, lameness is associated with both mechanical dysfunction and pain, such as occurs with fracture, luxation, and severe degenerative change.

Clinical Signs

Clinical signs associated with lameness include an abnormal gait characterized by gait asymmetry (including weight-bearing and non–weight-bearing lameness), altered stride length or limb motion, decreased range of motion, pain on direct palpation or joint manipulation, joint effusion, and limb or joint swelling. Head motion may be an aid to diagnosis; a patient with front limb lameness raises the head with weight bearing on the unsound limb and lowers the head with weight bearing on the sound limb. Joint laxity may be detected by observation of the weight-bearing patient for hyperextension or hyperflexion or by direct joint manipulation. Overall posture is noted to determine whether weight is being shifted from one limb to another. Patients with bilateral front limb lameness may move the hind limbs forward and under the body in an attempt to transfer weight from the front limbs to the hind limbs. The head may be raised to facilitate this transfer. A similar but opposite transfer of weight may be attempted if hindlimb lameness is present.

Diagnostic Plan

Historically, the onset of lameness may be acute or of a more insidious nature. Careful questioning about the possibility of trauma is important. Signalment often plays an important role, as age and breed predisposition may be important factors to consider in the diagnostic work-up. The presence of unilateral or bilateral abnormality can help distinguish between congenital and acquired conditions; many bilateral abnormalities are associated with congenital or systemic causes, and most acquired conditions involve unilateral abnormality. However, not all unilateral conditions are acquired, and not all bilateral conditions are congenital.

The diagnostic plan for all lameness evaluations begins with observation of the gait. Lameness may be observable in the examination room but at other times requires observation from a greater distance. Observation of the patient at various gait velocities is beneficial. Some lamenesses are more noticeable at a trot, whereas others are most noticeable at a slow walk. After gait observation, physical examination is performed. Complete physical examination is necessary, and the musculoskeletal system is specifically targeted for close examination.

On the basis of history and signalment, gait observation, and physical examination, a diagnostic rule-out list is formulated and a more thorough musculoskeletal examination is performed. If the patient is young and has a unilateral forelimb lameness, common disorders to rule out include trauma (including sprains and muscle strain), panosteitis, osteochondritis dissecans (shoulder and elbow), fragmented coronoid process, ununited anconeal process, joint luxation, angular limb deformity, hypertrophic osteodystrophy, and neoplasia. For unilateral hindlimb lameness in a young dog it is necessary to rule out trauma (including sprains and muscle strain), hip dysplasia, panosteitis, patella luxation, cruciate ligament rupture, Legg-Calvé-Perthes disease (avascular femoral head necrosis), osteochondritis dissecans (stifle and tarsus), joint luxation, and neoplasia.

The diagnostic rule-out list differs for the mature patient with single-limb lameness. Congenital and developmental conditions such as osteochondrosis dissecans, ununited anconeal process, or fragmented coronoid process can be present, but the manifestation of these processes, degenerative joint disease, is the actual cause of lameness. Panosteitis is unlikely to be the diagnosis for a patient older than 3 years. Differential diagnoses for front limb lameness in such mature patients include trauma (fracture or luxation), soft tissue injury, osteoarthritis, biceps tenosynovitis, carpal hyperextension, infection, neoplasia, and immune-mediated or infectious arthritis. Differentials for hindlimb lameness in mature patients include trauma (fracture or luxation), soft tissue injury, hip dysplasia, cruciate ligament rupture, patella luxation (medial or lateral), osteoarthritis, neoplasia, infection, and immune-mediated or infectious arthritis.

Once the region of pain or abnormality is identified, if further information is necessary it may be beneficial to sedate the patient to allow more complete palpation and radiographs if necessary. The majority of diagnoses are made with this degree of diagnostic work-up. If an answer is still not obtained, arthrocentesis is generally the next step. If arthrocentesis does not yield the diagnosis and life-threatening disease has been ruled out, allowing the patient to rest and re-examining the patient in 1 to 2 weeks may be an appropriate diagnostic action. If the condition does not resolve with rest, further diagnostic work-up such as repeating radiographs and arthrocentesis; more advanced radiographic procedures such as computed tomography; serologic testing; and exploratory surgery and biopsy may be indicated.

Multiple Joint Pain With Effusion

Multiple joint pain with effusion is an uncommon finding in the physical examination. Effusion of multiple joints is usually conspicuous when present. In the absence of effusion, joint pain may be difficult to localize. Clinical signs of diffuse pain related to joint involvement include reluctance to move or a stiff gait with a characteristic "walking on eggshells" appearance, pain and aggression with attempted manipulation of joints, and in some cases generalized swelling or distention of the capsules of multiple joints. Joints may have a decreased range of motion and may be palpably warm. The joints of the appendicular skeleton are more noticeably affected than are joints of the axial skeleton.

Pathophysiology

Multiple joint pain with effusion is often a manifestation of a systemic disease. Joint pain with effusion or swelling is usually associated with inflammation of the periarticular or articular tissues. Release of endogenous inflammatory mediators, such as prostaglandins, cytokines, leukotrienes, and metalloproteinases, results in vasodilation and increased fluid extravasation into the synovial cavity. These changes decrease the viscosity and lubricating qualities and increase the volume of synovial fluid. The changes lead to decreased biomechanical functioning of the joint, resulting in further cartilage injury. Damage to chondrocytes results in altered synthesis of cartilage matrix components and release of degradative enzymes, leading to more synovitis and perpetuation of this cycle. Thickening of the joint capsule associated with inflammation and synovitis causes pain and decreased range of motion with movement. Pain results from the stimulation of nociceptors present in the synovium, subchondral bone, ligaments, and other periarticular tissues.

Clinical Signs

Physical examination of these patients should be done carefully to minimize the pain response. Because these patients often have a systemic disease, clinical signs other than those associated with the joints are often present. In addition to observing the gait, close attention is paid to the overall body condition, mucocutaneous junctions, skin condition, close auscultation of the heart and lungs, and careful examination for any potential source of infection. The lameness may have either an acute or an insidious onset. It is important to determine whether trauma is a possibility or there has been a history of a penetrating wound to the joint involved. Temporal exposure to parasites, such as ticks, can play an important role, and knowledge of tick-borne diseases endemic to the area is important.

Diagnostic Plan

When multiple joint pain with effusion is identified, a diagnostic rule-out list is established. The patient is usually sedated to allow further palpation of the joints, and then radiographs of one or more joints are taken to determine the degree of change present. After radiography, with the patient still sedated, the area overlying the joint is aseptically prepared and arthrocentesis is performed. If a sufficient volume of fluid is obtained, it is best to submit samples for both cytologic evaluation and bacterial culture. Cell count and cell type are the most important parameters to be determined by cytology (see Diagnostic Procedures). Bacterial culture is most reliably performed by placing synovial fluid into blood culture medium at a dilution of 1:9. Bacterial culture is frequently needed to rule out sepsis.

If nucleated cell counts are greater than 5000/µL, a diagnosis of inflammatory joint disease is made. The differential diagnosis is then limited to immune-mediated or infectious disease. Immune-mediated diseases include erosive (rheumatoid arthritis) and nonerosive (systemic lupus erythematosus [SLE] and idiopathic immune-mediated arthritis) conditions. These are further distinguished by radiographic and serologic criteria. Infectious diseases include those with bacterial, rickettsial, and spirochetal etiologies. Bacterial causes are ruled in or out by cytology and culture. Patients with polyarthritis related to a rickettsial disease usually have other clinical signs such as systemic illness, skin lesions, and hematologic changes (see also Chap. 37). Arthritis associated with spirochetal organisms (Lyme borreliosis) is typically transient, may be associated with systemic illness or lymphadenopathy, and is difficult to confirm diagnostically (see also Chap. 36).

If erosive changes are noted on radiographs, the diagnostic rule-out list is limited to rheumatoid arthritis and bacterial infection. If bacterial culture and cytology are negative for causative organisms, a high degree of suspicion exists for rheumatoid arthritis. Confirmation is pursued through serologic testing (for rheumatoid factor) and synovial membrane biopsy. If after analyzing radiographic changes and synovial fluid changes a diagnosis cannot be made, the condition may be nonerosive and immune mediated. Serologic analysis is necessary to determine the etiology. Serum antinuclear antibody (ANA) and SLE preparations are made. If both these tests are negative, a diagnosis of idiopathic polyarthritis is made. If either test is positive and other clinical signs of SLE such as dermatitis, proteinuria, anemia, or thrombocytopenia are present, a diagnosis of SLE is made.

Bone Swelling and Pain

Bone swelling and pain can be defined as an abnormal enlargement of bone and a painful response when a typically nonpainful stimulus, usually in the form of direct pressure, is applied to bone. The swelling is typically firm because of the osseous or fibrous nature of this tissue.

Pathophysiology

Pain associated with bone swelling is usually due to disruption of surrounding soft tissues, such as periosteum, synovium, ligaments, or muscle, as all of these tissues are rich in nociceptors. Swelling or enlargement may be a normal response to disruption of bone, such as occurs in fracture healing, or may be due to a pathologic condition, such as neoplasia. Occasionally bone enlargement is due to bony proliferation as may occur with hypertrophic osteodystrophy or craniomandibular osteopathy.

Clinical Signs

Clinical signs include lameness, gross enlargement of the bone or limb, pain on direct palpation, warmth of the affected region, or angular limb deformity. Systemic illness may coexist. Historically the onset may be acute or chronic.

Diagnostic Plan

Diagnostic work-up is dependent on the physical examination findings, signalment, and history. The differential diagnosis for immature patients with bone swelling and pain includes fracture, hypertrophic osteodystrophy (if the distal radius, ulna, or tibia is involved), hypertrophic osteopathy, neoplasia, infection, and osteochondroma. The differential diagnosis for mature patients is similar but excludes hypertrophic osteodystrophy. Differential diagnosis of bone pain without swelling can include all these conditions and also includes the more common condition of panosteitis.

When bone swelling with pain is identified, radiographic evaluation is indicated. Neoplasia is characterized by osseous proliferation and destruction, whereas healing bone is characterized by proliferation. Infection can also be associated with both proliferation and destruction, but it tends to be associated more with proliferation and usually with pain or a draining tract. If a definitive diagnosis cannot be made radiographically, fine-needle aspiration can be attempted. Cytologic evaluation may provide evidence of neoplasia by demonstrating atypical cells, whereas infection is typified by inflammatory cells. If cytologic evaluation is inconclusive, bone biopsy is necessary (see Diagnostic Procedures). Specimens for bacterial or fungal culture or both should be submitted in case biopsy suggests osteomyelitis.

Diagnostic Procedures

Routine Laboratory Evaluation

A complete blood count, serum chemistry profile, and urinalysis typically contribute little to the diagnosis of orthopedic abnormalities. Abnormalities detected by these tests occasionally provide information regarding systemic disease. Increased white blood cell counts can be consistent with various disease conditions but are rarely diagnostic alone.

Special Laboratory Tests

A test for ANAs is useful for suggesting an immune-mediated etiology of certain joint disorders. The ANA test is an indirect immunofluorescence test that shows the presence of serum antibodies with specificity for nuclear antigens.[9] Although the presence of ANAs is considered to be a relatively sensitive indicator of SLE, both false-positive and false-negative results occur.[10] A positive ANA result can occur with other diseases, such as autoimmune skin disease, rheumatoid arthritis, and some infectious diseases.

Detection of lupus erythematosus (LE) cells can aid in the diagnosis of autoimmune conditions such as SLE. Unfortunately, interpretation of this test can be difficult, and it is considered an insensitive method of diagnosing SLE.[10]

Rheumatoid factor is an antibody against altered host IgG.[11] A change in the host IgG molecule that has bound to an unknown antigen renders the molecule immunogenic, and as a result activated B lymphocytes and plasma cells produce large amounts of rheumatoid factor (anti-IgG). Unfortunately, detection of rheumatoid factor is inconsistent in canine patients meeting other criteria of rheumatoid arthritis.[12] Furthermore, rheumatoid factor has been detected in normal dogs and in dogs with other chronic diseases, including osteoarthritis.[13]

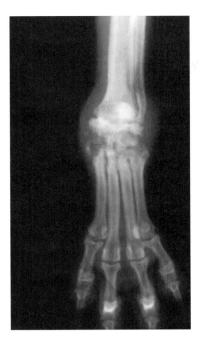

Figure 55-1
Craniocaudal view of the carpus demonstrating erosive change and soft tissue swelling typical of erosive arthritis. Note the lytic changes of the proximal aspect of the metacarpals; note also the small carpal bones and the narrowing of the joint spaces of the carpus.

Radiography

Radiographic evidence of systemic joint disease can range from minimal alterations early in the course of disease to quite severe lesions during the later stages. Early changes include periarticular soft tissue thickening and joint effusion with distention of the joint capsule. As the disease progresses, it is important to distinguish between erosive and nonerosive changes because these findings are important in differentiating between these two distinct classes of arthropathy. With nonerosive disease, the radiographic appearance of the joint may be normal or limited to joint effusion and soft tissue thickening, possibly with mild degenerative change (osteophyte production and subchondral sclerosis) as sequelae. Severe erosive disease is characterized by periarticular bone lysis, subchondral bone cysts or lysis, decreased joint space caused by cartilage destruction, subluxation or luxation, and demineralization (Fig. 55-1). Differentiation between infectious and immune-mediated causes of erosive arthritis is difficult on the basis of radiographic signs and is best done in conjunction with synovial fluid cytology and bacterial culture.

Joint neoplasia can usually be differentiated from the systemic arthritides by the aggressive appearance of the lesions, the severe degree of bone destruction, and soft tissue swelling associated with neoplastic conditions. All articular surfaces of a joint are typically involved in synovial cell sarcoma; other types of neoplasia may originate in the metaphyseal region of the bone and involve the joint only late in the disease process.

Arthrocentesis and Synovial Fluid Analysis

Synovial fluid analysis is commonly performed if a diagnosis cannot be made on the basis of history, physical examination, and radiographic findings. Synovial fluid is assessed grossly for color, clarity, and viscosity and microscopically to determine cell count, cell type, and the presence of any infectious agents. Normal synovial fluid is clear and colorless or pale yellow; it forms a 2- to 4-cm string when a drop is placed on a microscope slide and the needle is withdrawn or when a drop is placed between gloved fingers that are then separated. Alterations in these parameters suggest joint disease, with the major distinction being between noninflammatory and inflammatory disease. There can be considerable overlap in synovial fluid parameters in various disease processes, and the final interpretation is made in conjunction with the history and results of physical and radiographic examinations (see Table 55-1).

Arthrocentesis can be performed on many joints in the dog and cat. Because the small joints, such as the carpus and tarsus, are typically involved in systemic arthritides, these are the most frequently aspirated. Arthrocentesis can also be easily performed on the elbow, shoulder, and stifle. Although some patients with mild disease tolerate arthrocentesis without sedation, sedation and analgesia are beneficial for the patient in pain. Sedation is often required for radiographic evaluation, and arthrocentesis can be performed immediately after the radiographic examination is complete.

Equipment needed for arthrocentesis consists of a 1- to 1.5-inch, 20- to 22-gauge needle and a 3-mL syringe. Aseptic preparation of the site is appropriate to help prevent iatrogenic infection. Sterile gloves are worn to prevent iatrogenic contamination, as it may be beneficial to palpate the target area immediately before introducing the needle. The patient is properly restrained, the target site identified, and the needle placed into the joint. Gentle aspiration is performed. If no fluid is obtained, redirection of the needle is indicated. Aggressive aspiration and aggressive redirection of the needle are avoided to prevent iatrogenic hemorrhage. If blood is seen in the hub of the needle, aspiration is stopped and the needle withdrawn. Replacing the blood-containing needle with a new one before placing the fluid in a container or on a slide allows more accurate assessment of the sample. The fluid volume obtained varies depending on the disease present and the size of the patient. It is uncommon to obtain more than 0.5 mL from any joint in the normal dog, but diseased joints may yield many milliliters of fluid.

When fluid is obtained, color and turbidity are noted, a drop is placed on a microscope slide (without touching the needle to the slide), and a smear is made for evaluation. The length of the string of fluid that results as the needle is withdrawn from the slide is noted. After one or more slides have been made, the fluid is placed into a container for cytologic evaluation or into a bacterial culture medium. Changing the needle before placing the sample in the culture medium ensures that the sample is not contaminated, although it results in a slightly decreased volume for analysis.

Containers for synovial fluid should be obtained before collecting the sample, as clot formation can occur quickly once the sample is obtained (normal synovial fluid does not clot because of the lack of coagulation factors, but with inflammation or hemorrhage, coagulation factors are present and clots form). Appropriate containers include a tube with ethylenediaminetetra-acetic acid (EDTA) for samples submitted for cytology and a container with a blood culture medium (a commercial multipurpose nutrient broth medium such as tryptic soy, trypticase soy, or brain-heart infusion), at a ratio of one part synovial fluid to nine parts blood culture medium, for samples submitted for bacterial culture.[14] Allowing the blood culture medium to incubate for 24 hours with subsequent inoculation onto a blood agar plate results in the greatest success in identifying a bacterial organism responsible for septic arthritis.[14]

Synovial fluid is perhaps most easily obtained from the carpus. The most accessible site for carpal arthrocentesis is the radiocarpal space, although the intercarpal space is also accessible.[15] The target site is identified by gently flexing the carpus and directly palpating the junction between the distal radius and radiocarpal bone on the craniomedial aspect of the carpus. The space is readily palpable unless a large amount of soft tissue swelling is present. Once the space is identified, the needle is placed perpendicular to the skin, inserted into the joint, and gently aspirated (Fig. 55–2).

Other joints frequently aspirated include the shoulder, elbow, and tarsus. The scapulohumeral joint is most easily approached from the craniolateral aspect by using the acromion process as a landmark. With the patient in lateral recumbence and the shoulder slightly flexed, the needle is inserted from the craniolateral aspect, a few millimeters distal to the acromion process yet proximal to the lateral aspect of the greater tubercle of the humerus[16] (Fig. 55–3). The needle is

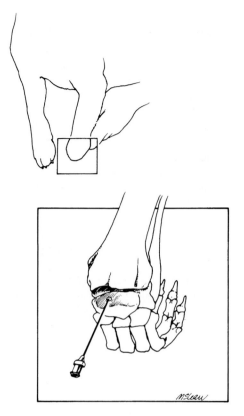

Figure 55–2
Antebrachiocarpal joint arthrocentesis. The joint is flexed and the needle inserted into the joint at its dorsal aspect just medial or lateral to the midsagittal plane. (From Lipowitz AJ. Synovial fluid. In: Newton CD, Nunamaker DM, eds. Textbook of Small Animal Orthopaedics. Philadelphia, JB Lippincott, 1985:1019. Copyright CD Newton.)

directed medially and caudally. It may be necessary to redirect the needle if bone instead of the joint space is encountered.

With the patient in lateral recumbence, the elbow is most readily approached from the caudolateral aspect. If joint effusion is present, a distended joint capsule may be palpable in the space delineated by the lateral humeral epicondyle cranially and the olecranon process caudally. To reach this fluid, the joint is placed in mild flexion and the needle penetrates the skin caudolaterally, slightly dorsal to the olecranon process (Fig. 55–4). The needle is directed cranially and distally toward the anconeal process so that the needle enters the joint between the anconeal process and the medial aspect of the lateral humeral epicondyle.[16]

Arthrocentesis of the stifle may be performed from the medial or lateral parapatellar region. This target area is the largest of all the readily accessible joints of the dog. With the patient in lateral recumbence and the joint slightly flexed, the patellar ligament is palpated and the needle placed just medial or lateral to this structure at a point approximately midway between the patella and tibial crest (Fig. 55–5). The needle is then directed toward the intercondylar space. Aspiration of fluid may be facilitated by applying digital pressure to the side of the patellar ligament opposite the point of approach.[15]

Arthrocentesis of the tarsus can be difficult because of the relatively small target site this joint provides. With the patient in lateral recumbence, flexion of the joint facilitates arthrocentesis. The space between the lateral malleolus, tibia, and talus is palpated. The needle is positioned so that it penetrates the skin caudal to the lateral malleolus and proximal to the calcaneus. The needle is advanced in a medial and distal direction parallel to the calcaneus so that it enters the joint space just medial to the lateral malleolus (Fig. 55–6).

In all instances, successful arthrocentesis is more likely if palpable joint effusion exists, as this

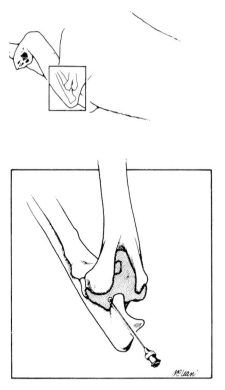

Figure 55–4
Elbow joint arthrocentesis. With the joint in partial flexion, the needle penetrates the skin laterally and caudal to the olecranon process and is directed downward and cranially toward the anconeal process. The needle enters the joint space between the anconeal process and the medial surface of the lateral humeral condyle. (From Lipowitz AJ. Synovial fluid. In: Newton CD, Nunamaker DM, eds. Textbook of Small Animal Orthopaedics. Philadelphia, JB Lippincott, 1985:1019. Copyright CD Newton.)

provides a greater fluid volume and facilitates identification of the target area. When the needle enters the joint, gentle aspiration results in the best sample. Vigorous aspiration or multiple attempts and redirection of the needle frequently result in iatrogenic hemorrhage, making interpretation of results more difficult.

Synovial Membrane Biopsy

If a diagnosis is not made through the combination of history, physical examination, radiographic examination, synovial fluid analysis, and ANA, LE, and rheumatoid factor testing, synovial membrane biopsy may be indicated. Synovial membrane biopsy aids in distinguishing immune-mediated or infectious disease from osteoarthritis. Synovial biopsy is most frequently performed by surgical arthrotomy, with sampling of both the synovium and the fibrous joint capsule. A cutting needle biopsy can be performed in

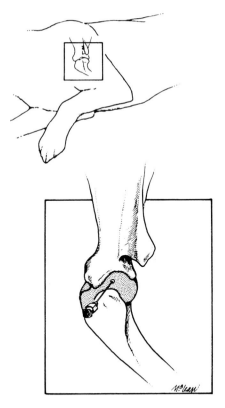

Figure 55–3
Scapulohumeral joint arthrocentesis. The needle enters the joint by passing proximal to the lateral aspect of the greater tubercle of the humerus, lateral to the supraglenoid tubercle of the scapula, and ventral to the acromion process of the scapula. (From Lipowitz AJ. Synovial fluid. In: Newton CD, Nunamaker DM, eds. Textbook of Small Animal Orthopaedics. Philadelphia, JB Lippincott, 1985: 1018. Copyright CD Newton.)

large joints, such as the stifle, but allows neither direct observation of the joint nor selective sampling of tissue.[17]

Bone Biopsy

Bone biopsy is performed to provide cytologic or histologic information about a bone lesion and to provide a sample for fungal or bacterial culture. As bone biopsy is most frequently performed when neoplasia is suspected, concurrent thoracic radiographs are frequently indicated.

Successful biopsy technique involves planning the procedure. The approach is made with consideration of the biopsy tract, which is made so that it

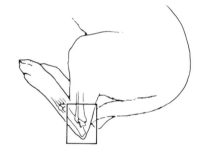

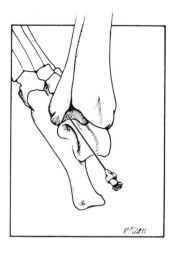

Figure 55-6
Talocrural joint arthrocentesis: caudal approach. The needle enters the joint from its plantar-lateral aspect and is advanced in a dorsomedial and distal direction, passing between the distal fibula and fibular tarsal bone. Joint flexion facilitates needle entry into the joint. (From Lipowitz AJ. Synovial fluid. In: Newton CD, Nunamaker DM, eds. Textbook of Small Animal Orthopaedics. Philadelphia, JB Lippincott, 1985:1021. Copyright CD Newton.)

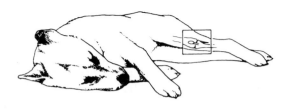

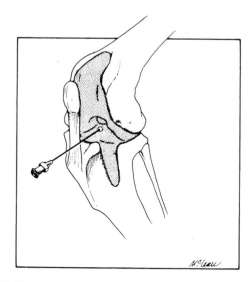

Figure 55-5
Stifle joint arthrocentesis. The joint is flexed sufficiently to cause tensing of the joint capsule. The needle enters the joint either just medial or just lateral to the patellar ligament midway between the distal end of the patella and the proximal articular surface of the tibia. Passing obliquely and caudally, the needle is directed toward the intercondylar space of the distal femur. The needle may also be passed directly through the patellar ligament. (From Lipowitz AJ. Synovial fluid. In: Newton CD, Nunamaker DM, eds. Textbook of Small Animal Orthopaedics. Philadelphia, JB Lippincott, 1985:1021. Copyright CD Newton.)

minimizes potential tumor cell seeding. This is particularly important if surgical excision is anticipated. It is less important if amputation follows biopsy. Major arteries, veins, and nerves should be avoided during the biopsy procedure.

Bone biopsy can be performed using a Michel trephine (usually 3/16 inch) or a Jamshidi needle. The Michel trephine is a saw-toothed instrument that results in a larger piece of bone than the Jamshidi needle. This provides a larger sample for histopathologic evaluation, but it usually results in fewer samples' being obtained because of concern about bone weakening. Jamshidi-type needles are useful when a lytic bone lesion is present and the biopsy site is relatively soft. However, it is difficult to drive these needles through thick, normal cortical bone. Because a small piece of bone is removed, multiple samples can be obtained when using a Jamshidi needle with less concern about weakening the bone.[18]

Regardless of the biopsy instrument used, multiple biopsy samples are beneficial, although they should be obtained with due consideration of potential bone weakening. Biopsy of the center of the radiographic lesion yields a diagnosis in approximately 84% of cases, whereas biopsy of the peripheral transition zone yields a diagnosis in nearly 55% of cases.[19] Biopsy of both the central area and the peripheral normal-abnormal junction increases the probability of diagnosis to approximately 93%.[18, 19]

Bone biopsy may be performed as a closed or open procedure. Open bone biopsy is done as an aseptic surgical procedure. The surgical approach offers the advantage of direct visualization and potential excisional biopsy. The disadvantages are that it requires general anesthesia and greater tissue disruption and results in greater potential morbidity.[20] A closed biopsy is done as an aseptic procedure through a small stab incision in the skin. Visualization is minimal, and radiographic confirmation of the needle or trephine position aids in obtaining an appropriate sample. The metallic portion of the biopsy instrument is easily identified on radiographs. If a Michel trephine is used, positioning is facilitated by first placing a small Kirschner wire into the lesion.[21] If appropriate positioning is confirmed radiographically, the trephine is placed over the Kirschner wire and advanced to the level of the bone. Closed biopsy results in less tissue disruption and potentially less morbidity. The major disadvantage is that it does not allow direct visualization of the affected tissues. Regardless of whether an open or closed approach is used, biopsy site placement should be confirmed radiographically.

Impression smears can be made from the sample obtained to provide immediate information cytologically, and then the sample is placed in buffered formalin in preparation for future histologic evaluation. Samples for culture are placed in a sterile container and immediately submitted for appropriate culturing. Anaerobic organisms are frequently isolated in osteomyelitis, and appropriate specimen handling is necessary to confirm this diagnosis (see Chap. 36).

Common Joint and Skeletal Diseases

Rheumatoid Arthritis

Rheumatoid arthritis is an immune-mediated condition that is classified as an erosive arthritis. It is a slowly progressive disease associated with destruction of articular cartilage and subchondral bone, along with weakening of the surrounding supportive structures. The incidence is unknown, but it is typically identified in middle-aged (median age approximately 5 years) small and toy breed dogs, although dogs of any age and larger breeds may be affected.[12]

Pathophysiology

The etiology of rheumatoid arthritis is essentially unknown. Suspected viral or bacterial causes of immune complex deposition exist, although a distinct cause-and-effect relation has not been demonstrated. Canine distemper virus has been implicated as a possible etiologic agent.

Immune complex deposition in the synovial tissues initiates a severe synovitis. This initiates the inflammatory cascade, with the production of various cytokines, prostaglandins, and other inflammatory mediators. Chondrocytes are induced to produce metalloproteinases, which are destructive enzymes that break down collagenase and proteoglycans. Chemotactic agents attract neutrophils, which release lysosomal enzymes and are associated with free radical production that results in further destruction of tissues. The loss of articular cartilage results in an abnormal force distribution in the joint, which leads to further damage to the articular cartilage and the subchondral bone. As the articular surface is damaged, granulation tissue invades the cartilage and spreads over the articular surface, resulting in a condition known as pannus. This leads to further breakdown of the articular surface. The inflammatory reaction in the synovial membrane results in thickening of this tissue. Neutrophil infiltration is followed by fibroblastic proliferation. The fibroblasts produce collagen, which eventually matures and contracts. The loss of the ability to produce normal hyaluronan to provide boundary lubrication, along with the gross thickening of the joint capsule and contraction of connective tissue of the joint capsule, results in great energy expenditure and pain associated with joint movement.

Clinical Signs

Clinical signs associated with rheumatoid arthritis include multiple joint swelling and pain, particularly involving the distal joints. Early stages may be characterized by only mild lameness or joint swelling, causing a low index of suspicion for this disease. Because the condition is frequently bilaterally symmetrical, lameness may not be discrete but instead may be manifest as generalized stiffness, a tentative gait, or recumbence. As the condition progresses, joint laxity caused by destruction of periarticular tissues can be so severe as to result in gross deformity or subluxation of the joint. Articular erosive changes may lead to joint collapse and palpable crepitus with manipulation. Onset of clinical signs occurs relatively slowly, although a small percentage of patients present with acute onset of signs.[12] The disease is usually progressive.

Diagnostic Plan

Definitive diagnosis of rheumatoid arthritis can be a diagnostic challenge. Specific criteria have been established for the diagnosis of rheumatoid arthritis in humans, and these have been extrapolated to apply to the dog[22] (Table 55–2).

The differential diagnosis for multiple joint swelling and pain includes infectious arthritis (including bacterial, fungal, rickettsial, and spirochetal etiologies) and immune-mediated nonerosive conditions. Diagnostic work-up consists of the methodical collection of data to confirm or refute any of these conditions. Radiographs of affected joints, arthrocentesis with cytology and culture, serology, and histopathology all may be necessary to reach a diagnosis. This work-up is frequently the same whenever a systemic arthropathy is suspected.

Erosive change on radiographs of the affected joints leads to a high index of suspicion for rheumatoid arthritis (see Fig. 55–1). Early in this condition, radiographic change may be limited to soft tissue swelling, joint effusion, and narrowing of the joint space. However, if erosive change is present, the nonerosive arthropathies are ruled out. Septic arthritis is then differentiated from rheumatoid arthritis through arthrocentesis, cytology, and bacterial culture.

Arthrocentesis of the affected joint results in a yellow to blood-tinged, moderately turbid fluid with moderately increased white blood cells (8–38 × $10^3/\mu L$) (see Table 55–1). Either neutrophils or macrophages may predominate. Rarely, ragocytes (poly-

morphonuclear cells that have phagocytized immune complex) are identified.[23] Serologic change, such as a positive rheumatoid factor test, is supportive but not necessary for diagnosis. Bacterial culture in rheumatoid arthritis is negative. Synovial membrane biopsy may be necessary to help confirm the diagnosis. Typical histopathologic changes include thickening of the synovium and infiltration with plasma cells and lymphocytes.[22, 24]

Treatment

Treatment is usually unrewarding but is attempted with corticosteroids, cytotoxic agents, or gold salts.[22] Treatment with nonsteroidal anti-inflammatory drugs alone is generally unrewarding. Treatment is usually initiated with prednisone at 1 to 2 mg/kg by mouth three times per day (t.i.d.) for 2 to 3 weeks, then reduced over weeks to months until the minimum effective dose is achieved.[25] If a satisfactory response is not obtained, combination therapy with corticosteroids and a cytotoxic agent, such as cyclophosphamide or azothiaprine, can be used in resistant cases.[25] Cyclophosphamide (1.5–2.5 mg/kg by mouth, with 1.5 mg/kg given to dogs >30 kg and 2.5 mg/kg given to dogs <15 kg and cats) is administered for four consecutive days each week for up to 16 weeks.[25] Azathiaprine is administered at 2.0 mg/kg by mouth every other day.[25] Both cyclophosphamide and azathiaprine can cause bone marrow supression and hematologic change, and therefore constant monitoring is necessary.[25] Chrysotherapy (gold compounds) is also useful in treating rheumatoid arthritis. Gold may be administered by either intramuscular injection (0.5 mg/kg per week for 6–8 weeks, then every 2–3 months as needed for maintenance) or by mouth (0.05–2.0 mg/kg twice per day [b.i.d.] with a maximum of 9 mg/day).[25] Gastrointestinal, hematologic, renal, and other side effects occur with chrysotherapy.[25]

Prognosis

The prognosis for recovery from rheumatoid arthritis is poor. At best, clinical signs are controlled and the disease enters a period of remission. Despite treatment, degenerative changes typically continue to progress and the clinical picture worsens. The quality of life can be maintained with treatment for a variable period of time, but eventually it deteriorates and the combination of disability and discomfort frequently results in the owner's electing euthanasia.

Systemic Lupus Erythematosus

SLE is classified as a nonerosive inflammatory joint disease. The incidence of disease is unknown, but the condition typically occurs in larger dogs of any age.

Table 55–2
Diagnostic Criteria for Rheumatoid Arthritis*

1. Stiffness after rest
2. Pain or tenderness on motion of at least one joint
3. Swelling of at least one joint
4. Swelling of one other joint within 3 months
5. Symmetric joint swelling
6. Subcutaneous nodules
7. Erosive changes on joint radiographs
8. Serologic test positive for rheumatoid factor
9. Abnormal synovial fluid
10. Histopathology of synovium
11. Histopathology of subcutaneous nodules

*Seven of these criteria must be met, including two of criteria 7, 8, and 10. For criteria 1 to 5, the condition should be present for at least 6 weeks to be considered positive.
Modified from Bennett D, May C. Joint diseases of dogs and cats. In: Ettinger SJ, Feldman EC, eds. Textbook of Veterinary Internal Medicine. Philadelphia, WB Saunders, 1995:2065.

Although joint involvement may be the primary presenting sign, multisystem involvement is an important aspect of this disease. The most frequent systemic conditions associated with SLE are autoimmune hemolytic anemia, immune-mediated thrombocytopenia, leukopenia, glomerulonephritis, dermatitis, polymyositis, pleuritis, central nervous system disease, and systemic polyarthritis.[22]

Pathophysiology

The pathophysiology of SLE is related to immune complex deposition in target tissues (type III hypersensitivity). This results in synovitis and initiation of an inflammatory response characteristic of joint involvement. Synovial fluid quality is decreased. Erosive changes typical of rheumatoid arthritis do not occur. Immune complex deposition leads to changes in the other involved tissue, such as the skin and kidney, that ultimately lead to multiple organ dysfunction.

Clinical Signs

Clinical signs are similar to those of rheumatoid arthritis but tend to be less severe. Involvement of other organ systems, including the hematopoietic, integumentary, and neuromuscular systems, is common. Integumentary involvement is common and is classically manifest as dermatitis or ulceration at the mucocutaneous junctions. Pale mucous membranes resulting from anemia may be present if the hematopoietic system is involved. Joint involvement is manifest as swollen, painful joints and is typically polyarticular and symmetrical, although monoarticular disease can occur. Lameness may point to specific joint involvement or may be manifest as a generalized stiffness or a tentative gait.

Diagnostic Plan

A diagnosis of SLE can be difficult to confirm but is usually made on the basis of multisystem involvement, a positive ANA test, and the presence of immunopathologic factors consistent with the disease, such as antibodies against red blood cells (positive Coombs test) or histopathologic evidence of immune complex deposition in skin, kidney, or joint capsule.[22]

Radiographic changes are mild and are characterized by the nonspecific signs of soft tissue swelling or joint effusion. Radiographic evaluation is most valuable in supporting a diagnosis of SLE in providing evidence to rule out another disease (trauma, congenital abnormality, osteoarthritis, neoplasia) or erosive joint disorders, such as rheumatoid arthritis, through the lack of erosive change. Synovial fluid examination reveals a yellow-tinged fluid that has poor viscosity and numerous nucleated cells ($4.4–371 \times 10^3/\mu L$) (see Table 55–1). Either neutrophils or macrophages may predominate. Negative bacterial culture is often necessary to rule out a septic joint, as early sepsis is considered with an inflammatory synovial fluid analysis.

A positive ANA test is considered by some to be necessary for diagnosis of SLE.[26] Detection of LE cells is considered valuable in the diagnosis of SLE, but absence of these cells is common and the test is considered insensitive.[10] Various criteria have been proposed for the diagnosis of SLE in dogs.[27] These criteria require that the patient have at least one of the following: skin disease with or without mucocutaneous ulceration, nonerosive arthritis, hemolytic anemia, thrombocytopenia, proteinuria, myositis, myocarditis, or pneumonitis.[27] Bennett[26] proposed that a definitive diagnosis of SLE requires at least one of the preceding conditions along with a positive ANA test and immunopathologic evidence (positive Coombs test, tissue biopsy positive for immune complex deposition on tissue fluorescent antibody testing) consistent with the disease. Others believe a positive LE cell test can be substituted for a positive ANA test.[9]

Treatment

SLE is treated with immunosuppressive agents such as corticosteroids. Prednisone, 1 to 2 mg/kg by mouth b.i.d., is administered initially. Treatment is continued for 10 to 14 days. If joint involvement is a prominent feature of disease, observing the degree of joint effusion or synovial fluid cell count can be a useful way to monitor treatment success. If corticosteroids alone do not control the condition, cytotoxic agents such as cyclophosphamide or azothiaprine may be added to the treatment regimen (see Rheumatoid Arthritis). Cytotoxic agents are used in addition to corticosteroids, not as single agents. An alternative treatment regimen has been reported using levamisole (3–7 mg/kg every other day for 4 months) as an immunomodulating agent.[28] Once the condition is brought under control, maintenance therapy may be decreased gradually by approximately 25% every 1 to 2 weeks, and some patients may be able to be weaned from medical therapy.

Prognosis

The prognosis for patients with SLE is guarded. Long-term studies of the treatment of SLE have not been completed.[27] In one study of 13 cases, 7 of the 13 responded to treatment with corticosteroids and cytotoxic drugs.[26] Of these seven, four have been successfully weaned from all drugs, and three require low-dose prednisone therapy (follow-up range, 5 months to 2 years).[26] Six of the 13 did not respond well to treatment and either died from or are severely affected by other systemic disease. Multiple organ system disease is a frequent cause of death with SLE.

Idiopathic Polyarthritis

Most nonerosive inflammatory arthritides that cannot be identified as SLE or infectious (bacterial, rickettsial, spirochetal) are included in this category. Because definitive diagnosis of rheumatoid arthritis or SLE is difficult, this diagnosis accounts for a large portion of patients diagnosed with inflammatory arthritis.

Idiopathic arthritis is typically divided into four subtypes based on the presence of associated conditions. Type I is polyarthritis uncomplicated by any other factor. Type II is polyarthritis associated with an infectious process remote from the joint, such as dental disease or skin infection. Type III is associated with enteric disease, such as ulcerative colitis. Type IV is associated with neoplasia.

Pathophysiology

Synovitis is the prominent histopathologic finding.[29] Immune complex deposition (typical of type III hypersensitivity) in the synovial membrane is a consistent finding.[22] Lameness is considered to be due to the synovitis along with an associated vasculitis.

Clinical Signs

Clinical signs are similar to those for SLE. Lameness and joint pain are typically milder than in rheumatoid arthritis. Lameness is typically acute in onset and may be manifest as either monoarticular lameness or generalized stiffness. Joints have soft tissue swelling and synovial fluid effusion. General signs of malaise, anorexia, and lethargy are frequently associated with this condition. Clinical signs of the primary or initiating disease in types II to IV may also be present.

Diagnostic Plan

Diagnosis is based on the lameness (commonly symmetrical), pain, and joint swelling associated with all the inflammatory arthropathies but without definitive evidence of other disease (except with types II to IV). Laboratory data reveal a negative ANA test, LE cell test, and bacterial culture. Radiographic evaluation is notable for the lack of erosive change or other diagnostic findings in the affected region. With type I disease, there is no evidence of other systemic organ involvement. Synovial fluid analysis reveals increased white blood cells ($3.2–106.3 \times 10^3/\mu L$) with a predominance of neutrophils.[29]

Treatment

Treatment is with an immunosuppressive agent such as prednisone, 2 to 4 mg/kg by mouth, divided b.i.d. for 2 weeks.[30] If remission occurs, the dosage is reduced by 50% every 2 weeks until the disease is controlled with 1 mg/kg every other day.[30] Some patients can be successfully weaned from all treatment, although a recurrence rate of 30% to 50% has been suggested.[31] If a positive response to corticosteroids is not recognized, cyclophosphamide can be added to the treatment protocol. Cyclophosphamide is administered at a dose of 50 mg/m^2 by mouth once daily for four consecutive days or every other day for a week until remission is attained, then for an additional month.[30] Remission generally occurs within 2 to 16 weeks.[30] If cyclophosphamide is used, weekly complete blood counts are recommended to monitor bone marrow suppression.

The primary condition, such as infection remote from the joint, should be treated appropriately. Treatment of the underlying condition is usually insufficient to resolve the lameness, and at least short-term treatment with corticosteroids is necessary.

Prognosis

The prognosis is relatively good; nearly 50% of patients can eventually be weaned from treatment. Remissions occur, and reinstitution of therapy may be necessary. Recovery is frequently reported for types I to III, although varying degrees of residual stiffness and relapses are reported.[29] The long-term prognosis with type IV is poor because of the severity of the underlying disease.

Panosteitis

Panosteitis is a benign, idiopathic bone disease characterized by shifting-leg lameness. German shepherds are classically affected with the condition, although it is reported in other breeds such as the Labrador retriever and golden retriever and is also common in the basset hound. The condition is typically recognized in young dogs (6–18 months), although it has been described in dogs up to 5 years of age.[32]

Pathophysiology

The increased medullary density recognized on radiographic examination is associated with replacement of hematopoietic and fatty marrow tissue by fibrous tissue.[33] This is followed by bone remodeling, with woven bone being formed in this fibrous tissue.[33] As the area of new bone production expands, there is increased congestion in the vascular sinusoids, stimulating an endosteal and periosteal response.[34] This new bone is eventually reabsorbed, with reestablishment of the normal marrow components (usually within 60–90 days).[34] The actual cause of lameness is unknown, although pain may be associated with vascular congestion in the medullary sinusoids.

The etiology of panosteitis is unknown. Speculation has focused on genetic, bacterial, or viral (particularly canine distemper) causes, but none has been confirmed.[33] There is no association with trauma.

Clinical Signs

Lameness is usually of sudden onset and of a single limb. Some dogs demonstrate mild signs of systemic illness, such as malaise, fever, anorexia, and lethargy. Lameness typically lasts for 2 to 3 weeks but can be present for much longer. Lameness may develop in another limb after a symptom-free period of varying duration. The severity of lameness ranges from mild to complete non–weight bearing.

Diagnostic Plan

Panosteitis is a diagnosis made by physical examination and confirmed via radiography. Pain is elicited with deep palpation of the long bones that are typically affected, which include the proximal ulna, distal humerus, central radius, proximal and central femur, and proximal tibia. [33]

Unfortunately, other conditions can present with similar lameness and pain on palpation, such as elbow dysplasia responding to palpation of the distal humerus and hip dysplasia responding to manipulation of the hind limb. Radiographs aid in differentiating these conditions but occasionally confirm the existence of both conditions. Panosteitis is associated with increased density of the medullary cavity of the affected bone, usually in the region of the nutrient foramen (Fig. 55–7). Endosteal and periosteal proliferation may be noted.

Treatment

The painful signs associated with this condition are palliated with nonsteroidal anti-inflammatory drugs. Aspirin is usually the drug of first choice, given at a dose of 10 to 25 mg/kg by mouth b.i.d. or t.i.d. If this treatment is ineffective, other nonsteroidal anti-inflammatory drugs or prednisolone (0.25 mg/kg by mouth b.i.d.) may provide relief. Appropriate caution should be used concerning long-term administration of corticosteroids, particularly in young dogs.

Prognosis

The long-term prognosis for recovery from panosteitis is excellent. Each painful episode typically lasts 2 to 3 weeks, although some patients demonstrate lameness for longer periods. If lameness is severe during painful episodes, some patients develop muscle atrophy because of disuse and weight loss because of

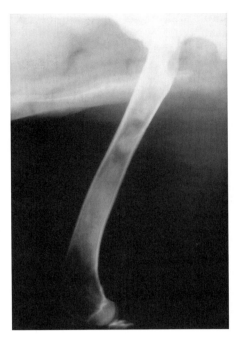

Figure 55–7
Lateral radiograph of a femur demonstrating increased density of the medullary cavity typical of panosteitis.

anorexia. This is a short-term setback, however, and when clinical signs resolve, body condition gradually returns to normal. Panosteitis commonly cycles through all limbs, with symptom-free periods of varying duration between episodes. When the condition has been present in a limb, it is uncommon for that limb to be affected again.

Hypertrophic Osteodystrophy

Hypertrophic osteodystrophy is a developmental disease that affects the metaphyseal region of the long bones of large and giant-breed dogs. The condition affects patients with open metaphyseal growth plates, usually between 2 and 8 months of age. Great Danes are classically affected, although the condition has been reported in many breeds. Males may be affected more commonly than females.[35]

Pathophysiology

Proposed etiologies for hypertrophic osteodystrophy include vitamin C deficiency, oversupplementation with calcium or vitamin D, overnutrition, infectious causes (bacterial and viral), and an inherited predisposition.[35] None of these, however, has been proved to be the cause.

It is believed that disturbance of metaphyseal blood flow in the region of the metaphysis leads to delay in ossification of the metaphyseal growth plate.[36] Hemorrhage, necrosis, and an inflammatory response of neutrophils and macrophages are found in this region adjacent to the metaphysis, which is identified radiographically as a radiolucent metaphyseal zone.[37, 38] The narrow zone of radiodensity between the metaphyseal growth plate and this radiolucent region is due to collapse of bony trabeculae and mineralization of trabecular hemorrhages.[38] Normal bone remodeling does not occur in this region because of disruption of normal endochondral ossification, resulting in widening of the growth plate to varying degrees.[38] Microfractures of the bony trabeculae may further compromise the condition and be associated with development of the periosteal response.[35, 36]

Clinical Signs

Clinical presentation is variable, with lameness ranging from a mild gait abnormality to complete recumbence. Many patients have systemic signs of fever, anorexia, dehydration, and depression. Muscle atrophy and weight loss are often found in severely affected animals.

The condition is usually symmetrical, and the affected metaphyses are warm and painful with firm swelling. The radius and ulna are the most commonly affected bones, although the condition has been recognized in the tibia. The condition is episodic, and relapses may occur at varying intervals.[35] However, most dogs recover after one episode.[39]

Diagnostic Plan

The condition is suspected in large and giant-breed dogs presenting with lameness and swelling of the metaphyseal region. Physical examination confirms pain with palpation of the metaphyseal region of the affected limb. The differential diagnosis includes panosteitis, hypertrophic osteopathy, infection, and retained cartilaginous cores. Diagnosis of hypertrophic osteodystrophy is confirmed by radiography, which demonstrates a flaring of the metaphysis and a radiolucent line proximal to the radial or ulnar metaphyseal growth plate (Fig. 55–8). Periosteal proliferation may be present in the metaphyseal region and may extend onto the diaphysis. In severe cases, angular limb deformity develops as a result of growth plate damage and is recognized radiographically.

Treatment

Treatment consists of palliation of pain. Support of the dehydrated and febrile patient with intravenous fluids and nonsteroidal anti-inflammatory drugs (such as buffered aspirin 10–25 mg/kg by mouth b.i.d. or t.i.d.) is appropriate. Good nursing care is imperative for the recumbent patient, as these large or giant-breed dogs may develop pressure sores or pulmonary con-

gestion. Although the influence of diet is inconclusive, abnormalities should be corrected. A high-quality diet is indicated, and vitamin or mineral supplementation should be avoided.

Prognosis

The overall prognosis is good if the patient is mildly affected. In these patients lameness is related to weight bearing, pain is moderate, the condition regresses spontaneously, and angular deformity is absent or minimal. When the animal matures and growth plates close, the condition does not recur.

Few dogs die of hypertrophic osteodystrophy if adequate supportive care is provided. However, some are euthanized because of the pain, recumbence, anorexia, and general morbidity associated with this disease. Disturbance of normal growth plate activity may lead to premature growth arrest and limb shortening (if both radial and ulnar growth plates are affected) or angular deformity (if one growth plate is affected), and this may be incompatible with a good quality of life.[35, 36]

If angular limb deformity develops, appropriate corrective osteotomy is indicated. Depending on the severity of deformity, the prognosis ranges from good to poor. Patients that develop angular deformity early in life, when deformity is potentially more severe because of the amount of remaining growth, have a

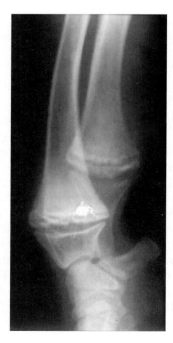

Figure 55–8
Lateral radiograph of the metaphyseal region of the radius and ulna demonstrating hypertrophic osteodystrophy. Note the radiolucent line proximal to both the radial and ulnar growth plates.

worse prognosis. Patients with arrest of both the radial and ulnar growth plates develop a severely shortened limb. Establishing normal limb length through distraction osteogenesis is difficult. Amputation may be indicated if severe growth deformity affects a single limb.

Osteosarcoma

Osteosarcoma is the primary neoplastic condition affecting bones of both the axial and appendicular skeletons. It typically occurs in large and giant-breed dogs but can occur in all breeds. More than 90% of these tumors occur in dogs weighing over 20 kg.[40] Osteosarcoma is most frequently identified in older patients (median age at diagnosis is 7 years), although a biphasic peak incidence has been reported, with the early peak at approximately 2 years of age.[41]

Approximately 75% of all canine osteosarcomas affect the appendicular skeleton.[42] The most common sites can be remembered as "away from the elbow, toward the stifle"; in descending order of frequency, they are the distal radius, proximal humerus, distal femur, and proximal tibia. Osteosarcoma of the axial skeleton, in decreasing order of frequency, occurs in the mandible and maxilla, spine, rib, and pelvis.[42]

Pathophysiology

Bone destruction is the primary pathologic process associated with neoplasia. This leads to weakening of the bone and frequently pathologic fracture. Tumor metastasis is common, not only to other areas of the musculoskeletal system but also to other organs such as the lungs and liver.

Clinical Signs

Patients most frequently are presented because of unilateral limb lameness, pain, or a palpable firm swelling of a bone. With appendicular osteosarcoma, lameness can be mild with slow progression to non–weight bearing, or there can be acute onset of non–weight bearing if associated with pathologic fracture. Pain is usually identified when pressure is placed over the involved site. When the axial skeleton is involved, presentation is typically due to dysfunction, swelling, or pain. This may be manifest as anorexia or oral bleeding with oral tumors, ataxia or paresis with spinal and pelvic tumors, or firm palpable swelling with rib tumors.

Diagnostic Plan

Definitive diagnosis is made by a combination of history, physical examination, radiography, and biopsy. Radiographs reveal a destructive lesion with varying degrees of osteoproliferation and periosteal

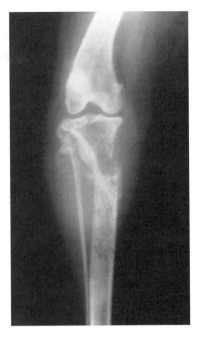

Figure 55–9
Craniocaudal view of the stifle demonstrating changes characteristic of bone neoplasia (osteosarcoma). Note the combination of lysis of the proximal aspect of the tibia and proliferation of the proximal portion of both the tibia and fibula. A pathologic fracture is present.

reaction (Fig. 55–9). If neoplasia is suspected, thoracic radiographs should be obtained to determine whether metastatic disease is present in the lungs.

Because most osteosarcomas originate in the metaphyseal region, the periarticular region may be swollen, and the differential diagnosis includes trauma or sepsis. Occasionally, it may be difficult to distinguish between neoplasia and osteomyelitis (particularly fungal osteomyelitis) radiographically. Fungal infection usually occurs at multiple locations, and thoracic radiographs may be helpful in distinguishing fungal disease from neoplasia. Metastatic pulmonary lesions frequently appear as relatively discrete neoplastic nodules, whereas fungal disease typically produces a more diffuse pattern.

Determination of the type of neoplastic process involving bone may be important for prognosis and therapy. Osteosarcoma is the most common neoplastic process involving bone, occurring in over 90% of cases. Other types of sarcoma, such as fibrosarcoma or chondrosarcoma, occur more frequently on the axial skeleton than the appendicular skeleton. Biopsy (see Diagnostic Procedures) is necessary to distinguish between various types of tumor and is also useful in distinguishing between osteomyelitis and neoplasia when a definitive diagnosis cannot be made radiographically.

Treatment

Osteosarcoma is treated by surgical resection. This can be done by amputation or limb-sparing procedures. The major advantage of amputation is that the source of pain is removed, and this often improves the quality of life. Limb-sparing procedures remove the source of pain and disease with the additional advantage of retaining function of the limb. Limb sparing is performed by resecting the affected bone and replacing it with an allograft. The allograft is held in place with a bone plate, and arthrodesis of the associated joint is usually done with this procedure.[43] Limb sparing is most successful when the tumor involves the distal radius or ulna.

Survival times are increased by a combination of surgical resection and chemotherapy, although complete cures are rare with any type or combination of therapy. Cisplatin is the chemotherapeutic agent most commonly used, although doxorubicin and carboplatin have also been used. Survival with carboplatin is similar to that with cisplatin.[44] An advantage of carboplatin is lack of nephrotoxicity, and administration is easier because saluresis is not required. Myelosuppression (neutropenia) is the dose-limiting toxicity of carboplatin.[44] The number of treatments with any of these agents is variable, but there is a trend toward increased survival with more than two treatments.

The timing of treatments is also variable. Generally the first treatment is given immediately after surgery or at the time of suture removal. Cisplatin is administered at a dose of 70 mg/m^2 and can be given every 21 days up to six treatments or until there is evidence of impaired renal function.[45] Cisplatin is given after 3 hours of saline diuresis (0.9% NaCl at 25 mL/kg per hour).[45] The cisplatin is diluted in 6 mL/kg of 0.9% NaCl and given as an infusion over 20 minutes, which is followed by another hour of saline diuresis.[45] Appropriate care must be taken when handling this drug and the urine of these patients. (See Chap. 17 for a further discussion of chemotherapy.)

Carboplatin is administered at a dose of 300 mg/m^2 IV (admixed with 5% dextrose in water) over 15 minutes, usually within 7 days of amputation.[44] Additional treatments are given at 21-day intervals for a total of four treatments.[44] Complete blood counts are recommended before treatment because neutropenia can be a dose-limiting factor.[44]

Prognosis

Prognosis for osteosarcoma is uniformly poor. Without any treatment, most patients are euthanized within 1 to 2 months of diagnosis because of severe pain.[45] Median survival is extended to approximately 5 to 6 months if amputation alone is performed.[46] Survival is approximately doubled if amputation or

limb-sparing procedures are combined with chemotherapy.[47] The complications of infection or tumor recurrence are associated with limb-sparing procedures. However, survival time is not decreased in these patients.[47]

Uncommon Joint and Skeletal Diseases

Craniomandibular Osteopathy

Craniomandibular osteopathy is characterized by bony proliferation of the mandible and tympanic bullae, causing pain when the animal moves its mouth. It is classically identified in immature Scottish and West Highland white terriers.[48]

Hypertrophic Osteopathy

Hypertrophic osteopathy is characterized by periosteal proliferation of the long bones typically associated with thoracic neoplasia, although it can occur with any space-occupying lesions of the thorax or abdomen.[37] The small distal bones, such as the metacarpals or metatarsals, are affected first, followed by progression proximally.

Nutritional Secondary Hyperparathyroidism

Nutritional secondary hyperparathyroidism occurs when a high level of parathyroid hormone is produced in response to a diet deficient in calcium, with a poor calcium/phosphorus ratio, or deficient in vitamin D.[49] Hyperparathyroidism may also be secondary to renal disease when chronic hyperphosphatemia, caused by renal insufficiency, leads to hypocalcemia.[49] The increased parathyroid hormone results in bone resorption, leading to bone weakness, lameness, and possibly pathologic fracture.

Chondrosarcoma

Chondrosarcoma is an uncommon tumor of bone. When present, it is typically identified in flat bones, most commonly the nasal cavity and ribs.[50] Surgical resection may be attempted. Median survival time for patients with chondrosarcoma of the ribs has been reported as 10.7 months[51] and 3 years.[52]

Synovial Cell Sarcoma

Synovial cell sarcoma typically affects the appendicular skeleton, with the stifle joint being the most common site.[53] Treatment is by amputation. The prognosis depends on staging at the time of diagnosis, but if staging is favorable, survival time may exceed 3 years.[53]

Chinese Shar-Pei Fever

Chinese shar-peis have been reported to develop tibiotarsal joint swelling and hindlimb lameness associated with renal or hepatic amyloidosis.[54, 55] The condition is typically episodic and lameness is associated with fever and systemic illness.

References

1. Evans HE. The skeleton. In: Evans HE, ed. Miller's Anatomy of the Dog, 3rd ed. Philadelphia, WB Saunders, 1993:123–125.
2. Rhinelander FW. Normal vascular anatomy. In: Newton CD, Nunamaker DM, eds. Textbook of Small Animal Orthopaedics. Philadelphia, JB Lippincott, 1985:12.
3. Evans HE. Arthrology. In: Evans HE, ed. Miller's Anatomy of the Dog, 3rd ed. Philadelphia, WB Saunders, 1993:219–220.
4. Mankin HJ, Radin EL. Structure and function of joints. In: McCarty DJ, Koopman WJ, eds. Arthritis and Allied Conditions. Philadelphia, WB Saunders, 1993:181–197.
5. Sledge CB. Biology of the joint. In: Kelley WN, Harris ED, Ruddy S, Sledge CB, eds. Textbook of Rheumatology, 4th ed. Philadelphia, WB Saunders, 1993:1–21.
6. Todhunter RJ, Lust G. Synovial joint anatomy, biology, and pathobiology. In: Auer JA, ed. Equine Surgery. Philadelphia, WB Saunders, 1992:844–866.
7. Johns RJ, Wright V. Relative importance of various tissues in joint stiffness. J Appl Physiol 1962;17:824.
8. Fox RI, Kang H. Structure and function of synoviocytes. In: McCarty DJ, Koopman WJ, eds. Arthritis and Allied Conditions. Philadelphia, WB Saunders, 1993:263–278.
9. Thompson JP. Immunologic diseases. In: Ettinger SJ, Feldman EC, eds. Textbook of Veterinary Internal Medicine, 4th ed. Philadelphia, WB Saunders, 1995:2002–2031.
10. Schraeder SC. The use of the laboratory in the diagnosis of joint disorder of dogs and cats. In: Bonagura JD, Kirk RW, eds. Kirk's Current Veterinary Therapy XII. Philadelphia, WB Saunders, 1995:1166–1171.
11. Lewis RM. Rheumatoid arthritis. Vet Clin North Am Small Anim Pract 1994;24:697–701.
12. Bennett D. Immune based erosive inflammatory joint disease of the dog: Canine rheumatoid arthritis. I. Clinical, radiological, and laboratory investigations. J Small Anim Pract 1987;28:779–797.
13. Bennett D, Kirkham D. The laboratory identification of serum rheumatoid factor in the dog. J Comp Pathol 1987;97:541–550.
14. Montgomery RD, Long IR, Milton JL, et al. Comparison of aerobic culturette, synovial membrane biopsy, and blood culture medium in detection of canine bacterial arthritis. Vet Surg 1989;18:300–303.
15. Werner LL. Arthrocentesis and joint fluid analysis: Diagnostic applications in joint diseases of small animals. Compen Contin Educ Pract Vet 1979;1:855–862.
16. Lipowitz AJ. Synovial fluid. In: Newton CD, Nunamaker DM, eds. Textbook of Small Animal Orthopaedics. Philadelphia, JB Lippincott, 1985:1015–1028.
17. Hardy RM, Wallace LJ. Arthrocentesis and synovial membrane biopsy. Vet Clin North Am Small Anim Pract 1974;4:449–462.
18. Powers BE, LaRue SM, Withrow SJ, et al. Jamshidi needle biopsy for diagnosis of bone lesions in small animals. J Am Vet Med Assoc 1988;193:205–210.
19. Wykes PM, Withrow SJ, Powers BE, Park RD. Closed biopsy for diagnosis of long bone tumors: Accuracy and results. J Am Anim Hosp Assoc 1985;21:489–494.
20. Tangner K. Bone biopsy. Semin Vet Med Surg (Small Anim) 1993;8:245–249.
21. Tangner CH. A modified technique for closed trephine bone biopsy. J Am Anim Hosp Assoc 1989;25:55–56.
22. Bennett D, May C. Joint diseases of dogs and cats. In: Ettinger SJ, Feldman EC, eds. Textbook of Veterinary Internal Medicine, 4th ed. Philadelphia, WB Saunders, 1995:2032–2077.
23. Palmer N. Diseases of joints. In: Jubb KVF, Kennedy PC, Palmer N, eds. Pathology of Domestic Animals, 4th ed. San Diego, Academic Press, 1993:178–179.
24. Lipowitz AJ. Immune-mediated arthropathies. In: Newton CD, Nunamaker DM, eds. Textbook of Small Animal Orthopaedics. Philadelphia, JB Lippincott, 1985:1055–1077.
25. Bennett D. Treatment of the immune-based inflammatory arthropathies of the dog and cat. In: Bonagura JD, Kirk RW, eds. Kirk's Current Veterinary Therapy XII. Philadelphia, WB Saunders, 1995:1188–1195.
26. Bennett D. Immune based non-erosive inflammatory joint disease of the dog. I. Canine systemic lupus erythematosus. J Small Anim Pract 1987;28:871–889.
27. Schraeder SC. Joint diseases of the dog and cat. In: Olmstead ML. Small Animal Orthopedics. St. Louis, Mosby-Year Book, 1995:437–472.
28. Fournel C, Chabanne L, Caux C. Canine systemic lupus erythematosus. I: A study of 75 cases. Lupus 1992;1:133–139.
29. Bennett D. Immune-based non-erosive inflammatory joint disease of the dog. 3. Canine idiopathic polyarthritis. J Small Anim Pract 1987;28:909–928.
30. Hopper PE. Immune-mediated joint diseases. In: Slatter D, ed. Textbook of Small Animal Surgery, 2nd ed. Philadelphia, WB Saunders, 1993:1928–1937.
31. Pederson NC, Wind A, Morgan JP, Pool RR. Joint diseases in dogs and cats. In: Ettinger SJ, ed. Textbook of Veterinary Internal Medicine, 3rd ed. Philadephia, WB Saunders, 1989:2329–2375.
32. Halliwell WH. Tumorlike lesions of bone. In: Bojrab MJ, ed. Disease Mechanisms in Small Animal Surgery, 2nd ed. Philadelphia, Lea & Febiger, 1993:932–943.
33. Muir P, Dubielzig RR, Johnson KA. Panosteitis. Compen Contin Educ Pract Vet 1996;18:29–34.
34. Van Sickle DC, Hohn RB: Selected orthopedic problems in the growing dog. Monograph, American Animal Hospital Association, 1975, 20.
35. Bellah JR. Hypertrophic osteodystrophy. In: Bojrab MJ, ed. Disease Mechanisms in Small Animal Surgery, 2nd ed. Philadelphia, Lea & Febiger, 1993:858–864.
36. Manley PA, Romich JA. Miscellaneous orthopedic diseases. In: Slatter D, ed. Textbook of Small Animal Surgery, 2nd ed. Philadelphia, WB Saunders, 1993:1985–1996.

37. Lenehan TM, Fetter AW. Hypertrophic osteodystrophy. In: Newton CD, Nunamaker DM, eds. Textbook of Small Animal Orthopaedics. Philadelphia, JB Lippincott, 1985: 597–601.

38. Muir P, Dubielzig RR, Johnson KA, Shelton GD. Hypertrophic osteodystrophy and calvarial hyperostosis. Compen Contin Educ Pract Vet 1996;18:143–151.

39. Grondalen J. Metaphyseal osteopathy (hypertrophic osteodystrophy) in growing dogs. A clinical study. J Small Anim Pract 1976;17:721–735.

40. Page RL. Musculoskeletal neoplasia: Biology and clinical management. In: Olmstead ML. Small Animal Orthopedics. St. Louis: Mosby-Year Book, 1995:417–426.

41. Brodey RS, Riser WH. Canine osteosarcoma: A clinicopathologic study of 194 cases. Clin Orthop 1969;62:54–64.

42. Heyman SJ, Diefenderfer DL, Goldschmidt MH, Newton CD. Canine axial skeletal osteosarcoma: A retrospective study of 116 cases (1986–1989). Vet Surg 1992;21:304–310.

43. Straw RC, Withrow SJ. Limb-sparing surgery for dogs with bone neoplasia. In: Slatter D, ed. Textbook of Small Animal Surgery, 2nd ed. Philadelphia, WB Saunders, 1993:2020–2026.

44. Bergman PJ, MacEwwen EG, Kurzman ID, et al. Amputation and carboplatin for treatment of dogs with osteosarcoma: 48 cases (1991–1993). J Vet Intern Med 1996;10:76–81.

45. Straw RC, Withrow SJ. Treatment of canine osteosarcoma. In: Bonagura JD, Kirk RW, eds. Kirk's Current Veterinary Therapy XII. Philadelphia, WB Saunders, 1995:506–511.

46. Spodnick GJ, Berg J, Rand WM, et al. Prognosis for dogs with appendicular osteosarcoma treated by amputation alone: 162 cases (1978–1988). J Am Vet Med Assoc 1992;200:995–999.

47. O'Brien MG, Straw RC, Withrow SJ. Recent advances in the treatment of canine appendicular skeletal osteosarcoma. Compen Contin Educ Pract Vet 1993;15:939–946.

48. Watson ADJ, Adams WM, Thomas CB. Craniomandibular osteopathy in dogs. Compen Contin Educ Pract Vet 1995;17:911–922.

49. Cavanaugh PG, Kosovsky JE. Hyperparathyroidism and metabolic bone disease. In: Bojrab MJ, ed. Disease Mechanisms in Small Animal Surgery, 2nd ed. Philadelphia, Lea & Febiger, 1993:865–875.

50. Popovitch CA, Weinstein MJ, Goldschmidt MH, Shofer FS. Chondrosarcoma: A retrospective study of 97 dogs (1987–1990). J Am Anim Hosp Assoc 1994;30:81–85

51. Matthiesen DT, Clark GN, Orsher RJ, et al. En bloc resection of primary rib tumors in 40 dogs. Vet Surg 1992;21:201–204.

52. Pirkey-Ehrhart N, Withrow SJ, Straw RC. Primary rib tumors in 54 dogs. J Am Anim Hosp Assoc 1995;31:65–69.

53. Vail DM, Powers BE, Getzy DM, et al. Evaluation of prognostic factors for dogs with synovial sarcoma: 36 cases (1986–1991). J Am Vet Med Assoc 1994;205:1300–1307.

54. DiBartola SP, Tarr MJ, Webb DM, Giger U. Familial renal amyloidosis in Chinese Shar Pei dogs. J Am Vet Med Assoc 1990;197:483–487.

55. Loeven KO. Hepatic amyloidosis in two Chinese Shar Pei dogs. J Am Vet Med Assoc 1994;204:1212–1216.

Index

ISBN 0-7216-4839-8

90071